Key Notes for the Student

The following features are highlighted within the text for your easy reference:

Keys for Learning. Each chapter begins with features to help you study information in the chapter. These include **Learning Objectives, Key Terms, Keys to Understanding This Chapter, Key Points, Key Topics Outline,** and **Key Learning Activities.**

- **Learning Objectives.** Objectives help you set goals for learning the material in the chapter.
- **Key Terms.** This list of important terms is defined in the chapter and in the Glossary.
- **Keys to Understanding This Chapter.** Chapters and units that will provide background information guide you in preparatory study.
- **Key Points.** This list highlights important information in the chapter.
- **Key Topics Outline.** This outline gives you an overview of the development of the chapter.
- **Key Learning Activities.** You may be assigned these experiential activities or pursue them on your own.

Keys for Review. Each chapter ends with features to help you review the information you learned. These aids include **Key Questions for Critical Thinking, Key Readings, Enrichment Keys, Keys to Learning More, Key Resources.**

- **Key Questions for Critical Thinking.** These statements help you think independently and apply your knowledge to situations you may encounter.
- **Key Readings.** This list contains books and journals the author used to supply facts for the chapter.
- **Enrichment Keys.** This list provides other reference materials for further knowledge.
- **Keys to Learning More.** These chapters or units later in the book relate to subject matter in this chapter.
- **Key Resources.** A list of agencies for your reference when working with individuals and families.

Key Concepts. Many of these little boxes occur throughout the text to review or summarize important information.

Nursing Alert. These boxes highlight vital information in patient care and will help you practice safe nursing.

Keys to Patient and Family Teaching. This boxed material lists key information you should teach to patients and families and will help you with this important nursing responsibility.

Special Considerations in Children and **Special Considerations in Aging.** These boxes help you adapt nursing care information in specific situations across the lifespan.

Sample Nursing Care Plans and **Nursing Process Overviews.** These boxes show nursing process in action, give you examples of how nursing process is used in a clinical setting, and outline information you may see on a Nursing Care Plan.

Keys to Nursing Assessment. These boxes summarize factors in nursing assessment for different body systems throughout the book.

Nursing Procedures. These highlighted boxes with illustrations outline common step-by-step procedures with rationale you will need to learn to provide patient care.

Nursing Skills. These other step-by-step skills with rationale are set off within the text.

Nursing Skill Guidelines. These boxed guidelines give general nursing information that will strengthen your knowledge and skills.

Key English-to-Spanish Healthcare Phrases. Phrases in Appendix A will help you communicate with your Spanish-speaking patients.

Key Abbreviations and Acronyms Used in Healthcare. This special glossary of abbreviations and acronyms appears in Appendix B and is in addition to charting abbreviations presented in the text.

Glossary. This Glossary, which helps you define important words used in the text, will become part of your nursing vocabulary.

Nursing Diagnoses. This list of NANDA-approved nursing diagnoses, which appears facing the back cover, will play a prominent part in your coordination of care with coworkers.

Universal Precautions. These precautions are vital to your nursing career. They are presented on the inside back cover. Following these precautions is critical for your safety, the safety of those with whom you work, and your patients' safety.

TEXTBOOK OF

BASIC NURSING

TEXTBOOK OF
BASIC NURSING

Sixth Edition

Caroline Bunker Rosdahl, RN-C, BSN, MA

Associate Education Specialist
University of Minnesota School of Nursing
Minneapolis, Minnesota

Staff Nurse, Hennepin County Medical Center
Minneapolis, Minnesota

Assistant Professor, Nursing
St. Mary's Campus, College of St. Catherine
Minneapolis, Minnesota

Instructor, Vocational-Technical Education
University of Minnesota
Minneapolis/St. Paul, Minnesota

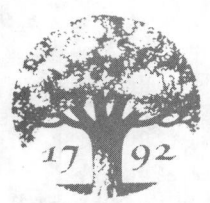

J. B. Lippincott Company
Philadelphia

Sponsoring Editor: Donna L. Hilton, RN, BSN
Developmental Editor: Eleanor Faven
Coordinating Editorial Assistant: Susan M. Keneally
Project Editor: Amy P. Jirsa
Indexer: Anne Cope
Design Coordinator: Doug Smock
Interior Design: Anne O'Donnell
Cover Designer: Ilene Griff
Production Manager: Helen Ewan
Production Coordinator: Kathryn Rule
Compositor: Tapsco, Inc.
Printer/Binder: Courier Book Company/Westford
Cover Printer: Lehigh Press Lithographers

6th Edition

6 5 4 3 2
Library of Congress Cataloging in Publications Data

Rosdahl, Caroline Bunker.
    Textbook of basic nursing/Caroline Bunker Rosdahl.—6th ed.
      p.   cm.
    Includes bibliographical references and index.
    ISBN 0-397-55109-6
    1. Practical nursing.   I. Title.
    [DNLM: 1. Nursing, Practical. WY 195 R794t 1995]
RT62.R58 1995
610.73—dc20
DNLM/DLC
for Library of Congress   94-30640
                                                                            CIP

Any procedure or practice described in this book should be applied by the healthcare practitioner under appropriate supervision in accordance with professional standards of care used
with regard to the unique circumstances that apply in each practice situation. Care has been
taken to confirm the accuracy of information presented and to describe generally accepted practices. However, the authors, editors, and publisher cannot accept any responsibility for errors or
omissions or for any consequences from application of the information in this book and make
no warranty express or implied, with respect to the contents of the book.

Every effort has been made to ensure drug selections and dosages are in accordance with current recommendations and practice. Because of ongoing research, changes in government regulations and the constant flow of information on drug therapy, reactions and interactions, the
reader is cautioned to check the package insert for each drug for indications, dosages, warnings
and precautions, particularly if the drug is new or infrequently used.

⊗ This Paper Meets the Requirements of ANSI/NISO Z39.48-1992 (Permanence of Paper).

This sixth edition is lovingly dedicated to:

my husband, Ron Christensen,
my son, Keith Bunker Rosdahl and his wife, Kim,
our other children, Gary and Kizzy, Mark and Tami, Kathy and Jeff,
and now, the grandchildren!

Contributors and Consultants

Becky L. Born Aftreth RN, BSN
School Nurse
Anchorage School District
Anchorage, Alaska
Chapter 67

Gerri M. Anderson RN
Clinical Manager, GI/Endoscopy Department
HealthEast Midway Hospital
St. Paul, Minnesota
Chapters 28 and 81
Unit 14 Coordinator

Donna M. Belitz RN, M.Ed.
Practical Nursing Coordinator/Counselor
Western Dakota Technical Institute
Rapid City, South Dakota
Chapter 92

Kathleen Prokott Borchert BA, RN, CETN
Enterostomal Therapist
ET Nurse Consultants PA
St. Paul, Minnesota
Chapters 15, 45, 81

Beverly E. Boyd BA, EMT
Rescue Consultant and Educator
Specialized Training Services
Farmington, Minnesota
Chapters 31 and 32

Frederick S. Brightbill MD
Professor, Department of Ophthalmology
University of Wisconsin Medical School
Madison, Wisconsin
Chapter 73

Marjana F. Callery MS, RN, MT (ASCP)
Consultant, Blood Banking/Transfusion Nursing
St. Paul, Minnesota
Chapter 75

Kathleen ''Kitty'' Carlson RN, BAN, OCN
Oncology Service Line Coordinator
North Memorial Medical Center
Robbinsdale, Minnesota
Chapter 76

Kathleen Casolino RN, BS, MSEd
Instructor, Practical Nursing
James L. Walker Vocational-Technical Center
Naples, Florida
Chapters 64–67

Marilyn R. Cheney-Stern RN, BS, MA, PhD
Vocational Coordinator-Special Populations
Jones County Schools
Trenton, North Carolina
Chapters 9–13, 52

Ronald L. Christensen BA, MA
Instructor
Anoka-Hennepin Technical College
Anoka, Minnesota
Chapters 57 and 93

Gwendelyn Combs-Marshall BS, RD, Lactation Educator
Nutritional Consultant
Little Dix Bay Hotel
Virgin Gorda, British Virgin Islands
Chapters 26–28, 60

Mary Jancaric Dierich MSN, RN, GNP
Geriatric Nurse Practitioner
HealthEast Corporation
St. Paul, Minnesota
Chapters 82 and 83

Carol J. Exum, Cancer Survivor
Lafayette, Georgia
Chapter 76

Nancy M. Glassgow RN, BA
Instructor, Practical Nursing
Western Dakota Technical Institute
Rapid City, South Dakota
Chapter 3

Andrea M. Groves RNC
Staff Nurse
Hennepin County Medical Center
Minneapolis, Minnesota
Chapter 71

Karen M. Gutierrez RN, MS
Staff Nurse, SICU
University of Minnesota Hospital
Minneapolis, Minnesota
Nursing Instructor
Anoka-Ramsey Community College
Coon Rapids, Minnesota
Chapters 73 and 77

Carrie J. Herkal RN, BAN
Orthopedic Nurse
Health One Unity Hospital
Fridley, Minnesota
Chapter 70

Jane A. Hurst RN
Instructor in Nursing
Upper Valley JVS School of Practical Nursing
Piqua, Ohio
Chapters 33–35

Judith Bond Johnson PhD, RN, FAAN
Speaker/Consultant, Oncology
Health Quest
Minneapolis, Minnesota
Chapter 76

Reid A. Johnson RN, BAN, CNA
Director of Nursing Services
Harbour Shores of Lawnwood
Fort Pierce, Florida
Chapter 93

Mary T. Kowalski RN, BA, BSN, MSN
Director, Medical Program
Platte College
Ontario, California
Chapters 12, 14–25, 85–86

William L. Lederman RN, BSN, MA
Professor of Nursing
Glen Oaks Community College
Centreville, Michigan
Chapters 58–62

Barbara Staley Lenta RN, BSN
Learning Coordinator
Onondaga-Cortland-Madison BOCES
Syracuse, New York
Chapter 37

Laurie Lopez RN
Instructor, Practical Nursing
Western Dakota Technical Institute
Rapid City, South Dakota
Chapter 4

Susan C. Lowe RN, BSN, MS
Staff Nurse, Psychiatry
Hennepin County Medical Center
Minneapolis, Minnesota
Chapter 87

Kimberly R. Malcolm RN
Staff Nurse
Fairview Princeton Home Care
Princeton, Minnesota
Chapters 53, 54, 57, 64–67

Eunice McClurg
Executive Director
Association for Retarded Citizens
Anoka, Minnesota
Chapter 67

Kathleen McCullough RN, BSN
Staff Nurse, Operating and Recovery Rooms
Hennepin County Medical Center
Minneapolis, Minnesota
Chapters 53 and 54

LeAnne E. Meier RN
Assistant Clinical Manager
Maternal and Child Care Unit
HealthEast Midway Hospital
St. Paul, Minnesota
Chapters 63 and 84

Judith L. Miller RN, BSN, MS
Director of Services
MCOSS Inc.
Red Bank, New Jersey
Chapter 7, 89

Paul A. Montague BA, RRT
Director, Respiratory Care Services
University of Wisconsin Hospital and Clinics
Madison, Wisconsin
Chapter 80

Alicia Rosales Olson BSN, RN, MPH
Clinical Nurse Specialist, Cardiovascular
Abbott-Northwestern Hospital
Minneapolis, Minnesota
Chapter 74

Edward R. Perl MD
Chapel Hill, North Carolina
Chapter 52

Carol A. Reilly RN
Practical Nursing Instructor
Rensselaer-Columbia-Greene BOCES
Hudson, New York
Chapter 36

Majorie L. Roark (Lofgreen) RN, BSN, M.Ed.
Instructor in Nursing
Angelina College
Lufkin, Texas
Chapters 38–50

MaryAnne Robinson RN, MS
Clinical Nurse Manager
Alzheimer's Disease Diagnostic Research Center
Irvine, CA
Chapter 86

Jennie Lee Rodlund RN, CGRN
Clinical Manager, Endoscopy
HealthEast Divine Redeemer Hospital
Education Coordinator, HealthEast GI Service
St. Paul, Minnesota
Chapter 69

Keith Bunker Rosdahl BS
CAD Designer and Estimator
Minneapolis, Minnesota
Chapter 57

Rosemary L. Rosdahl RPh, BS
Pharmacist
Waconia, Minnesota
Chapters 55 and 56

Susan Bold Schumacher RN, MS
Medical-Surgical Clinical Nurse Specialist
Methodist Hospital
St. Louis Park, Minnesota
Chapter 79

Donna L. Schuurman Ed.D.
Executive Director
The Dougy Center for Grieving Children
Portland, Oregon
Chapters 90 and 91

Tammy Scott RN, CDE
Program Director, Diabetes Resource Center
HealthEast Midway Hospital
St. Paul, Minnesota
Chapter 72

Pamela K. Sobotka RN
Staff Nurse
Hennepin County Medical Center
Minneapolis, Minnesota
Chapters 74 and 88

Linda St. Dennis SRN, RN, MS
Resource Analyst, Nursing Administration
Health One Unity Hospital
Fridley, Minnesota
Chapters 77 and 78

Frances S. Stoner RN, BSN
Instructor, Pacific Coast College
Santa Ana, California
Chapter 92

Amy K. Susag RN, MS, CCRN
Critical Care Clinical Nurse Specialist
Health One Unity Hospital
Fridley, Minnesota
Chapters 73 and 77

L. Craig Watson RN, CCDC
Chemical Dependency Counselor and CEO
Counseling Center of Waconia
Waconia, Minnesota
Chapter 88

Mary Jane Watson BS Pharm, Pharm D
Associate Director of Clinical Research
Associated Skin Care Specialists
Fridley, Minnesota
Chapter 68

Cynthia L. White M.Ed.
Training Director
The Dougy Center for Grieving Children
Portland, Oregon
Chapters 90 and 91

Carol Williams RN, BSN
Infection Control Practitioner
VA Medical Center
Syracuse, New York
Chapters 29, 30, 51

Karl S. Wittman PhD
Supervisor, Occupational Education
New York State Education Department
Albany, New York
Chapter 8

Dawn M. Yetter RN
Orthopedic Nurse
Health One Unity Hospital
Fridley, Minnesota
Chapter 70

Mary E. Zaccagnini BAN, RN
Staff Nurse
North Memorial Medical Center
Robbinsdale, Minnesota
Chapter 76

Transcultural Panel

Becky L. Born Aftreth RN, BSN
Anchorage, Alaska

Patricia Gauntlett Beare RN, PhD
New Orleans, Louisiana

Donna M. Belitz RN, MEd
Rapid City, South Dakota

Patti Brown-Winston RN
Minneapolis, Minnesota

Gwendelyn Combs-Marshall BS, RD, Lactation Educator
Virgin Gorda, British Virgin Islands

Carol Deneck MS, RD
Red Bank, New Jersey

Magna Diaz
Philadelphia, Pennsylvania

Jean A. Glynn RN, MA, PHN
Supervisor
Red Bank, New Jersey

Eugene Gomez, MHW
Minneapolis, Minnesota

Jane Hurst RN
Piqua, Ohio

Patricia A. Knecht RN, BSN
Coatesville, Pennsylvania

Katherine A. LaBonte RN, BSN
Rapid City, South Dakota

S. Colet Lahoz MS, RN
White Bear Lake, Minnesota

Lori Lopez RN
Rapid City, South Dakota

Eunice McClurg
Anoka, Minnesota

Nancy Etcheverry de Menendez RN, MA
Mayaguez, Puerto Rico

Judith L. Miller RN, BSN, MS
Red Bank, New Jersey

Alicia Rosales Olson BSN, RN, MPH
Minneapolis, Minnesota

Suzanne Resignola RN
Morgan City, Louisiana

Marjorie Roark BSN, M.Ed.
Lufkin, Texas

Carol Riley RN
Hudson, New York

Linda St. Dennis SRN (England), RN, MS
Fridley, Minnesota

Marilyn R. Cheney-Stern RN, BS, MA, PhD
Trenton, North Carolina

Nursing Care Plans and Nursing Process Overview

Mary Ann O'Brien RN, BSPA/HCA
Nurse Educator
Collier County School System, J.L.W. Vocational
   Technical Center
Naples, Florida

Nursing Procedures

Carol Lillis RN, MSN
Associate Professor

Department of Nursing, Delaware County
   Community College
Media, Pennsylvania

Clinical Editorial Consultants

Maryann Foley RN, BSN
Clinical Consultant
Flourtown, Pennsylvania
Lynne Conrad RNC, MSN
Clinical Nurse Specialist
Department of Obstetrics and Gynecology
Albert Einstein Medical Center
Philadelphia, Pennsylvania

Reviewers

Beth A. Beaudet, RN, BSN, MSEd, Head Instructor, Otsego Area School of Practical Nursing, Oneonta, New York

Gyl Ann Burkhard, RN, BSN, MSEd, Lead Instructor, OCM BOCES, Syracuse, New York

Gwendolyn R. Burton, PhD, Professor Emeritus, Microbiology, Anatomy and Physiology, Front Range Community College, Westminster, Colorado

Annice D. Conaway, RN, MS, Department Head/Practical Nursing, J. F. Drake State Technical College, Huntsville, Alabama

Mary Ann Cosgarea, RN, BA, BSN Coordinator, Portage Lakes Career Center, W. Howard Nicol School of Practical Nursing, Greensburg, Ohio

Monica DeCarlo, MSN, RNC, Coordinator, Practical Nursing Program at Indiana County Area Vo-Tech School, Indiana, Pennsylvania

Selma Durham RN, BSN, MS, Pediatric Nurse Practitioner, Ivy Tech School of Practical Nursing, Columbus, Indiana

Linda A. Ellsworth, RN, BSN, Clinical Instructor, Portage Lakes Career Center, W. Howard Nicol School of Practical Nursing, Greensburg, Ohio

Paul G. Engelkirk, PhD, Faculty, Department of Science, Central Texas College, Killeen, Texas

Janet R. Ericksen, RN, MA, Senior Instructor, University of British Columbia School of Nursing, Vancouver, BC

Anna Feldman-Rosen, MS, Instructor, Thomas Jefferson University, Department of General Studies, Philadelphia, Pennsylvania

Beth A. Garner, RN, BSN, (specialist in AIDS), Chesapeake Center for Science & Technology, Chesapeake, Virginia

Sheila Guidry, RN, DSN, Director of Practical Nursing, Wallace Community College Selma, Selma, Alabama

Margrit E. Hayes, RN, BSN, Otsego Area School of Practical Nursing, Otsego Area Occupational Center, Milford, New York

Sally R. Holland, RN, BSPA, MSEd, Coordinator, Health Occupations Department, J. L. W. Vocational Technical Center, Naples, Florida

Elizabeth Holman, RN, MS, Director, Community Health Services Clinic, Scottsdale, Arizona

Cheryl Lynn Morgan Hornbeck, Chairman, Practical Nursing Program, Rice Belt Vocational Technical Institute, DeWitt, Arkansas

Nancy Jo Kastor, RN, BSN, Instructor, W. Howard Nicol School of Practical Nursing, Portage Lakes Career Center, Greensburg, Ohio

Grace A. Kittoe, RN, BS, MEd, Instructor, Practical Nurse Program, Canton City Schools, Canton, Ohio

Patricia Laing-Arie, RN, Instructor, Practical Nursing, Meridian Technology Center, Stillwater, Oklahoma

Catalina Loya, RN, Vocational Nursing Instructor, The University of Texas at Brownsville in partnership with TSC, Brownsville, Texas

Elaine Mohn, RN, EdD, Nursing Faculty, Chemeketa Community College, Salem, Oregon

Mary Ann O'Brien, RN, BSPA/HCA, Nurse Educator, Collier County School System, J. L. W. Vocational Technical Center, Naples, Florida

Betty F. Owen, RN, BA, MEd, Chairman PN Department, South Arkansas Community College, El Dorado, Arkansas

Karen A. Paterno, RN, MSN, Director, Odessa College Vocational Nursing Program, Andrews Extension, Andrews, Texas

Maura P. Payne, RN, BSN, Instructor, Riverside School of Practical Nursing, formerly Surgery Staff Nurse, Laser Speciality Nurse, Riverside Regional Medical Center, Newport News, Virginia

Sally Roach, RN, BSN, MSN, CNS, Assistant Professor, School of Health Sciences, The University of Texas at Brownsville, Brownsville, Texas

Dianne C. Ruscoe, RN, BSN, Practical Nursing Instructor, Mississippi Delta Community College, Moorhead, Mississippi

Allene Shelton, RN, MSN, Director, Vocational Nursing, Cerro Coso Community College, Ridgecrest, California

Alice H. Sinclair, RNC, MSN, Health Occupation Coordinator, Burlington County Institute of Technology, Medford, New Jersey

D. Marie Stone, RN, BSN, MBA, Practical Nursing Instructor, Henry County Public Schools-Memorial Hospital School of Practical Nursing, Martinsville, Virginia

Maryfran McKenzie Stulginsky, RN, MS, Bon Secour of Howard County, Columbia, Maryland

Yvonne R. Wall, RN, Mississippi Delta Community College, Moorhead, Mississippi

Beverly Post Yeshion, RN, BSN, ACCE, Nursing Consultant, Nursing Instructor, Hillsborough Community College, previously with Hillsborough County School of Practical Nursing, Tampa, Florida

Preface

TEXTBOOK OF BASIC NURSING is unique in that it is designed to be a comprehensive textbook covering the entire curriculum for LPN/LVN. The sixth edition has been extensively revised and updated to provide the most usable format for teacher instruction and student learning. Nursing specialists, educators, and practitioners from across the United States and Canada have reviewed or contributed to this edition. This helps to make TEXTBOOK OF BASIC NURSING usable in clinical nursing areas all over North America.

The sixth edition retains features of previous editions that proved most useful. Many new features have been added to assist students to learn. Additionally, the sixth edition has more pages to accommodate expanded content and reworking of skills and procedures.

Key Concepts of This Text

Several underlying concepts were considered in the development of this textbook. They are:

Optimal learning takes place in a predictable sequence: from less complex to more complex. This book builds on an optimal learning sequence for maximum benefit to both students and teachers. Basic information is presented first with an emphasis on normal growth and development, anatomy, and body function. Deviations from normal are presented later. As the student progresses through the nursing program and through the book, the information becomes more complex and builds on previous learning.

Information about personal and environmental health and safety, and the healthcare system is prerequisite to studying nursing. The first chapters of the book present general information about nursing, today's healthcare delivery system, and legal and ethical aspects of nursing. Personal and environmental health are also presented as basic concepts. Safety, first aid, and cardiopulmonary resuscitation are presented early in the book as a prerequisite to clinical nursing experience.

A knowledge of normal human growth and development, body structure and function, and human behavior helps the student recognize deviations. Basic scientific information appears early in the book. It includes an introduction to microbiology, normal body structure and function, child and adult growth and development, and basic normal nutrition, as well as basic principles of homeostasis and elementary principles of chemistry and physics. It is important to understand these principles in order to successfully recognize change. Clinical applications are made throughout the remainder of the book in order to introduce the student to the concept of understanding illness and disease as a deviation from normal.

Many nursing skills are used throughout one's nursing career, regardless of the patient's age or physical or mental condition. Basic nursing skills and procedures are presented in the early chapters of the book. These skills are used throughout the nursing career, whether caring for infants and children or adults. More complex skills or those specific to a particular area of nursing are presented later in the book.

The nursing process is a systematic method of assessing and diagnosing patients' needs and planning, implementing, and evaluating care. Several chapters are devoted to a description of the nursing process. Nursing assessment is emphasized in a new chapter, so the student can recognize signs and symptoms of deviations. The nursing process is used as a guideline for the remainder of the book with sample nursing diagnoses and sample nursing care plans.

All people have physical and emotional needs. This book uses Maslow's Hierarchy of Needs which states that basic, life-sustaining needs (such as oxygen and food) must be met before a person can meet higher-level needs (such as love and self-fulfillment). Much of nursing is aimed at assisting patients to meet needs; sometimes because they are unable to meet these needs without assistance. By considering the needs of *both patient and nurse,* the nurse is better able to administer total patient care.

Each person is unique. Patients and nurses bring culture, beliefs, and past history to all life experience. Sociological and transcultural implications are discussed as they influence the delivering and receiving of healthcare. This includes cultural concepts such as nutritional beliefs, personal space, or anatomical differences among racial groups. The nurse must also consider his or her own personal cultural and religious beliefs, as well as those of the patient, in order to give competent care.

When frightened or ill, people may behave differently from how they would ordinarily behave. A child may regress to a previous level of development; an adult may behave more like a child. The nurse must understand the levels of normal development in order to understand the person at a level other than that which is expected.

Patients are assisted by nurses in a variety of settings—the hospital, the nursing home and the community, and the home. The nurse must be comfortable in varied settings. Throughout the book, consideration is given to people in various healthcare environments.

Reflection on Healthcare Reform

The ever-changing healthcare delivery system and the constant barrage of new medical information were carefully researched for the development of this book. This information helps make the book accurate, complete, and up-to-date. Healthcare reform and *Healthy People 2000* are discussed in the text. Environmental concerns as they relate to healthcare are considered.

The trend toward care being given outside the hospital and the use of hospitals for acutely ill patients is clearly described. The involvement of the family in care is illustrated in patient and family teaching. Because of the aging of the population more space is given to defining changes and needs of the aging.

Organization

There are four major parts to the textbook. Part A discusses *Foundations of Nursing* in Chapters 1 through 28. It includes introductory material to nursing, human growth and development, anatomy and physiology, and nutrition and diets. Specific *Nursing Care Skills* comprise Part B in Chapters 29 through 57. Safety, nursing process, communication, basic patient care procedures, surgical intervention, and pharmacology and administration of medications are presented. *Meeting Client Needs Throughout the Life Cycle,* Part C, involves Chapters 48 through 91. Using the life span approach, units include maternal and newborn nursing, fundamentals of pediatric nursing and care in dysfunctions, physical dysfunctions in the adult, the older person, special needs, and dying. Part D, Chapters 92 and 93, discusses *Personal Responsibilities of the Graduate Nurse:* trends, leadership skills, career opportunities, and job-seeking skills.

All sections and chapters of the book are presented in the same or similar order for ease in locating material. Thus the order of systems presented in Unit Four, Anatomy and Physiology, is followed in discussions of pediatric and adult disorders. The nursing assessment, using a systems approach in Chapter 50, also follows this order. In addition, all chapters in the normal anatomy and physiology unit follow a consistent format, as do the medical–surgical chapters in Unit Fourteen. This organization is discussed later in the Preface.

As in previous editions, headings within the chapters are clearly identified in four major levels. This helps the instructor in formulating lesson plans and helps the student easily outline each chapter and identify key topics and their relative importance.

Key Teaching-Learning Features

Teaching and learning features play a prominent role in the presentation of this material. Every attempt has been made to help the student learn and demonstrate knowledge of the chapter being studied. A "learning key" approach is used throughout.

Keys for Learning

Each chapter opens with **Keys for Learning,** a section that introduces learning factors before the student studies the chapter.

- *Learning Objectives* provide behavioral and learning goals to guide the student while studying the chapter.
- *Key Terms* is a list of terms used in the chapter. These terms appear in boldface where they are defined in the chapter. Definitions are also given in the Glossary at the back of the book.
- *Keys to Understanding This Chapter* refer the reader to previous chapters that will enhance information or serve as a prerequisite to the material in the current chapter.
- *Key Points* summarize the key concepts or critical information in the chapter, so the student can understand up front the concepts of the chapter and build from them.
- *Key Topics Outline* outlines the progression of the chapter.
- *Key Learning Activities* are a means for reinforcing the material through interesting and educational activities. Instructors may assign them or students may use them on their own to initiate further learning and experiences.
- *Key Nursing Procedures,* a list that appears in appropriate chapters, is a list of special nursing procedures appearing in that chapter. Nursing Procedures and Nursing Skills are discussed later in this Preface.

Keys for Review

At the end of the chapter, a section called **Keys for Review** summarizes chapter learning features. The review includes the following:

- *Key Questions for Critical Thinking* are thought-provoking review questions. Their purpose is to help the student make self-assessments and think through possible solutions to problems. There are no "right" or "wrong" answers.
- *Key Readings* includes the references used in preparing the chapter.
- *Enrichment Keys,* appearing in many chapters, offer additional bibliography for the student's personal reading or study.
- *Keys to Learning More* refers the reader to later supplemental chapters.
- *Key Resources,* appearing in some chapters, provides organizations and their addresses for further information or support.

Other Learning Features

Scattered generously throughout the text are additional features to enhance student learning. These include:

- *Key Concepts* are highlighted boxes that call out and review important concepts.
- *Nursing Alert* is important information that may present life-threatening or dangerous situations if not learned or if performed incorrectly.
- *Key Medications* are highlighted boxes that identify key medications and related nursing considerations for selected conditions.
- *Sample Nursing Care Plans and Nursing Process Overview* are two special types of Nursing Process material. Sample nursing care plans for selected common conditions provide a guide for students in understanding individualized nursing care plans for their own patients. The Nursing Process Overview summarizes actions in the nursing process steps for special situations.
- *Keys to Patient and Family Teaching* summarize teaching subjects to be taught in selected conditions. Because hospital stays are short, patient and family teaching and documentation of this teaching are increasingly important in nursing.
- *Special Considerations in Children* give key information for the nurse to consider when caring for the pediatric patient.
- *Special Considerations in Aging* give key information to consider when caring for the geriatric patient.
- *Nursing Assessment* boxes highlight factors in nursing assessments for various conditions or disorders.
- *Tables and boxed information.* Important information and guidelines are displayed prominently in boxes and tables for easier access and study. For instance, all of the anatomy and physiology chapters have a box called *Functions of the System* that summarizes functions of each system. When a chapter has a good many abbreviations and acronyms with which the student should be familiar, these are boxed near the beginning of the chapter.

As in the past, color is used throughout the book as a teaching feature: to emphasize points in art, to underscore organization of chapters, and to highlight features.

Presentation of Nursing Procedures

Basic to the practice of nursing are the various nursing skills performed in daily care of the patient. This textbook has always had a strong presentation of these skills. For the 6th edition most of these skills have been greatly revised, updated, and illustrated. Some are new. The majority of these procedures have been pulled into earlier chapters of the book where basic nursing care is covered. In this edition you will find nursing skills presented in four ways:

Nursing Procedures   About 38 of the most common procedures are placed in boxes identified as **Nursing Procedures** and are heavily illustrated. Each procedure has a list of Supplies and Equipment and a step-by-step approach to the procedure. Each step states the *rationale*. The student who understands why a procedure is performed in a certain way will be more likely to perform it correctly and safely and the graduate nurse who understands underlying rationale will be able to adjust more easily to practices used in individual healthcare facilities. Special considerations in the procedure may be listed at the end of the procedure.

Nursing Skills   These skills appear within the text but are set off for easy identification. They include Equipment and Supplies and the Procedure in step-by-step performance with Rationale. Many of these also include photographs.

Nursing Skill Guidelines   About 70 nursing skills appear in a boxed list called **Nursing Skill Guidelines.** Generally these are not presented in a step-by-step manner but give general nursing information in caring for patients.

Other skills are listed within the text with bullets. They identify key points in providing care. There are about 70 of these skills.

A **glove pictogram** (a drawing of a gloved hand) appears in each procedure or skill where gloves must be worn as a part of Universal Precautions.

Revised Material in the Sixth Edition

A new edition of a book always includes heavy revision of existing units to update information and to address changes in healthcare. This is true of the sixth edition of TEXTBOOK OF BASIC NURSING. Also, because more pages were added to this edition, many chapters have been expanded. The following major revisions were made.

◆ Chapters 3, *The Healthcare Delivery System*, and 7, *Community Health*, have been revised to reflect the latest in healthcare including *Healthy People 2000* and the proposed Clinton healthcare reform.

◆ Chapter 4, *Legal and Ethical Aspects of Nursing*. This chapter was reorganized and rewritten to present the latest in ethics and law as it pertains to the nurse.

◆ Chapter 8, *Introduction to Microbiology*, reviewed by microbiologists, was completely revised and illustrated.

◆ Chapters in the unit on normal anatomy and physiology have been revised. In addition to discussions of structure and function, a new section on "System Physiology" ties together the systems' actions. Information called "Effects of Aging" includes tables that present factors, results, and nursing considerations for that system.

◆ The Nutrition unit was revised by a Registered Dietition. The Food Pyramid and its use in diet planning play a prominent role. A great deal of new information was added by a GI Nursing Specialist regarding nutritional support such as tube feedings.

◆ Chapter 87, *Mental Health and Psychiatric Nursing*, was completely revised and updated and refers to the new DSM-IV.

◆ *The Aging Population*. As the population ages, nursing continues to be more and more involved in the care of aging citizens. Geriatric nursing is emphasized with a separate unit in the book, a section and table on aging in all chapters in the anatomy and physiology unit, and Special Considerations boxes throughout the book.

◆ The entire medical-surgical unit was extensively revised and updated. Each chapter is organized in a consistent format including anatomy and physiology review; laboratory, x-ray and other diagnostic tests; common medical and surgical treatments; and nursing process (nursing assessment, nursing diagnosis, planning and implementation, and evaluation). The reminder of chapter gives an overview of common disorders. Within the discussion of many disorders is included a description of the condition, signs and symptoms, specific diagnostic tests, medical and surgical treatment, nursing con-

siderations, key medications, and related patient and family teaching.

◆ The *Glossary* at the back of the book has been expanded to define new language in healthcare vocabulary. Around 300 new words or phrases have been added. Other definitions have been revised to accept the newest knowledge.

New Material in the 6th Edition

◆ A completely new chapter has been written on *Nursing Assessment and Physical Examination* (Chapter 50). This chapter is presented at a level appropriate to the beginning practitioner. It provides for the nurse who will help in the physical examination or perform some of the examination responsibilities.

◆ Some information has been separated out of other chapters to create the following new chapters in this edition: Chapter 15, *The Integumentary System;* Chapter 63, *Sexuality, Fertility, and Sexually Transmitted Diseases;* Chapter 78, *HIV, AIDS, and Autoimmune Disorders;* Chapter 75, *Blood and Lymph Disorders;* Chapter 76, *Cancer;* Chapter 79, *Respiratory Disorders;* Chapter 80, *Oxygen Therapy and Respiratory Care;* Chapter 83, *Male Reproductive Disorders;* and Chapter 84, *Female Reproductive Disorders.*

◆ Boxes called *Keys to Nursing Assessment* appear throughout the text. They appear in each chapter in Unit Fourteen as well as in other chapters.

◆ A new section of Chapter 55 is a review of *basic mathematics*. This information is prerequisite to the study of pharmacology and medication administration.

◆ All of the medication tables have been reviewed by a Registered Pharmacist and the material updated. In these tables, and throughout the book, whenever a medication is named, the generic name is given first with the trade name(s) following in parentheses.

◆ A new section on wound healing and special skin care was added by an Enterostomal Therapist Nurse to Chapter 45 in the basic skills unit.

◆ A new chapter has been added on Medical Asepsis and *Universal Precautions* (Chapter 30) as well as a separate chapter on *HIV, AIDS,* and *Autoimmune Disorders* (Chapter 78). Universal Precautions are also identified and summarized inside the back cover of the book.

◆ Appendix A, *Key English-to-Spanish Healthcare Phrases*, gives phrases that will help the nurse care for patients who are Spanish speaking.

◆ Appendix B, a special Glossary of *Key Abbrevia-*

tions and Acronyms Used in Healthcare has been added to this edition.

- ◆ Appendix C, *Normal Values and Reference Tables* gives information about norms for various blood and urine chemistries.
- ◆ Appendix D, *Exchange Lists for Meal Planning,* outlines the suggestions prepared by the American Diabetes Association and the American Dietetic Association.

Features of the 6th Edition

Materials included inside the covers, interspersed throughout the chapters, and at the end of the book provide quick information sources:

- ◆ Inside the front cover and on the front endpaper are the basic Table of Contents as well as an introductory section for the student called "Key Notes for the Student." Inside the back covers are the most recent NANDA nursing diagnoses and an overview of the most up-to-date Universal Precautions.
- ◆ Chapter 14 includes a box that introduces medical terminology (prefixes and suffixes) commonly used in medical terms.
- ◆ Chapter 37 contains a table of commonly-used medical abbreviations, symbols, and descriptive terms to be used in documentation.
- ◆ Chapter 56 contains tables of commonly used medications, with therapeutic indications, average adult doses, and special information.
- ◆ Pedagogic materials are spread throughout the book. Namely, **Keys for Learning, Keys for Review, Nursing Procedures, and Nursing Skills.**

General Considerations

"Readability" has always been one of the positive comments about TEXTBOOK OF BASIC NURSING. Every attempt has been made to maintain that readability in the sixth edition.

Transcultural aspects of nursing are emphasized throughout the book. More than 20 professionals from across the United States agreed to critique the chapters devoted to transcultural aspects of nursing and to make suggestions. Their suggestions were incorporated throughout the book and particularly in Chapters 17, 36, and 39.

Sexist language has been avoided by eliminating "he" and "she" when referring to nurses, patients, and physicians. If such a reference occurs, except in specialized areas such as maternal care, this is an oversight.

The term "patient" is used throughout most of the book, with the understanding that "client" or "resident" may be used in your facility. The important thing to remember is that whether you care for a "patient" or a "client" you are caring for a person who is unique.

The Ancillary Package

To strengthen teaching and learning concepts, several ancillaries are available in this package. *Study Guide to Accompany the Sixth Edition of Textbook of Basic Nursing* provides review questions and answers to strengthen learning. Each chapter also includes a "Critical Thinking Activity" to help students develop thinking and decision-making skills. This book helps the student review and prepare for classroom examination and the NCLEX licensing examination.

The *Instructor's Manual to Accompany the Sixth Edition of Textbook of Basic Nursing* provides the instructor with additional teaching ideas and resources and materials. A printed *Testbank to Accompany the Sixth Edition of Textbook of Basic Nursing* supplements test items. *Procedure Checklists* are a new supplemental feature this edition. The manual includes a checklist for each procedure to help the student with self-evaluation.

Caroline Bunker Rosdahl

Acknowledgments

Many people contributed to the completion of this book. Although it is impossible to thank them all, some require special mention. I would like to offer a special thank you to the following:

◆ my family, who were very patient and supportive; and, some of whom contributed to the book.

◆ students and instructors who took the time to give comments, corrections and suggestions—this is the only way we know what you want and need—please keep writing.

◆ contributors and consultants, who gave freely of their time and knowledge to make this book correct, comprehensive, and current.

◆ Pat Oatman and 3M Health Care for many photographs.

◆ reviewers who read sections of the book and evaluated them in terms of their own teaching needs and experiences.

◆ Gerri Anderson, RN, who coordinated a large portion of the book and who patiently worked out last-minute details.

◆ Donna Richardson, RN, BA, MA, who wrote the first several editions of the student workbook and who gave moral support throughout the preparation of this edition.

◆ Marge Roark, RN, BSN, MEd, Kathy Casolino, RN, BS, MSEd, and Mary Kowalski, RN, BA, BSN, MS, three new friends made with this edition. They each contributed a large portion of the book and all managed to maintain a sense of humor under great personal and professional duress and during "manuscript panic" situations.

◆ John Gray, who gave me the opportunity to gain first-hand clinical nursing experience in a hospital setting.

◆ Keith Rosdahl, Bill Frisch, and Maggie Hanson, who patiently listened to my screams, held my hand, and did repairs when the computer acted up or, worst yet, when it crashed.

◆ Mary Gortemacher, who cleaned around piles of manuscript in my house, so I would have more time to write.

◆ a special word of remembrance for Suzanne Resignola, Morgan City, Louisiana, who worked on part of the book but did not live to see its completion.

◆ and a word of remembrance for two others who planned to work on the book and died before they could begin—Jean Jung, Western Dakota Technical Institute, Rapid City, South Dakota, and Beverly Rambo, Mount St. Mary's College, Los Angeles, California.

◆ thanks to Carol Lillis, RN, MSN, for writing the Nursing Procedures; and to Cheryl Meyer, RN, BSN, MSN, for organizing and supervising the photo shoot to illustrate the Nursing Procedures.

◆ thanks to Mary Ann O'Brien, RN, BS, PA/HCA, for reviewing and writing Nursing Care Plans and Nursing Process overviews; to Patricia Dillon, RN, for writing the Instructor's Manual, Testbank, and Procedure Checklists, and to Marge Roark, RN, BSN, MEd, for revising the study guide. Thanks also go to Susan Blaker for coordinating plans for illustrations and photos for the 6th edition.

◆ very special thanks go to several people at the J. B. Lippincott Company, who authorized the new edition, came up with ideas for new features, and who painstakingly considered every word and illustration. Without them, there would be no book. I would particularly like to thank Diana Intenzo, Vice President/Publisher, for her continued vision of nursing, and Donna Hilton, Executive Editor, for her enthusiastic approach to the project. Very special thanks go to Eleanor Faven, Senior Developmental Editor, for her "key ideas" and for pulling it all together and making sure the book was concise and cohesive. Her hard work and guidance is rarely found in today's world. Susan Keneally, Editorial Assistant, is to be commended for her coordination of "behind the scenes" work with contributors and reviewers. No book can be published without the cooperation of an experienced and dedicated production department, in this case, Amy Jirsa, Project Editor; Kathryn Rule, Production Coordinator; Helen Ewan, Production Manager, and Doug Smock, Assistant Art Director.

Basic Contents

Expanded Table of Contents

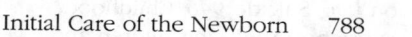

Unit 15
Assisting the Older Person   1337

85 Geriatrics: The Aging Adult   1338

86 Dementia-Type Disorders   1353

Unit 16
Meeting Special Needs   1370

87 Mental Health and Psychiatric Nursing   1371

88 Substance Abuse   1395

89 Rehabilitation, Ambulatory, and Home Care Nursing   1411

Unit 17
Assisting the Dying Person and the Family   1422

90 Death and Dying   1423

Summary of Special Boxed Displays

Nursing Procedures, Nursing Skills, and Nursing Skill Guidelines

Key: Nursing Procedures, NP; Nursing Skills, NS; Nursing Skill Guidelines, NSG.
Phrases with no initial abbreviation are in-text nursing skills and activities.

Sample Nursing Care Plans and Nursing Process Overviews

Sample Nursing Care Plans are listed by their titles. Nursing Process Overviews are dentified as "Overview."

Recurring Boxes

Several features in the book are called "Keys." The following list includes "Keys to Patient and Family Teaching" (identified here as "Keys to Teaching") and "Keys to Nursing Assessment" (identified here as "Keys to Assessment). Tables on aging are also listed from the anatomy and physiology unit.

Part **A**   Foundations of Nursing

Unit *1* The Nature of Nursing

1 The Origins of Nursing

Learning Objectives

♦ Describe some of the events in ancient and medieval Europe that influenced the development of modern nursing
♦ Identify some of the persons who have contributed to the history of nursing
♦ Discuss the influence of Florence Nightingale on modern nursing practice
♦ List at least 10 of Florence Nightingale's nursing principles that are still practiced today
♦ List two of the three pioneer practical nursing schools in the United States
♦ Compare and contrast the description of the first nursing insignia to the student's own school's nursing pin

Key Terms

Hippocratic Oath
insignia

Key Points

♦ Care of the sick in ancient times was performed by medicine men and women and later by religious orders.
♦ Florence Nightingale contributed a great deal to the development of nursing as we know it today.
♦ Establishment of nursing schools in the United States began in the late 19th century.
♦ The first practical nursing school in the United States opened in 1892 in New York.

Key Topics Outline

Ancient Medicine
   Hippocrates
Nursing's Heritage
   The Roman Matrons
   Christian Religious Orders
   The Reformation
   Fliedner in Kaiserswerth
   Florence Nightingale
Nursing in the United States
   The First Nursing Schools
   Notable American Nurses
   Collegiate Nursing Education in the United States
   The History of Practical Nursing Education
Nursing Insignia
   The Nursing School Pin
   The Nursing Cap

Key Learning Activities

♦ Interview the director of your nursing program. Write a report on the history of your program. What year did it start? Identify the important people involved in its establishment.
♦ Do a research/biographical paper on one of the leaders in the establishment of nursing educational programs. (Choose a person who is not described in detail in your textbook.)
♦ Look at the graduate pin from your nursing program. Can you identify all of the symbols? Ask your instructors to tell you the meaning of the symbols.

You have chosen to be a nurse. Whatever your personal motives, you are embarking on a career that combines scientific principles, technical skills, and personal compassion. People have been performing the skills of nursing for centuries. However, nursing as we know it today has been evolving for only the past few hundred years.

Ancient Medicine

In ancient times, illness was considered to be punishment for sins by God or as "possession" by an evil spirit. Most tribes and peoples had a medicine man or woman who performed rituals, using various plants and herbs, to heal the sick. By 500 B.C., the Greeks had begun to establish centers, sometimes called "hostels" or "hospitals," for care of the sick and injured. Pregnant women or people with incurable illness were not allowed in these hospitals.

Hippocrates

One of the early outstanding figures in medicine was Hippocrates, who was born in 460 B.C. and is credited with being the "Father of Medicine." Physicians still repeat the **Hippocratic Oath** when they enter the field of medicine, an oath based on the principles espoused by Hippocrates. (The Florence Nightingale pledge and the Practical Nurses' pledge are based on this oath). Hippocrates first proposed such concepts as physical assessment, medical ethics, patient-centered care, and observation and reporting. By emphasizing the importance of caring for the patient, he helped lay the groundwork for nursing.

Nursing's Heritage

A detailed history of nursing is beyond the scope of this book, but all nurses should be familiar with some important people in the history of nursing and medicine.

In earlier times, usually the men who cared for the sick were soldiers. They cared for their comrades on the battlefield. Women in healthcare concentrated on helping children and the poor and caring for the sick, usually in their own homes.

The Roman Matrons

The first recorded history of nursing begins with recordings in the Bible of women who cared for the sick and injured. Many were in the religious life. For instance, *Phoebe* was mentioned in the Epistle to the Romans, dated about 58 A.D. She is known as the first deaconess and the first visiting nurse.

Fabiola, a Roman woman, is credited with influencing and paying for the construction of the first free hospital in Rome in 390 A.D. Another Roman woman, *Saint Marcella*, converted her beautiful home into a monastery where she taught the skills of nursing. She could be considered the first nursing educator. *Saint Paula* is credited with establishing inns and hospitals to care for the pilgrims who were traveling to Jerusalem. She is said to have been the first to teach that nursing was an art rather than a service.

Saint Helena was the mother of the Roman Emperor, Constantine. She is credited with the establishment of the first geriatric facility, a home for the aged.

Christian Religious Orders

Monastic Nursing Orders

During the first century A.D., several monastic orders were established for the care of the sick. In some cases, the monastery became the refuge for the sick; in other cases, the religious order founded a hospital. Nursing was performed by both men and women of religious orders.

Military Nursing Orders

During the Crusades (1096–1291), the female religious orders in northern Europe were nearly wiped out, and nursing was performed by male military personnel, such as the Knights Hospitalers of St. John in Jerusalem. Because these military men were required to defend the hospital as well as to care for patients, they wore suits of armor under their religious habits. The symbol for this order was the Maltese cross, which later became the symbol of the Nightingale School. It was the forerunner of the nursing school pins worn today.

The Reformation

During the religious movement called the Reformation in Germany in the 1500s, monasteries were closed and the work of women in religious orders was nearly ended. The few women who cared for the sick during this time were prisoners or prostitutes. Nursing was considered the most menial of all tasks, and thus the least desirable. This period is known as the "dark ages of nursing."

Fliedner in Kaiserswerth

Fliedner in Kaiserswerth school for nursing was established in 1836 by Pastor Theodor Fliedner in his parish in Kaiserswerth, Germany. It was one of the first formally established schools of nursing in the world. Out of it grew the Lutheran Order of Deaconesses, directed by Fliedner. Its most famous student was Florence Nightingale.

By the late 1800s, there were many schools for "trained nurses" throughout Europe. The status of nursing was greatly improved and many women, including members of religious orders, were now involved in patient care.

Florence Nightingale (1820–1910)

Even during the days when nursing was considered menial and undesirable, some women continued to care for the sick. Probably the most famous of these was Florence Nightingale (Fig. 1-1). Nurses received little or no training or preparation, however. Not until Florence Nightingale helped reform these conditions did nursing become a respectable profession.

Florence Nightingale was born in Italy in 1820 to wealthy English parents. When she was still very young, her parents moved back to England. In 1844, an American doctor visited the Nightingale family, and Florence asked him if it would be appropriate for her to enter the field of nursing. (Nursing was not considered suitable for "high class ladies.") The reply from Dr. Samuel Gridley Howe to Nightingale has become a classic. He said:

> My dear Miss Florence, it would be unusual (for you to enter nursing), and in England whatever is unusual is apt to be thought unsuitable; but I say to you, go forward, if you have a vocation for that way of life; act up to your aspiration and you will find that there is never anything unbecoming or unladylike in doing your duty for the good of others. Choose your path, go on with it, wherever it may lead you, and God be with you!

And so it was that Florence Nightingale entered Deaconess School of Nursing in Kaiserswerth, Ger-

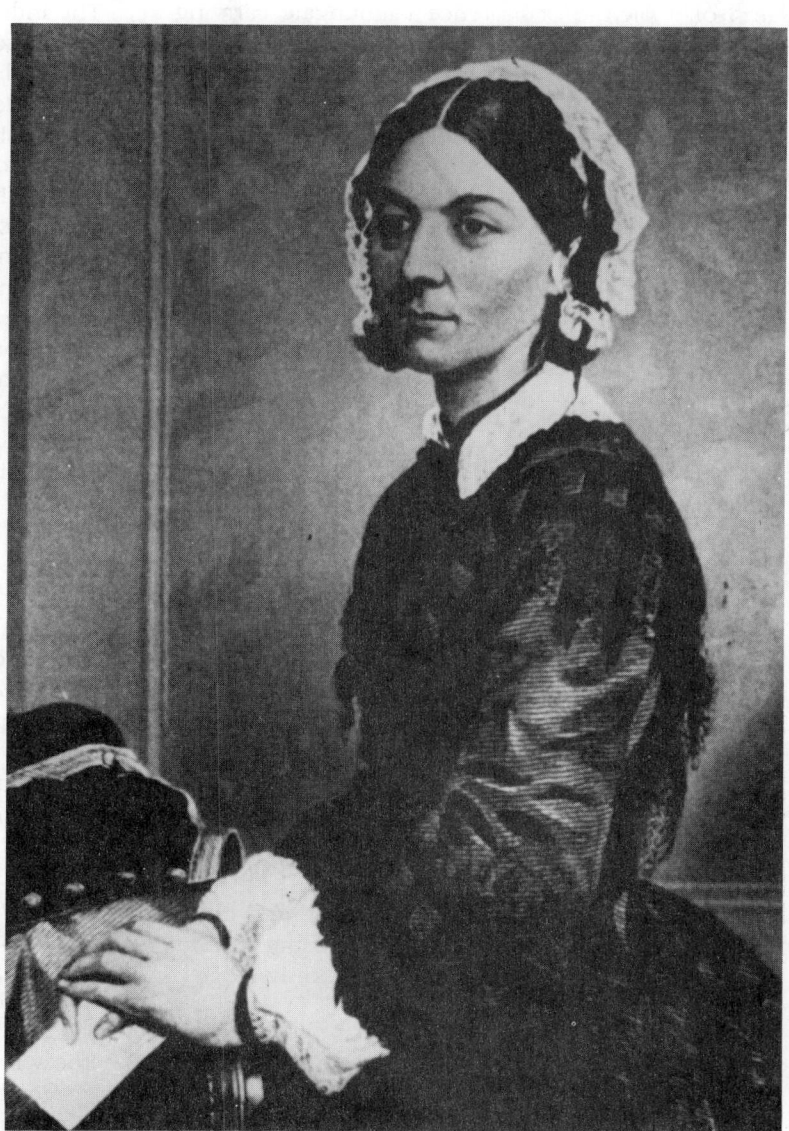

Figure 1-1. Florence Nightingale (Photo courtesy of the Center for the Study of the History of Nursing).

many, in 1851. She was 31 years old, and her family and friends were still strongly opposed to her becoming a nurse.

In 1853, after her graduation, she became superintendent of a charity hospital for governesses. She trained her attendants on the job and improved the quality of care. In 1854 the Crimean War began, and during this conflict Florence Nightingale gained fame. She entered the battlefield with 38 other nurses and cared for the sick and injured men. They had few supplies and little support from the other workers. Nonetheless, Nightingale insisted on establishing sanitary conditions and good nursing care for the soldiers. Her persistence made her famous, and her dedicated service both during the day and at night, when she and her nurses made their rounds carrying oil lamps, created a public image of "the lady with the lamp." In time the "Nightingale lamp" became the symbol of nursing. Today many schools of nursing display a model of the lamp or a picture of Florence Nightingale carrying a lamp.

The Nightingale School

In 1860, Florence Nightingale opened the first school outside a hospital for nursing in England. The course was one year in length and included both classroom and clinical experience, a revolutionary innovation at that time. Clinical experience in Nightingale's program was gained at St. Thomas Hospital in London.

Some of the principles taught in the Nightingale School for Nurses are still taught today. Examples include:

◆ Cleanliness is vital to recovery.
◆ The sick person is an individual with individual needs.
◆ Nursing is an art and a science.
◆ Nurses should spend their time caring for patients, not cleaning.
◆ Prevention is better than cure.
◆ The nurse must work as a member of a team.
◆ The nurse must use discretion, but must follow the physician's orders.
◆ Self-discipline and self-evaluation are important.
◆ A good nursing program encourages individual development of the nurse.
◆ The nurse should be healthy in mind and body.
◆ Teaching is a part of nursing.
◆ Nursing is a specialty.
◆ A nurse does not "graduate," but continues to learn throughout his or her career. The nursing curriculum should include both theoretical knowledge and practical experience.

Other innovations of the Nightingale School included:

◆ Separation of the school from the hospital to facilitate education, rather than service.

◆ Establishment of a nurses' residence.
◆ Entrance examinations and academic and personal requirements, including a character reference.
◆ Records of each student's progress—later known as the "Nightingale plan," a model for 20th century nursing programs.
◆ Records of employment of students after graduation—a formal "register"—the beginnings of nursing practice standards.

Nursing in the United States

Nursing in the colonial United States was primarily a family matter, with mothers caring for their own families or neighbors assisting each other.

The First Nursing Schools

The influence of Florence Nightingale and the Kaiserswerth school extended to the United States when Pastor Fliedner came to Pittsburgh, Pennsylvania with four nurse–deaconesses. In 1849, he became involved with the Pittsburgh Infirmary, which became the first Protestant hospital in the United States. Today it is known as the Passavant Hospital. These four deaconesses trained other nurses and began the movement to train nurses in the United States. This was the first real school of nursing in the United States although limited training existed in other hospitals in New York and Pennsylvania before 1849.

Formal establishment of three nursing programs based on the Nightingale plan took place in 1873. These included: Bellevue Hospital School of Nursing, New York; Connecticut Training School, New Haven; and Boston Training School at Massachusetts General Hospital.

Notable American Nurses

With the onset of the Civil War in 1861, the public need for nurses in the United States became more evident. *Dorothea Lynde Dix* (1802–1887) was appointed Superintendent of Female Nurses of the Union Army in 1861. Her job was to recruit volunteer nurses to treat men injured in the war. She was given instructions that the women were to be over age 30 and "plain-looking," and that they were not to curl their hair or wear any sort of ornaments. They were required to wear hoop skirts. Dorothea Dix is remembered for her campaign against the inhumane treatment of the mentally ill. One of Dix's volunteers was *Louisa May Alcott* (author of *Little Women*) and another was *Clara Barton* (1821–1912). Clara Barton later founded the organization now known as the American Red Cross in 1881.

Melinda Ann (Linda) Richards (1841-1930) was the first trained nurse in the United States. She graduated in 1872 or 1873 and organized the school of nursing at Massachusetts General Hospital (then called the Boston Training School).

Isabel Hampton Robb (1860–1910) was the founder of the school of nursing at Johns Hopkins University. She is credited with founding two national nursing organizations, one in 1911, which eventually emerged as the American Nurses Association (originally called the Alumnae Association). She and *Lavinia Lloyd Dock* (1858–1956) founded the American Society of Superintendents of Training Schools of Nursing, which later evolved into the Education Committee of the National League for Nursing. She wrote one of the earliest nursing textbooks, *Materia Medica for Nurses* and coauthored a four-volume *History of Nursing.*

Robb wrote extensively and founded *The American Journal of Nursing.* Robb introduced charting and nurse licensure to improve the continuity of patient care. She also initiated the idea of graduate study in nursing in the late 1800s.

Lillian Wald (1867–1940) is considered the founder of American public health nursing. She is best known for founding the Henry Street Settlement (Visiting Nurse Society—VNS) in New York City in 1893. The Henry Street Settlement was a neighborhood nursing service that became a model for similar programs in the United States and other countries. Wald also convinced the New York City schools to have a nurse on duty during school hours, persuaded President Theodore Roosevelt to create a Federal Children's Bureau, and insisted that nursing education occur in institutions of higher learning.

The first African American graduate nurse, *Mary E. Mahoney* (1845–1926), worked toward fair treatment of blacks in hospital care. She promoted integration and better working conditions for black patients and healthcare workers in Boston.

Mary Breckinridge (1881-1965) was a pioneer visiting nurse–midwife to the mountain people of Kentucky in the early 1900s, often making her rounds on horseback. She also started one of the first midwifery schools in the United States.

Collegiate Nursing Education in the United States

In 1907, *Mary Adelaide Nutting* (1858–1947), a good friend of Robb, was instrumental in establishing the first college-based nursing program, at Teachers College of Columbia University. She thus became the first nurse to be on a university staff. She was also instrumental in founding the International Council of Nurses.

In 1909, the University of Minnesota established the first program to educate nurses on the university level, with an enrollment of four students. Isabel Hampton Robb was instrumental in the organization of this collegiate program, which is considered the beginning of nursing as a *profession.* This program, however, did not

lead to a baccalaureate degree until 1919, when several other schools had also initiated college and university-based nursing programs.

The History of Practical Nursing Education

Practical nursing (also called vocational nursing) has been in existence for many years. Women often cared for others and called themselves "practical nurses," but it was not until the 1890s that formal education in practical nursing was available.

Pioneer Schools

Curricula in all of the early PN schools included child care, cooking, and light housekeeping, in addition to care of the sick at home.

Ballard School. In 1892, the first practical nursing school, the Ballard School, was opened in New York City by the YWCA. Practical nursing was one of several courses offered for women under the auspices of the school. Lucinda Ballard provided the funds for this venture. The practical nursing program was a 3-month course to train women in simple nursing care. The emphasis was on caring for infants and children, the elderly, and disabled in their own homes. The Ballard School closed in 1949 because of YWCA reorganization.

Thompson Practical Nursing School. Thomas Thompson, a wealthy man who lived in Brattleboro, Vermont during the Civil War, was disturbed to learn that women were making shirts for the army at only a dollar a dozen. In his will, he left money to help them. Richard Bradley, the executor, was a public-spirited man who saw that Brattleboro citizens needed nursing service. In 1907, some of Thompson's money was used to establish a practical nursing school in Brattleboro. This school is still in existence.

Household Nursing School. In Boston, a group of women were determined that something should be done to provide nursing care for people who were sick at home. They called on Richard Bradley for advice, and he encouraged them to follow Brattleboro's example. In 1918, the Household Nursing Association School of Attendant Nursing was opened. The school was later renamed the Shepard–Gill School of Practical Nursing in honor of Katherine Shepard Doge, the first director, and Helen Z. Gill, her associate and successor. This school operated until 1984.

American Red Cross Training

In 1908, the American Red Cross began offering "home nursing" training to lay women so they could care for illnesses within their own families.

Practical Nursing in Vocational Education

Nursing schools, training both practical nurses and professional nurses, were traditionally located in or affiliated with hospitals. In 1917, the U.S. Congress passed the Smith–Hughes Act, the funds from which gave impetus to vocational–technical and public education in the United States. In 1919, the first vocational school-based nursing program was opened, in Minneapolis. Today, the majority of practical nursing programs are located in vocational education settings or in community colleges.

Because of the great demand, 260 practical/vocational nursing programs opened between 1948 and 1954. Today there are more than 1,300 practical nursing programs in the United States.

Other Milestones in Practical Nursing Education

During World War II, people realized that nurses needed a consistent curriculum. In 1942, the first practical nursing curriculum was planned and advocated across the entire United States.

In 1914, Mississippi became the first state to license practical nurses (LPNs). By 1955, all states had laws to license practical nurses. The first state to have mandatory licensure for LPNs to practice was New York. (Permissive and mandatory licensure are described more fully in Chapter 2.)

In 1966, the Chicago Public School system's program was the first practical nursing program to be accredited by the National League for Nursing (NLN).

Key Concept

As you embark on your career as a nurse, you continue the history and heritage of nursing.

Nursing Insignia

An **insignia** is a distinguishing badge of authority or honor. The symbolism dates back to the 16th century in Europe, when only a nobleman could wear a coat of arms. Later this privilege was expanded to include the guilds. Certain types of training schools, including religious nursing orders, were also given the privilege. Until recently, female nurses wore nursing caps and all nurses were awarded a school pin at graduation. Some schools also had distinguishing capes.

The Nursing School Pin

You may receive a nursing pin at graduation. It is symbolic of your school of nursing.

Early nursing symbols were usually religious in nature, and today many nursing school pins bear some religious symbol, such as a cross or a Star of David, even though the school may not be directly affiliated with a religious organization. The Nightingale lamp is also a common component of the nursing pin.

The Nursing Cap

The nurse's cap was a functional piece of clothing in the Middle Ages, when neither the patient nor the nurse practiced habits of cleanliness. The cap, much like a dust cover or shower cap, covered the entire head and enclosed all of the nurse's hair. This protected both nurse and patient. Nursing caps are seldom worn by nurses today.

Keys for Review

Key Questions for Critical Thinking

1. Describe and discuss the influence of history on nursing and of nursing on history.
2. Discuss five people who were important in nursing history and explain why you feel they were important.
3. Discuss the contributions of Florence Nightingale and their importance to contemporary nursing.

Key Readings

Deming D (S Reverby, ed). The Practical Nurse. (History). New York, Garland, 1984 (Reproduction of 1947 Edition)

Dolan JA. Nursing in Society: A Historical Perspective. Philadelphia, W.B. Saunders, 1983

Ellis JR, Hartley CL. Nursing in Today's World: Challenges, Issues, and Trends, Ed 4. Philadelphia, J.B. Lippincott, 1992

Key Readings (continued)

Ellis JR, Nowlis EA. Nursing: A Human Needs Approach, Ed 5. Philadelphia, J.B. Lippincott, 1994

Kurzen CR. Contemporary Practical/Vocational Nursing, Ed 2. Philadelphia, J.B. Lippincott, 1993

Nightingale, F. Notes on Nursing: What It Is and What It Is Not (Commemorative Edition 1859). Philadelphia, J.B. Lippincott, 1992

Enrichment Keys

Kraegel J, Kachoyeanos M. Just a Nurse: The Hearts and Minds of Nurses in Their Own Words. New York, Dutton (Penguin), 1989

Enrichment Keys (continued)

Norman EM. Women at War: The Story of Fifty Military Nurses Who Served in Vietnam. Philadelphia, University of Pennsylvania Press, 1990

Keys to Learning More

Chapter 2: nursing education, code of ethics, and organizations

Chapter 3: healthcare facilities and payment

Chapter 4: legal and ethical aspects of nursing

Chapter 92: trends in nursing and leadership skills

Chapter 93: career opportunities

2 Beginning Your Nursing Career

Keys for Learning

Learning Objectives

♦ Compare the roles and education of the practical nurse and registered nurse
♦ Describe the various types of educational programs leading to licensure
♦ Identify at least one of the standards of the National Federation of Licensed Practical Nurses for licensed practical nurses in relationship to each of the following: education, legal status, and practice
♦ Define *permissive* licensure and *mandatory* licensure
♦ Discuss the reasons for a nurse to seek licensure
♦ Describe nursing organizations, their membership requirements, and benefits

Key Terms

accreditation
approval
clinical
ethics
licensure

mandatory licensure
permissive licensure
practical nurse
registered nurse

Keys to Understanding This Chapter

Chapter 1: historical background of nursing

Key Points

♦ Several types of nursing education lead to licensure as a registered nurse or as a practical/vocational nurse.
♦ Only graduates of state- or province-approved schools are eligible to write the licensure examination.
♦ Most states have mandatory licensure laws for nurses. Nurses must be licensed in all states, territories, and Canadian provinces.

Key Points (continued)

♦ Nurses promise to abide by a code of ethics.
♦ It is important to belong to a nursing organization. Such organizations keep the nurse up to date and act as advocates for the nurse.

Key Topics Outline

Types of Nursing Programs
  The Registered Nurse
  The Practical Nurse
Approval and Accreditation of Nursing Programs
  An Approved Nursing Program
  An Accredited Nursing Program
  Licensure of Nurses
A Code of Ethics for Nurses
  The Nurse's Pledge
Nursing Organizations
  National Organizations
  State Affiliates of National Organizations

Key Learning Activities

♦ Obtain a copy of your state's or province's nursing licensure laws. What type of education is required to take the licensure examination in your state or province? What is involved in establishing a nursing educational program?
♦ Ask your instructor for a copy of your school's "Philosophy and Objectives." How do these compare with your own personal philosophy of nursing?

Rosdahl CB: Textbook of Basic Nursing, 6th ed. © 1995 J.B. Lippincott Company

Nursing is a special kind of service that helps patients meet the daily needs of life that they have difficulty satisfying because of illness, injury, or age. The nurse assists individuals to achieve their maximum level of wellness. In addition, the nurse serves as a teacher to assist people to prevent illness or disability before it occurs.

The student brings certain knowledge, skills, attitudes, and abilities to nursing school. Further skills and knowledge are developed in school. The ability of a nurse to act independently will depend on his or her professional background, motivation, and work environment. It is difficult to define the roles of a nurse because roles constantly change. Among factors in nursing activity are the following: new discoveries in the biomedical field, development of new healthcare knowledge, changes in patterns of health services and payment, and the relationship among the healthcare team members.

This chapter discusses various programs for nursing education, approval and accreditation, licensure, a code of ethics, and nursing organizations. Chapter 3 covers information about the healthcare system, and Chapter 6 discusses opportunities for optimum health.

Types of Nursing Programs

There are four basic types of educational programs leading to a credential in nursing. Three of these allow the graduate to take the licensure examination and to become a registered nurse (RN). The fourth, a practical or vocational nursing program, allows the graduate to take the licensure examination and to become a licensed practical nurse (LPN) or a licensed vocational nurse (LVN).

The Registered Nurse

Registered nurses spend from 2 to 4 years learning their profession. In addition, they may have special training that teaches them to be public health nurses or to be specialists in fields such as surgical, psychiatric, maternal, or child care. RNs are responsible for the care of acutely ill patients; they teach professional and practical nursing students; they direct nurses and other people who work in hospitals and other healthcare facilities; and they are in charge in various healthcare settings. RNs also perform many duties today that only physicians performed 25 years ago. RNs may continue their education to become nurse anesthetists, nurse midwives, nurse clinicians, and nurse practitioners.

Three basic types of education lead to the RN license:

◆ The 2-year graduate attends a community or junior college and receives an associate degree (AD) in

nursing. This AD–RN is trained primarily as a bedside nurse.

◆ The 3-year program is located in a hospital and often does not carry college credits. Nearly all of these programs have closed in favor of 2- and 4-year programs that are conducted in a college setting.

◆ The 4-year program in a college or university leads to a baccalaureate (bachelor of science degree) in nursing. The graduate of this program may enter graduate school to study for an advanced degree (master's or doctorate). Most of these programs aim to prepare professional nurses who will be teachers or administrators or who will assume other leadership positions.

Some community colleges have "one-plus-one" or "career ladder" programs, which admit only LPNs. With approximately one additional year of education, the LPN becomes eligible to write the licensure examination and become an RN. Presently, all these programs lead to the RN license. In some states, such as Maine and Alaska, nursing groups are advocating different licensure for RNs who graduate from AD programs, as opposed to graduates of 4-year programs.

The Practical Nurse

The National Association for Practical Nurse Education and Service (NAPNES) gives this definition of the **practical nurse** (PN): "A trained practical nurse is a person prepared by an approved educational program to share in the care of the sick, in rehabilitation, and in the prevention of illness, always under the direction of a licensed physician and/or a registered professional nurse." PNs do many of the same things that RNs do for patients. The choice of the type of nurse assigned to a patient depends on the degree of the patient's illness.

The term "vocational nurse" is used in some states in place of "practical nurse." Do not confuse the person who is called a *nurse's aide* or *nursing assistant* with the PN. The nurse's aide or helper is a person who is taught on the job or in a very short program to assist in giving nursing care.

LPN/LVN Functions

In a 1991 statement, the National Federation of Licensed Practical Nurses (NFLPN) described the role of the LPN in today's healthcare system.

"In recent years, LPNs and LVNs have practiced in a changing environment . . . in expanding roles in the healthcare system. . . . These nursing practice standards (see accompanying box) are applicable in any practice setting. The degree to which individual standards are applied will vary according to the individual needs of the patient, the type

Licensed Practical/Vocational Nurses should adhere to the following standards:

Education

The Licensed Practical/Vocational Nurse

1. Shall complete a formal education program in practical nursing approved by the appropriate nursing authority in a state.
2. Shall successfully pass the National Council Licensure Examination for Practical Nurses.
3. Shall participate in initial orientation within the employing institution.

Legal/Ethical Status

The Licensed Practical/Vocational Nurse

1. Shall hold a current license to practice nursing as an LP/VN in accordance with the law of the state wherein employed.
2. Shall know the scope of nursing practice authorized by the Nursing Practice Act in the state wherein employed.
3. Shall have a personal commitment to fulfill the legal responsibilities inherent in good nursing practice.
4. Shall take responsible actions in situations wherein there is unprofessional conduct by a peer or other health care provider.
5. Shall recognize and have a commitment to meet the ethical and moral obligations of the practice of nursing.
6. Shall not accept or perform professional responsibilities which the individual knows (s)he is not competent to perform.

Practice

The Licensed Practical/Vocational Nurse

1. Shall accept assigned responsibilities as an accountable member of the health care team.
2. Shall function within the limits of educational preparation and experience as related to the assigned duties.
3. Shall function with other members of the health care team in promoting and maintaining health, preventing disease and disability, caring for and rehabilitating individuals who are experiencing an altered health state, and contributing to the ultimate quality of life until death.
4. Shall know and utilize the nursing process in planning, implementing, and evaluating health services and nursing care for the individual patient or group.
   a. *Planning:* The planning of nursing includes:
      1) assessment of health status of the individual patient, the family and community groups
      2) an analysis of the information gained from assessment
      3) the identification of health goals.
   b. *Implementation:* The plan for nursing care is put into practice to achieve the stated goals and includes:
      1) observing, recording and reporting significant changes which require intervention or different goals

2) applying nursing knowledge and skills to promote and maintain health, to prevent disease and disability and to optimize functional capabilities of an individual patient
3) assisting the patient and family with activities of daily living and encouraging self-care as appropriate
4) carrying out therapeutic regimens and protocols prescribed by an RN, physician, or other persons authorized by state law.
   c. *Evaluations:* The plan for nursing care and its implementations are evaluated to measure the progress toward the stated goals and will include appropriate persons and/or groups to determine:
      1) the relevancy of current goals in relation to the progress of the individual patient
      2) the involvement of the recipients of care in the evaluation process
      3) the quality of the nursing action in the implementation of the plan
      4) a re-ordering of priorities or new goal setting in the care plan.
5. Shall participate in peer review and other evaluation processes.
6. Shall participate in the development of policies concerning the health and nursing needs of society and in the roles and functions of the LP/VN.

Continuing Education

The Licensed Practical/Vocational Nurse

1. Shall be responsible for maintaining the highest possible level of professional competence at all times.
2. Shall periodically reassess career goals and select continuing education activities which will help to achieve these goals.
3. Shall take advantage of continuing education opportunities which will lead to personal growth and professional development.
4. Shall seek and participate in continuing education activities which are approved for credit by appropriate organizations, such as the NFLPN.

Specialized Nursing Practice

The Licensed Practical/Vocational Nurse

1. Shall have had at least one year's experience in nursing at the staff level.
2. Shall present personal qualifications that are indicative of potential abilities for practice in the chosen specialized nursing area.
3. Shall present evidence of completion of a program or course that is approved by an appropriate agency to provide the knowledge and skills necessary for effective nursing services in the specialized field.
4. Shall meet all of the standards of practice as set forth in this document.

Nursing Practice Standards, NFLPN, 1991.

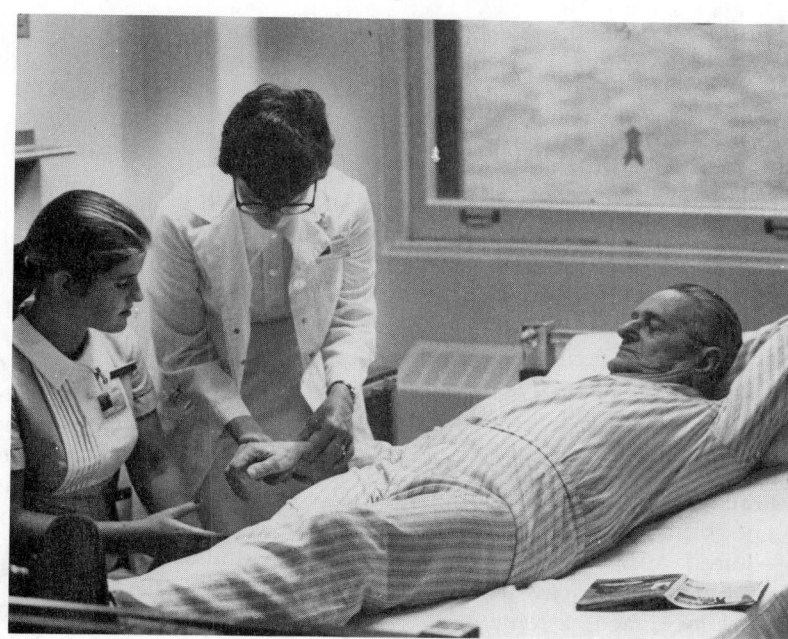

Figure 2-1. The instructor supervises clinical practice. (Photo by Bob Kalmbach, University of Michigan School of Nursing)

of healthcare agency or services and the community resources. The scope of licensed practical nursing has extended into specialized nursing services."[1]

The NFLPN goes on to state that

"Practical/Vocational nursing means the performance for compensation of authorized acts of nursing which utilize specialized knowledge and skills and which meet the health needs of people in a variety of settings under the direction of qualified health professions."

The NFLPN believes that

◆ "Practical/Vocational nursing comprises the common core of nursing and, therefore, is a valid entry into the nursing profession.
◆ Opportunities exist for practicing in a milieu where different professions unite their particular skills in a team effort for one common objective—to preserve or improve an individual patient's functioning.
◆ Opportunities also exist for upward mobility within the profession through academic education and for lateral expansion of knowledge and expertise through both academic and continuing education."

Practical Nursing Education

Most practical nursing programs exist under the auspices of a public education unit: a high school, a vocational institute, or a community college. Some programs are administered by hospitals. There are more than 1,300 state-approved practical nursing programs with

about 50,000 graduates annually in the United States. Canada also has a number of programs.

The curriculum is designed to include classroom theory in the various aspects of nursing. The student then has an opportunity to practice clinical skills in a hospital, nursing home, community health agency, or other health-related facility. The classroom theory and the clinical practice are correlated as closely as possible to ensure maximum retention of skills (Fig. 2-1). Most practical nursing programs are the equivalent of 12 to 18 months of full-time study. There are proposals to increase this to 2 years.

Approval and Accreditation of Nursing Programs

There is a difference between approval of a nursing program and accreditation of a program. It is important for the nursing student to understand this difference.

Approval is mandatory (required), meaning that schools must be approved or their graduates cannot be licensed. **Accreditation**, on the other hand, is voluntary and does not specifically concern licensure of graduates. A program can be approved without being accredited, but it cannot be accredited without being first approved by the state's Board of Nursing.

An Approved Nursing Program

When a school is on the approved list, it means that a nursing authority (usually the state, provincial, or territorial Board of Nursing) has visited it and is satisfied

---

[1] "Nursing Practice Standards for the Licensed Practical/Vocational Nurse." National Federation of Licensed Practical Nurses, Inc., 1991 Revision. Used with permission.

that the students are receiving an appropriate education. The word *approved* tells you that a school:

- Teaches the specific things a nurse must know
- Has stated objectives and teaches to those objectives
- Provides experience with the kinds of patients the nurse will care for when practicing nursing
- Employs qualified instructors to teach and supervise the students' practice in the classroom and in the hospital or other clinical facility
- Prepares graduates eligible for examination and licensure as LPNs or RNs
- Has courses of the required minimum length

Many nursing programs have liberal entrance requirements. Usually the entrant is required to be a high school graduate; certain high school courses may be required. Applicants must be considered for admission without regard to gender, age, marital status, sexual preference, race, or religion.

An Accredited Nursing Program

A nursing program may also be accredited by a national agency, such as the National League for Nursing (NLN). Application for accreditation is voluntary on the part of the program; accreditation is not given to all programs. The fact that a school is accredited gives further evidence of its excellence because the program must undergo a detailed evaluation to become accredited. A program need not be accredited for its graduates to become licensed.

Licensure of Nurses

Licensing laws protect the public from unqualified workers and establish standards for the profession or occupation. **Licensure** (licensing) helps the public to determine the difference between a qualified and an unqualified worker.

The first licensure laws for nursing were passed in 1903 in North Carolina, New York, Virginia, and New Jersey. The first LPN law was passed in Mississippi in 1914. In 1940, fewer than 10 states had LPN laws, but by 1955 all the states had LPN laws. Every state and the District of Columbia, Puerto Rico, Guam, American Samoa, the Virgin Islands, the Canadian provinces, and the North Mariana Islands now have licensing laws for both RNs and LPNs.

Any student who has been graduated from an approved RN or LPN/LVN nursing program is eligible to take the NCLEX licensing examination. Students who pass the examination can use the appropriate title (RN or LPN). (In Texas and California, the title is LVN—Licensed Vocational Nurse).

There are some differences in the licensing laws from state to state. For instance, in some states it is illegal for any nurse to practice nursing for pay without a license; violators can be prosecuted. This is called **mandatory licensure**. In some states only RNs are affected. In other states, the law does not forbid practicing nursing without a license, but does forbid using the title *Registered Nurse* or *Licensed Practical Nurse* if the nurse does not have a license. This is called **permissive licensure**.

Most states now have laws mandating (requiring) licensure of both LPNs and RNs. The mandatory law usually protects the functions of the nurse, as well as the use of the title. In other words, if a state has a mandatory licensure law, a nurse cannot perform the functions designed as being exclusively part of nursing without being properly licensed in that state.

Obtaining a license is no longer really a matter of choice because today a license is the passport to employment as a reputable nurse. It tells any employer that a prospective employee is a qualified person. The license is an important credential, and the time is quickly coming when a license will be essential if a person wants to practice nursing in any state.

A Code of Ethics for Nurses

All nurses are expected to abide by a code of ethics. **Ethics** is defined as the conduct appropriate for all members of a group. A brief code of ethics for practical nursing is listed in the accompanying box.

The nurse also accepts responsibilities within the role delineated by licensure. The roles and responsibilities of the LPN/LVN are to:

- Recognize the LPN/LVN's role in healthcare delivery and work together with other members of the healthcare team
- Maintain accountability for personal nursing practice within the ethical and legal limits
- Serve as a patient advocate
- Accept an appropriate role in maintaining and developing standards of practice for providing healthcare
- Take advantage of educational opportunities[2]

The Nurse's Pledge

Many of the principles found in a code of ethics are reflected in the Nurse's Pledge, frequently recited by students at graduation. Even if the pledge is not part of

[2] Adapted from a statement by the National Association of Practical Nurse Education and Service, 1981.

The Code for Licensed Practical/Vocational Nurses

"The Code, adopted by NFLPN in 1961 and revised in 1979, provides a motivation for establishing, maintaining and elevating professional standards. Each LP/VN, upon entering the profession, inherits the responsibility to adhere to the standards of ethical practice and conduct as set forth in this Code."

- Know the scope of maximum utilization of the LPN as specified by the nursing practice act and function within this scope.
- Safeguard the confidential information about the patient.
- Provide health care to all patients regardless of race, creed, cultural background, disease, or lifestyle.
- Refuse to give endorsement to commercial products or services.
- Uphold the highest standards in all ways.
- Stay informed about issues affecting the practice of nursing and delivery of health care.
- Accept the responsibility for safe nursing by keeping oneself mentally and physically fit and educationally prepared.
- Accept responsibility for membership in professional organizations.

Adapted from "Nursing Practice Standards," NFLPN, 1991

the graduation ceremony, it should serve as a guide for nursing practice. RNs recite the Florence Nightingale Pledge, and LPNs recite the Practical Nurse's Pledge (see accompanying box). The basic philosophy of nursing care espoused in both pledges is the same. Notice the similarity between them.

Key Concept

The nurse *always* practices within the Code of Ethics for Nurses. When you recite your pledge at graduation, you are promising to abide by this code.

Nursing Organizations

Nursing organizations provide educational programs and professional publications. They often participate in collective bargaining for nurses. The nursing organization allows members to keep up to date with trends in nursing and to discuss these with their peers. It is important for the nurse to belong to the appropriate organization.

There is great controversy over the educational qualifications for different levels of nursing, that is, the level of educational preparation that will be necessary to qualify a person to be a professional or practical nurse. Only by being a member of your appropriate nursing organization can you keep abreast of these and other changes and trends in nursing.

National Organizations

National Association for Practical Nurse Education and Service (NAPNES)

This group was the first national nursing organization to concentrate all its efforts on the development and improvement of practical nursing education, together with advancing the interests of PNs themselves. It was organized in 1941 as the Association of Practical Nurse Schools, with 20 members.

Nursing Pledges

Florence Nightingale Pledge

I solemnly pledge myself before God and in the presence of this assembly: To pass my life in purity and to practice my profession faithfully.

I will abstain from whatever is deleterious and mischievous, and will not take or knowingly administer any harmful drug.

I will do all in my power to maintain and elevate the standards of my profession, and will hold in confidence all personal matters committed to my keeping, and all family affairs coming to my knowledge in the practice of my profession.

With loyalty will I endeavor to aid the physician in his work, and devote myself to the welfare of those committed to my care.

The Practical Nurse's Pledge

Before God and those assembled here, I solemnly pledge:

To adhere to the code of ethics of the nursing profession.

To cooperate faithfully with the other members of the nursing team and to carry out faithfully and to the best of my ability the instructions of the physician or the nurse who may be assigned to supervise my work.

I will not do anything evil or malicious and I will not knowingly give any harmful drug or assist in malpractice.

I will not reveal any confidential information that may come to my knowledge in the course of my work.

And I pledge myself to do all in my power to raise the standards and the prestige of practical nursing.

May my life be devoted to service, and to the high ideals of the nursing profession.

Membership. NAPNES has three types of membership:

- *Individual*: open to RNs who are instructors and directors of practical nursing schools; LPNs; representatives of hospital, health, and education groups; and citizens interested in helping practical nursing grow and improve
- *Per capita*: open to members of state practical nurse associations voting a per capita assessment of dues
- *Future* (*student*): open to students in approved practical nursing schools on a divided payment basis while they are in the school (full membership is continued for a year after graduation at no extra cost)

Purposes. The purposes of NAPNES are to:

- Further the cause and image of practical nursing
- Improve practical nursing education
- Provide continuing education for practical nurses

The NAPNES national office answers inquiries about practical nursing. NAPNES sends consultants to state or other groups to help set up practical nursing programs. It publishes helpful booklets and other materials, including a newsletter, *NAPNES Forum*, and the *Journal of Practical Nursing*. NAPNES also publishes the "Declaration of Functions of the Licensed Practical/Vocational Nurse," which is updated regularly. It has helped PNs to organize their own state associations. Every year it holds a convention with special sessions for both practicing PNs and students. Scholarships are provided for students, as well as low-cost insurance programs for students and graduates.

National Federation of Licensed Practical Nurses, Inc. (NFLPN)

This group was organized in 1949 in New York State. This organization is "the professional organization for licensed practical nurses and licensed vocational nurses and . . . . students in the United States and Canada." It "provides leadership for [the] nearly one million licensed practical and vocational nurses. . . ."

Membership. "Membership is based on a three-tier concept of local, state, and national enrollment. It consists of LPNs, LVNs, and LPN/LVN nursing students. In September 1991, a new category of affiliate membership was established to allow those who have an interest in the work of NFLPN, but who are neither LPNs nor PN students, to join. Affiliate members receive all communications and may attend all NFLPN meetings, but do not have the right to vote or hold office. NFLPN has members in every state in the United States and in many provinces of Canada."[3]

Purposes. The stated purposes of NFLPN are to:

- Foster high standards of nursing education and practice so that the best nursing care will be available to every patient
- Encourage continuing education as a priority for the purpose of personal growth and improved patient care
- Achieve recognition for LPNs and LVNs and to advocate their effective utilization in every type of healthcare facility
- Interpret the role and function of the LPN and LVN for the public to win greater understanding and appreciation of the contribution of practical/vocational nursing to the healthcare system
- Represent practical/vocational nursing through relationships with other groups which share the common goal of improved patient care
- Serve as the central source of information regarding what is new and changing in nursing education and practice[4]

The NFLPN holds an annual convention to discuss matters involving practical nursing. At this convention, the policies of the organization are set and recommendations are made to the constituent state organizations. Their national office serves as a resource to members. The organization strongly urges members to attend continuing education programs at the national convention and in local communities.

The NFLPN publishes a bimonthly newsletter, *NFLPN Update*, which "includes reports of NFLPN activities on the national scene, news from the constituent states, book reviews, new product reviews, articles of professional and personal interest, health industry trends, career information, legislative notes, announcements of coming events. . .and continuing education opportunities." The NFLPN is also involved in legislation through relationships with regulatory agencies. In this way, the "policy makers can better understand the role of practical/vocational nursing in the nation's healthcare delivery system." NFLPN also sponsors legislative conferences for its members.

Rather than having its own accreditation process, the NFLPN supports the accreditation services of the National League for Nursing.

[3] "Facts About NFLPN." Published by NFLPN, Raleigh, NC, 1991. Used with permission.
[4] Adapted from "Facts About NFLPN." Published by NFLPN, Raleigh, NC, 1991.

American Association of Licensed Practical Nurses (AALPN)

This organization is smaller than the two other national LPN organizations. It has affiliates in about 16 states. The AALPN is mainly concerned with education and legislation. In some states, the AALPN participates in the collective bargaining process. The organization recently worked with the Joint Commission on Accreditation of Healthcare Organizations to help develop their policy statement. In this statement, the LPN/LVN is specifically identified as part of the healthcare team. The statement also states that the LPN/LVN can supervise the work of others in certain situations.

National League for Nursing (NLN)

Founded in 1952, the NLN is an organization whose members are interested in furthering nursing and nursing education. The NLN is open to individuals, such as RNs and LPNs, and to institutions, such as nursing programs and hospitals.

The NLN has various departments, among them the Council of Practical Nursing Programs (CPNP), which was originally established in 1961. Through its Department of Evaluation, the NLN has developed a number of tests that are used widely by nursing schools. Among their tests used by practical nursing schools are an entrance test called PACE (Pre-Admission and Classification Examination) and several achievement tests. The PACE test, consisting of aptitude and achievement sections, is used as a qualification for entrance to some nursing programs. The achievement tests are given to determine how well a student is doing after admission to the program. These tests stress pharmacology, maternal/child nursing, medical/surgical nursing, and psychiatric principles. Other tests are available for programs preparing for RN licensure.

One of the most important functions of the NLN is the voluntary accreditation of nursing programs, at both the RN and the PN levels. Accreditation signifies that a program has met or exceeded the basic minimum approval requirements of the state in which it is located. The NLN has many useful publications, among them its monthly publication, *Nursing and Health Care.*

American Nurses Association (ANA)

The ANA is an organization whose membership is made up of RNs. ANA often sponsors workshops for nurses, and it publishes several periodicals and a great deal of literature. The ANA's most widely circulated journal is the *American Journal of Nursing.* The ANA considers itself the "official voice" for professional nursing in the United States. The ANA assists with collective bargaining in many states.

State Affiliates of National Organizations

The national nursing associations usually have state affiliates and sometimes local chapters. This gives all nurses the opportunity to attend meetings and to become active in the nursing organization of their choice. Most national organizations also have student affiliates, so you can begin your professional membership as a student.

State organizations often publish newsletters of local interest. Sometimes scholarships are available to members.

Key Concept

It is important for nursing students and graduates to belong to an organization, so they will have a voice in the future of the profession.

Keys for Review

Key Questions for Critical Thinking

1. Discuss the differences between the educational preparation and the roles and responsibilities of the RN and the LPN.
2. Explain the difference between approval and accreditation of a nursing program. What is the status of your program?

Key Questions for Critical Thinking
(continued)

3. Describe the importance of a code of ethics for nursing practice.
4. Why is it important to belong to a professional organization?
5. Describe at least three nursing organizations open to your membership.

Key Readings

Carroll C, Miller D. Health: The Science of Human Adaptation, Ed 5. Madison, WI, Brown & Benchmark, 1991

Kurzen CR. Contemporary Practical/Vocational Nursing, Ed 2. Philadelphia, J.B. Lippincott, 1993

Thomas, CL (ed). Taber's Cyclopedic Medical Dictionary, Ed 17. Philadelphia, F.A. Davis, 1993

Enrichment Keys

Buckley CD, Walker D. Harmony: Professional Renewal for Nurses (J Stofman, ed). Chicago, American Hospital Association, 1989

Ellis JR, Hartley C. Nursing in Today's World: Challenges, Issues, and Trends, Ed 4. Philadelphia, J.B. Lippincott, 1992

Keys to Learning More

Chapter 3: healthcare in North America

Chapter 4: legal and ethical responsibilities of nursing

Chapter 6: basic health practices

Chapter 93: describes how to obtain your nursing license and how to transfer licensure from state to state

Key Resources

American Association of Licensed Practical Nurses
c/o Associated Resources Consultants
10100 West Sample Road, Suite 403
Coral Springs, FL 33065
Telephone: 305-341-7477

American Nurses Association
600 Maryland Avenue, SW
Suite 100 West
Washington, DC 20024
Telephone: 202-554-4444; 1-800-274-4262

National Association for Practical Nurse Education and Service
1400 Spring Street
Suite 310
Silver Spring, MD 20910
Telephone: 301-588-2491

National Federation of Licensed Practical Nurses, Inc.
1418 Aversboro Road
Garner, NC 27529
Telephone: 919-779-0046

National League for Nursing
350 Hudson Street
New York, NY 10014
Telephone: 212-989-9393; 1-800-669-1656

3 The Healthcare Delivery System

Learning Objectives

- Describe holism and holistic healthcare
- Discuss nursing criteria in healthcare reform
- Differentiate among various healthcare facilities
- State the differences between the acute care facility and the long-term care facility
- Describe the role of the patient representative or ombudsperson
- Discuss methods of payment for healthcare services
- Discuss current changes in healthcare that will affect healthcare and nursing through the decade

Key Terms

client

co-pay

diagnosis-related groups

Health Maintenance Organization

holism

holistic healthcare

incentive

prospective

payment

quality assurance

third-party payment

wellness

Keys to Understanding This Chapter

Chapter 1: historical background of nursing

Chapter 2: nursing programs and organizations

Key Points

- Holism, which was at the center of many ancient healthcare systems, has become accepted in North American society. It is a philosophy that views the "whole person."
- Types of healthcare facilities include hospitals, which now primarily treat people with acute conditions; extended care facilities, where care is given for a long period; and community services, which include outpatient care, walk-in care, home healthcare, and care in schools and industries. Employment opportunities for nurses exist in all these areas.
- Consumers are assured quality and appropriate care through standards established by the Joint Commission for Accreditation of Healthcare Organizations.

Key Points (continued)

- Many hospitals have established the position of patient advocate (representative, ombudsperson) to assist the patient and family in adapting to hospitalization.
- Third-party payment has been the method of payment for healthcare in the United States for a number of years. A variety of organizations provide this service.
- There will be many changes in the healthcare system by the end of the decade. New challenges await the nurse.

Key Topics Outline

Holistic Healthcare
    Teamwork
Healthcare Reform
Types of Healthcare Facilities
    Hospitals: Acute Care Facilities
    Extended Care Facilities
    Community Health Services
Quality Assurance
    Components of Quality Care
    Standards for Quality Assurance
Patient Representatives or Advocates
Financing Healthcare
    Health Resources
    Methods of Payment
    Prospective Payment and Diagnosis-Related Groups
Healthcare at the End of the Century

Key Learning Activities

- Interview a hospital administrator or a long-term care facility administrator. Discuss their feelings about the diagnosis-related groups and rules and regulations. How is current legislation affecting their agency?
- Interview a person representing a health maintenance organization. Describe the services offered by their organization.
- Search through current newspapers and magazines for information about the healthcare system and future changes. You may want to write a report for classes.

Rosdahl CB: Textbook of Basic Nursing, 6th ed. © 1995 J.B. Lippincott Company

Healthcare in the United States is changing dramatically. These changes include greater emphasis on wellness, with individuals assuming more responsibility for their own health. Agencies such as **health maintenance organizations** (HMOs) support these changes and are examples of managed care systems that offer healthcare on a co-pay basis. Another change in the delivery of healthcare is shorter hospital stays. This results in the need for extended care facilities (ECF) and home healthcare agencies. All of these changes in healthcare will affect the role of nurses in this decade, whether they practice in acute care settings or the community.[1]

This textbook discusses nursing in the context of the hospital. A variety of chapters, however, discuss nursing in community-based healthcare facilities. You may decide to practice nursing in a public health agency, a day surgery clinic, an emergency clinic, a hospice, a halfway house, or a nursing home. *Good nursing should be practiced anywhere.*

Because of rapid changes in healthcare and payment systems, information in this chapter can change within months of publishing. Your instructor will inform you of changes.

Holistic Healthcare

Although **holism** is at the center of many forms of ancient-based healthcare, it is only within the last half of this century that it has become accepted in North American healthcare. Holism is a philosophy that views the "whole person." The person is seen as a complete unit that cannot be reduced to the sum of its parts.

Holistic healthcare refers to comprehensive and total care of a person. Needs are met in all areas, such as physical, emotional, social, spiritual, and economic. Rather than defining health in terms of diseases, holistic health emphasizes wellness. **Wellness** not only includes absence of disease, but also the ability to cope with stress and achieve personal growth and contentment, as well as the freedom to be creative and avoid hazardous situations.

The holistic health movement says that an individual can be in control of his or her own life and health and that one can determine the quality of one's life. Sometimes, because healthcare recipients have control of their own situations, healthcare professionals refer to them as clients rather than as patients. The term **client** implies participation in decision making regarding one's own health. Patients (clients) have the right to participate actively in their own care. Rather than passively taking the physician's orders, the client considers the physician's advice and makes informed decisions about the care to be received. Part of the nurse's responsibility is teaching the client the steps of care and prevention.

Holistic nursing should be care provided in a supportive and positive fashion so that the patient's self-image as a worthy human being is maintained. By sincerely caring about the patient and respecting the patient's way of life, the nurse strengthens the client's feelings of self-respect and dignity.

Teamwork

Closely related to holistic healthcare is the concept of "teamwork." To give care to the whole person, the members of the healthcare team collaborate in their assessments, planning, and activities. They communicate with one another so services are not duplicated. Their goal is to help the client maintain wellness and when there is a problem, to restore the client to health. Throughout this book, various members of the team are discussed. As a nurse or a nursing student, you are part of the team providing healthcare.

Healthcare Reform

People are reacting across the country to President Clinton's healthcare reform plan, called American Health Security Act of 1993. To represent nursing's interest and responsibility in the Act, representatives of more than 60 nursing organizations met in August 1993. "Nursing's Agenda for Health Care Reform" focuses on primary care, prevention, and community outreach.[2] From this meeting came several key criteria that nursing organizations are using as reference points when analyzing the Act. They are listed in the accompanying box.

Types of Healthcare Facilities

The following is an overview of current healthcare facilities. Some of these agencies may serve as clinical facilities during your nursing program. As you near graduation, you will study the types of healthcare facilities in more detail, so you can make a decision about what type of facility interests you for employment.

---

[1] Sharp N. "Healthcare reform—where are we now?" Nursing Management 25(1):17-18, January 1994.

[2] Correspondence from Elizabeth Holmes, R.N., M.S., Director, Community Health Services Clinic, Scottsdale, AZ.

Hospitals: Acute Care Facilities

The hospital is the healthcare facility most commonly known. There are two major kinds of hospitals: general or specialized. A hospital is *general* or *comprehensive* if it cares for most ages and types of patients, including medical–surgical (care of people who have had surgical operations), obstetrics (care of mothers and babies at birth), and pediatrics (care of ill children). General hospitals are considered *acute care facilities*, because the patients are there for a short time, usually only a matter of a few days, and often are very sick.

Other hospitals are *specialized* hospitals, because they admit only one type of patient. Examples include mental health, pediatric, or obstetric hospitals.

Although the primary function of the hospital is to provide patient care, other functions exist as well. For example, your clinical facility has the added role of *education*, and many large hospitals, particularly those affiliated with a university, also play an important role in *research*.

Hospital Ownership and Funding

In addition to grouping related to types of patients served, healthcare facilities are classified in relation to their ownership and funding structure.

Governmental. Governmental, public, or official hospitals are owned by local, state, or federal units of government. These governmental agencies are also called *nonprofit, nonproprietary,* or *official* hospitals. Examples are given in Table 3-1.

Private. *Private* or *voluntary* hospitals are those owned and operated by individuals or by groups, such as churches, labor unions, and fraternal organizations.

These hospitals may be established for-profit or by not-for-profit organizations.

Profit Versus Not-for-Profit. A further classification of hospitals relates to distribution of their profits.

◆ *Proprietary*, investor-owned, or *for-profit* hospitals are those in which profits are returned to shareholders. Very few such hospitals exist today.
◆ *Not-for-profit* hospitals make up the majority of all hospitals today. In the not-for-profit hospital, profits are returned to the corporation or funding agency and are used for improvements to the facility, added equipment, and other related costs.

Hospital Administration

Hospitals are almost always governed by a board of directors or of trustees, or in the case of a university hospital, by a board of regents. This board appoints the administration of the hospital.

It is important for you to know the administrative structure of the hospital where you are a student or where you work. You will then know the appropriate "chain-of-command" to follow in various situations.

Hospital Accreditation. Just as your nursing program can be accredited, a hospital or other healthcare facility also can be accredited. The agency that gives this recognition to hospitals is called the Joint Commission for Accreditation of Healthcare Organizations (JCAHO). Other facilities have similar accreditation processes. It is important for you to find out the accreditation status of your hospital.

Extended Care Facilities

Some facilities admit clients for a longer period of time. These *ECFs* include nursing homes, inpatient rehabilitation centers, and facilities for chronic mental health care. Some of these facilities are attached to a general

Table 3-1. Examples of Hospitals and Types of Ownership

Type of Ownership	Hospitals
Federal public	Veterans Administration
	U.S. Army
	Bureau of Indian Affairs
	U.S. Public Health Service
State public	University hospital
	Regional or state mental hospital
Local public	City hospital
	County hospital

hospital; others are free-standing. More emphasis is being placed on returning people to their homes or other community-based living facilities as quickly as possible. Thus, the types of patients in long-term facilities are changing.

Nursing Homes

Nursing homes are divided into two categories by Medicare. A nursing home is classified as either a *skilled* nursing facility or an *intermediate* care facility. The skilled nursing facility (sometimes called an SNF) has 24-hour nursing care under the supervision of an RN. The intermediate care facility (ICF) has the 24-hour services of nursing assistants under the supervision of an LPN, with an RN on staff as a consultant. Many rules and regulations apply to nursing homes. There are many opportunities for employment for nurses in nursing homes.

Community Health Services

Community health services provide care for individuals and families within a specific area, such as a city neighborhood or a small town or rural county. Some of the features of community services are discussed here.

The current trend toward community healthcare is based on many factors. Some of these factors are as follows:

◆ The skyrocketing costs of in-hospital medical care, along with governmental limits and regulations, have forced many people to be cared for in the community rather than in a hospital.
◆ Many individuals are unemployed and do not have health insurance. These people cannot afford to be hospitalized for minor ailments, and they simply choose not to have voluntary (elective) surgery.
◆ Holistic health and preventive medicine are becoming more commonly practiced. Through holistic methods, many conditions can be prevented or lessened in severity; therefore, hospitalization is unnecessary.

Special Considerations in Aging
Home Care

The number of senior citizens is increasing rapidly. Many of these individuals prefer to be cared for at home because of the expense of hospitalization for people on fixed incomes.

Outpatient Services and Walk-in Care

More individuals are being seen in outpatient treatment centers because of the expense of inpatient hospitalization. Many surgical procedures are being performed on an outpatient basis in *day-surgery* centers. The patient is then sent home to recover.

Home Healthcare

With patients being sent home to recover from surgery or illness, the need for home healthcare is increasing rapidly. Nurses play an important role in teaching patients and their families to care for themselves and to document care. You may have a brief experience in home health nursing as a part of your nursing program. Opportunities for employment in home healthcare agencies are numerous for all types of nurses.

Because patients are discharged from the hospital earlier than in the past, the family needs to take responsibility for some of the care. The patient and family must be taught skills in patient care before a discharge (see patient teaching box).

Healthcare in School and Industry

Most school systems provide healthcare for students. A nurse may be on duty full time or divide his or her time among several schools. In addition to caring for ill children or children in emergencies, the nurse provides preventive care by performing regular assessments, teaching health information, and providing individual counseling as needed.

Industries in which machinery is operated usually have a full-time nurse for health promotion and interventions. Teaching is part of the nurse's responsibility in such a facility. Prevention of accidents is the goal.

Quality Assurance

Quality of care has become a major issue for *consumers* (patients) and *providers* (healthcare facilities).

JCAHO has set standards for an ongoing hospital **quality assurance** program. JCAHO requires objective and systematic monitoring and evaluation of the *quality* and *appropriateness* of patient care.

Keys to Patient/Family Teaching

Patient/family teaching for the patient who is being discharged for care at home must include the following:

◆ Patient care skills
◆ Importance of home documentation when directed
◆ Complications related to their disorder
◆ Side effects of medication and other procedures
◆ Importance of calling the health care provider when difficulties occur

Components of Quality Care

Quality management requires that healthcare services be well planned and delivered in a manner that assures good care. Adequate staff and support sevices must be available, which is the function of the nursing department. Quality control and quality assurance focus on the delivery of care. The process of care given is important, as is the outcome. (Process relates to *how* care is given; outcome relates to the *result*.) Nurse accountability is vital; this involves the delivery of quality care and the accurate documentation of that care.

Standards for Quality Assurance

Standards of quality are set up by each healthcare facility to guide the nursing staff in providing care. These include the following:

◆ Standards of *nursing practice*. These are the procedures used in the delivery of care, the hospital policy book, your textbooks, and other references. Sometimes the term *nursing protocol* is used. The standard of nursing practice focuses on the giver of care, the nurse, and on the nursing process.

◆ Standard of *patient care*. This activity is determined by the patient's expectations or personal standards of care. What did the patient expect the care to be like? How well did the nursing care given meet the patient's expectations? This standard focuses on the recipient of care, the patient. The patient participates in developing the nursing care plan.

◆ Standard of *performance*. This standard determines how well the nurse performs as compared with the job description. (How well you meet the standard of performance as a nursing student will change as you progress through the nursing program. As you become more experienced, you will be expected to provide more complex nursing care.)

The *nursing audit* (committee) evaluates care given to patients. *Peer review* allows nurses to constructively critique each other.

Patient Representatives or Advocates

Many hospitals have initiated the position of *patient representative, patient advocate, patient liaison,* or *ombudsperson*. The role of this person is to act as a "consumer advocate" and to assist the patient and family to make the hospitalization as comfortable and free of stress as possible.

A patient representative often welcomes the patient and family to the hospital and helps them to find needed services. The patient representative listens to the patient and family and answers questions. The representative can help the family find housing, restaurants, parking, child care, or chaplain services. During hospitalization, the patient has the right to contact the patient representative any time there is a problem or concern.

In preparation for discharge, the advocate can help the family locate home care and make sure the family knows where to purchase needed supplies and medications.

Many facilities have "patient discharge planning representatives" who assist the patient and family to plan for continuing care at home. Some patients will require assistance with treatments or dietary planning. The representative anticipates the patient's needs and assists in finding resources to meet these needs. They may use community services, or they may need rental equipment. Also, home healthcare may be needed.

Special Considerations in Aging
Patient Advocacy

Many older people who live alone may be confused or too frail to manage their care. Prior to hospital discharge, it must be determined if someone is available to evaluate them on a regular basis. Social services can assist in discharge planning and make arrangements for home healthcare.

Financing Healthcare

The costs of healthcare continue to skyrocket. Various programs and legislation have evolved to address these problems. Ethics committees work on determining who should receive what treatment.

Health Resources

Through the Health Planning and Resources Development in 1975, legislation was set up to govern the amount and types of facilities, services, and workers needed in each designated geographic area in the United States. It also was set up to prevent duplication and ultimately, to reduce costs in the administration of healthcare.

The initial act of 1975 identified the following priorities:

◆ Primary care services for medically underserved populations, especially those located in rural or economically depressed areas
◆ Multi-institutional systems for coordination or consolidation of health services that are very expensive or less used than medical or surgical units (eg, obstetrics; pediatrics, emergency, intensive, and coronary care; and radiation therapy)

◆ Group medical practices, HMOs, and other organized systems of healthcare delivery
◆ Training and increased use of assistants to physicians, especially nurse clinicians
◆ Multi-institutional arrangements for sharing of support services, such as purchasing and bookkeeping
◆ Improvements in the quality of health services
◆ Institutions to provide various levels of healthcare, to be developed on a geographically integrated basis to prevent excessive duplication of services, such as intensive and extended care
◆ Disease prevention, including studies of nutritional and environmental factors and provision of preventive healthcare services.
◆ Uniform cost accounting, simplified reimbursement, and utilization reporting systems
◆ Improved management procedures for health service institutions
◆ Effective methods of educating the general public concerning proper healthcare and effective use of available health services

Methods of Payment

Until recently, the majority of healthcare in the United States was a fee-for-service system. That is, the patient went to the physician and paid for each service performed. To help the family pay for a seriously ill patient when the family had limited funds, a **third-party payment** system developed. Various third-party payment systems exist, which are summarized below. Because the federal government is discussing a new program for healthcare, these systems may change greatly within this decade.

Private Insurance

Private health insurance is purchased by an individual or a family. Its cost is high, and the insurance company often refuses to insure anyone who is considered a health risk. Therefore, many people cannot afford or are not able to obtain private insurance.

Group Insurance

Group insurance offers insurance coverage for people belonging to a certain group. For example, many companies, institutions, and fraternal organizations offer members group insurance benefits. In this situation, the premium is fairly low, and usually people are insured without a physical examination.

In either private or group insurance policies, coverage may be purchased for medical bills, hospitalizations, and other related services, such as surgery or laboratory tests. People may purchase coverage only for themselves, or they may purchase family coverage for all members of the immediate family. It is also possible to purchase insurance that will pay a set amount if the person is not able to work because of illness or injury (*long-term disability insurance*).

Health Maintenance Organizations

An HMO is defined by the Department of Health and Human Services as "an organized healthcare delivery system, which includes health manpower and facilities capable of providing, or at least arranging for, all the health services a population might require." People and groups contract with this system for health services. Several features of HMOs are important:

◆ *Group practice.* Several physicians and specialists practice together in a clinic.
◆ *Prepayment.* A person pays a certain amount each month and then is entitled to whatever care is needed.
◆ *Prevention.* The emphasis is on preventing disease rather than treating it.
◆ *Treatment.* When diseases or disorders occur, they are treated.

Some states require that employees in large organizations be given a choice between group insurance and an HMO.

Some employers have initiated **incentive** programs to encourage employees to practice health habits. They are rewarded for stopping smoking, losing weight, and having regular physical examinations. Employees are encouraged to be seen in the urgent care center for routine illnesses, rather than in the emergency room. Usually the **co-pay** (the amount the employee pays) is much higher in the emergency room if the urgent care center was open at the same time.

Preferred Provider Organizations

The preferred provider organization (PPO) is somewhat like the HMO in that it is an organization used to deliver healthcare services. PPOs are made up of groups of physicians and nurses. They refer patients among their groups.

Medicare

Medicare, a federal health insurance program, is applicable to nearly everyone over age 65, no matter what a person's financial status. It is also available to younger people who are receiving social security disability payments. The insured person contributes to the monthly premiums. The hospital insurance portion of Medicare provides partial payment for inpatient care (in a hospital) and for extended outpatient care or home healthcare.

Medicaid

Medicaid, on the other hand, is a joint effort of federal and state governments. The federal government has set up guidelines for Medicaid, but individual states have designed their own programs. Therefore, regulations, eligibility requirements, and benefits of Medicaid vary greatly from state to state.

Generally, Medicaid is for people over age 65, those who are blind or disabled, or those who are members of families receiving assistance from Aid to Families with Dependent Children. States have assured access to preventive healthcare for women, infants, and children through their Medicaid programs (prenatal care, immunizations and health and developmental screening). Medicaid is a public health insurance program for which people must be eligible to receive benefits. These people do not pay a monthly premium; the program is tax supported.

Medicaid pays only for inpatient and outpatient services, including physician or nurse practitioner services; laboratory and x-ray services; and screening, diagnosis, and treatment for children. It also pays for home healthcare and family planning. In some states, services such as dental care and eye care, immunization clinics, well-child clinics, and various preventive medicine and rehabilitation programs are also available. Medicaid-waiver programs, including those for the chronically disabled, the elderly, and people with acquired immunodeficiency syndrome (AIDS), facilitate the ability of these participants to remain at home, within the community.

People who are eligible for Medicare and Medicaid can supplement one program with the other. Medicaid may pay expenses not covered by Medicare if a person is eligible for both programs.

Key Concept

Medicare and Medicaid benefits and payments change with each presidential administration and legislative year.

Prospective Payment and Diagnosis-Related Groups

In 1983 an amendment to the federal social security legislation again changed the delivery of healthcare. The amendment created a **prospective payment** system that originally affected Medicare payments but was later adopted by other agencies and insurance companies. Prospective payment is a reimbursement in which a predetermined amount is allocated for treating hospital patients with specific diagnoses.

Prospective payment is based on categories called **diagnosis-related groups** (DRGs) for hospitals. The term for nursing homes and ECFs is resource utilization groups (RUGs).

Key Concept

Patients should be assured that their care will not be compromised just to maintain lower costs.

The DRG system of prospective payment is based on medical diagnosis. It classifies patients according to the average cost of care for that particular diagnosis. In this system, a federal agency has predetermined how much it "should" cost to treat a certain condition in a particular area of the United States. This is the amount that is paid to the healthcare facility *without considering the actual cost.*

Because a preset or "prospective" amount of money is paid for each diagnosis, the healthcare facility *loses* money if an individual patient's care costs more than the average. However, the facility *gains* money if a patient's care costs less than the average. Healthcare at the beginning of the 1990s in the United States was big business, one of the top three industries in the country. With the DRG system, facilities must be run in a businesslike manner or they will not survive. Not all states, however, continue to use DRGs. For example, in 1993 New Jersey deregulated; this allowed the state to make more decisions.

Impact of DRG Laws

The prospective payment legislation has had great impact on the healthcare delivery system in the United States. Changes include the following:

- Decreased length of patient stay in hospitals
- More critically ill patients in hospitals and nursing homes
- Fewer patients admitted for inpatient care
- Sicker people discharged from hospitals, needing more care at home; the family and patient must take more responsibility for care
- More outpatient care needed; many procedures formerly done in the hospital are done on an outpatient basis.
- More community-based care and home health nursing
- More specialized care
- More diversified hospitals; rent out equipment, provide home care, have day-surgery centers, add ECFs
- Decentralized administration
- More cooperation required between departments to maximize resources
- Mergers of several hospitals to form a large corporation
- More computers used for information processing
- Advertising and marketing of hospital services as hospitals compete for patients

◆ More concern for consumers (patients) and their reactions to care
◆ More preventive medicine
◆ Many small hospitals closing because they can no longer compete

Healthcare at the End of the Century

Major governmental decisions related to healthcare and payment will be made during the remainder of this decade. President Clinton's proposed healthcare reforms are being discussed by all concerned groups, agencies, and legislators. Whatever system develops, it should meet the magnitude of problems facing this nation: uninsured and underinsured sections of the population; unequal services to the population; low immunization rates; high birth rates to adolescents; lack of primary care services; and the need for AIDS research and treatment.

Aikens states:

"It is not unreasonable to assume that a completely automated healthcare system will come into being in this decade and be more sophisticated in the next. Such a development will call for radical changes in the structure, preparation, and licensure of all healthcare personnel. The establishment of a national system of research and clinical knowledge as a basic foundation for the management of health is a very strong possibility. The main requirement for using all this knowledge correctly will be the ability to ask the right questions when dealing with all the issues surrounding each patient.[3]"

Managed care (discussed later in the book) and advanced nursing practice will be prominent in the future. Three goals proposed in *Healthy People 2000* (discussed in Chapter 7) will challenge policy makers to:

◆ Increase the span of healthy life for Americans
◆ Reduce health disparities among Americans
◆ Achieve access to preventive services for all Americans

[3] Aikens LH, Fagin CM. Charting Nursing's Future: Agenda for the 1990s. Philadelphia, J.B. Lippincott, 1992, p. 116.

As the healthcare system and methods of payment develop and change in the remainder of this decade, so will nurses' responsibilities and the facilities in which they work. Nurses are prominently involved in the planning for future healthcare service. Teamwork will remain important, but the methods of collaboration undoubtedly will change.

Terms and Abbreviations Commonly Used in the Prospective Payment System

DRG	Diagnosis-related groups. Groups of medical diagnoses on which payment for care is based.
HMO	Health maintenance organization. A system of health care in which the goal is prevention of illness, rather than care for crises.
HRA	Health Resources Administration
JCAHO	Joint Commission on Accreditation of Healthcare Organizations
MIG	Medicare insured group
OUTLIER	A patient who stays in the hospital longer than the average time for that DRG group. (The situation can be reviewed and the classification *might* be changed for that one patient only.)
PPS	Prospective payment system. The system of paying a certain amount for a certain diagnosis.
PRO	Professional review organization. Designed to safeguard the quality of care.
ProPAC	Prospective Payment Commission. A group of people representing business, industry, and consumers. This commission reviews the prospective payment system and reports back to the Secretary of Health and Human Services of the U.S. Government.
RUG	Resource utilization groups. Categories used in nursing homes for payment (instead of DRGs).
USPHS	United States Public Health Service

Keys for Review

Key Questions for Critical Thinking

1. Explain and describe the differences among the seven healthcare facilities discussed in this chapter.
2. Describe the role of the patient representative or ombudsman. Why is this role important?
3. Discuss healthcare reform in the United States and comment on how it will affect your future.

Key Readings

Allison S, Latham G. "Same day admission surgery." Canadian Nurse 87:25, 1991

Craven RF, Hirnle CJ. Fundamentals of Nursing: Human Health and Function. Philadelphia, J.B. Lippincott, 1992

Drew JC. "Health maintenance organizations: History, evolution and survival." Nursing and Health Care 1:145-149, 1990

Ellis JR, Hartley CL. Nursing in Today's World: Challenges, Issues, and Trends, Ed 4. Philadelphia, J.B. Lippincott, 1992

Gale BF, Steffl BJ. "The long-term care dilemma: What nurses need to know about Medicare." Nursing and Health Care 13:34-41, 1992

Healthy People 2000: National Health Promotion and Disease Prevention Objectives. U.S. Department of Health and Human Services, Public Health Service. DHHS Publication No. (PHS) 91-50212. U.S. Government Printing Office, Washington D.C.

Key Reading (continued)

Johnson PA. "A national health insurance program: A nursing perspective." Nursing and Health Care 11:416-429, 1990

Weingart M. "Commercially managed health care: An experience." Nursing Management 22:40-42, 1991

Enrichment Keys

Burckhardt J. Overview: Healthcare, the final frontier, going where no nurse has ever gone before. NSNA/Impint Vol. 40 #5, 11/12/95, pp. 33–36.

Rutherford G, Campbell D. "Helping people help themselves." Canadian Nurse 89(10):25-28, November 1993

Keys to Learning More

Chapter 7: community health and *Healthy People 2000*

Chapter 35: quality assurance in evaluation of nursing care

Chapter 92: leadership skills in nursing

Chapter 93: career opportunities

4 Legal and Ethical Aspects of Nursing

Learning Objectives

♦ State the important provisions of the Nurse Practice Act and the functions of the state Board of Nursing
♦ Define the terms mandatory and permissive in relation to nursing practice
♦ Define interstate endorsement
♦ State two legal reasons for revoking or suspending a nursing license
♦ Differentiate between a crime of commission and a crime of omission
♦ State the purpose of malpractice insurance and its limitations
♦ Describe precautions the nurse might take to prevent lawsuits
♦ Discuss advance directives and differentiate between living will, directive to physicians, and durable power of attorney
♦ Discuss the Code of Ethics for Nurses
♦ State some of the criteria for determining clinical death
♦ Discuss the meaning of "quality of life" as it applies to healthcare ethics
♦ Describe patient refusal of treatment and its relationship to the legal claim of battery
♦ Discuss termination of treatment and withholding of treatment and describe how these also apply to the concept of euthanasia

Key Terms

advance directive
assault
battery
brain death
crime
ethics
felony
informed consent
liability

libel
living will
malpractice
misdemeanor
negligence
slander
tort
values clarification

Keys to Understanding This Chapter

Chapter 1: historical events contributing to nursing
Chapter 2: nursing's Code of Ethics, the Nurse's Pledge, and some aspects of nursing licensure
Chapter 3: today's healthcare system

Key Points

♦ You are legally and ethically bound to practice nursing within the rules and regulations of your local Nursing Practice Act and within the laws of your state, territory, or province.
♦ Several types of advance directives allow the patient to plan ahead and make decisions in advance about the type of healthcare to be received.
♦ When you recite the Florence Nightingale Pledge or the Practical Nurses' Pledge, you are promising to abide by a code of ethics.
♦ The patient has the right to accept or refuse treatment, in most situations.
♦ There are many ethical decisions to be made in healthcare. Some of these require the assistance of an ethics committee.

Key Topics Outline

Regulations of Nursing Practice
    State Boards of Nursing
    Licensing Laws
Legal Responsibilities in Nursing
    The Nurse's Legal Rights
    Liability
    Safeguards for the Nurse and Student
    Overview of Relevant Legal Issues
    Patients' Rights and Responsibilities
Values Clarification
Ethical Standards of Healthcare
    Nurses' Role Regarding Ethics
    Selected Ethical Problems
    The Ethics Committee

Rosdahl CB: Textbook of Basic Nursing, 6th ed. © 1995 J.B. Lippincott Company

Key Learning Activities

◆ Make a list to compare ethical versus unethical behaviors.
◆ Obtain a copy of your state/territory/province's nursing law.

Key Learning Activities (continued)

◆ Does your area have mandatory or permissive licensure?

Standards of Practice and the Nightingale Pledge and Practical Nurses' Pledges were discussed in Chapter 2. That was your introduction to the ethical and legal practice of nursing. Additional topics are considered in this chapter. Laws applying to healthcare ethics, the Code of Ethics for Nurses, and the Patient's Bill of Rights are discussed.

The laws of the United States and Canada and the ethical standards of the profession are carefully designed to protect both you and your patients. It is your responsibility to become familiar with these concepts before caring for patients and to refer back to them if you ever have a question.

Regulations of Nursing Practice

In the United States the licensing law is called the Nurse Practice Act; in Canada it is the Nurses (Registered) Act. These laws define the title and the regulations governing the practice of nursing. In some states, territories, and provinces, a single nurse practice act covers regulations for both registered and practical nurses and is administered by a single board of nursing or nursing association. In other states, practical nursing is regulated by a separate act and administered by a separate board. In many states having a single board, the law requires that a specified number of practical nurses serve as practical nursing board members; this gives practical nurses a voice in affairs concerning them. The state practical nurse association makes recommendations for these appointments.

The law defines the regulations for practical and registered nursing, including:

◆ Definition of practical nursing and definition of registered nursing
◆ Requirements for an approved school of nursing (length of course, the curriculum, admission requirements)
◆ Requirements for licensure (age, graduation from an approved course, the passing score on the licensing examination)
◆ Conditions under which a license may be suspended or revoked and conditions for its reinstatement

◆ Procedures for becoming licensed in each state, territory, or province
◆ Procedures for transferring licenses from one state to another

The Nurse Practice Act also establishes state and provincial boards and associations of nursing, which are empowered to carry out the provisions of the Nurse Practice Act.

State Boards of Nursing

Sometimes state nursing boards are known by other titles, such as the Board of Nurse Examiners. These boards are responsible for approving schools of nursing, visiting the schools, administering licensing examinations, and issuing and renewing nursing licenses. They also have the authority to suspend or revoke a license. Boards are subject to legal conditions, but they usually have some leeway in interpreting these conditions.

Licensing Laws

The legal aspects of nursing begin with licensing laws that give the nurse the legal right to practice nursing and define nursing responsibilities. Every state and commonwealth, as well as the District of Columbia, Puerto Rico, Guam, Samoa, and the Virgin Islands, has a law covering licensing of practical and registered nurses. Canada has similar laws affecting each province.

Nurse licensing laws vary in other respects. The goal of nurse planners is to establish uniform requirements so that a license issued in one state will be recognized in all other states. This is not presently the case, but most states currently issue interstate endorsement without reexamination if the state board test score was high enough and without requiring additional education. The situation is similar in Canada.

The Licensing Examination

The nursing graduate's first responsibility is to pass the National Council Licensing Examination for practical nurses, NCLEX-PN or the NCLEX on successful completion of an approved nursing program and to obtain a license to practice either as an LPN or RN.

More and more states are requiring continuing education for license renewal. Individual nurses are required to maintain records of continuing education units (CEUs) received.

Cause for Revoking or Suspending a License

The law defines the conditions under which a license can be revoked. These include drug or alcohol abuse, fraud, deceptive practices, criminal acts, previous disciplinary action, and gross or ordinary negligence.

Legal Responsibilities in Nursing

In the course of your activities as a nurse, you will be held responsible for maintaining the established standards of nursing care for practical or registered nursing. You will encounter many situations involving legal responsibilities. You should know and understand basic legal terms.

The following four terms are used in legal matters. A **tort** is a wrong committed against another person or property. A **crime** is a wrong committed against a person or property but also against the public good. In a crime, intention to do wrong is also present. Crimes may be misdemeanors or felonies. A **misdemeanor** is not as serious as a felony. Punishment for misdemeanors usually are fines or imprisonment for less than a year; parole sometimes is given. A **felony** is a serious crime. Imprisonment occurs in a state or federal penitentiary for more than a year. Other common legal terms occur through the first section of this chapter.

The Nurse's Legal Rights

A nurse has a right to legal protection by contract (oral or written) that states the terms of employment in relation to duties and salary. If either party fails to live up to the terms, the contract can be terminated.

Liability

Liability is the legal responsibility for one's acts (and failure to act). It involves responsibility for financial restitution for harms resulting from negligent acts. The crime may be the deliberate *commission* of a forbidden act or *omission* of an act required by law.

Besides those acts that all citizens know are illegal, there are other laws that the nurse must be careful not to violate. For example, federal law requires that records be kept on dispensing narcotics. This law specifies that narcotics must be given under the direction and supervision of a physician, osteopath, dentist, or veterinarian. In a hospital all narcotics are kept double-locked, and every dose or tablet must be accounted for.

Violation of the Controlled Substances Act is a crime on the part of the nurse.

Examples of other nursing crimes include participation in an illegal abortion, participation in euthanasia ("mercy killing"), failure to report a case of child abuse or an animal bite, and practicing medicine without a license or beyond legal limits of nursing practice.

Negligence. One of the most common causes of lawsuits instigated by patients is negligence. **Negligence** is defined as harm done to a patient as a result of neglecting duties or procedures or not taking ordinary precautions. You may be found negligent for any of the following reasons:

◆ Performing nursing procedures that you have not been taught
◆ Failing to meet established standards for the safe care of patients
◆ Failing to prevent injury to patients, hospital employees and visitors (for which you may consequently be sued for damages)

Malpractice. **Malpractice** is the improper treatment of a patient that results in illness or injury.

> ### Key Concept
> *Acts of commission*: malpractice
> *Acts of omission*: negligence

Assault and Battery. Assault and battery are the threat of physical damage and the carrying out of that threat. **Assault** may be a violent act, either physical or verbal; **battery** is a physical striking or beating. Either of these acts may be cause for a lawsuit. In nursing, the offense may be subtle, such as calling the patient unkind names or physically restraining the patient with undue force. Giving an injection that the patient refuses is battery; forcing the patient to get out of bed can be assault and battery. False imprisonment or restraint of movement may be charged in certain situations, such as the use of unnecessary restraints or solitary confinement (as in seclusion in the mental health unit). By law, a person cannot be restrained against his or her will unless the person has been convicted of a crime, declared mentally incompetent, or determined to be a danger to self or others.

> ### Key Concept
> The nurse or physician also has the right to bring charges against a patient for an unlawful act, such as a physical attack.

Libel and Slander. Libel and slander relate to personal integrity. **Slander** is the term given to malicious verbal statements that might injure a person. **Libel** refers to a written statement or picture that might injure a person. Clearly, the nurse must avoid untrue and unwise statements at all times in reporting and documenting. This is another reason to avoid gossip and to preserve the patient's privacy; confidentiality is important. Violation of the confidentiality of the patient's care or the chart is a violation of privacy laws. If a patient requests anonymity, just acknowledging the person's hospitalization can be a *violation* of the law.

Safeguards for the Nurse and Student

Although a practical or technical nurse works under the direction of professional nurses and physicians, this nurse is personally liable for any harm a patient suffers as a result of the nurse's own acts. In a hospital or other healthcare facility, the employer may also be legally liable for the nurse's acts of negligence.

Legal actions involving negligent acts by a person engaged in a profession are generally known as malpractice suits. Many professional and technical personnel protect themselves from paying court-imposed settlements by carrying malpractice insurance.

Malpractice Insurance

Malpractice insurance is available through private insurance companies and sometimes through the hospital or a professional organization.

The wise nurse carries malpractice insurance. Even if the nurse is innocent of the charges, it still costs money to prepare a defense. Malpractice insurance will cover these charges if you have practiced within the limits of your job description and level of training.

Precautions

It is important to protect yourself from possible lawsuits. Always perform procedures as taught and as outlined in the procedure manual of your hospital or health facility. If these policies are incorrect or inadequate, work to improve them through proper channels.

Be Competent in Your Practice. You are always responsible for your own behavior. Refuse to perform procedures for which you have not been prepared. Ignorance is not a legal defense. Neither will lack of sleep or overwork be accepted as a legal reason for carelessness about safety measures or mistakes.

Ask for assistance when you are not sure how to do a procedure. Do not assume responsibilities beyond those of the graduate nurse or nursing student at your level. It is always better to admit that you do not know how to perform a procedure than to attempt to do it and to injure the patient.

> ### Key Concepts
>
> ◆ Always practice within the limits of practical or registered nursing as you were taught.
> ◆ Use good common sense and judgment.
> ◆ Ask if you are unsure.
> ◆ Report any errors made immediately.

Obtain the services of a good lawyer at the first sign that you may be involved in an illegal or negligent act or that you may be named in a lawsuit. Insist on your legal rights. If you remember your limitations and practice within the scope of your education, you will have no difficulty with lawsuits and your patients will be safe. The accompanying box gives examples of situations in which you may be liable.

Do Not Give Legal Advice to Patients. A nurse should never attempt to advise a patient on legal rights. The patient should be encouraged to confer with the family and to consult an attorney. The laws governing personal and property rights of an individual are many and complex.

Do Not Accept Gifts. The nurse should never accept gifts from patients. An exception to this would be in the event that the patient wishes to give candy or flowers to be shared by all the staff on the unit.

Do Not Help a Patient Prepare a Will. A nurse should *never* attempt to help a patient draw up a will. The law has formal requirements a will must meet to make it valid. As a graduate, you may be asked to witness the signing of a will. After the death of a patient, the nurse, as well as the other witnesses, may be asked to testify as to the mental competence of the testator or to other

Examples of Situations in Which the Nurse Can be Held Liable

- ◆ Burns, falls, incorrect medications
- ◆ Lack of common nursing judgment (such as using an oral thermometer in a confused or out-of-control patient)
- ◆ Failure to follow hospital policy to protect the patient and his or her belongings
- ◆ Allowing an unsafe condition to continue
- ◆ Damages that arise from violation of the patient's rights
- ◆ Treatment without patient consent (this can be assault and battery)
- ◆ Stories or photographs given without consent
- ◆ Revelation of confidential information

conditions prevailing at the time of the execution of the will.

Legal Responsibility in an Emergency

In some states, any person who witnesses an automobile accident is required by law to give aid to a person injured in that accident. In most states, a person who has medical or nursing education is required to assist, if needed.

In areas other than those to which this law applies, no person is legally obligated to render aid during an emergency. However, when one does so, he or she should act as a reasonably prudent person would, within the limits of education and experience. Thus, the nurse is expected to render a higher level of emergency care than is an untrained person.

A law called the *Good Samaritan Act* is in effect in most states. This law protects you from liability if you give emergency care within the limits of first aid and if you act in a "reasonable and prudent manner."

Documentation

It is impossible to overemphasize the importance of keeping exact records of all treatments and medications as well as a record of the patient's behavior. The patient's chart is the written and legal evidence of treatment during the hospital stay or of occurrences in the home. The chart reflects facts only and not judgments. *Careful* and *accurate* documentation is vital for the patient's welfare and your own (Fig. 4-1).

> **Key Concept**
>
> Careful documentation is perhaps the most important thing you can do to protect yourself against a lawsuit. If a treatment or medication was not documented, legally, the procedure is considered not to have been done or the medication not given.

Overview of Relevant Legal Issues

Many other laws relating to healthcare involve the nurse. Some of the most important legislation is about informed consent, advance directives, and vulnerable persons.

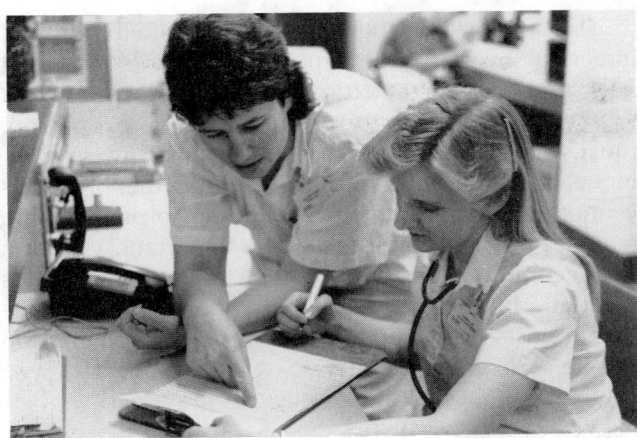

Figure 4-1. Careful documentation and reporting are nursing responsibilities and also maintain legal records (Craven RF, Hirnle CJ. Fundamentals of Nursing: Human Health and Function. Philadelphia, J.B. Lippincott, 1992).

Informed Consent

Before routine treatment, specialized diagnostic procedures, special medical or surgical treatment, or experimental therapy is used on a patient, the patient must give informed consent. **Informed consent** means that tests, treatments, and medications have been explained to the patient. Outcomes and possible complications along with alternative procedures must be discussed. The healthcare worker must be reasonably satisfied that the patient understands the directives. This teaching must be documented.

The consent form must be explained and signed by the patient or a legal guardian before the procedure is performed. In certain emergencies where death is a possibility, procedures can be performed without consent.

The person who will perform the procedure is responsible for obtaining the consent. The nurse confirms that the signed consent is in the patient's chart before the procedure is performed.

Advance Directives

To preserve a patient's rights, all healthcare workers need to be aware of a patient's wishes regarding continuing, withholding, or withdrawing treatment in the event the patient cannot make these decisions for himself or herself. An **advance directive** is a legal document in which a person either states choices for medical treatment or names someone to make treatment choices if he or she loses decision-making ability.

The Patient Self-Determination Act (PSDA) was passed by the federal government in 1991. This law requires all healthcare institutions to comply or forfeit Medicare and other types of funding. This legislation mandates patient rights, including the right to some sort of advance directive. The law *requires* that all adults admitted to the hospital be asked if they have an advance directive and assistance be given if the patient desires more information. The accompanying box describes the role of the nurse in carrying out the mandates of this legislation.

The three major types of advance directives are:

- Living will
- Directives to physicians
- Durable power of attorney for healthcare

Living Will. A **living will** is a written and legally witnessed document in which patients may indicate life-sustaining treatments they do or do not want used to keep them alive. Some form of living will legislation is in place throughout the United States. A great deal of controversy surrounds this issue. For example, in some states, the living will legislation states that artificial nutrition and hydration must be maintained, even though the patient has previously requested that no artificial means be used to sustain life. In addition, various states have slightly different formats for living wills and do not necessarily recognize documents written in another state.

It is the responsibility of the patient or family to present the living will to the healthcare facility on admission. A living will does not automatically expire in any certain length of time. It is in effect until the patient changes or revokes it.

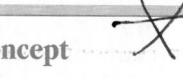

Key Concept

If there is no documented evidence to the contrary, the medical team will use all means available to keep any patient alive. Without a living will or other advance directive, a full "code" will be called on all patients who arrest, and full resuscitation efforts will be made.

Directive to Physicians. This is another type of written document that can be useful for terminally ill adult patients who have no other person they can name as their agent for making healthcare decisions. In this case, the person directs the physician to be the decision-maker. The physician must also agree, in writing, to accept this responsibility and to be the patient's agent.

Durable Power of Attorney for Healthcare. This is a written document in which a patient names another person to make healthcare decisions for him or her in the event that the patient is unable to make those decisions. This designated person does not need to be a relative. It is important to discuss one's wishes with this person in advance.

The Nurse's Responsibility in Determination of Advance Directives

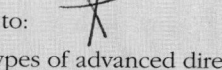

It is the nurse's responsibility to:

- Understand the different types of advanced directives
- Know the laws relating to the Patient Self-Determination Act
- Obtain assistance if the patient wishes to change an advanced directive, as the person's health or desires change
- Teach the patient so informed decisions can be made
- Inform patients that they have the right to refuse treatment or can refuse life-prolonging treatment, but still receive palliative care and pain control

On admission, the nurse must ask the patient if he or she understands the concept of advance directives and the Patient Self-Determination Act. The nurse needs to make sure the patient knows what a living will and durable power of attorney are. If the patient wishes to initiate an advance directive, the nurse must provide appropriate assistance (often in the form of a referral to another person). If the person has a living will, the nurse needs to make sure this information is placed on the chart, the physician notified, and the fact noted on the Kardex.

Mental Health Advance Declaration. In addition to the general advance declaration available to all hospitalized patients, the mental health declaration sets out guidelines for psychiatric care. In this case, the patient states his or her wishes about intrusive mental health treatment such as electroconvulsive therapy and special types of medications called neuroleptics. Even if the person who refuses these treatments is committed as mentally ill or mentally ill and dangerous, these treatments may not be given without a specific court order.[1]

Vulnerable Persons

Children and some adults can be considered vulnerable to deficient or harmful care. Reporting of suspected child abuse is mandatory in the United States and Canada. In addition, some states have laws protecting persons considered to be *vulnerable adults*. This includes any hospital patient but is particularly important when working with the mentally ill, mentally retarded, or confused person. The elderly can be vulnerable also. Vulnerable adults are protected by law from abuse or neglect while in the hospital or any other

---

[1] Adapted from "Questions and Answers Regarding Minnesota Law on Advance Directives." Minnesota Department of Health, Division of Health Resources, 1991.

health facility, a nursing home, a school, or their own homes.

Other Laws Relevant to Nursing

Examples of other laws and rules affecting nurses in a healthcare facility are:

◆ *Statutory definition of death*. With today's advanced life support systems, criteria other than breathing and heartbeat must be used to determine when biologic death has occurred.

◆ *Abortion and sterilization*. State laws differ as to what type of consents are required, who must be notified, and who must sign the consent.

◆ *Duty to provide treatment*. What happens if a person desires care but is unable to pay? Is the facility required by law to provide care?

◆ *Experimentation*. Does the hospital participate in research studies using human beings? What consents are required?

◆ *Release from liability*. What is the hospital's responsibility if a person leaves the hospital against medical advice? What is the responsibility if a person refuses treatment?

As you can see, the laws relating to healthcare are many and varied. You need to have a basic understanding of the laws that apply to your practice so that you can make informed decisions about your own practice of nursing.

Patients' Rights and Responsibilities

Patients also have rights and responsibilities. The concept of patients' rights stems from the rise of the consumer movement. The public demands the right to quality care.

Patients' Rights

In 1972, the American Hospital Association (AHA) adopted "A Patient's Bill of Rights," which states the rights of the hospitalized patient (see accompanying box). It serves as a basis for making decisions in regard to hospital patients. It helps ensure the concept of basic human rights that is widely accepted among healthcare providers.

Other groups have also formulated statements about rights of the health consumer, including the American Medical Association (AMA) and several nurses' associations. Local and national consumer groups constantly seek quality care and hospital accountability. President Clinton had, as one of his top priorities, the improvement of the healthcare system so that *all* individuals can receive equal care.

> **Key Concept**
>
> All patients have equal rights.

Right to Confidentiality. The patient also has the right to expect that his or her privacy will be protected. Privacy means that the information is available to the patient but not to the public. Information collected may be used "to provide effective medical/dental care and to develop treatment guidelines," to determine ability to pay for care and to bill third-party payors, and to do research studies. The patient may refuse to give information, but in this case, the quality of care may be limited by lack of information.

Patients' Responsibilities

The patient is an active participant in formulating his or her care plan and making healthcare decisions. Thus, the patient also has a responsibility to participate in and cooperate with care given. Certain cooperative actions can be expected of patients. It is the nurse's job to help patients understand their responsibilities and teach them how to enhance the recovery process. It is reasonable to request the following of a patient:

◆ Provide, to the best of your knowledge, accurate and complete information about matters relating to your health
◆ Be responsible for understanding your diagnosis/treatment
◆ Follow the recommended treatment plan
◆ Be responsible for your own actions if you refuse treatment, do not follow instructions, or leave the hospital against advice
◆ Report changes in your condition
◆ Keep appointments
◆ Meet financial obligations related to healthcare

> **Key Concept**
>
> The patient is an active participant in his or her own healthcare.

Values Clarification

Each of us, nurse and patient, brings values to the healthcare system. Our values include beliefs about such concepts as life and death, a higher power, who should receive healthcare and what kind of care, and complex issues such as abortion and euthanasia. Values are the culmination of heritage, culture, and one's fam-

A Patient's Bill of Rights

Introduction

Effective health care requires collaboration between patients and physicians and other health care professionals. Open and honest communication, respect for personal and professional values, and sensitivity to differences are integral to optimal patient care. As the setting for the provision of health services, hospitals must provide a foundation for understanding and respecting the rights and responsibilities of patients, their families, physicians, and other caregivers. Hospitals must ensure a health care ethic that respects the role of patients in decision making about treatment choices and other aspects of their care. Hospitals must be sensitive to cultural, racial, linguistic, religious, age, gender, and other differences as well as the needs of persons with disabilities.

The American Hospital Association presents *A Patient's Bill of Rights* with the expectation that it will contribute to more effective patient care and be supported by the hospital on behalf of the institution, its medical staff, employees, and patients. The American Hospital Association encourages health care institutions to tailor this bill of rights to their patient community by translating and/or simplifying the lanuage of this bill of rights as may be necessary to ensure that patients and their families understand their rights and responsibilites.

Bill of Rights*

1. The patient has the right to considerate and respectful care.
2. The patient has the right to and is encouraged to obtain from physicians and other direct caregivers relevant, current, and understandable information concerning diagnosis, treatment, and prognosis.

   Except in emergencies when the patient lacks decision-making capacity and the need for treatment is urgent, the patient is entitled to the opportunity to discuss and request information related to the specific procedures and/or treatments, the risks involved, the possible length of recuperation, and the medically reasonable alternatives and their accompanying risks and benefits.

   Patients have the right to know the identity of physicians, nurses, and others involved in their care, as well as when those involved are students, residents, or other trainees. The patient also has the right to know the immediate and long-term financial implications of treatment choices, insofar as they are known.
3. The patient has the right to make decisions about the plan of care prior to and during the course of treatment and to refuse a recommended treatment or plan of care to the extent permitted by law and hospital policy and to be informed of the medical consequences of this action. In case of such refusal, the patient is entitled to other appropriate care and services that the hospital provides or transfer to another hospital. The hospital should notify patients of any policy that might affect patient choice within the institution.

4. The patient has the right to have an advance directive (such as a living will, health care proxy, or durable power of attorney for health care) concerning treatment or designating a surrogate decision maker with the expectation that the hospital will honor the intent of that directive to the extent permitted by law and hospital policy.

   Health care institutions must advise patients of their rights under state law and hospital policy to make informed medical choices, ask if the patient has an advance directive, and include that information in patient records. The patient has the right to timely information about hospital policy that may limit its ability to implement fully a legally valid advance directive.
5. The patient has the right to every consideration of privacy. Case discussion, consultation, examination, and treatment should be conducted so as to protect each patient's privacy.
6. The patient has the right to expect that all communications and records pertaining to his/her care will be treated as confidential by the hospital, except in cases such as suspected abuse and public health hazards when reporting is permitted or required by law. The patient has the right to expect that the hospital will emphasize the confidentiality of this information when it releases it to any other parties entitled to review information in these records.
7. The patient has the right to review the records pertaining to his/her medical care and to have the information explained or interpreted as necessary, except when restricted by law.
8. The patient has the right to expect that, within its capacity and policies, a hospital will make reasonable response to the request of a patient for appropriate and medically indicated care and services. The hospital must provide evaluation, service, and/or referral as indicated by the urgency of the case. When medically appropriate and legally permissible, or when a patient has so requested, a patient may be transferred to another facility. The institution to which the patient is to be transferred must first have accepted the patient for transfer. The patient must also have the benefit of complete information and explanation concerning the need for, risks, benefits, and alternatives to such a transfer.
9. The patient has the right to ask and be informed of the existence of business relationships among the hospital, educational institutions, other health care providers, or payers that may influence the patient's treatment and care.
10. The patient has the right to consent to or decline to participate in proposed research studies or human experimentation affecting care and treatment or requiring direct patient involvement, and to have those studies fully explained prior to consent. A patient who declines to participate in research or experimentation is entitled to the most effective care that the hospital can otherwise provide.

11. The patient has the right to expect reasonable continuity of care when appropriate and to be informed by physicians and other caregivers of available and realistic patient care options when hospital care is no longer appropriate.

12. The patient has the right to be informed of hospital policies and practices that relate to patient care, treatment, and responsibilities. The patient has the right to be informed of available resources for resolving disputes, grievances, and conflicts, such as ethics committees, patient representatives, or other mechanisms available in the institution. The patient has the right to be informed of the hospital's charges for services and available payment methods.

The collaborative nature of health care requires that patients, or their families/surrogates, participate in their care. The effectiveness of care and patient satisfaction with the course of treatment depend, in part, on the patient fulfilling certain responsibilities. Patients are responsible for providing information about past illnesses, hospitalizations, medications, and other matters related to health status. To participate effectively in decision making, patients must be encouraged to take responsibility for requesting additional information or clarification about their health status or treatment when they do not fully understand information and instructions. Patients are also responsible for ensuring

that the health care institution has a copy of their written advance directive if they have one. Patients are responsible for informing their physicians and other caregivers if they anticipate problems in following prescribed treatment.

Patients should also be aware of the hospital's obligation to be reasonably efficient and equitable in providing care to other patients and the community. The hospital's rules and regulations are designed to help the hospital meet this obligation. Patients and their families are responsible for making reasonable accommodations to the needs of the hospital, other patients, medical staff, and hospital employees. Patients are responsible for providing necessary information for insurance claims and for working with the hospital to make payment arrangements, when necessary.

A person's health depends on much more than health care services. Patients are responsible for recognizing the impact of their life-style on their personal health.

Conclusion

Hospitals have many functions to perform, including the enhancement of health status, health promotion, and the prevention and treatment of injury and disease; the immediate and ongoing care and rehabilitation of patients; the education of health professionals, patients, and the community; and research. All these activities must be conducted with an overriding concern for the values and dignity of patients.

These rights can be exercised on the patient's behalf by a legally designated surrogate or proxy decision maker if the patient lacks decision-making capacity, is legally incompetent, or is a minor.
Reprinted with permission of the American Hospital Association. © 1992.

ily of origin, combined with life experiences. One's values evolve, as life situations change. The patient's values may change when faced with illness, injury, and possible death. To be of optimum support for patients, nurses must undergo their own personal **values clarification** process, but they must also allow patients the freedom to formulate and express their own values.

Ethical Standards of Healthcare

Ethics is defined as conduct appropriate for all members of a group. A brief code of ethics for PNs was given in Chapter 2. Many ethical issues confront healthcare workers today. These have arisen as a result of increased knowledge and technology, changing demographic patterns, and consumer demands. A few of the ethical issues are discussed here.

Nurses' Role Regarding Ethics

Nurses are expected to practice ethically. Because of their intimate work with patients, nurses often are the first to recognize that an ethical problem exists. Nurses are re-

sponsible for bringing forth these issues and participating in decision-making. The accompanying box presents several forms of a code of ethics for nurses. Whether the statements are made in the United States, Canada, or the international community, the basic ideas are the same.

Selected Ethical Problems

Examples of some of the major issues in healthcare ethics are presented here. Some of the issues mentioned in the legal section of this chapter are also ethical issues.

Organ Transplantation

Many organs are successfully transplanted from person to person. In some cases, as in heart transplant, the donor must be pronounced legally dead before the organ be can be removed. However, to keep the organ at its healthiest, it must be recovered at the moment the donor is pronounced clinically dead. (In most cases, circulation and ventilation are artificially maintained until the organ is removed.)

These situations involve such issues as defining clinical death and informed consent. Organ donation is a

Three Codes of Ethics for Nurses

International Council of Nurses Code for Nurses

The fundamental responsibility of the nurse is four-fold—to promote health, to prevent illness, to restore health, and to alleviate suffering.

The need for nursing is universal. Inherent in nursing is respect for life, dignity, and rights of humans. It is unrestricted by considerations of nationality, race, creed, age, sex, politics or social status.

Nurses render health services to the individual, the family, and the community and coordinate their services with those of related groups.

Nurses and People

The nurse's primary responsibility is to those people who require nursing care.

The nurse, in providing care, promotes an environment in which the values, customs, and spiritual beliefs of the individual are respected.

The nurse holds in confidence personal information and uses judgment in sharing this information.

Nurses and Practice

The nurse carries personal responsibility for nursing practice and for maintaining competence by continual learning. The nurse maintains the highest standards of nursing care possible within the reality of a specific situation.

The nurse uses judgment in relation to individual competence when accepting and delegating responsibilities.

The nurse, when acting in a professional capacity, should at all times maintain standards of personal conduct that reflect credit on the profession.

Nurses and Society

The nurse shares with other citizens the responsibility for initiating and supporting action to meet the health and social needs of the public.

Nurses and Coworkers

The nurse sustains a cooperative relationship with coworkers in nursing and other fields. The nurse takes appropriate action to safeguard the individual when his or her care is endangered by a coworker or any other person.

Nurses and the Profession

The nurse plays the major role in determining and implementing desirable standards of nursing practice and nursing education.

The nurse is active in developing a core of professional knowledge.

The nurse, acting through the professional organization, participates in establishing and maintaining equitable social and economic working conditions in nursing.

American Nurses Association Code for Nurses

1. The nurse provides services with respect for human dignity and the uniqueness of the client unrestricted by considerations of social or economic status, personal attributes, or the nature of health problems.

2. The nurse safeguards the client's right to privacy by judiciously protecting information of a confidential nature.

3. The nurse acts to safeguard the client and the public when health care and safety are affected by the incompetent, unethical, or illegal practice of any person.

4. The nurse assumes responsibility and accountability for individual nursing judgments and actions.

5. The nurse maintains competence in nursing.

6. The nurse exercises informed judgment and uses individual competence and qualifications as criteria in seeking consultation, accepting responsibilities, and delegating nursing activities to others.

7. The nurse participates in activities that contribute to the ongoing development of the profession's body of knowledge.

8. The nurse participates in the profession's efforts to implement and improve standards of nursing.

9. The nurse participates in the profession's efforts to establish and maintain conditions of employment conducive to high quality nursing care.

10. The nurse participates in the profession's effort to protect the public from misinformation and misrepresentation and to maintain the integrity of nursing.

11. The nurse collaborates with members of the health professions and other citizens in promoting community and national efforts to meet the health needs of the public.

Canadian Nurses Association Code of Ethics for Nursing Clients*

I. A nurse treats clients with respect for their individual needs and values.

II. Based on respect for clients and regard for their right to control their own care, nursing care reflects respect for the right of choice held by clients.

III. The nurse holds confidential all information about a client learned in the health care setting.

IV. The nurse is guided by consideration for the dignity of clients.

V. The nurse provides competent care to clients.

VI. The nurse maintains trust in nurses and nursing.

VII. The nurse recognizes the contribution and expertise of colleagues from nursing and other disciplines as essential to excellent health care.

VIII. The nurse takes steps to ensure that the client receives competent and ethical care.

IX. Conditions of employment should contribute in a positive way to client care and the professional satisfaction of nurses.

X. Job action by nurses is directed toward securing conditions of employment that enable safe and appropriate care for clients and contribute to the professional satisfaction of nurses.

Three Codes of Ethics for Nurses (continued)

XI. The nurse advocates the interests of clients.

XII. The nurse represents the values and ethics of nursing before colleagues and others.

XIII. Professional nurses' organizations are responsible for clarifying, securing, and sustaining ethical nursing conduct. The fulfillment of these tasks requires that professional nurses' organizations remain responsive to the rights, needs, and legitimate interests of clients and nurses.

Adapted from International Council of Nurses. ICN Code for Nurses: Ethical Concepts Applied to Nursing. Geneva, Imprimeries Populaires; 1973.

From American Nurses Association. Code for Nurses. Kansas City, MO, 1985.

* This represents only one element of the code—values. Obligations and limitations are provided with each value in the publication.

From Canadian Nurses Association. Code of Ethics for Nursing. Ottawa, Ontario, 1991.

difficult decision for a family to make at such a traumatic time. (A person can simplify this by designating during life that he or she wishes to be an organ donor.)

> ### Key Concept
>
> Even if you have designated yourself as a "donor" on your driver's license, your next-of-kin usually has to give permission after your death. Discuss this with your family *now*.

To ensure fairness in the receipt of donated organs, the United Network of Organ Sharing (UNOS) was established. This computerized network links all procurement organizations and maintains a list of potential organ recipients. Specific criteria have been established to determine which recipient will be eligible to receive a donated organ. It is not possible to purchase an organ, nor is it possible to guarantee that a particular recipient will receive a donated organ (except in the case of a living related donor).

Determination of Clinical Death

Great controversy surrounds the pronouncement of death. The Uniform Determination of Death Act was recommended to the states for enactment in 1980. State laws differ as to what constitutes death and how death is pronounced before the removal of organs or tissues for donation.

States use some or all of the following criteria for clinical death also known as irreversible coma or **brain death**:

◆ *Cessation of breathing* after artificial ventilation is discontinued (usually requires cessation for at least 3 minutes)

◆ *Cessation of heartbeat* without external stimuli

◆ *Unresponsiveness* to external stimuli

◆ *Complete absence of cephalic reflexes* (the lowest form of brain stem reflexes); in some states, some reflexes are allowed

◆ *Pupils fixed and dilated*; in some cases, pupils unresponsive to light but not necessarily dilated

◆ *Irreversible cessation of all functions of the brain*. In some states, this includes all functions of the brain stem as well. This brain and brain stem function can be assessed by the evaluation of reflexes. In some cases, an electroencephalogram (EEG) is done to *confirm* the diagnosis of clinical death.

In all cases, the following *exceptions* are identified:

◆ Marked hypothermia (core body temperature below 90°F [32.2°C], such as might follow time in a cold lake in a near-drowning episode)

◆ Severe depression of the central nervous system (CNS) after drug overdose with a CNS depressant, such as a barbiturate

You can see that the determination of death is complex and controversial. Check on the laws in your state.

> ### Key Concept
>
> There is no uniform definition of legal death in the United States. Each state has slightly different criteria.

Quality of Life

Quality of life is a complicated ethics issue. At what point does the healthcare team decide that a person should receive treatment or not? For example, there are not enough donated organs or specialized facilities to serve everyone who needs them. How then is the decision made as to who receives lifesaving treatment and who does not? This is where healthcare ethics comes into play.

Part of the discussion as to who receives treatment centers around the quality of life that can be expected following the treatment. Can the treatment measurably improve the quality of a person's life or the life expectancy? Would other patients benefit more? Who decides on the quality of another person's life? Who makes the decision as to who lives and who dies?

What determines quality of life? Some of the criteria suggested include ability to work, ability to be up and about, chronologic age, contributions to society, happiness or satisfaction with life, ability to care for oneself, and the patient and family's opinion.

Ethical Issues in Treatment

Who Should Receive Treatment? Other factors may have an impact on decisions to give or not to give treatment. Who will pay for the treatment, which sometimes amounts to hundreds of thousands of dollars? Do we make the decision to give treatment, even against the patient's will? (If the healthcare team makes this decision, it is called *beneficence*. If the patient makes the decision, it is termed *autonomy*.) Can a patient legally refuse treatment?

Patient Refusal of Treatment. Usually a person gives permission for treatment; thus, refusal is seen as the reversal of that permission. However, there is controversy among the states as to the patient's right to refuse lifesaving treatment. If there is any argument among family members or doubt on the part of the healthcare team, *treatment must be given* until the case is resolved in court. If there is controversy, a court order must be obtained before treatment may be withheld or removed. (If a person refuses treatment and it is illegally given, this may constitute battery on the part of the healthcare team.)

The only time the patient does not have the right to make the decision to refuse treatment is when the greater public interest would be in danger. For example, if a person has a communicable disease and refuses treatment, action may be taken.

> **Nursing Alert**
>
> Competent adults must speak for themselves. Another person cannot decide to withhold treatment, as long as the patient is able to make decisions. If the patient cannot talk, other means of communication may be used. This must be carefully documented, witnessed, and signed.

Withdrawal of Treatment. Termination of treatment involves the conscious decision to stop treatment, once it has been started. The treatment may be withdrawn at the patient's request or when the healthcare team determines that brain death has occurred. It is often legally more difficult to stop treatment once it has begun than to withhold treatment altogether.

Withholding Treatment. This involves the denial of treatment or care to a patient. It may be because the treatment has been deemed inappropriate for that person, because there is not enough of a particular treatment to go around (as in donor kidneys), or because the patient or family has refused.

Euthanasia

In the past, euthanasia was called "mercy killing." It meant the deliberate taking of a person's life to put the individual out of misery. This definition has been amended to include the withdrawal or withholding of treatment.

The Ethics Committee

Hospitals and other healthcare facilities have ethics committees. The chief functions are education, policy-making, case review, and consultation. These committees are important because they bring together a variety of healthcare workers from various disciplines. They are able to share their ideas and concerns related to their field. Nurses bring a unique voice to the committee because they are patient advocates and know their patients personally and intimately.

Keys for Review

Key Questions for Critical Thinking

1. Describe the differences between a crime of omission and a crime of commission.
2. Explain informed consent.

Key Questions for Critical Thinking
(continued)

3. Describe your personal values.
4. Describe *why* and *how* you plan to practice nursing.

Key Readings

American Nurses Association, Code for Nurses With Interpretive Statements. Kansas City, MO, 1985

Becker BG, Fendler T. Vocational and Personal Adjustment in Practical Nursing, Ed 6. St. Louis, C.V. Mosby, 1990

Benjamin M, Curtis J. Ethics in Nursing, Ed 3. New York, Oxford University Press, 1992

Canadian Nurses' Association. Code of Ethics for Nursing. Ottawa, Ontario, 1991

Husted GL, Husted JH. Ethical Decision Making in Nursing. St. Louis, C.V. Mosby, 1991

Kurzen C. Contemporary Practical/Vocational Nursing, Ed 2. Philadelphia, J.B. Lippincott, 1993

MacKay S. "Durable Power of Attorney for Health Care." Geriatric Nursing, March-April:99–108, 1992

Taylor C, Lillis C, LeMone P. Fundamentals of Nursing: The Art and Science of Nursing Care, Ed 2. Philadelphia, J.B. Lippincott, 1993

Enrichment Keys

Burke M, Walsh M. Gerontologic Nursing Care of the Frail Elderly. St. Louis, Mosby-Year Book, 1992

Keys to Learning More

The remainder of this book describes nursing and nursing procedures. A nurse practices within the guidelines of nursing protocols at all times.

Chapter 37: documentation

Chapter 56: accounting for "controlled" substances

Chapter 90: death and dying

Chapter 93: obtaining and renewing your nursing license

Unit 2 Personal and Environmental Health

5 Basic Human Needs

Learning Objectives

- Describe what is meant by a hierarchy of needs
- State the basic human needs as formulated by Maslow
- List at least five physiologic needs of all people
- Discuss the relationships between basic needs and nursing and between higher level needs and nursing
- Briefly describe how the needs of the family and community relate to the basic needs of the individual

Key Terms

hierarchy of needs	psychological	self-actualized
homeostasis	regression	self-esteem
physiologic	secondary needs	survival needs
primary needs		

Key Points

- All human beings are driven by physiologic and psychological needs.
- First level needs must be met before a person can address higher level needs.
- Illness or injury can interfere with a person's ability to meet needs.
- Illness or injury can also cause a person to regress to a lower level of functioning.
- Nursing can assist a person to meet needs or to eliminate potential threats to need satisfaction.
- Health is a state of physiologic and psychological well-being.

Key Topics Outline

Maslow's Hierarchy of Needs
Nursing's Relationship to Basic Needs
Overview of Individual Needs
   Basic Physiologic Needs
   Security and Safety Needs
   Social Needs (Love)
   Self-esteem Needs
   Self-actualization Needs
   Family and Community Needs

Key Learning Activities

- Tell a classmate about a time when you were unable to pursue higher level needs because one or more of your basic needs were not being satisfied.
- Interview a person who has recently been hospitalized. Discover some of the ways in which nurses helped that person to meet needs that he or she was unable to meet without assistance.
- Observe care of a patient who does not speak the same language as the nurse. Discuss in relationship to need satisfaction of the patient. Are his or her needs being met?

Rosdahl CB: Textbook of Basic Nursing, 6th ed. © 1995 J.B. Lippincott Company

In 1943, psychologist Abraham H. Maslow described a theory of basic human needs. This theory identified basic and higher level needs common to all people regardless of age, sex, race, social class, or state of health (well or ill). Maslow also stated that people respond to needs and *need satisfaction* as "whole" and integrated beings.

Nursing has been defined as a "helping relationship." Nurses help people to satisfy their basic needs and to reduce threats to this need satisfaction. Many nursing programs are based on the Maslow theory of needs. This chapter summarizes basic human needs and gives implications related to health and nursing care.

Maslow's Hierarchy of Needs

Maslow defined the basic needs of all people as a progression from simple physical needs (needed for survival) to more complex (aesthetic) needs. He called this a **hierarchy of needs**. On this hierarchy or ladder (Fig. 5-1), needs are ranked by their importance to the person's survival.

The needs at the bottom of the hierarchy must be met before a person can work toward meeting higher level needs. Thus, a person must meet needs at the first

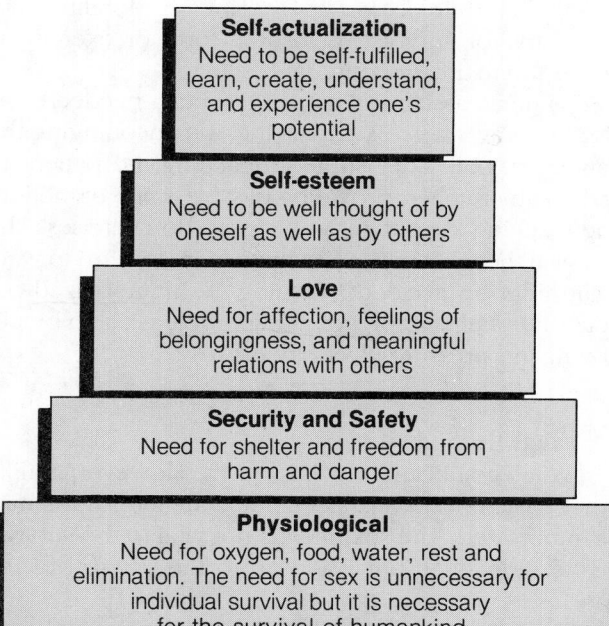

Figure 5-1. Hierarchy of needs. According to Maslow, basic physiological needs, such as food and water, must be met before the person can move on to higher level needs. Nursing is based on helping people to meet needs they cannot meet by themselves because of age, illness, or injury.

level, such as oxygen and food, before progressing to deal with needs such as safety, love, and self-esteem. People who are hungry will not be concerned about cleanliness or learning until they are fed. Individuals in pain will not be concerned about personal appearance until pain is relieved. Those facing surgery will not be able to learn about the operation unless they feel safe and secure. This is called **regression** to an earlier level of needs satisfaction and is common in illness or injury.

> **Key Concept**
>
> Maslow's hierarchy of needs has important implications for personal and family life, as well as for nursing.

Nursing's Relationship to Basic Needs

Illness or risk for illness occurs when people are not able to satisfy one or more of their basic needs. Much of your nursing career will center around assisting people to meet these needs. Much of your nursing care will involve avoiding risks to the patient's basic human needs. In other words, you will be helping the patient prevent complications before they begin.

There are many situations in which a nurse assists a patient to meet needs. The nurse may feed an infant, provide full range of motion for a person who has had a stroke, give a tube feeding to a person who cannot swallow, bathe a person who is in a full body cast, or play with a child. The nurse may encourage the recovering patient to attend to personal care, visit with someone who is lonely or frightened, or arrange for a social worker or a member of the clergy to visit a patient. This text discusses both needs common to all people and unique needs of the individual. Illness may modify a person's *perception* of his or her needs. As a result, the patient's *need priority* may differ from that of the nurse. Illness or injury may present a *block* or *obstacle* to the meeting of needs. Nursing tries to help remove those obstacles.

Meeting needs is a *process*; it is never static. In addition, needs are *interrelated* and some depend on others.

In many cases, the nurse can determine the patient's level of needs satisfaction by looking at the patient. For example, oxygenation can be estimated by looking for cyanosis and difficult breathing.

> **Key Concept**
>
> Basic needs are common to all people; needs are *universal*. Individuals of all cultures have basic needs; needs are *transcultural*. Needs can be satisfied or they can be blocked.

Overview of Individual Needs

Basic Physiologic Needs

First level needs are called **physiologic** needs, **survival** needs, or **primary needs**. They must be met to sustain life. Without them, the person will die. They take precedence over higher level needs. (**Secondary needs** are met to give *quality* to life.)

Oxygen

Oxygen is the most essential of all basic needs. Without oxygen circulating in the bloodstream, a person will die in a matter of minutes. Oxygen is provided to the cells by maintaining an open airway and circulation.

The nurse constantly evaluates the oxygenation status of the patient. Various situations can threaten the body's oxygen supply. For example, emphysema, paralysis, or secretions may make breathing difficult; circulation may be impaired, thus preventing oxygen from reaching the cells.

Water and Fluids

Water is necessary to sustain life. The body can survive only a few hours without water, although certain conditions may change this length of time. For example, the person in a very hot climate needs more water and fluids to sustain life than the person in a cold climate. The fluids in the body must also be in balance (**homeostasis**) to maintain health.

Examples of conditions requiring interventions for proper levels of fluids include unconsciousness, inability to swallow, and severe mental illness. If kidneys do not function, the body may retain water in the tissues (edema) or the body may not have enough water (dehydration). The nurse assists in these conditions by measuring intake and output, weighing the patient daily, and observing intravenous infusion of fluids.

Food and Nutrients

Nutrients are necessary to maintain life, although the body can survive for several days or weeks without food. Poor nutritional habits, inability to chew or swallow, nausea and vomiting, or overeating pose a threat to nutritional status.

Elimination of Waste Products

Elimination of the body's waste products is essential to maintain life and comfort. Wastes are eliminated in several ways. The lungs eliminate carbon dioxide and water; the skin eliminates water and sodium. The kidneys eliminate fluids and electrolytes, and the intestines discharge solid wastes and fluids. If wastes are allowed to build up in the body, many serious conditions can result.

A bowel obstruction, cancer of the bladder, kidney disease, and gallbladder disease disrupt normal elimination. Difficulty in breathing, poor circulation, acid–base imbalance, allergy, and infection also hinder adequate elimination. The nurse helps the patient eliminate wastes by giving an enema, by catheterizing a patient, or by assisting with dialysis. Surgery can eliminate a bowel obstruction, and medications can relieve diarrhea or constipation.

Sleep and Rest

Sleep and rest are important in maintaining health. People vary in the amount of sleep needed; factors such as pregnancy, age, and general health have an influence. The absence of sleep is not immediately life-threatening, but can cause various disorders if allowed to continue. For example, some forms of mental illness are aggravated by sleep deprivation.

The nurse assists the person to get enough sleep and rest by providing safe, comfortable, and quiet surroundings. Various treatments such as the soothing back rub, the warm tub bath, and certain medications can also promote sleep.

Activity and Exercise

Activity stimulates both the mind and body. Exercise helps maintain the body's structural integrity and health by enhancing circulation and respiration. Mobility is not necessary for survival, but some form of exercise is needed to maintain optimum health.

The nurse assists the patient to obtain needed exercise in many ways. Examples include encouraging the patient to walk after surgery, teaching the patient to walk with crutches, providing passive range of motion, and teaching the patient in a cast to do exercises. The physical therapist may assist the patient to learn to walk again after an accident. Turning the immobilized patient often helps to prevent lung problems, skin breakdown, and pressure ulcers (bedsores).

Sexual Gratification

Sexual gratification is important. However, unlike other basic physiologic needs, sexual gratification may be sublimated. The sex need is not vital to the survival of the individual, but it is vital to the survival of the species.

The nurse and patient are aware of sexuality issues when care is being given. However, the nurse helps the patient feel comfortable with the care. A patient may also wish to discuss sexual problems with the nurse. When the nurse is aware the patient has major sexual problems, the nurse should refer the patient for professional counseling.

Security and Safety Needs

The second level of Maslow's hierarchy of needs relates to safety. At this level, the needs contain both physical and **psychological** components.

Freedom From Harm

A person must feel safe and secure, both physically and emotionally, before being comfortable enough to move on to meet other needs. This includes freedom from harm, danger, and fear. Characteristics of safety include predictability, stability, and familiarity, as well as feeling safe and comfortable and trusting other people. Financial security is also a component of this need.

Safety adaptations must be made for the battered child or wife. In other cases, safety adaptations are made for age, whether the person is old or very young. The person who is physically challenged often needs special adaptations. The nurse may assist in removing threats to safety from the patient's environment. Examples include using proper handwashing techniques, preventing wound infections by using sterile dressings, disabling the gas stove in the home of a patient with Alzheimer's disease, and locking up poisons in the home to safeguard small children. Nurses teach the patient about the procedure before surgery; this makes the patient feel safer and aids in postoperative recovery.

Shelter

The lack of adequate shelter may not always be life-threatening but will thwart the ability of a person to progress toward a higher level of needs. A person's shelter should provide the warmth necessary to maintain an adequate body temperature, in addition to helping the person feel safe.

The nurse will meet homeless people in the hospital and can refer them to social service agencies for assistance.

Warmth

Several factors can threaten the body's need for temperature regulation. These include excessive external heat or cold or a high fever. The human body functions within a relatively narrow survival range of temperatures.

Core temperature *survival ranges* for the human body (under usual circumstances) are the following:

35°C to 41°C	"Normal" = 37°C
95°F to 106°F	"Normal" = 98.6°F

The body has mechanisms to assist in temporary regulation of body temperature. These include shivering, goose flesh, and perspiration. The nurse will assist patients to meet the need for temperature regulation in cases such as a severe burn, a high fever, or exposure to extreme heat (heat stroke) or cold (hypothermia, frostbite).

Social Needs (Love)

At the third level of Maslow's hierarchy, social needs, such as the need for love and belonging, are addressed. Love and affection begin with bonding at birth and must continue throughout life for the person to meet needs at this level. All people need to feel that they have meaningful relationships with others and that they belong to a group. People need the acceptance of family and friends.

When an ill or injured person is in the hospital, he or she is separated from friends and family. The nurse assists this person by encouraging visitors, cards, and phone calls and by visiting with the patient whenever possible (Fig. 5-2). The nurse explains to the family that the patient needs even more reassurance and acceptance if he or she is disfigured in any way. The elderly person and the young person in society often have much in common in that they may not feel a part of a group or may feel that they are not useful or appreciated:

Self-Esteem Needs

The term **self-esteem** (self-image, self-respect) is related to the person's perception of self. Positive self-esteem is a sense of personal worth. Esteem needs are met when the person thinks well or himself or herself (achievement, adequacy, competence, confidence) and

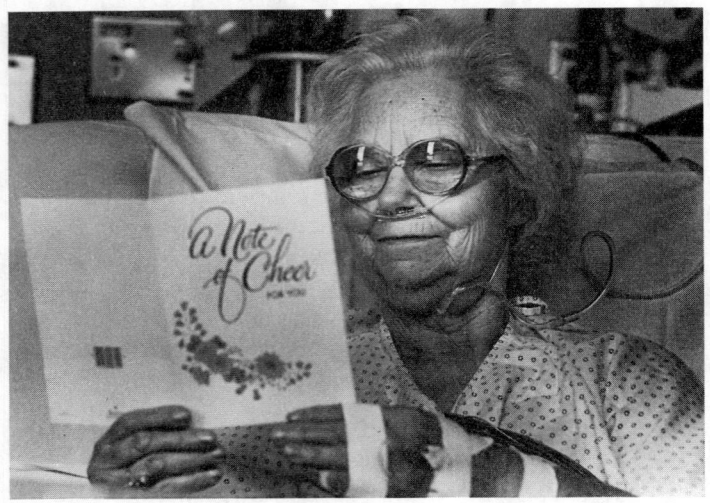

Figure 5-2. This woman's basic needs are being met. She is *resting* in the hospital, receiving *oxygen* by nasal cannula, and receiving *fluids* and *nourishment* by intravenous infusion. Therefore, she is able to enjoy secondary needs. Cards, phone calls, and visits from friends and family help her to meet some of her higher level needs: for *love, belonging,* and *self-esteem.* (© Bistram Photography. Photograph courtesy of Unity Hospital, Fridley, MN)

is well thought of by others (recognition, status, awards, prestige).

The person who is ill or injured or who has surgery may have an altered self-esteem. This is particularly true in situations such as amputation of a limb. Many women experience difficulty with their self-image following a hysterectomy or a breast removal. The nurse assists the patient to regain positive self-esteem by encouraging independence, rewarding for progress, and allowing the patient to do as much self-care as possible. The nurse observes the patient for depression, over-dependence, or a refusal to cooperate. Low self-esteem is directly related to disorders such as chemical dependency.

> ### Key Concept
>
> There is a danger in that the *needs of the nurse* can influence the level of nursing care. Be careful not to let this endanger your patient!

Self-Actualization Needs

Needs at this level are the highest order needs; the **self-actualized** person has "reached his or her full potential." The term self-actualized implies a *"fully functioning person."* Maslow described this state as a "more comfortable relationship with reality." Many psychologists believe that people continue striving to reach this level throughout life. It is commonly believed that very few people believe they are totally self-actualized.

The self-actualized person is able to cope with life's situations, to deal with failure, and to be free of anxiety. This person has a sense of humor, is self-controlled, and is not defensive. (One nursing instructor identifies Mother Teresa as an example of a person who seems to have achieved self-actualization.)

Nursing is one discipline that assists people to reach their fullest potential, given the person's individual limitations. It is important to restore as much functioning as possible to the person (rehabilitation). In some cases, people who have been severely physically challenged reach a higher level of intellectual functioning than they had previously imagined.

Family and Community Needs

The family unit has needs that must be met for life to run smoothly. The special needs of the family include developmental tasks and functions and goals. These needs are met in a variety of family structures.

The community has basic needs concerning the welfare of all its residents. Among these needs are public health measures (such as immunization programs), access to healthcare, maintenance services (such as water and electricity), environmental concerns (pollution), safety (police and highways), and emergency services.

> ### Key Concept
>
> Nursing is concerned with helping people meet their needs. Much of nursing deals with assisting the patient to meet basic physiologic needs.

Keys for Review

Key Questions for Critical Thinking

1. Describe the hierarchy of needs, including the components at each level.
2. Describe the relationship of Maslow's hierarchy to nursing.

Key Readings

Carroll C, Miller DF. Health: The Science of Human Adaptation, Ed 5. Madison, WI, Brown & Benchmark, 1991

Ellis JB, Nowlis, EA. Nursing: A Human Needs Approach, Ed 4. Philadelphia, J.B. Lippincott, 1990

Maslow AH. Motivation and Personality, Ed 2. New York, Harper, 1970

Enrichment Keys

Currer C, Stacey M (eds). Concepts of Health, Illness and Disease: A Comparative Perspective. Providence, RI, Berg, 1987

Sizer FS, Whitney EN. Making Life Choices: Health Skills and Concepts. Minneapolis, West Publishing, 1993

Keys to Learning More

Chapter 6: high-level wellness
Chapter 7: health needs of the community
Unit Three: human development
Chapter 27: nutritional needs
Unit Six: safety in the healthcare setting
Chapter 36: therapeutic communication skills
Unit Nine: basic nursing procedures
Chapter 53: needs of the surgical patient
Chapter 54: surgical asepsis
Unit Twelve: mother, newborn, and family needs
Unit Thirteen: young person with a dysfunction
Unit Fourteen: assisting adults meet needs
Unit Fifteen: assisting the older adult to meet needs

6 Optimum Health for All People

Keys for Learning

Learning Objectives

- State at least three definitions of health, including the World Health Organization definition of health
- List five components of health and describe how each is attained
- Describe the health–illness continuum
- Discuss stress and ways you and your patient can deal with it
- List at least five alternative healthcare therapies and summarize each
- Identify ways to avoid fraudulent medical treatments

Key Terms

body mechanics

fight-or-flight reaction

fraud

general adaptation syndrome

health

holistic

homeostasis

stress

wellness

Keys to Understanding This Chapter

Chapter 5: Maslow's hierarchy of needs

Key Points

- Although there are many definitions of health, optimum health includes physical, emotional, mental, social, and spiritual well-being.
- The concept of high-level wellness relates to the higher level needs in Maslow's hierarchy.
- The state of one's health is on a continuum and is dynamic, changing from day to day.

Key Points (continued)

- Some stress is beneficial, whereas too much stress can lead to physical and emotional disorders.
- Health habits, including good grooming, are important for nurses and their patients.
- Alternative healthcare can be a useful adjunct to traditional Western medicine.
- Fraudulent health claims can endanger the lives of innocent people; the nurse can help to teach recognition of fraudulent claims.

Key Topics Outline

Health and Wellness
  The Health–Illness Continuum
  The Impact of Stress
  General Adaptation Syndrome
  Practicing Healthy Habits
Alternative Healthcare
Consumer Fraud

Key Learning Activities

- Visit an acupuncturist, herbalist, or chiropractor. Describe how they see their role in the modern healthcare system.
- Attend a stress management seminar. Report back to the class healthy ways in which a nursing student can relieve stress.
- Cut out newspaper, supermarket, tabloid, or magazine ads that make claims for cures. What claims are made? What is the scientific proof? Cost? Discuss these in class.

Rosdahl CB: Textbook of Basic Nursing, 6th ed. © 1995 J.B. Lippincott Company

WHO Definition of Health

Health is a state of complete physical, mental, and social well-being and not merely the absence of disease or infirmity.

The enjoyment of the highest attainable standard of health is one of the fundamental rights of every human being without distinction of race, religion, political belief, or economic or social condition.

The human organism must continuously adapt to the environment to maintain a balance or **homeostasis**. Health in a **holistic** sense is total wellness—wellness of mind and spirit as well as body.

Health and Wellness

Carroll and Miller define **wellness** as: "involving good physical self-care, using one's mind constructively, expressing one's emotions effectively, interacting creatively with others, and being concerned about one's physical and psychological environment."[1]

The World Health Organization (WHO) was established to improve the health of all of the world's people. WHO's 1974 definition of **health** is given in the accompanying box.

Health is much more than physical well-being. It includes thoughts and feelings, and it influences work efficiency and relationships with other people. Health

[1] Carroll C, Miller D. Health: The Science of Human Adaptation, Ed 5. Madison, WI, Brown & Benchmark, 1991.

must be considered in its broadest sense, which includes:

◆ *Physical health.* Physical fitness, the body functioning at its best
◆ *Emotional health.* Feelings and attitudes that make one comfortable with oneself
◆ *Mental health.* A mind that grows and adjusts; in control, free of serious stress
◆ *Social health.* A sense of responsibility and caring for the health and welfare of others
◆ *Spiritual health.* Inner peace and security, comfort with one's higher power, as one perceives it

Notice how the aspects of health presented above fit into Maslow's hierarchy of needs, discussed in Chapter 5.

The Health–Illness Continuum

People do not tend to be totally healthy or totally ill at any given time. Your daily state of health falls somewhere on a continuum from high-level wellness to death (Fig. 6-1). Although the goal is to move toward high-level wellness, your status may vary daily.

Maslow's hierarchy relates to this continuum. If your needs are blocked or threatened, you move toward the "illness" end of the continuum. When your basic needs are satisfied and you are moving toward self-actualization, you move further toward the "wellness" end of the continuum. The body adapts to change in an attempt to maintain *homeostasis*. High-level wellness is *optimum health*. The remainder of this chapter describes ways in which you can move toward this goal. If you (as a nurse) are moving toward this goal, you can better assist patients to move toward the wellness end of the continuum.

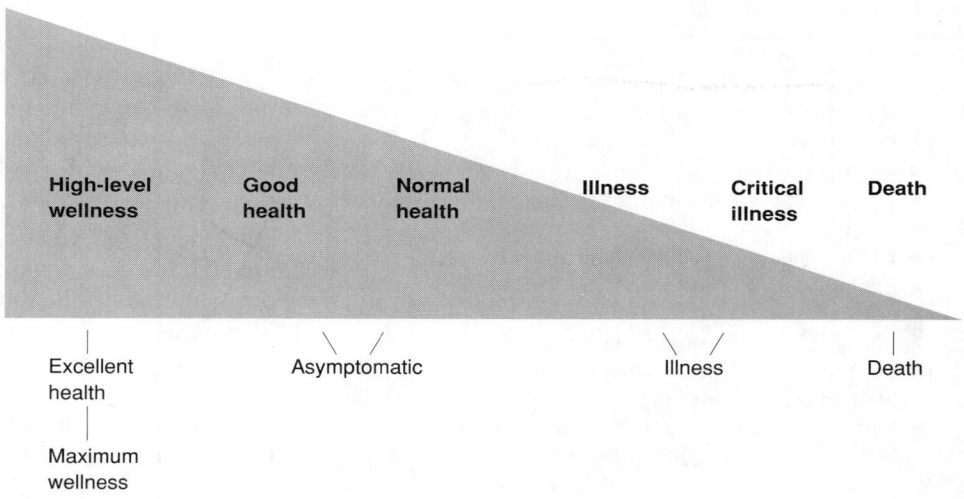

Figure 6-1. The health–illness continuum. (Adapted from curriculum of St. Mary's Campus, College of St. Catherine, Minneapolis, MN)

The Impact of Stress

If you are alive, you have stress. **Stress** is the normal wear and tear that is part of life, that is, the physical and psychological forces experienced by individuals that produce a strain on homeostasis. Examples of physical forces are gravity, mechanical forces, pathogens, and injury. Examples of psychological forces are fear, anxiety, crisis, and joy.

Stress can be beneficial. Many believe that people need a certain amount of stress to maintain well-being. Stress offers a challenge and spurs most people on to do more and better work. Stress can alert the body's defenses to danger and help the individual deal with emergencies.

Stress can be harmful. If people cannot deal with stress constructively, stress can become a problem. Some disorders, such as coronary conditions, chemical dependency, asthma, ulcers, and some mental illnesses, may result from unmanaged stress. Yet, the person with nothing to do and no goals in life finds life stressful simply because of lack of motivation.

Illness is a stressor. The nurse assists the patient in adapting to stressors, so that he or she can move to a higher level of wellness. Guidelines for helping reduce patient stress are given in the accompanying box.

General Adaptation Syndrome

Hans Selye explained the reaction of the mind and body to stressors in his **general adaptation syndrome** (Fig. 6-2). The response occurs in three stages:

- *Alarm*: The body recognizes the stressor and produces hormones necessary for either fight or flight. (**Fight-or-flight reaction** refers to the body's response to emergencies. It prepares the body to

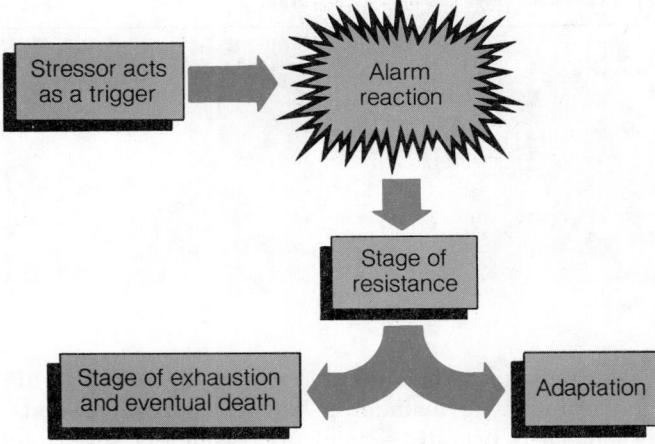

Figure 6-2. Selye's general adaptation syndrome. Once a stressor is present, an alarm reaction occurs. If the stressor is not so overwhelming that death results, the stage of resistance follows. Adaptation occurs, or if it does not, the stage of exhaustion arrives and death will eventually result when all adaptation energy is depleted.

"make a stand" or flee from the situation.) In this stage heart rate increases, blood sugar level increases, pupils dilate, and digestion slows.
- *Resistance* or *Adaptation*: The body begins to repair itself from the stress. Symptoms disappear. If stress continues, the body fails in maintaining a defense.
- *Exhaustion*: The body can no longer respond to the stress.

Key Concept

A person seeks professional healthcare when he or she is not able to meet basic needs without assistance. The person responds to threats that may be potential threats, perceived threats, or actual threats.

Practicing Healthy Habits

People who lead healthful physical and emotional lives are healthier and better able to deal with stress. Good health habits help to prevent disorders and enhance total wellness. Poor health habits can seriously affect efficiency. Guidelines for teaching basic healthy habits are given in the accompanying box. The following section summarizes healthy habits. More information on leading healthy lives appears throughout the textbook.

Diet

Everyone needs certain nutrients to keep the body functioning and in good repair. Individual nutritional needs vary, depending on body build, age, and activity.

Skill Guidelines for Helping to Decrease Stress

- Explain the features and operation of the bed unit, especially the location of the call signal.
- Place the call signal within easy reach.
- Answer the call signal promptly.
- Encourage the patient to do as much self-care as possible.
- Let the patient talk about fears and worries.
- Explain nursing procedures before you carry them out.
- Ensure privacy during nursing procedures.
- Perform nursing procedures efficiently with the least amount of discomfort.
- Before you leave the room, make sure the patient is comfortable and safe after a procedure.

As a nurse, you should understand and practice good nutrition to work comfortably and to teach others effectively. Eating regular and balanced meals, eating breakfast daily, and maintaining one's weight within the normal range are factors that contribute to wellness. Intake of salt, sugar, fats, and red meat should be limited. Plenty of fruits, vegetables, and grains should be included in the diet.

Elimination

The integumentary, respiratory, urinary, and digestive systems work to get rid of wastes. The woody fibers in vegetables and fruits supply bulk, or roughage, which stimulates proper elimination of solids. You can help your kidneys do their work of eliminating liquid wastes by drinking adequate amounts of water. Avoid smoking to maintain your lungs and cardiovascular system at their maximum efficiency.

Exercise

Exercise is necessary to maintain muscle tone, to stimulate circulation and respiration, and to help control body weight. All people need some sort of exercise daily. A person's age, occupation, and general condition help to determine the appropriate amount and kind of exercise.

A moderate amount of daily exercise is better than occasional spurts of strenuous activity. Walking is good exercise for most people. Isometric exercises (muscle tightening, which can be done while remaining in place) can be done while working, riding in a car, or lying in bed.

Sleep and Rest

Most people need 7 to 8 hours of sleep per night. You can tell if you are getting enough if you wake up rested. If you are chronically tired or have difficulty falling asleep, you need medical advice. Sometimes, after a day's work, rest is needed rather than sleep. Try lying relaxed and letting your thoughts drift. Some people find that meditation or "emptying the mind of all thoughts" is restful.

Personal Hygiene

Activities of personal hygiene are basic to normal functioning. Such activities help to protect the body from infections, make a good impression on others, and help to promote a positive self-image. It is important for the nurse to be well groomed. Your grooming indicates the type of care you might give the patient. How you attend to your personal grooming also is an example to your patient.

Key Concept

If you understand the concepts of healthy living, you will be better able to teach your patients.

Bathing/Showering

Regular bathing or cleansing removes perspiration, oil, and pathogens from the skin. It increases circulation and helps maintain muscle tone. Bathing is refreshing; it can help wake one up in the morning. It also is relaxing and can help one sleep at night.

Grooming

Hair, nail, and foot and hand care are important to one's appearance and well being. Shampooing removes dirt and oil and increases circulation.

Nails of both the hands and feet should be trimmed to a comfortable length. Bitten nails are unsightly and may lead to infection. A pale nail polish is better than a bright polish for those who are in the public eye. Hands should be massaged and hand lotion applied. Shoes should be comfortable, especially if the person stands or walks a good bit. They should also give the foot support without rubbing. Mobility can be jeopardized by corns, calluses, ingrown toenails, and other foot conditions.

Clothes should be clean, well fitting, and comfortable. They should be appropriate for the type of activity being performed. The appropriate mode of dress for nurses is prescribed by your healthcare facility and by the unit to which you are assigned. In many cases, street clothes are worn; in other areas, nurses wear scrub suits. All clothing, nails, and hair should be clean.

Guidelines for proper dress and grooming for the student nurse are given in the accompanying box.

> ## Key Concept
>
> The person who is ill is particularly sensitive to offensive odors and unusual clothing or makeup.

Dental Care

Teeth should be brushed regularly. Regular dental checkups are necessary to correct difficulties before they become major problems.

Many communities add fluoride to their water supply. Fluoride lessens tooth decay. It is estimated that one part fluoride to one million parts of water is an effective amount. Fluoride treatment can also be given by the dentist, who applies fluoride directly to the teeth two or three times a year.

Diet is important to dental health. For the first 6 to 8 years of life, the minerals calcium and phosphorus and vitamins A, C, and D are essential in forming normal teeth. If vitamin and mineral supplies are inadequate at any time in life, the jaw bones may become porous, the teeth may loosen, and the gum tissues may become diseased.

The single most common cause of dental difficulties is faulty diet. Americans in particular eat far too much sugar and meat and not enough fruits and vegetables. Sugar promotes tooth decay. The continuous eating of soft foods also affects the gums and teeth because you need to chew foods such as raw vegetables to maintain the tone and holding power of the gums and the strength of the teeth.

Eye Care

It is important to care for your eyes. You should have your eyes examined at least once a year. Danger signs that should send you to an eye specialist include persistent headaches; painful, watery, inflamed eyes; eye discharges; and visual disturbances. To take chances with your eyesight is to risk serious interference with your career and with your life. Hands should be washed before touching the eyes to avoid introducing infection. Do not put your contact lenses in your mouth! If something gets into your eye, do not rub it; you may scratch your cornea or embed a particle in the tissue. If tear secretions do not wash the object out, consult a physician. Eye doctors discourage the use of an eyecup because of the danger of infection. The preparations advertised as effective in brightening and rejuvenating the eyes are probably harmless in themselves. However, one danger in using eyewashes is that you may be lessening the symptoms of a disorder that requires medical attention. This may delay getting needed treatment for the problem.

Key Guidelines for Dress and Grooming for the Student Nurse

- ◆ Follow the protocol of your facility and area.
- ◆ Wear washable clothes and sweaters.
- ◆ Pants should be long enough to reach your shoe tops.
- ◆ Wear flat, comfortable shoes.
- ◆ Skirts should not be so short they preclude bending over.
- ◆ Hair should be clean and neat and usually should be pulled back from your face.
- ◆ Moustaches, sideburns, and beards should be kept neatly trimmed and clean.
- ◆ Use an absolute minimum of aftershave lotion or perfume.
- ◆ Make sure to brush your teeth and use mouthwash to avoid bad breath. (This is particularly important if you smoke.)
- ◆ Wear little or no jewelry (a ring might scratch a patient, tear gloves, collect bacteria, or hinder effective handwashing).
- ◆ Earrings should be small, if worn.
- ◆ Avoid very dark or bright red lipstick and extreme makeup.
- ◆ Keep fingernails short and clean; colored nail polish usually is not recommended.
- ◆ Carefully clip hangnails and cover with a Band-aid.
- ◆ Bathe or shower daily.
- ◆ Use an adequate deodorant to avoid body odors (additional protection might be necessary during menses).
- ◆ Wear your name tag; it is a required part of your uniform whenever you are giving patient care.
- ◆ CAUTION: In areas where patients may act out, such as mental health and detoxification units, the clothing you choose must also be considered for its safety. Necklaces, neckties, and long hair can be dangerous if a patient becomes violent.

Posture and Body Mechanics

The way you stand, sit, or move affects your efficiency and the impression you create. Good posture improves your health—you breathe better, and your circulation and muscle tone are improved. You also save energy, and you protect your health by preventing muscle strain and back disorders.

Posture is the position of your body, the way its parts line up when you stand, sit, move, or lie. You use your muscles to keep your body in good alignment. Think of your spine as a set of building blocks (the vertebrae) set one above the other and held together by strong bands of elastic tissue (the muscles), which can be made to stretch or contract to keep your body in line. Correct use of muscles is the secret of good posture. Nature has provided the appropriate muscles for every

Key Guidelines for Good Posture

Standing Posture

- ◆ Head erect with chin drawn in
- ◆ Chest lifted
- ◆ Shoulders back resting on spine
- ◆ Lower abdomen flat, upper abdomen full
- ◆ Natural curves of back
- ◆ Toes pointing straight ahead, weight on outer borders of feet

Sitting Posture

- ◆ Feet flat on floor
- ◆ Buttocks touching back of chair
- ◆ Back supported and straight
- ◆ Head erect

body movement, but their use is up to you. Poor posture overstrains some muscles and overrelaxes others.

The way you sit is as important as the way you stand. It is tiring to sit slouched in your seat; this position interferes with your breathing, strains your neck and back muscles, and throws your weight onto the end of your spine. Good posture is considerably more restful once it becomes a habit. Try sitting well back in your chair with your spine straight, your head erect, and your feet flat on the floor.

Body mechanics is the term that refers to the use of the body as a tool. You use proper body mechanics, as described in Chapter 43, to protect both yourself and the patient.

Healthy Environment

Everyone should be able to live in a safe environment. It is difficult to meet all of one's basic needs or to have optimum health if the environment is not safe. Fortunately, there is a growing concern about the environment, and people are banding together to address the issues.

A safe environment and various types of pollution are discussed in the next chapter as a community responsibility. The following discussion involves using a safe environment as a healthy habit.

Individuals need outdoor air and some sunlight (with protection from the rays). Swimming is a healthy exercise *if* the water is clean. Working smoke alarms in homes are important and help save lives. Regularly checking the batteries to see that they are functioning is a healthy habit.

Smoking is considered to be *one of the most significant health hazards* in the world today. Even second-hand smoke is considered dangerous. Smoking damages the lungs; contributes to heart, blood vessel, and gastrointestinal disorders; and aggravates many chronic

conditions. It is particularly dangerous to both mother and fetus during pregnancy.

Motor vehicles should not be operated by anyone under the influence of alcohol. Any kind of substance abuse is harmful to one's health. Among these substances are recreational drugs. Even prescribed drugs can be abused or become addictive. The interactions of a variety of drugs can be harmful, or the use of certain foods with certain drugs can be deadly. Over-the-counter drugs are harmful if overused.

Even one's choice of friends can create a healthy environment. It is good to surround oneself with happy people, people who are well adjusted and can cope with life in normal ways.

"Safer Sex"

During the last several decades the attitudes toward sex was "anything goes." However, countless deaths from acquired immunodeficiency syndrome (AIDS) and the rise in sexually transmitted diseases has affected the relationship between the sexes. It has been said that "no sex is safe," but many individuals and groups are trying to develop healthy habits related to sexual activity. This has been called "safer sex." It involves carefully choosing one's sexual partner and limiting the number of partners. Many people advocate a return to fidelity between two people. The use of condoms is another type of protection when participating in sexual activity.

Alternative Healthcare

Many people believe that diseases can be cured and optimum health achieved by other means than traditional Western medicine. Several of these modalities are discussed here. They may be used alone or in conjunction with other therapies. Only qualified practitioners should be visited. (Some of these therapists must be licensed to practice in the United States.)

Herbalists. *Herbalists* try to promote health through the use of herbs and other plants (botanicals). In many cases the use of herbs is combined with a healthful diet, exercise, and other health practices.

Acupuncture and Acupressure. *Acupuncture* is a healing method originating from Chinese medicine. It is based on "Chi," which is believed to be the energy of life. It looks at health and its functions as energy balance and disease as imbalance in the body. Acupuncture therapy includes the use of very fine needles inserted into specific energy points underneath the skin to balance the flow of energy. The use of this procedure is increasing in Western culture. It allows the body to heal naturally and does not involve the use of drugs. Acupuncture is often combined with other modalities, such as meditation and exercise. Acupressure (external pressure applied to the energy points) can be taught to the patient for pain and symptom control between treatments. (Physical therapy and chiropractic use many of the same energy/pressure points as acupuncture.)

Chiropractic and Physical Therapy. *Chiropractic* uses manipulation of the spinal column and joints. The therapy is based on structure and function of the body. It is believed that the relationships between the spinal column and nervous system are important. *Physical therapy* is a form of rehabilitation following disease or injury. Exercise, heat, cold, electricity, ultraviolet radiation, and massage are used to improve circulation and strengthen and retrain muscles.

Therapeutic Touch. *Therapeutic touch* grew out of the holistic care movement. It is a technique developed from the ancient practice of "laying on of hands." This therapy teaches that the patient is surrounded by an energy field. The practitioner assesses and treats the client's energy with the goal of restoring harmony. It is noninvasive, that is, it is not a procedure that requires entering the body or puncturing the skin. It may decrease the patient's need for medication.

Meditation, Relaxation, and Imagery. Meditation and relaxation are similar. They are the act of quiet thinking. They are practiced in some form by many religious groups. The person sits in a quiet place with eyes shut and the body in a relaxed position. Deep breathing is used and a word or phrase is repeated with the breathing. Hypnosis uses relaxation in its therapy.

Imagery involves calling up mental pictures or events. Although any of the senses can be used, the most prominent used in therapy is *visual imagery*. Imagery is used often in cancer therapy. It also is applicable to weight reduction and smoking cessation.

Laughter. The importance of laughter and humor cannot be overemphasized. Some hospitals have therapeutic laughter programs. There is a national organization related to therapeutic laughter for nurses.

Key Concept

Don't underestimate the role of humor in your own life. A good laugh can give you a much brighter outlook on the day and can also improve your health.

Consumer Fraud

An estimated $25 billion per year is spent on supposedly sure cures for every imaginable ailment. The result is that the ill person may run the risk of delaying vital treatment until it is too late. Cancer and arthritis "cures" are the most common. Cures for AIDS and chronic fatigue are on the rise.

It is illegal to mislead the public (**fraud**). A great deal of money is at stake, so new schemes continue to develop. Why are so many people taken in by claims for a drug or other magic cure? One victim remarked, "On your bed of pain, you will try anything at any cost." Also, the general public often cannot tell the difference between true and false claims. As a nurse, you might be asked for your opinion about a questionable medical practice. It is better for people to make their own decisions, rather than for you to tell them what to do. Encourage the person to find out all the facts. Some suggestions are given in the accompanying box.

Keys to Patient/Family Teaching
How to Detect Frauds

Patient/family teaching about fraud includes:

◆ Development of consumer awareness
◆ Membership in support groups
◆ Suspicion of advertising with the following:
   ◆ Special formula
   ◆ Claims of support by a physician or nurse (or includes photo of a woman in a nurse's uniform)
   ◆ Use of testimonials
   ◆ Attractive refund policy if not "completely satisfied"
◆ Discussion of treatment and prognosis with a qualified person (second opinion)
◆ Defense of your right for information

Keys for Review

Key Questions for Critical Thinking

1. Explain the various definitions of health. Discuss your definition of health.
2. Describe "high-level wellness."
3. Discuss the role of stress and its relationship to health and illness.
4. Describe how the nurse's state of health affects patient care.

Key Readings

Carroll C, Miller D. Health: The Science of Human Adaptation, Ed 5. Madison, WI, Brown & Benchmark, 1991

Cousins N. Anatomy of an Illness as Perceived by the Patient: Reflections on Healing and Regeneration. New York, Bantam, 1991

Craven RF, Hirnle CJ. Fundamentals of Nursing: Human Health and Function. Philadelphia, J.B. Lippincott, 1992

Murray R, Zentner JP. Nursing Assessment and Health Promotion Strategies Through the Life Span, Ed 4. Norwalk, CT, Appleton & Lange, 1989

Renner JH (L Vaughn, ed). Healthsmarts: How to Spot the Quacks, Avoid the Nonsense and Get the Facts That Affect Your Health. Kansas City, MO, Health Facts Publishers, 1990

Tenney D. Introduction to Natural Health. Provo, UT, Woodland Health Books, 1992

Key Readings (continued)

Thomas CL (ed). Taber's Cyclopedic Medical Dictionary, Ed 17. Philadelphia, F.A. Davis, 1993

Travis J, Ryan R. Wellness: Small Changes You Can Use to Make a Big Difference. Berkeley, CA, Ten Speed Press, 1991

Enrichment Keys

Fries JF. Take Care of Yourself. Menlo Park, CA, Addison-Wesley, 1990

McIlwain H, et al. The Fifty Plus Wellness Program. New York, John Wiley & Sons, 1990

Schwarz J. The Power of Personal Health. New York, Viking Penguin, 1992

Keys to Learning More

Chapter 7: community's participation in health factors

Chapter 26: importance of good nutrition

Chapter 43: body mechanics

Chapter 45: personal hygiene and skin care

Chapter 63: sexuality

Key Resources

Journal of Nursing Jocularity
5615 W. Cermak Road
Cicero, IL 60650-2290

7 Community Health

Learning Objectives

- Discuss *Healthy People 2000*
- Discuss healthcare on local and state levels
- Identify four federal agencies whose function is to protect the health of the public
- List two types of voluntary health agencies and name a service of each
- Identify the purpose of the American Public Health Association
- State one health-related activity of the United Nations
- List at least four types of pollution, their results, and their prevention
- Discuss the nurse as a member of many communities

Key Terms

bionomics

ecology

Keys to Understanding This Chapter

Chapter 3: today's healthcare system
Chapter 4: legal and ethical applications to healthcare
Chapter 5: basic needs of people
Chapter 6: optimum health for all people

Key Points

- Nurses are members of many communities and should serve as advocates and educators to protect those communities.
- Group action is an effective way to deal with health problems.
- Local, state, and national health efforts are measured against *Healthy People 2000*. Its goals are to increase the span of healthy life, reduce health disparities, and achieve access to preventive services for all Americans.

Key Points (continued)

- Federal agencies include the United States Public Health Service, with its many branches; the Food and Drug Administration; and the Social Security Administration, which supervises Medicare programs.
- Voluntary health agencies may be set up to provide direct service or may provide education and raise funds to combat a particular disease or disorder. The Blood-Borne Pathogen Standard, established by the Occupational Safety and Health Act has made significant impact on nursing procedures and delivery of other services in healthcare facilities.
- Community health is also concerned with the environment, including air pollution, water pollution, land pollution, noise pollution, radiation, and biohazardous waste disposal.

Key Topics Outline

Healthy People 2000
Healthcare on the Local Level
Healthcare on the State Level
Healthcare on the National Level
  Federally Sponsored Government Agencies
  Other National Agencies
  Voluntary Health Agencies
Healthcare Worldwide
The Environment

Key Learning Activities

- Review an issue of the *American Journal of Public Health*. Report to the class regarding current public health issues and describe the problem, locale, and disciplines involved.
- Attend a Board of Health meeting in your area. Identify the primary public health issues or decisions.
- Obtain a copy of *Healthy People 2000* and review it.

Rosdahl CB: Textbook of Basic Nursing, 6th ed. © 1995 J.B. Lippincott Company

As a nurse, you will be a citizen of many communities: your own family unit, the local town or city, the state or province, your nation, and the world. Health problems increase as the population grows, as the nation's economy changes, and as events refocus needs of the population. Thus, comes the requirement to form organizations and agencies to deal with problems and to set up health protection measures. The accompanying box will help you in understanding abbreviations and acronyms in community healthcare.

Healthy People 2000

Healthy People 2000 is a publication released by the United States Department of Health and Human Services (USDHHS) in 1990. All local, state, and national health efforts are measured against it. Its introduction states:

. . . the year 2000 will bring to its conclusion a tumultuous century, characterized by astounding scientific achievements, devastating world wars, and explosive population growth. It will inaugurate at once a new century and a new millennium, a future so vast in its human and historic dimensions that it defies prediction while posing momentous questions about social and economic viability and human vitality. . . .

. . . The beginning of the twenty-first century beckons both with challenge and opportunity for improved health of Americans. We began the current century with a sense of fatalism about the Nation's health problems. As we reach its conclusion, we do so with confidence in our ability to control many of the events that form our health prospects.

. . . New knowledge has brought with it both a keen sense of potential and a keen appreciation of how far most Americans, especially those with low incomes, are from that potential. Moreover, we are already feeling the effects of momentous new issues emerging on the horizon—the aging of our society, the prohibitive costs of many of the technologies developed for diagnosing and treating disease, and the ecologic consequences of industrialization and population growth.[1]

. . . Three overarching goals emerge from the complexity of the health challenge of the 1990s. They permeate the structure and the content of this report. They further define the challenge, especially for health planners, policy makers, and providers:

♦ Increase the span of healthy life for Americans
♦ Reduce health disparities among Americans
♦ Achieve access to preventive services for all Americans[2]

[1] Healthy People 2000: National Health Promotion and Disease Prevention Objectives. U.S. Department of Health and Human Services, Public Health Service. DHHS Publication No. (PHS) 91-50212. U.S. Government Printing Office, Washington, D.C., p. 1, 1991.
[2] Ibid., p. 43.

Key Abbreviations/Acronyms

AMA	American Medical Association
APHA	American Public Health Association
CDC	Centers for Disease Control & Prevention
DEP	Department of Environmental Protection
DOH	Department of Health
EPA	Environmental Protection Agency
FDA	Food and Drug Administration
HRA	Health Resources Administration
HSA	Health Services Administration
NIH	National Institutes of Health
OSHA	Occupational Safety and Health Act
UNICEF	United Nations Children's Fund
USDHHS	United States Department of Health and Human Services
USPHS	United States Public Health Service
VNA	Visiting Nurse Association
WHO	World Health Organization
WIC	Women, Infants, and Children

Healthcare on the Local Level

City, town, or county health departments deal with health protection of persons within their jurisdiction. Usually the Department of Health (DOH) operates under a Board of Health (BOH). Policies and regulations are carried out under the direction of a health officer. State regulations mandate requirements for health officer licensure; public health education is a prerequisite.

A health department provides services dealing with conditions affecting all residents. Its personnel inspect places where food is sold and people who handle food. They check water and milk supplies, housing, and sewage and other waste disposal facilities. They help control air pollution. They may provide school health services and health education, clinics, or hospital and nursing care. Public health nursing services are often provided through city or regional health departments.

Local public health agencies also work to alleviate poor health conditions in that particular community. For example, most large communities have programs to combat lead poisoning and to ensure access to prenatal care or immunization services.

Healthcare on the State Level

State health departments, through their divisions or bureaus, are responsible for health protection within a state. They are concerned with sanitation, food and water inspection, maternal and child health, public health nursing, laboratory services, vital statistics, and protection of the environment. State health laws must conform to federal laws, but states also have the right to make their own health laws, if necessary. For example, the state of Alaska works with the Indian Health Service (IHS) and native corporations to provide healthcare in remote villages. The state health department serves as an advisor or consultant to local health departments and exercises regulatory powers over them. Often, state health departments serve as surveyors for federal health requirements, as well as planners of health requirements for their own jurisdiction.

Healthcare on the National Level

Federally Sponsored Government Agencies

The federal agency concerned with health is the United States Public Health Service (USPHS), one of several agencies under the USDHHS. Some of the other national agencies are the Social Security Administration, Office of Vocational Rehabilitation, Department of Education, and Department of Agriculture.

United States Public Health Service

The USPHS is divided into regions. It has many responsibilities, including investigation and control of all communicable diseases, protection from disease carried by immigrants, control of sanitation and prevention of disease spread in interstate commerce, and control of the manufacture and sale of biologic products. USPHS also cooperates with state health departments in disease control and gives the states some financial assistance. This agency also publishes and distributes health information and collects statistics on various diseases.

The role of the USPHS in health planning is currently focused on achievement of the goals and objectives of the publication *Healthy People 2000*. In addition, President Clinton's healthcare proposals of 1994 are changing healthcare delivery in the United States. USPHS has several agencies. They are listed in the accompanying box. Some of them are discussed later in this chapter.

Food and Drug Administration

This federal agency is responsible for protecting the public from harmful drugs and false claims made about prescription and over-the-counter drugs. It regulates the release of new medications to the public. As the only agency overseeing legal drugs in many states, the FDA also enforces local laws. (Other federal agencies enforce laws relating to illegal drugs.)

The Social Security Administration

The Social Security Administration, also administered by the USDHHS, provides financial assistance for healthcare. Persons over ages 62 or 65 and those of any

Agencies of the USPHS

- ◆ Food and Drug Administration (FDA): regulation of legal drugs
- ◆ Health Services Administration (HSA): direct health services such as National Health Service Corps, Indian Health Service, Office for Migrant Health, and various types of local clinics aimed at diagnosis and treatment of specific diseases (such as sickle cell anemia, plumbism [lead poisoning], hemophilia, and tuberculosis)
- ◆ Health Resources Administration (HRA): comprehensive health planning
- ◆ National Institutes of Health (NIH): research in many separate institutes, exploring areas such as arthritis, cancer, child development, dental and eye disorders, neurologic diseases, stroke, and the important specialty of aging and its related effects
- ◆ Centers for Disease Control and Prevention (CDC): studies of communicable disease spread; development of immunization guidelines; administration of the Occupational Safety and Health Act (OSHA) and OSHA's research institute, the National Institute of Occupational Safety and Health (NIOSH)
- ◆ Alcohol, Drug Abuse, and Mental Health Administration (ADAMHA): supports local alcohol and drug treatment programs and funds research in mental health
- ◆ Maternal Child Health Bureau: assists in consultation with and supervision of state efforts on behalf of infants, children, and women

age with special disabilities or handicaps may receive financial support from this agency, as well as Medicare and Medicaid. Regular Social Security benefits are also available to persons under age 62 as a result of the death, disability, or retirement of a parent or spouse.

Medicare

Medicare is a federal program that provides partial payment for inpatient care and for extended outpatient care or home healthcare. It is discussed in Chapter 3.

Medicaid

Medicaid, in general, is for older adults, the disabled, or families receiving assistance. Medicaid is a public health insurance program that pays for inpatient and outpatient services, home healthcare, and family planning. The federal government pays from one-half to three-quarters of the cost of Medicaid, and the individual state and local units of government pay the rest.

Worker's Compensation

Another program is that of worker's compensation, which provides financial compensation to a worker who has been injured at work or who has contracted a disease that can be directly related to that job. The federal government supervises the program and the employer is required to contribute, based on the hazards of that particular occupation and place of employment.

Occupational Safety and Health Act

In 1972, the federal Occupational Safety and Health Act (OSHA) was passed. This act protects workers and students from job-related injuries and illnesses. The most significant change has been the passage of the Blood-Borne Pathogen Standard (see Chapter 30). Its purpose is to ensure education and protection of all levels of healthcare workers, in all settings, regarding blood-borne pathogens (particularly hepatitis B and human immunodeficiency virus [HIV], which causes acquired immunodeficiency syndrome). The Standard mandates that policies and procedures be developed to this end and encourages immunization of healthcare workers against hepatitis B. (This Standard ultimately serves as a protection to consumers as well.)

Office of Vocational Rehabilitation

This agency offers vocational rehabilitation services to disabled persons in many walks of life. In some instances, people are trained or retrained for employment. Services also include evaluation of vocational skills and aid in job seeking.

Other National Agencies

Federal Agencies

Many other departments of the federal government are involved in health protection. For example, the Department of Agriculture, through its various bureaus, is concerned with control of insect- and animal-borne diseases and with meat and other food inspection, as well as with school lunch programs. (The Department of Agriculture is also the agency that administers the supplemental nutrition program, called *Women, Infants, and Children* [WIC].) The Bureau of Internal Revenue (Alcohol, Tobacco, and Firearms), enforces narcotic laws.

National Safety Council

The National Safety Council and state councils promote safety by analyzing causes of accidents and suggesting ways of prevention. They disseminate information about accident prevention in industry, in the home, and on public highways. Highway and traffic laws protect everyone by requiring inspection of motor vehicles, driving licenses, speed regulation, and highway markings. All states now require seat belts and head rests as standard equipment in new motor vehicles. Building regulations and inspections reduce fire, accident, and health hazards.

American Red Cross

This well known organization, although not a federal agency, provides national services. For example, the local Red Cross chapter works with visiting nurse associations and public health departments to coordinate services during disasters such as floods, hurricanes, earthquakes, tornadoes, or plane and train crashes. The Red Cross also manages blood banks and tissue donation services (to recover skin, bone, heart valves, and other tissues for transplant). Red Cross volunteers often provide first aid coverage for public events, such as parades.

American Medical Association Council on Drugs

The group provides information to physicians about drugs and releases an annual list of new drugs. The Council has established a central registry in Chicago to provide up-to-date information about unfavorable effects of drugs or chemicals. (It is estimated that approximately one million people suffer every year from adverse effects of physician-prescribed drugs.)

American Public Health Association

This association was founded in 1872. Its purpose is to protect and promote personal and environmental health. It does this by providing leadership in development and dissemination of health policies. It represents all disciplines and specialties within public health and is the largest public health association in the world.

Voluntary Health Agencies

Voluntary health agencies include those that provide direct service and those national organizations that provide education and conduct fund-raising. Voluntary organizations have a great impact because of their appeal to public sentiment and large citizen participation.

Direct Service Agencies

Visiting Nurse Association. An example of a direct service agency is the Visiting Nurse Association (VNA). Throughout the country, VNAs provide both in-home and community-based healthcare services. Services are funded by third-party payors (public or private), grants, and fund-raised dollars. Health services may be provided in the person's own home or in a senior residence, board-and-care home, or homeless shelter. Services may be therapeutic or preventive in nature. For example, a VNA may conduct tuberculin screening (Fig. 7-1), immunization clinics for communicable diseases, or education programs about sexually transmitted diseases. VNAs collaborate with other health and social service agencies throughout the communities, setting up health linkages and networks.

Lillian Wald is recognized as the founder of public health nursing in the United States. She organized the

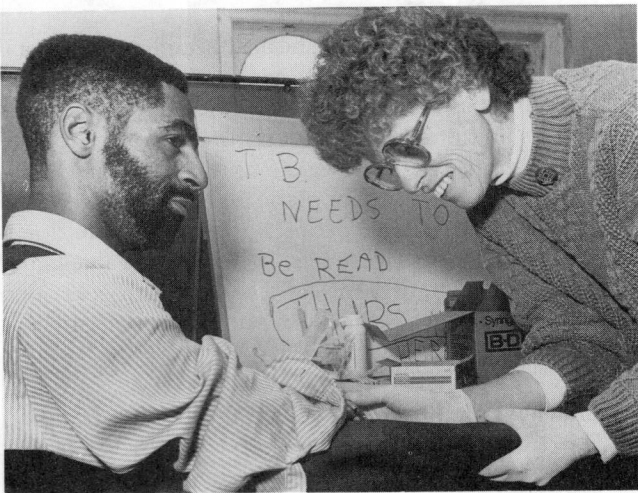

Figure 7-1. Tuberculin testing being done by a public health nurse at a local soup kitchen. This is part of an outreach program to prevent the spread of communicable diseases. (Photo courtesy of MCOSS Inc., Red Bank, NJ, Home News photo)

Henry Street Settlement, otherwise known as the Visiting Nurse Society (VNS) of New York City in 1893. Today's system of public health nursing evolved from this organization.

Organizations Related to Specific Disorders

These organizations often sponsor activities or conduct fund drives to raise money for treatment or research relating to their particular interest. They may also receive some funding from campaigns such as the United Way. Many organizations publish pamphlets or books to educate the public. Examples of such agencies are the American Cancer Society, the National Society for Prevention of Blindness, the American Heart Association, the Cystic Fibrosis Foundation, the National Easter Seal Society, the March of Dimes, and the Children's Defense Fund. These national voluntary agencies often have state or regional level affiliates.

Organizations Promoting Specific Health Goals

Some voluntary health agencies are concerned not with disease but with the promotion of one aspect of healthful living. For example, Planned Parenthood of America focuses on family planning and prevention of sexually transmitted diseases. Their counselors, physicians, and nurses assist people by genetic counseling, abortion counseling, infertility examination and counseling, and birth control and may provide prenatal care. Another such organization, La Leche League, advances the health of mothers and very young babies by encouraging breast-feeding.

Healthcare Worldwide

Health promotion is a worldwide concern, as evidenced by activities of certain international agencies created by the United Nations.

The World Health Organization (WHO), under the auspices of the United Nations, has conducted a great deal of research to reduce poverty, famine, and disease throughout the world.

The *United Nations Children's Fund (UNICEF),* another program sponsored by the United Nations, helps children, especially those in developing countries. Some of its accomplishments include nutrition instruction, development of low-cost food supplements, support of general education, childhood immunization programs, and infant rehydration programs.

The United Nations also tailors specific programs to meet a country's special needs, such as those that arise from a natural disaster. After events such as earthquakes or volcanic eruptions, a country may need assistance to prevent starvation and widespread disease.

The Environment

Humankind is but one part of a complex system of life, dependent on the balance of life, growth, and death of all living organisms on the planet. This growing recognition has awakened many concerned citizens to the need to preserve this balance. The study of mutual relationships between living beings and their environment is called **ecology** or **bionomics**. The federal Environmental Protection Agency (EPA) has been set up in an attempt to control problems relating to the environment and its ecology.

The task of preserving the ecologic balance, so we will have air to breathe, water to drink, and food to eat, is complicated. Technology has proven to be both a blessing and a curse. New sources of energy that will not pollute the air, land, or water are being sought. The nurse, as a member of the health team, will be called on to know about and work for the kind of study and action that contribute to a healthy environment.

Air Pollution

Air pollution is greatest in industrial areas, but every community has some air pollution problems, even though it may have comparatively few industries. Pollution also tends to drift from cities to nearby countryside. For instance, Philadelphia's air pollution drifts over New Jersey.

A great source of air pollution is exhaust from automobiles. The smog situation in Los Angeles, for example, is a result of the combined action of atmospheric conditions and specific geography with fog, smoke, and automobile exhaust gases. These materials combine to produce harmful substances that cannot be blown away because of the mountain range east of the city. This has happened in many major cities of the world surrounded by mountains.

Air pollution is responsible for increases in respiratory infections such as chronic bronchitis, asthma, and emphysema. Heavy pollution will cause irritation of the eyes, nose, and throat and may have other serious health effects not yet known. Polluted air damages plant life, including farm crops, and is destructive to building materials.

We are becoming more concerned with pollution inside buildings, as well. Persons who work in certain industrial environments must wear protective gear to prevent lung disorders.

Smoking and Air Pollution. Studies have shown that the risks of some disorders are almost as great, if not greater, for the person who is inhaling "second-hand smoke" as for the person who is actually smoking. Many companies, hospitals, schools, and even cities have become "smoke free."

Smoking is not allowed on commercial airline flights within the United States. Schools and hospitals often declare their buildings and grounds totally nonsmoking premises. Most restaurants have nonsmoking areas; hotels have nonsmoking rooms. This is an area of health importance for all people and particularly for families with infants and small children.

Water Pollution

Water pollution is a serious and increasing health hazard. A number of diseases are transmitted by contaminated water; noted examples include typhoid fever, dysentery, and infectious hepatitis. Water pollution not only affects people but also is a menace to recreation areas, wildlife, and fish. Millions of fish and shellfish are killed in the United States each year by polluted water. Increasing demands on the national water supply make it necessary to reuse water, thereby requiring that waste water be treated to make it safe for reuse. In many areas, this treatment is inadequate. Substances found in water also create health hazards. One example is lead. Lead in drinking water contributes to lead poisoning in children.

The federal government has responsibility for ensuring a safe water supply for its people. Until recently, the national government had little or no authority to do this; it was left to state and local governments. Legislation now gives the USPHS authority and funds to establish water treatment projects. The federal government has also enacted legislation establishing sanitary sewer districts around many lakes and along rivers. In this way, the quality of public waters will be maintained and improved.

Land Pollution

As the population grows, more garbage and trash is produced. Large cities are running out of places to dump their trash. People do not want dumps or incinerators in their neighborhoods. After shipping barges of trash and garbage to smaller nations or dumping in the ocean, the United States has become aware of its worldwide responsibilities. We cannot continue to pollute other people's lands or our large natural resource, the ocean, with our trash. As a result, many communities have developed recycling programs.

Noise Pollution

Many people are becoming aware of damage caused to hearing by extremely loud noises. Noise pollution also causes stress. Laws are in place that regulate noise. Workers in occupations that are very noisy are required by OSHA to wear ear protection.

Radiation

Citizens are concerned about radiation. Many disputes between the public and power companies using nuclear fuel have not been resolved. One problem is disposal of radioactive wastes. Accidents in the 1980s at Three Mile Island in Pennsylvania and Chernobyl in the Soviet Union raise the question of safety around the world.

Biohazardous Wastes

Proper and safe disposal of medical wastes is the responsibility of every institutional and individual healthcare provider. Policies and procedures dictate the process by which disposal occurs. This process must meet the multiple-standard regulations of OSHA, Department of Environmental Protection (DEP), and local and state health departments.

Other Types of Pollution

Other situations occur in the world that contribute to pollution and endanger the environment. An oil spill can kill many fish and animals and, thus, limit or contaminate food supplies. Insecticides and agricultural chemicals pose a threat to water and clean air. Substances may be brought home on work clothing, thereby endangering the health of family members. Asbestos particles on clothing contribute to chronic obstructive lung disease in spouses of workers, in addition to the cancer that affects the workers themselves.

> **Key Concept**
>
> You are part of the world community. All of us must participate in protecting the world in which we live. You, as a nurse, can teach others to protect the environment also.

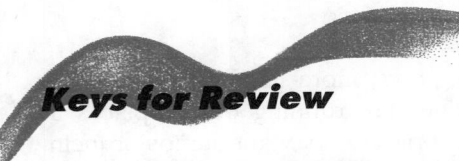

Keys for Review

Key Questions for Critical Thinking

1. Describe *Healthy People 2000*. Can you see evidence of its effect in your community?
2. Explain the acronym OSHA and its activities.
3. Describe services provided by the American Red Cross.
4. Describe pollution. What types of pollution are there? Which types are a problem in your local or state community?
5. Describe your responsibility as a nurse and a member of the worldwide community.

Key Readings

Abrahamson, L. Healing our Health Care System. New York, Grove Weidenfield, 1990

Healthy People 2000: National Health Promotion and Disease Prevention Objectives. U.S. Department of Health and Human Services, Public Health Service. DHHS Publication No. (PHS) 91-50212. U.S. Government Printing Office, Washington, D.C., 1991

Raffel MW, Raffel NK. The U.S. Health System: Origins and Functions, Ed 3. New York, John Wiley & Sons, 1989

Seinford P, Webster J. Promoting Wellness: A Nurse's Handbook. Rockville, MD, Aspen, 1988

Spradley BW. Readings in Community Health Nursing, Ed 4. Philadelphia, J.B. Lippincott, 1991

Keys to Learning More

Chapter 8: microbiology, the basis for the study of disease spread and infection control

Keys to Learning More *(continued)*

The remainder of this book studies health as it applies to individuals and groups.

Chapter 89: home care nursing

Key Resources

Administration on Aging
Department of Health and Human Services
330 Independence Avenue, SW
Washington, DC 20201
202-619-0724

American Public Health Association
1015 15th Street, NW
Washington, DC 20005
202-789-5600

American Red Cross
431 18th Street, NW
Washington, DC 20005
202-737-8300

Centers for Disease Control and Prevention
Department of Health and Human Services
U.S. Public Health Service
1600 Clifton Road, NE
Atlanta, GA 30333
404-639-3311

March of Dimes Birth Defects Foundation
1275 Marmaroneck Avenue
White Plains, NY 10605
914-428-7100

National Safety Council
1121 Spring Lake Drive
Itasca, IL 60143
708-285-1121

8 Introduction to Microbiology

Keys for Learning

Learning Objectives

- List at least three people who were important to the historical development of microbiology and describe their accomplishments
- Name and describe the essential factors that influence microbial growth
- Identify the means of studying microorganisms
- Describe the basic characteristics of the five main groups of microorganisms
- Describe the way in which bacteria are classified
- Describe three basic ways in which microorganisms are transmitted to people
- Describe the cycle of infectious disease and suggest ways in which the spread of disease could be stopped at each point in the cycle
- Define toxins and describe their effect on the body
- List and describe the four factors that determine if a pathogen will cause disease in a person
- Describe three lines of defense against infectious disease

Key Terms

antibodies	immunity	pathogenic
antigens	interferon	phagocytosis
communicable	microorganisms	sterile
contagious	mycosis	suppurative
endotoxins	nosocomial infection	toxins
epidemic	opportunistic	virulence
exotoxins	parasites	

Keys to Understanding This Chapter

Chapter 5: basic needs of all people
Chapter 6: health and health promotion
Chapter 7: health and health promotion for the community

Key Points

- Some microorganisms can cause disease in human beings, whereas others are beneficial in nature.
- All microorganisms, except viruses, engage in the same life functions as do other plant and animal cells, and their reproduction and infection of people depend on having the right set of conditions in the environment.
- Microorganisms are classified by their physical and biologic characteristics into a number of basic groups, each with distinguishing means of reproducing and, if they are pathogens, of infecting people.
- Viruses cause disease by taking over the host cell metabolism and genetic material and reproducing in extremely large numbers.
- Most common microbial diseases are communicable and are spread within the population by direct contact; contaminated air, water, or food; or by other animals.
- The chain of infection can be broken by healthcare professionals who practice antiseptic techniques and body substance precautions.
- The human body possesses many natural defenses against infection, including the skin and mucous membranes, cilia, normal secretions, fever, interferon, phagocytosis, and inflammation.
- Immunity is the body's response to the invasion of a specific pathogen; antibodies are produced to destroy the disease-causing microorganism.
- Immunity can be acquired artificially by vaccination with vaccines of dead or weakened microorganism.

Key Learning Activities

◆ Visit a microbiology laboratory and observe and describe three methods used to grow and culture microorganisms that are frequently used to classify pathogens.
◆ Using a microscope and a sample of pond water, observe common protozoa and draw your results.
◆ Prepare a sample of fungi by exposing a piece of bread to the air or dust, allowing it to generate mold. Observe the results using a microscope.

Every day, we hear and read about modern society being affected by diseases caused by **microorganisms** (minute living cells not visible to the naked eye). For example, we hear about people dying from acquired immunodeficiency syndrome (AIDS) caused by a virus called human immunodeficiency virus (HIV). Lyme disease, a disorder that is increasing in various parts of the United States and Canada, is caused by bacteria carried by tiny ticks.

Microorganisms are found almost everywhere in the environment. Although most microorganisms are important to life on earth, some microorganisms are **pathogenic** (they cause disease).

Microorganisms are so small, a magnifying device must be used to view them. Microbiology is the scientific study of organisms too small to be seen without the aid of a microscope. This chapter explores scientific discoveries related to microorganisms, types of microorganisms, how they were discovered and are now studied, and the types of diseases some of them produce. We will also learn about the spread of microbial diseases and the ways the body defends itself against microorganisms.

Historical Overview

Some of the major contributors to the field of microbiology are listed in Table 8-1. Little more than a century ago people had no real understanding of the relationship between disease and microorganisms. Why did food spoil and other matter decay? Why did wounds become inflamed? Why did pus appear? Why and how did disease spread, sometimes across continents?

Invention of the Microscope

A dramatic change in the understanding of living things occurred in 1655, when the English inventor, *Robert Hooke* (1605–1703) used a simple magnifying lens to discover that all living creatures consisted of cells. Although all future studies of microorganisms depended on this concept, Hooke's techniques did not detect microorganisms.

Anton van Leeuwenhoek (1632–1723), a Dutch businessman and scientist, developed the first single-lens microscope. With this device, van Leeuwenhoek observed many live microscopic organisms. He excitedly wrote the Royal Society of London of his "discoveries of animalicules," or little animals. He described and drew pictures of various types of bacteria, as well as of other microorganisms such as amoebae and other protozoa.

Early microscopes were crude and inadequate. During the early 1800s, the compound microscope (containing several lenses) was developed, and microbiology became a new field of study. Modern science has the powerful electron microscope, which uses an electron beam instead of visible light and provides a greatly enlarged image of extremely small objects.

Table 8-1. Early Contributors to the Field of Microbiology

Year or Period	Person	Contributions
1665	Hooke (1605–1703)	Discovered cells, using magnifying lens
1667	Van Leeuwenhoek (1632–1723)	"Father of Microbiology"
		Further developed magnifying lenses
		Described bacteria and protozoa
1796	Jenner (1749–1832)	Used cowpox vaccine to protect against smallpox (vaccination)
Mid-1800s	Pasteur (1822–1895)	"Father of Immunology"
		Stated: Life must arise from preexisting life
		Developed: sterilization and pasteurization
		• Germ theory of fermentation
		• Germ theory of disease
		• Vaccines
	Semmelweiss (1818–1865)	Promoted cleansing of hands between patients
Late-1800s	Lister (1827–1912)	Used antiseptics on dressings and in surgery
1876	Koch (1843–1920)	Culture research
		Germ Theory of Disease (Koch's Postulates)
		• Causative agent must be present in every case of disease
		• Pathogen must be isolated from host and grown in sterile environment
		• Same disease must be produced when culture is inoculated into a healthy, susceptible animal
		• Same pathogen must be recoverable again from the infected animals
1928–1929	Fleming (1881–1955)	Discovered penicillin
		Won Nobel Prize in 1945

The Concept of Biogenesis

People who lived before the mid-19th century believed that some living things created themselves or were produced from nonliving matter. Scientists of that age called this popular theory *spontaneous generation* and thought that flies could originate from putrefying food and animal manure and that lice came from dirty clothes and bed covers.

Opponents of spontaneous generation developed the theory of *biogenesis,* which stated that living cells can come only from other living cells. One of the outstanding scientists in the early days of microbiology was *Louis Pasteur* (1822–1895). In 1861, he proved that the theory of biogenesis was correct by demonstrating that spoilage of food and drink was caused by microorganisms present in air.

Pasteur also showed that microorganisms could be found in fluids and on the surfaces of objects and that these organisms could be killed by heat. Today, special healthcare procedures (*aseptic techniques*) based on Pasteur's work are used to prevent microbial contamination. His experiments also led to the process of pasteurization in which rapid heating of liquids, like milk, kills disease-causing bacteria.

Theory of Disease and Immunology

Prior to the work of Pasteur, many people believed that human disease was caused by evil spirits entering the body as punishment for sin. The efforts of Pasteur and other scientists of the 19th century gradually provided evidence for the *germ theory of disease*, which stated that microorganisms cause illness in all living things.

Pasteur's studies and the germ theory also influenced early medical procedures. It had been common practice for obstetricians to treat successive patients without effectively disinfecting their hands, thereby transmitting deadly disease from one mother to another. It occurred to *Joseph Lister* (1827–1912), an English surgeon, to use antiseptic-soaked dressings to kill the disease-causing microorganisms. His techniques significantly reduced wound infections. Another pioneer in this area was *Ignaz Semmelweiss* (1818-1865), a Hungarian physician. He initiated procedures to prevent disease transmission, including the use of chlorinated lime for cleansing hands. (The beliefs of these pioneer physicians were not always well accepted by other physicians of the time.)

Robert Koch (1843–1920), a German physician, was the first person to conclusively show that a bacterium caused disease. He developed a method for obtaining pure growths of bacteria (*cultures*). Using his techniques of cultures, Koch discovered that *Bacillus anthracis* bacteria found in the blood of cattle was the cause of the lethal anthrax disease. He also discovered that the tubercle bacillus causes tuberculosis.

The branch of medicine that studies immunity to disease (immunology) also owes its start to Pasteur. In the late 1700s, *Edward Jenner* (1749–1832), a doctor in England, learned that dairy maids who contracted cowpox were free from the risk of the lethal and epidemic disease of smallpox. In 1796, cowpox broke out at a farm near Jenner's home and a dairy maid was infected with the disease from her employer's cows. Jenner inoculated a healthy 8-year-old boy with some of the material from sores on the dairy maid's hand. After several days, the smallpox sores on the boys hand healed. To prove that the boy was protected against smallpox, Jenner later infected him several times with matter from a smallpox patient, but no symptoms of the disease occurred. The cowpox microorganism induced *immunity* in the patient. This means of protection from a disease is called *vaccination*, from the Latin word *vacca*, meaning cow. Pasteur later found that the smallpox-related cowpox microorganism was a less *virulent* form of the virus which causes smallpox. (Virulent means powerful or strongly pathogenic.)

Modern Microbiology

Key advances in microbiology in the identification and control of microorganisms and in the prevention and elimination of disease have occurred during the past century because of the work of pioneer microbiologists. Medical researchers and physicians are now able to look for and find the cause of disease, treat sources rather than symptoms, cure rather than simply relieve symptoms, and prevent such diseases as poliomyelitis and measles by immunization.

It is now often possible to prepare a culture of an organism, identify it, and then determine what drugs will kill it. The Scottish physician, *Sir Alexander Fleming* (1881–1955), discovered the first antibiotic in 1928. He found that a mold called *Penicillium notatum* limited the growth of bacteria and called the active ingredient produced by the mold penicillin.

Early microbiologists suspected that much smaller microorganisms than bacteria existed. Because these organisms possessed the unique capability of passing through the sheerest laboratory filters, they were named filterable viruses (after the Latin, *virus,* meaning poison). Not only were viruses invisible even under the compound light microscope, but also they could not be cultured by common means. Eventually, techniques were developed to permit these parasitic microorganisms to be grown in cultures of living tissues with chick embryos. With the invention of the *electron microscope*, viruses were visualized. This device enables scientists to see objects as small as 5 angstroms (Å), or 1/250 millionth of an inch.

An understanding of the methods of transmission of disease has given us the modern technology for preventing disease in conjunction with teaching sound personal, family, and community health practices to individuals. Healthcare personnel must have a basic comprehension of organisms that cause disease, their effects on the body, how they are transmitted, and how they can be controlled. Two important procedures in the prevention of disease spread are proper handwashing and universal precautions.

Much of nursing is concerned with caring for patients who have infectious or communicable diseases and with preventing the spread of disease. A patient in the hospital for treatment of one condition may actually contract another disease during the stay. Such hospital-acquired infection is known as **nosocomial infection** (see Chapter 30).

Facts About Microorganisms

Characteristics of Microorganisms

Despite their small size, the cell structures of many microorganisms are similar to the cell structures of larger organisms. Some microorganisms are identical in many ways to the cells of animals and plants. Bacteria are simpler and lack certain structures, such as membranes surrounding the genetic material or other organelles inside the bacteria. All these types of microorganisms carry on essential vital functions characteristic of living things: metabolism, growth, reproduction, irritability, motion, and protection. (Viruses do not have all of these characteristics.)

Many living organisms (eg, human beings) take in oxygen, use it to burn food for energy and growth, and then excrete wastes in a process called metabolism. (Chapters 14 and 17 describe metabolism more fully.) Many microorganisms also have this ability, and they can also increase in size, divide, and produce new members of their species. They react in various ways to changes in their environment, showing irritability or response to stimuli or changing conditions. Many microorganisms are able to move under their own power, as do animals. Some microorganisms safeguard themselves by forming protective capsules, or *spores*.

Pathogens and Nonpathogens

All human beings contain microorganisms in and on their bodies. These microorganisms most often are nonpathogenic. Often they are essential for life. For example, microorganisms are always present in the digestive system (microbiota or normal flora of the intestine) and some perform important digestive functions. Under usual circumstances, these microorganisms do not produce disease. They can do so, however, if they gain access to the bloodstream or various tissues of the body.

Thousands of species of nonpathogenic microorganisms exist in nature, and many are beneficial to people. Bread is raised or leavened by the action of the gas-generating yeast cells within it. Sharp, pungent cheeses owe their flavor to molds. Decomposition of animal and plant wastes depends on microorganisms and accounts for the fertile nature of soil.

On the other hand, microorganisms can cause disease. Such microorganisms are known as **pathogens**. Despite the many defenses individuals have against infection, some microorganisms can gain access to body systems. They have the potential for affecting health. **Opportunistic** organisms are those that usually do not cause disease, but can if the person is susceptible at that time (ie, has a compromised immune system). These otherwise nonpathogenic microorganisms become pathogenic to that person. The control of microorganisms is important in the techniques of healthcare workers. *Pathology* is the study of the cause and nature of disease and how it affects the body.

Key Concept

Diseases and disorders are caused by a relatively small percentage of microorganisms. Most microorganisms are helpful.

The Growth of Microorganisms

Microorganisms are said to *grow* when the number of individual microorganisms at a site increases. A group of bacterial cells at the beginning of an infection may consist of only a few hundred cells. As the bacteria reproduce, they form groups of many millions of individual cells, collectively called *colonies*. Certain factors in the environment promote or limit the growth of microorganisms. These include oxygen and nutrients, temperature, moisture, light, and proper pH.

Most microorganisms require oxygen for growth. Some microorganisms, called *obligate anaerobes*, cannot survive in the presence of oxygen. Most microorganisms require oxygen to live (*obligate aerobes*). Some microorganisms can live in either the presence or absence of oxygen (*facultative anaerobes*).

One of the key ingredients needed for microbial growth is the presence of organic, or carbon-containing, nutrients. Microorganisms also require other chemical elements, such as nitrogen for the manufacture of protein and sulfur for the synthesis of protein and vitamins. Some microorganisms can make their own food from raw materials, such as from carbon dioxide. Others must find their nutrition ready-made. **Parasites** are organisms that live on or within another living organism (the host). *Saprophytes* live off the organic remains of dead plants or animals.

The temperature at which a specific microorganism grows best is its *optimal temperature*. Most microorganisms with which we are concerned grow best at temperatures ranging from that of a cool room to slightly above normal body temperature. Pathogenic microorganisms flourish at normal body temperature. Cold temperatures often significantly slow the growth of microorganisms, which is why refrigeration is used to control bacterial growth in food. Some types of microorganisms prefer either extreme cold or hot environments.

All microorganisms require *water* or *moisture* to grow. The matter in or on which they grow must contain available moisture (such as jellies) or may be a liquid (such as milk or blood). The pH (acidity or alkalinity) also affects the growth of microorganisms. Generally, they survive well only when the pH is neither too acid nor too alkaline (pH is discussed in Chapter 16).

Green plants and some microorganisms need *light* for growth. Other microorganisms, however, grow well in darkness. Many microorganisms die when they are exposed to the sun's ultraviolet light rays, although moderately diffuse light does not affect them.

Key Concept

Microbial growth is influenced by oxygen, nutrients, temperature, moisture, light, and pH.

The Study of Microorganisms

Medical microbiologists can grow most microorganisms under controlled conditions in the laboratory. Studying microbial development assists them in devising methods to prevent microbial growth. (Antiseptics and disinfectants are chemicals that kill microorganisms; they are discussed in Chapter 30.). Common terms used in microbiology are shown in the accompanying box.

Cultures

A growth of microorganisms prepared for laboratory study is called a *culture*. Cultures are usually grown in test tubes or on small, flat, covered plastic plates called *Petri dishes*. The material in or on which the microorganisms are placed is the *culture medium*. Various types of culture media are used for different purposes. Solid media contain *agar*, which is obtained from a form of seaweed. Liquid media are called *nutrient broths*. All culture media contain specific nutrients designed to promote the growth of one or more types of microorganisms. Media must start out **sterile** (free from microbial contamination) for a valid study.

To see and study the individual characteristics of microorganisms grown in cultures, a small amount of the material to be examined is placed on a clean oblong piece of glass called a slide. The slide is prepared in a particular way, depending on the microorganism to be observed. The microorganisms can be viewed in their living, moving state in a drop of liquid culture placed on a slide.

Staining

Often, microorganisms are stained with a drop of dye to more easily see their features. Among the most common ways to stain microorganisms is the *Gram stain*. The Gram stain uses a series of dyes (described later). The ability to retain the different dye colors identifies the bacteria as gram-positive or gram-negative. This is a key distinguishing feature of microorganisms, and this characteristic is widely used to classify different species.

Another common characteristic for distinguishing bacteria is whether or not the microorganism is decolorized by an acid–alcohol mixture after staining with a red dye. *Acid-fast* microorganisms are not easily decolorized.

Types of Microorganisms

Microorganisms, like all living creatures, are categorized, based on a variety of physical and biologic characteristics. Each organism has a name consisting of two parts. The *genus* refers to a more general grouping and is listed first; the *species* defines a biologically unique category and is the second name. For example, the

Key Terms Common to Microbiology

Sterilization	Destruction of all microorganisms and spores
Clean technique	Technique in which many microorganisms are removed by washing ("medical asepsis")
Aseptic	Absence of infectious microorganisms on living tissue
Antiseptic	Inhibition of growth of microorganisms without destroying them
Disinfectant	Substance that removes infectious microbes from inanimate objects
Microbicide	Destructive to microbes
Germicide	Destructive to pathogens
Bactericide	Destructive to bacteria
Fungicide	Destructive to fungi
Virucide	Destructive to viruses
Microbistatic	Inhibition of metabolism and reproduction of bacteria
Sterile	Free of microorganisms ("surgical asepsis")
Universal body substance precautions	Specific procedures followed by health care personnel, designed to prevent the spread of disease (see inside cover of book)

common bacterium, *Escherichia coli*, is found in the colon. Microorganisms fall into a number of large groups: algae; fungi; protozoa; bacteria; and viruses.

Algae

Algae, of which there are many kinds, resemble plant cells. They produce their nutrients through *photosynthesis*, a process whereby they obtain energy from light. Algae are often found on sunlit water, appearing as green scum or green cloudy water. They are an important part of the environmental food chain. Algae rarely cause human disease.

Fungi

Fungi of concern in human medicine include the single-celled yeasts and the multicellular molds (Fig. 8-1). An infection caused by a fungus is called a **mycosis**. A type of ringworm, *tinea capitis*, is a lesion of the scalp often found in children. Another form of ringworm is *tinea pedis*, also known as athlete's foot. (Both are *fungal* infections.)

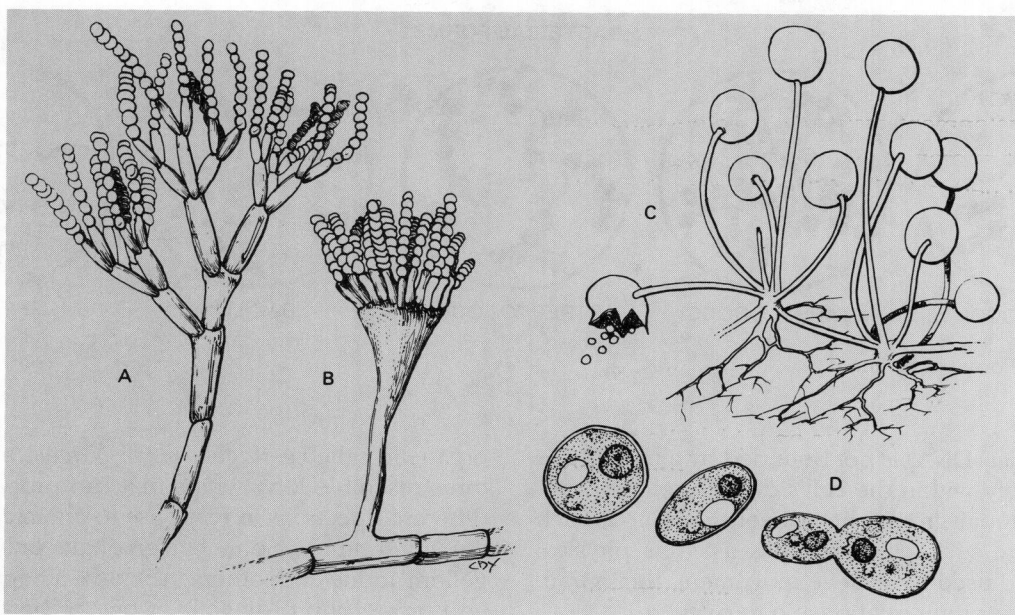

Figure 8-1. Typical fungi. **(A)** *Penicillium* mold, blue-green spores arranged like a brush. **(B)** *Aspergillus,* blue-green with yellow areas. **(C)** *Rhizopus,* white to dark gray with rootlike rhizoids. **(D)** *Saccharomyces* cerevisiae, a yeast. (From Burton GRW. Microbiology for the Health Sciences, Ed. 4. Philadelphia, J.B. Lippincott, 1992)

Yeasts

Yeast cells reproduce by a process called *budding.* Each parent yeast cell produces a "daughter cell" or bud that eventually breaks off and grows in the same manner as the parent cell. Yeasts require sugars in solution as their food. When yeasts metabolize sugars in the absence of oxygen, a chemical change called *fermentation* occurs, which produces alcohol and carbon dioxide. Many industries use controlled fermentation in manufacturing their products.

An example of a pathogenic yeast is *Candida albicans*, which can cause the disease known as thrush. Thrush produces a white growth in the mouth and on the tongue. *C. albicans* also causes approximately a third of the cases of vaginitis, an inflammation of the vagina.

Molds

Multicellular molds are common in our environment. Some familiar molds are seen as fuzzy patches on jelly and fruits, the greenish growth on spoiled breads, and the blue veins seen in some cheeses. Many molds grow best at room or refrigerator temperature and have a characteristic musty smell. They send threads or branches called *hyphae* throughout the material on or in which they are growing. Some hyphae extend beyond the surface of the host material and, when mature, produce at their tips rounded capsules containing *spores.* The spores give the molds their characteristic colors. The spores are wafted about by the slightest cur-

rents of air. When they find a suitable surface, they attach themselves and reproduce another colony.

Protozoa

Protozoa are single-celled microorganisms that can be seen with the ordinary laboratory microscope. The more common protozoa include the amoeba and paramecium. They are able to take in food and excrete wastes. They may reproduce sexually and generally live in a moisture-rich environment. Some protozoa capture and engulf their food and may even feed on bacteria.

Although most protozoa are not pathogenic, there are some notable exceptions. Amoebic dysentery is caused by *Entamoeba histolytica*, which forms ulcers in the colon and attacks red blood cells. This amoeba produces a capsule (cyst) to protect itself. It then infects people through fecal contact in contaminated food or water. Malaria is caused by a protozoa known as *Plasmodium malariae*. It reproduces in the *Anopheles* mosquito and its transmitted to people through the insect's bite. *Trichomonas vaginalis* causes vaginal infection in women and urinary tract infection in men. It is often transmitted by sexual intercourse from an infected individual to an uninfected partner.

Bacteria

The study of bacteria is called *bacteriology.* Bacteria are part of a group of single-celled organisms that are unique in that they do not have a true nucleus. Their

BACTERIAL FORMS

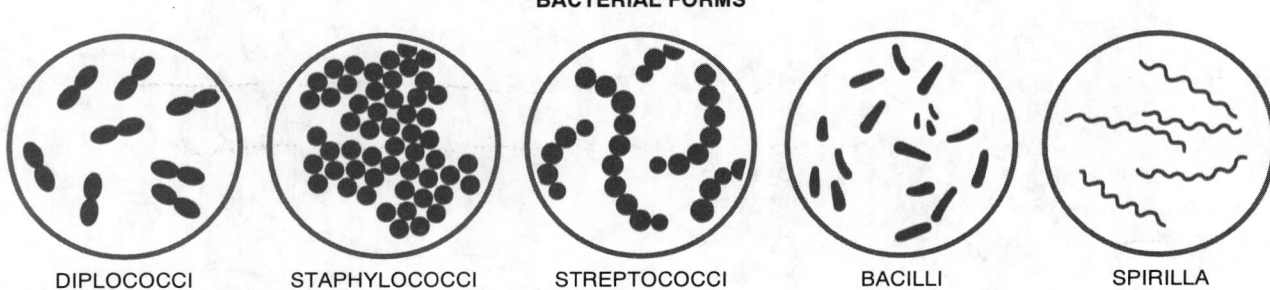

DIPLOCOCCI STAPHYLOCOCCI STREPTOCOCCI BACILLI SPIRILLA

Figure 8-2. Forms of bacteria.

genetic material (DNA) is not bounded by a membrane and floats freely within the cell's cytoplasm. Many varieties of bacterial groups have been identified, each categorized by such characteristics as their physical shape, method used to achieve movement, their Gram stain reaction, or their relationship to oxygen.

Classification of Bacteria

Classification by Shape. Most bacteria fall into one of three categories based on their shape, as illustrated in Figure 8-2 (see also Table 8-2 later in this section). A round or spherical bacterium is called a *coccus* (pl. *cocci*). A rod-shaped bacterium is known as a *bacillus* (pl. *bacilli*). A spiral-shaped bacterium has the name *spirillum* (pl. *spirilla*) or *spirochete*. The cells of cocci do not always separate when they reproduce. Sometimes they form pairs (*diplococci*), clusters (*staphylococci*), or chains (*streptococci*). Likewise, *diplobacilli* are paired bacilli and *streptobacilli* are chains of bacilli. Bacilli may have tapered ends (*fusiform* bacilli) or they may be shaped like long threads (*filamentous* bacilli).

Classification by Motility. Some bacteria are capable of locomotion. Movement is possible because of a cellular organelle called a *flagellum* (pl. *flagella*). These structures resemble long whips that can propel bacteria in different directions in response to chemical changes in the environment. Some bacteria have only a single flagellum at one end, others may have a flagellum at each end or a group of flagella at one or both ends, while still other species may have flagella distributed over the entire organism (Fig. 8-3).

Classification by Gram Stain. One of the chief tools a microbiologist has to identify different species of bacteria is the *differential stain* in which dyes react differently depending on the specific type of bacteria tested. Perhaps the most common differential stain is the Gram stain. As a result of Gram stains, bacteria may be classified as either *gram-positive* or *gram-negative* (see Table 8-2).

The first step in Gram staining involves staining all cells purple. The bacterial sample on a glass slide is next washed with alcohol to selectively decolorize the cells. Gram-positive bacteria have thick cell walls and do not lose their purple color. However, gram-negative bacteria lose their purple color. They would be difficult

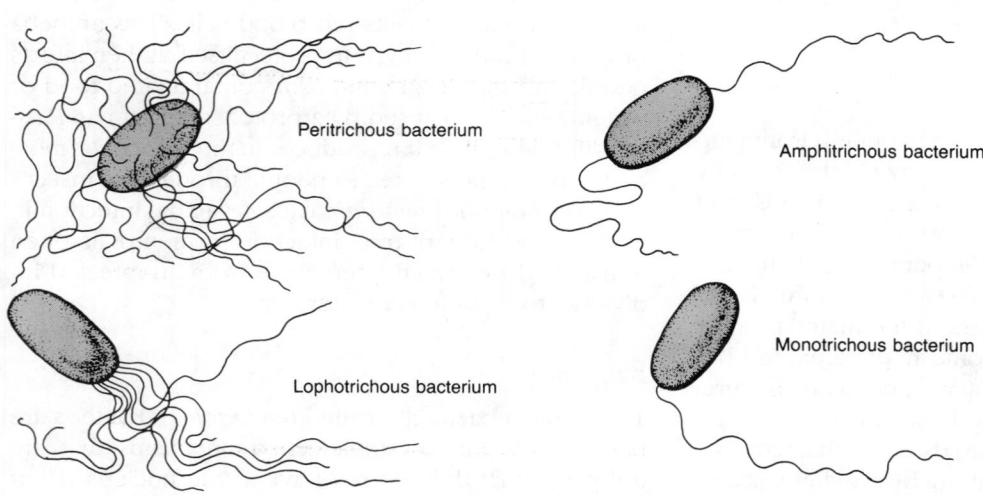

Peritrichous bacterium

Amphitrichous bacterium

Lophotrichous bacterium

Monotrichous bacterium

Figure 8-3. The four basic types of flagellation on bacteria: peritrichous, flagella all over surface; lophotrichous, a tuft of flagella; amphitrichous, flagella at each end; and monotrichous, one flagellum. (From Burton GRW. Microbiology for the Health Sciences, Ed 4. Philadelphia, J.B. Lippincott, 1992)

to see if another stain were not used. A counterstain turns gram-negative bacteria pink to red.

Classification by Relationship to Oxygen. Bacteria can be grouped according to the ways in which they use or react to oxygen. For example, some bacilli are obligate aerobes, others are obligate anaerobes, and still others are facultative anaerobes. Some bacilli are further divided into those that use oxygen to metabolize sugars (*oxidizers*) and those that metabolize sugars in the absence of oxygen (*fermenters*).

Key Concept

Bacteria may be classified by shape, by motility, by Gram stain, or by their relationship to oxygen.

Reproduction and Survival

A bacterium simply grows or increases in numbers by duplicating its genetic material and then splitting in two across the middle, sharing the DNA equally between the two new cells (binary fission).

Spores produced by molds in the fungi group are reproductive. Spores related to certain bacteria are for their protection. *Clostridium tetani* and *B. anthracis* are examples of spore formers. When conditions are unfavorable for their growth, these bacilli develop a protective covering (spore) and go into a nonactive (dormant) phase. The spore is resistant to the environment and can survive extreme conditions of light, drying, boiling, and many chemicals. When more favorable conditions return, the spore will germinate and the bacteria cell will become active again.

Spore-forming pathogens are the most difficult to control and destroy because of their added protection. All pathogenic bacteria are killed at the boiling point of water, which is 100°C (212°F), *except* the spore formers. Many items used in healthcare must be *sterile*. Because the lowest lethal temperature for pathogens varies widely, all healthcare providers can use an *autoclave* to ensure that equipment and other items are free from microorganisms. This device uses steam under pressure to raise the temperature above the boiling point of water, thus destroying spores and other pathogens.

Pathogenic Bacteria

Many bacteria are able to cause disease because of their capsule protection and the makeup of their cell walls. Some important pathogenic bacteria are summarized in Table 8-2. The following is a brief description of them by their staining qualities.

Gram-negative Bacilli. *Neisseria* is a genus of bacilli that are diplococcus in shape and cause gonorrhea, upper respiratory infections, and infectious meningitis. The bacillus, *Pseudomonas*, is responsible for **suppurative** (pus-forming) infections. Bacteria from the genus *Legionella* cause the infamous, pneumonia-like legionnaires' disease (*legionellosis*).

Rickettsiae are a special form of bacteria. Some are rod shaped and others are circular. They can grow only within the cell of another organism, or *host*. Rickettsiae are transmitted to people through the bite of an infected insect or tick. Resulting infections range from mild to fatal. A well known member of the spotted fever group of rickettsiae causes Rocky Mountain spotted fever. Members of the typhus group cause epidemic and endemic typhus.

Gram-positive Bacilli. Staphylococci are gram-positive cocci that are always present in the environment and are normal inhabitants of the human skin and respiratory tract. *Staphylococcus aureus* is the most dangerous of this group because it produces poisons called **toxins** and frequently is resistant to antibiotics. It can be responsible for serious or fatal infections of newborns or postsurgical patients. An outbreak of "staph" in a hospital is so serious that all hospital personnel constantly strive to prevent such nosocomial infections.

Streptococci are also gram-positive cocci; they are common inhabitants of the body. Members of this group cause "strep throat," pneumococcal pneumonia, and scarlet fever. Many gram-positive bacilli form spores, such as those from the genus *Clostridium*, which cause botulism (a form of food poisoning). These bacilli are particularly difficult to destroy. A respiratory tract infection, known as tuberculosis (TB), is caused by the tubercle bacillus, *Mycobacterium tuberculosis*.

Viruses

Viruses are protein-covered sacs containing either DNA or RNA and other organic materials. They lack most of the characteristics of living organisms. However, when a virus enters the cell of a living organism, the virus' nuclear material is activated. The host cell then becomes a culture medium for the reproduction of the virus. A virus must use the cell's ability to make protein and energy because a virus does not have its own means to perform metabolism.

Although scientists long suspected the existence of microorganisms smaller than bacteria, it was not until 1935 that the first virus was discovered. Since then, advances in electron and x-ray microscopy and biochemical technology have provided a clearer picture of these elusive structures. Scientists are now able to culture specific viruses, which can be maintained in the laboratory indefinitely.

Table 8-2. Some Important Pathogenic Bacteria

Bacterium	Diseases	Type	Gram Stain Reaction*
Bacillus anthracis	Anthrax	Spore-forming rod	+
Bordetella pertussis	Whooping cough	Rod	−
Borrelia burgdorferi	Lyme disease	Spirochete	
Brucella abortus and B. melitensis	Brucellosis, undulant fever	Rod	−
Chlamydia trachomatis	Lymphogranuloma venereum, trachoma	Coccoid	−
Clostridium botulinum	Botulism (food poisoning)	Spore-forming rod	+
Clostridium perfringens	Gas gangrene, wound infections	Spore-forming rod	+
Clostridium tetani	Tetanus (lockjaw)	Spore-forming rod	+
Corynebacterium diphtheriae	Diphtheria	Rod	+
Escherichia coli	Urinary infections	Rod	−
Francisella tularensis	Tularemia	Rod	−
Haemophilus ducreyi	Chancroid	Rod	−
Haemophilus influenzae	Meningitis, pneumonia	Rod	−
Klebsiella pneumoniae	Pneumonia	Rod	−
Mycobacterium leprae	Leprosy	Rod	+/−
Mycobacterium tuberculosis	Tuberculosis	Rod	+/−
Neisseria gonorrhoeae	Gonorrhea	Diplococcus	−
Neisseria meningitidis	Nasopharyngitis, meningitis	Diplococcus	−
Proteus vulgaris and P. morgani	Gastroenteritis, urinary infections	Rod	−
Pseudomonas aeruginosa	Respiratory and urogenital infections	Rod	−
Rickettsia rickettsii	Rocky Mountain spotted fever	Rod	−
Salmonella typhi	Typhoid fever	Rod	−
Salmonella species	Gastroenteritis	Rod	−
Shigella species	Shigellosis (bacillary dysentery)	Rod	−
Staphylococcus aureus	Boils, carbuncles, pneumonia, septicemia	Cocci in clusters	+
Streptococcus pyogenes	Strep throat, scarlet fever, rheumatic fever, septicemia	Cocci in chains	+
Streptococcus pneumoniae	Pneumonia	Diplococcus	+
Treponema pallidum	Syphilis	Spirochete	−
Vibrio cholerae	Cholera	Curved rod	−
Yersinia pestis	Plague	Rod	−

* +, gram-positive; −, gram-negative; +/−, gram-variable.
From Burton GRW. Microbiology for the Health Sciences, Ed 4. Philadelphia, J.B. Lippincott, 1992.

Pathogenic Viruses

A wide range of disease is caused by viruses. The common viruses are summarized in Table 8-3. Most pathogenic viruses cannot be easily controlled or destroyed. Immunization is the most effective means for preventing viral infections, such as measles and polio. Viruses affect every system and tissue of the body.

Infection with HIV often causes progressive loss of immune functions in the human body. People whose blood tests positive for the HIV antibodies often go on

Table 8-3. Common Pathogenic Viruses

Group	Name	Common Disorders Caused	Comments
Producing internal disorders	Picornavirus (enteric group)		
	Poliovirus	Poliomyelitis	At least three types Vaccine available
	Echovirus	ECHO syndrome (*enteric cyto-pathogenic human orphan*), aseptic meningitis, diarrhea neonatorum, paralytic disease	At least 30 types No vaccine
	Picornavirus (rhinovirus group)	Common cold, upper respiratory infections	No vaccine
	Coxsackievirus	Aseptic meningitis, myocarditis, pericarditis	At least 30 types No vaccine
Rash producers	Poxvirus	Smallpox	Has been eradicated
	Rubella virus	German measles (rubella)	Vaccine available Can cause birth defects
	Rubeola virus	"Red" measles (rubeola), encephalomyelitis	Vaccine available
	Erythema infectiosum	"Fifth" disease	No vaccine
	Varicella zoster (herpes zoster)	Chickenpox (varicella), shingles (herpes zoster)	No specific vaccine; may use gamma globulin
	Herpesvirus simplex	Cold sores (herpes simplex)	
	Herpesvirus type II	Herpes labialis (genital herpes), encephalitis, vulvovaginitis	No vaccine Two types
	Roseola infantum virus	Roseola infantum ("rose rash," exanthem subitum)	No vaccine
Respiratory	Influenza virus (myxovirus types A, B, C)	Influenza ("flu," grippe), croup, pneumonia	Three types Vaccine available (moderate effectiveness)
	Mumps virus (paramyxovirus)	Parotitis (mumps), orchitis (inflammation of testes), meningoencephalitis	Vaccine available
	Infectious mononucleosis virus (Epstein-Barr virus)	Infectious "mono"	No vaccine
	Adenovirus	Conjunctivitis	
Chronic (latent)	Hepatitis		
	Type A	Type A hepatitis (formerly called infectious hepatitis)	No vaccine
	Type B ("Dane particle")	Type B hepatitis (formerly called serum hepatitis)	No vaccine
	Type C (non-A, non-B)	Type C hepatitis (parenterally transmitted)	No vaccine
	Type D	Type D hepatitis (can be co-infection with Type B)	
	Papovavirus	Warts (verrucae)	
	Arbovirus		
	Group A	Equine encephalitis	Vaccine possible
	Group B	Yellow fever	Vaccine possible
	Diplovirus	Colorado tick fever	No vaccine
	Rabies virus (rhabdovirus)	Rabies (hydrophobia)	Vaccine available
Autoimmune disorders	Human immunodeficiency virus (HIV)	Opportunistic infections, such as pneumocystis pneumonia and Kaposi's sarcoma Can develop into full-blown AIDS	Virus has been identified No vaccine available Transmitted via body fluids, especially blood and semen

to develop opportunistic diseases. AIDS describes the last phase of HIV infection when the person is particularly susceptible to opportunistic diseases. HIV is transmitted through blood and certain body secretions.

Key Concept

Major types of microorganisms are algae; fungi (yeasts and molds); protozoa; bacteria; and viruses.

Infectious Diseases

An infection is a condition in which the body is invaded by pathogens. Diseases caused by microorganisms are called *infectious diseases*. The microorganisms increase in number and produce the symptoms of illness. Microbiologists use the term *etiology* to describe the specific cause of a disease. Many diseases caused by microorganisms are **communicable**, that is, they are spread from one organism (person) to another. **Contagious** diseases are communicable diseases that are transmitted to many individuals quickly and easily. When a large number of people in the same area are infected in a relatively short time, the disease is said to be **epidemic**.

Transmission of Microorganisms

Microorganisms are spread by several means: direct or indirect contact with the microorganism, transmission through contaminated substances, and transmission by animals (Table 8-4).

Knowledge of how pathogens enter and leave the body is essential in preventing the spread of disease.

Table 8-4. Transmission of Infectious Disease

Type of Transmission	Examples of Methods
Direct or indirect contact	Touching, kissing, shaking hands, sexual intercourse
Airborne	Dust particles and spores in the air, droplets from sneezing
Food-borne	Spoiled and uncooked food, food contaminated with feces or soil
Water-borne	Feces-contaminated water supply
Animals	Bites by infected insects, dogs, cats, rodents
Contaminated articles	Dishes, bedding, needles, syringes
Blood-borne	Transfusions, kidney dialysis, injections

Microorganisms can enter through the respiratory, gastrointestinal, urinary, and reproductive systems and through breaks in the skin or mucous membrane. Microorganisms may leave the body in any of the natural discharges: mucus, semen, sputum, saliva, urine, and feces. They may also leave the body in vomitus and in drainage or blood from breaks in the skin.

Transmission by Contact

Direct contact usually involves the spread of pathogens from one person to another through body contact, such as touching, shaking hands, kissing, or sexual intercourse. Many infectious diseases are spread in this fashion. *Indirect contact* implies that there is an intermediary object that harbors the microorganisms and carries them from the infected person to the new victim. Contaminated objects that might be found in a healthcare setting are bedding, tissues, used syringes, drinking cups, and dressings. A *human carrier* does not exhibit symptoms of the disease, but rather, carries the pathogens and transmits them to others.

Transmission Through Contaminated Substances

Airborne transmission is accomplished by dust particles or spores blowing from place to place. For instance, infectious diseases can be transmitted by contact with pathogen-containing moisture drops produced by sneezing or coughing and propelled far from the carrier. Common colds and other upper respiratory infections are easily spread by droplet infection.

Public water supplies contaminated with bacteria will produce *water-borne transmission* of diseases. Food poisoning can result from foods that have not been properly refrigerated or cooked. The spread of pathogens in this fashion is called *food-borne transmission*.

Transmission by Animals

Living carriers of pathogens are called *vectors*. Mosquitoes, flies, fleas, ticks, and lice are the most common vectors that transmit disease to human beings. These organisms spread disease by transferring microorganisms from insect feet, wings, or body to food. When the contaminated food is eaten, the microorganisms are further transmitted to the person. Another means of spread is when insects and other related organisms transmit microorganisms by becoming infected themselves and biting a victim, who then also becomes infected.

Cycle of Disease Spread

Communicable diseases spread easily. Scientists and healthcare workers use knowledge gained in *epidemiology* (the study of ways by which diseases are transmitted to people) to develop means of preventing the spread of microbial infections. Disease will spread if the cycle of transmission remains unbroken. The cycle is illustrated in Figure 8-4. To prevent the disease from spreading, the cycle must be broken. The cycle depends on the following elements:

- A *reservoir* in which the pathogenic organism can live and grow
- A *portal of exit* from which the organism can leave the reservoir
- A *vehicle* to transmit the organism
- A *portal of entry* through which the organism can enter the host
- A *susceptible host* in which the organism can find a reservoir

Some of these elements are controllable and some are not. The following section discusses each element, its presence in the healthcare facility, and the healthcare system's methods of breaking the chain of that specific element.

The Organism and Its Reservoir

A reservoir is any place where the organism can multiply or where it can survive until it is transferred to a place where it can multiply. Reservoirs usually are living, such as people, domesticated animals, wild animals, and insects, or they may be inanimate objects, such as air, soil, food, fluids, bedding, and eating and drinking utensils.

Hospital personnel can break the cycle at this point by destroying the organism or retarding its growth. Instruments and dressings used in the operating room must be sterilized; hospital floors and equipment are disinfected. Basic hospital items, such as thermometers and bedpans, are to be used only by one patient and sterilized or discarded after each use. Other types of equipment, such as catheters and syringes, are always disposable and are *never* reused.

Hospitals usually have infection control committees to oversee aseptic procedures, ensure that personnel frequently wash their hands, train staff in proper techniques, and take action when infections occur. Because microorganisms can survive in a wide variety of places, special precautions are instituted to make sure that contaminated waste materials are properly destroyed, air in patient areas is purified, and sterilized items are correctly stored. Even the healthcare staff is a potential reservoir. Hospital personnel, therefore, should not come to work when they might be a source of infection.

Portal of Exit

An organism must have a means of escape from its reservoir. Portals of exit in the human body include all body *orifices* (openings) and discharges from the skin.

The patient who has an airborne infection may be asked to wear a mask or be given medication to prevent coughing.

Vehicle of Transmission

A variety of vehicles are listed in Table 8-4 and in the discussion of transmission of microorganisms.

The cycle can be broken by burning all trash in non-residue incinerators, by removing linen without shaking it or allowing it to touch your clothing, by carefully covering all infected wounds, and by isolating infectious patients. Any paper tissues used by this patient should be burned. If the disease can be spread by body excretions, it may be necessary to disinfect the toilet after use or to use a toilet in an isolated room. Care should be taken with used syringes because a finger prick with a contaminated needle can spread disease to other patients or to hospital staff members.

Portal of Entry

There must be an avenue of entrance for a disease-causing organism to gain access to the body. An open wound, an incision area, a puncture site from an injection, or a body orifice into which a catheter (tube) or similar device is inserted are factors that predispose a hospitalized patient to infection.

Here, too, sterile technique will break the cycle of infection. Gloves are always worn by nursing and healthcare personnel to protect themselves when handling any body substances from the patient or other potential reservoir of pathogens (body substance precautions). On occasion, protective eye wear, masks, gowns, and shoe covers may also be worn if there is any danger of wider dispersal of body substances.

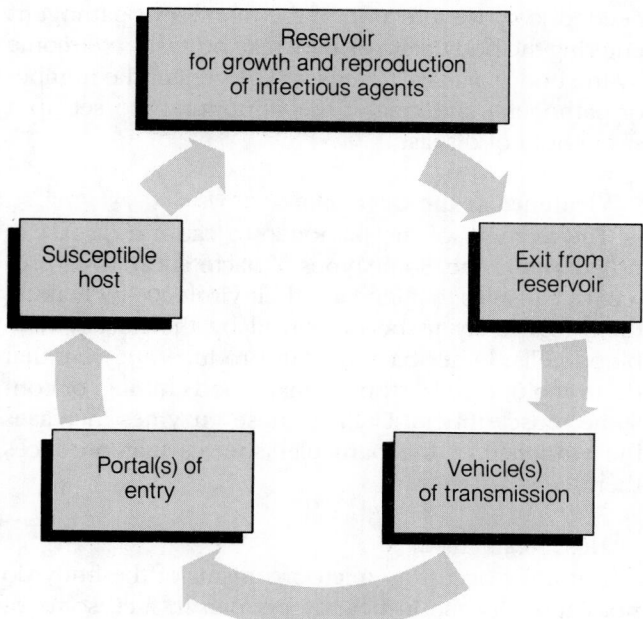

Figure 8-4. The chain of disease spread. To prevent a disease from spreading, the chain must be broken.

These precautions are particularly important to prevent infection by HIV and hepatitis-causing organisms.

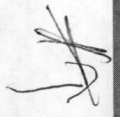

> **Nursing Alert**
> Body substance precautions are observed in *all nursing care.*

Susceptible Host

Healthy people normally have a variety of defenses against infection. Ill or inactive people or hospitalized patients, however, are more susceptible to infections. Their immune system may be compromised. Chronic fatigue and poor nutrition weaken the body's ability to respond to infection. Infants, young children, and the elderly are more vulnerable. Injury, wounds, shock, and trauma further weaken the body. Side effects of some medications also contribute to a person's susceptibility. Emotional factors, such as anxiety, may play a role in altering the body's defenses.

Nursing personnel can do little to directly change some of these factors. Nursing staff, however, must constantly be attentive to the control of infection. Preventing infection is every healthcare worker's daily job.

> **Nursing Alert**
> Proper handwashing is the single most useful and effective means of breaking the cycle of infectious disease spread.

Actions of Pathogens in the Body

Pathogenic microorganisms have two possible effects within the body: local destruction of tissue or production of poisonous substances that migrate. Although some microorganisms destroy the tissues in which they live, many organisms cause damage to host tissues far from the infection site. These microorganisms produce substances called **toxins**, which are poisonous.

Toxins may cause harmful effects by traveling through the circulatory system to damage other cells of the body. The wide variety of cellular effects include interrupting cellular metabolism, stopping protein synthesis, and destroying cell membranes. Toxins can cause many different symptoms.

Two types of toxins are produced by microorganisms. **Endotoxins** are part of the cell walls of gram-negative bacteria. When the microorganism dies, the cell wall decays and toxins are released. **Exotoxins** are toxins manufactured by a microorganism and excreted into the surrounding tissue. They are released into host

blood vessels, where they are carried to other parts of the body.

Response to Infection

Whether or not a pathogen will produce an active infection depends on both the organism and the host. A healthy individual often can muster physical defense mechanisms to ward off disease. Persistent and effective pathogens, however, can overwhelm even a healthy person.

Factors That Influence Infection

Several factors help determine whether or not disease-causing microorganisms will ultimately result in infection. These factors are the specific portal of entry, number of microorganisms, virulence of the organism, and host resistance.

Specific Portal of Entry

In general, microorganisms will cause disease only if they gain access to the body through a specific portal of entry. For example, *Streptococcus pneumoniae* will cause pneumococcal pneumonia only if they enter the respiratory system. Any other portal of entry will not result in infection. Likewise, the typhoid bacillus must enter the digestive tract, and meningococcus uses the nose as its chief portal of entry.

Number of Microorganisms

Usually, large numbers of microorganisms are needed to cause infection. If the number of pathogens entering the body is small, they may be easily overcome by the body's natural defenses. The greater the number of pathogens, the greater the opportunity to set up a stronghold of disease.

Virulence of the Organism

The strength of the pathogen to cause a disease is called **virulence**. Some types of bacteria can form protective capsules that increase their virulence by making them less likely to be destroyed by the host's white blood cells. Other bacteria can produce *enzymes* that destroy blood cells, stop normal blood clotting, or consume muscle fibers. Each of these enzymes increases the virulence of the particular species that produces them.

Host Resistance

Naturally occurring microorganisms of the body do not cause disease in healthy people. In fact, some of these microorganisms play a necessary role in resistance to disease. The ability of some species of microorganisms to live together is called *symbiosis.* An association in which one species of microorganism prevents the growth of another or actually destroys members of another species is called *antibiosis.* Some members of naturally occurring body flora possess an antibiotic relationship to pathogens and contribute to the overall health of an individual.

Normally, the body has a variety of defense mechanisms that contribute to its resistance to pathogenic infection. A number of mechanisms are general and not specific to any particular type of microorganism. The other common defense mechanism is specific to each species of microorganism and triggers a mechanism known as the *immune response.* These general protective methods, called nonspecific defense mechanisms and immunity, are discussed in the following sections.

Key Concept

Factors determining whether or not a pathogen causes disease in a particular host are: specific portal of entry, number of microorganisms, virulence of the organism, and host resistance.

Human Defense Against Disease

Humankind has survived because of its defense against disease. Although the individual is not aware of it, the human body is almost constantly defending itself against foreign invaders. Human beings have three lines of defense (Table 8-5). The first two lines are nonspecific, that is, the body attempts to destroy all types of substances that are foreign to it. The immune response is very specific.

First Line of Defense

The body defends itself against invaders of the body's orifices and, thus, its systems.

Intact skin covering the body surface and the intact mucous membranes lining its cavities (those open to the outside) serve as barriers to microorganisms. In addition, the sticky mucus secreted by the mucous membranes in some cavities traps the organisms and prevents them from journeying further into the body.

The cells lining the respiratory tract are covered with cilia. These hairlike projections are in constant motion and push a constant flow of mucus (and the foreign particles trapped within it) up and out of the lungs and trachea. These cilia offer significant protection against the common dust and other contaminants inhaled daily from our environment.

Some natural secretions help protect the body. Saliva, tears, gastric juice, and other secretions are foes of

Table 8-5. The Body's Defense Against Disease

Defense	Action
First Line of Defense	
Skin and mucous membranes	Prevent entry and eliminate microbes
Cilia	Push mucus and foreign particles out of lungs and trachea
Secretions	Destroy and wash out microbes
Expulsion of feces and frequent urination	Flush the gastrointestinal and genitourinary systems
Second Line of Defense	
Fever	Raises body temperature to destroy microbes
Interferon	Interferes with and prevents viral production process
Phagocytosis	Captures, engulfs, and destroys microbes
Inflammation	Destroys microbes through a complex reaction
Third Line of Defense: Immune Response	
Naturally acquired immunity	
Active immunity	Produces natural antibodies as a reaction to foreign antigens
Passive immunity	Protects infant temporarily with mother's antibodies
Artificially acquired immunity	
Active immunity	Provides long-term protection with the use of antigens or vaccines
Passive immunity	Provides temporary protection with antibodies received from another organism

microorganisms. Tears and saliva have antiseptic qualities and can wash away microorganisms by mechanical means. Gastric secretions, particularly hydrochloric acid, are so potent that they easily destroy most ingested pathogens. *Sebum* produced by oil glands of the skin slows the growth of microorganisms.

Normal body functions also are a means of defense. Expulsion of feces flush bacteria from the intestine; frequent urination flushes the urinary system. Blood during menstruation washes out the uterine and vaginal structures.

Second Line of Defense

Pathogens that escape the first line of defense are usually destroyed by the second line of defense. Major defense mechanisms include fever, interferon, phagocytosis, and inflammation.

Fever, an increase in body temperature, is an automatic response to infection. Elevated temperature checks the growth of most microorganisms until more effective bodily defenses are called on. In certain circumstances, therefore, it is not desirable to reduce fever.

Cells infected by viruses form a substance called **interferon**. These antiviral proteins protect the cell by interfering with and preventing the viral production process. Interferon is most effective with acute viral infections, such as those associated with flu.

When pathogens enter the body, white blood cells (*leukocytes*) increase in number and engulf invaders at or near their point of entry. Other microorganisms that have passed beyond the normal barricades of the body are shunted into the lymphatic vessels and carried in the lymph to the nodes, where they are destroyed by **phagocytosis**. This term describes the process of engulfing and destroying bacteria and other foreign particles by cells called *phagocytes*.

Inflammation is a complex set of responses to the invasion of microorganisms. The diameter of the small blood vessels surrounding the damaged area increases, causing the typical warmth and redness that often accompanies inflammation. Swelling of the affected area occurs, accompanied by pain and pressure. Various chemicals are released, including *histamine*. Phagocytes are then attracted to the damaged tissue and begin their work. Often *pus* accumulates at the site; pus is the collection of dead cells and fluids brought about by phagocytosis and other inflammatory reactions.

Third Line of Defense: Immune Response

The third line of defense is called immune response. Microorganisms and other material, such as pollen, that usually do not inhabit the human body are recognized as foreign invaders. The body's immune system responds in specific ways. Although the immune system protects against disease, it can also damage its host through hypersensitivity and autoimmunity.

Immunity

Immunity is the state of being highly resistant to a specific pathogen. Some immunity is inherited by all human beings. For example, people are usually immune to the "hoof and mouth" disease of cattle. However, people develop most forms of immunity to microorganisms in the course of living and are said to have acquired immunity. Immunity may be naturally acquired or artificially acquired.

Naturally Acquired Immunity. Once the individual is exposed to a microorganism, the body responds by producing specialized proteins called **antibodies** (Fig. 8-5). The foreign microorganisms that cause antibodies to form are known as **antigens**. Each antigen stimulates the formation of its own kind of antibody, and every pathogen and its toxic secretions act as antigens. Im-

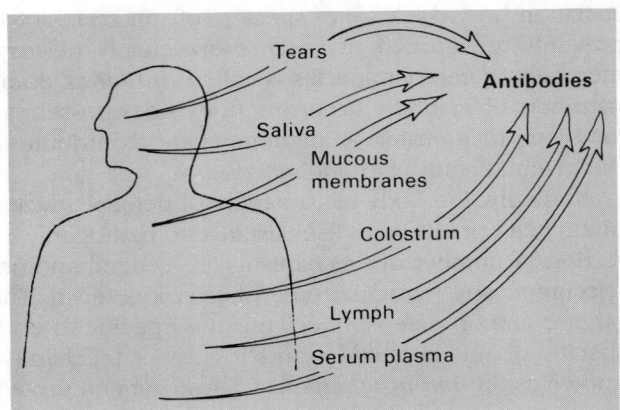

Figure 8-5. Body structures and sites in which antibodies are produced. (From Burton GRW. Microbiology for the Health Sciences, Ed 4. Philadelphia, J.B. Lippincott, 1992)

munity acquired in this manner is called *active immunity* because it is induced directly by the microorganism. Some types of *naturally acquired active immunity* last for the life of the person, whereas other types last only a short time.

Passive immunity occurs when an individual is given a substance containing antibodies or antitoxins that have been developed in another person. The substance is called either an *antiserum* or an *antitoxin*. The immunity is said to be passive because the body of the recipient plays no active part in response, but merely receives the antibodies. *Naturally acquired passive immunity* occurs when a fetus receives antibodies through the mother's placenta before birth. Thus, the neonate possesses immunity through the mother's antibodies. A newborn can also receive naturally acquired passive immunity through breast-feeding. Such passive immunity is temporary and lasts only until the infant's own immune system becomes operational.

Key Concept

◆ In naturally acquired active immunity, the person produces antibodies.

◆ In naturally acquired passive immunity, the person passively receives the antigen with no active response.

◆ In artificially acquired active immunity, the person is injected with weakened or dead microorganisms or an inactive form of its toxin.

◆ In artificially acquired passive immunity, the person is injected with antibodies derived from the blood of infected people.

Artificially Acquired Immunity. Artificially acquired immunity can also be either active or passive. *Artificially acquired active immunity* occurs when a person is injected with weakened or dead microorganisms or with an inactive form of a microbial toxin. These antigens are also called vaccines and the process of injecting the substances is known as vaccination or immunization. Although the vaccine does not produce the disease symptoms, it produces protective antibodies. Vaccination is commonly used to control polio, measles, mumps, and other infectious diseases.

Artificially acquired passive immunity is obtained by injecting people with antibodies derived from the blood of infected people or animals. These individuals already were immune to a specific disease and their protection is used to shield others. This resistance, like all passive immunity, is only temporary because the body does not produce new antibodies.

Autoimmunity. This situation occurs when the body mistakenly interprets its own cells as foreign and produces antibodies to its own tissues. Rheumatoid arthritis and AIDS are examples of autoimmune disorders (see Chapters 77 and 78).

Keys for Review

Key Questions for Critical Thinking

1. Describe how oxygen, food, temperature, moisture, and light affect the growth and reproduction of microorganisms.
2. Describe the factors involved in the spread of disease and how nurses can break this chain.
3. Describe how the skin, mucous membranes, and natural secretions of the body help provide a defense against infection.
4. Explain the difference between naturally acquired immunity and artificially acquired immunity. Give an example of each.
5. Discuss how vaccines protect the body against pathogenic microorganisms.

Key Readings

Balows A, et al., eds. Manual of Clinical Microbiology, Ed 5. Washington, DC, American Society of Microbiology, 1991

Baron EJ, Finegold SM. Diagnostic Microbiology, Ed 8. St. Louis, C.V. Mosby, 1990

Burton GRW. Microbiology for the Health Sciences, Ed 4. Philadelphia, J.B. Lippincott, 1992

Key Readings (continued)

Holt JG, Kreig NR, eds. Bergey's Manual of Systemic Bacteriology. Baltimore, Williams & Wilkins, 1984

Mills J, Masur, H. "AIDS-related infections." Scientific American, 263(2):48–57, August, 1990

The Lippincott Manual of Nursing Practice, Ed 5. Philadelphia, J.B. Lippincott, 1991

Keys to Learning More

Chapter 30: medical asepsis and universal precautions

Chapter 38: signs and symptoms of illness

Unit Nine: basic nursing care skills, all of which consider the principles of microbiology and aseptic techniques

Chapter 53: the person who has surgery

Chapter 54: use of surgical asepsis in nursing

Chapter 57: administration of medications. Sterile or clean technique is followed in these procedures.

Unit Thirteen: principles in care and disorders of infants and children

Unit Fourteen: care of the adult with various disorders

Unit *3*   Development of the Individual and Family

9 Infancy and Childhood

Keys for Learning

Learning Objectives

- State the characteristics and progression of growth and development
- Briefly describe Erikson's psychosocial development and discuss the challenges and virtues of each age
- Discuss the similarities and relationships between Havighurst's developmental tasks and Erikson's stages of development
- Name the four stages of human development, according to Piaget
- Describe the meaning of play to a child
- Discuss the ages at which various types of teeth erupt
- Describe physical and behavioral characteristics of the child at 6-month increments from ages 1 through 5 and of the school-age child at 1-year increments from ages 6 through 10
- Discuss areas of parental concern during childhood

Key Terms

bonding	fetus	masturbation
cephalocaudal	growth	neonate
cognitive	hereditary	proximodistal
development	interdependent	regression
environment		

Keys to Understanding This Chapter

Chapter 5: basic human needs

Key Points

- Infant and child growth and development is a continuing process throughout childhood.
- Growth and development progress in a particular sequence (*proximodistal*: center-outward; and *cephalocaudal*: head-to-toe).
- Theorists have identified specific tasks to be accomplished and stages an individual passes through on the way to becoming a mature, fully functional person.
- Most children pass through certain stages of growth and development at approximately the same ages.

Key Points (continued)

- To help their children comfortably progress through the developmental stages, parents need to understand certain areas of concern in childhood behavior.

Key Topics Outline

Growth and Development
Concepts of Growth and Development
Influences on Growth and Development
Growth and Development Theories
Role of Play in Growth and Development
Fetal and Neonatal Development

Infancy
Physical Growth
Developmental Tasks
Psychosocial Development
Cognitive Development

Toddlerhood
Physical Growth
Psychosocial Development
Cognitive Development

Preschool
Physical Growth
Psychosocial Development
Cognitive Development

School Age
Physical Growth
Psychosocial Development
Cognitive Development

Areas of Concern
Parental Guidance
Building Self-esteem

Key Learning Activities

- Visit a preschool nursery or day care center and observe normal children of various ages. What age-related differences did you observe? Report back to class.
- Compare the above observations with children of the same ages who are hospitalized. What differences can be observed? Explain the concept of "regression."
- Volunteer at a day care center to gain more understanding of the developing child.

Children are a country's stake in the future; they are the citizens of tomorrow. In this unit you will learn about growth and development during the life span.

Because the nurse may care for both healthy and sick children, it is important to understand normal growth and development. By knowing how most children can be expected to behave at any particular age, the nurse will be better prepared to care for any child. It is also necessary to understand normal behavior before one can understand abnormal behavior. It helps, for example, to know that, during illness, **regression** may occur. That is, the child's behavior may go backward to that of an earlier stage of development.

Growth and Development

You learned about the basic human needs in Chapter 5. An understanding of these basic needs is necessary before you attempt to study the development needs across the life span. The neonate and infant must have assistance to meet the most basic survival needs, such as food, water, and elimination. When these needs are met, the child can begin to meet needs for safety, security, and socialization.

Growth and development, which is considered a single process, go on constantly through childhood and into adulthood. **Growth** is defined as a change in body size and structure; **development** is a change in body function.

Concepts of Growth and Development

Growth and development occur in an *orderly sequence*; a developmental task must be accomplished before another can be attempted. Most children are able to perform certain tasks at about the same age although there are variations within the normal range.

In relation to the body, the process of growth and development follows *cephalocaudal* and *proximodistal directions* as shown in Figure 9-1. **Cephalocaudal** means "from head to tail"; babies can lift their heads before they can sit up; they can make sounds before they can walk. **Proximodistal** means "from the center to the outside"; babies can roll over before they can grasp small objects.

Growth and development progress from *simple to complex*; the baby learns to sit before learning to walk or to babble before learning to speak.

Growth and development are also *inclusive*, that is, they involve the "whole" child, family, and the child's culture. Growth and development, as a single process, may be divided into physical, physiologic, motor, intellectual, emotional, and social aspects. The last three are often considered together as *psychosocial* development.

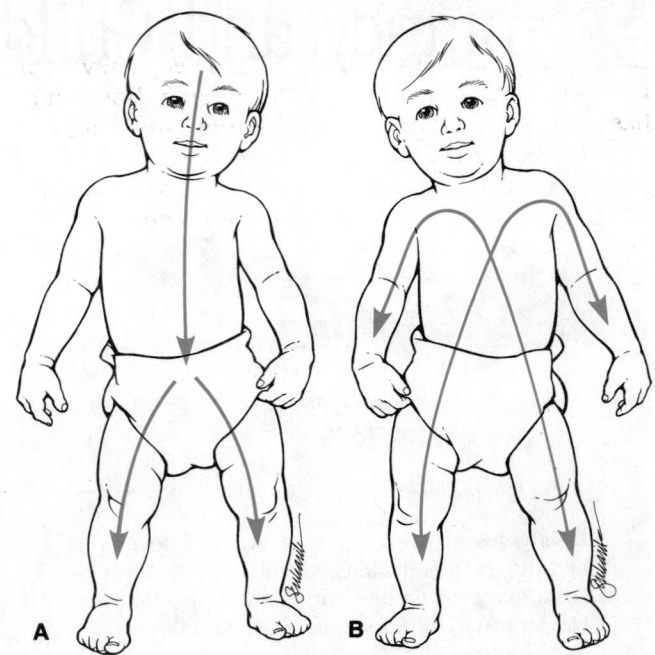

Figure 9-1. Principles of growth and development. **(A)** Cephalocaudal. Growth and development proceed from head to toe or tail. **(B)** Proximodistal. Growth and development proceed from the center outward (Jackson DB, Saunders RB. Child Health Nursing: A Comprehensive Approach to the Care of Children and Their Families. Philadelphia, J.B. Lippincott, 1993).

All aspects of growth and development are closely related and **interdependent**. For example, children cannot learn to control bowel movements (development) until their muscles are strong enough (growth) and until they can understand what is expected of them (development). Also, walking is controlled by motor development; motor development depends on normal bone and muscle growth (physical); normal growth depends on adequate food and energy (physiologic), whereas the nervous system exercises overall control (intellectual). If the baby is neglected, emotional development suffers; if the culture in which the child lives is too protective, social development suffers.

Key Concept

Growth is a change in body size and structure; *development* is a change in body function. They have the following characteristics:

◆ Orderly sequence
◆ Cephalocaudal
◆ Proximodistal
◆ Simple to complex
◆ Inclusive
◆ Interdependent

Influences on Growth and Development

Both heredity and environment influence the newborn. For a long time there has been a discussion about which has a stronger influence or whether they are of approximately equal importance.

Hereditary characteristics are inherited. These are often called *genetic* factors. Skin color, eye color, and body build are examples of hereditary characteristics.

Environment is the sum total of all the conditions and factors that surround the newborn. The kind of housing, the neighborhood, the number of siblings and placement in sibling order, and the amount of health-care available are examples of environmental elements. You can understand that the baby born into a wealthy family may develop differently from the one born into a poor family. Religious practices, nationality, and location of birth have a bearing on a child's development.

Growth and Development Theories

A number of scholars have studied various aspects of development. They have developed theories that can be used in understanding, explaining, and predicting behavior in children and adults. No one theory covers the whole spectrum of behavior; each theory concentrates on one aspect of development. The child and adult need to be considered by a combination of these views. The following are the major theories and their theorists:

♦ Psychoanalytic theory: Sigmund Freud
♦ Psychosocial development: Erik Erikson
♦ Developmental tasks: Robert J. Havighurst
♦ Cognitive development: Jean Piaget
♦ Moral development: Lawrence Kohlberg
♦ Spiritual development: James Fowler

There is not enough space to discuss all these theories here, but you especially need to know about developmental tasks, psychosocial development, and cognitive development. Adult development crisis theory is discussed in the chapters on the adult later in this unit.

Developmental Tasks

Physical growth occurs without personal effort, but development is an active process in which the person must participate. Havighurst theorizes that each stage of life has its own group of developmental tasks, as seen in the accompanying box.

To become a mature, fully functioning person, the developmental tasks of each stage of life must be met. The accomplishment of one task prepares a person for the next. Each person needs encouragement from family members, other caregivers, and school personnel to

Developmental Tasks of Childhood as Described by Havighurst

Birth to 24 Months

Learn to take solid food
Learn to walk
Learn to talk

Toddler and Preschool (18 Months to 6 Years)

Control processes of elimination
Learn sex differences and modesty
Get ready to read
Begin to form the conscience—to know right from wrong
Form concepts and be able to name them

Middle Childhood (6–12 Years)

Learn to get along with age mates
Learn fundamental skills of reading, writing, and figuring
Perfect physical skills and games
Develop a wholesome attitude about the self
Identify with a masculine or feminine role
Develop conscience, morality, values
Learn the difference between work and play
Develop industry and a pleasure in competition with others
Develop personal independence
Develop attitudes toward groups and social institutions

Theory concerning the adolescent appears in Chapter 10.

achieve the tasks leading to maturity, yet each must master the tasks himself or herself.

Psychosocial Development

Erikson's theory of human development focuses on the psychosocial and environmental aspects of personality as the person progresses from birth to death. Erikson stresses the uniqueness of each individual, the product of the interactions between the person's heredity, environment, and culture. Erikson emphasizes that the rate of development varies from child to child.

The major points of Erikson's theory, as outlined in Table 9-1, are:

♦ In each stage of development there is a *psychosocial challenge* or *critical period*, whereby the person has to deal with a major change in life. Erikson's theory states that if this challenge is not met, the person faces certain difficulty in achieving the next level of development. For example, if the infant does not achieve a sense of trust that needs will be met, the child will have difficulty later in achieving autonomy as a toddler.

♦ In each stage of development there is a *significant*

Table 9-1. Erikson's Theory of Psychosocial Development

Theory Concept	Infancy (Birth–1 Year)	Toddlerhood (1–3 Years)	Preschool (3–6 Years)	School Age (6–12 Years)
Erikson's Basic Tasks	Trust vs. mistrust	Autonomy vs. shame and doubt	Initiative vs. guilt	Industry vs. inferiority
Significant Other	Maternal person	Parents	Total family	School and neighborhood
Psychosocial Challenges	Develop trust	Learn appropriate behaviors / Learn right from wrong	Learn rules and regulations / Establish independence	Learn to get along with others / Learn school subjects
Virtues	Hope	Self-control / Will power	Direction / Purpose	Self-esteem / Competence
How Accomplished	Establish routines / Satisfy basic needs	Set limits / Let child make simple choices / Encourage curiosity / Gentle guidance	Consistent discipline / Explain things / Praise	Manage sibling rivalry / Give responsibility—tasks to do / Give recognition for away-from-home accomplishments
Developmental Phase	Oral–sensory	Muscular–anal	Locomotor–genital	Latency

Handwritten annotations on table: Not for yourself / Self driven / Autonomy – Doing what you / You want the child to be independent / Start on your own / Will Do useless / Peers – Friends, family / V initiative / You have to have Autonomy + initiative to have the purpose + direction / Cleanroom take out car / let them Explore / Freud / Piaget / V bowel movement / Walking / Latency ~ Something is About to happen

Theory concerning the adolescent and adult appears in Chapters 10 and 11.

---

person or group who exerts a lasting influence on the ongoing development of the child. For example, the parent who is primary caregiver is most significant to the infant, whereas the peer group has greater influence on the adolescent.

◆ Certain *psychosocial challenges* must be achieved at each stage. If the child does not achieve these tasks, he or she will have difficulty accomplishing the next stage's tasks.

◆ Certain *virtues* are appropriate for each developmental stage. The virtues are the beneficial, challenging, and exciting characteristics of the person that emerge if the task at that stage is successfully resolved.

◆ These tasks are *accomplished* by steps that the child, parents, and siblings share.

Cognitive Development

The term **cognitive** refers to knowledge, understanding, or perception. Throughout this chapter, the intellectual skills of the child at different ages are discussed. These represent cognitive skills.

Piaget stated that cognitive development "is a continuous progression" beginning with the *reflexes* of the newborn, which are spontaneous and automatic. The infant progresses to acquired *habits*. The child then goes on to acquire *knowledge* and to develop *intelligence*.

Cognitive development is *cumulative*, that is, what is learned is based on what has been known before. This theory is used in your nursing program—the information is presented to you in a progression from simple to complex, and you learn basic normal body structure and function and normal child development before you study deviations from those normal parameters.

Piaget's four major levels of cognitive development are summarized in the accompanying box and described here.

1. *Sensorimotor.* The infant learns by touching, tasting, and feeling. The infant learns to control movement of the body.
2. *Preoperational.* The child from 2 to 7 investigates and explores the environment and looks at things from his or her own point of view.
3. *Concrete operations.* The child from 7 through 11 "internalizes" actions and can perform them in the mind. The characteristics of cognition at the concrete operations level are:
   Reversibility. The child can walk to school and knows that by reversing the direction of the walk he or she can get home again.
   Seriation. The child can arrange things in a series, from big to little or in a numbered sequence.
   Conservation of matter. The child can begin to understand quantities, weight, or volume. The child

Stages of Cognitive Development (Piaget)

Stage I	Birth to age 2	Sensorimotor	(reflexes, habits)
Stage II	Ages 2–7	Preoperational thought	
Stage III	Ages 7–11	Concrete operations	↓
Stage IV	Ages 12–15	Formal operations	(knowledge → intelligence)

understands that 8 ounces of soda pop is the same amount whether it is in the can or in a glass.

4. *Formal operations.* The child can think in the abstract. Complex problem-solving is included in the formal operations category.

Role of Play in Child Development

Play is important to child development. It is through play that the child learns about the world. Experimentation, exploration, success, and failure are all a part of maturing at any age. Play with other children encourages peer cooperation, interaction, and sharing. It can enhance fine muscle or large muscle coordination and can strengthen muscles. It also "wears off" the excess energy that is characteristic of children.

Fetal and Neonatal Development

Fetal Development

The **fetus** is the unborn child in the uterus. Much is known about the sequence of development of the fetus. These stages of prenatal growth and development are described and illustrated in Chapter 58.

Neonatal Development

During the first month of life, an infant is referred to as a **neonate**. The average neonate weighs about 3.2 kg (7 lb) and is about 50 cm (20 in) in length. Although some of this birth weight may be lost during the first few days of life, it usually is regained quickly. The newborn cries lustily (crying is the neonate's only way of communicating), kicks vigorously, wiggles and squirms, and sucks often, even when not eating. For all the crying the newborn does, no tears are shed because the lacrimal or tear glands are not yet functional. Usually the neonate retains the fetal position, with the head tucked forward and the knees bent up to meet the chin. Indeed, all of the neonate, even the tiny fists, is curled into a ball.

The reactions to internal and external sensations and stimuli help to shape the child physically, intellectually, emotionally, and socially. Although neonates cannot focus their eyes, they respond to the person cuddling them and to moving objects, especially to white and black. Neonatal hearing is well developed; the neonate is easily startled and is disturbed by loud noises. The temperature-regulating mechanism is not stable. The neonate can chill easily.

Although the nervous system is not entirely developed at birth, the neonate is equipped with certain reflexes (involuntary responses) necessary for survival. The *sucking reflex* is vital to obtain nourishment, and the *rooting reflex* enables the neonate to search for and find the nipple. The *cough* or *gag reflex* prevents or helps to prevent choking (although the young baby chokes or gags often until this reflex is better developed). The *grasp reflex* causes the baby to grasp when something touches the palm of the hand. (This last reflex disappears as the baby grows older and begins to gain conscious control over movements). Further characteristics of the neonate are discussed in Chapter 60.

Infancy

Physical Growth

Weight and Height

During the first 3 months of life, the infant gains about 0.9 kg (2 lb) per month and grows about 2.5 to 5.0 cm (1–2 in.). From 3 to 6 months, the infant will gain about 0.45 kg (1 lb) per month. By the age of 6 months, the infant will have doubled the birth weight. By the end of 1 year, the infant will weigh about three times the birth weight and be about half again as tall as at birth.

Teeth

Teeth begin to erupt at about 6 to 7 months of age. The first to erupt generally are the two lower central incisors, followed by the four top central incisors. By 1 year of age most babies generally have these six teeth (Fig. 9-2). Because tooth eruption patterns vary greatly, parents should not be alarmed if the usual pattern is not followed.

The first teeth are known as *deciduous teeth*. The term *deciduous* literally means "falling off" or "subject to being shed." Like the leaves shed by deciduous trees, deciduous or baby teeth are lost later in life and are replaced by the permanent teeth.

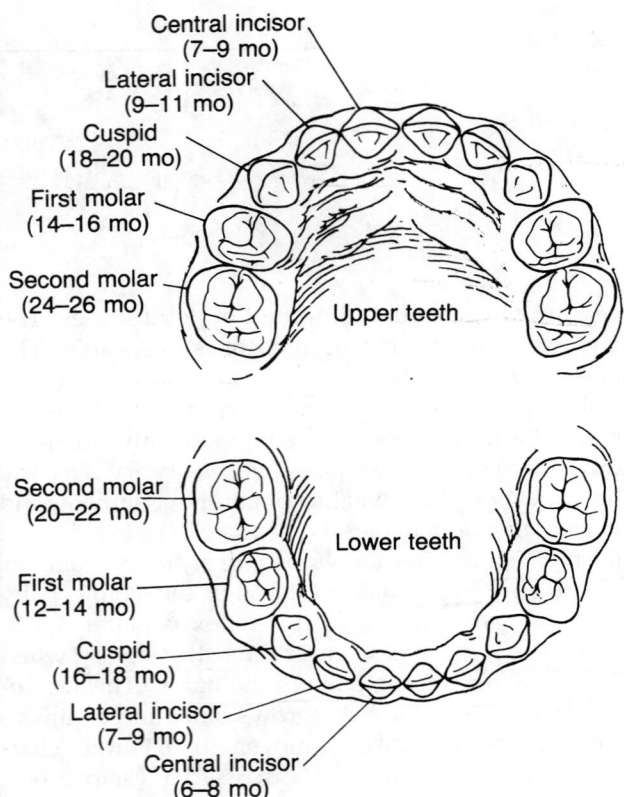

Central incisor
(7–9 mo)
Lateral incisor
(9–11 mo)
Cuspid
(18–20 mo)
First molar
(14–16 mo)
Second molar
(24–26 mo)

Upper teeth

Second molar
(20–22 mo)

Lower teeth

First molar
(12–14 mo)
Cuspid
(16–18 mo)
Lateral incisor
(7–9 mo)
Central incisor
(6–8 mo)

Figure 9-2. Approximate ages of eruption and locations of deciduous (baby) teeth. Refer to Chapter 23 for a diagram of the permanent teeth.

Ability to Eat Solids

There are a variety of opinions concerning the feeding of infants. Some child healthcare providers claim that infants should not have solids until 9 months to 1 year of age because their digestive tracts are immature. Others think that 6 months of age is the appropriate time to introduce solid foods. Most care providers agree that solids should not be introduced into the diet before 6 months of age.

Introduction of solids too early has been linked to food allergies. Research indicates that giving solids early does not help infants sleep all night. It is better for the child and easier for caregivers if solids are started later, so the infant receives the proper balance of nutrients and can quickly progress to table foods.

Introduction of new foods follows a logical sequence. Iron-fortified infant cereal, mixed with breast milk or human milk substitute, is the suggested first solid. It should be given by spoon, not bottle. New foods should be added weekly, so food allergies and intolerances can be identified. Foods are added in the following sequence: fruits, vegetables, meats. Although formula or breast milk may still be used, many infants drink cow's whole milk by age 1 year.

Babies should be fed *on demand* (when hungry). Breast-fed infants may eat every 2 hours and bottle-fed infants every 3 to 4 hours. Bottle-fed infants must not have the bottle propped; this practice has been linked to otitis media, sudden infant death, and pneumonia.

Developmental Tasks

Between the ages of 4 and 7 months, the infant undertakes many new activities (developmental tasks). As effort is made to succeed in these new tasks, failures inevitably occur, and the baby feels frustrated. Nevertheless, as physical development progresses, the baby begins to achieve success in many undertakings and becomes happier and more satisfied.

At 7 months, a baby can not only grasp the reached-for object but can also put it into the mouth. (The object may be baby's own toes). The baby is pleased with the accomplishment of transferring objects from one hand to another and will be entertained for some time at this task. The baby also enjoys the purposeful activity of bouncing or banging and makes many different sounds. Although babies can amuse themselves for long intervals, they welcome the company of others.

Psychosocial Development

Establishment of the infant's *trust* in the maternal figure (whether it's one of the parents or a primary caregiver) is clearly the most important challenge of infancy. The infant is a helpless being, entirely trusting the caregiver to meet basic needs. If trust is achieved, the infant will also achieve the virtue of this stage—*hope*—as summarized in Table 9-1. If trust is not established, later challenges of autonomy and initiative will be delayed.

Role of Caregiver. The infant's **bonding** (attachment to mother or a mother figure) is of primary importance. In today's economic climate, many mothers are employed and must seek day care to meet their child's day-to-day needs. Therefore, the "maternal person" may be some other caregiver or significant person.

Accomplishing Tasks. Being totally reliant on others for care, the infant must learn to develop trust—the feeling that basic needs will be met by the caregiver. The *basic needs* of the infant include holding, cuddling, feeding, stroking, and sucking (breast-feeding, bottle, pacifier). The infant, at this stage, is able to tolerate frustration only in small amounts. Distinctly, this period of development is "I want what I want when I want it!"

The primary caregiver (Erikson's "maternal person") must assist the infant in the establishment of *routines*. This system should include such items as feeding, playtime, and rest and sleep habits. This helps to establish the infant's feeling of trust in the caregiver.

Cognitive Development

The neonate progresses to the rank of infant by the time 4 weeks have passed. Piaget calls infancy the *sensori-motor* stage of development.

At 2 Months. At 2 months the infant can raise the head and turn the chin to the side although the lack of head control is still marked. The baby can stare directly ahead for a short time and may be able to focus the eyes on a light. The baby cries to signal needs and stops crying when comforted and satisfied. The baby has a preferred sleeping position, and although sleeping habits vary widely, will probably sleep from 18 to 20 hours a day.

At this stage, a baby's progress can be seen almost from day to day. When babies are 6 weeks old, they begin to make purposeful movements and stop crying when picked up; they are beginning to understand that someone will comfort them. As babies become aware of their surroundings, they smile, babble when spoken to, and follow lights within view.

At 3 Months. At 3 months the baby can reach for and grasp articles, but the automatic grasp reflex is now absent. The baby is able to turn over and can follow a moving object with the eyes.

At 4 Months. At 4 months, babies can sit with support and are beginning to coo and babble, especially when someone talks to them. The lacrimal glands have developed fully, and tears are shed. These babies usually sleep all night and take two or three naps during the day.

At 5 Months. The 5-month-old can hold the head steady, is able to recognize people, and, if bottle fed, tries to hold the bottle. The baby splashes in the bath and smiles at the reflection in the mirror.

At 6 Months. At this age, babies can pull up to sitting and sit for a short time without support. They turn over in bed without help, hold the bottle, and grab their own toes. If a toy is offered, the infant drops what he or she is holding to take the new toy. This baby now plays "peek-a-boo."

Some authorities feel that behavioral differences related to sex may be noted at 6 months; they observe that a boy may begin to be more assertive and a girl to be more passive. This issue is extremely controversial. Some researchers believe that role models are learned, whereas others believe that hereditary factors or differences in development of the endocrine system (particularly the hypothalamus gland) may be involved.

At 9 Months. By 9 months, the baby has learned to crawl and is "all over the house" and "into everything."

The baby responds when called by name, copies movements, and knows what "no" means.

At 1 Year. By about 10 months of age, the baby can usually pull up to standing while holding onto something and can walk with both hands held. The baby then learns to walk around furniture and to stand alone. At about 1 year of age, most children can take one or two steps alone. The 1-year-old can walk if one hand is held (Fig. 9-3).

The 1-year-old child can hold the bottle and drink out of a cup without difficulty. The child can say two or three simple words, such as "baby" and "bye-bye," and laughs aloud. The 1-year-old loves games such as simplified hide-and-seek.

Toddlerhood

Physical Growth

The toddler phase of growth and development encompasses approximately ages 1 to 3 years. The slowed physical growth of the toddler is reflected by the fact that, between 1 and 4 years of age, the child gains only 1.8 to 2.7 kg (4–6 lb) annually and grows only about 5.0 to 7.6 cm (2–3 in.) per year. However, great strides are made in physical and motor skills; the toddler can fit simple objects into appropriate holes and build a tower of two or three blocks.

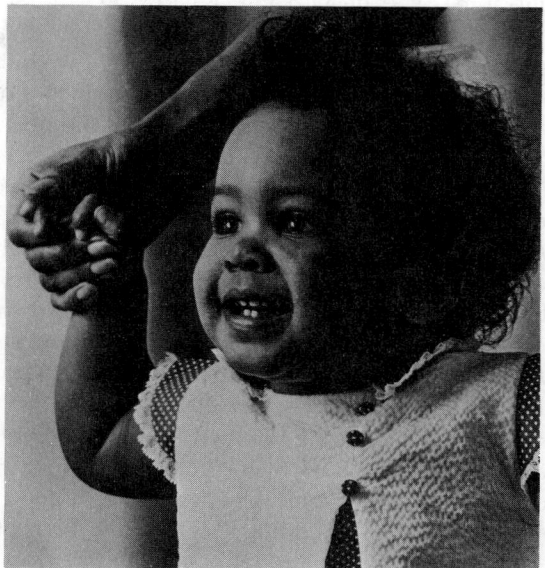

Figure 9-3. The 1-year-old takes her first shaky steps with assistance. Notice the normal tooth development for the 1-year-old child. She is bright-eyed and ready to conquer the world! (Courtesy of Gerber Products Company)

Psychosocial Development

The psychosocial challenge for this period is *autonomy* in independence versus shame and doubt. The mobile toddler begins to establish independence: walking, self-feeding, playing, and speaking.

The virtues of the toddler stage are *self-control* and *will power*, which evolve naturally as consistent discipline is given. Caregivers can foster the development of self-control and will power by allowing the child to make simple choices, thereby establishing independence. The development of self-pride and beginning positive self-esteem is enhanced by this process (see Table 9-1).

Accomplishing Tasks. Although curiosity should be encouraged, this is the stage of development in which caregivers must begin to establish *limit setting* for the child. At this young age, simple, consistent guidance is important. The child needs to know exactly what behaviors are expected and what is unacceptable. This guidance enables the toddler to learn right from wrong. It also sets a pattern for later years, when rules and regulations evolve into discipline.

Cognitive Development

Intellectual and social development becomes more evident as the toddler grows physically.

At 1 Year. The happy, mobile 1-year-old has passed through several peak stages of accomplishments (equilibrium) and several stages of frequent frustrations (disequilibrium). The growth rate is slowing, and social, physiologic, and psychological functions also advance at a slower rate. This does not mean that new skills do not appear—the creeping 1-year-old becomes a dashing, climbing explorer at 15 months—but the peak periods of accomplishment are farther apart.

Verbal skills also improve; toddlers, by 1½ years, have a vocabulary of about 20 to 30 words, although they understand many more, as shown by their ability to follow directions. Social contacts begin to broaden at this age as the toddler shares playtime with other children. However, the toddler seems to play next to playmates rather than with them. This *parallel play* will continue until social skills are better developed.

At 18 Months. At 18 months, the child is much more difficult to live with than is the 1-year-old. At age 1, the baby was sociable, cheerful, and friendly most of the time, but by 18 months the baby is beginning to sense that certain aspects of the environment can be controlled. The baby starts to take advantage of this to the fullest. The 18-month-old is a "no" creature in all respects and usually rejects all demands. This child is also a "now" creature who has no ability to wait. Sharing is beyond comprehension, and everything is taken to and for the baby. It seems that the greatest consolation and pleasures are gained from always being the opposition.

The 18-month-old can climb up the stairs without help but often crawls. Generally, this child cannot go down the stairs. The child runs on level ground, seldom falls, and can pull a toy along. The child can throw a ball to another person without falling down and can turn pages in a book two or three at a time. The 18-month-old can identify certain items in a book as well as indicate his or her own nose, eyes, and ears.

At 2 Years. The 2-year-old is good natured, warmly affectionate, and easily pleased, a joy to the family. As the mid-toddler learns to moves with more sureness and safety, the surroundings are explored with interest. However, because this child is accident prone, definite limits must be set.

Neuromuscular coordination has increased so that the 2-year-old can put on and take off simple items of clothing, such as slip-on shirts; can climb stairs without crawling (both feet on each step); and can throw or kick a large ball. The tower of blocks he or she builds is now five to seven blocks high; the toddler loves to knock it over and set it up again. The 2-year-old can string large beads, scribble with crayons, turn a doorknob, put on socks and pants, wash hands, and turn book pages one at a time.

The typical 2-year-old likes riding toys (Fig. 9-4). These children become frustrated with toys they cannot manage or with things they cannot do. Emotions are close to the surface—extremely happy or very sad. They love activity, noise, water, animals, and other people, as long as they get their own way. At the same time, they want to be accepted by the family.

Preschool

Physical Growth

Physically, the 3-year-old preschooler has a full set of baby (deciduous) teeth, consisting of 10 upper and 10 lower teeth. The child weighs about 13.6 to 15.6 kg (30–35 lb) and is 76 to 91 cm (30–36 in.) tall. Although the 3-year-old has achieved about half of the eventual adult height, the physical development is slowing. The child will probably gain less than 2.7 kg (6 lb) per year and about 7.6 cm (3 in.) annually, until entering school. Physical skills, however, are more refined. The 3-year-old can dress and undress almost completely, manage large buttons and zippers, form objects with clay, and draw recognizable forms, such as a square or a person.

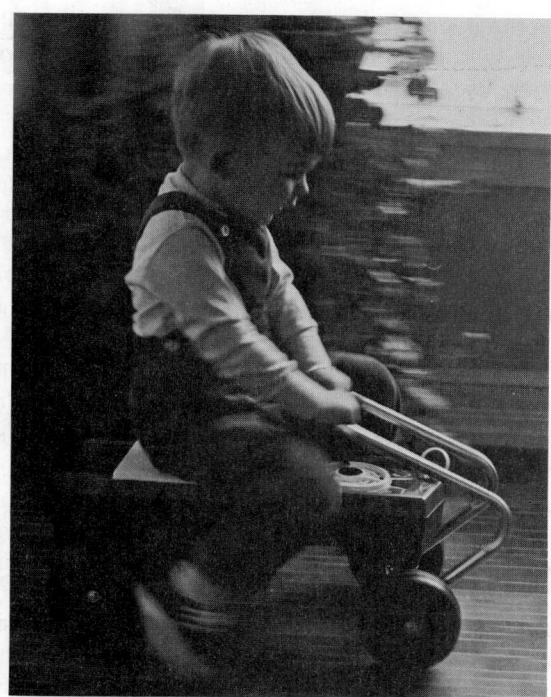

Figure 9-4. The typical 2-year-old likes toys to ride. He is a dynamo of constant activity; he never stops.

Psychosocial Development

The total family functions as the significant "person" in the life of the preschooler (ages 3–5). Individual independence continues to be important. Constant talking and questioning allow the preschooler to learn the "whys" and "what we can be." The child begins to learn sexual roles through fantasies and games. The child also becomes aware of and sometimes anxious about body differences.

Initiative Versus Guilt. According to Erikson, the preschooler must acquire *initiative*, the ability to take action without being told to. Otherwise a sense of guilt will prevail. The virtues for this age group are *direction* and *purpose* (see Table 9-1).

Cognitive Development

At 3 Years. The child at 3 years is in a stage of happy, conforming equilibrium. The "no" changes to "yes," and the routines become more flexible. The increased motor and language skills enable the 3-year-old to accomplish the developmental tasks required at this age, sometimes called the "trusting threes."

The 3-year-old child climbs up stairs, alternating feet, but must put both feet on each step while coming down; the child jumps off the bottom step. Three-year-olds can stand on one foot and ride a tricycle; they build towers with 9 or 10 blocks and can copy a circle on paper. Intellectually, growth has progressed to the point where the child can count to three or higher, identify objects in pictures, and tell which of several objects are alike. The vocabulary numbers about 1,000 words, which are used in incessant talk. The ability to use words also reflects the growing ability to reason; the child asks questions constantly.

The child of 3 years has a great desire to be independent and to do everything alone. The child can brush the teeth although muscular coordination and judgment are not developed to the point where the child can regularly perform this task properly. Parental supervision is essential. Three-year-olds are able to put on most of their own clothes and eat alone.

During this *oedipal stage*, when attention and interest focus on the parent of the opposite sex, the child may feel competitive and jealous toward the other parent; a boy talks of marrying his mother, and a girl of marrying her father. The child may copy the actions of the caregiver of the same sex as the child.

Generally, the child tries hard to do what is expected and to be obedient and helpful. The child is becoming sensitive to social interactions and is easily hurt by being scolded.

Socially, the child of 3 or 4 is beginning to play with other children, as well as next to them, and can make up simple games. The 3-year-old learns to share and to wait a turn. Play differences between boys and girls may develop. Some girls may show a preference for quiet play, such as card games, dolls, and coloring. In contrast, some boys may prefer rough and loud games; they play with trucks, balls, and hammers and other tools. (It is likely that these play preferences are caused by the different ways society expects girls and boys to act.)

The play and growth activities of the 3-year-old proceed with ease and delight. Wants and ability to carry out desires are well balanced; the child is pleased with self and playmates. This child is friendly and willing to share. Friendliness and interest in words and in sharing thoughts and knowledge make the 3-year-old an enjoyable and entertaining companion.

At 3½ Years. At age 3½, there is a great alteration in behavior; again, disequilibrium appears in many phases. The smooth motor functions of 3 may be replaced by clumsy actions or falling. Children commonly stutter at this age; they may seem to be tense and insecure; they may suck their thumb more and often are jittery and whiny. This new, uncertain child is in continual need of the sort of attention and affection lavished on the 3-year-old.

At 4 Years. At 4, the pendulum again swings to the opposite extreme. Uncertainty and insecurity are traded for the brashest self-confidence. The 4-year-old looks at a wider world (even if it does extend only to the corner of the block) and is sure it can be conquered. It is difficult for parents to preserve some of this confidence while firmly controlling it. The 4-year-old is described as being "out of bounds in most directions." The child now has a speaking vocabulary of at least 2,000 words and can probably count to 15 or 20. Four-year-olds can usually print part of their name and can state their age and full name. Many 4-year-olds also know their address and phone number.

In social relationships, the child tries hard to be a friend and get along with others. When quarreling, boys of this age often engage in physical fighting, including hitting, kicking, and biting; girls are more likely to yell at each other in their disagreements.

At age 4½, children like to draw and build with a purpose in mind. They want to be sure that things are "real" and enjoy talking about what they think and know.

At 5 Years. Many parents find it difficult to believe that their frustrating 4-year-old could be transformed into their "angel" of 5. The child is comfortable with self and with relations with others. The child is satisfied with the world of home and family although many 5-year-olds live in a land of make-believe, peopled by imaginary playmates and an imaginary family with fanciful names. The developmental tasks that have been mastered are sufficient for the moment. The 5-year-old is a "good" child, pleased with the equilibrium of his or her interests and skills.

School Age

Physical Growth

As the child approaches 6, the deciduous teeth are lost and the permanent teeth begin to erupt. From the time a child enters school, a slow, steady period of growth begins. The child will gain about 2.3 to 3.2 kg (5–7 lb) a year and will grow about 6.4 cm (2½ in.) a year until *puberty* (sexual maturity, from a Latin word meaning adult), at which time the young person will have a growth spurt. From age 6 or 7 until puberty, it becomes difficult to identify an "average" growth rate because the variations among normal children are wide.

Psychosocial Development

During the school years, the significant person for the child changes from the maternal person or caregiver to persons from the child's school or neighborhood. *Independence* is important. Learning to produce things (schoolwork, projects) takes precedence. The child ex-

plores the ever-expanding world and begins to collect pets, dolls, rocks, baseball cards, video games, books, or other objects.

Developing a Sense of Industry. The development of a sense of *industry* is the major psychosocial challenge for the school-age child (6–12 years). If this is not accomplished, the result is a feeling of inferiority.

Developing Self-worth. The school-age child needs recognition for accomplishments, such as school achievements, participation in groups (Cub Scouts, Girl or Boy Scouts, 4-H, sports, band, or orchestra). This will lead to feelings of *competence* and *self-worth*, the virtues of this stage of development.

Sibling Rivalry. Sibling rivalry, the competition between brothers and sisters, can lead to jealousy, trauma, and many verbal arguments, and sometimes physical fights. This is a natural occurrence. Brothers and sisters compete, whether as preschoolers or schoolchildren. Parents can become referees in their attempt to maintain a calm family atmosphere. Each child must be treated equally and fairly. As siblings progress through the school years, they should be responsible for resolving their own differences. Parents should be aware of the inevitability of sibling rivalry and intervene only when absolutely necessary.

Member of the Family. The school-age child should also have some responsibilities in the home. These may be as simple as cleaning the bedroom, setting and clearing the table, washing dishes or loading the dishwasher, taking out the trash, or walking the family pet. These tasks allow the child to acquire a sense of *responsibility* (see Table 9-1).

Cognitive Development

At 6 Years. Parents and family have been ousted from first place; the 6-year-old thinks that he or she is the most important and the best. Because the child of 6 always has to be first, it is difficult for the family. The eruptions now after the quiescent behavior of the 5-year-old is sometimes incomprehensible to parents. A squashy, squeezing "I love you" may be followed by "I hate you" 2 minutes later. Six-year-olds recognize no needs of others and insist that everyone yield to their demands. The saving grace is an eagerness to try new situations and an enthusiasm for learning and adventure. If self-development and reaching out from the family can be accepted by parents as a big step forward, understanding will soften the difficulties.

Because school occupies much of the child's waking hours, events at school begin to play a large part in the life of a 6-year-old. As children explore this new world beyond home, they become increasingly independent.

The child is interested in everything, is anxious to learn, and is eager to please the teacher. The teacher usually can do no wrong and is described in the most glowing terms. The 6-year-old asks questions in a never-ending search for information.

The child's reasoning and conceptual powers expand. Six-year-olds can tell time and can count to at least 40 or 50; typically, they can recognize the letters of the alphabet, the numbers from 1 to 10, and their own name. In fact, the child may be able to read simple words, and the speaking vocabulary numbers at least 2,500 words. As the year progresses, the 6-year-old will learn to read more, to count to about 100 and to subtract numbers up to 10.

At 7 Years. The child of 7 is sensitive and presents a changed picture. Often, the 7-year-old becomes quiet and thoughtful and tends to worry and daydream. Seven-year-olds crave adult approval and are sensitive to criticism; they are described by some authorities as moody. The child observes, listens, reads—this is an age of learning. The sense of touch becomes a source of knowledge; the child loves to feel things, to explore by touching, rubbing, and crumbling. The 7-year-old has a reasonable enjoyment of life, but seems to enjoy unhappiness too: "You don't love me"; "I'm going to run away"; "You're mean to me." Many children want a retreat of their own. Boys and girls of this age are aware of each other but typically prefer not to play together. In fact, they are usually antagonistic and may fight and call each other unkind names.

As these children approach 8, they gain self-confidence and poise and again become more stable and better able to cope with the world.

At 8 Years. If the 7-year-old is quiet and withdrawn, the 8-year-old bounces back into life. New facts and difficult tasks are joyful challenges for the child. Eight-year-olds are extremely active, daring, and unaware of danger; hence, they can be injured easily. Self-confidence is so great that they do not believe any harm can befall them. Enthusiasm and energy often cause the 8-year-old to undertake too much. Guidance is needed to prevent complex projects from becoming repeated failures and to prevent overexertion. Fortunately, at this age, children appreciate how others treat them and also are concerned about how they affect others. A child of 8 is good for the parent's ego because, although to the sensitive 7-year-old, the parent was a trial, the 8-year-old enjoys, needs, and wants the parents' company.

Friends occupy an important place in the life of an 8-year-old; the child will do almost anything for them (Fig. 9-5). The members of the "gang" or clique usually share secrets, including a favorite hangout. Boys and girls may fight openly at times.

At 9 Years. Nine-year-olds are independent and individual. At 7, children need to investigate and to learn about themselves. At 8, they need to measure relationships with the outside world. At 9, they begin to coordinate the developmental patterns of ages 7 and 8. Being self-reliant, the 9-year-old is able to make most decisions pertaining to customary activities. The family circle may seem too constricting, and the child wants to become involved in interests and activities outside the family.

Much time is spent with friends or with other clubs and groups. This age is sometimes referred to as "noisy nine." Despite all evidences of self-reliance, the 9-year-old worries a great deal and complains about tasks that involve responsibility, schoolwork, and home chores. However, the child often works hard at learning, for example, by experimenting with a chemistry set or by reading voraciously. Both boys and girls love stories of adventure and imagination and search endlessly for imaginary or real heroes to emulate. This is the age of

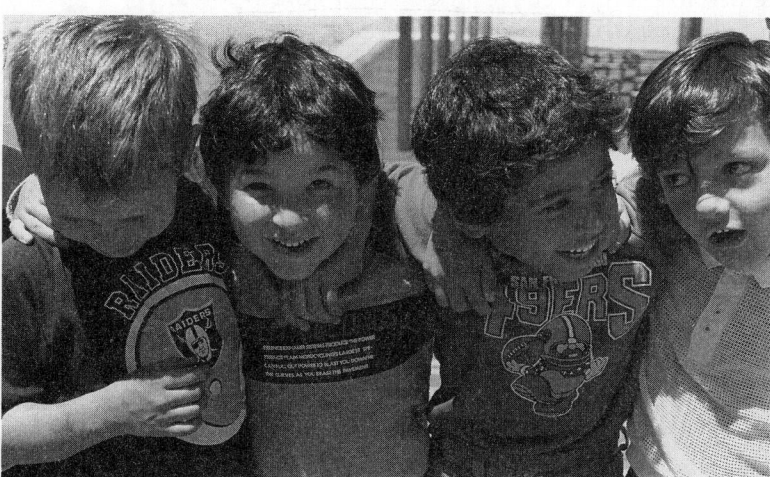

Figure 9-5. During the school years, identity is influenced by the peer group. (©1990, Kathy Sloane)

"hero worship," when photographs and stories of an outstanding athlete or movie star are collected and cherished. Many collect autographs.

At 10 Years. The child at age 10 is a more mature version of the delightful child of 5. Typical 5-year-olds accept themselves and others and are pleased with the world. Typical 10-year-olds are also satisfied children, enjoying the family, school, and life in general, as well as being obedient because it is reasonable and pleasing. Friendly and realistic, 10-year-olds accept themselves and life as it comes. Never again will parents enjoy such complete approval and acceptance of themselves both as parents and as people as that offered by their agreeable 10-year-old.

Areas of Concern

Parental Guidance

Most parents enjoy watching the progress of their children if they have a greater understanding of the developmental stages. Parents are happier if they see changes in their children as signs of growth and progress. The instinctive curiosity of children and their physical growth carry them to new fields to conquer. The challenge in being a parent is to allow the child to develop in such a way that the eagerness to learn is maintained.

Sincere concern for long-range development of their children leads many parents to seek knowledge that will foster greater understanding and happy parent–child relationships. Many cities have parenting classes as a regular part of the adult education curriculum. Such knowledge and understanding do not eliminate the need for parental discipline and guidance; rather, they enhance it and encourage mutual respect within the family. Understanding the needs and the problems of children will supply parents with clues to more effective methods of control or discipline for each stage and age. It will offer support to both parents and children in working toward their mutual goal of increased abilities, skills, self-knowledge, and self-discipline.

Certain areas of childhood behavior are of concern to parents. These concerns should be handled on an individual basis. Emphasis is placed on recognition of the child's pace of development and the natural ability of each child.

Bottle Feedings and Weaning

Infants should be held while being fed by bottle or breast. A serious dental condition known as *nursing bottle syndrome* can occur if the infant is placed in bed with the bottle propped for feeding. The sweetness of the liquid pools in the mouth cavities and emerging teeth develop caries (decay) as a result.

Weaning (changing from one form of feeding to another) usually begins around the sixth month. The caregiver slowly removes one bottle or breast feeding a day, using a cup in its place. To be ready for weaning from the breast or bottle, the infant should be able to sit up unsupported, have hand-to-mouth motions, and have head and neck control.

Sucking Reflexes and the Security Blanket

Infants need to develop their sucking reflexes. They will suck on their thumbs, fists, and fingers when they are not feeding. Sucking is a comfort and relieves tension and anxiety. A pacifier may be used for sucking when the infant is tired or fussy. Many parents allow the infant to use a pacifier beyond the age of 1 year.

Thumb-sucking may begin at around 3 or 4 months of age. Most infants pop everything into their mouths by the time they reach 7 months, and the thumb is a handy object. Usually by age 2, the child sucks the thumb only when tired or hungry. The 3-year-old often has a strong affection for the thumb and for a favorite blanket or soft toy. At 4, most children are ready to surrender the blanket.

Most dental authorities agree that damage can be done by thumb-sucking, especially during the eruption of the baby teeth. The long-term effects of the habit depend on factors such as frequency, duration, and intensity. The more frequent the sucking and the greater the percentage of time it is practiced, the higher the potential for permanent damage to mouth structure.

It is difficult to force a child to stop thumb-sucking. Suggestions include:

◆ Substitute a pacifier for the thumb. It is softer and less damaging to the teeth and does not provide sugar, as would a bottle.
◆ Try to redirect behavior into another activity.
◆ Praise the child when he or she avoids sucking the thumb for a period of time.
◆ Call the thumb-sucking to the child's attention (it is often an unconscious habit).
◆ Give the child a little extra attention; the thumb-sucking may reflect insecurity or loneliness.

Peer pressure may eventually embarrass the child and cause thumb-sucking to stop. The child who is ill, even when older, often gains comfort from the previously relinquished thumb, blanket, or stuffed toy.

Rocking and Head-Banging

Rocking and head-banging are also habits that usually lose their usefulness to the child as other outlets become available. If bed rocking has not stopped by the time a child is 3 or 4, moving to a bigger bed usually resolves it. Head-banging sometimes causes bruises, and therefore is worrisome to parents. Children who do this have many other characteristics in common, such as sleeping restlessly, having strong likes and dislikes, and resisting if not permitted to have their own way. Spanking, scolding, and other punishments do not stop head-banging. Picking up the child will be a momentary distraction. Because most children enjoy music, a record player or radio played softly in their room will sometimes help them to relax.

Masturbation

Even a 1-year-old infant likes to touch and handle things, finding that touching certain parts of the body gives pleasant sensations. **Masturbation** is the term given to the handling of the genital organs, usually to orgasm (climax). A preschool child may find that handling the genitals relieves tensions rising from conflict with parents. There is nothing abnormal or shameful about this practice if a child is taught that, if it is practiced, it should be done in privacy but never in public. Shaming, threatening, or punishing a child for masturbating may be damaging to later sexual expression. A happy, busy child is not likely to seek frequent comfort in masturbation.

Toilet Training

Toilet training is a major developmental accomplishment. It requires parental patience and encouragement. Toddlers are ready for toilet training when they can sit comfortably on a toilet or potty without assistance, can walk forward and backward, are able to remove clothing with elastic bands, and are able to stay dry for at least 2 hours. Behavioral changes before or after the child wets or soils indicate the child's emotional readiness. Readiness emerges usually between 18 and 30 months of age.

Bowel training is usually accomplished with less effort than bladder training, but this may not be true for some children (especially boys). Some perfectly normal children still do not have total conscious control by 5 years of age. Most parents are relieved, however, to find that toilet training, barring occasional accidents, is well under way by 3 years of age.

Bed-wetting

Bed-wetting (*enuresis*) is a problem more likely to occur in boys. In most cases, the underlying reason is simply physiologic or emotional immaturity. Getting the child up during the night or restricting fluids between the evening meal and bedtime sometimes helps. If the bed-wetting persists (and physical and psychol-

ogic problems have been eliminated), other measures can be tried.

Continued enuresis may be a sign of a dysfunctional family or child abuse. The nurse may need to refer the child for further assistance.

Some children have an "irritable" bladder, a condition in which a small amount of urine in the bladder produces the desire to urinate. In this case, the physician may order a drug to decrease the irritability. The child also can be encouraged to withhold the urine voluntarily during the daytime. This gradually distends the bladder, increasing its size and promoting retention.

Building Self-esteem

Probably the greatest single factor in chemical dependency, suicide attempts, and depression in later life is the lack of self-esteem. Self-esteem comes from a lifetime of feeling wanted and loved. In the book, *Self-Esteem: A Family Affair*, hints are given for building self-esteem and a feeling of worthiness.[1] Following are ways of telling children they are worthwhile and loved:

◆ Birth to age 6 months: The job of the infant is *being*. The baby needs to trust others, self, and the world. Parents should fulfill the baby's needs in a loving way; they let the baby be dependent now, so that independence can develop later.

◆ 6 to 18 months: The job of the toddler is *doing*. The toddler needs to explore; it is okay to let the child taste, chew, and feel safe in the environment.

◆ 18 months to 3 years: The job of the child from 1½ to 3 years is *thinking*. Children need to be allowed to express anger and to assert themselves, to think for themselves, to start to separate from parents, and to say "no."

◆ 3 to 5 years: The 3- to 5-year old child has to *learn who he is*. It is important to establish a personal identity; to expand imagination, but know what is real; and to become socially acceptable to others.

◆ 6 to 12 years: The job of 6- to 12-year-olds is to *do things their own way*. Adults need to allow school-age children to test rules and authority, to test their parents' personal values, and to receive answers and help with formulating their own internal values.

---

[1] Clarke JI. Self Esteem: A Family Affair. New York, Harper & Row, 1980. Quoted with permission.

Keys for Review

Key Questions for Critical Thinking

1. Explain the concepts of growth and development and describe the differences between them.
2. Describe some of the characteristics of the child at various stages: during the first year of life; at 1 year; at 1½ years; at 2 years; at 2½ years; at 3 years; at 3½ years; at 4 years; at 5 years; and during the early school years.
3. Discuss how play is related to child development.
4. Identify ways in which to build the child's self-esteem at various ages.

Key Readings

Castiglia PT, Harbin RE. Child Health Care: Process and Practice. Philadelphia, J.B. Lippincott, 1992

Craven RF, Hirnle CJ. Fundamentals of Nursing: Human Health and Function. Philadelphia, J.B. Lippincott, 1992

Erikson E. Childhood and Society, Ed 2. New York, Norton, 1963

Erikson E. Identity and the Life Cycle. New York, Norton, 1980

Friedman MM. Family Nursing: Theory and Assessment, Ed 3. Norwalk, CT, Appleton & Lange, 1992

Havighurst RJ. Developmental Tasks and Education, Ed 3. New York, David McKay, 1972

Key Readings (continued)

Hughes FP, Noppe LD. Human Development Across the Lifespan. New York, Merrill, 1990

Jackson DB, Saunders RB. Child Health Nursing: A Comprehensive Approach to the Care of Children and their Families. Philadelphia, J.B. Lippincott, 1993

Schuster CS, Smith-Ashburn SS. The Process of Human Development: A Holistic Life-Span Approach, Ed 3. Philadelphia, J.B. Lippincott, 1992

Scipien GM, Bernard MU, et al. Comprehensive Pediatric Nursing, Ed 4. St. Louis, Mosby-Year Book, 1990

Taylor C, Lillis C, LeMone P. Fundamentals of Nursing: The Art and Science of Nursing Care, Ed 2. Philadelphia, J.B. Lippincott, 1993

Wadsworth B. Piaget's Theory of Cognitive and Affective Development, Ed 4. New York, Longman, 1989

Whaley L, Wong D. Nursing Care of Infants and Children, Ed 4. St. Louis, C.V. Mosby, 1991

Keys to Learning More

Chapter 12: developmental tasks for adults

Unit Four: anatomy and physiology

Unit Twelve: fetal development; pregnancy; childbirth; newborns

Unit Thirteen: deviations from normal growth and development in children

10 Preadolescence and Adolescence

Keys for Learning

Learning Objectives

- State common characteristics of young people at ages 10, 11, and 12
- Describe the specific physical changes that occur in boys and girls between the ages of 10 and 18
- Describe the emotional development that occurs during adolescence
- Design a plan for presenting information concerning human sexuality to adolescents of different ages
- Discuss the appropriate disciplining for an adolescent

Key Terms

adolescence

peer group

preadolescence

puberty

Keys to Understanding This Chapter

Chapter 5: basic human needs

Chapter 9: growth and development theories; growth and development in infancy and childhood

Key Points

- The period of adolescence is a turbulent time, marked by rapid physical growth and frequent emotional upheavals.
- Great variation exists in physical and emotional maturity among young people of the same age during the period of preadolescence.

Key Points (continued)

- The developmental tasks of preadolescence and adolescence center around formulation of a self-image and establishment of goals for the future, as well as building relationships with other people.

Key Topics Outline

Growth and Development Theories
  Developmental Tasks
  Psychosocial Development
  Cognitive Development
Preadolescence
  Physical Growth
  Psychosocial and Cognitive Development
Adolescence
  Physical Growth
  Psychosocial and Cognitive Development
Areas of Concern
  Parental Guidance
  Building Self-esteem

Key Learning Activities

- Interview several adolescent mothers. What types of parenting classes are available? What other educational facilities are available to them? How do they support themselves? Who cares for their children?
- Interview a junior high and a senior high guidance counselor. What challenges do they identify among their students?

Developmental Tasks of Adolescence as Described by Havighurst

Adolescence (12–18 Years)

Develop appropriate and mature relationships with peers of both sexes

Achieve emotional independence

Accept physique and use body effectively

Develop social roles of one's culture

Prepare for adult life and for marriage or other relationships

Prepare for career, education, or other pursuits

Acquire values and ethics, develop ideology

Behave in a socially acceptable way

Childhood developmental tasks are discussed in Chapter 9.

Puberty is the period in life when a person becomes sexually able to reproduce. Adolescence is the period of development between puberty and maturity. Adolescence may be divided into preadolescence and adolescence and may range from around 11 years to 18 to 20 years, at which time the person enters early adulthood. Adolescence is marked by a rapid growth spurt, at the end of which the individual will have achieved adult height. Although tremendous physical growth occurs, emotional needs predominate during this period; the adolescent spends much time searching for meaning in life and for a sense of identity.

The adolescent is required to make critical choices that may well determine the outcome of the rest of his or her life. Some of these choices include the use of alcohol and other substances, moral obligations and respect for other people, school attendance, relationships (regarding friends, sexuality, and marriage), education after high school, and career choice.

Growth and Development Theories

Developmental Tasks

Developmental tasks for the adolescent, as described by the theorist Havighurst, are listed in the accompanying box. The ultimate task of the adolescent is to "grow up." The success of each child in progress to maturity is determined by heredity and environment, the culture in which he or she lives, and the young person's own self-determination and perceptions about self.

Although authorities define the components of achieving maturity in various ways, they generally agree on certain important steps. All tasks ultimately involve achieving independence from parental domination and the acceptance of individual responsibility.

For instance, emancipation from parental ties is seen in the form of intellectual, emotional, and economic independence. Further, to initiate and maintain satisfactory interpersonal relations with both sexes, the adult must have developed wholesome concepts of self-identity, self-respect, and self-control. To be free to decide on a course of action, the mature adult must develop and recognize the purpose of actions and be willing to accept personal responsibilities and social obligations.

Psychosocial Development

The emerging adult faces many decisions during preadolescence and adolescence. These decisions concern the future and the adult world. What vocation should I choose? Should I go to college? Can I afford further education? Do the courses I am taking in high school meet the college's admission criteria? Should I join the military? Should I get married? Should I have a baby even though I am not married? Should I live with my parents or move out?

You learned about Erikson's theory of psychosocial development in Chapter 9 and Table 9-1. Table 10-1 continues this list as it relates to the adolescent.

Table 10-1. Erikson's Theory of Psychosocial Development in Adolescence

Theory Concept	Adolescence
Basic Tasks	Personal identity vs. role confusion
Significant Other	Peer group Opposite sex Family
Psychosocial Challenge	Make life decisions Achieve personal identity Accept responsibility
Virtues	Independence, self-reliance, self-esteem, self-control, devotion, fidelity
How Accomplished	Provide privacy Encourage activities Support decisions Allow independence Give recognition, acceptance Good family relationships Facilitate information gathering

Erikson's theory for children is presented in Chapter 9. Adult psychosocial development is discussed in Chapters 11 and 12.

Personal Identity. The major challenge of adolescence, according to Erikson, is the achievement of *identity*. Who am I? Where am I going? With whom? And how am I going to get there? If this phase is not resolved, the result is *role confusion*.

Peer Group. The **peer group** is made up of contemporaries, a group of people with whom one associates. The peer group is extremely important to the adolescent, often more important than the family. The peer group influences the adolescent in many ways. Peer pressure to try cigarettes, alcohol, marijuana, or other drugs can be the first step to chemical dependency or drug abuse. The peer group can determine whether or not the young person gets good grades in school, joins the military, or buys a car.

A relationship with a member of the opposite sex is an important factor in the development of the young person's identity as a future adult. This also influences how the person will feel as an accepted member or nonmember of the peer group. Sexual identity may also be confusing.

Cognitive Development

According to Piaget's theory, the person from 12 to 15 years enters stage IV of cognitive development—formal operations. The child can think in the abstract and develops skills to participate in complex problem-solving.

Preadolescence

Preadolescence generally includes ages 11 through 13 years.

Physical Growth

Preadolescence is characterized by physical changes. Most boys at 11 do not yet show the changes of puberty. Some have started to grow rapidly again, but many have a heavier or more defined skeletal structure.

Girls show great variation in physical structure and sexual development. The average 11-year-old girl has begun a period of rapid growth and shows signs of approaching sexual maturity. Healthy curiosity and occasional embarrassment accompany awareness of female curves, with the beginning of breast development and an increase in the width of the pelvis. Most girls at 12 gain height and weight rapidly. Breast development is definite. Menstruation most commonly begins during the 12th or 13th year, but early periods frequently are irregular.

Physical growth is markedly varied in 12-year-old boys. The average boy shows some pubertal changes by the end of this year. Spontaneous erections and occasional ejaculations without external cause occur and are confusing to him. He should understand that involuntary discharge of semen while sleeping (*nocturnal emission*) is a normal part of reproductive health and is as natural as a change in voice or the appearance of chin whiskers. Twelve-year-old boys are often interested in sex from the viewpoint of their own development, rather than in relation to adult sexual activity.

Most young people have reached 90% of their adult height by age 12 or 13. They have at least tripled in height and gained 15 times in weight since birth.

By the completion of their 13th year, most girls have reached adult height and have established menstrual periods. Boys have begun a time of rapid growth and experience erections. Only about half will have had nocturnal emissions although most know about this. Thirteen-year-olds have all of their permanent teeth except the wisdom teeth.

Cognitive Development

At 11 Years. The difficulties and restlessness of the 11-year-old period are not regressions to earlier stages. The 11-year-old is an "adolescent in the making." Negativeness is a form of self-assertion, a beginning step in the establishment of the mature "I." Constant talk and arguments and seeming impudence and rudeness indicate inexperience in mastering new developmental tasks.

The typical child of 11 is a physical and emotional dynamo (Fig. 10-1). Even while apparently sitting still, the child is in constant motion, stretching, wiggling, jiggling, waving the arms, clicking the feet together, and generally finding it impossible to remain still.

Rebellion against parents, noisy and fault-finding quarrels with siblings, and constant evasion of household tasks are irritating to the family. Patience is necessary, and the child needs to be handled with both understanding and firmness. As this person attempts new undertakings to test independence and self-reliance, he or she needs strong support and guidance from parents. That the child behaves best away from home gives a clue to self-discipline and to other possibilities in the future emotional growth pattern.

At 12 Years. At 12, there is improvement in meeting the challenges of maturity. The typical 12-year-old is more controlled emotionally and better able to see situations in perspective. The psychological awareness of age 12 has broadened beyond self. A youth of this age has gained more objectivity toward self and others. This, along with a growing sense of humor, makes family associations much more pleasant.

Because the child of 12 is so enthusiastic, this young person brings spirit and buoyancy to all undertakings. Extensive projects in school show initiative and effort.

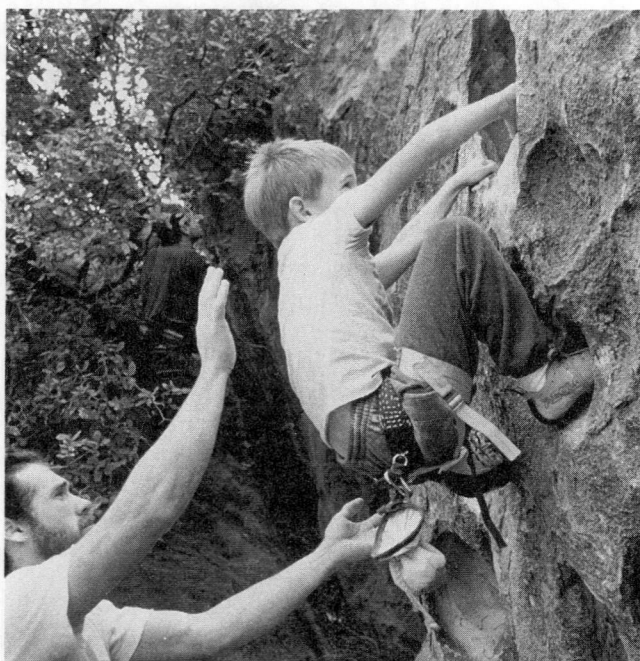

Figure 10-1. Risk-taking behavior often marks early adolescence (Castiglia PT, Harbin RE. Child Health Care: Process and Practice. Philadelphia, J.B. Lippincott, 1992).

However, this high pitch of enthusiasm and initiative may get out of hand. Planned parties and social events need adult supervision, or the boisterous activity of this age can wreck the event.

There is a slight improvement in attitude toward chores, which are now regarded as necessities to be endured, but frequent reminding by parents is still needed; the young person realizes this.

With the gradual displacement of the imbalances of age 11, age 12 foreshadows adult potential. The enthusiasm, the occasional self-discipline, the humor, the intelligence, and the self-knowledge are clues to the mature young person who is to emerge.

At 13 Years. In contrast to the open spirit of the middle years of childhood, the 13-year-old shows tendencies to seclusion and moodiness. At the same time, this young person has become aware of and takes pleasure in emerging reasoning ability.

The young adolescent reflects on self and others and assesses new experiences. Appraisal of interaction between self and the world needs a place as well as time, so the young teenager tends to spend more time alone. Assessment of the world naturally includes assessment of the family. Criticisms and withdrawals are often a source of puzzlement, as well as hurt, to parents. Both girls and boys have long associations with the mirror, which they use a prop for role-playing and for testing and measuring themselves in imagined situations.

The 13-year-old has taken further steps to social maturity. Some authorities think that at no other stage of development is there such a need for conformity to the group. At the same time, there is a tremendous need for individuality. Through this year and the remaining years of adolescence, the maturing adolescent takes frequent flights of independence but has a strong need to return to the "nest" for guidance and encouragement. As always in developmental progression, patterns are tempered and adjusted by the individual person.

Adolescence

Adolescence includes ages 14 through the late teen years.

Physical Growth

Glandular changes, alterations in body chemistry, developmental challenges, plus an ever-increasing capacity to consume food, provide a great supply of energy in the adolescent.

By the age of 14, most girls have the physical appearance of young women. Few will grow after age 14. Breasts and other secondary sex characteristics are those of an adult. Most boys grow more at 14 than at any other age. A strong, muscular appearance and continued deepening of the voice add to the impression of maturity. Nocturnal emissions have begun for most; if boys are properly informed, they accept it is a natural occurrence.

By 15, adult physical characteristics have already developed in most girls. The menstrual cycle has become regular. The girl of 14 to 16 is generally ready to accept menstruation as part of adult life. Most boys at 16 are close to their adult height.

Reproductive organs are adult size; secondary sex characteristics are pronounced. Sexual response is more directed and less subject to other stimuli, such as fear.

Cognitive Development

At 14 Years. The introspection of the 13-year-old gives way to the comparative ease of the 14-year-old, who experiences a relaxation of inner and outer tensions and greater self-assurance. The 14-year-old is more accepting of other people as individuals and more conscious of what makes other personalities unique. A sense of humor releases tensions that previously taxed family relationships. Although less critical and more tolerant of parents, the 14-year-old still tends to regard them and their ideas as antiques. The 14-year-old likes his or her brothers and sisters "more than he thought he did." "Talk, talk, talk, talk" is many an adult's version of this age. Some authorities state that this is a true growth characteristic and a developmental achievement of 14-year-olds (to verbalize ideas). They show increased natural ability in perceiving more than one side of a situation and are no longer frustrated by being unable to express or verbalize ideas. They are able to say what they *think*, a task of maturity.

At 15 Years. This "middle year" is baffling to many parents. It has been described as the phase when the nicest children behave in the "most awful way." The physical alterations, loud self-assertion, preoccupation with self, rapid shifts between dependent and independent attitudes, blithe spirit, and moody introspection are real challenges to even the most interested and conscientious parent.

The teenager is pulling away from childhood in a quest for *self-reliance* (see Table 10-1). Although the adolescent values the ability to depend on home and school, there is a need to counterbalance it with independence. Because the young person is searching for balance, immaturity frequently results in withdrawal, belligerence, or defiance. This first step into juvenile delinquency may be taken. All parental directions are viewed as efforts to control the young person completely, and the adolescent may seek guidance away from home.

The 15-year-old has ideas about the future and has begun to plan for more than present interests and activities. Vague ideas of marrying and of having a home and a career result in scrutiny of home and parents. Parents may feel that they have been rejected because they failed to meet the perfectionist standards of their observing 15-year-old. Yet the youth of 15 has a better relationship with siblings than before.

Increased independence and interest in the opposite sex now cause the young person to take more responsibility for self-care and personal cleanliness. At age 15, the adolescent likes to choose clothing and usually makes more clothing purchases than in previous years. There is general improvement in the care of clothes as well as in the care of the room. However, the typical 15-year-old is not a good helper at home. Interest is shown in working away from home because a job provides money. If the 15-year-old recognizes that money comes as a result of personal effort, a savings account may become important.

True attitudes of maturity are beginning to be evident in the middle teenager. In interpersonal relations, the young person is friendly and self-confident. Interest in people and an awareness and acceptance of social responsibilities make the middle teen years a companionable age, one with many friendships of both sexes.

The young person now recognizes sleep needs and makes plans to "catch-up" if tired, although school activities and part-time jobs may limit available "sleep time."

At 16 Years. The 16-year-old has made strides intellectually, as well as physically and emotionally. Judgment has been stimulated and developed by having accomplished the tasks of the preceding years. The older adolescent usually finds the ensuing years of adolescence happy and fruitful.

The next few years are those of further transition from adolescence through young adulthood, but there is no sharp line of demarcation to divide these years.

Areas of Concern

Preadolescents and adolescents develop physically and socially at various rates. As they take on more responsibilities, they may have special concerns, concerns that may be shared by their parents. These concerns deal with eating patterns, peer groups, skill development, sexuality and sex education, self-esteem, and family relationships. The nurse should be prepared to answer questions and give guidance similar to the items summarized in the accompanying box.

Nutrition

Boys, especially, have huge appetites, but occasionally the 15-year-old loses or gains weight for a specific purpose. Girls are often concerned about appearance and may go on a "starvation" diet. Anorexic or bulimic patterns of eating may emerge. (Bulemia is starving oneself by binge eating, followed by induced vomiting or excess use of laxatives.) The young person may indulge in a diet primarily of "junk food," high in fat, sugar, and empty calories.

Keys to Patient/Family Teaching
Adolescent Concerns

Patient/family teaching for the adolescent with concerns about growth and development includes:

◆ Development of healthy habits: cleanliness, balanced diet of food groups, sleep and rest, activity and exercise
◆ Safety measures with motor vehicles and bikes
◆ Importance of scholastic and skill achievement
◆ Importance and development of self-respect
◆ Selection of peers as friends
◆ Wise counseling about sex and sexuality
◆ Responsibilities resulting from sexual activity
◆ Problems that arise from substance use and abuse (cigarette smoking, alcohol, recreational drugs)

Peer Groups

Young people need to be part of a group of peers or close friends. Boys tend to be more tolerant and informal in groups, and their groups may be broadly inclusive. Girls, however, are often more selective or cliquish in forming peer groups.

Peer groups now take the place of the parents as sources of information and guidance. Peers can be a good or bad influence. Substance abuse or vandalism are examples of bad influences; examples of good influences are sports, music, drama, or scholastic achievement.

Skill Development

Skill development is part of cognitive growth, but it is also preparation for the future. Many skills developed in adolescent years will help in career choices. Many skills developed by young people are complex. Skill development may include such things as gymnastics, photography, writing, carpentry, auto mechanics, and dancing; acquiring leadership abilities and diplomacy; and participating in debate, school plays, science competitions, choral groups, orchestra, and band. Sports competition often becomes a primary interest. Cooking may appeal to both girls and boys. Some adolescents have never known life without computers, and they may develop a keen interest in experimenting with them. Adult encouragement and guidance are needed in skill development.

Sexuality, Sex, and Sex Education

Physical development is variable in adolescent years, but most preadolescents and adolescents have a curiosity about sex. If information is provided in a sensitive way by informed adults, adolescents can form healthy attitudes about sex (Fig. 10-2). If parents, teachers, or counselors do not give such information, adolescents will seek answers elsewhere. Unwholesome attitudes may develop from information they receive from their peers and older adolescents who appear to "have it all." The result may be early and unsafe sexual activities.

Dating may not be a routine practice, but mixed groups of young people may "hang out" together. Adolescents need to know that controls are necessary and why.

Sexual activity at a younger age is increasing. Even though birth control is available, many fail or refuse to use it. The number of births to adolescents is at an all-time high. In addition, the incidences of sexually transmitted diseases are on the rise. Gonorrhea, syphilis, genital warts, and acquired immunodeficiency syndrome are as serious a threat as pregnancy.

Further sex education is needed and accepted by adolescents. Parents may help to establish reasonable boundaries and, in doing so, present accurate information. Adolescents need the opportunity to discuss,

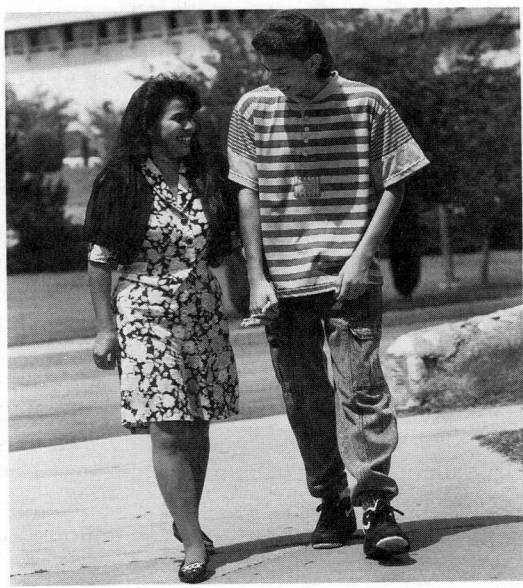

Figure 10-2. Establishing heterosexual relationships is a vital part of adolescence.

with both peers and concerned adults, the emotional conflicts involved with refusing and accepting sexual activity. Such discussions can help them make appropriate decisions. In instances where adolescents are sexually active, they should be counseled about "safer sex" and the use of condoms and birth control.

Nursing Alert

The adolescent should know that a condom is only about 80% effective against preventing sexually transmitted diseases and pregnancy. Only abstinence is 100% effective.

Family Relationships

Family relationships may be delicate in preadolescence. The attitude toward younger siblings may alternate between protectiveness and annoyance; the attitude toward parents varies and ranges from annoyance and criticism to genuine understanding. A wholesome family relationship at this time can influence lifetime interpersonal success because it fosters respect of self and others. The sense of self-respect is nourished by respect for and from others and is essential to psychological and emotional health. The parent's respect for the child's need for self-assertion, privacy, information, recognition, acceptance, experimentation, and growth in all developmental areas furnishes a firm foundation for the coming years. Family relationships may improve in adolescence.

The 15- or 16-year-old behaves so maturely that most parents naturally accept the attitude of independence.

The middle teenager has so many interests and associations outside the home that time spent with the family is limited, but the young person often consults parents about problems (if parents are willing to discuss them at the adult-to-adult level), and likes to feel free to have a home base where he or she can bring friends.

Parental Guidance

The importance of a wholesome family life is strongly supported by evidence. Homes are happy when family relationships are based on mutual respect and affection. Mutual respect recognizes the task of the parent to discipline the child, and the task of the child to adjust to discipline. The gradual growth to independence demands the development of self-discipline in the mature adult; children themselves agree that they need firm disciplinary measures, imposed fairly according to their age and the nature of their misbehavior. Many experts on child behavior agree that strict "discipline for discipline's sake" only stirs rebellion and undermines the child's self-respect. Parents need to be willing to "play the bad guy" for their children. For example, it is easier for an adolescent to say, "I have to go home at 10 because my mom said so," than it is to just go home at 10. Parents need to understand that this is a normal part of growing up; the adolescent is learning to make wise decisions and to take personal responsibility for those decisions. But the adolescent needs support from home, too.

The freedom of the adolescent to use the home as a base for friendships and personal activities, family conferences for planning or for problem-solving, wholesome companionship within the family, and acknowledged moral and ethical standards all furnish guidelines for learning to respect one's self and others and to live with others.

When the adolescent is loved, accorded a measure of freedom and responsibility, disciplined sensibly and respectfully, and encouraged to grow up and to achieve personal identity, he or she will naturally love and respect the parents, enjoy family life, and achieve a healthy, mature adulthood. In this way, the circle of parent-child relationships is successfully completed, and the relationships are oriented to a skillful and intelligent solution of the problems of adolescence. The future family life of young people, when they raise their own children, will probably be patterned after their past family experiences.

> ### Key Concept
> Parents need help in accepting their "child" as an "adult."

Building Self-esteem

Clarke's model for building positive self-esteem in young children was introduced in Chapter 9. Adolescents need positive self-esteem now more than ever in their development. The period of adolescence is filled with ups and downs; it is a time of upset and unrest. Adults can provide some stability and "positive strokes" to the young person who is searching for an identity in the world.

The adolescent must learn how to separate from the family. The young adult needs to emerge as an independent person with personal goals and values, to be responsible for his or her own future. Adults need to help the adolescent work through the previous stages of childhood, now with the added dimension of sexuality. Adults need to let the adolescent know they can accept all these adolescent shifts and still love him or her as a person.

Keys for Review

Key Questions for Critical Thinking

1. Describe the difference between the terms "puberty" and "adolescence".
2. Identify some of the key characteristics of the young person at each year of age between 11 and 16.
3. Discuss the role of the peer group to the adolescent.
4. Describe the differences in problems faced by preadolescents and adolescents.

Key Readings

Friedman MM. Family Nursing: Theory and Assessment, Ed 3. Norwalk, CT, Appleton & Lange, 1992

Hughes FP, Noppe LD. Human Development Across the Lifespan. New York, Merrill, 1990

Greenspan S, Pollock G (eds). The Course of Life. New York, International University Press, 1989; Vol. I: Infancy, 1989; Vol. II: Early Childhood, 1990; Vol. III: Middle and Late Childhood, 1991; Vol. IV: Adolescence, 1991

Key Readings (continued)

Jackson DB, Saunders, RB. Child Health Nursing: A Comprehensive Approach to the Care of Children and their Families. Philadelphia, J.B. Lippincott, 1993

Schuster CS, Smith-Ashburn SS. The Process of Human Development: A Holistic Life-Span Approach, Ed 3. Philadelphia, J.B. Lippincott, 1992

Keys to Learning More

Unit Four: anatomy and physiology

Chapter 25: puberty and menstruation

Chapter 63: sexuality, sexually transmitted diseases, fertility control, and infertility

Unit Thirteen: deviations from growth and development

11 Early and Middle Adulthood

![Keys for Learning]

Learning Objectives

- List at least five of Havighurst's developmental tasks for early adulthood and five for middle adulthood
- Describe Erikson's theory of psychosocial development as it applies to young adults and to middle adulthood
- Discuss how Levinson's "individual life structure" theory compares to Erikson's and Havighurst's theories
- Compare other theorists with Sheehy and her "phases of adulthood"
- Discuss the implications of life choices in early adulthood
- Take one aspect of life (eg, vocation, intimate relationship) and discuss its application across the middle adult life span

Keys to Understanding This Chapter

Chapter 5: basic human needs
Chapter 9: growth and development of infants and children
Chapter 10: growth and development of adolescents

Key Points

- Certain developmental tasks must be met for the adult to mature comfortably.
- Development continues throughout life and during adulthood, periods of stability alternate with periods of transition.

Key Points (continued)

- Because many adults choose to live with another person, it is helpful if they can integrate their individual goals into joint goals.

Key Topics Outline

Adult Growth and Development Theories
    Developmental Tasks
    Psychosocial Development
    Levinson's "Individual Life Structure" Theory
    Sheehy's "Phases of Adulthood"
Development in Early Adulthood
    At 20 to 30 Years
    At 30 to 40 Years
Development in Middle Adulthood

Key Learning Activities

- Enlist the aid of your family members to create a genealogy for yourself. Add as many photographs as possible. Present this information to the class. What did you learn?
- Interview people of various ages. What do they consider as "middle age"? How does this idea relate to their own age at the time?
- Interview several nurses who have been working at least 20 years. What types of nursing have they done? What are they doing now? What do they plan to do in the future?

A person continues to grow and develop throughout life. Periods of transition alternate with periods of integration. Although it is not possible to identify stages of adult life in terms of exact chronologic age, several stages of development can be identified.

This chapter continues the normal development and developmental tasks of the person following adolescence into early and middle adulthood. Late adolescence and the beginning of adulthood are interrelated and the individual may slip in and out of each. Aspects of physical change and aging are discussed in Unit Four.

Adult Growth and Development Theories

Researchers have been more active in establishing theories of child development than in studying the development of adults. Several persons, however, have proposed theories of adult development. Four major theories are summarized here.

Developmental Tasks

Havighurst's theory of developmental tasks was introduced in Chapters 9 and 10. To become mature and fully functioning, a person must continue to complete certain developmental tasks to set the stage for accomplishment of the next tasks. The tasks of early and middle adulthood are listed in the accompanying box.

Psychosocial Development

As discussed in Chapters 9 and 10, Erikson set forth theories related to the psychosocial development of various age groups. Table 11-1 continues his theory through early and middle adulthood.

Erikson established his theories as "positive" versus "negative"; here we consider them as opposites. No value judgments are placed on choices either way. These are choices we all must make. Choices can be *revised* as a person goes through life.

Intimacy Versus Isolation. The young adult is faced with choices related to occupation, further education, relationships, living environment, and independence. Often the young adult works hard at achieving financial and emotional independence from parents. Life goals and values are established although these may change later in life. Examples of opposite choices are:

◆ Choice to share a relationship or live alone
◆ Choice to work in a people-oriented occupation (such as nursing) or work in a quieter occupation (such as freelance work in one's home)

Havighurst's Developmental Tasks

Early Adulthood (18–40 Years of Age)

Select a mate
Learn to live with mate
Start a family
Raise the children
Manage a home
Begin occupation
Involve self in civic and church activities
Form social groups

Middle Adulthood (40–65 Years of Age)

Assist teenage children to become responsible adults
Achieve social and civic responsibility
Attain satisfying career
Develop leisure activities and hobbies appropriate to age
Strengthen relationship with spouse or companion
Accept and adjust to physical status of middle age
Deal with and assist aging parents

Generativity Versus Self-absorption. By the time a person reaches middle adulthood, a lifestyle has been chosen. The adult develops either in what is perceived by outsiders as "accomplishing a great deal" or in developing the "self." Many changes occur: children grow up and leave home, plans for retirement must be made, and some body processes begin to change.

Plans for retirement should be made so adults can continue to be productive and relaxed. The groundwork of good health, hobbies, leisure activities, financial security, and relationships with family and friends should be built in middle age in preparation for retirement. Examples of opposite choices are:

◆ Choice to climb the corporate ladder and make a great deal of money or develop the intellectual self by working on advanced degrees or pursuing extensive reading.
◆ Choice to spend more time with a significant other or pursue personal interests alone
◆ Choice to develop activities to be used after retirement or participate in activities for present satisfaction

Levinson's "Individual Life Structure" Theory

Daniel Levinson, a theorist of adult development, has formulated age-linked periods of adulthood (Table 11-2). His theory centers around the belief that life's patterns are formed by the interaction of three components:

◆ Self (values and motives)
◆ Social and cultural aspects
◆ Set of roles in which individual is involved

Table 11-1. Erikson's Developmental Tasks of Adulthood

Theory Concept	20–40 Years	40–60 Years
Developmental Tasks	Intimacy vs. isolation	Generativity vs. stagnation (self-absorption)
Psychosocial Challenges	Choose relationship style Occupation Establish independence	Accomplishments Develop self Plan retirement Raise family Enhance relationships
Virtues	Affiliation Love	Production Caring Cooperation
Developmental Phase	Young adulthood	Middle adulthood

When something changes in one of these components, a reorganization of the whole life structure occurs.

Sheehy's Phases of Adulthood

In 1987, Gail Sheehy published a bestselling book, *Passages.*[1] With the work of Erikson, Levinson, and others as background, Sheehy expanded and clarified the phases of adulthood. Table 11-3 outlines Sheehy's phases of adulthood. Whereas Levinson's theory was based largely on the male adult, Sheehy came forth with a woman's viewpoint of adulthood.

Development in Early Adulthood

The following section presents an integration of theories of major activities or decisions that occur in early adulthood. Some activities have been proposed by one theorist, and some are a combination of theories. The chronologic age line is muddled, but all or most adults go through these stages at some point.

At 20 to 30 Years

Leaving Home. One of the decisions the young adult makes relates to leaving the home of his or her parents. There is no correct way to leave home, simply different ways. In the current economic situation, many young people may encounter financial difficulties that force them to return to their parents' home temporarily. Leaving home can follow any of several patterns:

◆ The child leaves home and does not move back.

◆ The child stays at home until the parents finally force the child to leave.
◆ The child leaves, returns, leaves, returns, and continues a cycle of moving in and out.
◆ The child does not leave but lives with the parents as an adult or builds a house next door.

Choosing a Career. Choices of an occupation are closely tied to choices related to education. Both, in turn, are related to economic situations, goals, abilities, and interests. Individuals should be able to enjoy what

Table 11-2. Levinson's Classifications of Adulthood

Age	Periods	Transitions
18–22	Early adult transition	Adult choices Establishment of adult identity Career choice Intimate relationships Personal goals
22–28	Getting into the adult world	Balance of choices
28–33	30s transition	Possible change of lifestyle Late marriage Divorce Change of career
33–39	Settling down	Balance of choices
40–45	Midlife transition	Reappraisal of goals and values Self-identity Renegotiation of relationships Change of perspectives
45–65	Payoff years	Balance of choices
65+	Life review	Wisdom Stability Retirement

Source: After Levinson DJ, et al: The Seasons of a Man's Life. New York, Ballantine, 1986.

[1] Sheehy G. Passages: Predictable Crises of Adult Life. New York, Bantam, 1984.

Table 11-3. Sheehy's Phases of Adulthood

Age	Phase	Key Decisions and Issue	Virtues
20–30	"Trying Twenties"	Leaving home Adult relationships Seeking roots	Exploration and experimentation
30–40	"Catch Thirties"	Establish new home Career goals Women's issues Restlessness	Energy
Late 30s–50	"Deadline Decade" or "Time of Renewal"	Self-image change Midlife crisis Aging parents Facing own mortality	Experience

Sheehy G. Passages: Predictable Crises of Adult Life. New York, Bantam, 1984.
Sheehy G. Pathfinders: Overcoming the Crises of Adult Life and Finding Your Own Path to Well-being. New York, Bantam, 1982.

they do and feel they are doing the best with their abilities and making a contribution to society. Sometimes circumstances do not allow one to follow one's dreams, and adjustments must be made. Such adjustments will depend on how the person has made adjustments through childhood and adolescence. Many people have more than one interest and can make alternate choices. Although independence is important, the support of family and friends also is important.

Establishing an Adult Identification: Seeking Oneself. Sheehy describes the young person from 20 to 30 as seeking to establish roots. These people feel they "should" do a particular thing with their life. The family, peers, and surrounding culture influence what the "shoulds" are in any one person's life. A dilemma occurs when the young person feels that choices made at this stage of life cannot be changed. Young people may hesitate to enter into a certain lifestyle fearing that they will be forced to live that way or to do that job forever.

Sheehy states that two opposing impulses are at work during this time. The person wants to build a safe structure for the future, to have commitments, and to "be set." Yet, the person wants to explore and experiment, to keep the structure flexible. The *balance* between these two opposing forces determines how easily and how quickly the person passes through this phase of "provisional adulthood."

Establishing Adult Relationships. Young adults may find themselves lonely when they leave home. There are many ways of finding adult relationships. Choices include entering a religious order, living with a good friend of either sex, entering into a heterosexual marriage, entering into an intimate relationship with a person of the opposite sex without marriage, becoming a

member of an athletic team, or living in a homosexual relationship of love or convenience. Some people live with a relative or with their parents in an adult relationship.

People enter an intimate relationship for various reasons. Some marry to escape life with their parents. Others marry because they feel it is expected of them. Some people marry for protection or to be "taken care of" or for prestige. Many people marry because they find someone they love and want to spend their lives together.

Many couples live together without marrying. Some young people prefer to postpone marriage until after college or establishment of a career. Some young people do not want to commit to a long-term relationship. Others live together for the same reason others marry: protection, sharing expenses, or as a way of escaping the parental home.

Starting a Family. In general, society still expects young adults to marry and establish a family and home (Fig. 11-1). In today's society some couples postpone childbirth, preferring to establish careers or become financially secure before beginning a family. Yet many adolescent girls become pregnant and are thrust into adulthood before they are ready.

Modern young people who begin their families during their 20s usually share in child care. Fathers are entering into closer relationships with their children than ever before. The result is a stronger family unit.

At 30 to 40 Years

Settling In. In the early 30s, adults begin to "settle in." If they have not done so in their 20s, they now may purchase a home, establish themselves in a career, and

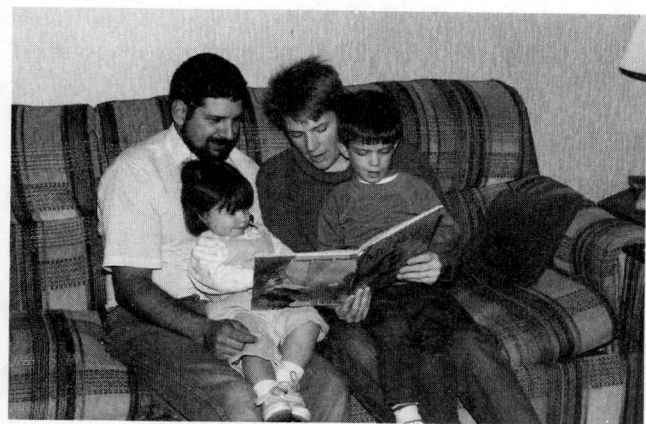

Figure 11-1. Many aspects of society still expect young adults to marry and start a family (Jackson DB, Saunders RB. Child Health Nursing: A Comprehensive Approach to the Care of Children and Their Families. Philadelphia, J.B. Lippincott, 1993).

become more comfortable with their intimate or other adult relationships. Life becomes more rational and orderly.

Reappraising Commitments. This stage of life is sometimes marked by restlessness, confusion, and doubt. The person asks, "What do I *want* out of this life, now that I'm doing what I *ought* to do?" From about 28 to 32, the person often must make new choices. A reappraisal of previous commitments occurs; the person may question whether or not to stay in a marriage or in a job. The person begins to realize that decisions should not be based on what other people feel they should do. Death, at this stage, is an abstract fear. Persons of this age feel they will never die.

Making Career Decisions. Career issues become important. Those who want to become upwardly mobile must follow the rules of the corporate culture. This may mean transfers from one city to another. In the case of the two-career couple, conflicts may arise. For example, if one member of the couple receives a desirable job offer in another state, the choice may involve whether to stay together as a couple, whether to move and have the second person seek a suitable job, or whether to have a commuting relationship.

As conditions change in industry and technology, many adults in their 30s or 40s may find themselves without a job. Companies are taken over by a bigger conglomerate, headquarters move to another city, trends change, and plants close. In some cases, a wife who has never worked outside the home is forced to supplement the family's income. Such circumstances— a husband laid off and a wife forced to work outside the home—can cause great hardships and difficulties in a marriage.

Addressing Women's Issues. Women in their 30s must make certain decisions. Many women feel they should begin a family now or it may soon be too late. Career goals and motherhood goals conflict. If the woman in the 30s never married, she may feel that she should hurry to get married or have a baby because life is "passing her by." Adoption and artificial insemination are options for the young woman today.

Facing Transitions. Many changes occur as the adult faces middle adulthood. As children enter adolescence, they spend more time away from home and are more interested in being with their peers. The person responsible for childrearing may have a great feeling of loss or loneliness. New interests must be found.

With career changes and transfers to other cities, home life and intimacy become less stable. Divorces may occur and adjustments to living styles must be made.

Development in Middle Adulthood

The following section is a summary of the main points of various theories related to middle adulthood. Although middle adulthood may be thought of as the years from 40 to 50 or 65, the following activities do not appear at any particular time in that age span.

Addressing Midlife Transitions. Erikson defines the developmental task of the age group from about 40 to 60 years as *generativity* (versus *stagnation*). This means the person is concerned now with guiding the next generation (Fig. 11-2). The person has a great deal to offer in the way of experience and advice and begins to see the younger generation as trustworthy and able to take over the world. Competition is not as important as before, and *cooperation* by this person is more evident in the workplace, particularly after age 50. The person is productive and knows how to "get the job done" quickly, accurately, and efficiently. A great deal of creativity is based on experience.

Some people at this stage of life are not able to accept aging and feel frustrated and unfulfilled. They may feel that they have failed. Some people brood and become mentally or physically ill. For this reason, the stage is also known as generativity versus *self-absorption.* Some of the problems that occur if this stage is not resolved are suicide, chemical dependency, and clinical depression.

Some theorists refer to these circumstances as the "midlife crisis." The midlife crisis involves some of the sense of failure in the person's chosen profession, as well as feelings of sexual inadequacy, of inevitable death, or of frustration with aging parents. Sometimes,

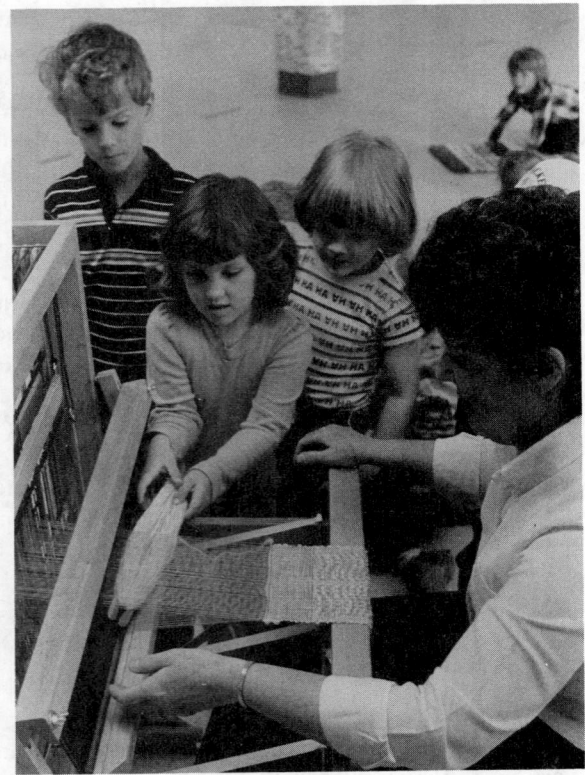

Figure 11-2. Generativity is expressed by sharing one's skills and interests with the next generation (Schuster CS, Ashburn SS. The Process of Human Development: A Holistic Life-Span Approach, Ed 3., J.B. Lippincott, Philadelphia, 1992).

the person just wants to "escape from it all" and acts out temporarily in an inappropriate way.

Reappraising One's Life and Goals. Sometimes as adults enter their 40s they feel panicky. They feel other people their age have achieved more. They feel they must achieve something now before it is too late. The person who has primary responsibility for childrearing begins to wonder what he or she will do when the children are gone. This may be a time when adults enter an educational program, finish high school, take college courses, or find new hobbies.

Adjusting to Role Changes. The person's view of self begins to change as children mature and change. This realization may occur when a child is taller than the parent, has more education, or is better at sports. Their child is becoming an adult.

The person's image of significant others also changes. As he or she looks at friends, it seems they are getting older. It is a difficult realization, however, to visualize oneself getting older as well.

Middle-aged adults often must face the aging of their own parents. Arrangements may need to be made for

a visiting nurse or for nursing home care. Roles are reversed and the former "child" becomes the responsible "parent."

Sometimes a person in the middle years is caught between caring for his or her aging parents, as well as for their own growing children. This has been referred to as the "sandwich generation."

The death of a spouse or significant other may occur in this period. The person becomes a widow or widower and significant adjustments must be made to such a role change.

On the positive side, grandchildren provide excitement and renewal. Grandparents often have more time to spend with their grandchildren than they had available when rearing their own children. Grandparents provide a special perspective in the life of young children.

Perceiving One's Own Mortality. Death becomes more of a reality as the person nears 50. Perhaps a relative or friend of the same age dies. The person begins to come to grips with his or her own mortality. The person may become frightened by the prospect of death or may experience a spiritual revival and become more comfortable with its inevitability.

Reestablishing Equilibrium. Nearing the end of the fourth decade, adults begin to look forward to new challenges. They can accept life as it is. Equilibrium is reestablished.

The couple's children often marry during the couple's 40s or 50s. The realization comes that life will be more peaceful when the children move out of the home, and the person or couple can plan for and look forward to retirement.

Sheehy refers to later middle age as a time of *renewal.* She comments that the "chief virtue traditionally associated with middle age is *experience.*" However, the person who has not successfully reassessed life in the previous stages of life and has not successfully achieved the developmental tasks may react in two ways. The first is the person who is resistant to change: the "protector of the status quo" or a "diehard." Others become "middle-aged kids" and inappropriately refuse to acknowledge their age.

Planning for Retirement. Some companies offer an early retirement package to employees; therefore, some people retire at an earlier age than in the past. In preparation for a productive and interesting retirement, hobbies should be developed in the middle years.

Financial planning is an important part of retirement planning. The trend seems to be for companies to give less in pension benefits. Many middle-aged adults have to plan their own retirement funds and investments. Other plans are made for the future: living arrangements and location or perhaps part-time work.

Keys for Review

Key Questions for Critical Thinking

1. Describe the major theories of the developmental tasks of early and middle adulthood. How do they relate? How do they differ?
2. Discuss the concept of "intimacy versus isolation" as it relates to life choices of the young adult.
3. Discuss the concept of "generativity versus self-absorption" as it relates to life choices of the middle-aged adult.
4. Discuss Sheehy's "phases of adulthood" and describe how these compare and contrast with the beliefs of the other theorists.

Key Readings

Hughes FP, Noppe LD. Human Development Across the Lifespan. New York, Merrill, 1990

Levinson DJ, et al. The Seasons of a Man's Life. New York, Ballantine, 1986

Schuster CS, Smith-Ashburn SS. The Process of Human Development: A Holistic Life-Span Approach, Ed 3. Philadelphia, J.B. Lippincott, 1992

Key Readings (continued)

Sheehy G. Passages: Predictable Crises of Adult Life. New York, Bantam, 1984

Sheehy G. Pathfinders: Overcoming the Crises of Adult Life and Finding Your Own Path to Well-Being. New York, Bantam, 1982

Taylor C, Lillis C, LeMone P. Fundamentals of Nursing: The Art and Science of Nursing Care, Ed 2. Philadelphia, J.B. Lippincott, 1993

Keys to Learning More

Chapter 12: growth and development of the older adult

Unit Four: anatomy and physiology

Unit Fourteen: deviations from normal growth and development

Chapter 86: dementia-type disorders

12 Older Adulthood and Aging

Learning Objectives

- Describe Havighurst's developmental tasks
- Describe the psychosocial development of the older adult as defined by Erikson
- Identify positive factors in development of the aging person
- Discuss stressors on the aged person
- Identify at least five implications for society related to the increase in the numbers of aging people
- Identify at least five challenges to future healthcare

Key Terms

ageism

aging

demographics

gerontology

Keys to Understanding This Chapter

Chapter 5: basic human needs

Chapter 9: growth and development theorists

Chapter 11: growth and development in early and middle adulthood

Key Points

- The process of aging is a continuation of earlier development. Each person differs in the speed with which they age, in adaptations to be made to aging, and in coping mechanisms.
- Ageism refers to discrimination against individuals as they grow older.
- Older people want to remain independent, maintain self-esteem, find some outlet for their energies and interests, develop a happy lifestyle within their financial means, continue positive relationships with others, meet all basic human needs, and deal with approaching death.

Key Points (continued)

- Physical and cognitive changes that occur in the older person are normal processes within aging. They should not be looked on as illnesses.
- Stresses are great on the aging population so it is important to develop healthy coping mechanisms.
- As the age of life expectancy continues to increase, society must find ways to address issues related to the aging population.

Key Topics Outline

Developmental Theories of Older Adulthood

Development as the Older Person Ages

Areas of Concern

Demographics and Population Trends

  Population Trends

Key Learning Activities

- Interview a couple who have been married at least 40 years. What are their suggestions for maintaining a marriage? How do they feel about growing older together?
- Talk to several people over age 65 and make a list of all the hobbies they have. Which of these hobbies are things you do now, at your age?
- Interview a couple over 65 who have recently married. How do they feel about marrying when they are older? If they have been married before, how do their children and other family members feel about their marriage?

Rosdahl CB: Textbook of Basic Nursing, 6th ed. © 1995 J.B. Lippincott Company

Developmental Tasks (Havighurst)

The Older Adult and Elderly
(Age 65 and Over)

Adjust to decreasing physical strength and declining health

Adjust to retirement and fixed income

Adjust to death of spouse or companion

Establish social relationships with persons of same age and with younger persons

Establish appropriate living arrangements

Make arrangements for care, if needed

Accept one's own mortality

Find satisfaction in one's family

Accept oneself as an aging person

Growth and development continue throughout the life span. During the last half of this century, society has recognized the importance of the process in children. The dimensions of growth and development in the older adult has had less recognition until more recently. The achievements, problems, and characteristics that occur during older adulthood are as important to an individual as were the milestones in younger years. And, as children differ, so do adults.

How does the study of aging relate to you as a nurse? Many of your patients in the hospital will be 55 years or older. Or you may use your skills in an extended care facility. In any case, you will need an understanding of the normal process of **aging**. Only by appreciating normal changes will you be able to recognize abnormal changes.

Developmental Theories of Older Adulthood

Developmental changes occur in the elderly but at variable rates. Development and maturation occur throughout older adulthood. Older age hastens the physical changes begun in middle adulthood, and there is a relationship between the physical changes and development.

Developmental Tasks

Havighurst's developmental tasks have been discussed throughout this unit. His theories related to tasks continue throughout the period of the older adult and elderly, as summarized in the accompanying box.

Psychosocial Development

One highly regarded theory of psychosocial adjustment to older adulthood is Erikson's concept of the eight stages of life. Erikson has delineated the last major

tasks to be *ego integrity* versus *despair*. Erikson's theory of the older adulthood is summarized in Table 12-1.

The older adult now realizes the "fruits of his or her labors." The person achieves a sense that life has meaning and that it has been worthwhile. The ego is comfortable with past resolutions; one does not regret past decisions. The goal of *ego identity* is to accept the accomplishments made in life. This acceptance may mean altering the goals set in youth.

If the developmental tasks of the older adult are not successfully mastered, the person will feel that time was too short. Regrets and feelings of failure may envelop the person. If the person does not accept the cycle of life and accept death as part of that cycle, the older adult enters *despair*.

Levinson's Theory

In Levinson's "individual life structure" theory, the period of 65 and over is a time of life review. Levinson says the transitions significant for this period are wisdom, stability, and retirement.

Sheehy's Phases of Adulthood

Sheehy says it is important to be comfortable with the changes that occur in the older person and to accept the dignity that comes with aging. Erikson means by *ego integrity* that the individual has arrived "at that final stage of adult development, in which one can give a blessing to one's own life," explains Sheehy. She calls *wisdom* the special *virtue* of this stage.

Development as the Older Person Ages

Ageism refers to labeling and discriminating against individuals as they grow older. It is a prejudice based on chronological age. But age is more than an accumula-

Table 12-1. Erikson's Developmental Tasks of Adulthood

Theory Concept	60 Years+
Developmental Tasks	Ego integrity vs. despair
Psychosocial Challenges	Balance choices
	Stability
	Retirement
	Evaluate life
	Accept life
Virtues	Renunciation
	Wisdom
	Dignity
Developmental Phase	Late adulthood

Lifestyle Changes in the Older and Aging Population

◆ General change in physiologic, psychological, and sociologic functions and roles
◆ Change in some body functions and abilities
◆ Adaptation to chronic physical or emotional disorders
◆ Change in employee or employer role
◆ Greater amount of leisure time for travel and hobbies
◆ Reduction of income
◆ Change of residence
◆ Change in parenting roles (sometimes a reversal)
◆ Adaptation to changed grandparent role
◆ Development of coping mechanisms to deal with accumulated changes
◆ Adaptation to possible changes in sexuality
◆ Reevaluation of self-worth
◆ Maintenance of self-esteem and independence
◆ More time for meditation and contemplation of life
◆ Adaptation to prospect of death

tion of years. People are affected by the aging process in different ways. Some people "age" faster than others. Some people never seem to age. Others are "old" at a young chronological age.

The study of the aging process is called **gerontology**. Gerontology includes all aspects of aging: physical, pathologic, psychological, economic, and sociologic. Factors in aging include such diversified things as heredity, congenital conditions, altered use of chemicals by the body, physical demands, environment, lifestyle (eg, smoking and exercise), and the lifetime nutritional status of an individual. A summary of the lifestyle changes is given in the accompanying box.

We have discussed holism as provision of care that sees the patient as a "whole person." This is true of aging. The aging personality cannot be separated from the aging body. The older person is seen as a whole. In the same way, all of the parts of the following discussion are interrelated.

Independence. The older person wants to remain independent as long as possible. If the individual is healthy and financially sound, it will be easier to remain independent. A strong support system is also a helpful factor. Self-care is an important aspect of independence. If one cannot provide for one's own basic needs, it may be difficult to live alone.

Maintaining Self-esteem. Going hand in hand with independence is self-esteem. In the aging person, self-esteem means to like oneself well enough to continue living with dignity. Self-esteem involves an acceptance of the aging process, but not giving in to it.

Working, Retiring, and Volunteering. The older person realizes that activity is necessary for life. Choices can be made and should be planned for. Some older people continue to work or may do consultant work from a home office. Others may plan to retire and travel, spend time with their spouse or grandchildren, or pursue a hobby. Participating in volunteer work is rewarding for others. Hospitals and healthcare and social agencies depend on volunteers to supplement a busy staff. Volunteerism can range from sitting in a rocking chair and talking to an ill neonate in an intensive care neonatal unit to driving a car to take elderly or disabled people to appointments.

Pursuing Interests. The wise person has begun a hobby before retirement so that it can be pursued following retirement (Fig. 12-1). All kinds of educational opportunities are open for older persons. One can follow interests as diverse as art and music appreciation, acting, astrology, and computers. Banks offer courses on how to manage finances. The International Elder-

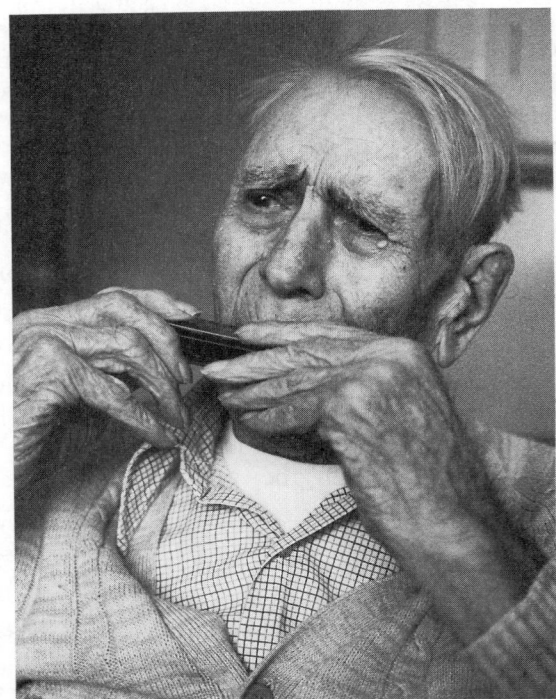

Figure 12-1. The development of hobbies in young and middle adulthood is important as the person ages. By maintaining his musical abilities, this man can entertain himself and others. (© Bistram Photography. Photograph courtesy of Unity Medical Center, Fridley, MN)

hostel* program offers opportunities to travel and study while participants engage socially with each other.

Adjusting to a Reduced Income. Most people after retirement have to adjust to a fixed income. Usually this means they have less money to spend than previously. At the same time, clothing and commuting expenses may go down. Plans for budgeting should be made before retirement so adjustments are easier to make. Living on a fixed income has made it difficult for some elderly people to move from homes in crime-ridden areas. They own their own home but its value has decreased and they have no resources to move to a safer neighborhood.

Relationships With Others. It is important that older people are not isolated from social contacts. As people become older, they usually need to make adjustments in their social activities. The health and attitudes of the spouse are a strong influence on social decisions. The couple may want to spend more time together (Fig. 12-2). Couples may enjoy one of the many social organizations that have arisen for senior citizens. If the wife is ill, the husband may have to learn to cook and clean, activities in which he had not participated previously.

At some point, the individual may have to give up driving. Certain areas may not be safe for walking alone. Individuals may need help getting to the grocery store, bank, healthcare facility, and place of worship. They become more dependent on friends and relatives or other support persons.

Spirituality. As people grow older, they can organize past experiences and thoughts into a "greater understanding of the universe." Although it may be more difficult to attend worship services outside the home, the older person now has more time to contemplate or meditate in private. If basic level needs are met, the older person is ready to move to the highest level of Maslow's hierarchy: self-actualization.

Accepting Death as Part of the Life Cycle. The deaths of a spouse and peers cause the older person to reflect on his or her own death. This attitude will be strongly influenced by the person's religious or spiritual beliefs.

People prepare for death in different ways. They may systematically verbalize about the past and may be especially interested in sharing family history and experiences with their offspring (Fig. 12-3). Some wish to do a life inventory. They may draw up a family tree,

* Elderhostel, 75 Federal Street, Boston, MA 02110.

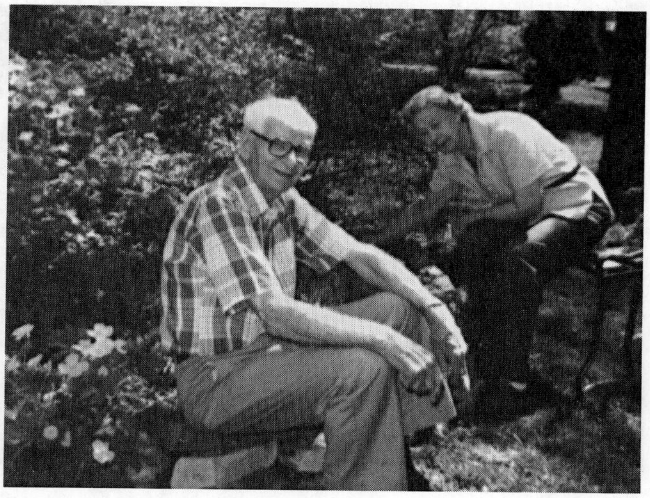

Figure 12-2. This couple, married 61 years, enjoy gardening together. They've found that they can continue most activities of middle age with only minor adjustments (Taylor C, Lillis C, LeMone P. Fundamentals of Nursing: The Art and Science of Nursing Care, Ed 2. Philadelphia, J.B. Lippincott, 1993).

create a scrapbook, organize photograph albums, or create an audio or video tape to share with grandchildren. They may make plans for their funeral, including choosing music and scripture to be used. This should not be considered morbid. It is part of a person's "organization" of his or her life.

Areas of Concern

The vast majority of elderly are active, healthy adults. Sometimes people consider normal aging processes to be signs of illness. This is not the case. The physical and cognitive changes that occur with aging are normal and require adaptation. The person's coping skills and attitudes toward life will, in part, determine if the changes are accepted or become harmful.

Space does not allow a detailed discussion of these areas of concern. Chapter 85, however, does continue the discussion about serious areas of concern and nursing care involved in care of the aging person.

Physical Changes

Many changes in aging are based on general physical changes. We (our cells) begin to age from the time we are born. A detailed presentation of the effects of aging on each body system is given in the text and in a table at the end of each chapter in Unit Four. For that reason, normal physical changes are not discussed here. However, major changes are summarized in the accompanying box.

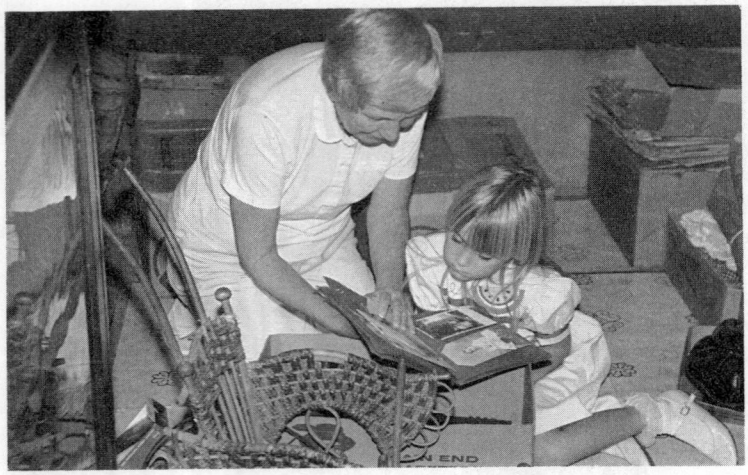

Figure 12-3. A confident older person enjoys sharing family history with a younger member of the family (Farrell J. Nursing Care of the Older Person. Philadelphia, J.B. Lippincott, 1990).

Cognitive Changes

Normal aging does not interfere with a person's intelligence, creativity, or ability to learn. Normally these mental functions continue. Psychomotor abilities may decrease, however, because of physical changes. As a result, the individual may need additional time to learn or respond. Short-term memory loss and delayed reaction time often accompany aging. Usually long-term memory is good.

Mental health problems often increase with age because of the accumulation of physical and psychological stressors. Stressors are discussed in the next section.

The Impact of Stress

Many stressors are evident in the aging population. The ability to adapt to stress and change is important. If individuals try to adapt to stress as they did in the past, they will find many of the options of youth are no longer available. Individuals with fixed habits and attitudes may have difficulty adjusting to change. The more adaptable a person is the easier it is to cope with stressors.

Generally the older person is less concerned about the opinion of others. Experience with past crises, not

Major Changes Related to Normal Aging Processes

- ♦ Decrease in functioning of organs
- ♦ Change in visual and auditory acuity
- ♦ Decreased reaction time
- ♦ Unsteady gait, decreased sense of balance
- ♦ Decrease in tactile sensations
- ♦ Stiff joints
- ♦ Increased emotional and physical losses
- ♦ Decreased capacity for recovery from injury or illness

necessarily age, influence how a person adapts to stress. An active lifestyle helps an older person to cope. It is important for the older person to choose and maintain social and civic activities and functions appropriate to his or her health, energy level, income, and personal interests.

Loss. One word summarizes many of the stressors: loss. Loss can begin subtly and continue to grow. Losses can be catastrophic or cumulative. The degree to which a loss becomes a stressor depends on the individual's attitude about it. For instance, one woman may accept the fact that she has gray hair and wrinkled and dry skin, whereas another may find much stress in this situation. Losses include such things as general appearance, physical ability and health condition, retirement, divorce, death of a spouse or other peers, and isolation from family.

Transcultural Factors. Many traditional ethnic patterns respect and revere the elderly. Support for the elderly may be sufficient to meet other stresses. As newer generations move further from some of the traditions of their cultural heritage, this attitude toward the aging may change. The elderly of minority groups generally are poorer than the general population.

Poverty. Some older people are on fixed incomes, may have little or no income if the supporting spouse has died, and may be separated from family and other support persons. Some of the elderly poor in the United States and Canada live in rural areas where limited social and healthcare facilities are available. Many of the homeless people in the cities are elderly. The lack of finances with which to meet basic needs creates major stress on the elderly.

Accumulation of Stressors. Just the accumulation of many stressors can be stressful in itself. It is easier to

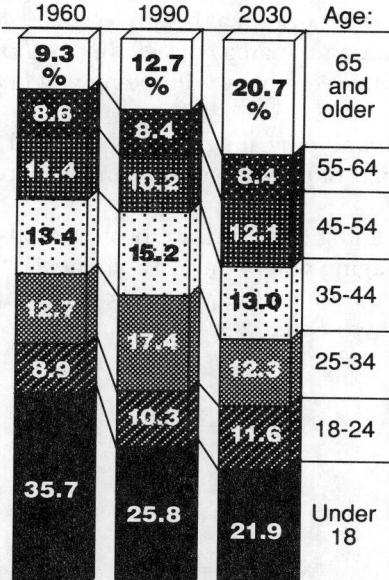

Age Distribution
of Total U.S. Population

Figure 12-4. Comparison of the growth of the population from 1960 through predictions of the early 21st century. (From the U.S. Census Bureau and Birchenall JM, Streight ME. Care of the Older Adult, Ed 3. Philadelphia, J.B. Lippincott, 1993)

deal with one stress at a time than to have them occurring rapidly or together. For instance, the loss of spouse is traumatic, but to lose a spouse, and perhaps a major source of income and the one who supplied transportation, can become overwhelming.

Demographics and Population Trends

Demographics is the study of characteristics and changes that bring about balance in a population. Demographics related to the aging population is important to industry, housing, social agencies, and the healthcare system.

Population Trends

Life expectancy is increasing in the United States and Canada. The fastest growing segment of the population is the group of people 75 years and older. The number of people who are more than 100 years old is increasing and will continue to grow. It is estimated that by the year 2000, more than 100,000 Americans will be over the age of 100.[1] Figure 12-4 graphically shows the in-

crease in the older population. A few facts about the aging population are given in the accompanying box.

As the number of older persons increases, society will be faced with problems different from those of the 20th century. Among the issues and challenges for the last half of this decade are:

◆ Consumers will expect quality, convenient, and cost-effective services. Groups like the American

Implications of the Aging Population on Society

◆ Many older people exist on a fixed income, which represents a reduction in resources for them. Income is from savings, investments, and retirement. A majority rely on Social Security, which was originally designed as a *supplement* to other income.

◆ About 6% of older people continue to work full-time; another 6% work part-time. Older workers have fewer accidents, are more reliable, can work more flexible hours (because of fewer outside commitments), use fewer sick days, and are more satisfied with their jobs than the younger population.

◆ The majority of the aging population own their own homes; most people do not move after retirement.

◆ Most older people live in urban areas. Trends in housing are toward group housing, shared housing, or retirement communities.

◆ Elderly minorities are more likely to face health problems because they are more likely to live below the poverty level.

◆ Many healthcare professionals have only begun to recognize that women's healthcare needs differ from those of men of the same age.

◆ About one-third of prescription medications are taken by seniors; often multiple drugs are taken by one person. Adverse drug reactions are five times more likely to occur in the elderly.

◆ Health problems and disabilities increase with advancing age. Approximately 31% of all healthcare expenses go to the elderly.

◆ Seven states contain 45% of the U.S. elderly population (California, New York, Florida, Illinois, Ohio, Pennsylvania, and Texas).

◆ Children of aging parents are frequently faced with responsibility for their parents. Some of these "children" are over 65 themselves.

◆ Men average twice the per capita annual income of women. Many widowed women are living at a much lower income level than when their spouse was living.

◆ Among the aging, women outnumber men. At age 65, the ratio is 3:1. At age 85, the ratio is 5:1.

◆ Nearly 80% of these men are married. Only 40% of the women are married; the majority are widows.

[1] Birchenall JM, Streight ME. Care of the Older Adult, Ed 3. Philadelphia, J.B. Lippincott, 1993, p. 3.

Association of Retired Persons (AARP) and the Gray Panthers have significant political influence.

◆ Financial planning should begin in early adulthood. The goal is to be self-supporting in one's old age.

◆ Urban transportation systems will assist the elderly in maintaining social contacts and provide easier access to preventive healthcare facilities.

◆ More flexible working and retirement schedules, opportunities for volunteer work, and recognition of past contributions will raise the resources within the elderly.

◆ Fitness programs designed for the elderly will promote better health, which will lower healthcare costs.

◆ Better nutrition in younger years will benefit people as they age. Nutrition will play a greater role in preventive healthcare, restoration of health, and maintenance of optimal health.

◆ Counseling in the areas of health, psychosocial situations, and economic well-being will be standard practice.

◆ The legal and ethical issues of death and dying will be part of the individual's and society's concerns.

◆ Better training of healthcare professionals in the areas of aging will be necessary. Special focus is needed to address the physical changes in older men and women.

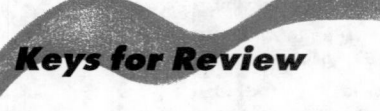

Keys for Review

Key Questions for Critical Thinking

1. Describe developmental theories related to older adulthood.
2. Define and discuss ageism and gerontology.
3. Describe the effects of stress on the aging process and discuss some of the stressors.
4. Discuss what you consider the major issues related to aging will be at the beginning of the next century.

Key Readings

American Association of Retired Persons. A Profile of Older Americans. Washington, D.C., AARP Pub. #PF 3049, 1990

Birchenall JM, Streight ME. Care of the Older Adult, Ed 3. Philadelphia, J.B. Lippincott, 1993

Burke MM, Walsh MB. Gerontologic Nursing: Care of the Frail Elderly. St. Louis, Mosby-Year Book, 1992

Clayton V. "Erikson's Theory of Human Development as it Applies to the Aged: Wisdom as Contradictive Cognitive," Human Development 18:119–128, 1975

Eliopoulos C. Gerontological Nursing, Ed 3. Philadelphia, J.B. Lippincott, 1993

Farrell J. Nursing Care of the Older Person. Philadelphia, J.B. Lippincott, 1990

Schuster CS, Smith-Ashburn SS. The Process of Human Development: A Holistic Life-Span Approach, Ed 3. Philadelphia, J.B. Lippincott, 1992

Sheehy G. The Silent Passage: Menopause. New York, Random House, 1992

Taylor C, Lillis C, LeMone P. Fundamentals of Nursing: The Art and Science of Nursing Care, Ed 2. Philadelphia, J.B. Lippincott, 1993

Keys to Learning More

Chapter 4: legal aspects of death

Unit Four: anatomy and physiology, including aging considerations

Chapter 85: disorders of aging

Chapter 86: dementia-type disorders in the aging population

Chapter 87: mental health deviations from normal aging

Chapter 90: death and dying

Chapter 91: hospice care

Key Resources

Alzheimer's Association
919 N. Michigan Avenue
Chicago, IL 60611
312-335-8700

National Council on the Aging
409 3rd Street, SW
Suite 200
Washington, DC 20024
202-479-1200

American Association of Retired Persons (AARP)
601 E Street, NW
Washington, DC 20049
202-434-2277

13 The Family Unit

Keys for Learning

Learning Objectives

- List functions and goals of families
- Describe the various types of family structure
- List at least five cultural aspects of courtship and marriage
- Briefly describe some of the cultural differences between families of different ethnic backgrounds; discuss these in terms of your own family of origin
- Discuss the impact on today's family of the mother working outside the home
- Discuss roles and relationships within the family
- Describe socioeconomic influences on the family
- List several factors that have an impact on marital success or failure
- Describe developmental tasks of the family at each stage of family life

Key Terms

blended family	nuclear dyad family
dysfunctional family	nuclear family
extended family	parenting
mixed marriage	siblings

Keys to Understanding This Chapter

Chapter 5: basic human needs as applied to family development

Chapter 6: family health as a family responsibility

Unit Three: growth and development of members of the family

Key Points

- The family is the basic unit of society, but it is a complex unit.
- All nursing care should involve the patient and family.
- Although functions and goals of families may be similar, each family is unique.
- Functions of the family help the individual meet basic human needs.
- Although there are many different family structures, all of them can be efficient and satisfying.

Key Points (continued)

- Roles and relationships within a family are many and varied; primary among these is the role of parenting and the relationship of siblings.
- Cultural and socioeconomic factors influence family outcomes. The family develops through a cycle, corresponding to the developmental tasks of various age groups. The family that can cope with stresses is functional; families that cannot cope are dysfunctional or at risk.

Key Topics Outline

Characteristics of the Family
  Functions and Goals
  Family Structure
  Roles and Relationships
  Cultural and Ethnic Features
  Socioeconomic Influences
Stages of Family Development
  Premarital Involvement Stage
  Establishment Stage: Marital Adjustment
  The Expanding Family: Childbearing Stage
  Childrearing: Socialization Stage
  Contracting Family: Child-Launching Stage
  The Postparental Stage: Empty Nest
  Aging and Retirement
Stress and Family Coping

Key Learning Activities

- Visit an adoption agency. Report back to the class regarding the criteria for an adoptive family and the suggestions made for assimilating the adoptive child into the family.
- Interview a parent and a child in a blended family. What have been their most important adjustments? What suggestions would they make for other similar families?
- Interview a person from a culture different from yours. What similarities and differences are there between your family and theirs?

The family is the basic unit of society. Even the most primitive people have rigid customs on establishing a family and maintaining its integrity. Throughout history, as family responsibility and relationships in great nations deteriorated and decayed, their civilizations crumbled from within. Just as you need to understand the development of the individual to provide quality nursing care, you need to understand the development of the family. In holistic nursing, each patient is a *person*, and each person should be considered *part of the whole* (in this case the family). All nursing care should involve the family, and family members should be shown how to give emotional and physical support to the patient.

Characteristics of the Family

Although the family is a basic unit, it is also a complex unit. It has varied functions, structures, roles and relationships, sociocultural aspects, and interests. Its members are in different stages of development at different points in the cycle. *Each family is unique.*

> **Key Concept**
>
> The patient and the family must *always* be considered when giving nursing care.

Functions and Goals

Reproduction is necessary for maintaining life on earth. Reproduction of the individual is the most important function of the family. Other functions and goals center around supporting individuals in their physical, emotional, and social growth. Duvall identified eight essential tasks for the family. Notice how they correspond to the basic human needs discussed in Chapter 5. Duvall's tasks are the following:[1]

◆ *Provision for physical needs* (food, shelter, clothing, safety, healthcare)
◆ *Allocation of resources* (careful planning and use of family money, material goods, space, and abilities)
◆ *Division of labor* (assigning the workload, including responsibility for household income and household management)
◆ *Socialization of family members* (guiding toward acceptable standards of elimination, food intake, sexual drive, respect for others and their possessions, sense of spirituality)

[1] Adapted from Duvall EM, Miller D. Marriage and Family Development, Ed 6. New York, Harper and Row, 1990.

◆ *Reproduction, recruitment, and release of family members* (bearing or adopting children, adding new members by marriage, and allowing members to leave)
◆ *Maintenance of order* (providing interaction and communication opportunities, discipline, affection, sexual expression)
◆ *Assistance of members in fitting into the larger society* (community, school, spiritual center, organizations)
◆ *Maintenance of motivation and morale* (recognition, affection, encouragement, family loyalty, help in meeting crises, philosophy of life, spirituality)

Each person within a functioning family unit must maintain individuality, establish a contributing role in the relationship with each of its members, and interact compatibly within the total group.

Family Structure

Modern society is more tolerant of social change than in the past. This, in part, counts for the variety in family structure. Some statistics about the changing American family are illustrated in Figure 13-1. Descriptions of a variety of family types follow.

Nuclear Family. This is the traditional family: a two-generation family of parents and children. In some cases, the mother stays home to care for the house and children while the father works. This is no longer the case in many nuclear families.

Extended Family. The extended family consists of grandparents, aunts and uncles, and cousins. The family may live together in a house, or they may live in close proximity. This type of family is also called a kin network or a three-generation family. Babysitting and discipline may be shared by various members.

Single-Adult Household. Some single adults prefer to live alone in their own apartment or home. There are no children involved, or there may be a divorce.

Nuclear Dyad Family. Such a family is made up of a male and female living together without children. This can be a young married couple without children or an older couple whose children no longer reside with them.

Single-Parent Family. This type of family is more prevalent today than in the past. It involves an adult head of the house with dependent children. The adult may be single as a result of separation, divorce, or death. Many unmarried women are opting to have children, and some single people are adopting children.

Nuclear Family vs. One-parent Family

☐ Two-parent family
▨ One-parent family

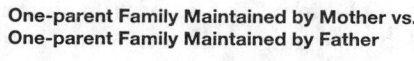

87.1%   78.5%   62.7%
12.9%   21.5%   37.3%
1970   1980   1990

**One-parent Family Maintained by Mother vs.
One-parent Family Maintained by Father**

☐ Mother
▨ Father

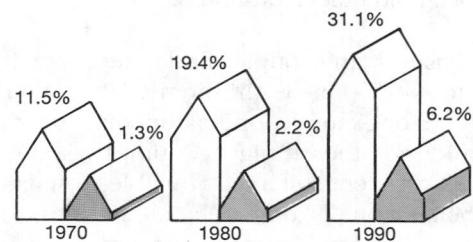

11.5%   1.3%   19.4%   2.2%   31.1%   6.2%
1970   1980   1990

Figure 13-1. The changing American family.

Cohabiting Family. This refers to individuals living together. This may include an unmarried couple living together, a gay or lesbian family, or a communal family.

Communal Family. In a commune, many people live together. They often strive to be self-sufficient and minimize contact with the outside society. Members share their financial resources, the work, and child care. An example of a communal family is the *kibbutz.*

Blended Family. As divorce and remarriage become more common in the United States, more children are living in blended families. If the newly married father and mother both have custody of their children, the two sets of children are placed together at a later stage in their lives, rather than being born into the situation. Such families are called blended or reconstituted families.

Homosexual Family. Partners of the same sex may live together or own property together. If one of them has children from a previous relationship or by adoption, they may share childrearing responsibilities. Artificial insemination is also an option for the lesbian couple.

Adoptive Family. A couple or single person may adopt one or more children. These children may be the only children in the family or may come into a family that has biologic children as well. Sometimes adopted children come into the family with special difficulties. The child may feel unwanted or insecure or may be a victim of abuse. The child may have lived in several foster homes.

There may be fewer children available for adoption today because of legalized abortion and single parenthood. Children with special needs or of mixed racial background are available in some localities. Some peo-

ple adopt children from other countries (Fig. 13-2). Adopting children into families of a different racial background is controversial.

Grandparent–Grandchildren Family. On the increase is the family in which children are being raised by grandparents for a variety of reasons. A simple one is that the parent, an adolescent, is at school or works. Divorce is another cause. In increasing numbers, parents are un-

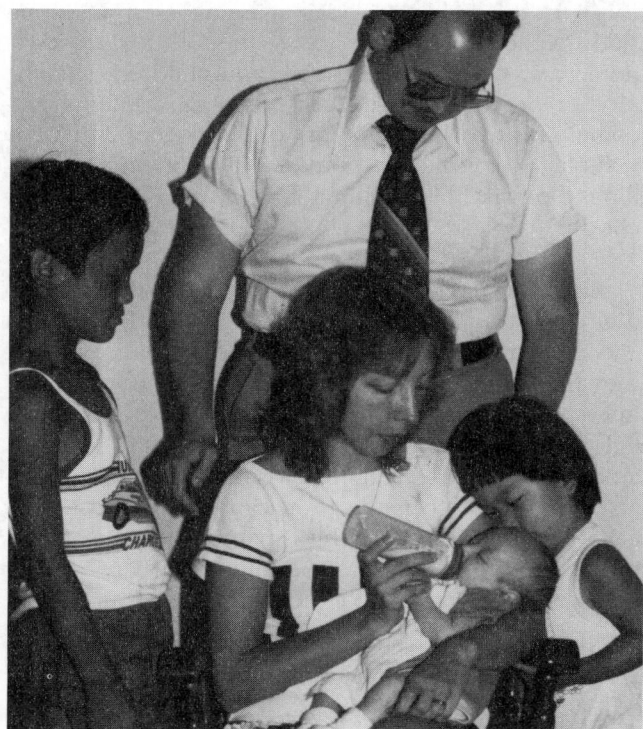

Figure 13-2. A family of parents, two adopted older children, and the new baby. The adopted children share in the joys of a growing family.

able to care for their children because of drug abuse or imprisonment. The changing acquired immunodeficiency syndrome statistics, which show that many women are now contracting the disease, are delegating child-care responsibilities to grandparents. Although family involvement is an asset, older grandparents may have difficulties meeting basic needs for the family because of financial difficulties or illness.

Two-career Family. Many couples find it necessary for both people to work outside the home. Work hours may be different; for example, one parent may work in the daytime and the other at night. Couples with children who work different shifts may be able to stagger their work hours so one is at home at all times to care for the children. Other families may need day-care services or may need to take the child to a babysitter.

Commuter Family. Somewhat new on the scene is the commuter family, in which both adults usually are professionals. Often one has been transferred to another city, but the other prefers to remain with the present employment. The situation may have occurred during their courtship and remains in their commitment. They have to commute a long distance, usually on weekends, to be together.

Role-Reversal Family. In the past the "traditional" family consisted of a working husband with a wife who cared for the children. Today, many women work outside the home. In some cases, the father remains at home and cares for the home and children, and the mother provides the major percentage of family income. This may be temporary or permanent. It may be voluntary, or it may be the result of unemployment, illness, or disability. The father who is a student may choose a "role-reversal" while attending school.

Mixed Marriage. Traditionally, families married within their own ethnic, racial, or religious group, but today it is common to find families of mixed marriage. That is, they may be from different ethnic groups, they may be interracial, or they may represent two very different religious or spiritual groups. Each brings into the family cultural factors representing his or her background. Adjustments must be made to acknowledge and accept each other's differences. This is particularly true of people of different religions, especially if they are actively involved in the practice of their religious group.

Roles and Relationships

The roles people play within a family may be many and varied. For instance, a woman may be a wife, mother, and daughter, while she also maintains roles as housekeeper, breadwinner, auto mechanic, tutor, and lawnkeeper. One of the major roles or relationships played out in a family is that of parent. Another is the sibling relationship.

Parenting

Parenting is the ability of one (or more) person(s) to help a child(ren) meet his or her needs and to guide that child or young person through developmental tasks. While the parent provides food, shelter, and safety, he or she is also helping the child develop identity, self-confidence, and creativity.

Parenting differs in each family. Some families may be strict in discipline, while others are lenient or even indifferent. Some parenting styles are guided by the parent's own upbringing. Others may be learned by watching role models or guided by moral or religious teaching. Parenting occurs while the parent is also working through adult developmental tasks.

Siblings

Because of forced interaction over the years of childhood, siblings exert powerful influences over each other. The sibling relationship is the first peer relationship, and usually it is a long-standing relationship. It may well last for 6 decades or more.

Siblings fill many roles for each other: protector, supporter, comforter, teacher, social planner, and disciplinarian. Although they share many of the same experiences, the experience is different for each sibling. The birth position plays a large part in sibling experience. The firstborn recalls experiences differently from the memories of the youngest in the family.

Cultural and Ethnic Features

Each culture or ethnic group sets up standards for that particular society. As people of a particular ethnic background move to the United States or Canada, they tend to live in communities of like-minded people. This "kinship" gives them support and helps them maintain their ethnic ideas. However, as families move into the general society (by relocation or as young people going to a school or college outside the ethnic community), some of their ethnic features may change. Examples of cultural factors relating to the family are the following:

- ◆ Choice of marriage partner (who chooses the spouse)
- ◆ Dating customs
- ◆ How many spouses a person may have
- ◆ Living arrangements
- ◆ Status of men and women
- ◆ Who makes decisions in the family
- ◆ Attitudes toward children
- ◆ Type of discipline, family disciplinarian
- ◆ Attitudes toward elderly people in the family

◆ Choice of vocation or occupation

Socioeconomic Influences

The characteristics of the family are greatly influenced by socioeconomic circumstances. A parent may have to work two jobs or several part-time jobs to provide for the family; this affects the amount of time spent with the family. Older siblings may be required to take on more household or babysitting responsibilities. Day care may replace home care. The choice of day care will be made, in part, by the level of income. In extended families, child care may be provided by grandparents or aunts or uncles.

Recreational pursuits will be determined by income. One family may be able to afford a vacation, while another family will find recreational opportunities in picnics and free community opportunities.

There are no ethnic boundaries to poverty. Millions of people in North America live in poverty. This includes the working poor; the homeless; migrant farm workers; residents of low-employment areas, including rural, mountain, and urban communities; and the elderly.

Families living in poverty may have a variety of health and social problems, including high infant mortality, malnutrition, anemia, lead poisoning, high dropout rates from school, fear of the environment, and shortened life span.

Key Concept

The problem of homelessness is increasing. Homeless people or families do not feel safe or secure and are not having their basic human needs met.

Stages of Family Development

The family develops through various stages, just as its members grow and develop through stages. Each stage has its own pleasures and rewards, as well as its sacrifices and duties. Socially accepted behavior in any area and aspect of life is based on the belief that rights bring corresponding duties, and duties bring corresponding rights. The duties of members of a family as they move through the various stages are called *developmental tasks*. The general pattern of family development is discussed in the following section and summarized in Table 13-1.

Premarital Involvement Stage

People meet in the neighborhood, at school, at a place of worship, at a social gathering, or at work. Because of the variety of cultural groups in North America and

Table 13-1. Stages of Family Developmental Tasks

Stages	Examples of Typical Tasks
Premarital involvement	Follow "rules of courtship"
	Choose a mate
	Continue self-socialization
Establishment	Set up budget
	Find a place to live
	Set up housekeeping
	Learn to live together
	Find career
Expanding Family	Revise budget (upward)
	Find bigger place to live
	Establish child care
	Learn to live together with children
	Find career
Childrearing	Revise budget (upward)
	Find bigger or better place to live
	Integrate children into family unit and community
	Revise child care setup
	Schedule family life
	Upgrade career
	Involve the family in community activities
Contracting	Revise budget (downward)
	Find smaller place to live
	Assist children with marriage or school and employment
	Adjust to children's marriage
	Learn to live together without children
	Consider retirement
Postparental	Revise budget or plan for retirement
	Adjust to grandchildren
	Downsize or stabilize career
	Develop hobbies and friendships with younger people
Aging	Learn to live on fixed budget
	Adjust to retirement
	Relocate to nursing home or retirement community
	Adjust to physical changes
	Adjust to widowhood
	Accept mortality

changing sexual relationships, premarital sexual behavior may vary. People may meet and date on their own, or they may be chaperoned, have their mate chosen for them, have sexual relationships before marriage, save sexual relationships for marriage, live together before being married, be monogamous, or have a variety of sexual partners.

Nursing Alert

The concern about sexually transmitted diseases and human immunodeficiency virus is changing sexual behavior. Some researchers state that more people are *monogamous* (one sexual partner) today than a few years ago. Some people equate this movement to the Victorian era when people were afraid of syphilis.

Courtship and Mate Selection. In general, people tend to marry others of the same social group, religion, age, and race. These factors are changing as families relocate, young people attend college away from home, and more people become involved in a variety of social and interest-related activities. Because there are more opportunities for socialization with people of different races and religions and because of a greater understanding and interest in people, mixed marriages are on the rise. These include not only interfaith and interracial marriages and relationships, but also relationships across social class and generations.

Establishment Stage: Marital Adjustment

The establishment stage begins with choosing a partner and setting up a household. This may or may not involve marriage. Some of the tasks of the establishment phase include setting up a home, working out a system of finances, and dividing the work and the routine chores that are a responsibility in family life.

A Place to Live. Finding a suitable place to live is usually one of the first tasks for a new couple. Typically, their first home or apartment is rented, close to their work, and often near family and friends.

A Financial System. The budget is not always as easy to establish as a place to live. Some young couples have worked and saved for the marriage, and some have become accustomed to living at home with all its comforts. They are not used to "doing without," which may come with unemployment, continued schooling, and so forth. Television also makes luxurious living look like a necessity.

Division of Work. Today's trend in many families is to share many household responsibilities, and to decide who will do what, according to individual interests, abilities, and time available. It is common today to find young couples doing the marketing together, buying household furnishings together, and sharing the responsibilities of cooking and cleaning.

Learning to Live Together. Some developmental tasks that begin in the establishment phase continue into the following phases of marriage. These tasks include achieving an effective system of communication, building a mutually satisfactory sexual relationship, forming an understanding relationship with in-laws and other relatives, and developing together a philosophy that recognizes individuality and "togetherness" in daily living and gives aim and purpose to married life. Qualifications couples should bring into relationships are listed in Keys to a Successful Relationship.

The Expanding Family: Childbearing Stage

Seldom is there a relationship as fulfilling as that of parent to child. No matter what the couple felt initially about the pregnancy, the arrival of a first child is usually an occasion of wonder and joy. The father and mother, finished with waiting, are ready for their new task: that of *parenting.* The family is now faced with new duties and responsibilities, which occur daily for parents.

Child Care. Child-care responsibilities vary for children of different ages: providing space for each child; assuring clean bodies, clothes, and surroundings; planning for a balanced diet; reorganizing family routines to accommodate the infant and toddler; toilet training; and interest in and guiding the growth of one or several children. All this is accomplished while maintaining a helpful, satisfying relationship with each other, relatives, and the community.

Keys to a Successful Relationship

- *Emotional maturity:* Self-discipline, self-objectivity, and self-responsibility
- *Love:* Genuine love based on realistic appraisal of the other person (erotic love is only part of love)
- *Compatability:* Similarity of interests, goals, energy, intellectual skills, and lifestyles
- *Skill:* Communication, negotiation, problem solving, empathy, and compassion
- *Effort:* Willingness to sacrifice and focus energies on solving problems
- *Commitment:* Determination to make it work and to "hang in there" during rough times
- *Support:* Relationship backed up by family, friends, and community
- *Flexibility:* Ability to adapt to changes, accept differences as stimulating and exciting
- *Caring:* Ability to be concerned about the welfare of the other, to desire to make life better for the other person

Adapted from Schuster CS, Ashburn SS. The Process of Human Development: A Holistic Life-Span Approach, Ed 3. Philadelphia, J.B. Lippincott, 1992.

Financial Challenges. Financial demands increase drastically, while income often grows at a slower pace. In some situations, the mother's income is discontinued, at least for the period of maternity leave, in which case the family must adjust to a lowered income. More of the financial burden then falls on the father. (If the woman did not work prior to having the children, the situation may not be as pronounced, except that the family's costs increase.) The father may choose to take a paternity leave while the mother supports the family.

Childrearing: Socialization Stage

Once children arrive in a family, life is forever changed. The members of the family learn to adjust to each other. They accept and integrate new members as they are added to the family.

Scheduling. Families in the childrearing stage often are pressured for time. Children's schedules must be taken into consideration as part of the family timetable. The parents' mealtime and sleep patterns must be changed when children arrive. As the children grow older, the scheduling of the family members becomes more hectic. Arrangements first must be made for babysitters, then often for car pools and attendance at school functions. The parents need to try to spend as much time as possible with their children.

Employment and Community Responsibilities. The parents' job responsibilities and community contacts usually increase in this active time of life. However, they must find time to encourage the growth tasks of all members of the family and combine them into a family design or plan.

To make ends meet, both parents often must work outside the home. In that case, adequate child care must be found. Each parent should spend a few minutes of uninterrupted time each day with each child.

Communication. Communication between father and mother, including sexual communication, may be sharply displaced as the family grows. Private conversation is difficult. Children are omnipresent; the baby jabbers, the preschooler talks loudly and endlessly, and the school child has many confidences and jokes to be appreciated. At this stage of the family cycle, communication is a family developmental task for all members. If the jabbering and jokes are enjoyed at least a good part of the time, it contributes to a happy family life.

Wise parents keep their avenues of communication as open as possible, spreading responsibilities for household tasks and arranging for some adult stimulation outside the home. The parents also need to plan times when they can be alone together without the children.

Stimulation and Encouragement. The family must stimulate the growth and development of all its members. It should encourage participation in community activities. (However, the family "taxi service" may seem never-ending as children are taken to and from their activities.)

Contracting Family: Child-Launching Stage

In the child-launching stage of the family cycle, the family has reached its maximum size. As each child leaves home, the parental task is to reorganize the family from a home full of children to a home again occupied only by the parents.

Assisting Children in Employment. Although the family has been preparing the child for future employment, part of the task of the child-launching stage is to guide the adolescent in making decisions regarding employment. Many families dream of their children attending college, but that step may not be realistic. The cost of college has risen considerably, and many families cannot afford it without scholarships and financial aid. The young person's abilities also must be realistically appraised. Aspirations above a possible achievement level can result in disappointment for both the parent and the child.

Furthermore, the young person's abilities and interests may lie in one of the trades. Technical training or on-the-job training may be satisfactory for the young person and may lead to a satisfying lifestyle. There are thousands of occupations from which to choose, but careful planning is needed because of the high potential for unemployment.

Finances and Responsibilities. As the children reach adulthood, the developmental tasks of other stages, such as financial obligations, budgeting, and sharing work responsibilities, continue but change. The philosophy of life that the parents have developed through two or more decades of rearing their children provides both parents and children with a feeling of achievement.

Marriage of Children. As older children marry, new "in-law" relationships enter the picture, and the family developmental tasks continue. A major task is to accept and appreciate, even if one does not always approve of, the differences in ideals, habits, and philosophies of the new generation. Changes in ways of living are inevitable.

The Postparental Stage: Empty Nest

Once the home is an "empty nest," habits of pressure (time, work, and finances) may be difficult to change. "Success" may be viewed in different ways. The person who devoted himself or herself entirely to progressing in business may be regarded by peers as eminently successful. The family's opinion of that person's success may be less satisfactory. The parent who is closer to the family may be viewed as a happier person. The woman who has been happy as a housewife and mother may have a great sense of satisfaction. On the other hand, some women who have not worked outside the house may feel they have not contributed to society.

Readjustment. Many people find their middle years a comfortable and serene period. Fewer demands allow more time to enjoy life. Financial burdens related to children are fewer, and time for shared activities increases.

Grandchildren give pleasure. However, grandparents must help without interfering, love without smothering, and be available without being intrusive. Limits in babysitting should be set. The middle-aged couple finds that the rewards of time allow both of them to come to terms with themselves and gain satisfaction in opportunities still available. However, readjustment to a period in which the children figure somewhat less prominently is necessary. If the couple shares common goals and interests, they will enjoy this period.

Preparation for Retirement. During this time, plans are made for financial security in later years. The expense of raising children has been lifted, and family income is usually at its peak, with more than 80% of the wives in the 45- to 54-year age group now working outside the home.

Financial planning for the later years indicates acceptance of the statistical fact that wives live longer than husbands. Therefore, both husband and wife should have a clear understanding of their financial standing.

Key Concept

Adjustment to retirement may be difficult if careful financial planning was not done or if hobbies and activities were not developed in earlier years.

Aging and Retirement

The aging family has several more challenges to meet.

Adjustment to Retirement. Retired people must have set goals. Some retired people lose interest in life because, as one man put it, "I don't have a reason to get up anymore." Social relationships are important, and friends are often younger.

A Place to Live. Deciding where to live is difficult for many older people. Often they have lived in the same home for 20 or 30 years or more. The place holds may memories, and it is hard to let go. The need for one spouse or the other to go to a nursing home makes the decision even sadder.

Financial Adjustments. Fixed retirement income is insufficient for many people because of inflation. Even though costs go up, the pension stays the same. Many older people have saved what they once thought would be enough money to take care of themselves in their retirement years. Unfortunately, even one short illness can wipe out a modest savings account. The couple then may be forced to sell their home or to seek financial assistance, an embarrassing situation for many older people.

Adjustment to Physical Status. As people get older, they may experience a decline in their physical faculties. A good sense of humor is probably the greatest asset in dealing with this deterioration. It is important for the older person to get some sort of exercise, to maintain an adequate diet, and to get enough rest. It may be difficult for the single person to eat adequately. The widowed man may not know how to cook; the widowed woman may not want to bother to cook just for herself. A regular physical examination is important to detect minor difficulties before they become major problems.

Acceptance of One's Own Mortality. The elderly person must face the fact that death comes as yet another stage of life. They need to plan their legal affairs and discuss finances for the future. If they have not yet made a will, they should do so now.

Widowhood. Many people will live alone at least part of their lives because of divorce or because their spouse has died. There are five times as many widowed women as widowed men in the United States. There are three reasons for this: Women live longer than men; women tend to marry men who are older than they are; and widowed men are much more likely to remarry than widowed women.

Key Concept

The developmental tasks of a family are the same, no matter what the type of family structure.

Stress and Family Coping

In addition to the normal changes, adaptations, and pressures of the family cycle, other socioeconomic, physical, and emotional stresses may occur. Some of these stresses may build on each other; that is, the stressor also may be the result of stress. Stressors to the family unit may include tension in the workplace, job relocation, unemployment, poverty, homelessness, the environment, divorce, death of a family member, dual careers, involvement with an older family member, single parenthood, adolescent parenthood, blended families, acute or chronic illness, boredom, inadequate communication, substance abuse, and family violence.

Many families are able to develop socially acceptable means of coping with stress. Other families cannot cope. The result is that as stressors build, coping systems disintegrate. The latter type of family is called a dysfunctional family or "at-risk" family.

Keys for Review

Key Questions for Critical Thinking

1. Identify at least six goals of all families and explain them.
2. Discuss the effect on families of employment of women outside the home.
3. Discuss the stages of family development.
4. Describe family stresses.

Key Readings

Duvall EM, Miller B. Marriage and Family Development, Ed 6. New York, Harper & Row, 1990
Friedman MM. Family Nursing: Theory and Assessment, Ed 3. Norwalk CT, Appleton & Lange, 1992
Giger JN, Davidhizar RE. Transcultural Nursing: Assessment and Intervention. St. Louis, C.V. Mosby, 1991

Key Readings (continued)

Jackson DB, Saunders RB: Child Health Nursing: A Comprehensive Approach to the Care of Children and Their Families. Philadelphia: J.B. Lippincott, 1993
Spector RE. Cultural Diversity in Health and Illness, Ed 3. New York, Appleton & Lange, 1991

Keys to Learning More

Throughout this text, the patient is considered a family member, and the family is taken into consideration when planning nursing care.

Chapter 39: transcultural considerations
Unit Twelve: maternal and newborn nursing

Unit 4

Normal Anatomy and Physiology

14 Organization of the Human Body

Keys for Learning

Learning Objectives

♦ Define and differentiate between anatomy, physiology, and pathophysiology
♦ Differentiate between a physical and a chemical change
♦ Discuss and give examples of the use of prefixes, root words, and suffixes in medical terminology
♦ Define and use the anatomic terms that apply to body positions, directions, cavities, and abdominal regions and quadrants
♦ Describe the organization of the human body in terms of cells, tissues, organs, and systems
♦ Identify the organs comprising each system and their locations
♦ Describe the role and actions of chromosomes and genes
♦ Briefly describe the activities of DNA and RNA
♦ Define terminology related to basic chemical concepts, to the cell, and to the various types of membranes and tissues in the body
♦ List the four major types of tissues, and give an example of each

Key Terms

anatomy	enzyme	nucleus
atom	frontal	organ
cell	gene	physiology
compound	homeostasis	protoplasm
chromosome	membrane	sagittal
deoxyribonucleic acid	mitosis	transverse
element	molecule	

Keys to Understanding This Chapter

Chapter 5: basic human needs

Key Points

♦ The human body is made up of solids, liquids, and gases that function independently but are interrelated. Homeostasis is the dynamic balance of an individual's physical and mental functioning.
♦ Medicine has developed a sophisticated system of describing anatomy and physiology called medical terminology. To assist the learner, much of this terminology can be broken down into prefixes, suffixes, and root words.
♦ Body directions, planes, and cavities are given specific names, using standard reference points.
♦ The body can be described in terms of a single cell, which collaborates with similar cells in groups called tissues. Similar tissues, functioning as a group, comprise organs. Groups of organs comprise the body systems.
♦ Each cell is composed of many complex structures. Each structure has a specific duty that relates to the body as a whole. Cells have similar abilities but have developed specialized functions.
♦ Genes, the controller of heredity, are found on chromosomes. Cells replicate (reproduce) through mitosis.
♦ There are four major types of tissues: epithelial, connective, muscle, and nerve.

Key Topics Outline

Anatomy and Physiology
Chemistry and Life
    Atoms, Compounds, and Mixtures
    Physical and Chemical Changes
    Energy
Medical Terminology
    Sources of Medical Terms
    Parts of Words
Body Directions
    Anatomic Position
    Body Planes

Key Learning Activities

◆ Using an anatomic model, locate the major organs of the body. Determine the body cavity in which each organ is located.
◆ Using the anatomic model, locate the quadrants and divisions of the abdomen and the regions of the spinal cavity.

The human body is a precisely structured arrangement of liquids, gases, and solids. These include atoms, molecules, chemicals, and approximately 60% water. Chemical reactions among these are organized into specific independent yet interrelated actions. This chapter comprises a summary of chemistry, medical terminology, and basic information about the anatomy and physiology of the human body.

Anatomy and Physiology

The study of body structure is called **anatomy**, and the study of how the body functions is called **physiology**. To understand our bodies, we must learn not only the structures of the body, but also how these structures are related and function. It is important to know normal anatomy and physiology to understand abnormal conditions, such as disease and illness. The study of disorders of functioning is called pathophysiology.

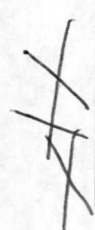

> **Key Concepts**
> ◆ *Anatomy* is the study of body structure.
> ◆ *Physiology* is the study of body function.
> ◆ *Pathophysiology* is the study of disorders of functioning.

Chemistry and Life

Before beginning any course in life science, a basic knowledge of chemistry and physics is important. Chemistry is the science concerned with the structure and composition of matter and the chemical reactions produced by these substances. Physics is the science of the laws of matter and their interactions with energy.

Why should a nurse learn about chemistry? Because chemistry is the basis for homeostasis. **Homeostasis** is the dynamic balance of anatomy and physiology. It is

the physical and emotional *equilibrium* the person strives to maintain. Homeostasis depends on the cumulative chemical reactions, the physical condition, and the emotional status of a person.

To begin a simplified discussion of chemistry, we must begin with the discussion of matter. Matter can be defined as anything that occupies space and has weight. There are three *states* of matter: solid, liquid, and gas. There are three *kinds* of matter: element, compound, and mixture.

Atoms, Compounds, and Mixtures

All matter, living and nonliving, can be broken down into a little more than 100 different elements. An **element** is a pure, simple chemical. Approximately 20 different elements are found in various amounts in the human body, although there are 92 naturally occurring elements. All elements have specific letter abbreviations, which frequently are used in medicine. Seven elements make up approximately 99% of the human weight. These elements and their symbols are carbon (C), hydrogen (H), oxygen (O), nitrogen (N), phosphorus (P), sulfur (S), and calcium (Ca). Elements found in very small amounts but vital to human life are sodium (Na), chlorine (Cl), potassium (K), iron (Fe), and iodine (I). An **atom** is the smallest part of any element. Atoms are composed of subatomic (smaller than an atom) particles or structures. The main subatomic particles are electrons, protons, and neutrons. They are arranged in relation to one another in somewhat the same manner as the earth and the other planets are arranged around our sun. An atom of one element differs from that of another element in the arrangement of its subatomic particles. For instance, a hydrogen atom has one proton and one neutron forming the **nucleus**, with one electron whirling around it. An atom of oxygen has eight electrons revolving about a central nucleus composed of eight protons and eight neutrons (Fig. 14-1).

Atoms of one element are able to interact with atoms of another element. When atoms of two or more elements react *chemically* with one another, they form a variety of substances called **compounds**. In every compound, the elements combine in definite propor-

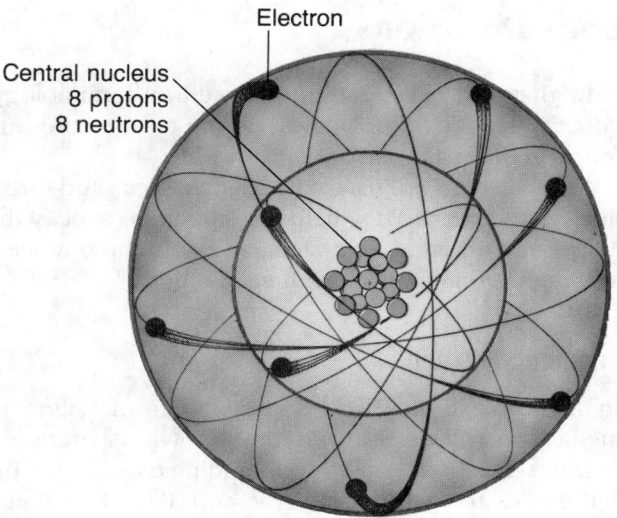

Figure 14-1. Representation of an oxygen atom. Eight protons and eight neutrons are tightly bound in the central nucleus, around which the electrons revolve.

Electron

Central nucleus
8 protons
8 neutrons

tions. For example, the most common compound found on the surface of the earth and in the human body is *water*. Water is formed when two atoms of hydrogen are combined with one atom of oxygen. In chemical shorthand, water is expressed as H_2O.

Not all elements or compounds combine chemically when brought together. A *mixture* is made up of two or more substances that have been mixed together without forming a new compound. Salt water (saline) is an example of a mixture. Both the salt and the water remain separate compounds. They can be brought together in any proportion, and they can be separated.

Physical and Chemical Changes

Water has a definite chemical structure, H_2O. Normally it is a liquid. If you lower the temperature of the water so that it freezes, it changes to a solid, ice; if you raise the temperature of the water so that it boils, it becomes water vapor, or steam. The water has undergone a *physical change*, that is, a change in its outward properties. However, the chemical composition is still H_2O, no matter in which of these three states it occurs. Its chemical structure remains unchanged.

However, if you pass a direct electric current through a sample of water, a different change occurs. The water gradually disappears, because the electric current causes it to break down into the two invisible gaseous elements, hydrogen and oxygen. A *chemical change* has occurred. Familiar types of chemical changes are the processes of burning (combustion) and the rusting of iron (oxidation). In those two types of chemical reactions, substances are changed into other substances that no longer have the same chemical structures as the original substances. Completely rusted iron no longer has the same characteristics as iron; burned wood is no longer wood, but ash and gases.

> **Key Concepts**
> ◆ *Chemical change:* One substance is changed to another, or the compound is broken down into atoms of elements, and is energy transferred (eg, water broken down into hydrogen and oxygen, and heat).
> ◆ *Physical change:* The chemical composition does not change (eg, water to ice).

Energy

Energy is the ability to do work. Energy can assume several forms, such as light energy, heat energy, mechanical energy, electrical energy, and chemical energy. One type of energy can be converted into another, but it cannot be created nor destroyed by ordinary means. For example, energy from the sun occurs in several forms: heat energy and light energy plus other types of radiation energy. The energy from the sun can be stored as chemical energy in natural fuels, such as oil and coal. The chemical energy in fuels can be transformed into electrical energy, which in turn can be transformed back into light and heat.

A chemical reaction is the process of chemical change by which one substance is changed into another substance or substances. All chemical reactions are accomplished by a transfer of energy. The *kilocalorie*, or kcal, is used as the unit for measuring the heat energy produced by food when oxidized, for example, when glucose is combined with oxygen in the body.

Medical Terminology

To study body structure and function, it is necessary to understand the vocabulary that is used in the medical and nursing fields. This is commonly called *medical terminology*. So much is involved in medical terminology that it can be regarded as a separate course of study.

Sources of Medical Terms

It is easier to learn the meaning of a medical term if you know the original source of the word. Most medical terms originated in ancient languages and have their roots in Greek or Latin words.

Modern language is another source of medical words. Some terms are *acronyms*, words formed by combining the first letter or letters of a word or phrase. For instance, MASH stands for mobile army surgical hospital. AIDS is an acronym for acquired immunodeficiency syndrome.

Eponyms are words based on the names of people. Examples include Parkinson's disease or Kaposi's sarcoma.

Parts of Words

Most medical terms consist of two or three parts: prefix, root, and suffix (Table 14-1). The prefix is at the beginning of a word. (Not all medical terms have a prefix). Prefixes are listed in Table 14-1 with a dash after the letters, for example, intra-, hypo-, or sub-.

The root of a word is the foundation of that word. All medical terms have at least one root word. The suffix is the word's ending. Most medical words have a suffix. Suffixes are listed in Table 14-1 with a dash before the letters, for example, -itis, -ic, or -pathy.

A combining vowel (usually O) joins a root to another root, or a root to a suffix. For example, note the combining vowel in the words electrocardiogram and thermometer. Medical terminology texts list roots combined with a vowel; this form is known as the *combining form*. Examples of combining forms are hepat/o, oste/o, and neur/o.

While the root is the core or main meaning of the word, its meaning can be totally changed by a prefix. A prefix introduces another thought or explains the root. For example, *epigastric* means "pertaining to on the stomach," while *hypogastric* means "pertaining to below the stomach." The suffix is added to clarify, to make a new word, or to change the meaning of the root.

Prefixes, roots, and suffixes can be used in various combinations. Sometimes a word may be a combination of two or three root words and connecting vowels. For example, *electrocardiogram* means a record (suffix: gram) of the electricity (root: electr-) of the heart (root: cardi-). Notice the two uses here of *o* as the combining vowel, joining the two root words.

To simplify a medical term, first break it down into its components. Start with the suffix, then go to the prefix, and end with the root. For example, the following is a breakdown of the term *intravenous:*

-ous (suffix) means pertaining to.
intra- (prefix) means within.
ven (root) means vein.

Thus, the word intravenous means "pertaining to within a vein." Table 14-1 lists many prefixes, suffixes, and root words for your reference.

Body Directions

Now that you have learned the medical terminology, you are ready to apply these terms to structure and function of the human body.

Several terms are used to designate areas and directions of the body. They help the student to specify the location of an organ or system, and help the physician and nurse communicate with each other.

Anatomic Position

In medical texts, the body is presented from a standard medical reference point of view known as *anatomic position*. The body is pictured standing erect with arms at the sides and palms turned forward (Fig. 14-2). When viewing anatomic pictures or diagrams, the right side of the body will be on the left side of the drawing. This is the same as looking at a person facing you.

Body Planes

A *plane* is an imaginary flat surface that divides the body into sections (see Figure 14-1). The following are planes of the body:

♦ **transverse** (horizontal plane)—passes through the body horizontally, dividing it into upper (superior) and lower (inferior) parts. Transverse planes may be imagined at *any level.*
♦ **frontal** (coronal plane)—the vertical plane that passes through the body longitudinally from head to toe, dividing it into front and back parts.
♦ **sagittal**—the vertical plane that passes through the body lengthwise and divides the body into right or left sides. *Midsagittal* passes through the midline from top to bottom dividing the body into right and left halves.

Other terms needed to describe relationships between parts of the body and positions of the body are described in Table 14-2.

Body Cavities

A body cavity is a space within the body that contains internal **organs**. Within the body are two groups of cavities that contain various organs. They are the *dorsal* (posterior) and the *ventral* (anterior) cavities. The dorsal cavity is subdivided into the cranial and spinal cavities. The ventral cavity is subdivided into the thoracic and abdominal cavities. The diaphragm, a large muscle, separates these ventral cavities. Often, the abdominal cavity is subdivided again into the abdominal and pelvic portions and is re-

(Text continues on page 135)

Table 14-1. Medical Terminology: Prefixes and Suffixes Commonly Used in Medical Terms

Prefixes	Meaning/Example	Prefixes	Meaning/Example
A- or AB-	*Away, lack of:* abnormal, departing from normal	CRANI-	*Skull:* craniotomy, surgical opening in skull
A- or AN-	*From, without:* asepsis, without infection	CRYPT-	*Hidden:* cryptogenic, of hidden or unknown origin
ACR-	*An extremity:* acrodermatitis, a dermatitis of the limbs	CUT-	*Skin:* subcutaneous, under the skin
AD-	*To, toward, near:* adrenal, near the kidney	CYST-	*Sac or bladder:* cystitis, inflammation of any bladder
ADEN-	*Gland:* adenitis, inflammation of a gland	✳ CYTO-	*Cell:* cytology, scientific study of cells; cytometer, a device for counting and measuring cells
ALG-	*Pain:* Neuralgia, pain extending along nerves	DACRY-	*Lacrimal glands:* dacryocyst, tear-sac
AMBI-	*Both:* ambidextrous, referring to both hands	DERM- or DERMAT-	*Skin:* dermatoid, skinlike
ANTE-	*Before:* antenatal, occurring or having been formed before birth	DI-	*Two:* diphasic, occurring in two stages or phases
ANTI-	*Against:* antiseptic, against or preventing sepsis	DIS-	*Apart:* disarticulation, taking a joint apart
ARTH-	*Joint:* arthritis, inflammation of a joint	DYS-	*Pain or difficulty:* dyspepsia, impairment of digestion
AUTO-	*Self:* autointoxication, poisoning by toxin generated in the body	ECTO-	*Outside:* ectoretina, outermost layer of retina
BI- or BIN-	*Two:* binocular, pertaining to both eyes	EM or EN-	*In:* encapsulated, enclosed in a capsule
BIO-	*Life:* biopsy, inspection of living organism (or tissue)	ENCEPHAL-	*Brain:* encephalitis, inflammation of the brain
BLAST-	*Bud, a growing thing in early stages:* blastocyte, beginning cell not yet differentiated	END-	*Within:* endothelium, layer of cells lining heart, blood and lymph vessels
BLEPH-	*Eyelids:* blepharitis, inflammation of an eyelid	ENTERO-	*Intestine:* enterosis, falling of intestine
BRACHI-	*Arm:* brachialis, muscle for flexing forearm	EPI-	*Above or on:* epidermis, outermost layer of skin
BRACHY-	*Short:* brachydactylia, abnormal shortness of fingers and toes	ERYTHRO-	*Red:* erythrocyte, red blood cell
BRADY-	*Slow:* bradycardia, abnormal slowness of heartbeat	EU-	*Well:* euphoria, well feeling, feeling of good health
BRONCH-	*Windpipe:* bronchiectasis, dilation of bronchial tubes	EX- or E-	*Out:* excretion, material thrown out of the body or the organ
BUCC-	*Cheek:* buccally, toward the cheek	EXO-	*Outside:* exocrine, excreting outwardly (opposite of endocrine)
CARCIN-	*Cancer:* carcinogenic, producing cancer	EXTRA-	*Outside:* extramural, situated or occurring outside a wall
CARDI-	*Heart:* cardialgia, pain in the heart	FEBRI-	*Fever:* febrile, feverish
CEPHAL- or CEPHALO-	*Head:* cephalic measurements	GALACTO-	*Milk:* galactose, a milk sugar
CHEIL-	*Lip:* cheilitis, inflammation of the lip	GASTR-	*Stomach:* gastrectomy, excision of the stomach
CHOLE-	*Bile:* cholecyst, the gallbladder	GLOSS-	*Tongue:* glossectomy, surgical removal of tongue
CHONDR-	*Cartilage:* chondrectomy, removal of a cartilage	GLYCO-	*Sugar:* glycosuria, sugar in the urine
CIRCUM-	*Around:* circumocular, around the eyes	GYNEC-	*Women:* gynecology, science of diseases pertaining to women
CLEID-	*Clavicle:* cleidocostal, pertaining to clavicle and ribs	HEM- or HEMAT-	*Blood:* hemopoiesis, forming blood
COLP-	*Vagina:* colporrhagia, vaginal hemorrhage	HEMI-	*Half:* heminephrectomy, excision of half the kidney
CONTRA-	*Against, opposed:* contraindication, indication opposing usually indicated treatment	HEPAT-	*Liver:* hepatitis, inflammation of the liver
COST-	*Rib:* intercostal, between the ribs	HETERO-	*Other* (opposite of homo): heterotransplant, using skin from a member of another species
COUNTER-	*Against:* counterirritation, an irritation to relieve some other irritation (eg, a liniment)	HIST-	*Tissue:* histology, science of minute structure and function of tissues

(continued)

Table 14-1 (continued)

Prefixes	Meaning/Example	Prefixes	Meaning/Example
HOMO-	*Same:* homotransplant, skin grafting by using skin from a member of the same species	ORTHO-	*Straight, normal:* orthograde, walk straight (upright)
		OSS-	*Bone:* osseous, bony
HYDR-	*Water:* hydrocephalus, abnormal accumulation of fluid in cranium (skull)	OSTE-	*Bone:* osteitis, inflammation of a bone
		OT-	*Ear:* otorrhea, discharge from ear
HYPER-	*Above, excess of:* hyperglycemia, excess of sugar in blood	OVAR-	*Ovary:* ovariorrhexis, rupture of an ovary
HYPO-	*Under, deficiency of:* hypoglycemia, deficiency of sugar in blood	PARA-	*Irregular, around, wrong:* paracystic, situated near the bladder
HYSTER-	*Uterus:* hysterectomy, excision of uterus	PATH-	*Disease:* pathology, science of disease
IDIO-	*Self or separate:* idiopathic, a disease self-originated (of unknown cause)	PED-	*Children:* pediatrician, child specialist
		PED-	*Feet:* pedograph, imprint of the foot
IM- or IN-	*In:* infiltration, accumulation in tissue of abnormal substances (such as an IV)	PER-	*Through, excessively:* percutaneous, through the skin
IM- or IN-	*Not:* immature, not mature	PERI-	*Around, immediately around* (in contradistinction to *para*): periosteum, sheath around bone
INFRA-	*Below:* infraorbital, below the orbit		
INTER-	*Between:* intermuscular, between the muscles	PHIL-	*Love:* hemophilic, fond of blood (as bacteria that grow well in presence of hemoglobin)
INTRA-	*Within:* intramuscular, within the muscle		
KERAT-	*Horn, cornea:* keratitis, inflammation of the cornea	PHLEB-	*Vein:* phlebotomy, opening of vein for bloodletting
LACT-	*Milk:* lactation, secretion of milk	PHOB-	*Fear:* hydrophobic, reluctant to associate with water
LEUK-	*White:* leukocyte, white cell		
MACRO-	*Large:* macroblast, abnormally large red cell	PNEUM- or PNEUMON-	*Lung* (pneum–air): pneumococcus, organism causing lobar pneumonia
MAST-	*Breast:* mastectomy, excision of the breast	POLIO-	*Gray:* poliomyelitis, inflammation of gray substance of spinal cord
MEG- or MEGAL-	*Great:* megacolon, abnormally large colon	POLY-	*Many:* polyarthritis, inflammation of several joints
MENT-	*Mind:* dementia, deterioration of the mind	POST-	*After:* postpartum, after delivery
		PRE-	*Before:* prenatal, occurring before birth
MER-	*Part:* merotomy, division into segments	PRO-	*Before:* prognosis, forecast as to result of disease
MESA-	*Middle:* mesaortitis, inflammation of the middle coat of the aorta		
META-	*Beyond, over, change:* metastasis, change in the site of a disease, spreading (often refers to cancer)	PROCT-	*Rectum:* proctectomy, surgical removal of rectum
		PSEUDO-	*False:* pseudoangina, false angina
MICRO-	*Small:* microplasia, dwarfism	PSYCH-	*Soul or mind:* psychiatry, treatment of mental disorders
MY-	*Muscle:* myoma, tumor made of muscular elements	PY-	*Pus:* pyorrhea, discharge of pus
MYC-	*Fungi:* mycology, science and study of fungi	PYEL-	*Pelvis:* pyelitis, inflammation of pelvis or the kidney
NECRO-	*Corpse, dead:* necrosis, death of cells adjoining living tissue	RACH-	*Spine:* rachicentesis, puncture into vertebral canal
NEO-	*New:* neoplasm, any new growth or formation	REN-	*Kidney:* adrenal, near the kidney
NEPH-	*Kidney:* nephrectomy, surgical excision of kidney	RETRO-	*Backward:* retroversion, turned backward (usually applies to the uterus)
NEURO-	*Nerve:* neuron, nerve cell	RHIN-	*Nose:* rhinology, knowledge concerning noses
ODONT-	*Tooth:* odontology, dentistry		
OLIG-	*Little:* oligemia, deficiency in volume of blood	SALPING-	*A tube:* salpingitis, inflammation of tube
		SEMI-	*Half:* semilunar, half moon-shaped valve
OO-	*Egg:* oocyte, original cell of egg	SEPTIC-	*Poison:* septicemia, poisoned condition of blood
OOPHOR-	*Ovary:* oophorectomy, removal of an ovary	SOMAT-	*Body:* psychosomatic, having bodily symptoms of mental origin
OPHTHAM-	*Eye:* ophthalmometer, an instrument for measuring the eye	STA-	*Make stand:* stasis, stoppage of flow of fluid, as in blood (hemostasis)

(continued)

Table 14-1 (continued)

Prefixes	Meaning/Example	Prefixes	Meaning/Example
STEN-	*Narrow:* stenosis, narrowing of duct or canal	TOX- or TOXIC-	*Poison:* toxemia, poisoned condition of blood
SUB-	*Under:* subdiaphragmatic, under the diaphragm	TRACHE-	*Trachea:* tracheitis, inflammation of the trachea
SUPER-	*Above, excessively:* superacute, excessively acute	TRANS-	*Across:* transplant, transfer tissue from one place to another
SUPRA-	*Above, on:* suprarenal, above or on the kidney	TRI-	*Three:* trigastric, having three bellies (muscle)
SYM- or SYN-	*With, together:* symphysis, a growing together, as symphysis pubis	TRICH-	*Hair:* trichosis, any disease of the hair
TACHY-	*Fast:* tachycardia, fast-beating heart	UNI-	*One:* unilateral, affecting one side
TENS-	*Stretch:* extensor, a muscle extending or stretching a limb	VAS-	*Vessel:* vasoconstrictor, nerve or drug that narrows blood vessel
THERM-	*Heat:* diathermy, therapeutic production of heat in tissues	ZOO-	*Animal:* zooblast, an animal cell

Suffixes	Meaning/Example	Suffixes	Meaning/Example
-ALGIA	*Pain:* cardialgia, pain in the heart	-OSIS (-ASIS)	*Being affected with:* arteriosclerosis, thickening and "hardening" of arteries
-ASIS or OSIS	*Affected with:* leukocytosis, excess number of leukocytes	-(O)STOMY	*Creation of an opening:* gastrostomy, creation of an artificial gastric fistula
-ASTHENIA	*Weakness:* neurasthenia, nerve weakness	-(O)TOMY	*Cutting into:* laparotomy, surgical incision into abdomen
-BLAST	*Germ:* myeloblast, bone-marrow cell	-PATHY	*Disease:* myopathy, disease of muscle
-CELE	*Tumor, hernia:* enterocele, any hernia of intestine	-PENIA	*Lack of:* leukopenia, lack of white blood cells
-CID	*Cut, kill:* germicidal, destructive to germs	-PEXY	*To fix:* proctopexy, fixation of rectum by suture
-CLYSIS	*Injection:* hypodermoclysis, injection under the skin	-PHAGIA	*Eating:* polyphagia, excessive eating
-COCCUS	*Round bacterium:* pneumococcus, bacterium of pneumonia	-PHASIA	*Speech:* aphasia, loss of power of speech
-CYTE	*Cell:* leukocyte, white cell	-PHOBIA	*Fear:* hydrophobia, fear of water
-ECTASIS	*Dilation, stretching:* angiectasis, dilation of a blood vessel	-PLASTY	*Molding:* gastroplasty, molding or reforming stomach
-ECTOMY	*Excision:* adenectomy, excision of adenoids	-PNEA	*Air or breathing:* dyspnea, difficult breathing
-EMIA	*Blood:* glycemia, sugar in blood	-POIESIS	*Making, forming:* hematopoiesis, forming blood
-ESTHESIA	*Relating to sensation:* anesthesia, absence of feeling	-PTOSIS	*Falling:* enteroptosis, falling of intestine
-FERENT	*Bear, carry:* efferent, carry out to periphery	-RHYTHMIA	*Rhythm:* arrhythmia, variation from normal rhythm of heart
-GENIC	*Producing:* pyogenic, producing pus	-RRHAGIA	*Flowing or bursting forth:* otorrhagia, hemorrhage from ear
-IATRICS	*Pertaining to a physician or the practice of healing* (medicine): pediatrics, science of medicine for children	-RRHAPHY	*Suture of:* enterorrhaphy, act of sewing up a gap in intestine
-ITIS	*Inflammation:* tonsillitis, inflammation of tonsils	-RRHEA	*Discharge:* otorrhea, discharge from ear
-LOGY	*Science of:* pathology, science of disease	-STHEN	*Pertaining to strength:* asthenia, loss of strength
-LYSIS	*Losing, flowing, dissolution:* autolysis, dissolution of tissue cells	-TAXIA or -TAXIS	*Order, arrangement of:* ataxia, failure of muscular coordination
-MALACIA	*Softening:* osteomalacia, softening of bone	-TROPHIA or -TROPHY	*Nourishment:* atrophy, wasting, or diminution
-OMA	*Tumor:* myoma, tumor made up of muscle elements	-URIA	*To do with urine:* polyuria, excessive secretion of urine

Definitions are in italic. Example terms with their definitions follow colons.

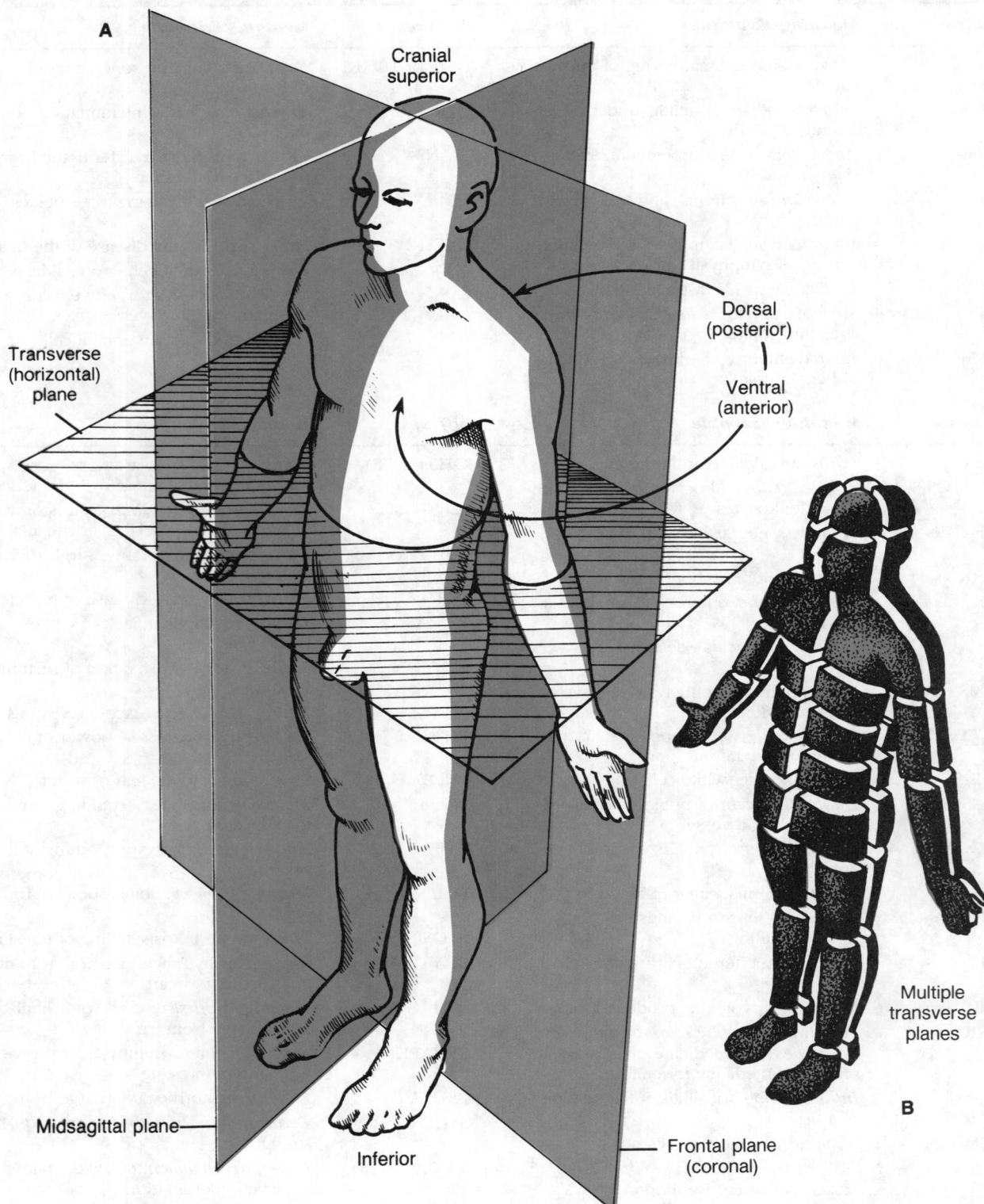

A

Cranial
superior

Transverse
(horizontal)
plane

Dorsal
(posterior)

Ventral
(anterior)

Multiple
transverse
planes

B

Midsagittal plane

Inferior

Frontal plane
(coronal)

Figure 14-2. **(A)** Body planes and directions. **(B)** Multiple transverse planes.

Table 14-2. Body Directions

Position	Definition	Examples
Superior	"Above" or in a higher position	The knee is superior to the toes but inferior to the femur.
Inferior	"Below" or in a lower position	The lips are inferior to the nose but superior to the chin.
Cranial	In or near the head	The brain is in the cranial cavity.
Caudal	Near the lower end of the body, (ie, near the end of the spine), "tail"	The buttocks, the muscles on which we sit, are located at the caudal end of the body
Anterior or ventral	Toward the front or "belly" surface of the body	The nose is on the anterior, or ventral, surface of the head.
Posterior or dorsal	Toward the back of the body	The calf is on the posterior, or dorsal, surface of the leg.
Medial	Nearer the midline	The nose is medial to the eyes.
Lateral	Farther from the midline, toward the side	The ears are lateral to the nose.
Internal	Deeper within the body	The stomach is an internal body organ.
External	Toward the outer surface of the body	The skin covers the external surface of the body.
Proximal	Nearest the origin of a part	In the upper extremity (arm), the upper arm above the elbow is proximal to the forearm below.
Distal	Farthest from the origin of a part	In the lower extremity (leg), the lower leg below the knee is distal to the thigh.
Central	Situated at or pertaining to the center	The brain and the spinal cord are part of the central nervous system.
Peripheral	Situated at or pertaining to the outward part of a surface	The peripheral nerves go out to the body parts and return to the central nervous system.
Parietal	Pertaining to the sides or the walls of a cavity	The walls of the abdominal cavity are lined with a membrane called the parietal peritoneum.
Visceral	Pertaining to the organs within a cavity	The stomach and intestines are visceral organs in the abdominal cavity
Supine	Lying with the face upward	A person lying on the dorsal surface of the body, or on the back, is supine.
Prone	Lying with the face downward	A person lying on the ventral surface, or the front of the body, is prone
Deep	Away from surface	The knife wound was deep in the abdomen.
Superficial	On or near the surface	The child had a superficial cut.

ferred to as the abdominopelvic cavity. (There is no specific anatomic division between the abdominal and pelvic areas). Table 14-3 lists the contents of each body cavity.

Divisions Within the Abdominal Cavity

The two methods of dividing the abdominal cavity for examination are *quadrants* and *regions* (Fig. 14-3).

Imaginary quadrants (fourths) help to describe signs and symptoms and locate the *viscera* (internal organs) from the surface. The quadrants can be located by drawing a line horizontally and vertically through the umbilicus. These lines create a right upper quadrant, right lower quadrant, left upper quadrant, and left lower quadrant. These quadrants are named as though being seen from the patient's point of view. They are often identified by initials in the patient's chart, such as *RUQ*, right upper quadrant; *LUQ*, left upper quadrant; *RLQ*, right lower quadrant; and *LLQ*, left lower quadrant.

Another way of dividing the abdominal cavity is by dividing it into nine regions: right and left hypochondriac, lumbar, and inquidan (iliac) regions, plus the epigastric, umbilical, and hypogastric regions in the middle.

Structural Levels in the Body

There are four basic structural levels within the body:

◆ *Cells*, the basic unit
◆ *Tissues*, made up of cells
◆ *Organs*, made up of tissues
◆ *Systems*, made up of organs

Table 14-3. Body Cavities and Their Contents	
Cavity	**Contents**
Dorsal (Posterior) Cavity	
Cranial cavity	Brain
Vertebral cavity (spinal cavity)	Spinal cord
Ventral (Anterior) Cavity	
Thoracic cavity	
Pericardial	Heart
Two pleural	Each contains a lung
Mediastinum	Large blood vessels, trachea, esophagus, and thymus gland
Abdominal cavity (abdominopelvic cavity)	
Upper abdominal cavity	Stomach, most of the intestine, liver, gallbladder, pancreas, spleen, kidneys, adrenal glands, and ureter
Pelvic cavity	Urinary bladder, remaining part of intestine, rectum, and internal reproductive organs

Cells

The basic unit of structure and function in all living things is the **cell**. A cell is living and carries out specific activities. The smallest forms of life are composed of a single cell. The human body, on the other hand, is made up of trillions of cells. The essential component of all living cells is a colloid material called **protoplasm**.

Although the human body has many different types of cells, all of them have the same basic chemicals and similar structural features. Despite being the smallest living subunit of the human body, the cell functions as a member of a highly organized team.

Special Properties of Cells

As team members, cells have become specialized in anatomic structure and physiologic function. Some cells have highly developed abilities for metabolism.

Metabolism is the ability to process foods, obtain energy from these foods, and create new products using the chemicals found in these foods.

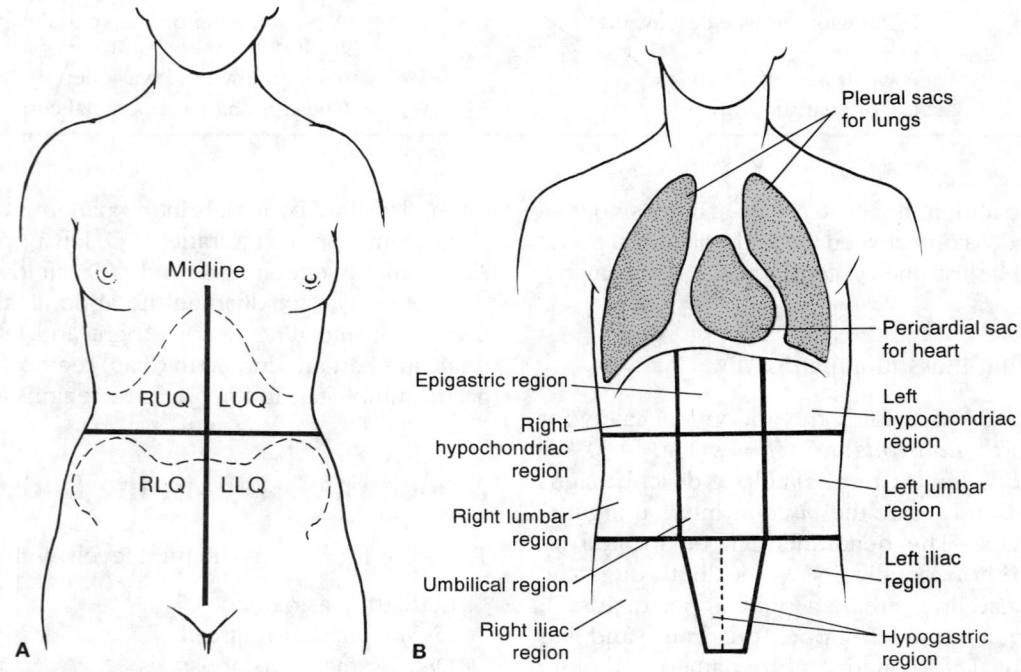

Figure 14-3. Divisions within body cavities used for examination. **(A)** Quadrants. **(B)** Regions.

There are two phases of metabolism: *anabolism* and *catabolism.* Anabolism is the building up, assimilation, or conversion of ingested substances. *Catabolism* is the breaking-down, disintegration, or tearing-down process of substances into simpler substances. By virtue of the breakdown of substances, particularly food, energy is released. The following are examples of other properties of cells:

◆ Muscle cells have the ability to move or contract; this is known as *contractility.*
◆ Nerve cells are specialized to send and receive impulses; this is known as *conductivity.*
◆ Cells are able to respond to stimuli; this process is called *irritability.*
◆ Cells have the ability to duplicate themselves, a process called *reproduction.*

The properties of metabolism, contractility, conductivity, irritability, and reproduction are present to some degree in all cells. Individual cells do not function independently. Rather, the cells have developed specialties interrelated to other cells. This teamwork permits the organism to have organization and adaptability, which is not possible in the single-cell microorganism.

Structure and Function of the Cell

Cytology is the science that investigates the formation, structure, and function of cells. From the study of various sample cells, a great deal can be learned about the general condition of an entire organism.

Cells are too small to be seen without a microscope, except for the egg cell or ovum, which is just visible to the naked eye. Human cells vary in shape, size, and function.

The shape of cells may be round, spherical, rectangular, or irregular. Some cells change shape as they move, but each category of cells retains its shape; for example, nerve cells will always look like nerve cells.

Most cells vary in size from 1 to 100 microns, abbreviated μ (1 micron = $\frac{1}{25,000}$ of an inch). Ten to 1,000 cells can be placed on the head of a pin.

Although cells have similar abilities, their functions are specialized. Nerve cells have filaments on their ends that carry or receive impulses. Muscle cells are long, thin fibers that permit contraction and relaxation of the cell. A fat cell is large with empty spaces suitable for storage of lipids (fat).

Cell Membrane. The parts of a cell are illustrated in Figure 14-4. The outer boundary of a cell is called the cell **membrane**. This membrane is a delicate film that is capable of permitting the entrance and exit of some materials, while excluding the transfer of other substances. This is called *selective permeability.* The cell membrane is an active participant in the life of the cell. Several mechanisms of cellular transportation across

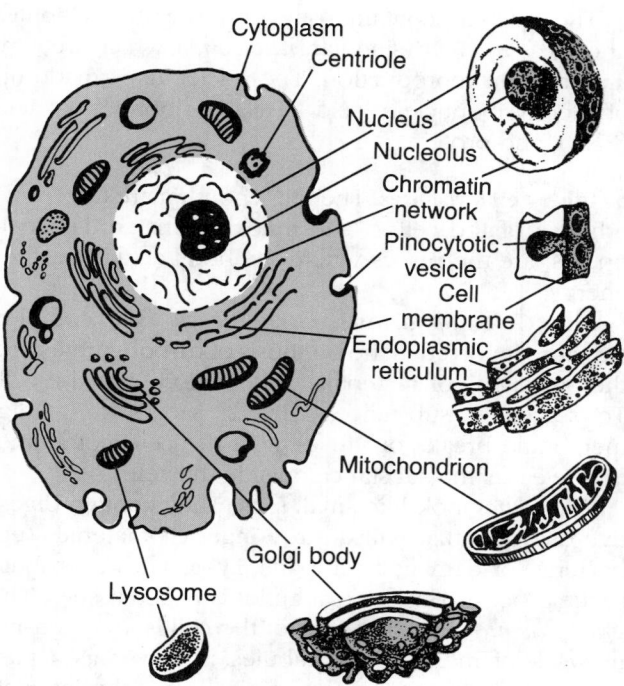

Figure 14-4. A typical cell. The nucleus is the control center of the cell. The organelles in the cytoplasm (the endoplasmic reticulum, mitochondria, Golgi bodies, and lysosomes) are the functional substances. Note that the cell membrane is more correctly called the *plasma membrane.* This plasma membrane is made up of lipids (fats) and proteins. There are also channels in the membrane, which are of vital importance in the transport of materials across the plasma membrane. Note that a pinocytotic vesicle is shown; this mechanism is explained in Chapter 16.

the membrane have developed. Cellular transportation is discussed in Chapter 16.

Nucleus. The control center of the cell is the nucleus. It is responsible for the reproduction (division) of the cell and the coordination of certain other cell activities. The nucleus is suspended in cytoplasm in or near the center of the cell and is surrounded by its own nuclear membrane.

Chromosomes. The human nucleus contains 46 chromosomes in the form of *chromatin.* When a cell divides, the chromatin uncoils its threads into visible chromosomes. The **chromosomes** contain the **genes** that transmit the specifications for the new organism. The new organism could be an enzyme, a red blood cell, a protein for tissue repair, or any of a thousand other proteins. Although normal human cells have 23 pairs, or 46 total chromosomes, the genes are present in the thousands. Genes determine whether a living organism is male or female, whether it has blue or brown eyes, and whether it has dark or light skin.

The nucleus contains one or more tiny globules known as *nucleoli* (singular: *nucleolus*), which are very important in reproduction. The nucleolus is made up of deoxyribonucleic acid (DNA), ribonucleic acid (RNA), and protein.

Other Cell Structures. The mitochondria are the "powerhouse of the cells." The mitochondria, rod-shaped bodies, are the places where the body actually makes energy.

The *Golgi apparatus* (Golgi body) is a complex structure involved in the synthesis of carbohydrates and the packaging of materials for secretion from the cell. To secrete a substance, a small sac of the Golgi membrane breaks off, fuses with the cell membrane, and releases the substance outside the cell.

Lysosomes look like small sacs. They contain digestive enzymes that will destroy ingested materials (eg, bacteria) or damaged cell parts. Lysosomes contribute to the process of inflammation in damaged tissues. The *endoplasmic reticulum* (ER) of the cell is an extensive network of membranous tubules. It serves as a passageway of materials within the cell. It is the intracellular roadway for the transport of materials used within the cell. The small dots on the ER are called ribosomes. They serve to manufacture enzymes and other proteins.

Ribosomes are the site of protein synthesis. While some are found in the ER, others float freely within the cytoplasm.

Cilia are hairlike threads that sweep materials across the cell surface. An individual cell has many cilia. Only one human cell has a flagellum, the sperm cell. The flagellum provides motility or movement for the sperm cell.

Cell Reproduction

Mitosis. Through a complicated process called **mitosis**, cells divide into two parts to reproduce themselves. Each of the "daughter" cells is an exact genetic duplicate of the original or "mother" cell. The body can be thought of as a group of cells, and mitosis is responsible for the body's growth and for repair and replacement of its injured and dead tissues.

The amazing process of mitosis occurs as a result of a rearrangement of particles in the nucleus (Fig. 14-5). Briefly, the centrosomes separate and are drawn toward opposite ends of the cell. The nuclear membrane then disappears. The chromosomes split, and half move toward each centrosome. The cell then begins to elongate, thinning in the middle with the cell membrane following the same shape. The cell finally splits into two parts, with half the cytoplasm, the nuclear material, and the cell wall in each new cell. Because of the genes, each new cell is identical to the original from which it was formed.

Mitosis is essential for the following:

◆ Growth of a single fertilized egg. After conception, the fertilized egg grows into trillions of cells.
◆ Repair of wounds by replacing damaged or dead cells
◆ Tumor formation in which abnormal cells, dividing by mitosis, result in more abnormal cells

Certain cells in the body are not able to reproduce in an adult. If muscle cells or neurons (nerve cells) die, their functions are lost. Loss of muscle cells in the heart due to a heart attack may damage the heart so severely that the heart may lose the ability to contract effectively, and the patient may die. Destruction of spinal cord neurons will result in paralysis and loss of sensation below the level of the injury.

Reproduction also refers to the division of the fertilized ovum (egg cell), which is responsible for the creation of new individuals. The sperm cell and the ovum reproduce by *meiosis*, a more complex process of cell division.

Deoxyribonucleic Acid. The chromosomes in the cell's nucleus are made up of **DNA**, which stores and transfers genetic information. All DNA **molecules** are composed of the same chemical compounds. The arrangement of these compounds within each molecule determines the genetic code of cell duplication (Fig. 14-6). The double helix formation and the specific arrangements of its basic chemicals create a chemical

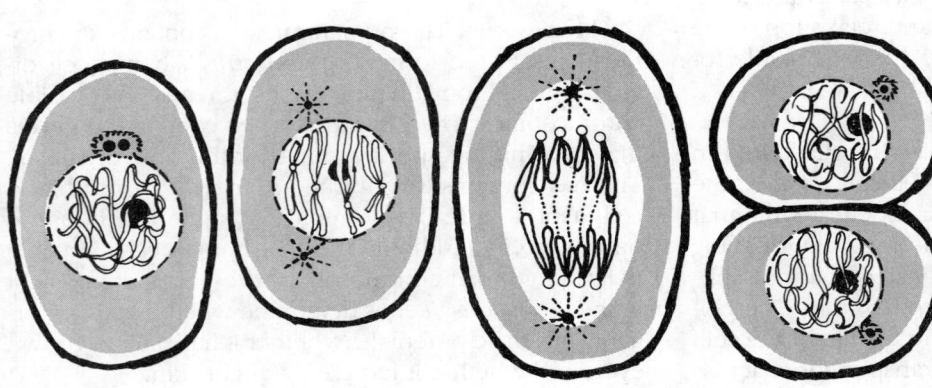

Figure 14-5. Mitosis (simplified sequence). The centrosome divides, the chromatin material of the nucleus changes into rod-shaped chromosomes, and two daughter cells form within the cell membrane.

blueprint. DNA molecules spell out genetic instructions that control the activities of a cell in general and the construction of complex protein molecules in particular. Because most of the molecules in every cell are proteins, their production is the key to life. Genes are segments of DNA. Genes are the genetic codes or specific recipes for proteins.

Enzymes are one type of the complex protein structures determined by DNA. Every one of the thousands of different chemical reactions that take place in our bodies requires a specific enzyme to speed it up. DNA directs the formation of thousands of different proteins to meet the needs of enzyme production.

Another of DNA's tasks is the formation of other proteins that make up skin, muscle, blood vessels, and all internal organs. DNA builds the body's protein from endless combinations of 20 amino acids. If all of the coded DNA instructions found in one single cell were translated into English, they would more than fill 100 volumes of an encyclopedia.

Ribonucleic Acid. For a protein to be formed, a gene must be duplicated. Protein synthesis occurs in the cellular ribosomes, which are formed in the cytoplasm. The specific gene must temporarily break from the DNA ladder and become duplicated. RNA is the chemical messenger that carries the duplicated gene away from the DNA to the ribosomes. The duplicated gene carried by RNA enters the cytoplasm and attaches to ribosomes.

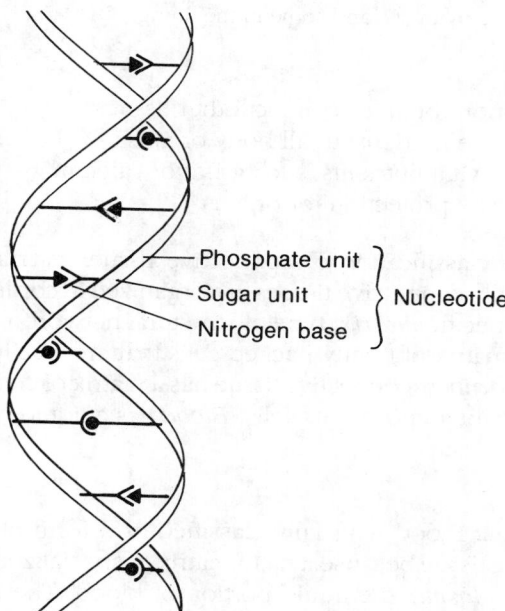

Phosphate unit
Sugar unit } Nucleotide
Nitrogen base

Figure 14-6. Schematic representation of the basic structure of a DNA molecule. Each structural unit consists of a phosphate group and a sugar group to which is attached a nitrogen base. The arrangement of nitrogen bases "spells out" the genetic instructions that control all activities of the cell.

The desired protein is made in the ribosomes. The newly formed protein can either leave the ribosomes by way of the canals in the ER or be packaged in the Golgi apparatus for secretion from the cell.

Tissues

Cells of the same type and structure form tissues. Each tissue has a special function. The list below identifies the four principal types of tissues and their basic functions:

♦ *Epithelial tissue* protects body parts and produces secretions.
♦ *Connective tissue* anchors and supports other body structures. Blood is a special type of connective tissue that carries food and oxygen to the cells and carries wastes away.
♦ *Muscle tissue* causes movement of the body.
♦ *Nerve tissue* conducts impulses to and from all parts of the body.

Epithelial Tissues

The main functions of epithelial tissues follow:

♦ Cover and protect all body surfaces, cavities, and lumina (hollow portions of blood vessels or body tubes)
♦ Absorb and secrete substances from the digestive tract
♦ Secrete substances from glands
♦ Provide filtration in the kidneys
♦ Form highly specialized epithelial tissues in the taste buds and nose
♦ Transport particles contained in mucus away from lungs

Generally, epithelial tissues are *avascular*, or without blood vessels. To receive nourishment, the tissues must receive nutrients from underlying tissue, such as connective tissue, through a process called diffusion.

In places where epithelium is subjected to much destruction, the tissues are modified to provide greater protection. For example, *calluses* form on the bottom on the feet or the palms of the hand. Because the outer layers of epithelial cells are constantly being worn off at the surface, the bottom layers of epithelium are continually producing new cells. Thus, epithelium is in a continuous state of regeneration.

Types. There are several types of cells that are called epithelial tissue. Each of these types of cells has a characteristic shape and may be found in single or multiple layers (Fig. 14-7). The term *simple* is used for a single layer of cells. The term *stratified* means that there are several layers of cells. For example, *squamous* (scaly) cells can be found in single layers, as in the alveoli (air

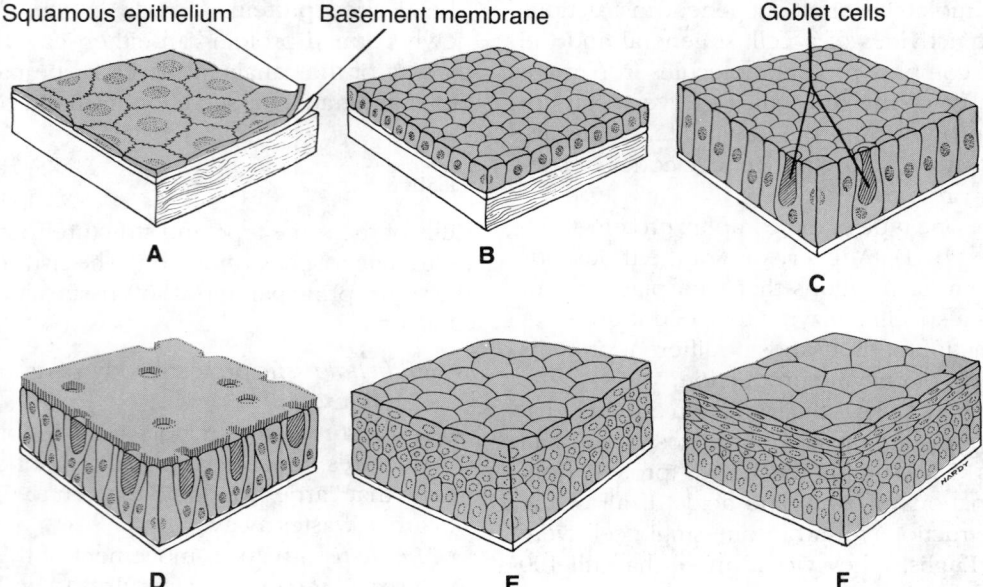

Figure 14-7. Types of epithelial tissue. **(A)** Simple squamous (basement membrane) tissue is found in the lungs. **(B)** Simple cuboidal tissue is found in the ovaries, thyroid, sweat glands, and salivary glands. **(C)** Simple columnar tissue is found in the stomach and intestines and in ducts of glands. **(D)** Pseudostratified columnar tissue (ciliated shown) is found as the mucous membranes of respiratory passages and eustachian tubes. It also exists as nonciliated. The nonciliated type is found in the ducts of some glands, such as the parotid salivary gland and the male urethra. **(E)** Transitional tissue lines the urinary bladder. It varies in shape, depending on whether the bladder is full or empty; when full, the cells slide and stretch. **(F)** Stratified squamous tissue makes up the epidermis of skin and the lining of the mouth, pharynx, ovaries, and vagina.

Types of epithelial tissue *not shown* include stratified columnar, which is found in the epiglottis, parts of the pharynx and anal canal, and the male urethra; and simple ciliated columnar, which is found in the lining of bronchi, the nasal cavity, the oviducts, and some in the lining of the uterus.

sacs) of the lungs, or they can be stratified, as in the mouth and the esophagus.

Transitional epithelium is a type of stratified squamous epithelium. It has the ability to change shape. In the bladder, it enables the bladder to fill and stretch without damaging its walls.

Ciliated epithelium is a type of columnar cell epithelium which has fine, hairlike extensions on its surface called cilia. The cilia move in waves and carry materials across the cell surface. A very effective protective mechanism, cilia sweep mucus with trapped dust and bacteria away from sterile areas, such as the lungs, toward nonsterile areas, such as the trachea and mouth. The stomach is also equipped to destroy bacteria with its hydrochloric acid.

Epithelial cells shaped like goblets have the ability to form secretions. They are called *glands* and are discussed in Chapter 19.

Connective Tissue

Connective tissue varies greatly in structure and function. The main functions of connective tissue follow:

◆ Support, bind, or connect other tissues
◆ Provide nutrients to all body organs
◆ Store vital nutrients, such as fat or calcium
◆ Provide protection for organs

The classification of connective tissues varies, but generally connective tissues are organized according to each specific *matrix* (type of structural network). *Bone* has a matrix of tightly packed cells that are rich in calcium. *Adipose* connective tissue has a matrix of collagen fibers and adipose (fat) cells. *Blood* has a liquid matrix called plasma.

Blood. Blood is usually classified as a form of connective tissue because it has a matrix of specialized cells called *plasma*, the liquid portion of blood. The major *formed elements* of plasma are the three types of blood cells: *erythrocytes* (red blood cells, or RBCs), *leukocytes* (white blood cells, or WBCs), and *thrombocytes* (platelets). RBCs carry the oxygen and carbon dioxide needed for cellular respiration or the formation of energy. WBCs destroy pathogens and develop immunity to some diseases. Platelets are cell fragments that provide a major step in the blood-clotting process.

Soft Connective Tissue. The three types of soft connective tissue are areolar (loosely structured), fibrous (densely structured), and adipose (fatty).

Areolar tissue (loose connective tissue) is the most abundant connective tissue in the body. It is like a packing material that holds things in place. It provides support for body parts and allows for some stretching in all directions. It is *highly vascular*, meaning that it contains numerous blood vessels; thus, areolar tissue plays an important role in cell nutrition. It is perfectly suited for the diffusion of nutrients and waste materials across cell membranes (see Chapter 16). Areolar tissues are located where the body can intercept pathogens before they enter the bloodstream, such as just underneath the skin and beneath the epithelial tissue that lines the digestive and respiratory tracts.

Fibrous connective tissue is found where a need for flexible strength exists, such as in the dermis layer of the skin and in *ligaments* and *tendons*. (Ligaments connect bone to bone; tendons connect muscle to bone.) The blood supply to fibrous connective tissue is poor, which is the reason it heals relatively slowly.

Elastic connective tissue can stretch to one and a half times its original size. Like a rubber band, it will snap back to its original size. It is found in areas that are stretched on a regular basis, such as in the large arteries, the larynx (voice box), the alveoli (air sacs), and the external ear.

Adipose tissue is fatty. It stores fat as a food reserve and is found throughout the body. It serves as a padding to protect various body structures, such as the eyeballs and kidneys. It insulates against heat loss. Researchers have noted that most of our body's adipose tissue is formed prenatally (before birth) and during the first year of life. While dieting and exercise may eliminate stored fat within the adipose tissue, the adipose tissue itself remains, waiting to be restocked with new energy stores (ie, new fat).[1]

Special Considerations in Children
Adipose Tissue

It has been suggested that increased amounts of fats during the child's first year of life will lead to an increase in adipose tissue, which may predispose a person to obesity in later years. This has not been proven but is held in high regard by many authorities.

---

[1] Van De Graff KM, Fox SI. Concepts of Human Anatomy and Physiology, p. 147. Dubuque, IA, W.C. Brown, 1992.

Hard Connective Tissue. Hard connective tissue includes bone and cartilage.

Bone is the hardest connective tissue. It gives the entire body structure, support, and mobility. Being well supplied with blood vessels (vascular), bone is also the site of numerous metabolic activities, such as the storage of calcium. Some bones contain red bone marrow, which is the site for producing red blood cells.

Special Considerations in Aging
Brittle Bones

Often during the aging process, the bones lose calcium and become brittle. This may result in fractures that do not heal easily.

Cartilage is tough, elastic tissue found between segments of the spinal cord (the vertebrae) and between the ends of the long bones. Cartilage (also known as *gristle*) gives shape to the nose, larynx, and ear. Between bones, cartilage serves as a shock absorber and reduces friction between moving parts. (Most bones are first formed as one type of cartilage and later convert into bone through a process known as *ossification*). Cartilage is poorly supplied with blood vessels; therefore, injured cartilaginous tissue will heal slowly, if at all.

Muscle Tissue

Muscle tissues contain unique fibers that can contract (shorten), thus bringing about movement. Chemicals sent to the muscles from the nervous system supply the stimulus to contract.

Muscle tissue may be classified in several ways. It may be classified according to function: skeletal, smooth, and cardiac. It may be classified according to appearance: striated and nonstriated. It also can be classified according to what controls its action: voluntary or involuntary (see Chapter 19).

Nerve Tissue

Nerve tissue is composed of *neurons* and *neuroglia*. Neurons are the actual working nerve cells that respond to stimuli. There are several types of neurons, but the two main types are the sensory (*afferent*) nerves and the motor (*efferent*) nerves. They send impulses to and receive impulses from all parts of the body (see Chapter 18).

Membranes

Membranes are sheets of epithelial or connective tissues that act together to cover surfaces, line surfaces, or separate organs or lobes. Some membranes produce secretions.

Epithelial membranes are subdivided into *mucous* membranes and *serous* membranes. *Connective tissue membranes* are subdivided into *skeletal* and *fascial* membranes.

Mucous membranes are also known as *mucosa.* They line body cavities that open to the outside of the body. The *mucus* secreted by the membrane lubricates and protects against bacterial invasion and other foreign particles. *Serous membranes* are also known as *serosa.* They line the cavities that do *not* open to the exterior. These membranes secrete *serous fluid,* which is thinner than mucus. It prevents friction when organs are in contact with one another. Serous membranes are divided into two layers: *parietal* and *visceral.* The *parietal* layer is the portion of the membrane attached to wall of the body cavity, while the *visceral* layer covers internal organs.

Skeletal membranes are connective tissue membranes that cover bones and cartilage. They act chiefly to support the body structures.

Synovial membranes are a type of skeletal membrane that lines joint cavities and secretes *synovial fluid.* Synovial fluid is a lubricant that provides for the smoother motion of bone; thus, friction is reduced between the moving parts. *Fascial membranes* are sheets of tissues that hold organs in place. The *superficial fascia* is a layer that connects the skin to underlying struc-

tures. *Deep fascia* binds muscles to tendons to anchor bones and separates muscles into functional groups.

Organs and Systems

An organ is a group of different types of tissues that formed in a specific manner to perform a definite function (Fig. 14-8). For example, the heart is a combination of muscle, nerve, blood, and epithelial tissues. Organs do not work independently but are associated with other organs and may have many functions.

These group associations are called *systems,* groups of organs in which each contributes its share to the function of the whole. Systems do specialized work in the body, but all systems depend on one another. Your understanding of the structure and the function of the systems is the basis for your own health habits and your care of patients. The structure and function of these systems and their organs are discussed in Chapters 15 through 25.

> **Key Concept**
>
> The body operates as an integrated whole. The optimum functioning of one body system is often dependent on the functioning of other systems.

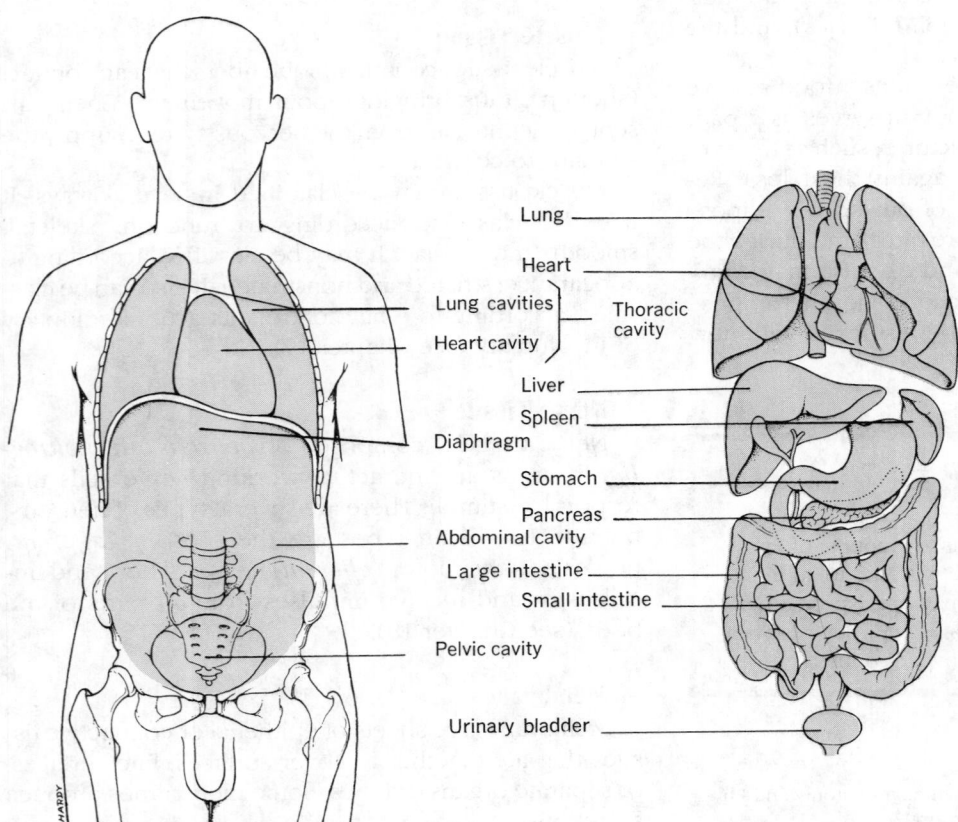

Figure 14-8. Major internal organs of the body and their relative positions. Each of these systems is discussed in more detail in Chapters 15 through 25.

Lung
Heart
Lung cavities
Heart cavity
Thoracic cavity
Liver
Spleen
Diaphragm
Stomach
Pancreas
Abdominal cavity
Large intestine
Small intestine
Pelvic cavity
Urinary bladder

Keys for Review

Key Questions for Critical Thinking

1. Discuss the concept of homeostasis.
2. Describe how information about prefixes, suffixes, and root words help you in studying to be a nurse.
3. Describe the following planes of the body: transverse, frontal, and sagittal.
4. Describe the functions of DNA and RNA.
5. Discuss the significant characteristics of muscle cells and nerve cells.

Key Readings

Chabner D. The Language of Medicine, Ed 4. Philadelphia, W.B. Saunders, 1991

Scanlon VC, Sanders T. Essentials of Anatomy and Physiology. Philadelphia, F.A. Davis, 1991

Thomas V. Life Sciences for Nursing and Health Technologies, Ed 5. Long Beach, CA, Technicourse, 1986

Van De Graff K, Fox SI. Concepts of Human Anatomy and Physiology, Ed 3. Dubuque, IA, W.C. Brown, 1992

Enrichment Keys

Memmler RL, Cohen BH, Wood DL. Structure and Function of the Human Body, Ed 5. Philadelphia, J.B. Lippincott, 1992

Keys to Learning More

Unit Four: normal anatomy and physiology

Unit Thirteen: deviations from normal body structure and function in children

Unit Fourteen: deviations from normal structure and function in the adult patient

Unit Fifteen: deviations from normal in the older adult

15 Integumentary System

Learning Objectives

◆ Name at least six functions of the integumentary system
◆ Identify the three major layers of the skin and their functions
◆ Name three factors that influence skin coloring
◆ Name the appendages of the skin and their functions
◆ State the function of glands
◆ Name at least five changes that occur to aging skin

Key Terms

carotene	desquamation	radiation
ceruminal	epidermis	sebaceous
collagen	evaporation	sebum
conduction	freckle	squamous
convection	integument	sudoriferous
corium	keratin	thermoregulation
dermis	melanin	

Keys to Understanding This Chapter

Chapter 5: basic human needs, including safety (protection)
Chapter 14: organization of the human body

Key Points

◆ The skin, the largest organ in the body, is vital for survival.
◆ The epidermis contains melanin (protects the body from ultraviolet rays) and keratin (protects the body from excessive water loss or gain) and is the outermost protective layer.

Key Points (continued)

◆ The dermis contains nerves, hair follicles, blood and lymph vessels, and glands. This is where skin reproduction takes place.
◆ The subcutaneous layer is made up of fat cells that insulate and protect underlying tissues.
◆ Glands are unicellular or multicellular structures of epithelial tissue that produce secretions.
◆ The skin plays a large part in the body's thermoregulation by convection, evaporation, conduction, and radiation.
◆ Skin problems are common in the elderly, and thorough daily inspection is necessary.

Key Topics Outline

Structure and Function
   Skin
   Accessory Structures of the Skin
System Physiology
   Thermoregulation
   Sensory Awareness
Effects of Aging on the System

Key Learning Activities

◆ Visit a burn unit, and discuss the healing process necessary when the skin has been badly injured.
◆ On a chart, identify the structures of the skin and its appendages. Describe the function of each.
◆ Write a report about pressure ulcers and their treatment.

Rosdahl CB: Textbook of Basic Nursing, 6th ed. © 1995 J.B. Lippincott Company

Skin forms the body's integumentary system. **Integument** means "covering." Because skin covers the entire outside of the body, it is the largest organ in the body. It is called an organ because it is composed of a variety of tissues, each of which has a specific purpose.

Several types of epithelial tissues are found in the skin. Epithelial tissues provide part of the skin's protective and absorptive functions. Glands, made up of epithelial tissue, provide secretions from the internal environment to the external world. Connective tissues attach the skin to the underlying muscle. Nervous tissue is integrated throughout the skin to help the body react to the world around it. Nerves in the skin are responsible for the sensations of heat, cold, pain, touch, and pressure. In addition, the integumentary system is interdependent with other tissues, organs, and systems of the body. The skin and its accessory structures create a dynamic surface for communication between internal and external forces.

> **Key Concept**
>
> The integumentary system is composed of the skin and its accessory structures: hair, nails, and glands. Integument means covering.

Structure and Function

Skin

The skin is composed of three principal layers: epidermis, dermis, and subcutaneous (Fig. 15-1). The epidermis makes up the outer layer of the skin. Below the epidermis lies the dermis. The dermal layer has the important structures of hair, glands, blood vessels, and nerves. The subcutaneous layer is a single layer below the dermis. It binds the upper layers to the underlying muscle tissues.

Functions of the skin are basically protection, metabolism, and sensation. The accompanying box lists these functions and the skin's methods of performing these functions. Substances produced by the skin aid in protection and metabolism. Secreted oil acts as a waterproofing material, while protecting the skin from drying and cracking. Perspiration helps the body get rid of certain waste products. The skin also has a role in the production of vitamin D from sunlight. (Vitamin D is important in the growth and repair of bones.)

The skin has some power of absorption. Scientists are learning how to adapt this mechanism to applying medications through the skin (transdermal).

Functions of the skin can be better understood with the following discussion of structures.

The Epidermis

The **epidermis** is the outermost protective layer of the skin. It is composed of **squamous** (scaly) epithelium. The innermost layer of the epidermis is composed of living cells and is called the *stratum germinativum* or *basal layer*. Here in the deepest level of the epidermis, mitosis (division and replication of cells) takes place. As the cells in the basal layer divide, they push up older cells toward the body's surface. Thus, the living inner cells of the epidermis are continually replacing the outer cells. The total replacement process takes about 6 to 8 weeks.

The outer layer, the *stratum corneum* or horny layer, contains all the dead cells from the layers below. These cells are rubbed off constantly by bathing, friction of movement, and so forth. This process is called **desquamation**.

All that is left of the cells after friction is a protein called keratin. **Keratin** is the true protector of the body. It creates a waterproof barrier. Most microorganisms cannot penetrate unbroken skin.

> **Key Concept**
>
> Damage to the dermis (such as a second- or third-degree burn) takes longer to heal because the mitotic (reproductive) structures of the skin have been lost.

The epidermis has no nerves or blood supply. It does not receive direct nourishment from the circulatory system.

Normally the epidermis and the dermis do not lie flat on one another. The dermis reaches up into the epidermis, causing ripples on the skin surface known as *fingerprints*.

Sometimes friction to the skin causes a separation of the epidermis and dermis. This leads to tissue fluid accumulation (blister). Areas of greater friction, such as the soles of the feet and the palms of the hands, will cause the epidermis to thicken and develop *calluses*.

Skin Color. Normal coloration of the skin is produced by a combination of three pigments: melanin, carotene, and hemoglobin.

Melanin is a brown-black pigment produced by melanocytes, found mostly in the basal layer of the epidermis. All races have the same number of melanocytes. The amount of melanin produced is a reflection of genetics and exposure to ultraviolet (UV) light. Melanin protects the body from the damaging effects of UV light. Occasionally, individuals, called albinos, are born without the ability to make melanin from the melanocytes. A true albino has totally white hair and skin. This person's eyes look red because of the lack of pigment in the iris and because of the reflection of the blood vessels in the eyes.

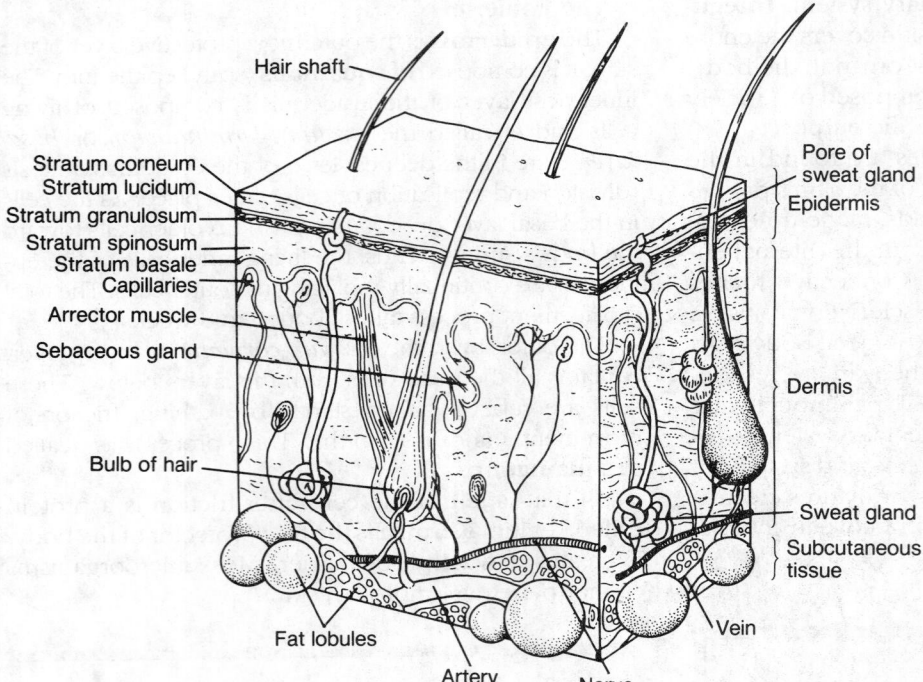

Hair shaft

Stratum corneum
Stratum lucidum
Stratum granulosum
Stratum spinosum
Stratum basale
Capillaries
Arrector muscle
Sebaceous gland

Bulb of hair

Fat lobules

Artery

Nerve

Pore of sweat gland
Epidermis

Dermis

Sweat gland
Subcutaneous tissue

Vein

Figure 15-1. Cross-section of structures of the skin.

Functions of the Integumentary System

Protection

♦ Provides barrier against microorganisms and foreign materials
♦ Helps prevent absorption of substances from outside the body
♦ Defends against many chemicals
♦ Protects against water loss or gain
♦ Protects underlying structures, such as fragile organs
♦ Protects against excessive sun exposure (ultraviolet rays) by production of melanin
♦ Provides thermoregulation (protection against excessive heat loss or gain)
♦ Cushions internal organs against trauma
♦ Produces secretions for protection and water regulation

Metabolism

♦ Provides insulation (skin hairs, subcutaneous fat)
♦ Helps produce and use vitamin D
♦ Helps the body eliminate certain waste products
♦ Absorbs medications
♦ Provides storage of fat

Sensation

♦ Perceives stimuli: heat, cold, pain, pressure, touch
♦ Provides social and sexual communication
♦ Allows for physical intimacy

Freckles are patches of melanin clustered together. Vitiligo is a skin condition in which the melanocytes stop making melanin, causing localized areas of distinct white spots.

Carotene is a yellowish pigment found in parts of the epidermis and dermis. Carotene is the precursor of vitamin A. It is abundant in the skin of Asian people.

Hemoglobin is a pigment found in red blood cells. Oxygen binds to the hemoglobin molecule and is carried by the red blood cells. The bright red color of oxygenated blood flowing throughout the dermis gives a pinkish tone to light-skinned people.

The Dermis

The **dermis**, also known as the **corium**, is the "true skin." It is composed entirely of live cells. The dermis contains blood and lymph vessels, nerves, hair follicles, sweat glands, and sebaceous glands.

Several types of connective tissue are found in the dermis. One of these is collagen ("colla" means glue). **Collagen** is a tough, resistant, and flexible fibrous protein. In youth, collagen is loose and elastic. It hardens and loses elasticity with age.

Special Considerations in Aging
Wrinkling of Skin

Wrinkles are due to the loss of collagen and elastic fibers. (Cigarette smoking has been linked to a more rapid destruction of these fibers and can lead to the development of wrinkles at a younger age.)

The Subcutaneous Layer

The subcutaneous tissue layer is the layer beneath the dermis and on top of the layer of muscle. Its purpose is to attach the epidermal-dermal layers to the underlying organs. It specializes in the formation and storage of lipocytes (fat cells). Functionally, the subcutaneous layer cushions and protects underlying areas. It also serves as a heat insulator. The amount of fat stored varies with the age, sex, region of the body, and the nutritional state of the individual.

The body genetically remembers ancestral times of famine and has become efficient at maintaining life-saving storage houses of energy (ie, the fat cells). Because modern civilization usually provides food on a regular basis, the body may not use its stored fat.

Accessory Structures of the Skin

The hair, nails, sebaceous (oil) glands, sudoriferous (sweat) glands, and ceruminal glands are the main accessory structures (appendages) of the skin.

Hair

The skin is covered with hair except for a few areas, such as the palms of the hands, soles of the feet, lips, nipples, penis, and labia minora. The scalp, axilla, and pubis are densely haired in a mature adult. Male hormones cause greater density of hair on the entire body of a male and influence the ability to grow a beard.

Hair is composed of keratinized cells. The visible, but dead, portion of hair above the skin is the shaft. The part lying below the skin is the root. Hair grows from a tiny sac or bulb within the hair follicles (see Figure 15-1). The dermal cell layer provides nutrients for the growing hair in much the same manner as the epidermis receives nutrients. (Hair care products do not affect hair growth, only the general appearance of the visible hair). Hair grows slowly (approximately 1 mm every 3 days). Each follicle contains a single hair root, which, as long as it is alive, will continue to grow a hair. We all lose 25 to 100 hairs per day. Each hair that is lost is actually pushed out by the growth of a new hair.

Baldness (alopecia) may be related to disease, high fever, emotional stress, surgery, pregnancy, chemotherapy, or hereditary factors. The male hormone testosterone contributes to baldness in men. Healthy females rarely become totally bald, although they may experience thinning hair.

Hair color is due to the type and amount of the pigment melanin in a layer of the hair. The greater the amount of melanin, the darker the hair. Red hair is due to a pigment with an iron base (trichosiderin).

Special Considerations in Aging

Melanin in Hair

As a person ages, melanin is lost, and the hair appears gray; with a total loss of melanin, the hair appears white.

Surrounding each hair follicle are small, smooth muscles called the *arrector pili* (singular; arrectores pilorum). Stimulated by cold or fear, these involuntary muscles contract, making the hairs stand erect. This gives the skin the appearance of "goose flesh" or "goose bumps." These erect hairs give the skin an "air cushion," which is a protective insulating mechanism of the body.

The primary function of hair is protection. Scalp hair protects from sunlight and insulates against cold. Eyelashes and eyebrows have the distinctive purpose of keeping dust particles and perspiration out of the eyes.

Clinically, hair can reveal several adverse conditions. A hair sample can reveal exposure to heavy metals or other poisons much more accurately than a blood specimen. Nutritional status is revealed in hair texture.

Attitudes and needs concerning hair vary among racial and ethnic groups. The Hispanic person may place a high regard on long hair in females. Native Americans may use hair as a method of identification of their cultural heritage. Hair is often associated with a person's individuality and sexual attraction by all races. Trauma or rubbing hair in an African American can cause a "wooling" effect. Black hair may spontaneously knot and may contain as much as 60% more sebaceous secretions than lighter hair. The person with very curly, dry hair may need to add grease to control or straighten the hair.

Nails

Nails protect the sensitive tips of fingers and toes. They help a person grab and pick up objects. Nails are tightly packed cells of the stratum corneum of the epidermis. They are keratinized dead cells. Table 15-1 summarizes parts of a nail.

Table 15-1. Description of Major Nail Parts

Part	Description
Nail root	Proximal portion of nail; live cells; mitosis occurs here.
Lunula	White, half-moon shaped area found at base of nail; white color is caused by air mixed with keratin.
Cuticle	Band of epidermis that covers nail bed; called "hangnail" when it splits.
Nail bed	Nail rests on this portion of epidermis.

Mitosis occurs in the nail root. The new cells push the older cells away from the nail bed at a rate of approximately 1 mm per week. A traumatically lost fingernail takes about 3 to 5 months to regrow, and toenails take about 12 to 18 months to completely regrow. A nail will continue to regrow as long as the live cells in the nail bed are undamaged.

The nails normally reflect a pinkish tone because of rich vascular areas in the fingers. When gentle pressure is applied and released, the nail becomes white but quickly returns to pink. Poor circulatory status and several nutritional deficiencies may be noted in unhealthy nails. Poor self-esteem and emotional difficulties may manifest in nail-biting, chewing and picking of cuticles, or poor nail hygiene.

The Sebaceous Glands

The **sebaceous** or oil glands, as shown in Figure 15-1, lie close to the hair follicles into which they usually drain. **Sebum** is the oily secretion of these glands; it travels to the surface of the skin through the hair follicles. Sebum helps to make the skin soft and the hair glossy. As a defense mechanism, sebum prevents drying of the skin, thus helping to protect it from cracking. Cracked areas in the skin are an invitation to invasion by microorganisms. Sebum also helps to waterproof the top layer of the epidermis (the stratum corneum).

The activity of the sebaceous glands increases in puberty. Sebum may trap bacteria in the skin's pores causing inflamed or infected glands, more commonly known as pimples or acne. Aging decreases the activities of these glands. Thus, older skin is dryer and more fragile.

Sudoriferous or Sweat Glands

The **sudoriferous** or sweat glands are located in the dermis. One type (apocrine sweat glands), which become active during puberty, secrete sweat into the hair follicle. The apocrine glands are most numerous in the axillae. The nominal odor from these glands gives each person an individual scent.

The second type (eccrine sweat glands), are distributed widely over the body, but are especially numerous on the upper lip, forehead, back, palms, and soles. They secrete sweat into numerous ducts that empty into pores. There are about 3,000 sweat glands in one square inch of the palm of the hands.

Perspiration secreted by the sudoriferous glands is nearly 100% water, with trace amounts of urea, uric acid, and salts and minute amounts of other elements. Urea and uric acid are breakdown or waste products of protein. The kidney, liver, and intestines normally excrete the majority of the body's wastes. In some diseased states, the skin can increase its capacity as an excretory organ and can become a noticeable clinical sign of pathology. (Diaphoresis refers to excessive perspiration.)

Ceruminal Glands

Ceruminal glands are specialized glands found only in the skin of the external auditory meatus, a passage that leads into the ear. The function of these glands is to protect the *tympanic membrane* (eardrum), which is essential to hearing.

Cerumen (wax) accumulates and impairs hearing or promotes infection in the ear canal. The moisture content of cerumen varies somewhat between the races, and this may affect hearing acuity or the tendency toward ear infections. Asians and Native Americans tend to have "dry ear wax." African American and white people have a tendency toward "wet ear wax."

System Physiology

One of the major functions of the integumentary system is protection, and especially protection of the internal organs. The internal temperature needs to remain almost constant for all the other systems to function. This is carried out through a process called thermoregulation. The skin also helps the individual experience the outside world through sensory awareness. The physiology of these two activities is discussed below.

Thermoregulation

A person's body temperature is an indicator of physiologic changes taking place in that person's body. That is why one of the important techniques nurses learn is how to take temperatures.

The body uses **thermoregulation** to regulate and balance the body's temperature and the body's system. The body accomplishes thermoregulation by four processes: convection, evaporation, conduction, and radiation, as shown in Figure 15-2.

The sweat glands are the primary aid to thermoregulation or control of the body's internal temperature.

When the Body is Too Warm

If the body becomes too warm, the dermal capillaries dilate (widen), and more blood flows to the skin surface. Because more blood is brought to the surface, body heat is lost to the surrounding air by convection, evaporation, conduction, or radiation.

Convection. In **convection,** heat is transferred from one surface (the skin) to the surrounding gases (the air) or to liquids (such as a swimming pool). Convection results in the loss of body heat.

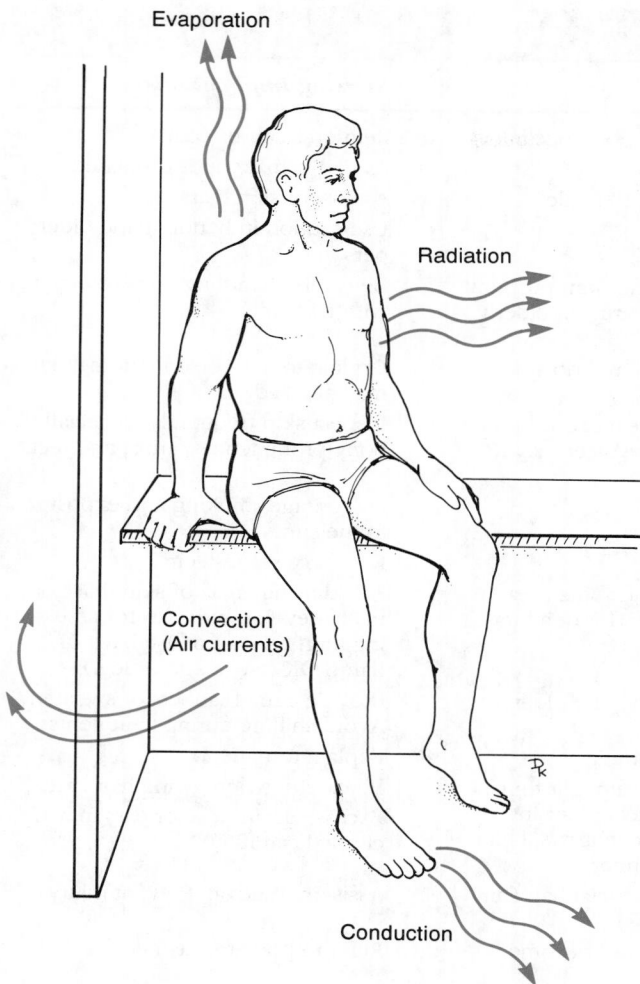

Figure 15-2. Heat is lost by four processes: radiation, conduction, convection, and evaporation.

Evaporation. Water on the body's surface can be perspiration (sweat), or water from an outside source. Such water is lost by **evaporation**, which causes a cooling effect. Evaporation is the returning of water to the air through vapor. The body normally loses about 500 mL per day with *insensible* (unnoticed) *evaporation*. Too much water loss can lead to dehydration.

Conduction. Conduction is the transfer of heat from one object to another by direct contact. When the body comes in contact with a cooler object, the body transfers heat.

Radiation. All objects give off infrared heat rays through **radiation**. We are able to feel a person's radiation energy when we stand next to them in a cool room.

When the Body is too Cold

Shivering and goose flesh are a means of thermoregulation. When the body becomes too cool, dermal capillaries constrict (narrow), thus reducing the amount of heat lost through the skin. The reflex action of shivering also helps to reduce the amount of heat lost by the body. The arrector pili muscles contract and cause the hair on the skin to stand erect. This action gives the body an insulating layer against cold.

Special Considerations in Children
Body Heat in the Newborn

Much body heat is lost through the head. This is particularly true of newborns; they are especially vulnerable because their thermoregulation processes are not fully functioning. Newborns in the nursery, particularly premature neonates, wear caps to protect them from excessive heat loss.

Sensory Awareness

The skin receives stimuli from the outside world, providing a dynamic interaction between the external and internal environments. Nerve endings in the dermis register pain and pleasure. The skin's sensation to heat and cold provides the original message to the brain and its response to withdraw the hand from a hot stove or a frozen piece of metal. (These unconscious reactions are discussed in later chapters.) This sensory awareness is part of the skin's protection of the body. The pain caused by other trauma creates bodily awareness in the same way.

The loving touch of a friend or family member is registered by the skin. The skin and blood vessels are involved in love making, foreplay, and sexual response (to be discussed in Chapter 63). Much of the communication between a newborn and its parents comes through the sense of touch. Nurses also use therapeutic touch in their care of patients.

Effects of Aging on the System

Table 15-2 summarizes major effects of aging on the skin. The skin has functional loss of abilities associated with aging. Normal changes are influenced by heredity, dietary habits, sun exposure, and general health.

With age, skin tends to become dry and appear scaly. It takes on a transparent appearance and, with the loss of subcutaneous (under the skin) fat, may sag and become wrinkled. The turgor (tone) of the skin is reduced; a pinched area does not return immediately into position. The glands in the skin decrease their secretions; thus, the older person has less perspiration and less oily skin. Hair becomes

Table 15-2. Effects of Aging on the Skin

Factors	Result	Nursing Implications
Melanin is either lost or migrates and clusters in the epidermal layer.	"Age spots" or "liver spots" occur.	Reinforce self-esteem. Available makeup is discussed.
Epidermal and dermal layers flatten.	The skin tends to tear ("fragile" skin).	Assess for skin tears. Use caution in handling the older person.
Capillary bed in dermis becomes more friable (fragile)—blood can ooze into dermis.	Dark red patches in the skin, purpura is commonly seen on arms of elderly.	Be careful handling arms of patients with purpura.
Capillaries leak small amounts of blood into tissues.	Petechiae occur (small red dots on skin).	Explain to the person that makeup may be used.
Individual may have loss of sensation and loss of abilities.	Unable to detect or treat cause of ulcerated areas; pressure ulcer may develop more quickly.	Inspect skin frequently, especially bony prominences, arms, and feet.
There is loss of elasticity in dermis and loss of subcutaneous layer of fat; loss of collagen fibers.	Wrinkles.	Discourage smoking and exposure to the sun. Reinforce self-esteem.
Turgor is lost.	Wrinkles. "Tenting" on some areas can give false positive (for dehydration).	Avoid using areas of skin that normally develop wrinkles for assessing turgor. (Do not use back of hand; OK to use arm or leg.)
Some insulating function is lost with loss of subcutaneous fat.	Heat lost more rapidly. The older person may be chilly.	Provide extra blankets or sweater. Avoid chilling during treatments.
Dermal layer thins.	Skin becomes transparent.	Explain to patient.
Changes occur in hair distribution influenced by heredity and other factors. General loss of body hair occurs.	Axillary, pubic, and scalp hair thins. Men may develop thicker hair in nose, ears, and over eyebrows; hair on head becomes thinner.	Be careful when giving hair care. Excess hair in nose or ears may be clipped carefully.
Female hormones are lost.	Women may develop facial hair (hirsutism).	Assist in removal. Prevent injury.
Nails grow more slowly and become thicker.	Nails, especially toenails, become thick and brittle.	Refer to podiatrist as needed.
The glands in the skin decrease their secretions.	Less perspiration and less oily skin than before causes skin to become very dry and may appear scaly.	Advise that daily shower or bath may not be needed (bath may dry skin more). Be sure skin is clean, because skin is more fragile and more subject to breakdown. Use lotion as needed.
Thermoregulation abilities are lost.	More susceptible to heat stroke.	Teach individual to avoid overheating. Observe in hot weather; encourage adequate fluids.
Circulation is reduced.	Wound healing takes longer—old or damaged cells are not readily replaced.	Provide careful wound care. Prevent further injury. Refer to physician as needed.

coarser and increases in areas such as the nose, ears, and eyebrows. Women may develop facial hair (hirsutism).

The skin of the older person is more fragile (friable) and more subject to breakdown than is the skin of the young person. Elasticity is lost, partly because of impaired circulation. The loss of subcutaneous fat removes some of the insulating function of the skin; heat is lost more rapidly. For this reason, older people often have difficulty keeping warm.

Keys for Review

Key Questions for Critical Thinking

1. Describe at least six functions of the integumentary system.
2. Explain the purposes of keratin and melanin. What are the advantages of their location in the epidermis rather than the dermis? How does keratin protect the body from excessive water loss or gain?
3. Name the major accessory structures or appendages of the skin and discuss the functions of each.
4. Describe the function of glands. Name the two major types of glands and discuss the differences in function.
5. Describe skin care in aging. How does it differ from skin care of a younger person?

Key Readings

Chabner D. The Language of Medicine, Ed 4. Philadelphia, W.B. Saunders, 1991
Castiglia PT, Harbin RE. Child Health Care: Process and Practice. Philadelphia, J.B. Lippincott, 1992
Eliopoulos C. Caring for the Elderly in Diverse Care Settings. Philadelphia, J.B. Lippincott, 1990

Key Readings (continued)

Farrell J. Nursing Care of the Older Person. Philadelphia, J.B. Lippincott, 1990
Scanlon V, Sanders V. Essentials of Anatomy and Physiology. Philadelphia, F.A. Davis, 1991
Smeltzer SC, Bare B. Brunner and Suddarth's Textbook of Medical-Surgical Nursing, Ed 7. Philadelphia, J.B. Lippincott, 1992

Enrichment Keys

Solomon EP. Introduction to Human Anatomy and Physiology. Philadelphia, W.B. Saunders, 1989
Memmler RL, Cohen BJ, Woods DL. Structure and Function of the Human Body, Ed 5. Philadelphia, J.B. Lippincott, 1992

Keys to Learning More

Chapter 45: how to assist a patient to maintain personal hygiene, including skin care
Chapter 53: normal and abnormal wound healing processes
Chapter 68: skin disorders

16 Fluid and Electrolyte Balance

Keys for Learning

Learning Objectives

♦ Define homeostasis, and relate it to nursing
♦ Define feedback, and state how it applies to homeostasis
♦ Differentiate between the intracellular and the extracellular water compartments and between interstitial and vascular fluid
♦ Explain three characteristics of water that make it the ideal medium for body processes
♦ Describe at least five major functions of electrolytes in the human body
♦ Name the most common electrolyte in the intracellular fluid and in the extracellular fluid
♦ Describe the role of the hydrogen ion in acid–base balance. Explain how acid-base balance relates to homeostasis
♦ Differentiate between freely permeable and selectively permeable membranes, and discuss factors affecting permeability
♦ Describe four methods of transporting substances across membranes
♦ Define intake, output, and edema

Key Terms

acid	extracellular	intracellular fluid
base	fluid	isotonic
buffer	feedback	ion
dehydration	filtration	osmosis
diffusion	homeostasis	permeability
edema	hypertonic	salt
electrolyte	hypotonic	solute

Keys to Understanding This Chapter

Chapter 5: basic human needs
Chapter 14: organization of the human body
Chapter 15: integumentary system

Key Points

♦ Homeostasis is a state of dynamic equilibrium; the body constantly adjusts to external and internal stimuli.
♦ Feedback is the relaying of information to and from organ systems (especially nervous and endocrine); it keeps the body's functioning capacity within normal boundaries.
♦ The body has two main fluid compartments: intracellular (within the cells) and extracellular. Extracellular fluid is located in blood vessels (plasma) and in tissues (interstitial fluid).
♦ Water acts as solvent and suspension agent. It helps regulate body temperature, pH, and fluid pressures inside and outside the cell. It assists and participates in chemical reactions.
♦ Ions or electrolytes are charged particles that circulate in the body fluids and take part in the body's chemical reactions.
♦ The body has buffer systems that help maintain the serum pH in the narrow range between 7.35 and 7.45. Acids and bases are important components of this system.
♦ Normal saline (0.9% NaCl) is an isotonic solution.
♦ Fluids are transported passively (without ATP energy), or actively (with ATP energy).
♦ The nurse monitors intake and output to assess the patient for fluid deficit (dehydration) or excess (edema).
♦ Minute changes occur constantly throughout the body, but the overall status in the healthy person is stability and equilibrium. To be healthy, a person's body must maintain this balance as much as possible.
♦ The processes by which the body maintains balance are discussed in this chapter. Most of the remainder of the book will be devoted in some way to fluid and electrolyte balance and its maintenance.

Rosdahl CB: Textbook of Basic Nursing, 6th ed. © 1995 J.B. Lippincott Company

Key Learning Activities

♦ Demonstrate to your classmates how skin turgor is determined. List some of the physical conditions that contribute to poor skin turgor.
♦ Demonstrate various means of transport across membranes, such as diffusion, osmosis, and filtration.

Homeostasis

Homeostasis is the process by which the body maintains balance. It is a dynamic process in which the body constantly adjusts to internal and external stimuli. (*Home/o* means constant or sameness and the suffix -*stasis* means stopping or controlling; thus, homeostasis means "controlling sameness.") The concept of homeostasis is the basis for the understanding of most physiologic processes.

For the body to maintain homeostasis, the body must be able to sense minute (tiny) changes and react appropriately to these changes. To do this, the body has sensors and integrating centers that involve the cells of all the body's systems.

Negative and Positive Feedback

All components of the body constantly send tiny signals that cause responses. Simply stated, **feedback** is the relaying of information about a given condition to the appropriate organ or system. The sum of these responses serves to keep the body in a stable condition: homeostasis.

In *negative feedback*, any deviation is resisted. Normally only a small variation is allowed. Illness is an interruption of negative feedback, while medical treatment is a plan to restore the negative feedback mechanisms. All of nursing is aimed at restoring and maintaining the individual's equilibrium (normal state) as much as possible.

In *positive feedback*, the body senses deviations, but the feedback generally is not homeostatic. In fact, with positive feedback, the body responds by making the deviation greater, leading to greater instability and frequently death.

The major systems involved in feedback are the nervous system and the endocrine system, discussed in Chapters 18 and 19, respectively.

> ### Key Concept
> An individual must maintain internal homeostasis to maintain health.

Body Fluids

A large portion of the body is made up of fluids. The fluids are divided into two main compartments: the intracellular fluid (ICF) and the extracellular fluid (ECF). The **ICF** is the fluid *inside* the cells and comprises about 60% to 65% of the total body water of the adult. **ECF** is *outside* the cells and comprises about 35% to 40% of the total body water.

ECF appears mostly as *tissue fluid* (*interstitial fluid*) and *intravascular fluid* (vascular fluid). Interstitial fluid is found between the cells. Vascular fluid is the watery fluid of the blood known as plasma. Specialized ECFs, such as fluid in the joint cavities, in the brain and spinal cord, the eyes, and lymph or plasma that has entered the lymph vessels, also exist. These are sometimes called *transcellular* fluids.

Fluids continuously exchange between compartments. The compartments contain slightly different components, and several homeostatic mechanisms work to maintain the correct balance of fluid to solid substance within each compartment. Table 16-1 sum-

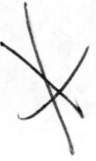

Table 16-1. Fluid Compartments and Body Fluids

Compartment	Fluid
Intracellular (ICF)	Water within cells (about 65% of total body fluid)
Extracellular (ECF)	Water outside of cells (about 35% of total body fluid)
Intravascular	Plasma—water component of blood
Tissue fluid	Interstitial or tissue fluid—water found in spaces between cells
Specialized ECF*:	
Lymph vessels	Lymph—tissue fluid found in lymph vessels
Joint spaces	Synovial fluid—fluid found within joint cavities
Eye	Aqueous fluid—fluid in anterior portion of eye
Brain and spinal cord	Cerebrospinal fluid—fluid circulating in brain and spinal cord

* Note: Some authorities list a third major fluid compartment with the following fluids: secretions and excretions, such as urine, cerebrospinal fluid, saliva, ocular fluids, peritoneal fluid, and gastrointestinal fluids.

Table 16-2. Average Percentages of Water In Relation to Body Weight in People of Different Ages in the Various Water Compartments of the Body

Water Compartment	Infant (% of body weight)	Adult (% of body weight)		Elderly Person (%)
		Man	Woman	
Extracellular	29	15	15	20
Intravascular	4	4	5	5
Interstitial	25	11	10	15
Intracellular	48	45	35	25
Total % body of which is water	77	60	50	45

Source: Craven RF, Hirnle CJ. Fundamentals of Nursing: Human Health and Function. Philadelphia, J.B. Lippincott, 1992.

marizes the fluid compartments and the names of their respective fluids.

Age, sex, and the individual structure of the body cause variations in the percentage of total body fluids to the total body weight. Children can be composed of more than 75% body water. Men are about 60% body water. Fat cells contain the least water of any cells in the body. Adult females have the lowest water content, about 50%, due to the presence of greater amounts of subcutaneous fat. Table 16-2 summarizes body water by body weight and locations.

Water

Certain properties of water make it important for body chemistry. An understanding of the properties of water will aid the nurse to understand the rationale behind numerous nursing interventions. The functions of water are identified in the accompanying box.

Special Characteristics of Water

A great difference in temperature is needed to bring about a physical change in water. Water boils at 100°C (212°F) and freezes at 0°C (32°F). This temperature span is great enough to allow many physical reactions to take place without affecting the chemical composition of the water itself. Water can become a solid, a liquid, or a gas with only a temperature change.

Water temperature, however, changes relatively slowly. It can absorb much heat before increasing its temperature, or it can lose heat before decreasing its temperature. Heat is required to change water from a liquid to a gas. The evaporation process (a change from liquid to a gas) will remove heat from the body.

Water directly and indirectly participates in all the chemical reactions that occur in the body. Chemically, each water molecule, H_2O, is made up of two elements, hydrogen (two atoms) and oxygen (one atom). During metabolism, numerous chemical changes in the body can separate the water molecule into its component elements for use elsewhere. Hydrogen is the main component of the pH system of the body, discussed later in this chapter. Oxidation is the process in which oxygen is used in the formation of new substances needed by the body. Indirectly, water acts as

Functions of Water

- Primary solvent within the body
- Primary compound in all body fluids
- Suspension agent
- Helps regulate body temperature
- Helps regulate body pH
- Helps regulate fluid pressures inside and outside cells
- Assists or participates in chemical reactions
- May be end product of chemical reactions

Water in Solution With Other Substances

- Transports nutrients and oxygen to cells
- Transports waste products away from cells
- Acts as "bumper" to protect cells and organs
- Lubricates to prevent outer walls (parietal) from rubbing against inner walls (visceral) of organs
- Participates in maintenance of blood pressure
- Helps regulate acid–base and fluid–electrolyte balance

the solution in which other chemicals ionize (dissociate). As ions, chemicals are available to participate in other chemical reactions.

Water is a good solvent. Many compounds, such as salts and sugars, are easily dissolved in water. A **solute** is a substance dissolved in a solvent. Nutrients and wastes are transported as solutes in water. Body water contains two main types of solutes: nonelectrolytes and electrolytes. Nonelectrolytes include proteins, glucose, carbon dioxide, oxygen, and organic acids. Electrolytes are solutes that generate an electrical charge when dissolved in water. Electrolytes are discussed in the next section.

Water functions as a suspension agent. Many larger molecules, such as lipids and proteins, are easily suspended in water. These suspensions must be kept in motion, or the larger molecules will settle to the bottom. Red blood cells will settle out of suspension unless kept in motion in the watery medium of blood. An individual's blood pressure partially depends on intravascular water as a suspension agent with specific amounts of proteins, electrolytes, and minerals as solutes.

Water exerts pressure against the walls or vessels that contain it. This pressure is known as *hydrostatic pressure*, and occurs because water has weight and volume. The amount of pressure depends on the depth of the liquid. Regardless of the amount, water in a tall, thin container exerts more hydrostatic pressure than water in a shallow container.

Osmotic pressure is pressure that develops when two solutions containing different concentrations of solutes are separated by a semipermeable membrane. In other words, *the amount of solutes in water affects the pressure that the water can exert against surrounding membranes.* The greater the amount of solutes, the greater the amount of pressure. This principle is normally maintained within very narrow limits. Human body cells have an osmotic pressure nearly equal to that of the circulating fluid of the blood. Solutions exerting equal pressures on opposite sides of the membrane are said to be **isotonic.** Stronger solutions, compared to an opposing side of a membrane, are said to be **hypertonic**. Hypertonic solutions will cause red blood cells to shrink because fluid will be drawn out of the blood cells by osmosis (discussed later). Weaker solutions are called **hypotonic**. Hypotonic solutions cause red blood cells to swell.

Key Concept

Water (H_2O) is vital to human life. Most of the body's activities cannot be carried on without it.

Ions

Each chemical element has an electrical charge, either positive (+) or negative (−). An element may be able to connect or "bond" to another element. This bonding ability or attraction between chemicals is determined by the chemical and its electrical charge.

Many elements gain or lose electrons that circle around them. An element that has lost one or more electrons is called an **ion.** Ions have acquired an electrical charge because they have gained or lost one or more electrons. Ions are atoms or groups of atoms that are in search of a bonding partner. Some ions have the ability to bond with one other ion; others can bond with two or more. This ability is expressed in terms of a positive (+) or negative (−) value and is called the *valence.* The valence would then be expressed as + or ++ and so forth. For example, sodium has a valance of +1 (Na+); sulfate has a valence of −2 (SO_4−−).

Cations and Anions

A positively charged ion is known as a *cation.* (Think of a positive ion as a ca+ion.) A negatively charged ion is known as an *anion.* The cation, because it has a positive charge, is attracted by a negatively charged ion. The anion, because it is negatively charged, is drawn toward the positive charge. In other words, opposites attract.

Examples of cations include Na+ (sodium), K+ (potassium), Ca++ (calcium), Mg++ (magnesium), Fe++ (iron), and H+ (hydrogen). Examples of anions include Cl− (chloride), HCO_3− (bicarbonate), SO_4−− (sulfate), and HPO_4−− (phosphate).

Ionization

Ionization is the dissociation of compounds into their respective ions. Ionization is an important process. The separation of chemical compounds into free-standing ions releases these chemicals for use in other chemical reactions. Ionization of the water molecule (H_2O or HOH) releases equal amounts of H+ (hydrogen ion) and OH (hydroxyl ion). Each of these two ions is now free to combine with another substance to form an acid or a base. The ionization of table salt (NaCl) will release a sodium ion (Na+) and a chlorine ion (Cl-). Each of these ions can recombine into new substances when needed by the body, such as hydrochloric acid (HCl).

Because of their ability to conduct electricity in a solution, ions are sometimes referred to as **electrolytes**. Health professionals commonly see the results of electrolytes, as in an electrocardiogram. Electrodes on the surface of the body detect electrical currents produced by the action of the heart. These electrical events can be graphically visualized. Laboratory tests are often done to determine blood levels of various electrolytes.

Electrolytes

Electrolytes are active chemicals or elements within the body. An electrolyte is an element or a compound that will dissociate into ions when dissolved in water. An electrolyte is able to conduct a weak electric current. Electrolytes are found in the form of inorganic salts, acids, and bases. They are found in all body fluids. Their concentration, however, will vary. Because electrolytes are active chemicals, their concentrations are measured according to their chemical activity, by milliequivalents (mEq). The major intracellular electrolytes are potassium (K+), magnesium (Mg++), sulfate (SO_4−−), and phosphate (HPO_4−−). The major extracellular electrolytes are sodium (Na+), chloride (CL−), calcium (Ca++), and bicarbonate (HCO_3−).

Sodium is the most important extracellular cation. Chloride is the most important extracellular anion. These two combine to form sodium chloride or NaCl (ordinary table salt), which is one of the most common compounds in the body. "Normal saline" (NS) is a salt solution (0.9% NaCl) and is the foremost compound of the body fluids. NS is referred to as *isotonic* because it has the same NaCl concentration as normal body fluids.

Inside the cells (intracellular), the most dominant cation is potassium (K^+). The most dominant anion is phosphate (HPO_4−−). ICF also contains sodium but in much smaller amounts than outside the cell. The balance of intracellular potassium to extracellular sodium is an extremely important aspect of energy production.

All of these electrolytes are needed for normal functioning of nerves and muscles, to develop the structures of the body cells, to clot the blood, and to coordinate the body's activities. The balance of electrolytes and fluids controlled by electrolytes is called homeostasis. A summary of the functions of major electrolytes is given in the accompanying box. Figure 16-1 compares plasma and intracellular electrolyte concentrations.

Salts, Acids, and Bases

An **acid** is a compound that contains the hydrogen ion (H+). A **base** (also known as an alkali) is a compound that contains the hydroxyl ion (OH−). A **salt** is created when the positive hydrogen ions of an acid are replaced by the positive ions (usually a mineral) of a base. A salt is an electrolyte that is made up of a cation other than hydrogen ion and an anion other than hydroxyl ion. For example, hydrochloric acid (HCl) can combine with the base sodium hydroxide (NaOH) to yield table salt and water HCl + NaOH → NaCl + HOH, or an acid plus a base yields a salt and water.

The body contains several important salts. These include sodium chloride (NaCl), potassium chloride (KCl), calcium chloride ($CaCl_2$), calcium carbonate ($CaCO_3$), calcium phosphate ($Ca_3[PO_4]_2$), and sodium sulfate (Na_2SO_4).

Acid–Base Balance

Acid–base balance is an important aspect of homeostasis. We have learned that salts that break up into ions are called electrolytes and that these electrolytes can combine and recombine to form acids, bases, and salts. We have discussed the ionization or dissociation of compounds. We have also mentioned that water (written as H_2O or HOH) contains the components of an acid (the hydrogen ion or H+) and a base (the hydroxyl ion or OH−). Pure water is considered a neutral solution. A neutral solution contains equal parts of hydrogen and hydroxyl ions.

Potential of Hydrogen (pH)

The symbol pH refers to the potential or power (p) of hydrogen ion (H+) concentration within a solution. The pH scale ranges from 0 to 14. Pure water, which is neutral, has a pH of 7. If the pH number is lower than 7, the solution is an acid. Acids contain more hydrogen ions than bases. If the number is greater than 7, the solution is basic (or alkaline). Basic solutions contain more hydroxyl ions. The pH scale is represented in Figure 16-2.

The change in the pH of a solution by one pH unit is a tenfold change in the hydrogen ion concentration.

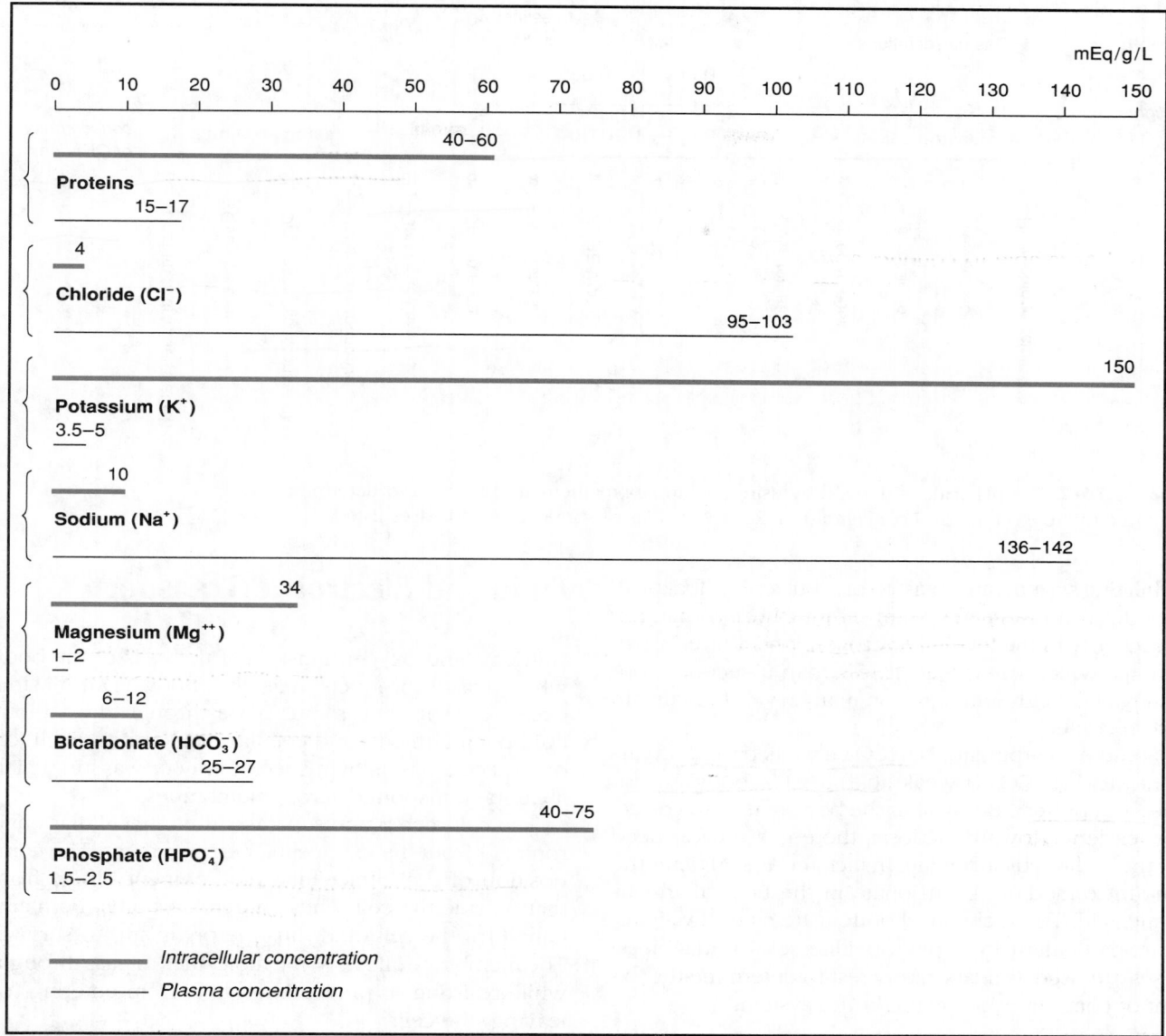

Figure 16-1. Comparison of electrolyte concentrations: intracellular versus plasma.

For example, a pH of 5 has 10 more hydrogen ions than a pH of 6. A pH of 5 has 100 times more hydrogen ions than a pH of 7. The pH of the ECF (for example, the blood and lymph) is normally slightly alkaline, about 7.35 to 7.45. The slightly alkaline pH of blood must be maintained within this narrow range. A decrease or increase of only one pH unit will result in a chemical disaster for the body. One of the normal negative feedback mechanisms of the body is to continually correct the body's tendency to develop acidosis and return the serum pH back into its alkaline state. The lungs and the kidneys are the organs of the body that are the most involved in H+ regulation.

Other body fluids have assorted pH values. The pH of ICF is approximately 6.8 to 7.0. Fluids that open to the environment may be more strongly acidic or alkaline and do not harm the body. Gastric juice is quite acidic with a pH of around 1. The pH of urine varies from about 4 to 8.

> ### Key Concept
> ◆ *Low* pH = high number of hydrogen ions
> ◆ *High* ph = low number of hydrogen ions

Buffers

Many acidic or basic ions are released in the chemical reactions that occur constantly in the body. Because of the constant changes in this mixture, a **buffering** or

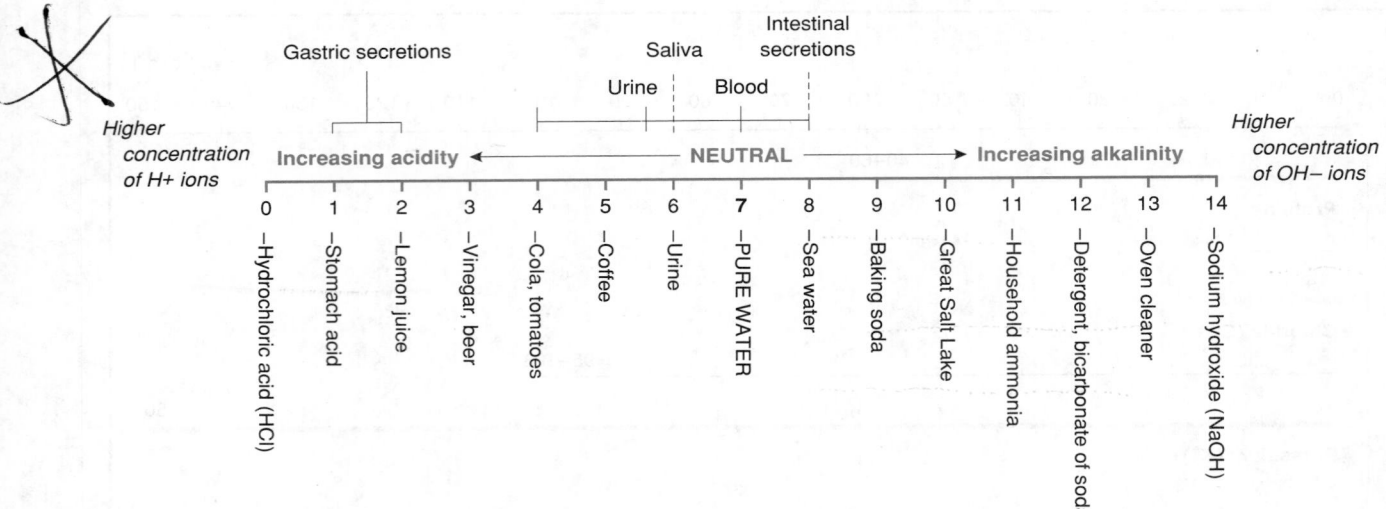

Figure 16-2. The pH scale is derived by using a complex mathematical formula to determine the free hydrogen ion (H+) concentration. Relative values of some acids and bases listed.

stabilizing system must exist to prevent a pH imbalance. A buffer is a chemical system set up to resist changes, particularly in the level of hydrogen ions. Buffering reactions, which can occur in less than a second, constantly alter acids and bases on many levels to maintain a correct ratio.

Sodium bicarbonate ($NaHCO_3$, a weak base) and carbonic acid (H_2CO_3, a weak acid) are the body's major chemical buffers. Because of the body's need to correct the tendency toward acidosis, there is a greater need for the sodium bicarbonate. In fact, there is 20 times the amount of sodium bicarbonate in the body than carbonic acid. These chemical buffers are clinically significant, particularly in respiratory illnesses. Arterial blood gases are used as a laboratory test to determine the extent of compensation by the buffer system.

> **Key Concept**
>
> The pH of the ECF must be maintained between 7.35 and 7.45 for health. Extremes (below 6.8 or above 7.8) are fatal.

Enzymes

Enzymes are biologic catalysts. They aid in chemical reactions without themselves changing. Enzymes are proteins and each acts in a "lock-and-key" manner with only certain chemicals. The clinical status of the patient influences enzyme activity; high body temperature or an imbalance in electrolytes may render an enzyme inoperable. Damage to certain organs shows up as excess enzymes in the blood, such as following a heart attack.

Fluid and Electrolyte Transport

Nutrients and oxygen must enter the cells of the body while waste products exit the body. During this exchange, substances must pass through the various fluid compartments and cellular membranes. Each ion or molecule has its own specific way or ways in which it can be transported across membranes.

The cell membrane separates the intracellular environment from the extracellular environment. The composition of the intracellular environment differs from that outside the cell. These differences must be maintained for the cell (and thus the organism) to survive. The membrane allows some molecules to pass through, while resisting or preventing others from entering (or leaving) the cell.

The ability of a membrane to allow molecules to pass through is known as **permeability.** Factors that affect permeability include the following:

◆ The size of the pores in the membrane
◆ The external and internal pressures exerted on the molecules (*osmotic pressure*)
◆ The pressure of the fluid against the membrane (*hydrostatic pressure*)
◆ The electrical charges of the molecule, the plasma membrane, or the body fluid
◆ The solubility of the molecules
◆ The size of the molecules

Freely permeable membranes will allow almost any food or waste substance to pass through. Freely permeable walls allow easy transfer of fluid and substances from the intravascular fluid to the interstitial fluid. Once the substances arrive in the interstitial fluid around the cells, they must still penetrate the cellular membrane to reach the ICF where the majority of the body's work occurs.

The cellular membrane is *selectively permeable.* The cellular membrane of each cell allows only certain specific substances to pass through. Movement across the cellular membrane occurs in one of four ways:

♦ Molecules dissolve through the cell membrane. These include oxygen, carbon dioxide, and steroids.

♦ Substances pass through membrane channels. These channels are of various sizes and allow only a certain size range and electrical charge to traverse the membrane.

♦ Carrier molecules in the membrane assist substances across the barrier.

♦ A vesicle (a membrane-bound sac) transports large molecules or whole cells across the plasma membrane.

Molecules may move passively through the membrane. This means they do not require any energy output by the body. This *passive transport* mechanism includes diffusion, osmosis, and filtration. Another form of transport uses energy and requires assistance. It is called *active transport.* This type of transport is used when molecules are too large or too specialized to pass through membranes without assistance.

Diffusion

Diffusion is the random movement of molecules from an area of higher concentration to an area of lower concentration. Atoms and molecules constantly move and bombard each other at random. The tendency of such movement is to equalize the number of molecules in any given area; this is the molecular equivalent of seeking homeostasis. If the molecules are highly concentrated, they will collide often and then tend to move to a place where there are few collisions. Diffusion means "to spread out." When diffusion occurs, equilibrium is reached, and there is no further movement or exchange of molecules. The molecules continue to move, but the number in each area or on each side of a membrane stays the same. (Heat speeds up the process of diffusion because the molecules move faster.)

Diffusion commonly occurs in liquids and gases. For example, when liquid cream or powdered creamer is added to coffee it spreads out (diffuses). Smoke or perfume diffuses in a room.

Diffusion is the most important mechanism by which nutrients and wastes pass across the cell membrane. In the body, oxygen and carbon dioxide diffuse across the alveoli of the lungs, as shown in Figure 16-3. There are more oxygen molecules on the inside of the alveoli; they are pushed passively toward the pulmonary cap-

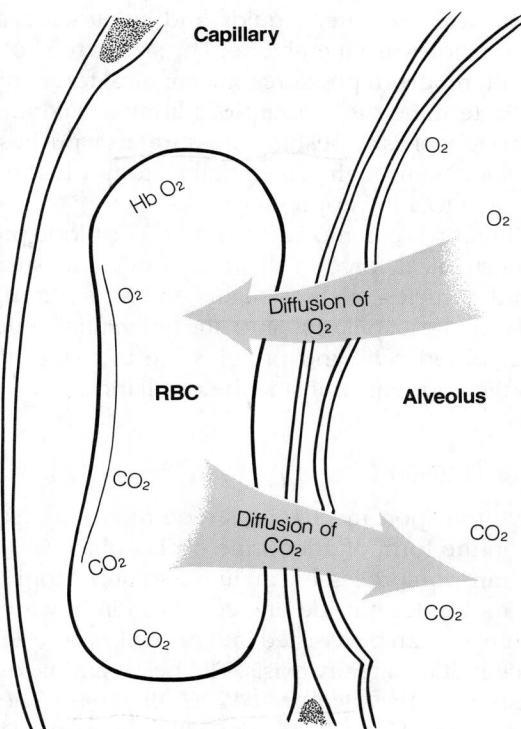

Figure 16-3. Oxygen is transported from the alveoli of the lungs into the circulating blood by the process of diffusion. There, a chemical process unites the oxygen with hemoglobin in the red blood cells. Carbon dioxide also is transported in the other direction by diffusion. Simple diffusion is an example of a passive transport of materials across membranes.

illaries where there are few oxygen molecules. The oxygen is then transported to the various body cells. Carbon dioxide gas is exchanged in the same manner, except in the reverse direction.

Osmosis

Osmosis is the movement of water across selectively permeable membranes. Water is passively moved from an area of more water, where there are fewer solutes, to an area of less water, where there are more solutes. The homeostatic mechanism of osmosis is to equalize the concentrations of salt or other solutes within the body. Water moves from an area of less salt content to an area of greater salt content (in an attempt to equalize the salt concentration). The salt itself does not move in this case. (Water "follows" salt.) Osmosis can be thought of as "pulling pressure."

Filtration

Filtration is the transport of water and dissolved materials through a membrane from an area of higher pressure to an area of lower pressure. Filtration requires mechanical pressure. Liquids and solutes are passed through holes in a membrane. The size of the holes and the differences in pressures (mechanical force) on each side determine the amount of filtration. Filtration can be thought of as a "pushing pressure" as it pushes water and solutes through a membrane from a higher pressure area to a lower pressure area.

Filtration is common in the body. The blood pressure (a mechanical force) will push water and small dissolved particles, such as sugars and salts, through the walls of the capillaries into the interstitial fluid. The larger blood cells and proteins are too large to pass through and remain inside the capillaries.

Active Transport

Active transport mechanisms require energy expenditure in the form of adenosine triphosphate (ATP). Active transport processes can move solutes "uphill." Specific molecules outside of a cell, even if they are fewer in number, can be assisted into the cell, where a greater concentration already exists. The best example of active transport is the *sodium–potassium pump*. There are more sodium ions outside the cell than inside. The natural tendency would be for sodium to diffuse across the cellular membrane into the cell. If this were allowed unchecked, the homeostatic mechanism governing nerve transmissions and muscle contractions would go berserk. Active transport mechanisms figuratively "pump" out sodium ions from inside the cell, while transporting potassium into the cell.

Another example of active transport involves the transport of glucose and amino acids into the cells lining the small intestine. The intestinal cells use ATP, even if the movement of solutes is from a higher to a lower concentration.

> ### Key Concepts
> If a transfer requires energy, it is *active* transport. If a transfer does not need energy, it is *passive* transport.

Fluid and Electrolyte Balance

Fluid and electrolyte balance is vital for all the body systems to function properly. The correct proportion of fluids to solutes in each fluid compartment must be maintained.

In this chapter, the body's various processes for maintaining balance are discussed. The body compensates for imbalances immediately. For example, if excess CO_2 (carbon dioxide) builds up, a person breathes faster to take in more oxygen. If the respiratory system cannot handle the imbalance, chemical buffers attempt a balance. Additionally the kidneys can adjust the ECF pH. Numerous hormones also act to influence water retention and excretion.

Many salts are needed by the body to regulate the acid–base levels and coordinate the water balance. Sodium is needed to maintain the electrical potential across the plasma membranes of the cells and to maintain acid–base balance. Potassium acts within the cells in much the same way that sodium acts outside the cells. Chlorine plays a major role in acid–base balance through its production of hydrochloric acid.

Electrolytes may be lost through vomiting, diarrhea, and hemorrhage, thus upsetting the fluid and electrolyte balance of the body. One of the important functions of the nurse is to assess fluid and electrolyte balance. The major assessments are listed in the accompanying box.

Water Intake and Output

Water Conservation
Water is conserved by the body and reused as much as possible. The kidneys, and to some degree the intestine, continuously filter and recycle water. Each day, we must take in approximately the same amount of fluid as we put out. The body can survive many days without food but only a few days without water.

Intake
The term health professionals use to monitor fluid gains and losses is "intake and output." Accurate intake and output records are vital when caring for patients with fluid deficits or excesses. Sources and approximate amounts for human intake and output are given in Table 16-3.

Intake refers to the water we take into our bodies each day. Water is obtained from three sources: liquid intake, the metabolism of food, and as the end product of cellular respiration. The average adult takes in approximately 2,000 to 4,000 mL per day (a little more than 2 to 4 quarts).

Output
On the other hand, to avoid an overload of water in the body, approximately the same amount that is taken into the body must be put out. Water output occurs normally through the kidneys, in sweat, as water vapor from the lungs, and in feces. Sweat may be sensible (visible) or insensible (nonvisible) water loss.

Causes of Loss. Many factors influence water loss. For example, water output increases with exercise, fever, some medications, and certain diseases. In illness, more fluids may be needed because of excess drainage from

Dehydration

Many disorders result in an excessive loss of water from the body (dehydration). Strictly speaking, **dehydration** refers to loss of water with an associated increase in sodium. *Fluid volume deficits*, a term for water loss with a proportional loss of electrolytes, may occur due to diarrhea, vomiting, decreased fluid intake, sweating, gastrointestinal suctioning, medications, or hemorrhage.

Edema

An accumulation of water in the interstitial fluid compartment of the body is called **edema** and may occur in conditions such as burns or ascites. Edema is an accumulation of fluid in the tissue spaces. It is sometimes referred to as "third spacing." Edema may be local, as in an injury (sprained ankle), or it can be systemic (throughout the body). Systemic edema is usually symptomatic of other more profound problems. The basic problem is that there is a disruption in the filtration and osmotic forces of the circulating fluids. Treatment of edema needs to be aimed at the cause of the underlying problem.

Effects of Aging on the System

Dehydration is a common and serious problem of the elderly. Normally the levels of electrolytes, acids, bases, and salts do not change as we age. However, in the older person, ICF levels are decreased by about 8% because muscle tissue changes to adipose tissue. (Fat cells contain less water than muscle cells.)

A nurse needs to be aware that as people age, the sensation for thirst decreases; therefore, the older person may not be aware of the need to consume fluids. Many medications cause fluid loss. Circulatory and renal problems and nutritional habits may cause sodium and water retention leading to edema. Exercise and activity levels also influence body fluid levels.

wounds, vomiting, or bleeding. A fever can cause a person to use about four times the amount of fluids that would be needed in normal homeostasis. *Diaphoresis* (profuse sweating) can cause considerable fluid loss. Each form of fluid loss also will alter the body's electrolyte concentrations.

Table 16-3. Normal Water Balances (Intake and Output)

Intake		Output	
Source	*Amount*	*Source*	*Amount*
Liquids	1,600 mL	Urine	1,500 mL
Foods	700 mL	Sweat	500 mL
Metabolism	200 mL	Water vapor	300 mL
		Feces	200 mL
Total	2,500 mL	*Total*	2,500 mL

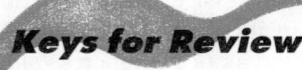

Keys for Review

Key Questions for Critical Thinking

1. Explain ICF. Discuss the two most important ions in ICF.
2. Explain ECF. Discuss the two major locations of ECF and the two most important ions.
3. Describe an acid, base (alkali), and a buffer. Discuss the importance of acid–base balance to health.
4. Describe fluid and electrolyte transport by each of the following means: diffusion, osmosis, filtration, and active transport.
5. Discuss the functions and special properties of water in the body.

Key Readings

Chabner D. The Language of Medicine, Ed 4. Philadelphia, W.B. Saunders, 1991

Metheny NM. Fluid and Electrolyte Balance: Nursing Considerations, Ed 2. Philadelphia, J.B. Lippincott, 1992

Scanlon V, Sanders V. Essentials of Anatomy and Physiology. Philadelphia, F.A. Davis, 1991

Seely R, Stephens T, Tate P. Anatomy and Physiology, Ed 2. St. Louis, C.V. Mosby, 1994

Key Readings (continued)

Smeltzer SC, Bare BF. Brunner and Suddarth's Textbook of Medical-Surgical Nursing, Ed 7. Philadelphia, J.B. Lippincott, 1992

Keys to Learning More

Unit Thirteen: deviations from normal body structure and function in children

Unit Fourteen: deviations from normal in adults

Unit Fifteen: deviations in older adults

Chapter 42: measurement of vital signs

Chapter 46: elimination

Chapter 47: procedures in intake and output measuring

Chapter 50: basics of physical assessment, including skin turgor, edema, and other signs related to fluid and electrolyte balance

Chapter 56: various types of medications, some used to aid in fluid and electrolyte balance

Chapter 69: discussion of disorders in fluid and electrolyte balance

17 The Musculoskeletal System

Keys for Learning

Learning Objectives

- List the four classifications of bones according to shape and give examples
- Locate and name the major bones of the body and describe their function
- Name three types of joints and give an example of each
- Differentiate between the axial and appendicular skeleton and give examples of bones in each
- List at least three functions of the skeletal system and of the muscles
- Describe and differentiate between skeletal, smooth, and cardiac muscles
- Locate and name on a chart the major muscle groups in the body and indicate the actions of each group
- State at least three factors that influence bone growth
- Define terms related to range of motion

Key Terms

articulation	hematopoiesis	periosteum
bursae	ligaments	sinuses
hyoid	lordosis	sternum
kyphosis	marrow	thorax
flexion	ossification	xiphoid process
extension	osteoblasts	

Keys to Understanding This Chapter

Chapter 5: basic human needs
Chapter 14: organization of the human body
Chapter 15: integumentary system
Chapter 16: fluid and electrolyte balance

Key Points

- The skeleton is the living framework of the human body
- There are four main shapes of bones: long, short, flat, and irregular.
- Red bone marrow is found in the ends of long bones, in the bodies of vertebrae, and in flat bones. Red bone marrow is responsible for the manufacturing of red blood cells, white blood cells, and platelets.

Key Points (continued)

- There are two divisions of the skeleton. The axial skeleton contains the bones of the center section, and the appendicular skeleton contains the bones of the extremities.
- There are three main types of muscle tissues: skeletal (voluntary), smooth (involuntary), and cardiac. Muscles are voluntary or involuntary.
- Ossification is the process by which bones become hardened through an increase in calcified tissue. Bones change in size and composition during one's lifetime.
- Muscles work in groups that have opposing actions. When one muscle contracts, the other relaxes. Most of the heat in the body is generated from the cellular muscle activity of adenosine triphosphate and oxygen.
- The musculoskeletal system loses its flexibility and strength as people age.

Key Topics Outline

Structure and Function
    The Skeleton
    Divisions of the Skeleton
    The Muscles
System Physiology
    Formation of Bone Tissue
    Muscle Contractions
    Mobility
Effects of Aging on the System

Key Learning Activities

- Visit a gym or health club, and interview one of the staff. Have them show you exercise equipment and describe exactly which muscle or muscle group each exercise is designed to strengthen. Have them indicate on their body each of the muscles as they are describing the exercises. Have them demonstrate the exercises using the equipment.
- Using your classroom skeleton, practice naming the bones of the body.

Functions of the Skeletal System

Support
- Supports the body
- Provides framework for the body
- Gives shape to the body

Protection
- Protects vital organs
- Protects soft tissues

Movement
- Provides locomotion (walking, movement) by attachments of muscles, tendons, and ligaments

Manufacture
- Produces red blood cells
- Produces white blood cells
- Produces platelets

Storage and Release
- Provides calcium
- Provides phosphorus

Most people take for granted the fact that their body can produce all kinds of motion and actions. By working in harmony, various components of the body produce actions that allow independence and discovery. The skeleton is the bony framework of the human body, but the muscles produce movement. The musculoskeletal system comprises the skeleton, joints, muscles, ligaments, and bursae.

Structure and Function

Functions of the skeleton are basically support, protection, movement, storage, and hematopoiesis (blood formation). The accompanying box lists these functions and the skeleton's methods of performing them.

The Skeleton

Not only is the skeleton the framework of the body, but it also is living. Each bone is made up of several types of tissue, and therefore bones are considered to be organs.

The Bones

Most sources identify 206 bones in the body. Bones, the marrow within certain bones, and the minerals with which bones are made contribute to the homeostatic functioning of the body.

Classification of Bones. Bones are classified according to their shape: long, short, flat, and irregular. Table 17-1 lists the classifications with their functions and examples.

Long bones have an extended shape and provide support and strength to the body. Short bones are irregular or cube shaped. Flat bones are shaped exactly as the name suggests. They provide broad surfaces for muscle attachments. Irregular bones are similar to short bones but are irregular in shape. The irregular classification includes small, rounded bones called sesamoid bones. They develop within joints or tendons. The patella (kneecap) is the largest sesamoid bone.

Structure of Bones. The **periosteum,** the outer bone surface, is hard and made up of a fibrous connective tissue membrane that covers most of the bone. It merges with tendons and ligaments, which attach to bones. The periosteum contains the blood vessels that supply oxygen and nutrients to the bone cells, keeping them alive. The blood cells also supply bone-building substances and minerals that harden the bone by filling the intercellular spaces.

The hollow inner part of the bone is filled with a soft substance called **marrow.** There are two kinds of marrow: yellow and red. The yellow, which is seen in soup bones, is found in the central cavities of the long bones and is mostly fat. The red marrow is found in the ends of long bones, in the bodies of the vertebrae, and in flat bones. Red bone marrow is responsible for the manufacturing of red blood cells, white blood cells, and platelets (hematopoiesis).

Two types of osseous (bony) tissue are involved in construction of the long bones of the extremities. The *diaphysis,* or shaft of the long bone, is hard and compact. The ends of the long bones, the *epiphysis,* are spongelike and covered by a shell of harder bone. The diaphysis and epiphysis do not fuse until full growth is achieved.

Table 17-1. Classification of Bones

Classification	Function	Example
Long	Act as levers, support frame	Arms, legs, hands, feet
Short	Facilitate movement, transfer forces	Wrists, ankles
Flat	Serve as muscle attachment and for protection	Cranial, ribs, shoulder blades, hips
Irregular	For attachment of other structures or articulations	Facial, vertebrae, patella

Bone Markings. The contour of bones resembles the configuration of an interesting landscape with its hills and valleys. There are hundreds of these bone markings, each type identified by special characteristics. A *facet* is a small plane or smooth area. A *condyle* is a large rounded projection, and a *tuberosity* is a large, elevated, knoblike projection. A flat projection is called a *plate*.

Any bony prominence or projection is called a *bony process*. A *spine* is a sharp process; a *ridge* or *crest* is a thin or narrow process; and a *tubercle* is a small, rounded process. The *trochanter* is the large process found on the femur.

Openings and depressions also occur in bones. A hole through which blood vessels, ligaments, and nerves pass is called a *foramen;* a long, tubelike hole is called a *canal* or *meatus.* A **sinus** is a spongelike air space inside a bone. A dent or depression usually is called a *fossa.*

Accessory Structures of the Skeleton

Joints. The points at which bones are attached to each other are called joints or **articulations**. Hundreds of motions are possible because of the way the bones are attached. Joints are classified according to the degree of movement they permit. The classification and examples are summarized in Table 17-2.

Synarthroses (fibrous joints) are immovable joints. Interlocking projections and fibrous connective tissue grow between the two articulating bones and join them together. Amphiarthroses (cartilaginous joints) are slightly movable joints. The articulating bones are connected by cartilage.

Diarthroses (synovial joints) are freely movable joints, allowing movement in various directions. A thin, smooth layer of cartilage covers and pads these joints. Synovial joints are further classified according to their structure and range of movement: hinge, ball-and-socket, pivot, gliding, condyloid, and saddle joints. Several of these joints are illustrated in Figure 17-1.

Bursae. Bursae are small, flat sacs lined with synovial membrane and filled with synovial fluid. Bursae help ease movement while reducing friction. Bursae are located around joints susceptible to pressure and trauma, such as the knee, shoulder, elbow, and hip.

Ligaments and Cartilage. Strong fibrous bands called **ligaments** hold bones together. Some ligaments do not move or stretch but produce stability in the joint. Others allow for great flexibility, stretching, and movement.

Cartilage is a type of connective tissue organized into a system of fibers. Articular cartilage covers the ends of the long bones. It helps to reduce friction in the joints and distribute weight-bearing. Cartilage makes a slick surface for rotation and absorbs shocks and jars.

Divisions of the Skeleton

There are two divisions of the skeleton: the axial skeleton and the appendicular skeleton. The axial skeleton contains the bones in the center or axis of the body. The appendicular skeleton contains the bones of the extremities (appendages) of the body. Figure 17-2 summarizes and illustrates divisions of the body and major bones of the skeletal system.

The Axial Skeleton

The axial skeleton is composed of the bones of the skull, the trunk (the vertebral column), and the thoracic (rib) cage.

Table 17-2. Classification of Joints

Type of Joint	Actions	Example
Immovable joints: synarthroses (fibrous)	No motion or only "give"	Bones of the skull fitted together with interlocking notches (see Fig. 17-3)
Slightly movable joints: amphiarthroses (cartilaginous)	Slight degree of motion or flexibility	Vertebral column (see Figs. 17-4 and 17-5) and pubic bones (symphysis)
Synovial or diarthrodial (freely movable)		
Hinge joints	Motion like a door on hinges	Finger, elbow, and knee joints (see Fig. 17-1)
Ball-and-socket joints	Rotation motions	Shoulders and hips (see Fig. 17-1)
Pivot joints	Motion like that of turning a doorknob	Elbow (turn forearm) (see Fig. 17-1)
Gliding joints	Gliding motion (past each other)	Wrist
Condyloid joints	Allow motions in two planes at right angles	Wrist, foot, hand
Saddle joints	Opposing surfaces reciprocally concavoconvex (fit together like two saddles with riding surfaces together); allow wide range of movements	Thumb, vertebrae, ankle

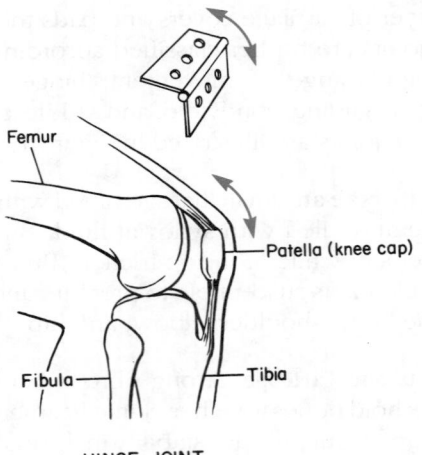

Femur

Patella (knee cap)

Fibula — Tibia

HINGE JOINT

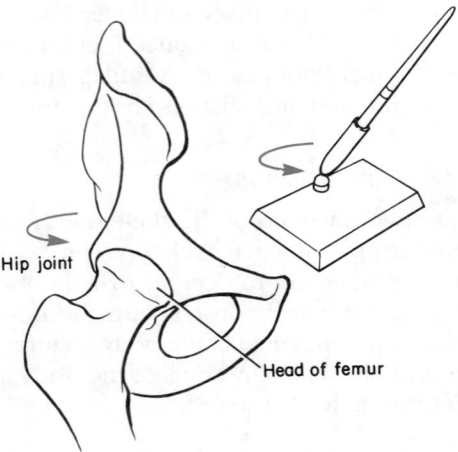

Hip joint

Head of femur

BALL-AND-SOCKET JOINT

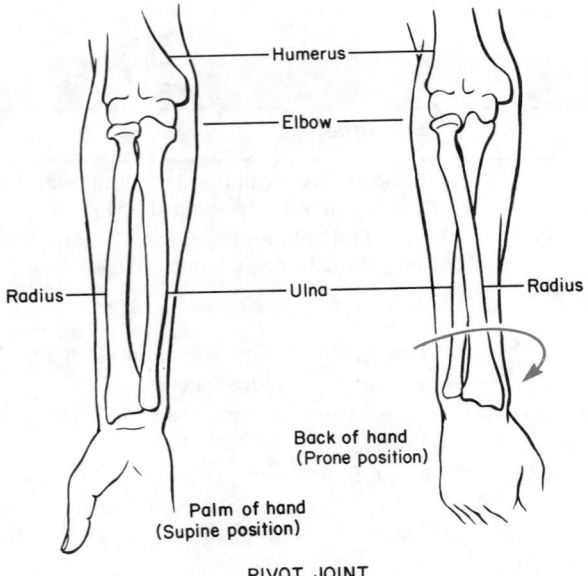

Humerus

Elbow

Radius — Ulna — Radius

Back of hand
(Prone position)

Palm of hand
(Supine position)

PIVOT JOINT

Figure 17-1. Some freely movable joints.

The Skull. The skull is made up of 28 separate bones. The eight flat bones of the cranium protect the brain, eyes, and ears. The 14 facial bones are lightweight, irregularly shaped, and generally small. The three pairs of bones of the middle ear (ossicles) are essential for hearing and are discussed in Chapter 20. The major bones of the skull are listed and illustrated in Figure 17-3. These bony surfaces are closely united by a thin fibrous membrane called a suture. Sutures do not permit movement.

The cranial and facial bones give the face its individual shape. The lower jaw bone, the mandible, is the only movable facial bone. The mandible can move up and down, as well as forward (protraction) and backward (retraction).

A small horseshoe-shaped bone, the **hyoid** bone, lies just behind and below the mandible and just above the larynx. It is not directly attached to any bone of the skull. Rather, it is attached by muscles and ligaments and seems to "float." Tongue muscles also are attached to the hyoid bone and assist in swallowing. Four pairs of cavities or sinuses in the cranial bones make the skull lighter and enhance voice sounds. The sinuses are named for the bones in which they lie: the frontal, the ethmoid, the sphenoid, and the maxillary. These sinuses are lined with mucous membrane that is continuous with the nasal mucosa; the sinuses drain into the nasal cavity.

The Trunk: Vertebral Column. The vertebral column is made up of 33 or 34 bones in the child and 26 bones in the adult. The vertebral column, or spine, holds the head, stiffens and supports the midportion of the body, and provides attachments for the ribs and pelvic bones (Figs. 17-4 and 17-5). It also protects the spinal cord, which passes from the brain down through the bony rings that make up the spinal canal. The vertebrae are constructed on a common plan; there are slight variations in their structure, but each one is made to adjust to the one beneath.

The top seven, or cervical, vertebrae are located in the neck. The first, or *atlas*, supports the skull, and the second, or *axis*, has an especially wide surface so that the head can be turned freely. The 12 below the cervical vertebrae are the thoracic vertebrae, to which the ribs are attached. The next five, the lumbar vertebrae, are in the small of the back. The five sacral vertebrae form one solid bone, the *sacrum*, which anchors the pelvis. The last four vertebrae, small and incomplete, form the *coccyx*. The sacrum and coccyx are commonly called the tailbone. The landmarks of the back are named correspondingly.

The vertebrae are separated anteriorly from each other by rounded plates of cartilage called *intervertebral disks*, which act as shock absorbers when you walk, jump, or fall. These disks have less dense ma-

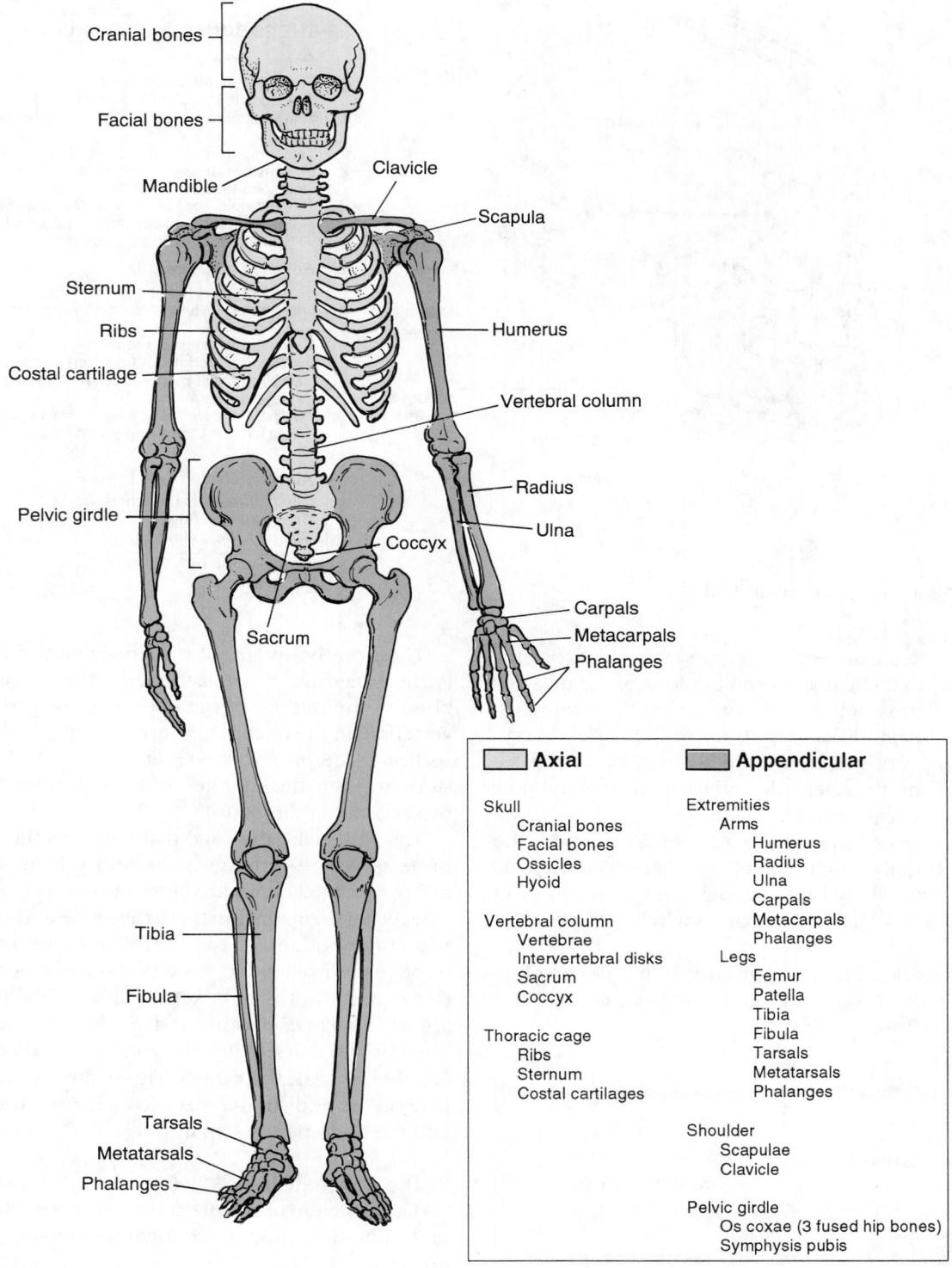

Figure 17-2. The divisions of the human skeleton.

terial in the center. A "slipped" disk refers to an intervertebral disk that has shifted out of position. A "ruptured" disk occurs when pressure forces some of the less dense tissue sideways, causing a protrusion of the walls of the disk (like a squashed grape). Either of these situations can cause pressure on a nerve and great discomfort.

On the inner side of the vertebrae is a bony structure called the *arch*, which forms an opening, or spinal foramen, through which the spinal cord passes. Jutting

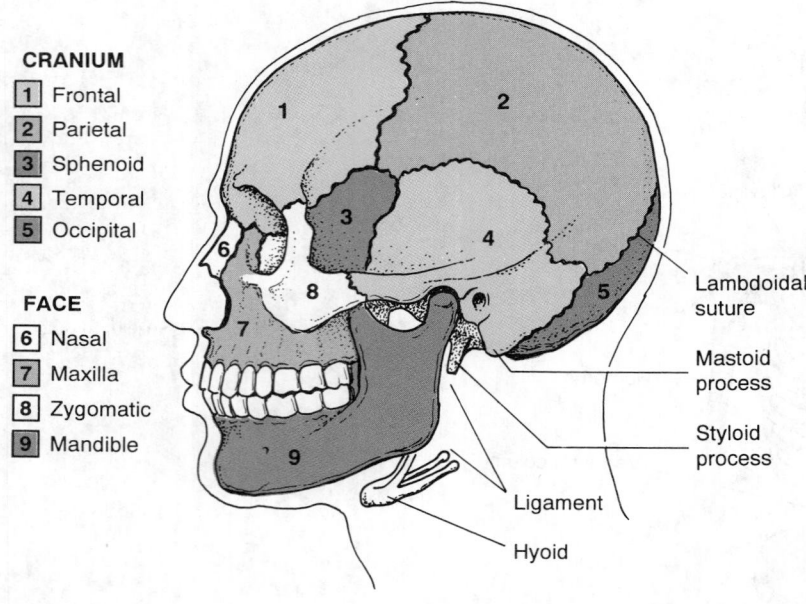

CRANIUM

1 Frontal
2 Parietal
3 Sphenoid
4 Temporal
5 Occipital

FACE

6 Nasal
7 Maxilla
8 Zygomatic
9 Mandible

Lambdoidal suture

Mastoid process

Styloid process

Ligament

Hyoid

THE 28 BONES OF THE SKULL

Bones of the Cranium (8)
Two parietal: top and sides of head
One occipital: back and base of head
One frontal: forehead, roof of skull and nasal cavities
Two temporal: sides and base of skull, contain ear cavities, mastoid cells in tip
One sphenoid: center of base of skull
One ethmoid: roof of nasal cavity, base of cranium, upper part of nasal septum (also includes the paired and fused superior and middle conchae)

Bones of the Face (14)
Two nasal: bridge of nose
One vomer: divides nasal cavity, as part of nasal septum
Two inferior turbinates (conchae): in the nostrils
Two lacrimal (orbitals): front part of eye sockets
Two zygomatic: prominent part of cheeks; base of eye sockets
Two palate (palatines): back of hard palate
Two maxillae: upper jaw, front of hard palate
One mandible: lower jaw, only movable bone in skull

Auditory Ossicles (6) in the Ear
One pair malleus (hammer)
One pair incus (anvil)
One pair stapes (stirrup)

Figure 17-3. Bones of the adult skull.

from the arch are several fingerlike extensions, or processes, on which ligaments and tendons of the muscles of the back are anchored. The muscles, the ligaments, and the cartilage disks help to make the vertebral column strong yet flexible. We are able to bend forward, backward, and to either side and rotate the central portion of the body considerably.

Between every two vertebrae is an area where the two bones lightly touch each other. This is called a *facet* (fah-set') joint. Many cases of back pain, particularly in the lower back, involve misalignment of these facet joints.

The normal spine has four curves that help to balance the body. Disease or injury and poor posture distort these curves.

Key Concept

The Vertebral Column

◆ *Cervical*—C_1 to C_7 ◆ *Sacrum*—S_1 to S_5
◆ *Thoracic*—T_1 to T_{12} ◆ *Coccyx*
◆ *Lumbar*—L_1 to L_5

The Thoracic (Rib) Cage. The **thorax** (chest) is a cavity formed by the ribs (costae), attached anteriorly to the sternum (the first seven pairs) and posteriorly to the thoracic vertebrae. The thoracic cage protects the heart, lungs, and great thoracic blood vessels. It is also a supportive structure for the bones of the shoulder girdle. The floor of the thorax is the diaphragm.

The front boundary of the upper part of the thorax is the **sternum** or breastbone, a flat, sword-shaped bone in the middle of the chest opposite the thoracic vertebrae in the back. The sternum is made up of three sections. The *manubrium* is at the top, the *body* of the sternum is in the middle, and the **xiphoid process** projects out at the bottom.

The ribs make the cage that supports the chest and protects the heart, lungs, liver, and spleen. These flat, narrow, bowed bones are arranged in pairs, 12 on each side. From their attachment to the spine at the back, the ribs curve out and to the front like barrel hoops. The upper seven pairs, the "true ribs," are attached to the sternum in front. The next three pairs, "the false ribs," are attached to each other and indirectly to the sternum. The last two pairs are free in front. These "floating ribs" are shorter than the others. The relatively elastic cartilage on the ends of the ribs allows leeway for the chest and the abdomen to expand.

The Appendicular Skeleton

The appendicular skeleton is composed of the bones of the shoulder, upper and lower extremities, and hips.

The Upper Extremities. The upper extremities include the shoulders and arms. The *shoulder girdle*, which anchors the arms, is formed by four bones. Two long, thin bones, the *clavicles*, or collar bones, are attached to the sternum and extend outward at right angles to it on either side. Opposite the clavicles at the back are the *scapulae*, or shoulder blades. They are flat, triangular bones attached to the outer ends of the clavicles on the

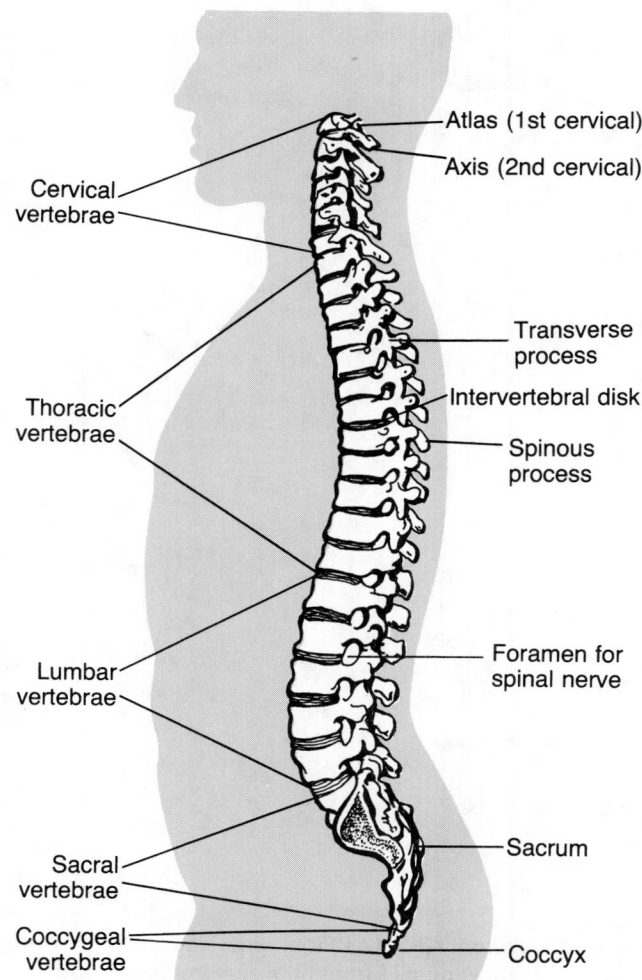

Figure 17-4. Vertebral column from the side.

Atlas (1st cervical)
Axis (2nd cervical)
Cervical vertebrae
Transverse process
Intervertebral disk
Thoracic vertebrae
Spinous process
Lumbar vertebrae
Foramen for spinal nerve
Sacral vertebrae
Sacrum
Coccygeal vertebrae
Coccyx

these bones in movement is shown in the illustration of a pivot joint in Figure 17-1.

More than one-fourth of the total number of bones in the human body are found in the *hands* and the *wrists.* Because of the many small bones, which allow for a great range of motions, such as twisting, bending, grasping, and squeezing, you can do such things as play a violin, write your name, and pick up minute objects with your thumb and forefinger.

Figure 17-6 illustrates the bones of the hand. The eight *carpal bones,* or wrist bones, are small, irregular bones that support the base of the palm and are attached to the radius, the ulna, and the five long, slender, and slightly curved *metacarpal bones* that form the palm of the hand. The other ends of the metacarpal bones are attached to the *phalanges,* or finger bones. There are three phalanges in each finger and two in the thumb.

The Lower Extremities. The *femur* (thigh bone), the upper bone of the leg, supports the weight of the trunk and is the longest and strongest bone of the body. Its upper end is attached to the pelvic bone in a ball-and-socket joint, where its rounded head fits into the depression (the acetabulum) on either side of the innominate portion of the pelvis; the other end of the femur is attached to the tibia in the lower leg. The head of the femur joins the shaft by a short length of bone called the neck. This area is a common site of fractures in older adults. Elevations on either side of the junction of the shaft and the neck are called the *trochanters* and serve as points of muscle attachment (see Fig. 17-1).

There are two bones in the lower leg, the *tibia,* or shin bone, and the *fibula.* The tibia is the weight-bearing long bone of the lower leg. The fibula is non–weight-bearing and is not a part of the knee joint.

The upper end of the tibia is attached to the lower end of the femur in the knee joint. The front of this joint is protected by a small bone, the *patella,* or kneecap, which is buried in a tendon that passes over the joint. The other bone in the lower leg, the fibula, is smaller than the tibia and is attached to it at the upper end. The lower end of these bones meets the bones of the ankle to form the ankle joint.

The *foot* is constructed to hold the weight of the entire body and at the same time, provide flexibility and resilience (Fig. 17-7). The seven *tarsal bones* of the ankle are compact and shaped irregularly; the largest of these bones (the calcaneus) is in the heel. They join the five *metatarsal bones,* or instep bones, to form two arches; the longitudinal arch, which extends from the heel to the toe, and the transverse or metatarsal arch, which extends across the foot. The weight of the body falls on these arches, and the many joints spring and give when a person walks. Weak muscles lessen this spring, and high spiky heels and poor posture upset the body balance, flattening the

skeleton. They are attached to the trunk of the body medially with the manubrium of the sternum and laterally with the scapula. This is why you can move your shoulders and arms so freely.

The *humerus* is the single long bone in each upper arm. The upper end is attached to the scapula, and the lower end meets the two forearm bones to form the elbow joint.

The larger forearm bone, the *ulna,* has two hollows in its upper end. The lower end of the humerus fits into one of these depressions. The upper end of the smaller forearm bone, the *radius,* fits into the other. The radius lies beside the ulna and is attached to it at the upper end. Both the radius and the ulna are attached to the wrist bones to form the wrist joint. The arrangement of these bones allows the palm to be turned forward (supine position) or backward (prone position).

The radius and ulna move so freely with the wrist bones and each other that when you turn your palm down, the radius crosses the ulna. The relationship of

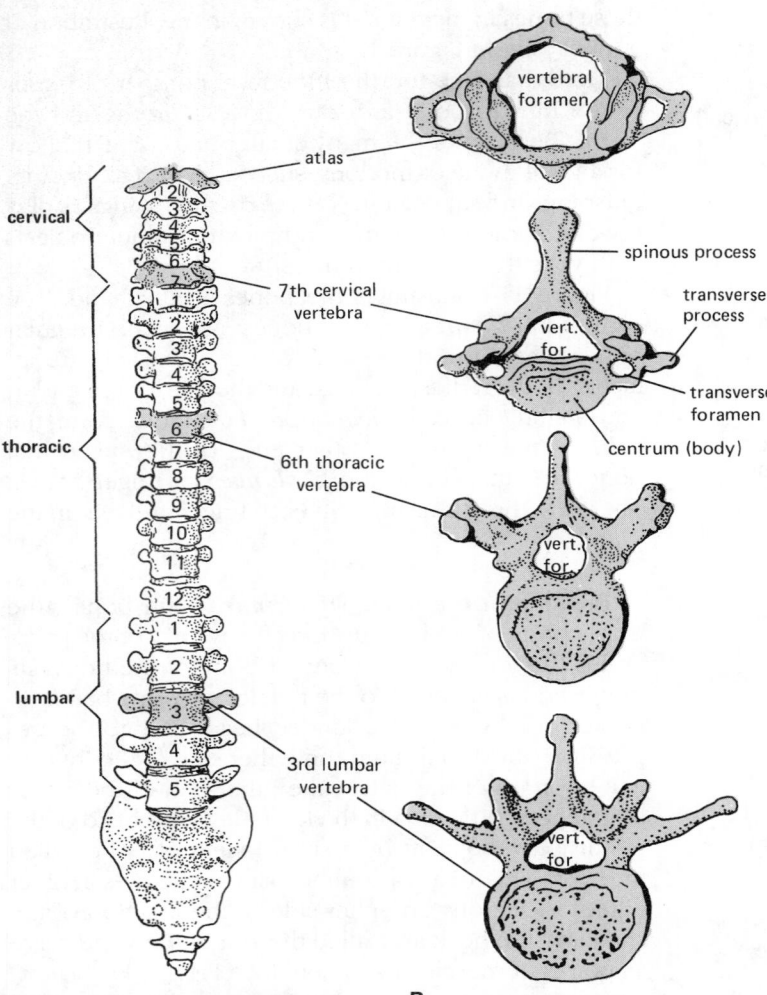

A front view of vertebral column

B vertebrae from above

Figure 17-5. **(A)** Front view of vertebral column **(B)** Vertebrae from above, Note the cartilage between the vertebrae; it is the intervertebral disk.

arches. The 14 bones of the toes, the *phalanges*, are attached to the metatarsal bones. The great toe has two phalanges, while each of the other toes has three.

In general, the hands and feet are built alike, but in the hands, the bones are finer and the joints more numerous (there are 29 in the wrist and hand and 26 in the ankle and foot). The hands are designed for fine and flexible movements and the feet for support. Together, these bones are about half the total number of bones in the body.

Key Concepts

◆ *Axial skeleton.* Skull, trunk (vertebral column), and thoracic (rib) cage
◆ *Appendicular skeleton.* Shoulders, hips, legs, and arms

The Pelvic Girdle. The pelvic girdle or pelvis is formed by the two large, irregularly shaped *innominate hip*

bones (or *os coxae*), attached posteriorly to the sacrum (Fig. 17-8). These bones spread outward at the top and become narrow at their front lower edges. In the fetus, these bones develop as three separate bones known as the *ilium*, the *ischium*, and the *pubis*, which usually fuse by the time growth is completed. The ilium is the upper flaring portion that one usually identifies as the hip bone. The ischium is the lower, stronger portion, which you may be conscious of only after horseback riding. The pubic bones meet in front and are joined by a pad of cartilage; this juncture is called the *symphysis pubis*. Connected to the sacrum and the coccyx posteriorly, these bones form the pelvic cavity, which houses the urinary bladder, the rectum, and in a woman, the reproductive organs. A woman's pelvis is larger and wider than a man's, which is nature's way of providing room for the development and delivery of the fetus. The angle of the pelvic opening (pubic arch) is less than a 90-degree angle in the man and greater than a 90-degree angle in the woman (see Figure 17-8).

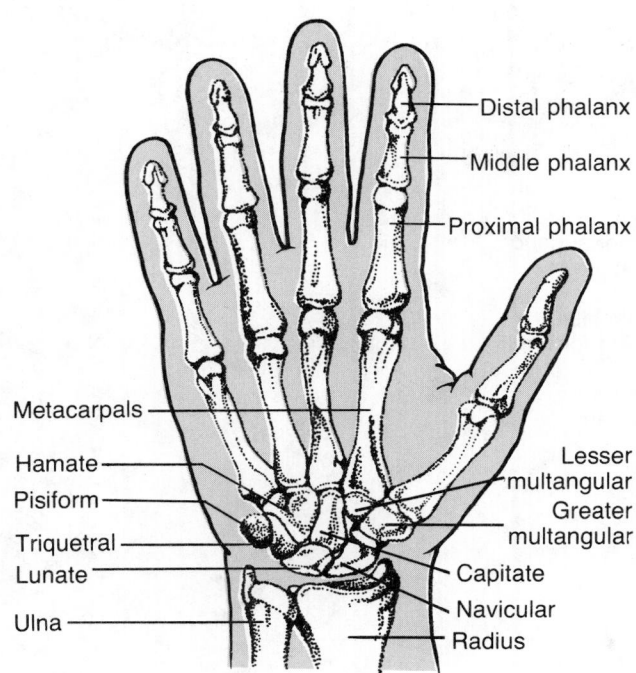

Figure 17-6. Bones of the right hand, ventral (anterior) view.

The Muscles

Functions of the skeleton include giving shape to the body and providing mobility, but without the aid of muscles, your body would be as immobile as the classroom skeleton. The skeleton also determines the size of the framework, but muscles and fat determine the body shape.

Functions of muscles are basically body movement, blood circulation, and heat production. The accompanying box lists these functions and the means of producing them.

Classification of Muscles

Three types of muscle tissue were listed in Chapter 14: skeletal, smooth, and cardiac. Each one is also identified as to its appearance. Skeletal and cardiac muscles are striated. That is, they consist of fibers marked by bands crossing it, giving a striped appearance. Smooth muscle is nonstriated. Muscles are further determined to be voluntary or involuntary (discussed later in this chapter). The classification of muscles and their functions are listed in Table 17-3.

Skeletal muscles, controlling movements of the skeleton, are muscles under voluntary or conscious control. They comprise approximately 40% of body weight. Their functions are locomotion, facial expression, and posture.

Smooth muscle controls involuntary motions inside body organs (viscera). It is also known as involuntary or visceral muscle. Smooth muscle is responsible for

propelling urine through the urinary tract, moving food along the digestive tract, dilating the pupils of the eyes, and dilating and contracting blood vessels to assist in circulation of blood.

Cardiac muscle is the middle layer of the heart (myocardium). It is responsible for propelling blood through the blood vessels. It works automatically and is called involuntary muscle. It is striated.

Compartments. Leg muscles are broken into compartments, as listed in Table 17-4. These muscle compartments are separated by connective tissue sheets. A condition known as *compartmental syndrome* involves swelling in muscle compartments of the leg or arm.

Structure of Muscles

Skeletal muscles are considered organs. They possess multinucleated cells and a connective tissue framework. Muscles lie in sheets and cords beneath the skin and cover the bones. Each fiber is comparable in size to a human hair and can hold about 1000 times its own weight. Fibers are wrapped together in bundles, and several bundles form a muscle.

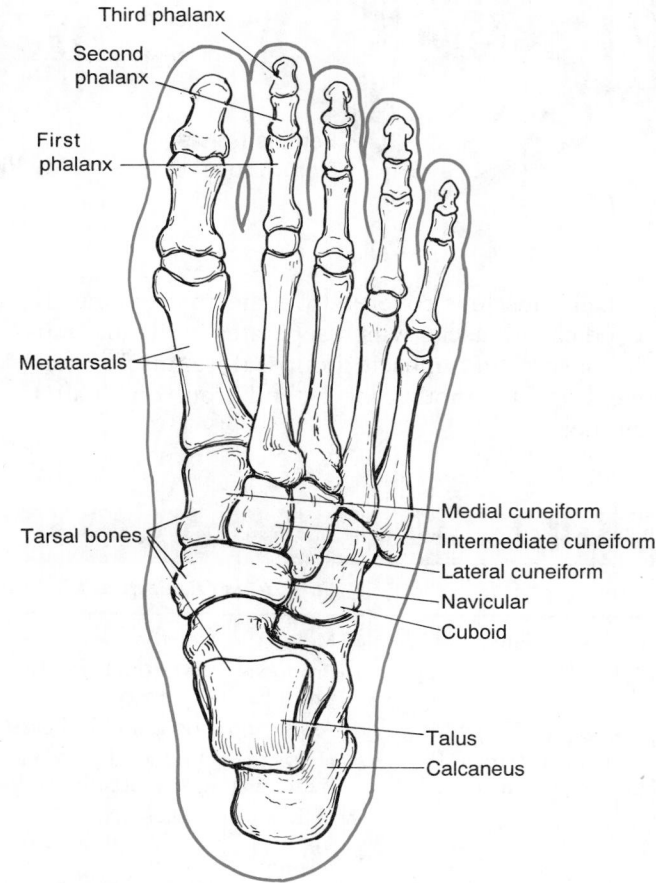

Figure 17-7. Bones of the right foot, dorsal aspect.

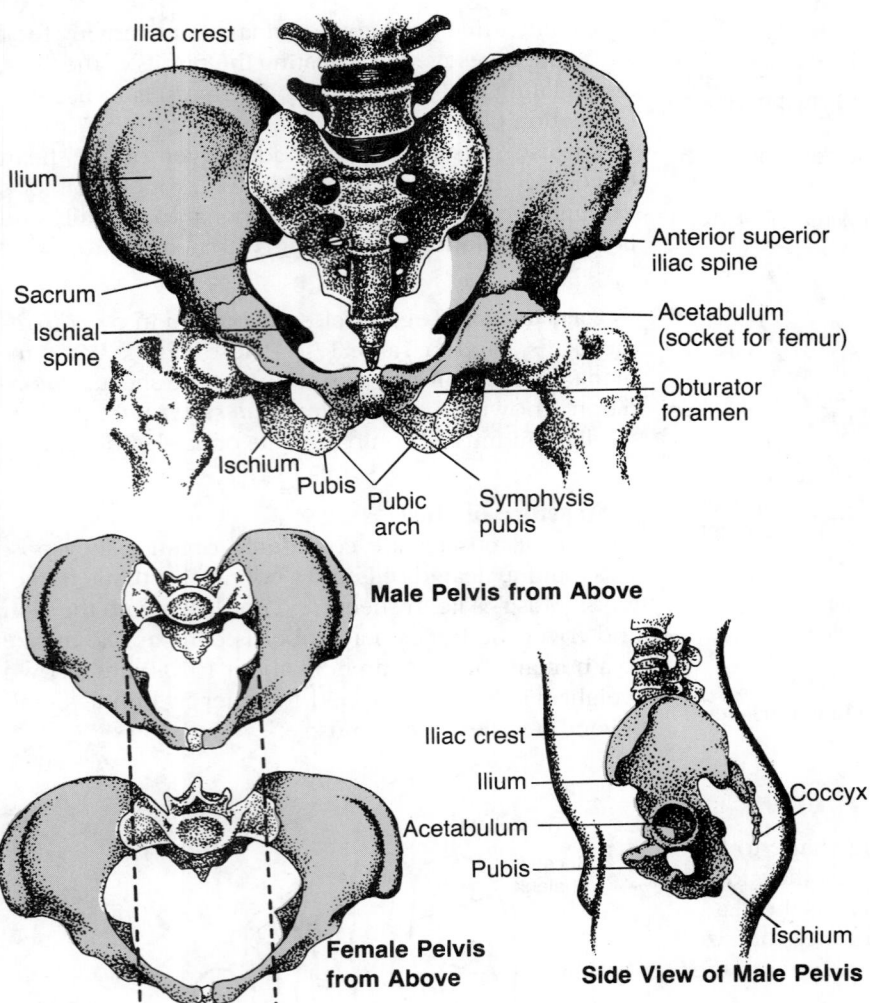

Iliac crest

Ilium

Sacrum

Ischial spine

Ischium

Pubis

Pubic arch

Symphysis pubis

Anterior superior iliac spine

Acetabulum (socket for femur)

Obturator foramen

Male Pelvis from Above

Female Pelvis from Above

Iliac crest

Ilium

Acetabulum

Pubis

Coccyx

Ischium

Side View of Male Pelvis

Figure 17-8. Pelvic girdle, showing male pelvis and female pelvis.

Each muscle is covered by a sheath of connective tissue called fascia, which separates individual muscles or surrounds muscle groups. Most muscles attach one bone to another or extend from one part to another.

One end of the muscle, the *origin*, is relatively immobile. It is attached to the more stationary of the two bones needed for movement. The *insertion* is the part of the muscle that attaches to the bone that undergoes the greatest movement. The main part of the muscle is called the *belly*. The fibrous muscle tissue that covers bone is called *periosteum*. It is continuous with collagen fibers that form tendons and ligaments.

Accessory Structures

Tendons. The ends of fascia lengthen into tough cords called tendons. Tendons attach muscle to bones. The tendons have sheaths lined with a synovial membrane that permit a smooth gliding movement.

To understand the anatomy of a muscle and its tendon, place your hand on the thick muscle at the calf of your leg. Located here are some of the strongest muscles in the body. Move your hand toward your ankle and you will find that as both the leg and the muscles become narrower, the tissues become tough, fibrous and ropelike. This occurs because approximately half-

Table 17-3. Classification of Muscle Tissues

Type	Functions (Examples)
Skeletal (striated and voluntary)	Moves the skeleton
	Produces heat through aerobic production of energy
	Assists in blood return to heart
Smooth (nonstriated and involuntary)	Helps maintain blood pressure by regulating size of arteries
	Maintains peristalsis by helping push food through the intestines
Cardiac	Pumps blood by contractions

Functions of Muscles

Voluntary Movement

- Enables walking, standing, sitting, and other movements
- Maintains body in upright position
- Participates in body balance

Involuntary Muscle Action

- Maintains heart beat to pump blood
- Provides arterial blood flow
- Promotes lymphatic and venous blood return to heart
- Dilates and contracts blood vessels to control blood flow
- Maintains respiration
- Performs digestion processes
- Performs elimination processes
- Participates in reflex acts
- Enables all other involuntary actions of body

Protection

- Protects body in emergency by reflex action
- Covers, surrounds, and protects internal organs (viscera)
- Supports internal organs

Miscellaneous

- Produces heat
- Assists in maintaining stable body temperature (shivering, goose flesh, muscles give off heat)
- Provides shape to body

way to the ankle, the muscle is attached to a tendon, the Achilles tendon, which extends down to the heel.

Major Muscles of the Body

Important muscles for the nurse to know are listed in Table 17-5. They are also identified in Figures 17-9 and 17-10.

Diaphragm and Intercostals. The *diaphragm* is one of the most vital muscles in the body. It is the dome-shaped muscle that forms the division between the thoracic and abdominal cavities. As the diaphragm contracts, it pulls downward, enlarging the thoracic cavity.

The *intercostal* muscles are located between the ribs. When they contract, the thoracic cavity is enlarged, both from side to side and from front to back.

The contractions of the diaphragm and the intercostals work together to form a negative pressure situation within the thoracic cavity. This causes atmospheric air to rush into the lungs. Relaxation of these muscles causes the thoracic cavity to become smaller, thus forc-

ing air out of the lungs and into the atmosphere (breathing).

Muscles of the Hands and Feet. The muscles and tendons of the hands and feet are arranged in a slightly different manner from those of the rest of the body. Many bones, muscles, and tendons in the hands and the feet are necessary to move the bones. Because bulky muscles would make clumsy motions, the larger muscles used to move the hands and feet are located in the forearm and lower leg. When you flex your fingers to clench your fist, you can feel the muscles move and tighten in your forearm. Other muscles begin at the wrist and extend into long, thin tendons that attach to the bones of the fingers. This placement permits accuracy and a variety of movements.

System Physiology

Formation of Bone Tissue

Bones are active, living organs that change greatly during a person's lifetime. The small, mostly cartilaginous bones of the baby grow in diameter and length and continue to harden until growth is complete, usually between the ages of 18 and 21. Although bone structure and size alter primarily to accommodate growth, change continues into later life when growth has essentially stopped. Bone cells multiply rapidly in the growing years. When the growth spurts have stopped, new cells form only to replace dead or injured ones and to repair breaks. With age, bones become harder and more brittle, breaking more easily.

Although bone tissue hardens by deposits of the minerals calcium and phosphorus, bones are made up of living cells. Bone-building cells are called **osteoblasts**. **Ossification** is the formation of bone by osteoblasts and is the process by which bones become hardened through an increase in calcified tissue. Ossification progresses from the middle of the shaft outward. Other cells, the *osteoclasts*, assist in the resorption (act of removal by absorption) or breakdown of bone. This process allows bones to grow and change shape. Bones continue the process of building up and resorption throughout life.

The following factors affect bone growth and maintenance:

- Heredity: genes and enzymes
- Nutrition: protein, vitamins (D, C, A), and minerals (calcium, phosphorus)
- Exercise: weight-bearing (provides "stress" for bones)
- Hormones: affect rate of bone growth, calcium metabolism, energy production, and overall mainte-

Table 17-4. Classification of Compartments of Muscles

Classification	Muscle or Muscle Groups	Attachments	Action
Compartments of Thigh			
Anterior (extensor)	Quadriceps femoris group	Femur and tibia	Extend leg and thigh
	Sartorius muscle		Flexes hip and knee
Posterior (flexor)	Hamstring group	Ischial tuberosity and tibia or fibula	Move hip and knee joints
Media (adductor)	Adductor magnus muscle		Adduct femur
	Adductor longus muscle		
	Adductor brevis muscle	Pubic bones and femur	
	Pectineus muscle		
	Gracilis muscle		Flexes and adducts legs
Compartments of Lower Leg			
Anterior	Tibialis anterior muscles	Tibia and metatarsals	Extend toes and dorsiflex ankle
Posterior	Superficial muscles:		Flex toes and plantar flex ankle
	Gastrocnemius	Femur and knee; helps form Achilles tendon	
	Soleus	Fibula, tibia: to Achilles tendon	
	Plantaris	Femur and Achilles tendon	
	Deep muscles (not discussed here)		Attach to Achilles tendon
Lateral (peroneal)	Peroneus longus	Tibia, fibula, and metatarsals	Evert foot and plantar flex ankle
	Peroneus brevis	Fibula and metatarsals	

nance (Hormones include growth hormone, thyroxine, calcitonin, insulin, parathyroid hormone, estrogen, and testosterone.)

Muscle Contractions

Some of the characteristics of muscle tissue are similar to those observed when stretching a heavy rubber band. Muscle tissue has the following unique characteristics:

◆ *Contractility:* the ability to shorten and become thicker
◆ *Extensibility:* the ability to stretch
◆ *Elasticity:* the ability to return to its normal length after use
◆ *Irritability:* the ability to respond to a stimulus

Usually the stimulus is a nerve impulse that originates in the spinal cord and travels to the nerve where it gives the message to contract.

Muscles operate under an all-or-none principle. An individual muscle fiber cannot partially contract. If a stimulus is strong enough to cause contraction, each fiber stimulated will contract as much as it can. If the stimulus is not strong enough, that fiber will not contract at all.

Contraction and Relaxation

Muscles are elastic, allowing them to work in pairs having opposite actions. When one muscle contracts, the other relaxes. A movement is initiated by a single muscle or a set of muscles, called the *prime mover.* When an opposite movement is to be made, another set of muscles called the *antagonist* takes over. Muscles that assist one another in the movement are called synergic or synergistic muscles. When you bend your elbow, you can feel the muscle in your upper arm contract, grow hard, and thicken as the muscle fibers shorten to raise the forearm (**flexion**). At the same time, the muscles on the back of your upper arm relax, lengthen, and pull against the front muscles. If you permit, they will pull your forearm straight (**extension**).

Power Source

Muscles need energy to move. Digested foods furnish carbon, hydrogen, and oxygen from which the body makes glycogen (sugar), a special form of stored glucose used by the body for fuel. Fatty acids also are broken down for fuel. This fuel is called adenosine triphosphate (ATP). Oxygen and ATP, brought to the muscles cells by the blood, react with each other, and the result of this oxidation, or burning, process is energy and heat. Most of the body's heat originates from

(Text continues on page 177)

Table 17-5. Important Muscles of the Body

Muscle	Location*	Action	Notes
Neck and Shoulders			
Sternocleidomastoid	Side of neck	Helps keep head erect	If diseased or injured, head is permanently drawn to one side (torticollis).
Deltoid	Shoulder	Moves upper arm outward from body	Site for intramuscular injections
Arm and Anterior Chest			
Biceps	Front of upper arms	Flexes forearm	
Triceps	Posterior to biceps	Extends forearm	
Pectoralis major	Anterior upper portion of chest	Help to bring arms across chest	
Pectoralis minor	Anterior chest, arising from ribs		
Serratus anterior			
Respiration			
Diaphragm	Between the abdominal and thoracic cavities	Assists in process of breathing	When it contracts, it moves downward, making chest cavity larger, forming a partial vacuum around lungs, and causing air to rush into them. When it relaxes, it pushes upward, and air is forced out of lungs
Intercostal	Between the ribs	Helps to enlarge the chest cavity (side to side and back to front)	Same actions as above
Abdomen			
Internal oblique	Flat bands that stretch from ribs to pelvis, overlapping in layers from various angles	Support abdominal organs	An opening in muscle creates weakness where a hernia (rupture) may occur.
External oblique			
Transversus abdominis			
Rectus abdominis			
Back and Posterior Chest			
Trapezius dorsi	Across back and posterior chest	Helps to lift shoulder	
Latissimus dorsi and other back muscles	Across back and posterior chest	Work in groups; help to stand erect, balance when heavy objects are carried, and turn or bend body; adduct upper arm	Also called "swimming muscle"
Gluteal			
Gluteus maximus	Form the buttocks	Help change from sitting to standing positions; help in walking	Frequently used as site for intramuscular injections
Gluteus medius			
Gluteus minimus			
Thigh and Lower Leg			
Quadriceps femoris group	Anterior thigh	Extend leg and thigh	Rectus femoris and vastus lateralis used as injection sites
Rectus femoris			
Vastus lateralis			
Vastus intermedius			
Vastus medialis			
Hamstring group	Posterior thigh	Flexes and extends leg and thigh	
Biceps femoris			
Semimembranosus			
Semitendinosus			

(continued)

Table 17-5 (continued)

Muscle	Location*	Action	Notes
Gracilis	Thigh	Flexes and adducts leg; adducts thigh	
Sartorius	Thigh	Flexes and rotates thigh and leg	Called "tailor's muscle" because it allows sitting in cross-legged position
Tibialis anterior	Anterior lower leg	Elevates and flexes foot	
Gastrocnemius	Calf	Flexes foot and leg	Give calf rounded appearance
Soleus	Calf	Extends and rotates foot	
Peroneus longus	Calf	Extends, abducts, and everts foot	
Achilles tendon	Attaches calf muscles to heel bone	Allows extension of foot and gives "spring" to walk	Term derived from Greek mythology
Hands and Feet (See text)			
Head			
Orbicularis oculi	Head	Move eyes and wrinkle forehead	Disorder may cause strabismus ("cross-eye")
Orbicularis oris	Head	Moves mouth and surrounding facial structures	
Masseter	Head	Assists in chewing by raising lower jaw	
Buccinator	Head	Moves fleshy portion of cheek for smiling	

* For placement of these muscles, see Figures 17-9 and 17-10.

Table 17-6. Effects of Aging on the Musculoskeletal System

Factor	Result	Nursing Implications
Bones		
Bone mass and strength is lost	Osteoporosis	*Assess for fractures
*Calcium is lost (greater in females)	Hunched posture (kyphosis-humpback; lordosis-swayback)	*Encourage Vitamin D and calcium supplements
	*Back pain	*Advise exercise to minimize bone losses
	*Brittle bones	*Teach safety and prevention of falls
Vertebral column shortens	Decrease in height	
Joints		
*Degeneration occurs in joints	Arthritis	Encourage person to increase mobility with active and passive range of motion exercises
	Osteoarthropathy	
	Joint stiffness	
Muscles		
Muscle cells are lost	Loss of muscle strength	Give suggestions on how to carry daily items (eg. groceries) when it becomes more difficult
Muscle cells are replaced by fat	Gain of fat tissue (and weight)	
Elasticity of fibers is lost	Loss of flexibility	Encourage person to control weight
	Easy fatigability	Suggest walking and swimming (good exercise for elderly); physical activity reduces loss of muscle and elasticity and increases flexibility
	Resting tremors may occur	Advise that exercise promotes psychologic stimulation
		Encourage proper nutrition, particularly adequate protein, vitamins, and minerals

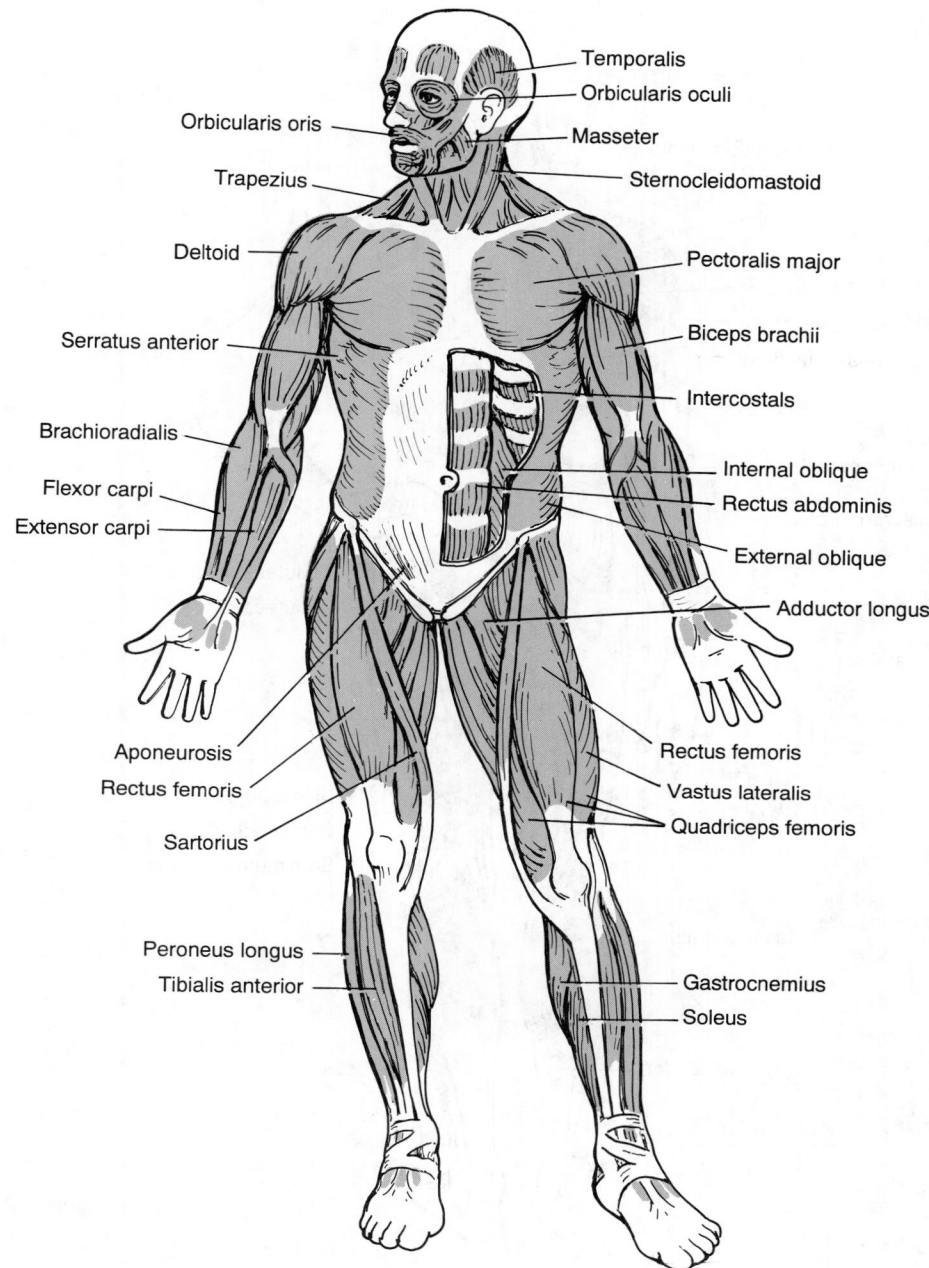

Figure 17-9. Muscles of the body, front (anterior) view.

muscle activity. When muscles are very active, they draw on the reserve glycogen stored in their cells. When the body is cold, it makes use of the ability of muscles to produce heat rapidly by the automatic device of general muscle action or shivering. To produce a great amount of heat in an emergency, the body produces the more violent action of chilling.

Waste Products. Carbon dioxide and lactic acid are waste products produced in the process of oxidation. The blood carries carbon dioxide to the lungs, where it is removed in breathing. Lactic acid is removed through the urinary system and the sweat glands. Vigorous or prolonged muscle action produces such a large quantity of waste products, especially lactic acid, that the blood cannot carry it away fast enough, and some of it accumulates in the muscle cells. Furthermore, it is not possible for skeletal muscles to remain in a contracted state for long periods of time without tiring. Gradually, due to a build-up of lactic acid and resultant lack of oxygen, a muscle will become fatigued. This is why your muscles are fatigued, ache, or feel sore after violent exercise or prolonged use. A simple formula helps to summarize the action of muscles:

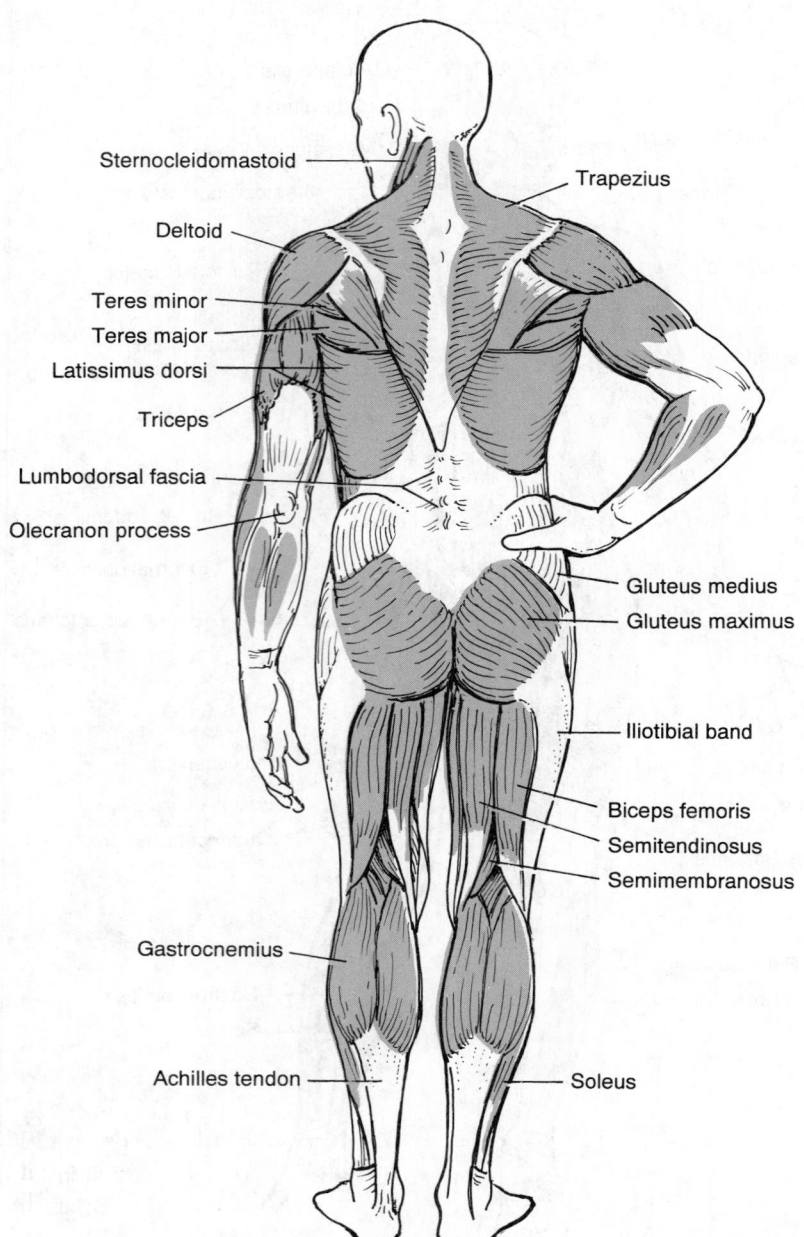

Sternocleidomastoid

Deltoid

Teres minor

Teres major

Latissimus dorsi

Triceps

Lumbodorsal fascia

Olecranon process

Trapezius

Gluteus medius

Gluteus maximus

Iliotibial band

Biceps femoris

Semitendinosus

Semimembranosus

Gastrocnemius

Achilles tendon

Soleus

Figure 17-10. Muscles of the body, back (posterior) view.

muscle cell + food and oxygen
↓
heat and energy
↓
by-products: lactic acid and carbon dioxide

Muscle Tone

Because we stand erect against the constant pull of gravity, many muscles are constantly in a mild state of contraction to help maintain balance. Even relaxed muscles are ready to go into action if they are in good condition. This state of slight contraction and ability to spring into action is called *muscle tone* (*tonus*). Physical exercise improves the tone of the muscles and increases their size. An idle muscle loses its tone and wastes away. If a patient does not use certain muscles or uses them very little, they become flabby and weak (atonic) and may atrophy (waste away).

Special Considerations in Children
Retaining Muscle Tone

It is important for children who sit in school all day to have an opportunity for vigorous play after school; their muscles need such stimulation.

Range of Motion in Body Movements

Flexion	Decreasing the angle between two bones or bending a part on itself, as in bending the elbow
Extension	Increasing the angle between two bones, as in straightening an arm
Hyperextension	Increasing the angle of an extremity beyond normal
Dorsiflexion	Bending a body part toward the dorsum (backwards), as in moving the foot so that the toes face toward the back
Plantar flexion	Bending the foot so that the toes are pointed downward
Abduction	Moving away from the midline of the body
Adduction	Moving toward the midline of the body
Circumduction	Moving an extremity in circles; the extremity draws a cone with the joint as the apex of the cone, as in moving or swinging an arm in circles
Rotation	Moving a bone on a longitudinal axis as in shaking the head "no" or to move in a circle from the waist
Supination	Turning the palm anteriorly or the foot inward and upward
Pronation	Turning the hand so the palm faces downward or backward
Inversion	Turning a part so that it faces medially or inside, such as turning your ankle so that the sole of the foot faces the opposite foot
Eversion	Turning an extremity laterally or outward, as in turning the foot to face away from the body
Protraction	Moving forward or anteriorly, as in jutting out the jaw
Retraction	Moving backward or back into anatomic position

Pressure on the nerves in muscles makes them sore. Patients who must often lie on their backs complain of aches and pains in these muscles. Strains or inactivity also affect them. For these reasons, a back rub can be comforting. It is also advisable to adjust the patient's body to positions that do not cause strain, change the position frequently, and support the patient the first time out of bed. The patient's position in bed should be the same *as if the patient were standing.* If this is not assured, the muscles may remain contracted because of the abnormal position (*contractures*).

Isometric and Isotonic Contractions. In addition to the constant muscle contractions we refer to as muscle tone, two other types of contractions are important. *Isometric* contractions do not increase the length of the muscle but do increase the muscle tension. For example, if you push against an unmovable object or tense the muscles in your upper arm, your muscles will tighten. *Isotonic* contractions shorten and thicken the muscle, causing movement. Exercises such as swimming, jogging, or bicycling are examples of isotonic exercises.

Rehabilitation. An injured or inactive muscle can be retrained to do its work. Retraining usually requires working with more than one muscle, because except for the simplest movements, muscles work in groups. Today people are being helped to recover the use of injured or inactive muscles. Rehabilitation activities are prescribed by physicians, and trained physiotherapists and occupational therapists carry them out. Nurses may work under the direction of these specialists to help the patient with selected exercises. Re-educating muscles is sometimes a long process. Improvement is likely to be so gradual that it is hardly noticeable from day to day, and the patient often needs encouragement to persevere.

Mobility

Purposeful coordinated movement of the body requires the integrated functioning of the skeleton, skeletal muscles, and nervous systems. Body mechanics is the efficient use of the body as a machine.

Newborns are uncoordinated in their movements. Maturation of the central nervous system is necessary to prepare the child to move purposefully. Neonates are born with crawling and stepping reflexes that need to be developed in later infancy. All children go through certain stages of development in which they learn to sit, stand, crawl, step with help, walk holding on, walk without assistance, and progress to stair climbing, running, skipping, and hopping.

Increased mobility allows for increased independence. An adult pattern of gait develops between ages 3 and 5. Gait is a manner of walking. Infants have a wide-based gait. As children mature, the base narrows, arms are swung in coordination, stride and walking speed increase, and movements become smooth and graceful.

Range of Motion
Range of motion (ROM) is the total amount of motion of which a joint is capable. Terminology and ROM movements of which the body and joints are capable are summarized in the accompanying box. ROM exercises are important in prevention and rehabilitation in musculoskeletal conditions (see Chapter 43).

Effects of Aging on the System

With aging, bone and muscle strength and endurance are gradually lost. The muscle cells atrophy (a deterioration in size and function of cells) and are replaced with fat cells. Bone tissue does not replace itself as quickly as in younger years. Osteoporosis and fractures are common because of mineral loss from within the bone. Women are affected with osteoporosis more than men because of the loss of female hormones in menopause. Joints commonly develop arthritis. Muscle aches and back pains are common due to the skeletal changes that cause **kyphosis** (hunchback) and **lordosis** (swayback). Table 17-6 summarizes major effects of aging on the musculoskeletal system.

Prevention of musculoskeletal problems is a nursing consideration. Appropriate exercise and a proper diet that includes adequate amounts of proteins and minerals are important. Safety is a major consideration. As a result of posture and balance adjustments necessary to compensate for the skeletal framework changes, the elderly are more likely to fall.

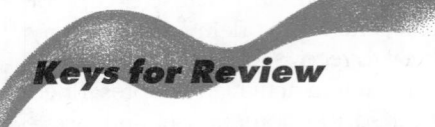

Keys for Review

Key Questions for Critical Thinking

1. Describe at least four functions of the skeleton.
2. Describe three types of joints in relation to their ability to move, and give an example of each.
3. Discuss the functions of the spinal column.
4. Describe three major types of muscle tissue.

Key Readings

Chabner D. The Language of Medicine, Ed 4. Philadelphia, W.B. Saunders, 1991

Eliopoulus C. Caring for the Elderly in Diverse Care Settings. Philadelphia, J.B. Lippincott, 1990

Farrell J. Nursing Care of the Older Person. Philadelphia, J.B. Lippincott, 1990

Hogstel M. Nursing Care of the Older Adult, Ed 2. Media, PA, Harwal Publishing, 1988

Jackson DB, Saunders RB. Child Health Nursing: A Comprehensive Approach to the Care of Children and Their Families. Philadelphia, J.B. Lippincott, 1993

Scanlon V, Sanders V. Essentials of Anatomy and Physiology. Philadelphia, F.A. Davis, 1991

Seeley R, Stephens T, Tate P. Anatomy and Physiology, Ed 2. St. Louis, C.V. Mosby, 1992

Smeltzer SC, Bare BG. Brunner and Suddarth's Textbook of Medical-Surgical Nursing, Ed 7. Philadelphia, J.B. Lippincott, 1992

Van De Graff K, Fox IF. Concepts of Human Anatomy and Physiology, Ed 3. Dubuque, IA, WC Brown, 1992

Enrichment Keys

Memmler RL, Cohen BF, Woods, DL. Structure and Function of the Human Body, Ed 5. Philadelphia, J.B. Lippincott, 1992

Keys to Learning More

Chapter 18: structure and function of the nervous system

Chapter 26: describes metabolism, providing energy for muscles

Chapter 38: basics of physical assessment, including gait, balance, and other aspects of musculoskeletal functioning

Chapter 43: body mechanics and positioning

Chapter 56: medications, some used in musculoskeletal disorders

Unit Thirteen: deviations from normal body structure and function in children

Unit Fourteen: deviations from normal in adults

Chapter 70: disorders in the musculoskeletal system

Unit Fifteen: deviations in older adults

18 The Nervous System

Learning Objectives

- Define the key terms and identify important abbreviations
- Locate the structures of the central nervous system on an anatomic chart
- List the functions of the spinal cord
- List the functions of cerebrospinal fluid
- State the divisions and functions of the peripheral nervous system
- List the cranial nerves and spinal nerves
- Describe what is meant by the action potential of a nerve cell
- Identify the functions of sensory neurons, motor neurons, and interneurons
- Describe the route followed by a reflex and state the homeostatic rationale for reflex arcs

Key Terms

afferent	meninges	neuron
axon	myelin sheath	neurotransmitter
cerebellum	nerve	plexus
dendrites	nerve tract	proprioceptors
efferent	neuroglia	reflex arc
interneurons	neurology	

Keys to Understanding This Chapter

Chapter 14: organization of the human body
Chapter 15: integumentary system
Chapter 16: fluid and electrolyte balance
Chapter 17: musculoskeletal system

Key Points

- Functions of the nervous system are basically communication and control.
- The basic structural and functional cell of the nervous system is the neuron. The neuron responds to chemical and physical stimuli.

Key Points (continued)

- The second type of cell in the nervous system are the neuroglia. They support and connect nervous tissue but do not transmit impulses.
- The nervous system is divided into major parts: the central nervous system and peripheral nervous system. The peripheral nervous system is further divided into cranial nerves, spinal nerves, and the autonomic nervous system. The autonomic nervous system has sympathetic and parasympathetic divisions.
- An action potential takes only milliseconds to reverse the cell's polarity and return to its original polarity. This is an electrical impulse.
- There are three types of neurons with specific actions: sensory, motor, and interneurons.

Key Topics Outline

Structure and Function
    Cells of the Nervous System
    Divisions of the Nervous System
    Central Nervous System
    Peripheral Nervous System
    Autonomic Nervous System
System Physiology
    Transmission of Nerve Impulses
    Reflexes
Effects of Aging on the System

Key Learning Activities

- Create a chart showing the interrelationships between the musculoskeletal and nervous systems.
- Using several resources, describe the types of learning believed to take place in the left and right hemispheres of the brain.

The nervous system takes impressions and information from the outside world (external stimuli) and selectively stores this information (memory) for future reference and application. It also coordinates messages from the internal body systems (internal stimuli), making it possible for the body to readjust constantly to changing internal and external environments. Thus, the nervous system is the director of all body activities.

The nervous system is often likened to a telephone system. Through a network of wires, messages come into a central switchboard, where the necessary connections are made to direct them to the right places. In similar fashion, the nervous system is organized to bring messages into a center that relays them to certain parts of the body. The brain and the spinal cord are the switchboard. The **nerves** are the wires that carry incoming and outgoing messages.

None of the body systems function alone. Activities of the various systems are interrelated, integrated, and coordinated by messages carried from one system to another. The nervous system is responsible for much of this communication. **Neurology** is the study of the nervous system.

Structure and Function

Functions of the nervous system are basically communication and control. The accompanying box lists these functions and the nervous system's methods of performing these functions.

To understand these functions, it is necessary to understand specialized cells of the nervous system. This chapter first discusses these cells and then the divisions of the nervous system.

Cells of the Nervous System

The nervous system has two types of cells: the neuron or nerve cell and the neuroglia. The basic structural and functional cell of the nervous system is the **neuron.** The neuron is specialized to respond to chemical and physical stimuli, and messages are conducted and transferred through it.

The human brain regulates more than 10 billion neurons at all times. There are five times as many neuroglia as there are neurons. **Neuroglia** support and connect nervous tissue but do not transmit impulses.

Neurons

Microscopic neurons perform many functions. Those in the brain influence thinking, affect memory, and regulate other organs and glands. Although neurons are microscopic, they can vary greatly in size and length.

Functions of the Nervous System

Communication

- ◆ Monitors impressions and information from external stimuli
- ◆ Monitors information from internal stimuli
- ◆ Responds to danger, pain, and other situations
- ◆ Responds to changes (internal and external)
- ◆ Helps to maintain homeostasis
- ◆ Responds to conscious decisions and thoughts
- ◆ Coordinates processing of new learning

Control

- ◆ Directs all body activities
- ◆ Maintains blood pressure, respiration, and other vital functions
- ◆ Regulates body systems (in coordination with endocrine system)
- ◆ Coordinates reflex actions
- ◆ Controls instinctual behaviors
- ◆ Controls conscious movement and activities
- ◆ Stores unconscious thoughts

A neuron is composed of three basic parts: one cell body and two processes (an axon and a dendrite). Figure 18-1 illustrates the structure of neurons.

Cell Body. Each neuron has only one cell body, which contains the nucleus. Cell bodies do not divide and reproduce by mitosis. Protein syntheses takes place in the cell body in specialized organelles unique to the neuron (Nissl bodies). The cell body may be quite a distance from its axon or dendrites.

Axons. An **axon** is an extension that carries impulses *away from the neuron cell body*. An axon may be as short as a few millimeters, or it may be longer than a meter. It may be myelinated (covered in a protective layer), or it may be bare. This structural difference is important.

If an axon is surrounded by a **myelin sheath** (a fatty covering), it is said to be myelinated. (Myelinated axons conduct impulses more rapidly than unmyelinated axons.) The myelin sheath electrically insulates one nerve cell from another. Without this sheath, these nerve cells would short circuit.

Key Concept

Multiple sclerosis is a disease that involves the deterioration of the myelin sheath of the central nervous system. When this occurs, impulses do not reach their intended destinations.

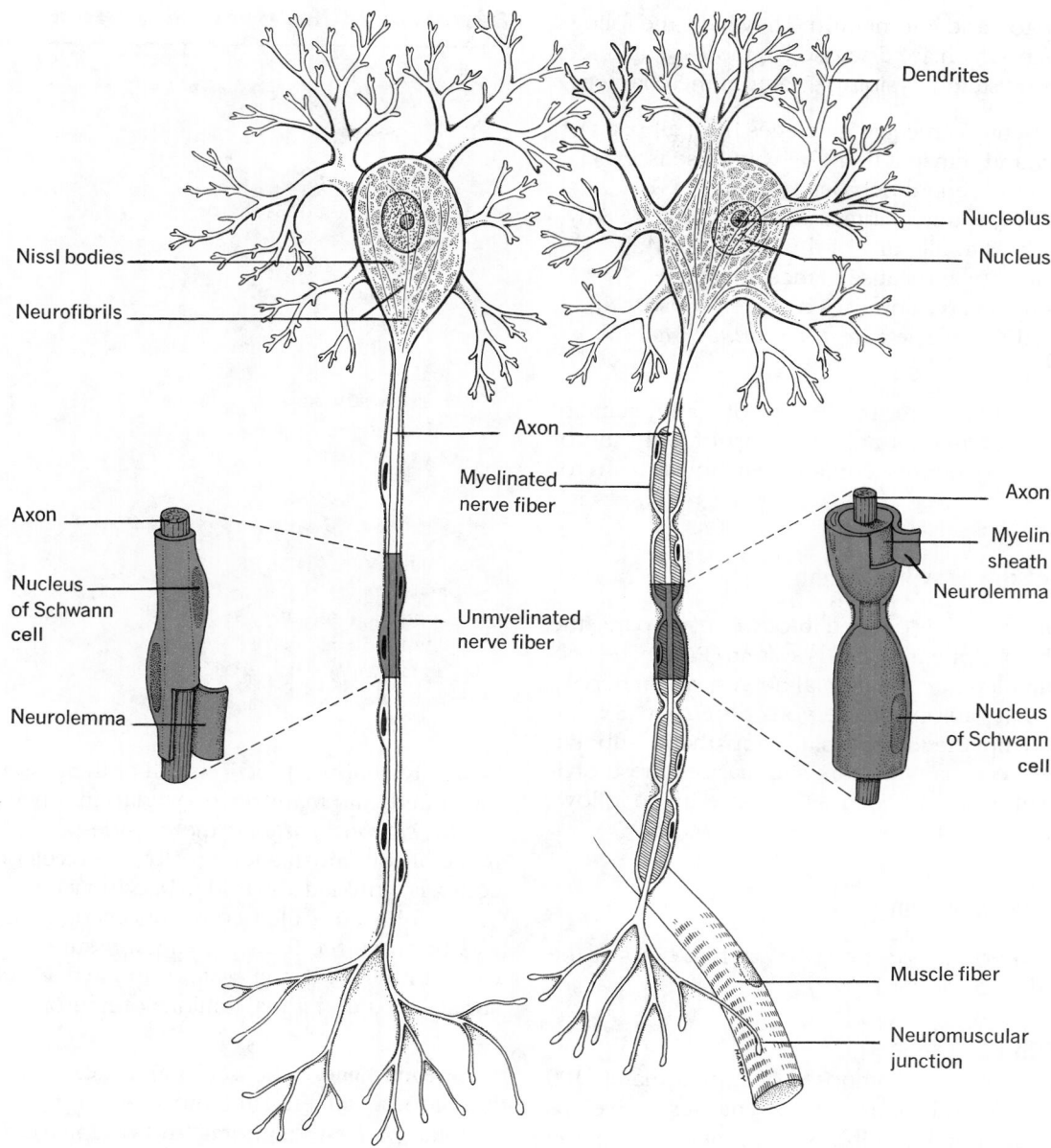

Figure 18-1. Structure of typical unmyelinated and myelinated neurons.

Dendrites. Dendrites are short, often highly branched extensions of the cell body. Dendrites receive impulses from axons of other neurons and transmit these impulses *toward the cell body*. Dendrites respond to chemical messages sent from across the tiny space that separates the neurons, the *synapse*.

The Synapse and Neurotransmitters. A synapse is the junction, or space, between an axon of one neuron and a dendrite of the next neuron. An electrical impulse is generated and carried down this neuron to the next. (The receiving cell quickly inactivates the neurotransmitter with a specific opposing chemical to prevent continuous impulses.)

A nerve can transmit impulses in only one direction because of the location of the neurotransmitters. (Cell bodies and dendrites do not have neurotransmitters.) An example of a **neurotransmitter** is *acetylcholine*, which is inactivated by cholinesterase. Dopamine, norepinephrine, and serotonin are also neurotransmitters. These names may be familiar to you, because many of their properties have been developed into useful pharmacologic products.

Classification of Neurons

Neurons can be classified according to their shape but are more commonly remembered by their function. According to function, there are three types of neurons:

sensory, motor, and interneuron. They have the following functions, which are discussed in more detail under the section "System Physiology" later in the chapter:

◆ Sensory neurons receive messages from all parts of the body and transmit them by way of sensory nerves to the central nervous system (CNS).
◆ Motor neurons transmit messages from the CNS by motor nerves to all parts of the body. They alter muscle activity and cause glands to secrete.
◆ Interneurons carry impulses between sensory and motor pathways. They are *interconnecting* neurons.

Sensory nerves are made up of only sensory neurons; motor nerves are made up of only motor neurons; mixed nerves contain sensory and motor neurons.

Divisions of the Nervous System

The nervous system is divided into two major parts; the CNS and the peripheral nervous system (PNS). The PNS is further divided into the cranial nerves, spinal nerves, and autonomic (automatic) nervous system (ANS). The ANS has sympathetic and parasympathetic subdivisions. The accompanying box summarizes these divisions and subdivisions. Each is discussed in the following section.

Central Nervous System

The central nervous system (CNS) is made up of the brain and the spinal cord.

The Brain
The human brain is composed of approximately 100 billion neurons and innumerable synapses. It weighs approximately 1.36 kg (3 lb), which is about 2% of the body's weight. However, the brain uses approximately 20% of the circulating blood flow or about 750 mL per minute. The brain has an extensive and specialized vascular supply. It has a higher metabolic rate than the rest of the body (which remains constant during physical or mental exercises). It must have a constant flow of oxygen and nutrients. A failure of blood flow for as little as 10 seconds will result in unconsciousness. The brain is particularly sensitive to toxins and drugs.

Although the brain has many parts, it functions as an integrated whole. The components and functions of the brain are summarized in the box.

Cerebrum. Eighty percent of the brain's volume is the cerebrum (Fig. 18-2), which fills the upper part of the cranium (skull cavity). The cerebrum is divided into two layers and two halves (hemispheres). Each portion

Divisions of the Nervous System

Central Nervous System

Brain
  Cerebrum
    Cerebral lobes
    Cerebral hemispheres
  Thalamus
  Hypothalamus
  Cerebellum
  Brain stem
    Midbrain, pons, medulla
Spinal cord
Accessory structures
  Meninges
  Cerebrospinal fluid
  Ventricles

Peripheral Nervous System

Cranial nerves (12 pairs)
Spinal nerves (31 pairs)
Autonomic nervous system
  Sympathetic nervous system
  Parasympathetic nervous system

has individualized functions. All of them, however, are integrated, and many areas overlap in functions.

The *cerebral cortex* is the outside of the brain. It is made of soft gray matter, mostly nerve cell bodies. The cortex is wrinkled and folded back on itself many times. These folds are called convolutions or *gyri*. The crevices between the folds are called fissures or *sulci*. Because of the folds, the cortex can have a much greater surface area and, thus, millions of neurons.

Cerebral Lobes. The cerebral cortex is divided into four lobes, named after the overlying cranial bones (frontal, parietal, temporal, and occipital). The special centers in the cerebrum enable humans to achieve higher mental functions; thus, we can associate impressions and information, which becomes knowledge. Other centers in the cerebrum are related to activities, including hearing, seeing, moving, and speaking. (The adjective, cerebral, pertains to the unique human abilities of learning and intelligent reasoning and judgment.)

Cerebral Hemispheres. The right hemisphere of the brain controls muscles and receives sensory input from the left side of the body. The left hemisphere controls muscles and receives sensory input from the right side. This phenomenon is a result of *decussation* (crossing) of the nerve tracts within the medulla of the brain. Some of the functional areas of the cerebrum are shown in Figure 18-2.

Components of the Brain and Their Functions

Cerebrum—center of conscious thought and higher mental functioning

Cerebral cortex: gray matter (nerve cell bodies), outer layer of cerebrum, has convolutions (grooves) and elevations (gyri) that increase surface area of brain

Lobes

Frontal: location of higher mental processes (intelligence, motivation, mood, aggression, planning), verbal communication, voluntary control of skeletal muscles

Parietal: location of skin, taste, and muscle sensations; understanding speech; formation of words to express thoughts and emotions; interpretation of textures and shapes

Temporal: location of sense of smell, auditory interpretation, storage of auditory and visual experiences, thoughts that precede speech

Occipital: location of eye movements, integration of visual experiences

Hemispheres—two halves of brain divided by longitudinal fissure

Corpus callosum: connects hemispheres internally

White matter: location of billions of connections due to presence of dendrites and myelinated axons

Thalamus—consolidates sensory input, influences mood and body movements; associated with strong emotions

Hypothalamus—temperature regulation centers; hunger and peristalsis centers; water, thirst, and electrolyte centers; control of heart rate and blood vessel diameter; influences on pituitary gland secretions; muscle control of swallowing, shivering, and urine release from bladder; sexual centers; sleep–wake cycle centers

Cerebellum—second largest part of brain; location of involuntary movement, coordination, muscle tone, posture, and equilibrium

Brain stem—connects cerebral hemispheres with spinal cord

Midbrain: located at top of brain stem; visual and auditory reflex center; righting reflex located here

Pons (bridge): nerve tracts that carry messages between cerebrum and medulla; respiratory centers to produce normal breathing pattern

Medulla: located at floor of skull; continuous with but not part of the spinal cord; vital for life; descending nerve tracts from brain cross here to opposite side; contains centers for many body functions (cardiac, vasomotor, and respiratory centers); swallowing, coughing, and sneezing reflexes

Spinal cord—conductor of impulses to and from the brain; reflex centers as substations that relieve the brain of routine work (such as some reflexes)

Meninges—connective tissue membranes

Dura mater: outermost layer, in contact with bone

Arachnoid membrane: delicate weblike middle layer

Pia mater: highly vascular layer, attached to surfaces of central nervous system (CNS); contributes to form choroid plexuses

Ventricles—four cavities in brain filled with cerebrospinal fluid

Cerebrospinal fluid—protective fluid of CNS

The corpus callosum is a band of approximately 200 million neurons connecting the right and left hemispheres of the brain. The corpus callosum allows one cerebral hemisphere to share information with the other. If this structure is severed, the right hand will literally not know what the left hand is doing.

Key Concept

Patients who have had a cerebrovascular accident (stroke) in one hemisphere have the symptoms or paralysis on the opposite side of the body.

Under the cerebral cortex is the white matter, the location of billions of synapses between axons and dendrites. It is white because of the myelinated axons and dendrites. These axons and dendrites connect the lobes of the cerebrum to each other and to all other parts of the brain.

The two hemispheres of the brain process information differently. The right side is associated with spatial perception, pictures, art, and musical ability. The left is believed to be concerned with analytic and verbal skills (reading and writing, words, symbols, mathematics, and speech).

Thalamus. The thalamus is located just inferior to the cerebrum and superior to the hypothalamus. It is a relay station between the cutaneous (skin) receptors and the cerebral cortex for all sensory impulses, except smell. The thalamus integrates the sensations so that we perceive the whole experience and not just individual impulses. For example, touching a snowball will produce sensations of cold, pressure, texture, and shape. The thalamus integrates all of these sensations so that we are able to understand the whole picture accurately. The thalamus also has some crude awareness of pain. It may suppress unimportant sensations to permit the cerebrum to concentrate on important aspects of daily activities.

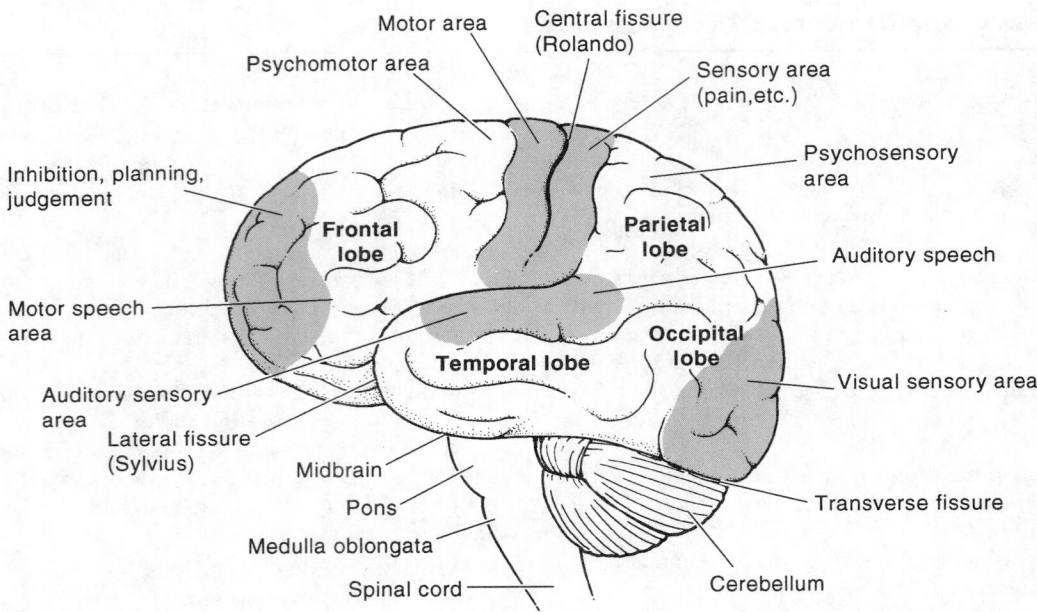

Figure 18-2. The human brain, showing the lobes and fissures of the cerebrum. Major functional areas also are indicated.

Hypothalamus. Although small, the hypothalamus is vital to human functioning. It is located below the thalamus. Most functions of the hypothalamus relate directly or indirectly to the regulation of visceral activities. It has a role in increasing or decreasing bodily functions and regulates the release of hormones from the pituitary gland (which regulates many of the body's hormones). It also fulfills emotional and instinctual functions.

Cerebellum. The **cerebellum** is the second largest part of the brain. All of its functions are concerned with movement; it is concerned with muscle tone, coordination, and equilibrium. It coordinates the action of voluntary muscles and adjusts to impulses from the proprioceptors within muscles, joints, and sense organs. (*Proprioceptors* relay information about balance and body position.) The adjustments made in the cerebellum help to maintain balance when walking, make movements graceful, and make it possible to throw a ball or roller blade.

Brain Stem. The brain stem connects the cerebral hemispheres with the spinal cord. It includes the midbrain, the pons, and the medulla.

The *midbrain* is located at the very top of the brain stem and functions as an important reflex center. Visual and auditory reflexes are integrated here. When you turn your head to locate a sound, you are using the midbrain. The righting reflex or the ability to keep the head upright and maintain balance is also located here.

The word *pons* means "bridge." The term reflects the fact that the pons contains **nerve tracts** that carry messages between the cerebrum and the medulla. The pons has respiratory centers that work with the medulla to produce a normal breathing pattern.

The *medulla* (also known as medulla oblongata) lies just below the pons and rests on the floor of the skull. It is continuous with, but not part of, the spinal cord. Nerve tracts that descend from the brain cross to the opposite side here. The medulla is vital for life; any injury to the occipital bone can be fatal because it can injure the medulla.

The medulla contains centers for many vital body functions, including the cardiac center (regulates heart rate), vasomotor center (regulates the diameter of blood vessels, thus regulating blood pressure), and respiratory center (regulates breathing). Other activities of the medulla are concerned with reflexes, such as swallowing, coughing, and sneezing.

The Spinal Cord

The spinal cord is a long mass of nerve cells and fibers extending through a central canal from the medulla to the approximate level of the first or second lumbar vertebra. Vertebrae were discussed in Chapter 17. It is well protected from shocks and injuries by its position within the vertebral column. This protection is essential because the nerve fibers of the spinal cord cannot regenerate after an injury.

The spinal cord has two main functions: It acts as a conductor of impulses to and from the brain and as a reflex center. The reflex centers in the cord receive and send messages through the nerve fibers. This "circle" is known as a **reflex arc** (see Figure 18-5). The reflex centers act as substations for messages and relieve the brain of routine work. Some nerve fibers in the cord are sensory; that is, they carry messages to the brain. Other nerve tracts are motor, carrying messages away from the brain.

Accessory Structures

There are three major accessory structures of the CNS: the meninges, the ventricles, and the *cerebrospinal fluid* (CSF).

The Meninges. The brain and the spinal cord (ie, the CNS) are covered with three protective membranes called the **meninges.** The *dura mater*, the outer layer, is a tough, fibrous covering that adheres to the bones of the skull. The middle layer is a delicate web of tissue called the *arachnoid*. The *pia mater*, the inner layer, lies closely over the brain and spinal cord. It is a thin vascular layer containing many blood vessels that bring oxygen to nourish the nervous tissue.

The space between the arachnoid membrane and the pia mater is the subarachnoid space. The subarachnoid space contains CSF, the tissue fluid of the CNS.

Cerebrospinal Fluid. CSF is a lymphlike fluid that forms a protective cushion around and within the CNS. It lets the brain "float" within the cranial vault, literally changing the effective weight of the brain from about 1500 g to about 50 g. The CSF removes cellular waste from the nerve tissue and lessens the damage caused by impact by spreading out the force of trauma. The CSF is also produced in a specialized capillary network (the choroid plexus) in the ventricles of the brain. About 800 mL are produced each day, although only 150 to 200 mL circulates at any one time. Some CSF is reabsorbed through arachnoid villi into the blood where it becomes blood plasma again. Laboratory study of CSF can reveal bleeding into the CNS and infections of the brain or its meninges. A physician may withdraw a small amount of CSF through the space between the vertebrae. This procedure is called a lumbar puncture or a spinal tap. Medications such as antibiotics or anesthetics may also be introduced into the CSF by lumbar puncture.

Ventricles. Deep within the brain are four ventricles, or cavities. These are lined with ependymal cells. They also contain many blood vessels from the pia mater, which make up the *choroid plexus*. The ventricles are filled with CSF.

There are two lateral (side) ventricles, right and left, which are large. Each lateral ventricle is divided into four parts: an anterior (front) horn, the body (middle), an inferior (temporal) horn, and an occipital (posterior)

Functions of Cerebrospinal Fluid

- Acts as shock absorber for brain and spinal cord
- Carries nutrients to the brain
- Carries wastes away from the brain
- Keeps brain and spinal cord moist, thus preventing friction
- Can be tested to determine the presence of some diseases
- Can be used to transmit medications

horn. The lateral ventricles connect to the third ventricle through foramina (openings) on each side.

The aqueduct of Sylvius (cerebral aqueduct) connects the third and fourth ventricles. If this aqueduct becomes plugged, the fluid cannot circulate, and the ventricles become distended or enlarged.

In some cases, fluid collects around the brain. Because the skull cannot expand, the accumulating fluid causes pressure on the brain (increased intracranial pressure). If not corrected, this can cause a variety of serious conditions.

Peripheral Nervous System

The PNS is made up of two nerve groups: cranial nerves and spinal nerves. The cranial and spinal terms simply imply that they begin either in the brain or spinal cord. The nerves of the PNS are sensory, motor, or mixed, depending on which direction or directions nerve impulses are being conducted.

The autonomic nervous system (ANS) and its subdivisions (the sympathetic nervous system and the parasympathetic nervous system) are also classified as part of the PNS.

The Cranial Nerves

The 12 pairs of cranial nerves attach directly to the brain. Most of the cranial nerves carry impulses to and from the brain and various structures around the head. However, some cranial nerves act on the organs of the thorax and the abdomen.

Cranial nerves are given Roman numerals. They are numbered in the order in which they orginate in the brain, from front to back. Most cranial nerves are classified as mixed nerves. Table 18-1 lists the cranial nerves and their functions.

Although all of the cranial nerves are important, one nerve deserves special attention. The vagus nerve (cranial nerve X) serves a much larger portion of the body than the others. It affects many body functions that are beyond a person's conscious control. Branches of the vagus innervate muscles of the pharynx, larynx, respiratory tract, heart, esophagus, and parts of the abdom-

Table 18-1. The Cranial Nerves and Their Functions

Number	Name	Functions (and Types)	Distribution
I	Olfactory	Smell (sensory)	Nasal mucous membrane
II	Optic	Vision (sensory)	Retina
III	Oculomotor	Eye movements (mixed)	Most ocular muscles
IV	Trochlear (smallest cranial nerves)	Voluntary eye movements (mixed)	Superior oblique muscle of eye
V	Trigeminal (largest cranial nerves)	Sensations of head and face; movement of mandible (mixed)	Skin of face; tongue; teeth; muscles of mastication (chewing)
	Ophthalmic branch	Sensations from front of head and face, eye sockets, and upper nose (sensory)	
	Maxillary branch	Sensations from nose, mouth, and upper jaw, cheek, and upper lip (sensory)	
	Mandibular branch	Sensations of tongue, lower teeth, chin (mixed)	
VI	Abducent	Eye movements (motor)	Lateral rectus muscle of eye
VII	Facial	Taste; facial expressions (mixed)	Muscles of expression; taste buds
VIII	Vestibulocochlear (acoustic)	Hearing and balance	Internal auditory meatus
	Cochlear division	Conduct impulses related to hearing (sensory)	
	Vestibular division	Conduct impulses related to equilibrium (balance) (sensory)	Inner ear
IX	Glossopharyngeal	Control swallowing; give information on pressure and oxygen tension of blood (mixed)	Pharynx, posterior third of tongue, parotid
X	Vagus ("wanderer") (Only cranial nerve not restricted to head and neck)	Somatic motor function; parasympathetic functions; speech (mixed)	Pharynx, larynx, heart, lungs, esophagus, stomach, abdominal viscera
XI	Accessory (spinal accessory)	Rotation of head; raising of shoulder (motor)	Arising from medulla and spinal cord
XII	Hypoglossal	Movement of tongue (motor)	Intrinsic muscle of tongue

inal viscera. Thus, the vagus has reflex control of the heart rate, sneezing, hunger, secretions from glands in the stomach, and constrictions within the respiratory tract. It is also involved in sympathetic and parasympathetic responses.

The Spinal Nerves

The 31 pairs of spinal nerves attach to the spinal cord, each group being named for the corresponding part of the spinal cord: the cervical (8 pairs), thoracic (12 pairs), lumbar (5 pairs), sacral (5 pairs), and coccygeal (1 pair). A group of spinal nerves forms a **plexus** (plural, plexes). Examples of plexes are the *cervical plexus,* where the phrenic nerve, which controls the diaphragm, arises; the *brachial plexus;* the *lumbosacral plexus,* from which the sciatic nerve arises; and the *pudendal plexus.* These nerves carry such impulses as temperature, touch, pain, muscle tone, and balance.

They also transport motor impulses to the skeletal muscles. In some situations, physicians prescribe medication to block these nerves to reduce pain or discomfort. For example, in childbirth, a local anesthetic is sometimes injected into the pudendal plexus (a "pudendal block").

Key Concept
Spinal Nerves
- Cervical, 8 pairs
- Thoracic, 12 pairs
- Lumbar, 5 pairs
- Sacral, 5 pairs
- Coccygeal, 1 pair

Spinal Cord Injuries. An injury to the spinal cord causes the cord to swell. This can result in temporary paralysis. If the spinal cord is cut through completely, paralysis below the level of injury is permanent. Paralysis results because nerve impulses are interrupted and can no longer reach the spinal nerves and brain. Damage is permanent because the spinal cord cannot regenerate itself.

Autonomic Nervous System

The ANS is composed of portions of the CNS and PNS. It is generally classified under the PNS, but the ANS is very specialized; it functions independently and without conscious effort. It innervates organs the functions of which are not usually under voluntary control, in particular the cardiac muscle, smooth (visceral) muscles, and glands. The ANS contains visceral motor neurons to these three areas. Figure 18-3 illustrates the ANS and the organs it influences. The body's ability to maintain homeostasis is largely due to the ANS.

The ANS has two divisions, sympathetic and parasympathetic. Stimuli to the structures illustrated originate in both divisions, but they often function in opposition to each other. For instance, sympathetic nerves increase heart rate and dilate the pupil of the eye; parasympathetic nerves slow heart rate and constrict the pupil. Effects of the ANS are summarized in Table 18-2.

Many chemicals are derived from the ANS; these are drugs that work in a similar manner to the action of the autonomic nerves. Simply stated, there are drugs that "turn on" or mimic either the sympathetic or parasympathetic nervous system. There are also drugs that "turn off" or lyse the sympathetic or parasympathetic subdivisions of the ANS. Some of these drugs have been duplicated chemically and can be administered to assist the patient.

Sympathetic Division

The sympathetic division of the ANS produces responses that prepare the individual for an emergency or for extreme stress or danger. This "fight or flight" response prepares us to defend ourselves or to run. During an emergency, the heart beats faster and the breathing rate increases. The skin becomes pale, secondary to the diversion of blood flow away from the skin. Blood flow is decreased to structures such as the external genitals and the abdominal organs. Thus, body processes, such as digestion, are slowed or stopped to allow more blood to flow to the more vital organs, such as the brain, lungs, and large muscles that move the body during the emergency. Involuntary defecation or urination can occur.

Obviously, the body can sustain an emergency awareness for only a limited time. The homeostatic mechanism that balances the sympathetic nervous system is the parasympathetic nervous system.

Parasympathetic Division

The parasympathetic division of the ANS is the predominant aspect of the ANS. The responses generally produced are the normal functions of the body while it is at rest or not under unusual or extreme stress. The effects are often the opposite of the sympathetic division. However, unlike the sympathetic division, it is not normally activated as a whole. For example, it can increase the body's heart rate without affecting other organs.

To return to homeostasis after a "fight or flight" episode with sympathetic responses, the parasympathetic nerves return the heart rate to normal, resume digestive processes, and restore blood flow to the skin and abdominal and genital organs. Previous patterns of defecation and urination return.

System Physiology

Transmission of Nerve Impulses

Messages from one part of the body to another can take several possible nerve pathways. As a rule, however, they will take the quickest route. (The body is thrifty in its use of body products and its automatic activities.) The same kind of messages tend to follow the same paths every time. Repeated motions become more or less automatic habits, which are patterns that have been built up by using the same nerve pathways over and over.

Simply stated, a neuron receives electrical and chemical impulses, which make it possible for the neuron to transfer a stimulus from one area of the body to another and to elicit a response. The electrical impulse is due to the positive and negative charges of electrolytes.

The Action Potential

Due to the polarity or electrical charge on a cell, a cell has the potential to create an electrical impulse. To create an electrical charge, there is an organized, rapid exchange of sodium and potassium ions across the cell membrane. A stimulus, such as a neurotransmitter, will bring about the needed adjustments in a cell membrane to cause a reversal of the cell's polarity. As quickly as this polarity takes place, it reverses itself back into its resting state. This action is called the "action potential." An action potential takes only milliseconds. Many neurons can transmit impulses over several meters per second. At a synapse, the electrical charge changes from electrical to chemical. Neurotransmitters are the chemicals responsible for the transfer of impulses from the axon of one neuron to the dendrites of another neuron. The alternating depolarization and repolarization move as a wave along the length of the neuron and become the transmitted message.

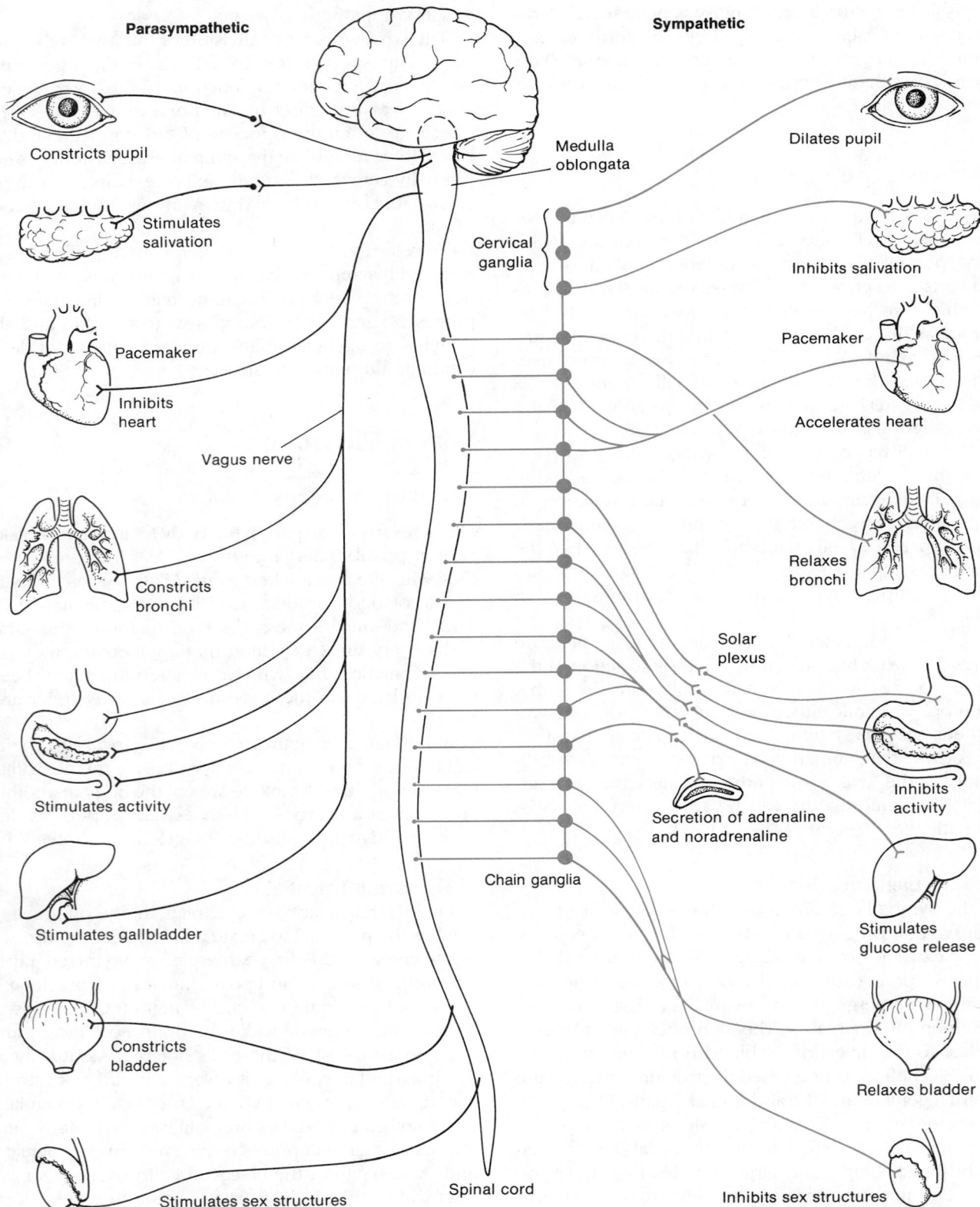

Figure 18-3. The autonomic nervous system and the organs it affects. The left side illustrates the actions of the sympathetic nervous system, which stimulates actions. The right side illustrates the parasympathetic nervous system, which inhibits actions.

Table 18-2. Effects of the Sympathetic and Parasympathetic Systems on Selected Organs

Effector	Sympathetic System	Parasympathetic System
Pupils of eye	Dilation	Constriction
Sweat glands	Stimulation	None
Digestive glands	Inhibition	Stimulation
Heart	Increased rate and strength of beat	Decreased rate and strength of beat
Bronchi of lungs	Dilation	Constriction
Muscles of digestive system	Decreased contraction (peristalsis)	Increased contraction
Kidneys	Decreased activity	None
Urinary bladder	Relaxation	Contraction and emptying
Liver	Increased release of glucose	None
Penis	Ejaculation	Erection
Adrenal medulla	Stimulation	None
Blood vessels to		
Skeletal muscles	Dilation	Constriction
Skin	Constriction	None
Respiratory system	Dilation	Constriction
Digestive organs	Constriction	Dilation

Memmler RL, Cohen BJ, Wood DL. Structure and Function of the Human Body, Ed 6. Philadelphia, J.B. Lippincott, 1992.

The All-or-None Law

Either a nerve impulse is transmitted across a particular synapse or it is not transmitted. There are no exceptions. Because an impulse cannot be partially transmitted, this is known as the all-or-none response of nerve tissue.

Electroencephalogram

An electroencephalogram is a visual record of the electrical activity of millions of neurons in the form of various waves within the brain. Brain wave activity is often diagnostic of neurologic problems. Cessation of brain wave activity has become one of the legal considerations in the determination of death in many states.

Actions of Three Types of Neurons

Sensory Neurons. The sensory neurons (neurons of sensation) are also known as **afferent** neurons because they carry impulses to the brain or spinal cord from the periphery of the body. They bring information to the brain by means of *receptors* (end organs that are the initial receiver of stimuli from outside and within the body; Fig. 18-4).

The receptors are usually classified as follows: The *exteroceptors* (related to the external environment) are involved in touch, cutaneous (skin) pain, heat, cold, smell, vision, and hearing; the **proprioceptors** carry sensations of position and balance or movement of the body in space; and the *interoceptors* (related to the body's internal environment) respond to changes in the internal organs of the abdomen (viscera), such as visceral pain, hunger, or thirst.

Once the receptors have picked up the impulse, the sensation is carried to the CNS by the fibers of the sensory neurons; it is sent by way of the connecting neurons through complex pathways to the CNS for interpretation.

Motor Neurons. If action is required after a stimulus is received, the CNS sends an impulse by the fibers of the motor neurons to a muscle or a gland to bring about the proper response. Motor neurons are also called **efferent** neurons because they carry impulses away from the center of the nervous system, brain, or spinal cord.

The structures that carry out activity are called effectors. The effector neurons are classified as *somatic–voluntary* or *visceral–involuntary*. For example, the initial sting of a mosquito bite is made known to the brain by a sensory neuron. The brain interprets the sensation for what it is. The brain, by motor neuron pathways, sends an order to the appropriate muscles to slap the insect away. This is a voluntary action; you control it at will. An example of a visceral–involuntary action is the peristaltic movement of food through the digestive system.

Interneurons. Neurons that serve to integrate signals between the neurons of various parts of the brain and spinal cord are called **interneurons.** Interneurons are found only in the CNS. They carry out or integrate sensory or motor impulses. They assist with thinking, learn-

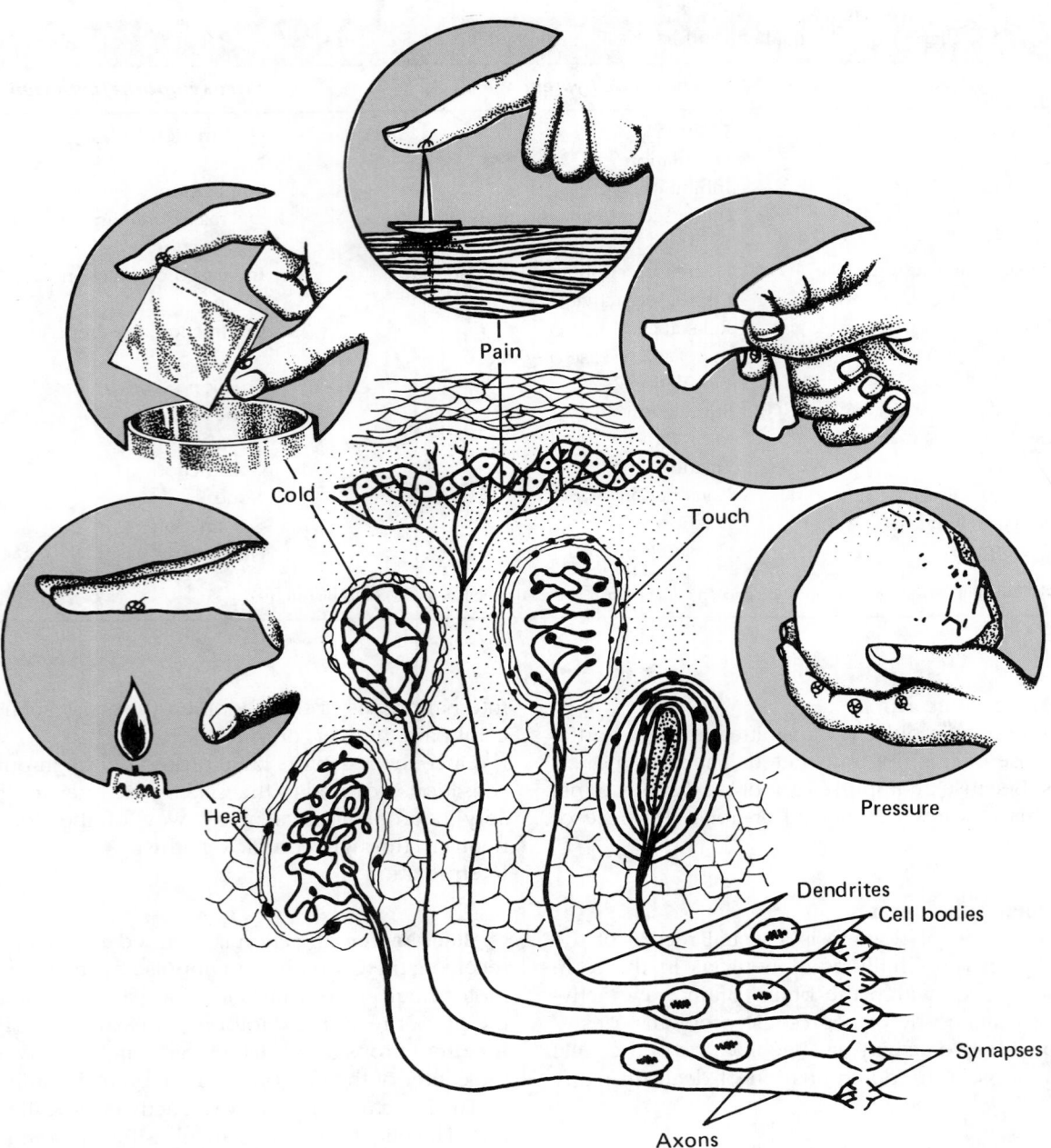

Figure 18-4. The receptors (exteroceptors) in the skin that receive stimuli related to temperature, pain, touch, and pressure. The afferent cell bodies and synapses, which are located in the dorsal root ganglia and spinal cord, are included in this drawing to suggest the continuity of sensory pathways from the skin to the central nervous system. The neurons in this case are sensory neurons.

ing, and memory. They can be thought of as a link between two other neurons.

Reflexes

A reflex is an automatic or involuntary response to a stimulus; a reflex occurs without conscious thought. Reflexes are homeostatic; that is, they try to maintain homeostasis. They move the body from danger, keep the body from falling, and maintain a relatively constant blood pressure, pH, and level of water reabsorption. Individual reflexes vary in complexity.

Reflex acts do not operate as isolated parts of the nervous system. True reflexes are integrated into the brain and spinal cord as a reflex arc; thus, the brain may inhibit or exaggerate a reflex. For example, you reflexively blink your eyes when danger approaches, but once the brain realizes the danger, you act as a whole unit and move away.

Other examples of reflexes include constriction of the pupil of the eye when exposed to light, the automatic increase in heart rate when the body senses a lowering of blood pressure, and the patellar (knee–jerk) reflex when the physician taps the patellar tendon just below the kneecap. Deep tendon reflexes are often tested as part of a clinical assessment to see if the nervous system is functioning properly. Figure 18-5 illustrates some reflexes.

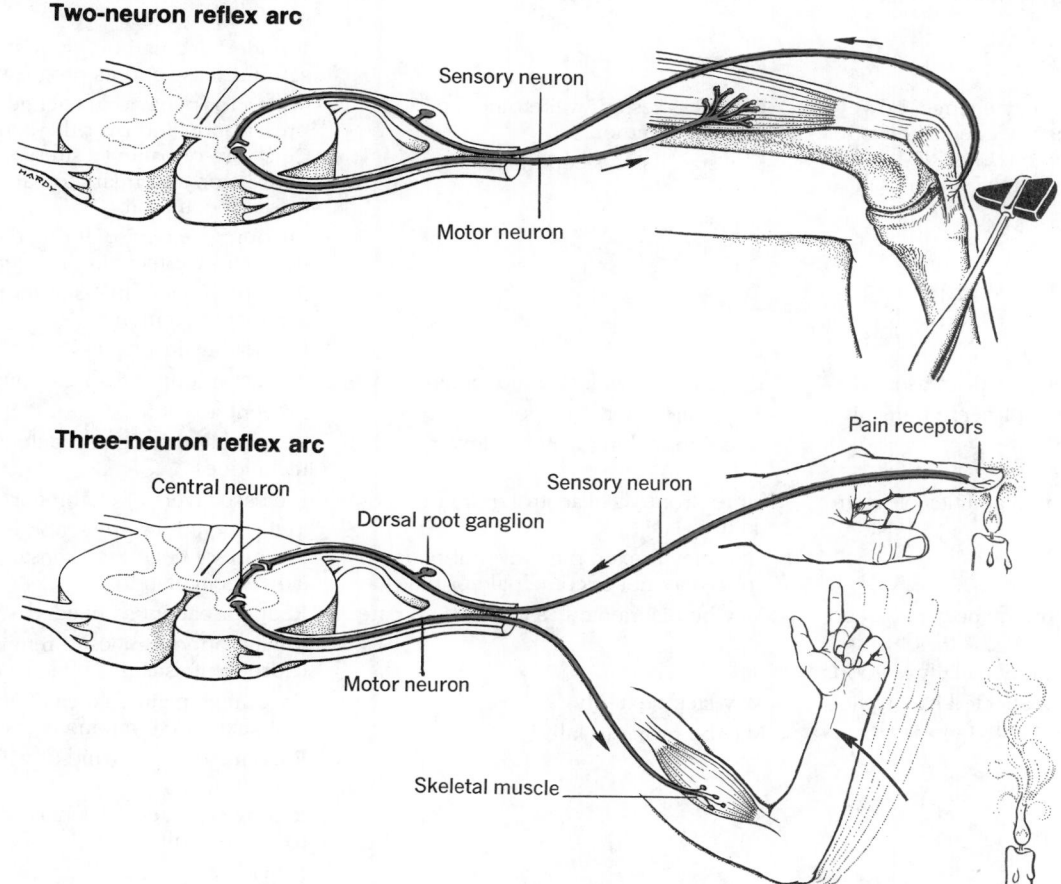

Two-neuron reflex arc

Sensory neuron

Motor neuron

Three-neuron reflex arc

Central neuron

Dorsal root ganglion

Sensory neuron

Pain receptors

Motor neuron

Skeletal muscle

Figure 18-5. Reflex arcs showing pathways of impulses in response to a stimulus. The cross-section of the spinal cord shows the simplest reflex, the knee jerk, which involves only sensory and motor neurons. The response to a painful stimulus, such as a flame, also involves a central neuron (a three-neuron reflex arc).

Effects of Aging on the System

Intelligence, memory, the capacity to learn, and personality do not normally change as a person ages. Changes are influenced by genetics, environmental conditions, physical changes resulting from disease processes, and psychological stressors. The ability to adapt often is limited more by one's physical body than by mental functioning.

Generally, the nerve cell cannot reproduce itself. Damage to brain cells may result in permanent loss of some or all mental functions. Common causes of such losses in older people include cerebrovascular accident (stroke and atherosclerosis, plaque deposits in blood vessels, diminishing bold flow to the brain). In addi-

tion, trauma, drugs, and degenerative disorders can cause irreversible organic brain damage in people of all ages.

Safety and preventive measures are priorities for nurses working with older people. Loss of equilibrium and changes in proprioception (spatial awareness) contribute to falling. Herpes zoster (shingles) is a very painful inflammation of nerve endings that often affects older people.

Sometimes confusion is reversible. It may be caused by electrolyte imbalances, hypoxia, small strokes, drugs, pain, stress, or anemia. The patient will be evaluated to see if the cause of confusion can be treated. True dementia (such as Alzheimer's disease) is not reversible. Table 18-3 outlines the effects of aging on the nervous system.

Table 18-3. Effects of Aging on the Nervous System

Factor	Result	Nursing Implications
Thought processes and ability to learn or reason should be retained.	Thought process, reasoning, or learning changes not normal	Treat elderly as normal, intelligent adults. Evaluate any changes in personality or thought processes. If underlying pathology exists, understand disease and its progression
Sleep patterns may change; however, amount of sleep needed often is relatively unchanged. Less REM (dream) sleep occurs.	Feels less rested; wakefulness periods at night common May start using sleeping aids	Watch for behavioral changes caused by prescription and over-the-counter drugs. Be aware of patient's stressors; clinical depression secondary to cumulative losses is common. Encourage exercise during the day and eating a light meal in the evening. Reassure patient that shorter periods of sleep are common. Caution against excess use of sleep aids.
Number of neurons decreases. Rate and spread of nerve transmissions decreases.	Decrease in voluntary movements Aggravated startle response Decision making may be slower	Allow for longer response time. Prevent accidents. Teach safe driving and defensive driving techniques.
Thermoregulation abilities often are reduced.	More prone to heat stroke or effects of cold Skin may remain pink, even if patient is cold (may not become pale or blue)	Increase layers of clothing in all weather. Tell patient foot protection is important because of decreased sensation and slowed circulation.
Some short-term memory loss is normal. Long-term memory usually is good.	May be disoriented as to time and date	Reorient patient as needed. Initiate opportunities to reminisce because reminiscing is beneficial.
Motor skills are affected by physiologic changes in other systems.	May lack dexterity May be prone to falls	Encourage maintenance of abilities by daily exercise (walking is excellent). Encourage use of cane or walker for stability if needed. Remove obstacles, such as scatter rugs, to prevent falls. Provide adequate lighting.

Keys For Review

Key Questions for Critical Thinking

1. Describe the major functions of the nervous system, including the specialized cells involved in these functions.
2. Describe and differentiate among CNS and PNS. Name the structures of each and describe their functions.
3. Differentiate among sensory and motor neurons and interneurons.
4. Describe the function of the ANS and discuss the difference in function of the sympathetic and parasympathetic divisions.
5. Describe reflexes and give examples.

Key Readings

Chabner D. The Language of Medicine, Ed 4. Philadelphia, W.B. Saunders, 1991

Eliopoulus C. Caring for the Elderly in Diverse Care Settings. Philadelphia, J.B. Lippincott, 1990

Farrell J. Nursing Care of the Older Person. Philadelphia, J.B. Lippincott, 1990

Jackson DB, Saunders RB. Child Health Nursing: A Comprehensive Approach to the Care of Children and their Families. Philadelphia: J.B. Lippincott, 1993

Scanlon V, Sanders V. Essentials of Anatomy and Physiology. Philadelphia, F.A. Davis, 1991

Seeley R, Stepphens T, Tate P. Anatomy and Physiology, Ed 2. St. Louis, C.V. Mosby, 1994

Smeltzer SC, Bare BG. Brunner and Suddarth's Textbook of Medical-Surgical Nursing, Ed 7. Philadelphia, J.B. Lippincott, 1992

Van De Graff K, Fox IF. Concepts of Human Anatomy and Physiology, Ed 3. Dubuque, IA, WC Brown, 1992

Enrichment Keys

Memmler RL, Cohen BJ, Woods DL. Structure and Function of the Human Body, Ed 5. Philadelphia, J.B. Lippincott, 1992

Keys to Learning More

Chapter 19: functions of the endocrine system, some hormones stimulating nerve responses

Chapter 20: interrelationships between the nervous system and the senses, especially vision and hearing

Chapter 50: basics of nursing assessment, including gross evaluation of some of the cranial nerves, level of consciousness, and the ability to speak, walk, and move normally

Chapter 56: various types of medications, some of which are used in neurologic disorders

Unit Thirteen: deviations from normal body structure and function in children

Chapter 67: the child with special needs; many of these children have neurologic disorders

Unit Fourteen: deviations from normal in adults

Chapter 71: specific discussion of disorders in the nervous system

Chapter 74: a discussion of stroke, which has many neurologic manifestations

Unit Fifteen: deviations in older adults, including disorders of the brain, such as Alzheimer's disease

Chapter 87: disorders in mental health

19 The Endocrine System

Learning Objectives

- Differentiate between exocrine and endocrine glands
- Define *hormone*
- On a chart, locate the major endocrine glands, and state what hormone(s) each secretes; list the chief actions of each hormone
- State the function of all glands
- List several clinical conditions caused by hormonal malfunction, and identify the hormone involved
- Relate the activities of the endocrine system to those of the other systems in the body
- Describe the relationship between the hypothalamus and the pituitary
- Discuss negative feedback in relation to the endocrine system
- Describe the effects of aging on the endocrine system

Key Terms

adenohypophysis	glycogen	parathyroids
adrenal glands	goiter	pineal gland
corticosteroids	hormones	pituitary gland
endocrine glands	insulin	prostaglandins
exocrine glands	islets of Langerhans	thymus
glucagon	neurohypophysis	thyroid gland

Keys to Understanding This Chapter

Unit Three: normal growth and development

Unit Four: dependence of systems on each other

Key Points

- Endocrine glands secrete hormones to target organs through the circulatory system. Exocrine glands secrete hormones into ducts.
- The pituitary gland is controlled by the nervous system tissue of the hypothalamus. The many hormones of the anterior and posterior pituitary have widespread effects on the body.
- The thyroid is responsible for controlling the rate of metabolism.
- The parathyroids regulate the amount of calcium and phosphorus in the blood.

Key Points (continued)

- The adrenal medulla secretes hormones that mimic the action of the sympathetic nervous system. They are active in emergencies or stressful situations.
- The adrenal cortex makes three types of steroid compounds from cholesterol: corticosteroids, mineralocorticoids, and sex hormones.
- As an endocrine gland, the pancreas secretes insulin, which lowers blood sugar, and glucagon, which raises blood sugar.
- Prostaglandins are hormonelike substances. Their effects are localized to the area in which they are produced.
- Hormones are chemical regulators. Hormonal blood levels are influenced by negative feedback mechanisms. Hormones are specific to target tissues and act in a "lock-and-key" fashion.

Key Topics Outline

Structure and Function
The Pituitary Gland
The Thyroid Gland
The Parathyroid Glands
The Adrenal Glands
The Gonads
The Pancreas
The Thymus and the Pineal Glands
Other Hormones
Prostaglandins
System Physiology
System Relationships
Information Relay to Target Cells
Negative Feedback
Effects of Aging on the System

Key Learning Activities

- Make a chart listing hormones, their source, their actions and functions, and deficiency disorders.
- Set up a contest between two teams. One team names a deficiency disorder, and the other teams names the hormone involved.

Key Medical Acronyms

ACTH	adrenocorticotropic hormone
ADH	vasopressin (antidiuretic hormone)
FSH	follicle-stimulating hormone
GH	growth hormone
LH	luteinizing hormone
MSH	melanocyte-stimulating hormone
PRL	prolactin, lactogenic hormone
T_3	triiodothyronine
T_4	thyroxine
TSH	thyroid-stimulating hormone

Functions of the Endocrine System

Growth and Maturation

◆ Regulates growth
◆ Regulates body response to stress

Metabolism

◆ Regulates metabolism
◆ Regulates absorption of nutrients
◆ Regulates use of glucose in cellular respiration
◆ Maintains body pH by maintaining fluid and electrolyte concentrations

Reproduction

◆ Produces sexual characteristics
◆ Controls reproductive processes
◆ Activates lactation

The endocrine system comprises a group of glands located in various parts of the body. Glands are a group of specialized cells that secrete a substance (in this case, hormones) in response to signals. The hormones produced are neither needed nor used by the gland itself.

There are two major types of glands in the body: endocrine and exocrine. Some glands, however, can perform both endocrine and exocrine functions. Table 19-1 compares these glands.

Endocrine glands secrete their hormones into the bloodstream directly. The hormones act on remote tissues (called target tissues). The major portion of this chapter discusses endocrine glands.

Exocrine glands secrete substances into a duct that opens onto the external or internal surface of the body. The substances secreted by the exocrine glands are usually protective or functional, whereas substances secreted by endocrine glands are usually regulatory. Exocrine glands include sweat glands, mammary glands, mucous membranes, salivary glands, and lacrimal (tear) glands. Examples of exocrine secretions are bile, tears, and pancreatic fluid.

Hormones secreted by the glands are chemical regulators, integrating and coordinating body activities. They speed up or slow down the activities of entire body organs, and some affect the rate of various activities of individual cells. Hormones also affect each other: Too much or too little of a particular hormone interferes with the actions of other hormones.

Hormones may be produced by nervous stimulation, the level of some substances in the blood, or other hormones. The hormones are discussed in this chapter with the glands that secrete them.

Structure and Function

The endocrine system provides a network for regulation and integration of all body cells. The main functions of the endocrine system are growth, maturation, metabolism, and reproduction. The accompanying box summarizes these functions.

The glands of the endocrine system include the pituitary gland, thyroid gland, parathyroid gland, adrenal glands, gonads, pancreas, and thymus and pineal gland. Their shape and location are illustrated in Figure 19-1. The following section describes the location of these glands, hormones they produce, and hormonal actions.

The Pituitary Gland

The **pituitary gland**, also called the *hypophysis*, is about the size of a pea. It is located in a saddle-shaped hollow in the sphenoid bone called the sella turcica.

Table 19-1. Comparison of Endocrine and Exocrine Glands

Gland	Definition	Action	Functions of Secretions	Examples
Endocrine	Ductless glands; glands of internal secretion	Secrete hormones into circulation	Regulatory	Insulin, ACTH
Exocrine	Secrete into a duct; glands of external secretion	Secrete substances directly into duct or body opening	Protective, functional	Digestive juices, tears, sweat

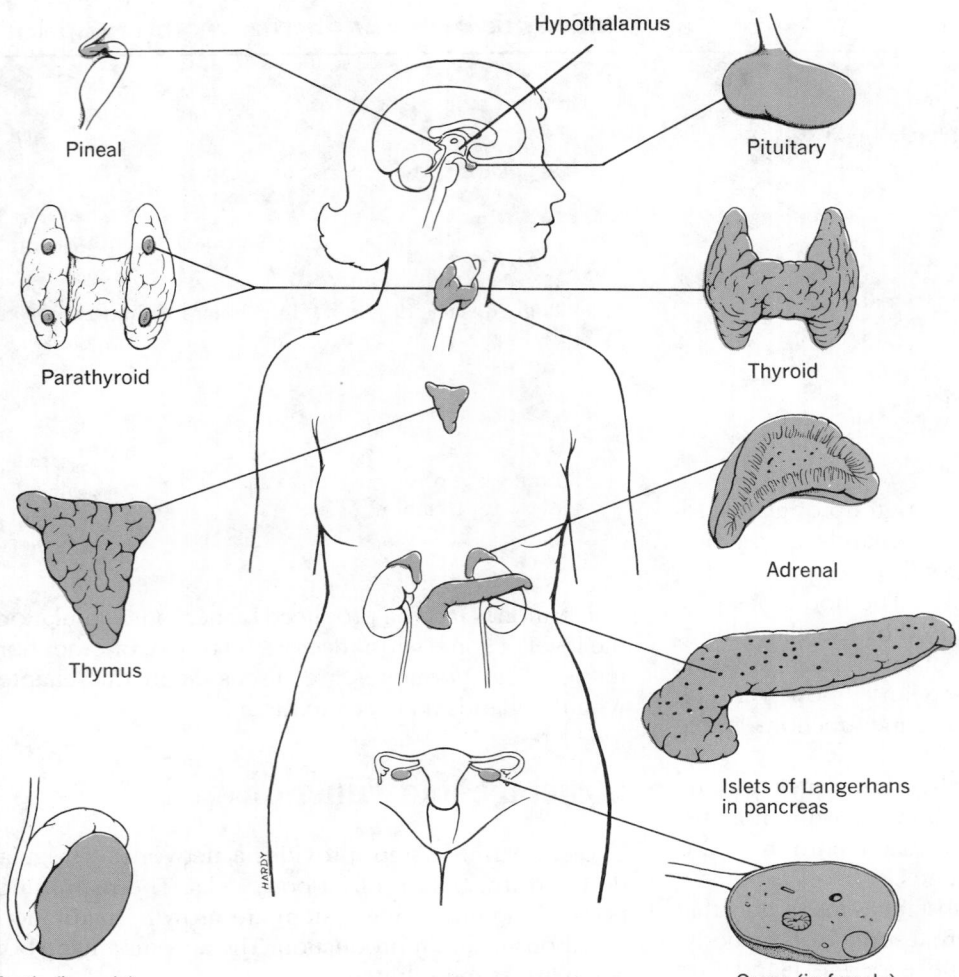

Hypothalamus

Pineal

Pituitary

Parathyroid

Thyroid

Thymus

Adrenal

Islets of Langerhans
in pancreas

Testis (in male)

Ovary (in female)

Figure 19-1. Location of the major endocrine glands in the body.

The sphenoid bone is located at the base of the brain. The pituitary is made up of two parts, the anterior lobe and the posterior lobe. It is sometimes classified as two separate glands, because the embryonic development and the function of the two sections are very different.

In the past, it was believed that hormones secreted by the pituitary were needed for all vital body functions. However, we now know that the hormones released by the pituitary are either secreted in, or their secretion is directly controlled by, the hypothalamus, a tiny but complex portion of the brain. The hypothalamus could be considered "the master controller" or the "master gland." Non-endocrine functions of the hypothalamus are discussed in Chapter 18.

The Anterior Pituitary

The anterior lobe, also called the **adenohypophysis**, releases several hormones, as shown in Table 19-2. Five of these (the tropic hormones) control the action of other endocrine glands. Many of these hormones are called *glycoproteins* because they are made of carbohydrates and proteins. The adenohypophysis is con-

trolled by the hypothalamus; therefore, these hormones are released by neural commands.

Adrenocorticotropic hormone (ACTH) stimulates the adrenal cortex to produce glucocorticoids, such as cortisol, which are vital in the metabolizing of carbohydrates. A chemically similar hormone, melanocyte-stimulating hormone, influences the pigmentation of the skin. ACTH binds to melanocytes in the skin and increases skin pigmentation. Addison's disease is a condition in which ACTH levels are chronically elevated, and the skin becomes noticeably darker.

Other hormones that are chemically similar to ACTH are the beta-endorphins. These hormones have the same effects as opiate drugs (such as morphine). Stress and exercise produce the stimuli for release of endorphins.

Thyroid-stimulating hormone (thyrotropin) stimulates the thyroid gland to produce and secrete thyroxine.

Growth hormone (GH or somatotropin) stimulates growth in all body tissues. It assists with the movement of amino acids into tissue cells and the transformation of amino acids into proteins needed by the body. It aids in the release of fatty acids from adipose (fat) tissue so that it can be used for energy. GH helps to regulate blood nutrient levels after eating and during periods of fasting. If the pituitary releases too much growth hormone during childhood, it causes giantism or excessive size and stature. Too little growth hormone in childhood results in dwarfism. The result of an excess of growth hormone in adulthood is a disorder called acromegaly.

Follicle-stimulating hormone (FSH) stimulates the growth and secretion of ovarian follicles in females and the production of sperm in the testes of males.

Luteinizing hormone (LH) in females stimulates ovulation and the formulation of the corpus luteum. In males, LH (ICSH) influences the secretion of testosterone and other sex hormones from specialized areas in the testes. LH and FSH are known as gonadotropic hormones because they influence the gonads (the reproductive organs).

Prolactin is a hormone secreted in males and females; however, its function is not well understood in males. Prolactin stimulates the production of milk following delivery in females.

Because the hormones released by the pituitary gland often control other endocrine glands and other organs, pituitary disorders can have widespread effects in the body.

The Posterior Pituitary

The posterior pituitary is actually an outgrowth of the hypothalamus and is embryonically derived from the nervous system. Thus, it is also called the **neurohypophysis.** (Notice in Figure 19-1 the close proximity of the hypothalamus and the pituitary gland.) The two posterior pituitary hormones, oxytocin and vasopressin, are actually secreted in the hypothalamus by neurosecretory cells and then released by the neurohypophysis (see Table 19-2).

Oxytocin stimulates the uterus to contract during delivery and helps to keep the uterus contracted after delivery (to prevent hemorrhage). It also stimulates the release of milk when the baby sucks. *Vasopressin* or *antidiuretic hormone* functions in several ways. It stimulates contraction of blood vessels to raise blood pressure, it influences the uterus, and it influences resorption of water by the tubules in the kidney.

The Thyroid Gland

The **thyroid gland**, the largest of the endocrine glands, lies in front of the neck, just below the larynx, with a wing (lobe) on either side of the trachea (Fig. 19-2). The thyroid secretes two hormones, thyroxine or tetraiodothyronine (T_4) and triiodothyronine (T_3). These hormones are made in the thyroid gland from iodine.

T_4 is more concentrated in the blood. T_3 is more potent. These hormones regulate body metabolism, controlling the rate at which the cells do their work.

Another hormone secreted by the thyroid is called *calcitonin* or thyrocalcitonin. It is involved in the maintenance of the calcium level within the body.

If the thyroid secretes too much thyroxine, all body functions are speeded up. The cells burn food too rapidly and produce more energy than is needed. This is termed *hyperthyroidism*, or *Graves' disease*, and causes such symptoms as nervousness, hyperactivity, irritability, and protrusion of the eyeballs (exophthalmia).

The thyroid removes iodine from the blood to make thyroxine; this iodine must be supplied in the diet. If the diet lacks iodine, the thyroid grows larger because it is overworking to make more thyroxine. An enlarged thyroid gland is called a **goiter**. The deficiency can be prevented by the use of iodized salt. Some seafood also contains iodine. *Hypothyroidism* (deficient thyroxine secretion) during childhood results in *cretinism*. Advanced hypothyroidism in the adult results in a condition called *myxedema*.

The Parathyroid Glands

The **parathyroids** are small glands, each about the size of a pea. They lie on either side of the undersurface of the thyroid gland (see Figure 19-1). Usually there are four, and despite their relatively small size, they are essential to health and to life itself.

The parathyroids secrete a hormone, *parathormone*, that regulates the amount of calcium and phosphorus in the blood, and this in turn affects nerve and muscle irritability. When the blood calcium is too low, parathormone is secreted. This stimulates the number and size of osteoclasts and causes calcium to leave the bones. (Thus, parathormone has the opposite action to calcitonin.)

Too little calcium (a result of hypoparathyroidism) causes *tetany*, a condition marked by muscle spasms and convulsions, sometimes causing death (not to be confused with the infection called tetanus or lockjaw). If the parathyroids secrete too much hormone (hyperparathyroidism), the diet cannot supply enough calcium, and the calcium salts are then drawn from the bones, making them soft and unable to support weight. Hyperparathyroidism also makes the person susceptible to forming calcium-based kidney stones.

The Adrenal Glands

The two **adrenal glands**, also known as the *suprarenal glands*, sit like hats, one atop each kidney (see Figure 19-1). Like the pituitary gland, the adrenal glands have two parts, each of which produces a different hormone.

(Text continues on page 202)

Table 19-2. Important Secretions of Endocrine Glands

Endocrine Gland	Hormone(s) Secreted	Actions	Results of Excess (↑) and Deficiency (↓)
Pituitary Gland			
Anterior or adenohypophysis	Adrenocorticotropic hormone (ACTH)	Stimulates adrenal cortex to produce cortisol	↓ Deficiency of adrenal hormones; ↑ Addison's disease
	Melanocyte-stimulating hormone (MSH)	Increases pigmentation of skin	↑ Excess pigmentation of skin
	Beta endorphins	Produces analgesia	
	Thyroid-stimulating hormone (TSH)	Regulates thyroid hormone	↑ Hyperthyroidism
	Follicle-stimulating hormone (FSH)	Stimulates growth and secretion of eggs in ovaries	
		Stimulates production of sperm in males	
	Luteinizing hormone (LH)—females	Helps to control ovulation and menstruation; important in sustaining pregnancy	
	Interstitial cell-stimulating hormone (ICSH)—males	Stimulates secretion of male hormones in men	
	Prolactin, lactogenic hormone (PRL)	Stimulates mammary glands to produce milk	
	Growth hormone, somatotropic hormone (GH)	Controls bone and tissue growth	↑ (Child) giantism ↑ (Adult) acromegaly ↓ (Child) dwarfism
Posterior or neurohypophysis	Oxytocin	Causes contractions of the uterus; stimulates milk production	
	Vasopressin (ADH)	Raises blood pressure; promotes reabsorption of water in kidney tubules	↓ Diabetes insipidus
Thyroid gland	Thyroxine (T_4) Triiodothyronine (T_3)	Regulate body metabolism (iodine required for synthesis of T_3 and T_4)	↑ Hyperthyroidism ↑ Graves' disease ↓ (Deficient iodine supply) goiter ↓ (Child) cretinism ↓ (Adult) myxedema
	Calcitonin	Stimulates calcium to leave plasma and enter bones	↑ Calcium imbalance

Gland	Hormone	Function	Disorder/Result
Parathyroid glands	Parathormone	Stimulates bones to release calcium and enter blood; Regulates phosphorus balance	↑ Soft bones; ↑ Kidney stones; ↓ Tetany
Adrenal Glands (Suprarenals)			
Adrenal medulla	Catecholamines; Epinephrine	Mimic actions of SNS, adapt to stress; Causes many body processes to speed up, especially in an emergency	
	Norepinephrine	Similar actions to epinephrine	
	Steroids		
Adrenal cortex	Glucocorticoids (such as hydrocortisone, cortisol)	Increase blood glucose; Break down nutrients; Decrease inflammation	↓ Hypofunction of total adrenal cortex; ↓ Addison's disease; ↑ Cushing's syndrome; ↓ Decrease in blood volume, shock
	Corticoids; Mineralocorticoids	Regulate electrolyte levels in extracellular fluid	
	Sex hormones; Androgens (males)	Produce male sex characteristics	↑ Adrenogenital syndrome; ↓ Lack of sexual development; ↑ (Girls) virilism
	Estrogens (females); Progestins	Produce female sex characteristics	
Gonads			
Testes (male)	Testosterone	Development of male sex characteristics (also influenced by androgens)	↑ or ↓ Abnormal sexual development in male
Ovaries (female)	Estrogen and progesterone (also produced in adrenal cortex)	Regulate female sex characteristics and function; regulate menstruation	↑ or ↓ Abnormal sexual development in female; ↑ Abnormally early menarche; ↓ Amenorrhea, difficult pregnancy; ↓ Early menopause
Pancreas			
Alpha cells (islets of Langerhans)	Glucagon	Speeds glucogenesis, raises blood sugar	
Beta cells (islets of Langerhans)	Insulin	Enables cells to use glucose, lowers blood sugar	↓ Diabetes mellitus
Delta cells (islets of Langerhans)	Somatostatin	Inhibits release of insulin and glucagon	
Thymus	Thymosin (thymic hormone)	Produces T-cell lymphocytes for cellular immunity	

The pituitary gland is controlled by the hypothalamus. Some pituitary hormones are secreted by the hypothalamus and released by the pituitary gland.

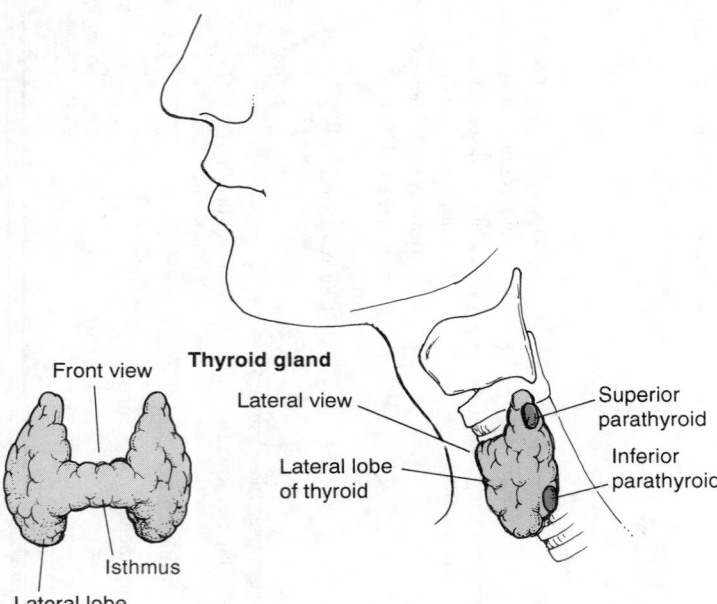

Thyroid gland

Front view

Lateral view

Superior parathyroid

Lateral lobe of thyroid

Inferior parathyroid

Isthmus

Lateral lobe

Figure 19-2. Thyroid and parathyroid glands.

The Adrenal Medulla

The central portion of the adrenal gland, called the medulla, secretes hormones called *catecholamines*, which are made from amino acids. Epinephrine and norepinephrine are the two hormones of the medulla. *Epinephrine* makes the heart beat faster, contracts blood vessels, raises blood pressure, and increases muscle power by causing the liver to release glucose for energy. The hormone *norepinephrine* has some, but not all, of the actions of epinephrine.

The hormones from the medulla mimic the action of the sympathetic nervous system. However, the adrenal medulla is not necessary for life, because its activities can be taken over by the sympathetic nervous system. The adrenals are active in emergencies; emotions of fright, anger, love, or grief stimulate them. They are said to prepare people for flight or fight. The functions of the medulla are important because they help us adapt to stress.

The Adrenal Cortex

The outer part of the adrenals, the cortex, secretes many compounds called **corticosteroids** or corticoids. There are three types of corticosteroids: mineralocorticoids, glucocorticoids, and the sex hormones (androgens). All of these compounds are derived from cholesterol.

Mineralocorticoids regulate the amount of mineral salts (also known as electrolytes) in the body. *Aldosterone* is the most important mineralocorticoid. Aldosterone stimulates the reabsorption of sodium into the plasma, which results in increased water reabsorption and therefore an increase in blood volume.

Glucocorticoids have an important influence on the synthesis of glucose, amino acids, and fats during the process of metabolism. They also decrease the inflammatory response. *Hydrocortisone* (cortisol) is the predominant glucocorticoid.

The sex hormones (*androgens* and *estrogens*) are supplements to the sex hormones secreted by the gonads.

Hyperactivity of the adrenal cortex is more common in females than in males. It can hasten sexual development in boys. In girls, it causes virilism, a condition with masculine sex characteristics. Excess cortisol (and in some cases androgens) from the adrenal cortex causes Cushing's syndrome. Table 19-2 identifies some of the steroids and their functions.

The Gonads

The gonads are the glands of reproduction: the testes of the male and the ovaries of the female (see Figure 19-1).

In addition to producing sperm, the testes produce testosterone, the male sex hormone. Other steroid hormones also produce masculinizing effects; as a group, they are called *androgens*. The ovaries produce estrogen and progesterone, which, in addition to regulating sex characteristics and functions, are responsible for menstruation. These hormones are also produced in the adrenal cortex.

Disorders relating to the hormones produced by the gonads show their effects by abnormal sexual development. In the female, this may be characterized by unusually early menarche, amenorrhea (absence of menses), early menopause, or difficulty in pregnancy and childbirth.

The Pancreas

The pancreas lies behind the stomach between the duodenum and the spleen. It is an endocrine and an exocrine gland. As an exocrine gland, it releases digestive enzymes into the duct system leading to the small intestine.

The endocrine portion of the pancreas exists in the 500,000 to 1,000,000 small islands (islets) scattered throughout the body and tail of the pancreas. Within the islets, called the **islets of Langerhans**, are cells that secrete one of three pancreatic hormones: insulin, glucagon, or somatostatin (see Table 19-2).

Approximately 75% of the islet cells are beta cells. They secrete the hormone **insulin**, which is a protein substance. The primary function of insulin is to control the glucose level in the blood. It accomplishes this task in several ways, as listed in the box. Approximately 20% of the cells in the islets of Langerhans are *alpha cells*. Alpha cells secrete the hormone **glucagon**, which is the opposing hormone to insulin. Glucagon raises blood sugar; insulin lowers blood sugar. Glucagon is needed to use the stored sugar, **glycogen**. Glucagon also stimulates the breakdown of fatty acids. (Fatty acids are large molecules that can be transformed into glucose and used as energy sources.)

Approximately 5% of the cells within the islets are *delta cells*, which secrete somatostatin. Somatostatin inhibits the release of both of the other hormones secreted in the islets, insulin and glucagon. The way this control mechanism operates is not yet known.

The most familiar disorder of the pancreas is *diabetes mellitus*. This condition is caused by a disorder in the islets of Langerhans. In diabetes mellitus, the islets are not making any insulin, or there is not enough insulin to meet body needs. Without adequate levels of insulin, most cells are unable to use glucose.

The Thymus and Pineal Gland

The **thymus** lies behind the sternum (breast bone). It produces *thymosin* (thymic hormone), a protein that stimulates production of small lymphocytes called T-cells (T-lymphocyte cells, T-helper cells, thymus-dependent cells). These lymphocytes are essential for the development of cellular immunity. The thymus secretes several hormones that are believed to stimulate T-cells after they leave the thymus. In infants and children, the thymus is relatively large. After puberty, the thymus atrophies, but little is known of the long-term effects of this phenomenon.

The **pineal gland** (pineal body) is a small cone-shaped structure lying just above the roof of the midbrain, between the two parts of the thalamus. It probably produces melatonin. Melatonin, or another pineal hormone, is believed to regulate the release of substances from the hypothalamus that stimulate and regulate the

Insulin's Actions to Control Glucose Level

◆ Insulin increases the cell membrane's permeability to glucose. Once in the cell, glucose is used in cellular respiration to produce energy.

◆ Insulin stimulates the liver to convert glucose into glycogen (glycogenesis) and helps the liver and muscles store glycogen. Glycogen is stored body sugar commonly referred to as animal starch.

◆ Insulin aids in the production of fat from glucose.

◆ Insulin increases the transfer of amino acids and fatty acids, which will be synthesized into lipids and proteins, across the cell membrane. (*Gluconeogenesis* is the conversion of excess amino acids or fatty acids into glycogen. The other major hormone of the islets of Langerhans, glucagon, is necessary to release the glycogen from storage, which then quickly becomes glucose. This process is called *glycogenolysis*.)

secretion of the pituitary hormone, gonadotropin. Thus, the pineal gland may influence reproductive functions. In animals, the amount of daylight is speculated to regulate pineal secretions and may therefore influence breeding seasons. The effect on humans is not well understood but is believed to affect the brain and influence the rate of gonad (ovary and testis) maturation.

Other Hormones

The stomach wall secretes a hormone called *gastrin*, which stimulates secretions of the gastric glands. The lining of the upper part of the small intestine secretes hormones that stimulate the pancreatic juices (pancreozymin, secretin) and another hormone that causes the gallbladder to contract (cholecystokinin). The placenta is also a temporary endocrine gland that secretes hormones that help to maintain pregnancy. These include estrogen, progesterone, and HCG (human chorionic gonadotropin). The presence of high levels of these hormones in the body provides the basis for the commonly used tests to determine whether a woman is pregnant.

The skin produces vitamin D, a hormone that is necessary for the absorption of calcium from the gastrointestinal tract. Vitamin D is necessary for proper amounts of calcium in the blood and bones.

A structure within the kidney called the *juxtaglomerular apparatus* produces a hormone called *renin* (renin-angiotensin-aldosterone), which acts on the vascular system to assist in blood pressure control. Another, *erythropoietin* (renal erythropoietic factor), is a glycoprotein (protein and carbohydrate combination) hormone that is produced in the kidney in the adult and the liver in the child. Erythropoietin stimulates red blood cell production.

The Prostaglandins

The **prostaglandins** are specialized fatty acids that were first isolated in the seminal fluid of the prostate from which their name is derived. They are actually widespread in the tissues of the body. They are not hormones, but rather hormonelike substances in that they share characteristics of the hormones and of the neural transmitters. Their effects are localized to the area in which they are produced. Generally, they stimulate either the contraction or relaxation of smooth muscles. The prostaglandins have an influence on blood pressure, respiration, digestion, and reproduction and actually have opposite effects on these functions in some cases. For example, one prostaglandin may cause dilation of the bronchioles, while another causes constriction of the same muscles.

Extensive research relating to prostaglandins is being carried out to determine their specific functions. It is possible that many disorders may be treated in the future by the control of prostaglandin secretion or by the administration of these substances.

System Physiology

System Relationships

There is a close relationship between the endocrine system and other body systems. Prominent among these is the relationship between the endocrine system and the nervous system. They cannot be separated anatomically or functionally. Each needs the other for optimum performance. They are similar also in that functions of both include stimulating and controlling actions of the body. Generally, the effect of nerve stimuli is immediate and lasts only as long as the stimulation is present, whereas the action of an endocrine gland is slower with a more prolonged stimulation and regulation. The hypothalamus is integral to the workings of the information relay to target cells, as discussed in the next section.

The dependency between the endocrine system and circulatory system exists because the hormones travel from the glands through the bloodstream and lymph. The endocrine system and digestive system are interdependent because of the secretion of insulin and the conversion of foods into glucose and glycogen.

Other systems are related to the endocrine system in that functions of many systems are stimulated and controlled to some extent by hormones of the endocrine system. These relationships are evident in Table 19-2.

Information Relay to Target Cells

The hypothalamus and the anterior pituitary are components of a unit that can be called an information relay system. Specialized cells in the hypothalamus respond to changes in the internal and external environments. Their response is to send messages (stimuli) to the glands to secrete.

Hormones are specific to certain target tissues. They bind to receptors on target tissues in a lock-and-key fashion. The target cells' response to the hormone involves acceleration or inhibition of certain biochemical processes.

Table 19-3. Effects of Aging on the Endocrine System

Factor	Result	Nursing Implications
Overall effects of aging are unknown.	Individualized changes	Monitor changes in metabolism or blood sugar levels.
There are few known changes.		Notify physician of abnormal laboratory values.
There are no generalized decreases, except in estrogen and testosterone.		
Reproductive secretions decrease.	Onset of menopause in middle age	Monitor for heart disease, which increases after menopause with loss of estrogens.
	Inability to become pregnant	
	Hirsutism in women	Advise about facial hair removal.
Sexual tissue atrophies.	Loss of pubic hair	
	Longer time needed for sexual orgasm	Explain that libido is essentially unchanged.
		Suggest ways older people may meet friends because they need companionship.
Decrease in thyroid hormones.	Decreased metabolic rate	Be aware that it may take longer to do daily activities.
	Thin hair	
	Dry skin	Listen to complaints of feeling cold.
Decrease in pancreatic secretions.	Decreased ability to metabolize glucose	Monitor weight. Counsel on exercise and proper nutrition.

Negative Feedback

The fine balance, called *negative feedback*, within the endocrine system regulates the rate and quantity of hormone secretion.

Negative feedback signals the controller (the specific gland) to correct a deviation from normal. Once the desired effect is achieved with the hormone, information is sent to the gland to halt secretion of the hormone. Likewise, feedback to the gland tells it to increase production when its level is below normal. Thus, the feedback system helps to promote homeostasis in the body.

Effects of Aging on the System

The decline of sex hormones is the most obvious effect of aging on the endocrine system. Estrogen and testosterone levels decline with obvious results. Table 19-3 summarizes the major effects of aging.

In women, the most obvious effect occurs with the reproductive organs. Menopause begins in middle age with a decrease in estrogen levels. As a result, breast tissue changes from glandular tissue to connective and adipose tissue. The elasticity of the tissue is reduced. The breasts begin to sag. The uterus, fallopian tubes, and external genitalia shrink with age. Hirsutism (facial hair) may occur.

In men, testosterone levels gradually decline from levels seen in young adulthood. Sperm production decreases. The ability to achieve an erection, orgasm, and ejaculation remain but may take longer than in earlier years.

Both men and women have a loss of pubic hair. Impotence in men and lack of sexual response in women are *not* natural results of aging. The desire for companionship, tenderness, and love remain as basic human needs.

Keys for Review

Key Questions for Critical Thinking

1. Differentiate between endocrine and exocrine glands. Name at least three of each and discuss their functions.
2. Describe at least four major functions of the endocrine system.
3. What hormones are released or secreted by the pituitary gland. Describe the function of each.
4. Discuss why the hypothalamus is called the "master controller".
5. Discuss the functions of epinephrine.
6. What are the prostaglandins? Describe their functions.

Key Readings

Chabner D. The Language of Medicine, Ed 4. Philadelphia, W.B. Saunders, 1991

Eliopoulus C. Caring for the Elderly in Diverse Care Settings. Philadelphia, J.B. Lippincott, 1990

Farrell J. Nursing Care of the Older Person. Philadelphia, J.B. Lippincott, 1990

Key Readings (continued)

Jackson DB, Saunders RB. Child Health Nursing: A comprehensive Approach to the Care of Children and their Families. Philadelphia, J.B. Lippincott, 1993

Scanlon V, Sanders V. Essentials of Anatomy and Physiology. Philadelphia, F.A. Davis, 1991

Seeley R, Stephens T, Tate P. Anatomy and Physiology, Ed 2. St. Louis, C.V. Mosby, 1994

Smeltzer SC, Bare BG. Brunner and Suddarth's Textbook of Medical-Surgical Nursing, Ed 7. Philadelphia, J.B. Lippincott, 1992

Keys to Learning More

Unit Four: interrelationships between body systems

Chapter 56: medications, including hormones given as medications

Unit Thirteen: deviations from normal body structure and function in children

Unit Fourteen: deviations from normal in adults

Chapter 72: specific disorders of the endocrine system

Unit Fifteen: deviations in older adults

20 The Sensory System

Learning Objectives

- Identify the sensory receptors of the body in terms of location and function, and identify the areas of the brain that interpret the sensations from each
- On a chart, locate the major structures of the eye, and state the function of each
- On a chart, locate the major structures of the ear, and state the function of each
- Define terms related to the eyes and ears
- Locate on the tongue the various types of taste buds that accept sweet, salty, bitter, and sour tastes
- Describe the functions of the olfactory nerve, and locate it on a chart
- Describe how the sense of touch functions, and locate at least one type of touch receptor on a chart
- Describe the effects of aging on the sensory system

Key Terms

accommodation	external auditory	retina
aqueous humor	meatus	sclera
auricle	iris	semicircular canals
cerumen	lacrimal glands	tympanic
cochlea	lens	membrane
conjunctiva	organ of Corti	vertigo
cornea	pinna	vitreous humor
	pupil	

Keys to Understanding This Chapter

Chapter 5: basic needs involve receiving information about the world around us

Unit Three: normal growth and development; if a baby does not have adequate sensory input, development will be altered or retarded

Chapter 18: Sensory information transmission to the brain
- A sense receptor in an organ or tissue responds to a stimulus and sends the information from this stimulus through nerve routes to the brain. There it is interpreted.

Key Points

- The eye has several protective structures, which include the bony orbit, eyelids, cilia, lacrimal glands, and antiseptic tears.
- The retina has rods, which function in dim light, and cones, which permit the perception of color and sharpness.
- The eyeball contains the sclera and cornea, choroid layer, and retina. Muscles help it move, and nerves carry messages.
- The ear has three divisions: the external, middle, and internal ear. Actual hearing takes place in the cochlea of the inner ear in the organ of Corti.
- Light transmissions occur because light rays enter the eye and are refracted (bent) by several eye structures, all of which help the light ray focus on the retina.
- The vestibule and semicircular canals maintain balance and equilibrium.
- Chemoreceptors in the taste buds detect chemicals in the solution of the mouth. The sense of taste is influenced by the sense of smell.

Key Topics Outline

Structure and Function
  The Eye
  The Ear
System Physiology
  Vision
  Hearing
  Balance and Equilibrium
  Taste
  Smell
  Touch/Tactile Sense
  Other Sensations
Effects of Aging on the System
  Eye and Vision Changes
  Ear and Hearing Changes
  Changes in Other Senses

Rosdahl CB: Textbook of Basic Nursing, 6th ed. © 1995 J.B. Lippincott Company

Functions of the Sensory System

Obtain General Information

♦ touch receptors receive information about the surrounding world (touch, pressure, hot, cold, pain)

♦ internal organs receive sensations of pain, pressure, fullness, etc.

♦ visual sense receives images (light)

♦ hearing receptors receive sound waves (auditory sense)

♦ chemoreceptors in nose receive sensations of odors (olfactory sense)

♦ chemoreceptors in mouth obtain information about tastes (gustatory sense)

Balance

♦ maintain sense of balance (proprioceptors, inner ear)

♦ maintain equilibrium

♦ identify position in space

Without your senses, you would know nothing about the world around you. Obvious sensory perceptions are those of seeing, hearing, smelling, tasting, and touching. You also can receive impressions of warmth, softness, pressure, and pain. A very important perception is the sense of equilibrium; you know whether or not you are moving and the posture and position of your body.

Structure and Function

The activities of the sensory system are composed of vision, hearing, taste, smell, and touch. Organs involved in these senses are eyes, ears, tongue, nose, and skin. These senses supply information to the inner body. By providing information, they help the body detect changes in the environment. The body can then respond to maintain homeostasis. Functions of the sensory system are outlined in the box.

Study of the nervous system shows that to be aware of information from the world around you, you must have the following:

♦ Receptors to receive the stimulus
♦ Nerve routes to carry the stimulus to the brain
♦ Centers in the brain to interpret the stimulus

This is also true of the sensory system. These steps, as related to vision and hearing, are summarized in Figure 20-1.

The senses of taste, smell, and touch are as interesting and as useful as sight and hearing, but because they are not as often involved in illness or disease, they are not mentioned in detail in this chapter. The tongue, as part of the digestive system, is discussed in Chapter 23; the nose is discussed with the respiratory system in Chapter 22; and the integumentary system is discussed in Chapter 15.

The Eye

The eye is the organ of vision. While the eye's anatomy is discussed here, vision itself is discussed in the System Physiology section later in this chapter.

The eye lies in a ball-shaped cavity of the skull, called the orbit. Between the eye itself and its bony surroundings is a protective cushion of fat. The eyelids, brows, and lashes (cilia) serve as further protection for the eye.

The eyelid is the cover for the anterior surface of the skull. (The medical prefix for eyelid is *blephar(o)-*). A reflex, the eye blink, protects the eye from foreign objects or blows. Also covering the anterior eye, beneath and lining the eyelids, is a transparent mucous membrane called the **conjunctiva**, which is supplied with blood vessels and nerve endings.

The surface of the eye is kept moist by the **lacrimal glands**, which produce tears (Fig. 20-2). The lacrimal glands are located at the outer edge of the corner (or lateral canthus) of the eye. Tears drain through a small opening in the inner (or medial canthus) corner of the eye, the nasolacrimal duct, into the nose. Tears help protect the eyes from infections and help to moisten

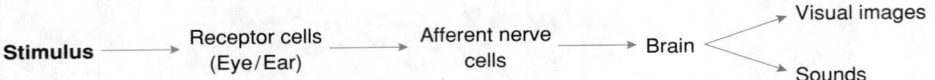

and lubricate the surface of the eyes. Normally about 1 mL of lacrimal fluid is produced per day. Irritating substances (eg, onions, dust) cause an oversecretion of the lacrimal glands. Humans are the only species that form tears in response to emotions.

Key Concept

Protection of the eye is provided by the bony orbit, fatty cushion, eyelids, eyebrows, eyelashes, eye blink reflex, conjunctivae, and lacrimal glands.

Eyeball

The eyeball is a hollow sphere made of three layers of tissue: sclera and cornea, choroid layer, and retina. The eyeball is illustrated in Figure 20-3.

Sclera and Cornea. The tough protective outer layer of the eyeball is the **sclera**. The sclera is also known as the "white" of the eye. To permit light rays to enter the front of the eye, the sclera is connected to a transparent section over the front of the eyeball, called the **cornea**. It is tough, yet transparent. The cornea has the ability to bend light rays, so the rays can focus on the light-sensitive cells in the posterior region of the eye.

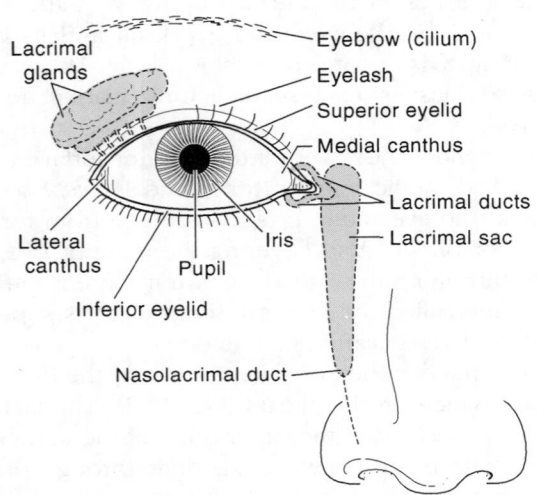

Figure 20-2. Details of the right eye and the lacrimal glands and ducts.

Key Concept

The cornea is often removed after death as a tissue for corneal transplant. Corneas were the first tissues used for transplantation and are used to restore vision to hundreds of people with defective corneas each year.

Choroid Layer. The middle layer, the choroid, is a vascular layer that brings oxygen and nutrients to the eyes. The choroid extends to the *ciliary body*. The ciliary body contains muscles that can adjust the shape and thickness of the lens. The ciliary body also secretes **aqueous humor** (5-6 mL/d), which flows through the anterior and posterior chambers of the eye, in the space between the cornea and the lens. The aqueous humor maintains intraocular (within the eye) pressure (normal is about 24 mm Hg). The aqueous humor also provides nutrients and oxygen to the avascular (without blood vessels) lens and cornea.

Over the front of the eyeball, the choroid develops into a pigmented section, the **iris**, which gives the eye its specific color. In the iris are muscles that control the size of the opening within its black center, the pupil. The **pupil** regulates the amount of light entering the eye.

The **lens** is a structure immediately behind the iris. It has a role in the focusing of the eye. The space behind the lens is filled with a transparent gelatin-like material called the **vitreous humor**. The vitreous humor helps maintain the shape of the eyeball and contributes to intraocular pressure. Loss of the vitreous humor causes blindness.

Retina. The inner layer of the eyeball, the **retina**, is an incredible structure. It contains the receptors of the optic nerve. The retina contains specialized neurons, called rods and cones, which permit the perception of light and dark and of color. Each retina contains between 100 and 120 million rods, which are dispersed throughout the retina. Because the pupil dilates in dim light, the light strikes all parts of the retina and thus activates the rods. Because they are suited to dim light, they are useful in night vision (*scotopic vision*). Each retina also contains approximately 6 to 7 million cones. The cones are concentrated in the center of the retina and function in daylight and bright light (*photopic vision*). They receive color and add to visual acuity (visual sharpness).

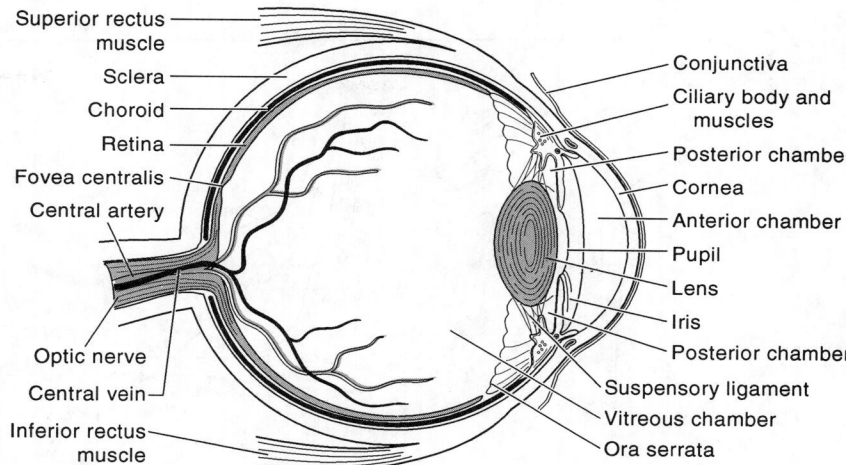

Superior rectus muscle
Sclera
Choroid
Retina
Fovea centralis
Central artery
Optic nerve
Central vein
Inferior rectus muscle

Conjunctiva
Ciliary body and muscles
Posterior chamber
Cornea
Anterior chamber
Pupil
Lens
Iris
Posterior chamber
Suspensory ligament
Vitreous chamber
Ora serrata

Figure 20-3. The eye and its appendages, lateral view.

> ## Key Concepts
> ◆ Rods permit perception of light and dark and are useful in scotopic (night) vision.
> ◆ Cones permit perception of color; they function in bright light (photopic vision).

Nerves and Muscles

The optic nerves carry the sensations from each eye. These stimuli are conducted to the occipital area of the brain. Figure 18-2 illustrates the site in the brain (visual sensory area) where these images are interpreted. At the optic chiasm, the optic nerves cross, continue as the *optic tract*, and enter the brain.

The ophthalmic nerve, a branch of the trigeminal nerve (fifth cranial nerve), carries sensations of eye pain and temperature to the brain. If a foreign object is in the eye, for example, this nerve carries that sensation.

Smooth muscles in the eye control pupil size and the action of the lens in accommodation. Three pairs of extraocular muscles, attached to its outer coat, move the eyeball. Another muscle, attached to the upper eyelid, holds the eye open; when the eyelids shut, this muscle is relaxed. The oculomotor nerves (third cranial nerve) innervate some of the voluntary muscles that move the eyeball and the eyelid. These nerves also are involved in some of the autonomic reactions of the eye, such as the accommodation of the pupil to varying degrees of light. The trochlear nerves (fourth cranial nerve) assist in some of the voluntary movements of the eyeballs. The sixth cranial nerves, the abducens, coordinate with the third and fourth cranial nerves to move the eyes.

The Ear

The ear is the organ of hearing and equilibrium. The anatomy of the ear is discussed here. Hearing is discussed later in the chapter in the section System Physiology.

The ear has three parts: the external, middle, and inner ear (Fig. 20-4). These lead to the auditory (acoustic) nerve and then to the center for hearing, which is located in the temporal lobe of the cerebral cortex.

External Ear

The external ear, also called the **pinna** or **auricle,** is the only readily visible part of the ear. It is composed mostly of cartilage and is shaped like a funnel to gather and guide sound waves into its small opening, which extends into a tube called the auditory canal. The opening into the auditory canal is called the **external auditory meatus**. The lining of the auditory canal is covered with tiny hairs and secretes a waxy substance called **cerumen**; the hairs and the wax aid in protecting the ear from foreign objects. The auditory canal is very short, approximately 1 inch (2.54 cm), and extends to the eardrum, a thin membrane also called the **tympanic membrane**. The tympanic membrane separates the external from the middle ear.

Middle Ear

On the other side of the tympanum is the middle ear, a small air-filled cavity in the temporal bone (see Figure 20-4). Within this cavity between the eardrum and the inner ear are three tiny bones: the malleus (hammer), the incus (anvil), and the stapes (stirrup). These three bones collectively are called *ossicles* and are so small that sound waves can set them in motion. The stapes transmit vibrations to the fluid-filled inner ear at the oval window. The oval window separates the middle ear from the inner ear.

There are two small muscles attached to the stapes and the malleus. These muscles contract at a sudden, loud sound; this is a reflex action. The purpose of this reflex is to stop the vibration of the ossicles and thus protect the vital internal organs of the middle and inner ear.

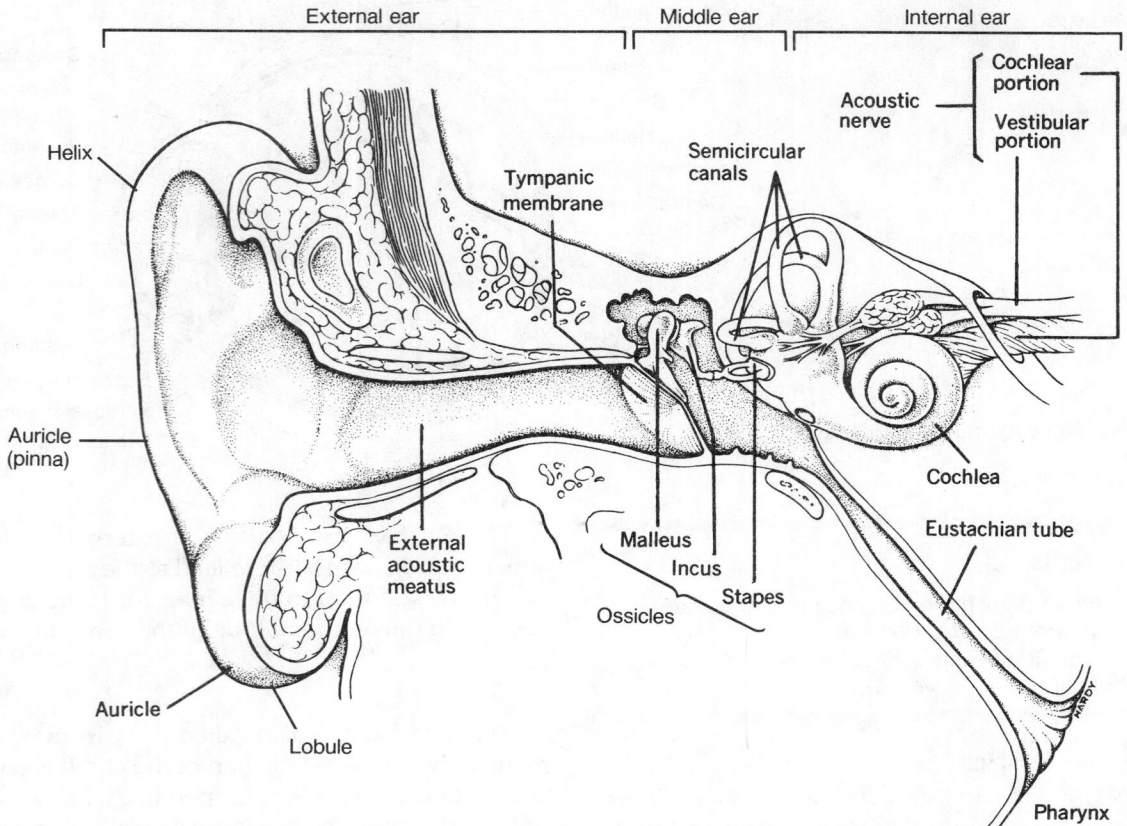

Figure 20-4. Diagram of the ear, showing the external, middle, and internal subdivisions.

Extending from the middle ear are two openings. One leads into the mastoid cells behind it and the other into the eustachian tube, or auditory tube, which communicates with the nasopharynx. To function properly, the pressure in the middle ear must be the same as the external atmospheric pressure. The eustachian tube opens during swallowing or yawning. Its function is to equalize the pressure in the middle ear with the atmospheric pressure, that is, to equalize the pressure on both sides of the tympanic membrane so that the drum can vibrate freely. It also helps to drain the middle ear. The middle ear, the eustachian tube, the nasopharynx, and the passage to the mastoid cells are lined with a continuous coating of mucous membrane.

Inner Ear

The inner ear is a bony labyrinth filled with a set of tunnels and also chambers called the *membranous labyrinth*. Both the bony and membranous labyrinth are filled with fluid. These fluids are similar to cerebrospinal fluid. They are important in the transmission of sound waves. There are three sections in the inner ear: cochlea, vestibule, and semicircular canals (see Figure 20-4).

Cochlea. The **cochlea** is shaped like a hollow snail shell buried deep inside the temporal bone of the skull. It is filled with fluid called *endolymph*. Inside the bony cochlea lies the **organ of Corti**, which is very small but intricate. It is approximately $1\frac{1}{2}$ in (3.75 cm) long and contains approximately 7,500 separate parts. This organ is referred to as the true organ of hearing, because the transmission of the nerve stimuli of hearing begins here.

Vestibule. The vestibule, the area between the cochlea and the semicircular canals, contains two membranous sacs called the *utricle* and the *saccule*. The utricle and saccule have specialized areas of hair cells that send information to the cerebellum and the midbrain. These areas of the brain are concerned with the subconscious information regarding body position at rest.

Semicircular Canals. Another section of the inner ear is the **semicircular canals**. Shaped like horseshoes, they lie behind the cochlea. They too contain hairlike nerve endings that are set in motion by fluid within the canals. Motion in the fluid is caused by head or body movements.

If you look at the semicircular canals in Figure 20-4, you will note that each is on a different plane, or angle, in space. Thus, the fluid (endolymph) in these semicircular canals can flow in various directions and can pick up more types of motion than would be the case if all of the canals were on the same plane. The sensory receptors for equilibrium (balance) while the body is moving are located in these canals.

Nerves

The nerve endings that are the receptors for hearing are located within the membranous cochlea in the organ of Corti. These hairlike receptors connect to the cochlear nerve, which becomes a division of the acoustic or auditory nerve (the eighth cranial nerve). This acoustic nerve is a combination of two divisions, the cochlear (for transmission of sound) and the vestibular (for transmission of signals relating to balance and position). Sometimes it is called the vestibulocochlear nerve.

Key Concept

Protective Devices Within the Ear
- Small muscles protect the delicate structures.
- The eustachian (auditory) tube helps to equalize pressure between the outer and middle ear.
- Ear wax helps to lubricate and protect the eardrum.
- Hairs within the auricle and auditory canal help keep out foreign matter.
- The mucous membrane provides lubrication.

System Physiology

Vision

Vision may be compared to a camera. Although this analogy is not totally accurate, the two have many parts with corresponding functions. Each eye registers a separate image. The visual areas of cerebral cortex fuse these separate images into a single image with a three-dimensional effect, called binocular vision. This binocular vision, which is responsible for depth perception, is possible because both eyes' coordinated muscles move the eyeballs in tandem.

Light enters the eye through the cornea and passes through the aqueous humor; the pupil, the opening in the iris that regulates the amount of light; the lens; and the vitreous humor before coming into focus on the retina. Refraction (bending of light rays) takes place within all of these components.

In the lens, the light rays are brought into focus to allow a clear image. The image is then reflected on the retina, the nerve center of the eye. Parallel rays of light passing through the lens are refracted (bent) so they focus on the retina. This adjustment by the lens to make

a sharp, clear image is called **accommodation** and is controlled by the autonomic nervous system. If the eyeball is too short, the light rays are focused behind the retina instead of on it; this causes farsightedness, which is known as *hyperopia*. In nearsightedness (*myopia*), the light rays are focused in front of the retina. This occurs because the muscles of the lens contract too tightly and do not allow enough light to enter the eye or because the eyeball is too long in relation to the muscles of the lens.

The receptors in the retina send the nerve impulses through the nerve fibers to the optic nerve, the nerve of sight. The optic nerve meets the retina at the optic disk. This optic disk is called the "blind spot" because it is the region of the eye that is not light sensitive.

The optic nerve, cranial nerve II, then carries the information to the brain. A summary of this pathway is given in Figure 20-5.

Hearing

Sound waves enter through the external auditory canal of the ear and strike the tympanic membrane. The tympanic membrane vibrates in response to various pitches of sounds. The bones within the middle ear (the hammer, anvil, and stirrup) act as a movable bridge to transmit these vibrations to the oval window.

The oval window is a small opening between the middle and inner ear, covered by a thin membrane. Because the oval window is so much smaller than the eardrum, the sound is concentrated onto a smaller space, thus amplifying the sound waves.

The base of the stirrup (stapes) fits into the oval window, the membrane between the middle and the inner ear. When stimulated, the stapes vibrates against this membrane, setting the fluid of the cochlea in motion.

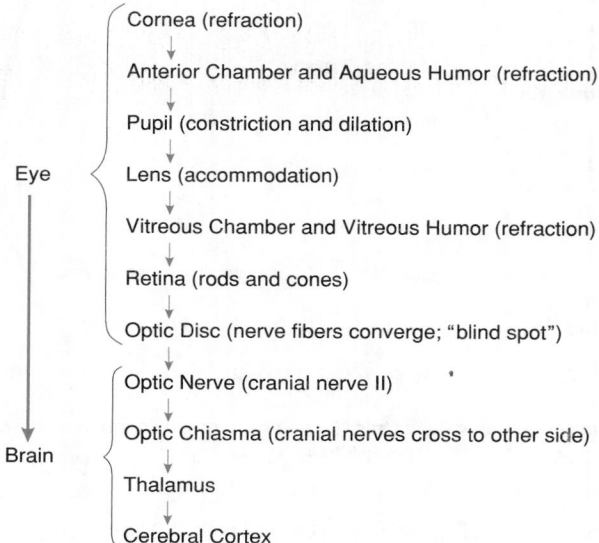

Figure 20-5. Pathway of light transmission.

The wavelike action of the fluid in motion passes the vibrations on to tiny hairlike nerve endings (receptors) in the organ of Corti. The stimulus from the nerve endings in the organ of Corti is sent to the auditory center in the cerebral cortex.

The pathway of sound transmission is summarized in Figure 20-6. Sound waves are amplified in three ways:

- ◆ The ear canal is open, and the resonance there approximately doubles the sound waves.
- ◆ The ossicles (hammer, anvil, and stirrup) act as levers. This mechanical advantage amplifies the sound approximately threefold. (This, when multiplied by the amplification in the ear canal, now equals a total of sixfold amplification.)
- ◆ The relative sizes of the eardrum and the oval window amplify or increase the sound waves approximately 30 times more. (This, when multiplied by the previous amplification, makes a total of approximately 180 times amplification of the original sound.)

Balance and Equilibrium

The sense of static balance is centered in the utricle and the saccule of the inner ear. Balance with movement is associated with the semicircular canals. The impulses of balance and position are transmitted to the brain by the eighth cranial nerve. Sensations of hearing and balance are interpreted within the sensory area of the brain.

Balance is a complex process. In addition to the receptors in the ears, there are *proprioceptors* in the mus-

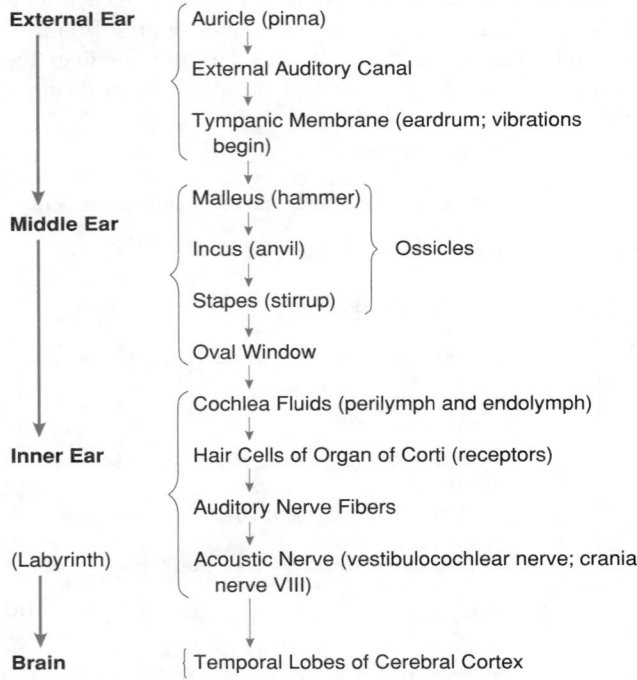

Figure 20-6. Pathway for sound transmission.

cles. Visual input and tactile skin receptors also contribute to our sense of position in space.

Sometimes the motion of the fluid in the ears confuses the mind if there is not an accompanying visual reference. For example, think of your sensation on a carnival ride if you close your eyes or in an airplane movie, even when you are not moving. The dizzy, sometimes ill feeling or the sense of being rotated is called **vertigo** (although vertigo does not have the same meaning as dizziness). True vertigo is caused by a disease of the inner ear or by a defect in the conductive pathways or central nervous system. Nausea often accompanies vertigo, as does tinnitus, a high-pitched buzzing sound or "ringing in the ears."

Taste

The sense of taste is based on the perception of sweet, salty, sour, and bitter flavors and combinations of these. The receptors of taste, located on the tongue, are called taste buds. Chemoreceptors in the taste buds detect chemicals in the solution in the mouth.

Basic tastes are perceived best by the taste buds in certain areas of the tongue (Fig. 20-7). Bitter tastes are sensed at the back of the tongue, sour on both sides, salty on the sides and the tip, and sweet at the tip (apex) of the tongue. (This information may be helpful when administering certain medications.)

Most foods are combinations of more than one taste sensation. Many characteristic tastes are combinations of taste and smell. For example, try tasting an onion while holding your nose; it usually does not taste like an onion.

The sensation of taste is carried to the brain by two cranial nerves: facial (VIII) and the glossopharyngeal (IX). The sense of taste is interpreted in the parietal–temporal cortex.

Smell

The nerve of smell or olfaction is the olfactory nerve, the first cranial nerve. The sensory chemoreceptors for smell are located in the upper nasal cavity in the olfactory epithelial tissue. These impulses are received by the sensory receptors in the olfactory nerve. The interpretation takes place in the olfactory center in the brain. The sense of smell and taste are strongly interrelated.

Touch/Tactile Sense

Your tactile receptors or tactile corpuscles are the receptors for the sense of touch, mostly in the skin. They are constantly receiving nerve impulses, allowing you to feel pain and the pleasures of softness and warmth and alerting you to the dangers of too much heat or cold. There are many more touch receptors in some

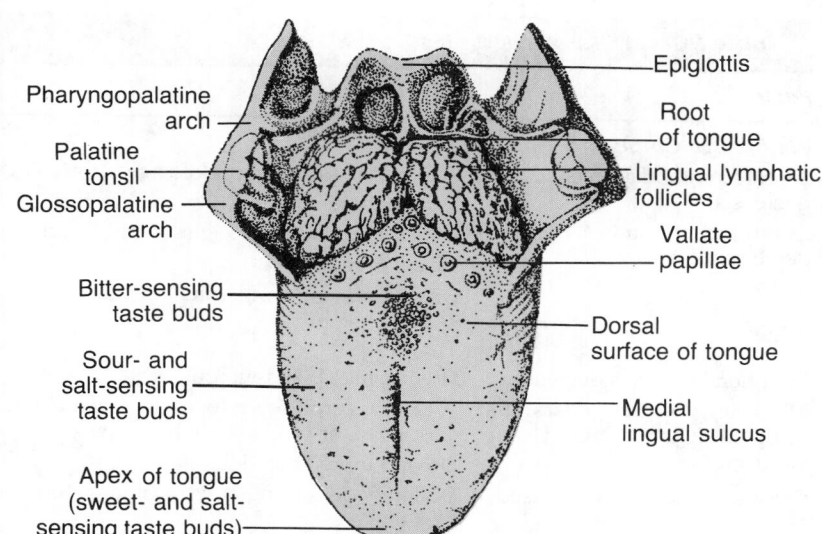

Figure 20-7. Surface of the tongue as seen from above. Note the location of various types of taste buds.

Labels (clockwise from upper left): Pharyngopalatine arch; Palatine tonsil; Glossopalatine arch; Bitter-sensing taste buds; Sour- and salt-sensing taste buds; Apex of tongue (sweet- and salt-sensing taste buds); Epiglottis; Root of tongue; Lingual lymphatic follicles; Vallate papillae; Dorsal surface of tongue; Medial lingual sulcus

areas, such as the fingertips and around the lips, than in other areas. Refer to Figure 18-4, which illustrates some of the sensations noted by the sensory receptors for touch in your skin. Note in this illustration that each of the sensory receptors for different sensations (eg, pain, temperature, pressure) are of a slightly different configuration (shape and size).

Other Sensations

Temperature

There are two types of temperature receptors, one for heat and one for cold. The sensation of heat is transmitted by heat receptors and cold by cold receptors. Temperature receptors are widespread in the body. There are 10 to 15 times the amount of cold receptors in the skin than heat receptors. The ratios between heat and cold receptors vary in different locations. They are abundant in the lips and mucous membranes of the oral and anal regions. The temperature sense is protective to the body, for instance, by preventing burns or by causing shivering or sweating.

Pain

Pain and its management are discussed in detail in Chapter 52. Pain is usually protective. It causes people to move away from a hurtful stimulus or to seek medical attention for an internal disorder. Pain that originates in an internal location but is perceived as a cutaneous sensation is called referred pain. Referred pain is extremely helpful in diagnosing many medical conditions. For example, a patient suffering a heart attack usually feels pain in the left arm, shoulder, or neck area. Pain receptors also respond to extremes in temperature such as pain from a decayed tooth when touched by ice.

Pressure

Mechanical forces that distort or displace tissue can be evaluated by the brain. Tactile receptors can detect fine or light touches. More tactile receptors are found in the hairless portions of the body, such as the eyelids, lips, fingertips, and external genitals. Pressure receptors within deeper tissues, some joints, and some visceral organs permit the sensations of deep pressure.

Proprioception

Location or position of the body depends on proprioceptors and the semicircular canals of the inner ear. Proprioceptors are located in muscles, tendons, and joints and relay information about the relationships of body parts to one another. The nerve fibers from these structures are located in the posterior portion of the spinal cord. The brain's interpretation of these relationships allows us to walk and perform other physical activities.

Effects of Aging on the System

The effects of aging are summarized in Table 20-1.

Eye and Vision Changes

The lens of the eye becomes less elastic with aging and is not able to accommodate well enough to see nearby objects. Reading material must be held at arm's length for it not to seem blurry. In some cases, a book may need to be held so far away to make the letters clear that they can no longer be identified; this condition is called *presbyopia*. Presbyopia is a gradual loss of the function of accommodation and usually begins to be noticeable between the ages of 40 and 45. Glasses, usually bifocal or trifocal lenses, will correct the situation.

Table 20-1. Effects of Aging on the Sensory System

Factor	Result	Nursing Implications
Vision/Eye Changes		
Lens accommodation is decreased.	Presbyopia (starts in middle age) More light needed	May need to advise having a vision check for corrective lenses.
Depth perception is decreased.	Difficulty in judging height of curbs and steps Falls common Driving may be dangerous	Encourage use of hand rails, canes, walkers. Advise to avoid fast moves or turns. Make patient aware of dangers. Encourage a defensive driving class.
Peripheral vision is decreased.	Driving may be dangerous.	Avoid standing at patient's side.
The ability to react to darkness or bright light and night vision are decreased.	Takes longer for eyes to adjust when entering dark room or bright sunlight Driving more hazardous	Advise use of night light. Advise person to avoid night driving if possible.
Color perception is decreased.	Difficulty discerning hues of blue, green, and violet May not be able to read signs Clothing may not match	Use yellow, red, or black for signs. Teach patient the configuration of traffic lights in your area.
A grayish-white ring (arcus senilis) forms around the iris.	Normal sign of aging; does not indicate disease May lower self-esteem and body image	Enhance self-esteem.
Tear formation is decreased.	Dry, itchy eyes Sjögren's syndrome More prone to infection	Advise about medication such as "artificial tears." Advise against rubbing eyes. Encourage regular visual exams.
Fluid circulation in the eye is decreased.	Increased risk of glaucoma	Encourage regular eye examinations, including intraocular pressure measurement.
Hearing/Ear Changes		
Numerous functional and structural changes occur in components of the ear.	Presbycusis Progressive hearing loss Loss of perception to high pitch, sound location, tracking sounds, normal conversation	Discuss hearing aid evaluation. Person may benefit from "helper" dog or special telephone volume controls. Face person when talking. Speak clearly but not too loudly. Advise against driving when it becomes dangerous.
	Increased incidence of vertigo (dizziness) and tinnitus (ringing in ears) Possible frustration and social isolation	Tell patients to use handrails and avoid sudden movement.
Structural changes affect balance and equilibrium.	Increased incidence of falls Dizzy on change of position	Advise about using hand rails. Advise person to change position slowly.
Increased build-up of cerumen.	Hearing loss	Suggest frequent ear examinations.
Taste Changes		
Taste sensation is decreased.	Decreased appetite (dentures also increase loss of taste)	Monitor nutritional status.
	May try to compensate by increasing salt and sugar intake, aggravating conditions such as hypertension and diabetes	Teach about proper nutrition.
Tactile Changes		
Efficiency and the number of sensory nerve endings (all sensations affected) are decreased.	Stronger stimulus needed for person to perceive sensation May not realize they are being burned or frostbitten Pain associated with some conditions may differ	Monitor patient's overall condition. Do not ignore complaints.

Clouding of the lens may occur at any age. The cloudy or opaque lens that results is called a cataract. However, it most often occurs by later middle age in people who are susceptible. As the condition worsens, surgery and corrective contact lenses or eyeglasses are usually required to restore some vision.

As people get older, they need more light to read. This is because the pupil is no longer able to dilate fully and cannot let in enough light. Loss of visual acuity may occur if debris (waste material) builds up within the eye. This process may occur at any time of life but is more common in older people because of their more extended exposure over the years to the ultraviolet rays of the sun.

The slowing of all body secretions may affect the lacrimal glands and may lead to extraordinarily dry eyes. Liquid tears can be used to help provide secretion to the eyes.

Ear and Hearing Changes

Many older people experience a degenerative loss of hearing, called *presbycusis*, which often begins at about age 60. There may be several causes, but the most common is deterioration of the cochlear structures. The specific difficulty most often is a result of the loss of hair cells in the organ of Corti. Usually the loss is most no-

ticeable in certain sound frequencies, particularly very high frequencies.

Other causes of impaired hearing in older people include fusing of the ossicles (small bones in the middle ear), an injury earlier in life, a disorder in the nerve pathway that carries the sound impulses to the brain or in the area of the brain where the impulses are received, or excess decalcification of bone to the point of impairing the sound-conduction qualities of the bone. A hearing aid may help many older people.

Changes in Other Senses

The senses of smell and taste gradually become less keen as a person ages. This is probably caused by loss of nerve function, which interferes with the transmission of the sensations to the brain. Another factor relates to the taste buds. The taste buds are gradually replaced by connective tissue cells as the person ages. At age 75, it is estimated that the person has approximately 40% of the taste buds that were functioning at age 30. With the loss of the sense of taste, the person does not feel hungry and may become emaciated.

The vocal cords of the older person may simply "wear out," making it difficult or impossible to speak. The person is able to whisper at first but may lose that ability as the condition progresses.

Keys for Review

Key Questions for Critical Thinking

1. Describe the five major senses. Describe the type of data gained through each sense.
2. Discuss three things that are needed to make the body aware of information.
3. Describe the effects of aging on the sensory system.

Key Readings

Chabner D. The Language of Medicine, Ed 4. Philadelphia, W.B. Saunders, 1991

Elipoulus C. Caring for the Elderly in Diverse Care Settings. Philadelphia, J.B. Lippincott, 1990

Farrell J. Nursing Care of the Older Person. Philadelphia, J.B. Lippincott, 1990

Memmler RL, Cohen BJ, Woods DL. Structure and Function of the Human Body, Ed 5. Philadelphia, J.B. Lippincott, 1992

Scanlon V, Sanders V. Essentials of Anatomy and Physiology. Philadelphia, F.A. Davis, 1991

Key Readings (continued)

Seeley R, Stephens T, Tate P. Anatomy and Physiology, Ed 2. St. Louis, C.V. Mosby, 1994

Smeltzer SC, Bare BG. Brunner and Suddarth's Textbook of Medical-Surgical Nursing, Ed 7. Philadelphia, J.B. Lippincott, 1992

Thomas CL (Ed). Taber's Cyclopedic Medical Dictionary, Ed 17. Philadelphia, F.A. Davis, 1993

Enrichment Keys

Ackerman D. A Natural History of the Senses. New York, Random House, 1990

McCutcheon M. The Compass in Your Nose and Other Astonishing Facts About Humans. New York, St. Martin's Press, 1989

Stoddart DM. The Scented Ape: The Biology and Culture of Human Odour. New York, Cambridge University Press, 1990

Vogel S. Vital Circuits. New York, Oxford University Press, 1992

Keys to Learning More

Chapter 50: basics of nursing assessment, including gross evaluation of some sensory functions, such as vision and hearing

Chapter 56: medications, some of which are used in the eye or ear

Chapter 57: administration of eye and ear medications

Keys to Learning More (continued)

Unit Thirteen: deviations from normal body structure and function in children

Unit Fourteen: deviations from normal body structure and function in adults

Chapter 73: specific discussion of sensory disorders

Chapter 85: disorders of older people and specific assistance required

21 The Cardiovascular System

Keys For Learning

Learning Objectives

- Describe the functions of the cardiovascular system
- Identify components of plasma
- Outline the structure and functions of the red blood cells, white blood cells, and platelets
- Describe the mechanism of blood clotting
- Identify the four blood groups, and explain Rh
- On a chart, trace the circulation through the heart, naming internal structures and the major arteries that connect to the heart
- Describe the lymphatic circulation and lymphatic tissues
- On a chart, trace blood through systemic and pulmonary circulation
- Describe the conduction system of the heart and how it stimulates a heartbeat
- Discuss the two mechanisms of immunity, cell-mediated and humoral

Key Terms

albumin	hematopoiesis	pericardium
atrium	hemoglobin	phagocytosis
endocardium	hemorrhage	plasma
epicardium	lymph	prothrombin
fibrinogen	lymphocytes	septum
globulin	myocardium	ventricles

Keys to Understanding This Chapter

Unit Three: normal growth and development

Unit Four: organization of the body and integumentary, musculoskeletal, nervous, endocrine, and sensory systems

Key Points

- The cardiovascular system consists of the blood, heart, and blood vessels. The lymphatic system is often included.

Key Points (continued)

- Blood is composed of plasma and formed elements.
- The function of the cardiovascular system is transportation, regulation, and protection by red blood cells, white blood cells, and platelets. Hematopoiesis, formation of blood cells, originates in stem cells in red bone marrow.
- All white blood cells fight infection. Each of the five types has different mechanisms to combat invaders.
- Platelets and numerous clotting factors must react in sequence before clotting can occur.
- The heart is a dual-muscle pump that has the ability to contract and relax in rhythm; the autonomic nervous system also regulates heart rate and influences blood pressure.
- Lymph drains interstitial fluid into lymphatic vessels and returns the fluid back to the veins. Lymph tissues filter blood, destroy pathogens, and develop antibodies against antigens.
- T-cells and B-cells are special lymphocytes that provide immunity to foreign antigens. Cell-mediated immunity uses the T-cells to physically combat invaders. Humoral immunity uses T-cells to activate B-cells, which develop antibodies against invaders.

Key Topics Outline

Structure and Function
  The Blood
  The Heart
  The Blood Vessels
  The Lymphatic System
System Physiology
  Blood Circulation
  Cardiac Conduction
  Cardiac Cycle
  Immunity
Effects of Aging on the System

The cardiovascular system is organized for transportation and communication throughout all parts of the body. In approximately 1 minute, a drop of blood will have traveled through the right side of the heart, the lungs, back through the left side of the heart, and through the systemic circulation and will complete its circuit by returning to the right side of the heart. In this brief time, the cells located at the tip of your toe or the end of your finger receive oxygen from the lungs and nutrients from the intestine and simultaneously send wastes to be excreted.

The cardiovascular system is composed of the heart, blood vessels, and lymphatic vessels and tissues. The cardiovascular system has many functions, which are listed in the accompanying box.

Structure and Function

The Blood

Blood is a versatile vascular fluid. Although it is a liquid, it can change quickly to form a solid clot. The term for that action is coagulation. The function of blood is to maintain a constant environment for the rest of the body's tissues. Thus, homeostasis is maintained because of the blood's liquid viscosity ("thickness"), its ability to carry dissolved substances, and its ability to move to all body parts.

Hematopoiesis (hemopoiesis) refers to the production and maturation of blood cells, the average adult body contains approximately 4 to 6 L of blood. Blood is considered a *connective tissue*. All formed elements in blood are manufactured in red bone marrow. Other hematopoietic tissues, such as lymph nodes and the spleen, produce at least one of the five types of white blood cells (WBCs). Blood is composed of plasma and formed elements, as shown in Figure 21-1. The composition of blood is discussed here, and blood circulation is discussed later in this chapter in the section "System Physiology."

Plasma

Blood **plasma** is the fluid portion of circulating blood. It constitutes 55% of blood volume and is 90% water. The remaining 10% consists of salts; antibodies; food elements; nitrogenous waste products; small amounts of gases, hormones, and enzymes; and plasma proteins.

Salts contained in plasma are sodium, calcium, potassium, and magnesium and the ions of other elements in the form of bicarbonates, sulfates, chlorides, and phosphates. These salts are absorbed by the plasma from food and used by the cells. The maintenance of these salts within the plasma controls the chemical and acid–base balance of the blood and contributes to the chemical and fluid balance of the entire body.

There are four groups of plasma proteins, which are manufactured in the liver. **Albumin** is the most abundant, accounting for 60% to 80% of plasma proteins. Its important function is to provide thickness to the circulating blood volume, thus providing osmotic pressure. (Osmotic pressure draws water from surrounding tissue fluid into capillaries.) Thus, osmotic pressure maintains volume and blood pressure. Loss of albumin can result in dramatic fluid shifts, edema, hypotension, and even death.

Fibrinogen and **prothrombin** are circulating proteins that are essential for blood clotting.

Globulin is the fourth group of plasma proteins. Two types of globulin (alpha and beta) are made in the liver and act as carriers for molecules such as fats. Gamma globulins (immunoglobulins [Ig]) are antibodies. Antibodies fight antigens to provide us with immunity. The section on immunity at the end of this chapter further discusses antigens and antibodies.

Formed Elements

The remaining 45% of blood volume consists of formed elements. These cells are red blood cells (RBCs), white blood cells (WBCs), and platelets.

Red Blood Cells. RBCs, also called *erythrocytes*, are flattened disks that are thinner in the center than at the edges (Fig. 21-2). When mature, they have no nucleus.

Functions of the Cardiovascular System

Functions of the Blood and Lymph

TRANSPORTATION
- Carries oxygen to body cells
- Carries carbon dioxide away from body cells
- Carries water, food, and nutrients to body cells
- Exchanges oxygen for carbon dioxide at cellular level
- Carries waste products away from body cells
- Moves blood to lungs to be oxygenated

COMMUNICATION
- Transports hormones throughout the body
- Transports electrolytes
- Transports enzymes

PROTECTION
- Fights disease and infection (white cells)
- Promotes clotting of blood (specialized cells)
- Provides immunity through antibodies and antitoxins (specialized cells)

REGULATION
- Contributes to regulation of body temperature
- Assists in maintenance of acid–base balance
- Assists in maintenance of fluid-electrolyte balance

Functions of the Lymphatic System

TRANSPORTATION
- Carries fluid away from tissues
- Carries wastes away from tissues

ABSORPTION
- Absorbs fats and transports fats to blood (lacteals)
- Stores blood (spleen)
- Destroys worn out red blood cells

PROTECTION
- Filters waste products out of blood
- Filters foreign substances out of blood (including dead blood cells, bacteria, smoke by-products, cancer cells)
- Destroys bacteria
- Participates in antibody production
- Functions as endocrine gland (thymus)

MANUFACTURE
- Manufactures lymphocytes and monocytes
- Manufactures red blood cells (spleen in fetus)

Functions of the Heart

PUMPING ACTION
- Pumps blood to body and lungs
- Receives blood from body and lungs
- Influences blood pressure

Functions of the Blood Vessels

TRANSPORTATION
- Provides channels through which blood and lymph travel
- Provides areas (capillaries) where transfer of gases, nutrients, fluids, electrolytes, and wastes can take place

RBCs are the most numerous of the blood cells. There are about 25 trillion RBCs in the body. Approximately 3,000 RBCs could be placed side by side within a 1-inch space. They are made from stem cells in red bone marrow. Old and fragile, RBCs wear out and are destroyed about every 120 days by the liver and spleen.

Each RBC contains molecules of the compound hemoglobin (Hgb or Hb). **Hemoglobin** is composed of the iron-containing pigment *heme* and a protein *globin*. (Iron is the pigment that makes RBCs appear red.)

As blood passes through the lungs, the iron in hemoglobin picks up oxygen in a loose chemical combination. When hemoglobin is saturated with oxygen, the blood is bright red. As blood circulates through the capillaries, the hemoglobin gives its oxygen to various cells of the body and picks up their carbon dioxide.

White Blood Cells. WBCs, also known as *leukocytes*, defend the body against disease organisms, toxins, and irritants. They differ greatly from RBCs. Leukocytes con-

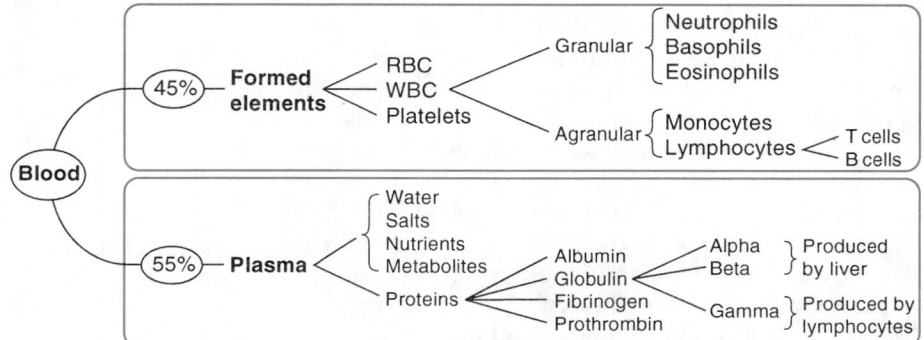

Figure 21-1. Composition of blood.

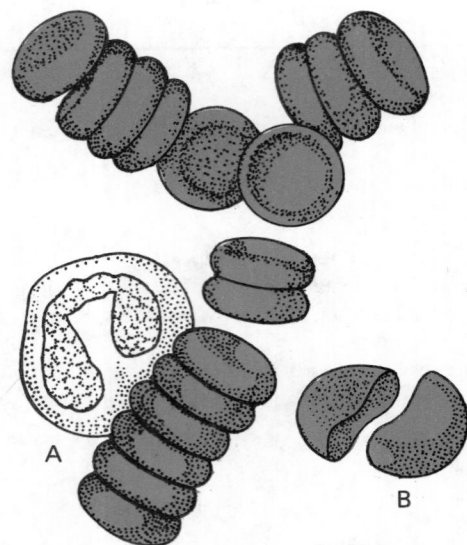

Figure 21-2. Grouped red blood cells. One *white blood cell* **(A)** also is shown. **B** shows a red cell split to show its biconcave shape.

tain nuclei and can move independently in an ameboid fashion. Because of their ability to move away from blood vessels, WBCs can move to sites of infection. They push or squeeze through the capillary wall and rush to the threatened spot. They find their way to foreign or damaged tissues by their attraction to certain chemical substances (*chemotaxis*). They are colorless unless they are stained to be visible under the microscope. Some types of WBCs engulf and devour invaders (**phagocytosis**). Phagocytosis is illustrated in Figure 21-3. Other types of WBCs develop specific mechanisms of defense.

There are two types of leukocytes: granular and agranular (Fig. 21-4). *Granular leukocytes* are divided into three subgroups: neutrophils, basophils, and eosinophils. They are characterized by a speckled or grainy cytoplasm and survive only about 12 hours to 3 days. The *agranular* (or nongranular) *leukocytes* are divided into two subgroups: monocytes and lymphocytes. Under normal conditions, agranular lymphocytes are functional for about 100 to 300 days.

Neutrophils are the most numerous of WBCs. They are considered to be first in the line of defense against bacteria. They increase in number, engulf, and devour invaders by phagocytosis and assist in repairing damaged tissues (see Figure 21-4). Sometimes they die during this activity and collect with bacteria to form pus.

Basophils contain heparin (an anticoagulant) and histamine. Histamine is important in the inflammatory process. *Eosinophils* are believed to detoxify foreign proteins in allergic reactions and parasitic infections.

Monocytes and **lymphocytes,** the two agranular leukocytes, are produced in the lymphatic tissue of the spleen, lymph nodes, and thymus, and in hemopoietic tissues in red bone marrow. *Monocytes* are transformed into macrophages, which are phagocytic cells. There are two types of lymphocytes: T-lymphocytes (T-cells) and B-lymphocytes (B-cells).

Platelets. Platelets, also called *thrombocytes (thrombo* means clot; *cyte* means cell), are the smallest of the formed elements of blood. They are not whole cells, but rather fragments of larger cells. They lack nuclei but are capable of ameboid movement. They are formed in red bone marrow. Platelets are essential for blood clotting.

Blood Clotting and Hemorrhage

Clotting. Blood protects the body from losing vital plasma fluid and blood cells by sealing off broken blood vessels through a process of clotting called coagulation. Otherwise, we would not survive minor cuts and wounds. The process of clot formation involves a number of complex activities within the blood, some of which are not totally understood. The clotting mechanism is illustrated in Figure 21-5.

When tissue is injured, platelets break down and cause the release of a chemical, thromboplastin. This interacts with prothrombin, a protein substance in blood, which

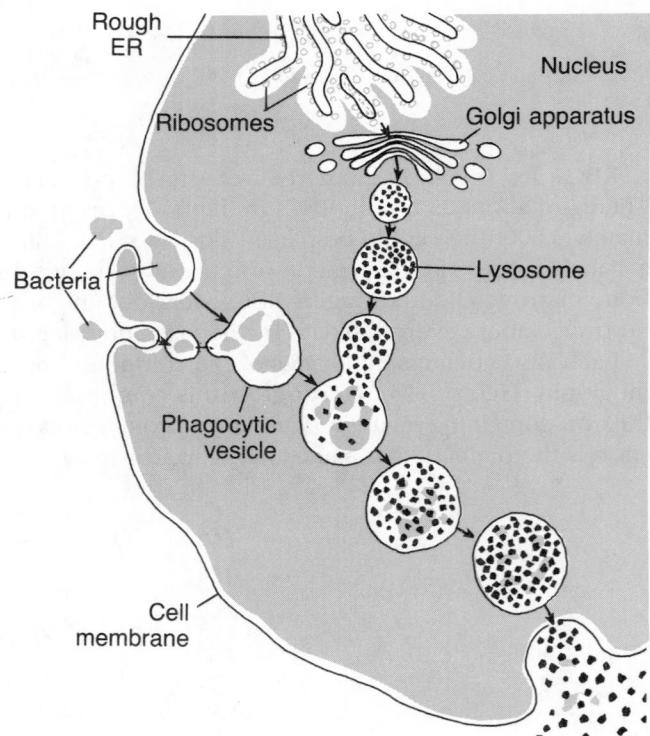

Figure 21-3. Phagocytosis. Bacteria engulfed by the white blood cell are enclosed in a membranous vesicle, which fuses with the cell's lysosome. Digested material is eliminated from the cell.

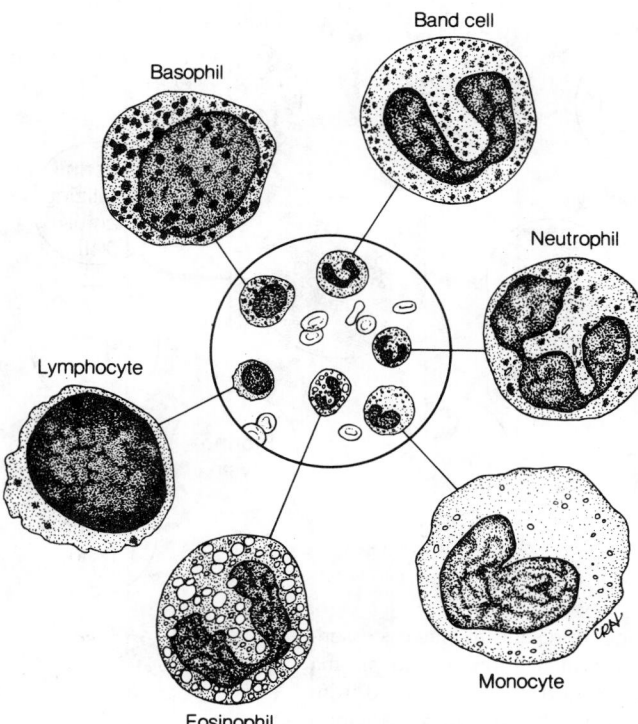

Figure 21-4. Types of white blood cells (leukocytes). Note comparison to red blood cells (the smaller cells in the center circle).

Basophil

Band cell

Neutrophil

Lymphocyte

Monocyte

Eosinophil

further reacts with *fibrinogen* to form threads of fibrin. The threads of fibrin form a net to entrap the cells that build up to form the clot. The clot acts like a plug in a hole and tends to draw injured edges together. As the clot shrinks, a clear yellow liquid called *serum* is squeezed out. Serum is like plasma except that fibrinogen and other clotting elements needed in the coagulation process are no longer present. Coagulation is a complicated mechanism that cannot take place if any necessary elements are missing. Vitamin K is necessary for the formation of prothrombin and other clotting factors. (Most vitamin K is produced by bacteria in the colon.)

A *thrombus* is a stationary clot. An *embolus* is a clot that is circulating. Both of these conditions can lead to death if the arteries to the heart, lungs, or brain are plugged. Several medications are available to treat blood clots.

Hemorrhage. The literal definition of **hemorrhage** is escape of blood from blood vessels, but hemorrhage is usually thought of as the loss of a considerable amount of blood. A cut or torn blood vessel allows blood to escape. As soon as a clot forms, bleeding stops. Therefore, once a blood vessel is broken, clotting becomes very important. Severe hemorrhage is serious because the body loses so much fluid and oxygen-carrying RBCs that death can result. Clotting can be influenced by a variety of factors: force behind the flow of blood, size of the wound,

volume of blood lost, or a deficiency in any of the coagulant substances. Severe hemorrhage is treated by replacing blood lost with blood from another person. This replacement of blood is called a *transfusion*.

Blood Groups

Blood falls into one of four groups A, B, AB, and O. Information about them is given in Table 21-1. These blood types are inherited combinations of antigens and antibodies. These antigens and antibodies (see Table 21-1) are found on the membrane of the RBC. Blood typing determines the ABO and Rh blood groups. Crossmatching is a laboratory test of donor and recipient cells to check for agglutination (clumping of cells). If an incompatible type of blood is given to a patient, a fatal transfusion reaction may result.

Except for blood types, there is no difference in the blood of healthy people of different races. Blood does not carry or transmit mental, emotional, or racial characteristics, and diseases such as acquired immunodeficiency syndrome (AIDS) cannot be transmitted to a blood *donor*.

Rh Factors. Rh factors are also antigens which are inherited, just as blood group is inherited. (The Rh system is named after the Rhesus monkey used in early experiments.) Of the several types of antigens that may be found on the surface of erythrocytes, more than 40 are loosely connected to the Rh system. The most commonly found Rh factor and the one most likely to cause a transfusion reaction is abbreviated D. Blood is tested for the presence of D antigen.

If a person's blood contains D factor, the person is said to be Rh-positive (Rh+ or D+); if this factor is absent, the person is Rh-negative (RH−). The percentage of Rh-negative people is lower in some races than in others; for instance, only approximately 2% to 7% of African Americans and 1% of Asians and Native Americans are found to be Rh-negative.

The presence of D antigen or significant amounts of the less common Rh and other red cell antigens can cause delayed hemolytic transfusion reactions, resulting in anemia in the recipient. When an Rh-negative person receives Rh-positive blood, he or she develops antibodies that could cause a severe reaction to subsequent blood transfusion or to an Rh-positive pregnancy in an Rh-negative mother. (The Rh factor and its effects on pregnancy are discussed in Unit 12.)

The Heart

The heart is a strong, muscular pump about the size of a doubled-up fist. It weighs less than 1 lb (approximately 250–310 g) and lies in the thoracic cavity behind the sternum and between the lungs. The heart is shaped like an irregular and slightly flattened cone.

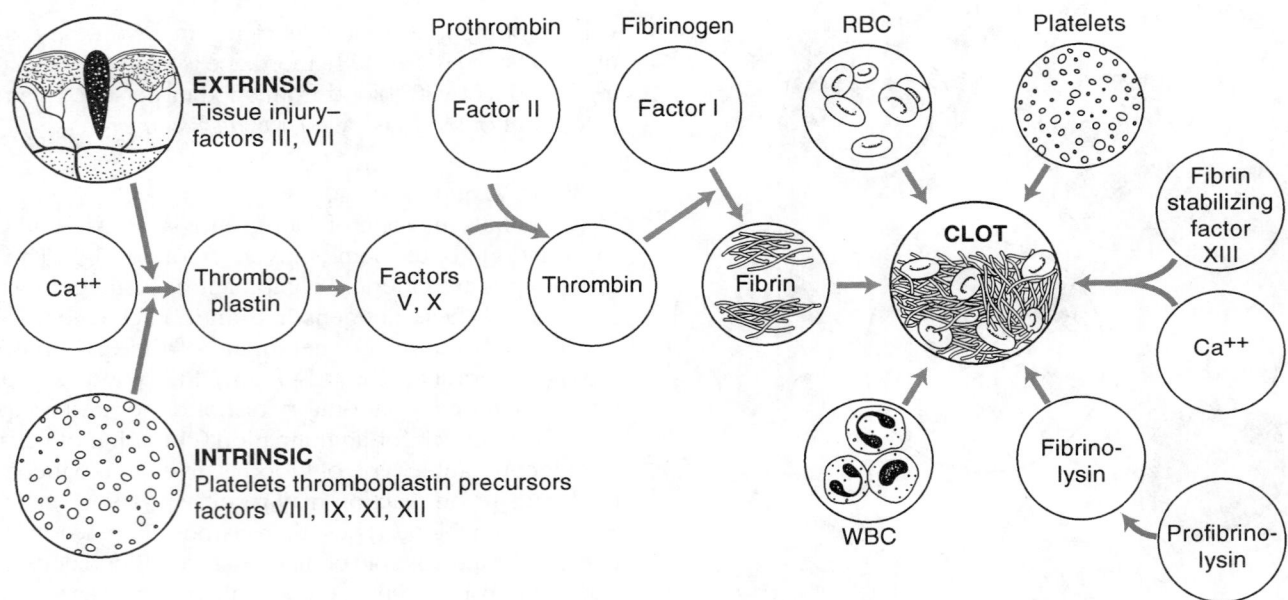

Figure 21-5. The blood-clotting mechanism. The schematic drawing represents the factors essential to change blood into a solid gel. The entire chain reaction in which fibrinogen (a plasma protein) is converted to fibrin (the clot) takes place at the site of vessel damage. (Adapted from Feller I and Archambeault C. Nursing the Burn Patient. Ann Arbor, The Institute for Burn Medicine.)

The heart wall has three layers: endocardium, myocardium, and epicardium. These are shown on the right hand side of Figure 21-6. The **endocardium** is a membrane lining the interior wall of the heart. Thick strong muscles make up the **myocardium,** the middle and thickest layer. Cardiac muscle, discussed in Chapter 17, is a unique type of muscle with striated cells. The **epicardium** is the thin outer layer of the cardiac wall. These three layers in the wall are called collectively **pericardium.**

Heart Chambers and Valves

The heart is divided into right and left halves by a complete muscular wall, the **septum**. The two sides are completely separated with no communication from right to left. Each side is a separate pump.

Heart Chambers. The heart is divided into four chambers, as shown in Figure 21-6. The two upper chambers are the right and left **atria** (singular, atrium). These chambers are the receiving centers for blood. The two lower chambers are the right and left ventricles. **Ventricles** pump the blood out of the heart. Because the left ventricle must contract with sufficient force to send the blood to the entire body, its muscle walls are thicker than the other chambers of the heart.

Heart Valves. Between the atria and the ventricles are one-way flaps of tissue called valves. Their purpose is to prevent back flow of the blood. The valve between the right atrium and the right ventricle is called the tricuspid valve, because it is formed of three flaps (cusps)

Table 21-1. Blood Groups and Compatibilities

Blood Group	Percent of Population	Antigen on Erythrocytes	Antibody in Plasma	Can Donate Red Cells to	Can Receive Red Cells From
A	41%	A	Anti-B (reacts against B antigen)	A or AB	A or O
B	10%	B	Anti-A (reacts against A antigen)	B or AB	B or O
AB	4%	A and B	None	AB	A, B, AB, or O*
O	45%	None	Anti-A and Anti-B (reacts against both A and B factors)	A, B, AB, or O†	O

* Blood group AB is known as the universal recipient, because people of this group may receive red cells from donors of any ABO group in an extreme emergency.
† Blood group O is known as the universal donor, because these red cells may be given to people of any ABO group in an extreme emergency.

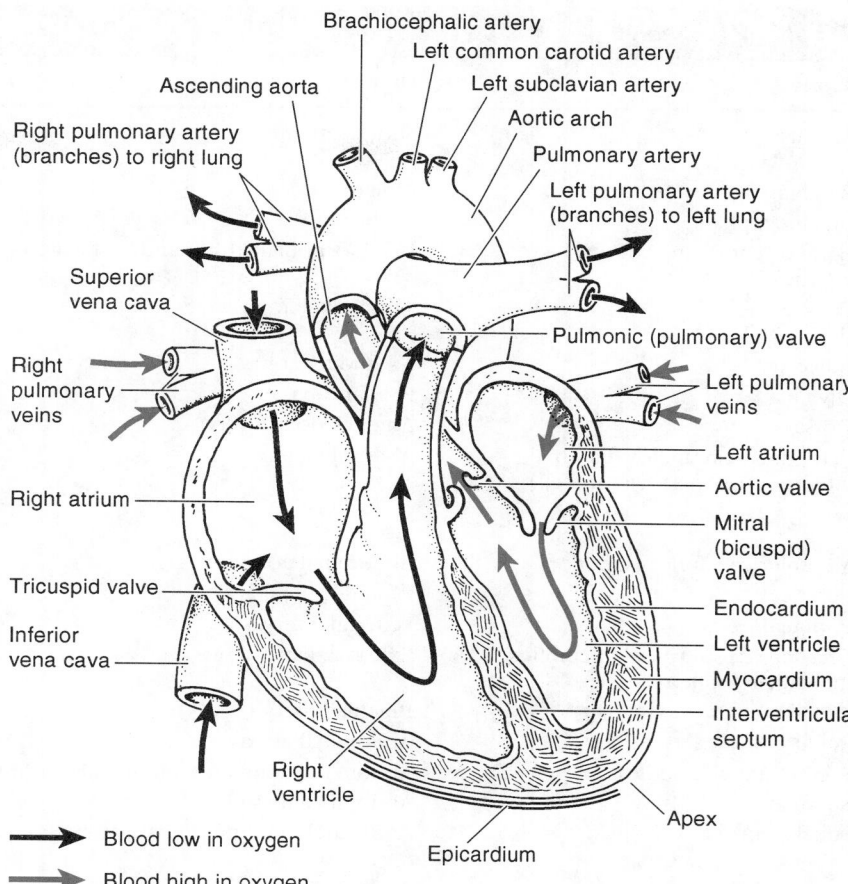

Figure 21-6. Heart and great vessels.

→ Blood low in oxygen

→ Blood high in oxygen

of tissue. The valve between the left atrium and the left ventricle is referred to as the bicuspid or mitral valve; it has only two flaps of tissue. Both of these valves are know as atrioventricular (AV) valves because they are between the artium and the ventricle on each side.

Each of the ventricles empties through a semilunar valve. The pulmonary semilunar valve separates the right ventricle from the pulmonary artery. The aortic semilunar valve separates the left ventricle from the aorta, the largest artery of the body. The semilunar valves prevent back flow from their respective arteries into their ventricles. Cardiac electrical conduction and the physiology of a heartbeat are discussed later in this chapter.

Coronary Arteries

The heart muscle has to have its own supply of blood, because none of the blood that flows through the heart chambers is absorbed for use by heart tissue itself. The first branches from the aorta are those that return to supply the heart tissue with oxygen and nourishment. They are called the coronary *arteries* because they fit over the heart like a crown (corona).

The ventricles receive their blood supply from the right and left coronary arteries, with the left ventricle receiving the greatest amount. (This ventricle does the most pumping, so it needs the most oxygen.) The atria receive much less blood. An important factor in heart physiology is that there are few places where the large coronary arteries join; thus, if one of these places becomes plugged, there is no way for the blood to detour. A blockage of these arteries causes myocardial insufficiency or myocardial infarction (a localized area of dead tissue caused by the lack of blood supply).

The coronary arteries drain into capillaries in the myocardium and then into a coronary sinus or directly into the right atrium.

The Blood Vessels

The blood is carried through the body in a set of tubes or blood vessels: arteries, capillaries, and veins. The arteries carry blood *away* from the heart, the capillaries serve as "in-between" channels, and the veins carry blood *toward* the heart.

Arteries

Arteries are elastic and smooth (involuntary) muscular tubes that carry blood (with oxygen and nutrients) to body cells. Major arteries are listed in Table 21-2 and

Table 21-2. Major Arteries

Name	Origin	Distribution
Axillary	Subclavian artery	Forms brachial artery and seven branches
Brachial	Axillary artery	Upper arm
Brachiocephalic	Aortic arch	Right side of head, neck, and arm
Carotid (common, external, internal)	Brachiocephalic trunk and aortic arch	Neck, thyroid, face, skull, anterior brain, eyes, forehead, nose
Celiac	Abdominal aorta	Stomach, liver, pancreas, duodenum, spleen
Coronary	Ascending aorta	Heart
Digital	Palmar arch	Fingers
Dorsal	Anterior tibial artery	Foot
Iliac (deep circumflex, external, internal, superficial circumflex)	Abdominal aorta	Pelvis, abdominal wall, muscles of abdominal skin, external genitalia and reproductive organs, lower limb
Mesenteric (inferior, superior)	Abdominal aorta	Small intestine, colon, rectum
Peroneal	Posterior tibial artery	Ankle, deep calf muscles
Popliteal	Femoral artery	Knee and calf
Femoral (deep, lateral circumflex, medial circumflex)	External iliac artery	Lower abdominal wall, hip joint, thigh muscles, femur
Radial	Brachial artery	Forearm, wrist, hand
Renal	Abdominal aorta	Kidney, suprarenal gland, ureter
Sacral (lateral, middle)	Abdominal aorta and internal iliac artery	Coccyx, sacrum, rectum
Spermatic	Abdominal aorta	Ureter, epididymis, testes
Subclavian	Aortic arch and innominate artery	Brain, meninges, spinal cord, neck, thoracic walls, upper limbs
Suprarenal	Abdominal aorta	Suprarenal gland
Temporal (middle, superficial)	External carotid artery	Temporal muscle, middle portion of foot
Thoracic (internal, lateral, superior)	Subclavian, axillary, and thoracoacromial artery	Shoulder muscles, axillary glands, muscles of chest, anterior thoracic wall, mediastinal structures, diaphragm
Tibial (anterior, posterior)	Popliteal artery	Leg, ankle, foot, heel
Ulnar	Brachial artery	Forearm, wrist, and hand
Vertebral	Subclavian artery	Muscles of neck, vertebrae, spinal cord, cerebellum, interior of cerebrum

illustrated in Figure 21-7. The largest artery, the aorta, is divided into the ascending aorta, aortic arch, thoracic aorta, and abdominal aorta. From the aorta, the arteries branch into smaller vessels, like branches from the central trunk of a tree. The smallest of the arteries are called arterioles.

Capillaries

From the arterioles, blood flows into the smallest blood vessels of all, capillaries. Capillaries are so small that the tiny RBCs must pass through them in single file. The walls of capillaries are one cell thick, allowing oxygen and food to pass through. (One estimate of the total length of blood vessels in the body is 60,000 miles, most of which is made up of capillaries.) Here, blood flows slowly and in a single file, allowing time for oxygen and nutrients to leave the blood vessels and enter body tissues. Ecchymotic areas (black and blue marks) are ruptured capillaries. Chapter 16 discusses transport of nutrients, salts, gases, and wastes across the plasma membrane of the cell and through the capillary wall. Exchanges through the capillary wall are due to diffusion and filtration. The osmotic pressure or pulling force of albumin (a plasma protein) within capillaries pulls interstitial fluid into capillaries. The fluid that is pulled back into capillaries has cellular waste products that are on their way to the kidneys for excretion.

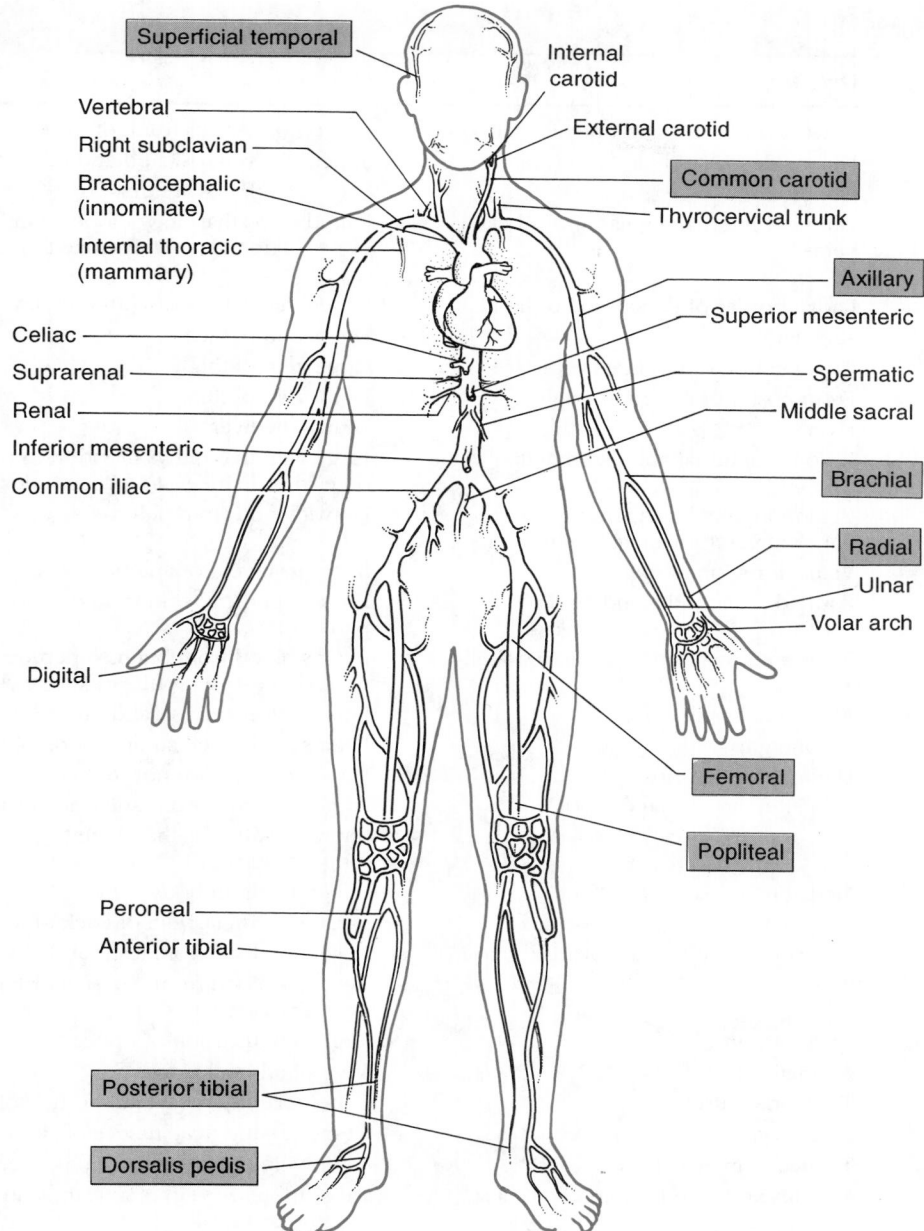

Figure 21-7. Schematic drawing of the arterial system. The arterial system carries blood away from the heart. The boxes indicate major pressure points (pulse points). These are used to count the pulse or to stop hemorrhage.

Veins

At the same time that materials are being delivered to cells, waste products are being picked up. From capillaries, the blood starts back toward the heart through venules, the smallest veins. The branches of the veins grow larger and fewer as they near the heart, until finally the blood reaches the superior and inferior venae cavae, two large veins that deliver blood to the right atrium. This blood is dark red because the oxygen has been replaced with carbon dioxide and other wastes. Major veins are listed in Table 21-3 and illustrated in Figure 21-8.

Valves contribute to efficient venous flow from the extremities and permit blood to flow in one direction only. Also contributing to venous return is the location of veins between skeletal muscles; muscle contractions squeeze the blood toward the heart. The blood in veins has lost the original force from the contractions of the

Table 21-3. Major Veins

Name	Origin	Description
Axillary	Junction of basilic and brachial veins	Portion of venous trunk of upper extremity
Basilic	Ulnar side of hand	Superficial vein of hand and forearm
Brachial	Upper arm	Each vein drains an arm
Brachiocephalic	Union of internal jugular and subclavian veins	Paired veins that draw blood from head, neck, and upper extremities (They unite to form superior vena cava.)
Cephalic	Radial border of dorsal side of hand	Superficial vein of arm and forearm
Facial	Angular vein	Deep vein of face
Femoral	Continuation of popliteal vein	Large vein of thigh
Femoral, deep	From posterior region of thigh	Deep vein of thigh
Hepatic	Liver	Drains the liver
Iliac, common	Union of internal and external iliac veins	Large vein that draws blood from pelvis and leg (One on each side meets to form inferior vena cava.)
Iliac (external, internal)	Behind inguinal ligament and near upper part of greater sciatic foramen	Draws blood from pelvis
Jugular, anterior	Veins in region of lower lip	Superficial vein of anterior neck
Jugular, external	Formed at parotid gland	Large superficial vein from exterior cranium and deep parts of face
Jugular, internal	From transverse sinus at base of skull	Drains blood from brain, superficial parts of face, and neck (largest vein of head and neck)
Lumbar	Abdominal wall	Four or five veins of abdominal walls
Phrenic, inferior	Diaphragm	Drains abdominal surface of diaphragm
Popliteal	Union of tibial veins	Large vein in posterior region of knee
Radial	Palmar arches of hand	Large deep veins on radial side of forearm
Renal	Kidneys	Short thick trunks that drain the kidneys (left is longer than right)
Saphenous, great	Medial marginal vein of foot	Longest vein in body
Saphenous, small	Marginal vein	Large superficial vein of back of leg
Spermatic	Testicular vein in male, ovarian vein in female	Receives blood from testis and epididymis in males Receives blood from pampiniform plexus of broad ligament in females
Subclavian	Axillary vein	Main venous trunk of upper extremity
Suprarenal	Adrenal gland	Vein of adrenal glands
Temporal, middle	Temporal muscle	Superficial vein of lateral portion of stomach
Temporal, superficial	Lateral scalp	Veins of superficial tissues of skull
Thoracic, internal	Tissues of intercostal spaces	Deep vein of chest that drains intercostal spaces
Thoracic, lateral	Muscles and glands of anterior chest	Large tributary vein of axillary vein that drains the lateral thoracic wall
Tibial, anterior	Leg tissue	Deep veins of anterior leg
Tibial, posterior	Deep leg tissues	Deep veins of posterior leg
Ulnar	Palmar arches of hand	Large deep veins of medial aspect of forearm
Vena cava, inferior	Right and left iliac veins	Returns blood from lower half of body
Vena cava, superior	Two innominate veins	Drains blood from upper half of body

heart during the slow journey through capillaries; therefore, veins do not pulsate. When a vein is cut, the walls collapse and blood flows in a steady stream, rather than pulsating like arterial blood.

In venous insufficiency, the pull of gravity reduces the return of venous blood. The extremities are the most affected by venous insufficiency. Blood can pool and stagnate in the lower legs, ankles, and feet. Skin coloring to these areas may look ruddy or cyanotic. Capillary refill is delayed. If left untreated, stasis ulcers may form. Patients with poor venous return should elevate their legs above their heart level whenever possible. To increase venous return (and permit fresh blood to enter), active or passive range of motion leg exercises should be done when standing or sitting still for long periods (see Chapter 43).

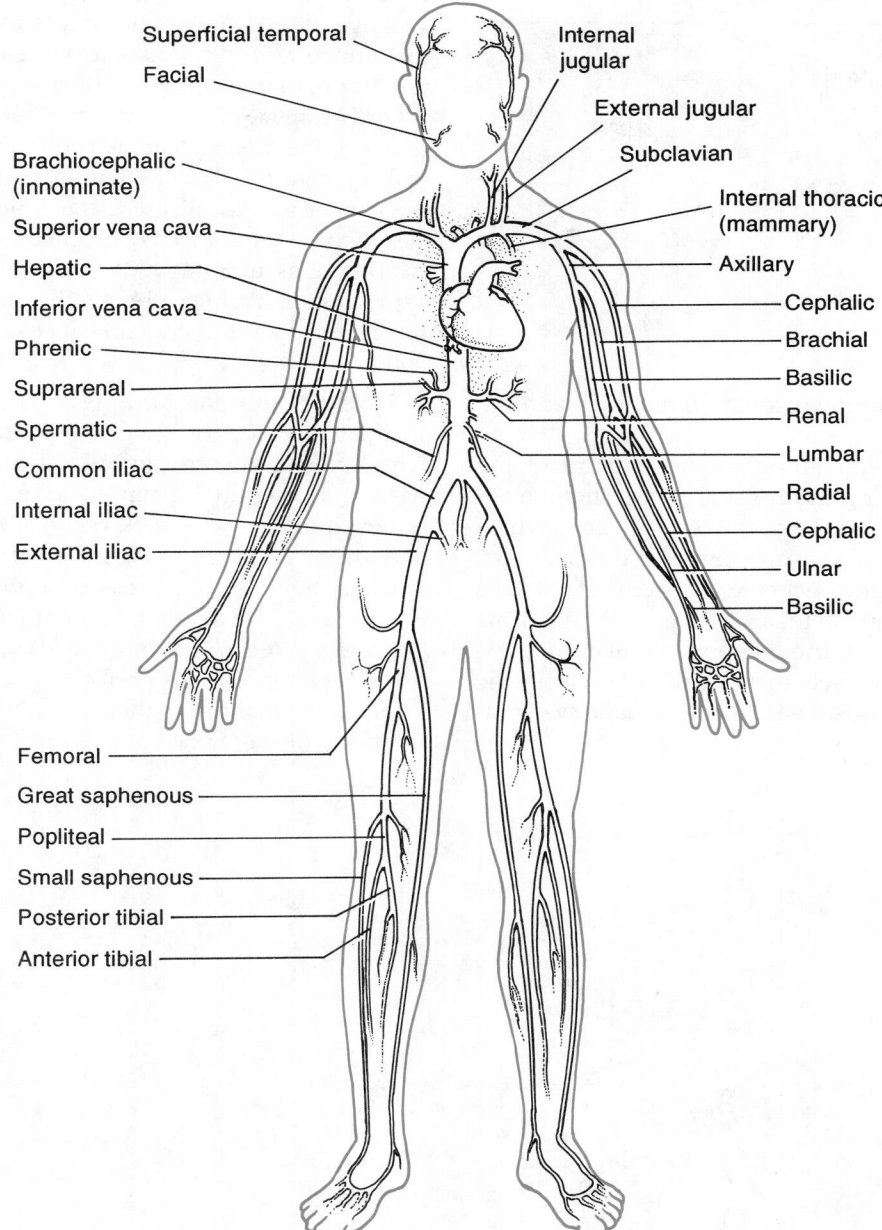

Superficial temporal
Facial
Internal jugular
External jugular
Subclavian
Brachiocephalic (innominate)
Internal thoracic (mammary)
Superior vena cava
Hepatic
Axillary
Inferior vena cava
Cephalic
Phrenic
Brachial
Suprarenal
Basilic
Spermatic
Renal
Common iliac
Lumbar
Internal iliac
Radial
External iliac
Cephalic
Ulnar
Basilic
Femoral
Great saphenous
Popliteal
Small saphenous
Posterior tibial
Anterior tibial

Figure 21-8. Schematic drawing of the venous system. The veins carry blood toward the heart.

The Lymphatic System

Body cells normally are bathed in tissue fluid. Some of this fluid drains into blood capillaries, which go directly to the veins. Another group of vessels, called the lymphatic system, also drains this fluid. The first group of these vessels is a network of tiny **lymph** capillaries in which excess fluid and certain other waste products collect to form the thin watery colorless liquid known as lymph. Because lymph originally is derived from plasma, its composition is much the same, except that lymph is lower in protein content.

Once these proteins have entered the lymphatic system, they will be deposited into veins and returned to the systemic circulation. Lymphatic capillaries called *lacteals* absorb digested fats in the small intestine. The lymphatic system also has several mechanisms to protect the body from infection and provide immunity. Functions of the lymphatic system are listed in the box.

Lymph only carries fluid *away* from tissues but does not have a pumping system of its own. Its circulation depends on the movement of skeletal muscles. Muscular contractions and pressure changes produced in

Functions of the Lymphatic System

- ♦ Filters out waste products and foreign substances (including dead blood cells and cancer cells)
- ♦ Transports digested fats to bloodstream
- ♦ Manufactures lymphocytes and monocytes
- ♦ Drains off excess tissue fluid
- ♦ Destroys bacteria
- ♦ Stores blood
- ♦ Destroys red blood cells
- ♦ Produces antibodies

the thoracic cavity during respiration assist with lymph circulation.

The lymph from the upper right quadrant of the body drains into the right lymphatic ducts. The remainder of the body is drained into the thoracic duct, which drains into the left subclavian vein. The thoracic duct and the right lymphatic duct enter the veins at the base of the neck where lymph mixes with the blood plasma and becomes part of the general circulation. It is through these two vessels that digested fats from the lacteal reach the bloodstream. The lymphatic system is illustrated in Figure 21-9.

Cancer cells can travel from their primary site of invasion to distant sites in the lymph nodes. Lymph nodes may function to filter out cancer cells or may inadvertently spread the cancer to other sites of the body. That is why when surgery is performed for cancer, the lymph nodes in the area also are tested. If there are no cancer cells present in adjoining lymph nodes, it is likely that the cancer was localized. If the cancer is spreading, it is said to be *metastasized*. In some cases, the adjoining lymph nodes are removed during surgery. This may be a precautionary measure, or the nodes may already have been found to contain cancer cells.

Lymph Nodes and Nodules

Small bundles of special lymphoid tissue termed lymph nodes (incorrectly called lymph glands) are situated in clusters along lymphatic vessels. Many of these nodes appear in the neck (cervical), groin (inguinal), and armpits (axial; see Figure 21-9). Before the lymph reaches the veins, it passes through these nodes. The lymph nodes are made up of lymphatic tissue, which is densely packed with lymphocytes.

These lymph nodes perform several vital functions. The most important is that of filtration. Lymph enters the node through several afferent ("bringing toward")

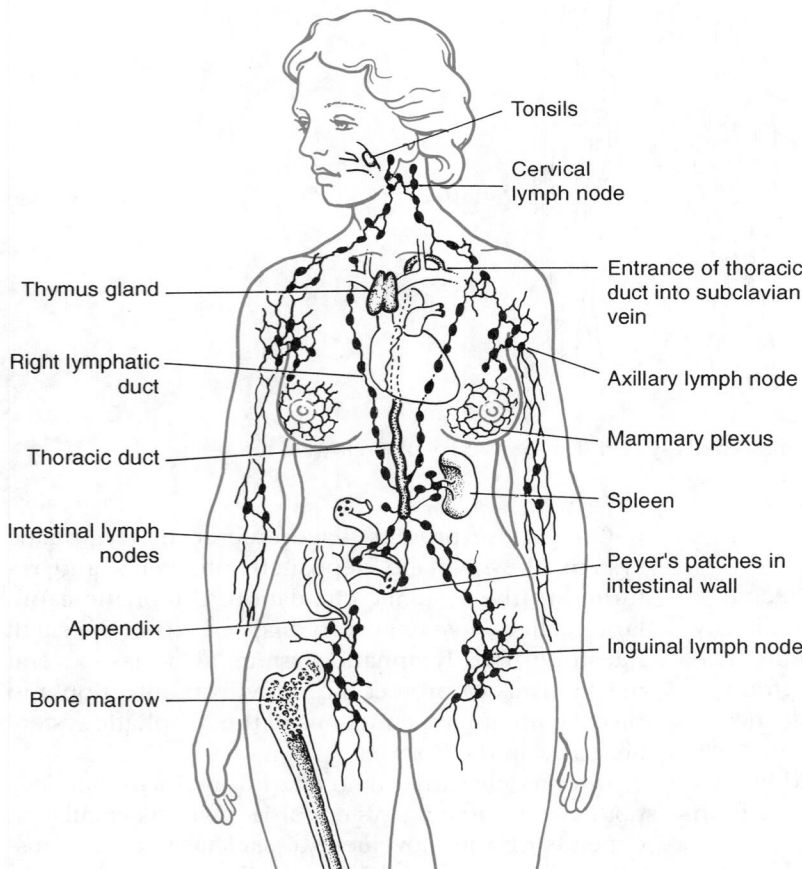

Tonsils

Cervical lymph node

Thymus gland

Right lymphatic duct

Thoracic duct

Intestinal lymph nodes

Appendix

Bone marrow

Entrance of thoracic duct into subclavian vein

Axillary lymph node

Mammary plexus

Spleen

Peyer's patches in intestinal wall

Inguinal lymph node

Figure 21-9. Lymphatic system showing the major lymphatic organs and vessels.

lymph vessels. Lymphatic tissue filters out dangerous substances (such as cancer cells and bacteria), dead RBCs, and foreign matter (such as smoke byproducts). The lymph then flows away from the node through one efferent ("taking away") lymph vessel and into the bloodstream. Lymph nodes manufacture lymphocytes and monocytes and add them to lymph for transportation to the blood.

The "swollen glands" that may appear in the cervical, inguinal, and axial regions are really lymph nodes at work. They are trying to filter and destroy pathogens. The nodes have enlarged as their macrophages (phagocytic cells) eat and destroy invaders.

Lymph nodules are small masses of lymphatic tissues of the epithelium of mucous membranes. Because membranes line cavities that open to the external environment, nodules are in strategic locations to filter substances entering the body.

Areas of Lymphatic Tissue

Some areas of lymph nodules or tissues have special names, for example, Peyer's patches in the small intestine.

Tonsils. Tonsils form a ring of lymphatic tissue around the pharynx. This tissue forms a protective barrier for substances entering the oral and respiratory passages.

Spleen. The spleen is a mass of lymphoid tissue and is usually considered part of the lymphatic system. It is a somewhat flattened, dark purple organ about 6 in (15.24 cm) long and 3 in (7.62 cm) wide, located directly below the diaphragm, above the left kidney, and behind the stomach (see Figure 23-4).

The spleen has several functions. In the fetus, the spleen produces RBCs (later produced by red bone marrow). In an adult, the spleen destroys old RBCs and forms bilirubin from the hemoglobin in RBCs. It also filters and phagocytizes pathogens and other foreign materials in the blood. It produces two types of leukocytes, lymphocytes and monocytes, which then enter the circulation and help fight infection. It contains specially treated B-lymphocytes, known as plasma cells, which are able to produce antibodies against foreign antigens. It also acts as a blood reservoir; it can release blood quickly in an emergency, such as a hemorrhage.

Although the functions of the spleen are very important, it can be removed without ill effects. A person without a spleen, however, is more susceptible to some bacterial infections, such as pneumonia and meningitis. After a splenectomy, removal of the spleen, its functions are taken over by the liver, bone marrow, and lymph nodes.

Thymus. The thymus is a small gland that weighs 1 oz at most. It is located in the mediastinum in the upper chest. With increasing age, the size of the thymus decreases. Little or no active thymus may be found in adults. It functions as an endocrine gland and is active in the production of immunologic competence. The thymic hormones enable specially treated lymphocytes, called T-cells, to participate in the recognition of foreign antigens. Colonies of T-cells that have seeded lymph nodes and other organs are apparently able to produce new T-cells under the stimulation of the various thymic hormones. T-cells physically attack other cells that are infected with viruses, fungi, cancerous cells, and transplanted human tissues. Without the benefit of the thymus and the T-cells that it created, we would have no immunity to diseases. This concept is important in the study of disorders such as AIDS.

System Physiology

Blood Circulation

Blood flows in a circuitous route throughout the entire body. Blood flow in and out of the heart is illustrated in Figure 21-6. Two other sections of the route are called systemic circulation and pulmonary circulation.

Systemic Circulation

The first part of the circulatory route is systemic (general circulation). Its purpose is to carry blood, and thus nutrients and oxygen, to cells of the body and to return with accumulated waste products. As blood leaves the left ventricle, it surges into the largest artery of the body, the aorta. The aorta is further divided into the ascending aorta, aortic arch, thoracic aorta, and abdominal aorta, which is divided into smaller arteries. The blood travels through smaller and smaller arterial branches. From the smallest arteries, the arterioles, the blood enters capillaries, where oxygen and food are exchanged for waste products. The blood then begins its journey back to the heart from capillaries to venules, then to larger veins, and finally through the inferior and superior venae caveae to the right artium, thus completing the circuitous route.

Hepatic-Portal Circulation. The hepatic-portal circulation is a subdivision of systemic circulation. It is an efficient method of transporting raw materials in the form of carbohydrates, fats, and proteins to the liver.

The hepatic-portal circulation is unique because it begins and ends with capillaries. The capillaries from the stomach, intestine, spleen, and pancreas empty into valves and then veins, which drain into a common vessel, the hepatic portal vein. The *portal vein* leads into the liver.

In the liver, blood again enters capillaries, called *sinusoids.* Here the liver extracts appropriate materials and makes chemical modifications on them. The liver synthesizes, stores, detoxifies, regulates, and transforms these raw materials into useful substances needed by the entire body. The useful substances and the blood then empty into the *hepatic vein*. The hepatic vein leads to the inferior vena cava.

Pulmonary Circulation

The phase of circulation in which blood is pumped through the lungs to get rid of waste products (particularly CO_2) and to pick up a supply of oxygen (O_2) is called pulmonary circulation. Blood in the general circulation flows from the right ventricle and into the pulmonary artery (the only artery in the body that carries *unoxygenated* blood). The blood continues to capillaries in the lungs where carbon dioxide, carried in hemoglobin, is exchanged for oxygen. The blood in the lung capillaries is collected by small veins that combine eventually into four pulmonary veins, which pour oxygenated blood into the left atrium. (The pulmonary veins are the only veins that carry *oxygenated* blood.)

Cardiac Conduction

There are special bundles of unique tissue in the heart (Fig. 21-10). The first of these bundles is embedded in the wall of the right atrium at the junction of the superior and inferior venae cavae. It is called the *sinoatrial node* (SA node), and it is the "pacemaker" of the heart. The heartbeat originates in the SA node. The SA node sets the pace, and the rest of the heart follows its bidding. The swift message is sent out through the muscular tissue of the atria, which causes them to contract. This contraction forces the blood through the triscupid and mitral valves down into the ventricles (see Figure 21-6).

The other bundle, the *atrioventricular node* (AV node), is found in the lower part of the septum between the atria. The AV node picks up the message like a receiving station. The impulse is then transmitted down the *bundle of His* (pronounced hiss). This bundle of fibers originates from the lower part of the septum and is sometimes called "the coordinator." The fibers in the bundle of His penetrate the ventricular muscle and terminate in the *Purkinje fibers*. When the Purkinje fibers pick up the message, they stimulate the ventricles to contract. When the right ventricle contracts, the blood is forced through the pulmonary valve into the pulmonary artery. When the left ventricle contracts, the blood is forced through the aortic valve, into the aorta (see Figures 21-6 and 21-10). The heart then rests for a short period between beats. (Failure of this electrical impulse results in *heart block*.)

After blood is squeezed from the atria into the ventricles, the tricuspid and mitral valves close to prevent the blood from flowing back into the atria when the ventricles contract. The aortic and pulmonic valves

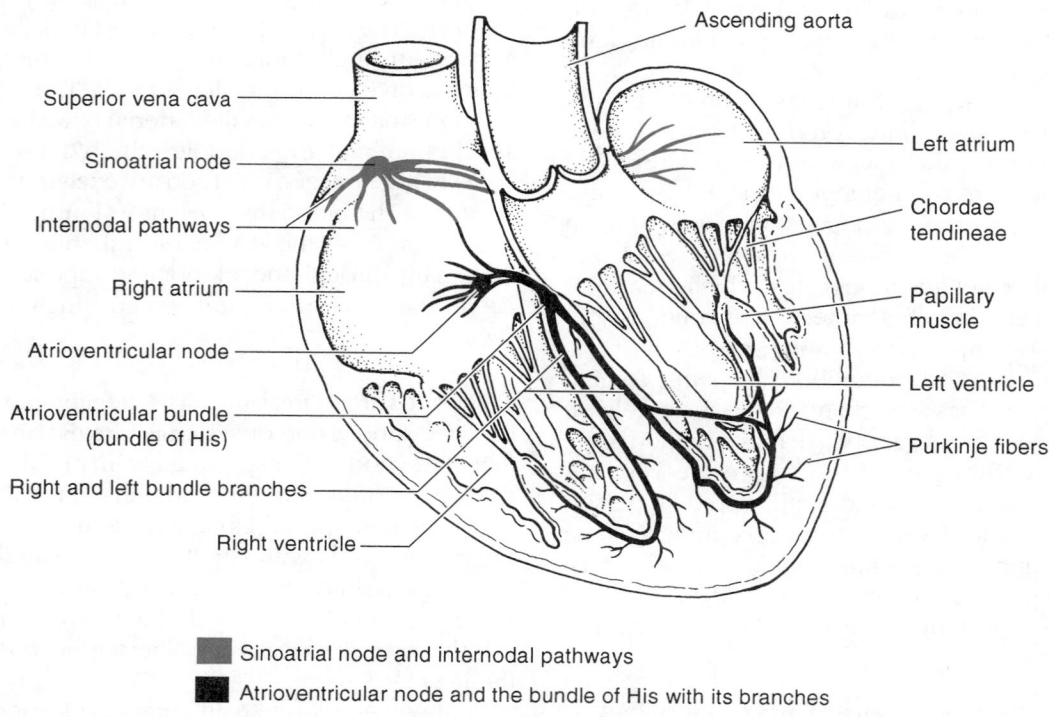

Sinoatrial node and internodal pathways

Atrioventricular node and the bundle of His with its branches

Figure 21-10. Conduction system of the heart.

close after the blood has been forced into the pulmonary artery and aorta.

Regulation of Heart Rate. The heart has several features that combine to regulate its rate. Cardiac muscles have autorhythmaticity, that is, the ability to contract spontaneously and regularly without neural input. The atria, septum, and ventricles can generate separate heartbeats.

To maintain homeostasis in individual situations, input from cardiac centers in the medulla is sent to the heart by way of autonomic nerves. A complex distribution, it has both accelerating and braking devices. Together, they permit an accurate and delicate control of heart rate.

> **Key Concept**
>
> Conduction system of the heart:
>
> ◆ SA (sinoatrial) node (pacemaker)
> ◆ AV node
> ◆ Bundle of His (AV bundle)
> ◆ Right and left bundle branches
> ◆ Purkinje fibers to muscles of ventricles

Cardiac Cycle

In less than 1 second, both atria contract as both ventricles relax, followed immediately by the contraction of both ventricles and the relaxation of both atria. This sequence of dual contractions, the atria followed by the ventricles, is called *systole.* The dual relaxation of the atria followed by the ventricles is called *diastole.* This is considered one cardiac cycle or one heart beat. The heart is really two separate pumps, the atrial "primer pump" and the ventricular "power pump."

> **Key Concept**
>
> The contraction that pumps the blood from the heart is called *systole,* and the period when the heart relaxes is called *diastole.* The heart is actually in systole twice, once for the atria and once for the ventricles. Additionally, both the atria and the ventricles have periods of diastole. If the terms systole and diastole are used without reference to either atria or ventricles, the reference implies the contraction and relaxation of the ventricles.

Pulse

Arterial walls are strong and elastic. They expand as the heart pumps blood to the body; this rhythmic expansion is the *pulse.* The pulse can be felt where arter-

ies are close to the surface. These locations are named for the artery in each area: radial (wrist), carotid (neck), popliteal (back of knee), femoral (groin), tibial (ankle), pedal (foot), and temporal (temple). These points are known as pressure points or pulse points and are shown in Figure 21-7.

Blood Pressure

Fluid always exerts pressure against the walls of its container. Blood pressure is the force that blood exerts against the walls of blood vessels. The force is greatest as blood leaves the left ventricle to start its journey through the aorta, the body's largest artery. The differences in blood pressure as blood flows through the systemic circulation are necessary for filtration of nutrients through capillaries to occur.

> **Key Concept**
>
> Blood flows from high pressure to low pressure.

Regulation of Blood Pressure. Many factors other than the force and rate of the pumping heart are related to maintenance of blood pressure. They include the amount and contents of circulating blood, elasticity and ability of smooth muscles in arterial walls to dilate and constrict, plaque build-up on arterial walls, kidney function, and hormones. The arteries become less elastic with age. Scientist believe that diet, physical and emotional status, smoking, and heredity influence blood pressure.

Heart Sounds

When heart valves close, sounds are produced. These sounds can be heard with a stethoscope. The first heart sound is called the "lubb" and is produced by closure of AV valves when the ventricles contract. The second sound is called the "dub" or "dupp" and is produced by the closure of semilunar valves when the ventricles relax. The first sound is loudest and longest.

Murmurs are extra heart sounds. A heart murmur may be of clinical significance. It may be caused by narrowing (stenosis) of a valve or blood regurgitation (going backward, leaking) through a valve that does not close properly. Many children and 10% of adults have nonpathologic murmurs, called "functional murmurs."

Immunity

Immunity is the body's ability to destroy pathogens or prevent infectious diseases. It is discussed briefly here because it involves the blood and lymphatic system, which are discussed in this chapter. Immunity is only one of several defense mechanisms in the body.

Nonspecific Immunity

Previous chapters have discussed several nonspecific defense mechanisms, including the following:

♦ The skin provides physical barriers and secretes enzymes that can kill bacteria.
♦ The stomach contains hydrochloric acid, which destroys pathogens.
♦ The respiratory tract contains cilia and macrophages (phagocytic cells) in its mucous membrane lining.
♦ Neutrophils and monocytes ingest and destroy bacteria and toxins and remove cellular debris.
♦ Interferon is a protein made by several types of cells that inhibit virus production and infection.

Specific Immunity

Specific immunity is the ability to recognize and respond to specific substances. These substances also are remembered later. Specific immunity is divided into two categories: cell-mediated immunity and humoral immunity. *Lymphocytes*, cells present in blood and lymphatic tissue, are the major means of providing capability for immunity. Lymphocytes are responsible for both types of specific immunity. *Cell-mediated immunity* results from activation of sensitized T-lymphocytes. *Humoral immunity* results from antibodies in body fluids that are synthesized and secreted by B-lymphocytes.

Special Considerations in Children
Immunity

Some childhood immunizations are not given until the child is 15 to 18 months old. This is because the thymus and immune system are not fully mature. They would not be able to recognize antigens in the vaccines as foreign. In addition, the fetus receives antibodies which pass across the placental barrier from the mother. The infant who is breast-fed receives additional antibodies via the breast milk.

Important to the understanding of immunity are the terms antigen and antibody. *Antigens* are foreign protein substances that stimulate the production of antibodies. Foreign antigens stimulate specific immune responses. Examples of foreign antigens are dust, pollen, and viruses.

The body responds to foreign invaders by producing *antibodies*. Antibodies are also called immunoglobulins or gamma globulins. Antibodies are derived from lymphocytes and are involved in humoral immunity. There are five groups of antibodies: IgG, IgA, IgM, IgD, and IgE. Each antigen (foreign invader) will stimulate the production of its own specific antibody. The body can

---

Table 21-4. Effects of Aging on the Cardiovascular and Immune Systems

Factor	Result	Nursing Implications
Metabolic rate is decreased.	Decreased body temperature	Offer blankets and keep room warm.
	Patient may be febrile, even though temperature is below 98.6°F	*Change* in temperature is often more significant than actual temperature.
Blood vessel walls are more rigid.	Increased blood pressure	Advise to decrease fat intake, increase potassium intake, and reduce sodium intake.
		Assess patient on multiple antihypertensive medications for hypotension.
Chest wall size may be reduced because of kyphosis and osteoporosis.	Inefficient coughing	Avoid exposure to cold or damp conditions.
	Susceptible to upper respiratory infections and pneumonia.	Encourage exercise and efficient coughing.
Elasticity of the tracheobronchial tree is lost.	Respiratory rate and total lung capacity may not change.	Assess for dyspnea, cyanosis, or other signs of oxygen deprivation.
Fibrotic changes occur in heart muscle and conduction system.	Decreased heart rate	Pace activities to provide rest periods.
	Irregular heart rate	Teach patient how to take own pulse and to be aware of his or her normal rate.
Ability of cells to absorb oxygen is decreased.	Heart rate takes longer to return to normal after exercise	Encourage rest periods.
Production of leukocytes is decreased.	Less response to infection	Watch for early signs of infection (increased fatigue, anorexia) because the body will not show fever or elevated white count.
	May feel less pain	
		Keep nutritional levels high.
Weakened blood vessels dilate.	Varicose veins	Prevent pressure ulcers.

make about 1 million individual antibodies. Antibodies do not destroy antigens; they label them for destruction. In the process of humoral immunity, macrophages destroy antibodies after they have been "prepared" for destruction.

Key Concept

Lymphocytes, formed in red bone marrow and lymphatic tissues, are able to transform into specialized cells called T-cells and B-cells. The thymus is responsible for formation of T-cells, which attack infected cells and provide cell-mediated immunity. B-cells react to the presence of antigens and transforming antibodies, which recognize and tag antigens for destruction. The bone marrow initiates the formation of B-cells.

Effects of Aging on the System

The cardiovascular system has functional loss of abilities associated with aging. Table 21-4 summarizes major effects of aging on the cardiovascular system. Normal changes also are influenced by heredity, hormones, dietary habits, lifestyle, and stress levels.

As a person gets older, the blood vessels often become less elastic. This depends, in part, on genetic factors and current lifestyle. This condition is known as arteriosclerosis (literally, hardening of the arteries). Because the vessels are less elastic, they cannot "recoil" as quickly between heartbeats. The heart is not as able to cope with exercise as in youth. When deposits called plaques attach to the walls of the blood vessels, the condition is called atherosclerosis. This build-up narrows the arteries and slows the blood flow.

Keys for Review

Key Questions for Critical Thinking

1. Describe and discuss the functions of the cardiovascular system.
2. Describe the components of the blood. Be specific about the functions of each component.
3. Describe the blood clotting mechanism.
4. Describe the functions of the lymphatic system.
5. Discuss at least four normal changes in the cardiovascular system caused by aging.

Key Readings

Berkow R (Ed). The Merck Manual of Diagnosis and Therapy, Ed 16. Rahway, NY, Merck & Co., 1992

Birchenall JM, Streight ME. Care of the Older Adult, Ed 3. Philadelphia, J.B. Lippincott, 1993

Chabner D. The Language of Medicine, Ed 4. Philadelphia, W.B. Saunders, 1991.

O'Toole M (Ed). Miller-Keane Encyclopedia & Dictionary of Medicine, Nursing, and Allied Health, Ed 5. Philadelphia, W.B. Saunders, 1992

Scanlon V, Sanders V. Essentials of Anatomy and Physiology. Philadelphia, F.A. Davis, 1991

Seeley R, Stephens T, Tate P. Essentials of Anatomy and Physiology, Ed 2. St. Louis, Mosby-Yearbook, 1994

Smeltzer SC, Bare BG. Brunner and Suddarth's Textbook of Medical-Surgical Nursing, Ed 7. Philadelphia, J.B. Lippincott, 1992

Key Readings (continued)

Taylor C, Lillis C, LeMone P. Fundamentals of Nursing: The Art and Science of Nursing Care, Ed 2. Philadelphia, J.B. Lippincott, 1993

Thomas CL (Ed). Taber's Cyclopedic Medical Dictionary, Ed 17. Philadelphia, F.A. Davis, 1993

Keys to Learning More

Unit Four: remaining chapters in this unit are concerned with interrelationships between body systems

Chapter 42: measuring vital signs, including pulse and blood pressure

Chapter 50: nursing assessment, including cardiovascular function

Chapter 56: medications, many of which affect the cardiovascular system

Unit Thirteen: deviations from normal body structure and function in children

Unit Fourteen: deviations from normal body structure and function in adults

Chapter 74: heart and blood vessel disorders

Chapter 75: blood and lymph disorders

Chapter 76: cancers, many of which are closely related to blood disorders or are spread through blood or lymph

Chapter 77: allergic and immune disorders

Chapter 78: human immunodeficiency virus, AIDS, and autoimmune disorders

22 The Respiratory System

Keys for Learning

Learning Objectives

- Differentiate between internal and external respiration
- Define key terms
- Locate and identify by name the major structures of the respiratory system
- Describe the anatomic relationship between larynx, trachea, and esophagus, and describe the function of the epiglottis
- Locate on a chart the areas of the lung, and differentiate between the right and left lungs in terms of structure
- Define pleura, and describe its action
- Explain the gas exchange that occurs in the lungs, and describe the mechanics of breathing
- Define tidal volume, inspiratory reserve volume, expiratory reserve volume, residual volume, and vital capacity

Key Terms

apnea	inspiration	respiration
bronchi	larynx	sinuses
diaphragm	lobes	surfactant
dyspnea	lungs	trachea
epiglottis	nares	ventilation
eupnea	pharynx	
expiration	pleura	

Keys to Understanding This Chapter

Chapter 5: oxygen is a basic human need
Unit Four: organization of the body and integumentary, musculoskeletal, nervous, endocrine, sensory, and cardiovascular systems

Key Points

- The functions of the respiratory system are to take in oxygen in exchange for carbon dioxide and to assist in maintenance of acid–base balance of the body.
- The nose warms, moistens, and filters air before it enters the lungs.
- The pharynx extends from the nose to the esophagus and is divided into three segments: nasopharynx, oropharynx, and laryngopharynx.
- The larynx is guarded by the epiglottis and contains the vocal cords.
- The trachea is the passageway to the bronchi and lungs. The bronchi divide into smaller bronchioles, which terminate in millions of alveoli.
- Breathing is controlled in the medulla and influenced by centers in the pons.

Key Topics Outline

Structure and Function
    The Upper Respiratory Tract
    The Lower Respiratory Tract
System Physiology
    Gas Exchange
    Breathing
    Regulation of Acid–Base Balance
    Respiratory Reflexes
Effects of Aging on the System

Key Learning Activities

- What laws exist in your community, state, or province related to clean air?
- Visit the American Lung Association for information and pamphlets.
- Read newspapers or magazines for articles on research related to smoking. Be prepared to discuss them in class.

Rosdahl CB: Textbook of Basic Nursing, 6th ed. © 1995 J.B. Lippincott Company

All body cells need oxygen. If breathing stops (apnea) for 4 or 5 minutes, a person will lose consciousness. If breathing is not established within 7 or 8 minutes, damage to brain cells is likely to occur. If apnea occurs for 10 minutes or more, death will occur.

Respiration is the exchange of gases between the external environment and the internal cells of a person. Respiration refers to three processes: **ventilation** (breathing), gas exchange, and oxygen use. The air you take in through your respiratory system is approximately 20% to 21% oxygen and under normal circumstances, provides an ample supply for your needs.

There are two types of respiration: external and internal. The exchange of oxygen for carbon dioxide (CO_2) within the alveoli of the lungs is called *external respiration* (lung breathing), because it is the part of the respiratory cycle involved with the environment external to the body. The trade of oxygen for carbon dioxide *within the cells* is called *internal* or *cellular respiration* (cell breathing). An increase in the level of carbon dioxide stimulates respiration. Carbon dioxide and water are the waste products of respiration. Some of the water is excreted as waste; some is recycled for use in the body. Cellular respiration can be reviewed in Chapter 16.

Key Concept

- External respiration (in lungs) is oxygen absorbed by hemoglobin; carbon dioxide is exhaled.
- Internal respiration (within body cells) is oxygen transferred into cells; carbon dioxide is removed from cells by hemoglobin.

Structure and Function

The functions of the respiratory system, summarized in the box, include taking oxygen from the atmosphere, exchanging it for carbon dioxide, and assisting with regulation of the body's pH. The respiratory system depends on the circulatory system to transport gases and the nervous system to receive chemical and nervous stimuli at respiratory centers in the brain. The respiratory system is illustrated in Figure 22-1.

The Upper Respiratory Tract

Nose

Air begins its journey into the body through the right and left external **nares** or nostrils. The internal nose is divided into two sides or cavities by the nasal septum, a structure consisting of bone and cartilage. The nerve endings in the septum and the nasal passages are re-

Functions of the Respiratory System

Oxygen–Carbon Dioxide Exchange

- Takes in oxygen from outside air
- Exchanges carbon dioxide for oxygen in lungs
- Eliminates carbon dioxide from body

Acid–Base Balance

- Assists in regulating pH of body
- Eliminates some water

Protection

- Warms air before it enters lungs
- Moistens air before it enters lungs
- Mucus in nose traps foreign particles
- Coughing and sneezing dislodge foreign particles
- Yawning helps equalize pressures between inner ear and atmosphere

Speech Production

- Air passes over vocal cords to produce sound

sponsible for the sense of smell. These nerve impulses are carried to the brain by the first cranial nerve, the olfactory nerve.

The nasal cavities are lined with mucous membrane richly supplied with blood vessels, which aid in warming and moistening the air before it reaches the lungs. The mucus is sticky and traps dust particles, dirt, and microorganisms from the air. The hairs at the entrance of the nostrils and the tiny hairlike projections (cilia) on the membranes serve as filters to remove some foreign particles that otherwise might be carried to the lungs. (Most of the mucus secreted is swallowed, where hydrochloric acid from the stomach destroys many pathogens.)

Three small bones, the turbinates or *conchae*, project into the nasal cavity to increase the surface area of the lining. This increased surface area helps to warm, filter, and moisten room air before it enters the lungs. The nasolacrimal ducts, or tear ducts, open into the upper nasal cavities, thus the "runny nose" that occurs when a person cries. The upper respiratory tract is illustrated in Figure 22-2.

Sinuses

There are four cavities, called **sinuses,** on each side of the nasal area. These sinus cavities are lined with mucosa that is continuous with the nasal mucosa. The names of the sinus cavities correspond with the facial bones in which they are situated. Sinuses lighten the skull and provide resonance for the voice.

The two largest sinuses are the frontal, one on each side above the eye socket, and the maxillary, one on each side of the nose, in conjunction with the maxillary

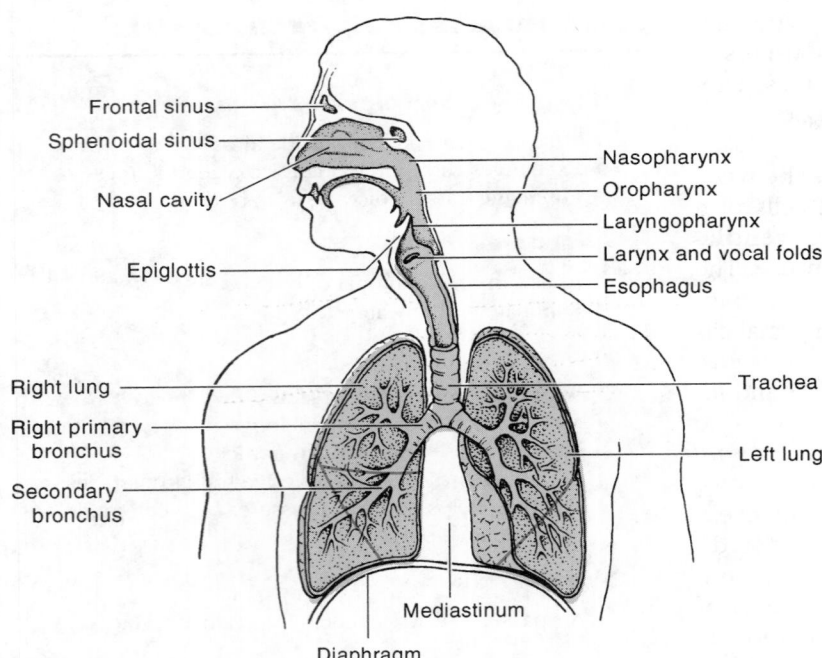

Figure 22-1. The respiratory system, showing the bronchial tree within the lungs.

bone. The ethmoidal and sphenoidal sinuses lie on each side of the nasal cavity in the area of the orbit (eye socket). Several sinus cavities are shown in Figures 22-1 and 22-2.

Because of the direct connection between the sinus cavities and the nasal mucosa, infection in one area can easily spread to the other. The sinuses drain directly into the nasal cavities, which drain into the throat.

Pharynx

Air travels from the nose to the pharynx, a tube-shaped passage for air and food. Figure 22-2 can be followed as you read the following descriptions.

Nasopharynx. The section of the pharynx that extends from the nares to the uvula is called the nasopharynx. It is a passageway for air only. In childhood, it contains

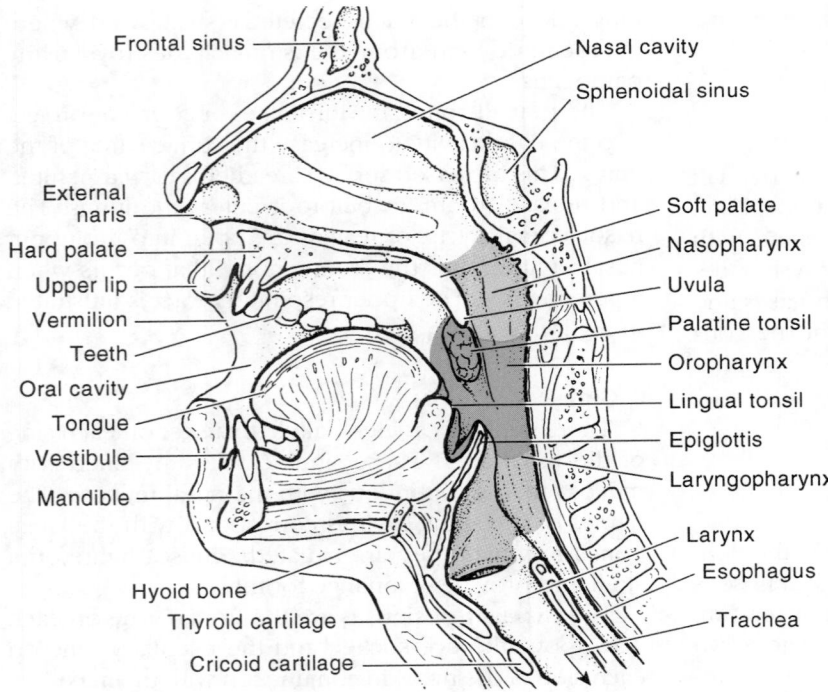

Figure 22-2. A sagittal section of the head, showing the structures of the upper respiratory tract.

the adenoids (pharyngeal tonsils). Only rarely does an adult have adenoids; when an individual approaches adulthood, the adenoids atrophy (waste away). During the act of swallowing, the soft palate and uvula are elevated to block the nasal cavity; this prevents food from entering the respiratory system. The auditory (eustachian) tubes connect the nasopharynx with the middle ear. The eustachian tubes permit air to enter or leave the middle ear cavities, which permits proper functioning of the eardrums (tympanic membranes).

Oropharynx. The oropharynx is the part of the pharynx that extends from the uvula to the epiglottis. Commonly called the throat, the oropharynx carries food to the esophagus and air to the trachea. Two sets of tonsils are in the oropharynx: the palatine tonsils on the lateral wall and the lingual tonsils on the base of the tongue.

Laryngopharynx. The laryngopharynx is the lowest portion of the pharynx. It extends from the epiglottis to the openings of the larynx and esophagus. The division of the laryngopharynx provides separate passageways for food and air.

Larynx (Voice Box)

From the pharynx, the air passes into the **larynx**, a boxlike structure made of cartilages held together by ligaments. It is located in the midline of the neck. (The largest and most prominent cartilage is the thyroid cartilage, commonly known as the "Adam's apple.") The function of these cartilages is to keep the airway open at all times.

The larynx serves as an air passageway between the pharynx and the trachea. The **pharynx** is a dual passageway for air and food, but only air is allowed to pass into the larynx. The entrance to the larynx is guarded by a lid or cover of cartilage called the **epiglottis** ("trap door cartilage"). The epiglottis automatically closes when you swallow, preventing food from entering the lower respiratory passage. The *glottis* is the opening on either side of the vocal cords. If a portion of food accidentally becomes lodged in the larynx, usually it can be dislodged by coughing. If not, the air passage may be blocked; such a blockage can be fatal unless proper emergency treatment is given.

Vocal Cords. Within the larynx are the vocal cords, two triangle-shaped membranous folds that extend from front to back. As air leaves the lungs and passes over the vocal cords, the cords vibrate, and the vibration produces sound. The size of the vocal cords and the larynx varies, accounting for the difference in people's voices. A man has a large larynx and therefore a deeper voice than a woman. Your voice becomes louder and stronger when you rapidly force out a lot of air.

Trachea (Windpipe)

Air passes from the larynx into the trachea. The **trachea** is a tube approximately $4\frac{1}{2}$ in (11 cm) long in the adult. It consists of cartilage and connective tissue. It extends from the lower end of the larynx into the chest cavity behind the heart. (Immediately posterior to the larynx and the trachea is the tube called the esophagus, which transports food from the pharynx to the stomach). The horseshoe-shaped cartilaginous rings of the trachea provide sufficient rigidity to keep the trachea open at all times for the air to pass through, yet they are flexible enough to permit bending of the neck.

The trachea is lined with ciliated mucous membrane. As in the nose, the mucus in the trachea traps inhaled foreign particles, which the waves of cilia carry out of the respiratory tract through the pharynx.

The Lower Respiratory Tract

The lower respiratory tract is illustrated in Figure 22-3.

Bronchi

As the trachea enters the chest cavity, it divides into two smaller tubes called the **bronchi**. One bronchus enters each lung. The right bronchus is shorter and wider than the left bronchus, which makes it a more common site for aspiration of foreign objects.

Each bronchus divides into smaller branches to form what is commonly called the bronchial tree, or tracheobronchial tree, which is spread throughout lung tissue. As the bronchi become smaller, their walls become thinner, the amount of cartilage decreases, and they become known as *bronchioles*. The bronchi and bronchioles continue to be lined with ciliated mucous membrane. The bronchioles branch first into *alveolar ducts*, which look like stems, and end in many *alveolar sacs*, which look like a cluster of grapes. Each lung contains millions of alveoli. These microscopic "balloons" give the lungs their spongy appearance. The walls of the alveoli are composed of a single layer of cells. The alveoli are lined with a chemical called **surfactant**, which helps to prevent the alveolar walls from collapsing between breaths.

Special Considerations in Children
Surfactant in Newborns

Surfactant is not formed until after the seventh gestational month. Premature newborns may have insufficient surfactant, which results in the collapse of alveoli. A newborn with this problem must exert tremendous energy to breathe. As a result, the newborn may die of fatigue of the respiratory muscles and inadequate ventilation. Mechanical ventilation and derived surfactant are used until the neonate can make his or her own surfactant.

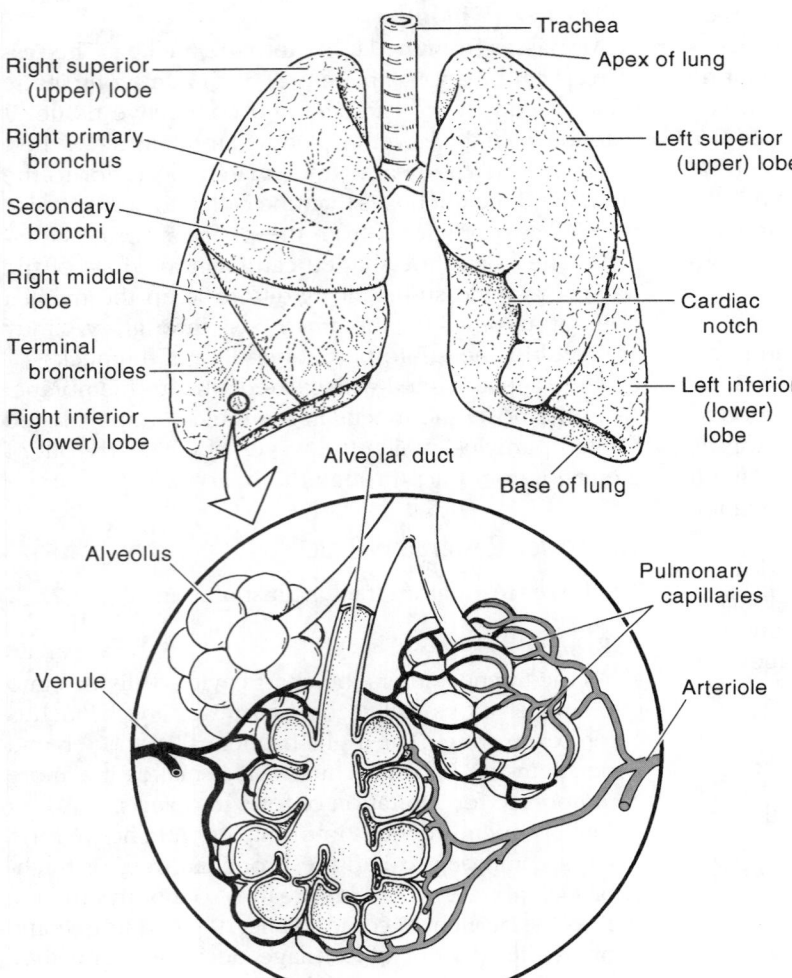

Figure 22-3. Anterior view of the lower respiratory tract.

Labels in figure:
Trachea
Apex of lung
Right superior (upper) lobe
Right primary bronchus
Secondary bronchi
Right middle lobe
Terminal bronchioles
Right inferior (lower) lobe
Left superior (upper) lobe
Cardiac notch
Left inferior (lower) lobe
Base of lung
Alveolar duct
Alveolus
Pulmonary capillaries
Venule
Arteriole

Lungs

The **lungs** are two cone-shaped organs that fill the chest cavity. They are the stations where the blood picks up oxygen and drops off its load of carbon dioxide. The top of each triangular cone is called the *apex*; the lower, wide portion that fits over the diaphragm is called the *base*. The lungs are spongy tissue filled with alveoli, nerves, and blood and lymph vessels. They are separated by the heart, the large blood vessels, the esophagus, and other contents of the *mediastinum*, the area lying between the lungs in the thorax.

The lungs are divided into sections called **lobes**. The right lung has three lobes, and the left has two (see Figure 22-3). On the inner surface of the lungs is an indented area called the hilum. The arteries, veins, bronchi, and nerves enter the lungs at the *hilum*.

Pleura. The lungs are covered with a smooth double-layered sac of serous membrane called the **pleura**. One layer covers the lungs (the visceral pleura), while the outer layer (the parietal pleura) lines the chest cavity. Their surfaces are in constant contact and are moist, as serous fluid is secreted. This allows the lungs to move without causing pain or friction against the chest wall. The space between the two layers of the pleura is called the *pleural cavity*. A vacuum normally exists within this space. Air or fluid accumulation in the pleural space causes a partial or total collapse of a lung.

Key Concept

♦ Pathway for air (external breathing): nose → pharynx → larynx → trachea → bronchi → bronchioles → alveoli (O_2 exchanged for CO_2)

♦ Pathway for oxygen distribution and carbon dioxide return (internal breathing): alveoli → capillaries (hemoglobin with oxygen) → cells → capillaries (CO_2) → alveoli

System Physiology

Gas Exchange

Exchange of gases (oxygen and carbon dioxide) takes place through the alveoli. The walls of the alveoli are one cell layer thick, and they are surrounded by equally thin blood capillaries. When oxygen enters the lungs, it travels through the walls of the alveoli into capillaries. Pulmonary circulation was discussed and illustrated in Chapter 21. Waste carbon dioxide in the lungs is exchanged for oxygen. The carbon dioxide is exhaled, fresh oxygen is inhaled, and the cycle begins again.

Breathing

Ventilation is the mechanical process of respiration that moves air to and from the alveoli. It is divided into inhalation and exhalation. Breathing air in is called **inspiration** or inhalation: breathing out is called **expiration** or exhalation. Adults usually average between 14 and 20 respirations per minute; the rate is much higher in children. Normal respiration is called **eupnea**; difficult breathing is known as **dyspnea**.

Normal breathing occurs as a result of stimulation of the respiratory center in the medulla. Because the lungs cannot move by themselves, they are inflated and deflated by actions of muscles surrounding them. The medulla sends impulses to the diaphragm and the intercostal muscles. The **diaphragm** is a dome-shaped muscle separating the thoracic and abdominal cavities. It contracts and flattens to increase chest space (Fig. 22-4). The intercostal muscles are located between the ribs; they contract to lift and spread the ribs during inhalation.

The actual movement of air from the external to internal environment occurs as a result of differences in existing pressures between the atmosphere and the lungs. A partial vacuum exists internally. The air goes in when the intrapulmonary (within the lungs) pressure is below that of the surrounding atmosphere (sub-atmospheric). Air rushes out when the pressures within the lungs rise above that of the atmosphere. The intrapulmonary pressure changes occur as a result of the changes in chest or thoracic volume. These volume changes are caused by the movements of the diaphragm and the intercostal muscles.

The depth and rate of respiration are controlled without conscious thought by the respiratory center in the medulla. The pons has centers that work with the medulla to produce a normal rhythm of breathing. The cerebral cortex gives some voluntary control to breathing to talk, sing, or change the rate of breathing. We can even stop breathing for a minute or two. The medulla, however, will take over control eventually.

Chemoreceptors in the medulla stimulate the muscles of respiration primarily in response to changes in carbon dioxide. Therefore, carbon dioxide, and not oxygen, is the major regulator of respiration because of the effects that CO_2 has on blood pH.

Nursing Alert

A certain amount of CO_2 is normal within the body. It stimulates breathing and causes the blood vessels of the brain to dilate, allowing proper oxygenation for the brain. An excess of CO_2 brings about cerebral vasoconstriction (constriction of the blood vessels in the brain). This causes neurologic symptoms, such as dizziness.

Lung Volumes and Capacities

Lung capacity varies with sex, size, physical condition, and age. Pulmonary diseases and other diseases that limit expansion of the chest cavity have a great influence on a person's comfort and ability to survive. The expansibility of the lungs and thorax also influences lung volumes and capacities. The accompanying box contains key terms with average measurements for a young, healthy male.

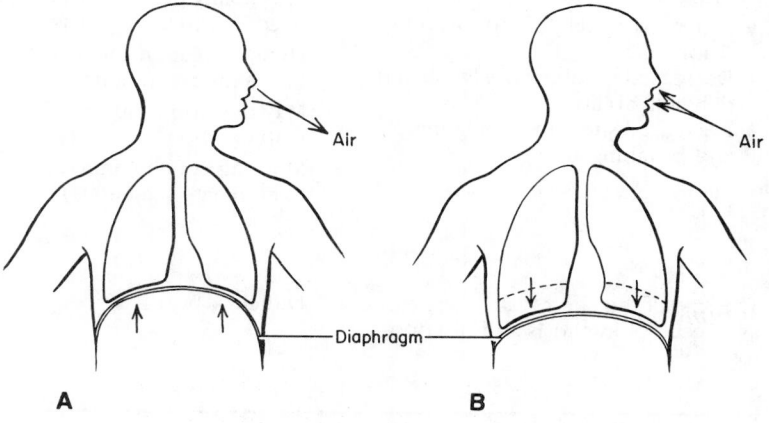

Figure 22-4. The mechanics of respiration (breathing). Arrows indicate the direction of air flow. **(A)** Chest space and lung size when air is exhaled and the muscles of respiration are relaxed. **(B)** Expansion of the lungs during inhalation. The ribs are lifted, and the diaphragm contracts and is pulled downward. These two movements cause an increase in the size of the chest and thus create a partial vacuum. The vacuum causes outside air to rush into the lungs.

Key Terms for Lung Capacity With Average Measurements[1]

- *Tidal Volume* (TV)—amount of air inspired or expired during a normal inspiration or expiration. Average = 500 mL (5–8 mL per kilogram of body weight)
- *Inspiratory Reserve Volume*—(inspiratory capacity)-amount of air that can be taken in with the deepest possible inhalation, beyond that of tidal volume. Average = 2,500–4,300 mL
- *Expiratory Reserve Volume*—amount of air that can be expelled with the most forceful exhalation, beyond that of tidal volume. Average = 1,200–1,500 mL
- *Residual Volume* (RV)—amount of air remaining in respiratory passages and lungs after the most forceful expiration. Average = 1,200–1,500 mL
- *Vital Capacity* (VC)—sum of inspiratory reserve volume and expiratory reserve volume. Average = 4,000–5,000 mL
- *Minute Ventilation* (MV)—tidal volume and respiratory rate per minute; the volume of air expired per minute
- *Total Lung Capacity* (TLC)—tidal volume plus inspiratory reserve volume plus residual volume. Average = 4,800–6,300 mL

[1] *These measurements vary according to age, sex, body build and weight. Data from Smeltzer & Bare. Brunner and Suddarth's Textbook of Medical-Surgical Nursing, Ed 7. Philadelphia, Lippincott, 1992, page 514 and Taylor, Lillis & LeMone. Fundamentals of Nursing, Ed 2. Philadelphia, Lippincott, 1993, page 951.*

Regulation of Acid–Base Balance

The primary function of the respiratory system is exchange of gases. However, another important function is regulation of the pH of all body fluids. The respiratory and renal systems interact to maintain homeostasis.

Carbon dioxide can alter pH, because it reacts with water to form carbonic acid (H_2CO_3). Carbonic acid can break down to form H+ and HCO_3− (hydrogen ion and bicarbonate ion). These ions are important to the buffer system, which helps the body maintain proper pH levels. (Refer to Chapter 16 for acid–base balance and the buffer system.)

Respiratory Reflexes

Coughing and sneezing are protective reflexes needed to dislodge materials from the respiratory passages. The bronchi and trachea have sensory receptors that initiate a cough in response to foreign particles or irritating substances. The reflex to sneeze is similar to coughing, except that the source of irritation is in the nasal passages.

Yawning is another respiratory reflex. While not well understood, it is conjectured that yawning is in response to lack of oxygen or an accumulation of carbon dioxide. (No one knows why yawning is contagious.) Yawning also helps equalize pressures between the middle ear and the outside atmosphere.

Table 22-1. Effects of Aging on the Respiratory System

Factor	Result	Nursing Implications
Functional capacity is decreased because of the following: ◆ Increased rigidity of thorax and diaphragm ◆ Decreased numbers of alveoli and diffusion ability ◆ Decreased strength in breathing and coughing	More energy needed to breathe Less ability to compensate for respiratory needs in stress or illness Hypoventilation can lead to respiratory problems and pneumonia May develop dyspnea (shortness of breath) with exertion Morning cough common (decreased ability to eliminate secretions)	Encourage good ventilation with daily exercise such as walking. Advise older person to avoid contact with children or others with respiratory tract infections. Advise patient to see physician early if symptoms occur. Encourage changing position slowly to avoid orthostatic vital sign changes. Advise to change position at least every 2 hours.
The size of the chest wall is decreased as a result of kyphosis and osteoporosis.	Difficulty breathing deeply	Help patient know his or her own ability. Encourage moving, coughing, and deep breathing.

Effects of Aging on the System

The organs of the respiratory system lose their elasticity with age. Table 22-1 summarizes major effects of aging on the respiratory system. The chest walls are stiffer, and the lungs cannot expand as much; thus, less air is exchanged with each breath. The ratio of the pressures of oxygen and carbon dioxide in the lungs may change; this causes difficulties in oxygenation of the blood and exchange of oxygen for carbon dioxide at the cell level.

The changes of aging also can make the older person more susceptible to respiratory disorders, such as pneumonia. This occurs not only as a result of decreased elasticity of lungs and bronchioles, but also because of reduced exercise, decreased ciliary action, and decreased secretion of mucus in respiratory tract linings.

Keys for Review

Key Questions for Critical Thinking

1. Define and describe the process of respiration. Explain the process of gas exchange.
2. Describe the upper respiratory tract, its components and their structure and function.
3. Describe the components and the process of voice production.
4. Describe the lower respiratory tract, its components and their structure and function.

Key Readings

Chabner D. The Language of Medicine, Ed 4. Philadelphia, W.B. Saunders, 1991

Eliopoulus C. Caring the Elderly in Diverse Care Settings. Philadelphia, J.B. Lippincott, 1990

Farrell J. Nursing Care of the Older Person. Philadelphia, J.B. Lippincott, 1990

Jackson DB, Saunders RB. Child Health Nursing: A Comprehensive Approach to the Care of the Children and their Families. Philadelphia, J.B. Lippincott, 1993

Scanlon V, Sanders V. Essentials of Anatomy and Physiology. Philadelphia, F.A. Davis, 1991

Seeley R, Stephens T, Tate P. Anatomy and Physiology, Ed 2. St. Louis, C.V. Mosby, 1994

Smeltzer SC, Bare BG. Brunner and Suddarth's Textbook of Medical-Surgical Nursing, Ed 7. Philadelphia, J.B. Lippincott, 1992

Enrichment Keys

Memmler RL, Cohen BJ, Woods DL. Structure and Function of the Human Body, Ed 5. Philadelphia, J.B. Lippincott, 1992

Keys to Learning More

Chapter 32: cardiopulmonary resuscitation (CPR) and management of blocked airway

Chapter 42: how to count respirations

Chapter 47: collection of specimens, including the sputum specimen

Chapter 50: nursing assessment, including respiratory function

Chapter 51: special respiratory isolation

Chapter 53: assisting with breathing exercises after surgery

Chapter 56: medications, many of which treat or affect the respiratory system

Unit Thirteen: deviations from normal body structure and function in children

Unit Fourteen: deviations from normal body function in adults

Chapter 79: discussion of respiratory disorders

Chapter 80: administration of oxygen and respiratory care

Chapter 85: disorders in older adults

23 The Digestive System

Keys for Learning

Learning Objectives

- State the functions of the digestive system
- Locate on a chart or model the small intestine, indicating the duodenum, jejunum, and ileum
- On a chart, locate the large intestine, indicating the ileocecal valve; the cecum; the vermiform appendix; the ascending, transverse, and descending colon; the sigmoid colon; the rectum; and the anal sphincter
- Describe the accessory organs of digestion, and state the functions of each
- On a chart, trace the digestive pathway, naming each major organ
- Describe the physiology of digestion in the stomach
- Describe the effects of aging on the digestive system

Key Terms

absorption	duodenum	mastication
bile	deglutition	peristalsis
bolus	esophagus	peritoneum
cardiac sphincter	gallbladder	rectum
chyme	ileum	rugae
defecation	jejunum	villi
digestion	liver	

Keys to Understanding This Chapter

Chapter 5: need for food, water, and elimination
Unit Four: normal anatomy and physiology

Key Points

- The gastrointestinal tract is lined with mucous membrane for protection and to lubricate food.
- The stomach is a storage and digestive pouch that makes hydrochloric acid, pepsinogen, intrinsic factor, and gastrin.

Key Points (continued)

- There are two types of digestion: mechanical (chewing of food) and chemical (breakdown of food into usable form).
- Most nutrient absorption occurs in the small intestine. The large intestine mainly absorbs water and produces Vitamin K. The liver has numerous functions that are vital for life.
- Metabolism is the total of all physical and chemical changes that occur in the body. This includes anabolism and catabolism.

Key Topics Outline

Structure and Function
  Mouth
  Teeth
  Tongue
  Pharynx and Esophagus
  Stomach
  Small Intestine
  Large Intestine
  Accessory Organs
System Physiology
  Digestion and Absorption
  Metabolism
  Elimination
Effects of Aging on the System

Key Learning Activities

- Use hydrochloric acid carefully to discover its action on various foods in the laboratory.
- Make a chart of the liver and all its activities.
- On a chart or body model, point out all of the structures of the digestive system, and name their functions.

Rosdahl CB: Textbook of Basic Nursing, 6th ed. © 1995 J.B. Lippincott Company

Because the body needs energy to perform its many tasks, it must have a supply of fuel and water. You breathe, your heart beats, and you talk, laugh, and move around. You can do all this because your digestive system converts food you eat into fuel for your energy demands.

The conversion of the mass of food to usable materials for energy is called **digestion**. The physiology of digestion is discussed near the end of this chapter, and this efficient food-processing machine is called the digestive tract. It is also called the alimentary canal, gastrointestinal (GI) tract, and GI system.

The GI tract or canal is like a tube, approximately 30 feet (9.1 m) long; it runs through your body and is open to the outside at both ends. The entire GI tract is lined with mucous membrane. Food travels through the GI tract in about 24 to 36 hours. The actions of the digestive system are subject to control by the nervous system.

The nutrients that provide fuel for the body are carbohydrates (starches and sugars), proteins, and fats. They are made up of carbon, hydrogen, and oxygen; proteins also contain nitrogen.

Structure and Function

The major organs or the digestive system are shown in Figure 23-1. You can follow this illustration as you learn about the functions of various organs.

The function of the organs of the digestive system is to break down food into simple forms that can be carried by the circulatory vessels and can pass through cell membranes to be used by cells. The cells use the simple forms of food molecules for energy and to build, maintain, and repair body tissues. The accompanying box lists these functions.

Mouth

The mouth is also called the oral cavity or buccal cavity. Food is taken into the body through the mouth, where digestion begins. The teeth cut, chop, and grind food so that the particles become smaller, and more surface is exposed to actions of digestive juices and enzymes.

The roof of the mouth is made up of the hard and soft palates. The hard palate is closest to the front and is made up of the palatine bones and parts of the maxillary bones. The soft palate is mostly muscle tissue. The palate separates the mouth from the nasopharynx, the area of the pharynx behind the nose. The soft palate is shaped like an arch in the back of the mouth and opens onto the oropharynx, the area of the pharynx behind the mouth. The structure that can be seen suspended in the back of the open mouth is the uvula.

The floor of the mouth is covered by the tongue. The walls of the mouth cavity are the cheeks and the teeth.

Salivary Glands. Three pairs of salivary glands pour 1 to 1½ L of saliva into the mouth per day. The names of these glands indicate their locations: sublingual (under the tongue), parotid (cheek), and submaxillary (jaw). Saliva is a thin, watery fluid that contains ptyalin, also called salivary amylase. It also contains water, mucus, and salts.

Saliva moistens food particles, makes food easier to swallow, and through the action of the ptyalin, begins the breakdown of starch into smaller sugar molecules. Saliva helps prevent oral infections, because it contains *lipozymes* (bacteriocidal enzymes) and immunoglobulins (IgA).

Teeth

The teeth are set in spaces or *sockets* in the upper and lower jaw bones: the maxilla and mandible. Humans have two sets of teeth: the deciduous or baby teeth and a permanent or adult set (Fig. 23-2). A baby's deciduous teeth usually begin to erupt between 6 and 8 months, and the 20 teeth are usually complete by 2½ years of age. When the child is about age 6, permanent teeth begin to appear. As they grow in, they push out the deciduous teeth, replace them, and fill in the spaces in the jaw. There are 32 teeth in the permanent set.

The chief function of teeth is to break food into small particles. This is accomplished through **mastication**, the act of chewing. The front teeth, the *incisors*, cut and tear food. The side teeth, *canine* or cuspids, hold and tear food. The back teeth, premolars (bicuspids) and *molars*, crush and grind food. The last permanent teeth, the wisdom teeth, sometimes do not appear before adulthood. If the jaw is small and the jaw space limited, they may not have room to erupt and become *impacted* in the tissue. Impacted wisdom teeth may need to be removed surgically.

Parts of a Tooth. A tooth has three parts: crown, neck, and root. The *crown* is the enamel-covered part of the tooth that is seen in the mouth. Tooth enamel is the hardest structure in the body. The tooth narrows into a *neck* at the gumline. The *root* of the tooth is in the bony socket. The root is covered by a substance called cement (or cementum). Beneath the enamel and the cement is a hard bonelike substance called dentin, which is the bulk of the material of the tooth. The center of the tooth is the pulp cavity. The pulp contains many nerve endings and blood vessels, which enter from a canal through the roots from the sockets. The teeth are embedded in and nourished by bone.

Tongue

The tongue is a tough skeletal muscle covered with mucous membrane. It is attached to four bones, the mandible, two temporal bones, and hyoid. On the bottom

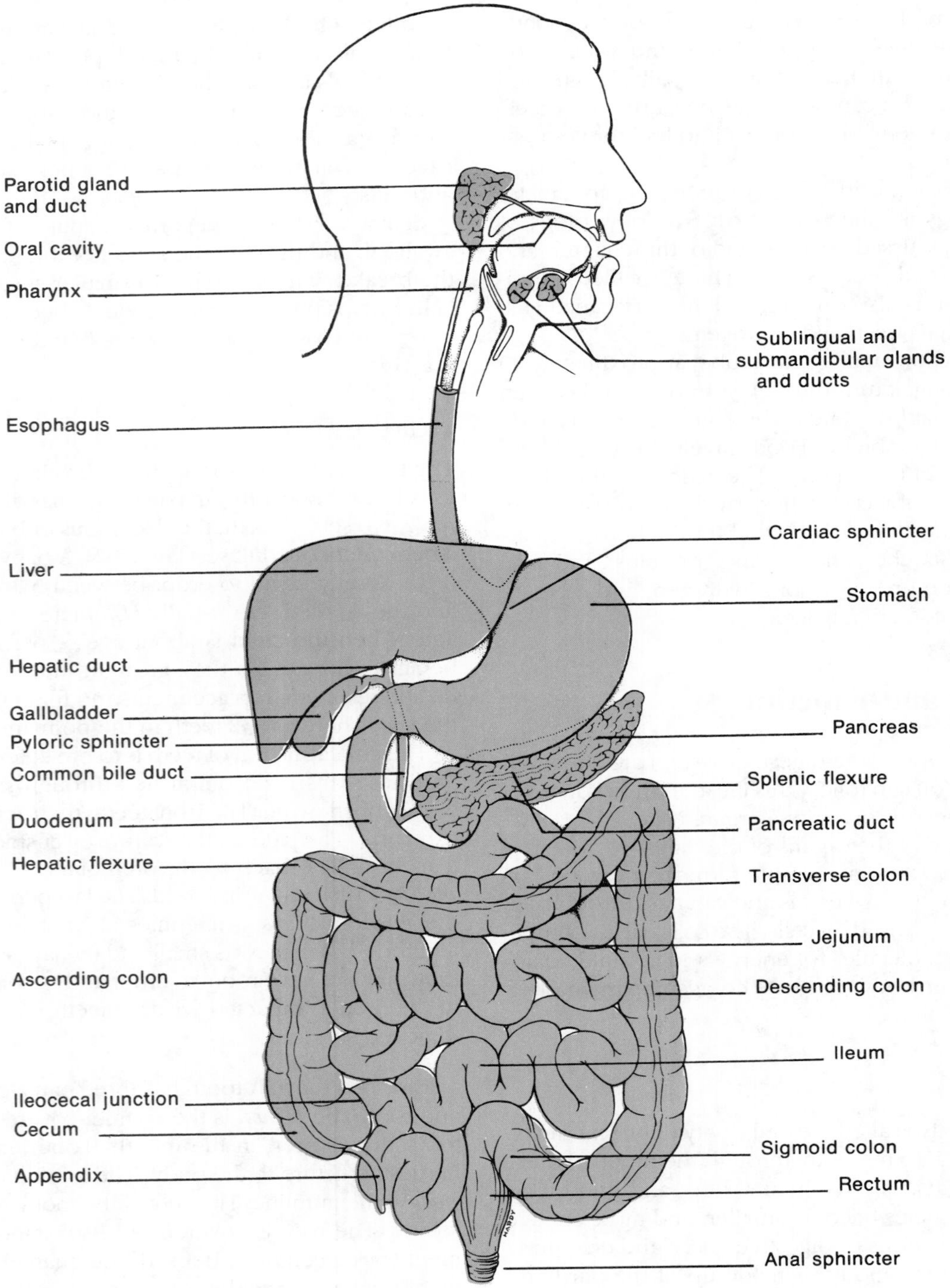

Parotid gland
and duct

Oral cavity

Pharynx

Sublingual and
submandibular glands
and ducts

Esophagus

Cardiac sphincter

Liver

Stomach

Hepatic duct

Gallbladder

Pancreas

Pyloric sphincter

Splenic flexure

Common bile duct

Pancreatic duct

Duodenum

Hepatic flexure

Transverse colon

Jejunum

Ascending colon

Descending colon

Ileum

Ileocecal junction

Cecum

Sigmoid colon

Appendix

Rectum

Anal sphincter

Figure 23-1. The digestive system, showing the digestive tube, or alimentary canal, and accessory organs.

of the tongue is a fold of mucous membrane called the frenulum. This structure helps to attach the tongue to the floor of the mouth. In some cases, the frenulum is short or too tightly attached. This makes speech difficult, and the person is said to be "tongue-tied." The situation can be surgically corrected.

The tongue has several functions. It senses the food's temperature and texture. It mixes food with saliva and moves food to be chewed. The voluntary movement of the tongue begins the swallowing process, called **deglutition**, by pushing food into the pharynx, the next portion of the digestive tube.

Functions of the Digestive System

Food Processing and Storage

- ◆ Breaks down foods into smaller particles (mechanical digestion)
- ◆ Converts food into substances that can be absorbed (chemical digestion)
- ◆ Moves food materials through the gastrointestinal tract (peristalsis)
- ◆ Stores food materials until needed

Manufacture

- ◆ Manufactures enzymes, hydrochloric acid, intrinsic factor, mucus, and other materials to assist in digestion
- ◆ Manufactures regulatory hormones in stomach
- ◆ Manufactures vitamin K in large intestine

Absorption

- ◆ Provides absorption of nutrients, mainly from small intestine, into capillaries

Reabsorption and Elimination

- ◆ Reabsorbs water to be reused by the body
- ◆ Reabsorbs minerals and vitamins
- ◆ Forms feces from remaining waste products
- ◆ Produces defecation

The upper surface of the tongue appears rough because of visible indentations (fissures) and projections (papillae). The taste buds are microscopic nipplelike projections located on the sides of the papillae. They are specialized nerve endings that allow us to detect various flavors. Figure 20-7 indicates structures of the tongue and areas of the tongue where specific taste buds appear.

The taste buds distinguish between flavors. Although there are all types of taste buds on most areas of the tongue, they are concentrated as follows: salty (tip and sides of the tongue), bitter (back of the tongue), sweet (tip and sides of tongue), and sour (sides of tongue). Alkaline and metallic flavors are sometimes considered distinct tastes as well. The taste of food also depends on the sense of smell.

Pharynx and Esophagus

The tongue lifts the ball of food that has mixed with saliva and is called a **bolus**, meaning lump or clod. The bolus is pushed into the muscular tube behind the mouth, the pharynx, where the movement of food becomes involuntary. The epiglottis covers the larynx and prevents food from entering the respiratory tract. The smooth or involuntary muscles pass the food along by waves of contractions called **peristalsis**, an alternate relaxation and contraction of muscles that sends food through the digestive tube. Contractions of the pharynx continue the act of swallowing and push food into the muscular esophagus.

The **esophagus**, or gullet, is approximately 10 in (25.4 cm) in length; it extends from the pharynx into the neck and thorax and, through an opening in the diaphragm, to the stomach. Its role in digestion is merely to serve as a passageway. The stomach opening, the cardiac orifice, is guarded by a muscle called the **cardiac sphincter**. Sometimes this muscle is called the esophageal-gastric sphincter. As waves of peristalsis push food through the lower esophagus, the cardiac sphincter opens and allows food to enter and closes to prevent food from being regurgitated (vomited).

Stomach

The stomach is a muscular, collapsible, pouch or sac capable of being greatly distended. It is located in the upper left side of the abdominal cavity and receives its blood supply from the celiac artery. The rounded por-

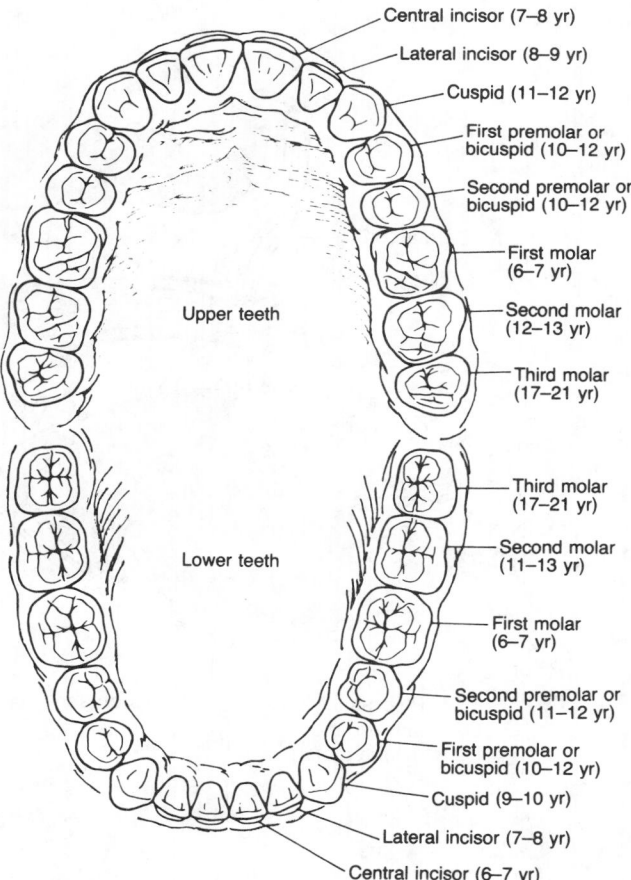

Figure 23-2. Approximate ages for eruption of permanent teeth. (See Fig. 9-2 for ages of eruption of deciduous teeth.)

tion above the level of the cardiac sphincter, containing the opening from the esophagus, is called the *fundus.* The central and largest portion is called the *body;* the lower narrow portion, which attaches to the small intestine, is called the *pylorus,* or pyloric portion (Fig. 23-3). The pyloric sphincter controls the opening between the stomach and the duodenum. (The prefix referring to the stomach is gastro-.)

The strong walls of the stomach consist of three layers of smooth muscle: a circular layer, a longitudinal layer (muscle fibers going the long way), and an oblique layer (muscle fibers on a slant or an angle). This spread of muscles in all directions allows much motion for stirring and churning food and breaking it into small particles. When the stomach is empty, it collapses and lies in folds called **rugae**. These rugae allow the stomach to distend (expand) greatly when food is eaten.

In the stomach, all foods are mixed with gastric juices and churned until they are in a semiliquid form called **chyme**. This process usually takes 3 to 5 hours. Peristalsis of the smooth muscles of the stomach normally moves food toward the pyloric outlet. The pyloric sphincter at the lower opening contracts to keep the food in the stomach until it is thoroughly mixed. The sphincter then relaxes to let peristaltic waves push food in small amounts into the small intestine. If the stomach is irritated or too full, sometimes the direction of the waves of peristalsis reverses and forces the material back into the lower end of the esophagus. Reverse peristalsis within the stomach combined with contractions of abdominal muscles and the diaphragm forces food back through the esophagus and out through the mouth, causing vomiting.

The stomach is lined with mucous membrane. Mucus coats and protects the stomach lining from mechanical and chemical injury. Chief cells secrete pepsinogen, an inactive form of pepsin, the enzyme necessary to break down proteins. Hydrochloric acid is secreted by parietal cells; its functions are to activate pepsinogen and kill most microorganisms in the stomach. When activated by hydrochloric acid, pepsinogen changes into the enzyme pepsin, which begins to break down proteins. Another secretion of the parietal cells is intrinsic factor, which is essential for life. Intrinsic factor is needed for absorption of vitamin B_{12}, necessary for development of red blood cells in bone marrow. The stomach also produces regulatory hormones, such as gastrin. Gastrin stimulates secretion of hydrochloric acid and pepsin.

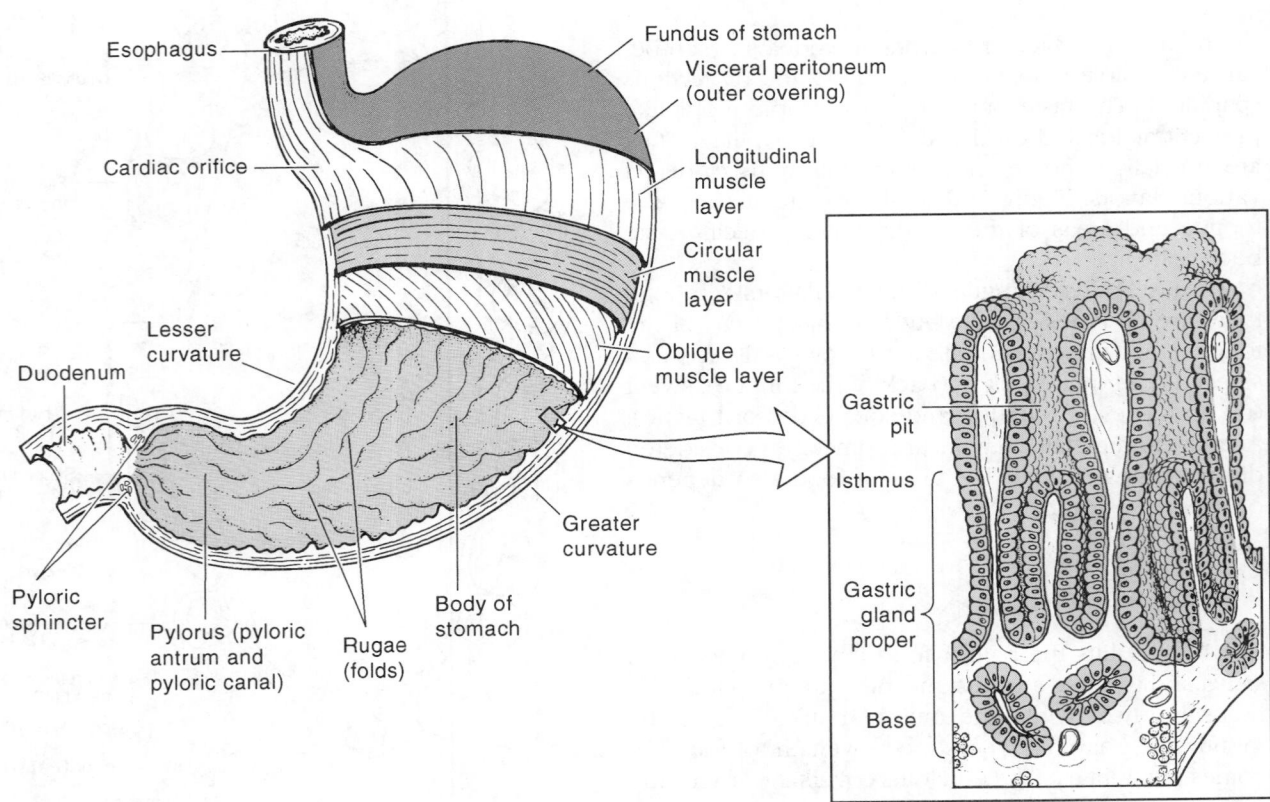

Figure 23-3. Longitudinal section of stomach and portion of duodenum. The art shows the interior with rugae and the three muscular layers.

Small Intestine

The small intestine is approximately 20 feet (6.1 m) long and $1\frac{1}{2}$ inches (3.81 cm) in diameter and lies coiled on itself in the abdominal cavity. It is about 18 feet longer than the large intestine, which follows it. (The prefix referring to the intestines is entero-.)

Intestinal glands in the small intestine secrete enzymes for the digestion of all foods. These enzymes break up the fats, carbohydrates, and proteins into materials that the cells can use. To be absorbed by the blood and lymph capillaries, the carbohydrates must be in the form of the simple sugars: glucose, fructose, and galactose. The proteins also must be digested into their simplest state, amino acids, and the fats must be converted to fatty acids and glycerol. Table 23-1 summarizes the action of the enzymes in preparing food for absorption.

The small intestine has numerous secretions. Mucus lubricates and protects the intestinal wall lining from the acidic chyme and digestive enzymes. Cholecystokinin is a hormone secretion that stimulates the pancreas to secrete pancreatic juice and stimulates the gallbladder to contract, resulting in the release of bile. Secretin is another hormone that influences other secretions in the stomach and pancreas.

Duodenum. The first portion of the small intestine is the 10- to 12-in C-shaped **duodenum**. As chyme enters the duodenum, more digestive juices are added. **Bile**, a greenish-brown liquid manufactured by the liver and

Table 23-1. Enzymes and their Actions

Area of Digestive System	Secretion	Enzyme	Action
Mouth	Saliva from salivary glands	Amylase (ptyalin)	Begins digestion of starch (CHO); breaks into simpler carbohydrates, such as dextrin
Stomach	Mucus		Protects lining
	Hydrochloric acid (HCl)		Destroys pathogens
			Changes pepsinogin to pepsin
			Hydrolyzes some CHO into glucose and fructose
	Gastrin (hormone)		Stimulates secretion of HCl
	Intrinsic factor		Necessary for use of vitamin B_{12} and growth of red blood cells
	Pepsinogen	Pepsin	Begins digestion of protein
		Lipase	Small amounts begin fat digestion
Liver	Bile		Stored in gallbladder; emulsifies fats
Small intestine	Receives bile and pancreatic juice	Peptidases	Converts proteins into amino acids
		Erepsin (protease)	
	Secretin		Influences stomach and pancreatic secretions
	Cholecystokinin		Stimulates pancreas to release enzymes
			Stimulates liver and gallbladder to release bile
		Sucrase, maltase, lactase	Completes CHO digestion
Pancreas (exocrine function)	Pancreatic juice	Amylase	Converts starch to maltose
		Trypsin (pancreatic protease) and chymotrypsin	Converts large proteins into smaller proteins (amino acids)
		Lipase	Converts emulsified fats to fatty acids and glycerol
		Bicarbonate ions	Helps neutralize chyme
			Provides proper pH for enzymes
Pancreas (endocrine function)	Insulin (hormone)		Enables cells to use glucose
	Glucagon (hormone)		Elevates blood sugar levels

stored in the gallbladder, pours in through the common bile duct to emulsify fats in preparation for further digestive action.

Jejunum and Ileum. The chyme travels through the remaining portions of the small intestine, the **jejunum** (about 8 ft), and the **ileum** (about 11 ft). (The word jejunum is derived from a Latin word meaning "fasting intestine;" it has been so named because, when dissected, the jejunum is almost always empty. The word ileum means "flank" or "groin.") Like the rest of the alimentary canal, the entire small intestine is lined with mucous membrane. There are numerous lymph nodules in the ileum called Peyer's patches.

Large Intestine

The large intestine is much wider than the small intestine (its diameter is approximately 2½ in, or 6.35 cm), but it is only about 5 feet (1.5 m) long. It does not coil but lies in folds and is divided into different areas by name. Water reabsorption is the colon's main function; 80% of it is reabsorbed. Vitamins and minerals also are absorbed. There are trillions of bacteria in the colon. Their function is to inhibit growth of pathogens. Some bacteria in the colon produce vitamin K, which is necessary for blood clotting.

Cecum and Appendix. The first portion of the large intestine is the *cecum,* a blind pouch about 2 to 3 inches (5–7.6 cm) long. A small fingerlike projection of the cecum is the vermiform (worm-shaped) appendix, which has no known function. (The word appendix is derived from the Latin word meaning "appendage.") It has the same lymphoid tissue as tonsils and like the tonsils, frequently becomes infected, a condition called appendicitis. It is prone to infection because fecal material enters and cannot always drain out. The cecum and appendix are located in the right lower quadrant of the abdominal cavity.

Colon. The next and longest portion of the large intestine is the colon, a continuous tube divided into three parts, taking their names from the course they follow: The *ascending* (going up) colon travels up the right side of the abdominal cavity; the *transverse* (going across) colon crosses to the left side in the upper part of the cavity; the *descending* (going down) colon goes down the left side into the pelvis. The next and last portion, which is called the *sigmoid* (sigma is the Greek letter S), ends at the rectum. The colon is illustrated in Figure 23-1.

Rectum and Anus. The **rectum** is about 5 inches (12.7 cm) in length and terminates at the anal canal; this is the terminal (end) portion of the large intestine. It is

about 1 to 1½ inches long (2.54–3.8 cm), and its opening to the outside, the anus, is guarded by internal and external sphincter muscles. The external sphincter is under control of the person and can be consciously contracted and relaxed.

> ### Key Concept
>
> The pathway of food materials through the body is as follows: mouth → pharynx → esophagus → (cardiac sphincter) → stomach → (pyloric sphincter) → small intestine (duodenum → jejunum → ileum) → (ileocecal valve) → large intestine (cecum → colon: ascending, transverse, descending, sigmoid, rectum) → anus.

Accessory Organs

Accessory organs include the liver, gallbladder, pancreas, and peritoneum. Table 23-2 lists secretions and functions of the first three of these.

Liver

Partially digested food that reaches the blood in the small intestine passes through the liver and undergoes vital changes.

The **liver** is the largest glandular organ in the body and lies just below the diaphragm in the upper right quadrant of the abdominal cavity (Fig. 23-4). It receives its blood supply from the hepatic artery and is divided into two major and two minor lobes. (The prefix referring to the liver is hepato-.) In humans, the liver weighs about 3 pounds (1.36 kg) and resembles calf liver in color and texture.

The liver plays such an important part in overall bodily functions that one cannot live long if it is severely diseased or injured. Only the brain is capable of more functions than the liver (Table 23-2).

Gallbladder

The **gallbladder** is a muscular sac 3 to 4 inches long (7.5–10 cm), resembling a small pear and located on the undersurface of the liver (see Figure 23-4). Some authorities regard it as an enlargement of the cystic duct through which it drains. (The prefix relating to the gallbladder is chole-.)

The main function of the gallbladder is to store and release bile as it is needed in the small intestine for the emulsification of fats. Another function of bile is to neutralize the pH of chyme that is leaving the stomach. This is necessary before pancreatic enzymes can function.

Cells within the liver manufacture bile. Small ducts from these cells emerge and join to form the hepatic duct, which then joins the *cystic duct* coming from the gallbladder. At this point it is called the common bile

Table 23-2. Accessory Organs of the Digestive System and Their Functions

Organ	Secretions	Functions
Liver	Bile	Emulsifies fats in stomach and duodenum
	Glycogen	Stores glucose
	Heparin	Anticoagulant
	Plasma proteins	
	Albumin	Provides osmotic pressure for blood pressure
	Fibrinogen	Necessary for blood clotting
	Prothrombin	Necessary for blood clotting
	Globulins	Forms immunoglobulins (antibodies) and other functions
	Other functions of liver	Filters blood
		Breaks down fat and protein
		Stores protein, fat, and carbohydrates
		Prepares wastes (urea)
		Regulates amino acids
		Produces body heat
		Detoxifies poisons
		Stores vitamins and minerals
		Forms vitamin A
		Stores vitamins A, D, and B complex
Gallbladder		Stores and releases bile
Pancreas (islets of Langerhans)	Pancreatic juice	Digests food
	Insulin and glucogen	Regulate sugar use

duct. This, in combination with the pancreatic duct, empties into the duodenum at the major duodenal papilla, an opening a small distance beyond the pyloric portion of the stomach.

As bile is produced, it flows down the hepatic duct and up into the cystic duct for storage in the gallbladder. With the appearance of fats in the intestine, the hormone cholecystokinin activates the gallbladder to release bile, which then flows through the cystic duct into the common bile duct to be deposited in the duodenum. This system of passageways for the transport of bile from the liver to the gallbladder to the intestine is known as the biliary apparatus.

Pancreas

The pancreas is a long fish-shaped glandular organ (about 6 in [15 cm] long) located behind the stomach (see Figure 23-4). This organ has two distinct functions: as an endocrine gland and as an exocrine gland. As an endocrine gland, it secretes the hormones insulin and glucagon into the bloodstream to regulate blood sugar levels. These functions were discussed in Chapter 19.

The exocrine function is to produce pancreatic juice, which is done by the acinar cells. The acinar cells secrete three main enzymes:

◆ Amylase, which digests starch

◆ Trypsin, which digests protein
◆ Lipase, which digests fats (in the form of triglycerides)

Most pancreatic enzymes are produced in inactive forms and are activated in the small intestine. The inactive forms help to minimize the risk of pancreatic self-digestion. In addition to the wide variety of digestive enzymes in pancreatic juice, bicarbonate and water are also present. Bicarbonate ions (HCO_3-) are secreted from small ductules in the pancreas; HCO_3- helps neutralize the hydrochloric acid in chyme. Enzymes work best in a pH solution between 5 and 8.

Pancreatic juice enters the duodenum through the pancreatic duct. Pancreatic juice is potent and necessary for life. Adequate digestion cannot take place without it. The common bile duct and pancreatic duct enter the duodenum a short distance beyond the pyloric sphincter of the stomach.

Peritoneum

The **peritoneum** is a large sheet of serous membrane that covers many abdominal organs (see Chapter 14). The peritoneum functions to protect abdominal organs. It also secretes a thin fluid that provides lubrication between its layers, the visceral and the parietal. Support is provided to the intestine by a fold of the

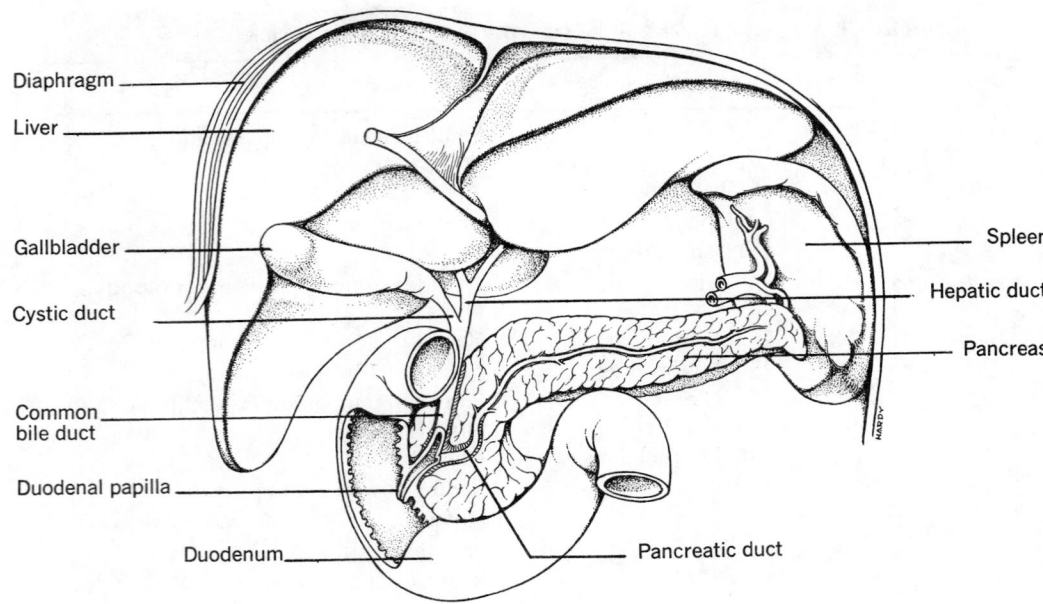

Figure 23-4. Liver and biliary system.

peritoneum called the *mesentery*, which consists of sheets of connective tissue. Some of the mesenteries have names (such as the greater and lesser omentum).

System Physiology

Digestion and Absorption

For nutritional elements to reach individual cells, food first must be broken down into small compounds. After food is broken down, absorption can occur.

Most digestion occurs in the stomach and duodenum, the first part of the small intestine. Most **absorption** (passage of liquids into the bloodstream for use by the cells) takes place in the jejunum and ileum, which makes up the remainder of the small intestine.

The body has two types of digestion: mechanical and chemical. *Mechanical digestion* is the physical breakdown of food caused by chewing and movement of food in the digestive tract. Breaking food into smaller pieces exposes more surface area to the effects of enzymes. *Chemical digestion* is the breakdown of the chemical bond in food with the addition of enzymes, acids, and water (H_2O).

Enzymes are the force of chemical digestion. They are secreted by the oral cavity, stomach, small and large intestines, liver, and pancreas. Enzymes derive their individual names from the substance on which they act, and they are each effective only on a specific nutrient. For example, proteases act only on proteins; lipases act on fats (fats are lipids); and amylases act on carbohydrates.

The GI tract uses other fluids to lubricate, liquefy, and digest food. Mucus, which is made by the mucous membrane lining of the GI tract, lubricates food and protects the lining of the tract from mechanical or chemical injury.

Water liquefies food, which makes it easier to digest and absorb. Water is also the solvent that follows electrolytes across the intestinal wall. Water moves by osmosis in either direction across the intestinal wall.

Digestion in the Stomach

Both mechanical and chemical digestion occur in the stomach. The fundus and body are mostly storage areas, while most stomach digestion occurs in the pylorus.

Saliva begins starch digestion in the stomach, but carbohydrates are not fully digested there. Very little fat digestion occurs in the stomach.

Digestion and Absorption in the Small Intestine

Most fat is digested in the duodenum. There the action of bile breaks down fat droplets into smaller particles.

Absorption of nutrients occurs as a result of active and passive transport mechanisms. Water travels by osmosis following absorption of mineral salts, mainly sodium.

Absorption of nutrients into the body occurs across the **villi,** the fingerlike projections of the intestine, into the capillary network (Fig. 23-5). To increase the surface area, villi also have microvilli, which are microscopic folds of the cell membrane. Unfolded and straightened out, the villi and microvilli could cover more than 2,000 square feet, or half a basketball court. They wave to keep food molecules thoroughly mixed

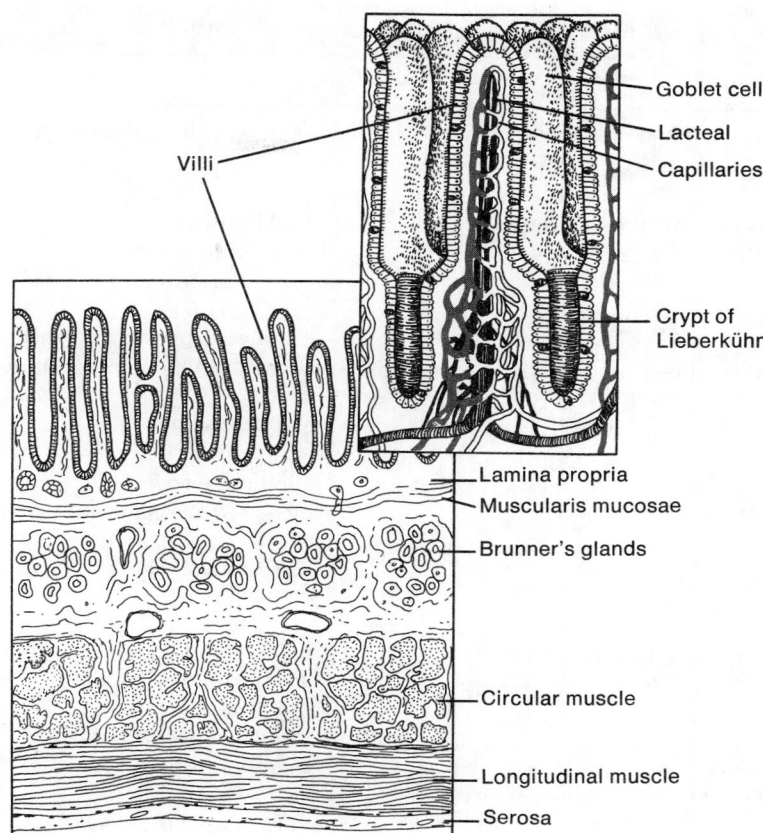

Figure 23-5. Structure of the small intestine villi (Jackson JB, Saunders RB. Child Health Nursing: A Comprehensive Approach to the Care of Children and Their Families. Philadelphia, J.B. Lippincott, 1993).

with digestive juices. Approximately 85% of the nutrients in foods are absorbed through villi into the bloodstream for delivery to cells. Because the villi play such an important part in absorption, they are heavily supplied with blood capillaries (see Figure 23-5). The capillaries in villi carry nutrients, by way of hepatic portal circulation, to the liver for further processing.

Once absorbed, fatty acids recombine with glycerol to form triglycerides, which then form cholesterol and proteins. Bile salts are necessary for absorption of fat-soluble vitamins and fatty acids. *Lacteals* are dead-end lymph capillaries within each villus that absorb fat-soluble nutrients. Due to the fat content in lacteals, their contents appear milky. The substance in lacteals is called *chyle*. Most digested fat is absorbed into lacteals and carried in lymph. Fats eventually reach the bloodstream by way of the thoracic and right lymphatic ducts.

After food has been in the small intestine for about 4 to 6 hours, it passes into the large intestine; all that remains of it is water and waste products. A sphincter-like muscle, located where the large and small intestines meet, acts as a valve to prevent backflow of material to the small intestine; it also regulates the forward flow. It is called the ileocecal valve, from the names of the two joining parts, the ileum of the small intestine and the cecum of the large intestine.

Key Concept

Absorption of nutrients into the bloodstream takes place in the digestive canal. However, these food materials cannot be used by the body until they are delivered to each cell by the bloodstream and transported across the plasma membrane of each cell.

Absorption in the Large Intestine

The large intestine and the remainder of the GI tract are lined with mucous membrane. As the contents move along, most of the water is absorbed through the walls of the large intestine into the circulation.

Metabolism

Metabolism is the term applied to the total of all physical and chemical changes that take place within the body. The physical conversions include chewing and breaking down food into smaller particles. Chemical conversions include the action of enzymes on food, which alters the food into chemically smaller substances. The liver is vital for metabolism. There are two major categories of metabolism: anabolism and catabolism.

Table 23-3. Effects of Aging on the Digestive System

Factor	Result	Nursing Implications
The mouth becomes drier.	More difficulty swallowing	Provide adequate fluids. Observe carefully for choking. Provide liquid with patient medications.
Bony structures are decreased around the mouth.	Mouth discomfort Poor eating habits Sunken appearance of mouth Low self-esteem, less desire for social contact	May need softer foods or ground foods. Assess fit and comfort of dentures. Reinforce self-esteem.
Tooth loss is not a normal function of aging but usually the effect of poor nutrition and hygiene.	Loose teeth, ill-fitting dentures, difficulty eating Mouth discomfort Periodontal disease	Monitor nutrient intake. Encourage high protein supplements. Puree or chop food as needed.
Taste buds are decreased, especially sweet and sour tastes.	Food not enjoyed Increased amounts of salt and sugar eaten Less desire to eat, leading to poor nutrient intake	Assess for eating patterns. Explain the harm of excess calories and salt. Teach about a balanced diet. Encourage programs such as "Meals On Wheels."
Cardiac sphincter is relaxed.	Reflux of undigested food into esophagus (heartburn common) May lead to excess use of over-the-counter (OTC) antacids.	Discourage overuse of OTC antacids.
Gastric mucosa is atrophied, and secretions, such as HCl, intrinsic factor, and enzymes may be decreased.	Digestion usually adequate	Monitor nutrient intake. Watch for signs of pernicious anemia.
Food stays in stomach longer.	Indigestion Bloating Excess gas	Tell patient to avoid foods that cause problems, such as spicy foods and gas formers.
Peristalsis is decreased.	Constipation Use of OTC laxatives or enemas	Encourage fluid and fiber intake. Encourage exercise. Avoid laxatives and enemas. Teach about fluid and fiber use. Check for impaction.
Occurrence of gall stones may increase.	May need gallbladder removal	Provide surgical care. Ensure lower fat intake postoperatively.

Anabolism involves synthesis of substances to form new, larger substances. Examples of anabolism include the synthesis of glycogen, triglycerides, or proteins, such as hemoglobin. Energy, usually in the form of ATP, is required for anabolism.

Catabolism is the breakdown of larger molecules into smaller ones. During catabolism, energy is often released. Cellular respiration is a series of catabolic reactions. The end-products of catabolism that appear during cellular respiration are carbon dioxide, water, and energy. The ATP formed from catabolism is used for anabolism.

The term *basal metabolism* refers to the amount of energy (calories) used by the body when at rest. This is measured by the amount of oxygen used or by the amount of energy released. Basal metabolism is the amount of energy needed to sustain life.

Key Concept

Metabolism

◆ Catabolism (destructive metabolism): breaking down of foods into usable substances (generates heat, carbon dioxide, water, and ATP)

◆ Anabolism (constructive metabolism): using the products of catabolism to build and repair body cells

◆ Catabolism (destructive metabolism): breaking down substances after anabolism (waste products)

Elimination

There are few enzymes in the colon; therefore, little digestion occurs there. Whatever nutrient is not reabsorbed and sent to the portal circulation is eliminated as waste. The process of eliminating intestinal wastes is called **defecation**.

As water is reabsorbed, plant fiber called cellulose, other undigested material, living and dead bacteria, and mucus remain. They mass together and pass into the rectum as solid waste or *feces*. As feces enters the rectum, it stimulates sensory nerve endings, causing sensation of accumulating bulk. Peristaltic waves push the contents against the anal muscle as a signal for tying the rectum. This defecation reflex continues as parasympathetic-controlled nervous activity causes strong contractions. The internal sphincter relaxes and pressure from peristalsis, along with that consciously exerted by diaphragm and abdominal muscles, brings about defecation. To expel feces, the external anal sphincter, a skeletal muscle, is relaxed voluntarily. If the defecation reflex is ignored, the impulse dies. Mass movements or strong peristaltic waves in the colon reinitiate the defecation reflex.

Effects of Aging on the System

The digestive system slows down with age, as do other systems. Major effects of aging on the digestive system are summarized in Table 23-3. Secretion of digestive juices and peristalsis are slowed. The result is a decreased ability to "eat anything and everything," as younger people can do. An indiscretion in eating often causes stomach upset, nausea, or diarrhea for the older person. In the aging person, more food is left undigested, and sometimes inadequate amounts of fluid are taken in, causing constipation. Some older people do not have a daily bowel movement because they do not take in enough food or get enough exercise.

The cells of the liver and pancreas are able to reproduce by dividing. Thus, these organs appear to age more slowly than some other body organs and systems.

Older people have often lost some of their teeth through accidents or tooth and gum disease. This may cause difficulty in chewing and may limit the types of food that may be comfortably eaten.

A person who has been overweight tends to gain even more weight with age. This is partly a process of aging, as muscle tissue is replaced by fatty tissue, but it is also a function of reduced exercise and poor diet. Weight gained in younger years now becomes very difficult to lose. However, reduced efficiency of the digestive system eventually offsets weight gain to some extent.

Many older people also are underweight. They may have difficulty chewing or swallowing, may digest or absorb nutrients insufficiently, may have a poor diet, lack appetite, or lack motivation to cook for themselves if they live alone.

Keys for Review

Key Questions for Critical Thinking

1. Name and describe the organs of the digestive system, including their functions.
2. Describe the accessory organs and their functions.
3. Describe the processes of digestion, absorption, and metabolism.
4. What effects does aging have on the digestive system?

Key Readings

Birchenall JM, Streight ME. Care of the Older Adult, Ed 3. Philadelphia, J.B. Lippincott, 1993

Chabner D. The Language of Medicine, Ed 4. Philadelphia, W.B. Saunders, 1991

Eliopoulus C. Caring for the Elderly in Diverse Care Settings. Philadelphia, J.B. Lippincott, 1990

Farrell J. Nursing Care of the Older Person. Philadelphia, J.B. Lippincott, 1990

Key Readings (continued)

Jackson DB, Saunders RB. Child Health Nursing: A Comprehensive Approach to the Care of Children and Their Families. Philadelphia, J.B. Lippincott, 1993

O'Toole M (Ed). Miller-Keane Encyclopedia & Dictionary of Medicine, Nursing, and Allied Health, Ed 5. Philadelphia, W.B. Saunders, 1992

Scanlon V, Sanders V. Essentials of Anatomy and Physiology. Philadelphia, F.A. Davis, 1991

Seeley R, Stephens T, Tate P. Anatomy and Physiology, Ed 2. St. Louis, Mosby-Yearbook, 1994

Smeltzer SC, Bare BG. Brunner and Suddarth's Textbook of Medical-Surgical Nursing, Ed 7. Philadelphia, J.B. Lippincott, 1992

Taylor C, Lillis C, LeMone P. Fundamentals of Nursing: The Art and Science of Nursing Care, Ed 2. Philadelphia, J.B. Lippincott, 1993

Enrichment Keys

Memmler RL, Cohen BJ, and Woods DL. Structure and Function of the Human Body, Ed 5. Philadelphia, J.B. Lippincott, 1992

Keys to Learning More

Unit Five: foods, their uses, transcultural aspects, assisting patients to eat, and diet therapy

Chapter 30: management of obstructed airway, such as choking on food

Chapter 46: assisting patients with elimination of feces

Chapter 47: collection of specimens, including stool specimens

Chapter 50: nursing assessment, including elements of digestive function

Chapter 51: special enteral isolation techniques

Keys to Learning More (continued)

Chapter 56: medications, many of which affect the digestive system

Chapter 57: intravenous administration of fluids and nutrients

Unit Thirteen: deviations from normal body structure and function in the infant or child

Unit Fourteen: deviations in the adult

Chapter 69: liver function as it influences fluid and electrolyte balance

Chapter 81: digestive disorders, including administration of tube feeding

Unit Fifteen: disorders in older adults

Chapter 88: alcohol abuse and its destruction of the liver

24 The Urinary System

Keys for Learning

Learning Objectives

- State the major functions of the urinary system and how these relate to homeostasis.
- Describe the effects of aldosterone and antidiuretic hormones on kidney function.
- Describe blood supply to and from the kidney.
- On a chart, identify major structures of the urinary system.
- Describe the anatomy and physiology of the nephron.
- List characteristics and components of normal urine.
- Describe filtration, reabsorption, and secretion as they relate to the formation of urine.
- Explain micturition.
- Describe effects of aging on the urinary system.

Key Terms

bladder	nephron
Bowman's capsule	nocturia
calyces (singular: calyx)	renal cortex
convoluted tubule	renal medulla
filtration	ureter
glomerulus (plural: glomeruli)	urethra
kidney	urination
micturition	voiding

Keys to Understanding This Chapter

Chapter 5: one of the basic needs is elimination of body wastes

Chapter 15: integumentary system, which is related to urinary system

Chapter 22: respiratory system, which is related to urinary system

Chapter 23: digestive system, which is related to urinary system

Key Points

- The urinary system eliminates wastes, controls water volume, regulates electrolyte levels, maintains pH balance, activates vitamin D, and secretes erythropoietin and renin.
- Kidneys lie behind the peritoneum (retroperitoneal).
- Nephrons are the functional unit of kidneys. Nephrons make urine; the rest of the urinary system expels it.
- Nephrons consist of renal corpuscles (glomerulus, Bowman's capsule) and renal tubules (proximal convoluted tubule, loop of Henle, distal convoluted tubule).
- Urine is 95% water and 5% solutes (salts, nitrogenous waste products, metabolites, hormones, toxins).
- Urine is formed by these three processes: filtration, reabsorption, and secretion.
- Micturition (voiding) is the release of urine; involuntary voiding is called urinary incontinence.
- As the body ages, the number of functional nephrons decreases.

Key Topics Outline

Structure and Function
   The Kidneys
   The Ureters
   The Urinary Bladder
   The Urethra
System Physiology
   Formation of Urine
   Micturition
Effects of Aging on the System

Key Learning Activities

- Interview a laboratory technician. What important urinary conditions can be discovered with blood testing?

As the body builds and repairs tissues and produces energy for life processes, waste products form and must be removed. The respiratory system and the skin, through the activities of breathing and perspiring, remove some of the water, carbon dioxide, and nitrogenous wastes; the digestive system removes the bulk wastes of food in the feces.

Another system, the urinary system or excretory system, is also involved in waste removal. Because waste is carried by the circulating blood from the cells to the kidneys for elimination in the urine, the urinary system has been called the body's "filtration and removal plant."

Although the anatomy of the urinary system is relatively simple, its action and influence on the total well-being of the body is complex. It has a great influence on the body's homeostasis.

Structure and Function

The urinary system has the ability to adapt to wide variations in diet and fluid intake. The composition of blood, tissues, and interstitial fluids also is adjusted and maintained by the urinary system. Functions of the urinary system are summarized in the accompanying box.

The urinary system helps control blood volume by excreting or conserving water. Blood pressure is affected by the volume of circulating fluids. An accumulation of water in the tissues is known as *edema*; an abnormal decrease is known as *dehydration*. Specific levels of electrolytes in body tissues and fluids are regulated by excretion or conservation of minerals, such as sodium and chlorine. The kidney can precisely regulate and adjust these levels. By regulating sodium chloride (NaCl), the volume of body fluids is controlled.

The pH (acidity/alkalinity) of blood, fluids, and tissues must be balanced. The kidneys can eliminate acids directly into the urine or can excrete acids bound to chemical buffers. Buffers enable the kidney to excrete large amounts of acid, without further lowering urine pH. As a result, urine is 1000 times more acidic than blood. The kidneys also have endocrine functions.

The Kidneys

The **kidneys** are two reddish brown, bean-shaped organs located in the small of the back at the lower edge of the ribs on either side of the vertebral column. The kidneys are said to be *retroperitoneal* because they lie behind the peritoneum (Fig. 24-1). This is important because it is possible to perform surgery on the kidneys from the back, without entering the abdominal cavity itself. The right kidney is slightly lower than the left because of the space taken up by the liver on the right. Renal is a descriptive term used for the kidneys.

Functions of the Urinary System

Maintenance of Homeostasis

◆ Controls water volume, controls blood volume
◆ Maintains blood pressure
◆ Regulates electrolyte levels
◆ Maintains pH balance (acid–base balance)
◆ Activates vitamin D (for calcification of bones)

Manufacture

◆ Secretes erythropoietin and renin

Processing of Wastes

◆ Forms urine (kidneys)
◆ Stores urine (bladder)

Elimination

◆ Eliminates protein wastes and toxic materials

The kidneys are about 4 inches (10 cm) long, 2 inches (5 cm) wide, and 1 inch (2.5 cm) thick. They are extremely vascular (heavily supplied with blood vessels). This blood supply is necessary so that the kidneys can do their work of removing wastes from the body. Approximately 10% of the circulating blood in the entire body circulates through the kidneys each day. Each kidney is embedded in fatty tissue surrounded by a fibrous capsule. This fibrous capsule continues downward, forming the outer layer of covering of the ureter. The fatty pads, plus the renal fascia, which is anchored to surrounding tissues, help to hold the kidneys in place. On the medial surface of each kidney is an indented area called the *hilum,* a notch through which the blood vessels, the nerves, and the ureter enter.

If the kidney is cut in half longitudinally (the long way) you can see that is divided into two parts: the outside called the cortex and the inner portion called the medulla ("middle").

Renal Cortex. The **renal cortex** is the outer reddish brown part of the kidney within the capsule (Fig. 24-2). The greater portion of the cortex is made of renal corpuscles (glomeruli and Bowman's capsules) and the proximal and distal portions of the convoluted tubules. These are discussed with the nephrons.

Renal Medulla. The **renal medulla** contains the remainder of the renal tubules, the loops of Henle, and collecting tubules. Within the medulla are cone-shaped structures called *pyramids*. These pyramids are arranged so that the base is on the outside near the cortex and the tip (renal papilla) points toward the renal pelvis. The renal pelvis is a funnel-shaped basin at the upper end of the ureter. Urine flows from the collecting tubules through the pyramids and into cuplike exten-

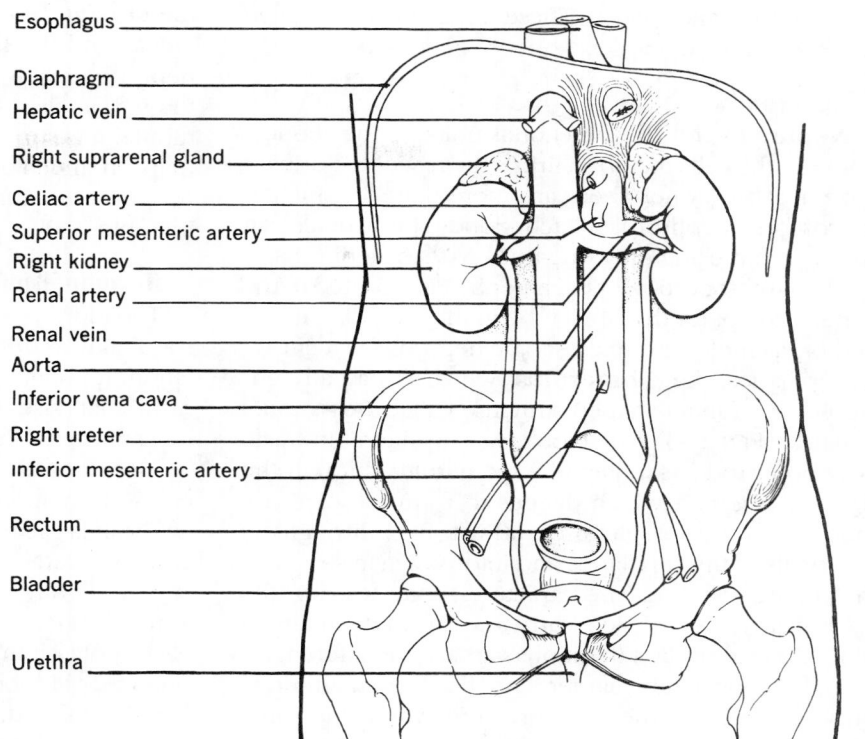

Esophagus
Diaphragm
Hepatic vein
Right suprarenal gland
Celiac artery
Superior mesenteric artery
Right kidney
Renal artery
Renal vein
Aorta
Inferior vena cava
Right ureter
Inferior mesenteric artery
Rectum
Bladder
Urethra

Figure 24-1. Anatomy of the urinary system showing the position of blood vessels, kidneys, and ureters. The relationships between the ureters, urinary bladder, and pelvic bones are also shown.

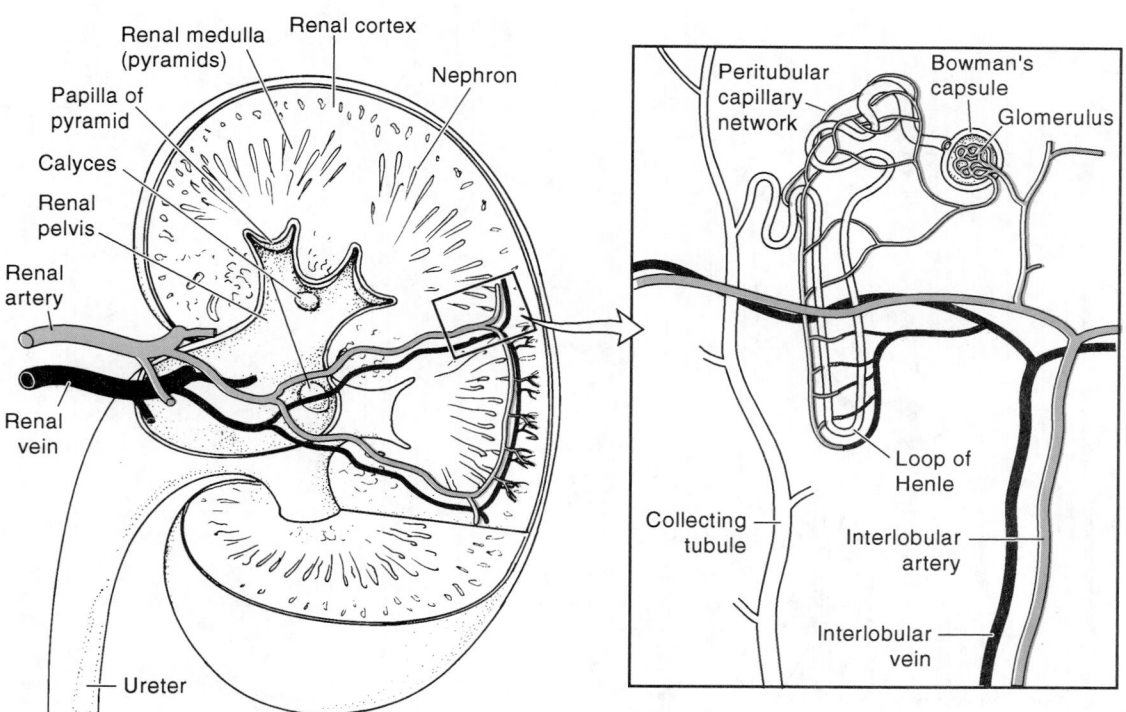

Renal medulla (pyramids)
Renal cortex
Papilla of pyramid
Nephron
Calyces
Renal pelvis
Renal artery
Renal vein
Ureter

Peritubular capillary network
Bowman's capsule
Glomerulus
Loop of Henle
Collecting tubule
Interlobular artery
Interlobular vein

Figure 24-2. Frontal section of the right kidney showing internal structure and blood vessels. An individual nephron is depicted in the upper part of the kidney.

sions of the renal pelvis. These extensions are called **calyces** (singular: calyx).

Nephron

Nephrons are the functional units of the kidney. They are the cells that *form* urine; the rest of the urinary system *expels* urine. There are more than one million microscopic nephrons in each kidney. Individuals can survive even using only one-third of their nephrons.

The largest portion of each nephron is located in the cortex, except for the small tube in the medulla. At one end of each of these microscopic nephrons is a cluster of capillaries, the **glomerulus**, which is partially enclosed in a funnel-shaped structure called **Bowman's capsule** (Fig. 24-3). The blood, with its filterable waste and food products, enters the glomerulus through the *afferent arteriole*, which divides to form the capillary loop. Water, wastes, glucose, and salts filter through the thin walls of the capillaries and into Bowman's capsule in a dilute solution. The capillaries unite to form the *efferent arteriole*, which carries away the remaining blood. It is important to emphasize that the afferent arteriole is considerably larger than the efferent arteriole. This accounts for the high pressure within the functional units of the kidneys and facilitates filtration.

Extending from Bowman's capsule is a long twisted tube called the **convoluted tubule**. The first portion is

the *proximal* convoluted tubule; the next is the *loop of Henle*; and the final portion (which is the end of the nephron unit) is the *distal* convoluted tubule. The water with its dissolved contents travels the length of this tubule. It is surrounded by capillaries whose job it is to reabsorb much of the water, salts, and all of the glucose. Nephron structures and their functions are summarized in Table 24-1.

Hormonal Influence and the Kidneys

The kidneys secrete two hormones; renin and erythropoietin. *Renin* is important in blood pressure regulation. It initiates a process (renin–angiotensin mechanism) that raises blood pressure. The renin–angiotensin mechanism is illustrated in Figure 24-4.

Erythropoietin stimulates red bone marrow to increase formation of red blood cells (RBCs or erythrocytes). It is secreted when hypoxia (low blood oxygen) is recognized.

Aldosterone is a mineralocorticoid hormone from the adrenal cortex. Aldosterone responds to high blood levels of potassium, low levels of sodium, and low blood pressure or blood volume. Aldosterone stimulates reabsorption of sodium ions and excretion of potassium. Sodium ions are returned to the blood; water follows the salt by osmosis. Potassium ions are excreted into the urine. The renin–angiotensin mechanism is acti-

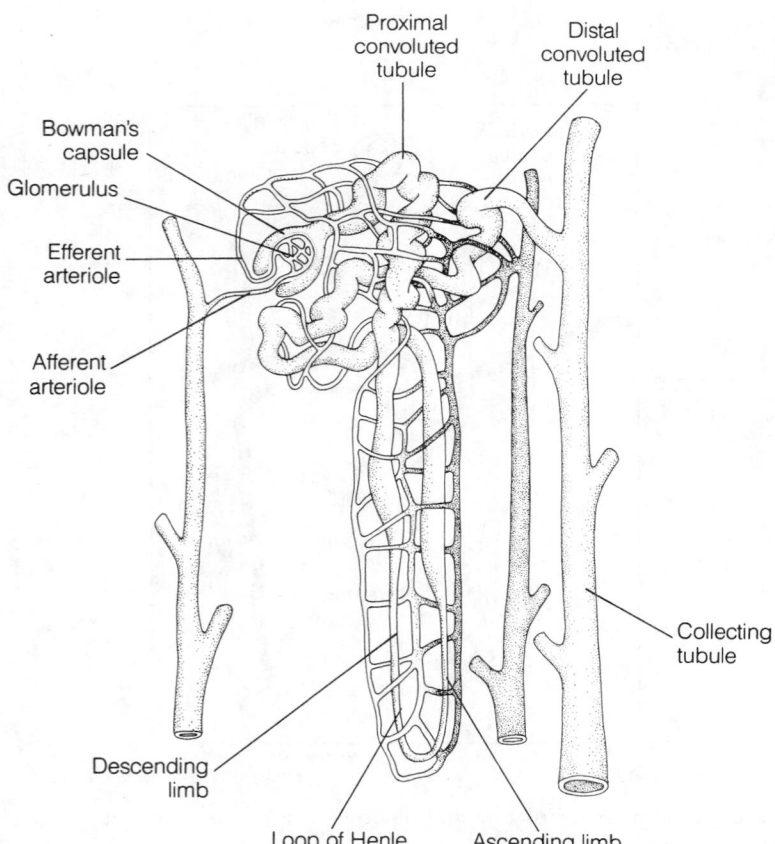

Proximal convoluted tubule

Distal convoluted tubule

Bowman's capsule

Glomerulus

Efferent arteriole

Afferent arteriole

Collecting tubule

Descending limb

Loop of Henle

Ascending limb

Figure 24-3. The nephron with blood supply.

Table 24-1. The Nephron Structures and Their Functions

Structure	Function
Glomerulus (within Bowman's capsule)	Filtration of water, wastes (urea), glucose, and salts (electrolytes) out of the blood (The filtrate consists of water plus all nonprotein components of the plasma.)
Convoluted tubules	
Proximal convulted tubule	Reabsorption of some needed electrolytes (potassium, chlorine), water, and glucose, as well as some amino acids and bicarbonate
Loop of Henle	Reabsorption of water, additional reabsorption of electrolytes
Distal convoluted tubule	Reabsorption of sodium, water, and remainder of glucose

vated by low blood pressure or low blood volume (see Figure 24-4).

Antidiuretic hormone (ADH) is released by the posterior pituitary. It increases the reabsorption of water by the kidney tubules. Thus, the amount of urine decreases. ADH responds to low water levels in the body. The effect is to maintain normal circulating blood volume and blood pressure.

Renal Blood Supply

The kidneys receive their generous blood supply from the renal arteries, which are early aortic branches. This blood flow is outlined in Figure 24-5. Because the blood arrives directly from the aorta, which carries freshly oxygenated blood directly from the heart, the renal blood is highly oxygenated. The renal arteries diverge, forming smaller arteries, until they become the afferent arterioles supplying blood to the glomerular capillaries of the renal corpuscle. These glomerular capillaries have a higher pressure than most capillaries (60 mm Hg versus 30 mm Hg), which is necessary to form renal filtrate (discussed later). Efferent arterioles arise from glomeruli and carry blood away. After the efferent arterioles exit the glomeruli, they branch off to become the peritubular capillaries (around tubes), surrounding the convoluted tubules. These capillaries drain into a system of veins, ending at the renal vein. This vein empties into the inferior vena cava for return of blood to the heart.

There are two sites of capillary exchange in the renal system: the glomeruli and the peritubular capillaries. The glomeruli begin the formation of urine. The peritubular capillaries carry substances from the kidneys back to the circulatory system for reuse.

The Ureters

Urine travels from the pelvis of the kidneys into the ureters. The **ureters** are narrow tubes about 1/5 inch (0.5 cm) in diameter and about 10 to 12 inches (25–30 cm) long (see Figure 24-1). They are attached to the kidney at the renal pelvis and carry the urine from the kidneys down to the urinary bladder. The ureters are lined with mucous membrane and contain a great many sensory nerves. In the walls of the ureters are smooth

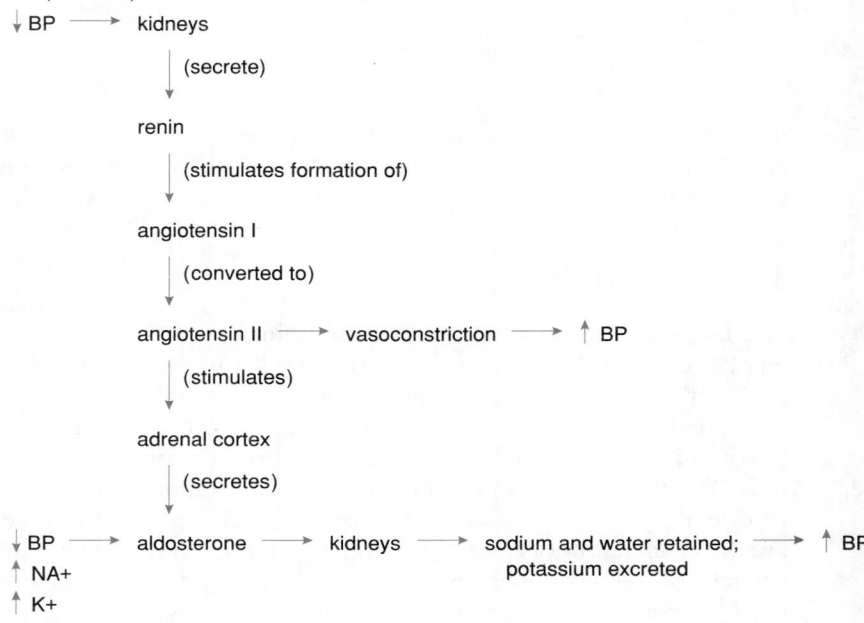

Figure 24-4. Renin–angiotensin mechanism.

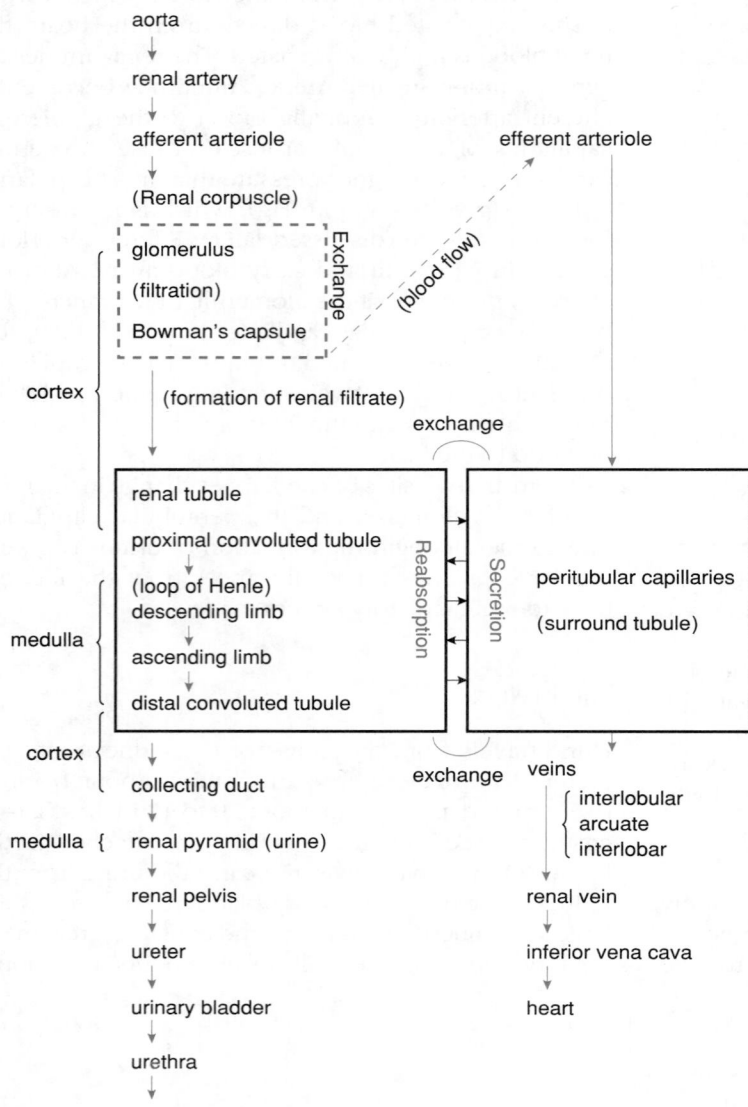

Figure 24-5. The formation of urine with renal blood flow.

muscles that contract in peristaltic waves (similar to peristalsis in the intestine) to carry the urine, drop by drop, to the bladder.

The Urinary Bladder

The **bladder** is a hollow muscular sac, which, when empty lies behind the symphysis pubis (see Figure 24-1). It is the reservoir where urine is stored. When full, it may extend well up into the abdominal cavity. It is lined with mucous membrane, as is the entire urinary tract. The *trigone* is a triangular area on the floor of the bladder that does not expand. The points of the triangle are the attachments of two ureters and the urethra. The capacity of the bladder varies, but usually the desire to empty the bladder (void) is present when it fills to about 200 to 400 mL. The muscles in the bladder's walls distend as it fills with urine and contract as it empties itself. A bladder can hold 800 mL or more. An involuntary internal sphincter relaxes as impulses to void are sensed.

The Urethra

The bladder wall contains three openings: two from the ureters and one into the **urethra**, the tube through which the urine passes to the outside (see Figure 24-1). In men, the urethra is about 8 inches (20 cm) long. It passes through the prostate gland where two ducts from the male sex glands join it, and then through the length of the penis, the male organ of copulation. The woman's urethra is short, about 1 1/2 inches (3.8 cm) long, and opens to the outside at the urinary meatus or urinary canal. In both male and female, the meatus is controlled by a voluntary sphincter or circular muscle band. The female urethra is a passageway for urine only. In the male, the urethra serves the reproductive system as well and is the passageway for both urine and sperm, the male sex cells.

> **Key Concept**
>
> The urinary system plays a vital part in the maintenance of homeostasis in the body.

System Physiology

Formation of Urine

Urine is formed in the nephron by three processes: filtration, reabsorption, and secretion (see Figure 24-5).

Filtration

Filtration is the process of removing particles from a solution by allowing the liquid solvent to pass across a barrier. The barrier allows certain solutes, which are small enough, to pass through. Larger solutes are kept in solution because they are too large to pass through the barrier. (Chapter 16 discusses filtration.)

In the kidneys, filtration is the movement of plasma across the glomeruli of the nephron into Bowman's capsule. Blood enters the glomerular capillaries and flows through smaller and smaller blood vessels. This causes increased pressure within the vessels and forces a fluid called *renal filtrate* out of the glomeruli into the capsule. Renal filtrate is similar to plasma, but it has no blood cells and less protein. The filtrate contains water, glucose, urea, creatinine, and numerous salts. About 125 mL of filtrate is produced each minute or about 180 L/day. Less than 1% of the filtrate becomes urine.

Reabsorption

As the filtrate leaves the renal capsule and flows through the proximal convoluted tubule, the loop of Henle, and the distal convoluted tubule, 99% of the filtrate is reabsorbed or recaptured. Useful substances such as water, salts, and organic molecules enter the interstitial fluid. Eventually, the reabsorbed fluid enters renal veins and is returned to the general circulation (see Figure 24-5).

Reabsorption occurs by active and passive transport mechanisms (see Chapter 16). The proximal tubules reabsorb most of the water that will be retained in the body. Water moves by osmosis. Sodium ions (Na+) are carried by active transport. The transport of all solutes is tied to the active transport of sodium ions. Many negative ions are returned to the blood following the reabsorption of positive ions because unlike charges attract.

Pinocytosis (a process in which a cell ingests substances) is responsible for reabsorption of large proteins; small proteins are reabsorbed by active transport. The specialized areas of the kidney tubules are permeable to different sizes, shapes, and types of molecules. Thus, certain substances, including water, can only be reabsorbed from certain portions of the kidney.

The kidneys have a limit or threshold of reabsorption to many substances. The tubules have a threshold level or an upper limit of a substance that can be removed from the plasma. When that point is reached, the plasma cannot hold any more of that substance and the kidney excretes it in urine.

Secretion

Secretion is the process by which substances are moved from the blood into the urine (the opposite of reabsorption). Secretion can occur by active or passive transport mechanisms. Molecules that are secreted in the peritubular capillaries move into the tubular cells, then into the tubular lumen. Secretions into urine include ions, such as hydrogen (H$^+$) and potassium (K$^+$), and end products, such as ammonia and bile pigments. Metabolites (end products) of drugs and ammonia are also secreted into the urine.

Characteristics and Composition of Urine

Characteristics. Fluids and dissolved substances are secreted by the kidneys, stored in the urinary bladder, and excreted through the urethra. The result is urine.

About 1000 to 1500 mL (2–3 pints) of urine is excreted from the body daily. The quantity is influenced by many factors, including the amount of fluid taken into the body, perspiration, hemorrhage, blood pressure, external temperature, drugs, fever, and various diseases.

Urine is initially a clear amber liquid, with a characteristic odor; it may become cloudy when exposed to air. It is acid in reaction; on standing it may become alkaline because certain substances in it break down into ammonia bodies.

The concept of *specific gravity* and its measurement is discussed in Chapter 47. The specific gravity of urine denotes the relationship between that urine and pure water. Normal urine is only slightly concentrated, with a specific gravity of about 1.010 to 1.025. A higher specific gravity can indicate dehydration (too little fluid in the tissues, a drying out) or urinary retention. A lower specific gravity may indicate overhydration.

Composition. Certain wastes are always present in urine, but careful analysis will show whether substances not normally found in urine are present. The composition of normal urine is as follows:

◆ *Water*, about 95% (water serves as a solvent)
◆ *Nitrogenous waste products* from the breakdown of

proteins; common protein wastes are urea, uric acid, and creatinine

◆ *Excessive minerals* from the diet, such as sodium, potassium, chlorides, calcium, sulfates, and phosphates
◆ *Toxins* and certain *drug metabolites*
◆ *Hormones* (especially those related to the sex of the person)
◆ *Yellow pigment* from certain bile compounds

In case of disease or malfunction, abnormal products such as blood, glucose, pus, casts, and albumin may be present in the urine. Urine is normally sterile (free from microorganisms.) Nonsterile urine implies disease or infection.

Micturition

The release of urine (**urination**) from the body is called **voiding**, or **micturition**; involuntary voiding is called urinary incontinence. The verb "to void" means to vacate, to make empty.

The urine flows from the collecting tubules into the renal pelvis, down the ureters, and slowly enters the

Table 24-2. Effects of Aging on the Urinary System

Factor	Result	Nursing Implication
There is 20% kidney weight lost and 30% decrease in number of nephrons.	Less ability to concentrate and form urine	Be aware of intake and output. Assess for dehydration or edema. Assess blood pressure. Daily weights may be needed. Measure intake and output q8h.
Nephron membranes thicken.	Decrease in rate of filtration, excretion, and reabsorption	Be aware that medications will concentrate in the blood. Watch for toxic levels.
	Rise in blood urea nitrogen (BUN), creatinine, uric acid. May be susceptible to gout	Watch lab reports for abnormal levels of BUN, creatinine, and uric acid
Blood flow to the kidney decreases.	Less urine formation	Watch intake and output. Offer fluids throughout day (maintain 2,000 mL minimum per day). Administer medications, such as Lasix, carefully.
The lining of bladder becomes fibrotic and muscles weaken in ureters and bladder.	Lessens capacity of bladder to about 200 mL, causing frequency and incontinence	Allow for frequent bathroom visits. Make available devices or pads to absorb leaks for ambulatory patients.
	Loss of muscle tone, causing bladder to retain urine because it cannot empty completely	Watch for bladder infection and urinary retention.
	Loss of tone, causing nocturia	Allow 3 h between last evening fluids and bedtime. Do not use evening fluids that stimulate voiding (coffee, tea, colas, alcohol). Make bathroom and bedroom safe for nighttime visits—move obstacles, keep a night light on.
Cancer or benign hypertrophy of prostate is common in men.	Frequent urge to void. Retention of urine. Sexual dysfunction	Encourage frequent testicular self-examination. Encourage medical evaluation.
Pelvic muscles weaken and relax (often due to childbirth) in women.	Incontinence. Uterine or bladder prolapse. Bladder infections common	Instruct in pelvic muscle exercises. Do not use incontinence pads for bed patients (to prevent pressure ulcer formation). Offer bedpan or assist to bathroom q2h. Provide adult incontinence pads or Attends for ambulatory patients. Assess symptoms of bladder infections. Teach proper feminine hygiene.

bladder. This sac, which is flat when empty, slowly fills. As the urine distends the bladder, it stimulates nerve endings in the bladder walls. The brain interprets the message that soon the bladder will have to be emptied. The internal and external sphincter muscles controlling the opening to the urethra are stimulated by the nervous system to relax. However, the external sphincter can be controlled voluntarily. Therefore, when the person wills, the external muscles in the bladder wall contract, and the urine that has accumulated within the bladder is forced out. If the bladder continues to fill without being emptied, voluntary control is lost.

Effects of Aging on the System

The ability to filter blood, reabsorb electrolytes, and secrete wastes is decreased with an aging kidney. Table 24-2 summarizes major effects of aging on the urinary system. Although the kidney can still function within normal limits, it has less ability to return to normal after losses of fluids and electrolytes. These losses occur during perspiration, surgery, trauma, or changes in food intake, for example. The loss of functioning nephrons decreases the glomerular filtration rate, resulting in a decreased clearance of protein waste products (urea, creatinine, uric acid). Drugs may reach toxic levels because they are not adequately filtered. Secretion and removal of substances such as ammonia are not as efficient. The threshold for glucose is decreased and higher blood sugar levels may be noted.

The bladder has a smaller capacity; thus, urinary frequency (inability to wait) and **nocturia** (waking up to void at night) are common. The bladder muscles are weaker, leading to urinary retention (abnormal holding), dribbling, and stress incontinence (involuntary voiding). Incontinence may need medical evaluation. Enlargement of the prostate (see Chapter 25) may also cause urinary difficulties in males.

Keys for Review

Key Questions for Critical Thinking

1. The body must constantly maintain homeostasis. Describe the influence of the urinary system on the body's homeostasis.
2. Describe the formation of urine in the kidneys. Include a discussion of the role of filtration, reabsorption, and secretion.
3. Describe micturition and compare to incontinence. Discuss causes of incontinence.

Key Readings

Birchenall JM, Streight ME. Care of the Older Adult, Ed 3. Philadelphia, J.B. Lippincott, 1993

Chabner D. The Language of Medicine, Ed 4. Philadelphia, W.B. Saunders, 1991

Memmler RL, Cohen BJ, Woods DL. Structure and Function of the Human Body, Ed 5. Philadelphia, J.B. Lippincott, 1992

O'Toole M (Ed). Miller-Keane Encyclopedia and Dictionary of Medicine, Nursing, and Allied Health, Ed 5. Philadelphia, W.B. Saunders, 1992

Scanlon V, Sanders V. Essentials of Anatomy and Physiology. Philadelphia, F.A. Davis, 1991

Seeley R, Stephens T, Tate P. Anatomy and Physiology, Ed 2. St. Louis, Mosby-Yearbook, 1992

Smeltzer SC, Bare BG. Brunner and Suddarth's Textbook of Medical-Surgical Nursing, Ed 7. Philadelphia, J.B. Lippincott, 1992

Key Readings (continued)

Taylor C, Lillis C, LeMone P. Fundamentals of Nursing: The Art and Science of Nursing Care, Ed 2. Philadelphia, J.B. Lippincott, 1993

Keys to Learning More

Chapter 46: specific techniques for assisting the patient with elimination

Chapter 47: collection of specimens, including urine specimens

Chapter 50: nursing assessment, including elements of urinary system function

Chapter 53: observation of bladder function after surgery

Chapter 54: urinary catheterization

Chapter 56: medications, many of which affect the urinary system

Unit Thirteen: deviations from normal in children

Chapter 69: disorders in fluid and electrolyte balance

Chapter 82: specific urinary disorders

Chapter 83: male reproductive disorders, many of which are closely related to the urinary system

Unit Fifteen: deviations in older adults

25 The Reproductive System

Keys for Learning

Learning Objectives

- Define *puberty* and describe hormonal influences on boys and girls during puberty.
- Identify the relationship between the hypothalamus, the pituitary, and the gonads.
- Locate the structures of the male reproductive system on a chart and describe their functions.
- Locate the structures of the female reproductive system on a chart and describe their functions.
- Describe the anatomy and physiology of the mammary gland in the nonpregnant woman.
- Describe the area classified as the perineum in the male and female.
- Describe the menstrual cycle, including menarche and menopause, and the three phases of the cycle.

Key Terms

cervix	ovary	spermatozoon
clitoris	oviducts	(pl: spermatozoa)
copulation	ovulation	testes (sing:
glans penis	ova (sing: ovum)	testis)
menarche	puberty	uterus
menopause	scrotum	vagina
menses	semen	vulva

Keys to Understanding This Chapter

Chapter 5: a basic human need is reproduction of the species

Chapter 18: nervous system and its relationship to copulation

Chapter 19: endocrine system and hormones

Chapter 20: urinary system and its close relationship to reproductive organs

Key Points

- Puberty begins when the anterior hormones, luteinizing hormone and follicle-stimulating hormone, stimulate the gonads to secrete increased amounts of sex hormones.

Key Points (continued)

- The primary sex organs (testes and ovaries) are called gonads. Gonads produce gametes (sperm and egg cells).
- The major male hormone is testosterone; the major female hormones are the estrogens.
- The testes produce spermatozoa, sperm cells, under the influence of testosterone.
- Spermatic ducts include the epididymides, the ductus deferentia, and the ejaculatory ducts, which propel the sperm into the urethra to be expelled.
- Spermatogenesis continues throughout a man's lifetime; a woman develops only about 400 ovum in her lifetime.
- The menstrual cycle is divided into three phases: follicular, luteal, and menstrual.

Key Topics Outline

Hormonal Influences on the Reproductive Systems
Structure and Function
    The Male Reproductive System
    The Female Reproductive System
System Physiology
    The Menstrual Cycle
    Copulation
Effects of Aging on the System

Key Learning Activities

- Interview a teacher who works with adolescent mothers. What type of sex education is given to them?
- Visit an office of Planned Parenthood or a similar organization. What services are offered, other than abortions? Obtain samples of their literature.
- Using a chart or body model, point out important structures of the male and female reproductive systems.

Rosdahl CB: Textbook of Basic Nursing, 6th ed. © 1995 J.B. Lippincott Company

The reproductive system is probably the most unusual and impressive of all body systems. Although other systems are designed to sustain the individual, the reproductive system specializes in continuing the species and in passing genetic material from generation to generation. Also, unlike other systems of the body, there are major differences between the two divisions: male and female reproductive systems.

Hormonal Influences on the Reproductive System

Unlike other systems of the body, the reproductive system develops during childhood and adolescence. It does not become functional until acted on by hormones during puberty. **Puberty** (or pubescence) is the stage of life during which the reproductive organs become fully functional. Puberty occurs around 10 to 14 years of age in girls and 12 to 16 years of age in boys, although this can vary a great deal.

Hormones from the hypothalamus, pituitary, and the gonads influence the reproductive system. Before puberty (*prepubescence*), the blood concentration of *androgens* (male hormones) and *estrogens* (female hormones) are the same in every person. During puberty, hormones from the anterior pituitary gland cause the reproductive glands to secrete increased amounts of sex hormones. As a result, the organs of the reproductive system (genitals) begin to function and secondary sex characteristics appear, differentiating between male and female.

The hypothalamus stimulates the secretion of both luteinizing hormone (LH) and follicle-stimulating hormone (FSH) from the anterior pituitary, which produces these hormones. LH is also called interstitial cell stimulating hormone (ICSH) in males. FSH and LH/ICSH are the gonadotropic hormones. These hormones have two main effects:

◆ They stimulate the formation of sperm in the male or ova in the female.
◆ They stimulate the primary sex organs (gonads) to secrete hormones.

Male Hormones. The gonadotropic (gonad-stimulating) hormones stimulate the testes to secrete androgens, the male hormones. The major androgen is *testosterone.* During puberty, male glandular development becomes very active. The youngster develops a beard, pubic and axillary hair, and an increase in hair growth all over his body. Musculature develops. His body becomes broader in the shoulders and remains narrow in the hips. His voice deepens. Testosterone also maintains the functioning of male accessory organs and stimulates protein anabolism. As a result, a man has larger and stronger musculature than a woman.

Female Hormones. Gonadotropic hormones also stimulate development of female sexual characteristics. The ovaries are stimulated to secrete female hormones, the *estrogens*. The estrogens include estradiol, estriol, and estrone. After puberty, another hormone, *progesterone*, is produced in the corpus luteum of the ovary. Progesterone has its primary function during pregnancy.

The young girl at puberty exhibits many changes as a result of estrogen production. The characteristic feminine contour appears: breast tissue develops and unique fatty deposits appear. The glands become active, and hair appears in the pubic and axillary areas. Although voice changes are not as marked as those in a boy, the voice does deepen and mature in tone and quality. As the glands of reproduction become active, menstruation occurs. All female secondary sex characteristics depend on secretion of estrogen and progesterone.

Structure and Function

The functions of the man are to produce sperm and to transfer them to the woman. The woman produces eggs and provides the environment necessary for growth and development of a fetus. Functions of the reproductive systems are summarized in the accompanying box.

Each system has both external and internal organs. In this chapter, the organs are discussed internally to externally.

The Male Reproductive System

The male reproductive system consists of the testes, ductal system, scrotum, penis, and accessory glands. The ducts are the epididymis, ductus deferens, ejacu-

Functions of the Male and Female Reproductive Systems

Development of Sexual Characteristics

◆ Secrete hormones that initiate puberty
◆ Maintain specific male and female sexual characteristics
◆ Secrete mucus, spermatic fluid, and other substances

Reproduction

◆ Produce ova (female) and sperm (male)
◆ Pass genetic information to infant
· ◆ Participate in copulation and fertilization
◆ Maintain and nourish fetus until birth (female)

Infant Nourishment

◆ Produce breast milk (female)

latory duct, and urethra. The glands are the seminal vesicles, prostate gland, and bulbourethral glands. The testes produce sperm, the ducts transport sperm, and the glands produce secretions.

The external structures of the male reproductive system are the penis and the scrotum. Internal structures include the ducts, glands, and supporting structures. The area between the scrotum and the anus is called the perineum. Figure 25-1 illustrates the male reproductive structures.

Testes

The **testes** (sing: testis), also known as the testicles, produce the **spermatozoa** (sperm cells) and secrete the sex hormones. Testosterone is the major male sex androgen. (The combining forms for testis in medical terms are: orcho/o, orchi/o, and orchid/o.)

The testes in the adult male are two small almond-shaped glands, one on each side of the scrotum. They are small, approximately 1.5 to 2 inches (3.7–5 cm) long and 1 inch (2.5 cm) wide and thick. Each testis is covered by tissue layers, one of which partitions the testis into 250 to 300 wedge-shaped lobules. Each lobule contains the functional units of the testis, which are called the *seminiferous tubules*. Each seminiferous tubule is tightly convoluted. The combined length of the seminiferous tubules is about ½ mile! Within these tubules the sperm cells are produced and mature. Between the tubules are small clusters of specialized endocrine cells, called *interstitial cells*, which secrete testosterone and other androgens. These cells lining the tubules produce sperm also.

Sperm Cells and Spermatogenesis. Around the age of 13 years and continuing throughout life, the male gonads,

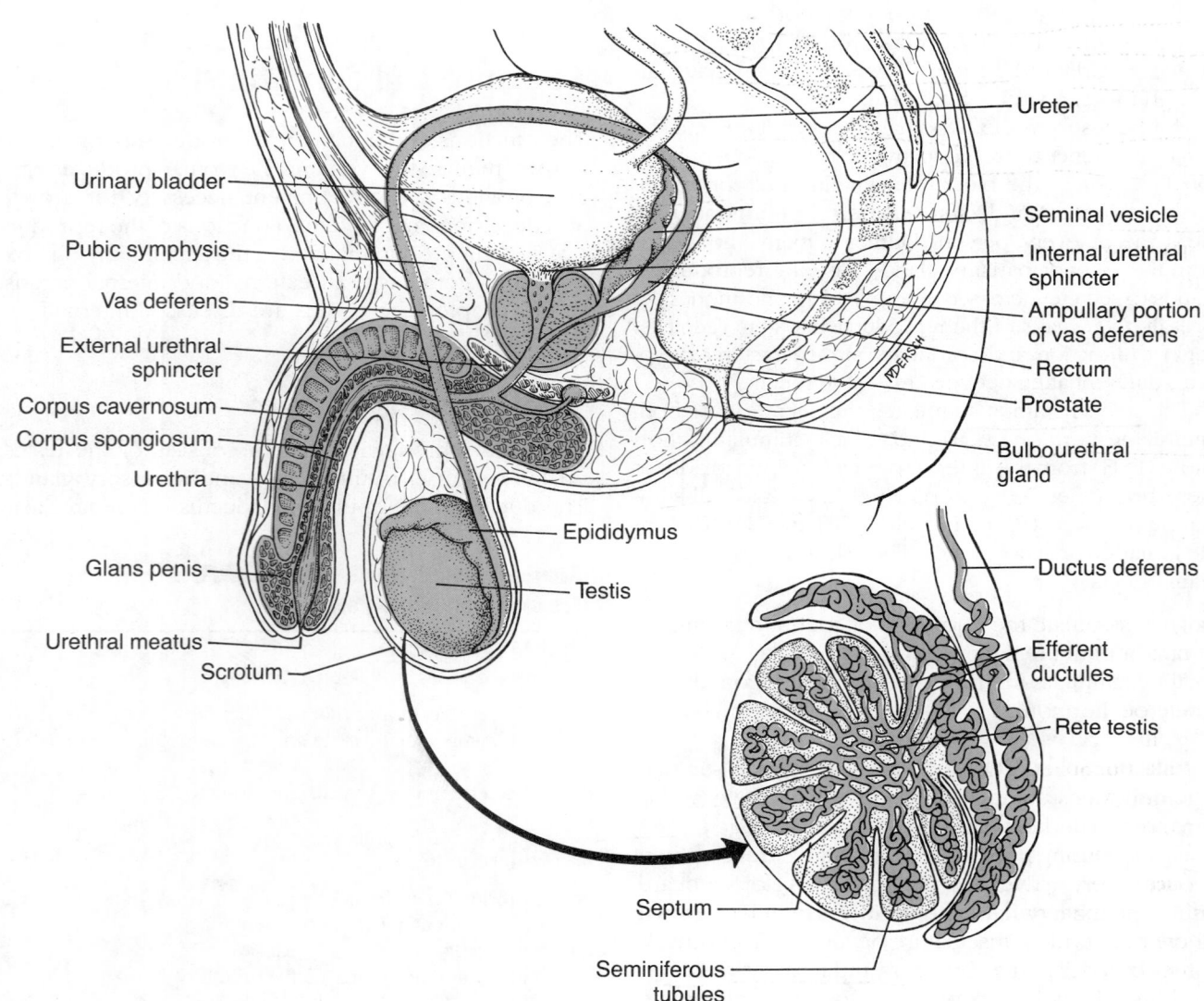

Figure 25-1. Organs of the male reproductive system. (Reeder SJ, Martin LL, & Koniak D. Maternity Nursing: Family, Newborn, and Women's Health Care, 17th ed. Philadelphia. JB Lippincott, 1992)

stimulated by testosterone, form sperm. This formation of mature and functional sperm cells (spermatozoa) is called spermatogenesis. Normal spermatogenesis does not occur if the testes are too warm or too cold, that is above or below 35°C (95°F).

Stem cells of sperm cell development are the *spermatogonia*. Spermatogonia divide by mitosis and then meiosis to form *spermatocytes*. (Mitosis and meiosis were described in Chapter 14.) The next form is called spermatids and they develop into spermatozoa. Millions of sperm are produced each day in the testes. It takes about 2 months from development of sperm cells until their storage in the ductus deferens.

Sperm cells (spermatozoa) are highly specialized. The sperm cell is made up of several divisions. The head contains 23 chromosomes. The tip of the head, the acrosome, contains enzymes that can dissolve the tough cell wall of the ovum. The body (middle piece) contains mitochondria, which provide the energy necessary for locomotion. The whiplike tail is a flagellum that propels the sperm with a lashing motion.

Sperm and semen combine in the ductus deferens. About 60 to 100 million sperm cells per milliliter are contained in the semen. A sperm count of less than 10 to 20 million per milliliter may have difficulty fertilizing an ovum.

The amount of semen ejaculated varies from about 2 to 5 mL. Most sperm degenerate after 24 hours. Of the average 250 million sperm cells ejaculated, only about 100 sperm survive to contact the ovum in the oviduct.

The Ductal System

The male reproductive organs have a system of ducts that store and transport sperm from the testicles to the urethra. These ducts include the epididymides, the ductus deferentia, and the ejaculatory ducts.

Epididymis. The epididymis (pl: epididymides) is a long, comma-shaped organ attached to the posterior surface of the testis. This tightly coiled tube is approximately 20 feet (6 meters) long but is so tiny that it can barely be seen with the naked eye. Within the epididymis, millions of sperm cells are in their final stages of maturation. Sperm cells are not able to fertilize an egg unless they mature in the epididymis. Smooth muscle propels sperm into the ductus deferens.

Ductus Deferens. The sperm continue their journey through a tube called the ductus deferens (pl: ductus deferentia), which is about 18 inches (45 cm) long. It transports sperm from the epididymis to the ejaculatory duct. The ductus deferens, also known as the vas deferens, passes on each side of the scrotum through the inguinal canal, which lies in the muscles of the abdominal wall. The ductus then enters the abdominal cavity

and continues over the top and down the posterior surface of the bladder, into the pelvic cavity. Peristaltic contractions propel sperm cells through the ductus. Each ductus deferens joins a duct from the seminal vesicles. These ducts, together with blood vessels, lymphatic vessels, nerves, and connective tissue coverings, make up the *spermatic cord*. The spermatic cord is covered with connective tissue.

The spermatic cord passes through an opening in the muscular abdominal wall called the inguinal canal. Normally the inguinal canal is closed. It is a weak spot, however, and a common site for herniation in men. It is the site where the testicles descend into the scrotum before birth.

Ejaculatory Ducts. These ducts are about 1 inch (2 cm) long. Each originates in the ampulla of the ductus deferens and empties into the urethra. The ejaculatory ducts receive secretions from the seminal vesicles and prostate gland.

Scrotum

The testes are enclosed in a saclike structure called the **scrotum**, which is suspended behind the base of the penis. The scrotum supports and protects the testes. The external appearance of the scrotum varies depending on environmental conditions and the contraction of its attached muscles. (The muscles involuntarily contract and bring the testicles closer to the body as external temperature lowers.) Temperature of the testes (35°C or 95°F) is lower than internal body temperature.

Penis

The *penis* is a cylindrical organ located immediately in front of the scrotum. It is composed of three masses of cavernous (erectile) tissue, each of which contains smooth muscle, connective tissue, and blood sinuses (large vascular channels). When blood flow through these sinuses is minimal, the penis is soft and flaccid. At the time of sexual excitement, blood fills the sinuses and the penis becomes firm and erect. The firm, erect penis is capable of penetrating the vagina to deposit sperm.

The smooth cap of the penis is called the **glans penis** and is covered by a fold of loose skin that forms the hoodlike foreskin (prepuce). Surgical removal of this foreskin, called circumcision, often is performed.

The urethra within the penis serves as a common passageway for both the urinary and reproductive systems. Urine and semen do not pass through the urethra simultaneously. This is because the nervous reflex during semen ejaculation automatically inhibits micturition.

Accessory Glands

Seminal Vesicles. The seminal vesicles are convoluted sac-shaped glands about 2 inches (5 cm) long; they are posterior to the urinary bladder. They secrete a sticky, alkaline, yellowish substance, called **semen**, which serves as a fluid medium for sperm. About 60% of all semen is secreted by seminal vesicles. The secretion contains many nutrients, citric acid, coagulation proteins, and prostaglandins. The duct from each seminal vesicle joins one of the two ductus deferentia to form the ejaculatory duct.

Prostate Gland. This gland is a doughnut-shaped muscular gland lying just below the bladder. It surrounds the neck of the urethra as it emerges from the bladder (see Figure 25-1). The glandular tissue adds an alkaline secretion to semen, which increases motility of sperm. The muscular portion of the prostate contracts during ejaculation to expel semen from the urethra.

Bulbourethral Glands. Located below the prostate glands are the bulbourethral (Cowper's) glands. They are approximately the size of a pea and secrete an alkaline mucus into tiny ducts, which empty into the urethra. This mucus coats the urethra to neutralize the pH of urine residue; it also lubricates the penis.

Sperm survive better in an alkaline than an acid medium. Alkalinity helps maintain sperm motility. The vagina is acid because of the normal flora (natural bacterial population) within it. The alkaline environment of seminal fluid helps to neutralize the acidic vaginal pH and maintain sperm motility.

Key Concept

Male reproductive structures:

◆ External: penis, scrotum
◆ Internal: testes (gonads) and seminiferous tubules, epididymis, ductus deferens (vas deferens), seminal vesicles, and ejaculatory duct, urethra, prostate gland, bulbourethral glands

The Female Reproductive System

The female reproductive system consists of the ovaries, oviducts, uterus, vagina, and external genital structures. The internal organs, the single uterus and vagina, and the paired ovaries, are located within the pelvis between the urinary bladder and the rectum. These structures are held in place by a group of ligaments, the most conspicuous of which is the broad ligament. The external structures consist of the vulva, with the clitoris. The mammary glands (breasts) are also considered female reproductive organs. The female reproductive system is illustrated in Figures 25-2 and 25-3.

Ovaries

The gonads (primary sex organs) in the female are the ovaries. The **ovaries** produce female gametes, the **ova** (sing: ovum) and secrete female sex hormones (estrogens). There are several estrogens. The primary one is estradiol, but often the entire classification "estrogen" is commonly referred to as a single hormone.

The ovaries are two almond-shaped glands, each about $1\frac{1}{2}$ inches (3.8 cm) in length, located within the brim of the pelvis, one on either side of the uterus (see Figures 25-2 and 25-3). (The combining form relating to ovary is oophor/o-.)

Egg Cells and Oogenesis. All the ova that an individual woman will produce in her lifetime are present as oocytes at her birth.

The development of the egg cell or oocyte is in different stages throughout a woman's life. About 5 to 7 million egg cells begin as oogonia in the fourth to fifth gestational month of fetal life. Before birth, most oogonia (sing: oogonium) degenerate or begin meiosis. With the start of meiosis, the oogonium is called a primary oocyte. A newborn girl has about 2 million oocytes. Between birth and puberty, the number of these primary oocytes decreases to 300,000 to 400,000, and of these, only 300 to 400 will eventually develop into mature egg cells (ova).

At puberty the primary follicle is stimulated by hormones to continue its development and become the secondary follicle (discussed later in the section on physiology). The many follicles in the ovary are in several stages of development. Normally only one follicle per month matures. The primary oocyte inside the follicle matures also and becomes the secondary oocyte. The secondary follicle, which when mature is known as the graafian follicle, enlarges and forms a bump on the ovary. From the time of puberty until menstruation ceases, at approximately monthly intervals, a mature graafian follicle ruptures the surface of the ovary. The mature oocyte, now known as the ovum, is expelled into the pelvic cavity near the duct that leads to the uterus.

Oviducts

Sometimes called the fallopian tubes, uterine tubes, or ovarian tubes, the **oviducts** are the passageway for the ovum between the ovary and the uterus (see Fig-

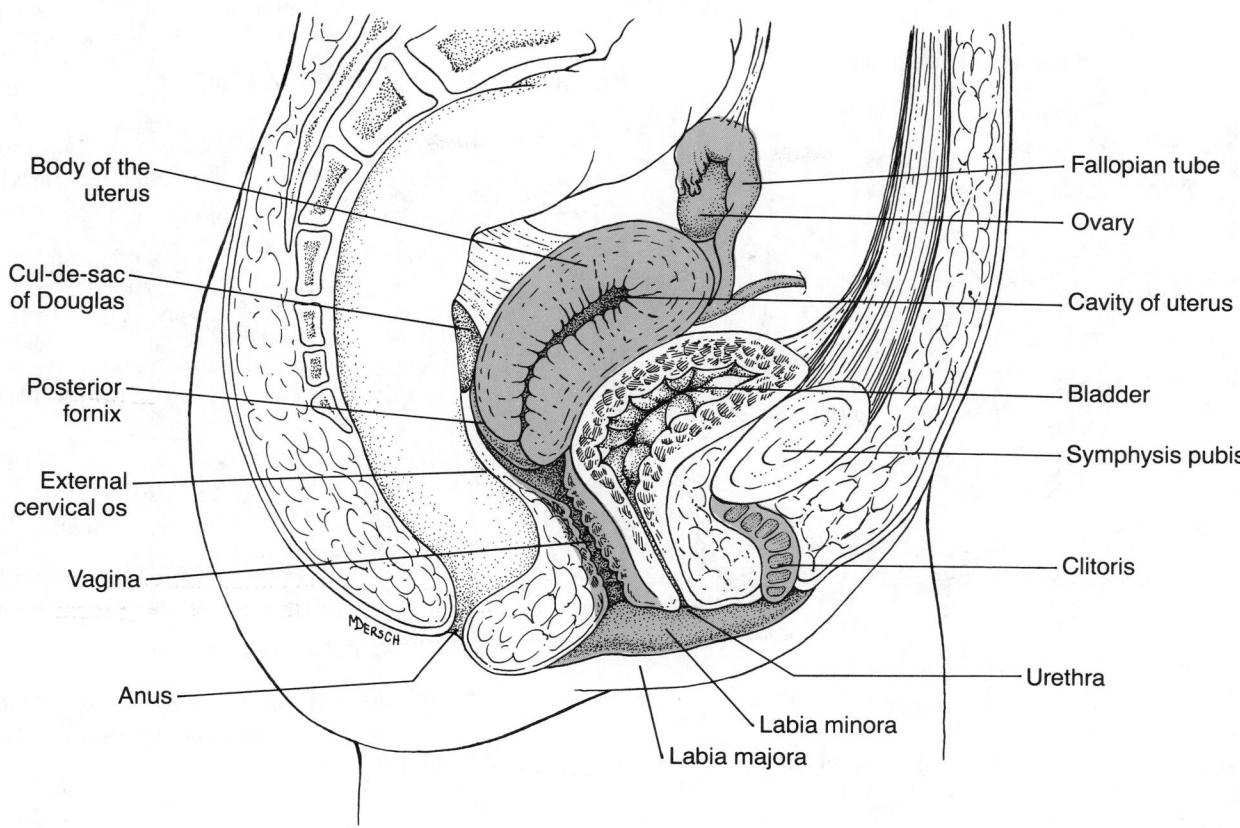

Figure 25-2. Female reproductive organs as seen in sagittal section. (Reeder SJ, Martin LL, & Koniak D. Maternity Nursing: Family, Newborn, and Women's Health Care, 17th ed. Philadelphia. JB Lippincott, 1992)

ures 25-2 and 25-3). The oviducts are 4 to 5 inches (10–12.5 cm) long. There are two oviducts, one on each side of the uterus; each is associated with one ovary.

As the ovum bursts from the ovary into the pelvic cavity, it is caught by the oviduct in structures called fimbriae. They are the fringelike ends of the oviducts. Cilia on the inner surfaces of the fimbriae and the lining of the oviducts help move the ovum toward the uterus. Smooth muscles of the oviducts contract in peristaltic waves, which also help to propel the ovum. The mucous layer of these tubes provides nutrients for the ovum (or developing embryo) as it travels in the oviducts.

Fertilization of the ovum (the meeting of the sperm and the ovum) normally occurs about midway in the oviduct. The fertilized ovum is called a zygote. The zygote travels to the uterus, where it becomes embedded in the uterine lining in preparation for growth into a new individual. (The process of normal pregnancy and prenatal development is covered in Chapter 58.)

Because there is no closed connection between the ovary and the oviduct, it is possible for the ovum to "escape" into the abdominal cavity. If fertilization does not occur, the ovum dissolves. It is possible, however,

for the ovum to become fertilized and enter the abdominal cavity or become lodged in the oviduct. Either situation is known as ectopic (outside the uterus) pregnancy. (Ectopic pregnancy is discussed further in Chapter 61.)

Uterus

The **uterus** is a hollow, muscular, upside-down, pear-shaped organ in the center of the pelvic cavity above and behind the urinary bladder (see Fig. 25-2). It is about 3 inches (7.5 cm) long, 2 inches (5 cm) wide, and 1 inch (2.5 cm) thick. It is also called the *womb*. The uterus normally is tipped forward (anteverted), but it is not uncommon for it to be tipped posteriorly (retroverted). Although movable, the uterus is held in position by strong structures, the broad and the round ligaments. During pregnancy it increases its size about 16 times (from about 60 g to about 1000 g); its capacity increases from about 2.5 mL to 5000 mL. After a term pregnancy, the uterus never returns to its original size.

The parts of the uterus are shown in Figure 25-3. The fundus is the round upper surface; the oviducts enter here. The body is the broad, large central portion. The **cervix** is the narrow lower end, which opens into the

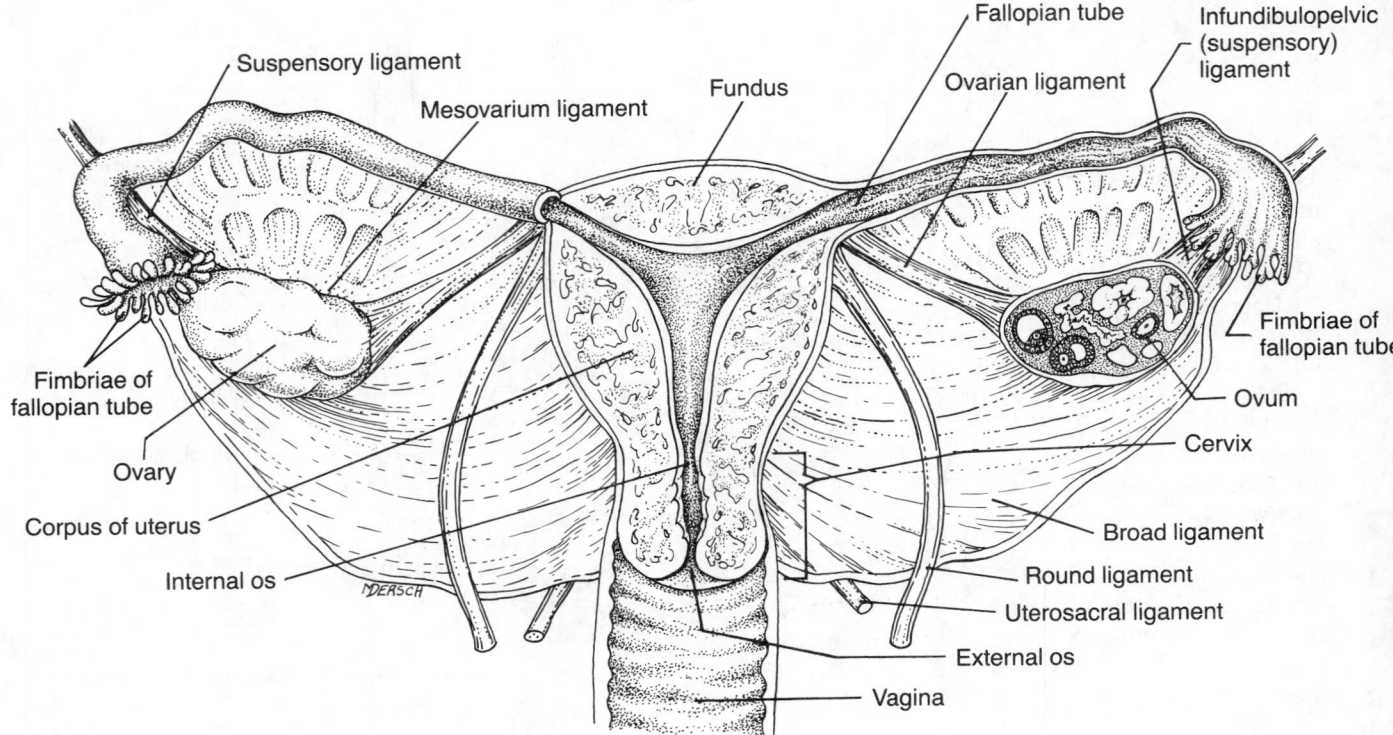

Figure 25-3. Anterior view of the uterus and related structures. (Reeder SJ, Martin LL, & Koniak D. Maternity Nursing: Family, Newborn, and Women's Health Care, 17th ed. Philadelphia. JB Lippincott, 1992)

vagina. The cervical os, or mouth of the cervix, is the opening of the cervix. It can be visualized during a vaginal examination. The size of the cervical os is about the diameter of the graphite in a pencil. The cervix feels like the end of your nose. (The combining form relating to uterus is hystero/o-.)

The uterus has three layers: serous, muscular, and mucous. The serous (outer) layer is called the perimetrium and is a fold of the peritoneum. The muscular layer is called the myometrium; it is the smooth muscle that increases in size during pregnancy and contracts during labor and delivery. The mucous layer is the endometrium. The endometrium forms the maternal portion of the placenta during pregnancy.

The uterus receives the fertilized ovum and provides housing and nourishment for a fetus. At the end of gestation, the uterus expels the fetus.

Vagina. The cervix of the uterus projects into a muscular canal, the vagina, which is about 4 inches (10 cm) long and opens into the vaginal orifice in the perineum (pelvic floor). The **vagina** is the female sex organ (see Figure 25-2). The superior, domed portion of the vagina has deep recesses, called the fornices (sing: fornix), around where the cervix extends into the vagina. The walls of the vagina are moistened by secretions of glands in the mucous membrane lining its walls. The mucus is acidic and retards microbial growth. (The

alkaline semen can temporarily neutralize the vagina's acidic environment.) Rugae are expandable folds within the walls, which accommodate the insertion of the penis and the passage of the fetus during childbirth.

The functions of the vagina are to receive sperm, provide an exit for menstrual flow, and serve as the birth canal.

The hymen is a thin mucous membrane over the vaginal opening. It may close the vaginal orifice completely or may be absent from birth. More commonly it may have one or more perforations. The hymen can be injured in various ways (during normal exercise, the use of tampons, or during the first sexual intercourse). The presence or absence of a hymen is not a reliable indicator of virginity.

External Genitalia

The external genitalia of the female are called the **vulva** (pudendum). They include the vestibule and its surrounding structures (Fig. 25-4). The vestibule contains the openings of the urethra and vagina and the Bartholin's glands. The external structures include the mons pubis, labia majora, labia minora, clitoris, and prepuce.

The mons pubis is a fatty pad over the symphysis pubis. Posterior to the mons pubis extend two rounded folds of skin called the labia majora. After puberty, the mons pubis and the labia majora are covered with coarse pubic hair. A thin pair of skin folds medial to the labia majora are the labia minora, which unite just above the clitoris to form the prepuce.

The **clitoris** is a small erectile structure that responds to sexual stimulation. The structure of the clitoris is similar to the structures of the penis; both become engorged with blood as a result of sexual excitement.

The vestibule floor contains Bartholin's glands (vestibular glands), which lubricate the vagina. If their openings become obstructed, Bartholin cysts result.

Perineum. The perineum is the space between the vaginal orifice and the anus. It is made up of strong muscles that act as slinglike supports for pelvic organs. Sometimes during childbirth the skin and muscles of this area are torn. To prevent such tearing, an incision (episiotomy) may be made. A clean, straight incision heals better than an irregular skin and muscle tear. Slow stretching of the perineum during delivery may prevent tearing and make an episiotomy unnecessary.

Accessory Structures

Mammary Glands. Before puberty, the breast structure in boys and girls is similar. Both have rudimentary glandular systems. With the onset of puberty, girls are influenced by estrogens and progesterone, which lead to breast enlargement. Both boys and girls may have some breast sensitivity in early puberty. Boys may even develop slight swellings, but symptoms disappear quickly.

The mammary glands are modified sweat glands (Fig. 25-5). They are located in the breast anterior to the pectoralis major muscles. They are stimulated by hormones (prolactin and oxytocin) to produce and release milk after childbirth. Each breast is divided into 15 to 20 lobes of glandular tissue, covered by adipose tissue, which gives the breast its shape. The lobes are made up of lobules, which consist of milk-secreting cells in glandular alveoli. From the alveoli, small lactiferous ducts converge toward each nipple like the spokes of a wheel. Each lactiferous duct forms a small reservoir for milk.

The structures of the breasts include nipple, areola, and the areolar glands. The nipple is a circular projection containing some erectile tissue. It is surrounded by the pigmented areola. Areolar glands, which are close to the skin's surface, make the areola appear rough. The secretions of the areolar glands keep the nipples from drying out. The breasts enlarge during pregnancy as a result of stimulation by estrogen and progesterone. The areola becomes more heavily pigmented and does not totally return to its previous pink color after pregnancy.

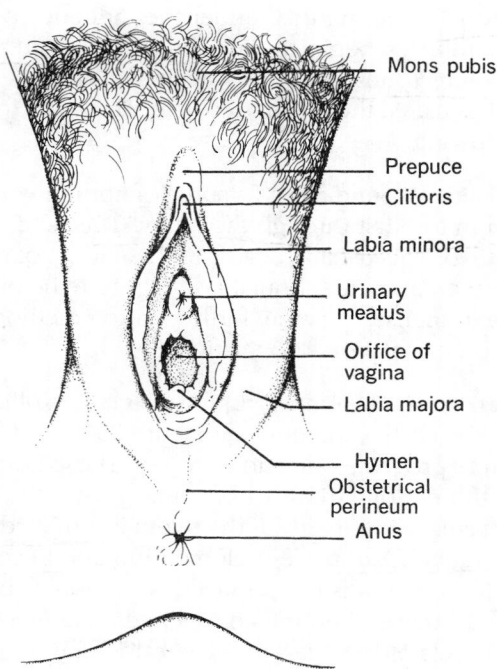

Figure 25-4. External genitalia of the female. The area lying between the orifice of the vagina and the anus is the obstetric perineum. Note the position of the urinary meatus (opening of the urethra); it is this meatus that is used for urinary catheterization.

Mons pubis
Prepuce
Clitoris
Labia minora
Urinary meatus
Orifice of vagina
Labia majora
Hymen
Obstetrical perineum
Anus

> ### Key Concept
>
> Female reproductive structures:
>
> ◆ External: vulva, mons pubis, clitoris, labia majora, labia minora, vestibule, urethral meatus, vaginal orifice, Bartholin's glands, perineum
> ◆ Internal: vagina, uterus, uterine tubes, ovaries
> ◆ Accessory organs: breasts

System Physiology

The Menstrual Cycle

The menstrual cycle is actually two interrelated continuous cycles: the ovarian cycle and the uterine cycle, as shown in Figure 25-6. These cycles are controlled by secretions released by the anterior pituitary. These changes occur in sexually mature, nonpregnant women and culminate in menstruation. Menstruation or **menses** is the flow of blood and other materials from the uterus through the vagina.

The first menstrual period is called **menarche** and marks the onset of puberty. This rhythmic series of changes occurs about every 28 days. Great variation

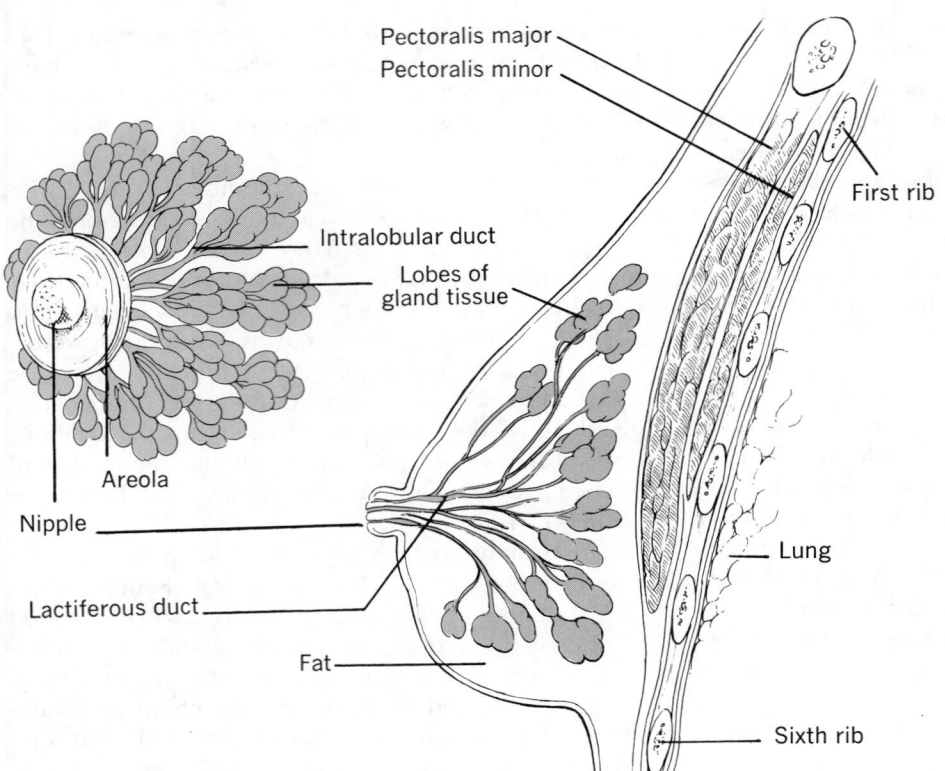

Pectoralis major
Pectoralis minor
First rib
Intralobular duct
Lobes of
gland tissue
Areola
Nipple
Lactiferous duct
Fat
Lung
Sixth rib

Figure 25-5. Glandular tissue and ducts of the mammary gland. (Reeder SJ, Martin LL, & Koniak D. Maternity Nursing: Family, Newborn, and Women's Health Care, 17th ed. Philadelphia. JB Lippincott, 1992)

occurs, however, among women and also within one woman's month-to-month cycle.

Menstrual cycles continue as long as ovarian hormones stimulate the uterine lining. Between 40 and 55 years of age, the ovaries become less active because they do not respond to FSH. Because of this, the eggs do not mature, and the ovaries stop producing estrogens. This decrease in ovarian function occurs gradually. The result is inability to become pregnant and **menopause** (cessation of menstruation). Menopause, a normal process, may occur abruptly, but usually it is gradual. It is often so gradual that the body adjusts without difficulty. However, because many hormonal changes are involved, some unpleasant symptoms such as headaches, irritability, insomnia, anxiety, or depression may occur. One of the most common symptoms is the sensation of heat (hot flashes). Hormonal imbalances affect the diameter of blood vessels; this causes their abrupt dilation or contraction. External indicators of menopause include a tendency to gain weight, thinning of hair, growth of hair on the upper lip, and dry, itchy skin.

Ovarian Cycle

The ovarian cycle is the cycle in which the ovum matures and is expelled from the ovary into the oviduct. While this is happening the maturation of another ovum is withheld until the next cycle. The three phases of the ovarian cycle are: follicular phase, ovulation, and luteal phase.

Follicular Phase. Following the steps in Figure 25-6, you can see that the follicular phase lasts from about days 4 to 14. During this, under the influence of FSH, several follicles begin to ripen and the ovum within each begins to mature. One follicle will become dominant; it is called the graafian follicle. The other follicles stop growing.

Ovulation. Around day 14 a surge of hormones causes the ovum to burst through the ovary. This act is called **ovulation**. This usually occurs in the middle of the 28-day menstrual cycle (about 14 days before the onset of the next menses). Some birth control methods are based on calculation of ovulation.

Luteal Phase. The empty, ruptured graafian follicle becomes the corpus luteum (see Figure 25-6) and begins to secrete progesterone and estrogen. These hormones cause the endometrium to become greatly thickened and vascular (engorged). If the ovum is fertilized, it becomes embedded in the endometrium and becomes a fetus. If the ovum is not fertilized, secretion of progesterone decreases, and the corpus luteum begins to decline. Levels of FSH start to rise around day 2 to begin preparation for the next cycle.

Uterine Cycle

The endometrium of the uterus has a similar cycle (see Figure 25-6). It can be called the uterine cycle or the endometrial cycle. The uterine cycle is controlled

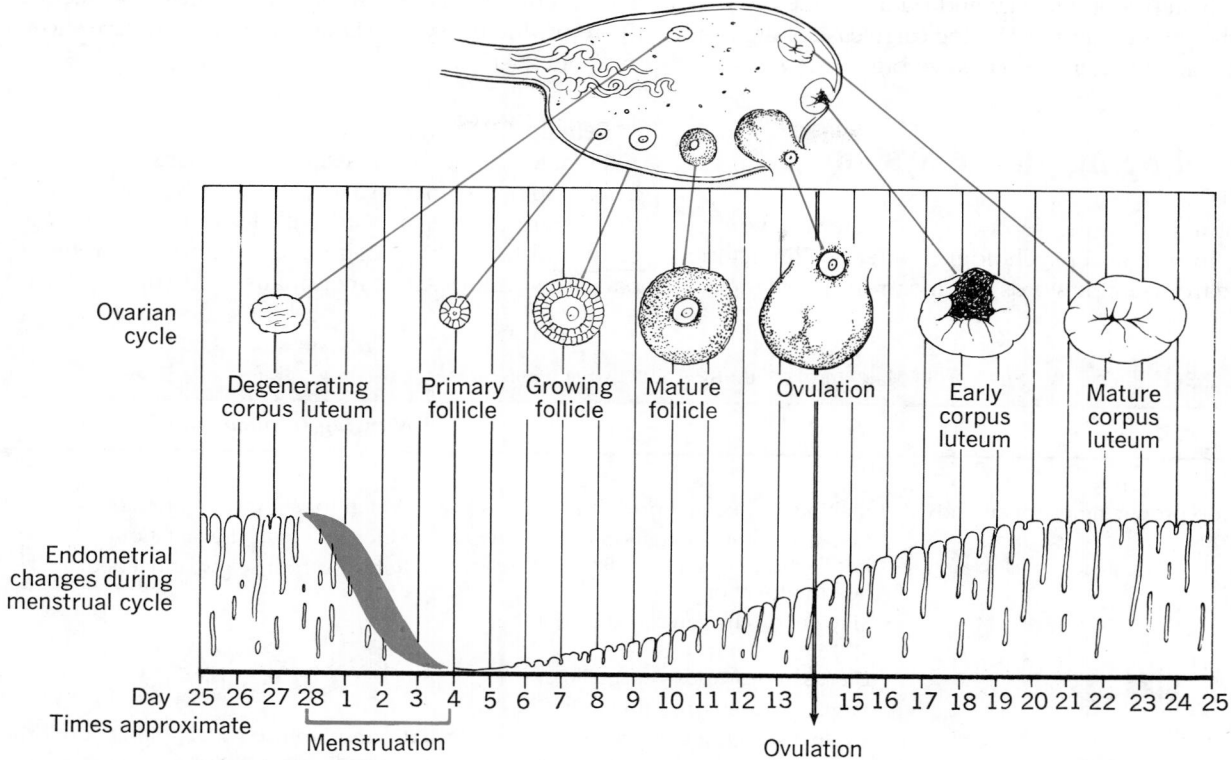

Figure 25-6. Schematic representation of one ovarian cycle and the corresponding changes in thickness of the endometrium. It is thickest just before the onset of menstruation and thinnest just as menstruation ceases. (Reeder SJ, Martin LL, & Koniak D. Maternity Nursing: Family, Newborn, and Women's Health Care, 17th ed. Philadelphia. JB Lippincott, 1992)

by the ovarian cycle and whether fertilization of the egg occurs. The three phases are: proliferative phase, secretory phase, and menstruation.

Proliferative Phase. While the ovarian follicles are producing increased amounts of estrogen, the endometrium prepares for possible fertilization. The endometrium thickens during days 1 through 14, as shown at the bottom of Figure 25-6.

Secretory Phase. As the endometrium prepares for implantation of the fertilized ovum, there is pronounced endometrial growth. If fertilization does not occur, the corpus luteum degenerates and hormonal levels fall. Withdrawal of hormones causes the endometrial cells to change, and menstruation begins.

Menstruation. The sloughing off of the endometrium causes menstruation. Menstruation averages 3 to 5 days but may last 2 to 8 days. While menstruation occurs, FSH levels are rising and several ovarian follicles begin to develop. This causes the beginning of the next uterine or endometrial cycle.

Copulation

Sexual intercourse or sexual union between a man and a woman is called **copulation** or coitus. The erect penis is inserted into the vaginal canal, and semen containing sperm is deposited.

The male sex act is a complex series of reflexes consisting of several components: erection, secretion, emission, and ejaculation. *Erection* occurs because nervous impulses from the spinal cord cause vasodilation of the arteries of the penis. When the arteries are dilated, venous return is obstructed and the cavernous tissue in the penis becomes engorged with blood. *Secretions* from the male glands lubricate the passageway for semen. *Emission* is the accumulation of sperm cells and secretions in the male urethra. *Ejaculation* is the forceful expulsion of semen from the ejaculatory ducts to the urethra. *Orgasm* is the physical and emotional, pleasurable sensation that occurs at the climax of sexual intercourse; in men it is accompanied by the ejaculation of semen.

Female nervous pathways involved in controlling the sexual response are the same as in the man. The erectile tissues within the clitoris and around the vaginal opening become engorged with blood. The vestibular glands secrete mucus before and during coitus. If the clitoris is stimulated with sufficient intensity and duration, the woman will feel the physical and psychological release of orgasm. A woman can experience successive orgasms.

Effects of Aging on the System

Effects of aging on the reproductive system have significant physical and psychological effects. Climacteric is derived from Greek words that mean "rung of ladder"

and "a critical time." It refers to changes that occur in the reproductive system later in life. Changes are shown in Table 25-1.

Female Climacteric

Female climacteric is called menopause (discussed in section on the menstrual cycle). Several physical conditions are also associated with loss of estrogen. Vascular and heart disease are less common in premenopausal women. After menopause the rate of heart

Table 25-1. Effects of Aging on the Male and Female Reproductive Systems

Factor	Result	Nursing Implications
Female		
Ovaries stop producing estrogen and progesterone.	Inability to become pregnant	Watch for signs of depression.
	Cessation of menstruation—may have hot flashes, headaches, dizziness, or heart palpitations	Refer for medical evaluation. Refer for counseling, if needed.
	May need estrogen replacement therapy	
	Uterus and ovaries get smaller	
	Vagina shortens and thins	
	Vaginal secretions decrease	Counsel to use water-soluble lubricant, if needed for comfort.
	Breasts get smaller and softer	Advise patient to wear a good support bra.
	Hair thins on scalp, axillae, and external genitalia	
	Hair grows on upper lip	Discuss removal by electrolysis or shaving.
	Muscles of upper arms and legs get flabby	Educate about exercise program.
	Weight gain around midline	Discuss need for fewer calories to maintain weight. Stress exercise.
	Skin dries	Use lotions and bath oils to maintain skin moisture.
Estrogen production is deficient.	Increase in atherosclerosis; thus, increase in heart disease	Educate about low-fat and low-salt diet. Encourage exercise program.
	Osteoporosis increases; bones become subject to fractures, as they become brittle	Educate about increased calcium intake. Encourage exercise. Encourage weight maintenance. Refer for physical examination and possible estrogen therapy.
Male		
Decrease in testosterone levels.	Degeneration of testicles	Educate as to normalcy of these changes.
	Decrease in sperm production	Refer to counseling, if needed.
	Difficulty in achieving and maintaining erection	
	Occurrence of erections decreases	
	Enlargement of prostate gland	Encourage testicular self-examination. Encourage medical examination to catch early prostate cancer.
Fibrosis, sclerosis, and vascular changes of penis occur.	Difficulty achieving and/or maintaining erection	Encourage medical examination. Refer to counseling, if needed.

disease between men and women is about equal. Osteoporosis is a condition in which bones become brittle and porous and fracture more easily. This condition worsens when hormones are absent. Estrogen replacement therapy (ERT) is commonly prescribed to lessen menopausal symptoms.

Older women may also suffer from urinary incontinence, the result of aging and childbirth trauma. Breast tissue may become smaller and more pendulous (sagging) as muscles relax and are replaced by fat. Loss of muscle tone causes external genital structures to sag; the vagina shortens and becomes less elastic. Intercourse may become painful (dyspareunia) as the vaginal mucosal wall becomes thinner and vaginal secretions decrease. In addition, the older woman is more

prone to vaginal infections. Changes in sexual response are relatively minor and are usually related to physical changes in the vagina.

Male Climacteric

Men may experience changes (andropause, male climacteric) but at a much slower rate. There is no sharp demarcation of beginning or end as in women. Men do not stop producing sperm, but the rate of sperm production decreases because of decrease in testosterone secretion. Men also tend to gain weight and become more prone to atherosclerosis and osteoporosis. Many men experience hypertrophy (enlarging) of the prostate gland. This may cause difficulty in urination, retention of urine, incontinence, or inability to have an erection.

Keys for Review

Key Questions for Critical Thinking

1. Describe what happens at puberty in males and females. Compare with the climacteric in males and females.
2. Describe the relationship between hormones and the reproductive system.
3. Describe the location of the perineum in the male and female. Describe the location of the urinary meatus in both sexes. Describe how these differences affect care?
4. Describe the menstrual cycle. Discuss the cycles and phases within the menstrual cycle. What happens and why during these phases?

Key Readings

Birchenall JM, Streight ME. Care of the Older Adult, Ed 3. Philadelphia, J.B. Lippincott, 1993
Chabner D. The Language of Medicine, Ed 4. Philadelphia, W.B. Saunders, 1991
Jackson DB, Saudners RB. Child Health Nursing: A Comprehensive Approach to the Care of Children and Their Families. Philadelphia, J.B. Lippincott, 1993
May KA, Mahlmeister LR. Maternal and Neonatal Nursing: Family-Centered Care. Philadelphia, J.B. Lippincott, 1994

Key Readings (continued)

O'Toole M (Ed). Miller-Keane Encyclopedia and Dictionary of Medicine, Nursing, and Allied Health, Ed 5. Philadelphia, W.B. Saunders, 1992
Scanlon V, Sanders V. Essentials of Anatomy and Physiology. Philadelphia, F.A. Davis, 1991
Seeley R, Stephens T, Tate P. Anatomy and Physiology, Ed 2. St. Louis, Mosby-Year Book, 1994
Taylor C, Lillis C, LeMone P. Fundamentals of Nursing: The Art and Science of Nursing Care, Ed 2. Philadelphia, J.B. Lippincott, 1993

Keys to Learning More

Chapter 50: gynecologic examination and nursing assessment related to the male and female reproductive systems
Chapter 56: medications, many of which affect the reproductive system
Unit Twelve: normal human reproduction and its complications
Chapter 63: issues related to sexuality, fertility control, infertility, and sexually transmitted diseases
Chapter 83: male reproductive disorders
Chapter 84: female reproductive disorders

Unit *5*   Nutrition and Diet Therapy

26 Food and Its Functions

Keys for Learning

Learning Objectives

- Define *RDAs, energy, kilocalorie, joules, empty calories, overweight, obese,* and *malnutrition.*
- Describe how RDAs are used.
- List major functions of carbohydrates, fat, and protein.
- Describe the need for water in the body.
- Name and state the functions of four important minerals.
- Name the fat-soluble and water-soluble vitamins.
- State the main functions and food sources of vitamins.
- Demonstrate an understanding of the Food Guide Pyramid by planning a day's diet for yourself.
- Discuss the special aspects of nutrition as related to various stages of life.

Key Terms

calcium	magnesium	potassium
carbohydrates	malnutrition	protein
cholesterol	minerals	saturated fats
chloride	obese	sodium
fats	overweight	triglyceride
iron	phosphorus	vitamin
kilocalorie		

Keys to Understanding This Chapter

Chapter 5: basic needs of all people, including food and water

Chapter 6: optimum health

Chapter 16: normal fluid and electrolyte balance in which nutritional status plays a part

Chapter 23: describes how foods are digested and used by the body

Key Points

- Five of the 10 leading causes of death are related to an overconsumption of nutrients.
- No one food or food group can supply all the nutrients needed.

Key Points (continued)

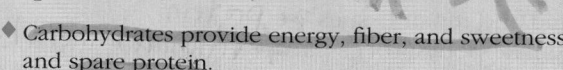

- Carbohydrates provide energy, fiber, and sweetness and spare protein.
- Fats supply energy, essential fatty acids, satiety, and flavor; carry fat-soluble vitamins; protect organs; and regulate body temperature.
- Proteins repair and build body tissues, contribute to fluid and acid–base balance, form hormones and enzymes, and provide immune functions.
- Fat-soluble vitamins are vitamins A, D, E, and K; water-soluble vitamins are vitamin C and B complex.
- Vitamins and minerals should not be supplemented in excess of the RDAs.
- Calcium, iron, and protein are important nutrients in the diets of infants, children, adolescents, and pregnant and lactating women.

Key Topics Outline

Nutrition
   Concepts Related to Nutrition
   Nutritional Problems
Specific Nutrients
   Carbohydrates
   Fats (Lipids)
   Protein
   Water
   Minerals
   Vitamins
A Healthy Diet
   The Food Guide Pyramid
Nutrition Across the Life Span

Key Learning Activities

- Plan a day's diet for yourself, using the Food Guide Pyramid.
- Plan two daily diets—one which is low cost and one which is higher in cost. Make sure both meet food pyramid requirements.
- Keep track of everything you eat for 3 days. Analyze it in comparison to the Food Guide Pyramid.

Food is vital to our lives. Although we eat because we enjoy food, we also eat to stay alive and be healthy. In fact, food is one of the most important items on the first level of the hierarchy of human needs you studied in Chapter 5.

In this chapter you will learn how important food is. Many aspects of normal nutrition are presented. These concepts can be used to assist people in meeting their nutritional needs.

Nutrition

The purposes of nutrition are to:

◆ Provide energy
◆ Build and repair tissues
◆ Regulate body processes

Good nutrition also contributes to health, happiness, enjoyable and productive work and play, and a long life relatively free of illness.

Concepts Related to Nutrition

Nutrients. The body is able to synthesize only a few of the substances needed for growth, maintenance, and repair of the body. The rest of the substances must be supplied by food. The foods we eat are made up of substances called *nutrients*, which are essential to the normal functioning of the body.

◆ Essential amino acids from protein
◆ Glucose from carbohydrate
◆ Essential fatty acids
◆ Vitamins
◆ Minerals
◆ Water

The body is able to synthesize certain vitamins; however, the body is not able to make these vitamins in the quantities needed. Therefore, the diet must include foods that contain these vitamins.

Recommended Dietary Allowances. Recommended Dietary Allowances (RDAs) are recommendations for average daily amounts of nutrients considered adequate in meeting nutritional needs of practically all healthy persons. These figures are "padded" by one-third to ensure a margin of safety. They are based on ongoing scientific research and study and are updated regularly.

Energy. The amount of energy a normal individual needs depends on age, sex, weight, and body composition. It also is influenced by the kind of work done. Children need a great deal of energy because they are growing and active. Older people use less energy. People at desk jobs need less than laborers, who are using

their muscles a great deal. Men often need more energy than women; large people use more than small people. Certain body disturbances, such as fever, increase the amount of energy the body uses. Other disorders can prevent the proper utilization of food. The *energy requirements* of an individual are the sum of the amounts necessary to keep body processes going and to carry on activities. This energy is provided by the food we eat.

Kilocalories. The unit of measurement that specifies the heat energy in a particular amount of food is called a **kilocalorie** (abbreviated kcal or C). The caloric value of foods can be determined in the laboratory. In this process, the heat that is given off by the burning of the test food raises the temperature of a known amount of water. The definition of kilocalorie is *the amount of heat required to raise the temperature of 1 kg of water 1°C.* The calorie values of energy-producing foods follow:

◆ 1 g protein yields 4 C
◆ 1 g fat yields 9 C
◆ 1 g carbohydrate yields 4 C

Guides have been published naming the foods and estimating the amounts of each that a normal individual needs for light, moderate, or heavy work. Calorie charts giving the number of kilocalories in a serving of average foods used are available without cost from a number of sources. The National Dairy Council has published many excellent booklets, obtainable from local dairy councils. The U.S. Government Printing Office is also a good source of nutrition information.

Joule Measurement. Energy furnished by food is sometimes measured in joules. One joule equals 4.2 C.

"Empty" Calories. Some foods, such as soft drinks, provide only "empty" calories, that is, they have no nutritional value. Whereas one egg provides about 75 kcal along with 7 g protein and many other nutrients, one 12-oz cola yields 140 to 210 calories but contains only carbohydrate. Although one 12-oz diet cola has no calories, it may yield high amounts of sodium and caffeine. Alcohol, another example of empty calories, supplies 7 kcal/g (199 kcal/oz) and no nutrients (except sugar).

Enzymes and Digestion. Thousands of chemical reactions occur in the body daily. Without enzymes these reactions would take much more time and use excessive energy. Enzymes are biologic catalysts made up of proteins. Each enzyme has a specific three-dimensional form that works with only matching shapes of other chemicals in a lock-and-key manner; each will catalyze only one specific reaction. Enzymes temporarily bond with the other chemicals until they form a new compound; then, the enzyme is released. Several factors influence enzymes: each works best in a particular pH and temperature controls are important. Temperatures greater than 106°F will destroy some enzymes.

A major area of enzyme action is *digestion*. With the exception of pepsin and trypsin, all enzymes end in the suffix *ase*. Several glands make enzymes. The pancreas makes numerous digestive enzymes; the salivary glands in the mouth make enzymes that help digest starches. Enzymes are discussed in the following section in relationship to each nutrient.

Nutritional Problems

The nutritional problems of most Americans are not due to deficiencies of single nutrients but to overconsumption of nutrients, particularly fat and calories. At the end of the 1980s, the Surgeon General of the United States issued his report on nutrition and health. This report revealed that, of the 10 leading causes of death, five are associated with dietary excesses and imbalances. These disorders are:

- ◆ Coronary heart disease
- ◆ Certain types of cancer
- ◆ Stroke
- ◆ Diabetes mellitus
- ◆ Atherosclerosis

Overnutrition also contributes to such conditions as hypertension, obesity, osteoporosis, dental caries, and gastrointestinal diseases.

Because of poor eating habits, a large percentage of the American population is overweight. A person who is more than 10% over the desirable weight for the body's frame size is considered **overweight**; a person 20% above desirable weight is considered to be **obese**. The physician may subdivide this classification by using terms such as mildly obese, moderately obese, and grossly obese. A person who is 100 pounds overweight or twice desirable weight is considered *morbidly obese*. Overweight or obese people may be malnourished even though they may overeat.

Although food seems plentiful in the United States, many Americans do not eat enough of the essential nutrients. Estimates are that 20% of the school-age population suffers from **malnutrition**, defined as a lack of necessary nutrients in the body. Although malnutrition may be due to some physical dysfunction, it can often be traced to poor eating habits.

Specific Nutrients

Table 26-1 summarizes the RDAs, sources, and functions of the major nutrients. The following text discusses structure, functions, food sources, and digestion of each nutrient. It also includes a discussion of types of the particular nutrient.

Carbohydrates

CHO   Come from plant   start in mouth

Carbohydrates are the most widely used energy source in the world. In many countries 80% of the total calories come from complex carbohydrates. Carbohydrates are summarized in Table 26-1.

Carbohydrates are made up of carbon, hydrogen, and oxygen. They include sugars, starches, and fiber. They are divided into groups depending on the complexity of their molecular structure. Simple sugars (glucose, sucrose, and galactose) can be absorbed directly into the bloodstream without being digested. Carbohydrates provide 4 C/g.

The major function of carbohydrates is energy production. The simple sugar, glucose, is a major source of energy for the body. Another important function of carbohydrates is the ability to "spare" protein. (If inadequate carbohydrate is available, the body will burn protein for energy. This may not leave enough protein available for the repair of body tissues. Protein is also a more expensive source of glucose than carbohydrate.) Carbohydrates add flavor and sweetness to foods and are the only source of fiber.

All plant foods, except plant oils (like corn, soy, and olive) contain carbohydrates. Milk is the only nonplant source of carbohydrate. Rich sources of carbohydrate include whole grain breads and cereals, legumes and dried beans, fruits, and vegetables.

Carbohydrate Digestion. Digestion of carbohydrates begins in the mouth. Here, the action of *salivary amylase*, an enzyme present in saliva, breaks starch into simpler carbohydrates. The most common of these simpler carbohydrates is *dextrin*. Little digestion of carbohydrates occurs in the stomach, but some carbohydrates may be hydrolyzed into units of glucose and fructose when subjected to hydrochloric acid.

In the small intestine, an alkaline secretion from the pancreas, called *pancreatic amylase*, converts complex carbohydrates into maltose, a disaccharide. In the intestinal wall the enzymes *sucrase*, *maltase*, and *lactase* are available to complete the digestion process.

Fiber in the diet is acted on by digestive enzymes but passes out of the body undigested. The final products of carbohydrate digestion are water, carbon dioxide, energy, and fiber. (The first three are also end products of fat digestion.)

Simple Sugars

Simple sugars have been blamed for causing obesity, diabetes, heart disease, and hyperactivity in children. These claims have not been proved by modern research. However, sugar, especially sticky sugar, can in-

Table 26-1. Summary of Carbohydrates, Fats, and Proteins in Nutrition

Nutrient	RDAs	Sources	Functions
Carbohydrate (Sugars and starch)	No RDA set; suggested intake 45–55% of total calories; minimum amount needed to supply calories for energy is about 100 g	Bread and cereals Potatoes, lima beans, corn Dried beans and peas Fruits, vegetables, milk Sugar, syrup, jelly, jam, honey	Major source of energy (glucose) Provides fiber Spares protein Excess is stored as fat
Fat	No RDA set; suggested intake no more than 30% of total calories; need small amount to carry fat-soluble vitamins and carry out other functions (approx. 15–20 g)	Butter and cream Salad oils and dressings Cooking and table fats Fat in meat Olives, avocados, other fatty foods Fried foods	Supplies large amount of energy in a small amount of food; excess stored as fat Conserves body heat Helps keep skin healthy by supplying essential fatty acids Carries vitamins A, D, E, and K (fat-soluble) Important in structure of nerve tissue; protects and insulates body parts
Protein	Adult: 44–56 g Child: 23–34 g Infant: 2–2.2 g/kg body weight Pregnancy: 60 g Lactation: 65 g	Meat, fish, poultry, eggs Milk and all kinds of cheese Dried beans and peas Peanut butter and nuts Bread and cereals	Builds and repairs all tissues Helps build blood and form antibodies to fight infection Supplies energy; excess stored as fat Assists in acid–base and fluid balance

crease the risk of dental cavities. Simple sugars contain few nutrients and should be limited to 10% of total calories.

Monosaccharides. *Glucose*, also called dextrose or grape sugar, is the most commonly occurring sugar in the body. Terms such as *hyperglycemia*, which means abnormally high blood sugar, or *hypoglycemia*, which means abnormally low blood sugar, refer to the levels of glucose in the blood. Other forms of sugar must be changed into glucose before they can be used. Sources of natural glucose are honey, fruits, and most vegetables.

Fructose (*levulose*, fruit sugar) is the form of sugar found mostly in honey and fruits and in some plants. Fructose tastes very sweet. Fructose and glucose often occur in the same food item.

Galactose is not usually found naturally, but it is an end product of milk digestion. The disaccharide in milk (lactose) is broken down into galactose and other end products.

Sorbitol is a sugar alcohol. It provides little energy value and is absorbed very slowly. It is often used in sugar-free or diet products.

Disaccharides. *Sucrose* is a mixture of fructose and glucose, which combine to form this "double sugar."

As crystallized sugar, brown sugar, or molasses, it is used on the table and in cooking. Sources of sucrose are sugar beets, sugar cane, maple sap, and most fruits and vegetables.

Lactose is the sugar found in milk. It is neither as soluble nor as sweet as sucrose. It is not found in plants but is formed only in the mammary glands. Lactose is split by an enzyme (lactase) into galactose and glucose. Virtually all infants can use lactose, but many adults cannot. This condition, known as *lactose intolerance*, is more common in African Americans, Native Americans, and Asians than in whites. If a person lacks the enzyme needed to break down the lactose, the ingestion of milk can cause bloating, gas, diarrhea, and in severe cases, death. The person with lactose intolerance usually can safely eat such foods as cheese and yogurt, in which the lactose has already been broken down by bacterial action.

Maltose is the product of young growing (sprouting) grain and the digestion of starch within the body. It is readily soluble and easily changed into glucose, so it is often used in infant formulas in preference to other sugars.

Trisaccharide. The "triple sugar" *raffinose* is composed of glucose, fructose, and galactose and is found in molasses.

Complex Sugars

Complex sugars are *polysaccharides*. They are broken down into starch, glycogen, and dietary fiber.

Starch. *Starch* is the form of carbohydrate stored in plants. It is the chief source of carbohydrate in the diet. Starch is made up of many glucose units linked together. The main sources of starch are grains, roots, bulbs, legumes, tubers, and seeds. Starch grains are encased in a tough covering that is broken down in the process of digestion. Cooking foods that contain starch speeds up their digestion. Enzymes in saliva can act on cooked starch but have little effect on raw starch. Starch must be broken down into glucose before it can be used by the body.

Glycogen. *Glycogen* is a reserve carbohydrate stored in the liver and muscle. It is converted to glucose and released into the bloodstream when needed. *Dextrin* is one of the intermediate stages of starch digestion. It is also a stage of sugar produced by toasting.

Dietary Fiber. Fiber is classified as a carbohydrate, but it has no actual energy value. Like starch, it is composed of many glucose units, but the fiber is put together in such a way that it is not digested or absorbed. The incidence of constipation and diverticulosis (a painful weakening of the large intestine caused by hard stools), can be reduced by a high-fiber diet. Diets high in fiber may also reduce the risk of some types of cancer. Current research has shown that pectins and gums may be protective factors against heart disease and diabetes mellitus. Experts suggest eating at least 20 to 35 g of fiber a day.

Cellulose and *hemicellulose* are the framework of plants and are *water insoluble*. This means that they cannot be broken down with water. Cellulose and hemicellulose occur in fruits; the skin, stalks, leaves, and pulp of vegetables; and seeds, grain, and legumes. Cellulose and hemicellulose hold water, produce bulk, and decrease the transit time of food through the intestines.

Pectin, gums, and *mucilages* are *water-soluble* fibers and absorb water to form a gel. They slow gastric emptying time and bind bile acids (which prevents the utilization of cholesterol). Pectins, gums, and mucilages are found in fruits, seeds, oats, and dried beans. *Lignin* is a noncarbohydrate polysaccharide found in woody portions of fruit, vegetables, and wheat bran.

Fats (Lipids)

Fats give flavor and texture to food. Fat is a concentrated energy source and is easily stored in the body. Table 26-1 summarizes information about fats and RDAs.

Fat is made of fatty acids and glycerol. It is comprised of carbon, hydrogen, and oxygen. Fat provides 9 C/g, more than twice as many calories as carbohydrate or protein.

The major function of fat is to provide energy to the body in a concentrated form. Fat carries fat-soluble vitamins in the body and provides essential fatty acids. Fat also cushions major organs to protect them from injury and insulates the body from extreme temperatures. Fat adds flavor and texture to food. It provides satiety (satisfaction) because it is digested very slowly.

Fat comes from animals and plant oils. Most foods of animal origin contain some fat. Meat, for instance, contains an outer layer of fat as well as internal marbling. Most fat in the American diet comes from meat. Fats are insoluble in water and need an emulsifier to be dissolved.

Fat Digestion. Because fats do not dissolve in water, there is no digestion of fats in the mouth and very little in the stomach. When fat reaches the small intestine, bile, released from the gallbladder, breaks up the fat into tiny droplets. Then the intestinal and pancreatic juices break up these droplets into fatty acids and glycerol, simple forms of fat that the body cells can use. As the body uses fatty acids, it breaks them down into other substances called *acetone bodies* or *ketone bodies*. These substances are further broken down into carbon dioxide and water and excreted as waste products.

Fatty Acids

Saturated Fats. Saturated fats (animal fats, butter, lard, hydrogenated shortening, and palm and coconut oils) are solid at room temperature because they already contain their full complement of hydrogen, either in their natural form or because hydrogen has been added by a process called *hydrogenation*.

Unsaturated Fats. The *unsaturated fats* (soft or liquid fats or oils) are capable of adding more hydrogen to their molecular structure. Manufacturers add hydrogen to liquid fats to make them solid. Many inexpensive vegetable oils, such as corn, cottonseed, soybean, and coconut oils are "hydrogenated" for this purpose. Margarine, which is also made in this way, is processed with cultured milk to give it a buttery flavor, and vitamins A and D are added. Fortified margarine has approximately the same nutritional and caloric value as butter.

You may hear the terms *monounsaturated* or *polyunsaturated* referring to fats. These terms refer to the number of double bonds in the chemical structure. *Monounsaturated fats* include olive, canola, and peanut oils. *Polyunsaturated fats* include corn, safflower, sunflower, and soybean oils. Both monounsaturated

[handwritten margin notes: HDL = Good, LDL = BAD]

and polyunsaturated fats will help lower blood cholesterol levels when used in place of saturated fats.

Essential Fatty Acids

Some of the fatty acids that are essential for normal nutrition (linoleic and linolenic) cannot be synthesized in the body from other substances. *Linoleic acid* is the most abundant in nature and the most important essential fatty acid. *Arachidonic acid* can be made in the body from linoleic acid. *Linolenic acid* appears to occur in adequate supply in conjunction with linoleic acid. These three fatty acids come from fats found only in animal fats, vegetable and seed oils, and soybean oil. (Olive, coconut, and palm kernel oils are poor sources of essential fatty acids.) Some fat sources containing essential fatty acids must be included in the daily food supply. Linoleic acid and the other essential fatty acids are a major component of the plasma membrane. A fatty acid deficiency causes, among other symptoms, a rash or dermatitis.

Cholesterol. Cholesterol is a member of a large group of compounds called *sterols*. It is found only in animal tissues. The body needs cholesterol to produce hormones, vitamin D, and bile acids. It is also a major component of the *myelin sheath*, which protects nerve tissue and the brain. The body makes cholesterol out of saturated fat in the liver. Research has established that high amounts of saturated fat in the diet increase blood cholesterol levels. High blood cholesterol levels promote atherosclerotic heart disease, especially coronary heart disease. Foods high in cholesterol include organ meats (such as liver, kidneys, and brains), whole milk products, butter, meat fats, and egg yolk.

[handwritten margin note: We need some Saturated fat]

Cholesterol is differentiated into two categories—high-density lipoprotein (HDL) and low-density lipoprotein (LDL). It is believed that the *balance* between these two is more significant for optimum health than is the total cholesterol count. HDL is sometimes called "good cholesterol" because it helps remove excess cholesterol from the body. HDL levels can be increased by exercise, weight loss, and smoking cessation.

Triglyceride. Triglyceride is probably the most commonly known fat in the body. It is stored in the body as body fat, after being converted by the liver from excess carbohydrate, fat, and protein in the diet. Fats slow digestion. Foods fried in fat, especially at high temperatures, are digested more slowly than foods boiled or baked. Although fats will produce about twice as much energy as equal amounts of carbohydrate, they are much more expensive as a source of energy.

Protein

[handwritten: CHO + Nitrogen —enable cell to repair tissue and cell]

Protein is the foundation of every body cell. Protein is the only nutrient that builds and repairs tissue. In the

absence of dietary protein, the body will begin to use protein from the bloodstream, muscles, and organs to carry on daily activities. Every major organ, except the brain, will shrink during a prolonged dietary deficiency of protein. Table 26-1 summarizes information about protein and RDAs. Protein comes from both animal and plant sources.

Proteins are made up of amino acids. Amino acids are made from carbon, hydrogen, and oxygen but also contain nitrogen. Some amino acids contain phosphorus, sulfur, cobalt, and iron.

Proteins produce and repair all major body constituents. They are needed for the formation of muscles, connective tissue, glands, organs, skin, and blood clotting factors. Every cell in the body contains some protein. Proteins also maintain the fluid balance of the body. Blood proteins called albumins and globulins help keep intracellular and extracellular fluids where they belong. If a person has a low intake of protein, edema may develop in the lower extremities because there is not enough protein in the blood to control fluid balance. Another important function is protein's contribution to the acid–base balance of the body. Proteins help to keep the body in perfect pH balance.

Hormones, such as thyroid hormone and insulin, are made from protein. Almost all enzymes are proteins. Proteins are also a key component of the body's immune system. Antibodies are also made up of protein. Proteins can be converted to glucose and burned for energy.

[handwritten margin note: Starts in stomach where an enzyme]

Protein Digestion. Protein digestion starts in the stomach, where an enzyme (*pepsin*) breaks down the basic structure of the protein. In the small intestine, pancreatic juices containing enzymes (*pancreatic protease* [or *trypsin*] and *chymotrypsin*) split some of the proteins into amino acids. These are absorbed directly.

The remaining dipeptides (two amino acids linked together) and tripeptides (three amino acids linked together) are further broken down into amino acids in the intestine and at the brush border of the intestinal walls.

Several amino acids are *essential amino acids*. They are called essential because they cannot be made by the body at a rate sufficient to meet its needs for growth and maintenance. Therefore, they must be supplied by the diet. The essential amino acids are valine, leucine, isoleucine, phenylalanine, threonine, methionine, lysine, tryptophan, and histidine.

Nonessential amino acids can be synthesized by the body if the protein supplied by the diet contains enough nitrogen. This synthesis involves the shifting of a portion of an amino acid molecule from the amino acid to another substance, to form a required amino acid. The more common nonessential amino acids are alanine, cystine, glutamine, glycine, and serine.

Complete and Incomplete Proteins

The number of amino acids and the amounts of each in individual proteins vary widely. Accordingly, proteins are classified as complete, partially complete, and incomplete. A complete protein can also be attained by correctly combining two or more partially complete proteins.

The *complete proteins* contain the essential amino acids in sufficient quantities for maintenance and normal growth. All animal proteins except gelatin are complete proteins. *with complete protein's high in fats*

Partially complete proteins will maintain life but will not promote normal growth. They are found in cereals and vegetables and are important in the diet to supplement the complete proteins.

Incomplete proteins will neither maintain life nor promote growth. The proteins in corn and gelatin are in this group. Incomplete proteins should be combined at the same meal to ensure that the protein is used.

> ### Key Concept
> Essential amino acids are needed to maintain life and normal growth.

Water

Except for oxygen, nothing is more essential to life than water. The human being can survive for weeks without food but only days without water.

In Chapter 16 we noted that about 60% of adult body weight is water and about 80% of an infant's body weight is water. We also stated that an adult loses about $2\frac{1}{2}$ quarts (2.37 liters) of water per day by perspiring, urinating, and exhaling. To maintain the fluid balance in body cells, the fluid lost must be replaced. Food provides some fluid, but it must be supplemented by drinking water and other liquids. Most authorities agree that the average adult needs 6 to 8 glasses of fluid a day.

Water comprises a large percentage of the cellular makeup. Nutrients are distributed to the cells by blood; water is one of blood's essential components. Water is the solvent in which vital chemical changes occur in the body and is also necessary for controlling body temperature. No organ of the body can function without water. Water is so necessary to life that nature has provided human beings with an inborn warning device: Thirst is our strongest appetite.

Minerals

Minerals are vital for building bones and teeth. They help to maintain muscle tone, to regulate body processes, and to maintain acid–base balance. Minerals are summarized in Table 26-2. Some minerals are used more readily by the body than others, and foods vary considerably in the amount of minerals they contain. Some minerals are lost in cooking, and some are lost in body wastes.

Calcium. Calcium, an important mineral, is the one most likely to be deficient in the ordinary diet. Calcium makes up about 2% of the adult human body; 99% of the calcium in the body is in the bones and the teeth. It has other important uses such as keeping the body fluids balanced, helping blood clot, and regulating heart and other muscle activity and nerve responses. An inadequate calcium intake can lead to osteoporosis (thinning of the bone), poor bone and dental health, slow blood clotting, and impaired function of muscles and nerves.

Milk contains more calcium than any other food. A quart of milk for a child and 2 to 3 cups for an adult will supply the body with its daily calcium requirement. Milk products are also high in calcium. Vegetables contain varying amounts of calcium but some of them in a form the body cannot use readily. Because of the high fat content in milk, many doctors today advise their patients to use nonfat or low-fat milk and milk products.

Phosphorus. Phosphorus is found in every body cell. It accounts for about 1% of adult body weight; 80% of the phosphorus in the human body is found in the bones and teeth. Phosphorus has more functions than any other mineral in the body. It helps the cells to use proteins, fats, carbohydrates, and vitamins, and it regulates the acid–base balance. It is also important to normal nerve and muscle functioning. So many ordinary foods contain phosphorus that the body almost certainly gets enough.

Iron. The body needs a relatively small amount of **iron**, but this amount is important because it is an essential part of every body cell and is also a constituent of *hemoglobin*, a substance in the red blood cells that carries oxygen. The body is thrifty with its supply of iron and uses it over and over, by salvaging the iron from worn out red blood cells. Young children, teenagers, and women require more iron than do men.

Sodium, Potassium, Magnesium, and Chloride. Sodium, potassium, magnesium, and chloride work together in a close relationship and have many similar functions. They are essential for maintaining the osmotic pressure balance between the cells and the surrounding cell fluids, for helping to maintain the normal acid–base balance, and for normal nerve and muscle functioning, as was discussed in Chapter 16.

Sodium is the major ion in the extracellular fl[uid] that is, the plasma and the interstitial fluids. Alth[ough]

Table 26-2. Summary of Minerals

Mineral	RDA or ESADDI*	Food Sources	Functions
Calcium	18–24 y: 1200 mg 25 and older: 800 mg Pregnancy and lactation: 1200 mg	Milk and dairy products, green leafy vegetables, whole grains, nuts, legumes	Forms and maintains bone and teeth Promotes blood clotting Stimulates nerve transmission Provides muscle function Activates enzymes Helps in cell membrane permeability
Chromium (Cr)	50–200 μg*	Brewers yeast, whole grains, eggs, vegetable oil, nuts, meats	Acts as cofactor for insulin
Copper (Cu)	1.5 mg–3.0 mg*	Organ meats, seafood, nuts, seeds, legumes	Provides integrity of heart and large arteries Acts in bone and blood formation
Fluorine (Fl)	1.5–4 mg*	Fluoridated water, tea, soy beans	Builds enamel of teeth Plays a role in bone formation and integrity
Iodine (I)	150 μg	Iodized salt, seafood, milk, eggs, bread	Helps form thyroid hormones, regulates basal metabolic rate
Iron (Fe)	Men: 10 mg Women: 15 mg Pregnancy: 30 mg	Liver, lean meat, dried beans, fortified cereals, dark green vegetables, dried fruits	Acts in oxygen transport via hemoglobin and myoglobin Helps form ATP Is a constituent of enzyme systems
Magnesium	Men: 350 mg Women: 280 mg	Green leafy vegetables, nuts, legumes, whole grains, seafood	Forms bone Acts in smooth muscle relaxation Regulates nerves Provides protein synthesis Acts in carbohydrate metabolism
Manganese (Mn)	2.0–5 mg*	Whole grains and cereals, fruits, vegetables, tea, nuts	Is a constituent of enzymes in mucopolysaccharide metabolism and in fat synthesis Needed to form urea Acts in growth, reproduction, and blood clotting
Molybdenum (Mo)	75–250 μg*	Milk, beans, breads, cereals	Is a component of enzymes and flavoprotein, and therefore important for normal body metabolism
Phosphorus	18–24 y: 1200 mg 25 and older: 800 mg	Meat, poultry, fish, eggs, legumes, milk and dairy products, nuts	Forms and maintains bone and teeth Acts in acid–base balance Acts in energy metabolism Acts in cell membrane structure Regulates hormone and coenzyme activity
Selenium (Se)	Men: 70 μg Women: 55 μg	Seafood, kidney, liver, meat, some grains	Protects against oxygen damage and heavy metals Assists in fat metabolism Is a constituent of an enzyme that acts as an antioxidant
Zinc (Zn)	Men: 15 mg Women: 12 mg	Meat, oysters, seafood, milk, egg yolks, legumes, whole grains	Used in tissue growth, development, and healing Used in sexual maturation and reproduction Is a constituent of many enzymes in energy and nucleic acid metabolism Constituent of insulin

* All information is RDA unless followed by an *. The * indicates Estimated Safe and Adequate Daily Dietary Intakes. Other trace minerals are also increased in pregnancy and lactation.

Source: Adapted from Dudek SG. Nutrition Handbook for Nursing Practice, Ed 2. Philadelphia, J.B. Lippincott, 1993, pp. 144, 151, 159.

sodium is needed by the body, most Americans eat far too much sodium. This has been identified as a major contributing factor in heart disease. Sodium is contained in many foods including monosodium glutamate, baking soda, and baking powder. Processed foods, fast foods, many diet soft drinks, and commercially canned foods are particularly high in sodium.

Potassium is the major ion inside the cells, in the intracellular fluid. People who are on certain diuretics require more potassium in their diet.

In addition to its function in the maintenance of homeostasis, **magnesium** is also combined with calcium and phosphorus in the bones; from 50% to 60% of the body's magnesium is in the bones. Magnesium also functions as an activator of enzymes and is involved with RNA in protein synthesis.

Chloride is needed for the production of hydrochloric acid in the stomach and is also one of the ions involved in the complex buffering system of the body.

Because the daily requirement of these minerals is relatively small and the minerals are found in so many foods, the ordinary diet provides adequate amounts. A case of deficiency may occur, however, as a result of a metabolic or absorption disorder.

Sulfur. Sulfur, an important mineral, is a constituent of the amino acids. It is most highly concentrated in bone, hair, and nails, although it is also present in all body cells.

Iodine. Although the amount of iodine in the body is small, the thyroid gland cannot function properly without it. Iodine is needed for production of the hormone *thyroxine.* Some parts of the United States have almost no iodine in the soil, especially near the Great Lakes and in parts of the Rocky Mountain regions. Because of this, food products from those areas lack iodine, so that goiter was locally common in the past. This deficiency can now be remedied by using *iodized salt,* a recommended practice in those parts of the country that lack iodine.

Trace Minerals. Some minerals, present in the body in very small amounts, are nevertheless important in body processes. These minerals are involved in absorption and synthesis of other minerals, production of enzymes, and metabolism within the cells. *Chromium* is found in brewer's yeast and grains; a deficiency may upset the function of insulin. *Copper* helps form hemoglobin. *Zinc* is important in producing hormones and RNA. Other trace minerals are *arsenic, aluminum, bromine, cobalt, fluorine, manganese, nickel, molybdenum, silicon,* and *selenium.* The ordinary diet usually provides an adequate supply. Table 26-2 gives the sources and functions of some of these minerals.

Vitamins

The word **vitamin** signifies the importance of these substances in food; *vita* is the Latin word for life. The body, with a few exceptions, cannot produce or store most vitamins. Therefore, an adequate daily supply of vitamins is essential for health and growth. General vitamin deficiency may not be the cause of a specific disease, but it does impair general health and efficiency. The accompanying box gives some general principles related to vitamins.

Foods are the natural sources of vitamins and should supply our vitamin needs. Table 26-3 identifies the major vitamins, sources, and their functions.

Vitamins are available in concentrated form, and physicians prescribe them for marked deficiencies. Foods differ greatly in the amount and number of vitamins they contain. Vitamins vary in their solubility and in the degree to which they are affected by cooking temperatures.

Fat-Soluble Vitamins

Fat-soluble vitamins are absorbed into the lymphatic circulation and must attach to a protein to be transported through the blood. They need fat to be absorbed and stored in the body and are not easily destroyed by cooking.

Vitamin A. Vitamin A is a group of related substances that promote growth, sustain normal vision, support normal reproduction, and maintain healthy skin and

(Text continues on page 288)

General Principles Related to Vitamins

- ◆ Some vitamins are lost by exposure to air or during storage of food. Fresh foods retain most vitamins; frozen foods are second; canned foods, third. (Canned foods should be processed carefully and should not be stored too long.)
- ◆ Some vitamins are soluble in fats and are stored in the body in this form. The diet must include enough fat to carry an adequate supply of these vitamins (15–20 g).
- ◆ Some vitamins are soluble in water. Foods should be cooked in a small amount of water and the cooking water should be used, if possible, in gravies, sauces, and soups.
- ◆ High temperatures destroy vitamins. Food should not be overcooked and should be served at once.
- ◆ In some foods, the vitamin content is in the portion that is likely to be thrown away, such as the outer leaves of lettuce and vegetable peel.
- ◆ A clinical condition called hypervitaminosis can occur as a result of an excess of a particular vitamin or vitamins.

Table 26-3. Summary of Fat-Soluble and Water-Soluble Vitamins

Nutrient	Adult RDAs	Food Sources	Functions
FAT-SOLUBLE VITAMINS			
Vitamin A Vitamin precursor: carotene Vitamin: retinol	Men: 1000 µg RE* Women: 800 µg RE Pregnancy: 800 µg RE Lactation: 1300 µg RE	Preformed retinol is found in egg yolks, liver, fish liver oils, whole + fortified milk and dairy products, fortified margarine, and fortified breakfast cereals. Carotenes are found in dark green and yellow vegetables, such as sweet potatoes, winter squash, carrots, broccoli, spinach, "greens," peaches, apricots, and cantaloupe	Helps the eye to adapt to dim light, helps maintain normal vision Promotes normal growth and development of bones and teeth Helps form and maintain skin and mucous membranes Helps maintain cellular (plasma) membranes Promotes normal reproduction
Vitamin D Vitamin precursors: ergosterol, 7-dehydrocholesterol Vitamins: D$_2$ (ergocholecalciferol), D$_3$ (cholecalciferol)	19–24-y: 10 µg After age 24: 5 µg Pregnancy or lactation: 10 µg	Fortified milk, margarine, and breakfast cereals; small amounts are found in butter, egg yolk, and liver. Concentrated in fish-liver oils, salmon, sardines, and tuna fish Sunshine on skin	Stimulates the intestinal absorption of calcium Mobilizes calcium and phosphorus from the bone Stimulates reabsorption of calcium by the kidney Increases reabsorption of phosphorus by the kidney Prevents rickets or osteomalacia
Vitamin E Tocopherol	Men: 10 mg α-TE Women: 8 mg α-TE Pregnancy: 10 mg-TE Lactation: 12 mg α-TE	Vegetable oils, whole grains, wheat germ, leafy vegetables, soybeans, corn, peanuts, pecans, walnuts, margarine and salad dressings made with vegetable oils, egg yolk, butter, and liver	Protects vitamins A and C from being destroyed by oxidation Protects cell membranes and red blood cells
Vitamin K Vitamin K$_1$ (phylloquinone) Vitamin K$_2$ (menaquinone)	Men: 80 µg Women: 65 µg Pregnancy or lactation: 65 µg	Green leafy vegetables, cabbage, cauliflower, spinach, cheese, vegetable oils, margarine, egg yolk, and liver. Synthesized by GI flora.	Forms 5 proteins necessary for normal blood clotting
WATER-SOLUBLE VITAMINS			
Vitamin C (Ascorbic Acid)	Men and women: 60 mg Pregnancy: 70 mg Lactation: 95 mg Smoker: 100 mg	Guava, broccoli, brussels sprouts, green peppers, strawberries, "greens," citrus fruits, potatoes, tomatoes, cabbage, cantaloupe, and yams.	Assists in wound healing and repair of bone fractures Helps form neurotransmitters Acts as an antioxidant Forms collagen Enhances intestinal absorption of iron; helps maintain bones and teeth Converts folate to its active form Involved in the metabolism of certain amino acids and steroid formation Prevents scurvy

blood clotting (handwritten annotation)

(continued)

Table 26-3 (continued)

Nutrient	Adult RDAs	Food Sources	Functions
Thiamine (Vitamin B₁)	Men: 1.2–1.5 mg Women: 1.0–1.1 mg Pregnancy: 1.5 mg Lactation: 1.6 mg	Pork, liver, organ meats, whole grain and enriched grains, nuts, legumes, potatoes, eggs, dried yeast, and milk	Provides energy metabolism, especially the metabolism of CHO; aids in CO_2 removal Promotes normal nervous system functioning Important in reproduction and lactation Prevents beriberi
Riboflavin (Vitamin B₂)	Men: 1.4–1.7 mg Women: 1.2–1.3 mg Pregnancy: 1.6 mg Lactation: 1.8 mg	Milk and dairy products, organ meats, eggs, enriched grains, and green leafy vegetables	Promotes CHO, protein, and fat metabolism Plays other metabolic roles Prevents cheilosis and glossitis
Niacin (Vitamin B₂)	Men: 15 to 19 mg NE Women: 13–15 mg NE Pregnancy: 17 mg NE Lactation: 20 mg NE	Kidney, liver, poultry, lean meat, fish, yeast, milk, peanut butter, enriched and whole grains, dried peas and beans, and nuts	CHO, protein, and fat metabolism Helps maintain body tissues Promotes oxidation of nutrients within cells Needed for DNA production Prevents pellagra
Vitamin B₆ (Pyridoxine)	Men: 2.0 mg Women: 1.6 mg Pregnancy: 2.2 mg Lactation: 2.1 mg	Chicken, fish, peanuts, oats, yeast, wheat germ, pork, organ meats, egg yolk, whole grain cereals, corn, potatoes, and bananas	Aids amino acid metabolism Helps in blood formation Helps to maintain nervous tissue Converts tryptophan to niacin
Folate	Men: 200 μg Women: 180 μg Pregnancy: 400 μg Lactation: 280 μg	Green leafy vegetables, asparagus, broccoli, liver, organ meats, milk, eggs, yeast, wheat germ, kidney beans, and orange juice	Aids amino acid metabolism Aids DNA and RNA synthesis; proliferation of cells Helps in blood formation Taken during pregnancy, helps prevent birth defects Helps prevent megaloblastic anemia
Vitamin B₁₂ (Cobalamin)	Men and women: 2 μg Pregnancy: 2.2 μg Lactation: 2.6 μg	Liver, kidney, fresh shrimp and oysters, beef, meats, milk, eggs, and cheese	Aids in RNA and DNA synthesis Helps form blood Helps maintain nervous tissue (especially the myelin sheath) Aids in CHO, protein, and fat metabolism Helps folate metabolism Helps prevent pernicious anemia
Pantothenic Acid	Men and women: safe and adequate intake 4–7 mg	Animal tissues, whole grain cereals, legumes, milk, vegetables, fruit	Promotes CHO, protein, and fat metabolism
Biotin	Men and women: safe and adequate intake 30–100 μg	Liver, organ meats, chicken, egg yolk, milk, whole grains, green leafy vegetables, and yeast. Synthesized by GI flora.	Promotes fat and CHO metabolism Forms glycogen Needed for enzyme function

*RE, retinol equivalents. 1 retinol equivalent is 1 μg retinol or 6 μg β-carotene. μg = microgram.

CHO, carbohydrate; GI, gastrointestinal; TE, tocopherol equivalent; NE, niacin equivalent.

Source: Adapted from Dudek SG. Nutrition Handbook for Nursing Practice, Ed 2. Philadelphia, J.B. Lippincott, 1993, pp. 112–113, 122–124.

mucous membranes, increasing resistance to infection. The best sources of vitamin A (also called *carotene*) are liver, spinach, and green and yellow vegetables. A bright yellow color identifies fruits and vegetables that are good sources. It is found also in cream, butter, and egg yolk in highly concentrated amounts. Preschool children and the elderly may be at risk for deficiency.

Vitamin D. Vitamin D (*calciferol*) is a group of sterols that are essential in regulating the use of calcium and phosphorus in the body. A marked deficiency of the vitamin D group hampers growth and affects the hardness of bones. This deficiency, which leads to an inadequate supply of calcium and phosphorus, causes *rickets*, a condition of childhood in which the bones do not harden as they should but bend into deformed positions, such as bowlegs. Before (and after, especially if the mother is breast-feeding) a baby is born, a mother must provide herself with enough vitamin D to prevent rickets from developing in the baby and to preserve her own bones and teeth. A vitamin D deficiency in an adult can cause a disorder known as *osteomalacia*. Vitamin D is also supplied by the sun in a complex reaction involving the skin, the liver, and the kidneys. The best food sources of vitamin D are the fish liver oils. Milk is not high in vitamin D, but milk bottlers increase the amount by irradiation and by adding vitamin D concentrate. It can be stored in the body to some extent, primarily in the liver.

Those most considered at risk for vitamin D deficiency are totally breast-fed infants or others who get little sunshine, such as prisoners or the elderly. Adequate sunlight and vitamin D-fortified dairy products provide sufficient vitamin D for most people. Excess vitamin D is toxic and should be supplemented only with physician approval.

Vitamin E. Vitamin E (*α-tocopherol*) is sometimes called "the reproductive vitamin" or the "antisterility vitamin" because it was first found to be necessary for reproduction in animals. There is no evidence that vitamin E has any effect on human reproduction or sexual function. Although the role of vitamin E is not fully understood, it is known to be a powerful antioxidant. In this role, it protects vitamins A and C, as well as some fatty acids and phospholipids in the cell membrane, from destruction by oxidation. Deficiency of vitamin E is rare, except in malabsorption disorders, such as cystic fibrosis, and in starvation. Good food sources of vitamin E include vegetable oils, margarine, leafy green vegetables, wheat germ, whole grains, egg yolk, butter, and liver.

Vitamin K. The body extracts vitamin K (*menadione*) from its food sources by the same route that it absorbs fats from the small intestine. Thus, any interference with fat absorption may result in a poor supply of any of the fat-soluble vitamins, including vitamin K. Vitamin K is essential in the formation of *prothrombin*, a substance necessary for the clotting of blood.

The average diet supplies an adequate amount of vitamin K, which is found in a variety of foods. Good sources are liver, cauliflower, cabbage, spinach, and other leafy green vegetables. Margarine and soybean and other vegetable oils are also sources. The limited amount stored in the body is found in the liver. Deficiencies of vitamin K produce hemorrhagic symptoms. Intramuscular administration of vitamin K is often used to overcome hemorrhagic tendencies.

Water-Soluble Vitamins

Water-soluble vitamins are absorbed directly through the intestinal walls into the bloodstream. They are easily absorbed, are not stored in the body in great amounts, and are easily destroyed by light, heat, acids, or alkaline solutions.

Vitamin C. Vitamin C, probably equally well known by its chemical name, *ascorbic acid,* is found in body tissues. Its function has been recognized for many years, but further uses are still being discovered. One of the functions of vitamin C in vital body processes is to aid in formation of *collagen*, a protein. Collagen is the most important protein in connective tissue; by holding cells together, it contributes to healthy tissue and to proper functioning of blood vessels, skin, gums, bones, joints, and muscles—indeed, of all tissues and organs of the body. Vitamin C is also important in the production of *steroids*, a group of compounds that include certain essential hormones. Iron absorption is enhanced by vitamin C, as is the synthesis of the neurotransmitters, serotonin, and norepinephrine. Vitamin C is also an effective antioxidant. Patients who have had surgery or have had extensive burns are frequently given large doses of ascorbic acid because it is essential to wound healing.

The classic disease of vitamin C deficiency, *scurvy,* is marked by bleeding gums, loose teeth, sore and stiff joints, tiny hemorrhages, and great weight loss. Lesser deficiencies affect health by causing listlessness, irritability, and lowered resistance to disease.

Vitamin C is probably the most unstable of the vitamins. It is destroyed by exposure to air and by being dried, heated, or stored. Because vitamin C survives longer in acid surroundings (it is an acid), baking soda (the alkali, sodium bicarbonate) should not be added to foods in cooking. Tomatoes retain vitamin C better than other vegetables because they contain acid. Freezing fruits and vegetables helps to preserve their vitamin C content, but they should be used immediately after thawing. Fruits and vegetables carefully canned commercially retain this vitamin because air is excluded during the canning process.

Because vitamin C is destroyed by heat and is water soluble, cooking should be done in as little water as possible. The cooking water or juices should be used for other preparations, and overcooking should be avoided. Many raw fruits and vegetables, especially citrus fruits, are high in vitamin C. Research has yet to confirm Linus Pauling's theory that vitamin C can prevent or cure the common cold. Because of its antioxidant properties, vitamin C may play an important role in cancer prevention.

Populations at risk for deficiency include elderly men and alcoholics. Smokers also may require supplemental vitamin C.

Vitamin B Complex. The B complex vitamins are generally known as thiamine (B_1), riboflavin (B_2), niacin, pantothenic acid, biotin, pyridoxine (B_6), folic acid, inositol, and B_{12} or cobalamin.

The B complex vitamins are all widely distributed in foods and soluble in water, but each one is chemically distinct. Each has functions that can be defined, and an extreme lack of any one produces distinctive deficiency symptoms.

Thiamine (B_1). Thiamine promotes general body efficiency. It is necessary for growth and cell metabolism. It functions as a coenzyme in many chemical reactions. It stimulates the appetite, aids digestion, regulates the nervous system, and aids reproduction and lactation. Signs of a deficiency of thiamine are poor appetite, fatigue, irritability, listlessness, loss of weight and strength, depression, and poor intestinal tone. A severe deficiency causes *beriberi*, a disease of the nervous system that leads to paralysis and death from heart failure.

The best food sources of thiamine are whole grain and enriched products, peas, beans and soybeans, pork, liver, meats from the glandular organs, and dried yeast. Some of the thiamine in milk is lost in pasteurization.

Thiamine is not stored in the body to any great extent; it is soluble in water and is heat sensitive. In acid foods, thiamine is quite stable.

The elderly and the poor probably have marginal thiamine intakes. Any diet high in processed food is likely to be lacking in adequate thiamine because thiamine is destroyed in processing.

Riboflavin (B_2). Riboflavin is part of several enzymes and coenzymes. It is essential for growth and plays a part in protein, fat, and carbohydrate metabolism. It is a part of a group of enzymes called *flavoproteins*. A deficiency of riboflavin leads to *cheilosis* (cracking at the corners of the mouth) and *glossitis* (inflammation of the tongue, with a smooth texture and purplish red color). Riboflavin is not stored in the body to any extent; therefore, a steady supply must be provided.

Riboflavin is available in a wide variety of foods but only in small quantities. The best sources are liver, meats, milk and milk products, eggs, leafy green vegetables, whole grain or enriched bread, and cereals. If riboflavin is exposed to light while in solution, it is destroyed.

Riboflavin deficiency is rare unless a person avoids all milk products. In that case, riboflavin could be supplied by an adequate intake of cereal grains.

Niacin. Niacin (nicotinic acid and nicotinamide) plays a vital role in the release of energy from carbohydrate, protein, and fat. It is also needed for the production of DNA.

A marked niacin deficiency in the body leads to the disease *pellagra*. The mucous membranes of the mouth and digestive tract become red and inflamed, and lesions appear on the skin. Symptoms of deficiency progress through the four Ds: dermatitis, diarrhea, dementia, and death. A lesser deficiency brings on these same symptoms in a milder form.

The best sources of niacin are lean meat, liver, whole grain and enriched products, and fresh and dried peas and beans. Niacin is a water-soluble vitamin, not readily destroyed by heat, and is stored in a limited amount in the body.

Niacin deficiency is rare, except in alcoholics. Nicotinic acid is sometimes prescribed by physicians to help lower blood cholesterol levels; however, intakes of over 100 mg are toxic. Symptoms of toxicity include flushing of the skin, hot flashes, headache, and itching.

Folate (Folic Acid). Folate plays a major role in the synthesis of DNA and RNA and in the formation of red and white blood cells. Good sources of folate include liver, meat, eggs, asparagus, green leafy vegetables, beans, seeds, and fruit, especially orange juice.

Deficiency results in megaloblastic (macrocytic) anemia, glossitis, diarrhea, poor growth, and impaired nerve function. Folate toxicity is not a problem because the Food and Drug Administration (FDA) limits the amount of folate in dietary supplements; folate masks the major symptom of vitamin B_{12} deficiency (pernicious anemia), which when left untreated, can cause death. New research has proven that folate, given during pregnancy, helps prevent some birth defects, particularly spina bifida.

Vitamin B_{12}. Vitamin B_{12} is a family of compounds all of which contain cobalt and are produced by microorganisms. For vitamin B_{12} to be available to the body, intrinsic factor must be present. *Intrinsic factor* is a proteinlike compound produced in the stomach in the presence of hydrochloric acid. Vitamin B_{12} is important in folate metabolism and blood cell formation. It is also involved in maintaining the myelin sheath (covering certain nerves).

Vitamin B_{12} deficiency leads to pernicious anemia and untreated, to death in 2 to 5 years. All foods of animal origin are good sources of vitamin B_{12}, especially beef. People most at risk of developing vitamin B_{12} deficiency are strict vegetarians who eat no animal products. Vegetarianism is discussed in Chapter 27.

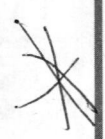

> ### Special Considerations in Aging
> ### Vitamin B_{12}
>
> The elderly may lack intrinsic factor or hydrochloric acid; antacid abuse can also cause a deficiency. In these cases, vitamin B_{12} must be given by injection.

Vitamin B_6. Vitamin B_6 is a family of compounds: pyridoxal, pyridoxine, pyridoxamine. The general name is pyridoxine. Vitamin B_6 is needed for enzyme activity in the metabolism of protein, carbohydrate, and fat. It is especially important in protein metabolism. Other functions include the formation of blood cells and the metabolism of neurotransmitters.

Good food sources of vitamin B_6 are meat, fish, and poultry. Most diets contain adequate amounts of vitamin B_6. Current research has shown that vitamin B_6 is not effective in the treatment of premenstrual syndrome although it is commonly prescribed by nonprofessionals.

A deficiency of vitamin B_6 results in retarded growth, confusion, headaches, and seizures. Vitamin B_6 is extremely toxic and can cause irreversible nerve damage. Symptoms include difficulty in walking and numbness of the feet and hands.

Biotin. Biotin is essential in the functioning of many enzymes. It acts as a coenzyme in the metabolism of carbohydrate and fat and aids in the removal of certain nitrogen groups from amino acids.

Biotin is found in almost all foods. Good sources of biotin include organ meats (such as liver), chicken, egg yolks, milk, whole grains, and green leafy vegetables.

Biotin deficiency is rare except when large amounts of raw egg whites are consumed. A substance in the egg white, avidin, binds biotin and keeps it from being absorbed. There is no RDA for biotin but the estimated safe and adequate daily dietary intake (ESADDI) is 30 to 100 μg for adults.

Pantothenic Acid. Pantothenic acid is involved in a number of metabolic processes in animals, especially in the metabolism of protein, carbohydrates, and fats. Because of its central role in energy metabolism, it is vital to all energy-requiring processes in the body. It is thought that the average diet supplies a sufficient amount. It is found in many foods. The word *pantothenic* means "widespread." Good sources include meat, milk, and many vegetables.

Like biotin, there is no RDA for pantothenic acid. The ESADDI for pantothenic acid is 4 to 7 mg for adults.

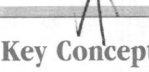

> ### Key Concept
> ◆ Fat-soluble vitamins: A, D, E, K
> ◆ Water-soluble vitamins: C, B complex

Vitamin-like Substances

The function of *myoinositol* in human beings is not known although it seems to be necessary for animals. It is abundant in the average diet and is also believed to be synthesized by the body in amounts sufficient for good health. It is closely related to glucose and is found in practically all plant and animal tissues.

Choline is associated with the metabolism of fat and its storage in the liver. Choline is a component of body cells, not a catalyst; thus, some scientists believe that it should not be classified as a vitamin, whereas others include it among the B complex vitamins. It is a precursor of the neurotransmitter, acetylcholine. Choline is manufactured in the body, and because it is also widely available in animal and plant foods, the average diet supplies adequate amounts.

Carnitine is involved in cell metabolism and is produced in the liver from amino acids. Vegetarians often have low intakes of carnitine, but they show normal blood levels. Except for times of recovery from disease or major trauma, carnitine may not be important to maintaining health.

Taurine performs many vital functions and is only found in foods of animal origin. No deficiency has been diagnosed in vegetarians, however. Taurine is needed during periods of rapid growth and is present in breast milk in large quantities. The manufacturers of infant formula have started adding taurine to formula.

A Healthy Diet

The amounts of nutrients present in individual foods vary considerably. Some foods contain a large amount of one nutrient and only a little of others; other foods have small amounts of several nutrients. The purpose of planning meals is to provide the essential nutrients in the amounts necessary to keep the body healthy. These food combinations make up an adequate diet. However, you also want meals to be appetizing and attractive.

What can be done to improve nutrition? Patients and their families may ask the nurse these questions. The nurse should have enough knowledge of nutrition and diets to be able to explain to a patient why a certain diet is required and why some foods are to be included or excluded.

The Food Guide Pyramid

A useful tool in helping people plan and eat a balanced diet is the Food Guide Pyramid, which was developed by the U.S. Department of Health and Human Services in 1992. The base of the pyramid represents foods that should be eaten in greater quantities. The top of the pyramid represents food to be eaten sparingly. The Food Guide Pyramid is described in the accompanying box. Explanations on how to use it are also given.

Daily Servings for Normal Healthy Persons

Table 26-4 lists the servings needed for the major food groups in the pyramid. These servings are spread out through the day.

Breakfast is an important meal because it follows a long period of fasting ("break fast"). It sets the pattern for the day. Eating a nutritious breakfast will help keep you alert until lunch time. If you skip breakfast, you will be hungry and sleepy in the middle of the morning and unable to concentrate. It is especially important for school children to eat a good breakfast.

Current research suggests that people who skip meals tend to overeat an hour or two later or at the next meal. To avoid feeling hungry by midmorning, include some protein in your breakfast.

The largest meal should be eaten at midday because afternoon activity will deplete the body's store of food. If the largest meal is eaten in the evening, the food may not be completely used, and extra calories will be stored in the body as fat. Working people need to adjust time of meals to suit their working hours, of course.

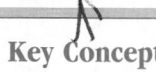

> ### Key Concept
>
> No one food provides all nutrients. Eating a balanced diet is the only way to provide the body with all the necessary nutrients.

Diet Planning

In the hospital or other healthcare facility, the diets probably will be planned by a dietitian. As a nurse you will need to understand dietary requirements to teach your patients effectively. It is important to select foods that offer adequate amounts of nutrients. At the same time, it is necessary to keep meals interesting. For ex-

How to Use the Daily Food Guide

What counts as one serving?

BREADS, CEREALS, RICE, AND PASTA
1 slice of bread
½ cup of cooked rice or pasta
½ cup of cooked cereal
1 oz of ready-to-eat cereal

VEGETABLES
½ cup of chopped raw or cooked vegetables
1 cup of leafy raw vegetables

FRUITS
1 piece of fruit or melon wedge
¾ cup of juice
½ cup of canned fruit
¼ cup of dried fruit

MILK, YOGURT, AND CHEESE
1 cup of milk or yogurt
1½ to 2 oz of cheese

MEAT, POULTRY, FISH, DRY BEANS, EGGS, AND NUTS
2½ to 3 oz of cooked lean meat, poultry, or fish
Count ½ cup of cooked beans, or 1 egg, or 2 tablespoons of peanut butter as 1 oz of lean meat (about ⅓ serving)

FATS, OILS, AND SWEETS
Limit calories from these, especially if you need to lose weight

Source: USDA's Food Guide Pyramid. Published by Human Nutrition Information Service. U.S. Department of Agriculture, Hyattsville MD, 1992. Home and Garden Bulletin #249.

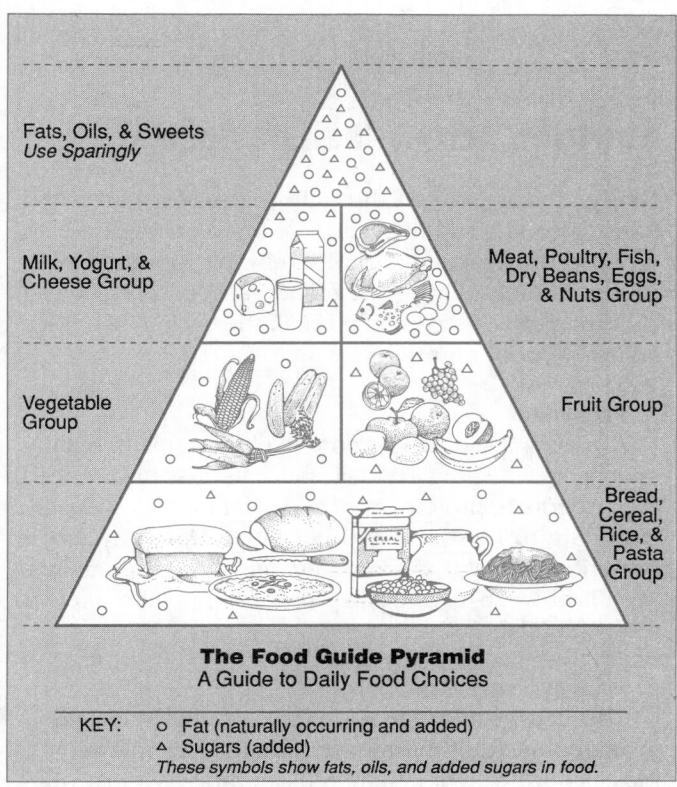

The Food Guide Pyramid
A Guide to Daily Food Choices

Fats, Oils, & Sweets
Use Sparingly

Milk, Yogurt, & Cheese Group

Meat, Poultry, Fish, Dry Beans, Eggs, & Nuts Group

Vegetable Group

Fruit Group

Bread, Cereal, Rice, & Pasta Group

KEY: ○ Fat (naturally occurring and added)
△ Sugars (added)
These symbols show fats, oils, and added sugars in food.

Table 26-4. Number of Servings Needed Daily

	Women, Some Older Adults	Children, Teen Girls, Active Women, Most Men	Teen Boys, Active Men
Calorie level*	About 1,600	About 2,200	About 2,800
Bread group	6	9	11
Vegetable group	3	4	5
Fruit group	2	3	4
Milk group	2–3†	2–3†	2–3†
Meat group	2, for a total of 5 oz	2, for a total of 6 oz	3, for a total of 7 oz

* These are the calorie levels if you choose low-fat, lean foods from the 5 major food groups and use foods from the fats, oils, and sweets group sparingly.

† Women who are pregnant or breast-feeding, teenagers, and young adults to age 24 need 3 servings.

Source: USDA's Food Guide Pyramid. Published by Human Nutrition Information Service. U.S. Department of Agriculture, Hyattsville MD, 1992. Home and Garden Bulletin #249.

ample, the body needs a considerable amount of calcium. Turnips contain calcium, but the amount is so small that you would have to eat a great many turnips to supply your body needs for one day. However, there is much more calcium in milk than in other foods, and milk is easily incorporated into the diet because you can use it in many ways. Therefore, it would be wiser to incorporate milk rather than turnips into the diet plan for each day.

In choosing foods that supply a particular mineral, select foods with the greatest amount of minerals, foods with minerals in a form that the body can use readily, foods with minerals that will remain in the body, and foods that are appetizing even in quantity. The accompanying box provides useful suggestions for teaching the patient and family about diet planning.

Nutrition Across the Life Span

Eating a balanced diet throughout the life span is the basis of good health. Because we often eat what we do because of our cultural and family background, educating mothers during pregnancy and parents during childrearing years will help break the cycle of diseases related to poor nutrition.

Pregnancy

A pregnant woman is more likely to remain healthy and bear a healthy child if she eats a well-balanced diet. Adequate protein, iron, and calcium are especially important to her body and her fetus. Most physicians prescribe prenatal vitamin and mineral supplements. See Tables 26-1 through 26-4 for specific dietary recommendations.

Infancy

The first year of life is marked by the most rapid growth outside of the mother's womb. An infant doubles its birth weight in 6 months and triples it in a year.

This explains the high need for energy, protein, vitamins, and minerals.

Breast milk is the best food for infants. Recent research indicates that breast-fed infants have less diarrhea and other infections than infants who are fed formula. Breast milk also has immune properties not found in formula. If breast-feeding is not possible, the physician usually recommends a human milk substitute. Infants should not be given cow's milk for the first year of life because they do not have the enzymes needed to digest the protein. Cow's milk given to infants frequently causes intestinal bleeding, which can lead to anemia and often contributes to colic.

Some parents give infants honey, but honey can contain botulism spores, which can kill an infant. It also contains antigens common to the bees' feeding area and may trigger allergies. Once an infant has reached his or her first birthday, honey can be tolerated with no ill effects.

Some physicians prescribe vitamin and mineral supplements during the first year of life. Breast-fed infants may need additional vitamin D if they don't get enough sunshine. Infants on a human milk substitute (formula), do not need additional supplements. All infants, however, begin to require a dietary iron source between 4 and 6 months of age. This is best supplied by iron-fortified infant cereals.

It is preferable to feed infants on demand (when they are hungry). If the infant is hungry, cries, and is fed and satisfied, then a sense of trust is created and frustration is prevented. It is important to take the time to hold the infant while feeding, even if using a bottle. Mealtime should be pleasurable. The infant reacts to the parents' emotions. Forcing food, withholding food, or adult tension will create tension and unhappiness in the child.

Children Aged 2 to 12

Parents with healthy eating habits set a good nutritional example for their children. Permanent eating habits usually develop during childhood.

Keys to Patient Teaching: Dietary Guide for North Americans

Eat a variety of foods. Include selections of

- Fruits—eat five servings a day.
- Vegetables—include those high in vitamins A & C
- Whole grain and enriched breads, cereals, and grain products
- Milk, cheese, yogurt (nonfat or low-fat)
- Meats, fish, poultry, (limit to 7 oz varieties/d)
- Legumes (dry peas and beans)
- Eggs, limit 3/wk

Maintain ideal weight.

- Increase physical activity.
- Eat less fat and fatty foods.
- Eat less sugar and sweets.
- Avoid too much alcohol.

Avoid too much fat, saturated fat, and cholesterol.

- Choose lean meat, fish, poultry, dry beans, and peas as protein sources.
- Moderate use of eggs and organ meat (such as liver).
- Limit intake of butter, cream, hydrogenated margarines, shortening, and coconut oil.
- Trim excess fat off meats.
- Broil, bake, or boil (rather than fry) food.
- Read labels to determine amounts and types of fat in foods.

Eat foods with adequate starch and fiber.

- Substitute starches for fats and sugars.
- Select foods that are good sources of fiber and starch, such as whole-grain breads and cereals, fruits, and vegetables, beans, peas, and nuts.

Avoid too much sugar.

- Use less of all sugar, including white sugar, brown sugar, honey, and syrup.
- Eat less of foods containing sugar, such as candy, soft drinks, ice cream, cake, cookies.
- Select fresh fruits or fruits canned without sugar or with light syrup (no heavy syrup).
- Read food labels to determine sugar content. (*Remember:* The first ingredient listed is the largest amount in the product.) Sucrose, maltose, dextrose, lactose, etc., are also sugars.
- Limit refined sugar to 10% of total calories.

Avoid too much sodium.

- Learn to enjoy unsalted flavor of foods.
- Cook with only small amount of salt.
- Add little or no salt at the table.
- Limit intake of salty foods (salted nuts, popcorn, soy sauce, pickles, prepared dinners, commercially canned foods, cured and smoked meats, etc.).
- Read labels to determine amounts of salt (sodium).
- *Remember:* Sodium is contained in some artificial sweeteners.

If you drink alcohol, do so in moderation.

- Pregnant women should be especially careful not to drink alcohol.
- Drink plenty of water.

Other

- Limit caffeine intake (colas, coffee, chocolate)

Source: Data from U.S. Department of Agriculture, Human Nutrition Information, 1990.

A child's rate of growth is not constant. Parents should understand that their child's needs will fluctuate. For the small child, the following plan may be used: add one additional tablespoon of each of the food pyramid groups per year of life at each meal. This will generally provide the child with the nutrients needed.

A child's likes and dislikes may change. Introduce new foods gradually in small amounts. Cut foods into small pieces. Cutting foods into attractive designs also encourages a child to eat. Limit the use of condiments such as ketchup and salt. Allow the child to assist with shopping and food preparation. Make mealtime a happy time. Provide snacks from the Food Guide Pyramid if the child's appetite is poor or if the child is hungry between meals. Children should not be required to "clean their plates" but should stop eating when they are no longer hungry. Try not to give empty calories. Good snacks include fruits, crackers, cheese, meat pieces, and raw vegetables. Make sure the child is able to chew the foods given and supervise carefully.

Children are more likely to enjoy mealtime if they can serve themselves. The understanding should be that they eat whatever they take. Use small plates, cups, and silverware to make eating more appealing and easier. Provide furniture that is comfortable and of appropriate size for the child. A high chair, infant seat, booster chair, or child's table and chairs next to the adult's table may encourage eating and make the child more comfortable.

> **Key Concept**
> Children should not be forced to eat. Usually children eat as much as needed.

Common nutritional problems during childhood are iron deficiency anemia and obesity. Anemia can usually be corrected by dietary changes combined with supplements prescribed by a physician. Obesity is harder to treat. Although obese infants do not necessarily grow up to be fat adults, an overweight 5-year-old may be on the road to lifelong weight problems. Childhood obesity has been linked to a sedentary lifestyle, especially long hours of television viewing. Treatment for childhood obesity is not food restriction but a change in dietary practices and an increase in physical activity.

Children, especially those under 2 years old, need fat in their diets. Children between the ages of 1 and 2 years should get whole milk. Children over 2 years should get low-fat milk, especially if the child is overweight for his or her height. Failure to thrive has been seen in children whose parents were overly concerned about avoiding obesity in their children and who severely restricted fat in the child's diet. Remember that fat is an important energy source for children because they have small stomachs and high energy needs.

Adolescence

The adolescent years are characterized by a period of rapid growth, accompanied by an enormous appetite. The young person needs extra food to meet the needs of growth and body development. When good eating habits have been developed in childhood, the adolescent is more likely to follow appropriate eating practices. It is important to have nutritional snacks available rather than "junk foods." This will make it easier for the young person to choose a good diet. Adolescent food fads are generally not harmful if good eating habits have been established previously. Adolescents, however, are influenced by their peers, and foods popular among young people tend to be high in calories, carbohydrates, fats, and salt.

Parents should allow adolescents to make choices. Sometimes, the foods chosen are not as harmful as you might think. Parents must realize that a slice of cold pizza for breakfast is better than no breakfast at all. Also, nagging is *not* effective!

> **Key Concept**
> Parents of adolescents need to be alert to disorders such as obesity, anorexia, and bulimia and to seek appropriate assistance for these disorders as soon as possible.

Iron deficiency anemia may be a problem for girls after the onset of menses and in boys during their growth spurt. Iron deficiency anemia can lead to fatigue and decreased ability to concentrate and learn. Treatment for iron deficiency anemia is an iron supplement, especially if a girl has heavy menstrual flow, and an increase in iron-rich foods. Calcium is another important mineral for adolescents, especially girls. It is thought that a low intake of milk and milk products during these years can lead to the development of osteoporosis later in life.

Young and Middle Adulthood

Nutritional needs are the same as at any other time of life. Calorie requirements may decrease, however, because the person is no longer growing and is less active. Using the food pyramid and choosing from a wide variety of foods will add interest to menu planning.

Being overweight can become a problem during this stage of life. This can be managed by carefully following the food pyramid and developing an active exercise program.

Older Adulthood and the Elderly

Although the body ages throughout the life span, proper nutrition can be the key to prevention of cell breakdown or disease. Eating a well balanced diet before senior years is often the key to preventing many chronic diseases. Calorie requirements in the senior years are decreased because the person is not growing and is often less active. All of the nutrients are still needed, however. Healthy eating habits from childhood help seniors continue to make wise food choices. Older persons can take advantage of services such as Meals On Wheels and senior center meals.

The Food Guide Pyramid may be offered in five or six small meals a day. Provide smaller portions and foods that are easily chewed. Whole grains, fruits, and vegetables are important. The person needs to be encouraged to drink plenty of water. Use eating utensils that are easy to handle. (For example, a cup for drinking soup may be easier to manage than a spoon and a bowl.) Remember not to serve very hot foods, so the person will not be burned. Companionship is important during meals.

> **Key Concept**
> Good nutritional habits should be practiced throughout a lifetime. Education is the cornerstone to good nutrition; good nutrition is the cornerstone to good health.

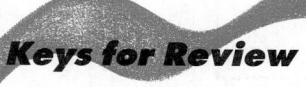

Keys for Review

Key Questions for Critical Thinking

1. Discuss the nutritional problems of Americans. Describe nutrition as it is related to leading causes of death. In what ways can these disorders be changed by eating habits?
2. Describe the difference between saturated fats and unsaturated fats. Give examples of each. Discuss their effect on health.
3. Describe the Food Guide Pyramid and its use.
4. Describe why you, as a nurse, should be familiar with nutrition and nutrients. Include you and your patients in your discussion.

Key Readings

Dudek S. Nutrition Handbook for Nursing Practice, Ed 2. Philadelphia, J.B. Lippincott, 1993

Eschleman MM. Introductory Nutrition and Diet Therapy, Ed 2. Philadelphia, J.B. Lippincott, 1991

Hamilton EM, Whitney EN. Nutrition Concepts and Controversies, Ed 5. St. Paul, MN, West Publishing, 1991

Krause MV, Arlin M. Krause's Food, Nutrition and Diet Therapy, Ed 8. Philadelphia, W.B. Saunders, 1992

Luke B. Principles of Nutrition and Diet Therapy. Boston, Little-Brown

Robinson C, Weigley E. Basic Nutrition and Diet Therapy. New York, MacMillan, 1989

Satter E. Child of Mine: Feeding with Love and Good Sense, Ed 3. Menlo Park, CA, Bull Publishing, 1991

Wardlaw G, Insel P. Perspectives in Nutrition, Ed 2. St. Louis, Times-Mirror/Mosby, 1993

Keys to Learning More

Chapter 27: transcultural considerations related to diet

Chapter 28: diet therapy and special diets; assisting a patient to meet nutritional needs when that person cannot meet his or her own needs

Keys to Learning More (continued)

Chapter 44: skin care and wound healing, as influenced by the patient's nutritional status

Chapter 46: elimination of wastes from the body

Chapter 50: nursing assessment of a patient, including nutritional status

Chapter 53: discusses surgery, as influenced by nutritional status

Chapter 58: importance of dietary intake during pregnancy

Unit Thirteen: disorders of children, including malabsorption disorders and other nutritional problems

Unit Fourteen: disorders of adults

Chapter 81: digestive disorders

Unit Sixteen: disorders in aging

Chapter 91: maintaining nutritional status in terminal illness

Key Resources

American Diabetes Association
  149 Madison Avenue
  New York, NY 10016
  212-725-4925

American Dietetic Association
  216 West Jackson Boulevard
  Suite 800
  Chicago, IL 60606
  312-899-0040

American Heart Association
  7320 Greenville Avenue
  Dallas, TX 75231
  214-373-6300

27 Social and Transcultural Aspects of Nutrition

Keys for Learning

Learning Objectives

♦ Relate the following factors to family food choice: financial, emotional, social, and physical factors and ethnic heritage.
♦ Identify several ethnic groups and discuss their common dietary practices.
♦ Identify at least three dietary practices related to each of the following religions: Islam, Jewish, Mormon, and Roman Catholic.
♦ Name the five general types of vegetarian diets and identify what types of foods are eaten by each type.
♦ Describe how the lacto-ovo vegetarian might meet needs for protein.

Key Terms

kosher
macrobiotic
soul food

tofu
vegetarians
Yin–Yang

Keys to Understanding This Chapter

Chapter 5: basic human needs, including food
Chapter 6: optimum health requires adequate nutrition
Chapter 26: classifications of foods, suggested requirements, and sources

Key Points

♦ The nurse plays an important role in helping patients meet nutritional needs.
♦ To provide optimum care, the nurse must understand the transcultural aspects of nutrition.
♦ Ethnic and religious factors may play an important part in food acceptance, especially during illness.
♦ The vegetarian diet is healthy and contains adequate protein if it is well planned and balanced.

Key Topics Outline

Regional Preferences
Ethnic Heritage
Religious Belief
The Vegetarian Choice
    Balancing the Vegetarian Diet
Other Sociocultural Factors

Key Learning Activities

♦ Explore sociocultural diversity in your classroom, specifically as related to food and eating practices.
♦ Have a "cultural dinner." Each student could prepare a dish from a specific culture or ethnic group to share with the class.
♦ Design a chart showing cultures/religions and dietary restrictions/practices that could influence nursing care.

Rosdahl CB: Textbook of Basic Nursing, 6th ed. © 1995 J.B. Lippincott Company

Our cultural backgrounds influence our eating patterns. Ethnic heritage and religious beliefs also influence what we eat and how we prepare food. The nurse should consider these influences when giving patient care: regional preferences, ethnic heritage, and religious belief.

The following factors influence people and their eating patterns:

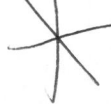

- ◆ Social aspects of eating
- ◆ Emotional attitude about food
- ◆ Food fads and fallacies
- ◆ Economic conditions
- ◆ Person's physical condition
- ◆ Personal choice (eg, vegetarianism)

Regional Preferences

Various regions of the United States have developed eating patterns. This is the result, in part, of availability of certain types of foods. These customs began before it was possible to economically, safely, and quickly transport foods from one part of the country to another or to adequately preserve fresh food. For example, people in the South tend to eat more fresh fruits and vegetables than do people in the North. Another influence on regional food patterns is the presence of many people with the same ethnic background in a specific geographic area. Thus, many West Coast cities have Chinatowns and Minnesota has Scandinavian smorgasbords. Regional dietary customs have become much less defined because of "fast food" chains and the fact that people relocate to the other regions.

Ethnic Heritage

Cultural habits affect the way a person thinks, feels, behaves, and eats. Food preferences may become particularly important during illness. When illness necessitates dietary changes, those changes should accommodate the person's ethnic and religious food preferences as much as is possible. Understanding these preferences enables the nurse to assist the patient in reaching optimum nutritional health.

Those cultural groups with representation in the United States in the largest numbers are identified and described in the following text. When people first immigrate to North America, they continue eating their native foods if they can buy or grow the ingredients. Eventually they may adapt American food habits. The second generation especially adapts to Western foods. With food changes many people also develop Western diseases. The accompanying box lists how ethnic diets may affect health and illness.

Ethnic Diets and Their Relationship to Health and Illness

- ◆ People of all ethnic groups have a source of starch or carbohydrate, whether it is pasta, potatoes, bread, or rice.
- ◆ Low intake of milk and dairy products may predispose to bone disorders, such as rickets or osteoporosis.
- ◆ Lactose intolerance in many people of a given race or ethnic group is reflected in their limited use of dairy products. Calcium needs must be met in another way (lactose-fermented cheeses or yogurt, for example).
- ◆ High sodium (salt) intake is often a factor in hypertension (high blood pressure).
- ◆ High caloric intake often causes people in certain cultural groups to be overweight. Obesity is a status symbol in some cultures.
- ◆ Intake of high amounts of fried foods and fats may predispose to atherosclerosis, gallbladder disease, and obesity.
- ◆ Long cooking of vegetables may cause deficiency of water-soluble vitamins.
- ◆ Foods high in saturated fat and cholesterol may predispose to blood vessel conditions, such as atherosclerosis and to obesity.
- ◆ High sugar intake may predispose to dental caries and diabetes mellitus.
- ◆ Many people find comfort in traditional ethnic foods when ill, even if they do not follow these traditions when well.
- ◆ The family or patient may insist on following religious or cultural practices during illness.
- ◆ Certain foods are ascribed as "hot" or "cold" by some properties unrelated to temperature and are eaten to offset or combat certain illnesses that are considered "hot" or "cold."
- ◆ Certain foods are believed to cause illness by some groups, who thus avoid these foods.
- ◆ Certain foods are believed to cure or prevent illness by some people.
- ◆ Hospital food might not be acceptable because it violates a cultural or religious practice. In some cases, the ill person is "exempted" from following religious food practices during illness.

In the following discussion related to ethnic heritage generalizations are made. *Not all members of a group observe a particular practice.* Material presented here describes many people who are members of a particular group.

African American

African Americans comprise many different cultural groups. Their food habits may be based on West Indian, African, or regional American influences.

African Americans who have recently immigrated to the United States eat different foods from those who have been in the country for many generations. The staple rice and bean combination, which has many variations from island to island in the Caribbean, is a basic and widely used dish that is considered by nutritionists to be a healthy alternative to meat. Another staple is cooked starchy tubers such as casava, yams, and plantains, which reflect African influence. Tropical fruits such as mango and papaya are also enjoyed.

African Americans who have been in the United States for several generations have similar meal patterns to other Americans. Some southern blacks are Seventh Day Adventists; some are lacto-ovo vegetarians and avoid meat, tea, coffee, and alcoholic beverages. Therefore, their diet is often heavy in greens, legumes (beans, peas) and cornbread. Some African Americans are Muslims and avoid pork, shellfish, and alcohol. A majority of African Americans are lactose intolerant and avoid fluid milk but can tolerate buttermilk, cheese, and yogurt. (In these foods, enzymes have already broken down the lactose.)

The term "**soul food**" is sometimes used to refer to foods originally prepared by southern blacks, who economized by using whatever was available. These foods include chicken wings, bacon ends, ribs, wild game, and chitterlings (chitlins). Greens (eg, collard, spinach) may be combined with pork. Diets of African Americans may be high in sodium, starch, and fat. Protein may be deficient and many children who eat a traditional diet are deficient in iron, vitamin A, and folic acid. Some West Indian blacks follow the voodoo dietary practice, which states that certain foods should not be combined.

Asian American

Chinese. Chinese people practice moderation in diet; extremes in texture or temperature are avoided. A common dietary principle throughout China is the "Fan-tsai" principle. Fan is the grain, and tsai are the vegetables or other items served at the meal. Chinese people obtain 80% of their calories from the fan (grains) and 20% from the tsai (vegetables, fruits, animal proteins, and fats). Rice is a staple food. The **Yin–Yang** (cold–hot) theory, not related to temperature, applies to foods and diseases. Yin conditions are treated with Yang foods and vice-versa to achieve a balance. Chinese believe it is important to leave the table when 70% satisfied. Most adult Chinese dislike milk and cheese; lactose intolerance is common. Meats are consumed in small quantities and are often stir-fried (which preserves vitamins). It is difficult to limit sodium because of the extensive use of soy sauce.

Japanese. In Japan, food is carefully prepared and enjoyed for its simplicity, purity, and beauty. Meals are light and little animal fat is used. A good protein and calcium source is **tofu** (soybean curd). The major starch is rice. Many vegetables (including seaweed, bamboo shoots, and bean spouts) are used. Commonly, meals contain fish, soup, fresh or pickled vegetables, and tea. Breakfast usually consists of a bowl of rice gruel. It is difficult to limit sodium because of extensive use of soy sauce and soy or rice oil. Many Japanese are lactose intolerant.

Korean. Korean food is heavily influenced by Chinese and Japanese cultures. Rice, noodles, or grains are served at every meal. Food is well seasoned. The first course of a meal often consists of vegetables, fresh in summer and pickled in winter. Meat and seafood are common. The fat intake of Koreans is high. Milk, milk products, and desserts are often avoided.

Cambodian. Cambodians use plates, forks, and spoons but consider knives at the table to be barbaric. Breakfast usually consists of noodles; rice is served with lunch and dinner. Raw vegetable salads are common, as are pungent sauces with meats and fish. Cambodians rarely snack between meals and hot water is the beverage of choice.

Laotian. Laotian cooking is similar to Cambodian, except the food is more highly spiced. Lemon grass and curries of pepper and coriander are often used. The eating utensils are the same as those used by Cambodians, but fingers are used too. Rice is served at all meals. Meals rely on fresh ingredients or long cooking time. Bananas and other fruits are commonly eaten. Coffee and tea are the beverages of choice.

Vietnamese. Vietnamese diets use poultry and cheaper cuts of pork; beef is rarely used. Fish is often used to make a sauce (which is high in sodium). Rice is used regularly, as well as soybeans and peanuts. Many vegetables are used. Tea is the most common beverage. Foods are not as likely to be deep fried as in other Asian cultures, although stir-frying is common.

Filipino. Food customs of Filipinos are a combination of Chinese and Spanish influences. The heaviest meal of the day is the evening meal. It involves the gathering of the family. The Filipino diet is often high in sodium and cholesterol. Various protein foods, vegetables, and fruits are used. Rice is a staple food eaten at every meal. Sugar is used liberally but not much milk is consumed.

Greek American

Lamb is the most commonly used meat among those of Greek ancestry. Other sources of protein include organ meats, poultry, fish, eggs, and legumes. Milk and cheese are popular, especially in cooking. Children are given hot, boiled milk with sugar; adults eat yogurt. Bread is eaten at every meal; rice and corn are widely used. Vegetables are well cooked; vegetables and legumes may be served as the main dish. Olive oil is widely used. Raw fruit is often eaten as dessert. It is difficult to restrict sodium because of the high sodium content of feta cheese and olives, which are used extensively.

Hispanic American

Hispanics represent the fastest growing population of the United States. They are a varied group, speaking over 21 different dialects of Spanish and other languages and having different food habits. The U.S. Hispanic population is thought to be 60% Mexican, 15% Puerto Rican, and 7% Cuban. The remainder are mostly Central and South American. The diets of these groups are high in complex carbohydrates and fat.

Mexican. Mexican Americans often serve corn or flour tortillas with all meals, along with rice and refried beans. Meats are usually marinated or heavily spiced and are often chopped or ground. Chorizo, a Mexican sausage, is popular. Adults use limited amounts of milk and milk products, except in sweet baked desserts, which are popular. Mexican Americans also enjoy sweetened beverages, such as hot chocolate, cafe con leche (coffee with milk), and carbonated drinks. Beer is often consumed with meals.

Cuban. Cuban Americans reflect predominantly Spanish influences in their cooking styles. Rice and beans are used extensively and meat is served as income allows. Fruits and vegetables are used liberally. Only children drink milk; adults use milk only in coffee. Food is not as highly spiced as in some other Hispanic cultures. Calcium may be deficient.

Puerto Rican. Although dietary practices are changing rapidly among younger people, the traditional diet is important, especially when a Puerto Rican is ill. Breakfast and lunch are light, with dinner served late. (This may require adaptation of hospital meal schedules.) The traditional diet consists of rice, beans, salted codfish and "viandas" (root vegetables, green cooking bananas [plaintains], and breadfruit). Some patients may refuse to eat hospital food. A dietary consultation and permission for the family to bring all food from home can be helpful. Chicken soup made from home-grown chicken is seen as healing food. Foods considered "hot" in the stomach cannot be eaten during certain illnesses. (Hot does not imply temperature; it refers to reactions in the stomach.) "Sour" foods should not be eaten during menses or during or immediately after childbirth. Calcium may be lacking.

Indian American

East Indian food varies greatly, depending on the province, climate, and religion. In northern India, wheat is the primary grain and meat dishes are popular. In southern regions, rice is the primary grain, the food is highly spiced, and the people are usually vegetarians because of their Hindu beliefs. Most Indians eat two meals per day. Sweets are very sweet and are eaten often.

Italian American

Bread and pasta are the major sources of starch. Protein sources include meats such as chicken, veal, beef, sausage, pork, and cheese. Vegetables often are cooked in a thick soup. Spices and condiments include garlic, wine, olive oil, and tomato paste. To limit sodium, sausage and preserved meats such as cold cuts should be eliminated.

Middle Eastern

These regions are more universal than diverse as a result of a long history of conquest. Traditions do vary, but the staples of these areas are similar. Staple foods include flat breads, legumes, olive oil, yogurt, cheese, olives, and tomatoes. Meats are cooked until well done. Lamb, chicken, fish, and rice are diet staples; all forms of pork are often forbidden. Calcium and protein intake may be low. Many different varieties of curry are used; these curries are the predominant spices used. Women are considered subservient to men and eat only after the men and children, even if they are ill. Traditional food beliefs are common and result in a high rate of stillbirths, low-birthweight infants, and maternal deaths. Only the right hand is used for eating.

Native American and Alaska Natives

Because there are more than 300 tribes in the United States, it is difficult to generalize regarding dietary practices. Several disorders are common, including hypertension. Therefore, it is advisable to limit sodium intake. Many Native Americans are lactose intolerant and they may be lacking in calcium. Riboflavin and vitamins C and A deficiencies are also common. Many spices are used, including the green chili (which contains vitamin C).

Religious Belief

Many people eat specific foods in certain combinations or refrain from eating certain foods because of their religious beliefs. Cultural and religious practices are often intertwined. Table 27-1 identifies some of the major religious customs relating to diet. Patients, particularly when ill, are often unwilling to deviate from their religious dietary customs. The nurse needs this information when caring for patients. Foods that must be prepared using special equipment or under certain conditions can usually be ordered in advance or arranged for by the patient's family. An example is the diet of some Jewish people. This diet is called **kosher**.

Table 27-1. Dietary Practices Based on Religious Belief

Belief or Practice

Jewish

The individual Jewish person chooses to observe or not observe the dietary laws. Separate dishes, pans, and silverware must be used to prepare and serve meat and dairy foods if the person "keeps kosher." Meat and milk may not be eaten at the same meal. Meats must be slaughtered by a ritual method and only the front quarter of the animal may be eaten. Some parts of beef, veal, lamb, mutton, goat, venison, chicken, turkey, goose, and pheasant are eaten. Pork products, rabbit, shellfish, and scavenger fish are not allowed. Food must be prepared ahead of time for the Sabbath (sundown Friday to sundown Saturday). Certain days of fasting are observed, but a rabbi may excuse an elderly or ill patient.

Church of Jesus Christ of Latter Day Saints (Mormon)

Mormons use no stimulants (coffee, tea, or caffeine-containing carbonated beverages) and no alcoholic beverages. Members observe "fast offerings," giving up two meals on the first Sunday of each month. (Money saved is used to feed the poor.) Mormons live by a health code and the Words of Wisdom; they are to preserve their bodies and maintain the best possible health. Meat is eaten sparingly and "in season" (winter).*

Roman Catholic

Dietary and fasting regulations are mostly voluntary. Some Catholics still abstain from eating meat on Fridays. Those aged of 14–59 must fast and abstain on Fridays during Lent. Ash Wednesday and Good Friday are observed as days of fast and abstinence (a priest may excuse the elderly or ill). Catholics do not eat or drink (except water) for 1 h before taking Holy Communion.

Seventh Day Adventists

Seventh Day Adventists are often lacto-ovo vegetarians or vegans. They use no stimulants (coffee, tobacco) and avoid pork, shellfish, and alcohol.

Hindu

Hindus believe that all life forms are sacred because they might be the reincarnation of an ancestor. Most are lacto-ovo vegetarians (no meat, fish, poultry), and they do not use alcohol. They eat eggs. Coffee, tea, and chocolate are widely used.

Muslim (Islam)

In Islam, dietary laws are similar to Jewish kosher laws. In addition, no alcoholic beverages are allowed, but tea is permitted. Moslems fast for a month each year, avoiding food from dawn until after dark. Foods considered healthy are honey, dates, and sweets.

* Some information from interview with Jill Itri.

The Vegetarian Choice

Some people have chosen to be **vegetarians** (not to eat any type of meat) for religious, ecological, or physical reasons. Some vegetarian diets are stricter than others. The lacto-ovo diet is the most liberal, whereas the vegan is a strict vegetarian. The range is as follows:

- ◆ *Lactovegetarian*—eats plant foods, plus dairy products (no eggs)
- ◆ *Ovovegetarian*—eats plant foods, plus eggs (no dairy products)
- ◆ *Lacto-ovo vegetarian*—eats plant foods, dairy products, and eggs
- ◆ *Fruitarian*—eats fruits, nuts, olive oil, and honey
- ◆ *Vegan*—eats only plant foods

A **macrobiotic** diet is one consisting of unprocessed foods, vegetables, beans, whole grains, and some fish and fruit.

Balancing the Vegetarian Diet

The most important concern of the vegetarian diet is that of attaining an adequate supply of complete protein. This is easy in the lacto-ovo vegetarian diet, but relatively difficult for the vegan. Among the sources of protein that can be used most efficiently by the body, meat actually ranks only third. The most efficient protein available is that found in dairy products, eggs, and fish. (Some vegetarians and health food advocates do not eat meat but do eat fish or poultry.) The second best supply of efficient protein is legumes, soybeans, nuts, and brown rice. Combinations of incomplete protein sources can yield complete protein. In Chapter 26, you learned that complete proteins are needed to sustain life and promote growth. Table 27-2 describes some of the combinations that provide a complete protein source. Several incomplete proteins, eaten at different times during the day, can also add up to yield complete protein. It may be difficult for a strict vegetarian who eats mostly vegetables and fruits to obtain adequate vitamins and minerals. Vegetarian diets are often deficient in calcium, iron, zinc, vitamin D, iodine, and riboflavin; vitamin B_{12} is probably entirely absent. These substances often need to be taken as supplements. It may also be difficult to obtain enough healthful calories for the energy needs of the body. See the

Table 27-2. Vegetarian Combinations That Yield Complete Protein*

Combinations	Examples
Grain with brewer's yeast†	
Grain and nuts with milk (or legumes)	Peanut butter sandwich and milk (or yogurt or soy milk)
Grain with milk or cheese	Cereal and milk
	Cheese sandwich
	Rice cooked in milk
	Vegetarian lasagna or pizza
Grain with dried beans or wheat germ (and/or nuts)	Baked beans with nut bread
Grain with egg	Poached egg on toast
Grain with cheese	Macaroni and cheese
	Tortilla with cheese
Beans with cheese	Meatless chili with beans and cheese
	Meatless tamali pie
Beans, legumes (peas, lentils), rice or soybeans (tofu) with milk, nuts, or eggs	Various combinations
	Rice and bean burrito
Textured protein product (TPP) or meat analog (meat substitutes made from soybeans)	

Note: The lacto-ovo diet replaces meat with legumes, nuts, grains, eggs, and milk. Other vegetarian diets may omit the eggs and/or milk and dairy products.

* The above foods are protein sources only. Other foods must be added to complete the adequate diet.

† Whole wheat grains and cereals are preferred.

accompanying box for suggestions on planning a vegetarian diet.

The Zen Macrobiotic Diet

The Zen macrobiotic diet (a diet followed by a particular religious sect) progresses through 10 steps. In the diet, various foods are limited or totally eliminated. The highest level of Zen uses only whole grain cereal, usually brown rice. It has been linked to vitamin deficiencies and death.

Other Sociocultural Factors

Social Factors

Most people prefer to eat with someone rather than alone and are probably used to eating meals with family or coworkers. When people are hospitalized, they suddenly find themselves alone in a hospital room with a dinner tray. They may have limited input into what foods are served. Illness and feelings of loneliness often result in poor nutritional intake. These factors are common in hospitals. Following are some guidelines to provide some sort of company for the patient during meals:

◆ The nurse could visit for a few minutes.
◆ Two patients may eat together.
◆ In a double room, the curtain can be opened.
◆ Patients may meet in a common lounge for meals.
◆ Family members can be encouraged to visit at mealtime.
◆ The TV or radio can be turned on.

Keys to Patient/Family Teaching
A Balanced Vegetarian Diet

Patient and family teaching regarding vegetarian diets includes:

◆ Selection from a wide variety of foods. The greater the variety, the greater probability of attaining an adequate diet.
◆ Information that diets containing dairy products and eggs have high-quality protein.
◆ Explanation that plant sources of protein help supply essential amino acids.
◆ Advice to combine proteins as indicated in Table 27–2.
◆ Use of the Food Guide Pyramid for information about food choices.
◆ Foods with low nutritive value should be minimized. Empty calories and alcohol should be avoided.
◆ Whole grain products should be used rather than refined foods.
◆ A food rich in vitamin C should be included with each meal. This enhances iron absorption.
◆ Strict fruitarians or vegans may need a vitamin B_{12} supplement.
◆ Include foods rich in minerals and vitamins that are likely to be missing in a meatless diet (especially calcium, riboflavin, iron, and vitamins A and B_{12}).
◆ Obtain vitamin D from sunlight or irradiated milk.
◆ Maintain adequate caloric intake (add oil and nuts).
◆ Provide a large quantity of food.
◆ *Vegans:* substitute fortified soybean milk or green leafy vegetables, and dried fruits, for milk.
◆ *Vegans:* eat at least *two* of the following to provide all essential amino acids:
    Grains or nuts and seeds
    Dried beans or soybean curd (tofu)
    Wheat germ
◆ *Vegans:* add brewer's yeast to the diet.
◆ Plan meals carefully.

Source: Data from Eschleman MA. Introductory Nutritional and Diet Therapy, Ed 2. Philadelphia, J.B. Lippincott, 1991.

◆ Flowers can be placed nearby.
◆ The patients can phone home and talk to family while eating.

Emotional Factors

Emotional factors have an influence on nutritional behavior and on total health. These factors may influence the eating patterns of the patient in a hospital. Food may become a reward. Purees of certain foods may be considered "for babies." The patient may feel guilty for not eating all the food on the tray or may overeat just because the food is there. The patient who is sad, lonely, or depressed may overeat or refuse to eat.

Food Fads and Fallacies

Many people follow food fads, fad diets, or the practice of eating only certain foods. Food fallacies (falsehoods) influence diet.

Economic Conditions

The family's financial status has an influence on eating habits. Food is relatively inexpensive in the United States. More affluent people tend to eat out more often and consume more vegetables, fruits, cheeses, meat, fish, and poultry (and thus, more fat). Diets higher in fat can be associated with heart disease, cancer, and other disorders. When income rises, people tend to eat fewer eggs, rice, or beans. People with lower incomes may skip meals. Street people may beg or look through refuse for food. If the nurse thinks the patient does not have enough money for food, a social work referral may be helpful.

Physical Condition

Hospitalized patients may not be well enough or strong enough to eat. If patients are not strong enough to eat, time must be taken to feed them. This is an excellent time to make physical and psychological assessments of patients. Absence of teeth, ill-fitting dentures, or difficulty swallowing should be considered when planning meals. A person who has been trying to eat a low-fat, low-calorie diet may not be able to obtain adequate nutrients to rebuild tissue. This can occur, for example, in the person who is having chemotherapy for cancer. Malnutrition is common among patients with acquired immunodeficiency syndrome (AIDS). In AIDS, emphasis is placed on foods high in protein, iron, zinc, and selenium. Preparation and serving of foods must be adjusted as the patient's condition changes.

> **Key Concept**
>
> You cannot change a patient's dietary beliefs. You can help the patient to adjust the diet, within the person's belief structure.

Keys for Review

Key Questions for Critical Thinking

1. Some cultures use soy sauce and fish sauce extensively in food. Describe the problems this entails. Describe how you would discuss this with the person from that culture who prepares the family meals. Describe what suggestions you might give for revising but maintaining the ethnicity of the diet.
2. Some cultures and religious groups forbid the use of common food and beverages. Give examples of cultures and religious groups and common foods and beverages forbidden. Describe how this could affect your care.
3. Your patient is a vegetarian. Describe the philosophy behind the patient's diet. Discuss any factors involved. Describe what you would ask or tell the patient about getting complete protein into his or her diet.

Key Readings (continued)

Boyle JS, Andrews MM. Transcultural Concepts in Nursing Care. Philadelphia, J.B. Lippincott, 1990
Dudek SG. Nutrition Handbook for Nursing Practice, Ed 2. Philadelphia, J.B. Lippincott, 1993
Eschleman MM. Introductory Nutrition and Diet Therapy, Ed 2. Philadelphia, J.B. Lippincott, 1991
Giger J, Davidhizar RE. Transcultural Nursing: Assessment and Intervention. St. Louis, Mosby-Year Book, 1991
Krause MV, Arlin M. Krause's Food, Nutrition and Diet Therapy, Ed 8. Philadelphia, W.B. Saunders, 1992
Moore MC. Pocket Guide: Nutrition and Diet Therapy, Ed 2. St. Louis, Mosby-Year Book, 1993
Spector R. Cultural Diversity in Health and Illness, Ed 3. East Norwalk, CT, Appleton & Lange, 1991
Wardlaw GM, Insel FM. Perspectives in Nutrition. St. Louis, Times-Mirror/Mosby, 1993

Enrichment Keys

Newman JM. Melting Pot: An Annotated Bibliography Guide to Food and Nutrition Information for Ethnic Groups in America, Ed 2. New York, Garland, 1993

Keys to Learning More

Chapter 28: diet therapy and special diets

Chapter 50: nursing assessment involves nutritional status

Keys to Learning More (continued)

Chapter 58: pregnancy may require dietary modifications

Chapter 66: eating disorders in adolescents

Chapter 81: nutritional and digestive disorders

Chapter 85: special nutritional considerations related to elderly people

28 Diet Therapy and Special Diets

Keys for Learning

Learning Objectives

- Describe procedures for serving a food tray.
- Describe means of assisting patients who are visually impaired, cannot swallow, or cannot chew.
- Identify common modified diets, listing foods included and a related disorder for each.
- List diet progression from liquid to regular.
- Describe high-fiber, low-residue, and bland diets.
- Discuss the purpose of the Diabetic Exchange List for Meal Planning.
- List items to be excluded in moderate sodium restriction.
- Discuss methods of administering a tube feeding.
- Describe total parenteral nutrition.

Key Terms

anorexia
bland diet
carbohydrate-controlled diet
dysphagia
edema
fat-controlled diet
hyperlipidemia
infusion
intravenous therapy
liquid diet
low-residue diet
polydipsic
soft diet
stoma
total parenteral nutrition
tube feeding

Keys to Understanding This Chapter

Chapter 5: basic needs of all people, including food and water

Chapter 23: digestion and utilization of foods

Chapter 26: basic classifications of foods, suggested requirements, and sources

Chapter 27: cultural dietary practices that might influence diet therapy

Key Points

- Modified diets are an important part of many patients' treatment.
- The nurse plays an important role in seeing that patients receive the diet ordered and that trays are correct.
- Documenting patient food and fluid intake is an important part of patient care.
- Some patients need special assistance to eat because of age or physical disorder.
- The diet progression for "diet as tolerated" is: clear liquid, full liquid, soft, regular (house).
- The Diabetic Exchange Lists for Meal Planning can be used for diabetic or weight loss diets and in many other situations.
- Fluid is required to maintain homeostasis; too much plain water can lead to electrolyte imbalance.
- Tube feeding is a commonly used means of providing nourishment to patients.

Key Topics Outline

Helping the Patient Meet Nutritional Needs
  The Patient Who Needs Assistance
  Documenting and Reporting
"House" Diets
Modified Diets
  Consistency Modifications
  Energy Value Modifications
  Nutrient Modifications
  Diets Modified by Small Amounts
  Diets Modified for Allergens
Nutritional Support
  Tube Feedings
  Intravenous Therapy
  Total Parenteral Nutrition
Food and Medication Interactions

Rosdahl CB: Textbook of Basic Nursing, 6th ed. © 1995 J.B. Lippincott Company

Key Learning Activities

◆ Write down everything you ate yesterday. Which foods would you have to eliminate if you were on a moderate sodium restriction (1,000–2,000 mg daily)? What foods might you choose instead?

◆ Interview a member of your class or family who is on a modified diet. Determine if the person follows the diet restrictions. Why or why not? What does the individual think of the diet?

Key Nursing Procedures

NP 28-1: Assisting the patient who is receiving a tube feeding

Nutrition is a vital component of therapy in many disorders. For example, in any condition involving healing of body tissues, such as after a burn or surgery, a high protein intake is essential to help rebuild and repair tissues. If the patient is perspiring profusely and has a high fever, or is hemorrhaging, vomiting, or suffering from diarrhea, fluids and electrolytes are needed to replace what has been lost.

Some disorders necessitate a special diet, either during a period of illness or throughout life. A person with diabetes mellitus usually is on a special diet. Persons with coronary or vascular disorders often must restrict sodium intake. People who are ill may need help in fulfilling their dietary requirements for food and fluids. Some of the means used to assist the patient meet the basic need for adequate nutrition are discussed in this chapter. The nurse can perform specific activities to help the patient. The nurse should be knowledgeable about diets so information can be shared with patients. Modified diets and nutritional support through tube feeding also are discussed in this chapter.

Helping the Patient Meet Nutritional Needs

Every hospital has its own system of food service. Trays are usually brought to the nursing station on a cart. Each tray is labeled with the patient's name, room number, bed number, and the appropriate diet. This information should be checked against the posted diet list before the patient is given the tray. The patient's name band is checked with the name on the food tray before the tray is served.

Eating is an event in the patient's long day and should be as pleasant as possible. See the accompanying box for suggestions for making the hospital mealtime more pleasant.

Serving Food

Food should be presented in as attractive and appetizing a manner as possible. Patients are encouraged to eat without force. They are encouraged to feed themselves so they don't feel helpless. The tray covers are removed just before the tray is placed on the overbed table. This allows diffusion of odors, which intensify while collecting under the cover. Strong odors can destroy appetite. Don't remove the cover too soon—the food will get cold.

If a patient is not hungry, you can remove items from the tray and "set" the overbed table as you would a table, with napkin, utensils, and plate. This simulat[es] the home environment and makes meals more ap[pealing]. The time used in serving food is a good [time for] "chatting" with the patient. Questions abou[t] can be answered and the person made co[mfortable be-]fore you leave the room.

Providing Between-Meal S[nacks]

Between-meal and bed[time snacks are an im-]portant part of the pa[tient's diet when pre-]scribed. The supple[ment is part of the total] dietary order. It i[s important for the patient] to eat it. Nouri[shment should be docu-]mented, as [well as]

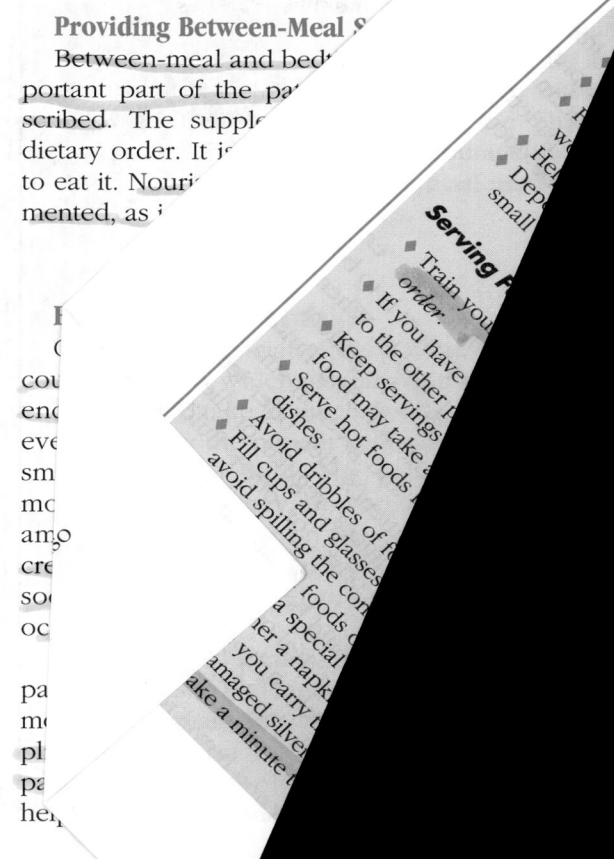

Nursing Skill Guidelines
Helping at Hospital Mealtimes

Preparing the Patient for Meals

♦ Give the person a chance to go to the bathroom or use the bedpan before the meal.
♦ Assist the person to wash the hands and face, and pehaps to rinse the mouth or brush the teeth.
♦ Help the patient into as normal a position as possible: sitting in a chair, sitting on the edge of the bed, or sitting with the head of the bed elevated.
♦ Put the overbed table in place; clear of unnecessary items.
♦ Bring the tray promptly when the patient is ready, to prevent overtiring the patient.
♦ Avoid unpleasant or painful treatments just before or after a meal.
♦ Try not to give unpleasant-tasting medications before or during a meal.
♦ If possible, give any prescribed pain medication ½ hour before a meal; this may provide some relief and allow the patient to eat more comfortably.
♦ Remove unpleasant odors (bedpan, commode) and litter (dressings, linens).
♦ Cover unpleasant things (wounds, blood, IV bags).
♦ Change linens and gown as needed.
♦ Give the person as much time as is needed.
♦ Offer assistance as needed.
♦ Encourage the patient to fill out the selective menu, so that preferred foods will be served.
♦ Explain special diets and their purposes.
♦ Consider cultural aspects.
♦ Arrange the tray attractively.
♦ Arrange foods for easy access. Help, as needed.
♦ Help arrange a towel or napkin so the patient won't worry about spilling.
♦ Help the patient to get some exercise during the day.
♦ Depending on type of diet, the family can bring amounts of favorite foods.

Food

♦ yourself to *check each tray with the diet*

a patient who must be fed, serve trays atients first.
small. The sight of large quantities of way the patient's appetite.
hot and cold foods cold. Cover hot

ood on the edges of dishes.
about three-quarters full, to tents.
on the tray are allowed for diet.
n, a spoon, or a glass is he tray to the patient.
ware or chipped glasses.
o chat with the patient.

Restricting Fluid

In some cases the physician orders a fluid restriction (eg, "restrict fluids to 1,500 mL/d"). This order might be seen in the psychiatric patient who is **polydipsic** (drinks excessive amounts of water) or in the person with end-stage renal disease. It may be easier to manage this restriction if about half the fluids are taken during the day and half in the evening. Intake of other substances (eg, caffeine) may also be restricted.

Nursing Alert

Serious toxicity and electrolyte depletion (especially of potassium) can occur if a person drinks excessive amounts of plain water.

Providing Teaching

Patients and their families want to know how they can achieve good health. Their education is an essential part of the nurse's provision of care. Handout sheets can be used for teaching along with charts and pictures of healthy foods. Diets must be explained and the patient should repeat the information so the nurse knows the patient (or family) understands the information.

One of the best times to teach is when the patient asks questions. That is why it is important for nurses to understand nutritional and diet information. When nurses do not know answers, they should tell patients they do not know, and then speak to the dietitian or physician and return with an answer as soon as possible. This helps patients build up confidence in nurses and other staff members.

The Patient Who Needs Assistance

You want to encourage independence whenever possible. In some situations, however, the patient will need to be fed the entire meal. In such cases, take time to make the patient comfortable, and encourage the patient to eat as much as desired. A family member may wish to feed the patient. This is relaxing for the patient and makes the family member feel he or she is helping to provide care. You are responsible, however, for seeing that eating is easy and safe for the patient. If this is not the case, take over or supervise the feeding.

Feeding the Patient

Even patients who can feed themselves may need assistance in spreading butter on bread, cutting meat, opening milk cartons, or pouring beverages. Always warn a patient about extremely hot foods to prevent burns, especially if the patient is using a straw. Encourage the person to do as much as possible to develop self-confidence and a sense of progress. Part of the nurse's responsibility in promoting good nutrition is to note any discomfort or digestive complaints expressed by the patient, during feeding or afterward.

Very young, helpless, or confused patients require special attention. You may have to feed them to make sure they ingest enough nutrients. It may be necessary to protect them from possible injuries or accidents.

Use your judgment about how much a patient can do—sometimes the person can hold a piece of bread but cannot manage other food. The accompanying box provides additional suggestions for feeding patients.

The Person With Special Feeding Needs

The Visually Impaired Person. Most nonsighted people can learn to eat without assistance if they are encouraged to be independent. When the patient is only temporarily blinded, following eye surgery, for example, the nurse may have to feed the patient every meal. The visually impaired patient needs to learn to locate the food on the plate. This may be done by describing the location of foods as if they were on the face of a clock (eg, "The meat is at 6 o'clock.") Be sure to warn the patient about very hot foods.

The Person With a Swallowing Disorder. Some patients have difficulty swallowing as a result of a neurologic or other disorder. **Dysphagia** is the medical term for a swallowing disorder. The patient is often given a semi-liquid diet. Elevate the head of the bed, feed the patient very slowly, and encourage swallowing after each portion of food.

The Person Who Cannot Chew. Some people have trouble chewing because of poor dental health, missing teeth, or poorly fitting dentures. These patients will need a modification in the consistency of their diets. The nurse should assess each patient's ability to chew and swallow. This information is given to the team leader or physician.

Documenting and Reporting

If a patient has a poor appetite or refuses food, has difficulty swallowing, or complains of nausea or vomiting, the nurse is responsible for observing and documenting such observations and calling them to the attention of the team leader. That person and the physician then give directions about how to provide the

---

> ### Nursing Skill Guidelines
> #### Feeding Patients
>
>
>
> ♦ Wash your hands first.
> ♦ Make the person comfortable.
> ♦ Arrange a napkin or towel to avoid spills.
> ♦ Arrange the tray conveniently.
> ♦ Do not rush.
> ♦ Sit down; take time to make the meal relaxing.
> ♦ Visit with the person (be careful that the patient does not choke).
> ♦ Use usual utensils (fork, spoon).
> ♦ Feed a small amount at a time.
> ♦ Ask the patient how he or she likes to eat; some people eat all of one food first, others rotate foods.
> ♦ Tell the person if something is very hot or cold; warn the person to test the food first.
> ♦ A straw or drinking cup may be helpful for sipping soup. Be very careful of hot liquids!
> ♦ Wipe the chin and face as needed.
> ♦ Let the person hold bread or otherwise help as much as possible.
> ♦ After the person has finished the meal, record intake and make the person comfortable.
> ♦ *Note*: In some states, the nurse is required to wear gloves when feeding patients.

---

patient with needed nourishment. The dietitian is also a valuable resource and should be consulted whenever problems with diet, nutrition, or patient food preferences are apparent. Other relevant observations must be documented in the patient's chart, including fluid intake, caloric intake, or the amount of a tube feeding taken.

> ### Key Concept
>
> Diet is an integral part of the patient's total treatment plan.

"House" Diets

General diets and menus in hospitals or long-term care facilities are called "house" or full diets. The *full diet* is the one most frequently ordered. It is served to patients whose condition does not require a special diet. You may hear it called a *general diet, house diet,* or *regular diet.*

The full diet is a normal diet. Because patients, especially in medical–surgical units, are relatively inactive, their caloric intake should be consistent with their level of activity. A full diet may be modified to meet individual needs. It allows a wide choice of foods and includes almost everything.

Modified Diets

A modified diet is an important part of therapy in many disease conditions. When planning a special diet, the physician and dietitian consider the disease process and patient's general condition. Always follow dietary orders carefully. When in doubt regarding a diet or when questions arise, always consult the dietitian and the facility diet manual.

A therapeutic diet may be prescribed as part of the treatment of more than one disease or condition. For example, a patient with a heart condition may also be overweight; a convalescent surgical patient may also be a diabetic. The following are general reasons for therapeutic diets and common examples of associated disorders.

♦ Regulating the amount of certain nutrients in disorders of metabolism (diabetes)
♦ Increasing or decreasing body weight by adding or limiting calories and fat (underweight or overweight)
♦ Reducing or preventing edema by controlling the level of sodium (cardiac conditions)
♦ Aiding digestion by avoiding foods that irritate the alimentary tract or interfere with stomach action (ulcer)
♦ Helping an overburdened organ regain normal function (nephritis)
♦ Eliminating a food that the body is unable to tolerate (allergies, phenylketonuria)
♦ Slowing overactive digestion (colitis)

A patient is far more amenable to diet restrictions if not constantly reminded of the disease by having the diet classified according to disease name. For instance: referring to a diabetic patient's diet as "controlled carbohydrate" deemphasizes diabetes and *concentrates attention on dietary habits you want the patient to develop.*

The following classifications indicate how diets are modified in treatment of patients:

♦ Diets modified according to consistency and texture (liquid, soft, high fiber, low residue, bland)
♦ Diets modified according to energy value (high and low calorie)
♦ Diets modified in one or more nutrients (controlled carbohydrate; high and low fat; protein, sodium, calcium, or potassium controlled)
♦ Diets modified in amount (six small feedings)
♦ Diets modified to eliminate specific allergens

These categories indicate the kind of diet prescribed although the amounts of specific nutrients may be varied for a patient, according to physician's orders. If there are no restrictions or special requirements, the patient may have any of the foods listed for that type of diet. The nurse must know in general what kinds of foods will be allowed. Although individual trays are checked carefully in the kitchen, mistakes can happen. The nurse should be able to recognize each type of diet and examine each tray with the patient's specific diet in mind.

Consistency Modifications

The consistency and texture of the diet may be modified with clear liquid, full liquid, soft, mechanical soft, pureed, low-residue, high-fiber, and bland diets. These are discussed in this section of the chapter. Tube feedings are a form of modified diet also. They are discussed at the end of the chapter.

Liquid Diets
A **liquid diet**, as the name suggests, consists entirely of liquids. (A liquid is described as a food that is fluid at room temperature or that becomes fluid at body temperature). Table 28-1 discusses liquid diets.

Liquid diets are prescribed after surgery as a patient's first step toward taking solid foods. They may be used during an acute illness or in certain body disturbances, such as irritation of the intestinal tract. Liquids are easily absorbed and do not overstimulate the digestive tract. According to a patient's needs, liquid diets may be clear, full, or limited and are often progressive. Feedings may be given every 2, 3, or 4 hours, as prescribed.

Clear Liquid Diet. Items in a clear liquid diet are listed in Table 28-1. The clear liquid diet is inadequate in calories, protein, and most other nutrients. It should not be used for more than 3 days, unless the patient is receiving nutrition support or other nutritional supplements.

Full Liquid Diet. Full liquid diet items are listed in Table 28-1. If a full liquid diet is to be used for a long time, other high-calorie liquids should be added. The nurse should be aware of side effects to these supplements.

> **Nursing Alert**
> The prolonged use of nothing by mouth (NPO) is a serious problem. A patient may be NPO for tests, after surgery, or because of vomiting. A patient who has been NPO for 3 or more days and is not receiving nutrition support is at serious nutritional risk. These patients should be brought to the attention of your team leader.

Table 28-1. Characteristics, Indications, and Contraindications for Liquid and Soft Diets

Diet Characteristics	Foods Allowed	Indications	Contraindications
Clear Liquid A short-term, highly restrictive diet composed only of clear fluids or foods that are fluid at body temperature. It requires minimal digestion and leaves a minimum of residue. Although it provides some electrolyte and carbohydrates, clear liquid diets are inadequate in calories and all nutrients except vitamin C.	Bouillon; fat-free broth Carbonated beverages; coffee, regular and decaf; tea Fruit juices, strained and clear (apple, cranberry, grape) Gelatin; popsicles Sugar, honey, hard candy	Initial feeling after surgery or parenteral nutrition; in preparation for surgery and various diagnostic tests of the bowel	Long-term use
Full Liquid Diet Composed of foods that are liquid or liquefy at body temperature. Full liquid diets can be carefully planned or supplemented to approximate the nutritional value of a regular or high-calorie–high-protein diet, making it suitable for long-term use. Full liquid diets may be inadequate in folic acid, iron, vitamin B_6 and fiber. If the diet is used longer than 2 to 3 days, modifications may be needed to increase calories and protein.	All the above plus: All milk and milk drinks, puddings, custards, and desserts All vegetable and fruit juices Refined or strained cereals Eggs in custard Butter, margarine, cream Dietary supplements such as Resource or Ensure	Used as a transitional diet between a clear liquid diet and a soft diet, and by clients who have difficulty chewing or swallowing	Severe lactose intolerance (diet relies heavily on milk and dairy products for protein and calories) Unless modified to decrease the cholesterol content, a liquid diet is not suitable for long-term use by clients with hypercholesterolemia
Soft Diet An adequate diet low in fiber, connective tissue, and fat. Restrictions vary considerably among institutions: Individual tolerances should determine the content of the diet.	All the above plus: Cooked vegetables as tolerated Lettuce in small amounts Cooked or canned fruit Avocado, banana, grapefruit and orange sections without membranes Whole grain or enriched breads and cereals Potatoes Enriched rice, barley, pasta All lean, tender meats, fish, poultry Eggs, mild cheese, smooth peanut butter Butter, margarine, mild salad dressings	Used for clients who have difficulty chewing or swallowing. A mechanical soft diet is used primarily by clients who have difficulty chewing because they are endentulous (without teeth) or have ill-fitting dentures. A regular soft diet is used as a transition between liquids and a regular diet.	None

Source: Adapted from Dudek SG. Nutrition Handbook for Nursing Practice, Ed 2. Philadelphia, J.B. Lippincott, 1993

Soft Diet

A **soft diet** includes semisolid food and is often supplemented with between-meal feedings. Usually, it is high in calories and easily digested. Gas-forming foods are avoided; mild seasoning is used. The soft diet is used as a transition between a liquid diet and the full or general diet. All needed nutrients can be obtained in this diet. Table 28-1 explains the soft diet. The physician may order a modification of the soft diet without some of the foods listed.

Key Concept

Progressive diets:
clear liquid → full liquid → soft → full diet

The *mechanical soft diet*, or dental diet, is used for the person who has difficulty chewing. All meats, fruits, and vegetables are chopped, ground, or pureed, depending on the patient's ability to chew and swallow.

High-Fiber Diet

A diet low in fiber may be one of the causes of constipation. Bulk is needed to stimulate peristalsis. Soluble fibers help lower serum cholesterol levels and improve glucose tolerance in diabetes. Potential problems with a high-fiber diet are cramping, diarrhea, and gas, especially if fiber is added too quickly or too much is added to a person's diet. A sample menu for a high-fiber diet is given in the accompanying box.

Low-Residue Diet

The **low-residue** diet is made up of foods that can be absorbed completely, so that little residue is left for formation of feces. This diet is also called a fiber-controlled diet. It may be prescribed in severe diarrhea, colitis, and other gastrointestinal disorders, in intestinal obstruction, and before and after intestinal surgery. This diet is adequate in most vitamins and minerals but may be inadequate in iron for women. Suitable foods on the low-residue diet include:

- Ground or well-cooked meats, chicken, or fish, or seafood
- Eggs (not fried) and plain cheese
- Fruit and vegetable juices without pulp
- Pureed or strained vegetables
- White rice, plain noodles, plain spaghetti, potatoes
- Refined white or rye breads and crackers
- 2 cups of milk or the equivalent (yogurt)
- Bouillon, broth, strained, or cream soups made from allowed foods
- Plain desserts in moderation

Foods to be avoided on the low-residue diet include:

Keys to Patient/Family Teaching

Sample Menu: High-Fiber Diet

Breakfast

Prune juice, bran cereal, milk, whole wheat toast with butter, orange, coffee/tea, salt/pepper/sugar

Lunch

Split pea soup, julienne salad made with cheese, egg, lettuce, tomato, carrots, and other vegetables as desired,
salad dressing, whole wheat crackers, apple, milk, coffee/tea, salt/pepper/sugar

Dinner

Roast chicken, brown rice, buttered peas, coleslaw, bran muffin with butter, fresh strawberries, coffee/tea, salt/pepper/sugar

Snack

Oatmeal raisin cookies, milk

Source: Dudek SG. Nutrition Handbook for Nursing Practice, Ed 2. Philadelphia, J.B. Lippincott, 1993.

- Coarse breads and whole grain cereals
- Nuts and seeds and anything containing them
- Potato skins, peanut butter, and popcorn
- Whole grain pasta and wild or brown rice
- Raw vegetables and gas-producing vegetables
- Tough, fibrous meats
- Spicy foods

Bland Diet

The **bland diet** is often prescribed for patients with ulcers, esophagitis (heartburn), gastritis, hiatal hernia, or other disorders of the gastrointestinal tract. The goal of this diet is to limit foods that cause secretion of excess stomach acid or cause gastric distress or irritation.

Foods to be avoided on the bland diet include:

- Alcohol
- Caffeine (including chocolate and cola drinks) and decaffeinated or regular coffee and tea
- Red and black pepper
- Any strong spices
- Fried foods and foods high in fat
- Peppermint and spearmint oils

Patients on a bland diet should also be encouraged to avoid other foods that cause them discomfort because intolerances are often individual. Instruct them not to lie down after meals, to maintain ideal weight, and to eat smaller, more frequent meals. If they smoke, advise them to cut down or stop. Milk-based diets are not commonly used because additional gastric acid must be secreted to help neutralize the alkaline nature of milk.

Energy Value Modification

Diets modified for energy value include high- and low-calorie diets.

High-Calorie Diet

Underweight occurs frequently in persons with prolonged illnesses. Such symptoms as lack of appetite, vomiting, diarrhea, and high fever can cause severe weight loss. A high-calorie diet may also be used in hyperthyroidism and general undernutrition. The person who has been severely burned needs large amounts of protein to rebuild lost tissue and calories to give energy. A high-calorie diet generally contains over 3,000 C and 130 g protein.

The successful high-calorie diet considers the patient's food preferences and eating habits. The high-calorie diet is high in proteins, carbohydrates, fats, vitamins, and minerals. Patients with depressed appetites may need smaller and more frequent feedings. Unless there is a definite reason for excluding solid food, patients are allowed to have solids if they can chew and digest them easily.

Low-Calorie Diet

When body weight is more than 10% above desirable weight for height and age, a low-calorie diet may be used. The standard tables of weight based on height and age may not apply in a specific instance because a person may be much more physically active than the norm. A reducing diet, or any other type of diet, should be prescribed by a physician because the physician will take these differences into account.

Recent research indicates that a high-fat diet, not excess calories alone, contributes to obesity. A safe reducing diet provides necessary protein, vitamins, and minerals and *reduces fat*. The Diabetic Exchange Lists for Meal Planning are often used for weight loss. These are in the appendix and are explained in the next section of this chapter.

Extreme fad diets are dangerous because they are almost always unbalanced. A balanced reducing diet provides enough calories to supply body needs while allowing for a weight reduction of 1 to 3 pounds (about 450–1,360 g) a week, a safe amount. Some guidelines for a low-calorie diet are given in the Patient Teaching box.

Nutrient Modifications

The modification of certain nutrients is necessary in some disease conditions. Your knowledge of nutrients contained in various foods will help you to explain

---

Keys to Patient/Family Teaching
Low-Calorie Diet

Patient and family teaching in low-calorie diets include:

- Advise to eat slowly and concentrate on the smell, taste, and texture of what you are eating.
- Food is placed on the plate in small portions. No seconds.
- Foods that require some preparation are chosen.
- Eat slowly.
- Number of places in the house where food is eaten are limited. Eat only at the kitchen or dining room table.
- Separate eating from other activities. Do not eat while doing other things.
- Fat should be restricted to 20–30% of total calories.
- A normal amount of protein is allowed; 1 pint (about ½ liter) of skim milk, 1 egg, or two servings of lean meat, poultry, fish, or low-fat cottage cheese will supply it.
- Encourage adequate fluid intake (eight 8-oz cups of water or other liquid).
- The balance is divided between fruits, vegetables, and whole grain cereals to supply minerals and vitamins. Liberal servings of low-calorie vegetables and fruits also help allay feelings of hunger.
- Cream and sugar are not allowed, and the amount of fat may be limited to 1 teaspoon (5 mL) per meal.
- Unrestricted salt unless there is a special reason.
- If the diet provides 1000 C or less, vitamin and mineral content becomes dangerously low, and a multivitamin, with mineral supplement, should be taken.
- Several diet formulas are on the market. Most of these are very low in calories. A physician must be consulted before one embarks on any very-low-calorie diet.
- Aerobic exercise (walking, jogging, bicycling, swimming, dancing) is encouraged at least three times per week, with physician's approval.

Information from a variety of sources.

---

these diets to your patients. Nutrient modifications include carbohydrate controlled, high- and low-fat diets, protein controlled, and controlled minerals and electrolytes.

Carbohydrate-Controlled Diet

Diet, exercise, and medication are important aspects of managing diabetes. The **carbohydrate-controlled diet** is based on the Diabetic Exchange Lists for Meal Planning. The lists have been devised by the U.S. Public Health Service and the American Diabetes Association. The lists are updated as further knowledge is gained about nutrients and diabetes. Foods are placed into one of six exchange lists: milk, meat, bread, fruit, vegetable, and fat. The Exchange List is given in Appendix D. The lists are helpful in planning other diet modifications also.

A serving of each exchange is assigned a value for calories, protein, carbohydrate, and fat. Serving sizes may vary (to standardize amounts of nutrients per exchange). This system provides the patient with a simplified meal plan and a wide variety of foods from which to choose. The patient's physician or dietitian sets up an individualized diet plan containing specified numbers of each exchange.

The goal of this diet is to distribute carbohydrate throughout the day, to achieve a constant blood sugar level. If the patient is overweight, weight loss will be a second goal. The carbohydrate-controlled diet is approximately 20% protein, 30% fat, and the balance carbohydrates.

Special dietetic foods are not needed for diabetics. Patients should eat foods in their natural form (whole fruits instead of juices, brown rice instead of white). This will help increase fiber intake. Fiber helps regulate blood glucose levels, by slowing gastric (stomach) emptying time. Processed foods and concentrated sweets (sugar, honey, molasses, jams, jellies, and desserts) should be avoided. Alcohol should be used only with the physician's approval. The diet should be individualized because most diabetic patients will be on the diet for life. The nurse should encourage the patient to follow the treatment plan to minimize the possibility of complications.

High- and Low-Fat Diets

Fat-Controlled Diet. A **fat-controlled diet** is often the first step in treating patients with elevated blood lipids (**hyperlipidemia**). These patients may have a high cholesterol level, a high triglyceride level, or both. Untreated hyperlipidemia can contribute to coronary heart disease, which often has serious consequences such as heart attack, stroke, or death. Hyperlipidemia may be caused by heredity or improper diet or may have a secondary cause, such as diabetes mellitus, hypothyroidism, nephrotic syndrome, or renal failure. In secondary hyperlipidemia, the primary goal is to treat the underlying disease.

The diet for hyperlipidemia consists of lowered fat intake (30% of total calories, with only 10% of this from saturated fats). Cholesterol intake is limited to 300 mg/d. Carbohydrates should account for about 50% to 55% of calories, with most of that percentage coming from complex carbohydrates such as whole grains and legumes. Overweight patients should lose weight and maintain ideal body weight. Diets of these patients may have a calorie restriction as well.

Fat-controlled diets are also used in malabsorption syndrome, where a high-fat diet causes diarrhea and nutrient losses. In these cases, fat is limited to 50 g/d. In hepatic, pancreatic, and gallbladder disease, high-fat foods are omitted and fat intake is limited to 25 to 50 g/d.

High-Fat Diet. High-fat diets are used in children with seizure disorders when anticonvulsant drugs and a balanced diet have failed to control seizures. This *ketogenic* diet is extremely low in carbohydrates and is sometimes as high as 80% to 90% fat. This diet must be supplemented with vitamins and minerals and loses its effectiveness over time.

Protein-Controlled Diets

High-Protein Diet. In conditions in which large areas of body tissue must be replaced, such as after a severe burn, in a high fever, or an infection, large amounts of protein are needed to aid tissue building. High fevers cause depletion of body fluids and proteins; in cirrhosis of the liver, large amounts of protein are needed to rebuild liver tissue. Sources of high-quality protein include eggs (highest quality), meats, poultry, fish, cheeses, and milk. High-quality protein contains all amino acids needed to form complete proteins. In some situations, liquid protein supplements are added to foods to increase protein intake. These liquids are also used in tube feedings.

Protein-Restricted Diet. In a person with a kidney or liver disorder, the amount of protein may need to be controlled. Protein is given in foods with high-quality proteins evenly spread over the meals of the day. In some kidney disorders, fluids and electrolytes will need to be controlled. Vitamins and minerals are usually supplemented.

Gluten-Restricted Diet. Grains such as wheat, rye, oats, and barley contain proteins called glutens. These glutens interfere with nutrient absorption in disorders such as celiac disease. In persons with celiac disease, gluten-containing grains are eliminated and proteins are obtained from other foods. Many foods must be omitted, including breads and cereals, as well as beer, ale, commercial chocolate milk, malted milk, cakes, cookies, commercial salad dressing (gluten is a stabilizer), and meat substitutes such as textured protein product. Rice cereals, breads, and grains are often used as a substitute.

Diets With Controlled Minerals and Electrolytes

Sodium-Controlled Diets. The *sodium-controlled diet* has different levels of restrictions, depending on the patient's disease and the amount of edema present. (**Edema** is an excess accumulation of water and salts in tissues, especially the lower extremities, which can often be controlled with a limited sodium intake). The sodium-controlled diet is prescribed for patients with cardiac disease, vascular disease (hypertension), and some kidney disorders. The accompanying box lists substances to be avoided.

A *mild sodium restriction* (3,000–4,000 mg sodium per day) is also known as a "No Added Salt" diet. A limited amount of salt is allowed in cooking, but no salt is added at the table. Overtly salty foods, such as canned soups, pickles, olives, potato chips, soy sauce, and cured meats, are discouraged. This diet is used when a patient has mild hypertension or stable kidney or heart disease.

A *moderate sodium restriction* (1,000–2,000 mg sodium per day) is used in cases of severe edema, hypertension, and heart disease. This diet omits foods listed in the "Dietary Substances To Be Avoided in Sodium Restriction" box. Minimal salt is to be used in cooking and no salt is added to foods at the table.

Strict and *severe sodium restrictions* (500 mg and 250 mg sodium per day, respectively) are unpalatable and hard to follow. They are only used in severe conditions and for short periods of time.

Salt substitutes are available but should only be used with a physician's approval. They often contain other electrolytes, such as potassium or calcium, which may also be restricted.

The diet for acute heart disease is sometimes divided into five or six small meals daily. Gas-forming foods, foods hard to chew or swallow, and stimulants such as coffee or tea are avoided. The overweight cardiac or hypertensive patient is usually also on a calorie-controlled diet because extra weight adds to the burden on the heart. These patients are also encouraged to quit smoking and to avoid alcohol.

Calcium- or Phosphorus-Controlled Diet. Specific foods are chosen to either increase or decrease the amounts of calcium or phosphorus in the diet. Calcium and phosphorus intake may be limited in the person with kidney disease. A woman with osteoporosis, however, needs to increase the amount of calcium in her diet. Good sources of calcium include milk, yogurt, cheese, and green leafy vegetables. Foods high in phosphorus include dairy products, protein foods, and green leafy vegetables.

Potassium-Controlled Diet. A high-potassium diet is given to patients who are on diuretics. Diuretics flush excess salt and water out of the body, but an unwanted side effect is loss of potassium. (Potassium is limited when patients are on kidney dialysis.) Potassium is found in most foods. Good sources of potassium include milk, fresh or dried fruits (especially bananas), fresh vegetables, dried peas and beans, cereals, fruit

Dietary Substances to be Avoided in Sodium Restriction*

(examples in parentheses)

- ◆ Table salt
- ◆ Vegetable salts (onion, celery, garlic salt); vegetable flakes (parsley, celery)
- ◆ Any smoked, processed, or cured meat or fish (ham, smoked fish, bacon, corned beef, cold cuts, frankfurters, sausage, tongue, salt pork, chipped beef, anchovies, pickled herring)
- ◆ Meat extracts, bouillon cubes, meat sauces
- ◆ Salty foods (potato chips, popcorn)
- ◆ Prepared condiments (relish, worcestershire sauce, steak sauces, catsup, pickles, mustard, olives, soy sauce)
- ◆ Prepackaged frozen foods, packaged sauce mixes, packaged gravy mix, soup mix; frozen peas and lima beans
- ◆ Prepackaged noodle, rice, or potato dishes
- ◆ Canned soups, chili, beef stews
- ◆ Prepared flour mixes (coating for frying chicken or fish)
- ◆ Packaged baking mixes (cake mix, frosting, pancakes)
- ◆ Frozen fish fillets and shellfish, except oysters
- ◆ Sauerkraut
- ◆ Canned meats, canned vegetables
- ◆ Butter, cheeses, peanut butter
- ◆ Some diet sodas

* Some of these foods are permissible if prepared without salt. Consult the label for dietary information.

Source: Krause MV, Arlin M. Krause's Food, Nutrition and Diet Therapy, Ed 8. Philadelphia, W.B. Saunders, 1992

juices such as orange or prune; sunflower seeds, watermelon, nuts, molasses, cocoa beans, fresh fish, beef, ham, and poultry.

Diets Modified by Small Amounts

Some patients do better with smaller portions of food served in more meals a day. Six small feedings is a common regimen. Any of the previously mentioned diets can be divided into six approximately equal servings. Such a diet would be used following gastric surgery, in a person with chronic obstructive pulmonary disease, or a person with **anorexia** (loss of appetite).

Diets Modified for Allergens

Sometimes people are allergic to certain food substances: milk, eggs, chocolate, and grains are common. Those foods can be eliminated from the diet, if necessary. Supplements for a particular nutritional element may be required.

Lactose (Galactose)-Restricted Diet. In the patient with an allergy to milk or with lactose intolerance, milk and dairy products must be controlled or eliminated. Small amounts of milk might be given to determine the level of allergy; the person with lactose intolerance can usually eat fermented dairy products, such as yogurt and cheeses and may be able to tolerate lactose-reduced milk. Milk in cooked breads and other foods are omitted in severe cases. An over-the-counter supplement, such as Lact-Aid, may be helpful.

Nutritional Support

Nutritional support is instituted when a patient is not able to meet nutritional needs normally. Nutritional support can be short or long term. It is not uncommon for a patient to be discharged on nutritional support or to maintain a tube feeding indefinitely. Nutritional support includes tube feedings, total parenteral nutrition, and administration of intravenous fluids.

Tube Feedings

A **tube feeding** is a means of providing liquid nourishment through a tube into the intestinal tract, usually the stomach. Tube feedings may be necessary in conditions that prohibit the person from taking adequate oral nourishment. Examples include loss of consciousness, inability to swallow (after stroke), esophageal cancer, oral trauma, mouth surgery, or anorexia. Supplemental nutrition may be needed in conditions such as burns, infection, cystic fibrosis, surgery, or fractures. In these cases, tube feeding will be necessary to supply or maintain adequate nutritional status.

Types of Formulas. The liquid formula for tube feedings contains amounts of protein, fat, carbohydrate, vitamins, and minerals adequate to maintain nutrition. The dietitian can be helpful to the physician in choosing the right formula for an individual patient. Ready-mixed formula is available in cans; powdered formulas are also available. In some cases, blenderized table foods are ordered. Major considerations in choice of formula are the type and amount of formula and the amount of extra water needed.

Placement Sites. Sites of access to the gastrointestinal tract may differ. If the tube is passed through the patient's nose and into the stomach, it is called *nasogastric tube* (NG tube). This method is uncomfortable and is not used for long-term administration. A tube may be placed directly into stomach through the abdominal wall, where it is called a *gastrostomy* tube (G tube) or into the small intestine, the jejunal tube (J tube).

Types of Tubes. Different types of tubes are used also. They are:

- ♦ *Percutaneous* (PEG): through the skin
- ♦ *Endoscopic*: placed with an instrument called an endoscope
- ♦ *Gastrostomy*: into the stomach
- ♦ *Button* feeding device: small silicone device used in place of a gastrostomy tube

Each of these has its own equipment, but the means of formula instillation is similar.

The PEG-type tube extends 12 to 15 inches beyond the skin and has a cap covering the end. A short cross-piece (bolster) is placed near the opening through the skin (**stoma**). It is important to note the level at which the tube enters the skin on the tube because if the tube migrates in or pulls out, you will know).

The PEG-type G tube may be replaced by a button, especially if long-term administration is anticipated. The function of the button is the same as for the PEG-tube; however, the button is level with the skin. It is less cumbersome and more difficult for the confused or agitated patient or the child to pull out.

Nursing Considerations

Steps in tube feeding are outlined in Nursing Procedure 28-1. The nurse is also responsible for washing the feeding bag and documenting care given.

Patients on tube feedings may continue to eat or drink by mouth, if the physician allows. The patient may need an extra water allowance, administered with feedings or in between. This is especially important if the patient has a fever or if signs of inadequate hydration develop. Document and alert the physician if untoward signs develop: dry mouth, poor skin turgor, complaints of thirst, illness, fever, or physical complaints.

Many patients go home with tube feedings. Teaching the patient and family how to mix formula, run the pump or use the gravity system, and care for equipment is an important teaching responsibility.

Problems in tube feeding and nursing actions are summarized in Table 28-2. Administration of medications via feeding tube is described in Chapter 81.

Intravenous Therapy

Intravenous therapy involves injecting into a vein any number of solutions that the body needs, including drugs and electrolytes. This is called an **infusion**. The peripheral intravenous process does not allow the administration of all nutrients needed to support life, as

(Text continues on page 318)

Administering a Tube Feeding

Supplies and Equipment

Gloves
Feeding solution
Feeding bag with tubing
Water
Feeding pump (optional)
Large catheter tip syringe (30 mL or larger)
Measuring cup
Clamp (optional)
Other optional equipment (disposable pad, pH indicator
   strips, water-soluble lubricant, paper towels)

Procedure

1. Gather equipment and supplies after checking physician's order for tube feeding.
   *(Rationale: Checking the order confirms the type of
   feeding solution, route, and prescribed delivery time.
   Organization facilitates performance of the skill.)*
2. Prepare formula:
   a) Shake can thoroughly. Check expiration date.
      *(Rationale: Feeding solution may settle and re-
      quires mixing before administration. Outdated
      formula may be contaminated or have lessened
      nutritional value.)*
   b) If formula is in powdered form, mix according to
      instructions on package. Prepare enough for 24
      hours only. Use a large enough container for the
      mixed amount and refrigerate any unused for-
      mula. Label and date the container. Allow formula
      to reach room temperature before using.
      *(Rationale: Formula loses nutritional value and
      can harbor microorganisms when kept over 24
      hours. Cold formulas can cause abdominal
      discomfort.)*
3. Explain procedure to patient.
   *(Rationale: Providing information fosters patient co-
   operation and understanding.)*
4. Wash hands prior to putting on gloves.
   *(Rationale: Hand washing prevents the spread of or-
   ganisms. Gloves act as a barrier.)*
5. Position patient with head of bed elevated at least
   30–40 degrees.
   *(Rationale: This position discourages aspiration of
   feeding solution into lungs.)*
6. Determine placement of feeding tube by:
   a) Aspirating stomach secretions
      ◆ attach syringe to end of feeding tube
      ◆ gently pull back on plunger
      ◆ measure amount of residual fluid (clamp tube
      if it is necessary to remove the syringe)

◆ return residual to stomach via tube and continue with feeding if amount does not exceed
agency protocol or physician's orders [if
greater than 120 mL or no return is obtained,
refer to "problem chart" in Table 28-2]
*(Rationale: Aspiration of gastric fluid indicates
that tube is correctly placed in stomach. The
amount of residual reflects gastric emptying
time and indicates whether the feeding should
continue. Residual contents are returned to the
stomach because they contain valuable electrolytes and digestive enzymes.)*

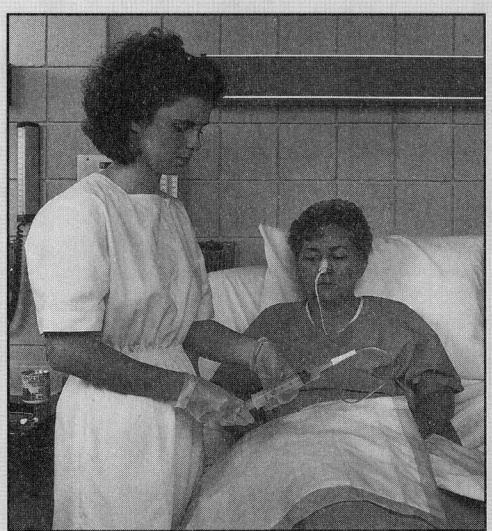

Step 6a.   Aspirating stomach secretions

b) Injecting 10–20 mL of air into tube (3–5 mL for
children)
   ◆ attach syringe filled with air to tube
   ◆ inject air while listening with stethoscope over
   left upper quadrant
   *(Rationale: A whooshing or gurgling sound
   usually indicates that the tube is in the stomach. This method may not be a reliable indicator with small-bore feeding tubes.)*

(continued)

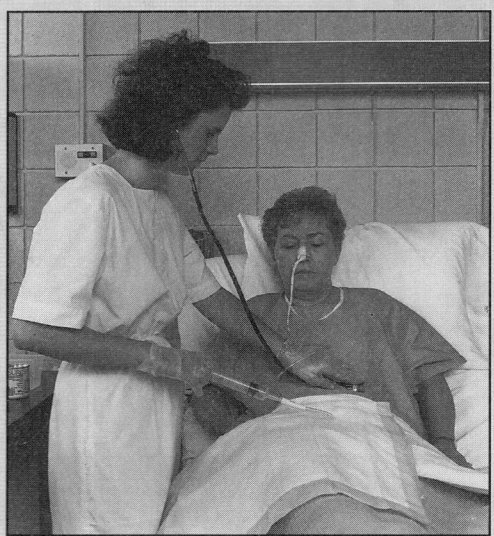

Step 6b. Checking tube placement by listening for the sound of air entering the stomach

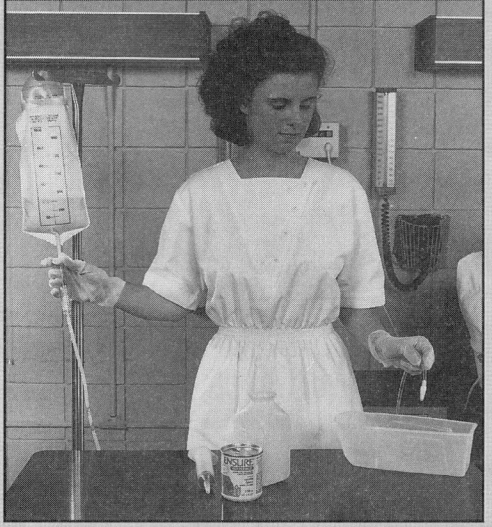

Step 7a. Priming the tubing

c) Measuring the pH of aspirated gastric secretions (*Rationale: Gastric contents are acidic and pH indicator strip should reflect a range of 1–4. Pleural fluid and intestinal fluid are slightly basic in nature.*)

d) An x-ray or ultrasound may be needed to determine tube placement.

Intermittent or Bolus Feeding

7. If using a feeding bag:

a) Hang feeding bag set-up 12 to 18 inches above stomach. Clamp tubing. Fill bag with prescribed formula and prime tubing by opening clamp allowing feeding to flow through tubing. Reclamp tube.
(*Rationale: Formula clears air from tubing and prevents it from entering stomach.*)

b) Attach end of set-up to gastric tube and open clamp. Adjust flow according to physician's order. (*Rationale: Rapid feeding may cause nausea and abdominal cramping.*)

c) Add 30–60 mL of water to feeding bag as feeding is completed. Clamp tube and disconnect feeding set-up.
(*Rationale: Water clears tube, keeping it patent. Clamping when feeding is completed prevents air from entering stomach.*)

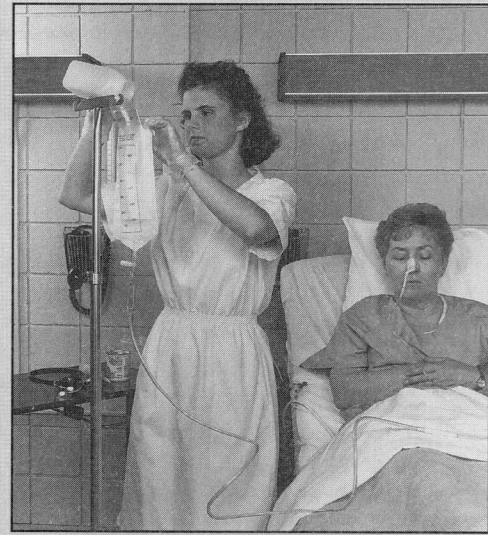

Step 7c. Flushing the feeding bag and tube with water

(continued)

8. If using a syringe:
   a) Insert tip of large syringe with plunger or bulb removed into gastric tube. Clamp gastric tube. Pour feeding into syringe. Raise syringe 12–18 inches above stomach. Open clamp.
   (*Rationale: Gravity promotes movement of feeding into the stomach.*)

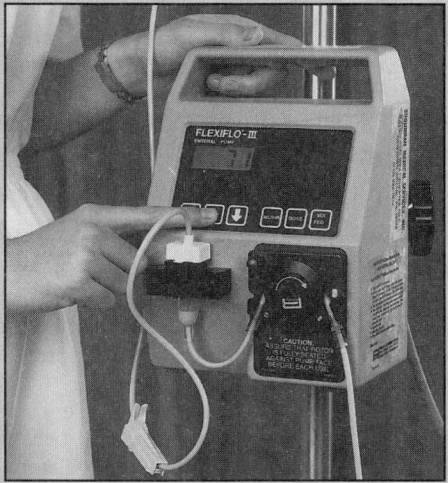

Step 9c. Setting the prescribed rate and volume (Photos © B. Proud.)

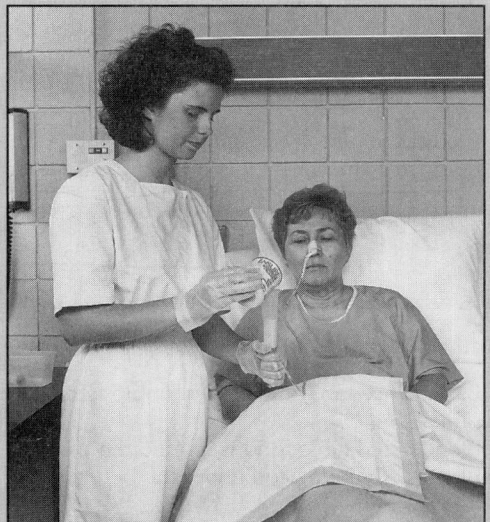

Step 8a. Adding feeding to the syringe

   b) Allow feeding to flow slowly into stomach. Raise and lower the syringe to control the rate of flow. Add additional formula to syringe as it empties until feeding is complete.
   (*Rationale: Controlling administration and flow rate of feeding prevents air from entering stomach and development of nausea and abdominal cramping.*)

Continuous Feeding

9. If using a feeding pump:
   a) Clamp feeding set-up and hang on pole. Add feeding solution to bag. Open clamp and prime tubing.
   (*Rationale: Formula clears air from tubing and prevents it from entering stomach.*)

   b) Thread tubing through or load tubing into pump, according to manufacturer's specifications.
   c) Attach end of set-up to gastric tube. Set prescribed rate and volume according to manufacturer's directions. Open clamp and turn on pump.
   (*Rationale: Pump controls rate of administration and volume of formula.*)
   d) Stop feeding every 4–8 hours and assess residual. Flush the tube every 6–8 hours.
   (*Rationale: The amount of residual reflects gastric emptying time and indicates whether the feeding should continue. Flushing the tube keeps it patent.*)
10. Terminate feeding when completed. Instill prescribed amount of water. Keep patient's head elevated for 20–30 minutes.
    (*Rationale: Elevated position discourages aspiration of feeding solution into lungs.*)
11. Assess skin around injection site of surgically placed tubes. Cleanse with mild soap and water and dry thoroughly. Check site for redness, swelling, pain or additional signs of inflammation.
    (*Rationale: Careful assessment and care can prevent infection and skin breakdown.*)
12. Provide mouth care by brushing teeth, offering mouthwash, and keeping lips moist.
    (*Rationale: These activities promote oral hygiene and improve patient comfort.*)
13. Clean and replace equipment according to agency policy.
    (*Rationale: This prevents contamination of equipment.*)

(continued)

14. Remove gloves and wash hands.
    (Rationale: Hand washing prevents the spread of organisms.)
15. Document time, amount of residual, amount of feeding, and patient's reactions to feeding.
    (Rationale: Documentation provides coordination of care.)

Nursing Alert

♦ If the patient becomes nauseated, chokes or vomits, stop the feeding immediately and consult the physician.
♦ Aspiration into the lungs is an emergency and may result in airway obstruction and/or a bacterial infection. Stop the feeding immediately and notify the physician.
♦ Diarrhea is a common complication. Report it promptly.
♦ Duodenal feedings can cause nausea and vomiting if accidentally delivered into the stomach.

Special Considerations in Children

♦ Children have smaller stomachs; therefore smaller amounts are given
♦ Feedings may take longer
♦ If stomach is too full, formula may leak around stoma, child may vomit or spit up; child may act "colicky"
♦ Decompression may be needed to relieve gas
♦ Include child in mealtimes with other children
♦ Use pacifier to provide sucking and to promote teething
♦ Protect the tube from being pulled out
♦ Because a smaller tube is used, it clogs easier

Home Care Adaptations

♦ Basic procedures and care of equipment is the same.
♦ Blenderized table food is more often used.
♦ Blocks may be placed under the bed, to raise the head.
♦ Unused formula can be stored in refrigerator. Discard after 24 hours. *(Rationale: Formula loses its nutritional value.)*
♦ Flush gastrostomy tube three times a week with 1–2 ounces of sugar-free cola or other soda. *(Rationale: The carbonation and mild acidity help keep the inside of the tube clean.)*

well as growth and repair of tissues. Therefore, intravenous therapy is not used for more than a few days without some sort of supplementation. This therapy is described in Chapter 57.

Total Parenteral Nutrition

Total parenteral nutrition (TPN) is a specifically formulated and calculated solution that is nutritionally complete to meet a specific patient's needs. Sometimes it is called hyperalimentation, although this term is not completely accurate. (See Fig. 81-3.)

Total parenteral nutrition is used when the gastrointestinal tract cannot be used, such as in stomach cancer, or when a patient has multiple trauma, severe infection or burn, or multiorgan failure. TPN is directly infused into the blood circulation and bypasses the digestive tract. Several types of catheters (tubes) are used. The large catheter is surgically placed into a large vein near the heart to allow the concentrated solution to be diffused quickly into the circulation. Use of a *large* peripheral vein is also possible for more dilute TPN solutions. TPN has grown in acceptance, as both a short-and long-term therapy modality.

Chapter 81 describes care of central line catheters and nursing implications of TPN. One of the most important considerations is prevention of infection at the catheter insertion site.

Food and Medication Interactions

Some medications and foods do not mix well or cause unwanted side effects. Some foods cause medications to be ineffective. Some medications should be given

Table 28-2. Problems and Nursing Actions in Tube Feeding

Problem/Symptom	Probable Cause	Nursing Action
Inability to instill formula	Tube blocked	Aspirate gently with syringe or instill small amount of water.
		"Milk" external tube with fingers.
Inability to aspirate stomach fluid from tube	May be normal (none present)	Check placement.
	Tube dislodged from proper position	Instill 10–20 mL tap water with syringe; quickly draw back (if discolored, tube is in stomach).
		Stop feeding and call physician if you think tube is dislodged.
Residual over 120 mL	Feeding too fast	Hold feeding for 2 h, recheck residual; if still more than 120 mL, call physician
	Stomach slow to empty	
Nausea, vomiting	Stomach emptying too slowly	Hold feeding for 2 h (or slow the rate of drip).
	Solution running in too fast	Check length, position of tube
	Gastrostomy tube has migrated to pylorus	Call physician if symptoms persist
Abdominal cramps, diarrhea	Formula too rich	Hold feeding for 2 h (or slow drip rate)
	Concentrated formula running too fast	Call physician if symptoms persist (physician may order formula to be diluted or changed).
	Formula intolerance	
	Formula spoiled	
	Change in formula or medications	
Gas	Too much air in stomach	Decompress as ordered.
Stoma bleeding (more than few drops), red, irritated	Gastric leakage	Call physician STAT if blood mixed with stomach contents, or fever, odor.
	Improper skin care	If persists, call physician
		Provide good skin care
Thirst, weakness, fever (over 100°F), reduced urine output (normal is more than 1.5 L/d)	Infection	Call physician (may increase amount of free fluids with or between feedings).
	Dehydration (body lacks fluids)	
	Formula intolerance	
Change in skin color (to pale or dusky), cough, noisy breathing, wheeze, restlessness, agitation, fever over 100°F	Aspiration (backup of water or feeding into lungs)	Position patient with head/upper body elevated 40°, keep elevated for 30 min. after feedings.
		Add small amount food coloring to formula (to determine if sputum coughed up is mixed with formula).
		Encourage person to cough and clear lungs.
		Call physician for further instructions.
Severe constipation (decrease in number of BMs expected, because less residue in feeding formulas)	Lack of fluids in body	Check for adequate fluid intake (I&O).
	Formula intolerance	Notify physician if more than 3 d.
	Inactivity	
	Change in formula or medications	
Formula will not drip with gravity system	Bag height too low	Raise bag to 3 feet above stomach level.
	Residue buildup in bag	Wash feeding bag and flush tubing with vinegar water (or replace).
	Residue buildup in tube	Flush tube with 50 mL warm water, diet soda pop, cranberry juice.
		Use a small syringe (3 mL or less) to provide greater pressure and unclog tube.
Gastrostomy tube becomes dislodged from stomach	Malfunction of balloon or device holding tube in place	Notify team leader or physician immediately for instructions (tract may close off).
Gastrostomy tube is longer or shorter than usual	Tube has become dislodged or migrated down into stomach or pylorus	Gently pull, push, or rotate tube to original position.
		Call physician if unable to relocate.

with food or water and some should be given between meals. Some medications react negatively to dairy products or alcohol. The nurse should know reactions of therapeutic medications when given with certain foods. Medication and food interactions are discussed in Unit Eleven.

Keys for Review

Key Questions for Critical Thinking

1. Your patient is not eating the meals served in the hospital. Describe the skills you can use to help the patient regain strength by eating.
2. Discuss patients who need special assistance with meals. Describe why assistance is needed and what assistance you can give.
3. Describe goals of the diabetic diet. Discuss the Diet Exchange List.
4. Discuss the need for nutritional support. Describe various types of nutritional support and nursing management of these feedings.

Key Readings

American Dietetic Association. Manual of Clinical Dietetics. New York, American Dietetic Association, 1992

Davis J, Sherer K. Applied Nutrition and Diet Therapy for Nurses, Ed 2. Philadelphia, W.B. Saunders, 1993

Dudek, SG. Nutrition Handbook for Nursing Practice, Ed 2. Philadelphia, J.B. Lippincott, 1993

Eschleman MM. Introductory Nutrition and Diet Therapy, Ed 2. Philadelphia, J.B. Lippincott, 1991

Krause MV, Arlin M. Krause's Food, Nutrition and Diet Therapy, Ed 8. Philadelphia, W.B. Saunders, 1992

Key Readings (continued)

Moore MC. Pocket Guide: Nutrition and Diet Therapy, Ed 2. St. Louis, Mosby-Year Book, 1993

Robinson C, Weigley E. Basic Nutrition and Diet Therapy. New York, Macmillan, 1989

Wardlaw G, Insel P. Perspectives in Nutrition, Ed 2. St. Louis, Times-Mirror/Mosby, 1993

Enrichment Keys

Hamilton EM, Whitney EN. Nutrition Concepts and Controversies, Ed 5. St. Paul, MN, West Publishing, 1991

Keys to Learning More

Chapter 46: special diet may be required to promote comfortable elimination

Chapter 50: nursing assessment includes nutritional status

Chapter 65: digestive/malabsorption disorders

Chapter 66: eating disorders in adolescence

Chapter 72: diabetes mellitus

Chapter 77: food allergies

Chapter 81: digestive disorders

Part B Nursing Care Skills

Unit 6   Safety and First Aid

29 Safety in the Healthcare Environment

Keys for Learning

Learning Objectives

- List at least three responsibilities of the healthcare facility safety committee.
- List at least 10 nursing measures that help to prevent accidents in the healthcare facility.
- Identify five potentially hazardous materials.
- Describe the use of a material safety data sheet.
- Describe the use of the emergency signal.
- Define *triage*.
- Explain what the acronym *RACE* means in relation to the fire plan.
- List four classes of fire extinguishers and their uses.

Key Terms

employee right-to-know laws

external disaster

internal disaster

triage

Keys to Understanding This Chapter

Chapter 2: licensure and ethics of healthcare facilities

Chapter 3: types of healthcare facilities

Chapter 5: safety and security of patients, coworkers, and visitors, a basic human need

Key Points

- The safety committee functions in evaluating accidents that have occurred and in planning to prevent future occurrences.
- The nurse not only should prevent accidents but also should know what to do if an accident occurs.

Key Points (continued)

- Staff members must be able to identify potentially hazardous substances and describe what to do if exposed to them.
- The facility's disaster plan is set up to deal with internal and external emergencies.
- Every staff member in a healthcare facility must be knowledgeable about fire safety and must make every effort to prevent fires.

Key Topics Outline

Safety and Preparedness
 The Safety Committee
 Patient Safety
 Employee Safety
 Emergency Preparedness
The Disaster Plan
 Internal Versus External Disasters
 Notification of Staff
 Implementation of the Disaster Plan
The Fire Plan
 Fire Prevention
 General Procedures in the Event of a Fire

Key Learning Activities

- Locate all fire alarms, fire extinguishers, and stairways in the area in which you are assigned; draw a map.
- Practice operating an ABC fire extinguisher.
- Design a safety poster for your healthcare facility.

Every person in the health facility is responsible for safety. Often the nurse or nursing student is the first person aware of an emergency. You are responsible for knowing exactly what to do in any emergency.

Safety and Preparedness

Safety extends to patients, employees, and visitors. The goal is twofold: to prevent accidents and to be prepared for emergency situations. Prevention is the key. The nurse is an important provider of safety and emergency care. In addition to prevention, the nurse must know where the emergency equipment is kept on each station or unit and how and whom to call in various types of emergencies.

The Safety Committee

Every healthcare facility is required to have a designated safety committee. The goal of the safety committee is to provide a safe environment for patients, employees, and visitors. Some of the responsibilities of the committee include establishing principles of worker safety, staff management, and occupational health nursing; analyzing job safety; investigating accidents; and tracking injury and illness rates. The committee usually includes representatives from the administrative, infection control, industrial hygiene, fire/safety, engineering, environmental management, and nursing departments.

Patient Safety

A patient has the right to expect that the environment of the healthcare facility will provide protection from injury or from other diseases. Safety measures in healthcare facilities include such essential precautions as fire safety and disaster and emergency evacuation plans. Other measures include provisions for emergency resuscitation and administration of correct medications and treatments. A more subtle aspect of hospital safety is proper waste disposal to prevent environmental contamination and patient or employee exposure.

Accident Prevention

There is little excuse for an accident in any healthcare facility. Most accidents can be prevented. All nursing staff should work together to prevent accidents. Guidelines for prevention are given in the accompanying box.

The nurse can help by observing potentially hazardous situations. For example, if the nurse notices a chipped glass on a patient's tray or a spilled substance on the floor, immediate corrective action should be taken. If an accident does occur, the circumstances

---

Nursing Skill Guidelines
Preventing Accidents

- Keep floors dry and clean to prevent falls. Know how to clean up various substances.
- Keep halls free of obstacles; promote good ward order at all times.
- Medicine carts should be locked and never left unattended on the floor. The nurse keeps the keys on his or her person at all times.
- Get adequate assistance to move and walk patients. Use a transfer belt when needed.
- Give medications properly; ask the head nurse, team leader, or primary nurse about any questions you may have. Know how to use reference books.
- Provide adequate lighting.
- Place the patient's necessary items within his or her reach; this includes the call light.
- Check temperatures of different solutions before they touch patients.
- Raise height of bed as necessary to prevent back strain when working with patients, and keep bed in low position when not working with patients.
- Use side rails for patients who are elderly, very young, disoriented, confused, or sedated.
- Do not perform procedures that are unfamiliar to you unless you have proper supervision. You are responsible for learning the specific procedures of your facility.
- Check all equipment routinely to make sure it is working properly. Be sure to check electrical cords for tangles, loose plugs, or fraying.
- Make sure sterile packages have not been opened and that medications are not expired or otherwise unfit for use.
- Check all patients frequently to make sure they are not having difficulty.
- Always be conscious of safety rules. (For example, never leave a patient unattended who has a rectal thermometer in place.)

---

must be documented in an official accident report or incident report. Some hospitals now use the term "variance report" because the wording is less negative sounding.

Shocks can be prevented. Water conducts electricity, so be sure your hands are dry before you insert a plug into an electric outlet; never turn appliances on or off when you are in contact with water. Always disconnect equipment by grasping the plug; do not pull on the cord. Always have frayed or worn cords repaired to prevent fires, short circuits, and blown circuit breakers. Disconnect the equipment or turn off the motor as soon as you have finished using an electrical apparatus. The maintenance department of the hospital keeps equipment in good repair. Notify maintenance people of any malfunction, including excess heat or burning odors from a running motor.

Employee Safety

Employee Right-to-Know Laws

Individual states have enacted **employee right-to-know laws**. This legislation is enforced by the Occupational Safety and Health Act (OSHA) of the Department of Labor and Industry. These laws state that employees have the right to be aware of dangers associated with hazardous substances or harmful physical or infectious agents they might encounter in the workplace, including healthcare facilities. Hazards include:

◆ Flammables (eg, alcohol)
◆ Poisons (eg, Chlorosorb)
◆ Skin/eye irritants (eg, Hibiclens)
◆ Carcinogens (eg, formalin)
◆ Harmful physical agents (eg, radiation)

The facility must have on file a material safety data sheet (MSDS) on each substance that is considered hazardous. The MSDS provides information about potential dangers of a substance and describes the product, its ingredients, physical properties, fire or explosion hazards, and reactivity. The MSDS also gives information on protective equipment required, safe handling information (in case of spill or leak), and first aid interventions for accidental exposure. All staff must be trained in the use of the MSDS. MSDSs for toxic substances must be kept for a period of not less than 30 years.[1]

Guidelines for Using Hazardous Substances

Hazardous substances are used daily in healthcare facilities. They were listed in the previous section on MSDS. Actions to take when using hazardous substances include:

◆ Read labels carefully
◆ Follow instructions
◆ Avoid spills
◆ Use protective equipment as recommended
◆ Do not use unlabeled substances
◆ Do not mix substances

Radiation is a potential source of accidents. Actions in radiation prevention should be followed closely.

> ### Key Concept
>
> It is the responsibility of every staff member to participate in accident prevention and in patient and employee safety.

[1] Adapted, in part, from materials published by Hennepin County Medical Center, Minneapolis.

Key Abbreviations/Acronyms in Hospital Safety

MSDS	Material Safety Data Sheet
OSHA	Occupational Safety and Health Act (Administration)
PASS	Pull pin. Aim nozzle. Squeeze handle. Sweep from side to side
RACE	Rescue/remove. Alarm. Confine/contain. Extinguish

Emergency Preparedness

The Nurse's Call Light and Intercom. The nurse's call light button should be within reach of the patient at all times. Remind the patient to use it whenever necessary. The patient should be told how to use the intercom to describe the problem and help needed. This will help the healthcare staff to respond appropriately in an emergency.

The Emergency Signal. In most hospitals, the signal light in the patient's bathroom causes a light to flash or a buzzer to sound at the nursing station. The nurse should also use this signal to request emergency assistance, for example, when a patient goes into cardiac arrest. This signal would probably result in the nurse receiving assistance sooner than would be the case if he or she were to use the signal light at the patient's bedside. If the patient is in a double room, the roommate can help by pressing the bathroom alarm button and then using the intercom to tell the nurse at the desk the nature of the emergency.

Emergency Resuscitation. The nurse must know where the emergency resuscitation equipment is kept. Each nursing station generally has an emergency cart with a variety of equipment. The nurse should learn where this is and how to use it. This cart must be checked regularly to make sure all items are there and in good condition. It is also important to know the procedure for calling the cardiopulmonary resuscitation (CPR) team in the hospital or the community emergency services team in the community. It is desirable for nurses and other healthcare personnel to become certified in CPR.

> ### Key Concept
>
> Each emergency situation will have its own code name in the facility public address system. The nurse *must* learn how to initiate and interpret the code system(s) used in the facility.

The Disaster Plan

A specific plan goes into effect in a disaster. It is every nurse's responsibility to know the disaster plan for the agency where he or she is employed. It is also important to carry out the plan calmly and effectively in the event of an emergency. Healthcare facilities are required to have regular, periodic fire and disaster drills to allow their staff to practice emergency skills. Each healthcare facility has a plan for natural disasters common to its area of the country. These disasters may include tornadoes, hurricanes, earthquakes, avalanches, floods, or mud slides. Be sure to find out what the plan is at your facility. In the event a disaster occurs, you will be prepared and will be able to protect yourself and your patients calmly.

Internal Versus External Disasters

There are two basic types of hospital disasters. The first is an **internal disaster**—one in which the hospital itself is in danger, such as a fire or an approaching tornado. An **external disaster** is a situation in which a large number of people are brought into the hospital, such as after an airplane crash or an earthquake. Specific plans are executed for each type of disaster.

Notification of Staff

Healthcare facilities usually incorporate the use of a *cascade call system* in the event of a disaster. This is a means of notifying staff by telephone that a disaster has occurred and that their assistance is needed immediately. The cascade system includes both on- and off-duty personnel. In the cascade system, key people are called and they, in turn, call others. This speeds up the process of notifying staff that they are needed. Personnel are expected to come, if at all possible, within 30 minutes.

Implementation of the Disaster Plan

The hospital disaster plan includes duties and responsibilities of each department. Staff nurses will be instructed to report to their general area of duty or to the nursing office for assignment. Persons working at the time of the disaster may be asked to assist in another department. Your charge nurse will notify you as to where you are to go or what your duties will be.

Triage. One of the assignments of the nurse may include assisting in triage. **Triage** is the process of sorting and classifying victims to determine priority of needs.

Patients must be identified, if possible. The next step is sorting and classifying patients by priority of needs. The triage person also assigns patients to the proper place for treatment. In the event of a major disaster, patients who are not badly injured may be asked to assist with patients who are in more critical condition. Triage is also discussed in Chapter 31.

The Fire Plan

Fire is a major hazard. Fires may be caused by improper management of flammable materials or gases or by careless smoking, frayed electrical wiring, or faulty equipment.

Fire Prevention

Nurses and other personnel must be constantly alert to prevent fires by detecting possible danger areas or dangerous situations. Personnel must also be alert to detect fires early so that preventive measures can be taken immediately. The following are general preventive actions:

◆ Enforce "no smoking" regulations
◆ Carefully observe any patients allowed to smoke
◆ Be sure no smoking occurs near oxygen
◆ Make sure all equipment is operating properly
◆ Practice electrical safety (no frayed cords, no three-prong adapters, no "cluster plugs," no extension cords)
◆ Be sure fire alarms, fire doors, and emergency stairs are clearly marked and not obstructed. NEVER prop open a fire door!
◆ Know procedures to follow in case of a fire

General Procedures in the Event of a Fire

If a fire does occur, every staff member must know exactly what to do to protect the patients and themselves. The nurse must know where the emergency equipment is kept and know the type of extinguisher appropriate for different types of fires and how to use them. The nurse must know the placement of fire alarms and the procedure for calling in a fire alarm and what to do to ensure the safety of the patients in the immediate area of the fire. It is most important for the nurse not to panic and to try to keep the patients calm. The goal is to protect the patient. Common sense should be used at all times.

It is important to know the code name for "fire" in the facility's public address system. RACE is an acronym that may help you to remember the general order of procedures for a fire.

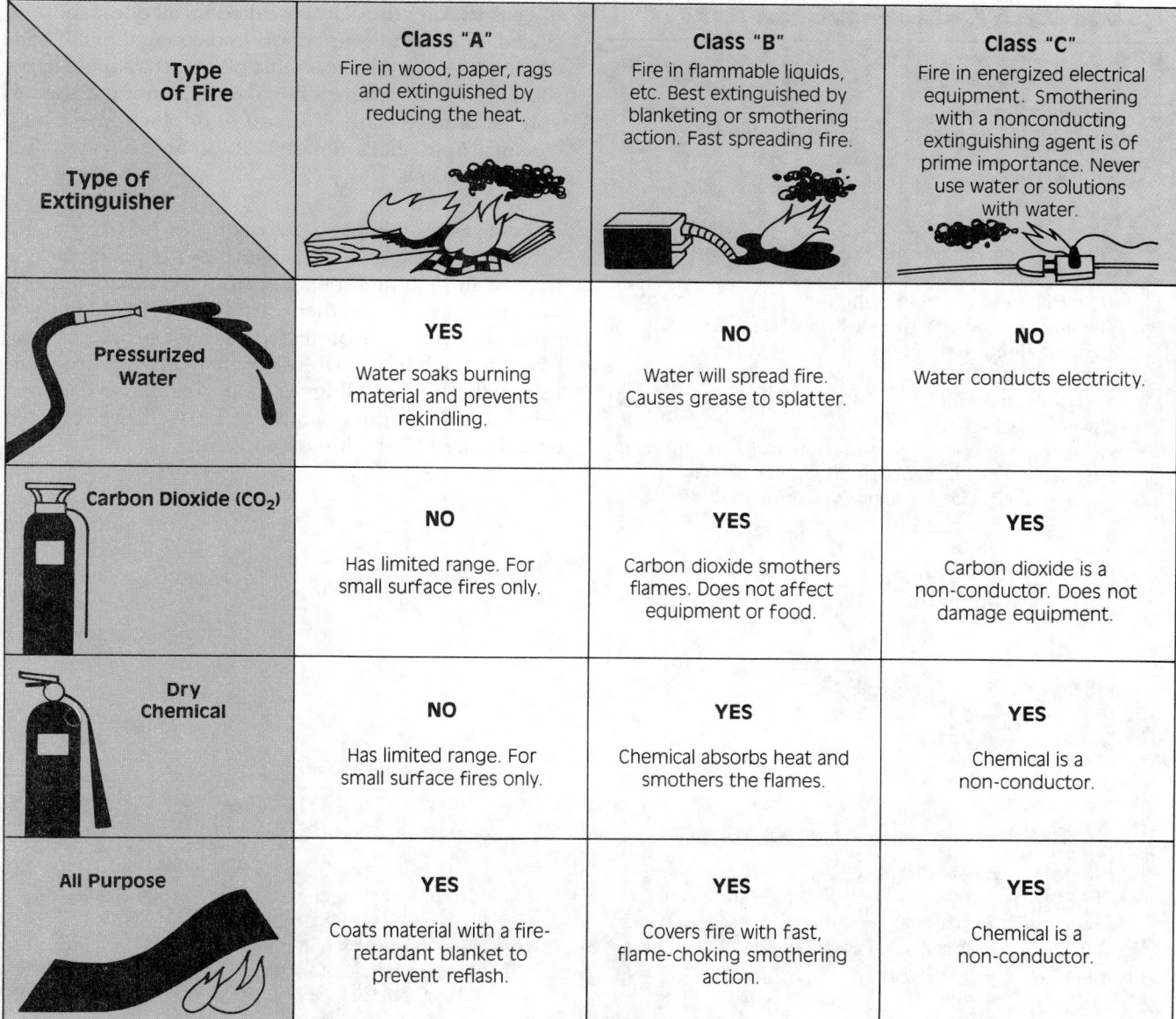

Type of Extinguisher / Type of Fire	Class "A" Fire in wood, paper, rags and extinguished by reducing the heat.	Class "B" Fire in flammable liquids, etc. Best extinguished by blanketing or smothering action. Fast spreading fire.	Class "C" Fire in energized electrical equipment. Smothering with a nonconducting extinguishing agent is of prime importance. Never use water or solutions with water.
Pressurized Water	**YES** Water soaks burning material and prevents rekindling.	**NO** Water will spread fire. Causes grease to splatter.	**NO** Water conducts electricity.
Carbon Dioxide (CO$_2$)	**NO** Has limited range. For small surface fires only.	**YES** Carbon dioxide smothers flames. Does not affect equipment or food.	**YES** Carbon dioxide is a non-conductor. Does not damage equipment.
Dry Chemical	**NO** Has limited range. For small surface fires only.	**YES** Chemical absorbs heat and smothers the flames.	**YES** Chemical is a non-conductor.
All Purpose	**YES** Coats material with a fire-retardant blanket to prevent reflash.	**YES** Covers fire with fast, flame-choking smothering action.	**YES** Chemical is a non-conductor.

Figure 29-1. Appropriate fire extinguisher usage for specific types of fires. (Taylor C, Lillis C, and LeMone P: Fundamentals of Nursing: The Art and Science of Nursing Care, 2nd ed. Philadelphia: J.B. Lippincott, 1993)

R = Rescue—remove patients from the general area
A = Alert/Alarm—sound alarm
C = Confine—contain fire (close doors, windows, make sure fire doors close)
E = Extinguish fire

Various facilities may use different acronyms, but the intent is the same.

Rescue. If a fire is in a patient's room, that patient must be rescued before anything else is done. If the patient can walk, have him or her walk into the hall, then close the door to the room, and sound the alarm. If the patient cannot walk, have him or her sit in a chair and remove it from the room or drag the patient out of the room on a blanket. (Do not try to carry a patient.)

Alarm. Use your facility's procedure to get help. This usually involves pulling a fire alarm or calling the switchboard operator. If it involves a telephone call, be sure to tell the person exactly where the fire is located. Make sure all other patients are in a safe place. Notify other staff if you need assistance.

How to Use a Fire Extinguisher: PASS

P = *Pull* the pin

A = *Aim* the nozzle

S = *Squeeze* the handle

S = *Sweep* from side to side

Special Instructions

♦ Rescue/remove patients and sound the alarm *before* fighting any fire.
♦ Use the proper type of extinguisher.
♦ Fight a fire only if it is small and not spreading. Be sure the fire is not between you and the exit.
♦ Aim the extinguisher nozzle at the base of the fire. Do not aim at smoke.
♦ Sweep back and forth to wet the entire area.
♦ Continue sweeping until the extinguisher is empty.
♦ Report any event involving fire or smoke in a healthcare facility to the fire department.

Confine. After the alarm is called in, all doors must be closed; this includes fire doors and room doors. If windows are open, they too must be closed. No elevators should be used during a fire alarm. Do not use the telephone unnecessarily. Turn off or unplug unnecessary electrical appliances. Report to the charge nurse for further instructions.

Extinguish. Attempt to put out a fire only if you are sure you can do it safely. Figure 29-1 explains the variety of fire extinguishers and the accompanying box describes how to use them. This is the last thing to be done after you have protected all other people and notified the authorities. Do not try to put out a fire yourself, without first calling for help. Again, use common sense. If you do put out a fire, it must still be reported and checked by the fire department.

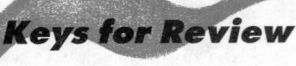

Keys for Review

Key Questions for Critical Thinking

1. Describe the healthcare facilities' safety committee. Discuss the makeup of the committee and goals. Describe differences in the committee's concerns if the facility is a hospital, a nursing home, a rehabilitation center, a walk-in clinic.
2. Describe the difference between internal and external disasters. Give several examples of each and discuss each.
3. Discuss the use of hazardous substances in a healthcare facility and identify such substances. Include a discussion of MSDS.
4. Identify OSHA, RACE, and PASS. Discuss each as related to health care.

Key Readings

Craven RF, Hirnle CJ. Fundamentals of Nursing: Human Health and Function. Philadelphia, J.B. Lippincott, 1992
Earnest VV. Clinical Skills in Nursing Practice, Ed 2. Philadelphia, J.B. Lippincott, 1993
Hayes G, Goodwin T, Miars B. "After Disaster." Am J Nurs 90(2):61–64, 1990

Key Readings (continued)

O'Toole M (Ed). Miller-Keane Encyclopedia and Dictionary of Medicine, Nursing and Allied Health, Ed 5. Philadelphia, W.B. Saunders, 1992
Taylor C, Lillis C, LeMone P. Fundamentals of Nursing: The Art and Science of Nursing Care, Ed 2. Philadelphia, J.B. Lippincott, 1993

Keys to Learning More

Chapter 30: prevention of infection spread within healthcare facilities
Chapter 31: first aid care usually outside the healthcare facility
Chapter 32: sudden death and CPR skills

Key Resources

National Safety Council
    1121 Spring Lake Drive
    Itasca, IL 60143
    708-285-1121

30 Medical Asepsis and Universal Precautions

Keys for Learning

Learning Objectives

- Review the chain of infection.
- Identify at least three organisms endogenous to the body.
- Discuss nosocomial infections and identify at least three factors that predispose the hospitalized patient to such an infection.
- Define medical asepsis and describe when it is used.
- State at least 10 points in universal precautions.
- Discuss the OSHA blood-borne pathogen standards.
- Perform skills in handwashing and in donning and removing both gloves and masks.
- Identify at least 15 examples of nursing care measures that help prevent infections.
- State the goals of an infection control committee.

Key Terms

asepsis	invasive
bacteremia	medical asepsis
body substance precautions	nosocomial infection
endogenous	opportunistic
exogenous	pathogens
immunosuppressed	universal precautions

Keys to Understanding This Chapter

Unit One: delivery of healthcare and legal aspects; rules and regulations designed to prevent spread of infections

Chapter 5: basic needs of people include safety and freedom from disease

Chapter 6: optimum health and ways in which an individual can remain healthy

Chapter 7: impact of communicable diseases on the community

Keys to Understanding This Chapter
(continued)

Chapter 8: introduction to microbiology

Chapter 15: most important barriers to infection in the body are skin and mucous membranes

Chapter 21: introduction to the concept of immunity and white blood cell activity

Key Points

- The nurse can prevent infection by becoming familiar with the chain of infection and ways to break the chain.
- Nosocomial infections are those acquired by patients while in the hospital. They are expensive in terms of added treatment and increased length of stay.
- Infections occur easily in hospitalized patients because their resistance is often lowered. Many pathogens are endogenous; they will not affect the body unless resistance is lowered.
- Medical asepsis helps lower the number of microorganisms in the environment and prevents and reduces their transmission.
- Handwashing is the single most important skill in prevention of disease spread.
- Universal precautions are recommended by the Centers for Disease Control and Prevention to reduce staff risks of infection from blood and certain body fluids.
- The Occupational Safety and Health Administration implemented a specific law in March 1992 to *enforce* procedures/practices that aid in prevention and transmission of blood-borne pathogen diseases to healthcare workers.
- One duty of an infection control committee is to monitor and evaluate infections in patients on admission to a facility and in staff who are exposed.

Key Learning Activities

◆ List common nosocomial infections that can occur in a healthcare facility.
◆ Interview a member of the infection control committee. Discuss methods of disease prevention.
◆ Attend a meeting of the infection control committee in your facility.

Key Nursing Procedures

NP 30-1: Handwashing

Control of microorganisms is vital to the operation of a healthcare facility. In Chapter 8 we discussed microorganisms and infectious diseases. A review of that chapter will prepare you for understanding this chapter, which has important information you need to know to control infection both in your life and in the lives of your patients and coworkers.

Infection Control

Diseases follow a cycle of development and spread. The cycle must be broken to stop the cycle and protect the public. The body has a defense system against infection, but the responsibility for infection control dwells with healthcare workers. As a student nurse and a practicing nurse, you are important in breaking the cycle and preventing the spread of infection.

The Chain of Infection

The chain of infection, as discussed in Chapter 8 and illustrated in Figure 8-4, involves the following elements:

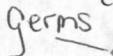

◆ Organism (eg, biologic, physical, or chemical)
◆ Reservoir (eg, patient, environment)
◆ Portal of exit (eg, blood; gastrointestinal, genitourinary, or respiratory system; skin)
◆ Vehicle of transmission (eg, direct, indirect, droplet)
◆ Portal of entry (eg, blood; genitourinary, gastrointestinal, or respiratory system; skin; transplacental—across the placenta)
◆ Susceptible host (eg, varies in relation to age, nutritional status, gender, socioeconomic status)

> **Key Concept**
>
> It is the responsibility of the nurse to recognize how diseases are transmitted and how to break the chain of infection.

Endogenous Organisms

Many organisms are normally found in the body. They are called **endogenous** organisms (arising within a cell). Without some of them our bodies would have difficulty maintaining homeostasis. For example, without the normal (endogenous) microorganisms in the digestive tract, we could not digest food. If these same organisms, however, invade the urinary tract, infection will occur.

In addition to those organisms that cause infection when they relocate, some endogenous organisms can actually become **pathogens,** that is, disease-causing organisms. They do not affect the body unless the body's resistance is lowered. They are called **opportunistic** organisms. This may occur when the body is **immunosuppressed**, that is, unable to form a normal immune response to an antigen. Such situations occur in cancer chemotherapy or in a disorder such as acquired immunodeficiency syndrome (AIDS).

Endogenous organisms include enterococci, lactobacilli, pseudomonas, staphylococci (skin, eyes, ears, intestinal tract), streptococci (perineal area), and yeasts. Table 30-1 lists the locations of some of these organisms and the disorders they can cause.

Nosocomial Infections

Nosocomial infections are serious problems in hospitals. They are infections acquired by the patient while *in the hospital.* In some cases, endogenous organisms

Table 30-1. Examples of Endogenous Microorganisms of Various Body Sites That May Become Opportunistic

Anatomic Site	Endogenous Organism	Possible Infection
Skin	*Staphylococcus aureus*	Impetigo, wound infection
	Staphylococcus epidermidis	Acne
Respiratory tract	*Streptococcus pneumoniae*	Pneumonia
	Neisseria species	Meningitis
Colon	*Escherichia coli*	Urinary tract infection (UTI)
	Pseudomonas species	Wound infection
Vagina	*Clostridium perfringens*	Diarrhea
	Yeasts	Moniliasis, pneumonia

The central nervous system, bladder, and blood are normally sterile and do not contain endogenous organisms.

may cause an infection. In many cases, **exogenous** organisms (those from outside the body) cause the infection. Nursing provides an important link in the prevention of nosocomial infections.

Lowered Resistance

Infections may occur in hospitalized patients because their resistance may be lowered. A variety of reasons are presented briefly here and will be discussed in detail later in the text.

Hospitalized patients may be predisposed to infection for the following reasons:

◆ *Trauma.* Injury, illness, or emotional shock lowers resistance as the body tries to rebuild itself. Trauma can cause a break in the skin, which provides an avenue for infection. Examples include burns, compound fractures, stab wounds, and lacerations (cuts).
◆ *Preexisting disease.* Before entering the hospital, the patient may have an infection that lowers the body's defenses.
◆ *Age.* The very young and the very old do not have as many defenses as do people of other ages. The newborn's immunity from the mother does not protect against all diseases. The older person often is poorly nourished, has fragile skin, or is inactive.
◆ *Inactivity.* The person in the hospital usually does not get much exercise, which leaves the body weakened.
◆ *Poor nutrition, inadequate hydration.* The ill person may be malnourished, dehydrated (not enough fluid in the tissues or the circulation), or overhydrated (too much fluid).
◆ *Fatigue.* The person who is extremely tired cannot fight off disease. A person who has had surgery, an illness, or an injury is often fatigued.
◆ *Invasive therapy.* **Invasive** refers to any therapy that enters or invades the body by a means other than normal, either through a break in the skin or

through an instrument that is introduced into an otherwise sterile area. The definition of invasive therapy includes any type of surgery, the injection of medication with a needle, intravenous therapy, the introduction of a catheter into the bladder, or a tracheotomy, which provides an airway.
◆ *Immunosuppressive therapy.* This type of therapy deliberately suppresses the natural immune system of the body. Examples are patients receiving chemotherapy for cancer or high doses of steroids.

> **Key Concept**
>
> Nosocomial infections increase the length of stay in the hospital, increase the cost of treatment, and can even cause death.

Common Nosocomial Infections

The most common nosocomial infections include:

◆ **Bacteremias** (blood infections)
◆ Gastrointestinal infections
◆ Genitourinary infections (the most common nosocomial infections)
◆ Respiratory infections
◆ Surgical site infections

Preventing Nosocomial Infections

Handwashing

The single most important skill or action performed by nurses in the prevention of disease spread is handwashing. You will be expected to wash your hands thoroughly *before and after* any direct or indirect contact with a patient or equipment. Gloves will be worn when you perform most procedures. Wearing gloves does not eliminate the need for thorough washing before and after donning gloves. Nursing Procedure 30-1

Supplies and Equipment

Liquid or bar soap
Paper towels

Procedure

1. Remove jewelry. Plain wedding band may remain in place.
   (Rationale: Rough places in jewelry can harbor microorganisms.)
2. Stand in front of sink and avoid leaning against it.
   (Rationale: Contamination from sink may be transferred to uniform.)
3. Turn on water and regulate flow and temperature. Knee or foot pedals may be available on some sinks.
   (Rationale: Controlling force of flow limits splashing. Warm water is comfortable and less irritating to skin.)
4. Wet hands and forearms with water, keeping hands lower than elbows.
   (Rationale: Water flows from less contaminated area toward hands which are more contaminated.)

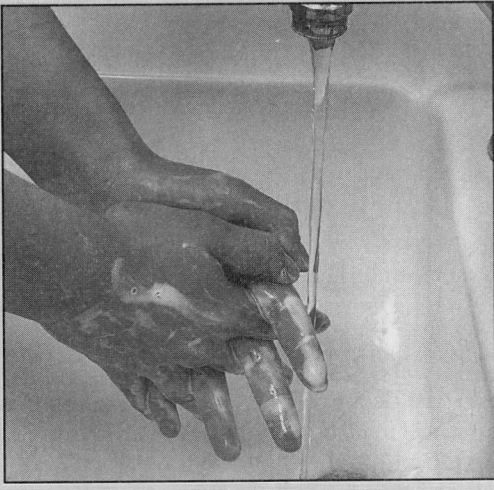

Step 4. Wetting hands, keeping the most contaminated area lower

5. Apply an antibacterial liquid soap. If bar soap, rinse before and after lathering and return to dish.
   (Rationale: Rinsing may reduce bacterial contamination on bar of soap.) Liquid soap with a foot-operated dispenser is the most sanitary.

6. Wash hands, wrists, and lower forearms for a minimum of 10–15 seconds, using a scrubbing motion. Interlace fingers and rub hands back and forth.
   (Rationale: Friction loosens dirt and bacteria on all surfaces.)

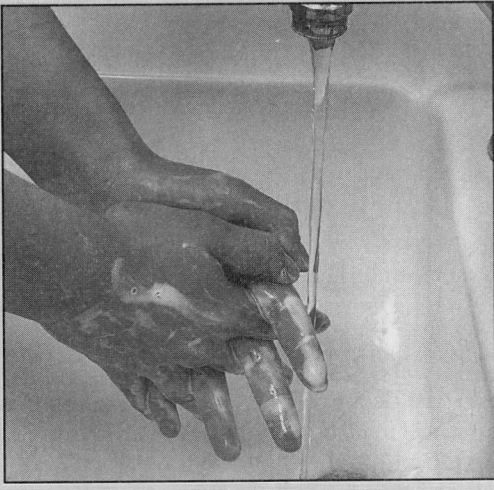

Step 6. Using scrubbing motion to wash hands

7. Insert fingernails from one hand under those of other hand using a sweeping motion. Repeat with other hand.
   (Rationale: Bacteria tend to accumulate under the fingernails.)

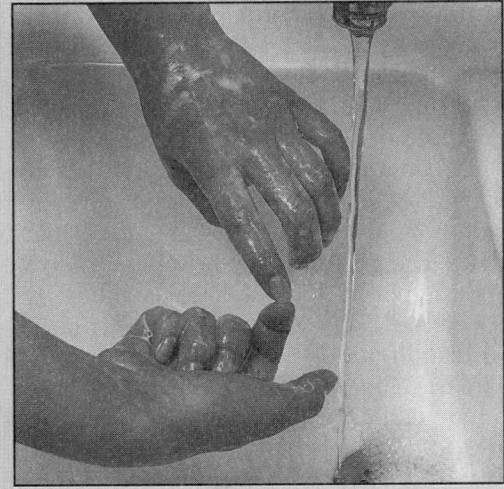

Step 7. Cleaning under fingernails

(continued)

8. Rinse thoroughly, keeping hands lower than fore-arms.
   (Rationale: This prevents soap lather from recontaminating clean areas.)
9. Repeat the procedure if hands are very soiled.
   (Rationale: This ensures thorough cleansing.)
10. Dry hands thoroughly with a paper towel. Discard towel.
    (Rationale: Drying thoroughly prevents chapping. Using paper towel prevents spread of organisms.)
11. Use clean paper towel to turn off faucets.
    (Rationale: Dry, clean towel prevents recontamination of hands with organisms on faucets.)

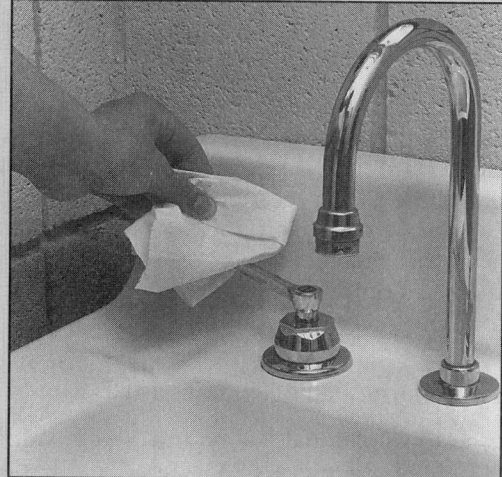

Step 11. Using a clean paper towel to turn off faucets (Photos © B. Proud.)

outlines *steps in handwashing*. Sometimes the nurse needs to teach the patient or family how to properly wash hands.

Asepsis means freedom form germs that can cause infection and disease. There are two kinds of asepsis: medical and surgical. Medical asepsis is discussed in this chapter; surgical asepsis is discussed in Chapter 54.

Medical Asepsis

Medical asepsis refers to the practice of reducing the number of microorganisms or preventing and reducing transmission of microorganisms from one person (or source) to another. This may also be referred to as "clean technique." Medical asepsis can be accomplished through:

♦ Reducing the number of skin microorganisms (handwashing)
♦ Using barrier techniques (gowns, gloves)
♦ Providing environmental controls to reduce transmission (special room ventilation, use of disinfectants)
♦ Using universal precautions. Universal precautions are discussed next in this text.

> ### Key Concepts
>
> ♦ Medical asepsis is *clean* technique.
> ♦ Surgical asepsis is *sterile* technique.

Universal Precautions

In an effort to control the spread of diseases, precautions have been established for all healthcare facilities. The precautions, called **universal precautions**, were prepared by the Centers for Disease Control and Prevention (CDC) in 1987. They are precautions against transmission of human immunodeficiency virus (HIV), hepatitis B virus (HBV), and other blood-borne pathogens in healthcare settings. A 1988 update specified the body fluids affected by universal precautions. The following was decided:

♦ Only blood, semen, vaginal secretions, and possibly breast milk are involved.
♦ Although the risk is unknown, universal precautions also apply to cerebrospinal fluid, synovial fluid, pleural fluid, peritoneal fluid, pericardial fluid, and amniotic fluid.
♦ Universal precautions do not apply to feces, nasal secretions, sputum, sweat, tears, urine, and vomitus (unless they contain visible blood).

Universal precautions further state that *all* patients must be considered as potentially infected with blood-borne pathogens. For that reason universal precautions must be used on *all* patients. The basics of universal precautions are given in the accompanying box. A more detailed outline is given on the inside back cover of this textbook. Every nurse should be familiar with these regulations. You protect not only your patients and co-workers but also yourself when you use universal precautions. More specific regulations relate to pregnancy, vaginal and cesarean delivery, neonatal care, surgical procedures, and other invasive procedures.

Body Substance Precautions

Other precautions are known as **body substance precautions**. They were originated with healthcare workers at Seattle Harborview Medical Center in 1985. They are similar to the CDC precautions but include the use of gloves when working around *all* body substances. Some healthcare facilities use body substance precautions rather than universal precautions, that is, they use gloves for almost all interventions.

OSHA Blood-borne Pathogen Standards

In 1992 the Occupational Safety and Health Administration (OSHA) implemented "Occupational Exposure to (BBP) blood borne pathogens" (Standard 29 CFR 1910.1030). This standard requires and enforces the implementation of policies, procedures, and control measures that will prevent employee exposure to patients' blood and body fluids. Violations of universal precautions carry a severe fine.

As of December 1991, as a part of OSHA regulations, employers must:

◆ Develop an infection control policy that conforms to OSHA guidelines. (This policy must identify when PPE [personal proetctive equipment] is required, how to clean up spills of blood or body fluids, how to take specimens to the laboratory, and how to dispose of infectious waste.)
◆ Educate staff about the policies
◆ Provide free hepatitis B immunizations to staff who might be exposed to blood/body fluids
◆ Provide follow-up to staff if exposed by accidental splash of blood/body fluids or needle stick
◆ Supply rapidly accessible protective equipment (gloves, gowns, eye protection, pocket masks)
◆ Provide proper sharps disposal containers and replace them regularly

---

Nursing Alert

Exposure to potential infection must be reported to the proper authorities immediately. Initial screening and follow-up of the exposure is required by OSHA.

Personal Protective Equipment

The OSHA regulations also relate to PPE. These are the gloves, gowns, masks, and eyewear that must be made available by the employer for the healthcare worker. Use of these in nursing is outlined in Table 30-2.

Gloves

Universal precautions and the BBP (blood-borne pathogens) standards require the use of (clean) gloves when there is reasonable anticipated exposure to blood or body fluids. The nurse should know how to don and dispose of gloves properly. Donning of sterile gloves is discussed in Chapter 54 because it is part of surgical asepsis. Gloves for universal precautions and general use do not need to be sterile. This is because the gloves are used to protect the nurse against body substances and not to protect the patient against infections. The skill for putting on and taking off clean gloves follows.

Nursing Skill
Donning and Disposing of Nonsterile Gloves

Supplies and Equipment
Appropriate size gloves

Procedure

Donning Gloves

1. Wash your hands. (*Rationale: Your hands must be as clean as possible.*)
2. Bunch the glove up and then pull onto your hand; ease into the fingers. (*Rationale: Gloves may be sticky if your hands are damp.*)

Disposing of Gloves

1. To remove gloves, grasp the *outside* of one glove, near the cuff, with the thumb and forefinger of the other hand. Pull it off, turning it inside out as you pull. (*Rationale: Confine contamination to gloves.*)
2. Hook your bare thumb *inside* the other glove and pull it off, turning it inside out. The two gloves will be rolled together, with the side that was nearest your hands on the outside. (*Rationale: Confine contamination.*)
3. Drop them into the prescribed glove container. (*Rationale: Prevent the spread of infection.*)
4. Wash your hands again. (*Rationale: Prevent the spread of infection.*)

Nursing Alert

◆ If the integrity of gloves is altered (eg, ripped or punctured), the gloves are no longer effective and must be discarded.
◆ Some nurses develop a severe allergy to latex and must use non-latex gloves. This presents a problem in some areas of the hospital.

Masks

Each hospital establishes its own policy about wearing masks. When you give nursing care to patients with communicable diseases transmitted through the respi-

Key Abbreviations/Acronyms Used in This Chapter

AIDS	acquired immunodeficiency syndrome
CDC	Centers for Disease Control and Prevention
HBV	hepatitis B virus
HIV	human immunodeficiency virus
OSHA	Occupational Safety and Health Administration (Act)
PPE	personal protective equipment

ratory tract, you may need to wear a mask. Everyone in contact with the patient, including visitors, may wear a mask, or only the patient may wear a mask.

The principal reason for wearing a mask is to keep organisms from entering and leaving the respiratory tract. Masks protect both the patient and healthcare personnel from upper respiratory infections.

Most masks are disposable to reduce the risk of cross contamination. A mask that, when not is use, dangles like a necklace beneath the nurse's chin is a menace, rather than a protection. The following nursing skill describes how to put on and take off a mask.

Nursing Skill
Putting On and Removing a Mask

Supplies and Equipment
Masks in container

Procedure

Putting on a Mask

1. Wash hands. (*Rationale: Your hands must be clean.*)
2. Remove the mask from the container or package, handling it as little as possible and by the strings only. (*Rationale: Too much handling will reduce its efficiency to screen out microorganisms.*)
3. Place the mask so that it completely covers your mouth and nose. If your wear glasses, be sure to bend the strip at the top of the mask so that it fits tightly around your nose (Fig. 30-1). (*Rationale: Your mouth and nose must be covered to prevent the transfer of microorganisms. If the strip is not tight over the bridge of your nose, your breath will fog up your glasses.*)
4. To tie the mask, loop the top ties over your ears and tie them under your chin in a bow, not a knot. (*Rationale: A bow is used because it is easy to untie.*)
5. Tie the bottom ties behind your neck in a bow. (*Rationale: By tying the mask in this manner, only one bow needs to be untied to take off the mask. If the top bow is tied behind your head, it may slip down and cause the mask to fall off.*)
6. Change the mask when it becomes damp. (*Rationale: A moist mask harbors and transmits organisms.*)

Removing a Mask

1. To remove the mask, untie the tie behind your neck. Touch the mask by the strings only. Be careful not to let the mask drop onto your clothes. (*Rationale: The mask is now contaminated.*)
2. Discard the mask in the proper receptacle. (*Rationale: Prevent infection spread.*)
3. Wash your hands. (*Rationale: Prevent infection.*)

Basic Outline of Universal Precautions

Prevention of Transmission of Human Immunodeficiency Virus, Hepatitis B Virus, and other Blood-borne Pathogens in Healthcare Settings

- ◆ Wear gloves whenever you come in contact with blood, body fluids containing blood, and other body fluids to which universal precautions apply. (*Rationale: Diseases can be carried in the body substance.*)
- ◆ Wear gloves *at all times* if you have any break in the skin of your hands. (*Rationale: You may be at risk of contracting a disease or you could spread disease.*)
- ◆ Change gloves after each contact with a client. (*Rationale: The gloves may be contaminated.*)
- ◆ Wash your hands and skin surfaces immediately and thoroughly if they are contaminated with blood or body fluids and after each contact with any patient. (*Rationale: Proper handwashing will help to stop the spread of infection.*)
- ◆ Wear a gown or apron when clothing could become soiled. (*Rationale: To prevent spread of infection to yourself or others.*)
- ◆ Wear a mask and eye protection if splashing is possible. Hospital protocol will determine what type of eye protection is required for each specific case. (*Rationale: Infection could enter your body through the mucous membranes of your mouth or nose or through your eyes.*)
- ◆ Do not recap or break needles. Needles and sharp objects are placed in a special container after use. Use the needleless system, and/or safety syringes, if available. (*Rationale: There is a possibility of accidental finger stick. It is important to protect yourself and housekeeping personnel.*)
- ◆ Report *any* exposure to blood/body fluids to your supervisor immediately. (*Rationale: Initial screening and follow-up of the accident is required by OSHA and is for your own protection.*)

Source: adapted from Centers for Disease Control and Prevention. "Recommendations for prevention of HIV transmission in health care settings." MMWR 36 (suppl 25). 1987. Centers for Disease Control and Prevention. "Update: Universal precautions for prevention or transmission of human immunodeficiency virus, hepatitis B virus, and other bloodborne, pathogens in healthcare settings." MMWR 37:24, 1988. (A more detailed summary appears on the inside back cover of this book.)

Table 30-2. Nursing Activities and Personal Protective Equipment Required to Decrease Blood-borne Pathogen Exposure

Procedure	Handwashing	Gloves	Gown	Mask	Eyewear
Talking with patient					
Hygienic care	*	*			
Feeding a patient	*	*			
Adjusting IV rate or noninvasive equipment	*				
Examining patient without touching blood, body fluids, mucous membranes	*				
Examining patient with contact with blood, body fluids, mucous membranes	*	*			
Drawing blood	*	*			
Inserting arterial or venous access devices	*	*	Gown, mask, eyewear are usually required		
Handling soiled waste, linen, other materials	*	*	Use gown, mask, eyewear if splattering is likely		
Operative and other procedures that produce extensive splattering of blood, body fluids	*	*	*	*	*
Handling lab specimens	*	*	Use gown, mask, eyewear if splattering is likely		

Adapted from the Centers for Disease Control and Prevention and other sources.

Eye Protection

Goggles, usually with side shields, are worn if there is any danger of the patient's body fluids splashing onto the nurse. Goggles, with and without masks are shown in Figure 30-1. Disposable goggles are often available in each patient unit. You may wear your own glasses with side shields. In some situations where extra protection is needed, such as in the operating room or morgue, full face shields are used. The specific situation dictates the type of eye protection to be used.

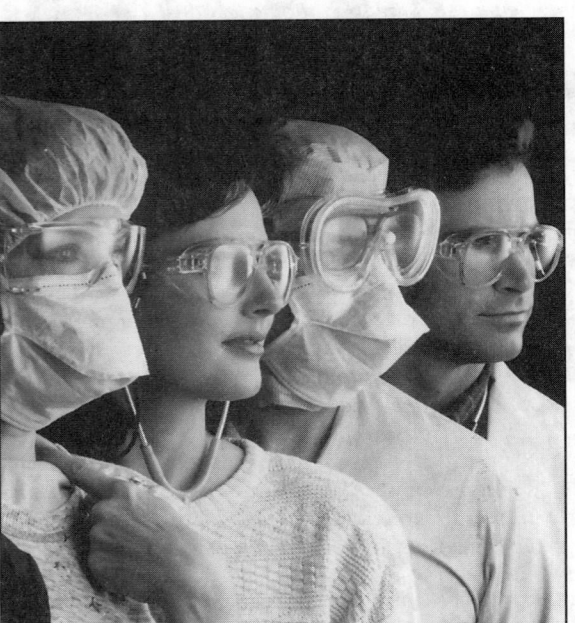

Figure 30-1. These nurses are shown wearing various pieces of personal protective equipment (PPE), including masks, goggles, hair protection, and disposable gowns. Gloves will also be needed when caring for their patients. The nurse second from the right is wearing goggles over eyeglasses. (Photo courtesy of 3M Health Care)

General Nursing Skills in Infection Prevention

Universal precautions have been planned for the use of healthcare workers in preventing spread of HIV, HBV, and other blood-borne pathogens. However, other good nursing practices help to prevent the spread of other infections. They are listed in the accompanying box.

The Infection Control Committee

Hospitals are greatly concerned about nosocomial infections. Each hospital has an infection control committee. The function of this committee is to monitor and evaluate any infection occurring in the facility. When causes are identified, steps can be taken to prevent them in the future.

Healthcare workers must report any infection that occurs. The infection control committee will investigate any case of infection and try to determine the cause. If a break in nursing technique is identified, the committee will propose different procedures to eliminate the problem. In many cases, the educational committee will

Nursing Skill Guidelines
Preventing Infection

♦ Get plenty of sleep, exercise, and eat nutritious foods.
♦ Practice good personal hygiene.
♦ Keep your immunizations up to date.
♦ Consult your clinical facility and physician regarding voluntary immunization to diseases such as hepatitis B and influenza.
♦ Attend in-service education classes related to infection control.
♦ Practice good nursing care skills and constantly review your skills.
♦ Report needle sticks or any breaks in the skin.
♦ Practice safer sex or abstain.
♦ Do not use non-prescribed drugs.
♦ Stay home from work if you have an infectious disease.
♦ Practice good handwashing.
♦ Wear gloves when in contact with any body fluids.
♦ Wear masks, goggles, gowns, shoe protectors, and hair covering when and as ordered.
♦ Isolate infected patients and practice good isolation skills (as discussed in Chapter 51).
♦ Practice sterile techniques for catheterization, injections, dressing changes, etc. (see Chapter 54).
♦ Do not use a sterile package if the seal is broken, if the wrapper is torn or wet, or if the indicator is not registered.
♦ Do not use a sterile package or medication if it has passed the expiration date.
♦ Keep cupboards closed where sterile materials, linens, or other supplies are stored.

♦ Change your clothes immediately if they become soiled with body substances from patients.
♦ Teach patients hygiene and good techniques of self-care.
♦ Do not shake linens or place linen on the floor when changing beds. Use covered linen hampers.
♦ Make sure sitz bath tubs and other common areas are carefully cleaned and disinfected between patients.
♦ Do not keep dinner trays for patients; some foods will spoil.
♦ Ensure that electronic temperature probes are covered and that the covers are disposed of correctly.
♦ Practice care when working with catheters or IVs.
♦ Use disposable equipment as much as possible.
♦ Follow procedures carefully for preoperative and post-operative patients.
♦ Use waterproof bags to send heavily soiled or moist linens to the laundry.
♦ Send items to be sterilized to CSR in plastic bags.
♦ Ensure that all trash is collected in heavy-duty plastic bags. Most is collected in special containers and incinerated.
♦ Make sure that any spilled body substances are cleaned up immediately, using the prescribed protocol.
♦ Report any infection *immediately*.
♦ Ask questions if you are not sure of something.

hold educational sessions to teach new techniques. You may be asked to serve on one of these important committees.

Goals of the Infection Control Committee

Some of the goals of the infection control committee are to:

♦ Provide a central place for reporting infections
♦ Investigate cases of infection
♦ Maintain total statistics related to the numbers and types of infections that occur in the hospital
♦ Determine the cause of infection
♦ Study current literature and identify effective national practices for prevention of infection
♦ Design local protocol and policies, following national guidelines, to control infection; the committee sets up universal body substance precautions and specific isolation procedures for that particular hospital

♦ Evaluate the effectiveness of protocols after they have been tried
♦ Offer continuing education for healthcare personnel to prevent infections
♦ Serve as consultants in cases of questions or concerns of healthcare personnel
♦ Review records of patients in an effort to identify organisms that have become resistant to drugs
♦ Assist in employee health and wellness programs of the hospital
♦ Prevent future infections

Key Concept

Handwashing is the single most important procedure for protecting yourself and your patients against disease transmission.

Keys for Review

Key Questions for Critical Thinking

1. Identify the steps in the chain of infection. Describe when and how this chain can be broken. Discuss how nurses can help prevent infection, identifying the single most important procedure for self and patient. Describe the importance of the infection control committee in breaking the chain of infection.
2. Discuss why hospitalized patients are more likely to contract infections than other people. Give reasons for your answers.
3. Discuss Universal Precautions and Body Substance Precautions. Describe the differences between the two. Give examples.

Key Readings

Becker SI. "Learning About Infection Control" in Controlling Infection section of Nurse's PhotoLibrary. Springhouse, PA, Springhouse, 1993

Centers for Disease Control. "Recommendations for prevention of HIV transmission in health-care settings." MMWR 36(suppl 25):, 1987

Craven RF, Hirnle CJ. Fundamentals of Nursing: Human Health and Function. Philadelphia, J.B. Lippincott, 1992

Department of Labor and Department of Health and Human Services. Joint Advisory Notice: Protection Against Occupational Exposure to Hepatitis B Virus (HBV) and Human Immunodeficiency Virus (HIV). Washington DC, U.S. Government Printing Office, 1987

Key Readings (continued)

Earnest VV. Clinical Skills in Nursing Practice, Ed 2. Philadelphia, J.B. Lippincott, 1993

Fritsch DE, Fredrick-Pilat DM. "Exposing Latex allergies." Nursing 93 23(8):46–48, 1993

O'Toole M (Ed). Miller-Keane Encyclopedia and Dictionary of Medicine, Nursing, and Allied Health, Ed 5. Philadelphia, W.B. Saunders, 1992

Smeltzer SC, Bare BG. Brunner and Suddarth's Textbook of Medical-Surgical Nursing, Ed 7. Philadelphia, J.B. Lippincott, 1992

Smith AJ, Johnson JY. Nurses' Guide to Clinical Procedures. Philadelphia, J.B. Lippincott, 1990

Taylor C, Lillis C, LeMone P. Fundamentals of Nursing: The Art and Science of Nursing Care, Ed 2. Philadelphia, J.B. Lippincott, 1993

Keys to Learning More

Unit Nine: all basic nursing skills require knowledge of medical asepsis

Chapter 51: isolation techniques

Chapter 54: surgical asepsis and sterile technique

Chapter 57: administration of medications requires use of universal precautions when there is exposure to certain body fluids

Unit Twelve: maternal and newborn care

Unit Thirteen: care of children and adolescents

Unit Fourteen: disorders of adults

Unit Fifteen: disorders of older people

31 Emergency Care: First Aid and Triage

Keys for Learning

Learning Objectives

- Define the Good Samaritan Law.
- Discuss why it is important to assess the safety of the emergency scene.
- Describe the medical identification tag and its purpose.
- List, in order, the steps for assessing a person in an emergency and describe how each step is performed.
- Describe emergency actions for a head, neck, or back injury.
- Describe first aid for injuries caused by exposure to cold.
- Describe the immediate first aid for a severe burn.
- Describe the removal of foreign objects from body orifices.
- Describe the emergency care for different types of hemorrhage.
- Describe actions to take when a person is poisoned.

Key Terms

anaphylaxis	heat cramps
antidote	heat exhaustion
bandage	heat stroke
caustic	hemorrhage
debride	hypothermia
dislocation	poison
emergency medical service	rabies
emetic	shock
epistaxis	sprain
fracture	tourniquet
frostbite	toxins

Keys to Understanding This Chapter

Unit Three: the study of normal human growth and development will assist the nurse in preventing accidents

Unit Four: knowledge of normal body structure and function is helpful in recognizing deviations from normal

Chapter 30: universal precautions

Key Points

- Universal precautions are practiced in administering first aid, whenever possible and to the extent possible.
- The nurse functions *only at his or her level of first aid training* in an emergency. Quickly evaluate the scene and determine the plan of action.
- Call 911 to summon the Emergency Medical Service system in almost all areas of the United States and Canada.
- If there is any doubt, call for help. Keep calm; enlist the aid of others.
- Make sure the patient is breathing and the heart is beating.
- Control bleeding.
- The injured person often should be treated for shock.
- Do not move an injured person, unless the situation is dangerous.

Key Topics Outline

Principles of Emergency Care
Assessing the Person in Emergencies
  A: Airway and Cervical Spine
  B: Breathing
  C: Circulation and Bleeding
  D: Disability
  E: Expose and Examine
Chest and Back Injuries
  Lifting and Moving Persons With Chest and Back Injuries
  Chest Injuries
  Head, Neck, and Back Injuries
Cold-Related Injuries
  Frostbite
  Hypothermia
Heat-Related Injuries
  Heat Cramps
  Heat Exhaustion
  Heat Stroke
  Burns

Key Learning Activities

◆ Visit a hospital emergency room. Discuss and observe the types of people who are brought in. What first aid care was given?
◆ With a partner practice locating pressure points on the body.
◆ Practice applying a sling, making an arm splint from a magazine, applying a bandage, and performing other first aid procedures.

Thousands of people lose their lives in accidents every year. A high percentage of accidents are motor vehicle accidents (MVA), but the occurrence of gunshot wounds is also on the rise. Most accidents are preventable. Trauma refers to a wound or injury and usually is caused by a force outside the person. This chapter describes the actions a first aid person should take in the event of trauma. Although anyone can assist at the scene of an accident, the text assumes the nurse is present.

Simply because you are a nurse, people expect you to be able to deal with emergencies. It is important that you be fully able to meet this expectation. Basic emergency care principles tell you what to do and what not to do when accidents happen. In a serious emergency, you must decide *quickly* what you are going to do. A confident, matter-of-fact manner will reassure the victim and onlookers. If you appear to be confident, others will follow your instructions and assist you.

Principles of Emergency Care

If brain cells do not have an oxygenated blood supply, they begin to die within 4 to 6 minutes. Therefore, it is vital for a person giving emergency care in a life-threatening situation to act quickly. Because the stress level is high at the scene of an emergency, it is helpful to have a plan of action and a predetermined, orderly method of assessment and care.

Assess Safety

Make sure the scene is safe before rushing to assist in an emergency. Check the environment and look for clues. Is there danger of fire or explosion? Is there dan-

Good Samaritan Laws

Most states have a law that protects the emergency care provider from legal liability, provided the rescuer gives *reasonable assistance* to the extent possible without danger or peril to the person or yourself. Some states consider the person guilty of a violation of the law, if aid is *not given* to someone who needs it.

As a nurse, you are required to assist in an emergency *to the level of your first aid training.* Do only what you are trained to do in an emergency. Familiarize yourself with the laws in the areas in which you work, live, and travel.

ger of being in the lane of traffic? Are there electrical hazards? Live wires? If the scene is unsafe, you may need to call for help *before assisting the person.* You may also need to move the person away from danger before you can begin your first aid care. The person, however, should not be moved if the area is safe.

Key Concept

Universal precautions should be followed whenever possible in administering first aid. The nurse should carry disposable gloves and a face mask.

Identify Problems

Is there anything unusual about the situation? Are there other clues? Are containers lying about that suggest attempted suicide, poisoning, or drug abuse? Could medication give you a clue to a medical problem? Are there signs of alcohol abuse?

Check for medical identification or a Medic Alert tag. The tag may be worn as a bracelet or on a chain around the neck. It signifies that the person has a specific medical problem that must be considered when administering first aid. Some emergency medical identification tags provide a 24-hour toll-free telephone number so that additional medical information can be obtained in an emergency. If these factors are not considered and treatment is not given accordingly, the patient may die. The nurse may need to look in an unconscious accident victim's wallet to see if it contains any medical information. The family should also be consulted, if possible.

If the nurse finds a card indicating that the person wishes to donate one or several tissues or organs after death, it is important to inform the emergency personnel of this at the scene of an accident. In many states, the fact that the victim wishes to be a donor is indicated on the driver's license.

Perform Triage

Triage is the process of sorting and classifying a person to determine priority of needs. Triage involves determining life-threatening situations and assisting those patients first. Triage in disaster situations was discussed in Chapter 29.

The nurse in a first aid situation will be expected to make decisions as to which person to assist first, when and how to call for help, and what to have the untrained bystanders do to assist. The nurse also uses triage in the emergency room or clinic, whether screening on the phone or on a walk-in basis.

Summon Assistance

Summoning help is an important part of emergency care. A victim's life may depend on rapid response. In most communities in the United States and Canada, the fastest way to summon the **Emergency Medical Service** (EMS) is by telephoning 911. It is your responsibility to know your local emergency number if it is not 911. You may be able to send someone to call, but make sure they have all the necessary information.

Treat for Shock

Shock results when the body loses its ability to keep an adequate supply of oxygenated blood circulating to all its components, particularly the brain. Many conditions can lead to shock in an accident. Shock usually occurs, however, because of problems with the pump (heart), blood volume, or blood vessels. If the heart is damaged, it cannot pump blood to the lungs to pick up oxygen or circulate enough blood volume to meet the body's needs. Either a loss of blood or a dilatation of the blood vessels will decrease the amount of blood volume available for the heart to pump. *Hypovolemic*

shock is the name given to shock caused by low blood volume from blood loss.

Because the central nervous system has the overall control of all body functions, it monitors changes and immediately implements compensatory circulation to maintain an adequate blood supply to vital organs, especially the brain and heart. This compensatory action can quickly adjust the rate and strength of the heart's contraction and the tone of the blood vessels in all parts of the body. It actually shuts down flow of blood to certain parts of the body and shunts (transfers) the blood to the vital organs. The compensatory action is a survival mechanism that ensures that the body's decision-maker, the brain and central nervous system, is adequately perfused until the last possible moment.

Shock may develop rapidly. Consequently, *every patient* should receive preventive and precautionary treatment for it. Anything that causes increased blood loss or that could contribute to shock should be avoided. This is particularly true of handling or moving the patient roughly or causing undue anxiety.

Shock is present in most cases of serious injury or illness, even though you do not see classic signs of it. Compensatory action may keep a person responsive, and in some cases, alert, even when massive blood loss has occurred. Look for signs of a change in the level of consciousness (LOC; see Chapter 71). Signs of shock

Key Signs of Shock

Early Signs of Shock

- Restlessness
- Panic
- Mental confusion
- Disorientation
- Weakness
- Anxiety

Common Signs of Shock

- Weak and rapid pulse
- Cold, clammy, moist skin
- Profuse sweating
- Skin pallor, then cyanosis (blueness)
- Shallow, irregular breathing; or labored, rapid, or gasping respirations
- Thirst
- Nausea or vomiting
- Shaking and trembling of the limbs
- A feeling of impending doom

Progressive Signs of Shock

- Confusion
- Disorientation
- Unresponsiveness
- Falling blood pressure

are listed in the accompanying box. Progressive signs indicate that circulation to the brain is not adequate. Falling blood pressure is a *late sign* of shock. If in doubt, treat for shock. A second box describes guidelines for emergency treatment of shock.

Key Concept

Look for all of the signs of shock. A falling blood pressure is a late sign of shock and is ominous.

Nursing Skill Guidelines
Treating Shock in an Emergency

- Keep the patient lying down and as calm as possible; reassure both the patient and bystanders. Have someone call for assistance. Avoid rough handling. *(Rationale: If the patient becomes excited, the oxygen needs of the body will increase, thus increasing the shock. The person may need advanced life support.)*
- Establish, maintain, and monitor the airway, breathing, and circulation. *(Rationale: These functions are vital to life.)*
- Administer high concentrations of oxygen, if available. Assist breathing as needed. *(Rationale: Administration of external oxygen increases the oxygen available in the blood and helps the person to breathe with less effort.)*
- Control bleeding. *(Rationale: Additional bleeding adds to shock, because of more blood loss.)*
- Maintain body temperature. Do not overheat the person. *(Rationale: Excessively low or high body temperature causes the heart to work harder.)*
- Give *nothing* by mouth. *(Rationale: The person could aspirate, choke, or vomit.)*
- Elevate lower extremities, unless contraindicated. (For example, in head injury, the body is kept level.)
- Use the position that is most comfortable for the patient and that is within medical limits for that injury. *(Rationale: Elevating the legs helps to drain blood toward the brain, where it is needed. Some people may need to have the head elevated, to breathe.)*
- Immobilize fractures. *(Rationale: To prevent further injury.)*
- Monitor level of consciousness. Take and record vital signs every 5 minutes. *(Rationale: It is important for the physician to know the person's reactions to the injury.)*

Adapted from Hafen B, Karren K: Prehospital Emergency Care and Crisis Intervention (Ed 3). Englewood Cliffs, NJ, Morton Series, Prentice-Hall, 1992

Key Abbreviations and Acronyms Used in Emergency Care

CPR	Cardiopulmonary resuscitation
EMS	Emergency Medical Service
IICP (↑ICP)	Increased intracranial pressure
LOC	Level of consciousness
MAST	Military Antishock Trousers
MI	Myocardial infarction
MVA	Motor vehicle accident
PERRLA	Pupils Equal/Round/React to Light/Accommodation OK
RICE	Rest/Ice/Compression/Elevation (for sprains)

Assessing the Person in Emergencies

Primary assessments are made as soon as you arrive on the scene. During this assessment you discover and deal with life-threatening problems or injuries. Unless there are life-threatening problems to correct, the primary survey usually can be completed in 60 seconds.

The secondary assessment involves taking and recording vital signs and continues with a head-to-toe assessment. This assessment should take from 1 to 2 minutes, unless injuries are found that require immediate intervention. If the person has life-threatening problems, the secondary assessment may be delayed until the person is being transported.

Use the letters A, B, C, D, and E to help you remember the order for assessing the person in an emergency situation.

A = Airway and cervical spine
B = Breathing
C = Circulation and bleeding
D = Disability
E = Expose and examine

A: Airway and Cervical Spine

The *patency* of the airway is evaluated to determine whether or not the airway is open (patent). As this is done, keep in mind the mechanism, location, and scope of the injury. If there is a possibility of a spinal injury, consider *stabilizing the person's cervical spine* before attempting other activities. If the *trauma* patient is not breathing, *open the airway*, using the jaw thrust maneuver (see Chapter 32). This technique opens the airway, but does not extend the neck. If the emergency does not involve trauma, it is appropriate to use the head tilt-chin lift method to open the airway (see Chapter 32). After opening the airway, quickly clear any visible foreign material from the mouth.

B: Breathing

Assess breathing by listening for breath sounds, by
watching for movements of the chest, and by feeling
for breath against your cheek and ear. If breathing is
not present, pinch the person's nose and give the person two slow mask-to-mouth breaths. Each breath
should be of sufficient force to cause the chest to rise
and should take from 1.5 to 2 seconds to deliver. Allow
the client to exhale *passively* between breaths.

If you are unable to ventilate the person on your first
attempt, reposition the airway and try again. If you are
still unable to ventilate the person, the airway is obstructed. Use the obstructed-airway technique to remove the obstruction and establish the airway. (See
Chapter 32 for a description of these techniques in more
detail.)

Maintain the Airway. It is important to *maintain the
airway* even if breathing is present. Blood, body fluids,
and vomitus may accumulate in the mouth and should
be removed. Be sure the person's tongue is out of the
way. (The tongue can occlude the airway in even such
a minor event as fainting.) Position the person on the
side if vomiting occurs.

Observe Respirations. As you assess breathing, note if
the *respirations* appear to be at normal rate and depth.
Examine the person's mouth, gums, lips, and nail beds
for color and moisture. Blueness (cyanosis) indicates a
lack of oxygen.

Look for Life-Threatening Chest Injuries. If indicated by
the mechanism of injury, examine the chest for life-
threatening injuries. Care for these injuries immediately
if they are present. Examples include a puncture wound
of the chest.

C: Circulation and Bleeding

Palpate the Pulse. Palpate the *pulse* for 5 to 10 seconds.
If there is no pulse, ask bystanders to call for assistance.
The person needs advanced life support as soon as

possible. Begin cardiac compressions and rescue
breathing. (Chapter 32 contains a description of these
procedures.)

Observe the Pulse. If pulse is present, note its rate and
regularity. Does it seem normal? Do *not* count the pulse
at this time; just try to get a sense of its quality. As you
palpate the pulse, also observe skin color, temperature,
and neck veins.

Reassess Breathing. A person may have a heartbeat
without having respirations; therefore, you must reassess breathing. Rescue breathing must be performed if
breathing is not present (see Chapter 32).

Assess for Shock. The nurse should consider the possibility of shock in any injury. Severe blood loss usually
causes shock. The treatment of shock is discussed
above. Use the *capillary refill test* to evaluate for *shock,*
as follows:

♦ Press your finger into the middle of the person's
   forehead until the spot you are pressing turns
   white.
♦ Remove your finger. Count the seconds it takes for
   the color to return. (Count: one-one thousand; two-
   one thousand, etc.)
♦ If it takes more than 2 seconds for color to return,
   shock is progressing.

Assess for Hemorrhage. The presence of a palpable
pulse indicates that the person's heart is beating.
However, you must also assess for major bleeding
(hemorrhage).

Stop Bleeding. Hemorrhage must be controlled *immediately* or the person will die from blood loss. With
your gloved hands, place sterile compresses over
wounds and apply pressure. If blood seeps through the
compresses, do not remove old dressings but place additional compresses over the top of the compress already in place. You may need to apply additional pressure over the wound.

Measures that can be used to stop bleeding include:

♦ Apply direct pressure (should be done first).
♦ Elevate a bleeding limb.
♦ Apply ice or cold pack, if available. (Place ice over
   several layers of dressing to avoid freezing the
   tissue.)
♦ Apply *indirect* pressure (press the vessel at a pressure point against a bone.
♦ If severe bleeding continues, reach into the wound
   and try to grasp the bleeding vessel with your
   fingers.
♦ Apply a tourniquet (final option). Mark the person
   with the time the tourniquet was applied.

D: Disability

Neurologic Assessment. It will be helpful to the receiving physician if a neurologic assessment has been conducted at the scene. The following levels can be identified:

- ◆ A: Alert; speaks and moves spontaneously; answers questions about name, place, and date correctly
- ◆ V: Responsive to verbal stimulus only; answers when directly addressed
- ◆ P: Responsive to painful stimulus only (such as rubbing the sternum or pressure on the nail beds)
- ◆ U: Unresponsive

Assess Eye Signs. Assess the person's pupillary responses. The pupils of both eyes should be the same (equal), should be round, and should constrict when a bright light is quickly shined into them. Reactions should be the same in both eyes and they should move together when following a moving object (eyes coordinated). This is abbreviated as PERRLA + C (see Chapter 71):

PE = Pupils equal
R = Round
RL = React to light
A = Accommodation OK
+C = Coordinated

E: Expose and Examine

Expose and examine any site of possible injury or area the person complains about even if examined previously. After you have controlled the immediately life-threatening problems, obtain a history, if possible. Your sources may be the person, the family, or bystanders. Try to find out what happened.

Vital signs (temperature, pulse, respiration, blood pressure) are taken every 5 minutes when life-threatening problems have been treated and are under control. Count the pulse and respirations for at least 30 seconds. Your recording establishes a *baseline* for further treatment.

Chest and Back Injuries

Lifting and Moving Persons With Chest and Back Injuries

The person *is not moved* until the EMS team arrives. A situation may arise, however, in which you will need to supervise the transporting of an injured person.

It is essential that any injured person be transported with utmost care. A back injury or other injury can be made more severe by careless transportation. When moving a person with a neck injury to the stretcher, immobilize the neck and back first, then keep the body straight. If the person is lying in an abnormal position, it is sometimes advisable to put the person on the stretcher in the position in which he or she is lying rather than to attempt to straighten the body. Enlist as many assistants as needed to move the person effectively and safely. *(Rationale: It is important to protect both the injured person as well as yourself.)* Transfer and lifting of an immobilized patient are discussed in Chapter 43.

In some cases, a person must be removed from a badly wrecked vehicle; however, only persons specially trained and having special extrication equipment should do this. The *only time* other people should attempt extrication is when there is great danger to the person if not moved. For example, in the event of an MVA in which there is great danger of fire or explosion, or if the vehicle is under water, the person must be removed from the car, even though this might aggravate the injuries.

Chest Injuries

Accidents such as blows, falls, or automobile collisions (falls against the steering wheel) are the most common cause of chest injuries. Fractured ribs may injure soft tissues by puncturing a lung or tearing blood vessels. If such complications are not present, fractured ribs can be treated by immobilizing the chest with an elastic bandage.

Compression of the chest as the result of an explosion or MVA may rupture a lung and cause death from hemorrhage or suffocation. Wounds that penetrate the chest are serious and require immediate first aid.

Emergency action must be taken in case of a puncture wound of the chest. An open chest wound allows air to enter, thus upsetting the negative pressure required for breathing. The wound must be sealed in any way possible, and the lungs reexpanded. (The person is brought to the hospital, and surgery is performed immediately so that chest tubes can be inserted for continuous, closed drainage).

In an emergency situation, *do not remove the article puncturing the chest* if it is still in place. *(Rationale: This will help to seal the hole and its removal may cause added damage.)* When transporting the person to the hospital, make sure that the object remains in place. If the wound is open, cover it at once with an occlusive dressing. Hold the dressing in place with your gloved hand. Oxygen may also be helpful and mask-to-mouth or manual breathing bag resuscitation may be needed. If the person seems to be getting worse, loosen the dressing to let out some of the air that is building up in the chest. Then reseal the wound.

Head, Neck, and Back Injuries

In automobile accidents, motorcycle accidents, and falls, one can suspect neck or back injuries. There is great danger of making the injury worse by moving the person without proper preparation. Always treat the person as though there were a back or neck injury if you have reason to suspect this. It is better to be too careful than to risk causing further injury. Immobilizing devices should be applied by specially trained personnel and should never be removed by a first aid person.

Laceration of the scalp causes profuse bleeding; even the smallest wound looks very serious. It is important to determine the extent and cause of the injury.

Emergency care includes having the person lie flat while restricting his or her movements. Keep the person warm and check for signs of increasing intracranial pressure (IICP; see Chapter 71). Serious complications are signified by dizziness, nausea, confusion, changes in LOC and headache.

If the person is moved, his or her head should be stabilized in a neutral position and kept in line with the back. Usually emergency personnel will bring special immobilizing equipment, such as cervical collars and short and long spine boards, which are used to prepare the person for transport. The first aid person should stabilize the person without moving the person until proper equipment and assistance arrives.

Cold-Related Injuries

Frostbite

Frostbite is the freezing of tissue caused by exposure to extreme cold. The body is so cold that ice crystals form in the spaces surrounding body cells; the cells then die. The body is more vulnerable when there is a high wind because blood rushes to the surface to warm it, then cools rapidly due to rapid loss of heat. The mathematical calculation of the combination of the temperature and the wind speed is called the *wind chill factor.* The skin can freeze when the wind chill factor is below the freezing point, even though the actual air temperature is considerably higher.

In frostbite, the extremities of the body and the nose, ears, and cheeks are most likely to be affected. The nose, ears, and cheeks are vulnerable because they are exposed, or in the case of toes and fingers, because circulation is slowed. However, larger areas of the body can be affected also.

If a part has become frostbitten, the area is first painful and then becomes numb. The frostbitten part is pale and cool to the touch and feels like a block of wood or marble. These symptoms exist initially regardless of how mild or severe the frostbite is. In later stages, hem-orrhage may occur; the part may swell and blisters may form. Degrees of frostbite are presented in the accompanying box.

Treatment. A person suffering from frostbite needs assistance immediately. *Do not rub* a frozen part to restore circulation. Rubbing, and particularly rubbing with snow, will only *increase* the damage and can lead to gangrene. Frozen parts should be protected; they should be handled gently. Tight clothing should be loosened. Do not allow a person to walk on a frostbitten foot. Fingers and toes may be separated by wedges of cotton. However, do not place bandages, ointments, salves, or anything else on the frostbitten part.

Frozen parts should be placed in water that is between 98°F and 104°F (36.6°–40°C). If you do not have a thermometer, keep the water temperature so that it feels tepid to the normal touch. Rewarming will take about 20 to 45 minutes in water. Some pain may be experienced as the part gets warm. It will turn pink or bright red as circulation resumes. Then protect from refreezing.

The person with severe frostbite needs medical attention. It sometimes takes physicians several days to assess the extent of the damage. If treatment is not successful, amputation may be necessary. In severe frostbite, blisters may form quickly. These should not be broken. Frostbite damage is often treated the same as a burn.

Nursing Alert

The nurse working in a public hospital is likely to see frostbite among homeless people. This is particularly true of persons who are mentally ill, inebriated, elderly, or physically debilitated.

Hypothermia

Hypothermia is a condition in which the person is exposed to extreme cold or is cold for a long enough time to lower the *core temperature* of the body dan-

---

Degrees of Frostbite

- First degree (*superficial*)—temporary tenderness, reddened skin—probably no permanent damage
- Second degree (*partial-thickness*)—blisters and some tissue and nerve damage—can result in permanent hypersensitivity to cold and increased risk of future frostbite
- Third degree (*full-thickness*)—tissue death—requires skin grafting or amputation

Adapted from "Frostbite—the Big Chill." Burn Center, Hennepin County Medical Center, Minneapolis, Minnesota, 1989.

gerously. Profuse sweating for a period of time can also cause this condition. When hypothermia results from one of these situations, it is known as *accidental hypothermia.* Hypothermia also occurs when the body's temperature regulation malfunctions. In addition, the temperature is sometimes intentionally lowered to perform surgery more safely; this is *induced* or *surgical hypothermia.* Induced hypothermia confined to one part of the body is called *local hypothermia.*

Lowering the core temperature (internal temperature) of the body even a few degrees can result in serious symptoms and even death. Symptoms include sleepiness, shaking, cardiac arrhythmias, loss of reflexes, and respiratory failure. In a first aid situation, the first symptoms the nurse should notice are confusion, disorientation, slurred speech, and lethargy. The person complains of blurred vision, dizziness, tiredness, and feeling cold.

Nursing Alert

If frostbite is accompanied by hypothermia, it is a medical emergency. Give *immediate* emergency care in any case of hypothermia.

Definitive diagnosis of hypothermia is based on an accurate measurement of body core temperature. Special monitoring equipment is needed because normal clinical or electronic thermometers often do not register low enough to measure the core temperature accurately.

Treatment. Gradual rewarming is necessary. *(Rationale: If the body is rewarmed too fast, cold blood is returned to the heart, causing severe arrhythmias and sometimes cardiac arrest.)* The person's cardiac status must be continually monitored during rewarming.

The core of the body is warmed to approximately 94°F (35°C); *then* the extremities are warmed. The body may be warmed with warmed blankets or by being placed in warm water. In addition, warmed oxygen and warmed intravenous infusions are often given. The blood may be circulated through the pump oxygenator and warmed before returning to the body's core circulation. Warm fluids may be instilled into the gastrointestinal system. Treatment continues until the body's core temperature is near normal.

Nursing Considerations. During the rewarming process, nursing care includes careful monitoring of vital signs and intravenous infusion, close observation of skin condition, special mouth and eye care, and measurement of oral/IV intake and urine output. The core temperature of the body is monitored with a special electronic thermometer. The person will have an intravenous infusion. Common complications are bleeding and gastric distention.

During first aid, the person's head, hands, and feet are covered. A ground cover provides a barrier against moisture and insulates materials under the person. Keep the person *awake* until medical assistance arrives.

Nursing Alert

Hypothermia can be a life-threatening condition. First aid treatment should be instituted immediately. The person needs to be rewarmed gradually. Seek medical attention.

More heat is lost through the head than any other part of the body; it acts like a chimney.

Heat-Related Injuries

Heat injuries are more likely to occur on days of high humidity, with temperatures from 95°F to 100°F (35°–37.8°C) and no breeze. *(Rationale: The body's major defense against heat accumulation is sweating; the evaporation of sweat helps cool the body. When humidity exceeds 75%, particularly if there is no breeze, evaporation decreases.)* Heat injuries typically occur early in the season, before people have an opportunity to acclimate themselves to higher temperatures. Such injuries can also occur inside enclosed areas when outside temperature is low but other heat sources increase the person's internal heat load. For example, on a bright day, a parked car can be a *fatal* enclosed area for children and pets because of the radiant heat produced by the sun. Heat produced in some work areas also can produce heat illness. Any enclosed area where equipment is producing large amounts of heat that is allowed to accumulate has the potential of causing heat illness.

Although people vary in their sensitivity to heat illness, certain individuals are more susceptible to it. Studies have identified infants, the elderly, persons with underlying illness, military personnel, and athletes as among those who are most at risk.

Heat Cramps

Heat cramps usually occur after hard exertion and are frequently found in physically fit young people, who usually have been sweating profusely and drinking plain water. These cramps occur in cool environments as well as hot ones and are usually located in the legs, arms, or abdomen. Along with heat cramps, a person may have signs of heat exhaustion.

Heat cramps are relieved by drinking salt solutions. The person should be given a mixture of up to ¼ teaspoon of salt per quart of water (or other balanced salt solution). If symptoms continue longer than an hour, medical advice should be sought. Salt tablets are not recommended because they are gastric irritants. It is helpful to move the person to a cooler environment, make sure the head is uncovered, and keep him or her calm.

Explain to the person what is happening. Tell the person to avoid exertion for the next 12 hours. The person is sometimes advised to put added salt on food during exertion.

Key Concept

Massaging cramping muscles does not cure heat cramps; in fact, it may increase pain.

Heat Exhaustion

Heat exhaustion often occurs in physically fit people who are exerting in a hot environment. Under such conditions, a person does not take in enough water and sodium to replace lost fluids, resulting in a serious blood flow disturbance, similar to shock. Pure forms of heat exhaustion are rare. However, if heat exhaustion has occurred quickly, it is likely to be related to *water depletion.* (Another type of heat exhaustion, called *salt-depletion* heat exhaustion, develops over a period of time.)

As large amounts of water and salt are lost through sweat and water is not replaced, blood flow decreases. This affects brain, heart, and lung functions. When a person has a loss of salt, as well as water, heat cramps may occur, along with signs and symptoms of heat exhaustion.

Headache, dizziness, nausea, and weakness are common in heat exhaustion. Other symptoms include faintness, hypotension, loss of appetite, and unconsciousness (usually brief). The skin is pale, cool, and usually sweaty; the body temperature may be subnormal. The eyes are dilated, breathing is rapid and shallow, and the pulse is rapid and weak. The person may have difficulty walking (see Table 31-1).

Treatment. Treatment for heat exhaustion includes cooling the person, without chilling. You may need to move the person to a cool place and remove and loosen as much clothing as practical. Apply cold, wet compresses to the skin. Fanning is helpful. Have the person lie down and elevate the feet 8 to 12 inches. *(Rationale: This will help increase circulation to the brain.)*

Water replacement and rest may relieve symptoms of heat exhaustion caused by water depletion. However, you may need to give sips of salt solution to the salt-depleted person suffering from heat exhaustion. If there is any doubt about the person's condition, transport the person to the hospital. *(Rationale: It is sometimes difficult to tell the difference between heat exhaustion and heat stroke.)*

Heat Stroke

Heat stroke is a potentially life-threatening condition. *Classic heat stroke* occurs when the body's heat-regulating mechanisms fail and the body temperature soars. As the body reaches temperatures of 105°F to 110°F, sweating stops and brain cells are damaged or destroyed, causing death. Classic heat stroke usually occurs during a summer heat wave, with its high temperatures and high humidity.

The people most often affected are the poor, living in poorly ventilated housing; the aged who may not take in enough water; and the chronically ill, who often are on medications that contribute to heat stress.

Exertional heat stroke develops because of increased internal heat load. This is caused by muscular exertion, along with high external temperatures and humidity. It usually occurs rapidly (within a few hours) in young, healthy, athletic individuals, simply because their heat-regulating systems are overwhelmed. In about half of these cases the person is sweating.

A heat stroke person has many of the same symptoms as the heat exhaustion person. However, there are some distinct differences as listed in Table 31-1. The heat stroke person has hot skin. (The person may be sweating, if it is exertional heat stroke, and dry, if it is classic heat stroke). This is important to note because the heat exhaustion person may be sweating but have cool skin. Another difference is body temperature. The heat stroke patient has a high temperature, often above 106°F (41.1°C). The heat exhaustion patient has normal temperature or even slightly below normal. The classic heat stroke person usually is brought to the hospital because of hypotension, fever, and coma. The person with exertional heat stroke is brought in because of bizarre behavior or collapse.

Treatment. Both forms of heat stroke can be life threatening. Each needs immediate medical care, without which death almost always follows, especially in heat stroke. (About 4,000 Americans die of heat stroke per year. About 80% of the deaths occur in people over age 50 years.) The longer a person goes without treatment, the greater the danger.

Treatment for heat stroke includes rapid cooling of the patient. Use ice, fans, cold water—anything that is available. Monitor the person's airway, breathing, and

Table 31-1. Differences Between Heat Exhaustion and Heat Stroke

Heat Exhaustion	Heat Stroke
Cool skin	Hot skin
May or may not be sweating	May or may not be sweating (dry = usually classic heat stroke; sweating = usually exertional heat stroke)
Normal or below-normal temperature	High temperature (often above 106°F)
Water depletion: occurs quickly	
Salt depletion: develops over period of time	
Symptoms: headache, nausea, dizziness, weakness, faintness, pale skin, weak pulse, tachycardia, anorexia, hypotension, brief periods of unconsciousness, rapid breathing	*Classic heat stroke*: hypotension, fever, coma
	Exertional heat stroke: confusion, bizarre behavior, collapse
Treatment: cool patient, without chilling; give water (water depletion) or salt solution (salt depletion type) Elevate feet	*Treatment*: rapid cooling of patient, monitor airway and circulation, observe seizure precautions
Seek medical treatment if in doubt	*Transport immediately to medical facility*. This is an emergency!

circulation. If necessary, begin CPR. Watch for seizures. Immediate transport to the hospital is crucial in heat stroke.

> **Nursing Alert**
>
> If the person suffering from any type of heat-related illness vomits, *stop giving fluids*. The person will need to be hospitalized for intravenous fluid replacement. (This is usually the only time a *heat exhaustion* patient needs to be hospitalized.) Any patient with *heat stroke* needs immediate medical attention.

Burns

Burns occur from many heat sources. Burns are discussed in Chapter 68 with classification and calculations. That portion of the text should be studied along with the discussion here.

The most common emergency cases are caused by thermal (radiant), electrical, and chemical sources. *Thermal burns* may be caused by flames, steam, hot liquids, heat objects, or the sun. *Electrical burns* may be caused by electrical power sources or lightning. Strong chemicals can cause severe chemical burns to the skin, respiratory system, or eyes.

Burns can be divided into several classifications, (see Chapter 68). *Superficial* burns are known as first-degree burns; *partial-thickness* burns are known as second-degree burns; and *full-thickness* burns are

known as third-degree burns. When a burn is so severe it invades the bone, it is sometimes classified as a fourth-degree burn.

The seriousness of a burn is estimated by its depth, percentage of the body burned, location, age of the patient, and any underlying complications. Examples of special considerations include:

- ◆ A full-thickness burn that involves more than 10% of the body surface is extremely serious.
- ◆ Burns to the hands, feet, mouth, throat, and perineum are serious. Full-thickness circumferential (all-the-way-around) burns to the limbs and chest are special problems because they can restrict circulation and breathing.
- ◆ Electrical current follows blood vessels and does severe internal damage, which may not be immediately apparent.
- ◆ Diabetic persons of any age have more difficulty recovering from a burn because they do not heal as fast; they may also have underlying circulatory or other difficulties.
- ◆ Any underlying injury can also affect the burn patient's recovery.

Hospital treatment of burns is discussed in Chapter 68. Immediate first aid care is summarized in the accompanying box.

Associated problems often cause more harm that the burn itself. Be alert for inhalation injuries and breathing problems, as well as for broken bones or other injuries. Signs of possible inhalation injury include:

Nursing Skill Guidelines
Providing Emergency First Aid for Burns

◆ Stop the burning process by removing the heat source. Make sure burning clothing is *cooled.* Do not remove burning fabric or other materials, unless they fall off. *(Rationale: Some materials continue to smolder or melt and must be neutralized. However, removing the clothing could tear the skin and damage it further).*

◆ If you arrive within a few minutes of the incident, flood the area with cool water. Do not apply ice. *(Rationale: The goal is to cool the area. This stops the burning and reduces the incidence of scarring.)*

◆ Continue to flood the area with cool water. *(Rationale: Cool water helps to control pain; discontinuation may increase pain temporarily because of damaged nerve endings.)*

◆ Flood most chemical burns with a gentle, continuous flow of plain water until emergency help arrives. *(Rationale: This will help stop the burning process and cool the area. It will also help to dilute and wash away caustic chemical.)* It is best to read the container for directions on emergency treatment. *(Rationale: Some chemicals react adversely when in contact with water.)*

◆ Watch for shivering if you are using water to cool a burn covering more than 10% of the body. Change to dry, sterile dressings if shivering occurs. *(Rationale: Exposure to cold may cause hypothermia.)*

◆ Do not put anything other than water or a specifically prescribed substance on a burn. *(Rationale: Materials such as salves, ointments, or butter occlude the burn so it becomes difficult to examine. Pain will be caused when they are removed. These substances also promote infection.)*

◆ Remove the patient's jewelry. *(Rationale: It can remain hot and continue the burning process. Swelling usually occurs later, making it impossible to remove rings or cutting off circulation.)*

◆ Monitor the airway, breathing, and circulation. Be prepared to initiate CPR. *(Rationale: Respiratory or cardiac arrest [or both] can occur from the shock.)*

◆ If the burn is extensive, cover it with a dry, nonstick, sterile dressing. Do not use gauze. *(Rationale: Gauze will peel off additional tissue and cause more damage.)* For all large burns, it is best to use only a dry, sterile dressing, following removal of the heat source and cooling down period. *(Rationale: The dressing will help to prevent infection.)*

◆ Keep dressings cool and wet. Be sure to keep person warm and monitor for hypothermia. *(Rationale: Wet dressings may promote hypothermia.)*

◆ Prevent contamination of the wound, as much as possible. *(Rationale: Infection is a major hazard in burns.)*

◆ Treat for shock. *(Rationale: Pain, loss of body fluids, and anxiety contribute to shock.)*

◆ Determine what first aid measures have already been given by others. *(Rationale: Some of these might be dangerous. The physician needs to be made aware of what has been done.)*

◆ Burned or singed nasal hairs or burns in or around the mouth
◆ Flecks of soot in the patient's saliva
◆ Smell of smoke on the patient's breath
◆ Hoarse voice

Nursing Alert

If the patient was trapped in a confined space and exposed to chemicals or smoke, suspect smoke or heat inhalation injury.

Musculoskeletal Injuries

Fractures, Sprains, and Dislocations

When a person has been involved in an MVA or a fall, these possibilities should be considered:

◆ **Fracture**: broken bone
◆ **Sprain**: twisting of a joint with rupture of ligaments and other possible damage
◆ **Dislocation**: displacement of a bone from a joint

Sometimes it is difficult to determine whether a sprain or a fracture has occurred. If in doubt as to the extent of the injury, assume that a fracture has occurred and treat the person accordingly until a definite diagnosis is made. Ice is the treatment of choice for a fracture or sprain until medical assistance is available. Usually the person will have pain on movement or weight-bearing after sustaining a fracture. It is dangerous to have a person stand or walk on a suspected fracture to check for pain. This is likely to aggravate the injury.

The cardinal rule of emergency care is *do not move the person.* Get emergency help. Question the person if he or she is conscious. Observe for obviously deformed limbs; cover with a blanket until adequate help can be obtained.

Never attempt to replace the ends of bones in a fracture where the skin is broken. Instead, cover the area with a sterile dressing and control excessive bleeding by direct or indirect pressure.

The acronym *RICE* will help in emergency procedures for sprains:

R = rest
I = ice
C = compression
E = elevation

Splinting a Fracture

Do not attempt to splint a fracture if emergency medical assistance is available. A *splint* is a device applied to *immobilize* a fracture or sprain. Any hard, straight item can be used. A good emergency splint for an arm is a magazine wrapped around the arm and tied. (Be careful not to tie splints so tightly as to cut off the circulation to the limb.) Numerous commercial splints are available. Traction splints should be used for most major leg fractures and should be applied only by specially trained members of the EMS team. Inflatable splints may also be used.

If you suspect a fracture of a knee or elbow, splint in the existing position. *(Rationale: Because of the close proximity to arteries, veins, and nerves, straightening of the joint can pinch these organs, cutting off circulation or sensation to the distal portion of the extremity.)* An effective splint for a fractured toe is the adjacent toe; digits can be taped together. The same is true for fingers.

Nursing Alert

When splinting a fracture, it is *important* to check distal pulses before and after splinting. If *no pulse* is present, this becomes a medical emergency. Obtain medical attention *immediately.*

Injuries Requiring a Bandage

Sterile Dressings. If emergency assistance is not available, the nurse may need to apply a dressing to an open wound. Many articles can be used as dressings in an emergency, but a sterile dressing should be used whenever possible. Sterile dressings are available in many sizes and thicknesses; the appropriate dressing should be chosen. If sterile dressings are unavailable, use the cleanest material at hand. A clean handkerchief or dish towel is suitable. Fresh newspaper can be used because it is clean.

Bandages. A **bandage** is a piece of material used to hold dressings or splints in place, to give support, or to

apply pressure. Generally, bandages are not applied by the nurse. However, if you do need to apply a bandage, guidelines should be followed:

◆ Apply bandages firmly but not so tightly that the circulation is cut off. Watch for evidence of tightness (blanching of skin, loss of sensation, absent pulses) and loosen the bandage if necessary.
◆ Always tie a square knot; it will not slip and is easily untied.
◆ If possible, leave the tips of the toes and fingers exposed. *(Rationale: You will need to check for impaired circulation.)* Look for pallor, lack of pulse, pain on passive motion, paresthesia, or paralysis.

Roller bandages of gauze, elastic, Kerlix, and other materials are available in various widths suitable for bandaging parts of the body. A roller bandage can be made to fit the extremities. Equal pressure should be exerted with each turn of a roller bandage. (If you make the turns progressively tighter as you progress, the bandage will constrict the body part. If you let the turns get looser, the bandage will slip and may come off.)

Cravat Bandages and Slings. A triangular or handkerchief bandage is made from a square of cloth and can be fastened without tape or pins, if necessary. A 36- or 40-inch square is an adequate size. It is folded diagonally through the center to form a triangle. The triangle can be folded several times to make a strip or *cravat bandage.* The triangular bandage is often used to make a sling to support an arm (Fig. 31-1).

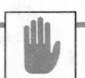

Nursing Skill
Applying a Sling

Procedure

1. Put one triangle end over the shoulder on the *uninjured* side, with the point of the triangle pointing toward the elbow of the injured arm and placed under it. *(Rationale: The injured arm will be supported by the sling around the neck.)*
2. Bring the other end of the triangle over the shoulder on the *injured* side and tie the two ends of the triangle together at the side of the neck. *(Rationale: The knot should be tied on the side of the injury, so it is pulled away from the neck, to avoid discomfort.)* If this is impractical because of the nature of the injury or of another situation, place some sort of padding beneath the knot.
3. Bring the point of the triangle backward around the elbow and pin it to the back of the sling. You can adjust the sling by adjusting the knot or by pinning a tuck in the front of the sling above the hand. The hand should be elevated 4 or 5 inches above the elbow level. *(Rationale: Elevation helps to prevent swelling and pain.)*

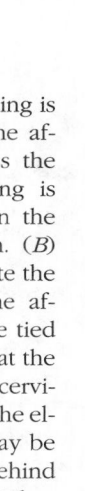
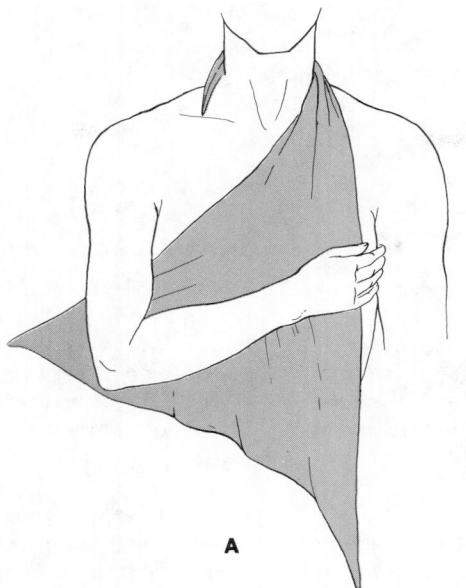
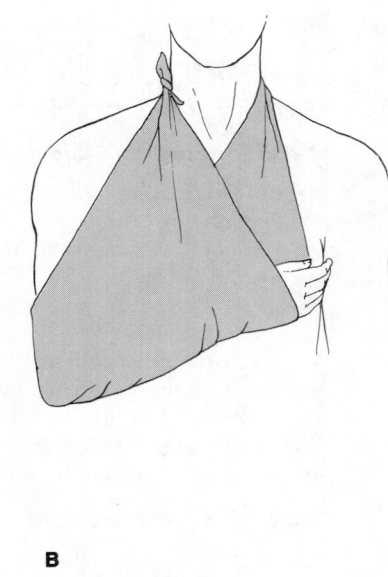

A   **B**

Figure 31-1. (*A*) An open sling is placed on the chest, and the affected arm is placed across the sling. One end of the sling is placed around the neck on the side of the unaffected arm. (*B*) The end of the sling opposite the shoulder is placed over the affected arm and the ends are tied at the side of the neck so that the knot does not rub over the cervical vertebra. The material at the elbow is folded neatly and may be secured with a pin placed behind the sling so that it is out of sight.

Dental Injuries and Missing Teeth

Teeth may be displaced or knocked out accidentally, particularly in children. If the tooth is pushed up into the socket, this is called an *intrusion injury.* If the tooth is knocked out, this is called an *avulsion injury.* In either event, *immediate dental care* is needed. In the case of an avulsion injury, the dentist may be able to reimplant and reposition the tooth. If an avulsed tooth is reimplanted within 30 minutes, it has a 90% chance of being saved. It *may* be saved if reimplanted within 2 hours. First aid for avulsed teeth is outlined here:

♦ Ask bystanders to look for the tooth. Instruct them to pick it up with a sterile piece of gauze by the crown and not to touch the root. (*Rationale: Touching the root may damage important structures.*)
♦ Call the dentist immediately. The person must be seen by a dentist or in an emergency room as soon as possible. (*Rationale: The sooner a tooth is repositioned, the more likely it is to be saved.*)
♦ Clean the patient's mouth with gauze. Using sterile gauze, have the patient gently bite down. (*Rationale: This will restrict bleeding and reduce pain.*)
♦ Instruct the person not to put pressure on adjacent teeth. (*Rationale: Adjacent teeth may have been loosened in the accident.*)
♦ Biting gently on a dry tea bag usually helps to stop bleeding. (*Rationale: The tannin in the tea acts as a natural coagulant.*)
♦ Do not allow the patient to suck on a straw or to smoke. (*Rationale: The sucking action will serve to suck out a blood clot and cause more bleeding.*)
♦ Place the tooth on sterile gauze. It may be cleaned by dipping in milk, while holding the crown. (*Ra-*

tionale: Use of water or any other solution may damage the root.)
♦ If the person will cooperate, have him or her hold the tooth under the tongue en route to the dentist. Otherwise, place the tooth in milk. (*Rationale: The patient's own saliva or the milk will help to preserve the integrity and viability of the root system.*)

Foreign Objects

A *foreign object* is any object or substance lodged in a place where it does not belong.

Foreign Object or Substance in the Eye

Foreign objects in the eye can be particles of dust or soot or an eyelash resting on the lining of the eyelid, or they can be particles that become embedded in the eyeball. Anything that lodges in the eye irritates it, especially when the eyelid is closed. A foreign object has a scratchy effect and causes tears to flow. **Caustic** substances are substances that are extremely irritating. Sometimes in an industrial accident, chemicals enter the eye. Quick action must be taken to flush the eye. The accompanying box summarizes skills in emergency care of eye injuries. If there is any question about the severity of the injury, a physician should be seen as soon as possible.

Emergency Removal of Contact Lenses
Most types of contact lenses used today can remain in the eyes for a few hours without incident. If lenses are left in place following an accident, the medical team must be aware of this fact. The corneas can become

Nursing Skill Guidelines
Giving First Aid for Patient Eye Injuries

First Aid for Foreign Objects in the Eye

◆ Instruct the person not to rub the eyes. Have the person keep the eye closed and avoid blinking. *(Rationale: Rubbing or blinking may drive a foreign object deeper into the eye.)*
◆ Never use an instrument, a toothpick, or a match to remove a foreign object. *(Rationale: These items are unsterile and may introduce pathogens into the eye.)*
◆ Never attempt to remove a foreign object if there is the slightest possibility that it is embedded in the cornea. *(Rationale: The object may be driven deeper into the eye and cause more serious damage.)*

When the Object is not Embedded

◆ Pull down the lower eyelid to see whether the object is on the eyelid membrane. *(Rationale: If the object is on the inside of the eyelid, you may be able to lift it off by touching it gently with the corner of a clean handkerchief or with a cotton-tipped applicator moistened in water.)*
◆ Always moisten cotton before touching it to the eye. *(Rationale: Small particles of dry cotton can become lodged in the eye.)*
◆ If object is under the upper eyelid, grasp the lashes of the upper eyelid with your forefinger and thumb; ask the person to look upward; gently pull the lid forward and downward over the lower eyelid. *(Rationale: Usually this dislodges the foreign body and the tears wash it away.)*

◆ Flush the eye with plain water. *(Rationale: Sometimes flushing washes an object out of the eye.)*

First Aid for Caustic Materials in the Eye

◆ Flush the eye with *large amounts* of water or normal saline solution. *(Rationale: The eyes are sensitive to chemical or thermal burns. It is vital to use a large amount of water to cleanse the eyes.)* You can do this with a *sterile* medicine dropper or a small *sterile* bulb syringe. Do not use an unsterile eye cup. *(Rationale: Eye cups may introduce infectious organisms into the eye.)*
◆ Use an eye wash sink or shower if possible. The person stands over the sink, with the eyes close to the jets. The person keeps the eyes open as much as possible. When the water is turned on, the jets direct a continuous stream of water into the eyes. *(Rationale: Large amounts of water are necessary; this is more easily provided with an eye wash sink.)*
◆ Do not instill another substance into the eye in an attempt to neutralize a caustic substance. *(Rationale: Putting another substance into the eyes could do more damage.)*
◆ Have the patient seen by a physician immediately. *(Rationale: Prompt action is necessary to prevent permanent eye damage.)*

---

ulcerated if the patient does not blink. Hard contact lenses are more likely to cause corneal ulcers than soft lenses.

In some cases, it is necessary to remove contact lenses at the scene of an accident.

Foreign Objects in the Nose, Throat, or Ear

Children often insert small objects into the nose. To remove the object, have the child blow the nose gently with *both* nostrils open. Unless the object is clearly visible and at the edge of the nostril, do not attempt to remove it with a finger or instrument. Call the physician.

Objects often become lodged in the throat. Children put coins or buttons in their mouths. Bits of food or bones can lodge in the throat or the esophagus. Do not attempt to remove the foreign object with your finger, unless it is an object that you can dislodge easily. If the foreign object is not visible but the victim is able to breathe adequately, call for emergency medical assistance.

If a foreign object lodges in the ear, do not attempt to remove it. Instead, transport the person to a medical center.

Obstructed Airway

If the person is not exchanging air and shows signs of respiratory distress, call 911 and use the obstructed airway techniques described in Chapter 32. The abdominal thrust maneuver is an effective means of dislodging a foreign object. Sometimes, rescue breathing is necessary, even though the object has been removed (see Chapter 32).

Cardiovascular Emergencies

Nosebleed (Epistaxis)

Another name for nosebleed is **epistaxis**. The following skill gives the basic steps for treating a nosebleed.

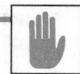

Nursing Skill
Giving First Aid for Nosebleed

Supplies and Equipment

Gloves
Cold compresses
Gauze

Procedure

1. Have the person sit down and lean forward slightly. If this position is not possible because of other injuries, have the person lie down, keeping head and shoulders elevated. *(Rationale: The head should be above the heart, to reduce pressure.)*
2. Apply pressure to the nostrils or the bridge of the nose with the thumb and forefinger, for 5 to 10 minutes, without releasing the pressure. *(Rationale: This location will put pressure on some of the blood vessels supplying the nose. Releasing the pressure too soon will allow the clot to break loose and bleeding will resume.)*
3. Place cold compresses on the nose and face. *(Rationale: Cold slows circulation to the area.)*
4. If bleeding continues, place small, clean pieces of gauze in one or both nostrils. Do not use cotton. *(Rationale: Cotton could stick to the bleeding area.)* Reapply pressure.
5. Apply pressure above the upper lip if the person is conscious. *(Rationale: To cut off some of the blood supply.)*
6. Seek medical assistance if bleeding is not controlled. *(Rationale: Continued bleeding may be a symptom of a more serious disorder and may also become life threatening.)*

> ### Nursing Alert
>
> If the person has a fractured skull, *do not attempt to stop the bleeding*, because this could cause an increase in ICP. In the case of severe hypertension, a nosebleed may be the body's safety valve against a cerebrovascular accident.

Fainting

Fainting is caused by an insufficient supply of blood and oxygen to the brain. Extreme hunger or tiredness, or being in a close, crowded, or smoky environment that is oxygen deprived can cause a person to faint. Fainting can occur as a result of emotional shock. Severe hemorrhage, excruciating pain, and standing in one place for a prolonged period of time, especially with the knees locked, are other causes.

The symptoms of imminent fainting are dizziness, blackness or spots before the eyes, pallor, and excessive perspiration. The person loses consciousness, the pulse is weak, and the breathing is shallow. The following skills can be used on the person who has fainted or who feels faint.

Nursing Skill
Giving First Aid for Fainting

Procedure

1. When someone complains of feeling faint, have the person sit or lie down and bend the head forward between the knees. Maintain the person in this position. *(Rationale: When the head is lower than the heart, more blood is carried to the brain.)*
2. Loosen tight clothing. *(Rationale: Tight clothing can restrict breathing, further reducing the amount of oxygen carried to the brain.)*
3. When the person has regained consciousness, help them to rise slowly, first to a sitting and then to a standing position. *(Rationale: The person may feel weak and could fall. A more serious condition could exist.)*
4. Do not allow the person to move until he or she has fully regained consciousness. *(Rationale: The altered LOC may be due to a more serious condition, such as a skull fracture, a concussion, cerebral hemorrhage, or shock.)*

Hemorrhage

When a blood vessel is cut or torn, blood escapes and bleeding occurs. The amount of bleeding depends on the number and size of the injured blood vessels. A great deal of blood can be lost if bleeding is excessive before clotting occurs.

If the bleeding is abundant or uncontrollable, the condition is known as hemorrhage. A severe injury to one large blood vessel can cause a serious hemorrhage; an injury to many small vessels or capillaries can cause an equally life-threatening hemorrhage.

Stopping severe bleeding is essential to life in an emergency situation. The most important first aid treatment, then, is to stop the bleeding. The second step is to treat shock that accompanies severe bleeding. Because blood is the chief means of transmission of human immunodeficiency virus, gloves must be worn.

The nurse quickly assesses for the type of bleeding:

♦ In bleeding from a capillary, the blood slowly oozes out of the wound.
♦ In bleeding from an artery, the blood comes in spurts with each heartbeat and is bright red or pink in color. Arterial bleeding is usually the more severe of the hemorrhages.
♦ In bleeding from a vein, the blood comes in a steady flow and is darker in color. Usually venous bleeding is minor and stops by itself unless a bleeding disorder is present.

- Internal bleeding is a major emergency and medical care is needed immediately.
- In any severe bleeding, the person should be placed on a flat surface with feet slightly elevated (unless there is a head injury).

Applying Direct Pressure

In external bleeding, clothes should be cut away to reveal the site and amount of bleeding. Direct, firm pressure is applied at the site. This will control bleeding in most injuries. The injured part is elevated, unless there is the possibility of fractures or other trauma to the area.

Applying Indirect Pressure

If direct pressure does not control hemorrhage, you may need to apply indirect pressure. This term means that the pressure is not applied directly to the wound but at a pressure point between the wound and the heart. Pressure points are illustrated in Figure 31-2. You need a firm surface to press against to cut off the flow of blood from the heart to the wound. Therefore, it is wise to choose a pressure point in which the supplying artery lies close to a bone.

If bleeding is severe enough to require use of a pressure point, maintain the pressure until medical assistance arrives. If you relieve pressure, the clot that formed may dislodge and bleeding will resume. There is also danger of embolism.

Methods of Applying Pressure

A sterile pad is placed directly over the wound. A prepared commercial adhesive bandage strip such as a Band Aid makes an adequate dressing for small cuts or scratches; these are packaged in various sizes and should be in every home medicine cabinet. Do not touch the part of a sterile dressing that covers the wound; put the dressing exactly where you want it; you cannot move it afterward without contaminating it. Be sure that the bandage or the adhesive is firm, yet not tight enough to cut off the circulation. Telfa (nonstick) pads are much less irritating on removal than conventional gauze bandages.

You can use a clean handkerchief or cloth if you do not have a sterile dressing. Press the dressing firmly on the bleeding area; then apply a firm bandage to hold the dressing in place. This should stop minor bleeding. If bleeding is more severe, a firmly rolled sterile pad can be applied under the dressing, which can be fastened securely in place. (A rolled pad allows for more pressure than a flat pad.) A dressing on an arm or leg may be fastened with an Ace-type roller bandage. Be sure that circulation is not shut off entirely. (An Ace bandage placed over the dressing may also help to control bleeding.)

An inflated blood pressure cuff or air splint can be used also to apply pressure and control bleeding.

Tourniquet. A **tourniquet** is a tie used on an extremity over a pressure point to stop bleeding. A tourniquet is used *only as a last resort.* The use of a tourniquet may mean the person will lose the limb as a result. The tourniquet must be tight enough to cut off completely the flow of blood in the artery. If it is too loose, it will only prevent the blood from flowing back through the veins and thus will increase the bleeding. The following skill outlines the use of a tourniquet.

Nursing Skill
Using a Tourniquet

Supplies and Equipment

Gloves
Piece of cloth
Small object such as a pencil or stick
Tightly rolled firm pad

Procedure

1. Try other methods (direct and indirect pressure) first. If everything else fails and bleeding is severe, prepare to apply the tourniquet. *(Rationale: Use of a tourniquet may necessitate later amputation of the limb.)*
2. Place a compact, rolled piece of material over the pressure point of the artery controlling the blood flow to the injury. Wind the tourniquet over this pad. *(Rationale: This applies pressure.)*
3. Tie a half knot at the side of the limb, place a stick or similar object over it, and tie a square knot over the stick. Twist the stick tightly enough to control bleeding. *(Rationale: The tourniquet has to be tight enough to inhibit bleeding.)*
4. Secure the stick firmly. *(Rationale: The tourniquet can loosen if not secure.)*
5. Do not cover the tourniquet; it should be in full view. *(Rationale: Medical personnel have to know it is there. If not, it could remain in place too long and severe damage could occur to the limb.)*
6. Do not loosen the tourniquet without a physician's order. *(Rationale: Clots may form, which, if dislodged, could cause embolism.)*
7. Tag the patient with a note stating the location of the tourniquet and the time of application. It is also a good idea to print a "T" on the person's forehead with a marker or lipstick. *(Rationale: It is vital for the physician to know that a tourniquet is in place. Prompt action may help to save the limb.)*
8. Keep the bleeding part immobile and elevate it if possible. *(Rationale: This action slows circulation.)*
9. Treat for shock and observe for cardiac arrest. *(Rationale: Patients with severe hemorrhage are candidates for cardiac arrest.)*
10. Transport the person to medical aid immediately. *(Rationale: Medical care is needed to save the extremity and to treat shock or other cardiovascular problems.)*

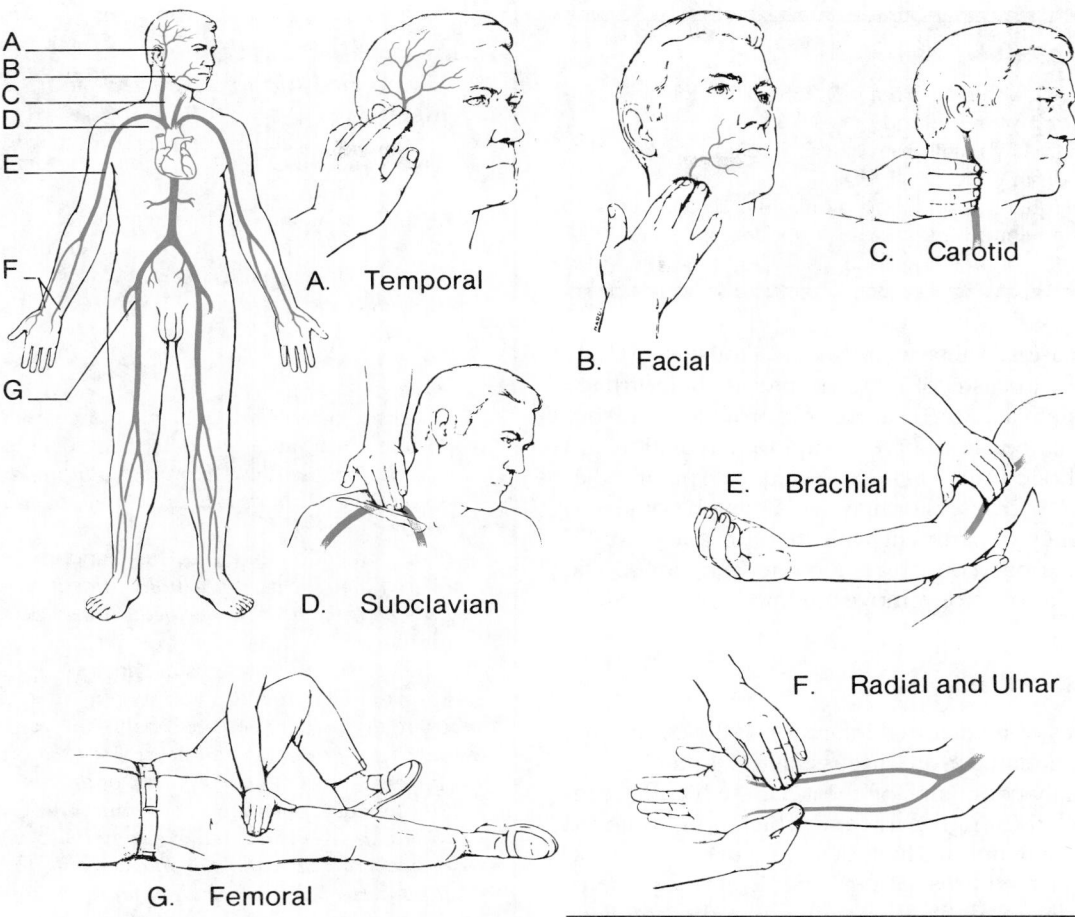

A. Temporal

B. Facial

C. Carotid

D. Subclavian

E. Brachial

F. Radial and Ulnar

G. Femoral

Figure 31-2. Pressure points for control of hemorrhage. Source: Smeltzer SC, Bare BG. Brunner and Suddarth's Textbook of Medical-Surgical Nursing, Ed 7. Philadelphia, J. B. Lippincott, 1992.

PRESSURE POINTS

Head and Neck

A *Temporal artery,* in front of the ear
B *Facial artery,* on the jawbone about 1 inch forward from the angle of the jaw
C *Carotid artery* in the neck, located beside the trachea (of questionable value for bleeding control, but may be used in an extreme emergency). **Note:** Do *not* apply pressure to both sides of the neck at the same time. (*Reason:* This would cut off the blood supply to the brain.)

Shoulder and Arm

D *Subclavian artery,* just behind the inner end of the collar bone (clavicle), exerting pressure down against the first rib
E *Brachial artery,* on the upper arm next to the body, halfway between the elbow and the shoulder

Lower Limbs

F *Radial artery,* on thumb side of wrist
G *Ulnar artery,* on little finger side of wrist
H *Femoral artery,* midway in the groin, where the artery passes over the pelvic bone

Nursing Alert

Never wipe blood clots from a wound. The clots act as plugs for ruptured blood vessels. If they break loose, death may result from external hemorrhage or from embolism.

A tourniquet should be used only in case of a life-threatening hemorrhage that does not respond to any other method of bleeding control.

MAST Trousers. Military Antishock Trousers (MAST) may be used in cases of massive internal hemorrhage or hypovolemia. MAST trousers provide pressure evenly to the body and serve to support circulation and to lessen shock (Fig. 31-3). You may see paramedics applying MAST trousers or may see a person come into the emergency department with them in place. MAST trousers are applied only by emergency personnel. The nurse never applies or removes them.

Suspected Heart Attack

The specifics of myocardial infarction (MI), commonly known as heart attack, are discussed in Chapter 74. The person usually complains of chest pain, which may radiate to the left (or right) arm and which is not relieved by rest. Other symptoms include pain radiating to back, neck, jaw, or teeth; restlessness; panic and a sense of impending death; difficulty breathing; and other signs of respiratory distress, as well as changes in pulse quality and rate. If a person has any of these symptoms, assume it is a heart attack. Call for help *immediately.*

Nursing Alert

The most frequent common denominator in heart attack is *denial.* The person cannot believe that he or she is having a heart attack.

Prompt action is the most important factor in whether a person lives or dies following an MI. First aid

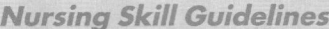

Nursing Skill Guidelines
Giving First Aid in Suspected Heart Attack (MI)

◆ Have someone call 911. *(Rationale: Prompt treatment is vital.)*
◆ Keep the person completely quiet. Do not allow the person to move about, no matter how much better he or she claims to feel. *(Rationale: Most people say they feel better. This is part of the denial system.)*
◆ Loosen any tight clothing. *(Rationale: This will make breathing easier.)*
◆ Cover the person with a blanket or coat. Put a ground cover under the person, if possible. *(Rationale: This will help to prevent chilling and shock. These complications add exertion to the already stressed heart.)*
◆ Place something under the head and upper back. *(Rationale: The person usually finds it easier to breathe if the head is elevated.)* It may be necessary for the person to sit up to breathe.
◆ If the person shows signs of shock, keep him or her flat, unless this prohibits breathing. *(Rationale: Lying flat helps to control shock.)* The person will become more panicky if he or she can't breathe, however.
◆ Be prepared to initiate CPR. *(Rationale: Cardiopulmonary arrest is a relatively common complication of heart attack. If the person can be maintained until arrival at the hospital, there is a chance of a positive outcome.)*

guidelines for a person suspected of having a heart attack are presented in the accompanying box. Emergency care for cardiopulmonary arrest is discussed and illustrated in Chapter 32.

Anaphylaxis

In a normal person, when the body senses the presence of an antigen (a substance foreign to the body), an antigen–antibody reaction occurs. This is a constant neu-

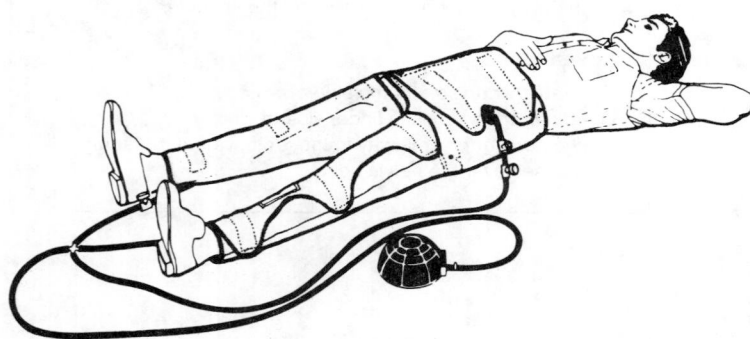

Figure 31-3. The medical antishock trouser (MAST) is a garment designed to correct internal bleeding and hypovolemia by the application of counterpressure around the legs and abdomen. This creates an artificial peripheral resistance and helps sustain coronary perfusion. It should be applied as soon as possible after injury, preferably before the patient is transferred to the emergency department. (Courtesy of David Clark Co, Inc, Worcester, MA.)

tralizing reaction that protects the person from toxins and infections. In the hypersensitive person, the antigen–antibody reaction works to the detriment of the patient. The release of chemicals, such as histamine, causes reactions affecting several body systems (systemic). This produces **anaphylaxis** (anaphylactic shock), a type I allergic reaction to a substance, which is a life-threatening situation.

Anaphylaxis is highly individualized; people can be hypersensitive to almost any substance. Common triggers for anaphylaxis, however, include:

♦ Bee stings
♦ Certain foods (such as peanuts and chocolate)
♦ Food additives or preservatives (such as sulfite)
♦ Medications (such as antibiotics)
♦ Chemicals
♦ Inhaled substances

Signs and symptoms of anaphylactic shock are given in the Keys to Nursing Assessment. The level of consciousness (LOC) of the person is also significant in anaphylaxis. The patient will be restless and panicky and may faint or have a seizure. Loss of consciousness often occurs early in the process if the anaphylaxis is severe. The time range for an allergic reaction is from a few seconds to several hours. The reactions are often generalized and violent. Each occurrence is more serious than the last. People who have severe allergies should carry medication such as IM epinephrine with them at all times. Their friends and relatives should be taught how to administer the medication in an emergency. Medications are listed in the accompanying box.

First aid care begins with securing an open airway. The EMS system is activated immediately. Ask the person if appropriate medication is available. If so,

the person may need assistance in administering this.

Animal Bites

Every year many people, particularly children, are bitten by domestic or wild animals. **Rabies** is a communicable disease that can be transmitted by an animal bite. Rabies is caused by a specific virus (*rhabdovirus*) that travels along the nerves to the spinal cord and brain. If untreated, it almost always is fatal. A specific **antidote** (a substance that neutralizes poisons) for rabies is available. The antidote is painful and expensive. Attempts are made to isolate and examine the animal because if it is not diseased, the injections are not needed.

After a person is bitten, the wounds are cleansed with warm, soapy water and rinsed thoroughly. Cleanse with Zephiran or alcohol. **Debride** (cut away) loose tissue. Flush with sterile normal saline if the wound is a puncture wound. Tetanus vaccine and antibiotics may be given to prevent infection. If injections are needed, *do not delay.* Follow the specific manufacturer's instructions for the type of serum used.

Obtain an accurate description of the animal and the circumstances. The law requires reporting the occurrence to the Public Health Department authorities and police.

Poisoning and Drug Overdose

A substance that affects health or threatens life when absorbed into the body or in contact with the surface is defined as a **poison**. Poisonous substances exist in abundance and are found in such substances as household cleaning agents, insecticides, antifreeze, furniture polish, kerosene, and nail polish. Accidental poisoning is a particular danger to children. The guidelines outline first aid care in poison-

ing. An additional box lists key medications used as antidotes in poisoning.

Nursing Skill Guidelines
Giving First Aid in Poisoning or Overdose

◆ Call for help: 911. *(Rationale: The treatment for poisoning depends on the poison ingested. You will need expert assistance.)*
◆ After calling 911, contact the nearest Poison Control Center. In some EMS areas, 911 dispatchers can connect the call to the Poison Control Center and monitor the call. *(Rationale: The Poison Control Center can instruct the first aid person in proper treatment. In some cases, vomiting is induced; in other csaes, this would cause more damage.)*
◆ Identify the poison. Question the person, if possible. Save all vomitus, urine, or stools and the remains of food or drugs that may have been responsible. Look for medication bottles or other containers. All of these materials should be brought to the medical facility with the person. *(Rationale: It is important to determine the nature and amount of poison or drug taken.)*
◆ Use your sense of smell to detect the odor of alcohol on the person's breath. *(Rationale: Many drugs are more dangerous when combined with alcohol. This could give you a clue to the seriousness of the patient's condition.)*
◆ In cases of suspected overdose, ask questions of the person and the family. Was this a suicide attempt or an accident? Was there a suicide note? Was the patient depressed or despondent? How many pills or how much alcohol was taken? *(Rationale: This information will be important to the medical team in planning emergency treatment and continuing medical care.)*
◆ Give supportive care. Keep the person warm. U[se] artificial ventilation if the person is having diffic[ulty] breathing. Maintain the heartbeat. If possible, k[eep] the person awake. Follow basic life support pro[ce]dures if CPR is needed. *(Rationale: This is a m[edi]cal emergency. It is important to maintain the [per]son in the most stable condition possible until [arri]val at the hospital.)*
◆ Follow the instructions of the Poison Control [Cen]ter. *(Rationale: They are the experts in treatm[ent of] poisoning or overdose.)*
◆ If syrup of ipecac or activated charcoal are pr[e]scribed, follow specific instructions. Do not g[ive ei]ther of these unless told to do so by the Pois[on] Control Center. *(Rationale: In some cases, yo[u may] be instructed to make the person vomit and [in] other cases, this would be very dangerous.)*

Nursing Alert
Never make the person who has ingested poison vomit unless specifically instructed to do so.

All drugs are potential poisons, but many do not have poisonous effects because they are given in small doses. Poisoning may be the result of misreading the label on a drug or taking a drug from an unlabeled bottle or from a medicine cupboard in the dark. Overdose of a drug may be accidental or intentional (as a suicide attempt).

Food Poisoning

Food poisoning is almost always caused by eating contaminated food. The normal action of bacteria on food causes decomposition, which causes the formation of **toxins** (poisonous substances). Other causes include the accidental eating of certain fruits, berries, or vegetables (eg, toadstools) that contain substances poisonous to humans.

The symptoms of food poisoning include abdominal pain, nausea, vomiting, and diarrhea. The onset is acute (within a few hours after eating the contaminated food).

Key Medications
in Poisoning and Drug Overdose

◆ All-purpose antidote: *activated charcoal* (Actidose-Aqua, Charcocaps)
◆ Emetic (causes vomiting): *syrup of ipecac*
◆ Acetaminophen overdose: *acetylcystine* (Mucomyst)

Nursing Considerations

◆ These medications are never combined.
◆ Activated charcoal and syrup of ipecac should be available to all first aid personnel and in every home medicine cabinet.
◆ The first bowel movement will be black with activated charcoal.
◆ Syrup of ipecac is an **emetic**; it induces vomiting. It should not be given if the patient is unresponsive, inebriated, having seizures, or in severe shock. It should not be given after ingestion of caustic substances (which would irritate the throat again when being vomited) or of volatile substances, such as gasoline (which could be easily aspirated into the lungs).

The symptoms usually disappear in 1 or 2 days, after the toxins have been excreted.

A more severe form of food poisoning is called botulism. This is caused by the specific organism *Clostridium botulinum*. About half of the cases result in death. Home-canned foods that have been improperly sterilized are a common cause. The symptoms of botulism are progressive: weakness, headache, muscular weakness, paralysis of the eye and the throat muscles, and finally, respiratory paralysis. Specific antitoxins are effective if given early. Rescue breathing is essential until the antitoxin takes effect.

> ### Key Concept
>
> In an emergency, use common sense and call quickly for emergency medical assistance.

Keys for Review

Key Questions for Critical Thinking

1. A motorcyclist has been hit by a car. Describe the scene and actions to be taken by persons on the scene. Give rationale for your answers. Discuss Universal Precautions and Body Substance Precautions in relationship to the accident scene.
2. An alcoholic street person is suffering from frostbite. Describe the actions to be taken and give rationale.
3. Discuss the differences among heat cramps, heat exhaustion, and heat stroke. Describe the emergency care for each and give rationale.
4. Discuss hemorrhage and emergency care. Differentiate between direct and indirect pressure. Give examples of each and describe methods of applying pressure for the examples you have given.

Key Readings

American Red Cross. Standard First Aid. New York, American Red Cross, 1988

Craven RF, Hirnle CJ. Fundamentals of Nursing: Human Health and Function. Philadelphia, J.B. Lippincott, 1992

Hafen BQ, Karren KJ. Prehospital Emergency Care and Crisis Intervention, Ed 3. Englewood Cliffs, NJ, Morton Series, Prentice Hall, 1992

Key Readings (continued)

Henry MD, Marck C, Stapleton ER. Prehospital Care. Philadelphia, W.B. Saunders, 1992

Smeltzer SC, Bare BG. Brunner and Suddarth's Textbook of Medical-Surgical Nursing, Ed 7. Philadelphia, J.B. Lippincott, 1992

Taylor C, Lillis C, LeMone P. Fundamentals of Nursing: The Art and Science of Nursing Care, Ed 2. Philadelphia, J.B. Lippincott, 1993

Thomas CL, ed. Taber's Cyclopedic Medical Dictionary, Ed 17. Philadelphia, F.A. Davis, 1993

Keys to Learning More

Chapter 32: sudden death and CPR

Chapter 38: signs and symptoms of injury

Chapter 42: vital signs

Chapter 48: bandages and binders

Chapter 50: physical examination and nursing assessment

Chapter 52: patient comfort and pain management

Chapter 65: trauma care as related to the younger child

Unit Fourteen: trauma to body systems in adults

32 Sudden Death and Cardiopulmonary Resuscitation

Keys for Learning

Learning Objectives

- Define sudden death and stage steps in dealing with it.
- Differentiate between clinical death and biologic death.
- State the ABCs of basic life support.
- Demonstrate the ability to perform rescue breathing.
- Perform the steps in CPR for one rescuer and for two rescuers.
- Demonstrate the ability to perform CPR on a child and on an infant.
- Demonstrate the abdominal thrust maneuver on a conscious patient, on an unconscious patient, and on yourself.
- Describe the differences in management of obstructed airway in an adult, a child, and an infant.
- State the procedure for calling a code in your health-care facility.

Key Terms

abdominal thrust

advanced cardiac life support

basic cardiac life support

biologic death

cafe coronary

cardiopulmonary resuscitation

clinical death

external chest compression

intubation

recovery position

rescue breathing

stridor

sudden death

sudden infant death syndrome

Keys to Understanding This Chapter

Chapter 21: the circulatory system

Chapter 22: the respiratory system

Chapter 31: general first aid assessment and procedures

Key Points

- Citizens (and particularly nurses) should know how to perform CPR in an emergency.
- Follow the ABC routine to evaluate the status of the patient and the need for resuscitation.
- It is impossible to do rescue breathing if the airway is blocked.
- The nurse is with the patient much of the time in the healthcare facility. Therefore, the nurse may be in the position to recognize and deal with cardiopulmonary arrest.
- The nurse has a responsibility to be trained in CPR and to keep up with the changes made in the techniques.

Key Topics Outline

Sudden Death and Life Support
  Basic Cardiac Life Support
  Advanced Cardiac Life Support
One-Rescuer CPR
  A Airway
  B Breathing
  C Circulation
Two-Rescuer CPR
  When CPR Is in Progress
  When CPR Is Not in Progress
Sudden Death and Basic Life Support in Children
  Sudden Death in Infants
  Differences in CPR for Children
Airway Obstruction
Assisting the Code Team

In Chapter 31 you learned the principles for emergency care and how to provide care in specific emergencies. This chapter goes a step further in describing the basics of cardiopulmonary resuscitation (CPR) and basic life support (BLS). To learn the detailed methods used in CPR, you need to take a specific course. Refresher courses are required every 2 years.

Sudden Death and Life Support

Sudden death takes place any time breathing and the heartbeat stop abruptly or unexpectedly. Causes of sudden death may include the following:

◆ Electrocution, severe electric shock
◆ Drowning, near drowning
◆ Anaphylaxis (severe allergic reaction)
◆ Drug overdose
◆ Poisoning
◆ Shock
◆ Myocardial infarction (heart attack)
◆ Stroke (cerebrovascular accident)
◆ Total airway obstruction or suffocation
◆ Adverse reaction to general anesthesia

There are two definitions for death: clinical and biologic. **Clinical death** occurs when breathing and the heartbeat stop. This type of sudden death may be reversible with prompt action by people trained in basic and advanced life support; a person often can be resuscitated. The term **biologic death** refers to permanent damage of brain cells due to lack of oxygen. Biologic death is final.

Basic Cardiac Life Support

Basic life support, also called **basic cardiac life support** (BCLS), includes rapid entry into the emergency medical services (EMS) system, performance of CPR, and use of techniques to clear an obstructed airway.

CPR is a technique that artificially supports circulation and ventilation (breathing) in a victim of cardio-

Key Abbreviations and Acronyms

ABC	airway, breathing, circulation
ACLS	advanced cardiac life support
BCLS	basic cardiac life support
AHA	American Heart Association
BLS	basic life support
CPR	cardiopulmonary resuscitation
EMS	emergency medical services (system)
EMT	emergency medical technician
SIDS	sudden infant death syndrome

pulmonary arrest. It helps to provide oxygen to the brain, heart, lungs, and other organs until advanced life support can be given.

CPR must be performed immediately after cardiac and respiratory arrest. If CPR is not begun immediately, sudden death will result in biologic death. The American Heart Association and the American Red Cross have established guidelines for CPR. Changes are made in CPR guidelines as new medical and emergency techniques are developed. Healthcare workers are expected to keep abreast of the latest techniques. Basic techniques are described in this chapter.

Nursing Alert

A one-way filtered breathing mask should be used for CPR, whenever possible, to protect the rescuer.

Advanced Cardiac Life Support

Emergency medical technicians, paramedics, and many nurses are trained in **advanced cardiac life support** (ACLS) techniques. Advanced cardiac life support includes starting intravenous lines, administering fluids and drugs, using defibrillation and cardiac monitoring, administering drug therapy and oxygen, and opening and maintaining the airway (sometimes by inserting a tube into the person's trachea, which is called **intubation**).

The nurse or professional rescue person will work under the supervision of a physician at the scene or will have standing orders previously established by a physician. If you do not have such orders, you must function as a *lay rescuer* or first aid person at the scene of an accident or sudden death.

One-Rescuer CPR

Emergencies create high anxiety levels. The person giving CPR must remain calm and remember the steps. One method used to recall the steps in BLS is referred to as the ABCs of BLS. Each phrase begins with an assessment of the person's response. If the person does not respond, steps are continued. The phases are as follows:

- ◆ **A** Airway
  - ◆ Assess for response.
  - ◆ Call for help.
  - ◆ Position the person.
  - ◆ Open the airway.
- ◆ **B** Breathing
  - ◆ Assess for breathing.
  - ◆ Manage an obstructed airway if necessary.
  - ◆ Perform rescue breathing.
- ◆ **C** Circulation
  - ◆ Assess for pulse.
  - ◆ Perform external chest compressions.

The following discussion of the one-rescuer method of CPR uses the method for adults and children older than 8 years. The techniques for CPR differ somewhat in infants and young children. Infants and children are discussed later in this chapter. Although this section is broken up into the ABCs and several skills and procedures, when CPR actually is performed, everything flows together.

A Airway

Determine Responsiveness

To establish unresponsiveness, shake the person's shoulder and shout, "Are you okay?" If the person does not respond, continue in the steps.

Activate the Emergency Medical Services System

Activate the EMS system immediately after unresponsiveness is determined. The number to call in most communities is 911. The person who calls should have basic information related to exact location, what hap-

pened, how many people need help, the person's condition, and what kind of aid is being given.

Position the Person

If the injured person may have sustained a back or neck injury, he or she must not be moved until help comes. In other situations, the person must be supine on a hard surface if you are to perform CPR. If the person is lying face down, the person performing CPR (called the rescuer) rolls the person over as a unit (head, shoulders, and torso rolling simultaneously). The rescuer should be at the person's side.

Open the Airway

The Jaw-Thrust Method. If the nurse has reason to believe that there may be a neck injury, the jaw-thrust method should be used to open the airway. This is done by positioning the hands at the angles of the person's jaw. The jaw is displaced forward while tilting the head backward. This usually can be accomplished without extending the neck. The head should be supported without moving it from side to side.

If ventilation is unsuccessful in this case, tilt the head back slightly. This should open the airway and effect ventilation.

The Head-Tilt Chin Lift. If there is no evidence of head or neck trauma, the nurse opens the airway by way of the head-tilt chin lift. The rescuer's hand closest to the person's head is placed on the person's forehead, pressing back and down. The fingers of the other hand are placed under the bony part of the patient's chin to lift it up, while pushing back and down with the top hand. This method makes the mouth-to-mouth seal easier to maintain for CPR.

Nursing Alert

The tongue is the most common cause of obstructed airway in an unconscious victim. In many cases all that is needed is to open the patient's airway to restore breathing.

The Finger Sweep. Any foreign matter, vomitus, or liquids should be removed from the person's airway before resuscitation can begin. In many cases removing the foreign body will restore breathing. If a foreign body can be seen in the mouth, it should be removed with the fingers; wear gloves whenever possible when attempting this. Such finger sweeps are performed *only on an unconscious person*. If a foreign body is strongly suspected but cannot be seen, abdominal thrusts may result in moving or dislodging it so that it is more accessible for removal. (Procedures for managing obstructed airways are presented later.)

Nursing Skill
Performing the Finger Sweep

Procedure

1. Don gloves. *(Rationale: This protects you.)*
2. With the person face up, perform the *tongue-jaw lift.* Open the mouth by grasping the tongue and lower jaw between your thumb and fingers and lifting. *(Rationale: This draws the tongue from the back of the throat and away from the foreign body.)* The obstruction may be partially relieved by this maneuver.
3. If you are unable to open the mouth with the tongue-jaw lift, the crossed-finger technique may be used. Open the mouth by crossing the index finger and thumb and pushing the teeth apart. *(Rationale: The mouth must be opened so the finger sweep can be done.)*
4. Insert the index finger of your available hand along the inside of the cheek and deeply into the throat to the base of the tongue. A hooking motion is used to dislodge the foreign body and maneuver it into the mouth for removal. Occasionally, it is necessary to use the index finger to push the foreign body against the opposite side of the throat to dislodge and lift it. *(Rationale: All maneuvers attempt not to force the object deeper into the airway.)*
5. If the foreign body comes within reach, grasp it and remove it. *(Rationale: It is important to remove the foreign body as quickly and completely as possible.)*

> ### Nursing Alert
> Do not finger sweep a child's mouth. It is likely to cause complications.

B Breathing

Determine Breathlessness

To assess absence or presence of breathing, the nurse's ear should be placed near the person's nose and mouth while holding the airway in an open position. Several procedures are used to determine if the person is breathing:

◆ Look at the chest to see if it rises and falls.
◆ Listen for sounds of breathing.
◆ Feel for any air exchange against your cheek.

This assessment should take 3 to 5 seconds. (Management of an obstructed airway is discussed in a separate section of this chapter.)

Perform Rescue Breathing

If the nurse determines that the person is not breathing, **rescue breathing** must be performed. In rescue breathing the person's lungs are inflated with oxygen from the rescuer.

> ### Nursing Alert
> It is important to use a one-way filtered mask whenever possible for rescue breathing. Although this chapter refers to "mouth-to-mouth" ventilation, which is used in an emergency, "mask-to-mouth" ventilation is used if a mask is available. The basic procedures are the same in either case.

Mouth-to-Mouth Ventilation. Mouth-to-mouth breathing is a quick and effective way to provide oxygen to a person. The nursing procedure for rescue breathing is given in Nursing Procedure 32-1.

Mouth-to-Nose Ventilation. If it is impossible to open a person's mouth or if an injury to the mouth makes it impossible to make a seal, the mouth-to-nose method may be necessary to replace mouth-to-mouth breathing. In this method, the hand that holds the chin gently presses and holds the mouth shut. The rescuer follows the mouth-to-mouth method but seals his or her lips over the person's nose and breathes in and out.

C Circulation

Check the Pulse

After establishing an airway and breathing for the person, the next step is to check for circulation at the carotid pulse in the neck.

The carotid pulse, rather than a peripheral pulse, is used in a rescue situation. *(Rationale: This pulse is close to the heart and is more easily found than the peripheral pulses.)* The nurse may use the femoral (groin) pulse in the hospital setting. If the patient is fully clothed, this is difficult to find.

To check the pulse, gently palpate the carotid pulse for 5 to 10 seconds, being careful not to compress the artery. (Note: If the pulse is thready, irregular, or slow, it is difficult to find.) The rescuer should avoid reaching across the patient to palpate the carotid pulse. *(Rationale: Pressure may be inadvertently placed on the trachea, obstructing the airway.)*

Take the pulse of only one carotid artery at a time. *(Rationale: Bilateral pressure on the arteries may accidentally restrict the flow of blood to the brain.)*

Resuscitate the Person Whose Heart Is Beating

Take time to do a proper assessment. If a pulse is present, ventilate the adult patient 12 times a minute or once every 5 seconds. The child should be ventilated once every 4 seconds. Continue to monitor the pulse, because it may stop. If spontaneous breathing resumes, place the victim in the **recovery position** if no trauma has been sustained or suspected. In the

Nursing Procedure 32-1

Performing Mouth-to-Mouth Rescue Breathing

Supplies and Equipment

CPR pocket mask (optional)
Gloves

Procedure

1. Position the patient's head to keep the airway open:
   a) Use the head-tilt/chin-lift maneuver.

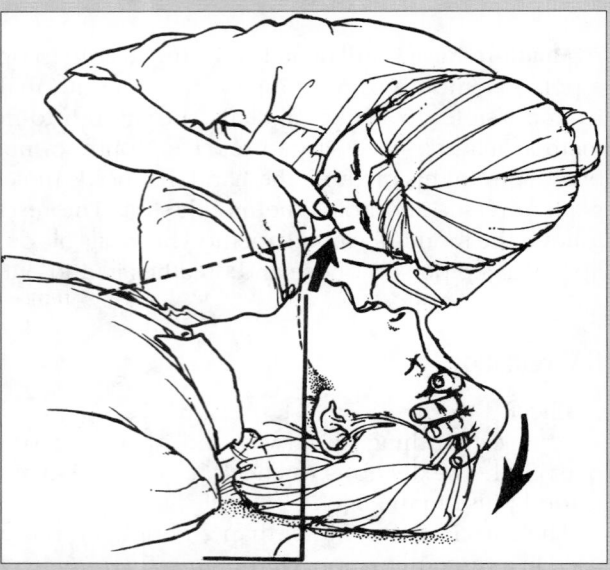

Step 1a. Using the head-tilt/chin-lift maneuver. Reprinted from Guidelines for Cardiopulmonary Resuscitation and Emergency Cardiac Care, Vol. 268, #16, October 28, 1992, p. 2187. Copyright 1992 American Medical Association.

- ◆ Place one hand on patient's forehead
- ◆ Place fingers of other hand under bony part of chin
- ◆ Apply backward pressure with palm on forehead while lifting the chin or jaw bone forward and upward with the other hand
  (Rationale: Moving the jaw forward lifts the tongue away from the back of the throat and opens the airway.)

b) Use the jaw-thrust maneuver if a neck injury is suspected.

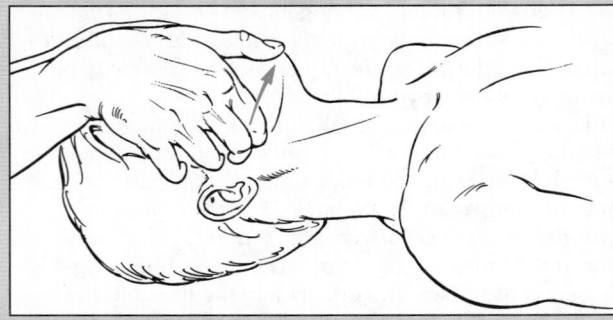

Step 1b. Using the jaw-thrust maneuver.

- ◆ Grasp the angles of the patient's lower jaw with both hands (one on each side)
- ◆ Displace the mandible forward while tilting the head backward
  (Rationale: This approach does not extend the neck, but opens the airway.)
2. Grasp the nose and pinch it closed with the fingers of the hand that is on the patient's forehead.
   (Rationale: This prevents air breathed into the patient from escaping through the nose.)
3. Take a deep breath and create an airtight seal with the lips around the outside of the patient's mouth.
   (Rationale: This seal prevents air from escaping that is breathed into the patient's mouth by the rescuer.)

(continued)

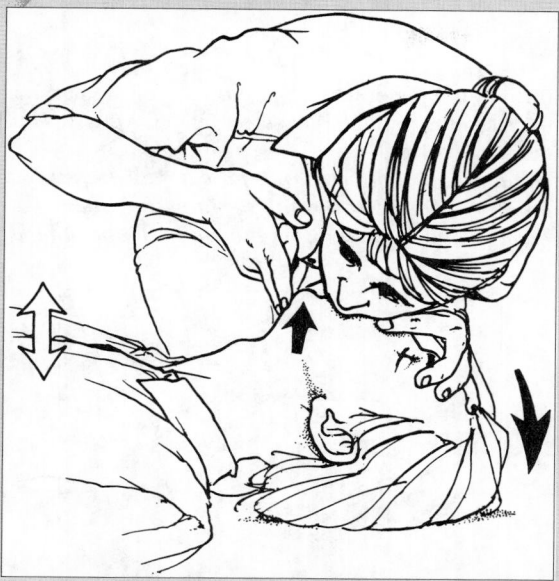

Step 3. Performing mouth-to-mouth breathing. Reprinted from Cardiopulmonary Resuscitation. Washington D.C.: American Red Cross 1981:25. Courtesy of the American Red Cross. All rights reserved in all countries.

4. Give two full breaths while watching for the patient's chest to rise. Each breath should take from 1 to 1 ½ seconds.
   (*Rationale: Adequate time provides good chest expansion and decreases the possibility of gastric distention.*)
5. Allow the patient to exhale passively between breaths.
   (*Rationale: The weight of the patient's chest and pressure within the chest aid in expelling the air.*)
6. Continue rescue breathing at the rate of 10 to 12 breaths per minute.
   (*Rationale: The exhaled air of rescuer breaths contains enough oxygen to support the life of the victim when delivered at this rate.*)
7. If first attempt at ventilation is unsuccessful, reposition the patient's head and try again.
   (*Rationale: Improper positioning of the airway can cause difficulty in ventilating the patient. The most common cause of airway obstruction is the patient's tongue; repositioning will help to move the tongue out of the way.*)
8. Use obstructed airway techniques to open the airway if ventilations are still not possible after repositioning.
   (*Rationale: Rescue breathing will be ineffective if airway is obstructed.*)

recovery position, the person is rolled onto the side moving the head, shoulders, and torso simultaneously without twisting.

Perform External Chest Compressions

If the heart is stopped, **external chest compressions** must be applied. These actions are listed in Nursing Procedure 32-2.

Two-Rescuer CPR

Nurses should learn the techniques of two-person CPR. In the hospital setting, the nurse often works as part of a team, with specialists establishing airways and providing ventilation for the patient and nurses and other healthcare providers giving chest compressions. Two-person CPR is less tiring than single-rescuer CPR; thus, it can be continued longer. Outside the hospital setting, the nurse may work with EMS personnel who are trained in two-person CPR techniques.

When CPR Is in Progress

When a second person comes to assist with CPR, it is important that the transition be made smoothly. The second person should enter after a cycle is complete and the pulse is checked by the first person. The new cycle begins with a ventilation by the first person and the compressions by the second person.

Taking Over from a Lay Rescuer. When two nurses take over CPR from one lay rescuer, allow the lay rescuer to complete a cycle of 15-minute compressions and two ventilations. Then one nurse goes to the patient's head, opens the airway, and checks for the pulse, while the other nurse locates the proper hand position for external chest compressions. This should take 5 seconds. The two rescuers then begin a new cycle of chest compressions and ventilations.

Roles of Two Rescuers. If no pulse is found, the *ventilator* gives one breath and the *compressor* begins external chest compressions at the rate of 80 to 100 compressions per minute, counting "one and, two and, three and, four and, five"; the ratio is five compressions to one ventilation.

At the end of each fifth compression, the compressor pauses to allow the ventilator to give one ventilation. The ventilation is given slowly, allowing 1 to 1½ seconds. The pause may be shorter if the patient is intubated with an endotracheal tube or if the airway is protected by an esophageal obturator airway or endotracheal tube.

Administering External Chest Compressions (Adult)

Supplies and Equipment

Hard surface (ground, floor, or board may be used)
Gloves

Procedure

1. Remove patient's clothing and locate the body landmarks before beginning external chest compressions:
   a) Kneel at the patient's side.
   b) Slide the index and middle finger of the hand nearest the patient's feet along the patient's lower rib margin closest to the rescuer.
   c) Move toward the center and locate the notch where the ribs meet the sternum.
   d) Place the middle finger on notch with the index finger next to it on the lower end of the sternum.
   (Rationale: Proper hand position prevents damage to the patient and is essential for effective CPR.)
2. Place the heel of the other hand on the sternum next to the fingers.
   (Rationale: This keeps the line of the force of compression on the sternum.)

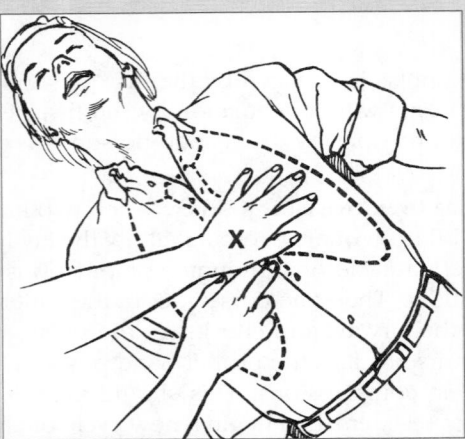

Step 2. Locating the correct hand position on the sternal notch. Reprinted from Guidelines for Cardiopulmonary Resuscitation and Emergency Cardiac Care, Vol. 268, #16, October 28, 1992, p. 2189, 2190. Copyright 1992 American Medical Association.

3. Pick up the lower hand, place on top of the hand on the sternum, and interlace these fingers with those of the hand below.
   (Rationale: Using two hands provides the pressure necessary to compress an adult sternum. Interlacing keeps them off the chest and prevents injury to the patient.)

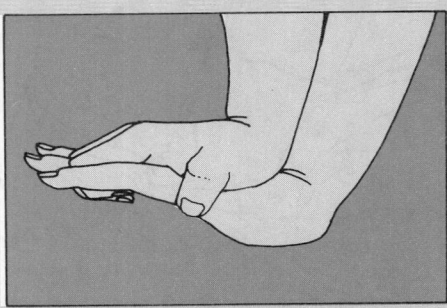

Step 3. Correct hand position for chest compression.

4. Move shoulders directly over hands while keeping arms straight and elbows locked (See Figure 32-4).
   (Rationale: This places rescuer in proper position to deliver the most force with the least amount of effort directly downward on the sternum.)

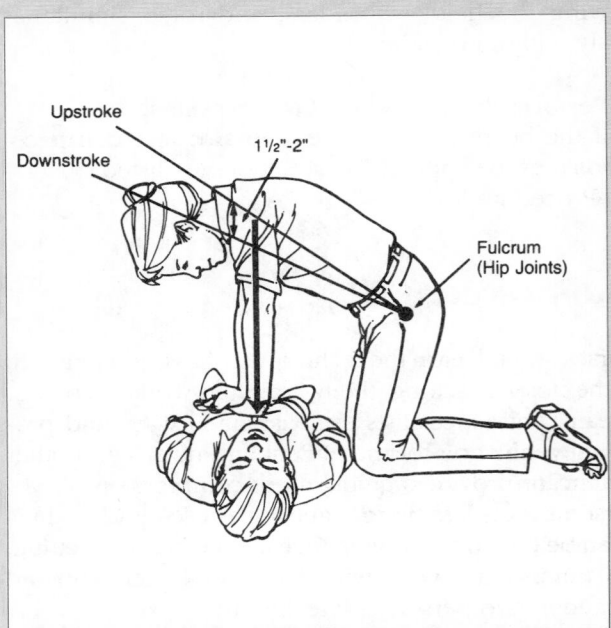

Upstroke
Downstroke
1½"-2"
Fulcrum (Hip Joints)

Step 4. Keeping shoulders over victim with fingers interlaced. Adapted with permission from Guidelines for Cardiopulmonary Resuscitation. Washington D.C.: American Red Cross 1981:25. Courtesy of the American Red Cross. All rights reserved in all countries.

(continued)

5. Using downward pressure, depress the sternum 1 ½ to 2 inches (3.8–5.1 cm).
   (Rationale: Compression on the sternum squeezes the heart between the sternum and the spine, simulating a heart contraction. Releasing the compression allows the heart to fill.)
6. Maintain a rate of 80 to 100 times a minute with a ratio of 15 compressions to 2 breaths (for one rescuer).
   (Rationale: This ratio simulates, as closely as possible, the pattern of human respiration and heartbeat.)
7. Keep hands in position on chest. Do not lift them between compressions.
   (Rationale: Correct hand position may be lost.)
8. Stop compressions and check carotid pulse after 1 minute (4 cycles of 15 compressions and 2 breaths). If pulse is not felt after 5 seconds, CPR is continued for 4 to 5 minutes before checking pulse again.
   (Rationale: It is important to deliver as much blood and oxygen to the victim as possible.)

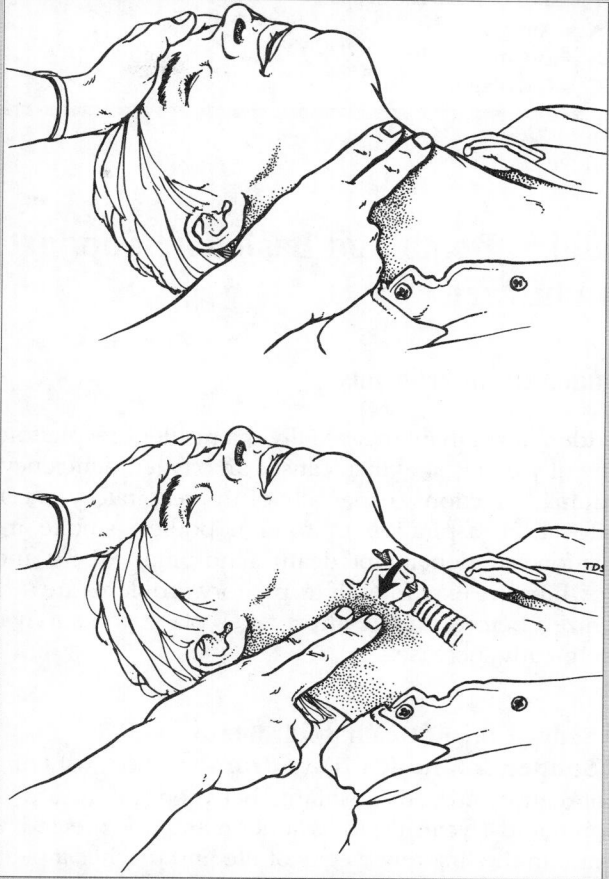

Step 8. Checking the carotid pulse. Reprinted from Guidelines for Cardiopulmonary Resuscitation and Emergency Cardiac Care, Vol. 268, #16, October 28, 1992, p. 2189, 2190. Copyright 1992 American Medical Association.

When CPR Is Not in Progress

If two nurses arrive at the same time, they assess the situation and begin care. If help has not been summoned, one nurse should make sure that the EMS has been notified. The other nurse should initiate one-person CPR.

If circumstances permit both nurses to proceed, the *first nurse* should go to the patient's head and determine unresponsiveness, open the airway, and assess breathing. If no breathing is found, that nurse should say, "No breathing" and give two ventilations. Next, the pulse is assessed for 5 to 10 seconds. If there is no pulse, the nurse should say, "no pulse." (The two rescuers should be on opposite sides of the patient for ease in reversing roles later.) The *second nurse*, at the same time, goes to the chest and locates the landmark for chest compressions, assumes the proper hand position, and begins compressions when told there is no pulse.

Changing Positions. To change positions smoothly, the compressor usually calls the signals. The compressor directs that a change be made after a five-to-one sequence. The ventilator gives a breath and moves into position to do compressions. The compressor moves up to check the pulse. If there is no pulse, he or she gives a ventilation and directs the compressor to continue CPR. If a pulse is found, this is also communicated.

Sudden Death and Basic Life Support in Children

Sudden Death in Infants

Sudden death in infants usually is a result of respiratory difficulty or arrest, which causes an oxygen deficiency. Trauma, infections (especially of the respiratory tract), suffocation, aspiration of foreign bodies, smoke inhalation, sudden infant death syndrome (SIDS), and drowning are examples. If respiratory problems are recognized before cardiac arrest takes place, the survival rate greatly increases.

Sudden Infant Death Syndrome

Sudden infant death syndrome is the most common cause of death in infants between the ages of 1 month and 1 year. Death is sudden and unexpected. It is rare in the first few weeks of life and reaches a peak incidence at 2 to 3 months; it becomes less frequent toward the latter part of the first year and is rare after 12 months. Although some high-risk factors have been identified, the cause of death is unknown. When a healthy infant is found not breathing and is successfully resuscitated with CPR, the incident is called a near-miss or aborted SIDS. These infants may be sent home with respiratory and heart rate monitors. Parents also are instructed in infant CPR.

Infant CPR

The steps in infant CPR are basically the same as for adults. Some adaptations are necessary because of the infant's smaller size. Differences are presented in Table 32-1. The steps are discussed in Nursing Procedure 32-3.

Differences in CPR for Children

Activating the Emergency Medical System. After the initial assessment, 1 minute of CPR is recommended for children before the EMS is activated.

Hand Position. The hand position for the child (ages 1–8) is similar to that for the adult. However, because the child is much smaller, only the heel of *one hand* is used to perform compressions.

External Chest Compression. Compressions are performed at the rate of 100 times a minute to a depth of 1 to 1.5 inches (2.5–3.8 cm). This is an approximate depth.

The ratio of compressions to breaths for a child is five compressions to one breath.

After 20 cycles of five compressions and one breath, (approximately 1 minute), recheck the pulse for 5 seconds. If no pulse is found, resume CPR. Recheck the pulse every few minutes.

Rescue Breathing. When the child is not breathing, but a pulse is present, only rescue breathing is performed. The child is given one breath every 3 seconds, or a rate of 20 breaths per minute.

Airway Obstruction

An airway obstructed by a foreign body will cause respiratory arrest in a short time. Anytime a person (particularly a child) becomes cyanotic, stops

Table 32-1. Differences in CPR for Adults, Children, and Infants

	Adults	*Children**	*Infant*
Pulse Location	Carotid	Carotid	Brachial
Hand Position	Find sternal notch	Find sternal notch	Line between nipples
Used for Compression	Two hands	One hand	Two to three fingers
Depth of Compression	$1\frac{1}{2}$–2 in	1–$1\frac{1}{2}$ in	$\frac{1}{2}$–1 in
Compressions Per Minute	80–100	80–100	100
Compression-to-Ventilation Ratio	15:2 (one rescuer) 5:1 (two rescuers)	5:1	5:1

* Child between 1 and 8 years old

Infant CPR

Supplies and Equipment

Hard surface (may be palm of rescuer's hand)
Gloves

Procedure

1. Assess for unresponsiveness. Call for help.
   (Rationale: This indicates need for beginning CPR.)
2. Position the baby on its back on a hard surface. Firmly support the head and neck when turning.
   (Rationale: The infant's size and the possibility of a head or neck injury require careful support and positioning.)
3. Open the airway using the head-tilt/chin-lift method. (Use the jaw thrust maneuver if a neck injury is suspected.) Avoid overextension of the head.
   (Rationale: This motion lifts the tongue away from the back of the throat and opens the airway. It is believed that the overextension of the head closes the trachea in small babies.)

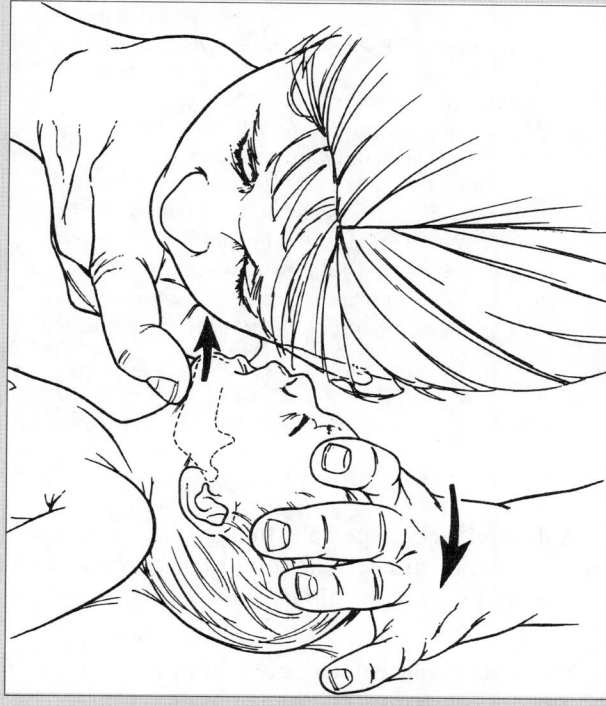

Step 3. Opening the airway. Reprinted from Guidelines for Cardiopulmonary Resuscitation and Emergency Cardiac Care, Vol. 268, #16, October 28, 1992, p. 2253-2256. Copyright 1992 American Medical Association.

4. Determine breathlessness by placing ear close to the infant's mouth and nose. Look, listen, and feel for breaths.
   (Rationale: This determines whether the infant is breathing.)
5. Seal your lips around the mouth and nose of the infant. Give two breaths (1 to 1.5 seconds for each breath). Allow deflation between breaths. Observe the rise and fall of the chest.
   (Rationale: A tight seal prevents the escape of air. Volume that is appropriate causes the chest to rise and fall. Giving the breaths slowly avoid gastric distention.)

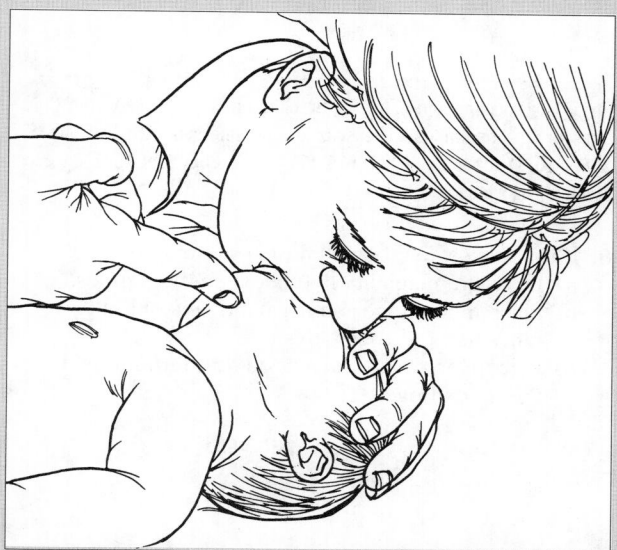

Step 5. Breathing with an airtight seal. Reprinted from Guidelines for Cardiopulmonary Resuscitation and Emergency Cardiac Care, Vol. 268, #16, October 28, 1992, p. 2253–2256. Copyright 1992 American Medical Association.

6. If the ventilation is not successful, reposition the head and try again.
   (Rationale: Improper positioning of the airway can cause difficulty in ventilating the infant.)
7. Assess circulation by feeling for a pulse in the brachial artery (in the upper arm) for 5 seconds.
   (Rationale: The short, chubby neck of the infant makes it difficult to palpate the carotid pulse.)

(continued)

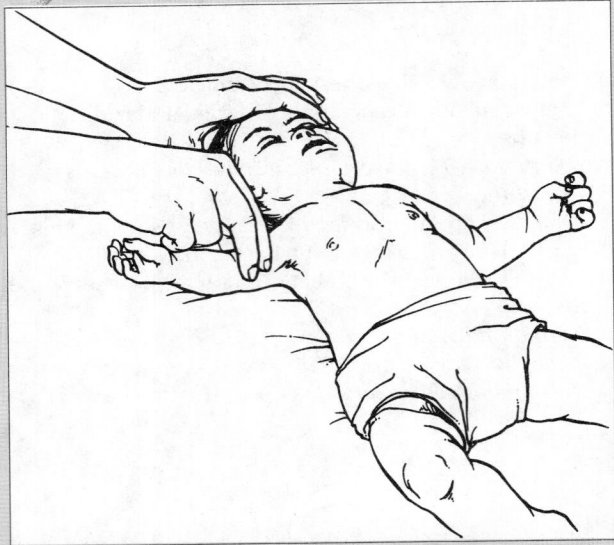

Step 7. Locating and palpating brachial pulse. Reprinted from Guidelines for Cardiopulmonary Resuscitation and Emergency Cardiac Care, Vol. 268, #16, October 28, 1992, p. 2253–2256. Copyright 1992 American Medical Association.

8. If no pulse is felt, begin chest compressions:
    a) Draw an imaginary line between the nipples.
    b) Place index finger on the hand closest to the infant's feet just below this line.
    c) Place 1 or 2 more fingers on the sternum next to the index finger.

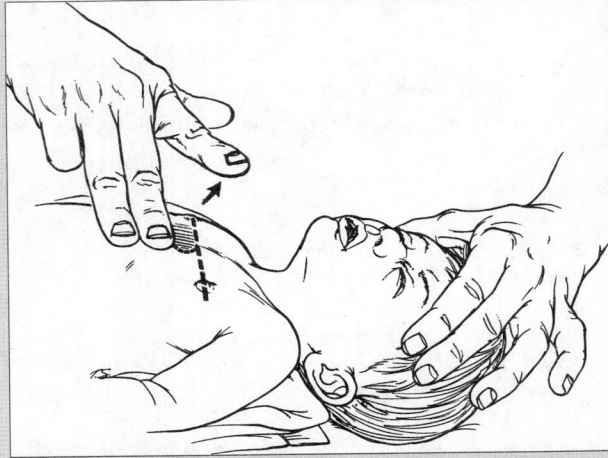

Step 8c. Locating finger position for chest compressions in an infant. Reprinted from Guidelines for Cardiopulmonary Resuscitation and Emergency Cardiac Care, Vol. 268, #16, October 28, 1992, p. 2253–2256. Copyright 1992 American Medical Association.

d) Using these fingers, compress the sternum ½ to 1 inch (1.3–2.5 cm) at a rate of at least 100 times per minute.
    (Rationale: This ensures proper placement for chest compression in the infant. Overcompression can damage the infant's heart. The infant's heart rate is faster than that of a child or adult.)

9. At the end of every fifth compression, pause to deliver a ventilation. Maintain a 5:1 compression/ventilation ratio for the infant. Reassess the infant after 10 cycles (approximately 1 minute) and every few minutes thereafter. Continue CPR if no pulse is present.
    (Rationale: External chest compressions and rescue breathing deliver as much blood and oxygen to the infant as possible.)

breathing, and collapses for no apparent reason, an obstructed airway should be suspected. It is important for the nurse to recognize this situation and take proper action.

Causes of Obstruction

In adults, the foreign body obstruction is usually caused by large pieces of food becoming lodged in the airway. Meat is the most common cause. The obstruction may be complete, with no air exchange. It also may be partial, with either a good air exchange or poor air exchange. Poorly fitting dentures and ingestion of alcohol also are associated with obstructed airways.

Although food, especially meat, is the most common cause of an obstructed airway in adults, children may choke on a variety of things.

The "Cafe Coronary." Obstruction of the airway often occurs in restaurants. The person is embarrassed by the incident and often leaves the table. The nurse should be highly suspicious of the person who may have been coughing and gasping, now looks frightened, and suddenly leaves the table. Follow the person, and ask if they are choking. If this person is allowed to go off alone, he or she may die. This is so common an occurrence that it is called a **cafe coronary.** The patient leaves the table, goes to the restroom, and is found not breathing and without a heartbeat (an apparent heart attack victim).

Partially Obstructed Airway

The patient with a partially obstructed airway with good air exchange will cough forcefully. Wheezing may be present, but adequate air exchange is obvious. Encourage the patient to cough. *Do not interfere* with attempts to expel the obstruction, and do not leave the person. Offer encouragement and continue to monitor the person. If the person's condition does not rapidly improve, activate the EMS.

Poor air exchange may be identified by ineffective coughing and sometimes by high-pitched wheezing sounds called **stridor.** The patient will experience increasing respiratory difficulty and may become cyanotic.

In a *complete airway obstruction*, the person will be unable to talk, breathe, or cough. The person may even indicate the condition by using the universal signal for choking. This involves clutching the neck between the fingers and thumbs of both hands. The nurse should ask the patient, "Are you choking?" In complete airway obstruction, no oxygen enters the lungs. The patient will soon become unconscious unless the obstruction is removed.

Administering Heimlich Maneuver

Heimlich maneuver, also called **abdominal thrusts,** is used in complete airway obstruction. The procedure may be used for a conscious or unconscious person and for an adult or child. The nursing skills for administering the Heimlich maneuver are given here.

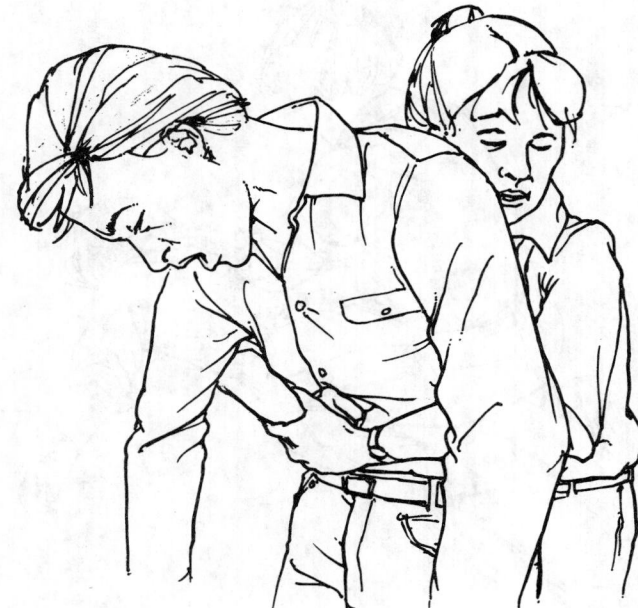

Figure 32-1. Heimlich maneuver administered to conscious victim of foreign-body airway obstruction who is sitting or standing. Reprinted from Guidelines for Cardiopulmonary Resuscitation and Emergency Cardiac Care, Vol. 268, #16, October 28, 1992, p. 2193. Copyright 1992 American Medical Association.

Nursing Skill
Administering Heimlich Maneuver (Abdominal Thrusts)

Procedure

Conscious Person

1. Assess the situation. Ask the person, "Are you choking?" Determine the person's ability to talk, breathe, and cough. *(Rationale: If the person is able to talk or cough, he or she is able to breathe.)*
2. If the airway is obstructed, stand behind the person and wrap both arms around his or her waist (Fig. 32-1.) *(Rationale: This position allows you to achieve maximum leverage. You also can support the person if he or she becomes unconscious.)*
3. Make a fist with one hand, placing the thumb side of the fist (with the thumb inside the fist) against the person's abdomen in the midline, slightly above the navel and well below the xiphoid process. *(Rationale: A thrust in this area will force residual air out of the lungs.)*
4. Grasp the fist with the other hand, pressing the fist into the person's abdomen with a quick upward thrust. *(Ra-*

tionale: *This is like an artificial cough and usually forces [pops] the foreign matter out of the airway.)*
5. Repeat the thrusts until the foreign body is expelled or the person becomes unconscious. Each thrust should be a separate and distinct movement. *(Rationale: The procedure is different for an unconscious person.)*

Unconscious Person

1. Gently ease the person down as he or she slumps to the floor. *(Rationale: Do not risk personal back injury, but protect the person's head.)*
2. Have a second person call for help. *(Rationale: You will need EMS aid.)*
3. Open the airway by head-tilt, chin-lift, or jaw-thrust method. *(Rationale: Use any method that opens the airway.)*
4. If the person is not breathing, attempt rescue breathing. *(Rationale: The person needs oxygen immediately.)*
5. If you are unable to ventilate, kneel astride the adult person's thighs. *(Rationale: This puts you in position to perform abdominal thrusts.)*
6. Place the heel of one hand against the person's abdomen, in the middle, slightly above the navel, and well below the tip of the xiphoid (Fig. 32-2). Place the second hand directly on top of the first. *(Rationale: This position provides maximum pressure with minimum potential for injury to the person.)*
7. Press into the abdomen with a quick upward thrust (see Figure 32-2). *(Rationale: This usually forces the foreign matter out of the airway.)*

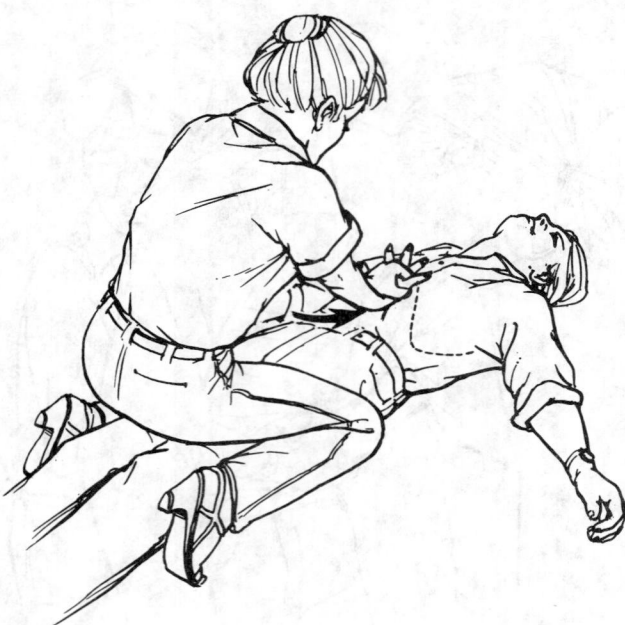

Figure 32-2. Heimlich maneuver administered to unconscious victim of foreign-body airway obstruction who is lying down. Reprinted from Guidelines for Cardiopulmonary Resuscitation and Emergency Cardiac Care, Vol. 268, #16, October 28, 1992, p. 2193. Copyright 1992 American Medical Association.

8. Repeat this thrust up to five times to clear the airway. *(Rationale: Repeated thrusts may be needed in order to move the foreign body up and out of the airway.)*
9. Open the adult's mouth, and perform finger sweep. *(Rationale: Finger sweep detects the expelled foreign body.)*
10. Attempt rescue breathing. *(Rationale: Now that the object blocking the airway is removed, the person should be able to breathe once ventilation is initiated.)*
11. If you have not found the foreign matter with the finger sweep, repeat the sequence (abdominal thrusts, finger sweep, and ventilation) as necessary until rescue personnel arrive. *(Rationale: Forceful ventilation may still enable oxygen to reach lungs despite the obstruction.)*

Nursing Alert

If the person is obese or pregnant, it may be impossible to do abdominal thrusts. In these situations only, the chest thrust may be used.

Self-Administered Abdominal Thrusts. If you act immediately, you can force a foreign object out of your own airway. The self-administered action simulates the Heimlich maneuver done by a rescuer. Several thrusts may be needed to clear the airway.

Make a fist with one hand; place the thumb side on the abdomen, above the navel and below the

xiphoid process. Grasp the fist with the other hand, and press inward and upward toward the diaphragm with a quick motion. If this is unsuccessful, press the upper abdomen quickly over any firm surface, such as the back of the chair, the side of a table, or a railing.

Obstructed Airway in Infants

A major cause of death and disability in infants is airway obstruction. Foreign bodies or infections (such as croup and inflammation of the epiglottis) may cause the obstruction. The nurse should learn to recognize the difference between an airway obstruction caused by a foreign object and one caused by swelling of the airway. Obstructed airway procedures will usually clear an airway obstructed by a foreign body, but these procedures could prove fatal if swelling is the cause. The actions for obstructed airway in infants differs from those for adults and children.

Nursing Skill
Managing an Obstructed Airway in an Infant

Procedure

1. Assess to see if the airway is obstructed. If the infant is able to cough and cry, the airway is not obstructed. *(Rationale: The child may be able to open the airway by coughing or crying. Coughing and crying indicate that air is being exchanged.)*
2. Monitor but do not attempt to remove the obstruction. *(Rationale: If the infant is exchanging air, you could drive the obstruction further into the airway and cause complete obstruction.)*
3. Call for help. *(Rationale: Trained EMS personnel should manage the airway.)*
4. If the airway is obstructed, support the infant's head and neck, holding the jaw. Hold the infant straddled on your forearm with the head lower than the body as in Figure 32-3. *(Rationale: The force of gravity will assist in removing the obstruction.)*
5. With the heel of your free hand, deliver five back blows, with force, between the infant's shoulder blades (see Figure 32-3). *(Rationale: Each blow should have the force to remove the object from the airway.)*
6. Supporting the head, sandwich the infant between your arms, and turn the infant over so he or she is face up. Keep the head lower than the trunk. *(Rationale: The infant is held between your arms to best support the body and head. The head is downward to facilitate drainage and prevent aspiration.)*
7. Deliver five chest thrusts in the same place and in the same manner as for chest compressions in an infant (but at a slower rate—3–5 seconds). Make sure your fingers are not on the tip of the sternum. *(Rationale: This will prevent further damage.)*

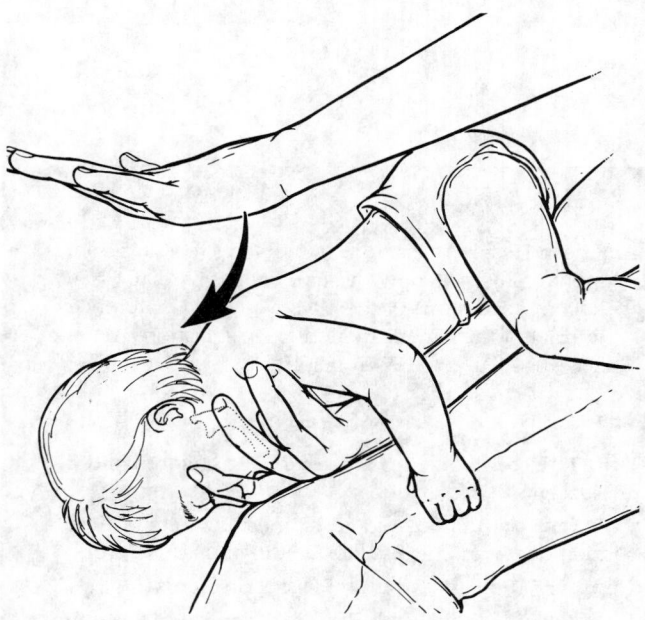

Figure 32-3. Back blows (top) and chest thrusts (bottom) to relieve foreign-body airway obstruction in the infant. Reprinted from Guidelines for Cardiopulmonary Resuscitation and Emergency Cardiac Care, Vol. 268, #16, October 28, 1992, p. 2258. Copyright 1992 American Medical Association.

8. Activate the EMS system. The infant or small child can be carried with you to the phone while you call 911. *(Rationale: EMS personnel should manage the airway.)*

9. Alternate back blows and chest thrusts (five each) until help arrives. *(Rationale: These alternating actions are usually effective in removing obstructions. Once rescue efforts are begun, they should continue until professional help is available.)*

10. Turn the infant back and forth from front to back, supporting him or her on your arm. *(Rationale: It is important to alternate back blows and chest thrusts, while preventing further injury.)*

11. Continue to attempt to ventilate between back blows and chest thrusts until the foreign body is removed and ventilation is successful. *(Rationale: The infant must be artificially ventilated until adequate oxygenation is achieved.)*

12. Check the pulse after the airway is cleared. *(Rationale: To make sure cardiac arrest has not occurred.)*

Assisting the Code Team

As soon as medical or paramedical assistance arrives, the nurse's role is to assist. If in the hospital, activate the signal for a "code" in your facility. Obtain the necessary emergency equipment: crash cart; manual breathing bag; emergency drugs; heart monitor; stethoscope; equipment for blood pressure, oxygen, intravenous (IV) line, and suctioning; and oral airways. If the resuscitation measures are successful, the pulse will be felt, the pupils will constrict, the patient's color will improve, and breathing will resume.

The patient may cough or move. If you are assisting a code team and suction is available, the patient's head should be turned to the side and suction used. Fingers should not be placed in a patient's mouth unless absolutely necessary. Always wear gloves.

Once the patient is resuscitated, a mechanical ventilator, IV therapy, or vasopressor drugs may be needed for maintenance. Until the physician decides that the person is out of danger, the patient will need to be watched closely in case another emergency resuscitation is required.

Document the entire procedure, including the time the arrest was discovered; your estimation of when the arrest occurred; the emergency measures you took; the time the code team arrived; the procedures performed from that time on; the drugs given, their dosage, and the time; the responses made by the patient; and the laboratory work done, as well as electrocardiograms, x-rays, and other tests. Finally, note the outcome of the resuscitation efforts and the subsequent nursing care if the attempt was successful.

Keys for Review

Key Questions for Critical Thinking

1. Discuss the difference between basic life support and advanced cardiac life support. Describe your responsibilities in both as a student nurse.
2. You are giving CPR to an infant. Describe how this differs from adult CPR.
3. Airway obstruction is an emergency situation. Describe common causes in infants, children, and adults. Describe how you would teach prevention to children and adults. Describe skills in managing obstructed airways in an adult and a pregnant woman.
4. A code is called in the healthcare facility where you work. Describe your responsibilities as a student nurse. As a licensed practical nurse.

Key Readings

American Heart Association. "Standards and Guidelines for Cardiopulmonary Resuscitation and Emergency Cardiac Care." Journal of the American Medical Association:2841–3044, June, 1986

Key Readings (continued)

American Heart Association. "Guidelines for Cardiopulmonary Resuscitation and Emergency Cardiac Care. Recommendations of the 1992 National Conference." Journal of the American Medical Association 268(16):2171–2302, October 1992

Keys to Learning More

Unit Thirteen: illnesses and injuries in children and adolescents

Unit Fourteen: illnesses and injuries that might cause sudden death and necessitate CPR in adults

Chapter 74: heart and blood vessel disorders

Chapter 79: respiratory disorders

Chapter 80: oxygen administration

Unit 7

The Nursing Process

33 Problem-Solving and the Nursing Process

Learning Objectives

- Review significant historical events that affected nursing as a profession.
- Define *nursing process* and state the reasons for using nursing process.
- List the problem-solving steps in the nursing process; define each step and state its place in patient care.
- List the seven steps of scientific problem-solving and the correlated steps of the nursing process.

Key Terms

North American Nursing
  Diagnosis Association
  (NANDA)
nursing process

patient-oriented care
scientific problem-solving
third-party payors
trial and error

Keys to Understanding This Chapter

Chapter 3: introduction to today's healthcare system
Chapter 4: legal and ethical aspects of nursing

Key Points

- Define key terms.
- Scientific problem-solving has been used for many years by scientists to systematize their research.
- The nursing process is built on the framework of scientific problem-solving.
- The nursing process is a systematic method that provides individualized care.

Key Points (continued)

- Steps in the nursing process include nursing assessment, nursing diagnosis, nursing planning, nursing implementation, and nursing evaluation.
- The nursing process can be used to identify not only the patient's actual problems, but also potential problems.
- The patient is involved in developing the nursing care plan.

Key Topics Outline

Problem-Solving
Historical Perspectives of Nursing Process
Nursing Process
  Steps in Nursing Process
  Characteristics of Nursing Process
  Nursing Process and Quality Care

Key Learning Activities

- Interview nurses in your healthcare facility. How are their nursing care plans developed? Are there "standard" nursing care plans for certain diagnoses to which individual patient information is added?
- Interview a person in an administrative position. What are the requirements of the Joint Commission on Accreditation of Healthcare Organizations (JCAHO) as related to the use of nursing process?

Rosdahl CB: Textbook of Basic Nursing, 6th ed. © 1995 J.B. Lippincott Company

One of the goals of nursing is to help individuals meet basic and higher level needs. When the patient and nurse meet, specific nursing behaviors result. These include communication, observation, support, education, and provision of care. Nurses support persons in their healthy habits and help patients solve problems. One of the ways in which nurses provide care is through a scientific problem-solving method known as the nursing process.

Problem-Solving

Problem-solving is a basic skill to be learned in life. It involves identifying a problem and taking steps to resolve the problem. Common sense helps us solve many problems in life.

Primitive human beings used trial and error to solve problems. **Trial and error** involves trying things (testing) and deciding which ideas work and which do not. Historical decisions about what medications to use or how to treat a person were based on trial and error. Often people died while plant berries, leaves, stalks, and roots were being tested on them.

Trial and error is still used in laboratory studies, but it is too dangerous to use in daily healthcare. It does not help the nurse determine how best to work with patients, and it is dangerous to the patient.

Science has developed a systematic means of investigating problems and arriving at solutions. This is called **scientific problem-solving**. The seven steps of scientific problem-solving are:

◆ *Gather information* relative to the problem.
◆ *Identify the problem.*
◆ *Formulate tentative solutions* (*hypotheses*); describe all possible solutions; choose preferred solutions.
◆ *Plan action* to test suggested solutions (*experiment* and observe the results).
◆ *Evaluate the solution* (*draw conclusions*); evaluate the results.
◆ *Formulate another tentative solution* if results are unsatisfactory.
◆ *Test solutions again.*

Scientific problem-solving requires both logical thinking and imagination. The person must use what has been learned from experience and must also know when a problem cannot be solved without help.

Scientific problem-solving was applied to nursing as nursing leaders and educators began a formal, critical evaluation of the purpose of nursing practice and of its traditionally intuitive nature. This application of scientific problem-solving to nursing is called **nursing process**. It is helpful to study historical perspectives in the development of nursing process before studying the process itself.

Historical Perspectives of Nursing Process

Nursing had its beginning in the simple acts of one person helping another during a time of physical or emotional need. These simple acts have evolved into a complex system known today as the *nursing profession* and involving the *nursing process*.

Early Beginnings of Nursing

When nursing first began, it reflected the ethic of "love thy neighbor" or a maternal instinct of a woman caring for the sick. No formal education for nursing existed, but learned skills were passed from generation to generation. The skills of a person practicing nursing were often based on trial and error, intuition, previous experiences, and advice of others.

Florence Nightingale's Influence

During Florence Nightingale's practice, nursing began to achieve some structure. She stressed knowledge and specific training for nurses, as well as compensation for their efforts. She also enforced specific rules, which helped to lend prestige to the profession.

Military and War Influences

Significant changes in healthcare occurred as a result of World War II (1939–1945). Clinical medicine benefited from important discoveries, such as new drugs, particularly antibiotics, that came into common use, as well as concepts of burn treatment and early ambulation following surgery. The increased demand for physicians and nurses resulted in new professions being added to the healthcare team.

The period from 1945 until the early 1960s saw rapid political and social change. The application of new scientific knowledge and technology to health and disease processes grew, and healthcare systems developed that reflected the public's awareness of health, wellness, and preventive medicine.

The Space Age

The space program has yielded many discoveries that have influenced modern medical practice. Many materials and pieces of equipment used in healthcare today were developed or discovered in the conquest of space.

Third-Party Payors

Third-party payors (such as Medicare, health maintenance organizations, and private insurance companies) require careful planning and documentation of care before they pay for it. This has greatly influenced the development of the nursing process.

Development of Nursing Process

In 1961, Ida Jean Orlando identified the nurse–client relationship and stressed deliberate nursing actions. In 1967, L. N. Knowles defined nursing that used the scientific approach as "discovery, delving, doing, and discrimination." Also in 1967, Helen Yura and Mary B. Walsh wrote the first comprehensive text describing the components of the nursing process based on the methods of scientific problem-solving.

By the 1970s most states had revised their nursing practice acts to reflect the components of nursing process, as published by the American Nurses Association in 1973. These components were called "Standards of Nursing Practice." Today state board licensing examinations test nursing knowledge about the components of the nursing process as it relates to the process of scientific problem-solving.

In 1973 a group that later became the **North American Nursing Diagnosis Association (NANDA)** formed a task force to define and refine nursing diagnoses for the benefit of client care. NANDA holds conferences every 2 years to review established nursing diagnoses and to formulate new diagnoses. (You will learn more about nursing diagnosis in the next chapter.)

Nursing Process

The nursing process is a systematic process based on the steps of scientific problem-solving. Nursing process is a framework that provides each patient with an individualized plan of care. When a nursing care plan is developed using the nursing process, the result provides guidelines for the individual patient. These guidelines help in time management and provide consistency of care.

The nursing process enables the nurse to identify not only actual problems but also potential problems. The ability to foresee problems may avert painful, as well as costly, complications.

The nursing process is used throughout the United States and Canada although its implementation varies from one area to another. The exact use of nursing process also varies between types of healthcare facilities and may be related to available staffing. In some situations, registered nurses are most concerned with diagnosing, planning, and implementing care. In other situations, licensed practical nurses are involved. It is important for you to determine what your role is expected to be (as a student and as a graduate) in your particular healthcare facility.

Steps in Nursing Process

Nursing process is a systematic method in which the nurse and patient work together to plan and carry out effective nursing care. The following are the five steps in nursing process:

◆ Nursing assessment (systematic and continuous collection of data)
◆ Nursing diagnosis (statement of significant data)
◆ Planning (development of goals and plans for care)
◆ Implementation (activities to meet goals)

Table 33-1. The Nursing Process as Compared to Scientific Problem-Solving

Steps in Scientific Problem-Solving	Related Steps in the Nursing Process	Activities to be Performed
Gather information relative to the problem	Nursing assessment	Identify assessment priorities; collect data; update data base
Identify the problem	Nursing diagnosis	Recognize significant data; recognize patterns or clusters; identify strengths and problems; reach conclusions; validate observations; write diagnostic statement
Formulate tentative solutions; describe possible solutions; choose preferred solutions	Nursing planning	Set priorities; establish expected outcomes; select nursing interventions
Plan action to test suggested solutions	Nursing planning	Write a Nursing Care Plan (NCP)
Test solutions	Nursing implementation	Put NCP into action; continue collecting data; communicate care to health team; document care
Evaluate the solution; evaluate the results	Nursing evaluation	Analyze patient's responses; identify factors that contributed to success or failure of the NCP
Formulate another tentative solution	Nursing evaluation	Plan for future nursing care; revise plan as needed

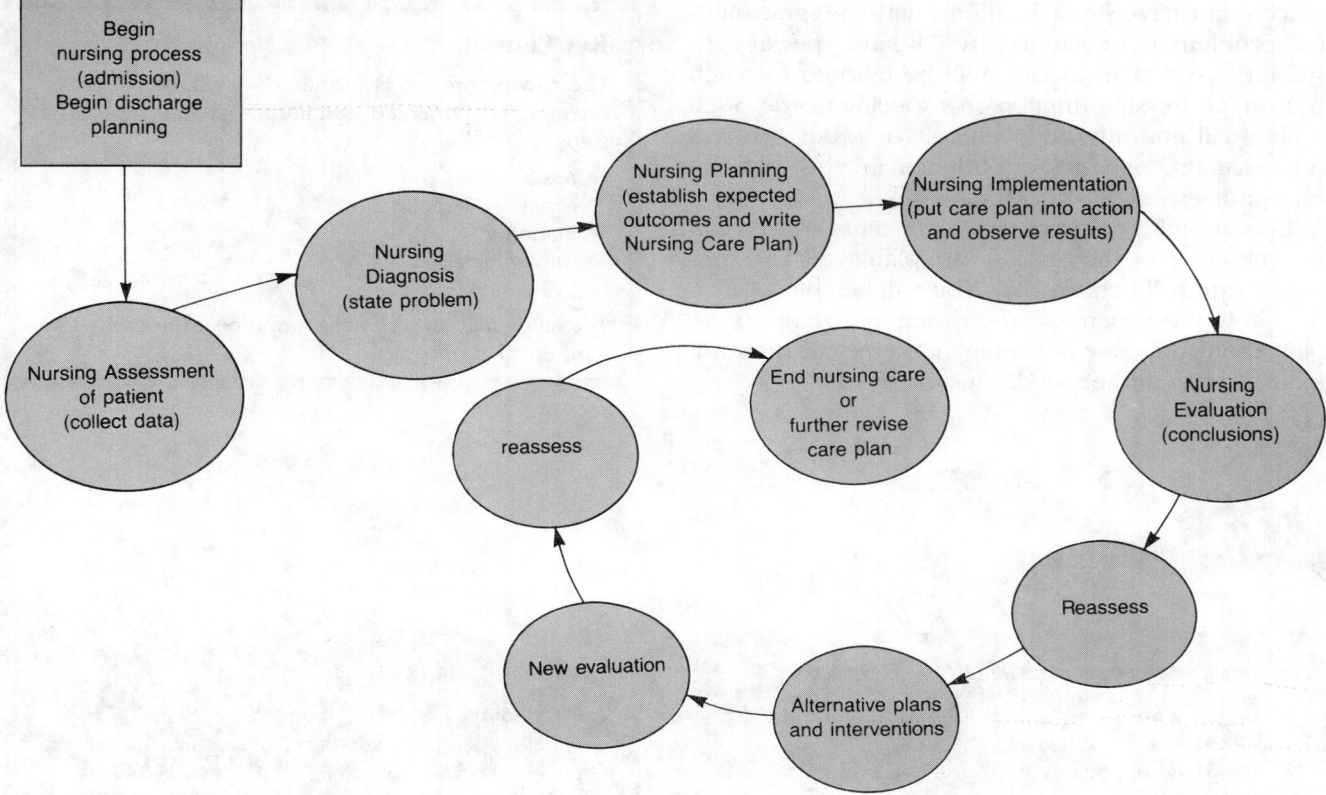

Figure 33-1. Nursing process is continuous, scientific, systematic, dynamic, patient oriented, and goal oriented. The patient and nurse work together to provide quality care.

◆ Evaluation (measurement of the effectiveness of nursing care)

The next two chapters expand on these steps of the nursing process.

Characteristics of Nursing Process

The series of five steps in the nursing process lead to the achievement of specific results. There are other characteristics of the nursing process.

Based on Scientific Problem-Solving. The five steps of the nursing process closely parallel the steps of scientific problem-solving. Table 33-1 shows the relationship between the steps of the nursing process and those of scientific problem-solving.

Systematic. One can follow definite steps in the progress of care.

Patient Oriented. By using the nursing process, the nurse focuses on meeting the needs of each patient rather than on performing specific skills or tasks. Nurs-

ing thus becomes **patient oriented**, rather than task oriented.

Goal Oriented. The patient, family, and nurse together determine what goals should be set and met in nursing care. These goals are prioritized.

Continuous. Nursing process is continuous or cyclic as shown in Figure 33-1. Problem-solving goes on throughout the total span of nursing the patient. There is continual reassessment, reevaluation, and revision of the nursing care plan.

Dynamic. The nursing process is dynamic (ever-changing). Although there are definite steps, they overlap. Sometimes they all occur at once. For example, in an emergency, the nurse may be performing an intervention, while evaluating its effect, while assessing another factor, while planning priorities of what to do next.

Nursing Process and Quality Care

Nursing process has become an important tool for providing *measurable* and *observable accountability* of nursing care given in any setting. Nurses are expected to be responsible for their actions.

You may have several patients with the same medical problem, but each person will have special considerations. A plan of care will be tailored for each person, addressing the person's specific needs. Such a plan will not only save valuable time but also will reinforce the patient's confidence in you and the other nurses.

Because all the nurses providing care for a certain patient will have the nursing care plan available, consistent care will be provided. You will be able to measure how the patient is progressing according to the plan. If outcomes are not being met, a reevaluation will indicate what further needs must be met.

> **Key Concept**
>
> The nursing process is scientific, systematic, patient oriented, goal oriented, continuous, and dynamic. The steps are:
>
> ◆ Assessment
> ◆ Nursing diagnosis
> ◆ Planning
> ◆ Implementation
> ◆ Evaluation
>
> The steps may overlap, change, repeat themselves, or happen all at once.

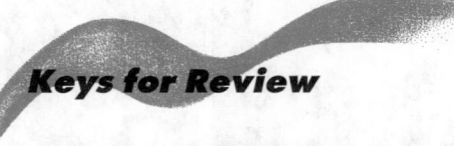

Keys for Review

Key Questions for Critical Thinking

1. Describe the scientific approach to problem solving. Discuss the advantages of such a system.
2. Describe how nursing process affects the quality of care received by the patient. Give examples and rationale.

Key Readings

Alfaro R. Application of Nursing Process: A Step-by-Step Guide to Care Planning, Ed 2. Philadelphia, J.B. Lippincott, 1990

NANDA Nursing Diagnoses: Definitions and Classification, 1992. St. Louis, North American Nursing Diagnosis Association, 1992

Key Readings (continued)

Shaffer FA (Guest Editor). "DRGs, Nursing and Health Care" Symposium in Nursing Clinics of North America. Philadelphia, W.B. Saunders, September, 1988

Yura H, Walsh M. The Nursing Process: Assessing, Planning, Implementing, Evaluating. Norwalk, CT, Appleton & Lange, 1988.

Keys to Learning More

Chapter 34: nursing assessment and nursing diagnosis
Chapter 35: planning, implementing, and evaluating
Chapter 36: therapeutic communication skills
Chapter 37: documentation and reporting
Chapter 50: basics of a head-to-toe nursing assessment

34 Nursing Assessment and Nursing Diagnosis

Keys for Learning

Learning Objectives

- Define *nursing assessment* and *nursing diagnosis.*
- Differentiate between subjective and objective data.
- Discuss methods of data collection.
- Describe techniques used in the health interview.
- Discuss the steps in nursing assessment.
- Differentiate between nursing diagnosis and medical diagnosis.
- State the purposes of nursing diagnosis.
- Explain the components of nursing diagnosis.

Key Terms

collaborative problems	nursing diagnosis
health interview	nursing history
independent nursing actions	objective data
medical diagnosis	observation
nursing assessment	subjective data

Keys to Understanding This Chapter

Unit One: the healthcare system and legal and ethical aspects of nursing

Chapter 33: basics of scientific problem-solving; steps of nursing process compared to scientific problem-solving

Key Points

- Nursing assessment is the systematic gathering of data about the patient, using observation (your senses), the interview, and the physical examination. Data collected include objective data (factual, measurable, what you can observe) and subjective (what the patient tells you, the patient's opinions and feelings).

Key Points (continued)

- Nursing diagnosis is a statement about the patient's actual or potential health concerns that can be managed by independent nursing interventions.
- A medical diagnosis is concerned with the disease process, but a nursing diagnosis is concerned with the person and how the disease affects the patient's functioning.
- Nursing diagnosis helps identify nursing priorities and aims to maintain quality of care and continuity of care.
- Nursing diagnosis is stated in terms of a problem (statement approved by the North American Nursing Diagnosis Association [NANDA]), its etiology, and signs and symptoms.

Key Topics Outline

Nursing Assessment
Types of Data Collection
Methods of Data Collection
Recognizing Significant Data
Validating Observations
Recognizing Patterns or Clusters
Identifying Strengths and Problems
Reaching Conclusions
Nursing Diagnosis
Nursing Diagnosis Versus Medical Diagnosis
Purpose of the Nursing Diagnosis
NANDA-Approved Nursing Diagnoses
Developing the Diagnostic Statement

All the steps of the nursing process depend on complete and accurate data on the patient. This information
is carefully collected by the nurse. This chapter discusses the first two steps of the process: assessment and
diagnosis.

Nursing Assessment

After the nurse enters the nurse–patient relationship,
the first step of the nursing process beings with assessment (see Figure 33-1). **Nursing assessment** is the systematic and continuous collection of data about the patient. Such data identify whether the person is well or
has problems. If the patient has problems, does he or
she have strengths to cope with those problems?

Types of Data Collection

Although information about the patient can be obtained
from many sources, the patient and family usually are
the best sources. The nurse also collects data from written materials, such as the patient's previous and present
chart, laboratory reports, and reference books dealing
with the patient's medical diagnosis or condition.

Objective Data. Objective data are all the factual,
measurable, and observable information about the patient and his or her overall state of health. The measurements must be precise and accurate. The term *objective* implies that only exact measurements are used,
not judgments or opinions.

Extent, rate, rhythm, amount, and size (as they relate
to body structure and function) are measurements included in the initial assessment of the patient (see
Chapter 50). These measurements are usually made by
instruments or are the result of laboratory tests. Urine
volume, vital signs, height, and weight are all measurements specific to each patient that are obtained by the
nursing staff. The laboratory contributes such measurements as blood chemistry and urine chemistry values.

What do the laboratory reports tell you about the
patient's condition? What are the patient's vital signs?
What can you observe? Have you read the physician's
history and progress notes? What do the other members
of the healthcare team have to say about the patient?

Be sure to read the patient's chart thoroughly; it plays
an important part in the nursing process. Without this
written documentation, the nursing process is handicapped. All information must be available to all members of the healthcare team.

Subjective Data. Subjective data consist of information on the patient's opinion or feelings about what is
happening, and for this you need to be a good listener.
Only the patient can tell you that he or she is afraid or
has pain.

What do you hear the patient saying about how he
or she is feeling? What does the patient say is the reason
for coming to the hospital or clinic? What is working
and what is not working in the home nursing care? How
is the patient coping with the immediate environment
(home, hospital, nursing home)? The patient's statements should be recorded in exact words, as a
quotation.

> **Key Concept**
>
> *Objective* data are what you *see* or *measure*.
> *Subjective* data are what the patient feels.

Methods of Data Collection

Achieving rapport with the patient or family is an important goal in nursing care. The result is a mutual verbal and nonverbal exchange of information between
the nurse and patient and family.

Methods used to collect data are *observation, interview,* and *physical examination.* To obtain complete
and accurate information, it is valuable to incorporate
all three components. This information should reflect

the *total patient*, as discussed in earlier chapters. Data must be objective, unbiased, and impartial.

Observation

Observation is an assessment tool that relies on the nurse's use of the five senses (sight, touch, hearing, smell, and taste) to discover objective information about the patient. This information relates to the characteristics of the patient's appearance, functioning, primary relationships, or environment.

Visual Observation. Sight provides an abundance of visual clues the nurse must continually process when assessing the patient. A few examples to consider are body movements, general appearances, mannerisms, facial expressions, mode of dress, nonverbal communication, family–friend interaction, use of space, redness or cyanosis of the skin, and cleanliness. As an example, the nurse may make statements that describe the patient's behavior objectively. Examples include "ambulated the length of the hall on Station 22 six times during this 8-hour shift," "patient requested pain medication four times this shift," or "smoked six cigarettes during a 1-hour interview."

Tactile Observation. Touch is used to collect information. Palpation of the skin can assess factors such as muscle strength, moisture, edema, or swelling. The temperature and moisture of the air can also be observed by touch.

Auditory Observation. Hearing allows the nurse to listen actively to the verbal expressions of the patient and family, as they interact with the nurse and the healthcare team. The nurse also uses specialized equipment to obtain data. For example, data collected by *auscultation* (listening to the heart, lung, or bowel sounds) depend on the nurse's sense of hearing and level of skill on interpreting these sounds. Similarly, the nurse must be able to hear the sounds of the pulse when taking blood pressure with the mercury manometer and stethoscope or the fetal heart sounds when using the fetoscope.

Olfactory or Gustatory Observation. The sense of smell identifies odors that can be specific to a patient's condition or state of health. This includes body and breath odors (which might indicate alcohol intoxication, poor hygiene, or metabolic acidosis). Chemicals in the air may also be detected by the sense of smell or the sense of taste.

The Health Interview

The **health interview** is a method of seeking information from the patient about himself or herself. This information may be called a **nursing history**. If its pur-

pose is part of the admission of a patient to a healthcare facility, it is called an *admission interview.* When the information is obtained by a physician it is called a *medical history.*

In some facilities, the patient interview is done by a registered nurse with the nursing student or practical nurse assisting. In other facilities, the practical nurse may do the health interview. A nursing student never does a patient admission interview alone.

Each facility has its own history form for the nurse and patient to complete. Forms may be focused for the specific needs of the patient (eg, if the patient wants to lose weight). The conversation may be controlled by the nurse with direct questions. The patient may be allowed to be in control by discussing health problems, symptoms, or feelings about the problem. (Techniques used in interviewing are discussed in Chapter 36.)

The nurse should have a plan for the interview before he or she enters the room. The patient is told that the purpose of the interview is to enable the nursing staff to plan effective care. Samples of questions asked at an initial interview are given in the accompanying box. Patients have the right to refuse to answer questions they feel are too personal. Sometimes you will need to talk with family members. Some patients are too ill to respond; some are too young. Even when you have a person who can respond, family members can provide you with additional information.

Patients are partners in their own care, and they need to feel they have an active role. At the initial interview, the nurse and patient determine what the patient can do alone and at what point the nursing staff needs to provide assistance.

Components of the Nursing History. It is important to obtain as complete a health history as possible. The nurse needs to obtain the following information:

♦ Biographical data (name, birthdate, spouse, support person, children, address, occupation, financial status, insurance, etc.)
♦ Reason for coming to the healthcare facility. This is also described as the patient's chief complaint or perception of the illness. What does the patient expect to happen in the care facility?
♦ Recent health history
♦ Important medical history (including family history of disease)
♦ Pertinent psychosocial information (family relationships, employment, living conditions, emotional stability, sexual relationship, substance use or abuse, medications, etc.)
♦ Activities of daily living (ADL). How well is the patient able to meet basic needs, including physiologic needs such as nutrition, sleep, oxygen, and

Sample Questions to Ask at the Initial Patient Interview

Use the following questions as a guide in interviewing the patient. Tailor the pace of the interview to what the patient can handle; if the patient is exhausted or in pain, you may wish to do the interview in several parts. If family members are providing the answers to any questions, indicate so in your notes.

◆ By what means did you come to the hospital? Who, if anyone, was with you? Did you come from another hospital? A nursing home? Another area of the hospital?

◆ Are you under the care of any other physician? If so, what is the physician's name? For what condition are you being treated?

◆ Have you been in a hospital before? For what? How long ago? In this hospital? If not, where? Have you had surgery? For what? How long ago? Have you ever had a bone fracture? When? Which bone? What happened?

◆ Are you on a special diet at home? If so, what is the diet and why was it ordered? When did you last eat? Have you had a recent sudden or unexplained weight gain or loss? Do you have any definite food dislikes? Does your religion prohibit you from eating certain foods? If so, what are they?

◆ Do you have any allergies to foods? To drugs? To other substances? If so, what are they?

◆ Are you taking any prescription drugs? Who prescribed the drug(s) you are taking? For what reason? What dosage? For how long have you been taking it (them)? Have you been taking them as ordered? Do you have them with you?

◆ Which nonprescription drugs, if any, do you regularly use? Home remedies? What do you take for pain? Headaches? Menstrual cramps? Upset stomach? Heartburn? Diarrhea? Constipation? Earache? A cold?

◆ Are you taking an iron preparation? Vitamins? Eye drops? Nose drops? Birth control pills? If so, what kind?

◆ Do you have difficulty sleeping? If so, what remedy do you take? Do you have any drugs with you? If so, which?

◆ Do you smoke? How many packs/day? Use smokeless tobacco? Do you drink alcoholic beverages, coffee, or cola drinks? If so, how much? Do you use marijuana, cocaine, recreational drugs?

◆ Do you drive regularly? Work around dangerous machinery?

◆ Have you had blood transfusions? When?

◆ Are you regularly exposed to strong solvents or pesticides? Other chemicals? Radiation?

◆ Do you have a history of diabetes? Heart trouble? High blood pressure? Asthma? Emphysema? Tuberculosis? Urinary problems? Cancer? Mental or emotional disorders? Rheumatic fever? Other diseases? What about other members of your family?

◆ Have you ever had a seizure? What were the circumstances? Are you taking anticonvulsive medications?

◆ Do you have any speech problems?

◆ Do you have any cold symptoms? Fever?

◆ Do you have any problems walking by yourself, or do you need assistance?

◆ Do you have a prosthesis (an artificial eye or limb, for example)? If so, please state what it is. Do you have it with you? (This also applies to crutches, canes, walker, and braces.) Do you wear glasses? Contact lenses? If so, do you have them with you? Do you have dentures, removable partial plates or bridgework, or a retainer? If so, do you have it (them) with you? Do you have a hearing aid? Is it with you? How is your corrected vision or hearing?

◆ Are you sexually active? Do you have any sexual concerns?

◆ When did you have your last menstrual period? Do you think you may be pregnant?

◆ When did you have your last bowel movement? Do you have difficulty with bowel movements? Do you regularly take laxatives? Enemas? Do you have any difficulty in voiding (urinating)?

◆ Have you ever passed blood in your stool or urine? Have you ever coughed or vomited blood?

◆ Do you have a family? Will they be visiting you here? Do you wish to restrict visitors or phone calls? Whom should we call in case of emergency? Phone number (day and evening)?

◆ Do you have any valuables with you? If so, describe them. Do you plan to lock them in the hospital safe or send them home with your family? (Do not give the patient any other choices.) What clothing and toilet articles do you have with you?

◆ Do you wish to see a member of the clergy or the hospital chaplain? Do you need assistance in telephoning?

◆ Do you need to see someone from the Social Service Department? Do you have a place to live? Do you need to apply for medical assistance?

◆ Is there any other way in which I can be helpful to you?

◆ Is there anything else I should know?

---

elimination, and higher-level needs such as cleanliness, mobility, safety, and love?

The Physical Examination

In Chapter 50 you will study how to assist with the physical examination. It is helpful to set up an organized system by which data are obtained. Nursing assessment also is further described in Chapter 50.

Key Concepts

Methods used to collect data are:

◆ Observation (use of the nurse's five senses)

◆ Interview (nursing history and assessment)

◆ Physical examination (general survey and specific examinations), usually by physician

Recognizing Significant Data

It is difficult to interpret the data if there is too much or too little information. As the nurse prepares to record the data, the nurse determines which items of information are pertinent to patient care and which are not. (As a nursing student, you need to discuss your assessments with your team leader or instructor.) As you gain experience, you will make more decisions on your own.

Validating Observations

One way to validate observations is to "check them out" with the patient. Do the nurse's observations tally with what the patient is experiencing or are they only interpretations? Sometimes it is helpful to think of a patient as a "team leader," directing the members of the healthcare team in his or her own care.

Recognizing Patterns or Clusters

Some data are similar or have a pattern. These data can be clustered for further analysis.

Identifying Strengths and Problems

While assessing the patient, the nurse looks for strengths the patient has that can be used in coping with problems. Actual or potential problems may be determined from the clusters formed above.

Reaching Conclusions

After the preceding steps, the nurse is ready to reach a conclusion. Four are possible:

- *The patient has no problem.* No further nursing care is needed; the nurse can reinforce the patient's health habits or recommend other health promotion activities.
- *The patient may have a problem.* The nurse needs to collect more data.
- *The patient has a problem or is at risk for a problem.* The nurse continues through the nursing process by planning, implementing, and evaluating. The patient may deny there is a problem or refuse treatment.
- **The patient has a clinical problem**; that is, the patient needs a medical, not a nursing, diagnosis. The nurse must consult a physician and they work together on the problem.

> **Key Concepts**
>
> Nursing assessment is the systematic and continuous collection of data about a patient. Steps in nursing assessment are:
>
> - Identify assessment priorities related to the nurse's purpose for the interview
> - Collect data about the patient from observation, interview, and physical examination
> - Continuously update data base
> - Recognize significant data
> - Validate observations
> - Recognize patterns or clusters
> - Identify strengths and problems
> - Reach conclusions

Nursing Diagnosis

Nursing diagnosis is a statement about the patient's actual or potential health concerns that can be managed through *independent* nursing interventions (see Figure 33-1). These are concise, clear, patient-centered, patient-specific statements.

Nursing Diagnosis Versus Medical Diagnosis

Nursing diagnosis is not to be confused with medical diagnosis. You are probably more familiar with medical diagnoses. A **medical diagnosis**:

- Identifies the disease a person has or is believed to have
- Is arrived at by studying the clinical manifestations of the illness and establishing the cause and nature of the illness
- Provides a basis for prognosis and medical treatment decisions

Medicine's emphasis is clearly on the *disease process.* Nursing's focus is on the *person*—the individual's response to his or her health. Nursing asks *how* the disease or illness influences the person's functioning and how needs can be met.

For example, a woman is admitted with pneumonia (a medical diagnosis). The nurse looks at the assessment data that has been obtained. The nurse is concerned about how the patient is functioning and what the nurse can do to help the patient improve functioning. The nurse realizes from the assessment data that the patient has abnormal breath sounds, an ineffective cough, and no sputum production (Ineffective Airway Clearance, a nursing diagnosis), fever (Hyperthermia, a nursing diagnosis), and Pain (a nursing diagnosis).

Purpose of the Nursing Diagnosis

The purposes of the nursing diagnosis are to:

♦ Identify nursing priorities
♦ Direct nursing interventions to meet high-priority needs of the patient
♦ Provide a common language and form a basis for communication and understanding among nursing professionals and the healthcare team
♦ Formulate expected outcomes for quality assurance requirements of third-party payors
♦ Provide evaluation as to whether or not nursing care was beneficial to the patient and cost effective
♦ Assist in making staff assignments

NANDA-Approved Nursing Diagnoses

Since 1973, NANDA has convened on even years to research new and established nursing diagnoses. This example of nursing as an organized body of clinical science directly and continually affects patient care outcomes and the nursing profession. The current NANDA-approved list of nursing diagnoses are listed inside the cover of this book. Most healthcare facilities have the list posted at the nurses' station.

Developing the Diagnostic Statement

Components of Nursing Diagnosis

Nursing diagnoses may be written as two- or three-part statements, depending on the healthcare facility. The three-part statement (as suggested by Gordon[1]) consists of:

♦ Problem
♦ Etiology
♦ Signs and symptoms

Problem. The problem statement describes the patient's health problems clearly and concisely. The problem is stated by using one of the NANDA-approved nursing diagnoses.

Recall the example given earlier of the patient admitted with pneumonia. After assessing the patient and taking the steps leading up to the diagnostic statement, the nurse has determined that one of the patient's problems is difficulty in breathing because the airway is filled with mucus. Following the NANDA guidelines

[1] Gordon M. "Nursing diagnosis and the diagnostic process." Am J Nurs 76:1298–1300, 1976.

and stating the problem concisely, the nurse states: *Ineffective Airway Clearance.*

Etiology. The etiology part of the statement gives the cause, which may come from physiologic, psychological, sociological, spiritual, or environmental factors. In the case of the patient with pneumonia, the etiology is: *increased secretions.*

Signs and Symptoms. Data collected earlier pointed to the nursing diagnosis. They are summarized in the third part of the statement. There may be several data (remember the clusters). For instance, the patient with pneumonia had abnormal breath sounds and an ineffective cough without sputum. The third part of the statement would be: *ineffective and unproductive cough.*

Key Concept

The three components of a nursing diagnosis are:

♦ P—problem
♦ E—etiology (cause)
♦ S—signs and symptoms

Writing the Statement

The problem, etiology, and signs and symptoms are connected in the diagnostic statement. The first two parts of the statement are linked by "related to, sometimes abbreviated R/T." The last two parts are linked by "as evidenced by, sometimes abbreviated AEB." Therefore the statement for the patient with pneumonia would read:

Ineffective Airway Clearance related to increased secretions as evidenced by ineffective and unproductive cough.

The nurse makes sure that the nursing diagnosis is something that can be managed by the nursing staff and the patient. (This is called **independent nursing actions**.) If management concerns something the nurse cannot do (such as prescribe medication for the cough), the problem is a collaborative problem. A **collaborative problem** is a problem in which the nurse will collaborate (work with) the physician. For instance, the physician will prescribe the medication, but the nurse will decide to administer a PRN (as needed) medication at bedtime.

Key Concept

Nursing diagnosis is a statement about the patient's actual or potential health concerns that can be managed through independent nursing interventions. Steps in making a nursing diagnosis are:

♦ Establish significant data
♦ Write a two- or three-part diagnostic statement

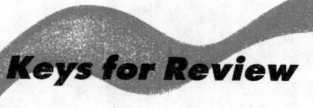

Keys for Review

Key Questions for Critical Thinking

1. You are asked to make an initial assessment on a woman entering the nursing home. Identify types of data collection you will use and describe the differences. Also describe the methods you will use in making assessments.
2. Explain the difference between medical diagnoses and nursing diagnoses. Give examples of each and explain why they are different.

Key Readings

Ackley BJ. Nursing Diagnosis Reference Handbook. St. Louis, Mosby-Yearbook, 1993

Alfaro-LeFevre R. Applying Nursing Process Diagnosis and Nursing Process: A Step-by-Step Guide, Ed 3. Philadelphia, J.B. Lippincott, 1994

Carpenito LJ. Handbook of Nursing Diagnosis, Ed 5. Philadelphia, J.B. Lippincott, 1993

Cox HC, Hinz MD, Lubno MA, et al. Clinical Applications of Nursing Diagnosis: Adult, Child, Women's Psychiatric, Gerontic and Home Health Considerations, Ed 2. Baltimore, Williams & Wilkins (Davis), 1993

Doenges M, Moorhouse M, Geissler A. Nursing Care Plans: Guidelines for Planning and Documenting Patient Care, Ed 3. Philadelphia, F.A. Davis, 1993

McFarland. Nursing Diagnosis and Intervention: Planning for Patient Care, Ed 2. St. Louis, Mosby-Yearbook, 1993

Key Readings (continued)

Murray R, Zentner J. Nursing Assessment and Health Promotion Strategies Through the Life Span. E. Norwalk CT, Appleton & Lange, 1993

NANDA Nursing Diagnoses: Definitions and Classification, 1992. St. Louis, North American Nursing Diagnosis Association, 1992

Taylor CM, Sparks. Nursing Diagnosis Cards, Ed 7. Springhouse PA, Springhouse, 1992

Weber J. Nurses' Handbook of Health Assessment, Ed 2. Philadelphia, J.B. Lippincott, 1992

Keys to Learning More

Chapter 35: completes the nursing process with planning, implementing, and evaluating

Chapter 36: basic communication skills used in interviewing patients

Chapter 37: methods of proper documentation and reporting

Chapter 50: description of head-to-toe assessment

The nursing process skills, as presented in these chapters, will form the basis for the remainder of your nursing program. All of the remaining chapters in this book use the nursing process.

35 Planning, Implementing, and Evaluating

Keys for Learning

Learning Objectives

- List the steps in planning patient care and describe how these steps might be carried out.
- List the major steps in nursing intervention (implementation) and describe ways in which these might be carried out.
- Compare and contrast intellectual (cognitive), interpersonal (affective), and technical (psychomotor) skills and describe how they apply to nursing.
- List the steps in evaluation of nursing care and describe how they might be accomplished.
- Describe at least three means used for evaluating patient care.
- Define *quality assurance*, *chart audit*, and *nursing peer review*.
- Describe discharge planning.

Key Terms

case manager	long-term objectives
chart audit	managed care
dependent actions	managed care path
discharge planning	nursing care plan
evaluation	nursing orders
expected outcomes	nursing peer review
implementation	planning
independent actions	quality assurance committee
intellectual skills	short-term objective
interpersonal skills	technical skills
Kardex	variance

Keys to Understanding This Chapter

Unit One: healthcare system and legal and ethical aspects of nursing, information basic to studying nursing process

Keys to Understanding This Chapter
(continued)

Chapter 33: introduction to problem-solving and nursing process

Chapter 34: first steps in nursing process: nursing assessment and nursing diagnosis

Key Points

- After establishing nursing diagnoses, planning of nursing care begins. Priorities, expected outcomes, and nursing interventions are selected; a nursing care plan is written.
- Implementation involves dependent (following physician's orders) and independent nursing actions (based on nursing judgment).
- Intellectual, interpersonal, and technical skills are used by the nurse to implement nursing care plans.
- During implementation, further data are collected and the nurse communicates with other members of the healthcare team.
- Some facilities use a system of managed care to increase cost effectiveness while maintaining quality care.
- The nurse evaluates patient responses and revises the nursing care plan as needed.
- The quality assurance program uses the nursing care plan and other documentation to evaluate quality of care given.
- Discharge planning and future planning are based on nursing care plans.

Rosdahl CB: Textbook of Basic Nursing, 6th ed. © 1995 J.B. Lippincott Company

Key Learning Activities

◆ If a facility in your area has managed care, obtain samples of "patient care paths" and present to the class. How do these relate to diagnosis-related groups (DRGs)?
◆ Interview an administrator. What suggestions have been made by the Joint Commission on Accreditation of Healthcare Organizations (JCAHO) related to nursing process? What was the result?

After nursing diagnoses have been identified, the process continues with planning, implementing, and evaluating (see Figure 33-1). These three steps of the nursing process are discussed in this chapter.

The cycle continues until the patient resumes self-care (alone or with assistance) and is discharged from the healthcare facility. The cycle continues if a nurse provides care in the home.

Planning Care

After the list of nursing diagnoses has been established, the planning of nursing care begins. **Planning** is the development of goals to prevent, reduce, or eliminate problems and identify nursing interventions that will assist in meeting these goals. Setting priorities, establishing expected outcomes, and selecting nursing interventions will result in a plan of nursing care.

Setting Priorities

Because some diagnoses have higher priority than others, they are more important than others. Nursing diagnoses are ranked in order of importance. Factors to consider are:

◆ Actual or imminent life-threatening problems must be addressed before actual or potential health concerns can be handled. (The physiologic needs for air, food, fluids, or sleep must be satisfied first, according to Maslow's hierarchy of needs). Needs such as safety, love, belonging, esteem, recognition, and self-actualization are met later.
◆ Material and human resource availability, as well as time limitations, affect the order of priority. (Equipment, supplies, and staff must be available.)
◆ The patient also determines the priority of health concerns. (A smoker may be fully aware of the health risks of smoking but may choose to continue smoking. In this case, plans to help the patient quit smoking will fail even though the need for oxygen is on the highest level in Maslow's hierarchy).

Establishing Expected Outcomes

You are familiar with learning objectives or behavioral objectives in your nursing program. A similar type of objective is established for the patient or client. **Expected outcomes** are measurable patient behaviors that indicate whether the person has achieved the expected benefit of nursing care. They may be called goals or objectives also, but expected outcomes are:

◆ *Patient oriented.* The patient, not the nurse, is expected to meet these outcomes. For instance, "the patient will walk around the room at least once a shift."
◆ *Specific.* Everyone, including the patient, knows what is to occur. For instance, the patient will walk up and down the hall for 5 minutes.
◆ *Reasonable.* The goal should be within the patient's capacity and abilities and the confines of the patient's condition. For example, if the patient is having trouble breathing, the amount of walking may be limited to walking to the bathroom.
◆ *Measurable.* The behavior can be observed to have occurred or not. The nursing staff can observe the walking or the patient can state that he or she walked for 5 minutes.

These outcomes should be set by the nurse and patient working together. Examples of some verbs used in expected outcome statements are given in the accompanying box.

A **short-term objective** is an expected outcome or goal that can reasonably be met in a matter of hours or a few days.

Long-term objectives are outcomes that patients hope ultimately to achieve but that are usually not accomplished in the hospital. The nurse can help patients put these objectives in writing. Then, as the patients work toward self-care, they may be able to identify their desired long-term goals or objectives and learn how to measure the progress they are currently making toward achieving their objectives. For example, the patient's long-term goal may be "to return to college," after self-care is achieved.

> ### Key Concept
> Expected outcomes are patient oriented, specific, reasonable, and measurable.

Selecting Nursing Interventions

Nursing interventions, also called **nursing orders**, are activities that will most likely produce the desired outcome or objective, be it short term or long term. Sometimes specific target dates are set by the patient and the nurse and checked off when they are completed. Nursing orders may include such things as further assessment, patient teaching, or referral.

The patient in Chapter 34 had a medical diagnosis of pneumonia. Her nursing care can be followed through the other steps of the nursing process. Her nursing diagnosis was Ineffective Airway Clearance related to increased secretions as evidenced by ineffective and unproductive cough. The nurse wants to help the woman cough up the sputum that makes her breathing difficult. An expected outcome could be "Woman will achieve a productive cough." Examples of nursing interventions are:

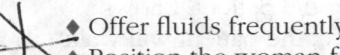

◆ Offer fluids frequently
◆ Position the woman for optimum breathing
◆ Teach the woman deep-breathing exercises
◆ Encourage correct use of the incentive spirometer.

Writing a Nursing Care Plan

The **nursing care plan** is formulated by the entire nursing care team at a meeting called a *nursing care conference* or *team conference*. Plans for patient care must be written. These written plans provide a baseline

Examples of Verbs Used in Expected Outcomes

◆ cough	◆ perform
◆ demonstrate	◆ relate
◆ describe	◆ share
◆ discuss	◆ sit
◆ express	◆ stand
◆ has a decrease in	◆ state
◆ has an absence of	◆ use
◆ has an increase in	◆ verbalize
◆ identify	◆ walk
◆ list	

that the total healthcare team can use for direction and communication.

The nursing care plan should include nursing diagnoses or patient problems (according to priorities), expected outcomes (short- and long-term objectives), and nursing orders (activities carried out by nurses which help the patient to achieve goals). The care plan is not a finished product, but a tool to guide the process of planned nursing actions. (See the sample Nursing Care Plan for a woman admitted to a long-term care facility.) The form for the written nursing care plan varies among healthcare facilities. Students and licensed nurses are expected to be familiar with the form used where they are practicing.

A **Kardex** care plan is used in some facilities. Plans are written on the master Kardex card for each patient. The Kardex also includes background information and care related to the patient's medical treatment.

The Kardex and nursing care plan usually become part of the patient's permanent medical record. The Kardex and nursing care plan are required by such agencies as JCAHO, nursing home regulators, and Medicare. These records are reviewed when a site visit is made to the facility. If a nursing care plan does not exist within 12 to 24 hours of the patient's admission, the hospital or nursing home is cited for noncompliance. The penalties can be severe.

> ### Key Concept
> Planning is the development of goals to prevent, reduce, or eliminate problems and identify nursing interventions that will assist in meeting these goals. Steps in planning are:
>
> ◆ Set priorities
> ◆ Establish expected outcomes
> ◆ Select nursing interventions
> ◆ Write a nursing care plan

Mrs Steel is an 86-year-old white, widowed female. She was admitted to a long-term care facility shortly after the death of her husband because of her inability to manage independently in her family home. Prior to the admission she was capable of self-care activities, such as hygiene, grooming, and feeding, but since admission she has become increasingly dependent on others for care. Her adult children believe she has "lost the will" to live. She has no major physical problems that would necessitate her being bathed, dressed, or fed by others.

Nursing Diagnosis: *Self-Care Deficit: Hygiene, grooming, feeding, related to decreased will to live as evidenced by lack of interest in self-care and increasing dependence on others.*

Goal 1: In one week (1/14/95) patient will demonstrate renewed interest in self-care activities: hygiene, grooming, feeding—with verbal encouragement.

Goal 2: By the end of the month (1/31/95) patient will routinely perform self-care activities independently without reminders.

Nursing Actions (assess/do/teach)	Rationale	Evaluative Statement
1. Continue to assess the patient's response to loss: husband, independent living, all that is familiar.	Depression is a common response to loss.	1/14 Goal 1 met; patient (with much direction) is performing own care.
2. Facilitate her transition to the long-term care setting by exploring new social contacts or other "reasons for living" that will provide incentives for self-care activities.	Without assistance some fail to resolve the grief related to loss and remain depressed.	
3. Verbally direct her in self-care (hygiene, grooming, feeding), but do not provide services she is capable of executing herself.	The patient must learn that independence is expected of her and that false dependence is not acceptable.	1/30 Goal 2 partially met; patient still requires verbal reminders for self-care activities.
4. Reinforce her accomplishments by praising her participation, appearance, efforts.	Knowing that someone cares about the efforts a person is making can be a powerful incentive to continue.	

Implementing Care

After the patient's needs have been assessed and nursing care plans made and documented, they must be carried out. This is called **implementation**, or implementing the plans. This can also be called nursing intervention.

"Do it," "share it," and "write it down" are the action phrases of this phase of care. You *do* nursing care with and for the patient. You *communicate* the results with the patient and with other members of the healthcare team, individually or in a planning conference. You *document* so the next healthcare provider can act with purpose and understanding. *Continuity of care* is facilitated by adequate communication and documentation.

Types of Nursing Action

Nursing actions may be *dependent* or *independent* as they relate to the medical plan of care. Physician orders regarding medication, treatment, activity, or diet are **dependent actions** the nurse will follow explicitly. **Independent actions** are nursing actions that reflect the steps of the nursing process and other actions based on the nurse's judgment. The nurse is legally responsible for such actions.

For example, the physician will leave an order for pain medication to be given every 3 hours as needed (PRN). Administering the medication is a dependent action. However, the nurse may choose to give the medication 30 minutes before ambulation, knowing the patient will be more comfortable and will be able to walk further. This is an independent action based on judgment. Additionally, the nurse may, independently, give a backrub or massage to relax the patient. Nursing orders may be written for actions such as "place side rails up at night," "assist to set up meal tray," or "encourage to attend support group."

Skills Used in Nursing

The implementation of the nursing care plan will be influenced by the nurse's ability to perform intellectual, interpersonal, and technical skills.[1] **Intellectual skills** involve *knowing* and *understanding* information such as basic sciences material before caring for a patient. **Interpersonal skills** involve *believing, behaving,* and *relating.* Communication techniques and patient encounters that promote the development of a trusting relationship (rapport) are interpersonal skills. Conducting oneself in a professional manner also involves interpersonal skill. **Technical skills**, such as changing a sterile dressing or administering a hypodermic injection, require the nurse to perform competently and safely.

Putting the Nursing Care Plan Into Action

The nursing team determines if the plan, as written, makes sense. Some of the criteria in making this decision are:

◆ It is important to protect the patient's *safety*.
◆ The plan should have been developed according to a *scientific problem-solving* approach and should be based on sound nursing knowledge.
◆ The nursing orders should logically be able to achieve the desired results and should be arranged in an *appropriate sequence*.
◆ The patient has an *active involvement* in this plan and should be able to give some input as to whether it is appropriate. (Many facilities encourage the patient to read and sign the nursing care plan after it is written.) How you manage your time, the patient's time, and your activities is important in determining what you and the patient accomplish during the day. Prepare a timetable so the patient can see the schedule of activities for a full day. Encourage patient participation in planning the timetable. Include the patient and the patient's family in the care.

Continuing Collection of Data

As care is given, you must observe the patients. Listen to what patients say; observe what they do; check their vital signs. Continue to evaluate your care and its effect on the patient and family.

[1] Yura H, Walsh M. The Nursing Process: Assessing, Planning, Implementing, Evaluating. Norwalk, CT, Appleton & Lange, 1988.

Communicating Care with the Healthcare Team

Periodically, a *patient planning conference* is held. If the patient is to be discharged, this conference will serve as a discharge planning conference. Interdisciplinary planning conferences offer an excellent way to coordinate your nursing care and teaching with other health disciplines. If you do not personally attend the conference, you are responsible for giving both verbal and written information to those attending. Then your plan of care not only will be coordinated with those of the other healthcare providers but also will be evaluated by them.

Documenting Care

Documentation is essential to communicate what changes are made in patient care as the nursing care progresses. Documentation is the basis for the next phase in the nursing process: evaluation of the appropriateness of nursing actions. By documenting or charting the patient's response to the care given, you can help to evaluate the effectiveness of the current nursing care plan. Chapter 37 discusses methods of charting (documentation) in more detail. (Any problems identified on the nursing care plan must be addressed in the nursing notes.)

Key Concept

Nursing implementation is the carrying out of the nursing care plan. Steps in nursing implementation are:

◆ Put the nursing care plan into action
◆ Continue the collection of data
◆ Communicate care with the health team
◆ Document care

Managed Care: Cost-effective Quality Care

Managed care and case management are two recent developments in healthcare delivery. The overall objective of both is cost effectiveness while maintaining quality care. Third-party payors have determined that if prescribed managed care is not received, they will have the right to refuse payment for a portion of care or deny payment of all charges for that patient.

Managed Care

Managed care focuses on coordinating the activities of health professionals to address the patient's physical, psychosocial, and family needs. Goals of managed care are to:

- Use available resources the most efficiently
- Deliver excellent quality care
- Prioritize needed services
- Manage outcomes, both in the acute facility and after discharge
- Contain costs
- Promote communication, teaching, and discharge planning with patient and family
- Promote communication among staff members—staff can identify where patient is in relationship to critical pathway (or anticipated patient outcomes)
- Avoid discharge delays
- Teach healthy life-style
- Avoid readmissions
- Identify and solve common problems within hospital (continuous quality assessment and improvement)

Variances. If a patient does not achieve an expected outcome by the designated time, a variance is written. The **variance** differentiates between expected outcome and actual occurrence. There are three types of variances:

- *Provider*—something the nurse or physician was not able to do (eg, nurse did not have time; physician did not order)
- *Patient*—patient refused; developed complications
- *System*—patient admitted at night/weekend when ordered services not available; patient cannot be discharged because no bed available at state hospital

Managed Care Paths. Managed care paths are similar to standardized care plans but, unlike standardized forms, the managed care path is used by *all* providers to determine how a particular patient is progressing.

Managed care paths are still being developed by healthcare professionals, and so a variety of forms are used. (They are also called by a variety of names including Anticipated Recovery Plan, Case Management Plan, Critical Pathway, Case Map, or Patient Care Pathway.) Basically managed care paths are developed by a team for selected DRG numbers. The length of hospital stay is determined (via DRGs). A problem list is developed with an accompanying time line and expected outcomes. Related assessments, activities, interventions, and participation by other team members are noted. Each patient is assessed regularly according to the time line. An example of a basic managed care path for one problem for one day appears in the accompanying box.

Particular procedures are stated and the time frame is noted. Some procedures must be performed each hour or more often (such as frequent vital signs). Others are designated to be done each shift (such as Accu-chek

for blood glucose) or each day (such as bed bath). Each item is checked off when it is performed. An example of such a form is given in the accompanying box. (You have not learned all the terminology and abbreviations given here. As you proceed through the chapters of this book you can refer back to this box.)

Case Management

In case management, the process of care is provided through the actions of a case manager. The **case manager** plans and coordinates patient care activities. This type of care may be most useful when the patient is high risk and care is more complex and costly.

Healthcare facilities are moving toward using nurses as case managers. These nurses are primary care nurses or nurses who are skilled clinicians.

Key Concepts

- Managed care and case management are two recent developments in healthcare delivery.
- They both provide cost-effective quality care.
- Time lines may be as short as 15 minutes or less (recovery room vital signs) or as long as several months (rehabilitation).
- A patient may have more than one managed care path. One is written for each major DRG classification.

Evaluating Nursing Care

Evaluation is the measurement of the effectiveness of assessing, diagnosing, planning, and implementing. The patient continues to be the focus of the evaluation. Steps in evaluation of nursing care involve analyzing the patient's responses, identifying factors contributing to success or failure, and planning for future care.

Means of Evaluating Care

The Patient. The *primary* source of evaluation criteria is the patient. The family may also be helpful in determining if care given was effective.

The Team Conference. The team conference is used not only to plan nursing care but also to evaluate the effectiveness of care and to design a discharge plan.

Community Health Agencies. Another way of evaluating care in terms of changes in patient behavior is to contact community agencies who are in touch with patients. Such agents are the public health nurse, the school health nurse, social workers, and the physician's office receptionist or nurse.

Sample of a Basic Managed Care Path Following One Problem

> ### Problem
>
> Impaired physical mobility related to recent surgery
>
> ### Day
>
> #1 postop
>
> ### Expected outcome
>
> Pain will be controlled
> Will tolerate increasing activity without distress
>
> ### MD Intervention
>
> Pain meds prescribed
> Up ad lib orders
>
> ### Nursing Intervention
>
> Offer pain meds 30 min before walking
> Assist to walk
> Check vital signs
> Check for bleeding
> Reapply TED socks each shift
> Patient teaching
> Encourage incentive spirometer, as ordered
>
> *Other therapy: Respiratory therapy (incentive spirometer)*

Analyzing the Patient's Response

The previously established goals and objectives of the nursing care plan become the *standards* or *criteria* on which the patient's progress is measured. Evaluation of care is based on these criteria. Was each goal met? The evaluation criteria also consider whether nursing care has helped the patient realize self-care goals.

Identifying Factors Contributing to Success or Failure

Various factors contribute to the achievement of goals. For example, the family may or may not be supportive. The patient may be too sick to perform activities, or the patient may have been uncooperative or may refuse treatments or medications.

The nurse may be a factor. For example, the nurse may not be fully knowledgeable about how to perform an action or may be thinking about personal problems and therefore not do a procedure correctly.

Planning Future Nursing Care

The nursing process is dynamic and cyclic. Problems may resolve or may change. As problems are resolved they are noted on the care plan as "resolved." As nursing goals for the patient are met, new goals are set. If goals were not

met, the nurse considers the reasons for goals not being achieved and suggests revisions in the nursing care plan.

> ### Key Concept
>
> Nursing evaluation is the measurement of the effectiveness of the assessing, diagnosing, planning, and implementing. Steps in nursing evaluation are:
>
> ♦ Analyze the patient's responses
> ♦ Identify factors that contributed to the success or failure of the care plan
> ♦ Plan for future nursing care

Quality Assurance

The Joint Commission for the Accreditation of Hospitals (JCAH; now called JCAHO) was formed in the 1970s, when the federally mandated Health Maintenance Act

Sample Checklist to Accompany the Managed Care Path

Diagnosis: _____	DRG #_____
DAY 1 DATE:	DAY 2 DATE:
Blood Tests	
☐ CBC/diff	☐ hgb
☐ electrolytes	
Nursing Procedures	
☐ VS q1h × 8	☐ VS q4h × 2, then
☐ VS q2h × 4	☐ VS q8h
☐ VS q4h until 2400	
☐ oximeter q1h × 4 h	
☐ neuro check q1h × 8, then	
☐ neuro check q8h	
☐ Accu-chek q8h	
☐ dressing check q2h × 4	☐ dressing check q8h
☐ dressing check q4h × 4	
☐ ACE/TEDS on	☐ ACE/TEDS on
☐ ambulate q4h with assist	☐ ambulate q2h per self
☐ TCH q2h	
☐ incentive spirometer q4h with assist	☐ incentive spirometer q4h per self
☐ I & O	☐ I & O
☐ diet as tolerated	☐ diet as tolerated
☐ Hep-Lock flush q8h	☐ Hep-Lock removed
☐ bed bath	☐ shower bath

was passed. One of the provisions was to develop guidelines for the evaluation of healthcare services.

Each hospital or ambulatory care setting accredited by JCAHO and other federal agencies is required to have a **quality assurance committee**. This committee sets standards of care that represent acceptable, expected levels of performance by nursing staff and other healthcare members, measured in terms of patient care outcomes.

A quality assurance program functions in the following manner:

◆ Establishes the desired standards of care and service that the healthcare agency is expected to provide to patients
◆ Gathers data systematically and regularly by chart audit, patient survey, or computer statistics and judges data against previously established standards
◆ Strengthens and reinforces quality outcomes; inadequacies or deficiencies can be recognized and changed

The Chart Audit and Nursing Peer Review

The chart audit and nursing peer review (nursing audit) are two currently established quality assurance mechanisms. The **chart audit** is an evaluation of outcomes of care from the patient's point of view. It is made by a representative sample of all members of the healthcare team. The **nursing peer review** is an audit specific to nursing activities and patient outcomes as they are reflected in the nursing documentation. The objective of the nursing audit, done by a nurse, is to improve patient care. The results of audits are shared with all persons who have been involved in the patient's care.

Discharge Planning

Discharge planning is a process by which the patient is prepared for continuation of care or independent living at home. Care may be provided by the patient, members of the family, or other healthcare workers. Planning for discharge begins as soon as the patient is admitted to the healthcare system. Because patients reach levels of care at different times, the discharge plan must be individualized.

Before the patient is ready for discharge from the facility, a conference is held with the healthcare team and the patient (and the family, if possible). In this conference, long-term goals still unresolved are identified

and plans are made for continued assistance to the patient (discharge planning).

New goals might be set at the discharge conference. The family is taught to help the patient meet the new as well as the former goals. The primary nurse, or team leader, is responsible for seeing that the patient or family has the necessary discharge instructions. All instructions, verbal and written/printed, given to the patient or family must be *carefully documented*. Discharge plans also include plans for follow-up. Components of discharge planning are given in the accompanying box.

Key Concept

Discharge teaching begins on admission. The patient and family cannot be expected to remember a large amount of teaching at one time, especially just as the patient is leaving the facility.

Components of Discharge Planning

A discharge plan includes specific components of patient teaching, with documentation as to exactly what was taught, who did the teaching and when, who was present (members of the healthcare team, patient, and/or family), and the patient's reaction or expressed level of understanding. Examples of specific components of discharge planning, which must be carefully documented, include:

◆ Equipment needed at home; documentation that the family has obtained it or knows where to get it
◆ Instruction in the use of any special equipment, including a return demonstration by the patient/family caregiver.
◆ Special diet, with documentation by the dietitian as to teaching the patient and family and their level of expressed understanding.
◆ Medications to be taken at home; documentation of instructions and special precautions
◆ Special procedures, such as a dressing change, to be performed at home; instruction must have been given several times and the patient allowed to practice under the nurse's supervision. Documentation that the family can get needed supplies.
◆ Referral to public health or home care services
◆ Appointment for next visit to the physician
◆ Danger signs and when to call the physician
◆ Instructions regarding activities allowed
◆ Documentation of verbal teaching and provision of a written instruction sheet for the patient describing what was taught

Keys for Review

Key Questions for Critical Thinking

1. Describe the nursing care plan and your responsibilities in following it. Describe the difference between short-term goals and long-term goals.
2. Describe various skills a nurse needs to implement care. Give examples of these skills and determine which skills you best perform. Draw up a plan to become more proficient in your weaker skills.
3. Healthcare should be cost effective. Describe managed care, managed care paths, and case management in relationship to cost effectiveness. Give examples.
4. The effectiveness of nursing care is measured. Describe the importance of evaluating care and methods to evaluate care.
5. Describe the importance of discharge planning and discharge teaching. Discuss how planning is done and who is responsible for performing teaching. Discuss documentation and follow-up in relationship to discharge planning.

Key Readings

Alfaro-LeFevre R. Applying Nursing Diagnosis and Nursing Process: A Step-by-Step Guide, Ed 3. Philadelphia, J.B. Lippincott, 1994

Bulechek GM, McClosky JC (Guest Editors). "Nursing Interventions" Symposium in Nursing Clinics of North America. Philadelphia, W.B. Saunders, June, 1992

Key Readings (continued)

Carpenito LJ. Nursing Diagnosis: Application to Clinical Practice, Ed 4. Philadelphia, J.B. Lippincott, 1992

Cox HC, Hinz MD, Lubno MA, et al. Clinical Applications of Nursing Diagnosis: Adult, Child, Women's Psychiatric, Gerontic and Home Health Considerations, Ed 2. Baltimore, Williams & Wilkins (Davis), 1993

Doenges M, Moorhouse M, Geissler A. Nursing Care Plans: Guidelines for Planning and Documenting Patient Care, Ed 3. Philadelphia, F.A. Davis, 1933

Kelly. Nursing Managed Care. St. Louis, Mosby-Yearbook (Series on Nursing Administration), 1993

McFarland. Nursing Diagnosis and Intervention: Planning for Patient Care, Ed 2. St. Louis, Mosby-Yearbook, 1993

Murray R, Zentner J. Nursing Assessment and Health Promotion Strategies Through the Life Span. E. Norwalk, CT, Appleton & Lange, 1993

Keys to Learning More

Chapter 36: basic communication skills

Chapter 37: importance and methods of proper documentation and reporting

Chapter 50: description of head-to-toe nursing assessment skills

Unit *8* Communication in Nursing

36 Therapeutic Communication Skills

Keys for Learning

Learning Objectives

- Define communication; list five components of effective communication.
- Discuss the three parts of the communication process.
- Describe rapport and its importance in nursing.
- Differentiate between verbal and nonverbal communication.
- List at least five nonverbal cues, and discuss each.
- Discuss factors influencing communication.
- Demonstrate the interviewing and communication skills of questioning, therapeutic silence, and clarifying techniques
- Demonstrate communication skills in special situations: toddler, elderly person, nonsighted person, hearing-impaired person, an unconscious patient, and an aphasic person.
- Demonstrate effective telephone communication skills.

Key Terms

aphasia

body language

closed questions

communication

eye contact

nonverbal communication

open-ended questions

personal space

rapport

therapeutic communication

verbal communication

Keys to Understanding This Chapter

Chapter 5: higher level needs cannot be met without effective communication

Unit Three: general development, much of which will not occur without effective communication

Unit Seven: introduction to the nursing process, which requires effective communication

Key Points

- Effective communication is the cornerstone to good nursing care. This is true regardless of the setting in which you are working.

Key Points (continued)

- For communication to occur, there must be a sender, a receiver, a channel, a message, and feedback.
- It is important to develop rapport with the patient.
- Verbal and nonverbal communication are significant.
- Consider the patient's cultural and religious background when communicating.
- The nursing interview is important, and specific communication techniques can assist you. Patients with special difficulties in communication are special challenges for the nurse.
- Accurate and ethical communication with the patient and healthcare team leads to effective nursing.

Key Topics Outline

Communication
    Components of Communication
    Types of Communication
    Factors Influencing Communication
Therapeutic Communication Techniques
    Interviewing
    Communication in Special Situations
Communications Among the Healthcare Team
    The Physician's Orders
    Telephone Communication
    Other Types of In-Hospital Communication

Key Learning Activities

- With a friend, role play effective use of the telephone.
- Practice communication techniques, such as paraphrasing, reflecting, and summarizing. Use appropriate eye contact.
- Simulate situations of patients with sensory impairments. Use a blindfold to simulate the nonsighted patients; earplugs for the hearing-impaired person.

Rosdahl CB: Textbook of Basic Nursing, 6th ed. © 1995 J.B. Lippincott Company

Communication is the giving, receiving, and interpreting of information directed to any of the five senses (sight, hearing, touch, taste, or smell) by two or more interacting people. **Therapeutic communication** is communication that is beneficial and healing for one or more of the interacting people. It requires self-awareness and interpersonal skills. It promotes patient coping and motivation toward self-care.

Effective communication will play an important role in your nursing career and your personal life. It is the foundation on which interpersonal relationships are built. The art of therapeutic communication does not come naturally. It is a learned skill. Guidelines for skill in therapeutic communication are listed in the accompanying box.

The purpose of this chapter is to help you develop these skills. The discussion covers components of communication, the communication process, types of communication, factors, techniques, and communicating with the healthcare team.

Communication

Harmony among individuals is sparked by personal characteristics of genuineness, caring, trust, empathy, and respect. This feeling of harmony is called **rapport.** When these attitudes are conveyed to another, it creates a social climate that communicates goodwill and empathy, even when fears or concerns cannot be fully expressed verbally. The nurse should develop the ability to convey appropriate nonjudgmental attitudes. This is especially true if the person's beliefs and values are different from the nurse's. Accept the person as an individual; respect each person's right to his or her own beliefs. Patients must feel this state of rapport if they are going to share personal, and sometimes embarrassing, information with you.

Components of Communication

For communication to occur, several components must be present, as shown in Figure 36-1.

◆ The originator or source of the idea (*sender*).
◆ The idea (*message*).
◆ A means of transmitting the idea (verbal and nonverbal).
◆ Someone to receive the message, interpret it (*receiver*), and provide feedback (*interaction*). The receiver responds to the message.

All senses can be involved in communication. Think of examples of a message you have sent or received by various senses. Communication can be distorted by various factors during the process. Noise is a major factor.

Nursing Skill: Guidelines for Using Therapeutic Communication

◆ Put the patient at ease, and develop rapport.
◆ Provide privacy.
◆ Respect your patient's rights.
◆ Do not invade the patient's "personal space."
◆ Respect confidential information.
◆ Begin the interview with general information; ask emotionally loaded questions after the patient gains confidence in you.
◆ Adjust your level of language to that of the patient.
◆ Do not use medical terms or "talk down" to the person. Obtain an interpreter if the patient speaks a language other than yours. (A smile is a "universal language.")
◆ Be attentive, and concentrate on what the person is saying.
◆ Make appropriate eye contact.
◆ Try not to write during the interview. Pay close attention, so you can remember later what the patient said. You can go back and clarify details later if you forget.
◆ Show your sincere interest in what the patient is saying.
◆ Ask for the patient's perception of the problems. Why did this patient come to the healthcare facility?
◆ Pay attention to the patient's choice of words, repetition, variations in tone of voice, silence, body language, assertivenss, behaviors, and so forth.
◆ Assess or ask the patient's attitudes about "touch" before using the technique.
◆ Include the family in conversations if the family and patient prefer this.
◆ Consider the patient's cultural background. Cultural practices can greatly influence how a patient may relate to you.

This is why it is important to conduct therapeutic communication in privacy or a quiet area.

Types of Communication

As a nurse, you will communicate with your patients often and in varied ways. Two types of communication are verbal and nonverbal. Ideally, you and your patient should feel comfortable with both. The following will assist you in communication skills.

Verbal Communication

Verbal communication is the sharing of information by written or spoken word. Nurses use verbal communication extensively. They share information with patients, write care plans, document information and

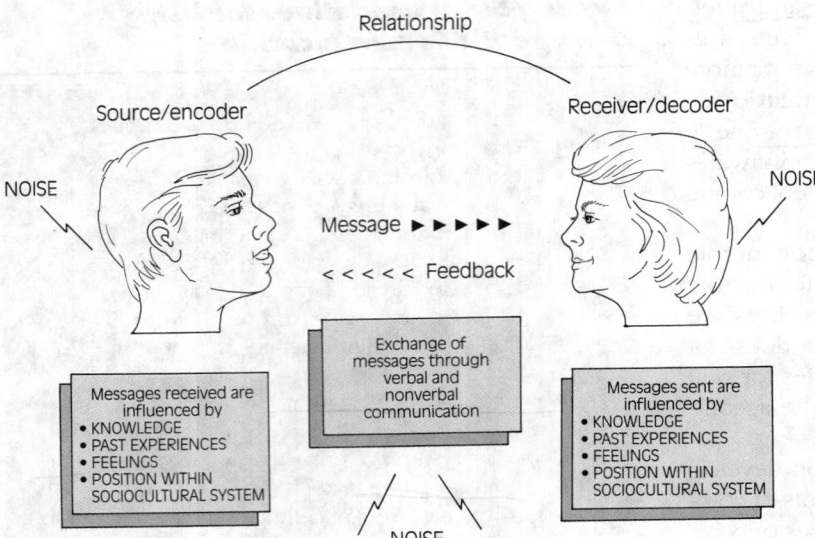

Figure 36-1. The various components in the process of communication. (Taylor C, Lillis C, and LeMone P: Fundamentals of Nursing: The Art and Science of Nursing Care, 2nd ed. Philadelphia: J.B. Lippincott, 1993)

assessments, chart, and give oral or written change-of-shift reports.

Much is related verbally through vocabulary, sentence structure, and pronunciation. People reveal their education, intellectual skills and interests, and ethnic, regional, or national backgrounds through verbal communication. Voice inflections or sounds reveal messages. The patient may say what you want to hear, but the patient's tone of voice might imply lack of sincerity. The person may make sounds that indicate true feelings. A snort, for example, may denote disgust.

Verbal Responses to Avoid. Negative responses stop the communication process. The following are examples of negative responses; appropriate responses are in parenthesis.

◆ Offering empty reassurance. (Reassure appropriately; be factual.)
◆ Changing the subject. (Help the patient ventilate feelings.)
◆ Trite clichés such as "the doctor knows best." (Involve the patient in decision-making.)
◆ Imposing your values on patients and giving advice according to your values. (Help the patient explore and choose an alternative.)
◆ Disapproving or judging the patient. (Accept each patient as unique; consider cultural practices and values.)
◆ Voicing personal experiences, especially those medically related. (Allow the person to discuss their concerns. Answer questions factually. Offer patient-oriented reference material.)

Nonverbal Communication
Nonverbal communication is the sharing of information without the use of words or language. It also can be called **body language.** Sometimes body lan-

guage differs from what the patient states verbally. For example, Mr. Hill, a young diabetic, begins clenching and unclenching his fists when you ask about his sexual expression. He says "everything is fine" through gritted teeth. Later, when he trusts you more, he admits that he has been impotent for the past 6 months.

Key Concept
The nurse must be sure his or her verbal and nonverbal communications are the same message. When verbal and nonverbal messages conflict, the patient is more apt to believe the nonverbal message.

Discussions of several nonverbal communications, as they relate to nurse–patient interactions, follow. It is important to realize that nonverbal behavior may have different meanings for different people or in different situations.

Personal Space. Each person has a space around him or her called **personal space.** That space should not be violated. If you come too close, you invade the person's space; if you are too far away, you give the person a feeling of isolation. When speaking with a person, you can sense the boundaries of their personal space. Try talking to a classmate from various distances; you can sense your own personal boundaries or personal space. Personal space boundaries vary greatly among cultures.

Eye Contact. If the person does not look at you, it may mean that he or she is nervous, shy, or lying. It also may be a sign of respect, as in the southeast Asian, Hispanic American, and Native American cultures.

Facial Expressions. An apparently happy expression, such as smiling, may be misleading; for example, the patient may laugh inappropriately throughout the interview. Practice acting out facial expressions with a classmate, and see if the person can tell what emotion you are expressing.

Body Movements and Posture. A twitching or bouncing foot may indicate anger, impatience, boredom, nervousness, or side effects of certain medications. A slouched appearance may indicate depression. Wringing hands may indicate fear or pain. Many other body positions and gestures also have special meaning.

Personal Appearance and Grooming. Personal hygiene, body weight, and general appearance relate information about the patient. These nonverbal messages may convey patients' true feelings about themselves, or they may be misleading, especially in illness. The person is trying to meet basic physiologic needs and may not have the physical or emotional energy to work on higher order needs, such as cleanliness.

Therapeutic Touch. Touch can say "I care" (Fig. 36-2). A firm touch may discourage a child from doing something dangerous; a light touch may be all that a person needs to have enough confidence to walk down the hall. In some cases touch may make the person anxious. Some people do not like to be touched; it invades their personal space. The nurse must be sensitive to the feelings of all patients. Sometimes it may be necessary to touch a patient to carry out a nursing procedure. In such a case, verbally convey your understanding of the patient's discomfort.

> **Key Concept**
>
> Nursing care revolves around communication: giving, receiving, and interpreting information. Communication is *verbal* and *nonverbal*.

Factors Influencing Communication

The effectiveness of communication is influenced by many factors. Some seemingly harmless factors may create barriers between people. A discussion of factors follows.

Attention. A listening barrier or attention barrier can occur because of lack of concentration or *selective* listening. In this case, the person hears only what he or she wants or expects to hear. The nurse may not hear because he or she is responding emotionally or may be mentally framing the next questions. Patients some-

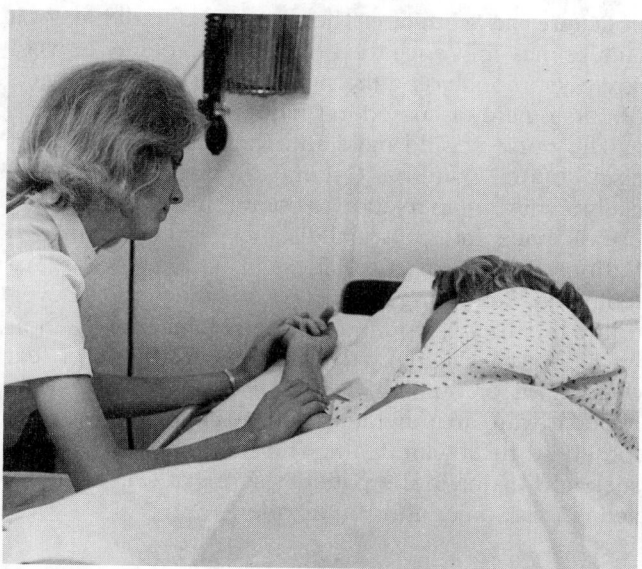

Figure 36-2. The communication technique of therapeutic touch is the most potent nonverbal communication technique of all. Many times words are not needed, just a gentle and reassuring touch.

times listen carefully. On the other hand, their pain may be so great that they will not comprehend what they are being told. Patients may also be preoccupied with internal stimuli (such as auditory hallucinations). If full attention is not given to the present communication, a good nurse–patient relationship may be halted.

Age. Your age may be an advantage or a disadvantage. Some patients would rather work with people close to their own age. Others refuse to follow instructions given by a person younger than themselves. The reverse also may be true.

Gender. Gender roles may influence patient–nurse interactions. For example, a man who is accustomed to "being the boss" may resent being told what to do by a female nurse. If you feel men should be tough, it may be difficult for a female nurse to see a male patient cry. A female patient may feel embarrassed to have personal care procedures performed by a male nurse. Approaching a personal situation professionally may eliminate embarrassment. If a patient sexually harasses you, consult with your instructor or team leader to curb this inappropriate behavior.

Family Situation. People who live alone may not be able to cope with illness because there are no loved ones at home to lend support. In their loneliness, they may not want to go home from the hospital and may resist getting well. Elderly patients are often lonely and may dwell on illness to obtain the attention they need for emotional survival.

Culture and Subculture. The norms and traditions of a culture may influence the behavior and perceptions of any person, including the nurse. Transcultural aspects of nursing are discussed in Chapters 27 and 39.

The nurse should have an awareness of his or her own cultural patterns. Cultural differences are especially significant in relation to communication involving use of space, interpersonal distance, and **eye contact.** Various cultures react to illness in different ways. Listening and accepting differences are the keys to developing therapeutic communication. Members of minority groups may initially demonstrate suspicion or fear of medical or nursing intervention. This may be directed toward an individual nurse or collectively toward the entire healthcare team. The nurse should actively seek and maintain the patient's sense of self-worth by acting in a nonjudgmental manner.

Social Factors. Social acceptance of a particular illness plays a role in a person's reaction to the illness. For example, a sexually transmitted disease may be more difficult for the patient to cope with than influenza.

Religion. Members of some religious groups do not go to physicians or hospitals (eg, Christian Scientists). Others do not believe in receiving blood transfusions (eg, Jehovah's Witnesses). Some religions believe in faith healing only. Such religious beliefs may be in direct conflict with procedures and goals of an institution. Such a person may speak out strongly about such matters. The nurse must be considerate and nonjudgmental.

History of Illness. People who have never been sick may feel threatened or incapacitated by a sense of loss of control. They may react by becoming depressed, hostile, or resistive to the people who want to help. Chronic or continuing illness can affect a patient's coping skills and motivation toward self-care and independence.

Body Image. How patients feel about themselves and their illnesses has a bearing on communication. For example, athletes who value a healthy body may see illness as a threat to self-image and their ability to function productively. The woman who has a mastectomy may worry about her appeal to her husband. The body part affected, its symbolic meaning, and the visibility of the bodily changes influence how the patient relates to others.

The Healthcare Team. An individual's attitude toward illness may be influenced by healthcare team members. The nurse must put aside personal needs and anxieties. For example, the nurse's pain threshold may be higher than the patient's. The nurse cannot pass judgment because of this difference. Therefore, he or she must set aside personal feelings, clarify what the patient

is experiencing, and offer appropriate pain-relieving measures.

Therapeutic Communication Techniques

Therapeutic communication techniques are strategies that facilitate the nursing process and enable you to be more perceptive of yourself and of others.

Interviewing

Open-Ended Questions. In the open-ended interview the nurse gradually takes control of the interview to obtain specific information. A simple yes or no seldom is informative. Open-ended questions encourage longer and more thorough answers. Consider the types of questions in the accompanying box.

Open-ended questions do not imply a certain answer. **Closed questions** may be used when you *do* wish to obtain just one bit of specific information. For example, after a woman says she has children, you may ask her how many pregnancies she has had and how many of her children are still living.

Use of Silence. Do not underestimate the value of silence. It gives you and your patient an opportunity to collect your thoughts and prepare to continue the conversation. Often, if you "wait it out," the patient will answer a question he or she was reluctant to answer before.

Examples of Closed and Open-Ended Questions

Closed

How well do you sleep?
How much do you like dairy products?
How many children do you have?
Do you have a normal sex life?
Does your leg hurt often?
Did you have a normal bowel movement today?

Open-ended

Tell me about your usual sleep patterns.
Do you eat foods in the milk and dairy products group? If so which ones, and how often?
Tell me about your family.
Tell me about your means of sexual expression.
Describe the pain in your leg.
What is your usual pattern of bowel movements?

Clarification. Clarification is necessary if the patient answers a question and you do not understand the answer. You can ask the patient to repeat what was said, or you can say, "Tell me more about it," or "Explain that to me." Other techniques, such as reflection, paraphrasing, and summarizing, also will aid in clarification.

Reflection. Reflection can be used in two ways. The nurse may echo the patient's words; this allows the patient to hear what was just said. In this way, the patient can reevaluate the words to determine if they expressed what he or she meant.

PATIENT: "My life has been one frustration after another."
NURSE: "Your life has been full of frustrations?"

Another reflection technique can be used to reflect the patient's behavior or attitude.

PATIENT: "I'm just a worthless old man, and no one cares about me!"
NURSE: "You say that as if you were very angry."
PATIENT: "I am angry. I raised six children and gave them the best years of my life. If they cared about me, they would come to visit me."

Paraphrasing. The use of paraphrasing will help the nurse clarify the interpretation of the message by restating it in other words.

PATIENT: "It was really noisy here last night. It was like Grand Central Station."
NURSE: "You didn't get a very good night's sleep?"

Summarizing. If you tell the patient what you heard, you will make sure that was what the person meant. Often the person will add more to the statement or will clarify what you say you heard.

PATIENT: "I was in the hospital 2 years ago, and I swore I would never come here again. The food was so tasteless I couldn't eat. My roommate died. The noise at night kept me from sleeping. I went home in worse shape than when I came to the hospital."
NURSE: "You were very uncomfortable and dissatisfied the last time you were here and are apprehensive about being admitted to the hospital again?"

Another example of summarizing is as follows:

PATIENT: "I don't eat meat. My son says I should, but I don't."
NURSE: "You don't eat meat?"
PATIENT: "That's right. I can't chew it any more."
OR PATIENT: "That's right. I can't afford meat."
OR PATIENT: "That's right. I have become a vegetarian."
OR PATIENT: "That's right. I am afraid of the cholesterol."

By allowing the patient to continue talking, you found out the real reason for not eating meat.

Use of Unfinished Statements. Sometimes, if you make an unfinished statement, the patient will finish it. For example,

NURSE: "You're going to live with your daughter . . . ?"
PATIENT: "Well, I don't know. She really wants to put me in a nursing home, but I don't want to go!"

Communication in Special Situations

Not all communication can be handled in the same manner. You may work with children, the aged, mentally ill people, or people with special problems of their senses or behaviors.

Communicating at Different Age Levels
The Young Child. Keep normal developmental stages in mind, and communicate at an appropriate level for age. Remember that children often regress to an earlier stage of development when ill. Role playing is one way to find out what a child is feeling.

The Elderly Person. Respect and treat elderly patients as you would expect to be treated. Communicate with older people at an appropriate level. Be considerate of their personal dignity.

Communicating With the Patient Who has Sensory Problems
The Nonsighted or Hearing-Impaired Person. Communication with sensory-deprived people is discussed in more detail in Chapter 73. There are two important points to remember:

♦ *Do not frighten the person.* The nonsighted person cannot see you coming; the hearing-impaired person cannot hear you. Make sure the person knows you are in the room before you touch them.
♦ *The person is more normal than abnormal.* The nonsighted or hearing-impaired person has strengths and likes and dislikes, just as you do. Take a little extra time to stop and communicate with these people. They are often lonely.

The Unconscious Patient. Tips for communicating with the unconscious patient are as follows:

♦ *Always* assume the patient can hear you.
♦ Introduce yourself.
♦ Explain what you are going to do.
♦ Do not talk about the patient.
♦ Treat the patient with kindness and consideration.

Many people who have been unconscious for some time remember, when they recover, everything that occurred while they were unconscious.

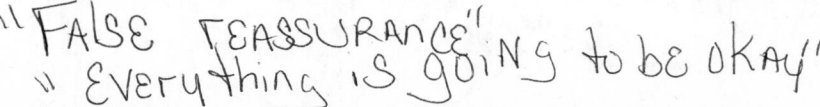
"FALSE reassurance"
"Everything is going to be okay"

The Aphasic Person. Aphasia is the inability to communicate verbally, usually because of a neurologic disorder or injury. Patients who have suffered a cerebrovascular accident often present with some type of aphasia. This can be frustrating for the patient, because intelligence is often unaffected. Some system or method of communication should be developed. This helps to prevent withdrawal and social isolation.

Key Concept

Set up some sort of communication system with all conscious patients.

Communicating With a Person Who Speaks a Different Language

Speaking a different language may be a barrier to total communication, but it certainly does not need to prevent communication and interaction. A smile is understood in all cultures, and people can usually communicate by hand signals for many needs. If you attempt to speak even a few words of another person's language, the person will appreciate it and will know that you care. For more technical communication, it is wise to have an interpreter. A member of the family may act as interpreter. Some healthcare facilities have staff members who can speak other languages. At the back of this book (Appendix A) is a brief list of Spanish and English words the nurse can use to help break the language barrier when working with Hispanics.

Dealing With Specific Patient Behaviors

Some of your patients may be anxious. Patients may be afraid of being in the hospital, afraid of dying, or generally depressed. Some people do not trust anyone and may be suspicious or paranoid. Some patients may question everything you do. Other patients regress and become dependent on the nursing staff. Others may become isolated and reject everything you try to do. Some people may be very fearful and may react with false bravado. These behaviors and suggested interventions are discussed in Chapter 87.

Communications Among the Healthcare Team

As a nurse you need to know how to interact with other members of the healthcare team.

The Physician's Orders

One form of in-hospital communication is the physician's order sheet. The physician depends on you to interpret orders correctly, make accurate observations concerning the patient, and document those observations. The physician's orders tell you *what* to do, and nursing protocols show you *how* to do it.

The physician may give verbal directions to explain written ones. The team leader or charge nurse should read the orders before the physician leaves to be sure they are understood. Some orders are absolute and positive; others may require the nurse's judgment. The nurse may need to decide when (or if) a PRN ("as needed") medication should be given, for example. Judgment is needed to decide what nursing procedures may be safe to perform without an order and what procedures require definite orders from the physician.

Telephone Communication

Answering the Phone. Wherever you work you will often be asked to answer the phone. When doing so, be sure to give the name of the department along with your name and position so that callers know to whom they are speaking. For example, you might answer the phone as follows: "Station Main 2 West, Sally Smith, nursing student speaking." The caller than knows if you can help or if someone else is needed.

Answer the phone as promptly as possible. The call may be an emergency, and the caller may become agitated while waiting for the answer.

Taking Messages. Don't trust your memory. Write down messages carefully. Repeating the message to the caller will help to clarify and verify the message. Write the date, time, and your name on all messages you take. Deliver messages promptly, especially in the case of laboratory, pathology, x-ray, or other reports.

Giving Information. Telephone information given out should be limited. If you are unsure, ask the team leader or charge nurse. For example, if someone calls to ask a patient's condition, generally you will be allowed only to state the condition listed on the Kardex. If someone wants more information, you should politely turn the call over to the team leader or charge nurse. It is illegal to give out information about patients without proper authorization.

Making Emergency Calls. There are times when you will have to make an emergency call. When you do, be sure to give all the necessary information. Above all, *do not panic.* Your prime responsibility in an emergency is to get assistance, but you will not be able to do so effectively unless you are calm and give all the necessary information.

Nursing Alert

Be sure you know the emergency numbers and code names for your facility.

Interoffice Calls. Whenever you telephone someone, be sure to state who you are and to whom you wish to speak. If you are calling a physician, you may need to explain to the office nurse what you want and whether it is an emergency. It is necessary for office nurses to screen the physician's calls.

General Telephone Protocol. The nurse does not chew gum while on duty, and this is especially true when conducting hospital or office business by phone. It is impolite to cover the receiver and continue a conversation with someone else. If you put someone on hold, be sure to return every few seconds, so they know they have not been forgotten.

Nursing Alert

The nursing student should *never* take verbal physician's orders, whether in person or on the phone. This is a legal responsibility you are not prepared to assume.

Other Types of In-Hospital Communication

You will facilitate communication between patients and members of the nursing team in various ways, including the following:

◆ Interviewing patients to determine their healthcare needs
◆ Teaching patients and their families certain aspects of care
◆ Documenting information on the nursing care plan and in the patient's chart
◆ Reporting the condition of the patient to other members of the healthcare team, either in person, on tape, or by written communication
◆ Participating in team conferences and patient care conferences

All these communications are important to patient care. How you handle this responsibility can have a direct bearing on the patient's recovery. Many of these subjects are discussed in Chapters 33, 34, 35, and 37.

Keys for Review

Key Questions for Critical Thinking

1. Describe the importance of rapport in therapeutic communication. Discuss ways of establishing rapport between the nurse and the person who is in the hospital for the first time. The person who is frightened about the medical diagnosis and prognosis.
2. Describe the differences between verbal and nonverbal communication. Give examples of each and an explanation of its interpretation by the nurse or the patient.
3. Describe situations in which special communication skills will be needed. Describe skills in communicating with people who have special difficulties.

Key Readings

Anderson C. Patient Teaching and Communicating in an Information Age. Albany, NY, Delmar, 1990
Bradley JC, Edinberg MA. Communications in the Nursing Context, Ed 3. East Norwalk, CT, Appleton & Lange, 1990
Dickson DA, Hargie O, Morrow NC. Communication Skills Training for Health Professionals: An Instructor's Handbook. New York, Chapman & Hall, 1991

Key Readings (continued)

Nussbaum JF. Communications and Aging. New York, Harper Collins College, 1990
Pagano MP, Ragan SL. Communication Skills for Professional Nurses. Newbury Park, CA, Sage, 1992
Ruben BD. Communicating with Patients. Dubuque, IA, Kendall-Hunt, 1992

Keys to Learning More

Chapter 37: methods of proper documentation and reporting
Chapter 39: transcultural considerations
Chapter 50: nursing assessment and the nursing interview
Chapter 73: communication with patients with sensory problems
Chapter 86: communication with a confused person

The remainder of your nursing career will be based on effective communication.

37 Documentation and Reporting

Keys for Learning

Learning Objectives

- State at least five reasons for maintaining a patient record.
- Name at least five items included in the patient record.
- Identify common methods of documentation, and demonstrate the ability to use the type done in your healthcare facility.
- Demonstrate a knowledge of the 24-hour clock.
- Demonstrate descriptive terminology for patient symptoms when documenting patient care.
- Demonstrate a knowledge of common abbreviations used in documentation of patient care.
- State the correct way to record a documentation error, and differentiate a documentation error from a patient care error.
- Describe change-of-shift reporting.

Key Terms

change-of-shift reporting

confidentiality

flow sheet

focus documentation

patient record

problem-oriented medical record

source-oriented record

walking rounds

Keys to Understanding This Chapter

Chapter 4: ethical and legal aspects of nursing

Chapter 5: accurate documentation to inform team members which patient needs are met

Unit Seven: introduction to nursing process that requires documentation

Chapter 36: communication skills used in documenting patient responses and interactions

Key Points

- All healthcare workers must maintain accurate and complete documentation of care given.
- Patient records serve as the legal record of care given and of patient reactions to that care.
- Approved abbreviations and terminology are used in documentation.
- Communication between healthcare workers is a key to continuity of patient care.
- Each healthcare facility determines the type of documentation to be used there. Certain guidelines must be met to obtain reimbursement.

Key Topics Outline

Purpose of the Patient Record
Documentation
    Documentation Formats
    Guidelines for Documentation
Reporting

Key Learning Activities

- Make flash cards of the abbreviations and terminology listed. Practice with a friend.
- Using your institution's format, retrieve data from a flow sheet, and practice writing nursing notes.
- Using a tape recorder and sample nursing documentation from your facility, simulate a change-of-shift report.

Rosdahl CB: Textbook of Basic Nursing, 6th ed. © 1995 J.B. Lippincott Company

Accurate and complete documentation in the patient record is important to patient care. Documentation is done by nurses and other healthcare team members who provide patient care.

Federal and state laws require adequate documentation for the agency to maintain its institutional accreditation and license. Requirements of the medical record include the following:

◆ Thorough documentation of each patient's condition
◆ What care was given and why
◆ The total plan of care
◆ Patient response to treatment
◆ A discharge plan

The Joint Commission on Accreditation of Healthcare Organizations (JCAHO) requires that documentation in the record meet particular standards for the agency to receive payment from Medicare and Medicaid. Most healthcare insurance companies require similar documentation.

Purpose of the Patient Record

There are several purposes for the patient record:

◆ Legal record
◆ Communication of care among the healthcare team
◆ Quality care record
◆ Baseline data record
◆ Reimbursement record
◆ Staff planning
◆ Research data

Legal Record

The **patient record** is a legal document that provides a written record of the patient's problem or condition, treatments, and teaching received, and the patient's reaction to that care. The patient record also documents discharge planning, which begins on admission and continues through discharge. The accompanying box describes the items that make up the patient record.

According to trial lawyers who handle bodily injury and medical malpractice cases, nursing notes contain the most significant statements in the chart as to whether medical orders were carried out. The total medical record, which contains the nursing notes, is often introduced as evidence in a lawsuit. It can substantiate or negate a patient's claim to malpractice damages. Nursing notes also document patient response to care. They usually contain more detailed information about the patient than is contained elsewhere in the chart. Nursing notes should include the date and time of events. They are written in chronologic order.

Communication of Care Among the Healthcare Team

The medical record contains all the information about a particular patient from the total healthcare team. Nurses, physicians, dietitians, social workers, physical therapists, occupational therapists, recreational therapists, respiratory care personnel, and others offer special expertise. These professionals each record their observations and actions in the medical record. The patients and their families benefit most from this, because all members of the team communicate through this ongoing written record.

The Nursing Care Plan and Patient Record. The nursing care plan, as described in Chapters 34 and 35, provides the framework on which healthcare workers base their care and treatment. Through the nursing care plan, nurses can provide consistent care or *continuity of care* for patients on a 24-hour, day-to-day basis. Consistency builds trusting relationships between the patient and the staff. The patient must trust the healthcare team to ensure the likelihood of successful treatment and a safe and timely discharge.

Quality Assurance Record

Healthcare professionals have the responsibility of monitoring their practice for safe, complete, up-to-date care. Nurses, physicians, and other healthcare workers, including federal and state monitoring agencies, use the medical record to monitor quality. Quality assurance programs are discussed in Chapter 35.

Baseline Data Record

The medical record is useful throughout the current hospitalization, but it also provides a baseline against which other health problems experienced by the same patient in the future may be evaluated. Thus, what is documented now can influence the patient's future care.

Reimbursement Record

Insurance companies, Medicare, and Medicaid require a written record for equipment used and services given before they pay the agency. Incomplete documentation may mean a loss of money for the healthcare agency.

Staff Planning

In some hospitals, patients pay for nursing services based on the number of hours of care they require from the nursing staff. This documentation is done on a plan sheet. Using data from patient records, nursing administrators justify nursing staffing patterns and plan future budgets.

Components of the Patient Record

◆ *Admission sheet:* Biographic and insurance information about the patient and family (and the discharge date and diagnosis after the patient leaves the hospital); also known as the *face sheet*

◆ *Initial nursing history* and patient assessment: Must be done by RN. Follow-up assessments may be done by LPN with RN supervision

◆ *Physician's orders:* Diet, activity level, medications, treatments, laboratory tests, x-rays

◆ *Physician's progress record:* The physician's impressions of the patient's progress toward resolving the illness or injury; written daily

◆ *Patient history and physical examination:* Documented by the admitting physician

◆ *Nursing note:* Nursing care plan (must be developed and signed by an RN), classification, or flow sheets (checklists) recording routine nursing care and nursing discharge summary

◆ *Records of any consultations:* Dietetics, social service, occupational therapy, and physical therapy; reports of physicians from services other than that which admitted the patient (eg, mental health, neurology, orthopedics, dermatology, gynecology). Often these reports are typed, but the consultant may put a hand-written note in the patient record as well.

◆ *Graphic sheets:* Detailed records of temperature, pulse, respirations, and blood pressure; may include amount of sleep, weight, diet, bowel movements (BMs), and other information in some facilities

◆ *Medication sheet:* Lists all medications ordered and given or refused/held

◆ *Laboratory reports:* All tests ordered and results

◆ *X-ray reports and reports of other diagnostic tests:* Interpretation of those examinations by specialists

◆ *Reports of other services* when applicable: Examples include reports from obstetrics (labor and delivery, postpartum, newborn), nuclear medicine, and renal dialysis.

◆ *Flow sheets:* Routine daily care, bath, ambulation, BMs, activity, diet, and so forth checked off

◆ *Surgical reports* describing any surgery: Anesthesia, pathology, and postanesthesia recovery room reports, as well as detailed graphic records made during and immediately following the surgery

◆ *Intake and output records* and records of any intravenous fluids given: Records of blood transfusions, tube feedings, and total parenteral nutrition

◆ *Physician's note or discharge summary:* Home care, referrals, and date of next appointment. All medications or prescriptions sent home with the patient are noted; discharge teaching of patient or family must be documented.

* Joint Commission on Accreditation of Healthcare Organizations, 1992.

Research Data

Medical record personnel and other healthcare professionals (eg, physicians, nurses, infection control practitioners) review records to determine trends. For example, a group of hepatitis patients may be studied to try to determine the source of their disease. It may then be possible to prevent the spread of hepatitis to other people. Medical records also can help scientists work toward a cure for specific diseases.

Documentation

Documentation Formats

Documentation systems and forms vary greatly. New and more efficient formats develop as the system becomes more sophisticated. The most commonly used methods of documentation include the traditional source-oriented record, the problem-oriented medical record, focus charting, and computerized charting. The new system of case management uses forms called by various names, including critical pathway, case management plan, or anticipated recovery plan. Some acronyms used in documentation are given in the box.

The Source-Oriented Record

The **source-oriented record** is a form with separate columns for each group of the healthcare team (eg, nursing, medical, laboratory, x-ray department). Chronologic notes are kept on each form. Each group can easily find its own record and continue documentation, but the record of care is fragmented, making it difficult to trace overall care. If the Kardex care plan is not retained, the written nursing care plan must be duplicated in a narrative format.

The Problem-Oriented Record

The **problem-oriented medical record** (POMR) may be called the patient-oriented medical record or the problem-solving medical record. It emphasizes the patient and his or her health problems. It also provides a logical way to organize information. A "problem" is a condition that requires further observation, diagnosis, assessment, intervention, and evaluation. A care plan is developed based on the identified problem.

"Soap" and "Soapier" Documentation. After care is given, it is documented on the patient record in chronologic order by the "SOAP" or "SOAPIER" method, as shown:

Key Acronyms Used for Documentation

PIE	problem, implementation, evaluation
POMR	problem-oriented medical record/ patient-oriented medical record
SOAP	subjective, objective, assessment, plan
SOAPIER	subjective, objective, assessment, plan, implementation, evaluation, reassessment

S: *Subjective* statements made by the patient or family that describe their perceptions of the problem (in quotes)

O: *Objective*, measurable data from interventions and staff observations

A: *Assessment* or nursing diagnosis (analysis of subjective and objective data)

P: *Plan* of interventions the nurse develops in response to the nursing diagnosis

Some agencies continue this format with three additional items:

I: *Implementation* of the interventions

E: *Evaluation* of the interventions

R: *Reassessment* of patient needs and care plan revision

PIE Documentation. Some facilities use the acronym PIE for documentation:

P: Patient or problem

I: Implementation by nurses

E: Evaluation of implementation

Focus Documentation

Focus documentation is a patient-centered approach to organizing the *narrative portion* of the medical record. Narrative notes include a description of the problem, nursing actions, and client responses. Focus charting uses a column format to separate topic words or "focus statements" from the body of the note. The column format enhances communication among healthcare team members and makes quality assurance auditing more efficient.

The following are the goals of focus charting:

◆ Improve the quality of data gathered at admission
◆ Reduce duplication of documented information
◆ Simplify the documentation system and yet continue to demonstrate use of the nursing process
◆ Identify specific concerns of the patient
◆ Create an "index" for quick reference to patient concerns

The body of the focus note is divided into three columns or categories: date and time, focus, and notes. The "problems" in focus charting are similar to those used in the POMR format. These are listed in the "Focus" column. The difference in focus charting is in the "Notes" column. Notes may fall under any of the following categories:

◆ Data: Subjective or objective data supporting the focus statement
◆ Action/Plan: Past, present, or future nursing interventions
◆ Response: Description of patient response to medical or nursing care

Information from all three categories may or may not be relevant for all documentation entries. Table 37-1 gives examples of focus entries. A sample workup of a single factor (focus) in a daily care plan using focus charting is also included on page 410.

Case Management Record

The concept and forms used in case management are introduced in Chapter 35. In case management the patient is expected to progress at a certain rate toward recovery. If this does not occur, a variance is written. Chapter 70 contains a sample of an anticipated recovery plan in the discussion of hip fracture. If your facility uses this method of documentation and management, you will need further inservice education.

Table 37-1. Examples of Focus Statements

Focus	*Example*
Nursing diagnosis	Altered Comfort—chest pain; Impaired Physical Mobility
Current patient concern or behavior	Chest pain, diabetes teaching
Sign or symptom of importance to nursing or medical diagnosis or plan	Fever, arrhythmia, elimination
Change in condition	Seizure, respiratory distress, fever
Significant event in patient care	Cardiac arrest, transfer off station
Key word reference from flow sheet	Patient teaching, bleeding
Key word indicating compliance with hospital policy	Postoperative assessment, transfer assessment
(Occasionally) Medical diagnosis, as used in critical care to determine nursing intervention	Bigeminy, atrial fibrillation

* Lampe S. Focus Charting: A Patient-Centered Approach. Minneapolis, Creative Nursing Management, 1988.

Example of Daily Care Plan (General Postoperative Care)

Date	Focus	Goal/Objective	Nursing Action/Plan	Note (Pt. Response/Date/ Nurse's Initials)
2/14	Elimination	◆ Pt. to have urine output of 400 mL q8H	◆ Due to void 8–10 h postop	2/14 120 mL 5 PM (DE)
				300 mL 8 PM (DE)
			◆ Monitor voiding q shift	3–11 PM (DE)
			◆ Check for bladder distention if not voiding	OK (DE)
		◆ Pt. will have BM or pass flatus by discharge	◆ Auscultate for bowel sounds until BM or flatus	2/14 Faint bowel sounds 10 PM (DE)

Computerized Documentation

Computerized documentation of nursing care is done in institutions that have installed computer terminals in each department. These are usually networked with the hospital's mainframe computer. Nursing personnel and other employees access records using a personalized code. The appropriate information is keyed in to formulate the patient record.

Flow Sheets

Flow sheets are used with almost all formats for documentation of routine care and repeated monitoring. Flow sheets are an efficient tool. They allow easy retrieval of data for quality assurance monitoring. At the end of each shift, or as outlined by agency policy, pertinent items from the flow sheet are summarized into the patient care record. Duplicate documentation is discouraged.

Guidelines for Documentation

The quality of your documentation says much about the kind of care you give. Accurate and complete documentation is important to effective communication. Regardless of the format used by your agency, you should use the following skills in documentation.

Describe What You See

Describe exactly what you observe, and document what you see. Descriptive terms used in documentation are given in Table 37-2. Describe your assessments in objective terms; do not give your opinions or interpretations. For example, when you observe bleeding, indicate how much blood there is; its color; whether it is gushing, oozing, or running; and its source. When you are describing patient response, describe the patient's activity, not what you think it meant. For example, "patient crying and rocking back and forth in chair" is objective and descriptive. If you try to interpret the pa-

tient's actions, one interpretation might be "patient lonely," another might be "patient out of touch with reality," and still another might be "patient in pain." Such interpretations may or may not be correct.

Is the patient having trouble moving? Does the patient stumble? Can the person stand in a normal fashion? Is speech coherent? Is speech clear and appropriate? Does the urine or stool smell foul? Does the patient's breath have a foul odor? These are the types of questions you need to ask yourself so your assessments will be accurate and your documentation informative.

Identify the patient's reaction to your action, whether it is to a medication given, patient teaching, or nursing intervention. Record patient response, as well as the time, dosage, description, and any adverse effects. Check the chart for previous adverse reactions to this medication or treatment.

Be Specific

Avoid ambiguous statements and generalizations. For example, "had an uncomfortable night" does not say anything specific, whereas "patient was up 10 times with diarrhea during the night" tells why the patient had an uncomfortable night and why sleep was interrupted.

Use Direct Quotes. Directly quote the patient, and differentiate the patient's words from what you observed. Enclose the patient's statement in quotation marks so others will know that this is exactly what the patient said. This statement, "Mrs. Chang stated, 'I have a throbbing pain in my head,'" is specific and describes how the patient interprets the pain.

Do not chart hearsay, such as what someone else has told you about the patient, unless you quote it. For example, "Mrs. Rodriquez's husband said, 'My wife does not like the food here.'"

(Text continues on page 415)

Table 37-2. Descriptive Terms Commonly Used in Documentation

Points of Observation	Observations to Be Charted	Specific Terms
Abdomen	Bloated; filled with gas	Distention, tympanites
	Hard; boardlike	Rigid
	Large; extends out	Protruding
Amount	Large amount	Copious, excessive, profuse
	Small amount	Scanty, light
Appearance (skin, mucous membranes)	Bluish discoloration	Cyanotic
	Skin appears yellowish	Jaundice
Appetite	Craves certain foods	Parorexia
	Eats everything served and asks for more food	Hearty appetite
	Appears never to get enough food	Insatiable appetite
	Loss of appetite	Anorexia
	Eats nonfood items	Pica
Arm or leg (extremity)	Appears puffy or swollen	Appears edematous; edema
Attitude	Afraid; worried	Anxious; fearful
	Fixed idea (right or wrong)	Obsession
	False belief insisted	Delusion
Baths	Given when patient arrives	Admission bath
	Entire body	Complete bath
	Face, neck, arms, back, and genitals	Partial bath
	Taken in bed	Bed bath
	Taken in tub or special tub	Tub bath or sitz bath
Belch	To expel gas from stomach through the mouth	Eructation; burp
Bleeding	In large amount and in spurts	Hemorrhage; spurting blood; profuse
	Very little	Oozing; minimal amount
	Nosebleed	Epistaxis
	Blood in vomitus	Hematemesis
	Blood in urine	Hematuria
	Blood in sputum	Hemoptysis
Breast	Large; hard	Engorged
	Nipple always depressed	Inverted nipple
Breath	Unpleasant odor	Halitosis
Breathing	Difficulty in breathing	Dyspnea
	Short time without breathing	Momentary apnea
	Rapid breathing	Hyperpnea
	Cannot breathe lying down	Orthopnea
	Snoring sounds made when breathing	Stertorous respiration
	Increasing dyspnea with periods of nonbreathing	Cheyne-Stokes respiration
Coma	Does not respond to stimuli	Coma (partially comatose or in profound coma); loss of consciousness
Consiousness (level of)	Aware of surroundings	Alert; conversant; fully conscious; oriented
	Level of consciousness	Evaluated by Glasgow coma scale
Consistency of drainage (exudate)	Watery (from nose)	Coryza, rhinorrhea
	Tears (from eyes)	Lacrimation
	Contains pus	Purulent
	Watery and bloody	Sanguineous, serosanguineous
	Thick and sticky	Concentrated, viscous and tenacious
	Mucuslike	Mucoid

(continued)

Table 37-2 (continued)

Points of Observation	Observations to Be Charted	Specific Terms
Cough	Coughs all the time	Continuous, spontaneous
	Coughs up material	Productive
	Coughs over a long period of time	Persistent
	Coughs without producing material	Nonproductive
	Coughs with a whoop	Whooping cough
	Coughs at certain times	Paroxysmal
	Various types of cough	Loose; deep; dry; painful; exhaustive; tight; hacking; hollow
Decay	Tissue	Necrosis; necrotic
Dizziness	Feeling of being unstable; unsteady; dizzy	Vertigo; (feeling of rotation) dizziness
Drainage	Fecal (contains bowel material)	Fecal
	Contains mucus and pus	Mucopurulent
	Vaginal discharge that occurs for 1 or 2 weeks after childbirth	Lochia
Dressings	New dressing applied over original one	Reinforced dressing
Ears	Wax in ears	Cerumen
	Ringing sensation	Tinnitus
Edema	Leaves a dent when pressed	Pitting
	Exists when body part is hanging down or lowered	Dependent
Emesis	Vomiting	Emesis
	Vomiting forcefully and without warning	Projectile
	Descriptive terms	Coffee ground, hematemesis (containing blood), color (describe), containing solid material (describe), amount
Expectoration	Coughing and spitting up sputum	Expectorate
	Spitting up blood	Hemopytsis
Eyes, vision	Dilation of pupil	Enlarged pupil, dilated pupil
	Small, pinpoint pupils	Contracted pupil; "pinpoint"
	Sees double (two images of a single object)	Diplopia
	Cross-eyes	Strabismus
	Drooping eyelids	Ptosis
	Appear to be staring; eyes appear not to move	Fixed
Face	Scars and pits	Pockmarked
Faint	Losing consciousness; fainting	Syncope
Feces	Resembling clay	Clay-colored BM
	Black (tarlike) color	Tarry BM, charcoal BM
	Inability to control (child)	Encopresis
	Inability to control (adult)	Incontinence (fecal)
	Bowel movement (BM)	Feces; stool; defecation
	Excessive; watery	Diarrhea
	Soft material	Soft, formless, or soft-formed stool; loose
	Constipated	Hard-formed stool expelled with difficulty; pellet like
	Condensed, retains shape	Formed
	Patient unable to expel	Impacted
Fever, body temperature	No evidence of fever	Atebrile
	Temperature above normal	Pyrexia

(continued)

Table 37-2 *(continued)*

Points of Observation	Observations to Be Charted	Specific Terms
	Temperature greatly above normal	Hyperpyrexia
	Elevated temperature suddenly returns to normal	Crisis
	Elevated temperature gradually returns to normal	Lysis (falling)
Fingers	Appear square across and curved at the end	Clubbed (as in some cardiac conditions)
Gas	Excessive amounts of air and gas in stomach or intestine, causing distention of organs, passing of gas	Flatus, flatulence
Gums	Pulling away from teeth	Receding; shrunken
	Other descriptive terms	Bleeding; spongy; firm; pink; cyanotic
Hair	Absence of hair; baldness	Alopecia
Hallucination	Abnormal sense perceptions not experienced by others	Hallucination
	Hearing	Auditory hallucination (voices, music, or sounds)
	Sight	Visual hallucination (visual images not observed by others)
	Smell	Olfactory hallucination (abnormal odors)
	Taste	Gusatory hallucination
	Touch	Tactile hallucination (feeling something on skin that is not there)
Heartbeat	Irregular beating	Arrhythmia
	Slow	Bradycardia (<60/min)*
	Fast	Tachycardia (>100/min)*
Hives	Hives (raised areas on skin)	Urticaria
	Itching	Pruritus
Lips	Tiny cracks	Fissured; cracked
Memory	Loss of memory	Amnesia
Mental state	Fails to accept reality; overly happy	Euphoric
	Indifferent; showing little or no emotion	Apathetic, flat affect
Muscle	Loss of normal tone or size	Atrophy
Odor	Spicy	Aromatic
	Like fruit	Fruity
	Unpleasant	Offensive; foul
	Belonging to a particular thing	Characteristic
Perspiration	Excessive perspiration	Diaphoresis
Pain	Descriptive terms	Dull; aching; faint; burning; throbbing; gnawing; grinding; squeezing; acute; chronic; generalized; superficial; excruciating; unyielding; cramping; shooting; darting; colicky; continuous; shifting; agonizing; piercing; intense; cutting; transient; localized; remittent; persistent; unremitting; intractable
Pulse	Number of beats per minute	Rate
	Rhythm	Regular or irregular (may describe arrhythmia)
	Beats missed; not continuous	Intermittent
	>100/min	Rapid, tachycardia*
	<60/min	Slow, bradycardia*
	Beats indistinct (rapid)	Running
	Beats hardly perceptible	Thready
	Rapid, distinct beats	Bounding, full
	Cannot be felt	Imperceptible

(continued)

Table 37-2 (continued)

Points of Observation	Observations to Be Charted	Specific Terms
Sensation	Feelings that are experienced	Tingling; burning; stinging; prickling; hot; cold
Skin	Descriptive terms	Pale; red; moist; dry; clear; warm; coarse; tanned; scaly; thick; loose; rough; tight; discolored; jaundiced; mottled; calloused; edematous; cyanotic; excoriated; abrasion; bruised; oily; painful; scarred; black; brown; white; pink; translucent; clammy; rash; wrinkled; smooth; poor turgor
	Fragile	Friable
	Bruise ("black and blue mark")	Hematoma, ecchymosis
Sleep	Inability to sleep	Insomnia
	Sleeps more than normal	Hypersomnia
Speech	Unable to be understood	Incoherent
	Meaningless	Rambling, loose, tangential
	Runs words together	Slurring
	Difficulty in speaking	Dysphasia
	Inability to speak	Aphasia
	Other descriptive terms	Stammering; stuttering; hoarse; feeble; fluent
Teeth	False teeth	Dentures
	Decayed	Caries
	Accumulation of material on teeth	Sordes
	Without teeth	Edentulous
Thirst	Excessive thirst	Polydipsia
Throat	Difficulty in swallowing	Dysphagia
	Inability to swallow	Aphagia
Tongue	Descriptive terms	Dry; furrowed; cracked; raw; coated; swollen; ulcerated; pink; inflamed; furry
Treatment	Preventive	Prophylactic
	Giving temporary relief but not curing	Palliative
Urination	Pass fluid from bladder	Void; micturate; urinate
	Unable to control	Incontinence; involuntary
	Unable to wait to void	Urgency
	Increased excretion of urine	Diuresis
	No urine passes	Anuria
	Frequent urination; large amount of urine	Polyuria
	Unable to start stream	Hesitancy
	Voiding during the night	Nocturia
	Pus in urine	Pyuria
	Blood in urine	Hematuria
	Sugar in urine	Glycosuria
	Albumin in urine	Albuminuria
	Scantiness of urine	Oliguria
	Bed-wetting	Enuresis
	Stones (in urine or elsewhere)	Calculi
	Other descriptive terms	Cloudy; with sediment; straw-colored; coffee-colored; foul-smelling
Weight	Overweight	Obese; morbidly obese
	Very thin; underweight	Emaciated; cachexic
Miscellaneous terms	Came on suddenly, as a symptom	Sudden onset
	Spreading from one part of body to another (eg, cancer)	Metastasis
	How long it (eg, infection) lasts	Duration of (state length of time); prolonged; intermittent; persistent

* Adult average rates.

Table 37-3. Common Abbreviations Used in Documentation

Abbreviation	Meaning	Abbreviation	Meaning
@	at	per	by
aa	of each	PM	afternoon
ac, Ac	before meals, ante cena	po (o)	by mouth (per os, oral)
ad lib	as desired, at liberty	P.R.N.*	when required, as needed, *pro re nata*
alt hor, QOH	every other hour	pt	pint, patient
AM	morning	pulv, pwd	powder
BID	twice a day (bidaily)	q	every
BRP	bathroom privileges	qd, QD	every day
c̄	with	qh, QH	every hour
cap	capsule	q (2, 3, etc.) h	every (2, 3, etc.) hours
cc	cubic centimeter	q.i.d., QID	four times a day
D/C	discharge, discontinue	QOD	every other day
dr	dram	qs	sufficient amount
dx	diagnosis	R, pr	rectally, per rectum
& (et) Ɛ	and	℞, Rx	take, prescription, treatment
elix	elixir	s̄	without
fx	fracture	2°	secondary to
Gm, gm, G, g	gram	Sig or S	write on label, instructions
gr	grain	SOS*	if necessary
gt or gtt	drop, or drops	spans	spansule
H, hypo	hypodermic	s̄s̄	one half
h (hr), H	hour	stat, STAT	at once, immediately
hs (HS)	at bedtime (hour of sleep)	subq	subcutaneously
hx	history	supp	suppository
IM	intramuscularly	susp	suspension
IV	intravenously	t.i.d., TID	three times a day (tridaily)
L	liter	tint, tinct	tincture
m, min, or m_x	minim, or minims	t, tsp	teaspoon
μg, Mcg	microgram	T, tbsp	tablespoon
mg	milligram	TPN	total parenteral nutrition
mL	milliliter	tx, TX	treatment
NPO	nothing by mouth	ungt, ung	ointment
od	right eye, oculo dexter	i	one
oint (ungt)	ointment	ii	two
os	left eye, oculo sinister	v	five
ou	both eyes	x	ten
oz	ounce		
PC	after meals (post cena)		

* Note the difference between these abbreviations: SOS (if necessary) means for one dose only; PRN (when needed, as often as necessary) means the nurse is expected to use judgment about repeating the dose. For instance, the doctor may leave a PRN order for a cathartic, but if the patient has an adequate bowel movement, a cathartic is not necessary on that day. Two days later it may be needed. Usually PRN orders specify the frequency (how often) the drug may be given and usually must be rewritten at specific intervals in order to be considered valid.

Be Prompt. Document immediately after giving all care, medications, and treatments. The chart does not have memory lapses, though you may. Always document *after* you give a medication or perform a treatment, never before. If you forget to document a pertinent fact and add it after other documentation has been entered in the chart, you must identify your entry as a "late entry."

Be Clear and Consistent

Correct spelling, punctuation, and sentence structure are essential. "Bathed in wheelchair in hall" is not clear. What the nurse means is "has had a bed bath given by the nurse and is now sitting in a wheelchair in the hallway."

Write or print neatly *in ink.* Make sure there is continuity to the record. Use the format specified by that particular agency. Indicate the date and time of each entry. (Most facilities use the 24-hour clock).

Use only standard abbreviations; common abbreviations are listed in Table 37-3. Do not invent your own. If you are unsure as to the institution's acceptance of an abbreviation, refer to the Policy and Procedure Manual. Sign the chart with your first initial, last name, and classification, such as M. Smith, LPN.

Do not leave vacant lines in the chart. Use of every line proves the chronology of charting. If you continue on the back of a sheet or on a new page, again write the date, time, and "(continued)" before continuing your entry. If a vacant line is left between entries, a line is drawn through it, to prove that the documentation is chronologic.

Finally, always replace the chart where it belongs. Do not remove it from the nursing station unless you have consulted the charge nurse or team leader.

Record All Relevant Information

Read the physician's notes. If any information is missing, you are responsible for documenting this in the nursing notes, so it will be brought to the physician's attention. Document all communications with other members of the health team. Other departments have policies and procedures also that must be followed to protect the patient. If, for example, the care plan notes that side rails must be up after 10 PM, document that this has been done. If it was not done, the reason must be stated.

Nursing Alert

If your charts are audited or you go to court, *if it wasn't documented, it wasn't done* in the eyes of the law.

Respect Confidentiality

Confidentiality means that your conversations with patients and your nursing observations and assessments are to be shared only with the appropriate healthcare givers in the proper setting. What you record and show to the patient and other health professionals is never to be shared with anyone else. Don't discuss patients "over coffee"; you may be overhead. You also may be held liable in court for "breach of confidentiality."

Record Documentation Errors

Erasures and the use of correction fluid on the patient's chart are illegal. This could be considered a cover-up for poor nursing care or for an error made in patient care. If you make an *error in documenting*, cross out the incorrect statement with a single line, en-

close it in parentheses, and write ERROR and your initials above it. (Your note must be readable). Some agencies recommend using RIE (recorded in error) instead. Then record the correct statement. (An *error in patient care* is an entirely different matter and must be reported to your instructor or team leader at once.)

Nursing Alert

The importance of careful documentation in healthcare cannot be overstated. Each nurse must make sure all nursing assessments and actions are documented completely and accurately.

Reporting

Several times during the day the nurse must "report off" to another nurse. It is important to do this efficiently and accurately to make good use of nursing time and to ensure continuity of patient care. (Communication between healthcare team members is discussed in more detail in Chapter 36.)

Change of Shift Reporting

Change-of-shift reporting is a means of communication between the outgoing and incoming staff on each shift. Guidelines for reporting are given in the box. It can be done in a variety of ways. The report may be

---

Nursing Skill Guidelines

Giving Change-of-Shift Reports

♦ Use the Nursing Care Plan as your guide.
♦ Identify the room number, admitting diagnosis, age (if relevant), physician's name, primary nurse or case manager's name, significant medical history.
♦ Report on each nursing diagnosis or problem listed.
♦ For each nursing diagnosis or problem, briefly identify
  ♦ Significant assessment data
  ♦ Related nursing and medical orders
  ♦ Medications
  ♦ Recently received test results
  ♦ Diagnostic tests or surgery scheduled
  ♦ Vital signs
  ♦ Significant events of day
  ♦ Short- or long-term goals met
  ♦ Teaching plans
  ♦ Discharge plans
♦ Prepare a written summary to give to the oncoming nurse if this is agency procedure.

by the team leader to the entire incoming shift or by caregiver to caregiver. The report may be recorded on a tape recorder or may be given in "walking rounds." In **walking rounds** the caregivers move from patient to patient. This encourages patient participation and en-

ables the new nurse to view equipment, dressings, and other treatments with the previous nurse. The outgoing nurse is able to introduce the incoming nurse to the patient. This personalizes patient care and helps to establish rapport.

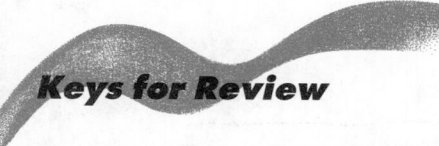

Keys for Review

Key Questions for Critical Thinking

1. Describe the patient record. Discuss its purposes and components.
2. Describe various formats for documentation. Describe advantages and disadvantages if there are any. Identify the format(s) used in your healthcare facility.
3. Describe reporting. Discuss its importance. Describe various ways it may be done. Relate reporting to the discussion of communication between healthcare team members discussed in Chapter 36.

Key Readings

Anderson C. Patient Teaching and Communicating in an Information Age. Albany, NY, Delmar, 1990

Bradley JC, Edinberg MA. Communications in the Nursing Context, Ed 3. Norwalk, CT, Appleton & Lange, 1990

Calfee BE. "Protecting Yourself from Allegations of Nursing Negligence." Nursing 91 21(12), December 1991

Dickson DA, Hargie O, Morrow NC. Communication Skills Training for Health Professionals: An Instructor's Handbook. New York, Chapman & Hall, 1991

Fischbach FT. Documenting Care: Communication—The Nursing Process and Documentation Standards. Philadelphia, F.A. Davis, 1991

Key Readings (continued)

Murray R, Zentner J. Nursing Assessment and Health Promotion Strategies Through the Life Span. Norwalk, CT, Appleton & Lange, 1993

Thomas E. Nursing Documentation Resource Guide. Gaithersburg, MD, Aspen, 1993

Enrichment Keys

Cordell B, Smith-Blair N. "Streamlined Charting for Patient Education." Nursing 94, 4(1):57-59, 1994

Keys to Learning More

Unit Nine: basic nursing skills, which are documented with patient reactions

Chapter 53: the patient having surgery requires careful documentation

Chapter 57: accurate documentation is important when administering medications

Accurate documentation will be stressed throughout your nursing career.

Unit 9 Basic Patient Care

38 Signs and Symptoms of Illness or Injury

Keys for Learning

Learning Objectives

- Differentiate between a functional and an organic disorder and between acute and chronic conditions.
- Define and give an example of each of the following classifications of physical disorders: hereditary, congenital, infectious, deficiency, metabolic, neoplastic, traumatic, and occupational.
- Discuss at least five factors that might predispose a person to a physical disorder.
- Differentiate between signs and symptoms, and give an example of each.
- Describe the PQRST method for categorizing, evaluating, and describing symptoms.
- List and define several objective words that could be written in the patient's chart to describe a cough, breathing, skin color or condition, emesis, hemorrhage, stool, or body temperature.
- List and discuss categories to be included in the observation of a patient.

Key Terms

acute disease	hereditary	organic disease
chronic disease	illness	orthopnea
congenital	infection	referred pain
disease	inflammation	signs
dyspnea	local	symptoms
edema	neoplastic	systemic
functional disease		

Keys to Understanding This Chapter

Chapter 5: basic needs of humans
Chapter 6: optimum health expectations

Keys to Understanding This Chapter
(continued)

Unit Four: normal body structure and function
Chapter 37: documentation and reporting

Key Points

- Illness, disease, and infections are deviations from the body's normal patterns of functioning, but each has a specific meaning.
- Classification of diseases may be described according to cause, body system affected, or the way in which they are acquired.
- Several factors predisposing illness are predictable. The body responds to disease by presenting signs (objective) and symptoms (subjective).
- Assessments of disease processes are based on a systematic method of recording.

Key Topics Outline

Illness and Disease
  Categories of Deviation from Normal
  Factors Predisposing to Illness
  The Course of Disease
Signs and Symptoms: The Body's Response to Disease
  Inflammation
  Assessments

Key Learning Activities

- Keep a daily journal of your clinical activities. Write your observations of your assigned patient. Express your own thoughts and feelings. Keep a journal for the duration of clinical rotation.

Previous units of this book have presented normal characteristics of physical and emotional health. Areas of normal values have been presented, which are necessary to study to be able to recognize deviations. This chapter briefly discusses some of these deviations; later chapters discuss deviations in greater detail.

Illness and Disease

Illness (the state of being sick) is a condition of pronounced deviation from the normal healthy state. **Disease** (lack of ease) is the deviation of bodily tissues, body systems, or human behavior from their normal state. **Infection** is a form of change in body tissues brought about by invasion of disease organisms.

Categories of Deviation From Normal

None of the various classifications of disease is satisfactory because categories overlap. For example, diseases may be classified according to their cause, the system of the body that is affected, or the way they are acquired. Classifying disease according to cause is not always satisfactory because the ultimate cause of many diseases is still unknown. Common classifications of disease and causes of illnesses follow.

Organic and Functional Diseases. A disease is described as organic or functional. **Organic disease** means that some detectable change has occurred in one or more organs, preventing them from carrying on their activities normally. **Functional disease** refers to a disorder for which a structural cause cannot be identified. A functional disorder interferes with the person's ability to continue normal activities of daily living. The person is said to be dysfunctional if normal activities cannot be carried out.

There also is an emotional response to physical illness. It may be exhibited in the form of a hysterical response or prolonged symptoms of physical illness after objective signs of the illness have cleared. Skillful observation is required to detect this situation and intervene.

Hereditary Disorders. A **hereditary** disorder is transmitted genetically by a parent or parents to the embryo, resulting in physical impairment. Hemophilia (prolonged blood clotting time) is inherited and is transmitted by the mother. It appears mostly in males, because it is almost always carried on the X chromosome. The mother is the "carrier" and is generally free of symptoms.

Congenital Disorders. Congenital disorders also are present at birth. Unlike hereditary disorders, they are not necessarily transmitted through the genes. Congenital disorders may be genetic or may be due to effects on the fetus of some unfavorable condition that interferes with normal development. For example, herpesvirus in the mother can be transmitted through the placenta and during the birth process. It can cause congenital defects. German measles contracted by the mother during pregnancy may cause body abnormalities or defects in the infant. Consumption of alcohol and smoking by the mother can have profound effects on the infant. Examples of abnormal fetal development are congenital heart disease and clubbed feet (deformities of bones in the feet).

Infectious Diseases. The most common cause of disease is invasion of the body by microorganisms, such as bacteria or viruses, or by animal parasites. As discussed in Chapter 8, microorganisms may or may not be contagious.

Deficiency Diseases. Deficiency diseases are disorders of nutrition that result from a deficiency of one or more vitamins or other nutrients in the diet. For example, lack of vitamin C causes scurvy. A deficiency of several vitamins, or general subnutrition, is more common in the U.S. than is a single vitamin deficiency. If the body doesn't use nutrients properly (malabsorption syndrome), various disorders result. Deficiency diseases also may be seen in the immune system. An immunodeficiency syndrome caused by the human immunodeficiency virus is often manifested in the body by infections, malignancies, and neurologic disease (AIDS).

Metabolic Disorders. Metabolic disorders are caused by a disturbance of one or more of the glands of internal secretion. These glands, known as endocrine glands, secrete hormones that regulate body processes. For example, the thyroid hormone affects the rate of metabolism for the entire body and insulin deficiency results in diabetes mellitus. Dysfunction occurs from hypersecretion or hyposecretion of a hormone.

Neoplastic Diseases. The term **neoplastic** is used to describe new growth of abnormal tissue, or tumors, which may be benign or malignant. A benign tumor is a growth of cells similar to the tissue in which it appears and is often surrounded by a capsule. Once removed, it usually does not recur. It may be disfiguring, but it is not dangerous unless it crowds other structures or robs surrounding tissues of their blood supply. A malignant tumor (eg, cancer) is a wild and disorderly growth of cells that is unlike the tissue from which it arises. This cell growth robs normal tissues of nutrients. The cells also tend to spread to other parts of the body, a process called *metastasis.*

Traumatic Injuries. Included in the category of traumatic injuries are physical injuries caused by external force, such as those incurred in automobile accidents or falls, and mental trauma, or shock, as from a personal loss.

Occupational Diseases. Certain occupational groups are subject to conditions peculiar to their jobs. Miners and oil field workers, for example, may be susceptible to lung conditions unless they wear proper protective gear. People working in noisy areas for prolonged periods of time must wear protective devices to prevent permanent hearing loss. The Occupational Safety and Health act was passed in an effort to protect American workers from occupational diseases and injuries.

Factors Predisposing to Illness

Some people are more susceptible to illness than others. A person's diet, mobility, age, weight, heredity, and gender influence whether illness will occur.

The presence of one condition may predispose the person to other disorders. Because of limited physical activity, a person with a severed spinal cord, for example, may experience such conditions as upper respiratory infections, pressure ulcers, urinary tract infections, and bowel obstructions more frequently than others.

Diet. The person who eats certain foods is more likely to contract certain physical disorders. For example, the person who eats a great deal of salt may be predisposed to cardiovascular disorders. The person who eats a great many fatty foods may develop inflammation of the gallbladder. It is believed that certain foods help to prevent colon cancer. Diseases also may result from a lack or an excess of a specific nutrient, such as vitamin C.

Immobility. The person who is confined to bed or to a wheelchair is more susceptible to certain disorders unless ambitious nursing care is practiced. Some of the disorders that must be prevented are pneumonia, pressure ulcer, contractures, and thrombophlebitis.

Age. Many disorders are associated with age. For example, older people are more likely to develop arteriosclerosis, cataracts, cerebrovascular accidents (stroke), osteoporosis, and diabetes. Young children are much more likely to have traumatic accidents, ingest poisons, or contract communicable diseases.

> ### Key Concept
> The age of a person can predispose to disease or disorders. Often, the people most likely to become ill or injured are the very young and the very old.

Obesity. Extremely overweight people are predisposed to heart attack, diabetes, gallbladder problems, and varicose veins in the legs. Other conditions, such as shortness of breath and dyspnea on exertion, may exist due to the person's inability to carry out physical activities.

Smoking. Cigarette smoking and the use of smokeless tobacco has been linked to lung and mouth cancers, emphysema, cardiovascular disorders, and birth defects. Smoking is the number one preventable health hazard.

Heredity. A person may be highly susceptible to diabetes mellitus, sickle cell anemia, or some types of cancer because of hereditary factors.

Sex-Linked Disorders. Some hereditary disorders, such as color blindness and hemophilia, occur almost exclusively in men. These are called sex-linked disorders, because the disorder is carried on the X or Y chromosome. Other disorders are not genetically sex linked but occur more commonly in one sex or the other. For example, leukemia is more common in men. Of course, certain reproductive disorders can occur only in men or in women; examples include prostatic hypertrophy in men and ovarian cancer in women.

The Course of Disease

An **acute disease** comes on suddenly and runs its course in days, whereas the course of a **chronic disease** may be prolonged for years or life. A subacute condition is classified between acute and chronic and may go on for weeks or months. Complications from chronic illness may occur at any stage. (The stage of a chronic disease may be described as early, continuing, late, and terminal.)

Diseases also may be described as independent (primary) or dependent (secondary). A *primary disease* occurs independently of another, such as a streptococcal sore throat. A *secondary disorder* is one that is the direct result of, or is dependent on, another disorder; an example is rheumatic heart disease, which is secondary to rheumatic fever. (Both are usually secondary to a streptococcal infection in the throat or tonsils.)

Signs and Symptoms: The Body's Response to Disease

Signs are *objective* evidence of disease that can be noted by an observer, such as a physician or nurse: a rash, swelling, pallor, pulse, and temperature changes. **Symptoms** are *subjective* evidence of disease, sensations that only the patient knows about and can report: pain, itching, nausea, fear, worry. Signs and symptoms are charted in the S (subjective) and O (objective) sections in SOAP documentation (see Chapter 37).

Signs may be **local,** that is, limited to the affected part (eg, swelling), or they may be **systemic,** affecting most or all of the body (eg, fever). A nurse must first know what is normal before deviations can be recognized, recorded, and reported.

Although a disease may be classified according to its seriousness as *mild, moderate,* or *severe,* people may react quite differently to the same disease.

Inflammation

Inflammation is the body's attempt to fight infection or cope with the damage to body cells resulting form an injury that has caused a break in the skin (wound). Inflammation is caused by the rush of white blood cells (leukocytes) into the area in an attempt to fight off an infection. Most words denoting inflammation end with the suffix *"itis."* Symptoms usually found in some degree where there is injury or infection, along with their causes, are listed in Table 38-1.

Inflammation may be *acute, subacute,* or *chronic.* In an acute inflammation, an excess of fluid and cells (*exudates*) is usually present in or issuing from tissues. Exudates may be clear (serum), such as discharge from a nasal cold; fibrinous, which causes adhesions to form as tissues are repaired; bloody, as a result of small hemorrhages in the area; or purulent (containing pus), because of bacteria. The formation of pus is called *suppuration.* In this process, the poisons of bacteria kill off white blood cells and destroy tissue. The death of tissue is called *necrosis.* Destroyed tissue may be cast off (*sloughed,* pronounced "sluffed"), leaving behind an area that needs to be filled in with new tissue (*granu-*

lation tissue). Sometimes there is a local unhealed area of epithelial tissue called an *ulcer.* A canal or passage leading to an abscess is called a *sinus.* A wound with a small, persistent tubelike opening that does not heal and that connects with an internal hollow organ is called a *fistula.*

A *chronic inflammation* is one that persists over a long period of time, often for the remainder of an individual's life, and does not follow the usual process of healing. A *subacute* inflammation is midway in severity between acute and chronic. The person may appear to be clinically well; the condition may be diagnosed by laboratory tests or by radiologic or computed tomography examination.

Assessments

Medical and nursing personnel gather information about the patient by several means, some of which are discussed in Chapter 34. Methods used include the following:

◆ Observation and visual inspection of the patient
◆ Interviews of the patient and the family (family history)
◆ Measurement of vital signs, such as temperature, pulse, and blood pressure
◆ Laboratory and x-ray procedures
◆ Examination by the physician
◆ Nursing assessment and diagnosis

You will learn how to perform many of these assessments during your nursing program. It is also important to document and report these assessments correctly.

Because the nurse is with the patient for extended periods, the nurse's assessments are invaluable to the physician. Your notes about each patient should create a vivid, individualized, and accurate picture. Patients are able to give only part of the information because they report only things that seem important to them. The nurse must be aware of signs that can be seen, heard, smelled, and felt. It is the nurses' responsibility to observe and report these signs. It is the physician's responsibility to decide what the signs and symptoms mean and to prescribe necessary treatment. The nurse, in turn, must understand the significance of certain symptoms to give intelligent nursing care.

Systematic Assessment

A detailed description of patient assessment is beyond the scope of this book. However, many aspects of assessment are presented throughout the remaining chapters, especially in Chapter 50.

PQRST. A general method of determining symptoms is known as PQRST (see box). These initials will guide

Table 38-1. Signs and Symptoms of Injury or Infection

Signs/ Symptoms	Cause (Examples)
Pain	Pressure of excess fluid on nerve endings
Redness	Increase in circulation to the part
Swelling	Fluid and leukocytes leave bloodstream to enter tissues
Heat	Increased circulation and increased chemical reactions in the area
Loss of function	The body's attempt to keep injured area at rest; also the result of pain
Pus	Bacteria destroy leukocytes and destroy tissue; decaying forms pus

PQRST Method of Nursing Assessment

P: Provocative/ Palliative	What causes it?
	What improves it?
	What makes it worse?
	Is it combined with any other symptom? Does it cause anything else?
	How is it controlled?
Q: Quality/Quantity	How much is there?
	What is it like? (How does it smell, taste, feel, sound, look?)
	How does it change?
R: Region/Radiation	Where does it start?
	Does it radiate from there?
S: Severity	Does it interfere with daily life? In what way?
	Is the person able to work?
	Rate it on a severity scale from 1 to 10. (How bad is it?)
	Has that rating changed recently?
	Is it bad enough to wake the person at night?
T: Timing	When does it begin (onset)?
	What is the person doing when it begins?
	How long does it last?
	Is there a time when it is worse or better? (When?)
	Does it ever go away?
	How often does it occur?
	Is it sudden or does it build up gradually?

(Adapted in part from Taking and recording a health history. In Assessment, p 25. Springhouse, PA, Intermed Communications, The Nurse's Reference Library, 1983.)

you in determining what you need to know about a symptom. Following this format when questioning the patient will help you remember each important component.

Review of Systems. The nurse may do a review of body systems or a "head-to-toe" assessment of the patient. These assessments are described in Chapter 50. The nurse must always use the procedures designated by the healthcare facility in which he or she is employed.

Common Signs and Symptoms

Signs and symptoms commonly associated with specific diseases are fully discussed under each disease in Unit Fourteen and are mentioned briefly here. A number of descriptive terms that can be used in documentation and reporting are presented in Table 37-2. It is helpful to think of body systems from head to toe when assessing the patient.

Cough. Cough usually indicates irritation somewhere along the respiratory tract. It is present in most respiratory diseases and in some heart conditions. A cough may be helpful or harmful. In some diseases, it aids greatly in draining an infected area. In the absence of pulmonary secretions, it serves no useful purpose and may be harmful.

Dyspnea and Orthopnea. Dyspnea (difficult breathing) and **orthopnea** (inability to breathe except when upright) usually indicate some difficulty in obtaining or using oxygen. These symptoms are frequently seen in cardiac and respiratory conditions.

Cyanosis. Cyanosis (blueness or grayness of the skin due to lack of oxygen in the blood) often occurs in cardiac and respiratory conditions. When oxygen is decreased, the bright red color in the blood diminishes and the patient's skin assumes a bluish or grayish pallor, especially noticeable in the lips or the fingernails. White or Asian patients with cyanosis usually appear bluish, whereas the condition in an African American person is observable as a dusky or ashen color (graying white) of the skin, nail beds, and lips.

Pallor. Pallor, or paleness of the skin, is easily observable in the light-skinned person. In a darker-skinned person, the skin appears to be a shade lighter than its normal tone. Pallor is caused by the absence of some of the blood that normally flows to the skin. An extremely frightening experience or an illness may cause pallor.

Jaundice. Jaundice is another change in the color of the patient's skin. The patient generally develops a yellowish color, first noticeable in the whites of the eyes.

Edema. Edema (swelling) is the result of an abnormal amount of water in the tissues, and there are several possible causes:

- If the return flow of blood and lymph to the veins is obstructed in some way, pressure on the capillaries increases, forcing more fluid into tissues.
- Obstruction of lymph vessels prevents them from carrying off tissue fluid.
- Injury to blood vessel causes them to lose plasma proteins and will cause edema.
- Normally, plasma proteins are retained in blood vessels and help maintain osmotic pressure, which keeps fluid in the blood vessels. If these proteins are reduced by disease, fluid escapes into the tissues.
- A high intake of salt keeps water in the tissues, because the body attempts to retain fluid to dilute the salt.

Edema frequently occurs in loose tissues, such as the eyelids and external genitalia, whereas dense tissues, such as large muscles or bones, resist edema formation. Edema also is more likely to occur in areas where the return flow of blood is slowest, as in fingers and ankles (dependent edema). *Pitting edema* is described as severe edema. When the swollen part is pressed with the finger, a "dent" remains after the finger is removed.

Emesis. Emesis (vomiting) has many causes. Sometimes it follows mental or emotional disturbance and has no apparent physical cause. It also may be due to disturbance, infection, or obstruction of the digestive (alimentary) tract. The form of the emesis varies according to the location of difficulty; the vomited material may tell much about this. Fermented, undigested food indicates that it has been returned from the stomach; bile-stained fluid is returned from the upper small intestine; fecal vomitus is returned from the colon. Blood in the vomitus indicates hemorrhage and is always regarded as a serious symptom. Projectile (very forceful) vomiting often indicates a brain disorder.

Special Considerations in Children

Projectile vomiting in the small child may be a result of a muscle spasm of the pyloric valve leading to the stomach.

Hemorrhage. Hemorrhage, or abnormal loss of blood, also may indicate a certain condition. In emesis or sputum, blood may be a sign of disease in the digestive or respiratory system. Bright red or blackish tarry blood in the stool indicates digestive tract disturbances. (The darker the blood in the stool, the higher up in the digestive tract is the bleeding. If blood is partially digested, it is darker. Fresh bleeding from the rectum, for example, will be bright red.) Blood in the urine (hematuria) indicates a urinary disorder. Hemorrhage from accidental or surgical wounds can be fatal in a short time if not controlled. A bleeding or clotting disorder may cause excessive bleeding from a small wound.

Diarrhea. Diarrhea, or frequent passage of liquid, unformed, watery stools, may be caused by physical or emotional difficulties. It is sometimes a protective mechanism that the body uses to get rid of irritating or toxic materials or poisons. Diarrhea may be an indication of constipation resulting from impacted fecal material in the bowel. Diarrhea also may have an emotional basis.

Fever. Fever is an elevation of body temperature above normal and is another sign of the body's attempt to fight disease. It may develop suddenly or gradually. Increased pulse and respiratory rate are associated with a rise in temperature and are two of the symptoms of body changes; both usually rise proportionately as body temperature goes up.

Fatigue. Fatigue, when it is a symptom of disease, is extreme tiredness for which no reasons can be found; sometimes it is due to toxic effects caused by a microorganism.

Other Symptoms. *Loss of appetite* (anorexia) or *general weakness* also may be symptoms of illness. *General malaise* indicates that the person is feeling "generally sick" or "sick all over."

A sharp increase or decrease in blood pressure (*hypertension* or *hypotension*) may indicate the presence of illness. Hypotension is one of the most common symptoms of hemorrhage.

Categories for Assessment

Various types of assessment can be made, depending on the seriousness of the person's condition or the reason for the person's visit. The following are types of assessments.

Discomfort and Pain. Pain has been defined as a disagreeable sensation elicited by a potentially harmful stimulus. Its purpose is mainly protective. Pain is characterized in a number of ways and is discussed in Chapters 37, 50, and 52. It is important to assess the patient in pain carefully and to report objectively. Pain may cause physical and emotional discomfort, which varies greatly in intensity among individuals. The sensitivity of various parts of the body also differs. Some patients will try to conceal pain; others will complain of pain when no cause for it can be found. Personality and culture have a bearing on reactions.

Pain may be *local*, that is, affecting one part of the body, or it may be *systemic*, affecting more than one part. Pain is sometimes felt in one part of the body, while the cause of it is located in another; this is **referred pain.**

Nutrition. When assessing nutrition and the following aspects in the patient, the nurse should ask himself or herself basic questions. Has the weight changed? Does the patient appear to be overweight or underweight? Are there obvious signs of malnutrition? Is the patient eating the food served? What is said about the food? Is the person nauseated? Is he or she vomiting? Is the person unusually hungry or thirsty? Does the person refuse to eat? Does the person eat nonfood items (perverted appetite, pica in pregnancy)? What is the condition of the mouth and teeth? Can the person chew and swallow?

Sleep and Rest. Sleep and rest also are important factors in illness. Excessive sleep or sleep deprivation can greatly influence the course of an illness. Does the patient complain of not being able to sleep? Does he or she seem tired, relaxed, or restless? Is it difficult for the patient to fall asleep or to stay asleep? What helps the person to fall asleep? Are noises in the hospital disturbing the patient during the night? What were the patient's sleep habits before coming to the hospital?

Body Function. Elimination habits can give you valuable clues about a patient. Can the patient control voiding and bowel movements? Are elimination habits regular? Does the patient complain about elimination? Is there something that the patient does or takes at home to regulate bowel or bladder activity?

The skin often reflects the internal environment of the body. Is the skin clammy, hot, or moist? Does the patient perspire profusely? Does the person complain about being too cold or too warm?

Other factors are also considered. Do you notice a cough, watering eyes, or runny nose? Are the face, legs, or feet puffy (edema)?

Reflex. Are reflexes appropriate? Do the eyes react to light? Does the person startle easily? Are responses equal on each side of the body? (See Chapter 50 for a description of neurologic assessment.)

Sensory. Does the person hear and see well? Is there a normal response to heat and cold and to pain or pressure on the skin? What is the response to heat and cold?

Activity. Can the person walk, sit, and stand without assistance? Does the person seem afraid to walk? Does the person look worried or anxious? Is the person expressionless? Is the person pale or flushed? Are movements jerky or very slow? Are there tremors or muscle spasms? Does the person walk standing straight or hunched over? Does the person need much encouragement to get out of bed?

Relationships. Does the patient visit with his or her roommate? Does the patient have visitors? Does the patient have some sort of diversional activity to pass the time? Are interactions appropriate? Does the family call and seem concerned? Has the patient requested *not* to have visitors?

Cognition and Perception. Is the person alert, disoriented, or unresponsive? Is there a language difficulty? Is the patient oriented to time, place, and person? Does the person make an attempt to keep clean and as well groomed as possible? Does the person cry a great deal? Is laughter and conversation appropriate and reality oriented? Does the person seem preoccupied or otherwise responding to internal stimuli (hallucinations)?

Reaction to Treatments. How does the patient react to nursing treatments? What do you observe about positive and negative effects of treatments? Is the patient cooperative when you are doing treatments? Does the person follow instructions for self-treatment? Does the patient have questions regarding his or her care?

Medication Effects. Are you aware of the expected effects and possible side effects of medications you are giving? Are there any undesirable side effects? Is the person experiencing the desired action of the medication (eg, relief)? Is the patient refusing medications? If so, what is the reason given? What are nursing actions that must be considered when giving drugs (eg, taking blood pressure, counting pulse)?

Blood, Urine, and Other Output. The blood and urine help indicate the condition of the internal environment of the body. Is the urine clear or cloudy? Does it contain sediment, blood, or pus? What is the color and amount of urine? How would you describe emesis, bowel movements, and other drainage? What do laboratory reports state about the patient's blood and other output? Does the person void abnormally often or abnormally seldom? (See Chapter 37.)

Observation of Objective Symptoms. Does the patient have bruises, cuts, or pressure ulcers? Does the skin color provide any information about the patient's condition? Is there any sign of redness or skin breakdown, cyanosis, or jaundice? What are the vital signs? How have they changed? Does the skin have natural turgor (elasticity)? Is there edema?

> ### Key Concepts
> ◆ Symptoms: Subjective data (what the patient feels)
> ◆ Signs: Objective data (what you see or measure)

Keys for Review

Key Questions for Critical Thinking

1. Discuss the difference between acute and chronic disorders. Give examples of each. Describe how an acute disease may become chronic.
2. Describe inflammation as a sign of disease. Describe various types of inflammation. Describe how you would assess for inflammation.
3. Review the difference between medical and nursing diagnoses as discussed in Chapter 34. Describe signs and symptoms that would help the physician in making a medical diagnosis and those that would help the nurse in making a nursing diagnosis.

Key Readings

Craven RF, Hirnle CJ. Fundamentals of Nursing: Human Health and Education. Philadelphia, J.B. Lippincott, 1992

Earnest VV. Clinical Skills in Nursing Practice, Ed 2. Philadelphia, J.B. Lippincott, 1993

Smeltzer SC, Bare BG. Brunner and Suddarth's Textbook of Medical Surgical Nursing, Ed 7. Philadelphia, J.B. Lippincott, 1992

Key Readings (continued)

Smith S, Duell D. Clinical Nursing Skills: Nursing Process Model, Basic to Advanced Skills, Ed 2. Norwalk, CT, Appleton-Lange, 1989

Swearingen PL. Photo Atlas of Nursing Procedures, Ed 2. Redwood City, CA, Addison-Wesley Nursing, 1991

Taber's Cyclopedic Medical Dictionary, Ed 17. Philadelphia, F.A. Davis, 1993

Taylor C, Lillis C, LeMone P. Fundamentals of Nursing: The Art and Science of Nursing Care, Ed 2. Philadelphia, J.B. Lippincott, 1993

Keys to Learning More

Chapter 39: transcultural aspects of patient care
Chapter 42: vital signs
Chapter 47: specimen collection
Chapter 50: head-to-toe physical examination
Chapter 52: pain management, including assessment
Chapter 69: edema

39 Transcultural Considerations in Nursing

Keys for Learning

Learning Objectives

- Define the terms *culture* and *transcultural nursing*.
- List and describe at least six cultural beliefs about illness and treatment.
- Describe specific characteristics of the Jewish, Protestant, Roman Catholic, Mormon, Christian Scientist, and Seventh Day Adventist religions as related to health care.
- Describe at least eight anatomic differences between races.
- Give examples of five disorders specific to certain cultural groups.
- Describe relationship of Eastern religions to Western medicine and nursing care.
- Describe at least eight sociocultural considerations in nursing care.

Key Terms

Buddhism	Imam	Muslim
Christianity	Hinduism	nirvana
Confucianism	Jewish	rabbi
culture	Judaism	Sabbath
curandero	karma	Taoism
Islam	Koran	transcultural nursing

Keys to Understanding This Chapter

Chapter 5: basic human needs of all people
Unit Three: individual and family development
Chapter 27: transcultural nutritional considerations
Chapter 36: therapeutic communication

Key Points

- Transcultural nursing is nursing that considers the religious and sociocultural backgrounds of patients. It is important to be nonjudgmental when working with patients of a culture or religion different from your own.

Key Points *(continued)*

- Cultural and religious traditions are not always followed by every member of that group. Furthermore, the patient should be treated as an individual.
- You should be acquainted with the predominant cultural and religious groups within the community where you work.
- You may suggest a visit from a spiritual leader, but do not call one without first asking the patient.

Key Topics Outline

Cultural Beliefs About Illness
Racial Anatomic Characteristics
Disorders of Cultural Groups
Religious Beliefs
    Judaism
    Islam
    Christianity
Nursing Considerations

Key Learning Activities

- Prepare an oral or written report on your own ethnic or religious heritage. Use as topics: beliefs regarding illness, methods of healing, beliefs relating to illness/death, procedures in dying/death, differences in communication.
- Design a chart showing cultural/religious groups and unique practices relating to nursing and medical care.
- Prepare a report on the dominant cultures or religious groups in your community. Outline their beliefs regarding illness and healing and how these affect nursing care.

Culture is the way we live, the way we behave as a social group. **Culture** has been defined by anthropologists and sociologists in various ways:

◆ A way of life for a group of individuals
◆ The sum total of "socially inherited" characteristics, handed down from generation to generation
◆ A group's "design for living"—socially transmitted assumptions about the physical and social world

All of these definitions include some common threads:

◆ Culture is *learned* (not genetic)
◆ Every society has a *unique* culture
◆ Human culture is *complex* and all-encompassing

Being a member of a cultural group means that certain components of that culture are common to all members. Common components include diet, language, customs and rituals, values and beliefs, traditions, and concepts of health and illness.

The patient's culture has a great influence on recovery from illness or injury. The nurse should consider all aspects of the total person.

Transcultural nursing is the nursing of patients while taking into consideration their religious and sociocultural backgrounds. The accompanying box lists a variety of factors involved in transcultural nursing.

This chapter gives examples of cultural beliefs about illness and healing, racial anatomic characteristics, dis-

orders common to specific cultural groups, religious beliefs, and nursing considerations. The information is stated in generalizations, and you should remember that not everyone in a particular group follows all the practices or has all the same characteristics of that group. Much more can be learned about these sociocultural and religious groups than presented here.

It is your responsibility as a nurse to become acquainted with the predominant cultural, racial, and religious groups in your community. Then you must view the people of these groups as individuals and provide care in a nonjudgmental way.

Cultural Beliefs About Illness

Causes of Illness

Some people believe that illness is the will of God or that illness is punishment for sins. Other cultural groups believe that illness is caused by external forces. The following are some examples:

◆ Many Chinese and Filipino people believe in Yin–Yang principles. Yin and Yang represent "unified opposites" that are interrelated. Yin (matter)–Yang (energy) examples include, respectively, cold–hot, weak–strong, female–male, night–day, hypofunction–hyperfunction, and expansion–contraction. A Yin condition requires a Yang treatment and vice versa.

Factors in Transcultural Nursing

◆ Cultural background of nurse; differences and similarities between patient and nurse (see Chapter 36)
◆ Definition of health and illness accepted by a specific culture, and concepts relating to causes of illness and injury
◆ Folk medicine practices
◆ Attitudes toward healthcare, relationships, and interactions (eg, personal space, eye contact)
◆ Economic level of patient/family (socioeconomic status)
◆ Environmental factors and related disorders (eg, ghetto living, lead poisoning)
◆ Specific names and terms related to illness and disorders; use of slang
◆ Language differences between healthcare staff and patient/family
◆ Modesty and concept of the human body
◆ Reactions to pain
◆ Reactions to aging and death
◆ Attitudes about childbirth, abortion, sexual expression
◆ Attitudes about mental illness or retardation
◆ Diets in relation to religious and cultural practices (eg, concepts of "hot" and "cold" foods and how these relate to specific illnesses); dietary taboos

◆ Attitudes about such factors as physical appearance, amputation, and obesity; adaptation to special therapeutic diets
◆ Importance of religion and religious practices
◆ Group identity: importance and type of family structure; cohesiveness within the group; traditional roles of men and women
◆ "Visibility" of ethnic background (eg, African American, Asian American)
◆ Disorders specific to a cultural group (eg, Tay-Sachs, sickle cell anemia)
◆ Attitudes about school; educational level and aspirations of most members of the group
◆ Predominant occupations within the group; role models
◆ "Americanization" of younger members
◆ Numbers of people belonging to that group in the same geographic area as the healthcare facility
◆ Prejudices within a cultural group relating to other members of the same group
◆ Stereotypes about other cultural/ethnic groups
◆ Mixed families (mixed races, religions, or cultural background)

- Many of these people also believe in a complex system of five basic energies/elements/substances in nature (wood, fire, earth, metal, water). This theory is an expansion of Yin–Yang and is also involved in the healing process.
- Japanese Shintoists believe that man is inherently good; illness is caused when the person comes into contact with pollutants.
- Native Americans often follow three concepts: prevention, treatment, and health maintenance. Health is defined in terms of the person's relationship with nature and the universe (wholeness).
- African Americans often believe that illness is caused by a lack of harmony or a conflict in the patient's life. They also may believe that trouble or pain is God's will.

Healing

Various cultures treat disorders in different ways. Examples are:

- African American and Hispanic cultures have long used roots, potions, and herbs for treating illnesses.
- Filipinos and Hispanic groups often believe that hotness, coldness, wetness, and dryness must be balanced to be healthy. Certain illnesses are considered hot or cold, wet or dry. Foods and medications, classified as hot or cold, are added or subtracted to bring about a balance.
- Chinese and Filipino cultures use massage, herbal medicine, and acupuncture to treat illness.
- Copper bracelets are worn by many groups as a preventive or cure for arthritis.

Diet

Dietary beliefs and cultural nutrition play a major role in the reaction of a patient to illness. For this reason, a separate chapter was devoted to social and transcultural aspects of nutrition (see Chapter 27).

Racial Anatomic Characteristics

Some characteristics of specific racial groups require adaptations in nursing care. The following are examples.

- The skin of African Americans tends to be very dry.
- African American people may have thinner skin folds than white people, which must be considered when assessing nutritional status.
- The pelvis in more than 1/3 of African American women shows a reduced transverse diameter and an increase in the anterior and posterior segments. This is a consideration during pregnancy, labor, and delivery.
- Dry ear wax (gray and brittle) occurs most often in Native Americans and Alaska Natives and people of Asian descent. Wet ear wax (brown and sticky) occurs in African Americans and whites.
- African American newborns tend to be larger than white newborns; Asian Americans and some Hispanics tend to be smaller.
- Several variations in tooth and bone formation occur among the races; the different appearance of the jaw should not be interpreted as an orthodontic problem. Nutritional deficiencies may result if the person is not able to chew adequately.
- Facial characteristics vary according to the part of the world from which the person's ancestors migrated. For example, the Asian American person usually has an epicanthic fold in the eyelid; small noses are seen in people from cold regions while people from dry areas, such as the Middle East, have a high bridge. Moist, warm areas tend to lead to the wide, flat nose of many people of African descent. Nasal shape may influence sinus and nasal disorders.
- Blood groups differ. Native Americans are most likely to be group O, with some A, and almost no B. Asians have almost equal percentages of O, A, and B type blood, and approximately 10% of AB. African Americans and American whites have about an equal percentage of blood types, with the majority being O, and with many being A. Fewer African Americans and whites are of AB or B types. Rh negative blood is most common in whites and rare in other races.

Disorders of Cultural Groups

Some disorders occur most often in particular cultural groups. Examples follow:

- More common in white than in African American people: psoriasis, congenital hip dysplasia, pyloric stenosis, cystic fibrosis, hemophilia, Huntington's disease, phenylketonuria, osteoporosis, and skin cancer.
- More common in African American than in white people: stomach cancer, esophageal cancer, sickle cell anemia, keloids, vitiligo. Hypertension is common in African Americans, especially men, and in Asian American people who use a great deal of salt and monosodium glutamate. African people rarely contract malaria.
- Asian Americans have a lower incidence of atherosclerosis than do people who eat large amounts of meat; however, those in the United States who follow the traditional American diet increasingly show atherosclerosis disease of the heart
- More common in Filipino and Malayan people:

gouty arthritis, diabetes mellitus, cancer of the liver, amyotrophic lateral sclerosis, and tuberculosis.

- ◆ Common in African Americans and Hispanics: pica of pregnancy. These two groups, in addition to southeast Asians, have a higher incidence of lactose intolerance (inability to properly digest the sugar in milk).
- ◆ Common in Native Americans: otitis media, cleft lip, nutritional problems, diabetes mellitus (especially gestational), fetal alcohol syndrome, emotional disorders of children, and infant death. This group tends to have higher incidence of alcohol abuse, suicide, and homicide. Tuberculosis is a problem, particularly in the Alaska Native groups (Eskimo, Indian, Aleut).

Religious Beliefs

Religion is a vital part of many people's lives. Because you will be caring for people of different faiths, you should be informed about differences among religions. Important points about major religions are presented here.

People who are injured or ill need reassurance, and they may talk to you about their illness and beliefs. Those confidences must be respected and a nonjudgmental attitude maintained.

You may suggest a visit from their spiritual leader, but do not contact such a person without first finding out if the patient wants spiritual counsel.

Judaism

The term **Jewish** refers to the total culture, religion, history, and philosophy of life shared by a particular group of people. Their religious belief is called **Judaism**. It comprises three forms: Reform, Conservative, and Orthodox. Reform Jews are the most liberal in their beliefs; Orthodox Jews are most strict in their adherence to their traditions. Within the Orthodox form are various elements. Orthodox men must have their heads covered at all times, and women may wear wigs on a shorn head.

The custom that is most difficult to follow during illness is that of conforming to kosher laws, which govern dietary practices. Although nonsectarian hospitals cannot prepare kosher meals, frozen kosher meals are available. The patient's family can bring food from home also. Observance of dietary laws varies among Jews. Ask Jewish patients if they observe dietary laws and notify the dietary department accordingly.

Circumcision of male infants is generally a religious ceremony. It is rarely performed in the hospital. The spiritual leader is called a **rabbi**. The Jewish **Sabbath** is observed from sundown Friday to sundown Saturday. Other than the Sabbath, the most important Jewish holidays are Yom Kippur, Rosh Hashanah, and Passover. The Jewish patient may wish to have a menorah, which is a special candelabra. An electric version is available for safety.

Islam

Muslims are believers in **Islam**, the religion founded by Mohammed. Islam is one of the largest and fastest growing religions in the world. There are several sects within Islam, some more strict than others. Muslims follow the teachings of the **Koran**, which influences their diet, attitudes about women, death, and so forth. They pray five times a day, facing Mecca. Their Sabbath is Friday. Pork and alcohol are prohibited. They do not believe in faith healing; there is no infant baptism. In case of death, prescribed procedures for washing and shrouding the body are followed by the clergy person, the **Imam**.

Many African Americans follow the basic teachings of the Koran. They call themselves members of the "Nation of Islam" or Black Muslims. They prefer to receive their healthcare from members of the African American community.

Christianity

Sunday is the major day of worship in most **Christian** sects. Easter and Christmas are the most important holidays, but other holy days are observed. Bible reading and prayer are important aspects of faith.

Roman Catholicism

Roman Catholics consider baptism, penance, Eucharist, and anointing of the sick as some of the basic sacraments of the church. During illness or an emergency, the patient may want a priest to hear confession and give communion. Most Catholics attend Mass at least once a week. The priest may also say Mass in the patient's hospital room. At such times, provide privacy.

A person may receive the sacrament of anointing of the sick many times; it is a service of comfort and consolation. If a Catholic patient dies suddenly, this sacrament can be administered conditionally, within 2 hours after death. To prepare the patient, loosen the covers at the foot of the bed.

Infant baptism is mandatory for Catholics and can be performed by a lay person in an emergency. If a Catholic patient is brought into the hospital, notify the hospital chaplain or priest. Many Catholics wear a crucifix or have an amulet attached to their clothing. They should be allowed to wear these in the hospital. Dietary practices are discussed in Chapter 27; most ill persons are exempt from fasting.

Eastern Orthodox

Theological differences in the 11th century resulted in the split between the Roman Catholic and Eastern Orthodox churches. Centers of the religion are head-quartered in each of the countries they represent. Churches may be Greek Orthodox, Russian Orthodox, and so forth. Their teachings are similar to Roman Catholicism, but their religious calendars differ.

Protestants

The many denominations in the Protestant faith came out of the Reformation in the 16th century. Their forms of worship vary from informal to highly ritualistic, but their basic beliefs are similar. Baptism and communion (the Lord's Supper) are important elements. In many denominations, baptism is performed on infants. Other denominations "dedicate" an infant but baptize only older children or adults. Following their belief in the "priesthood of believers," many Protestant denominations permit baptism by a lay person in an emergency. Some protestants believe in "faith healing" or healing by "laying on of hands." The ill person may wish to receive communion. Make every effort to contact the person's minister or the hospital chaplain in the event of illness.

Church of the Latter Day Saints

The Church of Jesus Christ of Latter Day Saints (LDS) is commonly called the Mormon Church. Members of the priesthood are revered as healers; one of them (bishop, elder) would be called during illness. The Mormon is not forbidden to receive healthcare; extraordinary life support is evaluated individually. Although there are no specific healers or regular healing services, Mormons often believe in divine healing. Baptism does not occur until a child is 8 years old; no specific religious rite is needed if an infant dies. However, baptism of the dead is important for adults. Sunday is observed as the Sabbath. During illness, a Mormon may wish to use one of four books for spiritual healing: The King James Version of the Bible, Doctrine and Covenants, Pearl of Great Price, and The Book of Mormon. The Mormon health code is called The Words of Wisdom. Adult Mormons wear a special undergarment, which may be worn under the hospital gown, but may also be removed at the individual's discretion. Chapter 27 describes special dietary practices.

Christian Scientists

Christian Scientists do not permit surgery or many other forms of medical care, such as blood transfusion or taking of medications. Alcohol, coffee, or tobacco are viewed as drugs and are not allowed. They believe that all illness is mental in origin and that illness can be cured by appropriate mental processes. Treatment consists of prayer and counsel for the ill person; healing is carried out by certified practitioners. There is no formal clergy and no baptism. In the event of death, there are no last rites. Autopsy is not allowed.

Seventh Day Adventists

Seventh Day Adventists believe that good health depends on an orderly life. They emphasize the holistic concept of health. They do not use alcohol, coffee, tea, tobacco, or over-the-counter drugs and do not eat pork. Many Seventh Day Adventists are vegetarian. Seventh Day Adventists will not allow blood transfusions. In the event of death, there are no last rites. Communion or baptism by the elder may be desirable in serious illness, but infants are not baptized. They observe the Sabbath from sundown Friday to sundown Saturday.

Jehovah's Witnesses

Jehovah's Witnesses believe that each person is a minister. They prohibit blood transfusions and will not eat anything containing blood. In case of death, there are no last rites. Infants are never baptized. Sunday is observed as the Sabbath.

Eastern Religions

The number of citizens from China, Korea, Japan, India, and Southeast Asia is increasing. Religions with an Eastern philosophy include Buddhism, Confucianism, Daoism (Taoism), and Hinduism.

Buddhism is a religion based on the teachings of Buddha. It teaches that "right living" will enable people to attain **nirvana**, the condition of soul that does not have to live in a body and is free from all desire and pain. If a Buddhist dies, the family will usually send for the Buddhist priest, who will perform last rites and chanting rituals.

In **Confucianism**, there is an appreciation of life. They desire to keep the body from untimely death. Public health solutions are emphasized in addressing health problems.

Taoism teaches that health results from harmony of the universe with proper balancing of internal and external forces. Following Tao is to know and live a natural life.

Karma is the force generated by one's actions that ethically determines one's destiny in the next life. In **Hinduism**, it is significant in promoting health or causing disease.

Eastern religions have a great influence on Western medicine. Within North America there is a growing acceptance of Eastern therapies: acupuncture, yoga, and biofeedback. Transcendental meditation influences hypnotherapy and relaxation practices also.

Nursing Considerations

The nurse must consider all these sociocultural aspects when implementing nursing care. Specific care is addressed in the following.

◆ Special techniques for assessing changes in skin color and condition are required for any dark-skinned persons. This includes African American, Hispanic, Filipino, Puerto Rican, Native American, and people of Mediterranean and Arabian descent who have darker skin pigmentation, and whites who are deeply suntanned. Some special considerations are also needed for Asian Americans, who have golden skin coloration.

◆ Special hair care is required in the African American patient with very curly/nappy hair. The hair is often dry; the person may wish to use oil or hair dressing. If no hair dressing is available, petrolatum may be used. Use a pick or comb with long, widely spaced teeth.

◆ Care must be taken in shaving an African American man with curly facial hair; the hair can curl back on itself, penetrate the skin, and lead to papules, pustules, and keloid formation. This is also true of some Puerto Ricans.

◆ The folk healer (**curandero** in Spanish) should be allowed to see the patient and administer herbs, if the patient so requests.

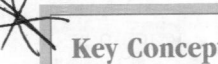

> ### Key Concept
> Puerto Ricans are citizens of the United States. They take offense if questioned about citizenship and usually do not wish to be referred to as persons of color.

◆ Many Catholics of Hispanic descent want a small statue of the Virgin Mary next to the bed and a Catholic medal pinned to their clothing. It is customary to burn candles and have altars with statues of saints. It may be possible to get permission to follow these practices in the hospital.

◆ The Native American/Alaska Native may request permission to burn plant substances as part of the religious healing process.

◆ Many Hispanic people use medicinal plants for kidney conditions, breaking up kidney or gallstones, colds, headaches, circulation problems, ulcers, and disorders of mental health. Even though people will take medicine prescribed by the physician, they will also continue to use home remedies. In other cases, people will buy prescribed medicines

but not use them. Follow-up on patients is extremely important.

◆ Family is important in many Hispanic and southeast Asian cultures. Many family members may come to visit the patient and some cultures insist on having a family member present day and night. Men from many cultures are uneasy about being bathed by female nurses, especially if the nurses are young. They prefer to wait until their wives visit to assist. Older women are often uncomfortable about being seen by male physicians.

◆ Native American and Chinese women may not seek early prenatal care. They believe that pregnancy is a natural process, whereas a clinic or a hospital is associated with illness.

◆ Many Hispanic patients believe that it is dangerous to bathe immediately after delivery. The nurse must remember this in postpartum care.

◆ Many cultural groups, such as Native Americans and Southeast Asians, believe that it is improper to look someone in the eye when speaking with them. Eye contact and facial expressions may be totally absent. The nurse must not interpret this as a "flat affect."

◆ Time may not be regarded as important by some cultures, including Native Americans and Hispanics. Be aware of this when scheduling appointments or giving instructions.

◆ Cultural groups react differently to pain. Some groups are stoic and do not complain, whereas others cry out with pain much of the time.

◆ It may be difficult for an Asian or Southeast Asian woman to have a male physician or nurse.

◆ The role of women in East Indian, Pakistani, and Arab cultures is subservient to men. A woman from one of these cultures may be more inclined to follow instructions from a male nurse or physician. Her husband or father may make decisions for her.

◆ Many cultures often do not observe personal space, as Americans from European origins do.

◆ Many people who speak only limited English try to be agreeable. They will nod and say "yes" when you ask if they understand, even if they do not.

◆ Amish or Mennonite patients may refuse to be shaved and may not have home telephones for emergency calls.

> ### Key Concept
> No matter how different your beliefs might be from those of your patients, it is important for you to respect each patient's personal values and cultural beliefs and to respond in a nonjudgmental manner.

Keys for Review

Key Questions for Critical Thinking

1. Discuss cultural beliefs about illness and health. How do they compare with your personal beliefs? If they are different, how can you adapt yourself to others' beliefs?
2. Your Chinese American patient follows the yin-yang principle. Describe the principle. How does this affect your nursing?
3. Describe the dietary laws of Jewish people. Discuss how you can help your Jewish patient keep kosher. Discuss similarities between kosher laws and dietary observances of other religions.
4. Identify the day of the week observed by each religious group. What may you expect to happen in your patient's room if that patient is religious? How can you help the patient observe his or her religious day?
5. Discuss the term "spiritual advisor." Discuss other names used for this person. How may the actions of these people differ from one another?

Key Readings

Boyle JS, Andrews MM. Transcultural Concepts in Nursing Care. Philadelphia, J.B. Lippincott, 1990

Dodson SM. Transcultural Nursing. St. Louis, Ishiyaku Euro, 1991

Giger J, Davidhizar RE. Transcultural Nursing; Assessment and Intervention. St. Louis, Mosby-Year Book, 1991

Pachter LM. Latino folk illnesses: methodological considerations. Med. Anthropol. 1993: 15:103–108.

Spector R. Cultural Diversity in Health and Illness, Ed 3. East Norwalk CT, Appleton & Lange, 1991

Enrichment Keys

Buchwald D, Panwala S, Hooton TM. Use of traditional health practices by southeast Asian refugees in a primary clinic. West J. Med. 1992, 156:507–511.

Diaz-Gilbert M. Caring for culturally diverse patients. Nursing 93. Vol. 23 #10, 1993, 44–45.

Grossman DC, Krieger JW, Sugarman JR, and Forquera RA. Health status of urban American Indians and Alaska natives. JAMA Vol. 271, #11, March 16, 1994, 845–850.

Grypma S. "Culture shock." The Canadian Nurse 89(8):33–36, Sept. 1993

Koss-Chioino J. Women as Healers, Women as Patients: Mental Health Care and Traditional Healing in Puerto Rico. Boulder, CO: Westview Press, 1992

Pachter LM. Folk illness beliefs and behaviors and their implications for health care delivery. JAMA Vol. 271, #9. March 2, 1994, 690–694.

Keys to Learning More

Unit Twelve: maternal and newborn nursing, where you will apply transcultural nursing

Unit Thirteen: care of infants and children, where the entire family is considered

Unit Fourteen: adult medical–surgical nursing, where you will meet people from a variety of cultures

Chapter 50: special skin assessment techniques used in persons with dark skin or golden-tone skin

40 The Healthcare Environment

Learning Objectives

- List and describe the articles included in the basic patient unit.
- Discuss the relationships between housekeeping procedures and patient safety.
- Identify the nursing procedures that constitute early morning care, morning care, afternoon care, and evening care.
- Summarize the guidelines for all nursing procedures.
- Describe at least four direct patient care departments.
- Describe the functions of at least two support departments.

Key Terms

autopsies	pathologist
hospice	patient unit
intercom	physical therapy
morgue	research laboratory
nuclear medicine	respiratory therapy
occupational therapy	

Keys to Understanding This Chapter

Chapter 3: the healthcare delivery system
Chapter 4: legal and ethical aspects of healthcare
Chapter 29: safety in the healthcare environment
Chapter 30: medical asepsis and universal precautions

Key Points

- The needs of patients include the basic needs every human being experiences plus special needs connected with illness or injury.

Key Points (continued)

- The patient unit is the area in which most nursing care is delivered.
- Certain guidelines are common for all nursing procedures.
- Hospitals offer a wide variety of services and are staffed with personnel who have special training.
- There are direct patient care departments, specialized patient care departments, and support services within the hospital.

Key Topics Outline

The Patient Unit
    Components of the Basic Patient Unit
    Restocking the Unit
    Cleaning the Unit After Use
    Unit Order and Housekeeping
Provision of Nursing Care
    Grouping Nursing Procedures
Hospital Personnel and Services
    Diagnostic and Treatment Departments
    Direct Patient Care Departments
    Specialized Patient Care Departments
    Support Services
    Provision of Nursing Care

Key Learning Activities

- Interview a hospital administrator about services provided for patient care.
- Describe the organizational structure of your healthcare facility. How many staff people are needed for the licensed number of beds?

Rosdahl CB: Textbook of Basic Nursing, 6th ed. © 1995 J.B. Lippincott Company

The needs of patients include the basic needs of every human being and special needs connected with illness or injury. The essential physiologic needs, as identified in Chapter 5, are intake and use of oxygen, intake and use of nutrients and water, elimination of wastes, sleep and rest, activity and exercise, and shelter. Higher-level needs include safety, emotional and spiritual support, and pleasant surroundings. Needs of the patient additionally include essential medical and nursing care, encouragement to return to normal function, and diversion. The patient's progress toward recovery and comfort and happiness depend on the extent to which these needs are satisfied. Meeting these needs involves teamwork among all who come in contact with the patient, including the patient's family.

You probably will practice skills in your school laboratory. Your first experience with actual patients may be in the hospital or in a nursing home. Wherever you begin, you will need to know the basic equipment found in the patient unit and understand the departments of the healthcare environment.

> ### Key Concept
> Allow the patient to do as much self-care as possible.

The Patient Unit

The **patient unit** is the area around the patient's bed. It includes the bed, other furniture, and equipment used in daily care. This unit may be in a private or a semiprivate room or in a ward containing four or more beds. Modern hospitals give a great deal of thought to providing patients with surroundings that are pleasant as well as practical.

Components of the Basic Patient Unit

The basic equipment for a patient unit includes:

◆ Furniture: bed, bedside table and chair, lamp, overbed table. Most beds have built-in side rails. The telephone and nurse call signal may also be built into side rails.
◆ Linens: sheets, pillowcases, blankets, spread, bath blanket, face towel, washcloth, bedpan cover, gown or pajamas
◆ Toilet equipment: washbasin, soap dish, toothbrush, toothpaste, toothbrush container, emesis basin, comb, bedpan, urinal for male patients
◆ Other articles: water pitcher and drinking glass, electronic thermometer, call bell or button, screen or curtain, TV, and often a telephone; many units have a built-in blood pressure set up

Equipment for nursing treatments may be kept outside the unit, in the treatment or utility room. The unit should always be complete and ready to use. This saves steps and prevents delay.

Furniture

The Hospital Bed. The hospital bed is specially constructed and equipped to provide maximum safety and comfort for the patient and the caregiver. Chapter 44 describes the bed, its attachments, and skills used for making the hospital bed.

The Overbed Table. The overbed table fits over the bed. It is useful when the patient is eating, reading, or grooming. The table can be opened, revealing a mirror and space for small toilet articles. The top is adjustable to permit the patient to place a book at a comfortable angle to read without having to hold the book.

The Bedside Stand. The hospital bedside stand/cabinet is durable and easy to keep clean. The top is covered with Formica or similar material that absorbs sound made by articles being placed on it.

Bedside tables come with a drawer and an enclosed storage space below, with shelves. The legs are metal or rubber tipped or have casters on which the table can be moved easily and quietly. The drawer provides a place for personal belongings.

Basins and bath blankets are stored on the top shelf of the table; if the patient's bedpan and urinal are kept at the bedside, this equipment and the toilet tissue go on the bottom shelf. In any storage arrangement, always keep the bedpan and the urinal apart from other personal things.

Other Components

The Intercommunication System. Each patient unit has an intercommunication (**intercom**) system, which the patient usually operates. It is often combined with TV and radio controls and buttons used to raise and lower the head and foot of the bed. (These may all be built into the side rails of the bed.)

The nurse demonstrates how to operate the equipment for the patient and family. It is frightening to the ill patient to be alone in unfamiliar surroundings and not to know how to obtain assistance. The nurse call button is the first button the patient should be taught to use. The patient should also be aware that the nurse may answer the nurse call light from the desk by using the intercom.

Safety and Nursing Care Equipment. Other equipment is available for the use of healthcare personnel. Many units have items such as nasogastric suction equipment, blood pressure apparatus, oxygen, and a hanger for the intravenous setups built into the wall or ceiling above the bed. Because this equipment may be frightening to the patient, it is important to explain that it exists in all patient units just in case it is needed.

If the patient is in a multibed room, there will also be a curtain for privacy. This runs in a track on the ceiling and can be pushed out of the way when not needed.

Ventilation and Air Quality. With concern for air quality, most hospitals have taken action to prevent pollution. Hospitals do not allow smoking although a special outside smoking area may be designated. Usually, the windows do not open and heating and cooling are controlled centrally. However, you will need to make sure each patient is comfortable. Air temperature affects comfort. There must be a balance between heat lost and heat produced. The room temperature that most effectively maintains this balance is between 68°F and 72°F. (20°–22.2°C).

Always protect your patient from chilling. An ill or injured person is often more susceptible to feeling cold. An ambulating patient can be protected by a warm blanket or bathrobe and slippers, and by placing the chair out of the way of drafts. When you give a bed bath, be sure to cover the patient with a bath blanket and protect from drafts.

Restocking the Unit

Replace used supplies promptly. Check equipment and inspect it for breaks, cracks, or rough places that might injure the patient or nurse. Replace broken or damaged equipment and report damage to the appropriate person so equipment can be replaced or repaired. It is customary in many hospitals to keep an inventory of equipment on each floor as a basis for ordering new articles or replacing damaged ones.

Cleaning the Unit After Use

Auxiliary personnel attached to the nursing or housekeeping departments are usually responsible for cleaning the unit. However, every nurse should know how to clean a unit according to the policy of the hospital and the principles of medical asepsis. In some situations, this procedure is supervised by the nurse.

Always make sure the unit is cleaned after a patient has been discharged from the hospital or transferred to another room or after a patient has died. Everything in the unit is considered contaminated and must be discarded or disinfected before it can be used by another patient. This prevents the spread of infection and helps allay the patient's concerns about the spread of diseases.

Unit Order and Housekeeping

The patient's unit should be kept neat and orderly at all times. Good housekeeping helps prevent accidents and infection and helps the nurse to carry out nursing care efficiently. Everything should be arranged so it can be located by all personnel. These measures help the patient to feel secure and make it less likely that staff or patient will fall or trip.

Odors. Illness may make a person extremely sensitive to odors. Bedpans, urinals, and soiled dressings should be removed from the patient's bedside immediately. Nurses should not use strong cologne or aftershave lotion. Smoking is offensive to most ill persons, so, if you smoke, be sure your breath is not unpleasant and your clothes do not smell of stale smoke. The hospital's smoke-free policy may need to be explained to the patient and visitors. Nurses will also be expected to abide by this policy.

Noise. Noise should be minimized or eliminated as much as possible. It may overstimulate the patient and produce fatigue. Slamming doors or dropping equipment startles the patient and causes restlessness and irritation. Radios and TV sets should be turned low. A headphone or an under-the-pillow speaker may be available and should be used whenever possible to prevent annoyance to other patients. Be especially aware of the noise level at night. Even the sound of two nurses talking can be irritating to the patient who is having difficulty sleeping.

Privacy. The nurse has an obligation to respect and preserve the privacy of *all* patients. In consideration of the patient's modesty, be sure to use screens, curtains, and bath blankets or other drapes to keep the person covered as much as possible during treatments. Shut the patient's door when procedures are performed. If a patient is confused and pulls off covers, pajamas may be more practical than a hospital gown.

It is also important to respect the patient's privacy when the patient is being visited by the family, a staff person, or spiritual leader.

Provision of Nursing Care

Most nursing care is provided in the patient unit. There are procedures the nurse is expected to follow. The accompanying box summarizes guidelines to be used in all procedures.

There are reasons certain steps in every nursing procedure must be followed to achieve desired results. These reasons (the rationale) will guide you in making a procedure effective. Individual procedures may vary,

Nursing Skill Guidelines
Performing Nursing Procedures

All Nursing Procedures

- Check physician's order; check Kardex; check Nursing Care Plan.
- Identify the patient.
- Perform the treatment on time.
- Follow guidelines of universal precautions.
- Wash your hands before carrying out a procedure and after it is completed. This cannot be emphasized 2enough! If in doubt, wash your hands!
- Wear gloves for most procedures. Follow your facility's procedures and protocols.
- Assemble all the necessary equipment so the procedure can be carried out as easily, quickly, and effectively as possible.
- Introduce yourself and explain the procedure to the patient to allay fears of pain or discomfort. Patients may be apprehensive about machines, sharp instruments or needles, applications of heat or cold, or apparatus that covers the face.
- Avoid using the words *hurt* or *painful*. Instead, say "You will feel some discomfort," or "you will have to lie in one position, but we will help to make you comfortable." Emphasize positive aspects: "It won't take long," or "It will make you feel better." A patient will be more cooperative knowing what to expect. Never tell a patient, "There is nothing to it," when you know a procedure has some painful or uncomfortable aspects.
- Make the person as comfortable as possible before beginning the procedure. A pain medication may be offered to the patient before an uncomfortable procedure is carried out
- Ensure the patient's privacy by closing the door or using cubicle curtains or screens. *Keep the person covered as much as possible.*
- Stay with the person during examinations and procedures as much as possible. Explain and answer questions as the procedure is done.
- Care for the equipment as necessary, and store it as indicated by hospital policies (wash, sterilize, store, or return to central supply department). Be sure to dispose of all dressings and disposable equipment in a manner that is safe for you, other staff members, and patients.
- Document the treatment, the time it is given, and results, including unusual patient reactions. Report any pertinent symptoms or observations to the appropriate person. Report emergency situations immediately.
- *Ask for help, if needed.*

Early Morning Care (Early AM Care)

Given before breakfast for health and comfort

- Offer bedpan or urinal
- Wash face and hands
- Brush teeth

Early Morning Care (Early AM Care) (continued)

- Adjust bed and bedclothes
- Take temperature, pulse, respiration, and blood pressure
- Change patient's position
- Adjust table for the breakfast tray

Later Morning Care (AM Care)

Given after breakfast for health and comfort

- Remove breakfast tray
- Offer bedpan or urinal
- Give bath (bed bath, tub, shower)
- Make bed with clean linen
- Change patient's position or help to ambulate
- Comb hair
- Care for nails
- Perform AM treatments
- Give backrub
- Tidy unit

Afternoon Care

Given to relax the patient in preparation for visitors

- Change patient's position or ambulate
- Offer bedpan, urinal
- Wash face and hands
- Perform afternoon treatments
- Give backrub

Evening Care (HS or "Hour of Sleep" Care)

Given for health and comfort and prepares the patient for the night

- Give evening treatments
- Offer bedpan or urinal
- Wash face and hands
- Brush teeth
- Comb and tidy hair
- Change patient's position
- Adjust bed and linens
- Give backrub
- Give HS medications
- Tidy up the unit (be sure all obstacles are out of the way so night nurses or the patient will not fall over equipment or furniture during the night)

The times for these procedures may vary. As often as possible, these procedures should be performed at a time that will be most comfortable and therapeutic for the patient, not necessarily at the nurse's convenience. For example, the patient may be accustomed to bathing at night; this may be possible. A painful procedure should be done first, then a backrub given, so the patient will be better able to rest after the procedure. Also, offer the bedpan before washing hands: Give HS medications after all other care has been given.

Key Abbreviations and Acronyms for Hospital Personnel and Services

ACU	acute coronary unit		NEURO	neurology
CCU	coronary care unit		NICU	neonatal intensive care unit
CDU	chemical dependency unit		OB	obstetric
CSR	central service room		OPD	outpatient department
CSS	central serivice supply		OR	operating room
ECF	extended care facility		ORTHO	orthopedics
ECG	electrocardiogram		OT	occupational therapy
EEG	electroencephalogram		PAR	postanesthesia recovery (room)
EMG	electromyogram		PEDS	pediatric
ER	emergency room		PSYCH	psychiatry
GU	genitourinary		PT	physical therapy
GYN	gynecology		REHAB	rehabilitation
ICU	intensive care unit		RR	recovery room
MRI	magnetic resonance imaging		RT	respiratory therapy

but as long as basic underlying principles are not violated, nursing care will be safe. As skills are presented in this book, the *rationales* for steps are given. These will guide you in adapting your care to an individual situation after graduation. As a student, you should follow procedures, as taught by your instructors, until you have a firm grasp on the *underlying principles* of nursing.

Each clinical faculty has specific procedures to be used in that facility. The "Procedure" or "Protocol" book is available in each institution and is to be used by employees and students in that facility.

Grouping Nursing Procedures

For efficiency, several procedures may be performed together, although each procedure is complete in itself. Some skills are grouped because they are associated with the same time of day or with a special kind of treatment. Many nurses know these blocks of nursing care by group names. See the nursing skill guidelines box for some examples.

You will have more than one patient to care for, and you will need to consider hospital routines when planning care. Meal hours, physicians' rounds, and patients' appointments for surgery, x-ray examinations, and laboratory procedures must also be considered when you prepare your work plan. You may be asked to assist temporarily with emergencies that come up on a busy unit. In all situations, your patients are your first responsibility.

Hospital Personnel and Services

Hospitals offer a variety of services; therefore, they are staffed with people with experience in a variety of specializations. Some of the abbreviations and acronyms for departments and services you will need to know are listed in the accompanying box.

Diagnostic and Treatment Departments

Laboratories. In the clinical diagnostic laboratory, numerous tests are performed to assist physicians in diagnosing the patient's disorder. The **pathologist** and associates have broad responsibility for determining the underlying nature of the patient's disease through their examination and study of specimens of tissue in the pathology laboratory. These specimens include blood, sputum, feces, and biopsied tissues.

Autopsies (examinations after death) are performed in the pathology laboratory. The **morgue** is under the direction of a pathologist and is the place where dead bodies are kept until identified or buried.

Some large teaching hospitals also include a **research laboratory**, where studies and experiments on animals are carried out in efforts to cure or prevent human disease.

Radiology and Nuclear Medicine. Diagnostic x-ray studies are performed in the radiology department to aid the physician in determining the exact location and nature of the patient's disorder. Radiation therapy is given in treatment of certain diseases. Sometimes this entire department is called **nuclear medicine**. Other procedures carried out in this department include computed tomography (CT) scans, xerography and mammography (breast studies), magnetic resonance imaging (MRI or NMR), and ultrasound studies. This department also supervises and carries out the implantation and injection of radioactive and opaque materials for treatments and examinations.

Other Diagnostic Departments. The *electroencephalography* (EEG) department, also known as the neurodiagnostic department, records a "brain wave" test on the patient. This test determines electrical activity within the brain. The EEG department also administers evoked potential examinations, does specialized sleep studies, and monitors patients who have seizures.

The electrocardiogram (ECG), a recording of the electrical activity of the heart, may be done by a specialized department or by the intensive care unit or EEG department. The electromyogram (EMG) is a recording of the minute electrical impulses within muscles; it may be done by the ECG, EEG, physical therapy, or respiratory care department, or in the clinical laboratory.

Direct Patient Care Departments

Therapies. The **physical therapy** (PT) department directs its efforts toward preventing physical disability. The PT staff assists the patient in regaining the best possible function of affected body parts through an individually planned program of exercise and activity, with emphasis on gross (large) motor muscle activity. Employees include registered physical therapists (RPT) and physical therapist assistants (PTA).

Through the use of diversional or craft activities in the **occupational therapy** (OT) department, the patient is helped toward rehabilitation, with attention to fine motor skills. The staff in the OT department may aid in job training, as well as therapy. Employees here include registered occupational therapists (OTR) and certified occupational therapy assistants (COTA).

The **respiratory therapy** (RT) department, also known as the respiratory care department or *cardiopulmonary* (CP) *department*, is responsible for carrying out measures prescribed by the physician to assist the patient who has certain cardiac or respiratory disorders. Many patients on regular units are treated by respiratory therapists and technicians in this department. Examples are patients after surgery and patients on ventilators, following accidents. All oxygen administered in the hospital may be under the supervision of the RT department. Often, this department draws blood for blood gas analysis and performs tests, including pulmonary function and vital capacity. The RT department may also administer other tests, including cardiac stress tests.

Some hospitals also contain facilities for *music therapy*, *recreational therapy*, and *play therapy*.

Surgery. The staff in the operating room (OR) and the postanesthesia recovery room (PAR), also called recovery room (RR), are concerned with care of the surgical patient immediately before, during, and immediately after surgery. This department may also manage a day surgery or ambulatory surgery unit.

Nursing Care Units. The head nurse may be called a coordinator or nurse manager. This person is responsible for the nursing station or unit. Other nursing staff are called by names such as team leader, primary nurse, and staff nurse. Nurses are licensed as RNs and LPN/LVNs, as described in Chapter 2. Various departments or units relate to specific kinds of care.

The *pediatric* (PEDS) *unit* is responsible for care of children. In large hospitals the department may be divided according to children's ages.

The *obstetrics* (OB) *department* provides care to mothers and neonates. This department is divided into the labor room; the delivery room, or birthing room; the newborn nursery; and the postpartum unit, where women receive care after delivery.

The *medical unit* has responsibility for caring for adults who have medical conditions or disorders that do not require surgery. The *surgical unit* is involved in care of patients before and after surgery. In a large hospital, the basic medical–surgical divisions may be further divided to include orthopedics (ORTHO), for musculoskeletal disorders; a urology or genitourinary (GU) unit, for disorders of the kidneys, bladder, liver, or male reproductive system; neurology (NEURO), for central or peripheral nervous system disorders, including disorders of the brain; geriatrics, for care of older people; dermatology, for skin disorders; oncology, for cancer patients; psychiatry (PSYCH) or mental health for mental and emotional disorders; and gynecology (GYN) for female reproductive disorders.

Specialized Patient Care Departments

Specialized departments and units are designed to give medical and nursing care for different degrees of illness. The following serve varied needs of patients:

◆ *Emergency Room* (ER)—where individuals involved in trauma or other persons requiring immediate attention are taken. The hospital ambulance service and cardiopulmonary resuscitation (CPR) service ("code team") are often components of ER functions.

◆ *Intensive care unit* (ICU)—provides care for critically ill patients. Many hospitals have specialized intensive care units, such as neonatal or newborn intensive care (NICU).

◆ *Coronary care unit* (CCU) or *acute coronary unit* (ACU)—where patients with serious heart disorders are attended by a specially trained nursing staff. After the crisis is over, the coronary patient may move into a *coronary step-down unit* or a *coronary rehabilitation unit*.

◆ *Dialysis unit*—for patients who need chronic renal (kidney) dialysis.

◆ *Mental health unit*—serves patients with emotional or psychiatric disorders.

- *Chemical dependency unit* (CDU)—serves persons who overuse or abuse chemical substances.
- *Intermediate care unit*—for patients requiring a moderate amount of skilled nursing care.
- *Self-care unit*—provides transition from the regular hospital to home. Patients care for themselves as much as possible; hospital staff provide assistance as needed.
- *Rehabilitation unit* (REHAB)—physical medicine and rehabilitation unit concerned with helping people who have a physical disability to regain as much of their capacity for activity as possible.
- *Hospice*—gives physical and emotional care to dying patients. The patients' families are given support and assistance in dealing with terminal illness. After the person dies, continued support is given by the hospice staff and hospice outreach staff.
- *Extended care facility* (ECF)—for elderly people, permanently disabled people, and persons with progressive degenerative diseases.
- *Outpatient department* (OPD)—cares for patients after discharge from the hospital or those patients who can be treated without being admitted to the hospital.
- *Home care*—for patients after they are discharged from the hospital. Many patients are discharged with special medical equipment or treatments that must be carried out at home.
- *Patient education*—to teach complex procedures to patients and their caregivers.

Support Services

The administration of the hospital sees that all departments operate efficiently. Most hospitals have a board of directors that employs one or more hospital administrators. Responsible to the hospital administrator are such people as the director of nursing service, personnel director, and medical director. Other support services in the hospital include:

- *Dietary department*—prepares all meals for patients, in accordance with diet instructions given by physicians. The dietitian is involved in teaching about special diets.
- *Pharmacy*—responsible for dispensing medications ordered by the physician.
- *Central service supply* (CSS) or *central service room* (CSR)—cleans and sterilizes equipment and instruments for use throughout the hospital. Most stock supplies are also processed through CSR.
- *Admissions department* and *business office*—processes patients when they enter and leave the hospital. Bills are paid through the business office.
- *Medical records department*—keeps medical charts for all patients who have ever been in that hospital. The department is responsible for making sure that all notations are made on the chart and the chart is complete. The medical record technician, or registered record administrator (RRA), may be called into court with the chart during a legal action.
- *Volunteer service*—assists the hospital in many varied ways. Volunteers may operate a gift shop; deliver mail, flowers, magazines, and books to patients; operate an information desk in the lobby; or run a coffee shop. They often bring patients to the nursing unit from the admitting department and transport the patient for discharge.
- *Chaplaincy service*—provides spiritual support to patients and families during illness, surgery, and death. Many hospitals have a chapel. Nondenominational worship services and religious rituals may be provided.
- *Social service department*—provides counseling and assistance to patients and families in matters of finances, home care, discharge plans, and living arrangements. The social worker may make a referral to an outside agency that can assist the family with special needs. This department may also assist at discharge or may help to refer the patient to a public health nurse or other specialized agency for continuing care after the patient leaves the hospital.

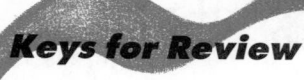

Keys for Review

Key Questions for Critical Thinking

1. Describe components of the patient unit. Describe how you would teach the new patient about the unit, including the purpose and operation of various components. Discuss maintenance of the unit.
2. Your patient is spending the first full day in your care. Describe the basic activities for that day. Discuss your responsibilities. How will your coordination of activities help your patient?
3. Your patient is a 35-year-old housewife and mother of three small children. She has broken her right arm and is soon to be discharged. Describe hospital support services that will be used in her care and discharge.

Key Readings

Earnest VV. Clinical Skills in Nursing Practice, Ed 2. Philadelphia, J.B. Lippincott, 1993
Smeltzer SC, Bare BG. Brunner and Suddarth's Textbook of Medical Surgical Nursing, Ed 7. Philadelphia, J.B. Lippincott, 1992

Key Readings (continued)

Swearingen PL. Photo Atlas of Nursing Procedures, Ed 2. Redwood City, CA, Addison-Wesley Nursing, 1991
Taber's Cyclopedic Medical Dictionary, Ed 17. Philadelphia, F.A. Davis, 1993
Taylor C, Lillis C, LeMone P. Fundamentals of Nursing: The Art and Science of Nursing Care, Ed 2. Philadelphia, J.B. Lippincott, 1993

Keys to Learning More

Chapter 41: admission, transfer, and discharge
Chapter 43: body mechanics and positioning
Chapter 44: beds and bedmaking
Chapter 45: skills to assist with personal hygiene
Chapter 46: skills to assist with elimination
Chapter 51: isolation techniques

41 Admission, Transfer, and Discharge

Keys for Learning

Learning Objectives

♦ Describe how to orient a new patient to the hospital.
♦ Describe how to take care of the patient's clothing and valuable items on admission.
♦ Discuss dehumanization and ways to avoid this phenomenon.
♦ List admission information that should be reported to the RN by the nursing student or the LPN.
♦ Demonstrate the ability to transfer the patient safely and effectively.
♦ Describe teaching that should occur when a patient is discharged from the hospital.
♦ Describe the procedure of discharging a patient.
♦ State the responsibility of the hospital, the physician, and the nurse toward a patient who signs out of the hospital against medical advice (AMA).

Key Terms

dehumanize   vital signs
litter scales

Keys to Understanding This Chapter

Chapter 4: legal and ethical aspects of nursing
Chapter 5: basic human needs
Chapter 29: safety in the healthcare environment
Chapter 30: medical asepsis and universal precautions
Unit Seven: nursing process
Chapter 36: therapeutic communication
Chapter 37: documentation and reporting
Chapter 38: signs and symptoms of illness or injury
Chapter 39: transcultural considerations
Chapter 40: healthcare environment

Key Points

♦ How the patient feels about the admission helps to determine the success of the hospital stay.

Key Points (continued)

♦ The patient is often apprehensive about his or her physical condition and about the unfamiliar procedures in the healthcare facility.
♦ The nurse is responsible for initial nursing assessment.
♦ Patients and their belongings must be properly identified.
♦ Careful documentation of the admission is important to establish a baseline and to give information to other members of the team.
♦ When a patient is transferred, explain this to the patient; take belongings, records, and medications; and safely transport the patient.
♦ Discharge teaching is individual and must be documented. The nurse makes sure the patient has all belongings at discharge and escorts the patient to the door.
♦ Some patients sign out against medical advice.

Key Topics Outline

Patient Admission
    The Admitting Department
    The Patient's Arrival on the Nursing Unit
    Assessment, Reporting, and Documentation
Patient Transfer to Another Unit
Patient Discharge
Leaving the Hospital Against Advice

Key Learning Activities

♦ Visit a local hospital. Secure copies of admission forms, consent forms, and inventory of property and valuables form.
♦ Role play an admission to the hospital. What feelings do you have about signing consent forms and giving up personal articles and clothing? What would you expect the nurse to do when caring for you?

Rosdahl CB: Textbook of Basic Nursing, 6th ed. © 1995 J.B. Lippincott Company

Hospital patients should be made to feel as comfortable as possible. Effective nursing care involves nurses who are aware of the patient's needs, attitudes, and emotions.

Knowledge of the stages of human development helps the nurse place the patient in a continuum of life experiences. Understanding basic human needs guides the nurse in planning care to meet those needs. Drawing on communication and interviewing skills, the nurse can help the patient express and work through emotions about hospitalization. The feelings of the patient's family also should be kept in mind.

Patient Admission

Key abbreviations used in this chapter are listed in the box on page 444.

The Admitting Department

Certain routines necessary to admit the patient are usually carried out in the admissions department. A member of the clerical staff records such information as age, sex, marital status, and whether the patient has a health insurance plan. This information is placed on the face sheet of the chart. An identification band is put on the patient's wrist. X-rays and blood work may be done at this time. During these preliminary procedures, every effort is made to put the patient at ease. The patient is then brought to the nursing unit.

The Patient's Arrival on the Nursing Unit

Before the patient arrives, the nurse should check to be sure that the unit is completely equipped. The nurse opens the bed. The patient may walk in or arrive in a wheelchair or on a stretcher. Introduce the patient to the charge nurse and staff before taking the patient to the room.

The patient's first impression of his or her hospital surroundings is formed the minute he or she is admitted. Routines that are commonplace to healthcare workers can become threatening and frightening to the newly admitted patient. Care is taken to explain routines to the patient.

Unless there are orders to the contrary, the patient undresses, puts on a hospital gown, and goes to bed in preparation for an examination by a physician, a routine procedure in most hospitals.

Removing the Patient's Clothes

Give the patient whatever assistance is needed in undressing. Sometimes a member of the family will assist, particularly if the patient is a child. A child may resist being undressed by a stranger, or may not understand the need for going to bed during the day. If the patient is unable to undress alone, you will assist.

Nursing Skill
Undressing the Immobile Patient

Supplies and Equipment

Hospital gown

Procedure

1. Push the patient's blouse or shirt off one shoulder. (*Rationale: One side is done at a time.*)
2. Push the sleeve on the same side down in a roll to the wrist. (*Rationale: This makes it easier to remove.*)
3. Slip the sleeve off. (*Rationale: Undress the patient on one side at a time.*)
4. Repeat on the other side. (*Rationale: By easing off one side at a time, you avoid straining the patient.*)
5. Put a hospital gown on the patient. (*Rationale: If you remove the garments from above the waist first and put on the gown, the patient will not be exposed while you take off the lower garments.*)
6. Unfasten the waistband, and push all lower garments down as far as you can around the hips. (*Rationale: This reduces strain on the ill patient.*)
7. Ask the patient to raise the hips while you pull the clothes down. (*Rationale: The patient is encouraged to help as much as possible.*)
8. If the patient cannot raise the hips, you may need assistance. (*Rationale: Avoid overtiring the patient or injuring yourself.*)
9. If garments must come off over the head, slip the arms from the sleeves, push the clothing up to the hips, and ask the patient to raise the hips. Pull the garments up to the shoulders. To get the clothing up over the shoulders more easily, you can turn the patient's shoulders first to one side and then to the other. (*Rationale: The goal is to undress the patient as easily and quickly as possible while preventing exposure.*)
10. Slip garments off over the face by raising the patient's head and gathering the clothes together into a roll behind the head. Do not cover the patient's face and avoid dragging clothing over the face. (*Rationale: Many people become frightened if their face is covered. Dragging clothing over the face may cause injury.*)
11. When putting the hosptal gown on the patient, cover the person with a bath blanket and work under it as much as possible. (*Rationale: To avoid undue exposure or embarrassment and to provide warmth.*)

Assisting the Patient Into Bed

If a patient is weak or tired when admitted, remove the shoes and outdoor clothing, and help the patient lie down on the bed immediately. Cover with a bath blanket or with bedclothes. Lying down will help to prevent more fatigue. The patient may have already exerted considerable effort in making the trip to the hospital.

Key Abbreviations Used in Admitting and Discharge

AMA	Against medical advice
BP	Blood pressure
BRP	Bathroom privileges
JCAHO	Joint Commission for Accreditation of Healthcare Organizations
MAR	Medication Administration Record
TPR	Temperature, pulse, respiration
VS	Vital signs

Orienting the Patient to the Hospital

The charge nurse or team leader will tell you what the patient is allowed to do. If the patient is allowed bathroom pivileges, indicate where the bathroom is. Check to see if the patient is to give a urine specimen or is on intake and output (a recording of all fluids taken in and urine expelled) before allowing use of the bathroom.

Allow the patient time to unpack. If the patient needs help, unpack and tell the patient where you are placing items. Place bathrobe and slippers in a handy spot. Arrange the patient's personal belongings. Place special items on the bedside table where they can be reached easily.

Adjust the shades, regulate the ventilation, and adjust the head or foot of the bed for comfort. Put the entire bed in *low position,* regardless of whether the patient is able to get in and out of bed without assistance. Explain how the bed works as you adjust it. Most hospital patients have access to the bed controls and can adjust the bed themselves.

Tell the patient the time that meals are served and that you will find out what he or she may have to eat or drink and when. The routines of admission often take a long time, and sometimes a newly admitted patient goes without a meal because the nurses have overlooked the person. Do not let this happen to your patient!

Introduce the patient who is in a semiprivate accommodation to the other patient. Do not leave the patient until you are sure all questions have been answered and the person is comfortable. Be sure the nurse call light is within the patient's reach.

The Intercom System. Show the patient how the communication system works, and put the "nurse call" signal where it can be easily reached. It is important for the patient to understand how to use the intercom and signal lights. Show the person where the signal mechanism is located in the bathroom. Explain that if this button is pushed, it signals an emergency. Ask the person not to use this signal unless it truly is an emergency. Taking time to show the patient will help to alleviate fear and anxiety in unfamiliar surroundings.

Many call systems are equipped with television controls. This can be confusing when the patient sees numerous buttons or controls to push. Turn on the television, and set it on a channel that is familiar and at a comfortable volume.

Toilet Articles. Every hospital has a means of supplying such essential toilet articles as toothbrushes, toothpaste, combs, tissues, and soap. Usually these supplies are sold in the hospital pharmacy or gift shop if the hospital does not provide them. Many patients have personal preferences and like to provide these articles themselves.

Many hospitals provide a new patient a packet of supplies, which usually contains soap and a plastic soap dish, backrub lotion, a plastic water glass and a water carafe, disposable tissues, and mouthwash. The articles may be discarded or taken home on discharge. Sometimes the packages also contain an emesis basin, bedpan, urinal, comb, toothpaste, and a toothbrush. You may need to provide other items for individual patients. If you provide a denture cup, be sure to label it. If you handle the patient's dentures or used tissues, wear gloves.

The Patient Gown. Patients usually bring their own pajamas or nightgowns, bathrobes, and slippers with them. Family is responsible for laundering these items. Most hospitals provide these articles if patients are unable to supply them. If the patient is bleeding, is incontinent, or has a large amount of drainage, it is advisable to use the hospital's supply. For bed patients, it is customary to use gowns provided by the hospital. They can be sent to the hospital laundry and are easy to put on and remove. Explain to the patient that the hospital gown is used for convenience, comfort, and economy. The gown opens in the back and is fastened with ties, Velcro, or snaps. The sleeves also may open to accommodate intravenous (IV) tubing. Be sure that the gown is long enough and large enough for the patient. Be sure the ties of the gown are not uncomfortable when the patient lies on them; tie with bows to the *side.*

Individual Equipment. Patients are informed as soon as possible that their equipment is for their use alone. Luxuries may be lacking in a ward, but necessities are provided. Point out which part of the closet and which drawers are for each patient's use. Point out towel rods to be used by each patient in a semiprivate room or in a shared bathroom.

Patient Identification. Be sure the patient has received and wears an identification band. Check the information on the band to see that it is correct. Check the tag on the bed or wall and door, and make sure the patient is properly identified. In addition to the patient's name, the bed tag should indicate whether the patient is allowed to be out of bed, the diet, and other pertinent information, such as intake and output or seizure precautions. This information can be checked with the physician's order sheet. A tag indicating the patient's name is often placed near the door of the room as well.

Care of the Patient's Personal Belongings

Clothing. A patient in a private or semiprivate room has more leeway with belongings than patients in a larger ward. Clothing can be hung in the closet. Each person has a place for a bathrobe and slippers, and dresser drawers provide space for other personal articles. The clothing of a patient in a ward may be sent to a special room for storage. It should be placed on hangers and protected from dust. It also can be sent home.

Fill out a property sheet, and list every item of clothing. It is important to follow the system the hospital has established; doing so protects the patient, the hospital, and you. Have the patient sign the property sheet, after checking the list.

Valuables. Valuables, such as jewelry, credit cards, and cash, should not be brought to the hospital. If they are, they usually are kept in the hospital safe. When patients learn they will not be able to keep these belongings at the bedside or wear them, they may prefer to send them home with family. The patient and family *must* understand that the hospital assumes *no liability* for articles left at the bedside. The patient usually keeps a small amount of change to buy newspapers and small items from the coffee or gift shop.

The patient keeps personal items, such as glasses, dentures, or a prosthesis. These items are noted on the admission sheet. Usually the patient signs a waiver verifying that the items are to remain at the bedside at the patient's own risk. The nurse must be careful not to lose the patient's personal items. All such items must be *carefully labeled* with the patient's name and room number.

If the patient goes to surgery or has a lengthy examination, items such as a watch or glasses may be locked in the narcotics cupboard for a short time. If this is done, it also must be noted, and the patient must sign later to verify that the items have been returned.

Preventing Dehumanization

The hospitalized person surrenders clothes, belongings, and individuality to follow orders about when to eat, sleep, take a bath, and even go to the bathroom. A stranger asks when the patient last had a menstrual period or a bowel movement. All these factors **dehuman-**

ize the person unless they are handled with utmost tact and respect for the person.

Whether care is given in a hospital, home, or physician's office, the nurse can do much to prevent the patient from feeling dehumanized. Always think of the patient as a person whose need for physical and emotional support is greater than normal because of illness, and emphasize the patient's strengths rather than weaknesses. In this way, you will be invaluable in assisting in the patient's recovery. Allow the patient to *maintain personal dignity.*

Anxiousness or Apprehension. Every hospitalized person is bound to feel anxious and nervous about the hospitalization and the family's welfare. What may be upsetting to one person may have no effect on another. The degree of anxiety may vary with severity of the illness. This anxiety may cause physical and emotional stress that can aggravate the patient's health problem.

Fear of the Unknown. Perhaps the most intense fear is fear of the unknown. The patient may be afraid of death or of a serious illness. Some people may feel that the medical staff is not telling the truth about their disease or condition and that it is really more serious than it actually is.

Fear of Body Image Changes. Patients react intensely to any threat to their body image. Many people feel threatened by an illness, especially if its treatment involves surgery. The threat exists even when surgery will not cause disfigurement. If the surgery involves amputation of a limb or removal of a breast, the threat of disfigurement is far more real. Disturbing fears arise about the spouse's response to disfigurement, how friends will react, or the possible loss of a job.

Financial Concerns. Another fear that haunts many patients is the fear of financial burden. Many patients cannot afford the expense of hospitalization and are concerned about how their families will manage while they are in the hospital. Such preoccupation with financial problems can affect the patient's reaction to illness.

Embarrassment. Many people are embarrassed if personal services have to be performed for them. Providing privacy and explaining what is taking place during the treatment is of key importance when performing procedures. Other difficulties may arise from superstitions or lack of knowledge of the body. A limited understanding of the English language also may be a problem for some patients.

Nursing Process Record

I.

Date:	Language:	Rel.:
Time:	Mode of Adm.:	ID Band On:

Occupation:

Glasses: Contacts: Hearing Aids: Dental Prosthesis:

Other Prostheses (List):

Local Phone:

Policies/Instructions Explained to Pt. or Significant Other (S/O) — (list names):

Answer Yes or No to the Following:

Valuables: Call Signals: TV: Smoking:

Bed Ht.:   Side Rails: Visiting Hours:

II. Chief Complaint (must include onset of symptoms, mechanism of injury, course prior to adm.):   Date   Initial

Phychosocial Needs:

Support System (list names):

Pt. (S/O) Expectation of Hospitalization:

Significant Past Medical/Surgical HX:

Allergies (include type of reaction):

MEDICATION REGIME AT HOME

Medication	Dosage	Frequency	Time of Last Dose	Sent Home	Locked Location	Date

Notification of Physician: PHYSICIAN: DATE: TIME:

Name: _____   Age: _____   Room # _____

	T	P	R
	BP	HT.	WT.

Initial	M	6
GLASGOW COMA SCALE	E V 4 5 R L	
	Pupils R L	

SIZE ● ● ● ● ● ● ● ●
1 2 3 4 5 6 7 8

LIMB STRENGTH (See Below)	RA	LA
	RL	LL

PULSES = Strong W = Weak Ab = Absent Ua = Covered unable to check	Rad.	DP	PT
R			
L			

SIGNIFICANT OBSERVATIONS/REVIEW OF SYSTEMS   Date   Initial

ENT.

Vision: (R)   (L)

Head & Neck:

Neuro: Mental Status: Alert _____ Oriented _____ Confused _____
Comatose _____ Other _____

Cardiovascular: Pulse _____ Reg/Irregular _____ Chest Pain _____
HX of Arrythmias: _____ SOB _____ Edema R/ _____ L _____

Respiratory:
Lungs Sound: Clear _____ Rales _____ Rhonchi _____
Wheezes _____

GI: Bowel Sounds: present _____ Diminished _____ Absent _____
Bowel Pattern: Last BM _____ Constipation _____ Laxative _____ Incont _____
GU: Voiding: _____ Freq. _____ Burning _____ Incont _____ Cath _____
Cath Care q Shift _____
Tarry Stools _____ Grey Stools _____ Rectal Bleeding _____
Hemorrhoids _____ Ostomies _____

ROM/Limitations: Amputee R ___ L ___ Paraplegic ___ Hemiplegic R ___ L ___
Specific For Pt   Leg Cramps _____
Smoking HX (When):
Sleep Pattern:
Alcohol/Drugs:
Diet (Freq., Type): Small meals _____ 3 x day _____ Tube Feeding _____
Restrictions: _____

RN/LVN:

**Nursing Process Record (NPR)
Admission Notes/Data Base**

Attending Physician: _____

(Form courtesy of AMI Nacogdoches Medical Center, Nacogdoches, Texas)

Assessment, Reporting, and Documentation

After the patient is oriented to the nursing unit and the hospital room, the admissions interview and history are taken.

Questions to ask on the interview are listed in a box in Chapter 34. You also will take vital signs and height and weight. You will collect urine, stool, or sputum specimens and may accompany the patient to the x-ray department or laboratory for tests. A sample form for admission notes and data base is shown at the top of the next four pages.

During the time you are with the patient, be observant. Be sure to report to your team leader if the patient complains of severe pain or seems to be very uncomfortable. Look for any physical signs or symptoms. Knowing the patient's diagnosis is helpful when observing signs and symptoms. Listen to what the patient says. Nursing skill guidelines for the admission of a patient are given in the box. The total nursing assessment is described in Chapter 50.

The assessment process can begin by learning a patient's likes and dislikes of food or television programs and his or her ability to use the equipment.

Special Considerations in Children
Hospital Admission Assessment

◆ Observe for signs of anxiety and fear of the unknown, as evidenced by crying and temper tantrums.
◆ Be knowledgeable of developmental stages to be better able to judge the child's physical and emotional needs.
◆ Determine if a parent or family member will be staying with the child.
◆ Determine how much self-care the child can perform.
◆ Be aware that regression often occurs when a child is ill.

Nursing Process Record (continued)

III. Teaching Potential: Memory: _____ Good _____ Poor _____ Coordination: Good: _____ Poor _____

Difficulty with Communicating: Aphasic _____ Dysphasic _____ HOH _____

Teaching Plan: Instruction in _____ given to pt./s.o. _____

Name

Nursing Problem: _____

PLEASE MARK THE FOLLOWING IF INDICATED ON THE CHART BELOW:

SCAR (S)   DRAINAGE WOUNDS (DW)   BRUISES (B)   DECUBITUS (D)-GRADE I, II, III EDEMA (+, ++, +++,)   IMPLANTS (I)   FRACTURES (FX)

Skin:

		Nail Beds:	
_____ Bruises Easily	_____ Cold	_____ Pale	
_____ Bleeds Easily	_____ Moist/Perspiring	_____ Pink	
_____ Itching/Rashes	_____ Pale	_____ Cyanotic	
_____ Skin Problems	_____ Pink	_____ Clubbed	
_____ Warm	_____ Ashy		
_____ Dry	_____ Cyanotic		

Signature RN: _____

Height and Weight. The patient's weight and height are recorded on admission. These measurements may indicate that the patient is retaining fluids or is overweight or underweight. They establish a baseline for further observations.

To be weighed, the patient may stand on a transfer paper or paper towel on the balance scales. An immobile patient is weighed lying down in a sling-type litter; this scale looks like a suspended hammock. You will need assistance to place the patient on a **litter scale.** A *chair scale* is also available for the patient who is unable to stand. The weight is documented on the flow sheet or graphic sheet (see Chapter 42), on the Kardex, and in the patient care or nursing notes. If daily weights are compared, the patient should be weighed on the *same scale,* wearing the *same amount of clothing,* and at the *same time* each day.

◆ Have the patient remove street clothes before weighing. *(Rationale: The weight will be more accurate if he or she is weighed in the hospital gown.)*
◆ After the admission weight is taken, weight is normally measured daily or weekly before the patient eats.
◆ Record on graphic sheet as soon as possible, because current weight is necessary for the physician to calculate dosages of medications or to determine effectiveness of total parenteral nutrition, a special feeding, for example.

Litter or Chair Scales. Patients who are unable to stand are weighed on chair scales or litter (bed) scales. The litter scale has slinglike or canvas straps on which the patient is positioned. The machine raises the patient from the bed surface. The weight is recorded on a balance or a digital electronic display.

The chair scale resembles the "step-on scale" but is equipped with a chair with arms for the patient's comfort. Weight is calibrated by the free moving balance arm. The scale is cleaned after each use.

When measuring height, have the patient remove shoes and stand on the scale with the back to the measuring bar. Ask the person to stand straight. Lower the L-shaped sliding bar so that it lightly touches the top of the patient's head. Record the height in inches or cen-

Nursing Process Record (continued)

IV. VITAL SIGNS (specify frequency)	Date Order	DIET	Date Order	TREATMENTS	Date Order
TPR: BP: NVS:		Type:		Urine Testing (method):	
Apical/Radial:		Nourishments:			
Peripheral Pulses:		Special Requests:		Resp. Therapy:	
Weights:		Assist:			
Other:		N/G Tube Feed:			
		Force/Restrict Fluids: 24° Total			
ACTIVITY (specify frequency and/or mode)		7-3 3-11 11-7		Anti-Emb. Hose:	
Comp. Bedrest: Reposition:		**IV FLUIDS**		P.T.:	
Bedrest c̄: BSC BRP		Type & Rate:			
Dangle: Chair:					
Amb. c̄ Assist. (specify):					
Up Ad Lib:				Traction:	
Exercise (specify):					
		INTAKE & OUTPUT		Dressing Change/Wound Care:	
Other:					
		I & O: Last BM:			
PERSONAL HYGIENE		Type Cath: Date Inserted:			
Bedbath: Shower: Tub:		Cath. Care: Date Change:			
Self: Assist:		G.U. Irrig.: Rate:			
Mouth/Denture Care: Peri Care:		Drains:			
Special Skin Care (specify):					
		Lab Procedures:	OB:	X-Ray Procedures:	
			Peri Care:		
			Fundal Massage:		
Other:			Anesthesia:		
SAFETY			Blood Type:		
			Breast Feeding:		
Side Rails:			DTV:		
Restrain (specify):					
Special Precautions:			Procedures/Tests:		
Blind Deaf					
Seizure					
Other					
Escort (transport): Amb. WC STR					
		Surgical Procedures:			
				Teaching Service:	
		Adm. Diagnosis:		Classification:	
			Admitting Physician:		
			Consults:	Date Revised:	
		Allergies:			

DATE REVIEWED (Must Be Reviewed Every 24 Hours)

timeters on the flow sheet or graphic sheet, according to hospital policy. Total height should be recorded in *inches* or centimeters (not feet or meters).

If the patient cannot stand, an approximate height can be obtained in bed. Have the patient lie on the back and stretch out as much as possible. Place a mark on the sheet under the person's heel and at the top of the head. Then measure between these two marks on the taut bottom sheet.

Vital Signs. The nurse measures and records the patient's **vital signs** during admission and as ordered while the patient is in the hospital. Vital signs include *body temperature, pulse* (rate of heartbeats), *respiration* (rate of breathing), and *blood pressure* (the pressure exerted by the blood against the walls of the arteries). These readings are abbreviated as TPR and BP. They are called vital signs because they all must be present for life to continue. Vital signs are so important to nursing that a separate chapter in this book is devoted entirely to their measurements (see Chapter 42).

Collecting Specimens. Usually a urine specimen is to be obtained. Give the patient instructions about the collection. Most often, a midstream or clean-catch specimen is to be collected; you will need to instruct the patient on how it is done. This procedure is described in Chapter 47.

The Chest X-Ray Examination. Some patients are given a chest x-ray on admission. This is done to rule out tuberculosis or tumors of the lungs. It also helps determine whether the heart is enlarged or lung disease is present. If x-rays or laboratory work are ordered, you may be asked to transport the patient to the x-ray department or laboratory. Be sure to follow the guidelines in Chapter 43 for transporting a patient by wheelchair or litter.

Reporting the Admission

The Joint Commission for Accreditation of Healthcare Organizations (JCAHO) requires that formal admission interviews, nursing diagnoses, and admission

Nursing Process Record (continued)

V.

Date	Initial	Social Service indicated Y — N —	DISCHARGE PLANNING

PATIENT STATUS AT DISCHARGE
(Refer to Audit Criteria Where Available/Applicable)

Date	Initial				LEGEND	
		Physical Status:		Initial	Full Signature	Title
		Psychosocial Status:				

VII.

Date	Initial	Instructions Given To/Discharge Med(2)-(list):	DISCHARGE INSTRUCTIONS
		Signs & Symptoms of Illness to Notify MD (specify):	
		Diet (specify):	
		Activity (specify):	
		Follow Up Visit (when, with whom):	
		Verbalizes/Demonstrates Understanding of Instructions (if no, explain):	

Discharge Date: _____ Time: _____ Belongings returned: _____ Meds: _____

Released to: _____ Glasses: _____ Contacts: _____ Hearing Aids: _____

Unit Dismissed From: _____ Room: _____ To Whom? _____

Mode of Discharge: Amb _____ WC _____ Stretcher _____ Valuables Returned: ☐ Yes ☐ No/explain _____

Ambulance _____ Private Car _____ To Whom? _____

Accompanied by staff member: Yes _____ No _____ Signature-Title: _____

charting be done by a registered nurse (RN). When a student or licensed practical nurse (LPN) has finished patient orientation and assigned admission procedures, the team leader or charge nurse is notified. Typically, the charge nurse is busy and may not know the patient has reached the unit. The charge nurse or team leader is responsible for seeing that the physician is notified of the patient's arrival. Later, it is important to determine that there are physician's orders for the patient and that the patient's diet order is sent to the dietary department.

The LPN reports preliminary observations and the patient's vital signs to the RN. Head-to-toe observations are important to the admissions interview (see Chapter 50). They give the RN a starting point for the interview, based on the observations. The nursing diagnosis can then be completed and the nursing care plan developed by the team. Guidelines for admission documentation are listed in the box.

Patient Transfer to Another Unit

There are a number of reasons for transferring a patient to another unit:

◆ When assignment to a certain unit is temporary
◆ When a change in condition necessitates placing the patient in another department
◆ When a quieter environment is required
◆ When the patient is disturbing others
◆ When the patient is transferred to an attached extended-care facility
◆ When the patient's condition becomes serious enough for the patient to be transferred to an intensive care unit (ICU) or when the patient leaves the ICU

Skills for preparing the patient to be transferred follow:

◆ Explain the transfer to the patient and family. Give

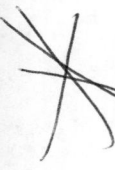

Nursing Skill Guidelines
Performing the Admissions Interview

- Gather necessary supplies (eg, patient record, physician's orders, charts).
- Become familiar with the patient information before you meet the patient.
- Introduce yourself; state that you will be taking information and explaining hospital routines.
- Observe patient's general appearance (eg, posture, ability to ambulate).
- Assess patient's general condition (eg, alert, oriented).
- Observe skin condition (eg, temperature, color, turgor, scars, lesions, abrasions, pressure areas, edema). Draw figure on interview form to describe location of above.
- Monitor respiratory status (eg, coughing, wheezing, shortness of breath).
- Assess psychological status, evidenced through verbal and nonverbal responses.
- Measure height and weight.
- Measure vital signs (temperature, pulse, respiration, and blood pressure).
- Obtain information on health history and current health status.
  - Reason for admission
  - Past illnesses and dates
  - Current medication routine
  - Allergies to medications, food, and other substances
  - Alcohol and tobacco usage
  - Daily routine for eating, sleeping, elimination, and exercise
  - Use of appliances or prostheses (eg, artificial limbs, hearing aids, contact lenses, dentures)
  - Family support systems (Will someone be visiting or staying in the hospital with them? For instance, will someone be available at mealtimes to help feed patient? Who should be contacted in an emergency?)
  - Employer or school

the reason for the transfer and when the transfer will take place. *(Rationale: Patients may become anxious and fearful when changed to an unfamiliar setting.)*

- Assemble all the patient's personal belongings. Double-check for all clothes and personal effects.
- Determine how the patient will be moved. *(Rationale: You are responsible for safely moving the patient. Type of transportation depends on the patient's condition. Seldom is the patient allowed to walk.)*
- Provide for patient safety. Take measures to accommodate IV bottles, drains, and catheters. Protect the patient from drafts, and cover him or her with a blanket for warmth and privacy.

- Collect all the patient's medications. Assemble routine medications, and check Kardex or MAR (medication administration record) for accuracy and completeness.
- Review the patient chart. Check documentation on the nurse's notes and graphic sheet for completeness.
- Record the transfer in a transfer note. Give the time, unit to which transfer occurs, type of transportation (wheelchair or stretcher), and physical and psychosocial condition of patient. A brief review of the patient's history is often included.

The following are skills for transporting the patient:

- Provide for safety during the move.
- Introduce the patient to the staff at the nurse's station (if condition permits).
- Give report to staff on new unit.
- Leave medications and records.
- Take the patient to his or her room.
- Assist the patient into bed, and make sure he or she is comfortable.
- When returning to the nursing unit, notify all necessary departments in the hospital of the transfer (eg, dietary, admitting, business, and pharmacy).

Patient Discharge

Planning for the patient's discharge begins at *admission.* Chapter 35 introduces you to discharge planning and patient teaching. The total nursing care team, the patient, and the family are involved in the planning for discharge and care at home.

Admission Documentation

Official interview information is documented by the RN, but students and LPNs will often be asked to record the following information:

- Weight and height
- Vital signs (temperature, pulse, respiration, and blood pressure)
- Whether laboratory tests were done, blood was drawn, or x-rays were taken
- Any other procedures performed
- Specimens sent to the laboratory; note the amount of urine voided and its appearance or inability of the patient to void.
- Whether the patient wears a prosthesis, dentures, contact lenses, glasses, or other devices; note what was done with these items.
- Location of the patient's valuables

Any other information should be reported directly to the charge nurse or team leader.

do a return demonstration of procedures. All discharge teaching must be carefully documented.

The Day the Patient Leaves

Before the day comes for the patient to go home, discuss the best time to leave. The family is instructed to bring clothing, pillows, or blankets if they are needed. If the person seems eager to leave and the condition permits, the patient can dress and rest on the bed until it is time to leave. Guidelines for discharging the patient are given in the accompanying box.

Discharge Documentation

In some healthcare facilities, discharge documentation is done by RNs. A student or LPN may be asked to assist with this documentation. In any event, your observations will be important, whether you are writing in the chart or reporting to another person.

The nurse who discharges the patient brings the chart up to date, records the hour of discharge, and records who accompanied the patient and whether the patient was in a wheelchair or required an ambulance. A nursing summary may be required. This includes the identified nursing problems and their resolution or revision.

Keys to Patient and Family Teaching
Discharge Teaching

Patient and family teaching for the patient preparing for discharge include the following:

- How to change dressings safely and why this is important
- Amount of rest needed and amount of activity allowed
- Dietary restrictions: foods that are allowed and in what amounts; foods that are "musts" each day and those that are not allowed (The dietitian most often does the instruction in the hospital and should be consulted if there are any questions.)
- If the patient will be confined to bed at home, how to make the bed, give a bed bath, move and turn the patient, give and remove the bedpan, adjust pillows, and maintain good body alignment and skin integrity
- How to operate the equipment and take care of tubes
- Informing the family if the patient has special preferences as to how treatments should be done
- Encouragement to patient to do as much self-care as possible. The family needs to understand that independence is beneficial for the patient's self-esteem and continued recovery.
- Information about public health and home nursing services. The Social Service department of the hospital can assist them in finding help. Some hospitals have home nursing departments.
- Where to buy or rent needed equipment, materials for dressing changes, hospital bed. If substitute equipment can be used, the family should be advised. For instance, in some cases a regular bed can be used if it is placed up on blocks.
- Administration of medications: how and when to take medications and information on undesirable side effects. Medications should be taken exactly as demonstrated by nursing staff. The patient should understand the need for accuracy.
- Danger signs of which to be aware
- Who and where to call if difficulties arise
- Date, time, and location of the next scheduled examination

Nursing Care Guidelines
Discharging the Patient

- Verify the discharge order:
  Check for written or telephone order.
  Check orders for "take home" medications, special treatments, or special equipment.
  Check orders for last-minute procedures, laboratory tests, or x-rays.
  Make sure the person has a place to go.
- Coordinate transportation if necessary. It may be necessary to make a telephone call to request an ambulance or taxi service or to call a neighbor.
- Determine what type of clothing is best suited for the patient to wear. (If he or she is being discharged to extended care, pajamas or robe may be appropriate rather than street clothes.)
- Assist the patient in packing and dressing for discharge.
- Check the closet and bedside stand for personal items.
- Arrange for a small utility cart or easy conveyance to the hospital exit.
- Secure release of any valuables checked into the hospital vault.
- Check and have the patient sign the property record.
- Notify necessary departments of the discharge. Unit clerk reports discharge to admissions, dietary, housekeeping, and business office.
- Escort the person from clinical unit.
- Accompany the patient to car or taxi.

As a nursing student and as a graduate nurse, you will assist with teaching a patient and the family prior to discharge. The accompanying box lists things to be taught to patients and their family. Follow instructions as to how much of the discharge teaching you are expected to do. Report to your team leader if you have any suggestions for patient teaching. The primary nurse or team leader also needs to know the patient's responses to teaching. To determine that the patient and family members understand, have them verbalize and

This completes the nursing record of the stay in the hospital. The physician is also required to write a discharge summary for the chart.

Leaving the Hospital Against Advice

Occasionally a patient leaves the hospital without the physician's permission. This is called "against medical advice" (AMA). Such a patient must sign a release form that absolves the physician and the hospital of all responsibility in the event that the patient suffers complications. If the patient refuses to sign, this must be noted on the form. The form is then signed by at least two witnesses. The nurse should report to the team leader any patients who say they are leaving the hospital against advice. The nursing student should *not* witness any legal papers, including the AMA form.

Keys for Review

Key Questions for Critical Thinking

1. An 81-year-old woman is admitted to the hospital for tests of the digestive system. Her mind is very clear. Describe what actions or skills you will use when she arrives on the unit, including assessments and reports.
2. Discuss dehumanization. Describe its causes, results, and methods of prevention.
3. Describe the concept of body image. Discuss implications of illness on body image. Discuss surgical implications to body image.
4. Using information from Chapter 35 and this chapter, discuss patient discharge. Include planning, teaching, the day of discharge, and documentation.

Key Readings

Craven RF, Hirnle CJ. Fundamentals of Nursing: Human Health and Function. Philadelphia, J.B. Lippincott, 1992

Earnest VV. Clinical Skills in Nursing Practice, Ed 2. Philadelphia, J.B. Lippincott, 1993

Kozier B, Erb G, et al. Techniques in Clinical Nursing, Ed 4. Redwood City, CA, Addison-Wesley Nursing, 1993

Smeltzer SC, Bare BG. Brunner and Suddarth's Textbook of Medical Surgical Nursing, Ed 7. Philadelphia, J.B. Lippincott, 1992

Key Readings (continued)

Swearingen PL. Photo Atlas of Nursing Procedures, Ed 2. Redwood City, CA, Addison-Wesley Nursing, 1991

Taber's Cyclopedic Medical Dictionary, Ed 17. Philadelphia, F.A. Davis, 1993

Taylor C, Lillis C, LeMone P. Fundamentals of Nursing: The Art and Science of Nursing Care, Ed 2. Philadelphia, J.B. Lippincott, 1993

Enrichment Keys

Stephan A. "Charting Tips: Documenting Your Patient's Valuables." Nursing 93. 23(10):31, October 1993

Keys to Learning More

Chapter 42: vital signs
Chapter 43: body mechanics and positioning
Chapter 45: personal hygiene and skin care
Chapter 46: elimination
Chapter 47: specimen collection
Chapter 50: head-to-toe physical examination

42 Vital Signs

Keys for Learning

Learning Objectives

- Identify the measurements that comprise the vital signs.
- Define the important terms and abbreviations in the chapter.
- Demonstrate the ability to record temperature, pulse, respiration, and blood pressure accurately.
- Identify reasons for changes in body temperature, and state the normal body temperature as measured in three different areas of the body.
- Define fever and its various courses.
- Demonstrate the ability to measure temperature by the various methods.
- Demonstrate the ability to measure accurately and describe a radial pulse, apical pulse, and apical–radial pulse.
- Demonstrate the ability to count accurately and describe the respiration of a patient.
- Demonstrate the ability to measure blood pressure by the various methods.

Key Terms

body temperature	Korotkoff sounds
bradycardia	lysis
cardinal symptoms	mean arterial pressure
Cheyne-Stokes respirations	orthopnea
crisis	pulse
cyanosis	pulse rate
diastolic	pulse rhythm
dyspnea	systolic
febrile	tachycardia
fever	vital signs

Keys to Understanding This Chapter

Chapter 4: legal and ethical aspects of nursing
Chapter 5: basic human needs
Chapter 8: microbiology
Chapter 30: medical asepsis and universal precautions
Chapter 37: documentation and reporting

Keys to Understanding This Chapter
(continued)

Chapter 38: signs and symptoms of illness or injury
Chapter 41: admission, transfer, and discharge

Key Points

- Temperature, pulse, respiration and blood pressure are called vital signs because they are indicators of vital functions of the body that are necessary to sustain life.
- Documentation of vital signs is essential to collect information regarding the patient's status and well-being.
- Temperature is the measurement of the heat inside the body. It is a balance between heat produced and lost.
- Pulse is the vibration of the blood through the arteries as the heart beats. It is measured by rate and rhythm.
- Respiration is the process by which the lungs bring oxygen into the body and remove carbon dioxide wastes.
- Blood pressure is the measurement of the pressure exerted by the blood on the walls of the arteries. The rate and force of the heartbeat determines the reading as the ventricles contract and rest.

Key Topics Outline

The Graphic Sheet
Assessing Body Temperature
  Regulation of Body Temperature
  Equipment
  Measuring Body Temperature
  Cleaning and Disinfecting Clinical Thermometers
Assessing Pulse
  Regulation of Pulse
  Methods and Equipment
  Measuring the Pulse
Assessing Respiration
  Regulation of Respiration
  Difficult Breathing (Dyspnea)
  Counting Respirations
Assessing Blood Pressure
  Regulation of Blood Pressure
  Methods and Equipment
  Measuring Blood Pressure

Rosdahl CB: Textbook of Basic Nursing, 6th ed. © 1995 J.B. Lippincott Company

Key Learning Activities

◆ Review the vital sign graphic sheets from different clinical units or facilities. Practice recording vital signs on each sheet.

◆ Discuss the value of vital signs with a licensed nurse. Why is it essential to be knowledgeable about the normal vital sign readings? What is the value in maintaining the record?

Key Nursing Procedures

NP 42-1: Measuring Oral Temperature With an Electronic Thermometer
NP 42-2: Measuring Radial Pulse
NP 42-3: Counting Respirations
NP 42-4: Measuring Blood Pressure

Body temperature, pulse, respiration (TPR), and blood pressure (BP) are important data collected by nurses. By using these data, assessments can reflect changes in the patient's condition. TPR and BP are called **vital signs** or **cardinal symptoms** because these measurements are indicators of vital functions that are necessary to sustain life.

Temperature, pulse, and respiration are usually observed together. It has been the practice in many acute care hospitals to require this observation at least morning and evening as a routine procedure for every patient. In some illnesses it is important to make more frequent observations of the cardinal signs. Changes in one of these signs may affect the others, which is one of the reasons for observing them at the same time. The physician will order the frequency for obtaining vital signs. The nurse, however, also may use nursing judgment in obtaining vital signs. Abbreviations used in taking vital signs are listed in the accompanying box.

The Graphic Sheet

The purpose of the graphic sheet is to have a record of reading that is easily accessible to all members of the healthcare team. The temperature, pulse, and respiration are recorded, and the chart shows their relationships. A sample graphic sheet is shown in Figure 42-1. Readings recorded throughout the patient's illness are indicated in unbroken lines across a page. Each reading is recorded as a dot in the proper space, with lines connecting the dots.

Every hospital has its own printed graphic form and method for recording the temperature, pulse, and respiration with space for recording other information, such as BP, the total intake and output of fluids, bowel movements, and weight. The vital signs should be recorded accurately and in a timely manner. Proper documentation ensures a data bank on the patient. The vital signs aid the physician in his or her diagnosis and serve as a reference for the nurse.

Key Medical Abbreviations for Recording Vital Signs

BP	Blood pressure
BPM	Beats per minute
CVP	Central venous pressure
ICU	Intensive care unit
MAP	Mean arterial pressure
PMI	Point of maximal impulse
TPR	Temperature, pulse, respiration
VS	Vital signs

Important activities in recording vital signs on the graphic sheet include the following:

◆ Locate the current date on the graphic sheet.
◆ Record temperature by making a dot on the scale under the appointed time. Connect dots from previous reading with a short line.
◆ Record respiration by making a dot on the scale under the appointed time. Connect dots from previous reading with a short line.
◆ Record respiration at the bottom of the graph with written numbers.
◆ Record BP with written numbers (eg, 120/80) or graph the numbers in a manner similar to temperature.
◆ Record other information, such as weight, bowel movements, and the totals for intake and output, with written numbers in the areas provided.
◆ Each clinical facility will have a different form to record vital sign information, but a general knowledge of transcribing written data is required to ensure accuracy. Always return the patient record promptly to the proper area of storage.

Sometimes blood pressure is stated on a graph with dots or check marks. The graph will be marked off in increments similar to the increments in the temperature graph. Many times a BP graph is superimposed on the temperature graph.

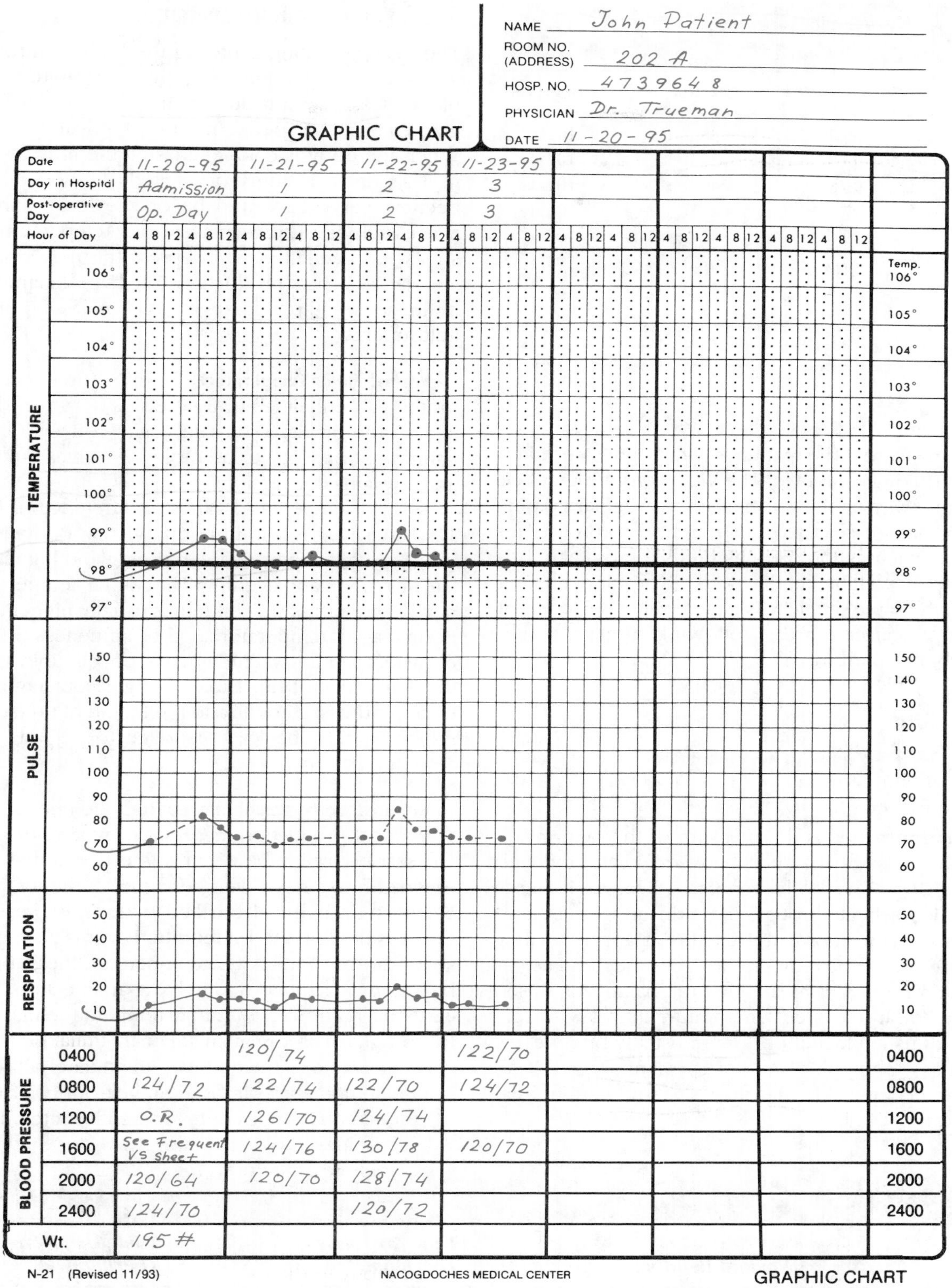

GRAPHIC CHART

NAME _John Patient_

ROOM NO. (ADDRESS) _202 A_

HOSP. NO. _473964 8_

PHYSICIAN _Dr. Trueman_

DATE _11-20-95_

Date	11-20-95	11-21-95	11-22-95	11-23-95				
Day in Hospital	Admission	1	2	3				
Post-operative Day	Op. Day	1	2	3				

BLOOD PRESSURE								
0400		120/74		122/70				0400
0800	124/72	122/74	122/70	124/72				0800
1200	O.R.	126/70	124/74					1200
1600	See Frequent VS sheet	124/76	130/78	120/70				1600
2000	120/64	120/70	128/74					2000
2400	124/70		120/72					2400
Wt.	195 #							

N-21 (Revised 11/93)   NACOGDOCHES MEDICAL CENTER   GRAPHIC CHART

Figure 42-1. Temperature graph. (Courtesy of AMI Nacogdoches Medical Center, Nacogdoches, Texas)

Table 42-1. Equivalent Celsius and Fahrenheit Temperatures*

Celsius	Fahrenheit	Celsius	Fahrenheit
34.0	93.2	38.5	101.3
35.0	95.0	39.0	102.2
36.0	96.8	40.0	104.0
36.5	97.7	41.0	105.8
37.0	98.6	42.0	107.6
37.5	99.5	43.0	109.4
38.0	100.4	44.0	111.2

* To convert Celsius to Fahrenheit, multiply by $^9/_5$ and add 32. To change Fahrenheit to Celsius subtract 32 and multiply by $^5/_9$.

"Frequent Vital Signs" Sheet

In many cases, the patient's vital signs are taken every 5, 10, or 15 minutes. The vital signs are graphed in the same way on this sheet as on the regular graphic sheet. In many cases there is space to record other information, such as intravenous fluids, oral intake, urinary output, weight, medications given, and nursing notes on the same sheet. This type of sheet is used most often in critical care areas, following surgery, or immediately postpartum.

Assessing Body Temperature

Body temperature is the measure of the heat inside the body; it is the balance between heat produced and heat lost. The body generates heat as it burns food. It loses heat through the skin and lungs, and body temperature normally remains at approximately 37°C or 98.6°F. If the temperature goes much higher or lower than normal, it means that the balance is upset. The signs of an elevated temperature are easy to recognize: a flushed face, hot skin, unusually bright eyes, restlessness, and thirst. A lifeless manner and pale, cold, and clammy skin are often signs of a subnormal temperature.

Regulation of Body Temperature

The heat-regulating center in the brain controls body temperature by controlling the temperature of the blood. Heat is a product of metabolism. Muscle and gland activities generate most of the heat in the body. When the body is cold, exercising the muscles warms it; if a person is angry or excited, the adrenal glands become very active and he or she feels warm. The process of digestion increases body temperature. Cold, shock, and certain drugs depress the nervous system and decrease heat production. The hypothalamus in the brain senses these changes and makes appropriate adjustments.

Normal Body Temperature. Temperature is measured on the Fahrenheit (F) or the Celsius (C) scale, depending on the facility. You can easily convert Celsius to Fahrenheit or vice versa. Table 42-1 gives equivalents and explains conversions.

Normal temperature varies; a difference of 0.5°F to 1°F either way is within normal limits. Body temperature is usually lowest in the morning and highest in the late afternoon and evening. The normal temperature for newborn infants and children is usually higher than the normal adult temperature. Other influences on normal body temperature include ovulation, childbirth, and individual metabolism. Table 42-2 gives average normal temperatures for adults and the length of time the thermometer must be kept in place to get an accurate reading.

Elevated Body Temperature. Body temperature rises when heat production increases or when heat loss decreases; both may be occurring at the same time. Everyone always has a "temperature." If the temperature is elevated, **fever**, also called *pyrexia,* is present, and the person is said to be **febrile.** Fever is a symptom of some disorder. It often accompanies illness, or it may be a sign that the body is fighting an infection. In some cases, a slightly above-normal temperature may be useful to fight microorganisms. For this reason, it isn't always desirable to treat a fever immediately.

Oral temperatures in fever range from 100°F to 103°F (37.8°C–39.4°C) Types of fever are illustrated in Figure

Table 42-2. Average Normal Temperatures

Route	Normal Reading	Time for Clinical Thermometer	Time for Electronic Thermometer
Oral (mouth)	98.6°F (37°C)	3–4 min	0.5–1.5 min
Rectal (anus)	99.6°F (37.5°C)	3–4 min	0.5–1.5 min
Axillary (armpit)	97.6°F–98°F (36.4°C–36.7°C)	8–10 min	1–3 min
Tympanic (auditory canal)	Convert to oral, rectal, or core equivalents	—	1–2 sec

42-2. A temperature that alternates between fever and normal or subnormal is called *intermittent fever*. A temperature that rises several degrees above normal and returns to normal or near normal is a *remittent fever*. A *constant fever* stays elevated. A sudden drop from fever to normal is called **crisis.** When an elevated temperature gradually returns to normal, it is called **lysis.** When temperature returns to normal for at least a day, and then fever occurs again, this is a *relapsing fever*.

Lowered Body Temperature. A temperature significantly below normal is called *hypothermia*. Such temperatures often precede normal death and may occur as a result of overexposure to the elements or cold water, as in drowning.

In some instances a body temperature that is slightly below normal indicates a desirable situation: The lowered body temperature slows body metabolism and thus decreases the need for oxygen. *Clinical hypothermia* may be used to perform some surgical procedures; *accidental hypothermia* is life threatening and must be treated immediately.

Nursing Alert

An extremely high or extremely low temperature can be fatal. Survival is rare if the core temperature is above 108°F (42.2°C) or below 93.2°F (34°C).

Equipment

The Clinical Thermometer

Body temperature is sometimes measured by a glass clinical thermometer, marked in degrees Fahrenheit or Celsius (centigrade) or in both scales. Glass clinical thermometers are rarely used in hospitals today except in isolation rooms, but they are sometimes used in nursing homes and in the patient's home. The nurse should know how to use and care for the clinical thermometer so that the patient and family can be taught this skill. The clinical thermometer is a hollow glass tube, or stem, with a mercury-filled bulb on one end; the other end is sealed. Heat expands the mercury, causing it to rise into the stem; the stem is marked off in full degrees and in two-tenths of a degree. The markings range from 93°F (33.9°C) or 94°F (34.45°C) to about 108°F (42.2°C). These ranges encompass the temperatures in living humans. The reading remains on the thermometer until you briskly shake it down.

There are two types of clinical thermometer tips: thin and slender and bulb shaped (Fig. 42-3). The thermometer with the bulb-shaped tip is used for taking rectal temperature because it makes insertion safer. The slender-tipped oral thermometer is used for taking tem-

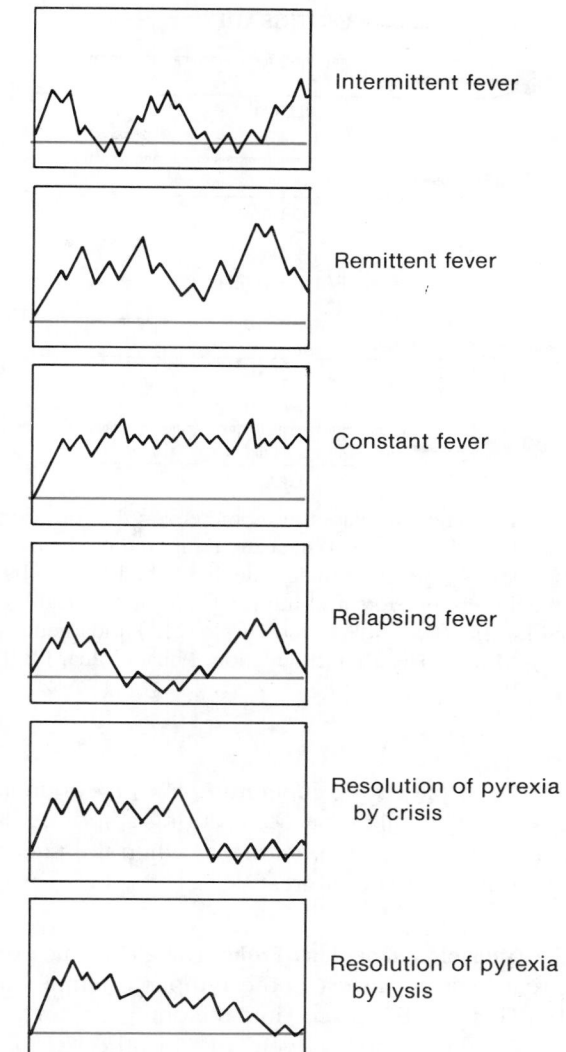

Figure 42-2. Common courses of fever and its resolution. The colored line represents normal temperature. (Taylor C, Lillis CA, LeMone P. Fundamentals of Nursing: The Art and Science of Nursing Care, Ed 2. Philadelphia, J.B. Lippincott, 1993.)

- Intermittent fever
- Remittent fever
- Constant fever
- Relapsing fever
- Resolution of pyrexia by crisis
- Resolution of pyrexia by lysis

perature by mouth. Oral and rectal thermometers must not be used interchangeably.

The Electronic Thermometer

Electronic thermometers are usually the only type of thermometer used in hospitals. The electronic thermometer is fast, accurate, and easier to use than the clinical thermometer. The temperature probe is placed in the patient's mouth, axilla, or rectum in the same manner as the bulb of the clinical thermometer (see Figure 42-3).

Electronic thermometers should be cleaned or sterilized following the maufacturer's instructions on a regular basis or after being used in isolation. During a treatment, the electronic thermometer can be left in

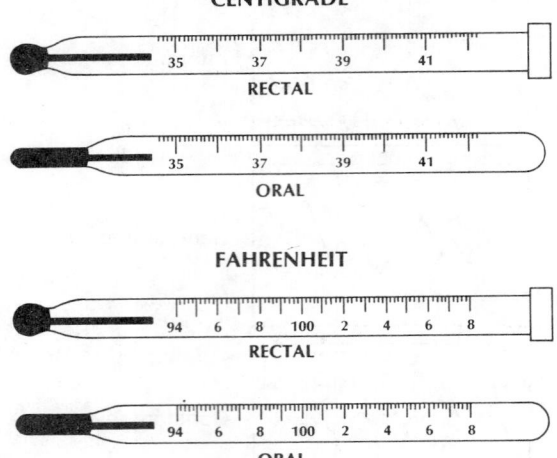

CENTIGRADE

RECTAL

35   37   39   41

ORAL

35   37   39   41

FAHRENHEIT

RECTAL

94   6   8   100   2   4   6   8

ORAL

94   6   8   100   2   4   6   8

Figure 42-3. The two glass thermometers on the top use the centigrade (Celsius) scale to measure temperature; the two on the bottom use the Fahrenheit scale. Note the blunt bulbs on the rectal thermometers and the long thin bulbs on the oral thermometers. (Craven R.F. and Hirnle C.J.: Fundamentals of Nursing: Human Health and Function. Philadelphia: J.B. Lippincott, 1992)

place so the patient's temperature can be continually monitored. This might be done during a sponge bath to reduce the body temperature or when the patient's temperature fluctuates a great deal.

The Tympanic Temperature Probe. The electronic probe that registers the fastest is the tympanic temperature probe. This probe is placed into the outer ear canal and measures the energy given off by the tympanic membrane. The tympanic thermometer is illustrated in Figure 42-4. It indicates the temperature in 1 to 2 seconds. The nurse can select a readout that is converted to the equivalent of the body's core temperature or to the rectal or oral temperature. This type of thermometer is used extensively in pediatrics and the intensive care unit because of its fast indication time. It is charged and cared for in a manner similar to other electronic thermometers.

Key Concept

All electronic temperature probes are covered with a new cover for each patient. One-time use covers also are available for glass clinical thermometers.

The Disposable Single-Use Thermometer

Temperature indicators made of paper are available. They are used only once. The wrapper is removed and the indicator placed under the patient's tongue. The reading appears on the paper. It can be a permanent record or discarded.

Measuring Body Temperature

No matter what type of thermometer or measuring probe is used, certain rules apply:

♦ The thermometer bulb or electronic probe is placed so as to be completely surrounded by body tissues.
♦ When the tympanic probe is used, it is surrounded by skin, rather than mucous membrane, so the risk of infection is less.
♦ Every hospital has an established routine for temperature taking. For instance, a hospital may require temperatures to be taken by rectum whenever possible to give the most accurate reading.
♦ Temperature probes and multiuse thermometers are covered when used. The cover is slipped tightly over the thermometer, the temperature is taken, and the cover is removed and discarded.
♦ Prelubricated covers are available for rectal thermometers.
♦ When the temperature is recorded on the patient's graphic chart, it is recorded to the even two tenths of a degree (unless the electronic thermometer is used).

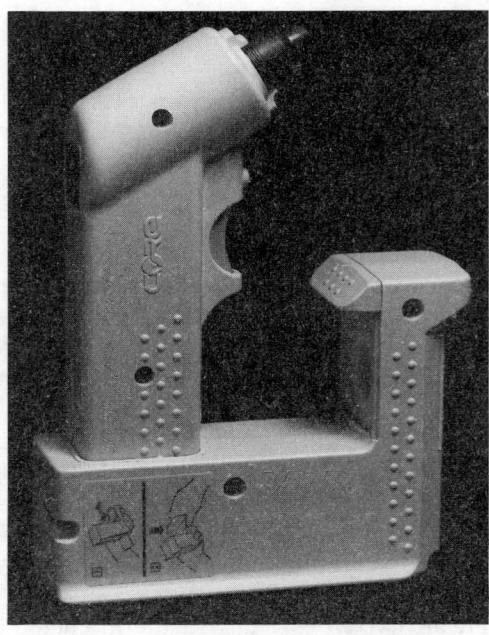

Figure 42-4. Tympanic thermometer. The probe is placed in the ear canal to seal the opening. (Fuller J and Schaller-Ayers J: Health Assessment: A Nursing Approach, 2nd ed. Philadelphia: J.B. Lippincott, 1994)

Sites for Assessment

Oral Temperature. The oral method is the easiest to use, and patients do not find it as uncomfortable as other sites. The oral method is not used if the patient is unconscious, delirious, or otherwise not responsible for his or her actions. This method also is not used with an infant or young child, because of the danger of injury from a broken thermometer. It is contraindicated in surgery or injury to the nose or mouth or in conditions in which the patient must breathe through the mouth. If a patient has had a hot or a cold drink, wait 15 minutes before taking a mouth temperature; the temporary effects of heat or cold will have disappeared from the tissues in that time. Chewing gum and tobacco smoke also can affect oral temperature. The skills used in measuring an oral temperature with an electronic thermometer are explained in Nursing Procedure 42-1.

Rectal Temperature. The rectal temperature is accurate because the thermometer is placed in an enclosed cavity. If there is any question about the accuracy of an oral temperature, it can be checked rectally. Some hospitals make it a policy to recheck oral temperatures by the rectal method when they are above a certain level. Rectal temperatures are always taken with unconscious or irrational patients and with infants and young children unless contraindicated. For easier insertion, a lubricated probe cover is used. To prevent injury, the nurse holds the thermometer in place. The method is contraindicated in such conditions as diarrhea, rectal disease, or following rectal surgery.

Nursing Skill
Measuring Rectal Temperature

Supplies and Equipment

Rectal thermometer
Wipes
Tissues
Water-soluble lubricant or lubricated probe cover
Disposable gloves
Graphic chart and pen

Procedure

◆ Wash hands and put on gloves. *(Rationale: To prevent the spread of infection.)*
◆ Turn the patient on one side. *(Rationale: Side position exposes the area for thermometer placement.)*
◆ Prepare the thermometer by lubricating the bulb and the area up to 1 in above it with lubricant placed on a wipe. Use a lubricated probe cover with an electronic thermometer. *(Rationale: Lubrication reduces friction and makes it easier to insert the thermometer or probe without injuring tissues. Applying the lubricant with a wipe prevents contamination of the lubricant supply.)*

◆ Fold back the bedclothes, and separate the patient's buttocks so that the anal opening is easily seen. *(Rationale: The area must be visible for easy insertion.)*
◆ As the patient takes a slow, deep breath, insert the thermometer about 1.5 in. *(Rationale: Deep, slow breaths allow the patient to relax the anal area. Insertion depth is needed to allow the probe to be surrounded by blood vessels in the rectum.)*
◆ Hold the thermometer in place for 3 to 5 minutes according to agency protocol. *(Rationale: The thermometer is held in place for safety and so it is not expelled. Adequate time is needed to give an accurate reading.)*
◆ Remove and wipe the clinical thermometer or dispose of the probe cover. *(Rationale: Fecal matter on the thermometer obscures the markings. Friction aids in cleaning.)*
◆ Read the temperature.
◆ Dispose of the equipment properly. Wash your hands. *(Rationale: Fecal material is especially contaminated.)*
◆ Record the temperature on the patient's graphic chart. Indicate that the temperature was taken rectally, which is often done by writing "(R)." *(Rationale: There is a difference in normal values between oral and rectal temperatures.)*

Axillary Temperature. Axillary (armpit) temperatures are taken only when conditions make it impossible to use any other method. The axillary method, however, is routinely used for newborns after the initial rectal reading. The axillary temperature is the least accurate because the skin surfaces in the axillary space may not come together to form a tightly closed cavity around the thermometer tip. The nurse also must hold the thermometer in place when using this method.

Nursing Skill
Measuring Axillary Temperature

Supplies and Equipment

Appropriate thermometer
Graphic chart
Pen

Procedure

◆ Wash your hands. *(Rationale: This prevents the spread of infection.)*
◆ Be sure the axilla is dry. If it is moist, pat it dry gently before inserting the thermometer. *(Rationale: Moisture will alter the reading.)*
◆ After placing the probe or bulb of the thermometer into the axilla, bring the arm down against the body as tightly as possible, with the forearm resting across the chest. *(Rationale: Close contact of the probe or bulb of the thermometer with the superficial blood vessels in the axilla ensures a more accurate registration of temperature.)*

Measuring Oral Temperature With an Electronic Thermometer

Supplies and Equipment

Thermometer with probe
Disposable probe covers
Paper or flow sheet
Pen

Procedure

1. Gather equipment.
   (*Rationale: Organization facilitates performance of skills.*)
2. Wash hands.
   (*Rationale: Handwashing prevents the spread of organisms.*)
3. Explain procedure to patient.
   (*Rationale: Providing information fosters patient cooperation and understanding.*)
4. Check that oral probe is attached to the portable thermometer unit. Slide disposable plastic cover onto probe until it snaps into place.
   (*Rationale: Disposable sheath prevents the spread of infection between patients.*)

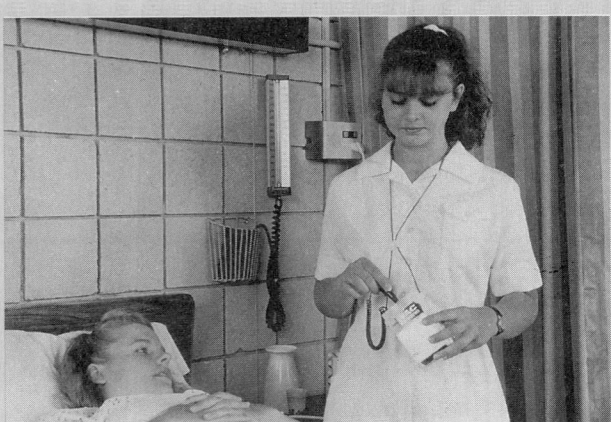

Step 4 Covering the probe with a plastic sheath

5. Place probe under patient's tongue at the base of the sublingual pocket on either side.
   (*Rationale: Heat from superficial blood vessels in the sublingual pocket produces the temperature reading.*)

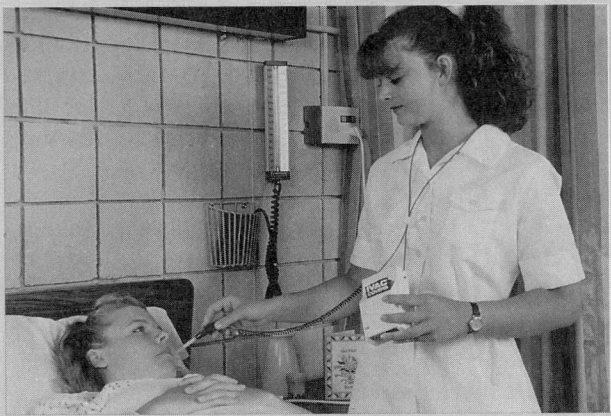

Step 5 Placing the probe under the patient's tongue

6. Instruct the patient to close lips (not the teeth) around the probe.
   (*Rationale: Closing the lips steadies and secures the thermometer. Injury may occur if the probe is bitten.*)
7. Remove the thermometer when "beep" sounds or numbers stop flashing and digital reading of temperature is displayed.
   (*Rationale: Signal indicates that temperature is registered and reading is recorded.*)
8. Remove the probe from patient's mouth and read displayed temperature.
   (*Rationale: Electronic instrument will display the patient's measured temperature.*)

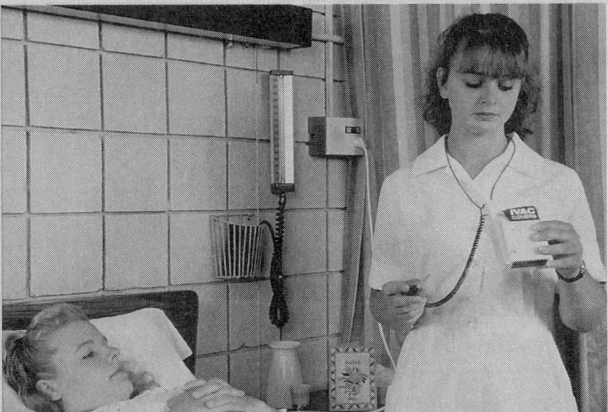

Step 8 Reading the displayed temperature

(continued)

9. Push "eject" button to discard plastic probe cover into waste basket. Return oral probe to portable unit. *(Rationale: Eject button allows nurse to dispose of cover without touching it.)*

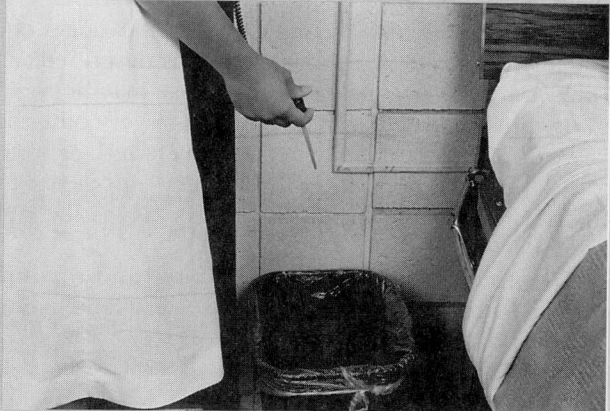

Step 9 Ejecting the plastic sheath (Photos © B. Proud.)

10. Wash hands. *(Rationale: Handwashing prevents the spread of organisms.)*
11. Record temperature on paper or flow sheet. Report any abnormal readings to the appropriate person. *(Rationale: Documentation provides ongoing data collection. Do not try to remember vital signs—write them down.)*

Note: A 15-second timer is usually available on the electronic unit. This can be used to count pulse or respiration. It is activated by pressing the "T" button on the unit.

◆ Hold the thermometer in place for at least 9 minutes. *(Rationale: It takes longer for the temperature reading to register by this method.)*
◆ Remove and read the thermometer. Dispose of the equipment properly. *(Rationale: To prevent the spread of infection.)*
◆ Wash your hands. *(Rationale: Proper handwashing prevents the spread of infection.)*
◆ Record the reading per agency procedures. Indicate that the axillary method was used by writing "(Ax)." *(Rationale: Axillary temperature readings usually are lower than oral readings and should be documented to avoid confusion in interpretation.)*

Cleaning and Disinfecting Clinical Thermometers

Each patient has an individual thermometer if glass clinical thermometers are used. Agency instructions are followed as to cleaning, disinfecting, and caring for clinical thermometers. If the patient uses a clinical thermometer at home, the nurse teaches the family how to clean and disinfect it. The principles for cleaning and disinfecting the glass thermometer are listed in the Patient Teaching box.

Patient/Family Teaching:
Cleaning and Disinfecting the Clinical Thermometer

◆ Wash in cold water. *(Rationale: Heat will break the thermometer.)*
◆ Wipe the thermometer with a soft tissue from the top down toward the bulb with a twisting motion. *(Rationale: Wipe from clean to dirty to prevent spread of microorganisms.)*
◆ Use detergent to remove lubricant from a rectal thermometer before it is disinfected. Rub any thermometer with a soap or detergent solution, and rinse under cold running water. *(Rationale: Lubricant interferes with disinfectant. Rubbing and soap loosen debris and organisms. Running water helps to rinse away soap residue, which would interfere with disinfection and would taste unpleasant. Water also rinses away organisms.)*
◆ Dry the thermometer, and place in prescribed disinfectant for the designated length of time. In some cases, thermometers are stored in a solution. Be sure to rinse before using. *(Rationale: Disinfectants have an unpleasant taste.)*

Assessing Pulse

Every beat of the heart produces a wave of blood that causes pulsations through the arteries. This vibration is the **pulse.** You can feel it through the nerves in your fingertips if you place your fingers over one of the large arteries that lie close to the skin, especially if the artery runs across a bone and has very little soft tissue around it. You can feel the pulse most plainly over the temporal arteries just in front of each ear, the mandibular artery on the lower jawbone, the carotid arteries on each side of the front of the neck, the femoral artery in the groin, and the radial arteries in the wrist at the base of the thumbs. These pulse points are illustrated in Figure 31-2.

Regulation of Pulse

Pulse Rate. The **pulse rate** tells how often the heart beats. The rate varies with patient's age, size, and weight. The normal rate for an adult is 60 to 80 beats per minute (BPM). Women have a slightly higher average rate than men. The pulse of a newborn ranges from 120 to 140 beats per minute. Rates for children are between the adult and infant rates, according to the size and age of the child.

Activity affects the pulse rate. The heart does not work as hard when a person is sleeping as when he or she is sitting or standing. After running, vigorous exercise, or heavy physical work, the heart beats faster, and the pulse rate increases. Excitement, anger, and fear increase the rate, as do some drugs. The pulse rate is more rapid if a person has a fever or the thyroid gland is overactive. It increases in proportion to the body's temperature: the pulse rate goes up about 10 beats for every 1°F (O.56°C) rise in body temperature. Many of the previously mentioned conditions cause a rapid rate temporarily. An abnormally rapid rate that persists may be a sign of heart disease, heart failure, hemorrhage, or some other serious disturbance. If the pulse rate is consistently above normal, the condition is called **tachycardia.**

Sometimes the pulse rate is continuously slow, below 60 beats per minute. This condition is called **bradycardia.** It may occur in convalescence from a long feverish illness. It is a sign in cerebral hemorrhage, indicating increased pressure on the brain. It also is a sign of complete heart block (nonfunctioning of the conduction system of the heart).

Pulse Volume. The volume of the pulse varies with the volume of blood in the arteries, the strength of the heart contractions, and the elasticity of blood vessels. When every beat is full and *strong*, a normal pulse can be felt with a moderate pressure of the finger (stronger pressure exerted by the finger could obliterate the beats). If a pulse is difficult to obliterate, it is called *full* or *bounding*. In hemorrhage, when a considerable amount of blood has been lost, every pulse beat may be *weak* or *thready*.

Pulse Rhythm. Pulse rhythm is the spacing of the beats. With normal or regular rhythm, the intervals between the beats are the same. When the pulse occasionally skips a beat, this irregularity is described as an *intermittent* or *irregular* pulse. A pulse may be regular in rhythm but irregular in force; that is, every other beat is weak. These beats may be so weak that they are not felt in the radial pulse at all. This is very serious because the heart is actually beating twice as fast as the pulse rate indicates.

The pulse may be irregular in force and rhythm, a sign of some forms of heart disease or overactive thyroid gland.

Methods and Equipment

Palpation. Palpation (feeling with the fingers) is used to assess a radial pulse. The area of strongest pulsation is located, and the pulse is then palpated with the first and second or third and second fingers (not the thumb) of one hand. The initial pulsation is counted as zero.

Ausculation With a Stethoscope. The most accurate assessment of pulse rate is made at the apical pulse (at the apex of the heart). An instrument called a stethoscope is used for this assessment. The stethoscope amplifies sounds in the head of the instrument, and they pass through the earpieces. Most stethoscopes have two heads: the diaphragm and the bell. The flat diaphragm is pressed firmly against the skin and is best for testing high-frequency sounds. These are breath sounds, normal heart sounds, and bowel sounds. The bell is cup-shaped and collects low-frequency sounds. It is placed lightly on the skin and is used in detecting abnormal heart sounds. (To change from one head to the other, turn the head until it clicks into place.)

The diaphragm of the stethoscope is placed over the apex of the heart to assess the apical pulse. Each heartbeat consists of two sounds. S_1, the first sound, is caused by closure of the mitral and bicuspid valves separating the atria from the ventricles. S_2, the second sound, is caused by the closure of the pulmonic and aortic valves. The result is a muffled "lub-dub." This is one heartbeat.

Doppler. An ultrasonic Doppler can be used to detect peripheral pulses. A conductive gel is applied, and the Doppler transmitter is placed over the artery being assessed. Sounds are amplified and heard through earpieces or a special speaker attached to the Doppler device.

Measuring the Pulse

Measuring a Radial Pulse. The radial artery is most commonly used to count the pulse because of its convenient location. The middle two or three fingers are used to take a pulse. *Do not use the thumb.* It has a strong pulse of its own, which may be stronger than the patient's pulse. This skill is shown in Nursing Procedure 42-2.

Measuring an Apical Pulse. The apical pulse should *always* be measured if there is any question about the rhythm or rate of the heart or if it appears the heart has stopped. In some cases, the physician orders apical pulses. The apical pulse is more accurate than the radial pulse. The following is the suggested procedure.

Nursing Skill
Measuring Apical Pulse

Supplies and Equipment

Stethoscope and watch

Procedure

◆ Wash hands. (*Rationale: This prevents the spread of infection.*)
◆ Expose the area of the chest while respecting the patient's privacy. (*Rationale: Noise from clothing and bedclothes will distort pulse sound.*)
◆ Locate the point of maximal impulse (PMI), the point over the apex of the heart where the apical pulse is best heard or felt. (This point can be felt in about half of adults.) It is near the pointed bottom of the heart. (*Rationale: A strong heartbeat is heard here.*)
◆ Warm the stethoscope's diaphragm in the palm of your hand. (*Rationale: A cold metal diaphragm is uncomfortable against the skin.*)
◆ Place the diaphragm of the stethoscope firmly over the PMI, and auscultate for the heart sound (lub-dub). (*Rationale: Lub-dub is the opening and closing of the heart valves to make one beat.*)
◆ Count for 1 full minute. (*Rationale: The heart rate is more accurate when measured for 1 full minute.*)
◆ Determine regularity. (*Rationale: Irregularity may indicate a need for further evaluation.*)
◆ Wash hands. (*Rationale: This prevents the spread of Infection.*)
◆ Record findings on vital sign sheet, and report abnormalities to the charge nurse. (*Rationale: Accuracy is needed in maintaining patient records.*)

Measuring an Apical–Radial Pulse. If an apical–radial (A–R) pulse measurement is ordered, two nurses are needed to carry out the procedure. Using the same watch, one nurse counts the patient's apical pulse for 1 minute, while the other nurse counts the radial pulse. Both nurses start counting at the same time. The nurses should agree to start counting at a specified time (eg, "When the hand is on 15 seconds..."). The two figures at the end of the minute are identified and charted, for example, A-R pulse 76/72 (apical/radial). If there is a difference between the two readings, it is called the *pulse deficit.* This information is important to the physician. Normally, these two readings should be the same. (Note: It is impossible for the apical pulse to be lower than the radial. If this occurs, you have made a mistake—check it again.)

Measuring the Pedal Pulse. The pedal pulse is felt over the dorsalis pedis artery of the foot. This site determines the status of circulation to the foot. A strong quality of pulse indicates that circulation to the lower extremities is unrestricted, while a weak and irregular pulse suggests impaired or restricted blood flow. The nurse should use caution in palpating the pulse site, so the pulse is not completely obliterated by excessive pressure. Inspect the feet for color, temperature, and presence of edema. The condition of the nails and cuticles also is observed.

Measuring Popliteal Pulse. The popliteal pulse is located posteriorly to the knee. It is palpated easily by placing the fingers behind the knee cap. This site is used to assess the status of circulation to the lower leg.

Measuring Carotid Pulse. The carotid pulse is located on either side of the neck directly over the carotid artery. This pulse can be palpated along the medial edge of the sternocleidomastoid muscle in the neck above the cricoid notch. The carotid artery is easily accessible to check the peripheral pulse and is used by individuals who must do self-checks or in cases of shock when other pulses are not palpable. It is used to determine the need for CPR.

The pulse can be counted on either side of the neck. The head is positioned in midline to the body. (*Rationale: It provides easier access to the pulse, which obliterates when head is turned to one side or the other.*) Never check carotid pulse on both sides at the same time. (*Rationale: This would cut off circulation to the brain.*)

Assessing Respiration

Oxygen keeps body cells alive; accumulated carbon dioxide kills them. Respiration is the process that brings oxygen into the body and removes carbon dioxide

Nursing Procedure 42-2

Measuring a Radial Pulse

Supplies and Equipment

Watch with second hand
Paper or flow sheet
Pen

Procedure

1. Wash hands.
   (Rationale: Handwashing prevents the spread of organisms.)
2. Explain procedure to patient.
   (Rationale: Providing information fosters patient cooperation and understanding.)
3. Position the patient's forearm comfortably with the wrist extended and the palm down.
   (Rationale: This position allows easier assessment of the radial pulse.)

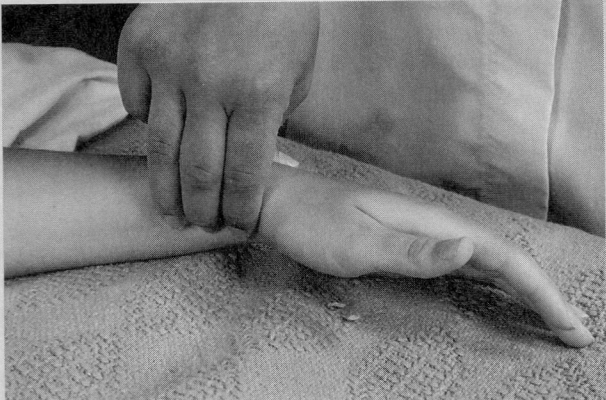

Step 4   Placing the fingertips over the radial pulse (Photos © B. Proud.)

5. Press gently against the radial artery to the point where pulsations can be distinctly felt.
   (Rationale: Excessive pressure will obliterate the pulse.)
6. Using a watch, count the pulse beats for 30 seconds and mulitply by two to get the rate per minute.
   (Rationale: This is sufficient time to assess the pulse rate when it is regular.)
7. Count the pulse for a full minute if it is abnormal in any way, or take an apical pulse.
   (Rationale: Counting a full minute permits a more accurate reading and allows assessment of pulse strength and rhythm. The apical pulse is the most accurate measure of the heart's contractions.)
8. Record the rate, beats per minute on paper or the flow sheet. Report any irregular finding to the appropriate person.
   (Rationale: Documentation provides ongoing data collection.)
9. Wash hands.
   (Rationale: Handwashing prevents the spread of organisms.)

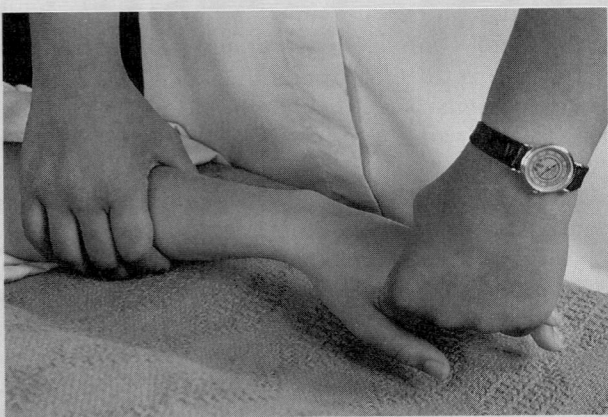

Step 3   Positioning the patient's arm

4. Place fintertips of first, second, and third fingers over the radial artery on the inside of the wrist on the thumb side.
   (Rationale: The fingertips are sensitive and better able to feel the pulse. The thumb should not be used because it has a strong pulse of its own.)

wastes. This exchange takes place in the lungs. Respiration must be observed closely to detect signs of interference with the breathing process.

Regulation of Respiration

Respiratory Control. Respiration is automatic; you breathe without thinking about it. You can control the action of your breathing apparatus to some extent by taking deeper or shallower breaths or even by holding your breath for a limited time. When the limit is reached, automatic control takes over, and your chest muscles relax in spite of your efforts. If this automatic resumption of breathing does not occur, a breathing disorder exists. An example is the apnea (cessation of breathing) that occurs in sudden infant death syndrome.

Respiration is controlled and regulated by the respiratory center in the brain and by the proportion of carbon dioxide in the blood. Injury to the respiratory center or to the nerves connecting it with the lungs will affect respiration; too little or too much carbon dioxide in the blood also affects it.

The organs that accomplish breathing include the lungs, the chest muscles, and the diaphragm; injuries to these parts of the body affect breathing.

Rate and Depth of Respiration. The rate of respiration for a normal adult is 14 to 18 breaths per minute, and women have a more rapid rate than men. For the new-born infant, the rate is approximately 40; for children, it varies from 25 to 30 per minute.

> **Nursing Alert**
>
> Rates of respiration below 8 or above 30 per minute in the adult are serious symptoms.

Normal breathing is called *eupnea.* When the rate of respiration is abnormally rapid (greater than 20 breaths per minute) *tachypnea* is present. When the respirations are abnormally slow and fall below 10 breaths per minute, *bradypnea* occurs. Abnormal breathing patterns are discussed in Table 42-3.

Excitement, exercise, pain, and fever increase the respiratory rate. Rapid respiration is characteristic in diseases that affect the lungs, such as pneumonia. Heart disease, hemorrhage, and nephritis also increase the rate, as do some drugs. Rapid respiration indicates that the body is making an increased effort to maintain the right balance of oxygen and carbon dioxide. The body also tries to adjust the balance by taking deeper breaths. Sighing occurs occasionally and cleanses the lungs and physiologically expands the small airways and alveoli that are not used during ordinary respiration. This type of respiration should not be confused with abnormal or difficult breathing.

Table 42-3. Abnormal Breathing Patterns

Abnormal Breathing Pattern	Description	Conditions
Bradypnea	Respiratory rate below 10 breaths per minute	Neurologic disturbances, electrolyte disturbances, narcotic or barbiturate overdose, postanesthesia
Tachypnea	Persistent respiratory rate above 20 breaths per minute	Trauma, injury, stress, pain; respiratory, cardiac, liver disease
Biot's	Cyclic breathing pattern characterized by shallow breathing alternating with periods of apnea	Neurologic problems (meningitis, encephalitis), head trauma, brain abscess, heatstroke
Cheyne-Stokes	Cyclic breathing pattern characterized by periods of respirations of increased rate and depth alternating with periods of apnea	Congestive heart failure, drug overdose, increased intracranial pressure
Kussmaul's	Increased rate (above 20 breaths per minute) and depth of respirations	Metabolic acidosis, diabetic ketoacidosis, renal failure

Source: Craven RF, Hirnle CJ. Fundamentals of Nursing: Human Health and Function. Philadelphia, JB Lippincott, 1992.

If a patient takes in and breathes out small amounts of air, the respirations are described as *shallow.* Pressure on the respiratory center in the brain decreases the rate of respiration; cerebral hemorrhage has this effect. Some drugs, such as opium preparations, depress the respiratory center, and poisons that accumulate in the body in uremia and diabetic coma also slow the rate of respiration. In Kussmaul's respirations the patient's respirations are abnormally deep, much like a gasp. This condition is associated with severe diabetic acidosis and coma.

Sounds of Respiration. Snoring can occur when the air passageway is partially blocked. This commonly occurs during sleep when the person's tongue falls back because of relaxation.

Stertorous breathing occurs when air is passing through secretions in the air passages. These bubbling noises or rattles (rales) are characteristic before death, when the air passages fill with mucus. Obstruction near the glottis causes a hissing, crowing sound.

Difficult Breathing (Dyspnea)

When a person is making a definite effort to get more oxygen and get rid of carbon dioxide, breathing is difficult. The term for difficult or painful breathing is **dyspnea.** This may be a temporary condition, such as when a runner breathes in gasps at the end of a race or when a person runs upstairs and pants to get his or her breath at the top. Obesity also can cause dyspnea, especially on exertion. In some cases, breathing difficulty is more or less constant, as in the acute stage of pneumonia, emphysema, or some types of heart disease. When the difficulty is so marked that the patient can breathe only when in an upright position, it is called **orthopnea.**

Obstructions of the air passages by secretions or a foreign object interfere with breathing. Asthma causes difficult breathing because of spasm and edema of the small bronchi.

Normally, the proportion of respirations to heartbeats is 1 to 5 in adults. Respirations usually increase if the pulse rate increases but not always in a definite proportion. Usually the pulse rate increases faster than the respiration rate. However, the respiration rate increases faster in respiratory diseases.

The characteristic signs of breathing difficulties are heaving of the chest and abdomen, a distressed expression, and **cyanosis** (bluish tinge) in the skin, especially in the lips and mucous membranes of the mouth.

Cyanosis (Blueness). In severe conditions, cyanosis spreads to the nails and the extremities and eventually becomes apparent over the entire body. The bluish tinge of the skin and mucous membranes in cyanosis is caused by an excess of carbon dioxide. Cyanosis also may be the result of a circulatory or blood disorder. Cyanosis is much easier to detect in white and Asian people. The condition shows as a dusky gray color in the African American.

Cheyne-Stokes Respirations. Cheyne-Stokes respirations are slow and shallow at first and gradually grow faster and deeper, then taper off until they stop entirely. Periods of apnea may last several seconds and then the cycle is repeated. The length of the period of apnea should be documented in seconds. Usually the patient experiencing Cheyne-Stokes respirations is not cyanotic. Cheyne-Stokes respirations constitute a serious symptom and usually precede death in cerebral hemorrhage, uremia, or heart disease.

Counting Respirations

Respirations are the easiest to assess of all the vital signs. Each time assessments are made, the nurse checks with the baseline information. The skills used in counting respirations are given in Nursing Procedure 42-3.

Assessing Blood Pressure

Assessing BP is especially important for patients who have abnormally high or low readings, for postoperative patients, and for patients who have sustained serious injury or shock. The BP reading gives significant information about patient status and is one of the most important parts of the nursing assessment. In routine patient care, BP is measured at least once or twice daily.

Regulation of Blood Pressure

As the heart forces blood through the arteries, there is a certain amount of pressure exerted on the arterial wall. Two things determine the degree of pressure: the rate and force of the heartbeat and the ease with which the blood flows into the smallest branches of the arteries. If normal elasticity of the arteries and the arterioles is maintained, if the volume and composition of the blood is normal, and if contraction exerts normal force, the BP will be within normal limits (about 120/80).

If the heart rate or force is increased by exertion or illness, the BP will increase. If the quantity of blood within the circulatory system is reduced with the other factors remaining the same, the BP will fall. By

Supplies and Equipment

Watch with second hand
Paper or flow sheet
Pen

Procedure

1. Prepare to count respirations by keeping fingertips on the patient's pulse.
   (Rationale: A patient who knows you are counting respirations may not breathe naturally.)
2. Observe the rise and fall of the patient's chest or one inspiration and one expiration. Respirations can also be counted by placing a hand lightly on the patient's chest or abdomen.
   (Rationale: One full cycle of respiration consists of an inspiration and an expiration.)
3. Count the number of respirations for 30 seconds and multiply by 2 to get the rate per minute.
   (Rationale: This is sufficient time to assess respirations when the rate is regular.)

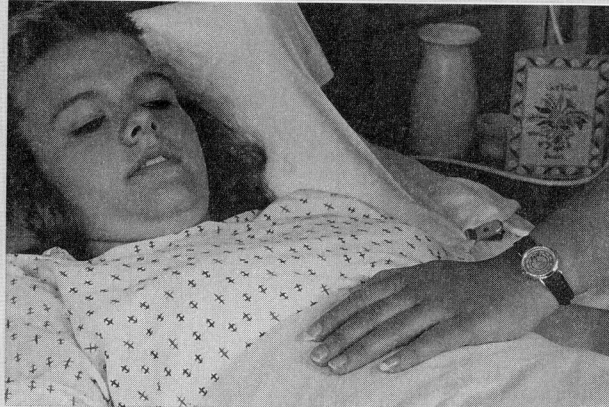

Step 2   Counting respirations by placing a hand on the patient's chest (Photo © B. Proud.)

4. Count respirations for 1 full minute for an infant, a young child, or an adult with an irregular, more rapid rate.
   (Rationale: Children normally have an irregular, more rapid rate. Adults with an irregular rate require more careful assessment including depth and rhythm of respirations.)
5. Record the rate on paper or the flow sheet. Report any irregular finding to the appropriate person.
   (Rationale: Documentation provides ongoing data collection.)
6. Wash hands.
   (Rationale: Handwashing prevents the spread of organisms.)

---

contrast, if the blood volume is normal but the elasticity or caliber of the arteries is reduced, the BP will rise. High BP is called *hypertension;* low BP is *hypotension.*

Systole and Diastole

BP is highest with each heartbeat during contraction; this is the **systolic** pressure or systole. The pressure diminishes as the heart relaxes and is lowest when the heart is relaxed before it begins to contract again; this is the **diastolic** pressure or diastole. The difference between the two readings is called the *pulse pressure.* A value called the **mean arterial pressure** (MAP) is calculated using a complex mathematical formula. It is approximately the value of the diastolic pressure plus ome-third of the pulse pressure. MAP denotes the average pressure within the arteries. An

electronic device determines the accurate average pressure or MAP.

Normal Blood Pressure

Normally, the difference between the systolic and the diastolic pressures is a number equal to one-third to one-half of the systolic pressure. Both readings give information; a wide difference between the two indicates some sort of problem. Normal systolic pressure for an adult at the age of 20 is approximately 120, and diastolic pressure is approximately 80. BP increases gradually with age. At 60, the normal systolic pressure can be expected to reach 130 to 140, as a result of the effects of aging on the heart and the arteries. This pressure may be considered alarming in a 20-year-old person. Any pressure that is much higher than normal for the person's age *(hyperten-*

sion) is a sign of a circulatory problem. A very low BP (*hypotension*) may indicate hemorrhage or shock.

Nursing Alert

The normal range of BP for an adult is:

Systolic: 90 to 140
Diastolic: 60 to 85

Shock or other difficulty is usually indicated by a systolic reading of 80 or less. A diastolic reading over 100 is usually considered dangerously high.

Methods and Equipment

BP may be measured *directly* by means of a probe or catheter inserted directly into the blood vessel or the heart. Usually BP is measured *indirectly* with a sphygmomanometer.

The sphygmomanometer consists of an inflatable bladder enclosed in a cuff. An inflating mechanism, such as bulb or pump, with a deflating mechanism is used. The cuff is wrapped around the arm. Cuffs come in various sizes, as indicated in Table 42-4. It is important to use the correct size. Cuff size and bladder placement are illustrated in Figure 42-5.

You obtain the indirect BP reading with a manometer by listening to the heartbeat with a stethoscope, which you place over the brachial artery on the inside bend of the elbow. The stethoscope magnifies the sound of the beat within the arteries. Many nurses carry their own stethoscope instead of using the one at the station. A sphygmomanometer may be of two types: mercury or aneroid. The placement of the arm wrap and stethoscope is the same in each.

Mercury Manometer. The manometer tube is connected to a glass tube that contains mercury and has markings to indicate BP level. The mercury manometer is fastened to a stand or case. Most hospitals have a wall-mounted mercury sphygomomanometer in each patient room. The pressure readings are watched on the glass tube at eye level for accurate readings.

Aneroid Manometer. With the aneroid manometer, the arm wrap is attached to a dial rather than to the mercury manometer. This method is considered less accurate but more convenient. Pressure readings are watched on the dial; the level is not important as in the mercury manometer. The systolic pressure can be estimated in an emergency with this method, because it is possible to see heartbeats as the needle deflects.

Electronic Blood Pressure Apparatus. The cuff of the electronic BP apparatus is applied and manipulated in basically the same manner as with the mercury manometer. It is important to place the microphone under the cuff so the arrow that indicates the artery is in the correct location. Hold the microphone in place while you apply the cuff. Systolic and diastolic pressures will be printed out on the screen within a few seconds. The nurse should use the stethoscope also as a double check. The cuff is sometimes inflated and deflated automatically. The electronic device may be left in place and used to monitor BP.

Palpatation. When electronic equipment is not available, palpation may be used. Pulsations of the artery are palpated by the nurse as pressure is released from the cuff. The systolic pressure is estimated when the pulsation is first felt. When the pulsation is no longer felt without applying pressure over the artery, the diastolic pressure is estimated.

Pulmonary Artery Pressure Monitoring. The pulmonary artery (PA) catheter is a special balloon-tipped catheter introduced into the subclavian or jugular vein that leads to the right atrium. Here the central venous pressure or right atrial pressure and the PA systolic and diastolic pressures may be measured. This is a means of direct BP measurement and is called internal invasive monitoring. The Swan-Ganz catheter is an example of this type of catheter.

Table 42-4. Recommended Bladder Dimensions for Blood Pressure Cuff

Arm Circumference at Midpoint* (cm)	Cuff Name	Bladder Width (cm)	Bladder Length (cm)
5–7.5	Newborn	3	5
7.5–13	Infant	5	8
13–20	Child	8	13
24–32	Adult	13	24
32–42	Wide adult	17	32
42-50†	Thigh	20	42

* Midpoint of arm is defined as half the distance from the acromion to the olecranon.

† In patients with very large limbs, the indirect blood pressure should be measured in the leg or forearm.

From Frolich E, Grim C, Labarthe D, et al. Recommendations for Human Blood Pressure Determinations by Sphygmomanometers. Dallas, Texas, American Heart Association, 1987.

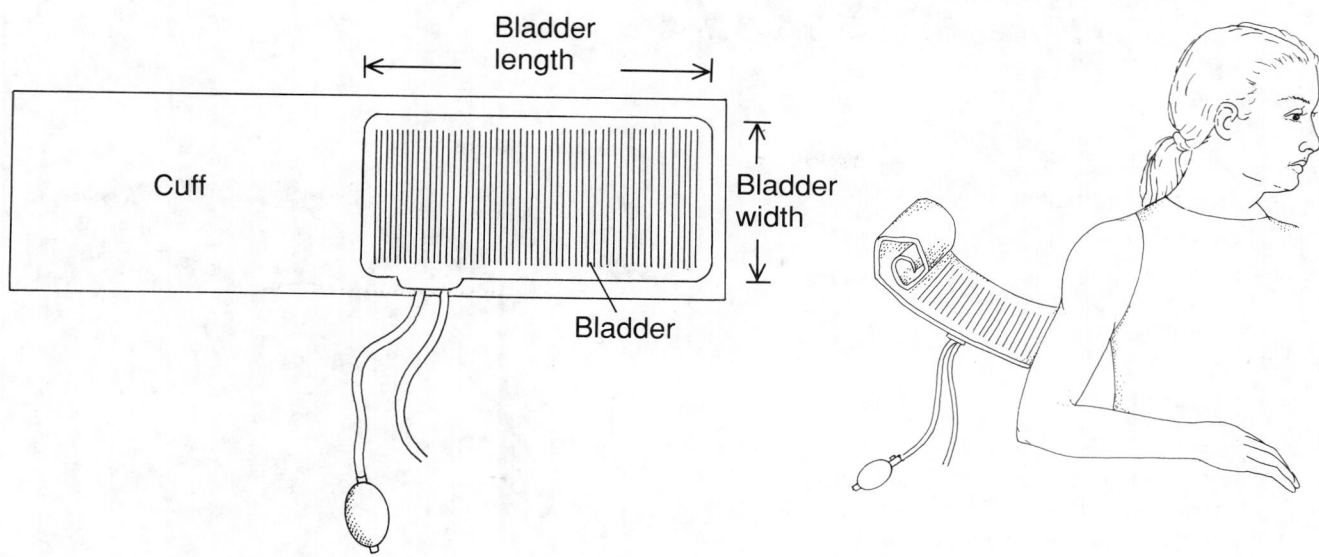

Figure 42-5. Proper cuff size is important in obtaining accurate blood pressure measurements. The bladder length should be 80% of the limb circumference or about twice the bladder width. (Craven R.F. and Hirnle C.J.: Fundamentals of Nursing: Human Health and Function. Philadelphia: J.B. Lippincott, 1992)

Measuring Blood Pressure

Whenever you take a BP with a manometer, you must listen to the heartbeat through the stethoscope and *watch* the manometer at the same time. When the cuff is deflated, blood returns through the artery. **Korotkoff's sounds** are heard in the stethoscope. There are five phases of Korotkoff's sounds (Fig. 42-6). The onset of phase I is the recorded systolic pressure. The onset of phase IV indicates diastolic pressure in children, and phase V indicates diastolic pressure in adults.

When using the electronic device, you do not always need to listen; the systolic and diastolic pressures are read out for you. However, it is still more accurate to listen. The BP also may be estimated in an emergency by watching the beats on the aneroid manometer.

Take the BP when the patient is resting and quiet. Physical exertion or emotional stress will affect the BP. Prepare the patient by explaining that the cuff on the arm may feel tight for a second or two, that otherwise the procedure will not be bothersome, and that it will only take a few minutes.

Nursing Procedure 42-4 explains how to take a BP reading. The slight differences between the mercury and the aneroid manometer are stated in the procedure.

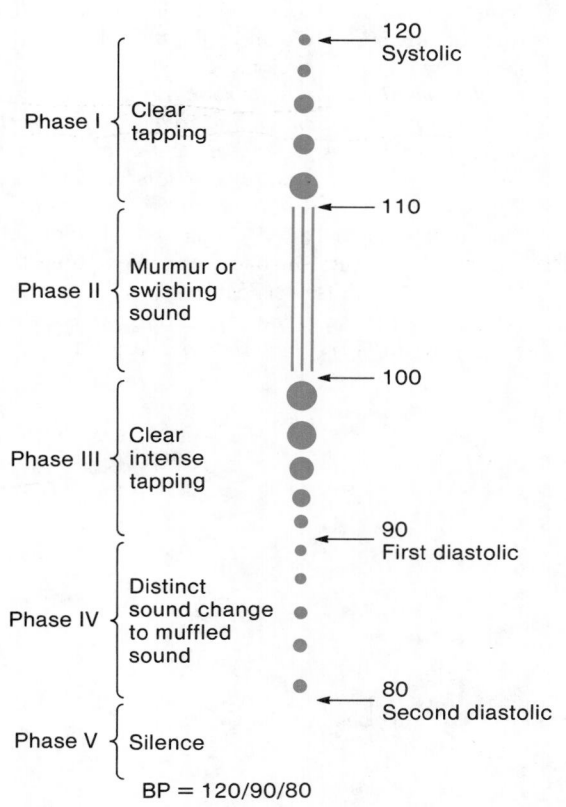

Figure 42-6. Five phases of Korotkoff sounds. (Craven R.F. and Hirnle C.J.: Fundamentals of Nursing: Human Health and Function. Philadelphia: J.B. Lippincott, 1992)

Measuring Blood Pressure

Supplies and Equipment

Stethoscope
Sphygmomanometer
Blood pressure cuff (appropriate size)
Alcohol wipe
Paper or flow sheet
Pen

Procedure

1. Gather equipment. Select cuff that is appropriate size for patient. Cleanse ear pieces and diaphragm of stethoscope with an alcohol wipe.
   (Rationale: Organization facilitates performance of the skill. Incorrect cuff size may give inaccurate reading. Cleansing a stethoscope that may be used by others prevents the spread of infection.)
2. Wash hands.
   (Rationale: Handwashing prevents the spread of organisms.)
3. Explain procedure to patient.
   (Rationale: Providing information fosters patient co-operation and understanding.)
4. Assist the patient into a comfortable position with the selected arm supported and palm turned upward. Remove any constrictive clothing.
   (Rationale: Ideally, the arm should be at heart level for accurate measurement and rotated so the brachial pulse is easily accessible and not constricted by clothing. An arm where circulation is compromised in any way should not be used to measure blood pressure.)
5. Palpate the brachial artery. Center the bladder of the cuff approximately 1 inch (2.5 cm) above the site where brachial pulse was palpated.
   (Rationale: Centering the bladder ensures even inflation of the cuff over the brachial artery.)

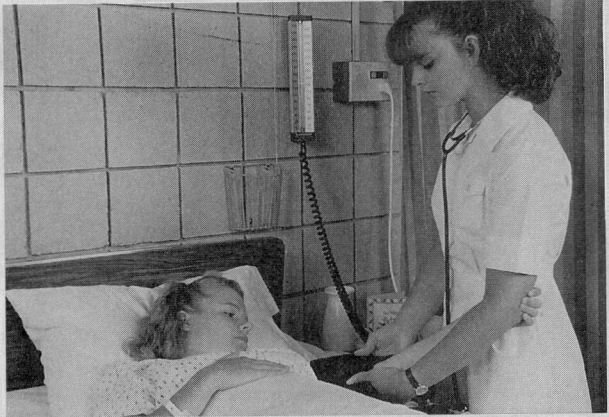

Step 5   Positioning the cuff over the brachial artery

6. Wrap the cuff snugly around the arm and secure the end appropriately.
   (Rationale: The blood pressure reading will be inaccurate if cuff is applied too loosely.)
7. Check that the mercury manometer is vertical and at eye level and level with the patient's heart.
   (Rationale: Improper height can alter perception of reading.) (When using the aneroid manometer, it does not need to be at eye level.)
8. Palpate the radial or brachial pulse with one hand. Close the screw clamp on the bulb and inflate the cuff while still checking the pulse with the other hand. Observe the point where pulse is no longer palpable.
   (Rationale: Palpation identifies the approximate systolic reading.)

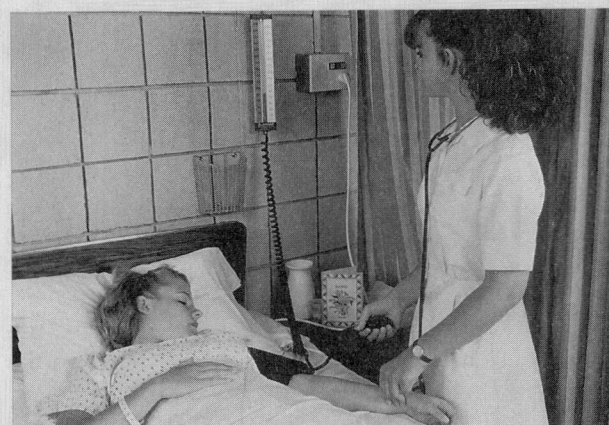

Step 8   Estimating the systolic reading

(continued)

9. Open the screw clamp, deflate the cuff, and wait 30 seconds.
   (Rationale: Short interval eases any venous congestion that may have occurred.)
10. Position stethoscope earpieces comfortably in ears and place diaphragm or bell over the brachial artery.
    (Rationale: Blood pressure is easier to hear when stethoscope is placed directly over artery.)

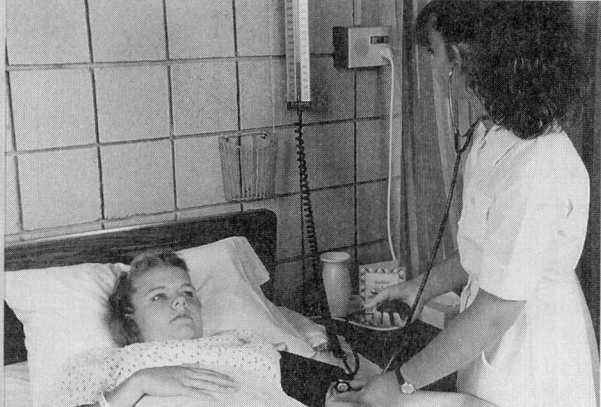

Steps 13–14 Listening for the systolic and diastolic pressure readings (Photos © B. Proud.)

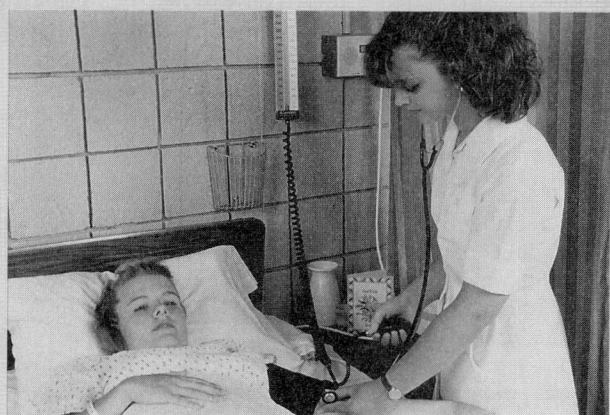

Step 10 Placing stethoscope diaphragm over the brachial artery

11. Close the screw clamp on the bulb and inflate the cuff to a pressure 30 mm Hg above the point where the pulse had disappeared.
    (Rationale: This ensures that the systolic reading will not be underestimated.)
12. Open the clamp and allow the mercury column or aneroid dial to fall at 2–3 mm Hg per second.
    (Rationale: If deflation occurs too rapidly, reading may be inaccurate.)
13. Note the point on the column or dial at which you initially hear a distinct sound.
    (Rationale: The first sound that is heard represents the systolic pressure or the point where the heart is able to force blood into the brachial artery.)
14. Continue deflating the cuff and note the point where the sound disappears.
    (Rationale: This is the diastolic pressure and represents the pressure exerted on the blood by the walls of the arteries with the heart at rest.)

15. Release any remaining air in the cuff and remove it. If reading must be re-checked for any reason, allow 1 minute interval before taking the blood pressure again.
    (Rationale: This interval eases any venous congestion and provides for an accurate reading when measurement is repeated.)
    If there is any question, repeat procedure on the other arm.
    (Rationale: This allows for comparison of pressures to assess for circulatory problems.)
16. Assist patient to position of comfort. Advise the patient of the reading.
    (Rationale: This indicates interest in the patient's well-being and allows the patient to participate in the care.)
17. Wash hands.
    (Rationale: Handwashing prevents the spread of organisms.)
18. Record the blood pressure on paper or the flow sheet. Write the systolic pressure over the diastolic reading (using even numbers). For example, record a systolic of 120 and a diastolic of 70 as 120/70. Indicate site where blood pressure was taken. Report any irregular findings to the appropriate person.
    (Rationale: Documentation provides ongoing data collection.)

Nursing Skill
The Flush Method of Estimating Blood Pressure

This procedure is used when other methods are not available. It is most easily used in the small child or infant. This method is the least reliable and is only used when Korotkoff's sounds cannot be heard and electronic equipment is not available. A change in skin color is the determining factor as to the pressure when blood flow returns to an extremity. (This method is particularly unreliable if the patient has vascular disease.)

Estimating Blood Pressure, Using the Flush Method

♦ Wrap the blood pressure cuff around the arm or leg.

♦ Wrap the rest of the limb with a roller bandage. *(Rationale: This restricts blood flow to the extremity.)*
♦ Inflate the blood pressure cuff and remove the bandage.
♦ As the pressure is released from the cuff, watch the manometer. The blood pressure is estimated when the extremity flushes. *(Rationale: This indicates the return of blood flow.)*
♦ This blood pressure estimate is assumed to be the midway point between systolic and diastolic pressures (**mean blood pressure**).

Measuring Orthostatic Blood Pressure and Pulse

Some patients, particularly older adults and patients taking certain medications, will experience a drastic drop in BP and an increase in pulse when changing from lying to sitting or from sitting to standing. A drop of as much as 25 mm Hg systolic pressure and 10 mm Hg diastolic pressure or more can occur. When there is a severe drop in BP, the condition is known as *orthostatic hypotension.*

The pulse rate may be affected with the drop in BP. The pulse rate may decrease, but often it increases. If a person has orthostatic hypotension, he or she may be dizzy or lightheaded when standing up and may be prone to falling. Measures should be carried out to ensure the patient's safety. Instruct the person to rise slowly to adjust to each new position. A decrease in BP, with an accompanying rise in pulse, also may indicate low circulating blood volume, as in hemorrhage.

BP Measurement in Other Sites. If the BP cannot be taken in the arm, the thigh may be used. Wrap the cuff at mid-thigh with the bladder of the cuff in the back. Auscultate over the popliteal artery in the back of the knee. The lower arm also can be used, with auscultation over the radial artery in the wrist. If an alternate site is used, this must be identified and always used, to maintain comparability of data.

> ### Key Concept
> BP and pulse should initially be taken in both arms, especially if there is known vascular disease or if the reading is not within normal range. It is common for a difference of 5 to 10 mm Hg to exist between arms. Readings of greater than 10 mm Hg difference indicate arterial occlusion in the arm with the lower pressure.

Keys for Review

Key Questions for Critical Thinking

1. Identify measurements that comprise vital signs. Describe how each measurement is made and documented. Discuss normal and abnormal readings and their indications.
2. Discuss reasons for changes in body temperature. State normal body temperature as measured in three different areas of the body. Discuss the reasons for the variations. Describe in what instances each area is used.
3. Using information you studied in Chapter 22 and this chapter, describe respiration and its control. Describe normal and abnormal breathing patterns. Include their indications.
4. Blood pressure is one of the most important parts of nursing assessment. Describe normal pressure and its regulation, and low and high blood pressure. Explain orthiostatis hypotension, what it may indicate, and nursing actions.

Key Readings

Craven RF, Hirnle CJ. Fundamentals of Nursing: Human Health and Function. Philadelphia, J.B. Lippincott, 1992

Earnest VV. Clinical Skills in Nursing Practice, Ed 2. Philadelphia, J.B. Lippincott, 1993

Sheehan MM: "Blood pressure monitoring." Nursing 90 20(4):79-81, 1990

Smeltzer SC, Bare BG. Brunner and Suddarth's Textbook of Medical Surgical Nursing, Ed 7. Philadelphia, J.B. Lippincott, 1992

Swearingen PL. Photo Atlas of Nursing Procedures, Ed 2. Redwood City, CA, Addison-Wesley Nursing, 1991

Taber's Cyclopedic Medical Dictionary, Ed 17. Philadelphia, F.A. Davis, 1993

Taylor C, Lillis C, LeMone P. Fundamentals of Nursing: The Art and Science of Nursing Care, Ed 2. Philadelphia, J.B. Lippincott, 1993

Enrichment Keys

Tourangeau A, MacLeod F, Breakwell M. "Tap in on ear thermometry." The Canadian Nurse 89(8):24-28, September 1993

Keys to Learning More

Chapter 50: head-to-toe physical assessments

Keys to Learning More (continued)

Chapter 54: surgical asepsis
Unit Thirteen: nursing care of children and adolescents
Unit Fourteen: medical–surgical nursing

43 Body Mechanics

Learning Objectives

- Describe the three principles underlying good body mechanics.
- Describe various ways of assisting a patient out of bed.
- Demonstrate how a partially or totally immobile person might be moved up in bed.
- Describe how the immobile patient is moved to the side of the bed.
- Describe and demonstrate how to move an immobile patient from bed to chair and back to bed.
- Demonstrate the ability to use the litter safely.
- Describe and demonstrate the ability to use the three-carrier lift.
- State the reason for range-of-motion exercises.
- Demonstrate the ability to perform and supervise range-of- motion exercises.
- Demonstrate the ability to position a patient safely for various examinations.

Key Terms

abduction	extension
active range of motion	flexion
adduction	gravital plane
body alignment	hemiplegic
body mechanics	inversion
center of gravity	paraplegic
circumduction	passive range of motion
continuous passive motion	range of motion
contractures	rotation
eversion	supination

Keys to Understanding This Chapter

Chapter 6: optimum health:
Unit Three: child and adult development
Chapter 17: musculoskeletal system
Chapter 29: safety in the healthcare environment
Chapter 36: therapeutic communication

Keys to Understanding This Chapter
(continued)

Chapter 37: documentation and reporting
Chapter 40: the healthcare environment

Key Points

- It is easier to pull, push, or roll an object than it is to lift it. Often less energy or force is required to keep an object moving than to start and stop it.
- Rocking backward or forward on your feet uses your body weight as a force for pulling or pushing.
- A patient may become dizzy or faint whenever you first get him or her out of bed.
- Do not let the patient grab you around the neck while transferring him or her. Such a force can seriously injure you.
- A hospital bed should be in low position except when care is given.
- The patient's body alignment when lying down should be approximately the same as if the person were standing.
- Do not force joint movement when doing PROM.

Key Topics Outline

Proper Body Mechanics
Body Mechanics in Patient Positioning
  Assisting the Mobile Patient
  Mobility Devices
  Moving Patients Who Are Paralyzed
  Using the Wheeled Stretcher
  Assisting the Patient Confined to Bed
  Positioning of Patients
Joint Mobility and Range of Motion
  Passive and Active Range of Motion
Positioning for Examinations
  Preparing the Patient for Examination

Rosdahl CB: Textbook of Basic Nursing, 6th ed. © 1995 J.B. Lippincott Company

Key Learning Activities

◆ Practice correct lifting of a box or heavy object from the floor.
◆ Team up with a partner, and practice positioning each other in the bed using Table 43-2 as a guide.
◆ Practice PROM exercises on a partner.

Key Nursing Procedures

NP 43-1: Helping the Patient Into a Wheelchair or Chair
NP 43-2: Assisting the Immobile Patient to Move up in Bed
NP 43-3: Turning the Patient to a Side-Lying Position
NP 43-4: Performing PROM Exercises

A nurse is expected to help patients use good body mechanics. The first step is for *you* to practice good body mechanics. People (patients and nurses alike) differ in weight, size, and ability to move. How strong you are is not as important as how efficiently you use your body. Efficiency determines how effective and safe you will be moving patients.

Proper Body Mechanics

The use of the safest and most efficient methods of moving and lifting is called **body mechanics:** the use of mechanical principles as applied to the human body.

Principles of Body Mechanics

Certain ways of moving objects and carrying them are more effective than others. Movement is governed by laws of physics, and from them we have learned the general principles of body mechanics, as shown in the box.

The principles underlying good body mechanics involve three major factors: the center of gravity, the base of support, and the line of gravity (Fig. 43-1).

Basic Principles of Body Mechanics

◆ It is easier to pull, push, or roll an object than it is to lift it. The movement should be smooth and continuous, rather than jerky.
◆ Often less energy or force is required to keep an object moving than it is to start and stop it.
◆ It takes less effort to lift an object if you work as close to it as possible. Use your leg and arm muscles as much as possible and your back muscles, which are not as strong, as little as possible. Avoid reaching.
◆ Rocking backward or forward on your feet uses your body weight as a force for pulling or pushing.

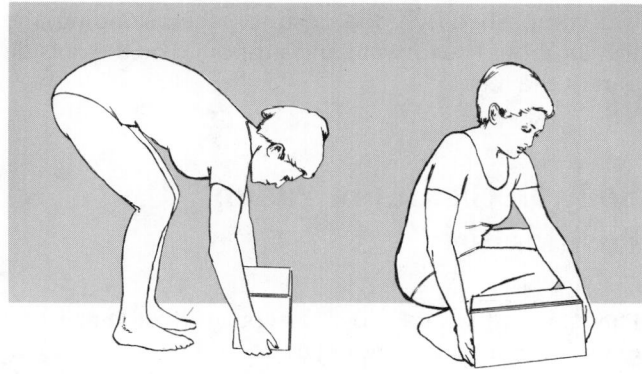

Figure 43-1. (*Left*) Poor position for lifting. Pull is exerted on the back muscles, and leaning causes the line of gravity to fall outside the base of support. (*Right*) Good position for lifting, using the long, strong muscles of the arms and legs and holding the object so that the line of gravity falls within the base of support.

Center of Gravity. The **center of gravity** is located in the pelvic area; approximately half the body weight is distributed above that area and half below. When lifting an object, bend at the knees and hips, and keep your back straight. With this method, the center of gravity remains over the base of support (the feet), and it is easier to keep your balance.

Base of Support. Your feet are your base of support. Good body mechanics dictate that you keep a wide base of support to avoid tipping over. Spread your feet when lifting; this will give side-to-side stability. Put one foot slightly in front of the other; this will give back-to-front stability. Distribute your weight evenly between both feet. Flex your knees slightly to absorb jolts. Do not twist your body; move your feet to turn an object you are moving.

Line of Gravity. If you draw an imaginary line through the top of your head, through the center of gravity, and through the base of your support, you will have determined the line of gravity, or the **gravital plane.** For the most efficiency, this line of gravity should be a straight vertical (up and down) line from the top of the head, through the center of gravity, and through the base of support with equal weight on each side.

Body Alignment

When lifting, walking, or carrying out any body activity, good **body alignment** is vital. When your body is in good alignment, your muscles work together. To be in proper alignment is to stretch the body tall. This is accomplished by good posture: when standing, the weight should be forward and supported on the outside part of the feet.

Body Mechanics in Patient Positioning

Patients may be able to help you move them if you explain what you are going to do and how they might help. Get help from another person if the patient is heavy or if you are not sure that you will be able to move the person alone. No matter how difficult it is to get help, it is always better to wait than to risk injury to yourself or the patient.

Assisting the Mobile Patient

Some patients are allowed out of bed for the entire day; others are up for a certain length of time each day as their condition permits. The patient usually views being up and dressed as a hopeful sign. A change of position helps to strengthen muscles and prevent deformities.

When a patient is encouraged to get out of bed, several purposes will be served. Patients readily assume more of the "sick role" or helplessness when they are constantly cared for. By assisting the patient to maintain or regain mobility, the nurse fosters good self-care practices.

Basic principles in assisting the patient out of bed follow:

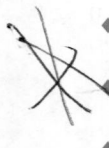

◆ A specific physician's order is required for any change in activity.
◆ Being up is tiring after an illness; be sure not to overtire the patient.
◆ If the patient complained of pain when up previously, it may be a good idea to offer PRN (as needed) medication approximately ½ hour before the person is to get up.

Dangling

Dangling legs over the side of the bed is the transitional procedure followed before the patient is ready to get up in the chair. The person will need to dangle his or her legs for a few minutes before being assisted out of bed. A patient may be strong enough only to dangle and then to lie down again.

Nursing Skill
Dangling

Procedure

1. Put the bed in low position, and explain the procedure.
2. Fan-fold the bed covers to the foot of the bed, and cover the patient with a bath blanket. *(Rationale: Protect the patient's privacy.)*
3. Measure and record pulse and blood pressure. *(Rationale: This procedure is often done to evaluate how well the patient might tolerate being up.)*
4. Elevate the head of the bed as high as it will go. *(Rationale: Elevating the head of the bed raises the patient up without your having to lift.)*
5. Place one arm around the patient's shoulders and the other arm under the knees. *(Rationale: This allows the patient's body to be turned as a unit.)*
6. Turn the patient toward you so the feet touch the floor or provide a foot stool. *(Rationale: The patient's feet must be supported.)*
7. Roll a pillow and tuck it firmly behind the patient's back. *(Rationale: This will help to support the person in the sitting position.)*
8. Dangle the patient's legs for as long as ordered if tolerated. Stay with the person at all times. Help the person to lie down if he or she becomes dizzy or feels faint. *(Rationale: When the person sits up for the first time, the blood rushes into the legs. The patient may feel faint, caused by orthostatic hypotension.)*
9. When the procedure is completed, help the person to lie down again by supporting the shoulders and knees and turning back around.
10. Measure and record the pulse and blood pressure immediately following the procedure. *(Rationale: These readings, compared with the baseline measurements, will help the physician determine how well the patient tolerated sitting up.)*
11. Wash your hands, and document the procedure: how long the patient dangled, how the procedure was tolerated, and any unusual occurrences.

Helping the Mobile Patient Out of Bed
According to the physician's order, help the patient out of bed. Skills to accomplish this follow.

Nursing Skill
Assisting the Mobile Patient Out of Bed

Procedure

1. Get assistance if you need it. *(Rationale: It is vital to prevent falls.)*
2. Position the patient as described for dangling.
3. Reassure patients before getting them out of bed that they will be protected, and explain how. *(Rationale: Patients worry about falling.)*
4. Protect the patient with clothing and blankets, and keep out of drafts. Have the person wear few clothes and use more blankets. *(Rationale: This will cause less exertion.)*
5. Lift or support the person while moving. *(Rationale: Being in bed, even for a short time, can make a person very weak.)* You will need assistance in moving immobile, weak, or unusually heavy patients.
6. Choose a chair that will not slide for the patient to sit in; keep the footstool steady. Use extra care if the floor is slippery. *(Rationale: Most hospital injuries are caused by falls.)*
7. Check your patient's pulse rate before and after putting him or her into a chair. *(Rationale: The change in position affects circulation and blood supply to the brain; the patient may feel faint.)* Watch for signs of fatigue.
8. Place signal cord within easy reach. *(Rationale: The patient must be able to call for assistance if he or she has pain or feels faint.)*
9. Check on the patient frequently. Provide diversion (eg, television, a book, mail). *(Rationale: This will encourage the person to stay up longer.)*

Nursing Alert

A patient may be dizzy or faint whenever you get him or her out of bed.

- If the patient becomes dizzy, help him or her sit on the bed.
- If the patient is in a chair, have him or her bend over at the waist and lower the head.
- If you are walking with the patient, help him or her to lean against a wall and bend over. If this does not help and no one else is there, you may need to help the patient sit on the floor.

The Transfer Belt

You should use a transfer belt whenever you assist a weak or unsteady person to walk. The use of a transfer belt is illustrated in Figure 43-2. A transfer belt is a sturdy webbed belt with an easily used buckle. Explain to the patient that the belt is used to provide safety and protection for you and the patient.

- Place the belt securely around the patient's waist

before he or she gets up. It must be tight enough to support the patient's weight if he or she begins to fall but not be uncomfortable. Fasten the buckle securely, with the loop back through the gripper teeth.

- Keep one hand inside the back of the belt at all times when transferring or walking with the patient. *(Rationale: You must be prepared to support the patient if he or she begins to fall.)*
- Always insert your hand into the belt from the bottom with fingers pointing upward and the bottom of the belt in the palm of your hand. *(Rationale: If the patient slumps or slips, you will be able to support the weight. If you grasp the belt from the top, it would slip out of your hand from the patient's weight.)*
- If the patient is likely to soil the belt, give him or her a personal belt to keep in the room.
- Store the belt outside the room if a patient is depressed or suicidal or may assault someone else.

The patient is assessed for good body alignment when the transfer is completed. If the body is twisted or misaligned and the patient is left sitting for long periods of time, pressure on certain muscle groups and nerves can cause damage.

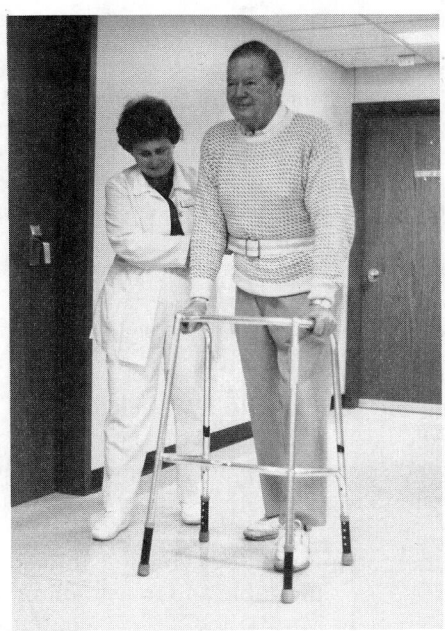

Figure 43-2. The nurse grasps the transfer belt as the patient walks with a walker. The transfer belt gives the patient more confidence and will help the nurse if the patient begins to weaken or fall. Always grasp the transfer belt with the fingers inside the belt and pointing upward, with the palm of the hand under the bottom edge of the belt. (Craven RF and Hirnle CJ: Fundamentals of Nursing: Human Health and Function. Philadelphia: J.B. Lippincott, 1992).

Helping a Patient From Bed to Chair

Some patients cannot provide much help in transfers. The following skill explains how to help the patient from bed to chair.

Nursing Skill

Helping the Patient From Bed to Chair

Procedure

1. Position the patient as described for dangling.
2. Place the bed in low position. *(Rationale: Safety is important.)*
3. Move a comfortable armchair close to the bed. *(Rationale: The shorter the distance, the safer the move.)*
4. Place a pillow on the chair seat, and cover it with a moisture proof pillowcase if the patient is likely to soil it.
5. Spread a blanket across the seat, and leave enough at the lower end to wrap around the patient's legs and feet as needed. *(Rationale: Keep the patient warm.)*
6. Get the patient's stockings, slippers, or shoes for him or her to wear. *(Rationale: Keep the patient comfortable.)*
7. Transfer the patient to the chair in the same manner as that for the wheelchair.

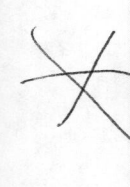

Nursing Alert

Do not let the patient grab you around the neck, because your neck cannot withstand the force if the patient falls. If the patient grabs for your neck, *put your head down* so that the patient cannot get a grip on your neck. *Lower* the *patient* to safety, and explain why you reacted in that manner.

Mobility Devices

Helping the Patient Into a Wheelchair

A wheelchair is used to move patients who cannot walk or who should be spared fatigue as much as possible. Nursing Procedure 43-1 explains the transfer into the chair.

Once the patient is in the wheelchair, check to see that he or she is comfortable and not straining any muscles. If the patient is to be left alone, secure the signal cord within easy reach. You may need to apply a protective device, called a restraint, so that the person does not fall out of the chair. Usually an order is required for the use of a patient safety device. Safety devices are discussed later in the chapter and two samples are illustrated in an accompanying box.

Because the patient in a wheelchair may become weak, the patient must be checked frequently. Carefully

assist the patient back into bed, remembering the patient's weakness. Be sure to lock the wheels for transfer.

Pushing a Wheelchair or Litter

Sometimes the nurse needs to push the patient's wheelchair to another area for examinations or tests. Skills in pushing a wheelchair are given in the accompanying box. The same skills are used when the nurse is required to push a litter. A litter is a four-wheeled cart with a moisture-proof mattress. It is often used in the emergency department or when transferring a patient to surgery.

Nursing Skill Guidelines
Pushing a Wheelchair or Litter

- ◆ Secure restraint straps or safety belts and side rails. *(Rationale: Prevent the patient from falling.)*
- ◆ Push from the back; do not pull. *(Rationale: This prevents back strain.)*
- ◆ Look for clear traffic path ahead (*eg,* people approaching, equipment left in hallway, or wet floors.) *(Rationale: This prevents accidents.)*
- ◆ Negotiate corners slowly. *(Rationale: This will prevent the patient from falling and prevent hitting someone coming the other way.)*
- ◆ Use slow to moderate speed in pushing litter or chair. *(Rationale: It is more difficult to stop a faster moving object.)*
- ◆ Secure the patient's equipment (*eg,* IV stands, ventilatory machines, and drainage apparatus). *(Rationale: This prevents injuries to the patient and self.)*
- ◆ When approaching a downward incline, walk in front of the litter or chair. Wheel the chair backward. *(Rationale: This prevents the litter or chair from going too fast.)*
- ◆ When approaching an upward incline, turn the litter or chair around, so you pull the patient head first. *(Rationale: It is easier to pull than to push uphill.)*
- ◆ When approaching a curb or single stair, tip the chair back, and put the small wheels up on the curb or step. Move ahead by lifting or pushing the back wheels over the curb or step. *(Rationale: This prevents jarring the patient.)*
- ◆ Do not attempt to go up or down a curb with a litter. To go *down* a curb with a wheelchair, turn the chair around and ease the large back wheel off the curb first. *(Rationale: This prevents the possibility of lurching the patient forward. The large wheel is easier to roll over the curb and the front wheels are likely to spin sideways and get stuck.)* Use an elevator or "bridge" if available. *(Rationale: This will provide for the patient's safety and avoid injury to you.)*
- ◆ Take the patient's chart when transporting from one station to another. *(Rationale: The chart helps identify the patient and other departments often need the information.)*

Helping the Patient Into a Wheelchair

Supplies and Equipment

Wheelchair
Slippers or shoes (non-skid soles)
Robe
Transfer belt (optional)

Procedure

1. Wash hands.
   (*Rationale: Handwashing prevents the spread of organisms.*)
2. Explain procedure to patient.
   (*Rationale: Providing information fosters patient co-operation and understanding.*)
3. Position wheelchair next to the bed or at a 45 degree angle to the bed. Lock the wheel brakes and remove the foot rests or move them to the "up" position.
   (*Rationale: Positioning the wheelchair carefully and locking the wheels provides for patient's safety.*)

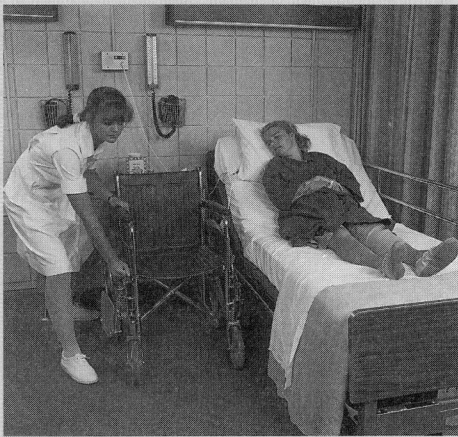

Step 3   Locking the wheelchair brakes

4. Prepare to move the patient:
   a) assist with putting on robe and slippers.
   b) obtain another person if patient is immobile, heavy, or connected to multiple pieces of equipment.
   (*Rationale: Slippers with non-skid soles ensure safety and stability. Requesting assistance prevents accidents.*)
5. Raise the head of the bed so patient is in sitting position.
   (*Rationale: A sitting position facilitates movement out of bed.*)
6. Assist the patient to sit on side of the bed:
   a) support the head and neck with one arm.
   b) use other arm to move the patient's legs over the side of the bed.

   c) allow feet to rest on the floor.
   d) maintain in this position for a short time.
   (*Rationale: A gradual change in position lessens the chance of developing orthostatic hypotension.*)

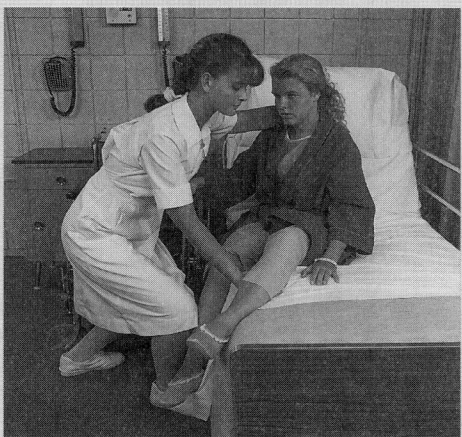

Step 6   Assisting the patient to the side of the bed

7. Prepare to raise patient to a standing position:
   a) apply transfer belt if necessary.
   b) spread feet and brace knees against patient's knees.
   c) place arms around patient's waist.
   (*Rationale: This position provides stability for the transfer.*)
8. Use rocking motion of legs to assist patient to stand. Patient may use hands to help push upward from bed.
   (*Rationale: Nurse uses large muscle mass to lift patient.*)

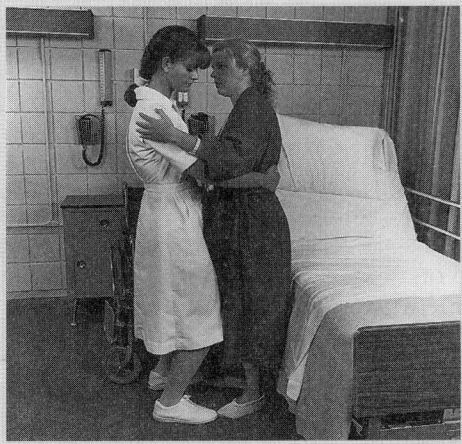

Step 8   Assisting the patient to stand

(continued)

9. Pivot patient into position immediately in front of wheelchair. Encourage patient to use arm rests for support while lowering him or her into chair. *(Rationale: This position supports and stabilizes patient as he or she moves into the chair.)*

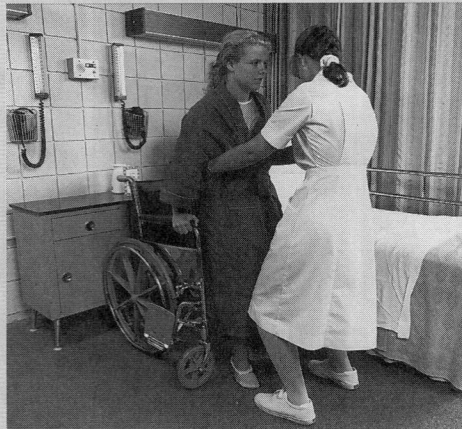

Step 9   Lowering the patient into the wheelchair (Photos © B. Proud.)

10. Reposition foot rests. Secure patient in chair with safety belt if needed. Cover with blanket. Provide nurse call button. *(Rationale: Safety belt prevents accidents, blanket ensures warmth. The patient must be able to call for help.)*
11. Wash hands. *(Rationale: Handwashing prevents the spread of organisms.)*
12. Check on patient frequently. *(Rationale: You could then assist if the patient feels faint. This provides a feeling of security.)*
13. Document transfer and patient response. *(Rationale: Documentation provides ongoing data collection.)*

Use of a Cane

A cane is a slender curved stick or device that is held in the hand and is meant to give support while walking. The three basic types of canes are the standard straight-legged cane, the tripod cane (three feet), and the quad cane (four feet). The cane should have a sturdy handle grip and rubber-tipped feet. Canes support balance and ability to walk and provide additional support when one side of the body is weak. The following are skills for using a cane:

♦ Adjust cane height to allow for a slight bend in the elbow (approximately at hip level).
♦ Instruct the patient to hold the cane on the *strong side* (unless specifically contraindicated).
♦ Check the patient's balance.
♦ Move the cane and the weak side at the same time while the weight is carried on the strong side.
♦ Move the stronger leg forward while the weight is carried on the weak side and the cane.
♦ Continue walking in this manner.
♦ The nurse should walk on the patient's *affected side*.

Use of a Walker

The standard walker is made of aluminum and is a molded tubular device that supports the front of the body. A moderate amount of upper body strength is required to pick up the walker and move it along the floor. Some walkers have rubber-tipped feet; others have wheels in front. The patient must feel secure when walking and should stand upright (see Figure 43-2). Skills for using the walker follow:

♦ Position the walker in front of the patient.
♦ Have the patient pick up the walker and move it ahead approximately 6 in at a time, with weight equally on both feet.
♦ When both sides are weak, move the right foot forward while the weight is shifted to the left side and arms.
♦ Next, move the left foot forward while the weight is shifted to the right side and arms.
♦ Continue moving forward in this manner.
♦ When only one side is weak, first move the walker and weak leg together while the weight is carried by the strong side.
♦ Next move the strong or unaffected side while the weight is carried by the weak side and the walker.

Crutchwalking

Crutches must be adjusted correctly for the patient. If they are too long, they will cause pressure in the axilla. Weight bearing must be on the hands; if not, a condition called *crutch palsy* or *brachial paralysis* can occur. If crutches are too short, the patient will slump.

The bottom of the crutch should be placed about 6 inches (15 cm) to the side of the foot. The top of the crutch should be two to three finger widths from the axillae when the elbows are flexed approximately 30 degrees. The placement of the handbar is just as important. It should be at a height that allows the patient to extend the arm almost completely when leaning on the palms. Even if crutches are the correct length, individual arm lengths are different. Thus, if crutches are shortened more than 1 inch, the position of the handbar will most likely also need to be changed.

The crutch tip should be make of sturdy rubber. It should fit snugly. A large vacuum tip is a necessity. *(Rationale: This gives confidence to the severely disabled person who must place his or her crutches wide to provide a firm base and prevents slipping.)*

If the crutch fits and is used properly, there will be no pressure under the arm. The tops of the crutches are not padded. *(Rationale: A patient may tend to lean on the crutches if the tops are padded.)* Once the patient learns how to use the crutches, rubber pads can be used to protect the patient's clothing; sponge rubber covered with a soft material or rubber pads made to fit the crutch are inexpensive. Properly fitted crutches are comfortable to use.

The patient should wear shoes that fit well, with low, broad heels and straight inner borders. *(Rationale: An old pair of comfortable shoes is excellent, but bedroom slippers should not be worn. They give no support and may seriously damage the foot. They also may have slippery soles.)*

Nursing Alert

A serious disorder called brachial paralysis or crutch palsy can be caused by leaning on crutches. To prevent this condition, the weight of the patient's body must be borne by the hands and not in the axillae.

The first steps in using crutches come before the patient tries to use them to stand or walk. The nurse assists the patient in conditioning. Patient teaching and assisting in using crutches and canes is another nursing responsibility.

Conditioning Exercises. Reconditioning exercises prepare the body for action. The patient dangles, sits in a chair, and learns to stand by the side of the bed. As the patient does this, he or she practices good posture; head and chest are up, and the abdomen is in. If allowed, the patient may be encouraged to press the feet down on a footstool to get the feeling of standing again. While sitting with the arms extended, the patient may be shown how to press the palms down on the bed to

exercise the arm muscles or may lie on the stomach and do bed push-ups. Short crutches may be used so the patient can practice and build up strength while still in bed. Push-ups can be done in a wheelchair. These exercises are described in more detail later in this chapter.

Crutchwalking Gaits. The patient's strength and type of disability are guides to the best possible crutchwalking gait. The patient should use muscles and joints as much as possible. There are four crutchwalking gaits as listed in Table 43-1. The physician and physical therapist will instruct you as to the gait to be used for each patient.

In *two-point gait*, the patient puts his or her body weight on one leg and the *contralateral* crutch (the crutch on the other side), brings the other crutch and leg forward together, and shifts the weight to them. The patient then brings the other leg and crutch forward. This gait is faster and less boring than the others, and the patient can change the gait as muscle power improves. This gait is used following spinal cord injury, when both legs are about the same strength, and the patient is learning to walk again.

In *three-point gait*, the weak leg and both crutches are advanced together, the weight is balanced on them and the *unaffected* leg is advanced. The steps should be of equal length and timed so that there is no pause before the unaffected leg is advanced. This gait is used when one leg is disabled, and the other is strong enough to bear all the patient's weight. This keeps most of the weight off the weak leg. However, a small amount of weight can be placed on the weak leg. This gait is one means of strengthening the weak leg without endangering the patient.

In *four-point gait,* one crutch is placed forward, and the contralateral foot is advanced; the second crutch is brought forward, and the contralateral foot follows. Rhythm and short, equal steps are important. Counting helps to develop rhythm: *one*, right crutch forward; *two*, advance left foot; *three*, left crutch forward; *four*, advance right foot. This is the easiest gait and the safest (the patient always has three points of support). The patient must be able to bring each leg forward and clear the floor with each foot. Those who are partially paralyzed and those with fractures of both legs or with arthritis can use this gait.

In *swinging or tripod gait*, the patient stands on the strong leg, advances both crutches the same distance, rests his or her weight on the palms, and swings forward slightly *ahead* of the crutches. The patient then rests the weight again on the good leg and balances for the next step. Because this is a fast gait, the patient should learn to balance before attempting it. This gait is often used following a fracture when *no weight bearing* is allowed on one leg. It also is used following amputation, when the prosthesis is not in place (particularly in young people). The patient who is allowed to

Table 43-1. Crutch-walking Gaits

Gait	Walking Pattern
Two-point gait	Weight bearing is permitted on both feet. The pattern is a speeded up version of the four-point gait. *Pattern:* Right crutch and left foot forward at the same time, left crutch and right foot forward at the same time.
Three-point gait	Weight bearing is permitted on only one foot. The other foot cannot support but acts as a balance. *Pattern:* Both crutches and the nonsupportive leg go forward, then the weight-bearing leg comes through; the crutches are brought forward immediately, and the pattern is repeated.
Four-point gait	Weight bearing is permitted on both feet. *Pattern:* Right crutch forward, left foot forward, left crutch forward, right foot forward.
Swing-through gait	Weight bearing is permitted on only one foot. *Pattern:* Unaffected foot bears weight while both crutches are brought forward; then both legs swing through between the crutches, and weight bearing returns to the unaffected leg. (Swing-through gait also can be used by the paraplegic client with weight bearing on both feet.)

Source: Taylor C, Lillis C, LeMone P. Fundamentals of Nursing: The Art and Science of Nursing Care, Ed 2. Philadelphia, J.B. Lippincott, 1993.

put weight on only one leg must hold the other up, *bending the knee*, not the hip. This gives better balance. It is the best method for an amputee, a patient with a recent fracture, or a patient with little leg power. Bending the knee is tiring, and the patient should rest frequently with this leg elevated.

Climbing Stairs. When going up stairs, the patient holds the handrail on the unaffected side and has both crutches on the affected side. The stronger leg advances first, followed by the affected leg and crutches. When descending stairs, the patient reverses the process.

Using One Crutch. When the patient progresses to using only one crutch, the crutch is placed on the side of the stronger leg, because it is natural to walk reciprocally. That is, when the affected leg moves forward, the crutch will naturally swing forward with the contralateral hand (the hand on the other side).

The Lofstrand Crutch. This type of crutch is a single bar, with a cuff that fits around the arm. It is popular with people who use crutches for a long time. The person can drop the hand bar and grasp a hand rail or do work, without losing the crutch. Although the Lofstrand is more convenient than traditional crutches, it does not offer as much stability.

Use of the Patient Lift

A hydraulic lift is a mechanical device that allows the totally immobile patient to be transferred from the bed, stretcher, wheelchair, tub, or toilet without the nurse lifting the patient. The lift is equipped with a cloth sling apparatus that supports the body and holds it in alignment while the transfer takes place. Eyelets are located in each corner of the sling, allowing the sling to be attached to the swivel bar with canvas straps. The lift is pressure driven and works much like a car jack as the lever is pumped up. As the patient is lifted from one surface to another, the sling actually holds the body securely. When the next surface is reached, pressure is released and the patient is lowered to the new surface. Safety precautions must be maintained at all times to prevent falls or injuries. Check to make sure that equipment and tubing (eg, catheter drainage tubing) are secure.

Safety Devices

The patient's environment must be safe and accidents or injuries prevented. One way to prevent accidents is to use safety devices. Any number of devices may be used. The most common protective devices are restraints. The Nursing Skill Guidelines explain the use of some of these restraints.

The nurse must be aware of legal implications in using restraints and must know the facility's policy regarding them. Restraints are applied *only* on the physician's order or on order from the charge nurse who has made an independent decision *within policy guidelines* to apply them. Certain procedures must be followed regarding their application and release so that the patient's body can be assessed. Be sure to check your facility's policies and procedures before applying any safety devices.

The patient may view the devices as a threat, especially when a body part is immobilized. When patients are confused, dangerous, or disoriented, the situation becomes even more pronounced. Explain their purpose to help allay the patient's fear and anxiety. The family also may misunderstand the use of restraints, so their use should be explained to the family also.

Moving Patients Who Are Paralyzed

As more vehicle and swimming accidents occur, more paralyzed patients are being seen in healthcare facilities. Some patients have control over parts of their bodies, and others are immobile.

Nursing Skill Guidelines
Using Restraints

◆ Use restraints according to physician's order. *(Rationale: There are legal implications in restraint use.)*
◆ Explain the procedure to the patient and family. *(Rationale: This relieves fear and gains cooperation.)*
◆ Document use of restraints and reasons for use. Verbal intervention *must* be attempted first and documented.
◆ Restraints must be loosened periodically, the limbs exercised, and the condition of the skin checked. *(Rationale: To prevent skin breakdown.)*

Upper Body Restraints

There are two types of safety vest: Posey vest and jacket restraints. It is important to determine which type of safety device you are using. If you have any questions, ask your team leader or instructor. *(Rationale: Improper application can be dangerous and can cause death from suffocation.)*

Criss-Cross Vest

◆ Place the vest on the patient with the opening in the front.
◆ Pull the long tie on the end of the vest through the slit on the opposite side.
◆ Cross over the patient's abdomen. Be sure to cross the two sides of the vest in the *front*.
◆ Bring one tie down on each side and tie to chair.

Posey Jacket Restraint

◆ Another type of restraint looks like a jacket with sleeves and an opening down the back. It has an attached belt around the waist.
◆ Put the jacket on with the opening in back. The side seams should be under the arms.
◆ Close with zipper, ties, or hooks. Some types have extra ties. *(Rationale: Ensure a snug fit.)*
◆ Tie shoulder loops around the push handles of a wheelchair. *(Rationale: This prevents the patient from falling forward.)*
◆ Use the loops; never tie anything around the patient's neck. Do not use this jacket on a bed. *(Rationale: It does not allow the patient to turn over in the bed. Shoulder loops may choke the patient who struggles in bed.)*
◆ Tie the waist straps to the bars at the bottom back of the wheelchair. *(Rationale: To prevent the patient from sliding out of the chair.)*

Soft Wrist Restraints

◆ Apply the padded portion of the restraint around the wrist. *(Rationale: This prevents skin breakdown.)*
◆ Protect the wrist with thick gauze or padded dressing under the restraint. *(Rationale: This prevents skin breakdown.)*
◆ Pull the long tie through the slit in the restraint; apply the velcro, or close the buckle.
◆ Bring both ends of the long tie together, and attach to the *movable* portion of the bed frame or to the chair post.
◆ Measure distance of the tie to allow for range of motion of the arm, while protecting tubes or equipment from hands. *(Rationale: Total restraint is frightening and can add to a patient's confusion, therefore making the patient combative.)*

Fastening Restraint Straps

◆ If the patient is in a wheelchair, tie the straps on each side to the restraint posts in the bottom at the back. Be sure knots are out of the patient's reach.
◆ If the patient is in bed, tie the straps to the movable part of the bed, and tuck any extra length up under the bed springs. *(Rationale: If straps are tied to a stationary part of the bed, the patient could be injured if the bed is raised. The restraint must be able to move with the patient.)*
◆ A quick-release knot or a square knot should be used.

Other Types of Restraints

◆ If the patient struggles, locked or unlocked leather restraints may be necessary. They are described in Chapter 87.
◆ If the patient slides forward, a restraint with a crotch piece is necessary.

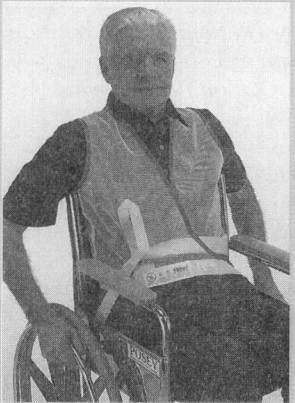
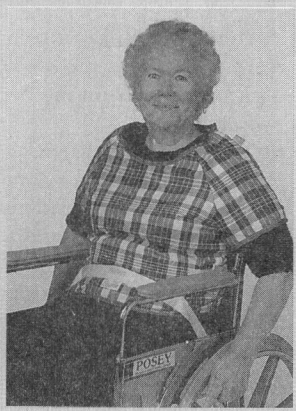

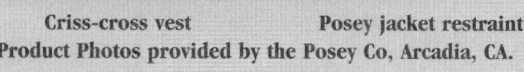

Criss-cross vest　　　　Posey jacket restraint
Product Photos provided by the Posey Co, Arcadia, CA.

Helping the Hemiplegic or Paraplegic Person

The person who is paralyzed on one side (**hemiplegic**) often can be moved from bed to chair with assistance of one nurse. The person is assisted to stand. Your foot and knee are placed firmly against the patient's foot and in front of the knee on the disabled side. Pivot the person around, and assist him or her to sit in the chair; you should be bracing the chair. (*Rationale: Provide support for the paralyzed side, because the person can usually stand on the other side. The most important factor is to prevent the paralyzed foot from slipping or the knee from buckling.*)

The **paraplegic** person is paralyzed from the waist area down. This person has limited or no use of the legs but usually has strong arms. When assisting this person with a transfer, you will have to move the legs, but the patient can help lift with his or her arms. Figure 43-3 illustrates how to move this patient.

Sliding an Immobile Patient From Bed to Chair

The sliding technique is especially useful when an immobile patient is too heavy for one person to lift, and no other help is available. It also can be used to transfer a person to a chair or commode. The procedure should always be explained to the person. If the nurse feels the task is too much to handle alone, it is his or her responsibility to report to the charge nurse and ask for help. It is important to deliver safe nursing care.

Nursing Skill
Sliding an Immobile Patient From Bed to Chair

Procedure

1. Place the bed in low position. (*Rationale: This position is safest for the nurse and patient.*)
2. Lock the wheels on the bed. (*Rationale: A moving bed is a hazard.*)
3. Be sure there are no obstacles in the area. (*Rationale: Protect the patient and yourself.*)
4. Place a chair facing and against the bed opposite the patient's buttocks. (*Rationale: The bed and chair should be at the same level.*)
5. Slide your arms under the patient's head and shoulders. (*Rationale: This position supports the patient.*)
6. Advance one foot. (*Rationale: Give yourself support.*)
7. Rock backward, drawing the upper part of the patient's body to the edge of the bed. (*Rationale: Momentum will bring the patient's body forward for easier sliding.*)
8. Standing behind the patient at his or her head, reach under the shoulders, and put one arm well under each axilla, resting the head and shoulders against you. (*Rationale: Your body provides support for the patient's head.*)

9. Move carefully behind the chair, drawing the patient into it as you move. Rock back, pulling the patient into the chair, and brace yourself by leaning against the chair back. The chair is supported against the bed. (*Rationale: Support the patient's body as much as possible, and use good body mechanics.*)
10. Grasp the seat of the chair, and slowly pull the chair back until only the patient's feet and ankles are resting on the bed. Be careful not to drop the feet to the floor. (*Rationale: Injury could result.*)
11. Flex the patient's knees and legs as you lower the feet to the floor, keeping your own knees flexed. (*Rationale: This provides passive exercise for the patient's legs, and it simulates normal sitting position.*)

Moving an Immobile Patient From a Chair to an Elevated Bed

The following procedure is slightly different from that when the bed and chair levels are the same. In this instance, the hospital bed is higher than the chair.

Nursing Skill
Moving an Immobile Patient From a Chair to an Elevated Bed

1. Bring the chair with the patient in it to the side of the bed, and keep the patient facing the center. If the chair does not roll, slide it to the bed rather that lifting it. (*Rationale: Protect yourself.*)
2. Stand in front of the patient on one side of the chair, and place your arms under the patient's axillae, drawing the person close against you. (*Rationale: Supporting the upper portion of the patient's body on your body reduces the weight to be moved.*)
3. Standing with the foot near the chair drawn back and the other foot forward, rock the patient's trunk strongly upward, lifting the entire trunk and buttocks onto the bed. (*Rationale: Using the weight of your body to move the patient is an application of body mechanics.*)
4. Support the patient's thighs by resting against them. (*Rationale: This position prevents falls.*)
5. Slide the chair away with your foot. (*Rationale: You need room for the next step.*)
6. Pivot the patient onto the bed. (*Rationale: It is important to brace the patient's knees and thighs so they cannot buckle.*)
7. Lift the patient's legs onto the bed, and roll and slide the patient into proper position. (*Rationale: It is easier to lift the patient in "sections" than all at once.*)
8. Make sure the patient is comfortable, and the call light is within reach.

Using the Transfer Board or Bridge

The transfer board (sliding board) or bridge may be used for patients who are unable to stand. The board is made of hard plastic, approximately $\frac{1}{2}$ to $\frac{3}{4}$ inches

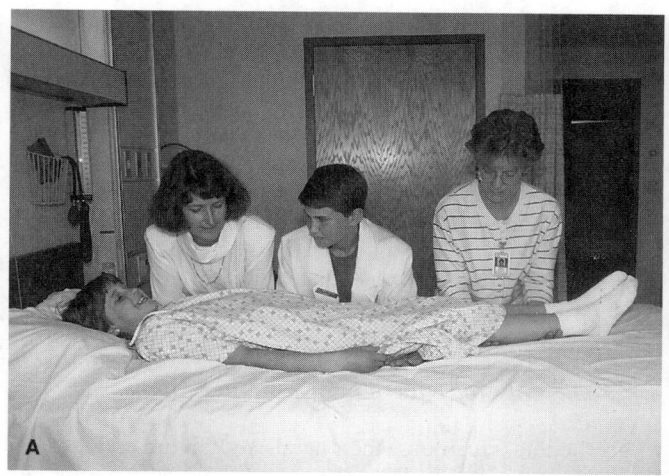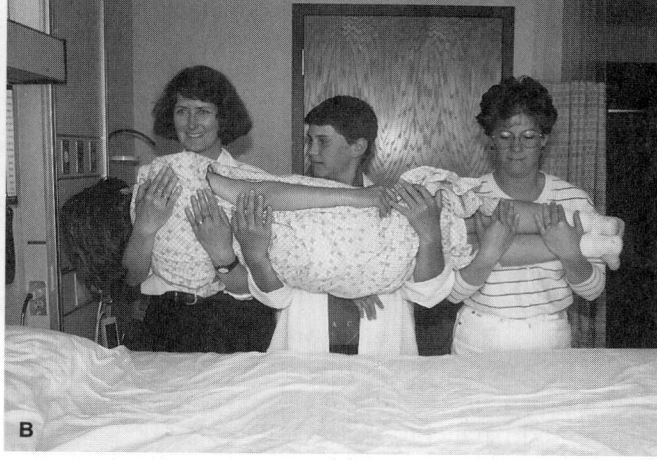

Figure 43-3. Three-Carrier Lift. **A.** In preparation for the three-carrier lift, the carriers place their hands under the immobile patient, as per the accompanying procedure. When the person at the head calls the signal, all three carriers rock backward and gently move the patient to the side of the bed. **B.** After repositioning their hands, on a second signal, the carriers logroll the patient onto their chests. They can then pivot and reverse the procedure to place her on a litter or operating table. (Even though it is better to have the tallest person at the patient's head and the next tallest in the middle, this patient is small and will be easily lifted anyway. In the case of a larger patient, each lifter may also cross arms with the next lifter, for more stability.) (Photos by Kimberly Malcolm, Courtesy of Fairview Northland Regional Home Care, Princeton, Minnesota)

thick and long enough to reach from the side of the bed to a chair. The surface of the board is smooth and allows for ease in sliding the body. Transferring a patient in this manner promotes self-esteem and independence and conserves the nurse's energy. The procedure is explained to the patient. If you are assisting in the transfer, you will supervise the procedure and guide the patient.

Nursing Skill
Using the Transfer Board or Bridge

1. Lock the wheels on the bed. *(Rationale: Prevent bed movement.)*
2. Position the chair, commode, or wheelchair close to the head of the bed. Lock the wheelchair brakes. *(Rationale: This prevents movement of the chair.)*
3. Remove the arm rest from wheelchair or commode. *(Rationale: This accommodates transfer.)*
4. Assist the patient to an upright position in the bed. *(Rationale: This position prevents orthostatic hypotension.)*
5. Insert one end of the board under the buttocks. *(Rationale: The board serves as a wedge to accommodate body weight.)*
6. Position the other end of the board on the chair. *(Rationale: This establishes the bridge.)*
7. Guide the patient across the board from the bed to the chair. *(Rationale: This helps control the transfer.)*

8. Assess the patient for good body alignment. *(Rationale: This prevents pressure on bony prominences and allows for good circulation.)*
9. Apply a seat belt or other restraint if needed. *(Rationale: This provides for patient safety.)*

Using the Wheeled Stretcher

Sometimes patients are moved by stretcher or litter. This is a four-wheeled cart that is used for the following purposes:

- ◆ To move patients who cannot sit up
- ◆ To move patients with appliances or casts that do not fit into a wheelchair or that would be disarranged if they were put in a wheelchair
- ◆ To move patients to the operating room or the x-ray department or to other rooms for special tests, treatments, or examinations, especially if they are sedated
- ◆ To transfer patients from one unit to another

Safety precautions related to the use of a litter are the following:

- ◆ The rubber tires should be intact so the patient is not jarred.
- ◆ The stretcher covering should be clean and enough blankets provided to keep the patient warm.

◆ Patients should be protected from injury by lifting them correctly and putting them down carefully on the stretcher, using enough people to lift the patient.

◆ A patient should never be left alone on the stretcher unless restrained or unless the side rails are up.

Guidelines for pushing a litter and wheelchair are presented in a box earlier in this chapter.

Helping a Mobile Patient Move From Bed to Litter or Litter to Bed

If the patient is able to help, place the litter tight against and parallel to the bed. Raise the bed, so it is level with the litter. Lock the wheels of the litter and the bed. Cover the patient with a blanket, and turn back the bedclothes. (Rationale: *This prevents tangling in bed linens.*)

Steady the litter, and assist the patient to move onto it. (Rationale: *It is important for the nurse to prevent falls.*) During the move, brace your body tightly against the litter, holding the litter tightly against the bed. Make sure there is no space between them. (Rationale: *This prevents the patient from falling through.*) A bridge may be used if the patient has difficulty moving.

Moving a Nonresponsive Patient From Bed to Litter

It takes at least three people to move an immobile or nonresponsive patient to a litter. Another person also may be needed to move a cast or traction apparatus or the legs of a person who has had spinal anesthesia. The three-carrier lift works well.

Three-Carrier Lift. The purpose of the three-carrier lift is to move an immobile patient, while keeping him or her in a horizontal position with the back straight.

Nursing Skill
Using the Three-Carrier Lift

Procedure

1. Lock the bed wheels, and raise the bed to high position. (Rationale: *This provides safety for the patient and nurse.*)
2. Lock the stretcher wheels. (Rationale: *This provides safety for patients and nurses.*)
3. Place the stretcher at a right angle (90-degree angle) to the bed. (Rationale: *This position allows safe movement of patient.*)
4. Three nurses of near equal height stand side by side near the patient's bed. (Rationale: *Nurses of equal height can maintain the patient's body alignment.*)

5. Each carrier assumes responsibility for one of three areas (the area where he or she stands): the head and shoulders, the hips, and the thighs and feet. (Rationale: *Body weight must be distributed evenly.*)
6. The carrier at the head calls the signals. (Rationale: *One person is in charge; this provides for continuity.*)
7. The carriers will place their arms under the patient's head and shoulders, the hips, and the thighs and legs. The adjoining arms of the carriers should be touching (Fig. 43-3A). (Rationale: *It is important to maintain the patient's body alignment.*)
8. The carriers assume a broad-based stance and gently move the patient to the side of the bed. (Rationale: *It will make the patient more accessible and easier to lift.*)
9. The lifters rearrange their hands and on the count of three, the carriers lift up the patient and hold him or her against their chests (Fig. 43-3B). (Rationale: *The patient's body weight is distributed evenly.*)
10. On another count of three, the carriers take one step backward, turn and pivot toward the stretcher. They step forward if necessary. (Rationale: *Timing is important.*)
11. On a count of three, the carriers gently lower the patient to the stretcher by flexing their legs and thighs. (Rationale: *This distributes the body weight of carriers and patient.*)
12. Assess patient's body alignment and position safety devices as needed. (Rationale: *This prevents injury to the patient's musculoskeletal system.*) Wash your hands before and after the lift.
13. Record the procedure in the nurse's notes. (Rationale: *This provides a record of completion of procedure and tolerance of procedure.*)

Assisting the Patient Confined to Bed

Patients confined to bed need exercise and regular change in body position to preserve muscle tone and morale. A schedule must be set up and followed whereby the patient is turned at regular intervals to prevent musculoskeletal deformities, respiratory complications, circulatory disorders, and skin breakdown.

This section describes how to move and make the patient more comfortable. It discusses measures and exercises in which the person can participate to help maintain muscle strength and prepare to get out of bed.

Key Concept
Always apply body mechanics principles. They will prove extremely valuable to you.

Adjusting the Backrest and Pillows

If a patient is in a bed that can be adjusted to different positions, it is no problem to raise or lower the backrest. However, to adjust the pillows, the patient's shoulders and back must be lifted. The steps in this procedure are explained in the following nursing skill.

Nursing Skill
Adjusting the Backrest and Pillows

Procedure

1. Stand facing the patient with one foot forward and the body bent forward from the hips. (*Rationale: This position helps you maintain good body alignment.*)
2. Put one arm under the shoulders, and put the patient's nearer arm over your shoulder and around your neck.
3. Put your other arm under the patient's other arm and across the back.
4. Tighten your thigh and hip muscles, and bring your body and the patient's body upright together. (*Rationale: The use of good body mechanics makes moving the patient easier.*)
5. Continue supporting the patient while you adjust the pillows or backrest with your hand under the patient's back.

Assisting the Patient to Move Up in Bed

Nursing Procedure 43-2 applies to moving all bed patients. The nurse assesses the patient's ability to participate, encourages the patient to help as much as possible, and gives detailed instructions. The nurse must realize his or her own strength and ask for assistance if the patient is too heavy to move alone.

Alternate Procedure. When absolutely necessary, you can move a patient up in bed by yourself by standing at the head of the bed and pulling the patient up. Stand on the bed frame or a footstool. Put one hand under each armpit. Rock backward, pulling the patient up in bed. (*Rationale: The rocking motion, using your body weight, maximizes your strength and is an example of good body mechanics. By straight-up pulling from the head of the bed, you keep the patient's body in good alignment. By grasping under the patient's arms, you move the person in a straight line.*)

The Lifting-Sheet Method

Another method for moving the totally immobile patient is the two-person draw sheet or "lifting-sheet" method. This method is easier for everyone. The following describes the actions.

First lock the bed wheels. Slip a wide draw sheet or folded large sheet under the patient from the head to below the buttocks. Roll the sides of the sheet close to the patient's body. A piece of plastic under the lift sheet helps to make it slide easier and prevents dragging. (*Rationale: The sheet will serve as a "handle" to grasp on each side of the patient.*)

You and your assistant stand opposite each other, near the patient's shoulders. Face toward the foot of the bed, with the leg nearest the bed behind the other leg. Together, grasp the sheet near the neck and near the lumbar region, lean forward, and rock backward. Then, slide toward the head of the bed. Your combined weight lifts the patient off the bed and then slides the draw sheet and patient up toward the head of the bed. This method helps to prevent sheet burns or irritation to the patient caused by being pulled up in bed. It also helps to prevent patient injury, which may be caused by pulling on the patient's shoulders or by the nurses placing their hands under the patient's body. This procedure also saves strain on the nurses. Special care is necessary to guard against injuring the elderly or ill person.

Assisting the Immobile Patient to Move to the Side of the Bed

It is often necessary to move the patient to the side of the bed so the patient will be closer to you for a treatment or injection or in preparation for rolling the patient to a side-lying position. One nurse, using proper body mechanics, can move any patient to the side of the bed. Whenever possible, the patient should be encouraged to assist in the movement. This action can be carried out by lifting the body while holding onto the raised side rail or by using the overhead trapeze. The nurse serves as a support to the patient. The nurse must assess the patient's ability to understand the instructions for the move and must judge the patient's size and weight based on the nurse's own strength. The following skill is used in assisting the immobile patient to move to the side of the bed.

◆ Support the patient's head and shoulders with one arm and the middle back with the other arm. (*Rationale: By placing your hands in this manner, you will move the largest area of the patient's body.*)
◆ Do all lifting and moving gently. (*Rationale: It is important to prevent injury or irritation to the patient's skin.*)
◆ Bend at the knees, and move from front foot to back foot to prevent injury to yourself. Do not lift.
◆ After you have moved the patient's shoulders, repeat the same procedure with the hips and legs.

Assisting the Immobile Patient to Move up in Bed

Supplies and Equipment

Pillows
Side rails
Overhead trapeze (optional)
Draw sheet (optional)

Procedure

1. Wash hands.
   (Rationale: Handwashing prevents the spread of organisms.)
2. Explain procedure to patient.
   (Rationale: Providing information fosters patient co-operation and understanding.)
3. Adjust the bed to a comfortable height.
   (Rationale: Bed at proper height prevents back strain.)
4. Lower a patient's bed to as flat a position as can be tolerated and lower the side rail.
   (Rationale: A flat bed eliminates the need to pull against gravity.)
5. Lock the wheels on the bed.
   (Rationale: This action prevents the bed from rolling.)

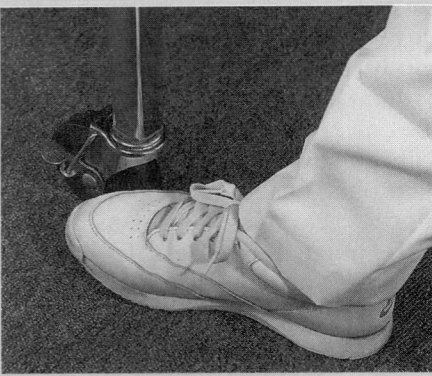

Step 5   Locking the bed wheels

6. Remove pillow under patient's head and place it against the head of the bed.
   (Rationale: Repositioning the pillow prevents injury to the patient's head when moved upward.)

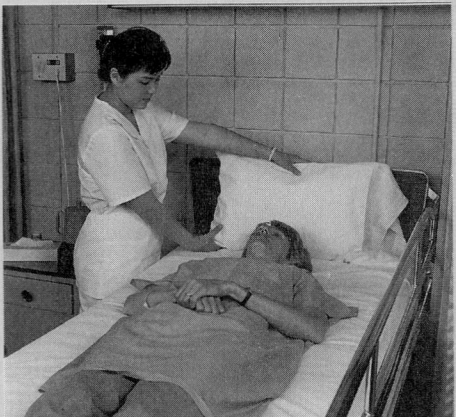

Step 6   Repositioning the pillow at the head of the bed

7. Assist patient to flex the knees and hips with feet flat on the bed.
   (Rationale: This allows the patient to assist with the lift using the strength in his or her legs.)
8. Ask patient to assist with move by:
   a) folding arms across the chest.
   b) using overhead trapeze (if available) to lift and pull body upward.
   c) pushing upward with feet.
   d) grasping top of bed and pulling with both hands.
   (Rationale: Encouraging patient to assist with movement fosters independence. Keeping arms off the bed prevents friction rub of sheets when moving upward. Using large muscle groups increases the force of upward movement.)
9. Assume a broad-based stance by flexing your knees and hips with feet spread and turned toward the head of the bed.
   (Rationale: This position lowers the center of gravity and provides a broad base prior to moving the patient.)

(continued)

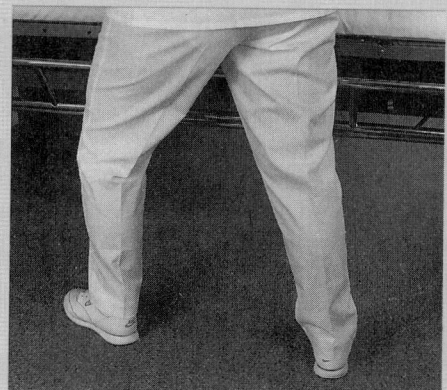

Step 9   Assuming a broad-based stance

10. Slide arms under the patient's shoulders and thighs. *(Rationale: This supports and evenly distributes the patient's weight.)*
11. Rock weight back onto back leg and shift upward with the patient's assistance on the count of three. Repeat steps if necessary to advance patient further up in bed. *(Rationale: Rocking motion assists the forward motion of the patient.)*

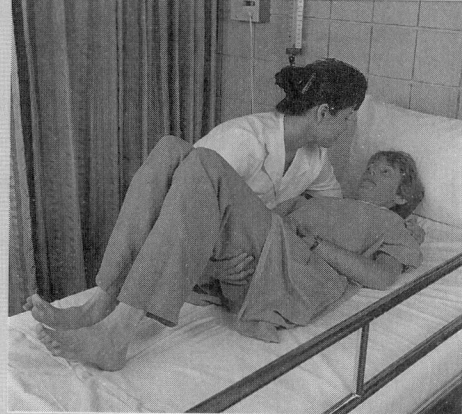

Step 11   Moving the patient up in bed (Photos © B. Proud.)

12. Replace pillow under head. Lower bed and elevate head as tolerated. Raise side rail. *(Rationale: Repositioning provides for patient's comfort. Side rails ensure safety.)*
13. Wash hands. *(Rationale: Handwashing prevents the spread of organisms.)*
   Note: Be sure to get assistance if needed.

♦ When moving a very large patient, two nurses are more efficient than one.
♦ Use good body mechanics at all times, but do not be afraid to ask for help if necessary.

Positioning of Patients

The position of a patient's body may be changed to promote comfort, restore body function, prevent deformities, relieve pressure and prevent strain, stimulate proper respiration and circulation, and give treatments. See the Nursing Skill Guidelines for positioning.

Explain to the patient why you are changing the position and how you will do it. The patient's understanding is important, because then he or she will be more likely to maintain the position. Tell the patient who can help what they can do. The patient's assistance will save strain on you and will give the person some exercise and a feeling of self-worth.

Sometimes turning the patient is such an important part of treatment that the physician specifies how often to do it. This is especially important for elderly or immobile patients. In certain conditions, it may be impossible to turn the patient, for example, if the patient has fractures that require traction appliances. In addition, turning may be harmful, as with spinal injuries. In this case, you need to rub the back by lifting the patient slightly off the bed and massaging with your hand held flat. *(Rationale: It is especially important to prevent skin breakdown in the person who lies on the back for long periods of time.)* You may want to turn a patient only to wash or rub the back or change the bed. If a patient cannot turn, he or she usually is placed in a special bed. These beds are discussed in Chapter 44.

Turning the Patient to a Side-Lying Position

When turning a patient to the side, he or she must be kept in good alignment. When a person is to be maintained in the side-lying position, turn as you would if the person were to be temporarily on the side—to rub the back, for instance. Then prop the person into that position. Nursing Procedure 43-3 outlines steps in turning the patient.

In an alternative side-lying position (modified Sims' position), the patient's knees may be bent more and the bottom arm placed behind the person's back. This po-

◆ Maintain good patient body alignment. (Think of the patient in bed as though he or she were standing.)
◆ Maintain patient safety.
◆ Reassure the patient to promote comfort and cooperation.
◆ Properly handle the patient's body to prevent pain or injury.
◆ Keep in mind proper body mechanics for the nurse.
◆ Obtain assistance, if needed, to move heavy or immobile patients.
◆ Follow specific physician's orders.
◆ An order is needed for a patient to be out of bed.
◆ Do not use special devices (eg, splints, traction) unless ordered.

sition may be used for variety, but the patient will probably be uncomfortable if left for very long.

Supporting a Patient in a Sitting Position

A patient may sit up for a short time to eat meals, work at a table, or change position, or the person may need to be in this position continuously to make breathing easier, as in cardiac conditions. Support is needed when the body is resting in a sitting position. Pillows support the back, neck, and head to keep the spine in its normal curves. Folded pillows support the arms and keep the shoulders up. Pads in the hands support the wrists and keep the fingers bent slightly and the thumb out, which is the grasping position. The knees are supported in a comfortable position. A slanting footrest is comfortable for the feet and prevents footdrop.

There is tendency for the mattress to slip to the foot of the bed when the head of the bed is raised. This makes it difficult to keep the body in good alignment. To avoid this, a pillow or rolled blanket is sometimes placed in the space between the edge of the mattress and the lower end of the bed.

When a patient is placed in the sitting position for the first time during an illness, do so only on the physician's order. Observe the patient closely for signs of fatigue and faintness until the patient has adjusted to the change.

Promoting Good Body Alignment With the Patient on the Back

Typically, patients lie on their backs much of the time. Some patients may stay in that position throughout a long illness. It is important to make such a patient

as comfortable as possible and to prevent body deformities. Use pillows to support the patient's head, neck, arms, and hands and a footboard to support the feet. This position gives respiratory and digestive organs room to function normally. The footboard is slanted to support the feet at right angles to the legs (a normal angle) and prevent footdrop.

If the patient's trunk must lie flatter than the upper part of the body, the person will have only one pillow to support the head and neck. A knee-roll may be used under the knees, and the person may have a pad under the ankles to prevent pressure on the heels. The footboard will be more nearly upright.

The Protective Prone Position

The person may be positioned on the stomach for short periods of time to provide variety. This position is called the "protective prone" position. This position, however, is not comfortable for any length of time. Having the head turned sideways can be a great strain on the neck and can cause headache.

Key Concepts

The patient's body alignment when lying down should be approximately the same as if the person were standing.

If in doubt about moving any patient, ask for assistance.

The Logroll Turn

The logroll turn is a method of turning the patient that keeps the body in straight alignment (like a tree log). This method is used on patients who have spinal cord injuries or surgery. Because the goal is to turn the patient as one unit, caution must be exercised to prevent further injuries to the back and spine. Two or three nurses are required to turn the patient properly in this fashion; however, one nurse may perform this procedure in an emergency, such as the patient who is vomiting.

The logroll turn is used to reposition the patient to allow for bed linen changes, change of body position, or to give nursing care. This position is helpful in relieving pressure areas over bony prominences and generally adds to the patient's comfort by allowing the change of positions. In patients who have a cervical injury, one nurse is required to maintain the stability of the neck and keep it in alignment. Assess the patient's ability to understand instructions and to be cooperative in the turn.

Nursing Procedure 43-3

Turning the Patient to a Side-Lying Position

Supplies and Equipment

Pillows
Side rails
Cotton blanket or towels, rolled for support

Procedure

1. Wash hands.
   (Rationale: Handwashing prevents the spread of organisms.)
2. Explain procedure to patient.
   (Rationale: Providing information fosters patient cooperation and understanding.)
3. Adjust the bed to a comfortable height.
   (Rationale: Bed at proper height prevents back strain.)
4. Lower the patient's head to as flat a position as can be tolerated and lower side rail.
   (Rationale: A flat bed eliminates the need to pull against gravity.)
5. Move the patient to the side of the bed. Raise side rail. Move to other side of bed.
   (Rationale: Positioning patient near the far side allows adequate room to turn. Raised side rails keep the patient safe.)
6. Lower side rail. Place one hand on the patient's far shoulder and the other on the far hip.
   (Rationale: Turner is positioned near patient's center of gravity.)
7. Assume a broad stance with abdominal and gluteal muscles tensed. Roll patient toward you.
   (Rationale: This action provides a wide base of support and uses large muscle masses to move the patient.)

8. Position the patient's legs comfortably:
   a) flex the lower knee and hip slightly.
   b) bring the upper leg forward and place a pillow between the legs.
   (Rationale: This helps prevent strain on the hip joint and minimizes pressure on bony prominences.)

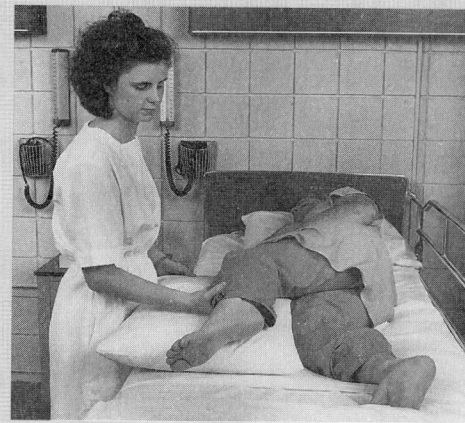

Step 8   Positioning the patient's legs

9. Adjust the patient's arms:
   a) shift the lower shoulder toward you slightly.
   b) support the upper arm on a pillow.
   (Rationale: This supports the upper body and prevents pressure on body prominences.)

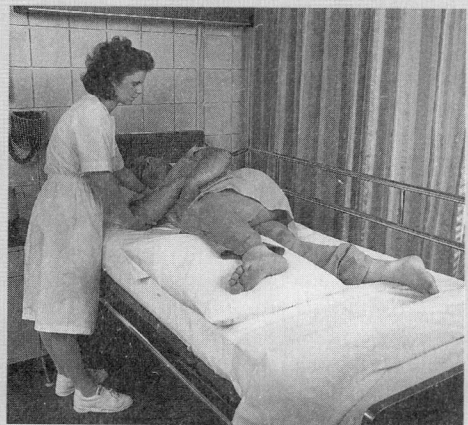

Step 9   Adjusting the patient's arms

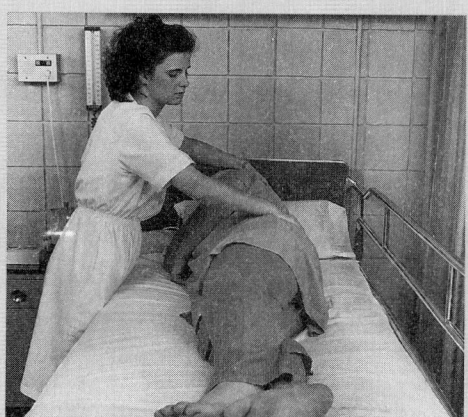

Step 7   Rolling the patient toward you

(continued)

10. Wedge a pillow behind the patient's back. Use rolled blankets or towels as needed for support. *(Rationale: Pillow helps keep patient on the side.)*

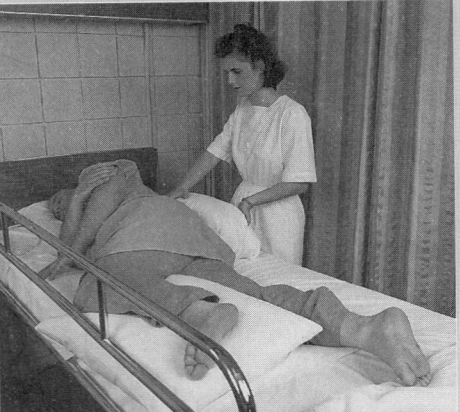

Step 10 Supporting the patient's back (Photos © B. Proud.)

11. Lower bed, elevate the head as tolerated, and raise the side rail. *(Rationale: Repositioning provides for patient's comfort. Side rails ensure safety.)*
12. Wash hands. *(Rationale: Handwashing prevents the spread of organisms.)*

Nursing Skill
The Logroll Turn

Procedure

1. Determine number of nurses needed for move. *(Rationale: Large patients may require the help of three nurses.)*
2. Position yourselves together on the same side of the bed assuming a broad-based stance with one foot slightly ahead of the other. *(Rationale: This provides easier access to the patient and aids nurses in weight distribution.)*
3. Position the patient's arms on his or her chest. *(Rationale: This prevents the arms from becoming entangled under the body during the turn.)*
4. Shift the weight of your trunk and flex the knees, thighs, and ankles. *(Rationale: This position enables nurses to use their large muscle group.)*
5. Slide arms under the patient. If two nurses are turning, one should lift the neck region and upper body, the other should lift the hips and thighs. In the three-nurse lift, each nurse should take a smaller region of the body. *(Rationale: This allows for even distribution of body weight and prevents possible cervical injury.)*
6. The nurse at the head of the patient will call the signals. *(Rationale: This ensures organization and control in the turn.)*
7. On the count of three, move the patient to the side of the bed. *(Rationale: This maintains body alignment.)*
8. On the count of three, roll and position the patient on his or her side. *(Rationale: This provides position change.)*
9. Place a small pillow under the patient's head. *(Rationale: The pillow will help stabilize the neck.)*
10. Place one or two pillows under the patient's legs. *(Rationale: Pillows help keep the legs aligned.)*
11. Place a pillow to the back (optional). *(Rationale: This supports the back and provides for comfort.)*
12. A turning sheet may be used in the logroll turn. *(Rationale: This allows for ease in turning the patient, especially if only one nurse is available.)* Care should be taken to carry out all safety precautions in the turn.

Joint Mobility and Range of Motion

Parts of the body may be elevated to improve circulation, relieve congestion or pain, or check hemorrhage. Pillows are used to elevate a leg or an arm. If necessary, pillows may be protected with plastic covers. Sandbags also may be used to keep a body part in position. Do not elevate any part of the body without a physician's order. (In emergencies, such as a hemorrhage, a part may be elevated without an order. In such an instance, notify the physician immediately, and report what you have done and why.)

Joints are capable of specific movements, they cannot be pushed past these movements without risking injury. The body movement is divided into three planes: sagittal, transverse, and frontal. They are illus-

Key Medical Abbreviations and Acronyms in Positioning

AROM	Active range of motion
CPM	Continuous passive motion
PRN	*Pro re nata,* as needed
PROM	Passive range of motion
ROM	Range of motion

trated in Figure 14-2. **Range of motion** (ROM) is the range of movement that is possible to the point of resistance for that joint. The individual's range is determined by such factors as body development, genetic inheritance, presence or absence of disease processes, and amount of exercise the person usually gets through daily activities. Abbreviations used in ROM discussions are given in the accompanying box.

It will be helpful to review terms related to basic body movements in Chapters 14 and 17. A boxed display in Chapter 17, called Range of Motion in Body Movements, will help you review the various motions the body can perform. These basic movements include the following:

- **Flexion**, decreasing the angle between two bones, and its opposite, **extension**, increasing the angle
- **Abduction,** moving a part away from the midline of the body, and its opposite, **adduction**, moving toward the midline
- Circular movements, such as **circumduction** and **rotation**
- **Supination (inversion)**, turning the foot so its sole faces the other foot, and its opposite, **eversion**

The ability to move a joint is controlled by ligaments, muscles, and tendons that connect the bones. For example, if the patient has an injury to the tendon, muscles, or ligaments, the joint will have limited movement.

Passive and Active Range of Motion

Every joint must be moved regularly several times each day to prevent deformities. This must be done by a nurse or therapist for patients who cannot move by themselves. The following joints should be exercised unless contraindicated: neck, shoulder, elbow, wrist, finger, thumb, hip, knee, ankle, and toe.

The patient is assisted by the nursing staff with activities called *ROM exercises.* If the patient does his or her own exercises, the procedure is called **active range of motion**. Nursing supervision may be necessary to assure that the patient moves all joints and muscles to the fullest extent possible. If the nurse moves the patient's extremities, the procedure is called **passive range of motion** (PROM). Guidelines for providing PROM exercises are given in the accompanying box.

The patient who does not exercise the body and move the joints regularly may develop joint deformities. **Contractures,** caused by the continuous pull of the strongest muscles in any muscle pair, may cause such deformities. Exercise also is necessary to prevent hypostatic pneumonia, thrombophlebitis, footdrop, circulatory difficulties, skin breakdown, and fecal impactions. A patient ordered to remain on bedrest should not be subjected to further and unnecessary physical damage. Good nursing care is essential to prevent such complications. As many ROM movements as possible should be applied to each body joint during ROM exercises.

Passive Range-of-Motion Exercises

Performing Passive Range-of-Motion Exercises. The nurse, under the direction of the physical therapist, performs PROM exercises. Skills in performing PROM exercises are summarized in Nursing Procedure 43-4.

Continuous Passive Motion Machine. Mechanical devices to provide continuous motion to a specific joint, usually the knee, are called **continuous passive motion** (CPM) machines. These machines are commonly used after orthopedic surgery. The leg is moved without effort on the part of the nurse or the patient. The exercises

Nursing Skill Guidelines
Performing Passive Range of Motion Exercises

- Check the physician's order. A physician's order is needed for complete range of motion exercises. The physician also may order range of motion exercises for specific joints only.
- Practice good personal body mechanics to prevent injury to yourself. For example, put the bed in high position, and move the patient close to you so you need not stretch and bend.
- Move slowly and gently so you do not injure the patient.
- If the patient complains of extreme pain, stop and report it to your team leader. *Do not force joint movements!*
- Support the dependent part of each extremity while performing passive joint exercises.
- Repeat each movement three times.
- Perform limited range of motion movements during treatments, such as the bed bath.
- If the patient becomes tired, allow reasonable rest periods between exercises.

Supplies and Equipment

None required

Procedure

1. Wash hands.
   (Rationale: Handwashing prevents spread of organisms.)
2. Explain procedure to patient.
   (Rationale: Providing information fosters patient co-operation and understanding.)
3. Adjust bed to a comfortable height. Select one side of bed to begin PROM exercises.
   (Rationale: Bed at proper height prevents back strain and eliminates reaching across bed.)
4. Uncover only limb to be exercised.
   (Rationale: This ensures warmth and protects patient's privacy.)
5. Support all joints during exercise activity.
   (Rationale: Cradling joints prevents injury and discomfort.)
6. Use slow gentle movements when performing exercises. Repeat each exercise 3 times. Discontinue if patient complains of pain or discomfort.
   (Rationale: Repetitive motion maintains joint mobility. Discontinuing exercises, if they cause pain, prevents injury to joint.)
7. Begin exercises with patient's neck and work downward.
   (Rationale: Performing procedures in a systematic manner ensures that all joints will be exercised.)
8. Flex, extend, and rotate the neck. Support the head with your hands.
   (Rationale: This prevents flexion contracture of the neck.)
9. Exercise shoulder and elbow:
   a) support the elbow with one hand and grasp the wrist with the other hand.

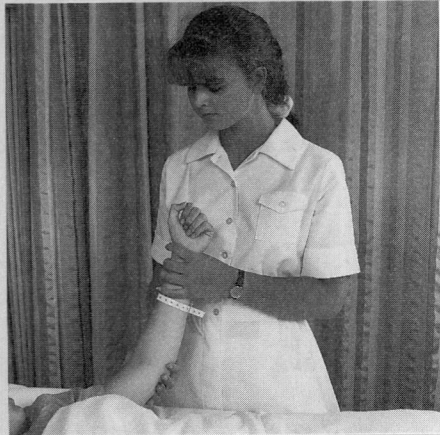

Step 9a Supporting the joint

b) raise arm from side to above head.
   c) perform internal rotation by moving the arm across the patient's chest.
   d) externally rotate the shoulder by moving the arm away from the patient.

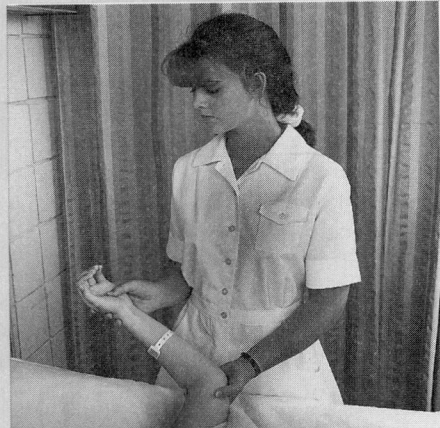

Step 9d Externally rotating the shoulder

e) flex and extend the elbow.
   (Rationale: This maintains strength in the deltoid muscle and prevents contractures.)

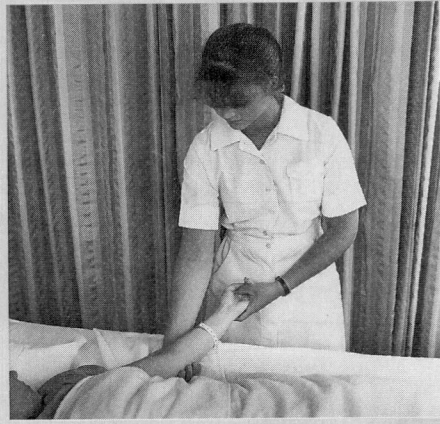

Step 9e Extending the elbow

10. Perform all exercises on wrist and fingers:
    a) flex and extend wrist.
    b) abduct and adduct wrist.
    c) flex and extend fingers.
    d) abduct and adduct fingers.
    e) rotate the thumb.
    (Rationale: This maintains strength and flexibility in the wrist and fingers.)

(continued)

11. Exercise the patient's hip and leg:
    a) flex and extend the hip and knee while supporting the leg.
    b) abduct and adduct the hip by moving the straightened leg toward you and then back to median position.

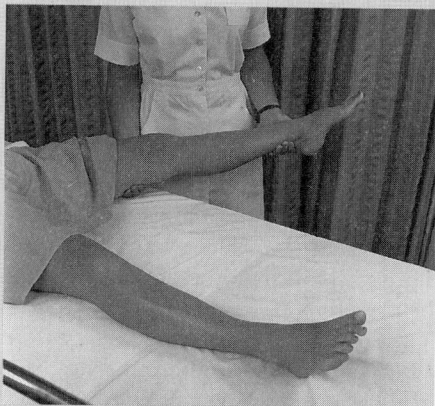

Step 11b   Abducting the hip

c) perform internal and external rotation of the hip joint by turning the leg inward and then outward.
   (Rationale: A contracted hip or fixed knee severely limits ability to ambulate.)
12. Perform exercises on the ankle and foot:
    a) dorsiflex and plantar flex the foot.

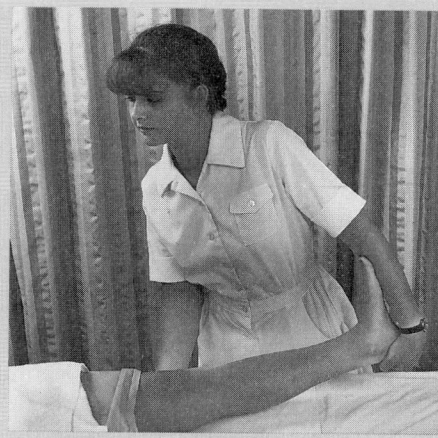

Step 12a   Dorsiflexing the foot

b) abduct and adduct the toes.
c) evert and invert the foot.

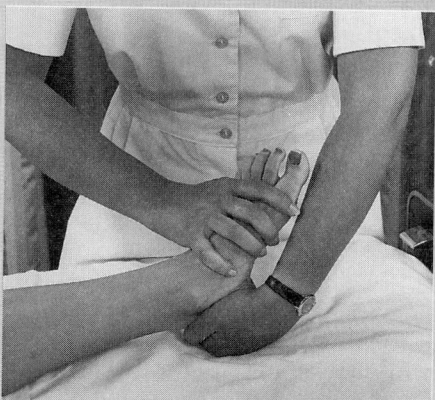

Step 12c   Everting the foot (Photos © B. Proud.)

(Rationale: Feet support body and allow patient to walk.)
13. Move to the other side of the bed and repeat exercises.
    (Rationale: This ensures that all joints are exercised.)
14. Reposition and cover patient. Return bed to low position.
    (Rationale: Repositioning provides for patient comfort. Lowering bed prevents accidents.)
15. Wash hands.
    (Rationale: Handwashing prevents the spread of organisms.)
16. Document completion of PROM exercises.
    (Rationale: Documentation provides ongoing data collection.)

promote joint mobility and speed rehabilitation. The purpose of the machine must be explained to the patient, because the machines can cause some degree of discomfort.

The CPM machine is electric with a padded rack to hold the extremity. The machine is set for the number of movements per minute it is to move, as ordered by the physician. The patient's leg is secured into the rack, with the knee joint far enough away from the end of the rack to allow flexing without rubbing the skin. The call light should be placed within the patient's reach. Instruct the patient to call if there is too much discomfort. You may give a PRN medication for pain approximately 15 minutes before the CPM treatment begins. *(Rationale: Medication may allow freer movement to the affected joint.)*

> **Key Concept**
>
> Do not force joint movement when doing PROM. If the patient complains of extreme pain, *stop* and check with your team leader.

Active Range-of-Motion Exercises

Muscle-Setting Exercise. Muscle-setting *(isometric)* exercises are those that the patient performs by tightening and releasing certain muscle groups. These exercises are helpful for strengthening abdominal, gluteal, and quadriceps muscles necessary for the patient to ambulate. Because the exercises only preserve muscle mass, they are not useful in preventing contractures. Therefore, isometrics are useful in preparing the patient for crutchwalking, maintaining tonus in a casted limb, or teaching bowel training. The routine that achieves the best results is repetition of five sets of exercises, each lasting 5 seconds with 2-minute rest periods between repetitions. (For example, tighten the abdominal muscles; count 1-1,000, 2-1,000, 3-1,000, 4-1,000, 5-1,000. Rest for 2 minutes. Repeat until five sets have been completed.)

Other Bed Exercises. Other exercises include sitting up in bed or a wheelchair. The patient lifts the hips by pushing the hands down into the mattress. For push-up exercises, the patient lies face down with the hands placed flat on the mattress next to the shoulders with the elbows bent. The patient extends the elbows stiffly to raise the head and chest up off the bed. The thigh and leg muscles can be strengthened by having the patient contract the quadriceps femoris, the large muscle on the anterior thigh; the patient will feel as though he or she is pushing the popliteal space behind the knee downward into the mattress and pulling the foot forward. Some of these exercises prepare the patient for wheelchair use or crutchwalking.

Some daily activities can be turned into useful exercise (eg, reaching for objects on the bedside table, pulling the overbed table forward and pushing it away, and brushing the hair). Many patients confined to bed are given a trapeze. The patient can use it to pull up in bed, thus exercising the arms. Usage strengthens muscles, and the patient will often create his or her own exercises when their importance is explained.

The physical therapist may introduce the exercises, but the activities are repeated several times a day, and the nurse must be able to supervise them. Occupational therapy also provides muscle exercises, often for smaller muscle groups.

Positioning for Examinations

Patients are sometimes put into special positions as part of their treatment or examination; many different positions are used for a physical examination, for nursing treatments and tests, and to obtain specimens. Because you will put patients in some of these positions and will see other positions used, you should know how to assist the patient and adjust the necessary drapes. Important positions are horizontal recumbent, dorsal recumbent, prone, Sims', Fowler's, knee-chest, and dorsal lithotomy. Their descriptions, uses, and illustrations are given in Table 43-2.

Preparing the Patient for Examination

Although Chapter 50 describes physical examination in detail, a few hints are included here. Prior to draping the patient for examination, several key points should be carried out by a nurse:

◆ Urge the patient to empty the bladder. *(Rationale: This helps the person feel more relaxed and helps the physician to better palpate the area being examined.)* Collect a specimen for possible laboratory studies. The specimen can always be discarded if not needed.
◆ Encourage the patient to defecate before a rectal examination.
◆ Provide the patient with an examination gown or bath towel to cover the chest.
◆ Provide a bath blanket or sheet for warmth and privacy.
◆ Explain the examination procedure to the patient.
◆ Drape the body appropriately.
◆ Stay with the patient during the examination.

Table 43-2. Patient Positioning for Examinations and Treatments

Horizontal Recumbent Position

Required for most of physical examination. Patient is on back with legs extended. Arms are above head, folded on chest, or alongside body. One small pillow may be used. Cover with bath blanket. *Caution:* May be uncomfortable for a person with back problem.

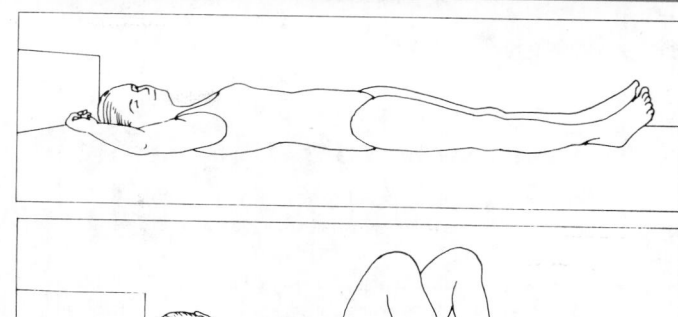

Dorsal Recumbent Position

Used for variety of examinations and procedures. Patient is on back with knees flexed and soles of feet flat on bed. Cover with sheet or bath blanket folded once across chest, second sheet crosswise over thighs and legs. Wrap lower ends of sheet around legs and feet; fold sheet so genital area is easily exposed. Keep patient covered as much as possible.

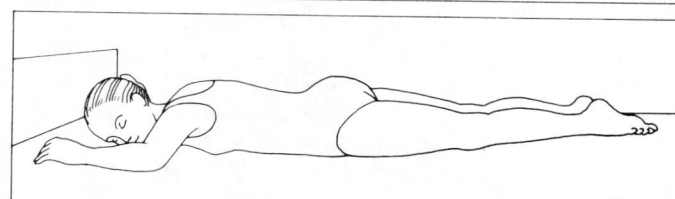

Prone Position

Used to examine spine and back. Patient is on abdomen, head turned to side for comfort. Arms are above head or alongside body. Cover with bath blanket. *Caution:* Unconscious patients, pregnant women, patients with abdominal incisions, or patients with breathing difficulty usually cannot lie in this position.

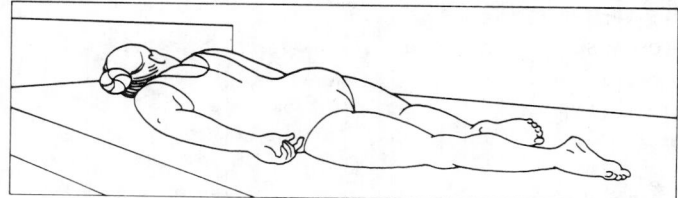

Sims' Position

Used for rectal examination. Patient is on left side with or without pillow under head. Right knee is flexed against abdomen, left knee is flexed slightly, left arm is behind body, and right arm in comfortable position. Cover with bath blanket. *Caution:* Patient with leg injuries or arthritis often cannot assume this position.

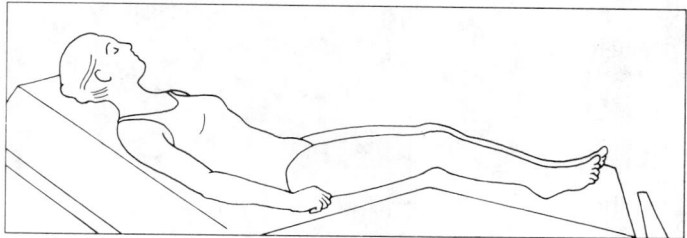

Fowler's Position

Used to promote drainage or make breathing easier. Head rest is adjusted to desired height, and bed section (Gatch bed) is raised slightly under patient's knees. Rolled pillow can be placed between patient's feet and foot of bed as brace. *Caution:* Observe for signs of dizziness or faintness when head is raised.

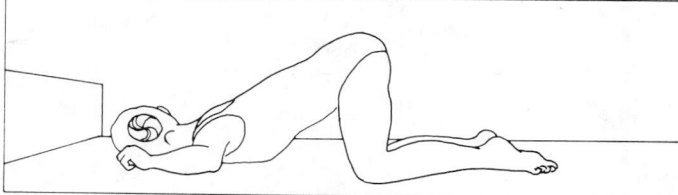

Knee-Chest Position

Used for rectal and vaginal examinations and as treatment to bring uterus into normal position. Patient is on knees with chest resting on bed and elbows rested on bed, or with arms above head. Head is turned to one side. Thighs are straight up and down and lower legs are flat on bed. *Caution:* Patient may become dizzy or faint and fall. Do not leave patient alone.

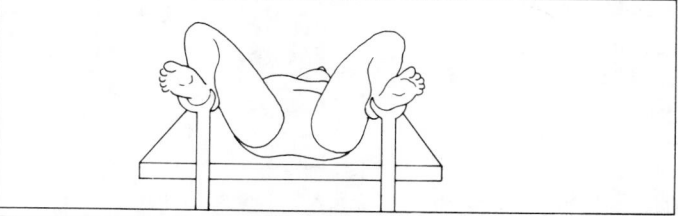

Dorsal Lithotomy Position

Used for examinations of pelvic organs. Similar to dorsal recumbent position, except that patient's legs are well separated and thighs are acutely flexed. Feet are usually placed in stirrups. Keep patient covered as much as possible.

Keys for Review

Key Questions for Critical Thinking

1. Discuss principles of mechanics in relationship to the human body. Discuss each as it pertains to nursing care of patients. Describe how you would teach these principles to a 30-year-old housewife with a toddler.
2. Your patient is recovering from cardiac arrest and has been in bed for two weeks. He will soon be able to get out of bed and learn to walk again. He is curious about various kinds of walking aids. Describe your answer.
3. You are caring for an 88-year-old man in the nursing home. The physical therapist has advised the patient to do isometric exercises. The patient is not sure why exercises are important. Explain to him the purposes of his exercises. Describe how you would lead him through some exercises.

Key Readings

Craven RF, Hirnle CJ. Fundamentals of Nursing: Human Health and Function. Philadelphia, J.B. Lippincott, 1992

Earnest VV. Clinical Skills in Nursing Practice, Ed 2. Philadelphia, J.B. Lippincott, 1993

Smeltzer SC, Bare BG. Brunner and Suddarth's Textbook of Medical Surgical Nursing, Ed 7. Philadelphia, J.B. Lippincott, 1992

Smith S, Duell D. Clinical Nursing Skills: Nursing Process Model, Basic to Advance Skills, Ed 2. Norwalk, CT, Appleton-lange, 1989

Key Readings (continued)

Taber's Cyclopedia Medical Dictionary, Ed 17. Philadelphia, F.A. Davis, 1993

Taylor C, Lillis C, LeMone P. Fundamentals of Nursing: The Art and Science of Nursing Care, Ed 2. Philadelphia, J.B. Lippincott, 1993

Timby BK, Lewis LW: Fundamental Skills and Concepts in Patient Care, Ed 5. Philadelphia, J.B. Lippincott, 1992

Enrichment Key

Leger-Krall S. When restraints become abusive. Nursing 94, March 1994, 24:3, 54–56.

Keys to Learning More

Chapter 44: beds and bedmaking

Chapter 45: skin care

Chapter 49: application of heat and cold

Chapter 50: head-to-toe physical examination

Chapter 52: patient comfort and pain management

Chapter 67: the child with special needs, including orthopedic disorders

Chapter 68: skin disorders

Chapter 70: musculoskeletal disorders

Chapter 89: rehabilitation

44 Beds and Bedmaking

Keys for Learning

Learning Objectives

- State the purposes of hospital bedmaking.
- Demonstrate the ability to make an unoccupied bed, an occupied bed, and a postoperative bed.
- Demonstrate the ability to open a bed for a patient.
- Describe the use of a bed cradle.
- Discuss the need for side rails. Demonstrate the ability to safely adjust side rails.
- Describe the least three other devices that may be added to the hospital bed.

Key Terms

bed cradle	footdrop
CircOLectric bed	Gatch bed
closed bed	mitered
egg crate mattress	open bed

Keys to Understanding This Chapter

Chapter 5: basic human needs
Chapter 15: epithelial tissues and skin
Chapter 29: safety in the healthcare environment
Chapter 30: medical asepsis and universal precautions
Chapter 40: the healthcare environment
Chapter 43: body mechanics and positioning for the nurse and patient

Key Points

- Organize work. Gather all supplies before making the bed. Strip and make one side of the bed at a time to conserve time and energy.
- To prevent spread of microorganisms, never shake linen or put it on the floor.
- Hold soiled linen away from your uniform, and never place soiled linen from one patient's bed on another patient's bed.
- Place soiled linen in a pillow case or on a chair while continuing work.

Key Topics Outline

Bedmaking
Methods of Bedmaking
Attachments and Accessories
Special Beds

Key Learning Activities

- Practice making an unoccupied bed, which includes stripping and replacing linens.
- With your lab partner, practice making an occupied bed.

Key Nursing Procedures

NP 44-1: Making a Closed or Unoccupied Bed
NP 44-2: Making an Occupied Bed

Most hospitalized patients are so ill they are totally or partially confined to bed. The hospital bed is a specialized piece of equipment that aids in safe and convenient patient care. This chapter describes its use.

The bed must be arranged for comfort and good posture. A good bed is durable, lightweight, easy to move, and easy to clean. One modern hospital bed is the **Gatch bed,** equipped with a spring frame and motor so it can be adjusted to different positions. Hi-lo hospital beds are equipped with an electric mechanism to lower and raise the entire bed so the patient can get in and out easily and to lower and raise the head and foot of the bed. The patient who is being encouraged in self-help can operate this mechanism. The **CircOLectric bed** is used occasionally. It makes it possible to place the paralyzed or unconscious patient in an upright position or to turn the patient easily.

Bedmaking

The objective in bedmaking is to make the patient comfortable. This means using clean linen, a tight cover sheet to prevent wrinkles that might irritate the skin, and upper bed clothing that does not weigh on the patient's body or restrict movements but still covers the shoulders. Adjustments in bedmaking may be necessary for comfort and convenience of individual patients and to suit individual patient conditions.

Making the bed is a routine nursing skill that follows the patient's bath or morning care. Exceptions are made if changing the bed may prove harmful to the patient. For example, a patient may be bleeding, may be having a special treatment, or may be too weak or exhausted to be disturbed. The schedule for changing the bed varies with patients and hospital policy. If the sheets are stained, they are changed immediately. In some cases, beds are not changed every day. Even if a bed is not changed, the nurse tucks in sheets and blankets to get rid of wrinkles and fluffs the pillow.

Methods of Bedmaking

It is important for the nurse to know the principles of bedmaking. Good body mechanics are essential. Put them into practice by following the guidelines in Chapter 4.

Making a Closed or Unoccupied Bed

A **closed bed** is made when preparing the unit for a new patient. An unoccupied bed may mean the patient can sit in the chair or walk with help. An **open bed** allows bed linens to be turned down, making it easier for the patient to get into bed. The

bed, the linens are drawn completely up to the top of the bed, with the pillow resting on top of the linens to keep the bed clean. After the bed is made, step back and survey your work to see if the linens are straight, firmly tucked under the mattress, smooth and without wrinkles, and not hanging on the floor. Steps in making a closed or occupied bed are given in Nursing Procedure 44-1.

Making an Occupied Bed

Some patients are unable to get out of bed. This may be the result of their specific medical condition or generalized weakness. To preserve the patient's strength, the nurse may change bed linens with the patient in the bed. Work quickly, and disturb the patient as little as possible. This task of bedmaking may be done alone; however, if the patient is large or the medical condition is unstable, you may ask a coworker to assist you. Nursing Procedure 44-2 gives the steps in making an occupied bed.

This method used to make an occupied bed should require minimum exertion for patient and nurse. Some patients need extra blankets for additional warmth, and some may have fractures or injuries that necessitate their being turned or moved in a special way.

> ### Key Concept
> The patient needs to have a smooth bed for comfort. Any wrinkles or crumbs can make the patient uncomfortable and can cause skin breakdown.

Opening a Bed for a Patient

A bed is opened for a new patient or may be left open when the patient is out of bed for a short time. The skills in opening a bed follow:

◆ Turn the spread down from the top, and fold it around and over the top edge of the blanket. (*Rationale: This protects the blanket, keeps the rougher blanket away from the patient's skin, and makes it easier for the patient to handle the bedclothes.*)
◆ Turn the top bedding down to the foot of the mattress, and fold it back on itself. (*Rationale: This shows the patient that the bed is ready. It is also easier to help the person into bed when it is open.*)
◆ Always leave the bed in low position. (*Rationale: It is vital to prevent falls.*)

Making a Postoperative Bed

When a patient is to return from the operating room or from another procedure that will require lifting him or her into bed, a postoperative bed is often used.

(Text continues on page 506)

Supplies and Equipment

Gloves (optional)
2 sheets (either 2 flat sheets or 1 flat sheet and 1 contour bottom sheet)
Draw sheet (optional)
Blanket
Bedspread
Pillowcases
Linen hamper or bag
Mattress pad
Bedside table or chair

Procedure

1. Gather linens and supplies.
   (Rationale: Organization facilitates performance of the skill.)
2. Wash hands.
   (Rationale: Handwashing prevents the spread of organisms.)
3. Adjust bed to a comfortable height. Remove call bell if attached.
   (Rationale: Bed at proper height prevents back strain.)
4. Wear gloves if linens are soiled. Loosen all soiled linens. Remove, roll up, and place in linen hamper or bag. Never place soiled linens on floor or hold against your uniform.
   (Rationale: Many organisms are present on the floor. Soiled linens from bed or floor contaminate uniform which may come in contact with other patients.)
5. Refold spread or any item that is to be reused and place on table or back of chair.
   (Rationale: Agency policy indicates which linens are reused if not soiled.)
6. Remove soiled pillowcases and place in linen hamper. Move pillows to chair.
   (Rationale: Removing pillows from bed simplifies the bed-making task.)
7. Slide mattress to head of bed. Place mattress pad on bed.
   (Rationale: Moving mattress up provides more foot room for the patient.)
8. Place bottom sheet on bed. Open lengthwise with center fold along center of bed. Fold back upper layer of sheet toward opposite side of bed. Slide sheet upward over top of bed leaving bottom edge of sheet even with the edge of the mattress. If fitted (contour) sheet is used, tuck over mattress at upper and lower end of that side.
   (Rationale: Unfolding sheet in this manner allows bed to be made on one side.)

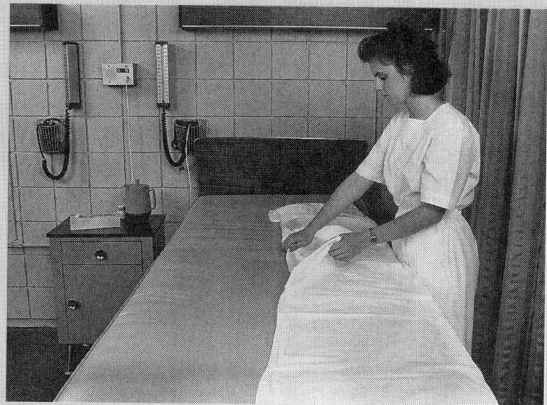

Step 8 Centering the bottom sheet on the bed

9. Tuck sheet securely under the head of the mattress. Make a diagonal or **mitered** corner if sheet is not fitted:
   a) pick up selvage edge with hand nearest the foot of the bed.

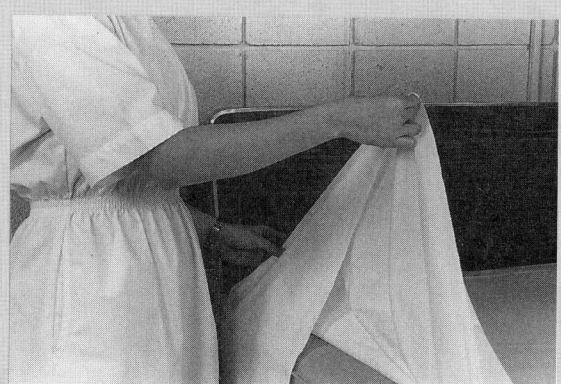

Step 9a Picking up the selvage edge

(continued)

b) lay a triangle back on the bed.

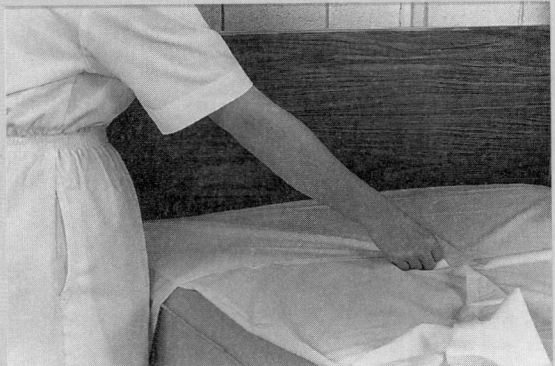

Step 9b   Laying a triangle back on the bed

c) tuck the hanging part of the sheet under the mattress.

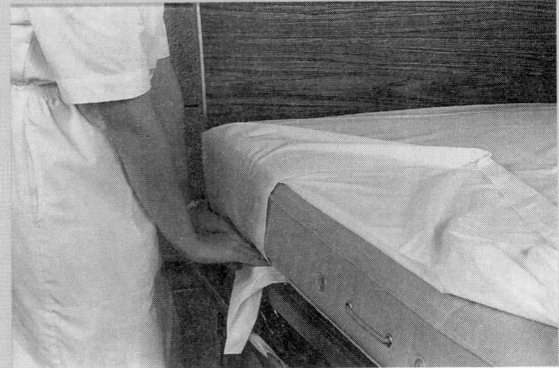

Step 9c   Tucking the hanging part

d) drop the triangle over the side of the bed.

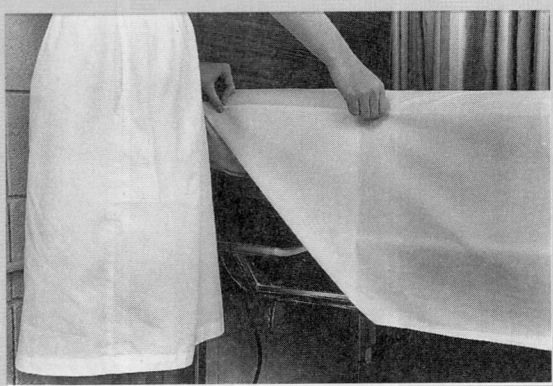

Step 9d   Dropping the triangle over the side of the bed

e) tuck hanging edge under the mattress.
(Rationale: Mitered corner has neat appearance and keeps sheet securely under the mattress.)

10. Tuck sheet under entire side of bed.
(Rationale: Bottom sheet is secured on one side of bed.)

11. Place draw sheet on bed if used, folded in half, with fold in center of bed. Lift top half backward toward other side of bed. Tuck draw sheet under mattress.
(Rationale: Draw sheet is additional protection for the bed and serves as a lifting or turning sheet for an immobile patient.)

12. Place top sheet on bed, centering in the same manner as bottom sheet. Upper hem of top sheet should be level with top of mattress. Drop lower end of sheet over end of mattress.
(Rationale: Staying on one side of the bed until it is completely made saves steps and time.)

13. Cover top sheet with blanket and/or bedspread. Tuck all these together under bottom of mattress. Miter the corner.
(Rational: Tucking all these together saves time and provides a neater appearance.)

14. Move to the other side of the bed. Tuck in bottom linens in the same manner. Brace knee against bed and pull draw sheet taut prior to tucking under mattress. Smooth top sheet, blanket and/or bedspread and secure under mattress. Miter corners. Fold back cuff at head of bed with sheet and bedspread if patient will be returning to bed. (Pull covers up to top of bed when making a closed bed.)
(Rationale: Blanket provides warmth and bedspread ensures a neat appearance. Cuff makes it easier to fold the linens back.)

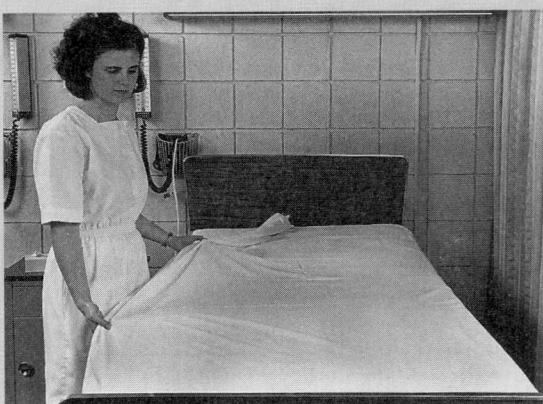

Step 14   Pulling the drawsheet taut

(continued)

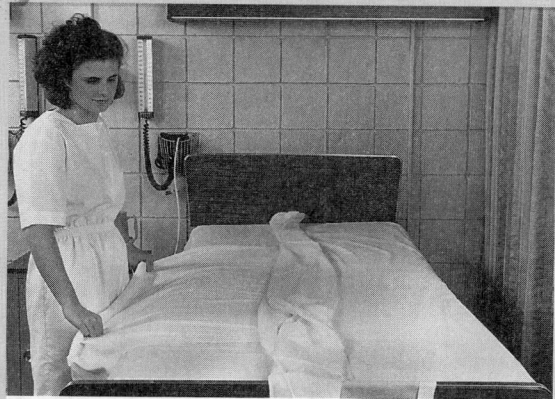

Step 14   Smoothing the top sheet

15. Put a clean pillow case on the pillow:
    a) rest the pillow on a flat surface.
    b) grasp the pillow case in the center on the closed end.
    c) turn the pillowcase back over your hand.
    d) grasp pillow through the pillow case.
    e) pull pillow case over pillow.
    f) adjust pillow case smoothly over pillow. An alternate method is to put one hand inside the pillow case and pull the pillow corners into the corners of the pillow case.
    (Rationale: Using this method minimizes shaking of the pillow excessively.)

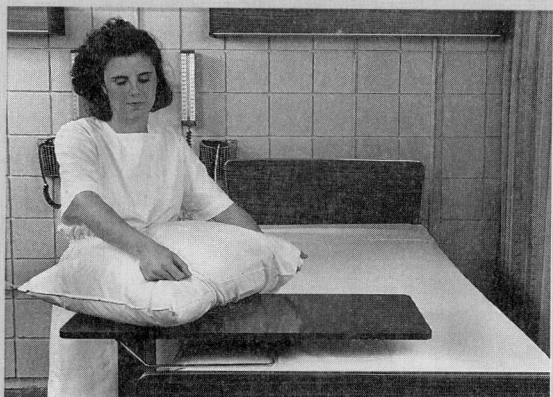

Step 15   Sliding the clean pillow case over the pillow (Photos © B. Proud.)

16. Place pillow at top of bed in center with open end away from door.
    (Rationale: Pillow is comfort measure for patient. Open end may collect dust or organisms.)
17. Make a toe pleat at the foot of the bed:
    a) for a horizontal pleat gather the linens to make a fold approximately 5 to 10 cm (2 to 4 inches) across the foot of the bed.
    b) for a vertical pleat gather the linens to make a fold approximately 5 to 10 cm (2 to 4 inches) perpendicular (up and down) to the foot of the bed.
    (Rationale: Toe pleats allow for freedom of movement of the feet.)
18. Fan-fold the top of the linens to the bottom third of the bed.
    (Rationale: This allows patient easier entry into the bed.)
19. Replace call signal on the bed and secure it in place.
    (Rationale: This allows patient to call for the nurse.)
20. Move overbed table next to the bed.
    (Rationale: Bedside necessities will be within easy reach for the patient.)
21. Return bed to low position if patient is ambulatory or high position if patient is returning to the room by stretcher.
    (Rationale: Bed is prepared for patient's return.)
22. Discard linens appropriately. Wash hands.
    (Rationale: Handwashing and proper linen disposal prevent the spread of organisms.)

Pediatric Nursing Alert

When changing linens on a crib, leave crib sides up in high position.

Making an Occupied Bed

Equipment and Supplies

Gloves (optional)
2 sheets (either 2 flat sheets or 1 flat sheet and 1 contour bottom sheet)
Drawsheet (if needed)
Blanket
Bedspread
Pillowcases
Linen hamper or bag
Mattress pad
Bedside table or chair
Bath blanket (optional)

Procedure

1. Gather linens and supplies.
    (Rationale: Organization facilitates performance of the skill.)
2. Explain procedure to patient.
    (Rationale: Providing information fosters patient co-operation and understanding.)
3. Wash hands prior to putting on gloves.
    (Rationale: Handwashing prevents the spread of organisms. Gloves act as a barrier and should be worn if linens are soiled with body fluids or drainage.)
4. Adjust bed to a comfortable height. Remove call bell if attached to linens. Lower side rail on near side while keeping the other side rail raised.
    (Rationale: Bed at proper height prevents back strain. Raised side rail prevents the patient from falling out of bed.)
5. Lower the head of the bed if patient is able to tolerate this.
    (Rationale: Bed is easier to make when it is in the flat position.)
6. Loosen top bed linens. Remove spread, refold if it will be used again, and place on table or back of chair.
    (Rationale: Agency policy indicates which linens are reused if not soiled.)
7. Place bath blanket over the top sheet and ask patient to hold onto the upper edge. Remove the top sheet and place in linen hamper or bag. If bath blanket is not available, leave the top sheet in place.
    (Rationale: Bath blanket or top sheet keep the patient warm and protect privacy.)

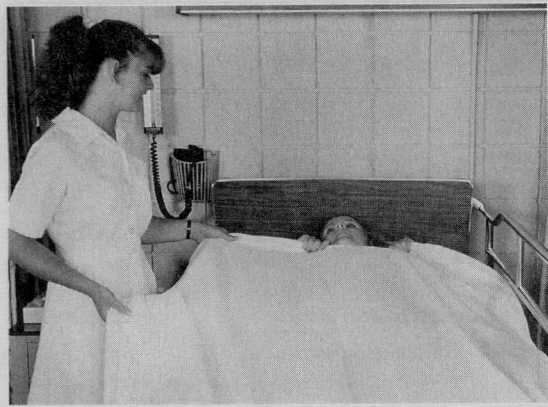

Step 7   Placing the bath blanket

8. Slide mattress to head of bed if necessary. Request assistance to do this.
    (Rationale: Moving mattress up provides more foot room for the patient.)
9. Assist patient to turn toward the other side of the bed. Adjust the pillow. The patient can help by hanging onto the side rail, if able.
    (Rationale: Moving the patient as close to the other side of the bed as possible gives you more room to make the bed.)
10. Loosen bottom bed linens. Fan-fold soiled linens from the side of the bed and wedge them close to the patient. Leave mattress pad in place unless soiled.
    (Rationale: Placing folded soiled linen close to the patient allows more space to place the clean bottom sheets.)

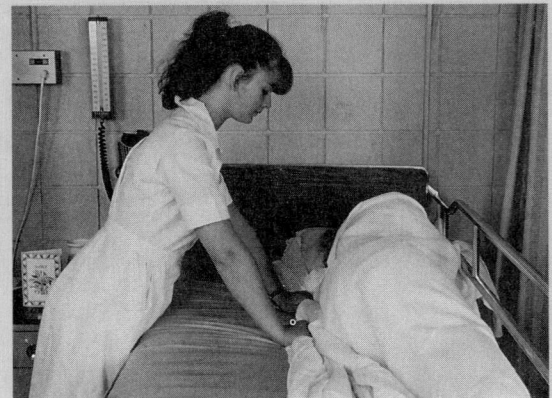

Step 10   Fan-folding soiled linens toward the patient

(continued)

11. Place clean bottom sheet on the bed folded length-wise with the center fold as close to the patient's back as possible. Adjust sheet, miter upper corner, and place draw sheet (optional) as in Procedure 44-1, steps 8, 9, and 10. If fitted (contour) sheet is used, tuck over mattress at upper and lower end. Fold upper half of sheet and drawsheet back toward center and tuck under patient and under soiled linens.
(Rationale: Soiled linens can easily be removed and clean linens are positioned to make the other side of the bed.)

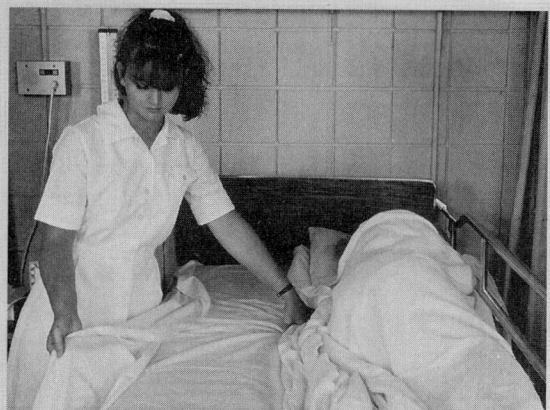

Step 11 Unfolding the clean linen (Photos © B. Proud.)

12. Raise the side rail. Move to other side of bed. Help patient to roll over folded linen to other side of bed. Lower side rail on your side. Readjust pillow and bath blanket.
(Rationale: Side rails maintain the patient's safety. Moving the patient to the other side of the bed allows the bed to be made on that side.)

13. Remove the soiled bottom linens. Hold away from uniform and place in hamper or bag. Straighten the mattress pad.
(Rationale: Soiled linens can contaminate nurse's uniform which may come in contact with other patients.)

14. Grasp clean linens and gently pull out from under patient and spread over unmade side of bed. Pull taut and tuck in bottom sheet and miter corner. If a contour sheet is used, tuck in both the top and bottom corners. Brace knee against the bed and pull bottom sheet and drawsheet taut prior to tucking under mattress.
(Rationale: Wrinkled linens can cause skin irritation.)

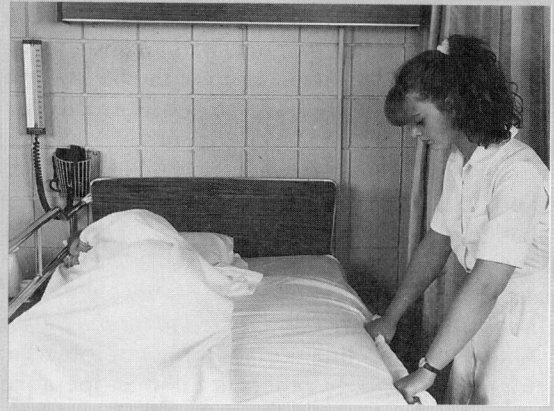

Step 14 Tucking in the bottom sheets

15. Assist patient back to center of bed. Remove pillow. Replace soiled pillow case with clean one and return pillow to bed under patient's head.
(Rationale: Pillow is a comfort measure for patient.)

16. Place the top sheet over the bath blanket and ask patient to hold onto upper edge. Remove bath blanket and place in linen hamper or bag or in patient's closet. Unfold spread over top sheet. Tuck lower ends securely under mattress and miter corners.
(Rationale: Tucking these together saves time and provides a neat, tight corner. Bath blanket can be reused.)

17. Turn the top edge of the spread back over the sheet.
(Rationale: This provides a neat appearance.)

18. Make toe pleat or loosen top linens over patient's feet (see Procedure 44-1, step 17).
(Rationale: Toe pleats allow for freedom of movement of the feet.)

19. Raise side rail. Lower the bed and adjust the head to a comfortable position. Replace call signal on bed.
(Rationale: These measures provide for patient safety.)

20. Discard linens appropriately. Remove gloves and wash hands.
(Rationale: Handwashing and proper disposal of soiled linens prevents the spread of organisms.)

◆ If the patient has had surgery, the entire bed should be made up with clean linen.

◆ Wash your hands. *(Rationale: To help prevent postoperative infection, as much contamination should be removed from the area as possible.)*

◆ Make the bottom (or foundation) of the bed as you normally would. The postoperative bed usually requires a draw sheet under the patient's hips. You also may wish to place several disposable pads on the bed. Usually another draw sheet is placed under the patient's head. *(Rationale: If the patient has emesis or is incontinent of urine or stool, it will not be necessary to change the entire bed, only the soiled drawsheets. They may also be used to lift the patient.)*

◆ In some cases, top linens are simply fan folded to the foot of the bed. In others, a full postoperative bed is made. In this event, put the top linens over the foundation, but do not tuck them in. Fold down the top as you would for an occupied bed. Then fold the bottom of the linens up so that the fold is even with the bottom of the mattress. Do not tuck the linens in. Fanfold the top linens to the side so that they are on the opposite side from where the litter with the patient will be placed. Alternatively, the linens may be fanfolded to the foot of the bed. You may leave a tab on top for easy grasping. *(Rationale: Keeping the linens all to one side or folded to the bottom keeps them out of the way so that the semiconscious patient can easily be transferred into the bed. The tab on top makes it easy to pull the covers over the patient once he or she is in bed.)* Figure 44-1 illustrates one type of completed postoperative bed.

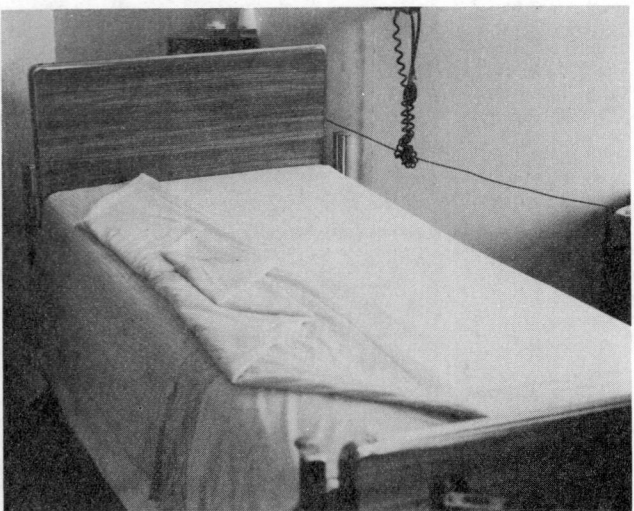

Figure 44-1. Example of one type of postoperative bed. Covers are folded out of the way so the patient can easily be helped into bed. The bedside table and other pieces of furniture also are pushed out of the way. (Photo by Paul Montague.)

◆ Have one or two pillows available, but do not put them on the bed. *(Rationale: Having a pillow may be contraindicated for a patient; usually the physician or charge nurse will determine when it is safe for the patient to have one.)*

◆ Be sure all furniture is out of the way so the litter can be brought to the bedside easily. Also, be sure the call light is available, but do not put it on the bed until the patient is in bed.

◆ For the convenience and safety of the postoperative patient, the following items should always be available: tissues, an emesis basin, a blood pressure cuff and stethoscope, a blood pressure graph, an "intake and output" sheet, an intravenous (IV) stand, side rails, and other items according to the patient's specific requirements. You will need to know what surgical procedure your patient has had before you can determine what special equipment is needed. You also will learn from the nurse's report whether your patient needs such items as suction machine, a chest drainage setup, or other special equipment.

Attachments and Accessories

A Bed Cradle

A **bed cradle** is a frame used to prevent the bedclothes from touching all or part of the patient's body. It is used for fractures, extensive burns, and open or painful wounds. A wide cradle fits across the bed. A narrow one fits along the bed lengthwise; it can be used over one arm or leg. Bed cradles are usually made of metal or plastic. Bed linens are arranged over the cradle. In some instances, the linens may be pinned to the cradle or frame. The linens should be left long enough at the top to cover the patient's shoulders comfortably. Side rails should remain up for safety. Patients are encouraged not to adjust the bed controls for fear of displacing the cradle and causing injury to themselves.

Nursing Skill
Using a Bed Cradle

Supplies and Equipment

Linens used for changing a bed
Extra top sheet
Extra blanket
Extra bedspread
Bath blanket

Procedure

◆ Make up the bed as for any patient. *(Rationale: A smooth foundation is especially important for the patient who spends a great deal of time in bed.)*

- Tuck the top sheet under the foot of the bed. *(Rationale: To hold it in place.)*
- Draw the top sheet over the cradle. *(Rationale: The cradle protects the patient's limb.)*
- Place another top sheet over the first top sheet, overlapping the two as much as is necessary. *(Rationale: This will make the linens long enough to cover the patient's shoulders when the bed is completed.)*
- Hold the bottom of the second sheet and the top of the first sheet, with hems lined up, off the bed. Roll them over each other, making a flat fold crosswise to the bed. Repeat this process as many times as is necessary to obtain the correct length of sheeting. *(Rationale: The goal is to keep the patient warm. The double fold will hold the sheets together, and they will seem like one long sheet.)*
- Tuck the blanket in at the bottom of the bed and pull it up over the bed cradle. Add a second blanket, and fold it over in the same manner as you did the sheets. Follow the same procedure for the bedspread, folding the covers at the head of the bed as for an open bed. *(Rationale: When all three layers of covers are folded together, the covers will be long enough to cover the patient's shoulders and will be secure enough to be pulled up without separating.)*
- Place a bath blanket under the cradle, covering the patient as much as is tolerated and desired. *(Rationale: This will further prevent chilling and discomfort.)*
- Be sure the signal light is within reach of the patient. *(Rationale: The person needs to be able to call you for help. The cradle restricts the patient's movements, so he or she will need assistance with daily needs.)*
- If you are using a cradle that applies heat, you will need special instructions. *(Rationale: Burns must be prevented.)*

Side Rails

Side rails not only prevent the patient from falling out of bed, but also are assistive devices for changing positions while the patient is in bed. Sometimes, however, bed rails confuse and alarm elderly or confused patients. Most facilities have a standard policy regarding the use of side rails. Make it your practice to be aware of these policies and follow the protocol, always keeping in mind the safety of your patient and using nursing judgment regarding safety restraints of any type.

It is natural for a patient to resent side rails. Most people have a fear of being shut in or being treated as irresponsible. Explain to the patient and family that side rails are used for protection. If it is necessary to protect the patient from pressure or possible injury, pad the bedsides with a mattress pad, bath blanket, seizure pads, or pillows. Restless, confused, or seizuring patients may press or throw themselves against the hard metal.

Other Equipment

The Footboard. A footboard may be attached to the foot of the bed to prevent a deformity called **footdrop.**

The Bed Board. A board may be placed under the mattress to provide greater support.

The Trapeze. A trapeze may be necessary so that the patient can pull up to a sitting position. These devices are usually attached to a large overhead frame, which is attached to the bed.

Traction Equipment. The patient may be placed in traction. The ropes and pulleys must be maintained in straight alignment. Traction weights should not be removed without supervision of the instructor or charge nurse. (See Chapter 70.)

The IV Stand. Most hospital beds are equipped with a means for attaching a standard that holds bags for IV or blood therapy.

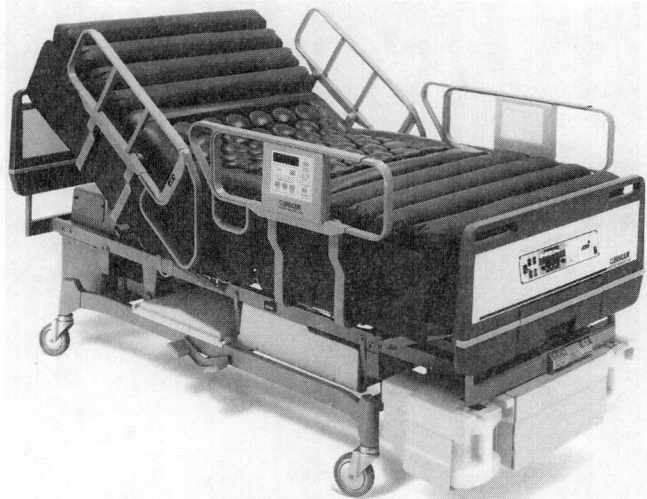

Figure 44-2. This special bed not only greatly lessens the possibility of pressure area development, but also manages incontinence in the immobile patient. It provides drainage for body fluids into the receptacle at the foot of the bed, where it can be measured. It also provides a cleansing and vacuuming system for skin care. (Photo courtesy of Support Systems International Inc. and Hillenbrand Industries, Batesville, IN.)

The Emergency Headboard. Most hospital beds are equipped with a detachable headboard or separate cardiopulmonary resuscitation (CPR) board that may be placed under the patient in the event that emergency CPR is needed.

Special Beds

Sometimes the patient requires a special type of bed or mattress. Examples include the **egg crate mattress**, which is foam rubber and shaped like an egg carton and the flotation mattress or pad (for a specific area of the body). These mattresses provide comfort, prevent skin breakdown, and promote cleanliness.

Several types of beds are designed for management of the immobile patient. Many of these are based on the theory of air fluidization. The bed continuously changes its configuration, so pressure is not on one body area for more than a few minutes. One of these beds is designed to manage the immobile patient who is incontinent. In addition to relieving pressure, the bed detects moisture, sounds an alarm, and captures and drains moisture into a receptacle where it can be measured. It also provides a charcoal filter to eliminate odors, a warm water spray for cleansing the patient, and a suction tip to pick up excess moisture. This bed helps turn the patient, so the nurse's hands remain free for patient care (Fig. 44-2).

Keys for Review

Key Questions for Critical Thinking

1. Relate the importance of good body mechanics to bedmaking.
2. The patient argues about bedrails being placed in an "up" position. Describe your explanation of bedrail use to the patient and the family. Discuss the possible need for restraints also.
3. Identify other attachments for the bed, explaining their use and advantages and disadvantages.

Key Readings

Craven RF, Hirnle CJ. Fundamentals of Nursing: Human Health and Function. Philadelphia, J.B. Lippincott, 1992

Earnest VV. Clinical Skills in Nursing Practice, Ed 2 Philadelphia, J.B. Lippincott, 1993

Key Readings (continued)

Smith S, Duell D. Clinical Nursing Skills: Nursing Process Model, Basic to Advanced Skills, Ed 2. Norwalk, CT, Appleton-Lange, 1989

Swearingen PL. Photo Atlas of Nursing Procedures, Ed 2. Redwood City, CA, Addition-Wesley Nursing, 1991

Taylor C, Lillis C, LeMone P. Fundamentals of Nursing: The Art and Science of Nursing Care, Ed 2. Philadelphia, J.B. Lippincott, 1993

Keys to Learning More

Chapter 45: personal hygiene and skin care

Chapter 52: patient comfort and pain management

Chapter 65: nursing care of children

Chapter 68: skin disorders

Chapter 70: musculoskeletal disorders, including management of traction

45 Personal Hygiene and Skin Care

Keys for Learning

Learning Objectives

- State at least five reasons for giving mouth care to the patient.
- Demonstrate the ability to help a patient do oral self-care.
- Demonstrate the ability to clean and care for dentures.
- Describe and demonstrate skill in caring for the patient's fingernails, toenails, and hair.
- Describe how to assist a male patient to shave.
- Describe and demonstrate skills in giving a backrub.
- State three types of cleansing baths and the situation in which each is used.
- Demonstrate the ability to safely assist a patient with each type of cleansing bath.
- Discuss causes, development, and care of pressure areas and skin breakdown.

Key Terms

cerumen

debridement

decubitus ulcers

eschar

nits

pediculosis

pressure sores

pyorrhea

sloughing

sordes

Keys to Understanding This Chapter

Chapter 5: basic needs of individuals

Chapter 6: obtaining optimum health

Chapter 15: anatomy and physiology of the integumentary system

Chapter 17: anatomy and physiology of the musculoskeletal system

Chapter 30: medical asepsis and universal precautions

Chapter 38: signs and symptoms of illness or injury

Chapter 43: body mechanics and positioning

Key Points

- The patient should be encouraged to provide as much personal hygiene self-care as possible.
- The skin is one of the body's defenses against disease and infection.
- Certain conditions, such as hemorrhage, heart attack, and phlebitis, contraindicate vigorous rubbing of the skin and scalp.
- Shampooing the patient's hair allows the nurse to inspect the scalp for disease.
- The backrub relaxes the patient and provides an opportunity for the nurse to observe the patient's skin.
- The patient's position should be changed frequently to relieve pressure.
- The bed bath provides an opportunity for the nurse to observe the patient's skin.
- Aggressive nursing care is required if a patient shows any sign of skin breakdown.

Key Topics Outline

Care of Mouth, Eyes, and Ears
  Oral Hygiene
  Routine Eye Care
  Ear Care
Grooming
Hair Care
  Daily Hair Care
  The Shampoo
Skin Care
  The Backrub
  The Hand Massage
  Bathing
  The Bed Bath
  Skin Breakdown and Healing

It is important for people to have personal cleanliness to be more comfortable. This chapter describes how to assist patients to meet this need when they cannot do this alone.

Care of Mouth, Eyes, and Ears

Proper mouth care is especially important in the ill person for several reasons.

◆ Many disease organisms enter the body through the mouth.
◆ Food particles lodged between the teeth cause decay, breath odor (*halitosis*), and inflammation of the tooth sockets (**pyorrhea**).
◆ Some illnesses cause irritation or dryness or brownish deposits on the tongue and the mucous membranes of the mouth.
◆ Some infections of the gums are communicable.
◆ A mouth condition can interfere with a person's appetite and with proper nutrition.
◆ Some oral conditions cause infection or pain in other parts of the body.
◆ Breath odors or decayed teeth make people self-conscious.

Oral Hygiene

Some people have not learned good oral health habits. You can help them by teaching them. The patient who learns to perform good oral hygiene in the hospital may continue to do so at home. Teach the patient:

◆ How to do proper oral hygiene
◆ That good oral hygiene improves appearance
◆ That good oral hygiene improves appetite and makes food taste better
◆ That total health is improved by healthy teeth and gums

Offer the patient the opportunity to brush the teeth before and after each meal and in the morning and evening. In caring for the patient's mouth, observe its condition and that of the teeth and record the effect of brushing. Note on the chart such factors as bleeding, swelling, and unusual mouth odor. If the gums or teeth are unusually sensitive, it may be necessary to use applicators or a tongue depressor wrapped in gauze, rather than a toothbrush, for oral hygiene. While assisting the patient, foster good future self-care.

Assisting With Routine Daily Mouth Care. Assemble all supplies and equipment before assisting the patient. Disposable gloves should be worn by the nurse as a protection against body fluids and microorganisms.

◆ Assist patient to a comfortable upright position.
◆ Protect the gown and bedclothing with a towel.
◆ See that the patient brushes the teeth effectively by placing the bristles at a 45° angle against the teeth. The tips of the bristles are directed under the gum line; moving the bristles back and forth using a vibrating or jiggling motion until all outer and inner surfaces of the teeth and gums are cleaned. The biting surfaces of the teeth and the tongue are brushed next. (*Rationale: This cleans all surfaces and stimulates the gums.*)
◆ Assist the patient to floss the teeth. Teach the technique of moving the floss on the outer edge of each tooth surface between teeth. (*Rationale: Prevent cutting gums with floss.*)
◆ Observe the condition of the teeth, gums, and tongue.
◆ Caution the patient not to swallow the mouthwash.
◆ Wipe the mouth and chin. Rinse the toothbrush and put away supplies.
◆ Remove gloves and wash your hands.
◆ Document procedure.

The Patient Who Needs Special Mouth Care. Some patients will need assistance with mouth care. Special mouth care is needed if:

◆ Brownish material (**sordes**) has collected on the tongue and teeth (caused by some illnesses)
◆ The patient breathes through the mouth
◆ The patient cannot take fluids by mouth or has fluids restricted
◆ The patient needs to be encouraged to take food (cleansing the mouth before meals makes food more palatable)
◆ The patient is unresponsive or paralyzed

Hygiene procedures will sometimes remove oral secretions from the dependent patient and thus help to prevent choking. In such cases, special mouth care is needed often. In the unresponsive patient who is breathing through the mouth, for example, special oral hygiene is often ordered every hour (spec OH qh).

Each clinical facility differs in its procedures regarding special mouth care and the time it is given. A basic procedure is given in Nursing Procedure 45-1.

Giving mouth care to unresponsive patients is important because their mouths become dry and are open portals for infection. Position the unresponsive patient in a side-lying position with the head of the bed slightly lowered. In this position, gravity causes saliva to run out of the mouth and prevents the patient from choking. This position also allows for the patient to be suctioned. Inspection of the mucosa of the mouth and the gums may be done while giving oral hygiene.

The Patient Who Wears Dentures. A patient's privacy should be respected when the dentures are cleaned. If the dentures are left out of the mouth, put them in an opaque container, preferably covered, out of sight. Keep them in water. Dentures must be kept moist to preserve their fit and general quality.

Wash your hands carefully before and after handling dentures. Wear gloves. Handle dentures carefully. Dentures are fragile and expensive. You can avoid breakage by holding them over a basin of water with a washcloth folded in the bottom. Do not hold them over a hard surface. Label the denture container and take care not to lose them.

If a patient constantly removes dentures, look for an irritated area in the patient's mouth. The dentures may fit poorly. Poorly fitting dentures are often the reason for poor eating habits and poor nutrition.

The mouth needs the same care when dentures are worn as it does with natural teeth. Specially designed brushes and preparations for soaking dentures are available to remove deposits. Dentures are brushed in the same way as are natural teeth. Be sure to rinse them. The denture cleaner may have a disagreeable taste.

Most dentists encourage their patients to wear their dentures all the time. If dentures are removed for long periods, the gum line changes and the dentures do not fit. If the dentures must be removed, they should never be stored in cups or glasses that are used for drinking because they may be accidentally swallowed or cause the patient to choke.

Remove dentures if a patient is unresponsive, irrational, having seizures, or going to the operating room. If dentures are removed, document that fact.

Nursing Skill
Caring for Dentures

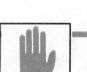

Supplies and Equipment
Gloves
Tissue or gauze square
Denture container
Washcloth
Toothbrush
Denture cleaner
Tap water
Mouthwash
Curved emesis basin
Towel

Procedure

1. Position patient in upright or side-lying position.
2. Wash hands and don gloves. *(Rationale: Protect the nurse from infection.)*
3. With tissue or gauze square, grasp the upper plate with thumb and index finger. Gently move the denture up and down. *(Rationale: Break the suction that holds the denture in place.)*
4. Remove the upper plate from the mouth and place it in the denture container. *(Rationale: Dentures must be protected from breakage.)*
5. Remove the lower plate from the mouth by turning it to a slight angle. *(Rationale: Break suction to remove.)*
6. Place the lower plate in the denture container. *(Rationale: Dentures must be protected from breakage.)*
7. Carry denture container carefully to sink. *(Rationale: Dentures must be protected from breakage.)*
8. Place washcloth in the sink or in the emesis basin. *(Rationale: This will prevent damage if dentures are dropped.)*
9. Pick up dentures one plate at a time and scrub with denture cleaner that has been applied to the toothbrush.
10. Rinse dentures with tap water. *(Rationale: Remove food particles and denture cleaner.)*
11. Soak dentures in commercially prepared solution at the patient's request.
12. Rinse with tap water. *(Rationale: Remove solution.)*
13. Inspect dentures for breaks, rough edges, missing teeth, and other damage.
14. Inspect mucosa of the patient's mouth for redness or irritation. *(Rationale: Dentures may rub and be uncomfortable. It is important to locate irritation immediately.)*
15. Assist patient to rinse the mouth with mouthwash. *(Rationale: This is refreshing.)*
16. Apply denture adhesive, if the patient requests this. Return dentures to the mouth, one plate at a time. Hold plates at a slight angle while inserting. *(Rationale: Prevent injury to the lips.)*
17. Wipe patient's mouth and chin with towel. *(Rationale: Always keep the patient as comfortable as possible.)*
18. If the patient chooses not to wear the dentures or is unable to wear them, store the dentures covered with water in the denture container. *(Rationale: Moisture helps preserve dentures.)*
19. Label the container with the patient's name and room number. *(Rationale: Identification is important if dentures are misplaced.)*
20. Remove and discard gloves and wash hands. *(Rationale: Prevent spread of infection.)*
21. Document the procedure on the patient's record.

Giving Special Mouth Care

Supplies and Equipment

Gloves
Toothbrush or sponge toothette
Tongue blade padded with 4 × 4 gauze sponge
Water, mouthwash, or hydrogen peroxide (H_2O_2)
Towel
Emesis basin
Water-soluble lubricant for lips
Suction catether with suction apparatus (optional)

Procedure

1. Gather supplies.
   (Rationale: Organization facilitates performance of skill.)
2. Explain procedure to patient.
   (Rationale: Providing information fosters patient cooperation.)
3. Wash hands prior to putting on gloves.
   (Rationale: Handwashing prevents the spread of organisms. Gloves act as a barrier.)
4. Close the curtain or door to the room.
   (Rationale: This protects the patient's privacy.)
5. Raise the bed to a comfortable height. Lower the near side rail. Turn patient on his or her side toward the nurse with the head tilted down toward mattress.
   (Rationale: Bed at proper height and patient closer to nurse prevents back strain. Head tilted downward encourages fluid to drain out of mouth.)
6. Place towel and emesis basin under patient's chin. Have suction catheter and apparatus available if needed.
   (Rationale: Towel protects the patient and bed. Emesis basin and suction equipment facilitate drainage from mouth.)
7. Open the patient's mouth and insert padded tongue blade toward back molar area. Nurse's fingers should never be inserted in patient's mouth.
   (Rationale: Tongue blade assists in keeping the mouth open. As a reflex mechanism, the patient may bite the nurse's fingers if they are placed in the mouth.)

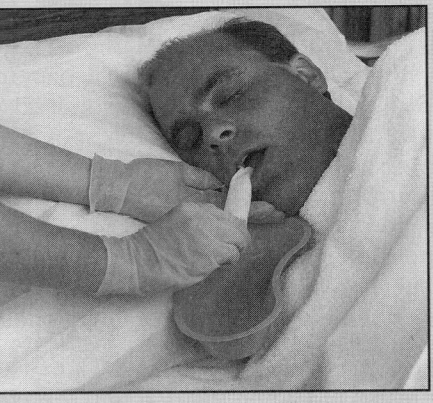

Step 7 Positioning the mouth open with a padded tongue blade

8. Dip toothette sponge, soft toothbrush, or another padded tongue blade in water, mouthwash, or diluted hydrogen peroxide. Move back and forth gently across teeth and chewing areas. Cleanse roof of mouth and inner cheek area.
   (Rationale: Friction cleanses the teeth. Cleaning solutions aid in removing residue on teeth and softening encrusted areas.)

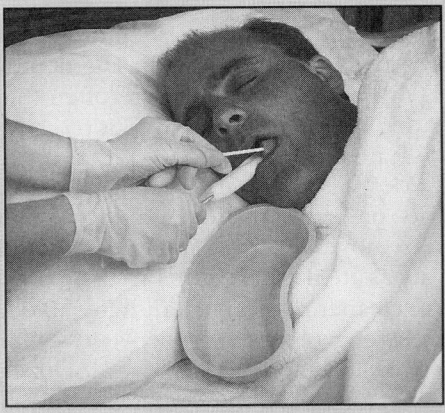

Step 8 Cleansing the teeth and mouth with a toothette sponge

9. Rinse areas using clean toothette or padded tongue blade in moistened water. Suction any drainage if necessary.
   (Rationale: Rinsing or suctioning removes cleaning solution and debris.)
10. Apply water-soluble lubricant to lips.
    (Rationale: This prevents lips from drying or cracking.)
11. Reposition patient. Lower bed and raise side rail.
    (Rationale: This measure provides for patient's comfort and safety.)

12. Remove gloves and wash hands.
    (Rationale: Handwashing prevents the spread of organisms.)
13. Document assessments made during mouth care on chart.
    (Rationale: Documentation provides coordination of care.)

Routine Eye Care

As a result of decreased function of the lacrimal ducts, dried secretions may accumulate on the lids and lashes of the patient's eyes. These secretions can be removed by applying a cotton ball or gauze square moistened with sterile water or normal saline to the eyelids. Special eye care must be provided for the patient who cannot blink. Care of the prosthetic eye is discussed in Chapter 73.

The following routine eye care is given:

♦ Wash hands and don gloves.
♦ Clean the eyes with sterile water or normal saline solution and cotton balls or gauze square.
♦ Wipe the eyelid from the inner canthus (next to nose) to the outer canthus. *(Rationale: Prevent reinfection or contamination of the eye.)*
♦ Repeat steps on other eye using clean supplies.

If the patient wears contact lenses:

♦ Determine type of contact lens worn by patient and the patient's usual cleaning practices.
♦ Provide necessary materials.
♦ Notify the charge nurse or team leader if the patient is unable to remove the lens by himself or herself.
♦ If lenses are removed, they must be stored according to the manufacturer's specifications. Be sure to label *separate* containers for *each eye* and include the patient's name and room number.

Special eye care in the patient who cannot blink includes:

♦ Clean the eyes with sterile water or normal saline solution with a cotton ball or gauze square.
♦ Wipe from the inner canthus outward.
♦ Use a clean cotton ball or gauze on each wipe. *(Rationale: Prevent cross-infection.)*
♦ Instill lubricating drops in the eye or ointment into the lower lids as ordered by the physician. *(Rationale: Keeps eyes moist.)*

♦ Close the patient's eyelids.
♦ Cover the eye with a saline soaked eye pad, if ordered.
♦ Document all procedures on the patient record.

Ear Care

The ears are cleaned during the bed bath. **Cerumen** (ear wax) may need to be removed to prevent hearing difficulty. *Be sure to receive special instruction before doing wax removal.* Patients should be warned never to use bobby pins, Q-Tips, or toothpicks to clean the ears. These objects can injure the ear canal or puncture the eardrum.

The hearing aid is a battery-operated, sound-amplifying device used by people who have impaired hearing ability. It consists of an ear piece that fits into the ear and amplifies sounds. Hearing aids may be very small and may fit entirely into the outer ear.

The nurse may be required to help care for the hearing aid.

♦ Clean the ear piece regularly with saline or the prescribed solution (to prevent buildup of cerumen).
♦ Check and replace batteries regularly.
♦ Adjust volume to meet the individual's needs.
♦ Turn off aid when not being used.
♦ Remove batteries if aid is not used for extended periods.
♦ Do not clean with alcohol.
♦ Avoid exposure to heat and moisture.
♦ Turn volume down completely before inserting aid into ear.

Grooming

Caring for the Fingernails

The patient's general condition and health habits affect the nail condition. Brittle, broken nails may be due to improper diet or fever. Emotional tension may cause nail or cuticle biting. Some occupations cause nails to be stained or broken. Water, strong soaps, and washing powders make nails and cuticles dry. Well cared for nails are pleasing to look at and are a health protection. Convalescent patients may be able to care for their own nails.

Conditions such as torn cuticles are an invitation to infection. Therefore, reddened areas or breaks in the cuticles should be reported. Dirty nails can spread infection. It is better to file nails than to cut them. Filing prevents rough edges that catch on clothing and cause the nail to break. Cutting may result in cutting the skin.

Cleaning beneath the nails and pushing back the cuticle are essential to daily care. The best time to do this is after the patient's hands have been in water. Soap and water loosen dirt and temporarily soften cuticle. Oil on the nails and the cuticle softens dry, tight cuticles and dry nails. Use an orangewood stick to clean nails and push back cuticle. The stick is blunt and smooth and less likely to injure the nails than is the tip of a metal nail file. Clip hangnails with manicure scissors or snippers to keep them from tearing more.

Check your agency procedure book to see if you should wear gloves while caring for a patient's nails. Supplies and equipment needed are: a basin half full of warm water, soap, lotion, towel, nail brush, and orangewood stick. The female patient may have other items, such as nail polish, cuticle oil, and an emery board (a metal file should not be used).

Never give equipment that has a sharp point or that is used for cutting to a patient who has unsteady hands or who is depressed or self-injurious. Injury may occur. The person who is going to have surgery or who is experiencing respiratory distress usually is asked not to wear nail polish.

Skills used in caring for the fingernails are:

- ◆ Assist the patient to a comfortable upright position.
- ◆ Remove nail polish.
- ◆ Soak fingers in basin of warm water and mild soap.
- ◆ Scrub nails with nail brush.
- ◆ Dry hands thoroughly.
- ◆ Trim fingernails straight across.
- ◆ Shape fingernails with a file, rounding the corners.
- ◆ Clean under nails with an orangewood stick.
- ◆ Apply lotion to hands and gently massage. (See procedure later in this chapter.)

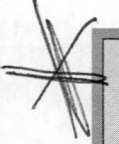

Nursing Alert

Special orders are required before cutting nails or cuticles of a patient with diabetes.

Caring for the Toenails

Cutting toenails is not a nursing measure unless specifically ordered. Do not cut the patient's toenails without the physician's permission. Never cut toenails of patients with diabetes or hemophilia or the nails of newborns because these patients are particularly susceptible to injury. Chapter 72 describes special foot care for the diabetic patient.

Follow the same procedure as when caring for the fingernails, with some exceptions. If toenails are thick and hard, you may have to cut them first (with a physician's order), then smooth them with a file or emery board. Cut toenails straight across and do not round off the corners. If you cut into the corners, you encourage ingrown nails. If the nails tend to grow inward at the corners, place a wisp of cotton under the nail to prevent pressure on the toe. A notch cut in the center will pull the edges and corners in. Sometimes, very thick, hard toenails must be surgically removed.

Toenails need the same care as fingernails. Long toenails may scratch the skin or catch on bedclothes and break. Dirty toenails may cause infection if they scratch the skin.

While caring for toenails, observe whether corns or calluses are present. If they are, you can apply oil to soften them, but nothing else. If the patient is distressed by corns, calluses, ingrown nails, or bunions, report the condition. Corns and calluses may become infected as a result of cutting them with razor blades or using corn removers that contain salicylic acid. You may cover an infected area with a sterile dressing, but the physician will prescribe any other treatment. Be sure to report and document any such situation.

The following skills are used in caring for toenails:

- ◆ Assist the patient to a sitting position or lying position with head of bed elevated.
- ◆ Place feet in basin of warm water and soak.
- ◆ Gently dry feet.
- ◆ Scrub nails with nail brush.
- ◆ Trim nails straight across.
- ◆ Do not shape corners.
- ◆ Clean under the nails with an orangewood stick.
- ◆ Apply lotion to feet and gently massage.

Shaving a Patient

Men who are unable to shave every day may feel or look untidy. In many hospitals, electric razors are used because they are easier and safer than blade razors. If your patient cannot shave himself, it may be necessary for you to shave him. When using an electric razor, read the instructions carefully.

If your healthcare facility uses blade razors, caution must be taken with certain patients. A patient with unsteady hands or poor eyesight should not be allowed to shave himself with a blade razor, nor should a patient who is depressed, suicidal, or assaultive.

If the patient can shave himself, you can get the equipment ready, provide a mirror, and see that the room is well lighted. If you are shaving a patient with a safety razor, follow your facility's recommended procedure. Be sure to wear gloves because you may nick the patient's face or neck and expose yourself to blood.

Some women shave also. Allow as much privacy as possible for the woman to carry out this part of her care. If she is unable to shave and needs assistance, you need to provide this care. Follow the steps of the procedure for both men and women.

Nursing Skill
Shaving a Patient

Supplies and Equipment

Razor: safety or electric
Wash basin
Warm water
Disposable gloves
Shaving cream or soap
Aftershave lotion
Towels

Procedure

1. Explain procedure to the patient. *(Rationale: Gain patient's confidence.)*
2. Have patient in a position that is comfortable for both you and the patient. *(Rationale: Allow easy access to face.)*
3. Place a warm wet washcloth on face for a few seconds. *(Rationale: Moisture softens the beard.)*
4. Apply shaving cream or soap to face. *(Rationale: Make the hair easier to cut.)*
5. Hold the skin of the face and neck taut while making strokes. *(Rationale: Helps preventing cutting the skin.)*
6. Holding razor at 45° angle to the skin, move razor across skin in short strokes in the direction the hair grows.
7. Make short downward strokes over the lip.
8. Wash face thoroughly with clean, warm, moistened washcloth. *(Rationale: This will remove any cream or soap and stray hairs.)*
9. Pat the face dry. *(Rationale: Patting rather than rubbing prevents skin chaffing.)*
10. Apply aftershave lotion if the patient prefers. *(Rationale: This stimulates and tones capillaries in the epidermis.)*
11. Properly dispose of gloves and document the procedure in the patient record. *(Rationale: To maintain the client record and note any unusual skin observations.)*

Hair Care

Brushing and dressing one's hair is part of daily care. It keeps the hair in condition and makes the patient feel better. Part of our self-image is related to how our hair looks. Encourage patients to comb their own hair; it is good exercise for the shoulder joints and enhances self-esteem.

Daily Hair Care

Daily hair care will give the nurse an opportunity to assess the hair and scalp. Brushing stimulates the scalp circulation and distributes oil over the hair to give it sheen. Short hair should have the same care as long hair. In some hospitals, beauty parlor and barber services are available. Although you will not have time to do elaborate hair arrangements for patients, try to arrange a patient's hair as becomingly as you can in the time you have. Comb one strand of hair at a time, holding the strand firmly and leaving it slack between your hand and the patient's head to avoid pulling. Hair ribbons may help to raise the spirits of both women and girls.

Braid long hair to prevent tangles. Start braids toward the front so the patient does not have to lie on them. Fasten them at the end with rubber bands or ribbons. A male patient with long hair may wish to have his hair tied in a pony tail. Be sure the braid or pony tail will not be uncomfortable when the patient is lying in bed. Avoid using hairpins or bobby pins; these might be uncomfortable or injure the patient's head.

Wash the brush and comb frequently. This will help to keep the hair clean and prevent reinfection of the scalp in infectious conditions. Report and document such conditions as excessive dandruff, falling hair, lice, crusts, or sores.

Hair Care for the African American Patient. In caring for patients with very thick, curly, dry hair, frequent use of shampoo and water is harmful because it dries out the hair. Warmed mineral oil is usually effective in cleaning the hair. In some cases, alcohol may be used, but it is drying. Ask the patient what cleansing method is preferred.

After oil is warmed, pour it into the hair, massaging it into the hair and scalp with the fingertips. Apply it along the entire length of the hair strands. While the hair is wet, gently comb it with a pick comb with teeth that are long and far apart; the curlier and coarser the hair, the larger the comb should be. Towel dry the hair after combing.

Routine daily hair care for the African American patient often includes an application of baby oil, hair oil, or olive oil. Excess oil is removed with a towel.

The Shampoo

A shampoo may be needed after lotions or other medications have been applied to the scalp, after an electroencephalogram for which a paste is used, as part of the treatment for lice, or for cleanliness during a long-term illness. Guidelines are given in the accompanying box.

Giving a Shampoo to an Ambulatory Patient

The simplest method of shampooing is for the patient to shampoo during a shower or bath. The patient who is ambulatory can have a shampoo in the bathroom, using the lavatory sink. Choose a chair low enough to let the patient's head rest comfortably on the edge of the bowl. The person may prefer to sit facing the sink, resting the forehead on the edge and holding a folded towel over the eyes. If a spray is used, adjust the temperature of the water before you begin. If the patient feels faint, stop the procedure, wrap the head in a bath towel, and get the patient back to bed.

The patient who can be moved on a stretcher can be wheeled to a convenient sink for a shampoo. The shampoo is done while the patient is lying on the stretcher.

Giving a Shampoo to a Bed Patient

If a patient cannot ambulate, you will have to shampoo while the patient is in bed.

Nursing Skill
Giving a Shampoo to a Bed Patient

Supplies and Equipment

Comb and brush
1 bath towel, 1 hand towel, 1 washcloth
Plastic for floor and chair
1 large pitcher of water
Cotton balls
1 small pitcher for pouring
Shampoo
1 pail
Shampoo trough
Moisture-proof pillowcase
Gloves
Conditioner and hair dryer (optional)

Procedure

1. Wash hands and wear gloves as ordered in your facility.
2. Cover the patient with a bath blanket and turn back the bedclothing. (*Rationale: This keeps bedclothing dry while covering and warming the patient.*)
3. Cover the pillow with a moisture-proof case and place it under the patient's head. (*Rationale: This will prevent soiling and wetting of bed linen.*)
4. Raise bed to the highest position and place in the flat position. (*Rationale: This protects you from back strain.*)
5. Gently move the patient's head and shoulders toward you to the edge of the bed. (*Rationale: Both the nurse and patient need to be comfortable for the procedure.*)
6. Comb and brush hair thoroughly. (*Rationale: Hair is easier to wash when it is combed and brushed.*)
7. Place plastic on the floor. (*Rationale: For safety reasons you want to keep the floor dry.*)

Nursing Skill Guidelines
Shampooing

- ◆ The goal of the shampoo is to cleanse the hair and scalp.
- ◆ A physician's order is required for a bed shampoo.
- ◆ The shampoo should *not* be given if the patient is weak or very tired or if the patient has a respiratory infection or fever.
- ◆ A shampoo is not usually given unless the patient has been in the hospital for some time. However, a shampoo may be needed if the patient's hair is very greasy or dirty on admission.
- ◆ The procedure for giving a shampoo is determined by the equipment available in the hospital. (Some larger institutions have beautician services available; equipment similar to that used in beauty salons may be provided.)
- ◆ Wear gloves if the skin is not intact or if you suspect a condition such as pediculosis (the presence of lice).
- ◆ Usually a mild soap solution or shampoo is used. Ask the patient about preferences.
- ◆ Soap and water and soapless or dry shampoos remove oil from the hair; however, if used too frequently or too lavishly, they may remove too much oil.
- ◆ Protect the patient from drafts and be sure that the room is comfortably warm.
- ◆ Use warm water, 105° to 110°F (40.6°–43.3°C).
- ◆ Protect the patient's eyes and ears.
- ◆ Use enough solution to make a thick lather.
- ◆ Lather and rinse twice.
- ◆ Rinse and dry the hair thoroughly.
- ◆ Ensure continuous drainage for shampoo water.

---

8. Place the pail on a covered chair. (*Rationale: Water will splash if it falls a great distance.*)
9. Place shampoo basin under patient's head with trough directed to side of bed. It should flow into the pail. (*Rationale: Water will need to drain continuously.*)
10. Cover the patient with an extra bath blanket. (*Rationale: Chills must be prevented.*)
11. Pin a folded towel around the patient's neck. (*Rationale: This absorbs drips and keeps the water from running down the patient's back.*)
12. Cover the patient's eyes with a damp washcloth and place cotton in the patient's ears. (*Rationale: This protects eyes and ears from soapy water. These areas cannot drain normally when patient is in a back-lying position.*)
13. Place a towel over the patient's chest. (*Rationale: Protect the patient from water.*)
14. Wet hair thoroughly with warm water (about 105°–110°F, 40.6°–42°C). (*Rationale: Warm water prevents burns to face and scalp.*)
15. Apply shampoo and rub it into a lather, massaging scalp as you do so (Fig. 45-1). (*Rationale: Friction loosens particles and soap and water will wash them away.*)

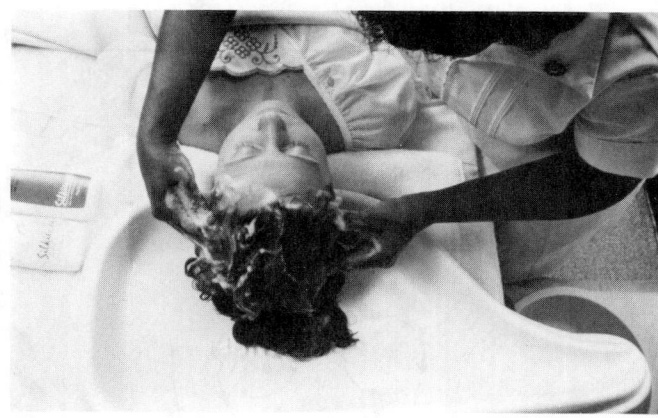

Figure 45-1. Using a trough supplied by the hospital, the nurse shampoos from the front to the back of the head with the tips of the fingers.

16. Rinse well. *(Rationale: It is important to rinse out soap and dirt particles.)*
17. Reapply shampoo, massage, and rinse thoroughly. *(Rationale: Oil may collect in the hair of a bedridden patient. Blood or vomitus may collect.)*
18. Rinse with conditioner. *(Rationale: Conditioner prevents drying and makes combing easier.)*
19. Squeeze excess water from hair and wrap a towel around the patient's head. Gently pat or rub to dry hair. *(Rationale: Removing extra moisture helps prevent the patient and bedclothes from getting wet.)*
20. Remove wet towels and equipment. *(Rationale: Prevent chilling the patient. Make area comfortable and clean.)*
21. Use hair dryer, comb and brush, as needed. *(Rationale: Individuals have preferences on how their hair is styled.)*
22. Dispose of gloves and wash your hands.
23. Document the procedure and note how the patient tolerated it.

Giving Hair Care After an Accident

After an accident, a patient may come to the hospital with dirt, blood, or glass in the hair. If no scalp wounds are apparent, you may be asked to shampoo the patient's hair. The shampoo removes debris from the patient's hair and makes the patient more comfortable. It also gives the nurse an opportunity to examine the head. Gloves are always worn for this procedure. Be careful not to cut yourself on glass or debris in the patient's hair.

Brush or comb the hair first; combing will help to remove larger pieces of debris. Check at that time for scalp wounds. If scalp wounds are discovered, report them before you proceed with the shampoo. Scalp wounds need attention before a shampoo; they might become infected and the shampoo would be irritating.

If the patient cannot tolerate a shampoo with water, dry shampoo can be used instead. Follow the instruc-tions on the package of dry shampoo, being sure to keep the powder out of the patient's eyes.

Treating Pediculosis

Pediculosis is caused by lice, tiny insects that suck blood from the person they infect. They are found on the hairy parts of the body. Head lice are found on the hair and scalp. They are tiny oval, grayish insects. The eggs, called **nits**, look like dandruff but are solid specks, not flakes. They cling tightly to the hair and are hard to destroy.

Body lice are found on the body and clothing. Crab lice are found on the hairy parts of the body, especially the pubic area (pediculosis pubis). The nurse should be suspicious of scratches in these areas of the patient's body.

Lice spread diseases. They cause itching, and the resulting scratches may become infected. They spread from person to person on clothing, bedding, and combs and brushes. Part of your observation of a patient on admission to the hospital is to notice signs of skin irritation and lice.

Both nits and adult lice can be destroyed by a routine treatment, often a shampooing with a special shampoo or a shower with a special medicated soap. If you observe lice, report it to your team leader. The physician will order specific treatment. Specific care of patients with parasitic skin infestations is covered in Chapter 68.

Skin Care

The skin is a defense against disease and infection. If that defense system is to be effective, the skin must be kept unbroken and nonirritated. The skin also helps regulate body heat; a break in the skin could upset that balance. When giving nursing care, observe for any skin irritation.

Good skin care is essential to keep the skin intact and remove dirt, excess oil, and harmful bacteria. If the skin is oily, frequent cleansing is needed; if the skin is dry, a daily bath may be harmful. However, the face, underarms, and perineum need daily cleansing. Also remember that body discharges, such as perspiration, vomitus, urine, and feces, are irritating.

The Backrub

Give a backrub when you give a bath and as part of evening care. Do it at other times during the day and night when it is a necessary part of treatment or for patient comfort. You will not be expected to give a massage because that is a task for someone with special training.

Specific Techniques in Backrubs

These four movements are the simplest and most effective for the kind of light massage you will give to stimulate circulation and relax contracted muscles. Perform all four patterns at least three times.

◆ *Stroking.* Stroke the large surfaces of the back with the palms of your hands. Stroke in the direction of venous circulation, *toward the heart.* You can use your thumb and fingers on smaller surfaces. Keep the strokes and pressure even. Begin and end the backrub with stroking.

◆ *Kneading.* Press on muscle groups or single muscles, picking them up and squeezing them gently. Use the palms of your hands for the large muscles; use your fingers and thumbs for single muscles. Use this movement for the outer aspects of the back.

◆ *Tapping.* A light tapping with the edge of the hands (the edge further from the thumb) is sometimes used to stimulate the circulation.

◆ *Friction.* Rub around the bony prominences of the body, such as at the end of the spine and along each shoulder blade.

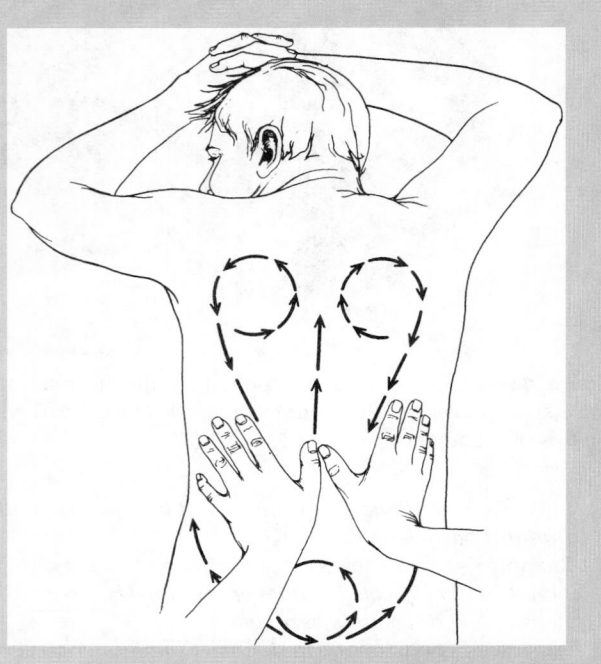

The backrub is often the highlight of the day for the patient who is confined to bed. It can be relaxing for the patient, and it gives you a good chance to observe skin condition and converse with the patient.

Alcohol may be used for the backrub. Skin breakdown is more likely to occur if the skin is wet; alcohol dries and toughens the skin. Backrub lotion is most often used because it soothes and softens the skin.

Warm your hands and the lotion to prevent chilling the patient. You can float the bottle of lotion in the warm bath water during a bed bath to warm the lotion. Be sure your nails are short enough to rub the back effectively, and do not wear jewelry. Long fingernails and jewelry can scratch the patient, and both can collect lotion, skin debris, and microorganisms.

The backrub is given by applying pressure and friction to the back with your hands. It may be given to stimulate or soothe. Light pressure is soothing; heavier pressure is stimulating. Techniques used in backrubs are discussed in the accompanying box. Use long, firm strokes and give extra attention to pressure areas.

Nursing Skill
Giving a Backrub

Supplies and Equipment
Backrub lotion or alcohol
Gloves, if ordered

Procedure

1. Wash your hands. Wear gloves, if ordered.
2. Make sure the room is warm enough. *(Rationale: A large portion of the patient's body will be exposed.)*
3. Provide privacy for the patient by closing the door or pulling the curtain.
4. Place the patient comfortably on the side, or face downward, with the entire back and buttocks exposed.
5. Apply lotion all over the back after warming it in your hands or in warm water.
6. Stand with one foot slightly forward and your knees bent slightly.
7. Have the patient as near your side of the bed as possible.
8. Rock on your feet as you rub. *(Rationale: Using this position allows your strong arm and shoulder muscles to do the work and helps prevent back strain.)*
9. Using the first three fingers of both hands, rub the neck under the hairline with a circular motion. *(Rationale: This helps to relax the neck, a frequent source of tension and headaches.)*
10. Using the first three fingers of one hand, rub in the hollow at the back of the neck with a circular motion. *(Rationale: This also helps to relax the neck.)*
11. Separating the thumb and the fingers of one hand, place the thumb on one side of the neck and the fingers on the other. Beginning at the hairline, rub the length of the neck with a circular motion.
12. Using the first three fingers of both hands, continue the circular motion down each side of the spine to the coccyx. *(Rationale: Tension builds up along the spinal column. The coccyx is a bony prominence with very little*

fatty covering; thus, it is in great danger of skin break-down. The rubbing motion stimulates circulation.)

13. Using the flat of both hands, with the fingers extended toward the front, rub the shoulders with a circular motion. *(Rationale: The shoulder blades are also bony prominences that need stimulation of the circulation.)*

14. Continue the circular motion with the flat of the hands down the entire surface of the back and the buttocks.

15. Separating the first and second fingers of one hand, place the hands on either side of the spine and run them lightly up from the coccyx to the hairline and firmly down.

16. Repeat steps 9 to 15 three times.

17. If you have used alcohol for a rub, finish by applying a dusting of powder.

18. Wash your hands after the procedure, and dispose of gloves in the prescribed manner.

19. Document any pertinent observations.

> **Nursing Alert**
>
> Certain conditions, such as hemorrhage, heart attack, and phlebitis, contraindicate (negate the use of) vigorous rubbing.

The Hand Massage

Massage of the hands and feet is a valuable tool in relaxing and calming patients. The circulation improves as blood vessels dilate from the warmth of friction. Muscle tone is improved so the muscular system functions better. The patient begins to feel better about the body. This positive attitude produces a feeling of calmness and vitality. Hand massage may be performed by the nurse. The patient can be taught to administer self-massage. Part of the healing process is the patient's acceptance of the massage.

The nurse may take the following actions in hand massage:

♦ Take either of the patient's hands in both of your hands.

♦ Shake out the hand. *(Rationale: Relieve tiredness.)*

♦ Rotate and twist each finger with the whole of your hand bending it back and forth. *(Rationale: Redistribute the synovial fluid around the finger joints.)*

♦ Massage the palm of the hand with your thumb and fingers. Rotate in a circular motion. *(Rationale: According to acupuncture, this massage relaxes the heart.)*

♦ Massage the back (dorsum) of the hand with your thumb and fingers. Rotate in a circular motion.

♦ Massage the webbed area between the thumb and first finger. *(Rationale: Pressure points for sinuses and intestines are located here. Massaging this area helps headaches, constipation, and menstrual cramps.)*

♦ Gently shake out the hand or quietly place it on the table.

♦ Repeat steps on the other hand.

♦ Teach steps to the patient for self-massage.

♦ Document the procedure on the patient record.

Bathing

A bath is given to remove the waste products of perspiration, to stimulate circulation, and to refresh. A complete daily bath is not essential or even advisable for every patient. Personal bathing habits have an influence on the frequency of hospital baths. It is important to consider the patient's comfort and personal preference rather than hospital routine. If a patient has had an uncomfortable, sleepless night, a rest after breakfast may be more appealing than a bath.

Three types of cleansing baths are the bed bath, tub bath, and shower. The patient's condition and physician's order determine which bath is the safest and best. A bed bath is the least tiring for the patient and is the safest if the person has any difficulty in moving or is suicidal or irresponsible. Showers and bathtubs equipped with self-help devices allow patients to bathe themselves when they are able to do so. In some cases, the patient is ill and only a sponge bath can be given. All patients should at least have the face and hands washed, if possible.

Washing the Patient's Face and Hands

Wash the patient's face and hands before breakfast, during a bath, and before dinner. You may also do it at other times for the patient's comfort. Always see that the person's hands are washed after a bedpan or urinal has been used. The following actions are involved in washing the patient's face and hands:

♦ Gloves are worn for this procedure, if ordered.

♦ Arrange the equipment conveniently on the overbed table. Allow the person to do as much self-care as possible.

♦ Wring out the washcloth to prevent dripping.

♦ If you will be washing the patient's face, wrap the washcloth around your hand and tuck in the ends to form a mitt. *(Rationale: If loose ends are allowed to remain, the washcloth can drag over the patient's face, possibly in the eyes.)*

♦ Wash carefully around the patient's nose and ears. *(Rationale: These areas collect perspiration, oils, and dirt.)*

♦ You may carefully sponge the patient's closed eyelids with clear water unless they are wearing contacts. *(Rationale: Soap stings the eyes; if contacts are in place, the eyes are sensitive to rubbing or pressure.)*

◆ Do <u>not</u> use soap on the face unless the patient wants it. *(Rationale: Soap is drying, especially to the face.)*

◆ The patient's hands are washed in the basin of water. Allow them to soak for a few minutes in the basin. *(Rationale: Soaking is very soothing.)*

Giving a Foot Soak

A foot soak is of particular importance to the patient who has edema, tenderness, or some form of infection. The foot may be soaked in warm water or a variety of commercially prepared salts and solutions. Warm water helps dilate blood vessels to promote improved circulation and relaxes the feet and legs. Salts contain medication or chemicals that are absorbed by the skin during the soaking time. The length of time varies for the soak. Usually you start with a warm solution (105°–110°F) and allow the feet to remain in the solution approximately 10 to 20 minutes until the water cools.

Nursing Skill
Giving a Foot Soak

Supplies and Equipment

Wash basin
Warm water or commercially prepared salts or solutions
Towels
Protective pad for bed or floor
Gloves (optional)
Detergent (optional)

Procedure

1. Position patient in comfortable upright position with feet uncovered. If patient is too weak to sit in a chair, patient may recline in bed with head of bed elevated if tolerated. *(Rationale: Easy access to feet is necessary.)*
2. Place protective pad on bed or floor. *(Rationale: For safety and to prevent water damage.)*
3. Place wash basin of warm water on protected bed or floor. *(Rationale: Make sure patient is comfortable and can tolerate position.)*
4. Place both feet in wash basin, if basin size accommodates them. Otherwise, soak one foot at a time, using fresh water or solution for each foot. *(Rationale: Promote comfort.)*
5. Allow feet to soak for 10 to 20 minutes *(Rationale: Soaking is comfortable for feet. Medications must have time to act.)*
6. Dry feet thoroughly with blotting or patting motion. *(Rationale: Harsh rubbing could damage skin.)*
7. Dry between each toe. *(Rationale: Prevent cracking between toes and eliminate a growth medium for fungi.)*
8. Apply lotion and gently massage each foot. *(Rationale: Lubricate dry skin and provide comfort.)*
9. Apply foot powder if preferred. *(Rationale: Absorb moisture and cool the feet.)*

10. As you dry feet, carefully assess skin integrity. Check for lesions, corns, and calluses. *(Rationale: Methodical drying of feet allows for excellent evaluation of feet.)*
11. Document procedure and note any foot problems that were assessed *(Rationale: Maintain the patient record and document any unusual findings.)*

Assisting the Patient with a Tub Bath

A tub or shower bath is a step toward resuming normal habits. Patients gain independence and feel they are recovering. However, a physician's order is required for a tub bath, especially if patients have previously been receiving bed baths.

It is better not to give a bath immediately after a meal because a bath draws blood to the skin and away from the digestive organs. The nurse must judge how much assistance the patient will need in bathing; the nurse is responsible for the patient's comfort and safety. It is important to observe carefully to see that patients do not overexert themselves.

The sitz bath as a treatment is discussed in Chapter 49. The therapeutic bath for allergies or specific skin disorders is discussed in Chapter 68.

Nursing Skill
Assisting With a Tub Bath

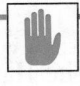

Supplies and Equipment

Blanket
Bath mat
Bath towels
Soap
Clean gown or pajamas
Clean bed linen
Bath thermometer
Disinfectants for cleaning the tub

Procedure

1. Check the temperature of the bathroom. *(Rationale: Prevent chilling.)*
2. Make sure the tub is clean. Scour it carefully with prescribed disinfectants. Unless using a long-handled swab, gloves are worn when cleaning the tub. *(Rationale: It is important to prevent cross-contamination for patients and nurses.)*
3. Rinse well. *(Rationale: Rinsing prevents the harsh cleanser or disinfectant from coming in contact with the patient's skin.)*
4. Place a chair near the tub with a bath blanket opened over it. *(Rationale: The blanket is convenient for the patient to towel dry. It also allows the patient to keep part of the body covered to prevent chilling and exposure.)*
5. Place towels, washcloth, and soap where the patient can reach them easily. *(Rationale: Everything should be convenient for the patient's use.)*

6. Fill the tub about halfway (less for a child). *(Rationale: Prevent drowning should the patient slip or faint.)*

7. Test the water with a bath thermometer. The temperature of the water should be warm to very warm, never hot or over 105°F (40.6°C). *(Rationale: The bath thermometer is the only accurate way to measure temperature.)*

8. Place bath mat in front of the tub. *(Rationale: The person needs a clean, dry place to stand.)*

9. Bring the patient to the bathroom. Help the person to remove clothing and, if necessary, to get into the bathtub. *(Rationale: It is vital to prevent falls.)*

10. Show the person where the bathroom call light is located. Explain that this signal sounds an alarm; instruct the person not to use it unless help is urgently needed. *(Rationale: The call light will help the patient feel more secure.)*

11. Check often, so the patient will not be tempted to use the signal. *(Rationale: If the patient uses the bathroom call light, the emergency code team will probably respond.)*

12. Ask the patient not to lock the door unless you have a key or unless it is a special "safety" door, which can be easily opened from the outside. Tell the person that you will see that no one comes in and that you will be near if help is needed. Place the "occupied" or "in use" sign on the door. *(Rationale: The nurse must be able to get in the door, in case help is needed.)*

13. Don't leave a child, a depressed person, or a person who is unsure or unsteady alone. *(Rationale: A child may easily and quickly slip under the water; a depressed or suicidal person may use this means to commit suicide.)*

14. When the bath is finished, help the patient out of the tub and help dry the body, if assistance is needed. After dressing, assist the patient back to bed. *(Rationale: The bath is tiring; the person will probably need to rest.)*

15. Carefully clean the tub after the patient has completed the bath, using the procedure listed in steps 2 and 3. *(Rationale: It is important to prevent cross-contamination.)*

16. Dispose of gloves and wash your hands. *(Rationale: Prevent cross-contamination.)*

17. Document the procedure, describing any unusual patient reactions. *(Rationale: It is necessary to keep accurate records.)*

The Shower Bath

Guide rails both inside and outside the shower stall are essential. Two sets of rails are better than one. One set of rails is needed at a level the patient can reach for support when sitting on a stool, and the other higher up for support when standing. Some people need to hang on with both hands.

When the shower is in the bathtub rather than in a separate stall, the suggestion to use a stool in the tub is often welcomed by apprehensive or weak patients. It is safer for most patients to sit down while taking a shower, especially if they are elderly or weak (Fig. 45-

2). No patient who is weak or unsteady should be permitted to take a shower unattended. The patient should have the necessary assistance, and the same precautions should be taken for safety as with a patient taking a tub bath.

Giving Perineal Care

Perineal care is commonly referred to as "pericare." Perineal care is an important part of the bed bath. Some patients may find it embarrassing to have nurses assist them in cleaning the perineal area. Nurses may be required to provide perineal care to members of the opposite sex. A professional attitude should be maintained at all times. Provide a wet washcloth, soap, rinse water, and a towel for the patient who is able to do self-care. You may need to speak in simple terms for the patient to understand your instructions of bathing the genitals. For example, the nurse can say, "I'll give you a washcloth so you can wash between your legs" or "You can finish your bath."

Perineal care is given to patients after any perineal surgery and after delivery. Many patients will need instruction in special perineal care. The female patient should be taught to cleanse from front to back with tissue or sponges. A perineal bottle ("peribottle") is filled with warm tap water, sterile water, or saline, and the perineal area is thoroughly sprayed to keep it free of infection. Sometimes, cotton balls or Zephiran sponges are used. The patient should use each cotton ball or Zephiran sponge only once. The patient should be taught to wipe the outside areas first, saving the last sponges for the urethral area. Nursing Procedure 45-2 outlines steps in giving perineal care.

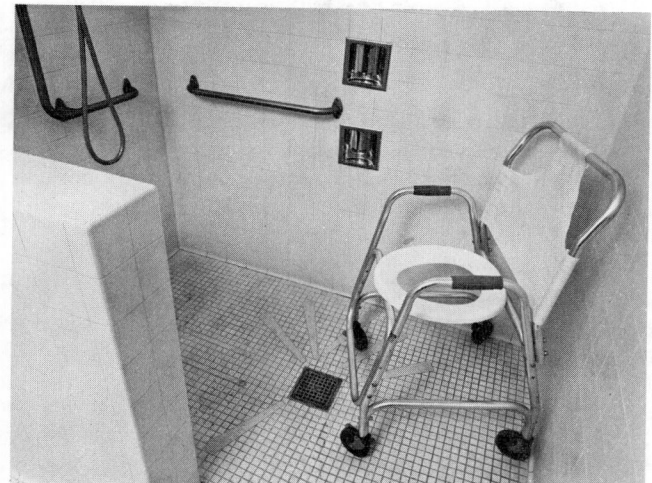

Figure 45-2. This shower can be used by the ambulatory patient or by one who can be transported by and remain in the shower chair.

Giving Perineal Care

Supplies and Equipment

Gloves
Wash cloths
Basin
Waterproof pad
Towels
Bath blanket
Soap
Toilet tissue

Procedure

1. Gather supplies.
   (Rationale: Organization facilitates performance of the skill.)
2. Explain procedure to patient.
   (Rationale: Providing information fosters patient cooperation.)
3. Wash hands prior to putting on gloves.
   (Rationale: Handwashing prevents the spread of organisms. Gloves act as a barrier.)
4. Close the curtain or the door to the room.
   (Rationale: This protects the patient's privacy.)
5. Raise the bed to a comfortable height. Lower near side rail.
   (Rationale: Bed at proper height prevents back strain. Lowering the side rail near the nurse provides for patient safety.)
6. Uncover perineal area. Place towel or waterproof pad under patient's hips.
   (Rationale: Towel or pad protects bed. Towel can be used to dry the perineal and rectal area.)
7. Make a mitt with the washcloth. (See instructions for making a mitt in bed bath procedure.) Cleanse upper thighs and groin area with soap and water. Rinse and dry. Wash the genital area next.

Female Patient

a. Use a separate portion of the washcloth for each stroke. Change washcloths as necessary.
b. Separate labia and cleanse downward from pubic area to anal area.

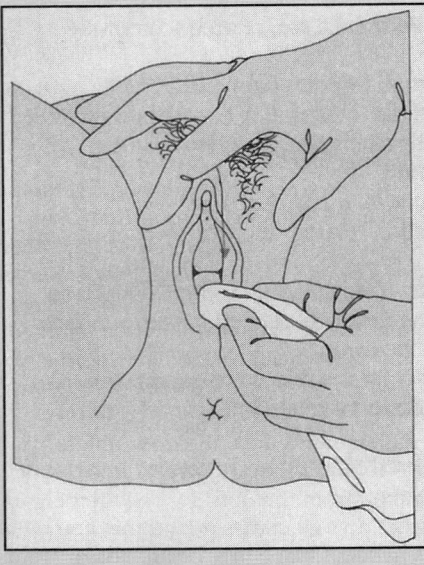

Step 7b Cleansing downward from the pubic area to the anal area

c. Wash between labia including the urethral meatus and vaginal area.
d. Rinse well and pat dry.
(Rationale: Cleansing from the pubis toward the anus, or washing from a clean area to a dirty area, prevents contaminating the vaginal area and urinary meatus with organisms from the anus.)

Male Patient

a. Gently grasp the penis.
b. Cleanse in a circular motion moving from the tip of the penis backward toward the pubic area. In an uncircumcised male, carefully retract the foreskin prior to washing the penis.

(continued)

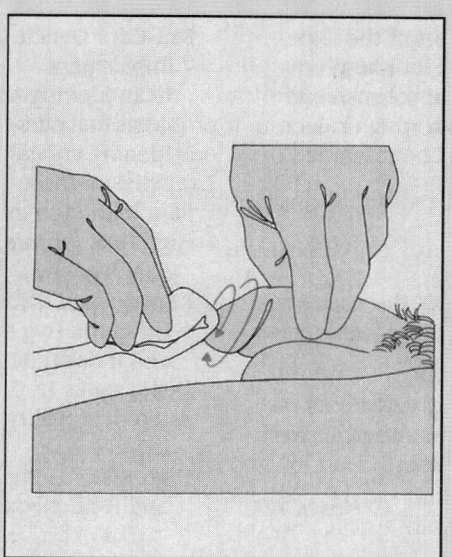

Step 7b Cleansing in a circular motion from the tip of the penis backwards toward the pubic area (Pick up from Taylor)

   c. Rinse well and dry.
   d. Return the foreskin to its former position.
   e. Wash, rinse, and dry the scrotum carefully.
   (Rationale: Cleansing from the tip of the penis backward toward the pubic area prevents transferring organisms from the anus to the urethra. Secretions that collect under the foreskin can cause irritation and odor. Returning the foreskin to its normal position prevents injury to the tissue.)

8. Assist patient to turn on the side. Separate the buttocks and use toilet tissue, if necessary, to remove fecal material.
   (Rationale: Removing fecal material provides for easier cleaning.)
9. Cleanse the anal area, rinse thoroughly, and dry with towel. Change washcloths as necessary.
   (Rationale: Keeping the anal area clean minimizes the risk of skin irritation and breakdown.)
10. Apply skin care products to area according to need or physician's order.
    (Rationale: Ointments can provide a moisture barrier. Lotions may be prescribed to treat skin irritation.)
11. Return patient to a comfortable position. Lower bed and raise side rail.
    (Rationale: These measures provide for patient comfort and safety.)
12. Remove gloves and wash hands.
    (Rationale: Handwashing prevents the spread of organisms.)
13. Document the procedure, describing skin condition.
    (Rationale: Provide continuity of care.)

Nursing Alert

Perineal care for the female may also be accomplished by using a "peri-bottle" for irrigation. The patient can be positioned on the toilet or a bedpan. Care may vary for specific situations (ie, woman after childbirth, patient with an indwelling catheter, or patient recovering from surgery).

The Bed Bath

Preparation is particularly important in giving a bed bath; you should not have to leave the unit for forgotten equipment once the bath is begun. If the bath is interrupted, the patient may become chilled and the bath water will become cold. The accompanying box presents guidelines for giving a bed bath.

Key Concept

The bed bath provides an opportunity for the nurse to look closely at the condition of the patient's body. The nurse should record the type of bath given and any significant observations.

Giving a Partial Bed Bath

The patient should have a partial bath on days when he or she does not have a complete one. A partial bed bath consists of bathing the face and hands, axillae, back, buttocks, and genital area, and under the breasts in the female patient. Some patients are able to bathe themselves, except for the back. Every patient should be encouraged to do as much as possible; the person will be using muscles and become more self-sufficient. Follow the steps of giving the bed bath, bathing only those areas that require attention. Elderly patients and some bedridden individuals need only partial bathing. After the bath, remove equipment and make the bed.

Giving a Towel Bath

Research has shown that simply giving a bath with a dry or damp towel helps improve circulation and in-

- Check the physician's order each day. (*Rationale: The bath order may have changed.*) In some instances a bed bath may be harmful for a patient (eg, one in pain, hemorrhaging, or weak); you may need to defer the bath.
- Depending on the patient, a bath is most refreshing in the morning or at night before sleep. (*Rationale: If, for example, the person perspires a great deal or feels hot and uncomfortable, a bath at night may help to induce sleep.*)
- It is not always possible to give every patient a complete bed bath every day. A common procedure is to give a patient two or three complete baths a week and partial baths on the other days. Very sick patients and those who are perspiring profusely, vomiting, or incontinent may have a complete bath every day. (*Rationale: The patient must be kept clean to avoid skin breakdown and discomfort.*)
- Allow time to give an unrushed bath. You will be able to give the bath in about 20 minutes when you become skillful. (*Rationale: You have to allow additional time for the accompanying procedures; preparing the patient, collecting equipment, making the bed, and caring for used equipment, soiled linen, and the patient's unit.*)
- Plan your time according to the condition of the patients to whom you are assigned and the number of complete or partial baths you will give. (*Rationale: Nursing always includes planning, so that each patient receives necessary care.*)
- The bed bath is given in such a way as to achieve the desired end with the least exertion for the patient and without chilling the patient. (*Rationale: Water hastens the loss of body heat.*)
- Reassure a patient who is hesitant to have a bed bath.
- Some patients can help with the bath; they can turn and move themselves. Others must not be allowed to make any effort.

crease energy. In this procedure, the nurse often does not use water on the body. A dry towel is rubbed against the dry body, thereby creating friction. Friction produces warmth to the area, causing blood vessels to dilate. Dilation of the vessels, in turn, helps improve circulation and promote a revitalized feeling in the patient. Gentle to mild pressure in rubbing the body is all that is required. While you are performing the procedure, take the opportunity to assess the patient's skin and bony prominences. Note any irritation, redness, swelling, or discharge. Always check your patient's medical diagnosis before performing a procedure of this nature. Certain medical conditions may contraindicate the massage of body parts. Gloves may be worn if desired.

The Complete Bed Bath

The steps in Nursing Procedure 45-3 assume the patient cannot move without assistance. However, allow the person to do as much as possible.

Skin Breakdown and Healing

As the nurse inspects the skin while giving skin care, he or she may see and assess different types of skin breakdown. Special care, called wound care, is needed in skin breakdown.

The most common type of skin breakdown the nurse will see in the hospital patient are trauma or accidental wounds, surgical wounds, and pressure sores. Other types of skin breakdown include infection, rashes, lesions, and burns. This section concerns pressure sores; other skin lesions are discussed in Chapter 68.

Pressure Sores

Pressure sores, sometimes called **decubitus ulcers** or bedsores, are potentially serious skin lesions caused by pressure of any kind on the skin. They can lead to death in underlying tissues of the skin. Continuous pressure on any part of the body makes a patient uncomfortable, hampers circulation, and causes skin breakdown. The main pressure areas include bony prominences, such as shoulder blades, elbows, end of the spine, hips, knees, sides of the ankles, and back of the head as well as areas such as the buttocks, heels, and ears. These areas are subject to pressure sores because they are not covered by pads of fat. The skin breaks down and tissues beneath are destroyed. Examples of common sites of pressure are illustrated in Figure 45-3.

A thin patient is often more susceptible to pressure areas than a heavier person. The skin is more likely to break down if an area is continually moist or is not kept clean. An inadequate diet, especially one low in protein, will render the skin prone to breakdown. In the patient who must remain in bed, circulation is affected and pressure on bony prominences is increased. The danger of developing pressure areas is increased if a patient must lie in one position, or has a cast or splint, or a disease condition that affects circulation.

Classification of pressure sores is made related to their stage of development. There are four stages, as shown in the accompanying box. In the fourth stage a leathery black crust of dead tissue, called **eschar**, may develop around the edges. When eschar separates from the living tissue, it is called **sloughing**. Removal of this dead tissue is called **debridement**. Debridement allows healthy tissue to grow, progressing from internal tissue to external tissue.

Giving a Bed Bath

Supplies and Equipment

Gloves (optional)
Bath blanket
Towels
Washcloths
Basin
Gown or pajamas
Personal items (deodorant, powder, etc.)
Bedpan or urinal
Linen hamper or bag
Soap

Procedure

1. Gather supplies.
   (Rationale: Organization facilitates performance of the skill.)
2. Explain procedure to patient. If alert and oriented, question patient about personal hygiene preferences and ability to assist with bath.
   (Rationale: Providing information fosters patient co-operation. Encouraging patient to assist with care promotes independence.)
3. Wash hands prior to putting on gloves.
   (Rationale: Handwashing prevents the spread of organisms. Gloves act as a barrier and are optional, but must be worn for perineal and anal care.)
4. Close the curtain or the door to the room.
   (Rationale: This protects the patient's privacy.)
5. Provide opportunity to use bedpan or urinal.
   (Rationale: Voiding before the bath begins prevents interruption of the procedure and promotes comfort.)
6. Raise the bed to a comfortable height for you.
   (Rationale: Bed at proper height prevents back strain.)
7. Remove the bedspread, fold it, and place it on a chair or table. Cover the patient with a bath blanket and remove top sheet while patient holds onto bath blanket.
   (Rationale: Bedspread may be reused based on agency policy. Bath blanket provides warmth for patient. Top sheet may be used if bath blanket is not available.)
8. Fill the basin about two-thirds full with quite warm water. (43°–46°C or 110°–115°F) and place on bedside table.
   (Rationale: Water, at the proper temperature, is relaxing and provides warmth for the patient. Water will cool during the procedure.)

9. Lower the side rail. Remove the patient's gown and keep the bath blanket in place covering the patient. If IV is present on upper extremity, thread IV tubing and bag through sleeve of soiled gown and rehang IV solution. Recheck the IV flow rate or activity of pump.
   (Rationale: Removing the gown permits easier access when washing the upper body. IV delivery is uninterrupted and sterility of setup is maintained.)
10. Assist patient to move toward side of bed where you will be working. Usually you will wish to do most of the work with your dominant hand.
    (Rationale: Keeping patient near the nurse limits reaching across the bed and prevents back strain.)
11. Open a bath towel across the patient's chest. Make a mitt with the washcloth. A mitt is formed by holding the top two corners so the washcloth is around the back of your hand, with the open side across your palm. Then tuck the loose end into the top, enclosing your fingers.
    (Rationale: Towel provides privacy and warmth. Making a mitt prevents water from dripping across the patient and gives you better control.)

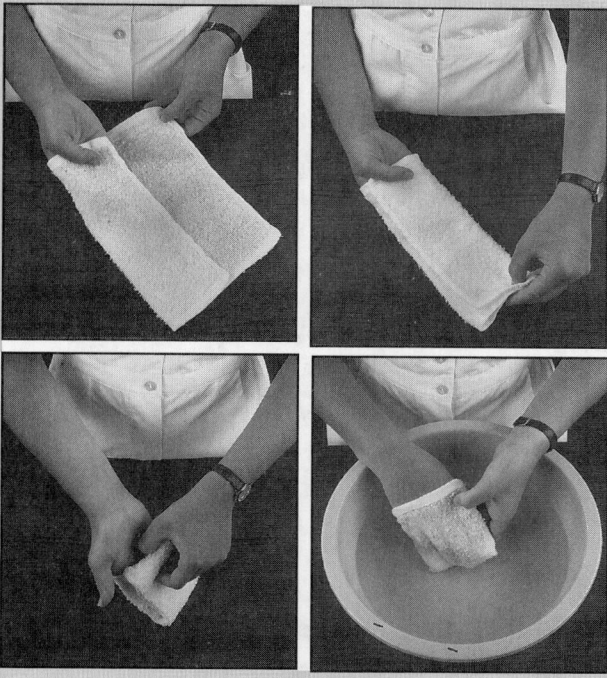

Step 11 Making a mitt (Photos © B. Proud.)

(continued)

12. Moisten the mitt with plain water and wash the patient's eyes. Cleanse from the inner canthus to outer corner (near nose) using a different section of the mitt to wash each eye.
    (Rationale: Soap is irritating to the eyes. Washing from inner to outer corner, prevents sweeping debris into the eye where the nasolacrimal duct is located. Using a separate portion of the mitt for each eye prevents the spread of infection from one to the other.)

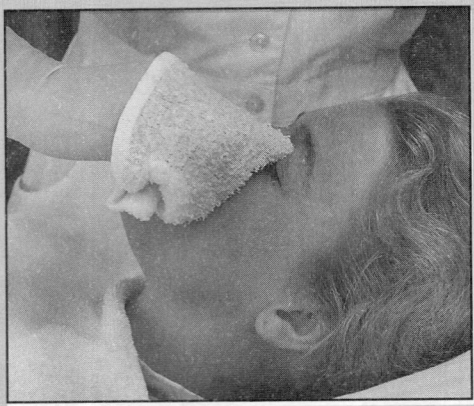

Step 12 Cleansing the eye, moving from the inner toward the outer corner

13. Wash the face, neck, and ears. Use soap on this area only if the patient prefers it. Dry these areas carefully.
    (Rationale: Soap is particularly drying to the face.)
14. Uncover the patient's far arm. Place bath towel under arm. Wash with long strokes, rinse, and dry arm with special attention to the axilla.
    (Rationale: Washing far side first prevents dripping bath water on a clean area. Long strokes improve circulation by facilitating venous return.)

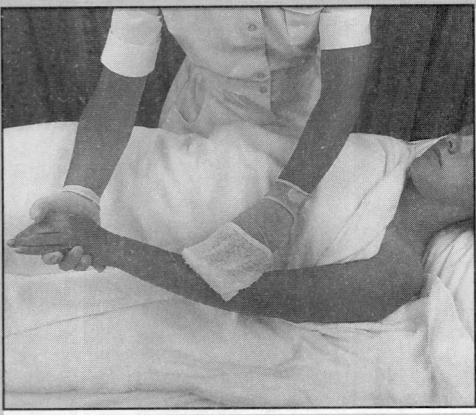

Step 14 Washing the arm

15. Place basin on folded towel under far hand and immerse hand in water. Wash, rinse, and dry the hand. Recover arm with bath blanket. Repeat for the near arm and hand.
    (Rationale: Soaking the hand is comforting and aids in cleansing under the fingernails.)
16. Put the towel over the patient's chest and fold the bath blanket back. Wash, rinse, and dry the chest. Wash, assess, and dry carefully the skin under the breasts. Apply powder if the patient desires.
    (Rationale: Moisture collects in the skin folds under the breasts and may cause irritation. Powder is soothing and helps keep area dry.)
17. Keeping the towel over the chest, lower the bath blanket to just above the pubic area. Wash, rinse, and dry the abdomen, paying special attention to the umbilicus or any skin folds. Recover chest and abdomen with the bath blanket. Patient gown may be put on at this time leaving it untied at the neck.
    (Rationale: Bath blanket and towel continue to provide warmth and privacy. A patient who is chilled may feel warmer once gown is applied.)

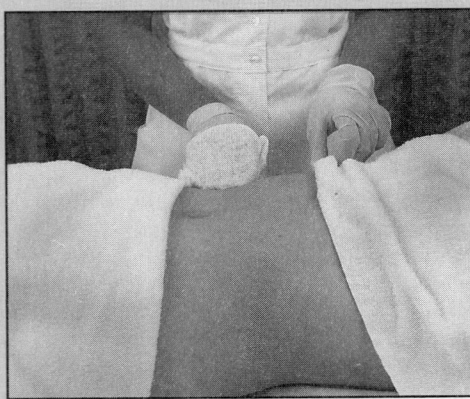

Step 17 Washing the abdomen

18. Uncover the patient's far leg. Wash with long strokes, rinse, and dry the leg. Place a towel under it.
    (Rationale: Washing far side first prevents dripping bath water on a clean area. Long strokes improve circulation by facilitating venous return.)
19. Place basin on folded bath towel and carefully immerse far foot in water. Wash, rinse, and dry the foot, paying particular attention to the area between the toes. Recover leg and foot with bath blanket. Repeat this on the other side.
    (Rationale: Soaking the foot is comforting and aids in cleansing between the toes and beneath the toenails.)

(continued)

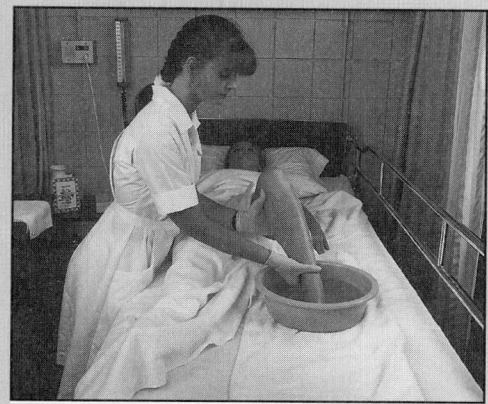

Step 19   Soaking the foot

20. Raise side rail and change bath water at this point.
    (Rationale: Cool bath water is uncomfortable for patient. The water is probably unclean. Water may be changed earlier if necessary to maintain the proper temperature.)
21. Lower side rail. Assist patient to turn away from nurse onto the side. Uncover the back and the buttocks area. Place opened towel on bed at patient's back. Wash, rinse, and dry this area. Assess for reddened areas or any skin breakdown.
    (Rationale: Skin breakdown usually occurs over bony prominences, and the sacral area and back must be carefully observed for any indication of this.)

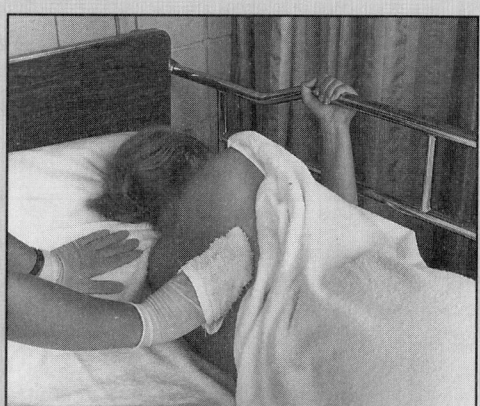

Step 21   Washing the back (Photos © B. Proud.)

22. Give a backrub at this time. Tie or snap patient gown at the back of the neck.
    (Rationale: Backrub stimulates circulation and is a comfort measure for the patient.)
23. Return patient to his or her back and adjust bath blanket so patient is covered. Use side rails for safety and change bath water again. Use clean washcloth and towel to wash the perineal area if the patient is unable to do so. Otherwise, place the necessary equipment within easy reach and allow the patient to complete this care. Provide privacy. Recover with blanket. Remove gloves and discard in proper receptacle.
    (Rationale: Cleaning the perineal area prevents skin irritation and breakdown and decreases the potential for body odor. Self-care may eliminate embarrassment for the patient.)
24. Put on gown or pajamas if this was not done earlier in the bath. Assist with personal hygiene such as deodorant and cologne. Assist with hair care and oral hygiene.
    (Rationale: Gown provides warmth. Helping with specific hygiene needs personalizes the patient's care.)
25. Make the bed with clean linens. Lower the bed and raise the side rails.
    (Rationale: These measures provide for patient's comfort and safety.)
26. Dispose of gloves properly. Wash hands.
    (Rationale: Prevents the spread of organisms.)
27. Document assessments made during bath on flow sheet and chart.
    (Rationale: Documentation provides coordination of care.)

Wound Healing

Wound healing differs according to how much tissue has been damaged. Wound healing takes place by first, second, and third intention.

First intention healing occurs in wounds with minimal tissue loss such as in surgical incisions or sutured wounds. Edges are approximate, which means they are close to each other; thus, they can seal together rapidly. Scarring and infection rates are low.

Second intention healing occurs with tissue loss such as in deep lacerations, burns, and pressure sores. Because edges do not approximate, the opening fills with

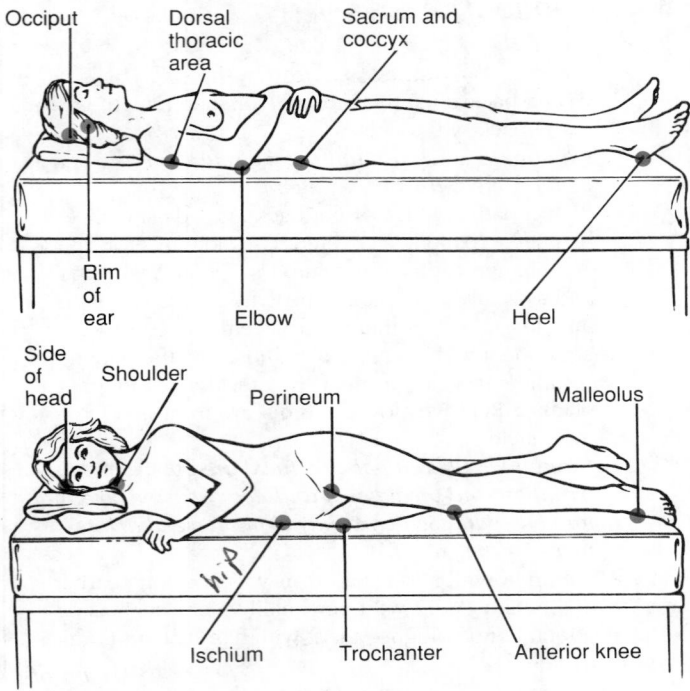

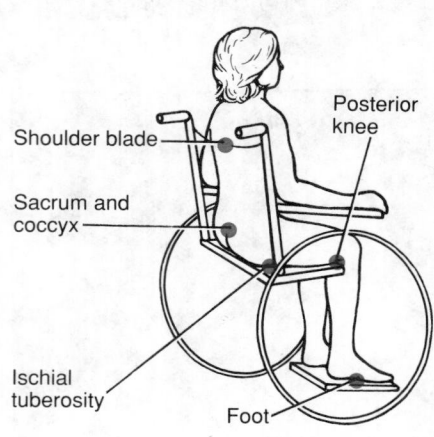

Figure 45-3. Common locations for pressure sores when person is supine and sitting. (Craven RF and Hirnle CJ. Fundamentals of Nursing: Human Health and Function. Philadelphia: J.B. Lippincott, 1992.)

granulation tissue, that is, soft pinkish tissue. Later, epithelial cells will grow over the granulation tissue. Scarring may occur and the risk of infection is increased.

Third intention healing occurs when a wound is intentionally left open temporarily. In the meantime, wound surfaces have started to granulate. An example of this type of healing is an abdominal wound left open at the time of surgery and closed later. Scarring is common.

Nursing Care in Skin Breakdown

Prevention. The nurse should always be alert for signs of pressure on the body, especially when bathing a patient or rubbing the back. The patient may also tell you about painful spots. Report signs of pressure and be suspicious of reddened areas that stay red after being rubbed. Preventive treatment is most important. As soon as a break in the skin occurs, the way is open to infection.

Stages of Pressure Sore and Ulcer Classification

Stage 1: Inflammation and redness; does not blanch when pressed with finger: only epidermis is involved; reversible process if pressure is relieved

Stage 2: Loss of epidermis with damage into dermis; appears as shallow crater or blister; swollen and painful; takes several weeks to heal once pressure is relieved

Stage 3: Subcutaneous tissues involved; not painful; may have a foul-smelling drainage; may require months to heal after pressure is relieved

Stage 4: Extensive damage to underlying structures including tendons, muscles, and bones; wound may appear small on surface but have extensive tunneling underneath; foul-smelling discharge; may take months or years to heal

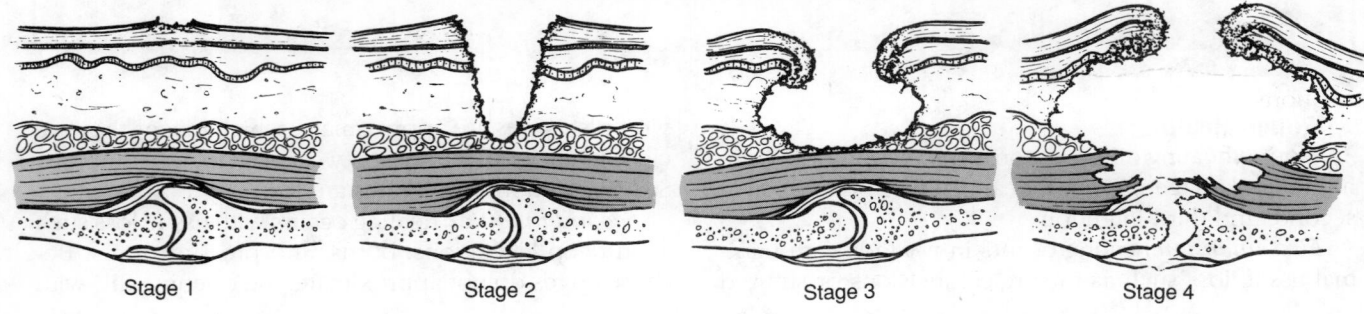

Stage 1   Stage 2   Stage 3   Stage 4

Keys to Nursing Assessment
Wound Care

◆ Anatomic location
◆ Duration of wound (how long has it been there?)
◆ Size: width, length, and depth (in mm/cm)—(a cotton tipped applicator may be inserted and then measured)
◆ Color of wound bed and surrounding tissue
◆ Presence of undermining or tunneling tracts
◆ Areas of wound, using clock as comparison
◆ Type of tissue (granulation, subcutaneous, muscle, eschar, leathery, slough and so forth)
◆ New tissue formation in margins
◆ Presence or absence of exudate (drainage) and its description (odor, amount, color, general appearance)
◆ Feeling of warmth, coldness, hardness, etc. around wound.
◆ Complaints (and description) of pain or other symptoms.
◆ Presence of any foreign bodies (sutures, gauze, dressings, medications)
◆ Appearance of skin surrounding wound
◆ Draw diagram of wound, if irregular in shape
◆ Other objective assessments (body temperature, blood tests, etc.)

The condition of an individual patient and the probable length of the illness will help you decide whether to use aids to prevent pressure sores. An airfoam mattress or special bed helps distribute pressure evenly on every part of the body. Smooth, tight undersheets also help eliminate skin irritation. In some cases lamb's wool is prescribed. Lamb's wool is effective because it is soft and gives off oils (such as lanolin) that help to keep the skin soft. Air spaces in the lamb's wool also help keep the skin dry.

At the first sign of redness, washing the area with soap and water and rubbing with lotion are the best actions. The area should be covered with large wool or cotton pads, which are changed frequently. Table 45-1 lists measures for preventing common causes of wounds. It is particularly important to prevent skin irritation in the person who is slow to heal, such as the person with diabetes mellitus, or one who is immunocompromised, such as in AIDS or cancer therapy.

Cleaning and Assessing the Wound. If, despite your precautions, a pressure sore does develop, two points in treatment are most important:

◆ Protect the broken area with sterile dressings.
◆ Relieve pressure on the area as much as possible.

The ulcerated area must be kept clean and dry. Moisture, combined with continuous pressure, pre-disposes the skin to breakdown. Pathogenic microorganisms from an infected wound or feces can be dangerous, particularly when there is a break in the skin. The nurse always wears gloves when treating a pressure sore. Hands are washed thoroughly before and after the treatment. The following interventions are performed by the nurse for the patient with pressure sores:

◆ Explain procedure to the patient.
◆ Close door or pull bedside curtains for privacy.
◆ Wash hands and don disposable gloves. (*Rationale: Prevent spread of infection.*)
◆ Position patient comfortably.
◆ Drape patient but expose area around pressure sore or ulcer.
◆ Assess the ulcer and surrounding skin.
◆ Wash the skin around the ulcer with warm water and washcloth. (*Rationale: Bacteria around the ulcer must be reduced.*)
◆ Rinse the skin with water.
◆ Dry the skin by patting with towel. (*Rationale: Gentle patting will prevent further breakdown of skin.*)
◆ Clean ulcer with prescribed solution.
◆ Apply prescribed topical ointment.
◆ Cover ulcer with type of dressing ordered. (*Rationale: Dressing prevents bacteria from entering open wound.*)
◆ Place patient in a position that is comfortable but prevents pressure on the ulcer. (*Rationale: Further breakdown of the skin is prevented.*)
◆ Discard soiled dressings, remove gloves, and wash hands. (*Rationale: Prevent spread of microorganisms.*)
◆ Document findings of the ulcer's appearance. Report to the team leader. (*Rationale: Evaluation of need for additional treatment can be made.*)

Assessment of the wound is important, as outlined in the accompanying box. Observations are documented and reported.

Moist Dressings. Many products, such as Tegasorb, use a control gel formula that provides a moist healing environment. These dressings aid in healing, while providing a seal around the wound. Often, they are covered with a transparent dressing, such as Tegaderm.

Other types of wound coverings include absorptive (absorbs the drainage and debris but is nonadherant) and gauze (dry gauze removes drainage from the ulcer, whereas moist gauze retains moisture while it removes drainage from the ulcer).

The physician will prescribe the specific treatment to be provided. Because there are a variety of ways to treat a pressure sore, the nurse should follow the guidelines of the healthcare facility.

Table 45-1. Nursing Preventive Measures for Common Causes of Wounds

Causes of Wounds	Location	Prevention
Pressure External force great enough to occlude blood in capillaries resulting in tissue anoxia	Bony prominences	Establish a turning schedule at least q2h. Use relieving support. Keep pressure off elbows and heels by elevating them with pillows and by padding.
Shear Interaction of gravity and friction against the skin's surface	Surfaces exposed to bed or chair, especially if poor skin turgor; coccyx most common site	Use draw sheets. Limit elevation of head of bed to 30°. Position feet against footboard before head elevation.
Friction Superficial abrasion resulting from the skin rubbing another surface	Surfaces that rub on bed or chair surfaces	Apply transparent dressings to areas of friction. Move patient carefully; avoid dragging across bed. Use heel or elbow protectors. Keep skin adequately hydrated.
Stripping Unintentional removal of the epidermis by mechanical means such as with adhesive removal	Surfaces where applied	Use only porous tapes and apply without tension. Remove tape by slowly pulling tape away with one hand, while supporting surrounding skin with the other. Use alternatives to tape such as Montgomery straps, Kerlix to wrap a limb, or stockinette.
Urine or Stool Urinary and fecal incontinence	Perianal skin	Use containment equipment: absorptive products, condom catheters, or fecal pouches. Keep perianal skin cleansed, moisturized, and protected with barrier ointments. Investigate cause (ie, urinary infection, need for toileting schedule, impaction, organisms in stool, tube feeding intolerance).
Perspiration	Areas where moisture can get trapped (ie, skin folds)	Keep areas of skin folds dry. Use barrier ointments. Use antifungal powder (not cream), if yeast noted.
Arterial Insufficiency Arterial perfusion jeopardized	Feet, toes, and lower leg	Avoid compression. Protect from mechanical, chemical, or thermal injuries. Provide adequate remoisturizing. Take special care with diabetics, paralyzed persons, or persons with a bleeding disorder.

Key Concept

- ◆ Change patient's position frequently to relieve pressure.
- ◆ Keep patient's skin dry and clean.
- ◆ Observe area carefully.
- ◆ Check for reddening around pressure areas.
- ◆ Document clearly.

Drug Application. When applying a drug, several steps must be followed. First, gently cleanse the area with normal saline or other prescribed solution. If infection is present, an antibiotic powder may be used. Apply the drug to the wound only; do not fill the crater unless ordered. Place a sterile gauze pad or DuoDERM, as ordered, over the ulcer. If it is to be taped in place, put tape across the middle of the pad and not at the edges, so air can reach the wound. DuoDERM is self-adhering.

Diet. Adequate nutrition is vital in both treatment and prevention. A high-calorie, high-protein, high-vitamin diet is usually given, along with large quantities of fluids. Protein supplements may be given; multiple vitamin capsules and extra vitamin C are usually given.

Pressure-Relieving Devices. Various pressure-relieving devices may be used in prevention and treatment. Such devices include air mattresses, egg-crate mattresses, air–fluid support systems, and low–air-loss bed systems (eg, Clinitron or Kin-Air).

> **Nursing Alert**
>
> Authorities do not recommend the use of doughnuts, air cushions, or air rings for most patients because, rather than relieving pressure, these devices themselves create a circle of pressure and constrict circulation.

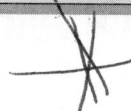

Keys for Review

Key Questions for Critical Thinking

1. You are caring for a depressed patient. Describe how you would encourage the patient to perform self-care personal hygiene.
2. You are performing personal hygiene on a patient. Describe your opportunities for assessment.
3. Describe your reasoning for repositioning a patient frequently.
4. You have a patient with a pressure sore. Describe how you would assess and provide care for this patient.

Key Readings

Craven RF, Hirnle CJ. Fundamentals of Nursing: Human Health and Function. Philadelphia, J.B. Lippincott, 1992

Earnest VV. Clinical Skills in Nursing Practice, Ed 2. Philadelphia, J.B. Lippincott, 1993

Smeltzer SC, Bare BG. Brunner and Suddarth's Textbook of Medical Surgical Nursing, Ed 7. Philadelphia, J.B. Lippincott, 1992

Smith S, Duell D. Clinical Nursing Skills: Nursing Process Model, Basic to Advanced Skills, Ed 2. Norwalk, CT, Appleton-Lange, 1989

Swearingen PL. Photo Atlas of Nursing Procedures, Ed 2. Redwood City, CA, Addison-Wesley Nursing, 1991

Key Readings *(continued)*

Taber's Cyclopedic Medical Dictionary, Ed 17. Philadelphia, F.A. Davis, 1993

Keys to Learning More

Chapter 46: elimination

Chapter 48: bandages, binders, and personal hygiene

Chapter 49: applying heat and cold for comfort

Chapter 50: head-to-toe nursing assessment

Chapter 51: isolation techniques

Chapter 52: patient comfort and pain management

Chapter 53: wound care in surgery

Chapter 54: surgical asepsis

Chapter 56: classification of medications, including those used for skin care

Chapter 68: skin disorders

Chapter 70: special skin care when a patient has a cast or traction

Chapter 76: special skin care in cancer chemotherapy or radiation therapy

Chapter 81: special skin care when a person has an "ostomy"

Chapter 89: skin care in rehabilitation

Chapter 91: personal hygiene during hospice care

46 Elimination

Keys for Learning

Learning Objectives

- State the importance of proper elimination of body wastes.
- Demonstrate the ability to assist a patient to the bathroom, to use a urinal and bedpan, and to use the bedside commode.
- Demonstrate the ability to care for the patient who has had a urinary catheter inserted.
- State basic principles for giving an enema and explain why these principles exist.
- Differentiate between the cleansing enema and other types of enemas.
- Demonstrate the ability to administer various enemas accurately.
- List two procedures for removing feces and flatus other than by enemas.
- Describe similarities and differences in bladder and bowel retraining.
- Describe the nursing care of a patient who is nauseated or vomiting.

Key Terms

anuresis	dysuria	oliguria
anuria	emesis	polyuria
calculi	enuresis	pyelonephritis
Credè's maneuver	flatus	retention
cystitis	impaction	void
diarrhea	incontinence	vomitus
distention	nocturia	

Keys to Understanding This Chapter

Chapter 5: basic human needs
Chapter 8: microorganisms and infections
Unit Three: child and adult development
Chapter 16: fluid and electrolyte balance

Keys to Understanding This Chapter
(continued)

Chapter 23: anatomy and physiology of the digestive system
Chapter 24: anatomy and physiology of the urinary system
Chapter 30: medical asepsis and universal precautions
Chapter 37: documentation and reporting
Chapter 38: signs and symptoms of illness or injury
Chapter 45: personal hygiene and skin care

Key Points

- Adequate elimination is a basic function critical to life.
- Always wear gloves when coming in contact with body secretions or drainage from the patient.
- Good handwashing technique is important.
- Assist the patient to as comfortable a position as possible for elimination and allow for privacy.
- In caring for an indwelling catheter, precautions should be taken not to allow the drainage bag to be elevated above the bladder.
- Diarrhea may be a symptom of impacted stool.
- Retraining of the bladder and bowel aids the patient in health and emotional state.
- Projectile vomiting is a significant symptom that should be reported at once.

Key Topics Outline

Urine and Feces
  Urine
  Feces
Assisting With Elimination
  The Indwelling Catheter
  The Incontinent Patient
  Enemas
  Impacted Feces
  Flatus
Nausea and Vomiting

Rosdahl CB: Textbook of Basic Nursing, 6th ed. © 1995 J.B. Lippincott Company

Elimination, a basic function of the body, is taken for granted. Most people don't think about these functions until dysfunction occurs. The importance of adequate elimination cannot be overemphasized. If the bowel or bladder is not properly evacuated, severe discomfort, physical disorders, and even death could result.

Nursing Alert

Body substance precautions require the nurse to wear gloves when coming in contact with any body secretion or drainage from the patient. Good handwashing techniques are also important.

Urine and Feces

Urine and feces provide information about a patient's condition, especially digestive and urinary disturbances. The nurse should always observe the contents of a bedpan or urinal carefully and note any unusual appearance. He or she may receive orders to save specimens of urine or feces. Save the entire specimen if you note anything unusual. Show it to the team leader or send a specimen to the laboratory. Document and report any difficulty the patient has in voiding or defecating.

Urine

About four-fifths of the excess water, some carbon dioxide, some of the solid wastes of the body, and poisons that appear in the blood are removed from the body in the urine. The normal amount of urine voided in 24 hours averages from 500 to 2,500 mL. The total output is influenced by the fluid intake and by the amount removed by the lungs, skin, and intestinal tract. In hot weather or when a patient perspires freely, the amount of urine is less than in cold weather. It is less in illnesses in which perspiration is present or fluid is retained in body tissues. To keep a normal balance of fluid in the body, from six to eight glasses of fluids are required every day. If this amount is supplied and other

conditions are normal, between 1,000 and 1,500 mL would be a normal output of urine. The normal output for an adult naturally will be more than that for a child. The processes of fluid balance and urinary waste removal are detailed in Chapters 16 and 24. In disturbances of the urinary system, the urine tells a great deal about the condition of the kidneys and the bladder.

Visual Observation

The first assessment related to the urine is observation of its physical appearance.

Color. Freshly voided normal urine is transparent and light amber in color. When urine stands, decomposition from bacterial activity gives it an ammonia-like odor.

Abnormal Components. Certain substances in urine indicate disorders. For example, it is abnormal to have the following in urine:

◆ Blood—*hematuria*
◆ Pus—*pyuria*
◆ Protein—*proteinura* (this may also occur in healthy joggers or marathon runners)
◆ Albumin—*albuminuria*
◆ Ketone bodies—*ketonuria*; seen in starvation, very severely restricted and unbalanced diets, uncontrolled diabetes mellitus, and sometimes in alcoholism
◆ Sugar or glucose—*glucosuria*; most common in diabetes mellitus

The presence of many of these abnormal components of urine can be determined by means of a simple dipstick test. The nurse is often asked to perform this procedure on the nursing unit. Instructions are given on the bottle for the particular test being done.

Urinary Tract Disorders

The basic factors in assessing for urinary disorders are given here. Report any of these conditions. The collection of specimens is discussed in the next chapter. These factors help in assessing and forming nursing diagnoses. The causes and treatment of urinary tract conditions are discussed in detail in Chapter 82.

Polyuria. A great increase in the amount of urine (an output of more than 2,500–3,000 mL/d) is called **polyuria**. It may be the result of drinking excessive amounts of fluids, or it may be a symptom of diabetes mellitus, diabetes insipidus, or nephritis (at some stages). It is often the result of the inability of the kidneys to concentrate urine.

Oliguria. A marked decrease in the amount of urine excreted, below 500 mL/d, is called **oliguria**. It may be due to the amount of fluid taken into the body. Disorders that result in oliguria include kidney failure and, in some cases, a urinary tract obstruction, which may be correctable.

Anuria. Anuria is the absence of urine secretion by the kidneys (secretion of less than 100 mL/d). It is also known as *urinary suppression*. (The cessation of any secretion is called suppression.) This condition occurs if both kidneys are injured or destroyed by disease or if a poison stops their work. Other signs of suppression that may appear with the failure to void urine are headache, dizziness, puffiness beneath the eyes, spots before the eyes, nausea, and dim vision.

Retention. Usually, when the bladder contains about 200 to 250 mL of urine, a person is aware of **distention** (a full and bloated feeling). The person also has a desire to **void** (urinate, also called micturition). Failure of the bladder to expel the urine is called **retention**. If the amount of urine increases, the bladder muscles stretch, with the danger of weakening them or making them less sensitive. One cause of retention is an obstruction of the bladder outlet or the urethra. This may be due to swelling in the tissues or to masses of fecal material in the rectum pressing on the urethra. Fear or pain may cause tension in the muscles controlling the urethral opening so that they will not relax to expel urine. Another common cause of retention is the position of the bladder when the patient is lying down.

Incontinence. Incontinence is the opposite of retention. Loss of muscle tone, injury, or paralysis destroys the ability of the urethral muscles to constrict and keep the urinary outlet closed; thus, urine dribbles constantly or the muscles relax without the person knowing it or controlling it. If the nerve pathways to the control center in the brain are injured, the patient either does not feel the impulse to urinate or is unable to control the outlet muscles and voids involuntarily. Weak muscles can be retrained. Bladder retraining is a tedious process but can achieve excellent results.

Poor Hydration. Poor hydration means there is too much or too little water in the blood or tissues. These symptoms will be discussed in Chapter 69. Some of the symptoms are the following:

- *Overhydration:* puffiness, abnormal swelling, edema, sudden weight gain, difficulty in breathing, and bounding or irregular pulse
- *Dehydration:* dry skin, extreme thirst, poor skin turgor (tone), low blood pressure, increased urine specific gravity, and elevated temperature

Other Signs of Urinary Tract Disorders. The following are additional signs of tract disorders:

- *Frequency:* the need to void more often than an average of four to six times per day, without an increase in total urine volume
- *Urgency:* inability to wait to void; may be accompanied by involuntary voiding
- **Nocturia:** waking up to void during the night
- **Enuresis:** involuntary voiding in bed, or wetting the bed, more commonly seen in children than in adults
- **Anuresis:** retention of urine in the urinary bladder
- **Dysuria:** pain on voiding, which may be in the form of cramping, burning, or shooting pains

Calculi

Calculi may be present in the kidney or urinary system. These crystalline stones are waste products from the kidneys. Certain conditions such as infection, urinary stasis (standstill), or periods of decreased activity can cause these substances to form into stones. The stones may vary in size in the bladder and kidney from microscopic sand to accumulations in size larger than a marble. As the stones move along in the kidney or urinary tract, occasionally they cause an obstruction of the urine flow. This obstruction causes a kidney infection called **pyelonephritis** or a urinary bladder infection called **cystitis**. Symptoms are chills, fever, dysuria, severe pain, and discomfort.

The nurse caring for a patient with possible kidney stones will need to strain the urine for calculi. Encourage the patient not to discard the urine until it has been examined. The following steps should be done each time the patient voids:

- Don gloves.
- Provide a graduated container to measure the urine.
- Provide a fine wire strainer in which a clean gauze has been placed.
- Poor urine through the strainer and gauze.
- Check for the presence of visible stones.
- Inspect any blood clots for the presence of stones by pressing them against the sides of the urinal or bedpan.
- Retrieve any stones and place them in a specimen

container to be sent to the laboratory for examination.

Treating Suppression

Anuria or urinary suppression is fatal if not treated. The medical treatment for suppression includes the following measures:

- Stimulate skin and bowels to eliminate wastes more freely.
- Rest and relieve the kidneys by diet (low sodium).
- Force fluids to dilute wastes.
- Give medications that stimulate the kidneys to secrete urine.
- Remove (medically or surgically) an obstruction to the urine flow.
- Use dialysis (discussed in Chapter 82) to remove wastes from the body.

Relieving Retention

The nurse may use a number of measures to help relieve retention. The sound of running water, putting the patient's hands in warm water, or pouring warm water over the genitalia of the female patient helps to stimulate the muscles to function. If the female patient is permitted to sit up in bed or on a commode, she may be able to void. The male patient will be more likely to void if he is able to stand.

Feces

Feces, also called stools or bowel movements (BM), are an important source of information about the digestive system. They provide information about digestion, inflammation, or obstruction and the presence of parasites or blood. Their appearance tells much about the way food moved through the digestive tract. Because the food mass loses water as it moves along, liquid feces indicate a rapid movement, whereas hard feces indicate that slower passage has occurred or that the feces have been in the rectum for some time. The process of expelling stool or feces is called *defecation* (see Chapter 23).

Intestinal Disorders

The portion of the physician's order requesting information on stool elimination may read *TAC stool*, which means the physician wants to know the time, amount, and character of the stool. Any unusual stool should be reported to the team leader. Save the bedpan specimen for inspection.

Time. Note the time the patient passes a stool, especially if an intestinal disorder is suspected. This observation includes frequency of stools.

Amount. The size of the mass indicates the amount of roughage or waste material in the diet and the time during which it has accumulated. The feces must always be considered in relation to diet. In some disorders, the size of the stool is not consistent with the amount of intake. For example, in some malabsorption disorders in children, the stools are abnormally large.

Color. Normal feces are a greenish brown; this color comes from bile. Clay-colored stools show that the normal amount of bile is lacking, which may be a mark of gallbladder disturbance, caused by undigested fat. A dark, tarlike stool is a sign of hemorrhage, either in the stomach or high up in the intestine. Bright red blood in the stool or streaked on the outside of the stool indicates hemorrhage lower in the intestinal tract, perhaps in the rectum; this blood is free, not mixed with stool and not yet digested. Blood is a danger signal that should be reported at once. Blood in the stool is sometimes called *melena*. Some foods and medications affect the color of the stool.

Consistency. Normal feces are soft and formed. Hard, dry stools point to constipation. It may be the result of lack of roughage in the diet or of ignoring the impulse to empty the rectum, thereby allowing feces to become dry and hard. Lack of fluids or exercise can contribute to constipation, as can lack of peristalsis, sometimes following surgery. Some medications, such as barium and codeine, are constipating.

Diarrhea is defined as frequent, loose, watery stools. The consistency of stools in diarrhea is more important than their frequency. Diarrhea may be a symptom of an intestinal infection, a parasitic infestation, or a chronic irritation of the intestine. Some intestinal disorders, such as colitis, also have an emotional component. Constipation and diarrhea may also be symptoms of *fecal impaction*, a hard mass of feces that cannot pass through anal sphincter. In this case, only the liquid stool can get past the obstruction. This person feels constipated but has diarrhea.

Odor. Feces have a characteristic odor. Unusual odors should be noted. Some medications and disorders affect the odor. Protein decay in accumulated feces also affects it.

Shape. The normal stool is cylindrical. A decrease in diameter of the stool may indicate a mass in the colon. An increase in the diameter of the stool may indicate a relaxation of colonic muscles in the walls of the lower intestine. Sometimes, a mass can cause stool to be a specific shape consistently.

Floating. A floating stool is probably indicative of undigested fats. This occurs in disorders such as gallbladder disease and cystic fibrosis.

Pus or Mucus. Pus in the stool may be due to intestinal infection or rupture of an abscess into the intestinal tract. Mucus indicates irritation of the lining of the intestinal tract.

Foreign Objects. A patient may be admitted to the hospital after having swallowed a foreign object. This is especially common in the pediatric department. You will be expected to save each fecal specimen, break it down from the solid mass, and examine it carefully to see if the object has been passed. Placing a small amount of warm water in the bedpan and using wooden tongue blades to stir the mass will facilitate examination.

Bowel Sounds. If bowel sounds can be heard, this indicates that peristalsis is occurring. This is a significant observation, for example, after surgery or a spinal cord injury. The proper technique to listen for bowel sounds is to auscultate the different quadrants of the abdomen with a stethoscope. Bowel sounds are described in the accompanying box. Skills used in listening for bowel sounds are:

◆ Wash your hands and position patient in a dorsal recumbent (supine) position. *(Rationale: Major part of the abdomen must be accessible to examiner.)*
◆ Expose the abdomen, but keep other areas of the patient's body covered.
◆ Warm the stethoscope in your hands.
◆ Place the flat side of the stethoscope against the abdomen.
◆ Imagine the abdomen to be divided into four quadrants or regions (see Fig. 14–3). Begin at a particular quadrant and continue in a clockwise fashion around the abdomen. Always use the same pattern.
◆ Listen to peristalsis, which makes a gurgling sound that occurs every 5 to 20 seconds. A sound may last for several seconds.
◆ If sounds are difficult to hear, listen for 3 to 5 minutes before deciding that they are absent. *(Rationale: This period of time confirms the absence of sounds.)*
◆ Wash your hands and document procedure on the patient record. *(Rationale: Establish a data base for intestinal motility.)*

Abnormal Girth. Assessment of abdominal girth is important if distention is present or suspected. The nurse measures the circumference around the patient's waist, usually on a daily basis. This information is valuable to the physician. Distention can point to major complications in the lower digestive tract. Actions in measuring abdominal girth are:

Description of Bowel Sounds

Audible: heard every 5–20 seconds.
Decreased and soft: hypoactive, occurs only about once per minute.
Increased and rapid: loud and high-pitched, occurring at more frequent intervals (every 3–5 seconds)
Absent: no movement of intestine heard after listening for at least 3 minutes; may result from surgery, bowel obstruction, inflammation, spinal cord trauma, and other conditions

◆ Wash your hands and position the patient in a supine position. *(Rationale: This position makes it easier to obtain the measurement.)*
◆ For repeated examination, measure the girth at the same time each day, usually before breakfast. *(Rationale: Consistency is needed in comparing measurements.)*
◆ Use a paper tape measure. *(Rationale: Paper tape will not stretch and is accurate.)*
◆ Measure the patient in the same area of the waist each time, usually at the umbilicus. *(Rationale: This enables accurate comparison of measurements.)*

Other Observations. Other observations of feces include the presence of gas and pain on defecation. Such occurrences should be noted and reported. Abdominal distention, which is a swollen, hard abdomen, may indicate an overfull colon from an intestinal obstruction, fecal impaction, or lack of peristalsis. The stool may also be sent to the laboratory for tests including the presence of occult (hidden) blood or ova and parasites (which indicates intestinal worms or other parasites).

> **Key Concept**
>
> The patient may be embarrassed about elimination processes. Give the patient privacy and treat the person with consideration.

Assisting With Elimination

Many urologic patients become dehydrated because the kidneys do not function properly. Therefore, special attention must be paid to encouraging fluid intake. The mouth may become dry and sore as a result of dehydration; appropriate hygiene and moistening agents should be given.

Sitz baths or warm, moist packs may be ordered to offset pain and discomfort and encourage voiding. Fluid intake should again be emphasized; this will help dilute the urine and lessen the burning sensation that accompanies inflammatory conditions.

The nurse keeps in mind the general complications that can arise from prolonged bed rest. It is also important to be aware of more serious problems related to urologic factors, such as hemorrhage, shock, and associated changes in blood pressure.

Helping the Patient to the Bathroom

Before assisting the patient to the bathroom, verify that he or she has permission to be up. The order "up ad lib" means that the patient can be up as much as desired. BRP means "bathroom privileges," which means that the patient has permission to get up and go to the bathroom only. Find out if the patient is on "intake and output" (I&O). If the person is on recorded output, you may place the patient's bedpan on a chair to use and then measure the urine, or you may place a collecting "hat" under the toilet seat in the bathroom so the patient can collect the specimen or use a commode. Chapter 47 describes the method for measuring urine output and determining specific gravity.

Assist the patient as needed. Explain that the nurse's call button in the bathroom will activate an alarm at the nurse's station.

Giving and Removing a Bedpan or Urinal

If the male patient is confined to bed, he will use the bedpan for defecation and the urinal for voiding. Female patients use the bedpan for both defecating and urinating; a female urinal is also available, however. The nurse wears gloves when working with bedpans. Nursing Procedure 46-1 outlines the steps in giving and removing a bedpan.

A full bladder makes a patient uncomfortable. In a hospital it is customary to offer bedpans to the patients before meals and visiting hours and when they settle down for the night. It is harmful to keep a patient waiting repeatedly for a bedpan; it weakens sphincter tone in the urethra and rectum and is physically and emotionally distressing. If a patient is forced to wait when a bedpan is needed and does not have prompt attention after using it, the person may try to walk to the bathroom alone or may upset the bedpan or be incontinent and soil the bed.

Bedpans are usually made of metal or plastic. If they feel cold, they should be warmed before being placed under the patient. Some bedpans are made of nylon resin, which feels warmer to the touch; they are less noisy in handling and can be cleaned and sterilized by conventional methods. Most are disposable.

The position that the patient must assume often makes it difficult to get on and off the bedpan; often the person needs assistance. Male nursing personnel may be available to help male patients who cannot manage by themselves. It is essential to provide privacy

for the patient. If a patient is confused or unable to follow directions, protect the bed with a pad and stay with the person.

A female patient may be allowed to sit up on the bedpan or even to dangle her legs over the edge of the bed if she is having difficulty voiding. However, she must have whatever back support is necessary and should not be left alone.

A child's bedpan is smaller than the standard size. You may be able to use a small bedpan for an adult who is helpless or unable to lie on the larger pan. A fracture pan or slipper pan, which is small and flat, is also available. The fracture pan has much less capacity and spills more easily, however.

Using a Commode

Some patients find it difficult to urinate and defecate when using a bedpan. If a patient is unable to go to the bathroom, the physician may permit the use of a commode at the bedside. A commode is a straight-backed chair, with an open seat and a receptacle beneath.

The nurse wears gloves for this procedure. Transfer the person from bed to commode as you would from bed to chair (see Chapter 43). Stay with the patient if there is any chance that the patient will become faint. The directions for using a bedpan also apply to using a commode. Wash the patient's hands, note the contents of the commode container, clean the commode after use, and wash your hands. Properly dispose of gloves. If the commode cannot be kept out of sight, it may be closed and kept at the bedside.

Using the Urinal

The urinal is used by a male patient for voiding. Wear gloves and carefully wash your hands when handling the urinal. Cover the urinal when you bring it and remove it. Help the patient to position the urinal if necessary and provide needed articles for handwashing. It is often easier for a man to void while standing at the bedside, if this is allowed. After he urinates, measure the urine, if ordered. Then rinse the urinal, first with cold, then with hot water. (*Rationale: Hot water causes protein substances to coagulate.*)

The Indwelling Catheter

Occasionally you will take care of patients who have retention catheters inserted for urine drainage. It is your responsibility to care for the equipment that is used and to see that the drainage apparatus is working properly. The equipment considered here consists of the drainage tubing attached to the catheter and the container for the urine. *Never remove the catheter without an order.* If it should fall out, report the incident to the team leader immediately. *Do not attempt to replace it without*

Nursing Procedure 46-1

Giving and Removing the Bedpan

Supplies and Equipment

Gloves
Bedpan
Cover for bedpan
Toilet tissue
Handwashing supplies
Air freshener (optional)

Procedure

1. Obtain bedpan if one is not available in bedside cabinet.
   (Rationale: Organization facilitates performance of the skill. Each patient has a separate bedpan.)
2. Explain procedure to patient.
   (Rationale: Providing information fosters patient cooperation.)
3. Wash hands prior to putting on gloves.
   (Rationale: Handwashing prevents the spread of organisms. Gloves act as a barrier.)
4. Close the curtain or door to the room.
   (Rationale: This protects the patient's privacy.)
5. Raise the bed to a comfortable height. Lower near side rail.
   (Rationale: bed at proper height prevents back strain. Lowering side rail near the nurse provides for patient's safety.)
6. Fold the bed linen away from the patient, exposing as little of the body as possible.
   (Rationale: This protects the patient's privacy and provides access for placing the bedpan.)
7. Assist the patient onto the bedpan. If patient is able to help, encourage him or her to flex the knees and lift hips:
   a. Place the bedpan under the buttocks with the rounded curved end toward the patient's back and the narrow, open end toward the feet.
      (Rationale: Placing a regular bedpan in this position fits the contour of the body, alleviates discomfort, and prevents spilling of waste materials.)
   b. Place the fracture pan under the buttocks with the flat end toward the patient's back if the patient cannot use a regular bedpan.
      (Rationale: A fracture pan exerts less pressure on the hips and spine and is easier to place under the patient.)

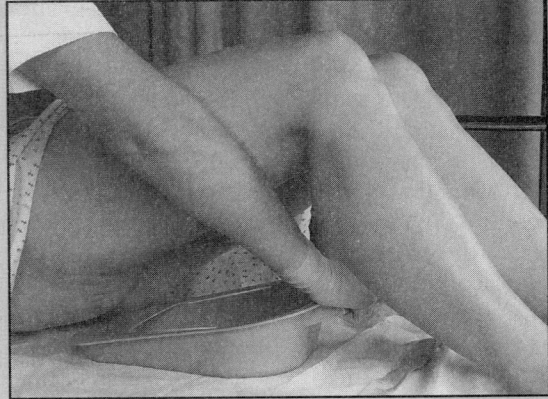

Step 7b   Placing a fracture pan under a patient

8. If patient is immobile, roll the patient on the side away from the nurse. Position the bedpan against the buttocks, hold firmly in place, and turn the patient onto his or her back. Check the location of the pan.
   (Rationale: Bedpan is properly positioned to avoid spillage.)

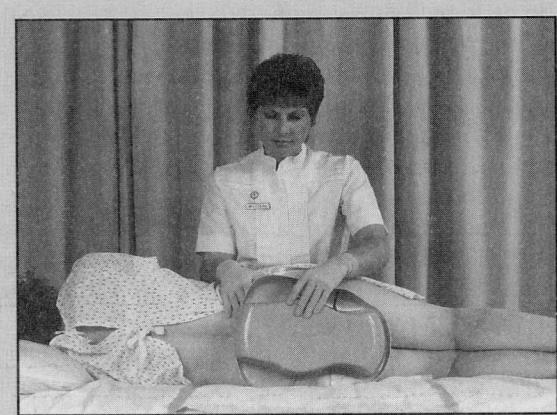

Step 8   Positioning the bedpan against the buttocks while the patient is on the side

9. Replace the bed linen over the patient.
   (Rationale: This protects the patient's privacy.)
10. Elevate the head of the bed to semi-Fowler's position if tolerated.
    (Rationale: This most closely resembles the normal position for elimination and uses gravity as an additional force.)

(continued)

11. Place call light and toilet tissue within reach and leave patient alone if possible. If leaving the bedside, raise the side rail, remove gloves, and wash hands. *(Rationale: Call bell and raised side rail provide for patient's safety. Leaving the patient alone allows for privacy.)*
12. Remove the bedpan:
    a. Wash hands and put on gloves.
    b. Lower the side rail and the head of the bed.
    c. Uncover the patient.
    d. Fold the toilet tissue and wipe from front (pubic area) to back (anus) if patient is unable to do this independently.
    e. Steady the bedpan as the patient either lifts hips or is assisted to turn away from the nurse.
    f. Place the bedpan on the chair and cover it.
    g. Cleanse area with soap and water if necessary. Shaving lather works well and is soothing. Dry carefully.

(Rationale: Holding the bedpan steady and assisting the patient off it prevents spillage of its contents. The skin must be kept clean and dry to prevent skin breakdown.)

13. Offer handwashing supplies to patient. *(Rationale: Handwashing prevents the spread of organisms and teaches good hygiene.)*
14. Return patient to a comfortable position. Lower bed and raise side rail. Use air fresheners if necessary. *(Rationale: These measures provide for patient comfort and safety.)*
15. Empty pan into toilet and rinse. Remove gloves and wash hands. *(Rationale: Handwashing prevents the spread of organisms.)*
16. Document results according to agency policy on flow sheet, intake and output summary, or chart. *(Rationale: Documentation provides coordination of care.)*

---

a specific physician's order. A new, sterile catheter must be used, or the catheter may be discontinued.

There are several types of retention catheters such as the Malecot four-wing catheter and the dePezzer mushroom catheter, but the Foley catheter is most frequently used. Indwelling catheters of the Foley type are multilumened, which means there are several channels within the catheter. One is connected to the balloon; another is for urinary drainage. A third lumen is present in some catheters to provide a means for continuous bladder irrigation. Sterile water or sterile normal saline is usually used for inflating the balloon in an indwelling catheter. The amount of solution used follows the manufacturer's recommendation.

Catheters such as the Malecot and the dePezzer are inserted by the urologist, using a stylet. The stylet is removed after the catheter has been inserted. These catheters are self-retaining and do not have a balloon to inflate.

Catheter Insertion

The method of inserting a catheter is described in Chapter 54. This is a *sterile* procedure that must be performed with utmost care to avoid introducing bacteria in the bladder. (If bladder surgery is done, the catheter is inserted in the operating room by the urologist.)

The disposable drainage bag is already connected to the tubing, to avoid contamination. The bag is lightweight and can easily be fastened to the patient's gown while the person is out of bed. The closed drainage system collection bag must *never* be higher than the level of the patient's bladder. *(Rationale: This would*

cause urine in the bag to flow back into the bladder and could lead to infection.)*

Catheter Care

The catheter is considered a closed, sterile system. If the catheter is to be changed, the entire drainage set is changed. The nurse must be sure that there is no pulling on the catheter and that the tubing is not kinked. The tubing should go over the patient's leg when the patient is in bed. To prevent pulling, the catheter is taped to the thigh in the female patient and to the abdomen in the male patient, as ordered by the physician. Guidelines for catheter care are given in the accompanying box.

Emptying the Urinary Drainage Bag. The nurse will be asked to empty the drainage bag, using sterile technique.

Nursing Skill
Emptying the Urinary Drainage Bag

Supplies and Equipment

Disposable gloves

Procedure

1. Wash hands and don gloves. They need not be sterile. *(Rationale: Gloves are worn when handling any body fluids. You can avoid touching the sterile part of the catheter, so your gloves only need to be clean.)*

Nursing Skill Guidelines
Catheter Care

- A catheter should be used only when absolutely necessary and the catheterization procedure itself should be done only by trained personnel under sterile conditions. *(Rationale: Catheterization is an invasive technique.)*
- The catheter drainage system should consist of a closed sterile system. *(Rationale: Catheterization is a sterile technique.)*
- Wash hands and wear gloves when working with catheters.
- Tubing is not disconnected unless there are specific orders.
- Catheters are *not* irrigated unless the physician writes specific orders to do so.
- If the patient ambulates, the bag goes along.
- Sterile urine specimens may be obtained from most indwelling catheter systems by using a syringe with a small-gauge needle and aspirating from a designated specimen port area that has been cleansed with alcohol or povidone iodine (Betadine).
- Catheters should be secured externally. *(Rationale: This prevents pressure on the urethra and prevents the catheter from being pulled out.)*
- The urethral meatus and the catheter near the meatus should be cleansed at least twice a day with alcohol or pHisoHex soap. *(Rationale: This prevents infection.)*
- Many facilities recommend application of an antimicrobial ointment to the meatal area after the bidaily cleansing.

- Urine is secreted constantly and should drip constantly through the drainage tube.
- The tubing should be *over* the patient's leg, not under. *(Rationale: The weight of the patient's leg might slow or stop drainage.)*
- Some slack in the tubing should be allowed above bed level. Fasten the tubing to the bed. *(Rationale: The patient should be allowed to turn freely. If the tubing is loose above the level of the bed, drainage will not be impaired. Fastening the tubing to the bed keeps it from falling over the side.)*
- The tubing should fall straight down from the bed to the drainage bag. (This is called straight drainage.) It should not hang down or be kinked. *(Rationale: If the tubing is kinked or hangs down, drainage will be slowed and infection can occur.)*
- The level of the bag must always be kept *below* the level of the bladder. *(Rationale: If urine flows back into the bladder, infection often results.)*
- Drainage systems are closed systems. Do not open bag except to drain it from the bottom. Follow the instructions for the particular bag being used. *(Rationale: Ensuring the integrity of the system is vital to maintain sterility.)*
- Measure and record output in the proper manner. *(Rationale: The volume of urine is an important piece of information in the care of the catheterized person.)*
- Dispose of gloves properly and wash hands after catheter care. *(Rationale: This procedure follows all patient contact, especially those involving body fluids.)*

2. Carefully pull the drain tube, located on the bottom of the bag, out of the storage pocket, without touching it below the level of the clamp.
3. Hold the tube over the container and release the clamp, making sure that the drain tube does not touch anything. *(Rationale: You avoid touching the lower part or the inside of the drain tube because pathogenic organisms can travel up the system and cause a bladder infection.)*
4. When the urine has drained out, clamp the tube and carefully replace it into the storage pocket. Be sure the clamp is far enough up the tube to allow most of the tube to fit into the pocket. Do not move the clamp up on the tube. *(Rationale: These procedures help maintain the sterility of the catheter's closed drainage system.)*
5. Collect the urine in a graduated container and measure it.
6. Observe the color, odor, and other characteristics of urine. *(Rationale: The nurse's observations are important to the healthcare team when they evaluate the patient's illness and response to treatment.)*
7. Rinse the graduate with cool water and dispose of it in the toilet.

8. If the person will be going home with an indwelling catheter, teach him or her what you are doing as you do it. *(Rationale: Patient and family teaching are important for accuracy of procedures.)*
9. You may ask the patient to do a return demonstration after you have demonstrated the procedure. *(Rationale: Patient teaching and its documentation are important components of the nursing care plan.)*
10. Properly dispose of your gloves and wash your hands.
11. Record output on the appropriate sheet and document and report any special observations about the urine.

Catheter Irrigation

If the physician orders catheter irrigations, the nurse must remember that the bladder is sterile and that any solution injected into the bladder must also be sterile. Because the drainage tubing is usually disconnected for irrigation, organisms can travel up the tubing into the bladder after the tube is reconnected. Therefore, catheter irrigation is performed only when absolutely necessary and only using strict sterile technique (see Chapter 54).

Catheter irrigation is usually done to remove clots, to fight infection (by using an antibiotic or bacteriostatic agent), or to ensure that the catheter is patent (open).

The Patient With a Suprapubic Cystocath

The suprapubic cystocath is a type of bladder drainage often used after gynecologic and other genitourinary types of surgery. The catheter is inserted surgically through a small incision just above the pubic bone. This area is the suprapubic region. It is inserted through an adhesive body seal to prevent drainage around the catheter. It is then connected to a drainage bag. The advantage of this method is that the patient can void naturally while the catheter is still in place. Recatheterization is avoided. The patient also does not feel annoying irritation from the catheter in the urethra. If perineal surgery has been done, this type of catheter eliminates urinary drainage that might contaminate the surgical area. As in any other instance in which a catheter is inserted into the bladder, sterile technique and proper precautions are observed. The physician must remove the cystocath.

The Incontinent Patient

Causes and treatment of urinary incontinence are discussed in Chapter 82. You will care for these patients in all areas of the hospital or nursing home.

The Patient With an Appliance

Appliances for collecting urine are available, particularly for the male patient. Such an appliance consists of a bag that slips over the penis and is attached to a belt. The patient wears the appliance under his clothes. The bag has an outlet at the lower end, which can be opened. A condom catheter may also be used. This fits over the penis like a condom.

Because no effective appliance is available for collecting urine in a woman, the problem of urinary incontinence is more difficult to manage. She can wear a perineal pad, although perhaps a better solution is a disposable incontinent brief.

The following actions are taken in caring for the incontinent patient:

◆ The buttocks and genitals should be cleansed frequently and the area dried. Shaving cream is excellent because it cleans and disinfects. An antiseptic may be applied to the skin. (*Rationale: These measures help to prevent irritation and infection.*)
◆ Cleanliness and prompt attention to removing soiled pads or incontinent briefs is important. (*Rationale: This helps eliminate urine odor and skin irritation.*)

◆ Any appliance or protection device should be washed thoroughly inside and out with soap and water at least once a day. (*Rationale: Eliminate odor and prevent buildup of dangerous bacteria.*)
◆ Carefully assess the condition of the skin in the perianal area to detect early signs of skin breakdown.

> **Nursing Alert**
>
> The incontinent patient should *not* have limited fluids.

Bladder Retraining

It is possible to control some types of incontinence by establishing a voiding routine. It takes patience and experimenting, but it can be successful. The nurse can start by documenting when the patient's bladder empties. (The patient's voiding routine may follow a pattern.) The patient should either be given the bedpan or should go to the bathroom just before these times so a routine can be established for emptying the bladder. This will also aid in keeping the patient dry. The time span between voidings can be gradually increased, thus building up the tone of the bladder muscles and increasing the capacity of the bladder. The bladder eventually becomes trained to empty at regular intervals with the assistance of the Credè's maneuver (pronounced cru'da').

In **Credè's maneuver**, the nurse applies firm, gentle pressure to the bladder, with hands held flat, starting at the umbilicus and moving down to the symphysis pubis. This procedure is repeated several times, with the final pressure being applied directly over the bladder itself.

Various incontinence patterns can be managed with Kegel exercises, discussed in Chapter 84. These exercises are designed to increase sphincter tone. The patient will need to wear a disposable pad during the training period to catch the urine. If after one year this conservative mode of treatment is not effective in retraining the bladder, the patient may opt for surgery.

> **Key Concept**
>
> The goal of all rehabilitation is to restore the patient to functioning that is as normal as possible.

Bladder incontinence is more difficult to control than bowel incontinence, but with perseverance, control can be established for many patients. Timing is essential to bladder retraining. The bladder must be emptied the first thing in the morning and the last thing at night, as well as in between. Plenty of fluids and exercise must be provided. During the night, the male patient may wear a condom catheter. Women usually wear adult incontinence briefs.

Be prepared for incontinent episodes during the training period. Assure the patient that bladder control takes time and that incontinence is to be expected and is not a sign of failure. Keep a careful record of fluid intake and output to maintain a balance and to be sure that urine is not being retained. Adequate fluid intake helps prevent urinary stasis, and thus prevents infections. Complete bladder control is not possible for every patient, but many do accomplish it. Bladder control is especially important because a permanent catheter in the bladder greatly increases the danger of bladder infection.

Home Care Adaptations
The Incontinent Person

Many patients are released from the hospital without having overcome incontinence. This becomes a family concern. The nurse has an obligation to do aggressive patient and family teaching. Demonstrate how to keep the patient dry without changing the entire bed. Absorbent pads, covered by a liner, are placed next to the skin. The pads can be changed easily, and the liner helps to prevent irritation. Disposable pads on the bed or chair should be used when possible. If the patient has established a routine for voiding, the family should be taught to understand the importance of maintaining this routine. The use of disposable incontinent briefs should be explained and demonstrated. The nurse should also emphasize the importance of fluids, diet, and cleanliness.

Bladder Retraining on the Closed Drainage System. Bladder retraining may be started while the catheter is connected to the closed drainage system. Some techniques temporarily disconnect the catheter from the drainage tube, but these methods increase the possibility of microorganisms ascending the catheter to the bladder. The following procedure does not disconnect the catheter but clamps it.

Nursing Skill
Retraining the Bladder With Catheter in Place

Supplies and Equipment

Protective pad for bed
Catheter clamp
Sterile 4 × 4 pads
Disposable gloves

Procedure

1. Explain the procedure to the patient. (*Rationale: You need the patient's cooperation.*)
2. Don disposable gloves. (*Rationale: Prevent the spread of infection.*)
3. Position the patient in supine position with head of the bed slightly elevated. (*Rationale: Prevent pressure on the bladder.*)
4. Place protective pad under the patient. (*Rationale: Protect the bed from becoming wet.*)
5. Clamp off the catheter and leave catheter clamped for 1 to 2 hours. (*Rationale: This allows time for the bladder to fill*).
6. Open clamp and allow bladder to drain by gravity into drainage bag. (*Rationale: This empties bladder and prevents urine stasis.*)
7. Repeat the procedure, as ordered by the physician.
8. Dispose of gloves properly and wash your hands carefully. (*Rationale: Prevent the spread of infectious organisms.*)
9. Record the procedure on the patient record, including urinary output. (*Rationale: chart the progress toward gaining bladder control.*)

The time the bladder is clamped off is increased to 3 or 4 hours as ordered. The goal is to help the patient regain the sensation to void.

Enemas

Normal bowel movements may be hampered by poor diet, lack of fluid, lack of exercise, and certain illnesses. An enema can help clean out the colon in the preceding situations or can be used to administer medications.

A physician's order is required for an enema. The order will state the type of enema to be given, as well as how often it is to be given. The order may be PRN (as needed). In the facility, the nursing student or new graduate must consult the instructor or team leader about carrying out a PRN order.

An enema may be given with a commercially prepared, disposable enema unit or by the bag-and-tubing method. With the bag-and-tubing method, the solution flows from a bag through a length of tubing, which is attached to the rectal tube by a connecting tip. Both units are disposable.

Types of Enemas

Cleansing Enema. The cleansing enema may also be called a purgative enema. The purpose of this enema is to inject enough fluid into the colon to soften feces, stimulate peristalsis, and produce a bowel movement that empties the rectum and lower colon. This procedure often is a necessary part of treatment when body functions are disturbed or before surgery.

Usually, after a meal, a peristaltic wave is set up that moves feces from the colon into the rectum. The fecal mass stimulates nerve endings in the rectum and brings the desire to empty it. If this impulse is ignored, it disappears, the feces become dry and hard, and defecation is difficult. Other situations also cause constipation. The colon and rectum become distended and lose muscle tone as feces accumulate. An enema provides an artificial stimulus and helps to remove feces, but unless normal stimulation and regular defecation are established, taking an enema could become a habit.

The most common enema solution used for the cleansing enema is plain tap water (TWE). Other solutions include normal saline, hypertonic saline, or a soap solution (SSE). A small amount of oil (such as cottonseed, mineral, or olive oil) may be given as a retention enema to cleanse the bowel. Action may result immediately or it may take longer; usually it occurs in less than 15 minutes.

Adding prepackaged soap concentrate to water is the method of mixing a soap suds enema (SSE). Soap irritates the mucous membrane of the colon and stimulates peristalsis. Mild soap is used to avoid excessive irritation and is usually not used before rectal examinations or for patients known to have rectal disease. The commercially prepared, disposable enema unit contains a hypertonic solution in small amounts, usually 4 oz (120 mL) for an adult. Acting on the principle of osmosis, it draws fluid from the tissues in the colon to create fluid bulk. The solution is not irritating; it easily brings good results in less than 10 minutes. It is especially useful for patients who are unable to retain larger quantities of fluid or who have anal incontinence. It helps to prevent anal impaction in patients who must lie in one position or who are unable to sit up. The disposable enema unit is also widely used in preparing a patient for radiographic or rectal examinations.

Carminative Enema. The carminative enema is given to stimulate peristalsis so that gas may be expelled from the intestine.

Anthelminthic Enema. Anthelminthic drugs help destroy intestinal parasites. They usually are given orally, but because they are toxic drugs, they are unsafe for some patients to take orally. In such instances, a solution of an anthelmintic drug may be instilled into the rectum to be retained.

Emollient Enema. An emollient enema consists of a small amount of olive or cottonseed oil, given to protect or soothe the mucous membrane of the colon. This enema is to be retained.

Oil Enema. The enema is given in small amounts because it must be retained to be effective. Sometimes, if an oil solution has not been effective after several hours, it is necessary to follow with an enema of soap or saline solution.

Medicated Enema. The medicated enema, in which a drug is inserted into the rectum, is sometimes the only way to give a patient a drug. It may also be the best way to make a drug take effect quickly. Some drugs are rapidly absorbed by the mucous membranes. The drug is combined with a small amount of oil or saline to reduce its irritating effect on the mucous membranes and to lessen the desire to expel it, because it is given to be retained.

Administering the Enema

Principles for administering any type of enema are indicated in the accompanying box. Nursing Procedure 46-2 explains how to give a cleansing enema by the bag-and-tubing method.

Self-contained disposable enemas, such as Fleet's, are frequently used. General principles for administration are the same as for any other enema. Specific instructions are on the package. The person administrating the enema must be sure to use the correct solution and the correct child or adult size. Fleet's enemas are usually stored and administered at room temperature; however, warming the solution in a container of warm water or under running warm water is comfortable for the patient. The patient often self-administers the enema prior to surgery or x-rays. It is easy to discard.

Special Circumstances

The Patient Unable to Retain an Enema. If the patient is unable to contract the anal sphincter muscles, it will be necessary to give the cleansing enema with the patient on the bedpan. Elevating the head of the bed slightly and placing a pillow in the lumbar region help to prevent back strain. In some cases, the enema tubing is passed through a ball, and the ball is held against the rectal opening to hold the fluid inside. The advantage of the disposable enema unit for this patient is that only a small quantity is required.

The Patient Unable to Expel an Enema. When the sphincters do not respond to stimulation and the patient is unable to expel an enema, the solution must be withdrawn. The bedpan is placed on a chair at the bedside, beneath the level of the rectum. When the rectal tube is directed into the pan, the force of gravity helps to drain off (siphon) the fluid.

Colostomy Irrigation. The method of removing fecal material from the bowel after a colostomy has been performed is known as colostomy irrigation. This procedure is described in Chapter 81.

Nursing Skill Guidelines
Administering an Enema

♦ Wash your hands *before and after* giving an enema. Be sure to wear gloves. (*Rationale: Prevent the spread of microorganisms.*)

♦ The height at which the solution is instilled affects the force and speed of its flow; the higher the bag is held, the greater the force. The bag is *never* held more than 18 inches (45 cm) above the mattress. (*Rationale: This prevents injury.*)

♦ The bag-and-tubing enema is given by way of a rectal tube, which is smooth and flexible so it will not irritate the rectum. Rectal tubes come in different sizes. (*Rationale: The larger the catheter, the faster and the more forcefully the fluid can flow. The faster the fluid is instilled, the harder it is to retain and the faster it will be expelled.*)

♦ The amount of solution used for a cleansing enema (bag-and-tubing method) for an adult usually ranges from 750 to 1000 mL, whereas the amount used for a retention enema ranges from 150 to 200 mL. (*Rationle: The larger amount will stipulate rapid expulsion; the smaller amount will be retained longer.*)

♦ The nurse must judge when to stop instilling fluid based on the patient's statements and reactions. (*Rationale: Each person has a different limit in the amount of fluid he or she can retain.*)

♦ The temperature of the solution should be only slightly higher than body temperature. Measure the temperature with a thermometer. The temperature must *never* exceed 105°F (40.5°C). (*Rationale: Avoid injuring the lining of the intestine.*)

♦ Disposable enema units are usually stored at room temperature; these units should never be stored in a cold place. You may also wish to warm the solution slightly. (*Rationale: Instillation of cold solution is uncomfortable and can cause shock.*)

♦ The patient lies on the side (preferably, the left side) for the cleansing enema. (*Rationale: The position of the colon within the body makes this the most effective position.*) If the patient is in traction or in a cast, the enema can be given with the patient lying on his or her back. The person may be placed in a knee–chest position for a retention enema, if the patient can tolerate it. (*Rationale: This position helps to encourage retention of the fluid for a longer period of time.*)

♦ Drape the patient, covering the body as much as possible. (*Rationale: It is important to preserve the patient's privacy and dignity.*)

♦ The enema cannot be effectively given if the patient is sitting up. (*Rationale: Without the aid of gravity, great force must be exerted to instill the fluid into the colon and it is difficult to retain.*)

♦ The rectal tube is lubricated and inserted carefully. Prepackaged units have prelubricated enema tips. Insert the tube about 3 to 4 inches (7.5–10 cm). Do not attempt to force the tube against the resistance. Instruct the patient to take a few short, panting breaths and relax. (*Rationale: The anus has an inside and an outside sphincter muscle which, together, control the opening to the outside of the body. The tube should be inserted past both of these muscles.*)

♦ The solution is usually given slowly. Instruct the patient to retain the enema as long as possible. (*Rationale: Both the cleansing and the retention enema can be retained longer if given slowly. Longer retention enhances the effectiveness of the enema.*)

♦ Carefully dispose of all materials after the enema is completed. Wash your hands. (*Rationale: Fecal material is contaminated and carries many microorganisms.*)

♦ Record that the enema was given and document the results and the patient's reactions. Chart the type of solution used, as well as the temperature of the solution. (*Rationale: It is important to communicate to other healthcare team members. This is part of the nursing care plan.*)

Giving an Enema to a Child. This procedure is described in Chapter 64. This amount of solution and technique used depend on the child's age and size.

Giving an Enema to a Paralyzed Person. Giving an enema requires a special approach if the person is paralyzed. The paralyzed patient is unable to retain the enema solution. If the patient must have an enema, it should be given at the same time every day. Later, a suppository at this time may be all that is necessary to stimulate a bowel movement, until finally the patient needs neither of these aids. Manual digital pressure to the abdomen or manual disimpaction may also be applied to assist in evacuation.

Impacted Feces

Sometimes, the feces become tightly fixed in the rectum or colon, so that the patient cannot expel them. This is called an impaction and develops because of frequent, incomplete evacuation of feces. As feces accumulate in the colon or rectum, water continues to be absorbed from them through the intestinal wall. The fecal mass becomes large, very dry, and difficult to move. Conditions that cause constipation may lead to fecal impaction, a patient's inactivity usually being the greatest offender. (Diarrhea may be a symptom of impaction if only loose, watery stools are able to pass around the accumulated feces.) In the event that an impaction does

Giving a Cleansing Enema (Bag-and-Tubing Method)

Supplies and Equipment

Gloves
Disposable enema setup
  or
Enema container with tubing and clamp
  (Approximate rectal tube size:
  adult 22–30 Fr, child 12–18 Fr)
Solution as prescribed by physician
Bedpan and cover
Toilet tissue
Waterproof pad
Water-soluble lubricant
Bath blanket
Cleansing supplies
IV pole

Procedure

1. Gather supplies.
   (*Rationale: Organization facilitates performance of the skill.*)
2. Explain procedure to patient.
   (*Rationale: Providing information fosters patient cooperation.*)
3. Wash hands prior to putting on gloves.
   (*Rationale: Handwashing prevents the spread of organisms. Gloves act as a barrier.*)
4. Prepare the enema:
   a. Fill enema bag with prescribed solution at proper temperature (adults, 100°–110°F; children, 100°F).
   b. Open clamp and allow fluid to flow through tubing.

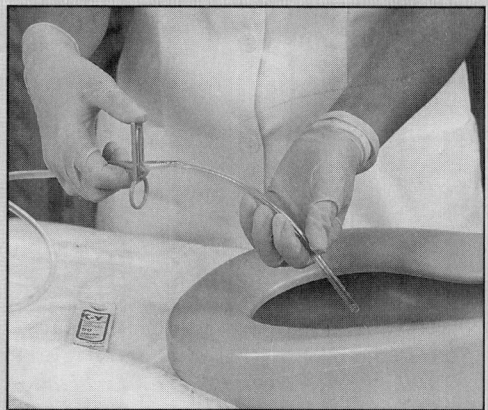

Step 4b   Clearing the air from the enema tube

   c. Reclamp tubing.
   (*Rationale: Enema solution clears tubing of air.*)

5. Close the curtain or door to the room.
   (*Rationale: This protects the patient's privacy.*)
6. Raise the bed to a comfortable height. Lower near side rail.
   (*Rationale: Bed at proper height prevents back strain. Lowering side rail near the nurse provides for patient's safety.*)
7. Place a waterproof pad under the patient's buttocks.
   (*Rationale: This prevents moistening or soiling the bed linens.*)
8. Assist the patient to turn onto the left side with right knee flexed. Place bedpan in bed close to patient. If patient is unable to retain enema solution, place on bedpan.
   (*Rationale: Gravity facilitates the flow of solution when the patient is on the side. Poor anal sphincter control makes it difficult to retain enema solution.*)
9. Lubricate the tip of the rectal tube for 2 to 3 inches.
   (*Rationale: Lubricant allows for smooth insertion of the rectal tube without injuring bowel mucosa.*)

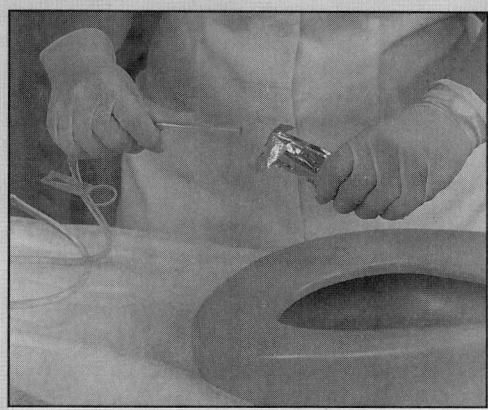

Step 9   Lubricating the tip of the tube

10. Place the enema bag on an IV pole or raise container 18 inches above the anus.
    (*Rationale: Gravity aids in the instillation of the enema solution.*)
11. Separate the buttocks. Ask the patient to take a deep breath. Gently insert the rectal tube 3 to 4 inches toward the umbilicus (2–3 inches for a child).
    (*Rationale: Taking a deep breath helps to relax the anal sphincter. Inserting the rectal tube too far can damage or perforate the rectal mucosa.*)

(continued)

12. Hold tube in place with one hand while opening clamp with the other hand and allowing solution to flow into rectum. Enema should be delivered over a 5- to 10-minute period. If patient complains of cramping, lower the bag or temporarily clamp the tubing.
    (Rationale: The higher the container is positioned, the more rapid the flow of enema solution. Halting the enema for a brief time aids in retention of the solution.)

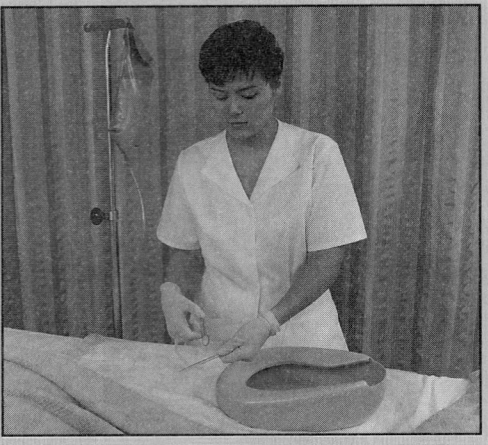

Step 12   Preparing to give the enema (Photos © B. Proud.)

13. Apply clamp and remove rectal tube when enema is completed. Ask patient to retain the solution as long as possible.
    (Rationale: this facilitates effective results from the enema.)
14. Assist the patient into the bathroom or onto the bedpan with the head of the bed elevated. Place the call bell within easy reach.
    (Rationale: Contracting the abdominal and perineal muscles is easier in a sitting position.)
15. When enema solution has been expelled, assist patient back to bed or off bedpan. Inspect enema results.
    (Rationale: Some diagnostic tests require that enemas be given until results are clear. Observing results of enema confirms its effectiveness.)
16. Return patient to a comfortable position. Lower the bed and raise the side rail.
    (Rationale: These measures provide for patient comfort and safety.)
17. Remove gloves and wash hands.
    (Rationale: Handwashing prevents the spread of organisms.)
18. Document enema results and type of enema administered to patient on flow sheet or chart.
    (Rationale: Documentation provides coordination of care.)

not respond to an enema, the physician may order the nurse to remove the feces manually, a procedure known as *manual disimpaction* or digital removal. Many patients with permanent paralysis perform manual disimpaction as part of their activities of daily living program.

Nursing Alert

Digital removal of feces is contraindicated for most cardiac patients; after gynecologic or male reproductive system surgery; and after abdominoperineal repair, rectal surgery, a colostomy, or other genitourinary surgery. It should not be done in patients who are receiving radioactive isotope therapy (especially in the abdominopelvic area) or perineal perfusion of anticancer drugs. Patients who have a bleeding tendency, especially in the rectal or vaginal area, should not receive this treatment and neither should pregnant women. *(Rationale: The procedure could aggravate the existing condition or could cause damage.)*

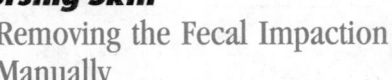
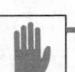

Nursing Skill
Removing the Fecal Impaction Manually

Supplies and Equipment

Disposable gloves
Bedpan
Toilet tissue

Procedure

1. Don gloves. You may wish to wear two pairs.
2. Explain to the patient what you are doing and why.
   (Rationale: Patient cooperation and relaxation help to make the procedure more comfortable.)
3. Position the patient on the left side, with the knees, especially the upper knee, drawn up as far as possible.
   (Rationale: The position is comfortable for the patient and allows easy view of and access to the area for the nurse.)
4. Drape the patient. *(Rationale: Preserve the patient's privacy as much as possible.)*

5. Place a disposable waterproof pad under the buttocks. *(Rationale: A pad helps to prevent soiling the bed.)*

6. Instruct the patient to take short, panting breaths during the procedure. *(Rationale: Panting helps relax the anal sphincter.)*

7. Using clean disposable gloves, lubricate one or two fingers well. Insert one or two fingers *carefully* into the rectum until you feel the stool; then, rotate the finger gently. *(Rationale: This helps break up the stool.)*

8. Before removing your finger, gently stimulate the anal sphincter with a rotating motion. *(Rationale: This stimulation helps cause a natural response to defecate.)*

9. Dispose of your gloves properly and wash your hands. *(Rationale: Prevent spread of microorganisms from intestinal tract.)*

10. Assist patient to bathroom, commode, or bedpan as needed. *(Rationale: Patient may be uncomfortable and need assistance.)*

11. Leave the patient's signal cord within reach. *(Rationale: The person may need the bedpan again in a short time.)*

12. Provide a washcloth and soap for the patient for cleansing the rectal area or the nurse should do the cleansing if the patient cannot. Leave the waterproof pad in place for a few minutes to protect the bed. Dispose of gloves and wash hands. *(Rationale: The patient and bed area should be kept clean to prevent spread of microorganisms.)*

13. Document the procedure, noting any special patient re[...] ll as the amount, color, consistency, and [...] ool obtained or expelled.

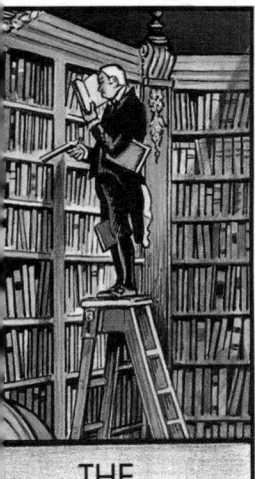

e should be stopped immediately if the [...]s of pain, faintness, or nausea, or if you [...]rd effect, such as bleeding. Usually, [...] broken into pieces, the patient will be [...] The patient may be given an enema for [...]me cases, the nurse may be instructed [...] articles of feces after breaking up the [...]s removed in as noninvasive a manner

[...] *is a woman*, the following procedure [...]e. Apply a *sterile* glove to one hand, [...]r, and insert it into the vagina. Insert [...]to the rectum. The two gloved fingers [...]same time, work to break up the stool. [...]ed into the vagina must be kept sterile. [...]ific order before doing this procedure. [...]use the vaginal method is a more in-[...]t must be done carefully and with a [...]r. The uterus is considered sterile; care [...] not to introduce infection-causing

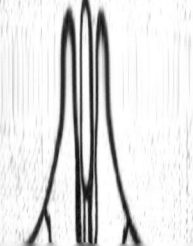

THE BOOKSTORE FOR MEDICAL PROFESSIONALS

[...]ning

[...]g are important factors in bowel

◆ Timing: Elimination should be done at the same time each day.

◆ Fluid intake: A high fluid intake is recommended.

◆ Diet: A diet to assist in maintaining a fairly solid consistency without causing constipation or diarrhea is recommended.

◆ Physical activity: The more exercise the patient receives, the more likely the person will be able to achieve bowel control.

The nurse can assist by providing a large quantity of liquids and bulk foods in the diet, such as fresh fruit and vegetables, and avoiding those foods that have been found to produce loose stools and excess gas (flatus).

If possible, the patient should be assisted into the bathroom, rather than using a bedpan or commode. *(Rationale: Moving about helps to stimulate a bowel movement and gives the patient satisfaction.)*

A successful bowel retraining program includes the following suggested procedure:

◆ Don gloves.

◆ Choose a time that is convenient for the patient within the daily schedule. *(Rationale: It is important to establish a daily routine.)*

◆ Administer oral stool softeners daily, as ordered, or insert a cleansing suppository at least 30 minutes before the scheduled time for elimination. *(Rationale: Initiates retraining of the bowel to react to softeners or a suppository on a regular basis.)*

◆ Offer a warm cup of liquid or fruit juice. *(Rationale: This stimulates peristalsis.)*

◆ Assist the patient to the toilet, bedpan, or bedside commode at the designated time.

◆ Provide for privacy. *(Rationale: Elimination is a private matter.)*

◆ Instruct the patient to apply pressure to the lower abdomen, and bear down. *(Rationale: This action stimulates colon to empty.)*

◆ Empty and cleanse the elimination receptacle. Wash your hands.

◆ Document results of bowel movement on the patient record. *(Rationale: Progress in bowel retraining is monitored.)*

The patient always is given positive reinforcement for any progress that is made. Bowel retraining is a long process. Sometimes it takes as long as 4 to 6 weeks to establish a successful routine.

Flatus

Sometimes a rectal tube or an Evac-u-sac is used to aid the patient in expelling **flatus** (gas) from the intestine. Inserted in the rectum, the device provides an outlet for accumulated gas and relieves the discomfort of intestinal distention.

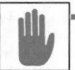

Nursing Skill
Inserting the Rectal Tube

Supplies and Equipment

Rectal tube
Lubricant
Evac-u-sac or cardboard
Disposable gloves

Procedure

1. Don gloves.
2. Ask the patient to lie on his or her side (preferably the left). *(Rationale: This position promotes comfort for the patient and ease of the nurse in inserting the tube.)*
3. Wash hands and put on gloves. *(Rationale: Prevent transfer of micoorgnisms.)*
4. Lubricate the tube. *(Rationale: This promotes easy insertion and prevents friction in the intestine.)*
5. Insert the tube 3 to 4 inches (7.5–10 cm) into the rectum. *(Rationale: The tube is inserted far enough to pass any stool in the lower rectum and reach the gas above the stool.)*
6. Determine the patency of the tube. If the tube is patent, gas or feces will return. *(Rationale: The tube can become plugged with stool; it must be kept open.)*
7. Place the outer end of the tube in an Evac-u-sac. *(Rationale: An Evac-u-sac or cardboard container helps to absorb odor and sound and helps to minimize embarrassment for the patient.)*
8. Leave the tube in the rectum from 20 to 30 minutes. *(Rationale: After that time the sphincter muscles become numbed and the tube ceases to stimulate peristalsis.)*
9. Properly dispose of your gloves and wash your hands. *(Rationale: Prevent the spread of infection.)*
10. Document the result on the patient's chart; the duration of the insertion, the amount of gas and feces expelled, if any, and whether the patient felt relief.

Nausea and Vomiting (N & V)

Nausea is an unpleasant sensation in the abdomen, sometimes followed by vomiting. Vomiting, also called **emesis**, is an involuntary action that expels contents from the stomach. Other symptoms of nausea leading to vomiting include weakness, frequent swallowing, profuse perspiration, dizziness, pallor (paleness), and shakiness. The pulse and blood pressure may drop during vomiting.

In some cases, vomiting is *projectile*, that is, expelled with great force. Projectile vomiting is a significant symptom and must be reported at once.

In some situations, such as following eye surgery, prevention of vomiting is advisable. A violent action, such as vomiting, could disrupt the delicate suture line.

Vomitus is stomach contents; its appearance and odor tell something about the cause of emesis. Assess for particles; assess the color, odor, and consistency. Vomitus may contain bright red blood, a sign of gastric (stomach) bleeding. It may contain coffee-ground material, a sign of bleeding in the lower digestive tract. Does vomitus contain mucus or pus? Vomitus containing bile is a yellowish or greenish color. If the vomitus is material that has been forced back into the stomach from the intestine, it has a fecal odor.

Always save for inspection any unusual vomitus. Measure and document the amount, if possible. The physician may want the entire specimen sent to the laboratory for examination. As with other specimens, vomitus should be placed in a moisture-proof covered container and properly labeled. It should be taken to the laboratory immediately. (See Chapter 47.)

Note the nature of the vomiting. Was it violent or projectile? How does the patient describe the episode? If the patient is on intake and output measurement, vomitus is considered output. Report the vomiting to your team leader. Carefully document all your observations on the patient's chart.

Assisting the Nauseated or Vomiting Person

The person who is nauseated or vomiting feels miserable and helpless. He or she cannot talk. Rather than ask questions, assist the person in comfort measures. The following actions may be taken when a patient is nauseated:

♦ Wear gloves.
♦ A cool, damp washcloth on the patient's forehead will be comforting and may relieve nausea.
♦ Tell the patient to take slow, deep breaths through the nose. Talk the patient through the breaths. *(Rationale: This helps relax the patient and distracts from the nauseated feeling. Adding oxygen to the blood, and thus, the control center in the medulla of the brain, helps relieve nausea.)*
♦ Have the patient lie on the right side. *(Rationale: This moves gastric contents toward the bottom end of the stomach and away from the cardiac sphincter, and may relieve irritation.)*
♦ Give antiemetic drugs by injection or rectally, as ordered. *(Rationale: Antiemetics may be ordered in special situations. The drugs cannot be given by mouth because that might cause vomiting.)*
♦ Offer something dry, such as a bite of soda cracker or unbuttered toast. Do not give the food until the worst of the nausea has subsided. *(Rationale: The dry food may soak up some of the excess acid in the stomach. It also helps to remove the disagreeable taste from the mouth.)*

Add the following if vomiting occurs:

st wear gloves when the patient is
e vomiting is projectile or if there is
y that the vomitus will splash, you
r eye goggles. *(Rationale: It is impor-
t yourself.)*

sis basin directly under the chin of
Rationale: This helps catch all of the

e patient should sit up; if the patient
make sure he or she is lying on the
*le: Lying on the back while vomiting
because vomitus could be aspirated
.)*

under the basin or use a draw sheet
the bed. *(Rationale: Protect the pa-
g and the bed linens.)*

s the vomitus. *(Rationale: The appear-
s and nature of vomiting can be im-
physician in making a diagnosis.)*

as subsided, allow the patient to
h with mouthwash or a weak salt so-

lution. Tell the patient not to swallow any of the
solution. *(Rationale: Vomiting leaves a disagreeable taste in the mouth. Gastric contents are also irritating to the throat and mouth. Swallowing fluid
could cause more nausea.)*

◆ Remove soiled linen and wash the patient's face
and hands if necessary. *(Rationale: Make the patient comfortable.)*

◆ Empty the emesis basin and measure vomitus. *(Rationale: The sight and smell of vomitus is very disagreeable to patients and staff. Knowing the amount
of vomitus will help the physician in making a
diagnosis.)*

◆ Wash the emesis basin in cold water. *(Rationale:
Hot water will cause protein material to
coagulate.)*

◆ Dispose of gloves and wash your hands. *(Rationale: To prevent spread of organisms.)*

◆ Carefully document the event and your observations. *(Rationale: To assist the physician in treatment of the patient.)*

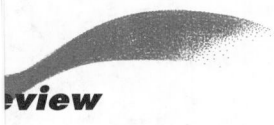

view

ons for Critical Thinking

en assigned to teach a patient about the
of proper elimination and personal hy-
be how you would teach the importance
care activities.

en asked to give an enema to a patient.
reasons for and principles in giving an
e the different types of enemas and ex-
pes of patients will need them.

bladder retraining and bowel retraining
escribe how they are different.

rming care of a patient who begins to
be what you would do and give

gs

le CJ. Fundamentals of Nursing: Human
unction. Philadelphia, J.B. Lippincott,

ical Skills in Nursing Practice, Ed 2. Phila-
Lippincott, 1993

e BG. Brunner and Suddarth's Textbook
rgical Nursing, Ed 7. Philadelphia, J.B.
92

Photo Atlas of Nursing Procedures, Ed 2.
y, CA, Addison-Wesley Nursing, 1991

Key Readings (continued)

Taber's Cyclopedic Medical Dictionary, Ed 17. Philadelphia, F.A. Davis, 1993

Taylor C, Lillis C, LeMone P. Fundamentals of Nursing:
The Art and Science of Nursing Care, Ed 2. Philadelphia, J.B. Lippincott, 1993

Keys to Learning More

47 Specimen Collection

Keys for Learning

Learning Objectives

- Describe normal color, appearance, and odor of urine.
- Describe some of abnormalities of urine.
- Describe how intake and output records are kept.
- Demonstrate the ability to correctly measure urine volume and urine specific gravity.
- Identify some of the reasons for laboratory examination of the urine.
- Demonstrate the ability to collect correctly a midstream specimen, an accumulated 24-hour specimen, a fractional 24-hour specimen, and a specimen from an indwelling urinary catheter.
- Demonstrate the ability to collect a stool specimen.
- Demonstrate the ability to collect a sputum specimen.

Key Terms

expectorate	specific gravity
guaiac	urinalysis
Hemoccult	urinometer
hydrometer	venipuncture

Keys to Understanding This Chapter

Chapter 8: microbiology
Chapter 21: cardiovascular system including description of blood components
Chapter 22: anatomy and physiology of respiratory system
Chapter 23: anatomy and physiology of digestive system
Chapter 24: anatomy and physiology of urinary system
Chapter 30: medical asepsis and universal precautions
Chapter 37: documentation and reporting
Chapter 38: signs and symptoms of illness or injury

Key Points

- Body substance precautions must be us working with body fluids.
- Careful handwashing is important in pr spread of disease.
- Routine specimen collection is usually early in the morning.
- Nurses do not draw blood unless they instructions.

Key Topics Outline

The Urine Specimen
   Intake and Output Records
   Measuring Urine Specific Gravity
   Collecting Urine Specimens for Examir
   Measuring Urine Glucose and Acetone
   Collecting a Specimen From an Indwel
The Stool Specimen
The Sputum Specimen
The Blood Specimen

Key Learning Activities

- Keep a 24-hour record of your own in Analyze the record to see if intake and balanced.

Key Nursing Procedure

NP 47-1:   Collecting a Urine Specimen Fr
                ing Catheter

ans by which nurses collect data is by
, stool, sputum, and blood specimens
y. Nurses may be responsible for col-
ecimens. They may observe specimens
o the laboratory for examination. You
he specific protocols for collection of
ur facility. This helps preserve the spec-
vides consistency in interpretation of
s for collecting all specimens are pre-
companying box.

t

ays worn whenever you work with
is includes urine, stool, sputum, wound
lood. Careful handwashing is also im-
enting the spread of disease.

Specimen

a great deal of data about the patient's
ack of it.

ut Records

patient's status, often the physician
ctly how much fluid (and sometimes
food) the patient consumes and elim-
Over a 24-hour period the normal
fluid volume intake and output (I&O)
nately balance. When a person be-
id I&O may become unbalanced. Con-
from this imbalance may become life-
ords are kept to verify I&O. This helps
ons regarding increasing or restricting
ements. The nurse may refer to these
s the effectiveness of medication that
is well as to establish elimination pat-
ls are usually collected every shift and
our period. To measure *total* food and
order is given to "record food and fluid
+ calorie count." In this case, all food
e being served. The nurse must then
hat was eaten, as well as what fluids

es, I&O records are recorded in milli-
entimeters (cc). These two measure-
timately equal (1 cc = 1 mL). A sample
en in Figure 47-1. Generally, the I&O
he patient's bedside, and each nurse is
ecording the intake and output as it is
ecords may be maintained. A tempo-
nay be kept by the bedside or on the

Nursing Skill Guidelines
Collecting Specimens and Samples

◆ Specimen bottles are labeled with the patient's name and other data before the specimen is collected.
◆ Always wash hands before and after collecting the specimen.
◆ Always observe body substance precautions when collecting specimens.
◆ Collect the sample according to individual facility policy and procedure.
◆ Clean the area involved for sample collection.
◆ Observe sterile technique if needed for sample or culture collection.
◆ Place all specimens in "biohazard" bags to protect staff.
◆ Transport the specimen to the laboratory immediately.
◆ Be sure specimen is accompanied by appropriate request or laboratory cards.
◆ Record the collection and forwarding of the sample to the laboratory on the patient's record.

patient's bathroom door. This worksheet records the I&O for each shift. The 24-hour totals are recorded on the permanent record.

Measuring Fluid Intake

Fluid intake includes all fluids taken by mouth, as part of intravenous (IV) therapy, by total parenteral nutrition (TPN), nasogastric (NG) tube feeding, hypodermoclysis, or proctoclysis.

Generally, when a patient is on I&O, all fluid intake must be measured. Such items as gelatin, ice cream, and thin cereal are considered liquid intake. Each hospital has a list describing the quantities of liquid found in various containers and in different foods. The nurse follows this when recording. Record all fluids taken. Ice is counted as 50% water (eg, 200 mL of ice would count as 100 mL [or cc] of fluid intake.)

Be sure to find out the policy of your facility concerning recording of water intake from the bedside water pitcher. In some agencies it is recorded when it is filled and in others, when it is empty. Do not fill a pitcher or empty one unless you are sure of the procedure. Do not empty a bedpan or urinal without first finding out if the patient's I&O is being recorded.

Measuring Output

Output includes urine and such fluid as wound drainage, emesis, and bleeding and NG suction tube. As part of the record, it is also noted when the patient has a bowel movement. Sometimes all stools are weighed so the physician knows more closely what the total output was.

DAILY INTAKE AND OUTPUT BEDSIDE WORKSHEET

Date: 11/27/94

John Menendez
3987624
Dr. Gomez
Green Medicine Service

Record Shift totals on 24 Hr. Nurses Progress Notes

Approximate Measures in cc's (mL's)

1 oz.	30 cc's
8 oz. water glass (tea)	240 cc's
8 oz. glass of ice (melted)	135 "
Soup bowl	150 "
Jello (1 serving)	100 "
Small milk carton	240 "
8 oz. ice cream cup	90 "
Small juice glass	120 "
6 oz. hot styrafoam cup	180 "
12 oz. tea glass	360 "
Coca-cola paper cup	240 "
Insulated coffee cup	220 "
Canned 12 oz. drinks	360 "

FOR ISOLATION PATIENTS

9 oz. disposable cups (tea and water)	240 cc's
6 oz. styrafoam cup	180 "
5 oz. plastic glass	150 "

	INTAKE			OUTPUT			
	ORAL		I.V. FLUIDS	URINE	EMESIS	SUCTION	STOOLS
7-3 0700-1500	Juice 120 Milk 240 H₂O 120 " 200 Jello 50 Coffee 100		D₅W 420	0830-200 1045-225 1300-300 1400-125	0930-50	Paracentesis 350mL	
Total	830		420	850	50	350	
3-11 1500-2300	Juice 240 Coffee 240 Milk 140 Soup 100 H₂O 300 Ensure 200		D₅W 400 +50 piggyback 2 meds.	1530-275 1630-125 1845-200 2100-125 2200-Incont. (lg. amt.)	1545-50		
Total	1220			725+ incont	50	0	
11-7 2300-0700	Water 100		D₅W 375	0030-200 0245-325 0600-350			
	100		375	875	0		
Total 24 Hr.	2150		1245	2450	100	350	

Figure 47-1. Examples of Intake and Output (I&O) Forms. (A) *Bedside worksheet.* When the patient is given fluids or uses the bedpan, amounts are recorded on this worksheet. At the end of each shift, the nurse figures a total. This patient was incontinent at 2200 (10 pm), so the nurse estimated the amount ("large"). This estimate is recorded as output, along with measured amounts. Note that emesis and paracentesis are recorded as output and IV fluids are recorded as intake. (B) *Permanent Chart Record.* At the end of 24 hours, the totals for that day are recorded in the patient's permanent chart. (In some hospitals, these totals are done at 12 midnight; in others, this is done at 7 am.) You will notice that this patient's intake and output are approximately equal, which is normal. (The permanent record in this case has spaces for two days of I&O recording.) (Forms courtesy of AMI Nacogdoches Medical Center, Nacogdoches, Texas.)

Johnathan Menedez
3987624
Dr. Gomez
Green Medical Service

ogdoches Medical Center
AKE and OUTPUT RECORD

	INTAKE					OUTPUT				
te: 11/27/94	7am 3pm	3pm 11pm	11pm 7am	TOTAL	Date:	7am 3pm	3pm 11pm	11pm 7am	TOTAL
al	830	1020	100	1950	Urine	850	725 +incont	875	2450+inc
al supplement	✓	200	✓	200	Emesis	50	50	✓	100
S. snack	✓	✓	✓	✓	Wangensteen-gomco	✓	✓	✓	✓
be feeding	✓	✓	✓	✓	Stool	✓	✓	✓	✓
er/tf,gastro	✓	✓	✓	✓	Hemovac's	✓	✓	✓	✓
od products	✓	✓	✓	✓	Chest tubes	✓	✓	✓	✓
/IVPB	420	450	375	1245	Thor/paracentesis	350	✓	✓	350
her	✓	✓	✓	✓	Other	✓	✓	✓	✓
TOTAL INTAKE	1250	1670	475	3395	TOTAL OUTPUT	1250	775	875	2900 +

+incont   incontinent

	INTAKE					OUTPUT				
e:	7am 3pm	3pm 11pm	11pm 7am	TOTAL	Date:	7am 3pm	3pm 11pm	11pm 7am	TOTAL
l					Urine				
l supplement					Emesis				
. snack					Wangensteen-gomco				
e feeding					Stool				
er/tf,gastro					Hemovac's				
od products					Chest tubes				
IVPB					Thor/paracentesis				
er					Other				
TAL INTAKE					TOTAL OUTPUT				

All charting must be in cc's. (mL's)

e 47-1. (Continued)

nd Recording Urine

uipment

oilet hat

Procedure

1. Wash hands and don gloves. (Rationale: Protect yourself from infection.)
2. Ask the patient to void in the bedpan, toilet hat, or urinal. The toilet hat, urinal, or bed pan is labeled with the patient's name, if there are two or more patients in the room. The toilet hat is positioned in the toilet with the collecting receptacle toward the front. (Rationale: All urine output must be measured. Placing the toilet hat in this manner allows collection of urine without stool, if the

patient has a BM. Labeling prevents cross-contamination.)

3. Pour the urine into the graduated measuring container and read the urine volume in milliliters. *(Rationale: It is important to obtain an accurate measurement.)*

4. Pour the urine into the toilet and flush, unless the urine is to be saved. *(Rationale: Sometimes more than one test will be made from one urine sample.)*

5. Rinse the bedpan or urinal and the graduate in cool water. *(Rationale: Hot water will cause any protein substances to coagulate and will break down the urine faster, releasing ammonia.)*

6. Allow the patient to wash the hands. *(Rationale: It is important to reinforce habits of good hygiene.)*

7. Properly dispose of gloves and wash your hands. *(Rationale: To prevent cross-contamination.)*

8. Record the urine volume on the output sheet. *(Rationale: It is important to have an accurate reading for the day.)*

Intravenous Records

Many facilities have a separate I&O record for intravenous fluids. These record specific types of intravenous fluids, additives, amount of intravenous fluid absorbed, and amount remaining per shift. Intravenous fluids, however, should be included in the 24-hour total. Chapter 57 describes IV administration in more detail.

Measuring Urine Specific Gravity

Often when a urine output recording is ordered, a specific gravity measurement to determine the *concentration* of urine is ordered at the same time. Generally the order calls for urine volume and specific gravity (abbreviated as *vol & spec*) to be recorded at specified intervals. **Specific gravity** is the urine concentration as compared with that of pure water.

The reading is measured in decimal increments above 1.000, which is the reading for pure water. Because the increments are in thousandths, it is important to be very accurate. The normal range of urine specific gravity is from 1.010 (dilute) to 1.025 (highly concentrated). Urine must be tested as soon as possible after obtaining it to avoid inaccuracies in results.

Nursing Skill

Measuring Urine Specific Gravity

Supplies and Equipment

Specific gravity beaker
Hydrometer
Gloves
Bedpan, urinal, or toilet hat

Procedure

1. Maintain body substance precautions. *(R... infection.)*

2. Measure urine for urine volume, as descr... nursing skill. *(Rationale: Volume must be ... fore other tests are made.)*

3. Fill the specific gravity beaker. Gently dro... suring instrument, called a **hydrometer**... twisting it gently as you do. *(Rationale: I... is rotating, it will be easier to keep away ... the beaker. Handle the hydrometer gently ... breakage.)*

4. Be sure the hydrometer is floating freely ... ing the side of the beaker. *(Rationale: If ... touches anything, the reading will not be ...*

5. Hold at eye level and read at the *bottom* ... cus, the slight bulge or curve seen on th... liquid. *(Rationale: Liquids must always ... this way for accuracy and for consisten... illustrates the correct method to read the... gravity.*

6. Rinse the beaker and hydrometer in cool ... ale: In addition to coagulating the protei... break the instrument.)*

7. Properly dispose of gloves and wash han...

8. Record the results.

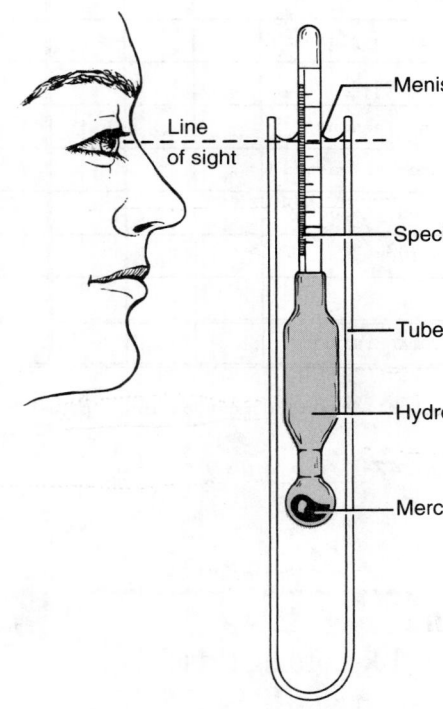

Figure 47-2. Specific gravity of urine is meas... for accuracy. It is read at the bottom of the ... is the slight bulge or curve seen on the liqui... ven RF and Hirnle CJ. Fundamentals of ... Health and Function. Philadelphia: J.B. Lipp...

Specimens for Examination

btains urine specimens to send to the
alysis, the analysis of urine samples, is
nation of every patient at the beginning
ness. Simple urine tests, such as tests for
e, and the Keto-Diastix for ketone bod-
tors are often performed by the nurse
or by the patient at home. Follow the
structions on the package for perform-
g these tests. Brief guidelines are pre-
his chapter. Guidelines for collecting
are listed in the accompanying box.

ngle-Voided Urine Specimen. A single-
(clean-catch specimen) may be used
nces, such as sugar, acetone, and al-
or for specific gravity and pH. Some-
are done to determine the efficiency

Single-Voided Urine

uipment

bottle or container (wide-mouthed bottle

or urinal

guidelines for collecting urine specimens.
with the date, patient's name, room, and
ntification, and physician's name.
d don gloves. *(Rationale: Prevent*

ent to void in a clean receptacle. *(Ratio-*
oss-contamination.)
cimen as soon as possible after the pa-

mL of urine into the labeled specimen
r the bottle. *(Rationale: It is important to*
ine for the required tests. The bottle is
d decomposition and to prevent added
) Place in a biohazard bag.
es properly and wash hands.

stream Urine Specimen. Midstream urine
most common method of obtaining
from adults, particularly men. By this
men not contaminated from external
btained without catheterization. If bac-
the laboratory tests, they most likely

Nursing Skill Guidelines
Collecting Urine Specimens

◆ The amount and the content of a urine specimen
vary with the time of day, and the food and fluid intake. The physician may ask for specimens at different times in the day. The urine specimen collected for
part of a day is called the *single fractional specimen.*

◆ Label specimen bottles before the patient voids.
*(Rationale: Reduce handling after the bottle is con-
taminated.)* Include patient's room or department
and physician's name.

◆ Wake a patient in the morning to obtain a routine
specimen. *(Rationale: If all specimens are collected
at the same time, the laboratory can establish a
baseline. Also this voided specimen usually represents urine that was collecting in the bladder all
night, usually the longest period of time the patient
goes without voiding.)*

◆ It is important to note on the specimen label if the
patient is menstruating at that time. *(Rationale:
One of the tests routinely performed is a test for
blood in the urine. If a woman is menstruating at
the time a urine specimen is taken, a false-positive
reading for blood will be obtained.)*

◆ To avoid contamination and the necessity of collecting another specimen, soap and water cleansing
of the genitals immediately preceding the collection
of the specimen is advocated. Single, prepackaged
wipes are available for this purpose. *(Rationale:
Bacteria are normally present on the labia or penis
and the perineum and in the anal area.)*

◆ Half pans (toilet hat) are available for use in the
toilet. *(Rationale: This allows the patient to have a
bowel movement while collecting only urine.)*

◆ Body substance precautions are maintained when
collecting all types of urine specimens. *(Rationale:
To maintain safety.)*

◆ Wash your hands before and after the procedure
and instruct the patient to do the same.

◆ Be sure to document the procedure in the designated place and mark it off on the Kardex to avoid
duplication.

will be from urine in the bladder. Nursing actions in
collecting a midstream urine specimen are:

◆ Instruct the patient to cleanse the urethral area
thoroughly. *(Rationale: This will prevent external
bacteria from entering the specimen.)* Use prepackaged wipes, if available. Label the container before
giving it to the patient.

◆ The female patient must cleanse from front to back
and cleanse each side with a separate wipe, saving
the last for the urethral area itself. *(Rationale:
Women should always wipe from front to back to
avoid contaminating the vaginal and urethral
areas from the anal area.)*

◆ The male patient is instructed to cleanse the penis using a circular motion. The first cotton wipe is for the urethral meatus. The next wipe cleanses the end of the penis, and the last wipe again cleanses the urethral opening. *(Rationale: The urethral area should be kept the cleanest.)*

◆ Instruct both male and female patients to void a small amount into the toilet to rinse out the urethra.

◆ Next the patient voids to catch the *midstream urine.*

◆ Finally the patient voids the last of the stream into the toilet. *(Rationale: The midstream urine is considered to be bladder and kidney washings; this is the portion that the physician wants tested.)*

◆ Take the specimen to the laboratory without delay. *(Rationale: Especially when bacterial determinations are to be made, delay could cause a false result.)*

Collecting an Accumulated Urine Specimen. An accumulated specimen of urine gives more detailed information than a single specimen because it shows what total amounts of wastes the kidneys are eliminating and the amount of each. The urine may be collected for 24 hours or for some part of that period, depending on the specific information desired. The following actions are performed in collecting an accumulated urine specimen:

◆ Collect additional supplies.

◆ Maintain body substance precautions and follow guidelines for urine collection given earlier in the chapter.

◆ Label the large bottle with the patient's name and pertinent data before beginning. *(Rationale: Prevents contamination.)*

◆ Give the bedpan, toilet hat, or urinal to the patient and ask the patient to void. Discard this urine and record the time on the patient's chart. *(Rationale: Collection begins with an empty bladder.)* If this collection is made from an indwelling catheter, proceed following the same timetable.

◆ Measure each specimen of urine voided and pour into an iced brown bottle; record each amount.

◆ Cover with a towel. Label with the patient's name and the time the test started.

◆ Continue for 24 hours from the time the urine was discarded. *(Rationale: It is important to save all urine for the 24-hour period to obtain accurate results.)*

◆ At exactly 24 hours after beginning the collection, ask the patient to void. Save this voiding. *(Rationale: The last voiding completes the 24-hour total; collection ends with an empty bladder.)* Pour the specimen into the bottle.

◆ Add the time collection ended to the [...] with the total amount of urine. Cover [...] tightly and place it in a clean bag. La[...] hour urine collection, maintaining cl[...] the outside of the bag.

◆ Dispose of gloves and wash hands.

◆ Take to the laboratory immediately.

Collecting the 24-Hour Fractional U[...] Twenty-four hour fractional specimens [...] determine amounts and characteristics [...] various periods of time during the day. [...] lecting the 24-hour fractional urine spe[...]

◆ Follow all procedures as for other ur[...]

◆ Depending on the order, determine [...] tles you will need. Often the fraction[...] are obtained for 6-hour periods or "f[...] the day: 12 midnight to 6 AM; 6 AM to[...] noon to 6 PM; and 6 PM to 12 midnig[...] case, you need four specimen bottle[...] labels. Label all bottles before you b[...] times.

◆ Begin by asking the patient to void. [...] Each new time slot begins with an e[...]

◆ Collect all urine from the first fractio[...] bottle #1. Ask the patient to void at t[...] time period. *(Rationale: Each new t[...] with an empty bladder.)*

◆ Continue for the other "fractions" of [...] with an empty bladder. Store all spe[...] during the 24 hours. Take the specim[...] oratory immediately at the end of the[...] lection period. Document the proce[...]

Measuring Urine Glucose and Acetone

Normal urine is free from sugar, aceton[...] but any of these may be present in t[...] person with diabetes or kidney disease[...] ability of a variety of sophisticated, b[...] blood glucose monitors, urine testing [...] quently. The most common need for uri[...] test for ketones.

Keto-Diastix. This convenient test me[...] and acetone at the same time. Acetone i[...] that is present when the body cells are s[...] of faulty metabolism. Buildup of aceto[...] tosis, which in turn leads to acidosis. V[...] tion diets, excessive intake of plain wat[...] perspiration can alter the electrolyte bal[...] measuring urine glucose and acetone a[...]

◆ Follow procedure as for other urine [...]

◆ Obtain a freshly voided sample.

◆ Dip the test strip quickly into the uri[...]

dings for glucose and acetone by fol-
irections on the container.

risons of the color chart with the urine

tle tightly closed between use.
Moisture can render the dipstick

sults.

n teach the patient how to use tests.

. A double-voiding technique must be
ests in diabetic patients to obtain a true
the amount of sugar and ketones spilled
y particular time. The patient should void
specimen because the procedure begins
bladder. One-half hour later, another
ecimen should be collected and used for
schedule is used for the patient with a
ecimen from a catheter must be obtained
and not from the bag.
stance that Keto-Diastix are ordered, the
taught to check the fasting urine result
a fasting blood sugar. This is done to
enal threshold. If a discrepancy exists,
ld be encouraged to ask the physician
a blood glucose monitor.

etone is especially important if the pa-
g, has a fever, or if a high concentration
ent in the blood (above 235 mg/dL).

ecimen From an Indwelling Catheter

ecimen will most likely be obtained from
is unconscious or who has a catheter.
idstream or clean-catch method is used.
adder is a sterile area. Any contamination
e indwelling catheter system can cause
ause microorganisms can travel up the
bladder. Therefore, when collecting a
cimen you must be particularly careful
the patient by causing contamination of
should be taken not to allow the Foley
ed above the level of the bladder. This
ult in urine possibly flowing back into
n carrying with it microorganisms. Also
ould not be allowed to touch the floor,
y contaminated area. Nursing skills are
accompanying box and the procedure
dure 47-1.

e-Time Catheterized Urine Specimen. Oc-
heterized urine specimen will be or-

Nursing Skill Guidelines
*Collecting a Urine Specimen
from an Indwelling Catheter*

♦ Use body substance precautions. Carefully wash hands
before and after the procedure and wear gloves.
♦ Drain all urine from the small collecting area of the
closed drainage bag. Then, clamp off the catheter
for a few minutes before the specimen is needed,
unless contraindicated. You will be collecting a
current sample.
♦ If the unit has a stopcock, turn it to collect urine in the
small collection bay. *(Rationale: If you take the specimen from the larger bag, it will not be representative of
the appropriate time slot. The bag may also be previously contaminated or you may contaminate it.)*
♦ If the system has a drain for the small collection
area, open it and collect the specimen in a sterile
container.
♦ Otherwise, use a sterile, small-gauge needle inserted into the *sample port*. Cleanse the port first
with an alcohol wipe. Then insert your sterile needle. Draw the urine out into a syringe, above the
clamped area or at the stopcock. *(Rationale: A sterile syringe and needle may be safely introduced
into the system without contaminating it. Using the
syringe is safer than detaching the drainage tubing. The sterile syringe/needle and container and
cleansing the port will help to ensure that microorganisms in the specimen came from the urine in
the bladder and not from faulty technique.)* In
some hospitals, a needleless system is available.
♦ Do not leave the tubing clamped for more than 15
minutes. *(Rationale: Excess urine backing up in
ureters and kidneys can cause damage.)*
♦ Dispose of gloves and wash your hands. *(Rationale: Prevents transmission of organisms.)*
♦ Take specimens to the laboratory immediately.
♦ Document the procedure, noting any pertinent observations.

dered. Generally, catheterization is not done for urine
collection unless the patient is catheterized for some
other reason. The procedure for performing a urinary
catheterization is presented in Chapter 54.

The Stool Specimen

The stool specimen yields information related to functioning of the gastrointestinal system and its accessory
organs. Many examinations of the feces are carried out
in the laboratory. The most common is the test for ova
and parasites (O&P). This test indicates the presence of
intestinal parasites and/or their eggs (ova).

Stools are often tested for blood using **guaiac** or
Hemoccult tests. The test is sometimes done at the

Collecting a Urine Specimen From an Indwelling (Syringe and Needle System)

Supplies and Equipment

Gloves.
Container with label
Alcohol prep or disinfectant swab
Laboratory request slip
10–20-mL syringe with 21–25-gauge needle
Clamp or rubber band
Biohazard bag for transportation of specimen

Procedure

1. Gather supplies. Label the container.
   (Rationale: Organization facilitates performance of the skill.)
2. Explain procedure to patient.
   (Rationale: Providing information fosters patient cooperation.)
3. Wash hands before putting on gloves.
   (Rationale: Handwashing prevents the spread of organisms. Gloves act as a barrier.)
4. Clamp drainage tubing or bend tubing and secure with a rubber band below the collection port. Allow adequate time for urine to collect; no longer than 15 minutes.
   (Rationale: Collecting urine from the tubing guarantees a fresh specimen.)

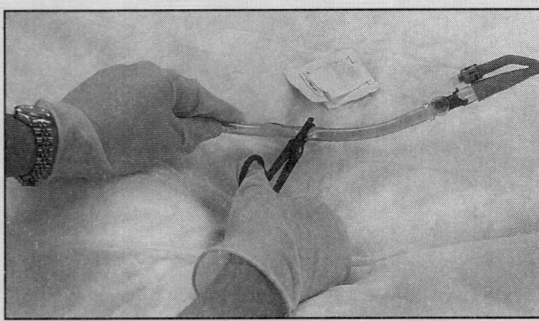

Step 4   Clamping the drainage tubing

5. Cleanse aspiration port with alcohol prep or Betadine swab.
   (Rationale: Disinfecting the port prevents organisms from entering the catheter.)

6. Insert needle into aspiration port and w
   into the syringe. The laboratory test de
   amount of urine to be collected.
   *(Rationale: This technique provides an
   nated urine specimen and prevents co
   the bladder.)*

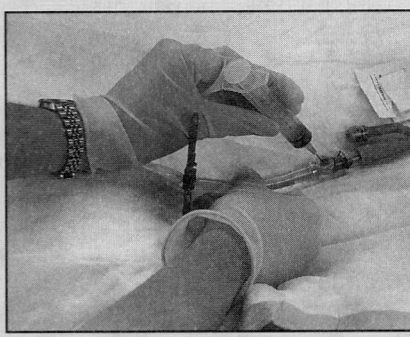

Step 6   Inserting the needle into the aspiration

7. Transfer urine to labeled specimen co
   lid on container. Container must be st
   ture and clean for a routine urinalysis.
   *(Rationale: Careful labeling and trans
   contamination or confusion of urine s*
8. Unclamp catheter.
   *(Rationale: Catheter must be unclamp
   flow or urine and prevent urinary stas*
9. Prepare container according to hospita
   transport to laboratory.
   *(Rationale: Proper packaging ensures
   is not an infection risk.)*
10. Dispose of used equipment. Remove g
    wash hands.
    *(Rationale: Handwashing prevents the
    organisms.)*
11. Send container to laboratory immedia
    *(Rationale: Organisms grow quickly in
    ature urine.)*
12. Document on flow sheet or chart that
    obtained.
    *(Rationale: Documentation provides c
    care.)*

with test cards or Hemastix, or it may
laboratory. If it is done at the nursing
ions should be kept with the reagents
r is often written "guaiac stools × 3."
done, they are crossed off the Kardex.

are placed in leakproof containers. The
container must be clean and dry. The
r is placed into a plastic biohazard bag
the laboratory. Containers are labeled
some facilities, the bag is labeled as
include requests or lab cards, so the
what tests to do.

Stool Specimen

quipment

l cover or toilet hat
container and cover

lades
r used tongue blades and the specimen

substance precautions. Wash your hands
ves.
cedure to the person and ask the person
n the urge to have a bowel movement is
: *Most people cannot have a bowel move-
and.)*
iner.
n when the patient is ready. If you are us-
place it with the collecting receptacle to-
of the toilet. *(Rationale: You are most
a usable specimen at this time. The toilet
to collect stool without urine.)*
dpan. Use the tongue blade to transfer a
eces to the container. Do not touch the
ionale: It is grossly contaminated.)
of feces from three different areas of the

ainer. Note any special examination

se of gloves and wash your hands.
iner immediately to the laboratory. *(Ra-
should be examined when fresh. Examina-
ites, eggs (ova), and organisms must be
e stool is warm.)* Sometimes, the examina-
ade of the entire stool. In this case a larger
ed.

The Sputum Specimen

In some respiratory disorders, a specimen of sputum
("sputum spec") is obtained and sent to the laboratory
for culture or other examination. It often is done for 3
days in a row. It is difficult to cough up enough sputum
for a specimen; therefore, an organism might be missed
if only one culture is done. For two reasons, the best
time to obtain a specimen is soon after the patient
awakens: the sputum will have had a chance to collect
during the night and it will be easier for the patient to
expel the sputum. The specimen must be obtained before the patient eats, uses mouthwash, or brushes the
teeth.

Body substance precautions are observed when collecting sputum. Keep the inside of the specimen container sterile. A sterile container ensures that any organisms cultured from the specimen will be from the
specimen and not from a contaminated container. Keep
the cover on as much as possible to prevent contamination by particles from the air and to prevent the
spread of organisms from the sputum specimen.

Consuming adequate amounts of fluid and breathing
humidified air or aerosolized medications often help to
loosen and liquefy secretions, making it easier for the
patient to cough them up. If aerosolized medications
have been used, this fact should be documented in the
nursing notes, along with the fact that you collected a
specimen.

Nursing Skill
Collecting a Sputum Specimen

Supplies and Equipment

Sterile covered sputum container
Labels
Tissues
Gloves

Procedure

Collecting the Specimen

1. Wear gloves when handling the specimen and facial
   tissue.

2. Explain the procedure to the person. *(Rationale: If the person understands the procedure he or she will more readily cooperate.)*
3. Label the container. *(Rationale: Careful labeling ensures accuracy of the report and alerts the laboratory personnel to the presence of a contaminated specimen.)*
4. Ask the patient to cough up secretions from deep in the respiratory passages. *(Rationale: A sputum specimen should be from the lungs and bronchi and it should be sputum rather than mucus.)*
5. Have the patient **expectorate** (spit) directly into the sterile container. *(Rationale: Avoid any chance of outside contamination to the specimen or any contamination of other objects.)*
6. Cover the specimen immediately. *(Rationale: Prevent contamination.)*
7. Dispose of gloves and wash hands. *(Rationale: Wash your hands to prevent contamination of other objects, including the label.)*
8. Transport specimen to the laboratory immediately. *(Rationale: Prevents proliferation of organisms.)*

Measuring the Specimen

1. If the order is to measure the sputum, you may do so in one of two ways: 1) If there is enough sputum and the specimen container is graduated, you can read the amount directly; or 2) you can pour an equal amount of water into an identical container and measure the water.
2. Weigh the specimen if ordered. Do so on a balance scale, subtracting the initial weight of the container.
3. Take the specimen to the laboratory immediately after collection. *(Rationale: A delay may alter the result of a culture.)*
4. Call the attention of the laboratory personnel to the fact that this is a sputum specimen.
5. Document the amount (copious, moderate, small), color, and consistency of sputum.

> **Nursing Alert**
>
> ◆ The sputum specimen is considered highly contaminated and is treated with caution.
> ◆ Paper tissues used by any patient are considered contaminated and must be disposed of properly.
> ◆ Gloves must be worn when handling tissues and sputum specimens and when providing nursing care if the patient is coughing up sputum.

The Blood Specimen

A blood specimen usually is taken when a person is admitted to a healthcare facility. This is done to assess the blood's normal cells and other components and to determine the presence of abnormalities or disease organisms.

In some body disturbances, differen
increase in number or change in shap
the number and the shape of the red
mation about anemia; the number and
leukocytes give information about infe

> **Nursing Alert**
>
> The nurse who draws blood needs spec

Assisting With Venipuncture

Venipuncture is the obtaining of blo
often on the inside surface of the forea
bow, called the antecubital space. He
near the surface and are easy to see or
where the veins stand out prominently
instead. If only a few drops are need
pricked with a lancet, and the blood i
a pipette, dropped onto a test strip, or
onto a glass slide. Blood for glucose te
tained with a lancet.

The primary caregiver or the labora
(phlebotomist) usually collects the blo
venipuncture. The nurse with special t
form this procedure. The skill is explain
you may be asked to assist with draw
sembling equipment.

◆ Observe universal precautions. Alw
  gloves.
◆ Have the patient lie on the back wi
  ing comfortably on the bed, or sit in
  the arm resting on the overbed tabl
◆ Place a protective sheet under the a
◆ A tourniquet is applied around the
  tightened, and secured with a slip k
◆ The area over the vein is cleansed f
◆ The needle is inserted into the vein
  Vacutainer tube often is used. This
  into the tube without the need for a
  the required amount of blood has b
  the tourniquet is released.
◆ A sterile gauze square or cotton ba
  the needle and the needle withdraw
◆ The patient bends the elbow, using
  cotton ball as a compress.
◆ Properly dispose of gloves and nee
  oughly wash your hands.
◆ Label the specimen and take it to th
  immediately.

Assisting in Obtaining Blood for C

Sometimes a blood culture is done
to identify a disease-causing organis
specimen is often ordered drawn if the

as a routine on a certain day ("blood for
and drug sensitivity). If the blood is to
you must have the equipment located
o that it is ready when needed. In some
uipment for a blood culture is kept on
ion; in others it is sent up from the lab-
rdered.

hat of assistant. It is your responsibility
oper person when the culture is to be
all the materials, and explain the pro-
tient. The following actions are used in
lood cultures:

abel the proper tubes or bottles.
sh your hands. *(Rationale: Prevent*
on of the culture and spreading

ersal precautions. Don gloves and
es for the person you are assisting.
ed with a pad under the patient's arm.
arefully "prepped" to make sure it is
ossible. Use the skin prep protocol
your facility.

echnique is maintained when drawing

the blood sample and when placing it in the specimen container.

◆ Assist the person drawing blood. The blood may
be placed into two or more tubes or bottles.
◆ Place a gauze pad, folded into a compress, tightly
over the venipuncture site and secure firmly with
tape. Check a few minutes later to make sure all
bleeding has stopped.
◆ Properly dispose of gloves, bed pad, and syringes.
◆ Carefully wash your hands.
◆ Document that the procedure was done and by
whom.
◆ Take the specimen to the laboratory immediately.
This is especially important with cultures.

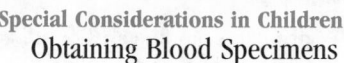

Special Considerations in Children
Obtaining Blood Specimens

A blood specimen from an infant or a young child
may be obtained by puncturing the jugular vein in the
neck. A mummy restraint is used. The nurse holds the
child with the head over the edge of the treatment table and steadies the child, while a second person obtains the specimen. (See Chapter 64.)

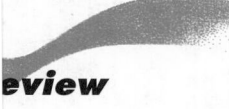

eview

ions for Critical Thinking

ies are involved in making an accurate in-
tput record? Describe activities involved in
ccurate intake and output record. Discuss
ce of such records.

nurse's responsibility and skills needed in
ine, stool, sputum, and blood specimens.
v documentation is made for each type of
llection.

ngs

le CJ. Fundamentals of Nursing: Human
Function. Philadelphia, J.B. Lippincott,

nical Skills in Nursing Practice, Ed 2. Phila-
Lippincott, 1992

re BG. Brunner and Suddarth's Textbook
urgical Nursing, Ed 7. Philadelphia, J.B.
992

D. Clinical Nursing Skills: Nursing Process
to Advanced Skills, Ed 2. Norwalk, CT,
nge, 1989

Key Readings (continued)

Taber's Cyclopedic Medical Dictionary, Ed 17. Philadel-
phia, F.A. Davis, 1993
The Lippincott Manual of Nursing Practice. Philadelphia,
J.B. Lippincott, 1991

Enrichment Keys

Smith-Temple AJ, Johnson JY. Nurses' Guide to Clinical
Procedures, Ed. 2. Philadelphia, J.B. Lippincott, 1994

Keys to Learning More

Chapter 50: head-to-toe nursing assessment
Chapter 54: sterile technique
Unit Thirteen: pediatric nursing
Chapter 69: disorders in fluid or electrolyte balance
Chapter 72: blood glucose testing
Chapter 75: blood and lymph disorders
Chapter 79: respiratory disorders
Chapter 81: digestive disorders
Chapter 82: urinary disorders

48 Bandages and Binders

Keys for Learning

Learning Objectives

- State the purposes of applying binders and bandages.
- State the reasons for applying the elastic roller bandage.
- Describe the T-binder.
- Describe the use of Montgomery straps.
- Describe evaluation of an extremity in the patient who has an arm or leg wrapped or who is wearing antiembolism stockings.
- Demonstrate the ability to apply the bandages and binders described in this chapter.

Key Terms

antiembolism stockings   Montgomery straps

maceration   T-binder

Keys to Understanding This Chapter

Chapter 30: medical asepsis and universal precautions
Chapter 31: first aid, including slings
Chapter 37: documentation and reporting
Chapter 43: body mechanics and positioning
Chapter 45: personal hygiene and skin care

Key Points

- Elastic roller bandages encourage and support circulation after surgery.
- Elastic roller bandages stop bleeding by application of direct pressure.

Key Points (continued)

- Binders supply support for specific body parts.
- Binders and bandages must be rewrapped every few hours.
- Never allow an antiembolism stocking to "bunch up" or cease circulation in the leg.
- Apply even pressure over the leg when applying an antiembolism stocking or elastic roller bandage.

Key Topics Outline

Bandages
Binders
     The T-Binder
     Tape
     Montgomery Straps
     Antiembolism Stockings

Key Learning Activities

- Familiarize yourself with elastic roller bandages, T-binders, Montgomery straps, and antiembolism stockings.

Key Nursing Procedure

NP 48-1: Applying Antiembolism Stockings

Rosdahl CB: Textbook of Basic Nursing, 6th ed. © 1995 J.B. Lippincott Company

n When Bandages Are Used

r fingers

pink or an appropriate color for race; not
ite, cyanotic, or mottled
y pressing lightly. Skin tones should im-
y return to normal; if the area touched
lighter the skin is *blanched*
ility
ld be able to move toes or fingers freely
pain
nsation
ld be able to feel your touch on toes and

bjective feelings; tingling, numbness, or
complaint of pain (report pain and follow
mplication of extreme tightness is signif-

elling
or foot is pressed, indentation should not
mprint indicates edema
the toes or fingers
arm like rest of the body

---

ed bandages or binders, and the nurse
to apply them. It is important to un-
s for their use and principles of

upport and hold dressings in place.
ed in various widths and can be strips
or elasticized material.
r elastic stocking is applied to an arm
ulation must be assessed regularly.
sensitivity (CMS), and temperature
e accompanying box describes this

sign should be noted and the team
t once. The elastic roller bandage,
an ACE bandage, is commonly used
ressure to a part of the body to stop
support, or hold a dressing in place.
he following actions in applying an
lage:

ges must be ordered by the

s order will indicate the specific part
and how often this is to be done.
he bandage used is determined by
wrapped. Generally, a bandage

---

wider than 3 inches (7.5 cm) is difficult to keep in place on an arm or leg. Wider bandages may be used on the chest or abdomen. More than one roller bandage may be used, if necessary. Simply overlap ends.

◆ Explain to the patient what you plan to do. (*Rationale: The patient will be more cooperative.*)

◆ The extremity to be wrapped should be elevated or level with the recumbent lying body (Fig. 48-1). (*Rationale: This will help to prevent congestion of the blood and lymph in the leg.*)

◆ When you begin to wrap, the bandage must be rolled. (*Rationale: This will help ensure that even pressure is applied.*)

◆ The roller bandage is applied to the leg or arm from the toes or fingers up toward the hip or shoulder. (*Rationale: Wrapping from the toes or fingers up provides support for the circulation.*) Wrap the bandage firmly, but not too tightly. Do not stretch the bandage while wrapping.

◆ Overlap each layer about half the width of the strip. Proceed to wrap from distal to proximal.

◆ Anchor the top with tape. (*Rationale: Pins or clips may scratch the patient.*)

◆ Assess the circulation of the toes or fingers after the bandage is in place. (*Rationale: A bandage that is too tight can cut off circulation and cause permanent problems.*)

◆ Document the procedure, noting the patient's reactions.

◆ Release the bandage at least once every 4 hours, unless you are ordered otherwise. At this time, the leg or arm should be exercised and skin care

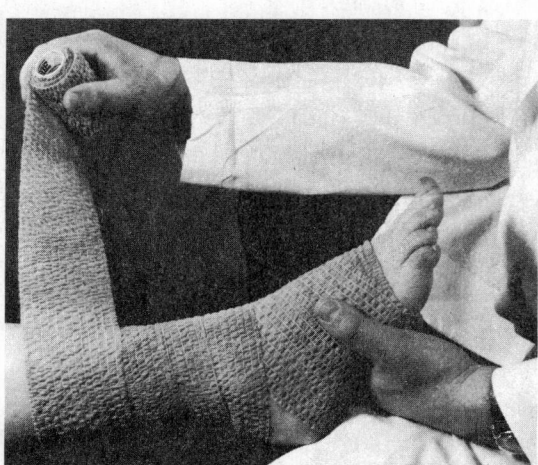

Figure 48-1. An example of applying a roller bandage. During the wrapping procedure, the foot is elevated to the level of the body or higher. Firm, even pressure is applied on the bandage as it is applied. Each successive wrap covers about half the previous part of the bandage. (Courtesy of 3M Company, Medical Products Division)

given. (*Rationale: This increases circulation and helps to prevent deformities and discomfort.*)

Binders

Binders supply support for specific body parts or hold a dressing in place. They include slings and T-binders. They may be made of cloth or elasticized material and are often fastened with Velcro. Guidelines for applying binders are listed in the accompanying box.

The T-Binders

A **T-binder** gets its name from its shape. It is made of two strips of material, 3 or 4 inches (7.5 or 10 cm) wide, which are fastened together, forming a T. The T-binder is used to hold rectal or perineal dressings in place. The perineal strap is split through the middle to make a T-binder for a male patient. T-binders are shown in Figure 48-2.

Wear gloves when you apply the T-binder. Place the band around the patient's waist, bring the perineal strap between the legs, and pin the band and the strip at the midline. Be sure to get the binder on tightly enough to hold the dressings, but not so tightly that it is uncomfortable.

Tape

Strips of hypoallergenic tape are often used in place of bandages and binders to hold dressings in place. Tape may be used also to give support, as in sprained ankle,

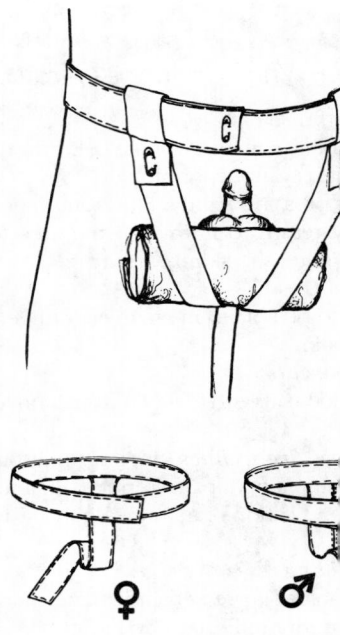

Figure 48-2. The T-binder may be adapte[d] or female patient to hold dressings in plac[e]

fractured ribs, or fractured toes. The shaved before large dressings of tape cause hairs stick to the tape and r painful.

Tape such as 3M Micropore tape and helps to prevent maceration of t **tion** is softening and breakdown du move tape in the direction of hair gr comfort. If tape is difficult to remove, applied to the skin at the edge of the a to remove it. Keep moistening the sk hesive as you peel the tape off gently

> ### Nursing Alert
>
> Be careful with acetone and other sub remove tape marks. *Never* use these li open flame or on an open wound!

Montgomery Straps

If a dressing needs to be changed ver[y] or **Montgomery straps** may be use adhesive ends of the straps are tape the dressing is held in place by the of the straps, which are either tied, b[u] with Velcro over the dressing. The be changed as often as needed wit[h] tape from the skin each time. This h

> ### Nursing Skill Guidelines
> #### Applying Binders
>
> ◆ Wash your hands before and after applying or adjusting a binder. Use universal precautions (gloves are not usually needed if the patient's skin is intact).
> ◆ The binder should be applied firmly enough to give support, but not too tightly. If the dressing is not held firmly in place, bleeding could occur or the area could be irritated by the dressing's movement. If a binder is used to hold a body part in place or to support, it must be firm enough to be effective. A binder applied too tightly might cause unnecessary discomfort or cut off circulation.
> ◆ If a binder is pinned from the bottom up, it will give upward support. If it is applied from the top down, it will exert a downward pressure.
> ◆ The binder must be a size appropriate to the body part and size of the patient.
> ◆ Binders should be rewrapped every few hours. (*Rationale: The patient's movements tend to loosen the binder. When the binder is rewrapped, you can assess the skin and check the dressing.*)

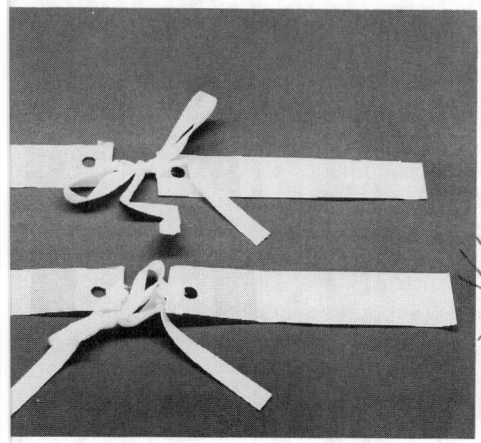

bulky dressing. (*Rationale: Two sets provide more support.*)
- Untie for dressing changes.
- Leave straps in place until they become soiled or need to be changed or removed.
- Document procedure and condition of wound on patient record. (*Rationale: Inform other caregivers of their presence for future dressing changes.*)

> **Nursing Alert**
>
> If the patient complains of pain or itching while any bandage is in place, assess the area immediately.

ntgomery straps or ties are used to prevent
from frequent tape removal when dressings
;ed often.

 ways: dressings can be changed more
 conveniently, and the tape remains in
ing skin integrity. The following nursing
l in applying Montgomery straps.

Wear gloves.
l precautions. Properly dispose of
gs. (*Rationale: They are highly
d.*)
n with dressing. (*Rationale: Keep the
of microorganisms.*)
ercial product or fashion strap by plac-
of a strip of tape or adhesive-backed
e skin, folding the other half onto it-
ile: *Make a flap to secure ties or pins.*)
e other side of the dressing. (*Ratio-
orresponding strap.*)
eed to be cut into the ends of the
idhesive-backed strip does not contain
nale: *This allows strings to be inserted
 be pulled together.*)
ids of the straps with ties across the
tionale: *This secures the dressing.*)
iore sets of straps and ties for a large,

Antiembolism Stockings

Many physicians routinely order **antiembolism stockings** (also called TED socks) for all postoperative patients. These are firm stockings that cover the foot (not the toes) and the leg, up to the knee. They support the blood vessels in the leg, helping to maintain adequate blood pressure and prevent emboli (blood clots).

The stockings should fit tightly enough to give support, without binding the leg or cutting off the circulation. Stockings are available in various sizes. Measurements must be taken to ensure proper fit. Elastic stockings do not release, as do roller bandages, and can be very tight.

Periodic circulation checks must be made and documented. Most antiembolism stockings are made with a small opening near the toes, which allows for easy assessment of the extremity. (See Chapter 70.)

The procedure for applying the stockings in described in Nursing Procedure 48-1. It is *important* the stockings be applied before the patient gets out of bed or after assuming the recumbent position for at least 15 minutes to avoid pooling of fluid in the tissue and to promote circulation. Stockings should be removed each shift, the condition of the leg checked, and the stockings reapplied. The patient's legs should be washed each day or more often and clean stockings applied.

Applying Antiembolism Stockings (TED Socks)

Supplies and Equipment

Support stockings
Talcum powder
Tape measure

Procedure

1. Explain procedure to patient.
   (*Rationale: Providing information fosters patient cooperation.*)
2. Use tape measure to decide on proper stocking size for patient.
   (*Rationale: Stockings that are too tight may interfere with circulation. Stockings that are too loose do not encourage venous return.*)
3. Gather supplies.
   (*Rationale: Organization facilitates performance of skill.*)
4. Wash hands. Wear gloves if skin is not intact.
   (*Rationale: Handwashing prevents the spread of organisms.*)
5. Assist patient to supine position. Allow at least 15 minutes before applying stockings if patient has had lower extremities in a dependent position.
   (*Rationale: Stockings are best applied early in the morning before a sitting or standing position is assumed; otherwise, veins become distended and edema occurs.*)
6. Apply small amount of talcum powder to feet and legs if not contraindicated.
   (*Rationale: Powder reduces friction and allows easier application of the stockings.*)
7. Grasp heel of stocking and turn inside out.
   (*Rationale: This minimizes bunching of stocking on patient's foot.*)

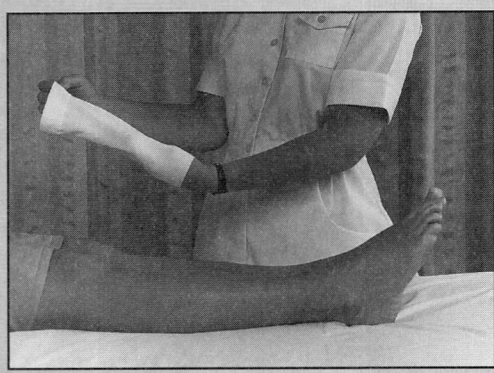

Step 7   Preparing to put on the stocking (Photos © B. Proud.)

8. Slip the foot, toes, and heel into the sto the heel in the heel pocket of the stock stocking over the foot.
   (*Rationale: Stocking will be properly po foot.*)
9. Support the ankle and ease stocking sm the calf and remainder of leg.
   (*Rationale: This prevents wrinkles from which can impede circulation.*)

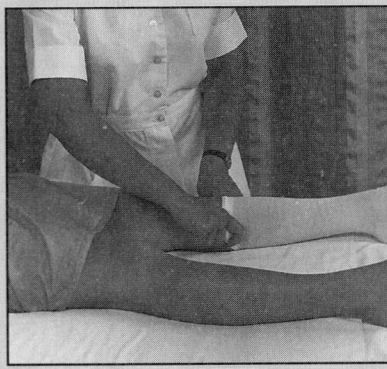

Step 9   Easing the stocking over the calf (Photo ©

10. Pull forward slightly on toe section.
    (*Rationale: This eases pressure on toes*)
11. Instruct patient to report any extreme d
    (*Rationale: Complications can occur.*)
12. Wash hands.
    (*Rationale: Handwashing prevents the organisms.*)

Nursing Alert

If TED socks are allowed to bunch up, can be occluded. Serious complications amputation and death, can result.

eview

tions for Critical Thinking

ve important elements in checking circula-
bandages are used. Describe the signifi-
ese elements.

e difference in the female and male T-

r what situations you would use a T-binder
nery straps. Describe application of each.

ings

rnle CJ. Fundamentals of Nursing: Human
Function. Philadelphia, J.B. Lippincott,

inical Skills in Nursing Practice, Ed 2. Phila-
3. Lippincott, 1993
. Photo Atlas of Nursing Procedures, Ed 2.
City CA, Addison-Wesley Nursing, 1991
edic Medical Dictionary, Ed 17. Philadel-
Davis, 1993

Keys to Learning More

Chapter 49: heat and cold application
Chapter 50: nursing assessment
Chapter 52: patient comfort and pain management
Chapter 53: the person who has surgery
Chapter 54: surgical asepsis
Chapter 64: care of children
Chapter 70: musculoskeletal injuries, traction, and cast care
Chapter 74: cardiovascular disorders, including embolism and phlebitis
Chapter 89: rehabilitation and home care

49 Heat and Cold Application

Keys for Learning

Learning Objectives

- State the purposes of heat and cold application to the body.
- State the precautions involved in heat and cold applications to the body.
- Demonstrate the ability to administer a leg soak, a sitz bath, and an aquathermia pad.
- Demonstrate the ability to use the cooling blanket and apply an ice collar.

Key Terms

aquathermia pad

hypothermic blanket

icecap

infrared rays

sitz bath

ultrasound

ultraviolet rays

Keys to Understanding This Chapter

Chapter 15: epithelial tissues and the skin
Chapter 30: medical asepsis and universal precautions
Chapter 31: first aid, including burns and hypothermia
Chapter 37: documentation and reporting
Chapter 45: personal hygiene and skin care
Chapter 48: bandages and binders

Key Points

- Whenever you apply heat, take measures the patient from possible burn injury.
- Moist, hot applications heat the skin more than applications of dry heat.
- Moist cold compresses are applied to sma parts.
- The water temperature for a soak should than 105°F.
- A sitz bath applies heat and water to the p
- Cold constricts the surface blood vessels.
- Giving a tepid water sponge bath helps to body temperature.

Key Topics Outline

Heat and Cold
    Heat Application
    Cold Application
Heat and Cold Therapies

Key Learning Activities

- Give yourself a warm foot soak. Express y reaction.
- Review your facility's policies for heat and applications.

Rosdahl CB: Textbook of Basic Nursing, 6th ed. © 19

cal conditions require the application of
cold. The nurse will often be asked to
erapeutic measures. Because of compli-
n occur from extreme heat or cold, the
be knowledgeable in using these two
y. This chapter will assist you in learning
d moist heat and cold safely.

Cold

on

mmonly used for the following reasons:

cal pain or aching
circulation to an area
wound healing
chilly patient more comfortable
temperature of the body
drainage (might be used to draw in-
ial out of a wound)

t must be fairly intense to produce the
there is one great danger in using it: *the*
s. Whenever you apply heat, take mea-
t the patient from possible burn injury.
heat applications are listed on the pre-

d moist heat are usually applied for their
ommon methods for applying dry heat
pad, warm-water bag, Aqua-K (aqua-
eat lamp, or electric cradle. Moist, hot
at skin more quickly and are more pen-
plications of dry heat because water is
nductor than air.
ion must be hot enough to accomplish
t must be kept within the safety range.
er a large area affords more warmth and
ous than heat applied over a small area.

on

of cold is constriction of surface blood
events escape of heat from the body by
tion, which also relieves congestion and
nuscle pain. Cold applications are com-
the following reasons:

feverish patient more comfortable
terial activity in infection
top bleeding
ain following throat surgery or tooth
d in headache
eristalsis in abdominal inflammation
ain in engorged breasts
painful swelling in injured tissues, in-
ins, fractures, and as first aid for burns

Nursing Skill Guidelines
Applying Heat and Cold Therapy

Heat Application

◆ Heat is applied only on a physician's order, and
with utmost caution.
◆ The nerves in the skin are numbed easily, and the
patient may not feel the pain of a burn, especially
if heat has been applied often.
◆ Some body parts are especially sensitive to heat:
eyelids, neck, and inside of the arm.
◆ Each person should be tested for sensitivity before
you apply heat. *(Rationale: You need to determine
how much heat is safe and for how long.)*
◆ Infants, older people, and those with fair, thin
skin have less resistance to heat. Lowered body
resistance also makes body tissues less resistant to
heat.
◆ Be especially careful with patients who are unresponsive or anesthetized and some patients suffering from cerebral disorders or dementia.
*(Rationale: They cannot tell when heat is too
intense.)*
◆ Impaired circulation and some metabolic diseases
make people more susceptible to burns (eg, the
patient who is in shock or who has diabetes).
◆ Patients receiving radiation therapy or chemotherapy for cancer and those with any degree of paralysis are particularly susceptible to burns. *(Rationale: Their immune system or skin integrity is already compromised.)*

Cold Application

◆ If the patient complains of numbness in the area
where cold has been applied, and the skin looks
white or spotty, discontinue application. *(Rationale: Cold numbs nerve endings.)*
◆ As cold decreases the flow of blood in one area of
the body, flow is increased to other areas. (This explains why cold or chilling drafts striking the body
often cause congestion in the nasal passages.)
◆ Continued application of cold affects deeper tissues. Prolonged exposure to extreme cold may
cause actual freezing (frostbite).
◆ Cold often is applied to a sprain, strain, fracture, or
burn. *(Rationale: This helps to remove blood and
lymph congestion in the area and reduces pain.)* If
in doubt, apply cold.

In a sprain or similar injury, a cold application is
much more appropriate than heat. Cold is applied to
sprains or bruises to prevent swelling (edema); however, it will not reduce edema already present. Cold
is applied to the body by means of icecaps, ice
collars, compresses, cool sponge baths, or cooling
blankets.

Guidelines for cold application are listed on the preceding page.

Heat and Cold Therapies

An Icecap or Ice Collar

An **icecap** is a flat, oval rubber bag with a leakproof, screw-in top. Its opening is wide so it can be easily filled with ice chunks. An ice collar is a narrow rubber or elastic bag, curved to fit the neck. The physician prescribes the application of an icecap or ice collar to specific parts of the body. However, you may usually apply an icecap for headache or in an emergency, such as a sprain or nosebleed, without an order.

Cold may have harmful effects on a weakened or undernourished person although it is stimulating to a healthy person.

Nursing Skill

Applying an Icecap or Ice Collar

Supplies and Equipment

Icecap or ice collar
Safety pins or paper tape
Basin of chipped ice
Bath blanket (if needed)

Procedure

1. Wash your hands.
2. Inspect the stopper or closure of the bag and test for leakage. *(Rationale: A leak would cause the bedclothes to become wet and chill the patient.)*
3. Fill an icecap or collar about three-fourths full, using small pieces of ice. *(Rationale: It will be easier to fit the bag closely to the body if the ice pieces are small. Small pieces of ice cool faster because they have more surface area.)* Sometimes cold water is added to increase the cooling effect further.
4. Flatten the bag on a hard surface, and press on it to expel air. *(Rationale: A flat icecap or ice collar is easier to fit to the body.)*
5. Screw in the top or fold over the end, making sure that the top is firmly in place. *(Rationale: Prevent leaks as ice melts.)*
6. Dry the icecap or collar and cover with a towel. *(Rationale: Prevent moisture from condensing on the outside of the bag, which would make the patient uncomfortable.)*
7. Secure the towel with a pin or tape, being careful not to puncture the bag.
8. Adjust bag on the part of body to be treated (Fig. 49-1).
9. Leave icecap or ice collar in place for 30 minutes to 1 hour, as directed. Keep icecap or ice collar off for 1 hour before reapplying it, unless directed otherwise. *(Rationale: Prolonged applications of cold could dan-*

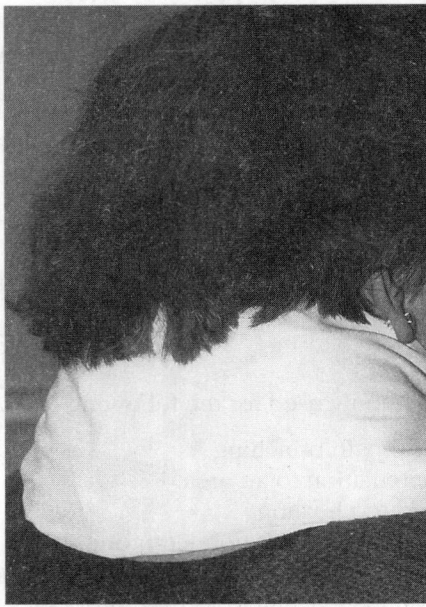

Figure 49-1. An ice collar may be used to and reduce swelling following a neck in Crushed ice is used because it provides be the collar is wrapped in a towel or soft cloth ding and to prevent overchilling. The air is the collar is closed to allow it to fit closer patient is cautioned to notify the nurse if th unusually uncomfortable. (Photo by Kimbe

gerously slow circulation and may cau The ice will melt in this length of time c

10. Wash your hands after applying the ice and after removing it.
11. Document the treatment on the patient "on" and "off" periods and patient's rea

---

The Single-Use and Refreezable Ice

Many hospitals provide ice packs fil tion and kept frozen in a refrigerator rea erally, disposable ice packs are used. Ar available for one-time emergency use. which, when broken, releases a chem the bag. Once it thaws it cannot be refr filled packs are available, which can be heated. Thus, they can be used as eithe an ice pack, and may be reused.

Nursing Alert

Use extreme caution when you apply co tient's skin becomes blanched (white) or red, discontinue the treatment and checl team leader.

Compresses

compresses are applied to relieve pain
on in eye injuries or after a tooth extrac-
be helpful in sinus congestion. Some-
applied to hemorrhoids. Nursing activi-
cold, moist compresses are:

presses in a basin containing pieces of
all amount of water. (*Rationale: The
ses the speed with which the com-
ooled.*)

e patient that the treatment will relieve
(*Rationale: A relaxed patient will feel
than a tense patient.*)

mpress thoroughly and apply. (*Ration-
ter drips, it may startle the patient.*)

presses frequently. (*Rationale: Com-
absorb body heat.*)

e treatment as ordered, usually for 15 to
to be repeated every 2 to 4 hours. If
s able, he or she could apply the

reatment on the patient's chart, noting
d the patient's reaction.

t Compresses and Packs

t compresses and packs apply heat to an
te circulation, to ease pain, and to pro-
from infections. They may also be used
ations.

gauze *compresses* apply heat to a small
oist, *packs* of cotton or terry cloth apply
area. Covering the pack with heavy ma-
retain heat longer, and application of the
r a pack will enable the pack to remain
ndefinitely. Compresses and packs do not
ile, unless there is a break in the skin.
n prescribes the type of application, how
and the length of time the application is
ce. The physician also prescribes the so-
ed; often it is water, a mild antiseptic so-
2% boric acid), or normal saline.
re applied as hot as the patient can com-
them. Apply the pack slowly so the pa-
ou how it feels. The patient is the best
rt. During the procedure, the patient may
recautions should be taken to keep the
nd protected from drafts. Nursing activi-
rm, moist compresses and packs are:

hands before and after treatment. Wear
re is a break in the patient's skin. (*Ra-
vents cross-contamination.*)

ack machine set at the proper tempera-
ise, immerse the compress or pack in
r (or heat in a microwave for one-time
. (*Rationale: Using the hot-pack ma-

chine ensures a particular temperature. Because it
has an attached wringer, you do not have to wring
out the packs by hand.*)

◆ Petroleum jelly may be applied before the pack.
(*Rationale: Protect the skin.*) *Caution:* It may become overheated.

◆ Place plastic or a dry pack over the moist compress. (*Rationale: This covering will keep out air,
which could cool the pack. The extra pack also provides insulation against heat loss and helps protect
the bed.*)

◆ Wring the compress or pack with forceps or
wringer, removing as much water as possible. (*Rationale: Hot water dripping on the patient's skin
could cause a burn.*) To wring out packs with forceps, clamp one forceps onto each end of the pack
and twist them in opposite directions.

◆ Shake the pack lightly, and apply it to the area
gently at first, gradually pressing it against the skin.
(*Rationale: Shaking the pack cools it a little. Because air is a poor heat conductor, eliminating air
spaces between the compress or pack and skin will
make the treatment more effective.*)

◆ Believe the patient if he or she says the pack is too
hot.

◆ Cover the moist compress or pack with the dry
pack and moisture-proof cover. (*Rationale: The
pack is covered to insulate against heat loss and
evaporation of moisture.*) Omit this step if the
Aqua-K pad is used.

◆ Change the pack as often as necessary to keep the
area heated. (*Rationale: The pack must be kept
warm for the specified length of time to ensure that
the physician's order is carried out.*) Small applications will cool more quickly than large ones. Using
an Aqua-K pad on top of the large warm, moist
pack will keep it warm.

◆ Check the condition of the patient's skin at least
every 30 minutes. (*Rationale: Continued exposure
to heat and moisture can cause the skin to break
down.*)

◆ Continue treatment for the prescribed time, then
remove the applications. Packs are used for one
patient only. They are then discarded or laundered.

◆ Dry the skin and cover it, as ordered.

Applying Warm, Moist Compression to the Eye. The eyelid
and the skin around the eye are thin and delicate structures. Precautions to prevent burning the eyelid and the
skin around the eye are especially important when applying warm, moist compresses. Be sure to wash your
hands carefully before and after applying eye compresses (the eye is very susceptible to infection). If the
eye is draining, discard each compress when you remove it. All equipment is sent for sterilization after the
treatment. If compresses are applied to both eyes, use

separate equipment for each eye to prevent spreading infection from one eye to the other. Eye treatments must be given very carefully. They may be the deciding factor between preserving and losing sight.

The Aquathermia Pad

The aquathermia pad, which produces heat, is used in muscle sprains, mild inflammations, and to relieve pain. Temperature-controlled distilled water flows through the waterproof pad. The control unit can be placed on the bedside table. The receptacle is filled two-thirds full with distilled water (Fig. 49-2). It is checked periodically and refilled as water evaporates. The pad is not placed directly against the patient's skin; it is covered with a pillowcase or towel, or placed over a pack. It should always be placed on top of a body part; the patient should be told not to lie on it.

The pad is applied according to the physician's order. The nurse checks the pad to make sure it is heating properly and not overheating. Any malfunctions are reported to the maintenance department.

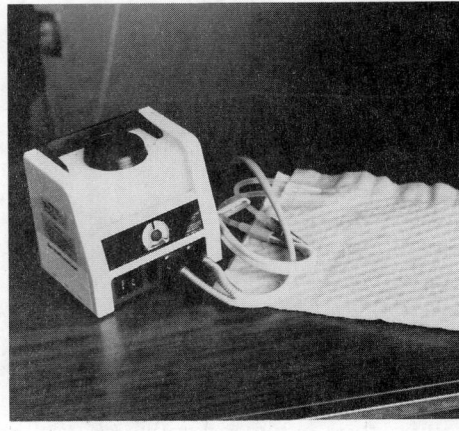

Figure 49-2. Aqua K (aquathermia) pad.

Nursing Skill
Applying the Aquathermia Pad

Supplies and Equipment

Pad
Cover for pad
Control unit
Distilled water

Procedure

1. Wash hands before and after procedure. Fill control unit receptacle two-thirds full with distilled water. (*Rationale: Distilled water will not damage the unit as tap water might.*)
2. Set temperature control on 105°F. (*Rationale: This temperature will deliver heat to the body without burning the area.*)
3. Cover the pad with the cover, sheet, pillowcases, or towel. (*Rationale: Protect the skin.*)
4. Plug the control unit into electrical outlet, and place the control unit on bedside table.
5. Apply the pad to specific body part, as ordered.
6. Use tape or roller bandage to secure the pad in place. Do not use safety pins. (*Rationale: Pinpricks can cause the pad to leak and possibly short circuit.*)
7. Instruct the patient to not lie directly on the pad and to avoid changing temperature settings on the control unit.
8. Place call signal within reach. (*Rationale: The patient must be able to get attention if uncomfortable.*)
9. Assess area for redness after 5 minutes.
10. Remove pad after 20 to 30 minutes or as directed.
11. Store pad until next treatment.
12. Document procedure on patient record.

Lamp Treatments and Ultrasound

Lamp treatments are given by trained cause exposure to light rays must be reg to prevent injury to the patient.

Infrared rays are used to relax mus circulation, and relieve pain. They hav fect on the body as other forms of dry **olet rays** are not as penetrating as infr light provides mild ultraviolet radiati exposure to the sun, however, will skin. Ultraviolet rays are used to treat and wounds.

Ultrasound is used to apply deep h and body tissues. Before treatments, sure that the timer is working correct burns, it is also important to keep the u dle or wand moving at all times during A lubricating gel is applied to the skin t movement.

Nursing Alert

Do not perform any type of lamp treatme physician's order and special training in t lamp.

The Heated Bed Cradle

Some medical conditions of the low must be treated with heat, while being the pressure of bed linens. In instances a heated bed cradle is used. The device i described in Chapter 44; however, the h dle is equipped with low wattage lamps *heat to the lower extremities.* Nursing when caring for a patient using the hea are:

lle over the foot of the bed.
att (eg, 15–25 watt) lamps in unit.
o electrical outlet.
ent not to touch lamp because it will

linens over the cradle.
; observe time for treatment to be

and remove cradle from the bed, un-
for continued use.
efully for overheating.

can be applied by immersing a body
ater or a solution for a prescribed time.
is called a soak. The soak may be
ve circulation, to increase blood sup-
ted area, to aid in breaking down into apply medication, to cleanse dis-
ds, or to loosen scabs and crusts from
nds. Often a soak is combined with a
. The physical therapy department
ath.
not considered necessary to sterilize the
ld be cleaned thoroughly with soap, a
water, as per facility protocol. Persons
often have open wounds. It is impor-
he spread of infection between patients.
ed for soaks unless otherwise specified.
other substance often is added to the

ture of the water should be no higher
°C). The physician may prescribe a def-
e. The temperature of the water should
ntly, and hot water be added *slowly* to
; the patient. Stir the water to distribute
The usual length of a soak is 15 to 20
g actions for giving an arm or leg soak

with a bath towel. (*Rationale: Pad-*
bruises.)
ient with a protective sheet.
vater in the tub (100°–105°F, 37.8°–
s otherwise specified). Always use a
neter.
round, remove the dressing (wear
are to dispose of the dressing

ver the body part into the water.
dding on the edge of the tub for the
w to rest on; support the body part
pillow if necessary.
perature of the water frequently with a
neter. Add hot water carefully as
stir the water.

◆ Remove the body part from the bath in 15 or 20
minutes, or as ordered, and dry the skin.
◆ If there is a wound, apply a sterile dressing. In the
case of a discharging wound, sterilize equipment
after use. Properly dispose of gloves.
◆ Document treatment and patient reactions.

Sponge Bath

A tepid water sponge bath may be ordered to reduce
a patient's elevated temperature. The first effect of cold
water on the skin is constriction of blood vessels. Alcohol is rarely used because it cools too much (because
it evaporates so fast).

A cool (tepid) sponge bath is often given for its temporary soothing effect and may not produce a marked
temperature drop unless used for a period of time. The
minimum time is about 30 minutes. If elevated temperature is a threat to the patient's life, more dramatic
means must be taken to bring it within a manageable
range more quickly and permanently. In conditions associated with a dangerously high temperature an "ice
mattress" or hypothermia blanket (a plastic mattress
pad through which very cold water flows continuously)
can be used.

Tepid sponge baths are not advisable for older people with inelastic arteries, for arthritic patients, for patients with lowered resistance to disease, or for very
young children. Cold has a depressing effect on the
body at first. Guidelines are listed in the accompanying box.

Nursing Alert

The nurse should constantly assess the patient's
core body temperature with an electronic thermometer during the sponge bath. If the patient begins to
shiver or if the core temperature falls to within 1.5°F
of normal, discontinue the treatment and report the
situation.

The Sitz Bath

The purpose of a **sitz bath** is to apply heat to the
pelvic area. The patient is placed in a tub containing
enough water to cover the perineal area. A regular
bathtub can be used, but a special sitz tub (Fig. 49-3)
or seat built to accommodate hips and buttocks may
be provided if the baths are ordered frequently. Disposable type tubs are used commonly for maternity
patients and patients who have undergone rectal or
perineal surgery. The tub fits on the inside of the
commode and is equipped with a bag, tubing, and
nozzle to allow the water to flow freely to the perineal
area.

Nursing Skill Guidelines
Giving a Tepid Sponge Bath to Reduce Body Temperature

◆ Explain the procedure to the patient. (*Rationale: If the patient is nervous and fearful, the bath is less likely to be effective.*)

◆ Give the patient an opportunity to use a urinal or bedpan before the bath. (*Rationale: The patient will become more comfortable with an empty bladder, and once the bath is begun its effectiveness is lessened if it is stopped and restarted.*)

◆ Take the patient's temperature. (*Rationale: You will have a baseline temperature to guide the treatment.*)

◆ Note whether the patient has had an antipyretic to reduce fever. (*Rationale: Such medications may influence the effects of the sponge bath.*)

◆ Add tepid water to the bath basin (70°–85°F or 21.1°–29.4°C). Use thermometer. (*Rationale: This temperature is below normal body temperature, so it will lower body temperature, yet it is not so cold as to be dangerous. It is vital to be accurate.*)

◆ Place moist, cool cloths—wrung out just enough to prevent dripping—in the axillae and groin. (*Rationale: In these areas, the large blood vessels lie close to the skin and evaporation of water will cool the body efficiently.*)

◆ The patient's first reaction to a cool sponge bath is a sensation of chilliness, which disappears as the body adjusts to the temperature. Therefore, the bath must be continued long enough to allow for this adjustment, at least 25 to 30 minutes. The patient's body temperature should be constantly monitored electronically during the procedure to determine the effect of treatment. (*Rationale: There is a danger of reducing the core body temperature too much. The temperature will continue to drop for a while after the completion of the sponge bath.*)

◆ Sponge each limb for at least 5 minutes and the back and the buttocks for at least 10 to 15 minutes. (*Rationale: Sponging for this length of time is necessary to reduce fever.*)

◆ Stop the procedure if the patient becomes very chilled or begins to shiver. (*Rationale: People respond differently. Prevent hypothermia.*)

◆ Stop sponging as soon as the temperature approaches the normal range (about 100°F or 37.8°C, orally). Give the patient a bath blanket. (*Rationale: Otherwise the temperature will drop too low.*)

◆ Take the patient's temperature 30 minutes after the procedure is completed. (*Rationale: It takes 25 to 30 minutes for the body to totally respond to cold applications.*)

◆ Document the treatment on the patient's chart, noting reactions. Be sure to record the beginning and ending temperatures on the graph sheet. A separate temperature record should also be kept during the procedure. (*Rationale: It is vital to record how the patient responded to the treatment, especially if it needs to be repeated.*)

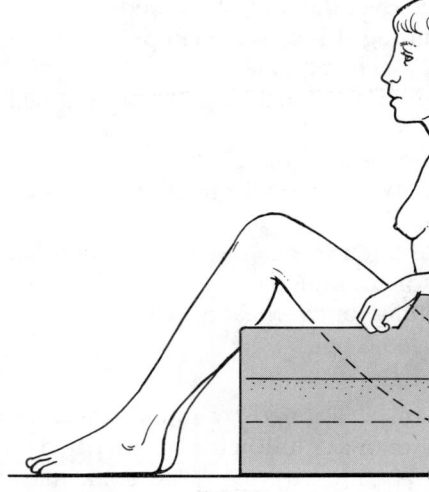

Figure 49-3. Sitz bath.

Nursing Skill
Giving a Sitz Bath

Supplies and Equipment

Bathtub or sitz tub
Cotton bath blanket
Bath towels
Bath thermometer

Procedure

1. Make sure the tub is clean. Use gloves the tub. (*Rationale: Because the tub is patients, it must be sanitized between use the solution and methods as direct cal facility.*)

2. Check the order. The physician will pr of the treatment, which usually is from

3. Fill the tub to the required depth with ified temperature. The patient's body w in proportion to size.

4. Place a large bath towel in the bottom needed, place the drain adapter in plac continuously drain. (*Rationale: The tou tub more comfortable and easier to cle*

5. Help the patient in the bath. A short pa stool under the feet (*Rationale: The sto pressure on the blood vessels in the legs towel in the lumbar area. (Rationale: ʼ port the back and keep the patient's bo alignment.*)

6. Instruct the patient to sit far enough fo so the drain is not occluded.

7. Cover the upper and lower part of the ton bath blanket. (*Rationale: Many pe during this procedure. It is also import person from drafts.*)

8. Set the water temperature gauge on th tain the required temperature. You car supply and drain so a constant circulat

(Rationale: Water of the correct temperature ...herapeutic and safest.)

...the bath is to apply heat, the temperature ...at 95°F (35°C) and be gradually increased to ...of 105°F (40.5°C). If given to cleanse and ...ling, the bath temperature should be from ...(34.4°–36.7°C). *(Rationale: Extremely hot ... may damage tissues, rather than promoting ...pital sitz bath tubs are set so that the tem-...! not exceed 105°F.)*

...tient closely for signs of fainting or weakness. ...ient get out of the bath after he or she has ...d to the heat. *(Rationale: The person may ...en standing or walking.)*

...ient to bed after the bath. *(Rationale: Heat ...large area of the body may make the pa-...k or faint because blood is drawn away ...in. Resting in bed will allow circulation to ...rmal.)*

...tient adequately in bed. *(Rationale: Protect ...nd chilling.)*

...g gloves, clean the tub, according to the ...licy for the patient's specific condition. ...ands. *(Rationale: Prevent transmission of ...sms.)*

...e treatment on the patient's chart, noting ...reactions.

...ity

...ty is commonly ordered for the patient ...y breathing. In most hospitals air con-...eating systems provide a constant level ...t if the level is not high enough, an aux-...r may be placed in the room.

...ts need constant cold humidity in high ...A child may be placed in a croupette or ...t. Oxygen administered to the patient ...ified to prevent drying of the mucous ...he nose and throat. If the patient has a ..."trach mask" may be placed over the ...vide humidity, either with or without

auxiliary oxygen. A face tent is also available, which may be used to provide a high concentration of moisture in the inhaled air.

The Hypothermic Blanket

Hypothermic blankets are used to decrease a patient's body temperature. They are used primarily in surgery to prevent complications resulting from unstable regulation of body temperature. Hypothermic blankets are also used in cases of extremely high body temperatures that are uncontrolled with medications. The blanket has the possibility to be used to increase a patient's body temperature. The blanket is equipped with an electrical control unit on which the desired temperature is set and the patient's core temperature is registered.

The Electric Heating Pad

Because of its dangers, the dry electric heating pad is seldom used in hospitals. Occasionally it is used in nursing homes. It is described here so you can teach people who will use an electric heating pad at home.

An electric pad is a covered network of wires that gives off heat when an electric current passes through them. Pads with a waterproof covering are the safest. *Never* put pins into a heating pad; if a pin touches the electric wires, it can cause shock. If wires are crushed or bent, the pad can overheat and cause burns or a fire. There is a great danger of burning the patient with an electric heating pad. A heating pad's temperature is constant or may rise. Electric heating pads are not safe to use for children, the elderly, irrational and unresponsive persons, or those with spinal cord injuries.

Before applying the pad, connect it to an electric outlet and turn the heating switch to high to see whether the pad heats promptly. Then turn it off and disconnect it. Cover the pad, connect it to the bedside outlet, adjust it to the proper temperature, and apply it. Inspect frequently to prevent burning the patient. Leave setting on low at all times.

...eview

Key Readings

Craven RF, Hirnle CJ. Fundamentals of Nursing: Human Health and Function. Philadelphia, J.B. Lippincott, 1992

Earnest VV. Clinical Skills in Nursing Practice, Ed 2. Philadelphia, J.B. Lippincott, 1993

Swearingen PL. Photo Atlas of Nursing Procedures, Ed 2. Redwood City, CA, Addison-Wesley Nursing, 1991

Enrichment Keys

Smith-Temple AJ, Johnson JY. Guide to Clinical Procedures, Ed 2. Philadelphia, J.B. Lippincott, 1994

The Lippincott Manual of Nursing Practice. Philadelphia, J.B. Lippincott, 1991

Keys to Learning More

Chapter 50: head-to-toe physical examination
Chapter 52: patient comfort and pain management
Unit Twelve: maternal and child nursing
Unit Thirteen: pediatric nursing
Chapter 68: skin disorders
Chapter 70: musculoskeletal disorders
Chapter 89: rehabilitation and home care

50 Nursing Assessment and Physical Examination

Keys for Learning

Learning Objectives

♦ Describe the tools the physician uses in making a medical diagnosis.
♦ Describe the functions of the nurse when accompanying the physician on patient rounds.
♦ Describe the activities performed by the nurse when doing a basic head-to-toe nursing assessment.
♦ List the components of a health history as related to specific body systems.
♦ State the duties of the nurse when assisting with a physical examination of an adult patient.
♦ State the main components of the following special examinations: neurologic, cardiovascular, respiratory, gastrointestinal, gynecologic, and rectal.

Key Terms

auscultation	hemoptysis	rhonchi
crackles	keloids	spastic
electrocardiogram	otoscope	tenacious
electroencephalogram	palpation	tinnitus
endoscope	percussion	turgor
flaccid	purulent	wheezing

Keys to Understanding This Chapter

Chapter 6: optimum health as related to the physical examination
Unit Three: child and adult physical development
Unit Four: normal body structure and function
Chapter 30: medical asepsis and universal precautions
Unit Seven: nursing process, including nursing assessment

Keys to Understanding This Chapter
(continued)

Chapter 36: therapeutic communication during assessment
Chapter 37: documentation and reporting
Chapter 38: signs and symptoms of illness or injury
Chapter 41: initial assessment in male or female patient on admission
Chapter 42: vital signs
Chapter 43: positioning during the physical examination
Chapter 47: specimen collection, included in assessment

Key Points

♦ Proper positioning of the patient is necessary to ensure accuracy of the physical examination.
♦ Nursing assessment and physical examination provide baseline data, which assist the physician in making a medical diagnosis.
♦ Cooperation of the patient is particularly important when examining an infant or child.
♦ The nurse who is interested in learning more takes advantage of the learning experience when making rounds with a physician.
♦ The physical examination is performed when the patient first seeks care and on an ongoing basis thereafter.
♦ The physical examination and nursing assessment can be organized from head-to-toe or by body systems.
♦ Any disorders or untoward symptoms discovered during assessment must be called to the attention of the primary caregiver as soon as possible.

Key Learning Activities

♦ Practice positioning an assigned patient [ ]
  examination.
♦ Volunteer to make rounds with a physic[ ]
♦ List sequences in head-to-toe and systen[ ]
  aminations. Compare and list similarities[ ]
  differences.

The nurse is often asked to assist during a physical examination. It is important for the nurse to know the basics of the examination so the patient can be placed in the proper position and draped correctly and so appropriate equipment is available.

The primary caregiver relies on the physical examination and the patient history for much of the information about the patient. The history gives information about possible genetic problems, past illnesses, habits, and present complaints. From the physical examination specific and general observations are made. The examination includes the body from head to toe, including eyes, ears, nose, mouth, throat, neck, chest, breasts, abdomen, and extremities. The examiner listens to the heart and lung sounds. A vaginal or rectal examination is performed, as are other internal examinations as indicated. Certain laboratory tests are often included routinely as part of the physical examination.

Establishing a Medical Diagnosis

A medical diagnosis is based on *objective observations,* that is, those that can be seen or measured, and *subjective data,* that is, what the patient or family says.

Examinations Performed by the Primary Caregiver

Inspection. The condition of the ears, nose, and throat can be determined by use of special instruments such as the otoscope or laryngoscope. By looking at

the blood vessels in the retina of the e[ ] thalmoscope, the physician can infer t[ ] blood vessels in other parts of the bo[ ] structures of the body can be evalu[ ] observation.

Palpation, Auscultation, and Percussion. [ ] normal structures can be felt by **palp[ ]** the examiner's hands are used to apply[ ] The examiner listens to the heart, lung[ ] with a stethoscope. This type of exan[ ] **cultation**. A light tapping or thumpir[ ] called **percussion.** Some vital signs are[ ] methods. Of these three procedure[ ] should be done first to obtain the mos[ ] ysis. Palpation and percussion ma[ ] conditions.

Abdominal structures, the neck, bre[ ] are often assessed by palpation. The u[ ] ital organs of the patient are examine[ ] the presence of pathology. This exami[ ] palpation for hernias or testicular [ ] breast abnormalities. Bowel, heart, [ ] can be assessed by auscultation. The[ ] learn a great deal about cardiovascu[ ] tory status by auscultation and percuss[ ] and back.

Other Routine Diagnostic Examinations. [ ] dures such as the rectal or gynecolog[ ] may be done during the physical exam[ ]

Laboratory Tests

Many laboratory tests are done as part of the physical examination. Results of these tests are used in planning patient care. Some laboratory tests are done as a routine screening during all physical examinations and others are specific for certain disorders. Many of these tests are discussed in relationship to disorders throughout the remainder of this book. Commonly accepted normal values for some of the more frequently performed laboratory tests are given in Appendix C.

Examples of laboratory tests include urinalysis, complete blood count, stool examinations for blood or parasites, and blood tests for specific antibodies, chemicals, or abnormal blood components. Specimens of body fluids may be cultured to isolate a pathogenic organism and determine the appropriate antibiotic for treatment. Respiratory status can be determined by blood gas analysis or analysis of a sputum specimen. Damage to heart (cardiac) muscle can be determined by specific blood tests. Specific diseases can often be diagnosed by blood tests. The patient's blood may be typed and crossmatched for later blood transfusions. Blood or urine may be tested for levels of various drugs to evaluate situations such as driving under the influence of alcohol or the amount and identification of a drug used in a suicide attempt by overdose.

Special Diagnostic Procedures

Many other diagnostic procedures are done to determine abnormalities or disorders of various body systems. Preparation of the patient and results obtained with many of these examinations are discussed throughout much of the remainder of this book.

Endoscopy. An **endoscope** is a long tube with a fiberoptic scope on the end. The tube is passed through a body orifice so internal areas of the body can be examined without surgery. Using endoscopes, samples of tissue can be taken, bleeding can be stopped, and some surgical procedures can be done.

Digestive structure and function are often determined by use of endoscopes. Specially trained physicians examine areas such as the esophagus (esophagoscopy), stomach (gastroscopy), large intestine (colonoscopy), or rectum (sigmoidoscopy). The trachea, bronchi, and lungs are examined with the bronchoscope.

Surgery on the abdomen is also done using the laparoscope; joint surgery uses the arthroscope. These procedures are more invasive than the diagnostic procedures, but they are less invasive than traditional incisional surgery.

Biopsy. If a growth or body tissue appears suspicious, a biopsy may be done. A piece of tissue or small

Key Abbreviations and Acronyms for Examinations

CT scan	Computed tomography
ECG/EKG	Electrocardiogram
EDR	Electrodermal response
EEG	Electroencephalogram
EER	Electroencephalographic response
EMG	Electromyogram
GI	Gastrointestinal
ICP	Intracranial pressure
LOC	Level of consciousness
MRI	Magnetic resonance imaging
PERRLA	Pupils equal, round, react to light, accommodation

amount of fluid is obtained and sent to the laboratory, where it is examined microscopically. In this way, cancer and other disorders can be diagnosed. A biopsy specimen may be obtained with an endoscope or needle or by making an incision through the skin. A biopsy specimen of the cervix may be obtained during the pelvic examination.

X-ray, Ultrasound, and Other Examinations. An examination can yield valuable information about the status of the body's internal organs and structures without requiring surgery. These procedures include x-ray and fluoroscopy examinations of all areas of the body, including upper and lower GI series, kidney films, or x-rays of bones to determine fractures and other pathology. Other tests performed for diagnostic purposes are ultrasonography (ultrasound), CT scan, MRI, and EEG to evaluate brain function. Respiratory status may be evaluated by spirometry or pulmonary function tests. Cardiovascular status may be determined by use of tests such as the ECG and the treadmill stress test. These procedures are, for the most part, noninvasive; there are no incisions or injections. In some cases however, dye is injected or a scope is passed into the body through a body orifice. The accompanying box describes precautions needed when dye is used.

Lumbar Puncture. A lumbar puncture, also called a spinal tap, may be done to determine the status of the neurologic system. The lumbar puncture can determine intracranial pressure and the presence of abnormal components such as blood or pus in the spinal fluid, or it can be done to inject drugs or spinal anesthesia. This test is discussed in more detail in Chapter 71.

Nursing Considerations

Preparing the Patient for Diagnostic Procedures

It is important for patients to completely understand what is to be done. Informed consent is required for most procedures. In addition, if patients know what to

Precautions When Tests Are Performed Using Dye

In any procedure in which a dye is used, a skin test is often done first to determine if the patient is sensitive to that drug. Ask if the patient is allergic to shellfish or iodine. The nurse must be alert for signs of anaphylaxis (an exaggerated allergic reaction). Nursing assessment includes noting untoward signs such as:

◆ Restlessness, apprehension, weakness
◆ Perspiration, cold, clammy skin
◆ Sneezing, nose itching
◆ Rash, pruritus (itching)
◆ Difficult breathing, wheezing, choking sensation
◆ Rapid, thready, or irregular pulse
◆ Lowered blood pressure
◆ Incontinence
◆ Seizures
◆ Coma

If you observe any of these symptoms, it is important to notify the team leader or the physician *immediately*. Death can result if the allergy is severe and if it is not treated at once.

expect, they will be less apprehensive and more relaxed during the examination.

Nurses should be mindful of universal precautions to protect themselves, their patients, and the examiners. In areas of high radiation exposure (eg, radiology department), nurses must wear a lead shield to protect vital organs from overexposure to radiation.

Positioning a Patient for Examination or Treatment

Patients are sometimes put in special positions as a part of their treatment or examination; a number of different positions are used for a physical examination, for nursing treatments and tests, and for obtaining specimens. Because you will put patients in some of these positions and will see other positions used, you should know how to assist the patient and adjust the necessary drapes. Important positions are horizontal recumbent, dorsal recumbent, prone, Sims', Fowler's, knee–chest, and dorsal lithotomy. Their descriptions, uses, and illustrations are given in Table 43-2.

Assisting with the Adult Physical Examination

When you assist in a physical examination, do everything you can to make the patient feel comfortable. You should already have told the patient that the examination will occur and explained the reasons for it. Examinations are done in various ways, but the following nursing skill outlines basic steps.

Nursing Skill
Assisting With an Adult Physical Examination

Supplies and Equipment

Hospital gown
Sheet or disposable paper drapes
Bath blanket
Gooseneck lamp or hospital light
Tray with flashlight, gloves, lubricant, and tissues
Extra gloves
Tongue depressors
Ophthalmoscope
Otoscope
Blood pressure apparatus and stethoscope
Percussion hammer
Small speculum
Temperature probe
Tape measure
Scale and height-measuring device
Basin for soiled instruments
Waste container for paper goods
Other equipment as needed
Vaginal speculum (optional)
Slides, blood tubes, and syringes as needed

Procedure

Before the Examination

1. Explain to the patient what is to be done. (*Rationale: The patient who knows what to expect will be more relaxed and cooperative.*)
2. Assist the patient to put on a hospital gown. (*Rationale: The hospital gown allows free movement and makes the patient's body more accessible for examination.*)
3. Offer the bedpan or urinal, or encourage the patient to use the bathroom. (*Rationale: The patient will feel more at ease; the examination could be hindered by a full bladder or colon.*)
4. Wash your hands. Wear gloves if the patient has a draining wound, is bleeding, is vomiting, or has an infection. (*Rationale: prevent spread of infection.*)
5. Assist the patient onto the examining table. Use a sturdy step stool. (*Rationale: Be sure the patient will not fall from the examining table.*)
6. Arrange needed equipment and supplies. Make sure you have everything you need and that everything is operating correctly. (*Rationale: Valuable time is wasted if you have to leave to get something in the middle of the examination.*)
7. Measure the patient's vital signs and height and weight. (*Rationale: This provides baseline data for the physician and saves time.*)

During the Examination

1. Stay with the patient during the examination, if possible. Usually, if a male examiner examines a female patient, or vice versa, the nurse must stay in the room. (*Rationale: This protects the patient, the examiner, and the hospital and offers support and reassurance to the patient.*)

2. Assist the patient to assume the proper position for each part of the examination. *(Rationale: By assisting the patient to get into position, you will speed up the examination.)*

3. Adjust the drapes whenever the patient assumes a new position. *(Rationale: Provide continuing privacy for the patient.)*

4. Assist with specific procedures as needed. For example, hand instruments to the examiner, receive and care for specimens. *(Rationale: Your assistance will speed up the examination.)*

After the Examination

1. Help the patient with the gown.

2. If the patient was examined in bed, draw up the bedclothes, remove the bath blanket, and make the patient comfortable.

3. If the patient was in an examining room, see that he or she is returned safely to the room and is in bed or seated comfortably, as ordered. *(Rationale: The patient may feel weak or tired following the examination.)*

4. Place the call signal within reach.

5. Wash your hands. *(Rationale: Prevent cross-contamination.)*

6. Make sure any special activity orders from the physician are carried out. *(Rationale: Untoward effects may occur if these orders are not followed.)*

7. Change the cover on the examining table and dispose of all wastes. Place all instruments in the proper area for disinfection or sterilization. Replace all equipment. *(Rationale: Prevent the spread of infection and make the room ready for another examination.)*

8. Label and handle all specimens properly.

9. Take specimens to the laboratory promptly. *(Rationale: Delay in processing a specimen can alter the test and can cause false results.)*

10. Document the examination, by whom, and any special procedures performed. *(Rationale: Documentation is vital to ensure communication among members of the healthcare team.)*

Assisting With the Gynecologic Examination

The gynecologic examination is also called a pelvic or vaginal examination. Its purpose is to examine the external genitalia and pelvic organs for signs of irritation, growths, displacement, or other abnormal conditions. Vaginal and cervical smears are taken and evaluated for the presence of cancer or other abnormalities. The Papanicolaou (Pap) test is one of these. Biopsy of the cervix and other areas may also be done.

Some women are nervous about the pelvic examination. The nurse should be matter of fact and calm. Reassure the patient and explain what is being done. An informed patient is more relaxed; relaxation aids the physician and promotes patient comfort. Additional information regarding the gynecologic examination is contained in Chapter 84.

Nursing Skill
Assisting With the Gynecologic Examination

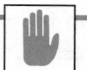

Supplies and Equipment

Hospital gown
Draw sheet
Examination tray
Speculums of various sizes
Lubricant jelly
Applicators and glass slides
Fixatives (or hair spray)
Gloves

Procedure

1. Give the patient a gown and a drawsheet. *(Rationale: Facilitate proper draping.)*

2. Ask the patient to empty her bladder before being examined. *(Rationale: The examiner cannot feel all structures if the patient has a full bladder.)*

3. Wash your hands and don gloves. *(Rationale: Prevent the spread of infection.)*

4. Place the examination tray nearby. Warm and lubricate the speculum. *(Rationale: A lubricated and warm speculum reduces discomfort.)*

5. Assist the patient into the lithotomy position and adjust the drape. *(Rationale: Proper positioning maximizes the examination.)*

6. Hand the lubricated speculum to the gloved examiner when he or she indicates it is needed. *(Rationale: The physician inspects the vagina and cervix after inserting the lubricated speculum. If the examiner wants to take smears of vaginal or cervical secretions, applicators and glass slides are usually used.)*

7. Follow the specific procedure for specimens. Fixative is usually applied to the Pap smear slide.

8. Wipe traces of the lubricating jelly from the perineum when the examination is over.

9. Adjust the patient's position.

10. Provide her with a sanitary pad if necessary.

11. Help her off the examining table if assistance is needed.

12. Dispose of gloves and wash hands. *(Rationale: Prevent cross-contamination.)*

13. Care for the equipment as indicated in your facility.

14. Dispose of all trash and disposable equipment; put items to be sterilized in the proper place. *(Rationale: Prevent the spread of infection.)*

15. Label specimens and send or take them to the laboratory. *(Rationale: The specimens must be taken to the laboratory immediately to avoid inaccuracy.)*

16. Document the procedure. *(Rationale: It is important to record pertinent information to ensure communication among members of the healthcare team.)*

Assisting with an Infant's or Child's Physical Examination

The equipment for an infant's or child's physical examination is the same as for an adult except that some items may be smaller. One of the most important aids in this examination is the child's cooperation. Do your best to get a child to cooperate without restraint.

If the child is too young or too ill to cooperate, you may have to use restraint for parts of the examination. An infant or a small child may be restrained by positioning the child's arms alongside the body and then wrapping the child in a blanket.

The nurse may restrain a child for an anterior chest or abdominal examination in the following way. With the child in a back-lying position on the examining table, hold the child's arms above the head at the wrists with one of your hands, and with your other hand hold the child's feet at the ankles. You will need to stand on the opposite side of the table from the examiner. For examination of the spine and the chest, hold the child upright, with one of your arms around the legs, the other supporting the lower end of the spine, and the head against your shoulder. More detail is given in Chapter 64.

Making Rounds

The nurse may have the opportunity to accompany the physician while he or she is "making rounds" of patients. During rounds, the physician will talk to patients while reviewing the chart to determine recent progress. In teaching hospitals residents and medical students will also be included in rounds, and teaching at the bedside is often done. If you have an opportunity to take part in medical rounds, take advantage of this valuable learning experience. You may also be requested to assist with procedures or to follow up on physician's orders as a part of making rounds.

Nursing Assessment

Nursing assessment is an important nursing responsibility. As you progress through your nursing program and as a graduate nurse, you will have the opportunity to assist or to perform nursing assessments. This may be done informally as a part of your routine daily nursing observation, or it may be done formally to establish a baseline when the patient is admitted to the healthcare facility.

You must continue to upgrade your observational skills throughout your nursing career. The remainder of the information in this chapter is presented as a guideline for you; it is not intended to be a complete course in nursing assessment. A great deal of background information important to nursing assessment is presented throughout this book. For instance, you need to know normal physiology and anatomy to perform an examination. It is important for you to become familiar with related topics before doing an accurate and meaningful nursing assessments.

Although ongoing nursing assessment occurs throughout the patient's hospitalization, a formal nursing assessment is done when the patient is first seen. The nursing history and nursing assessment are often obtained prior to the primary caregiver's examination. The physician uses this information in formulating a medical diagnosis. The nursing assessment also serves as baseline information to assist the healthcare team to evaluate the course of the patient's recovery and to plan ongoing interventions.

The Nursing History

Part of the initial nursing assessment is the nursing history. In most cases, this formal nursing assessment is done by a registered professional nurse. The nursing student or practical/vocational nurse may assist.

The nursing history is important. By obtaining information from the patient and family, you can determine the patient's past and current concerns and health conditions. You learn about the patient's health habits. The admission questionnaire presented elsewhere in the book serves as an outline for the interview. Components of a nursing history are given in Chapters 34 and 50.

The Physical Examination

The physical examination usually takes place after the interview and history. The nurse or examiner explains the purpose of the examination. Important information is gained from the physical examination.

The two major methods of conducting the physical examination are body systems and head-to-toe. The difference is illustrated in the accompanying box. This book is organized by body systems, and the rest of this chapter follows that outline.

Each method is adjusted to the examiner, the purpose of the examination, and the seriousness of the person's condition. Some examiners may prefer to do a certain portion before another. A pregnant woman's examination will concentrate largely on her pregnancy although all systems are relevant to a healthy pregnancy. A person admitted to the emergency department with a heart attack will require other priorities in the examination.

Sequence of Major Methods of Physical Examination

Systems Approach	Adult Head-to-Toe	Infant and Children Head-to-Toe
General survey	General survey	General survey
Integumentary system	Vital signs	Vital signs
Fluid and electrolyte balance	Hair, scalp, cranium, face	Weight
Musculoskeletal system	Eyes and vision	Skin
Head and neck	Ears and hearing	Heart sounds
Extremities	Oral cavity	Lung sounds
Nervous system	Cranial nerves	Head, scalp, cranium
Endocrine system	Thyroid gland	Eyes
Sensory system	Neck veins and nodes	Oral cavity
Cardiovascular system	Upper extremities	Neck
Immune system	Nails	Ears
Respiratory system	Breasts	Musculoskeletal system and reflexes
Digestive system	Precordium	Upper extremities
Reproductive system	Anterior thorax	Chest and back
	Abdomen	Abdomen
	Back	External genitals
	Lower extremities	Lower extremities
	Genitals and pelvis	
	Anus and rectum	

Assessment of the Integumentary System

Information about the internal status of body organs can be learned by observing the skin, hair, and nails. The accompanying box outlines some of the components of this assessment. Skin disorders themselves are discussed in Chapter 68.

Skin Assessment

Usually the skin is the first part of the body you are able to observe. Many dermatologic disorders can be assessed with the naked eye. Sometimes the fluid and electrolyte balance of the body can be assessed through the skin. Several factors are indicators of the condition of various body systems.

Objective Signs. The nurse must be able to describe in detail what the skin disorder looks like, how it feels, its size, its location, whether it is draining, what the drainage looks like, and if other *objective* symptoms are present. A skin lesion can be a problem in itself or it can indicate the existence of an underlying, possibly more serious, condition. Five terms can be used to describe the primary lesions of nearly all skin diseases: macule, papule, vesicle, wheal, and purpura. (See Chapter 68 for definitions of these terms.) Keys to nursing assess-

ment of the skin/integumentary system are presented in the accompanying box.

Subjective Symptoms. In addition to obtaining objective signs, the nurse listens to the patient's subjective complaints. The most common dermatologic symptom is itching, also called *pruritus*. Other subjective symptoms include pain, numbness, or tingling. Ask if the person bruises easily.

The patient may be able to identify the cause of the skin disorder. The patient's medical history is of great importance. The nurse may also observe for an elevated temperature and other symptoms.

Interrelationships Between the Skin and Other Body Systems

Many systemic disorders have skin manifestations. Chapter 68 describes some of these disorders.

The Circulatory System. Local and systemic changes in the circulation are reflected by changes in skin tones of a person. Examples of this interdependence between the skin and the circulatory system are:

◆ Local skin changes can be associated with the stages of pressure areas or skin breakdown.
◆ Skin moisture, temperature, or *diaphoresis* (profuse perspiration) may be indicators of circulatory status.
◆ *Turgor* refers to skin elasticity, which can reflect

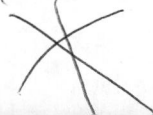

Assessment for these conditions is discussed later in this section of the chapter.

The Nervous System. Examples of interrelationships between the nervous system and the skin are:

- The nervous system can be assessed by checking the skin's sensory receptors.
- Symptoms such as numbness, tingling (*paresthesia*), and pain are abnormal.

The Digestive System. Examples of the interrelationships between the skin and the digestive system are:

- The skin reflects the type and amount of wastes being excreted. For example, the amounts of electrolytes, urea, and bilirubin in the circulation can be reflected in the skin color and condition.
- *Jaundice* (yellow coloration) can occur in digestive disorders. For example, jaundiced skin is an indicator of hepatic (liver) problems.

Hydration Level Assessment

The correct amount of body fluids (*hydration*) must be maintained in all areas of the body. If this balance is upset, the patient can encounter several problems, including overhydration or underhydration (*dehydration*). Symptoms of overhydration and dehydration are listed in the accompanying box. These conditions and related nursing care are discussed in Chapter 69.

Evaluation of Edema. Edematous areas often appear to be puffy and swollen. The presence of edema can be determined by pressing lightly in the edematous area (Fig. 50-1). If a "dent" remains, edema is present. This is called *pitting edema.*

Assessment of Skin Turgor. Fullness and elasticity, which is called skin **turgor**, can indicate a great deal about the hydration status of a patient. Nursing actions in assessing skin turgor are:

- Gently pinch and lift a fold of skin on the forehead, sternum, arm, or back of the hand between your thumb and forefinger, as shown in Figure 50-2.
- Observe how quickly the skin returns to its normal contour. If the skin immediately returns to normal, skin turgor is documented as "good or adequate." If the skin makes a "tent" that remains for 2 seconds or more, this is interpreted as "poor skin turgor." (*Rationale: Poor skin turgor may be an indication of dehydration; this must be documented and reported immediately.*)
- In the elderly person, the skin may normally resume its shape more slowly. (*Rationale: This is

the patient's hydration status. Nursing skills in assessing skin turgor appear later in the chapter.

- Systemic circulatory status can be assessed by observing the patient's overall skin coloring. *Pallor* (paleness) represents a decrease in normal pigmentation. This can indicate severe pain, fear, or a deficiency in red blood cells. An extremity might be pale and very cool to the touch, indicating a block in circulation to that limb. *Cyanosis* (bluish coloring) also indicates poor tissue oxygenation.
- The terms *ruddy* and *erythema* also describe skin tones. Do not confuse these terms. Erythema is a bright red color associated with capillary dilation; this can indicate fever or infection. A ruddy color is a dark red to red-purple color associated with stagnant or poorly oxygenated blood.

The Urinary System. The presence of *edema* or *dehydration* can indicate circulatory or urinary disorders.

Keys to Nursing Assessment
Overhydration and Dehydration

Symptoms of Overhydration

- Obvious swelling, including pitting edema, increase in circumference of wrist or ankle
- Sudden weight gain
- Bounding pulse or arrhythmia
- Elevated blood pressure
- Changes in venous and arterial pressures (hypertension)
- Puffy eyelids
- Fluid intake greater than output; (sometimes) elevated urine specific gravity; (often) lowered specific gravity
- Distended neck veins (with head elevated 45°)
- Weakness, anorexia
- Confusion, slow responses, apathy
- Pulmonary congestion and shortness of breath (dyspnea)
- Orthopnea (must sit up to breathe)
- Sodium retention, causing low sodium in urine
- Abnormal electrolytes, serum creatinine, blood urea nitrogen (BUN), decreased hemoglobin and hematocrit
- Edema (sometimes)—check sacrum when patient is sitting

Symptoms of Dehydration

- Hypotension
- Decrease in venous filling
- Weak, thready, rapid pulse
- Elevated temperature
- Rapid weight loss (overnight)
- Dry skin, pale skin
- Dry mucous membranes or sticky mucous membranes
- Patient complains of thirst
- Poor skin turgor
- Lethargy, disorientation (late stage) and coma
- Sunken eyes
- Intake and output not equal sometimes (output greater)
- Urine output below 50 mL/h
- Increased urine specific gravity
- Increased packed plasma protein level
- Increased BUN level
- Elevated hemoglobin, hematocrit
- Abnormal electrolyte levels

caused by reduced elasticity and may be normal for the person's age.)
- If pits or dents remain where the skin was pinched, this should also be reported and documented. (*Rationale: Pitting indicates edema, retention of fluid in the tissues.)*

Skin Assessment of Persons of Color[1]

You have learned about assessing pallor, cyanosis, jaundice, and many other descriptions of skin. These are based primarily on skin tones of white people. When the person is tanned, has an area where skin tones are darker, or is of another race, assessment directives must change. These people are called persons of color for lack of a better term.

Because it is more difficult to observe some of these signs, other skills must be learned. This section has that purpose in mind. For instance, some lesions may be palpated if they cannot be visualized.

The skin of the African American person often has a reddish undertone; the lips, nailbeds, and mucous membranes are often pink; and the fingernails may have dark lines running through them.

Cyanosis is evidenced by a dusky gray color, sometimes described as ashen. Check especially the mucous membranes of the mouth, lips, cheekbones, and earlobes. Also, look for physical signs that indicate lack of oxygen, such as lowered blood pressure, anxiety, and rapid pulse.

Jaundice may be more evident in the whites of the eyes than in the nailbeds or skin. Laboratory tests also are used to determine liver disorders manifested as jaundice.

Erythema is often indicated by a purple or dark gray skin color. Observe for excess warmth of the skin or enlarged lymph nodes, both of which indicate infection.

Dermatitis can be determined by stretching the skin in the affected area, which enables the rash to stand out; it can then be felt by the nurse. In some rashes, the tip of the earlobe will be redder than usual. Flaking of the skin should also be observed for and reported.

Hypopigmentation and *hyperpigmentation* (less or more skin color than usual) may occur following an injury. An extremely dark-colored nasal crease below the eye may indicate allergy.

The dark-skinned person may have any skin disorder but is less likely to have skin cancer. Dark-skinned persons are more prone to **keloids** (benign tumors that sometimes are formed from scars) than white persons.

Key Concept
Additional lighting may be helpful in assessing the skin in a person of color or with deeply suntanned skin.

[1] Adapted from information in Smeltzer SC, Bare BG. Brunner and Suddarth's Textbook of Medical-Surgical Nursing, Ed 7. Philadelphia, J.B. Lippincott, 1992.

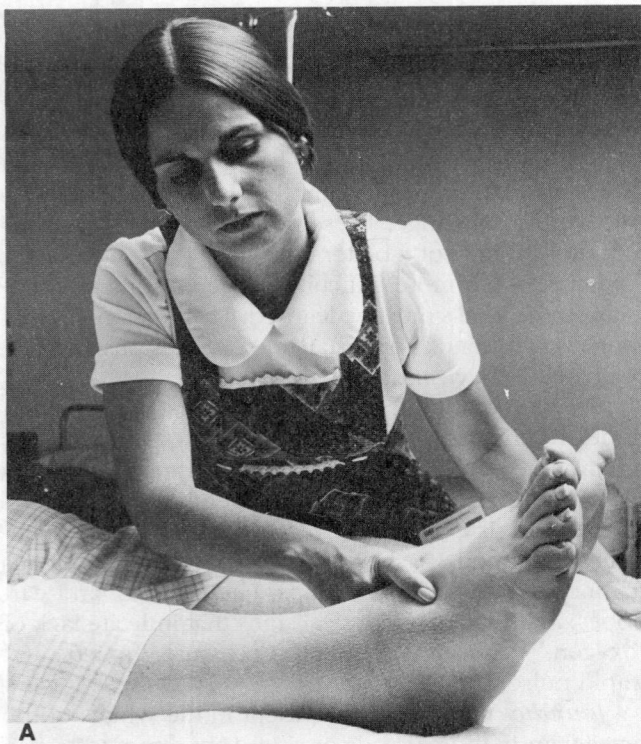 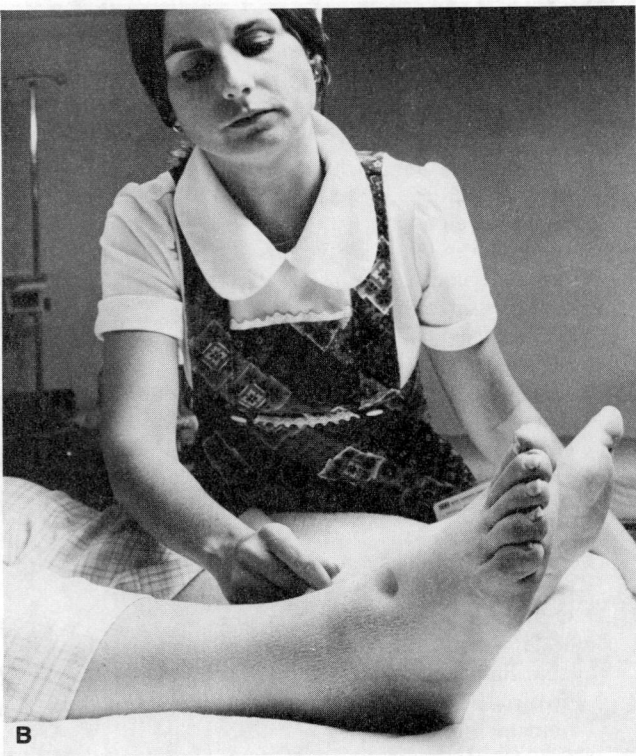

Figure 50-1. (A) The nurse depresses an area near the ankle of the patient where edema is present. **(B)** An indentation remains, indicating edema. This is called pitting edema and indicates excess fluid in body tissue.

Nail Assessment

Observe the condition of the fingernails and toenails. Are the nails dry or split? Are the nails discolored or thickened? Are the nails clean and filed evenly? Are there hangnails present? Is there evidence of cuticle or

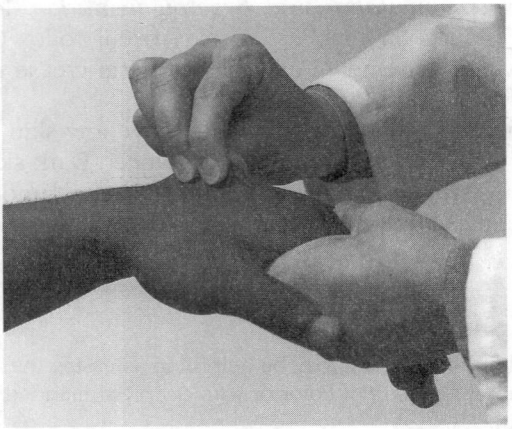

Figure 50-2. Evaluation of skin turgor (fullness) is done by gently pinching up a portion of skin, pulling upward, and releasing. This provides a quick evaluation of the tissue hydration of the body. Normally, the skin will resume its former shape immediately. (Fuller J and Schaller-Ayers J. Health Assessment: A Nursing Approach, 2nd ed. Philadelphia: J.B. Lippincott, 1994.)

nail biting? Are the toenails cut straight across and kept short? Is there evidence of ingrown toenails?

Hair Assessment

It is important to observe the condition of the hair. Is it excessively oily or dry? Are the ends split? Does it appear to be clean and freshly shampooed? Is oil or grooming gel being used? Is there flaking or scaling present? Is there abnormal hair loss (*alopecia*)? Is the hair distribution normal?

Check for evidence of lice (pediculosis). Pubic hair can also harbor lice.

Skin Tests

The primary caretaker may take a skin biopsy to determine a disorder. A procedure called "culture and sensitivity" is done to determine what organism is causing an infection and what drug will combat the causative organism. The physician may apply patch tests to determine allergy. Intradermal testing may be performed to determine if the person has previously been exposed to an allergen. Skills in interpreting various tests are given here.

Skin tests are given to determine immune response to an antigen. They can be used to determine if a person has been exposed to a disease such as tuberculosis or if a person has an allergic reaction to a substance such as a bee sting or a drug. These tests can be administered by the scratch or patch method or intradermally. The procedure for intradermal administration is in Chapter 57, and a special two-step test, which is often done, is discussed in Chapter 77.

To evaluate the results of *any allergy/immune response test:*

♦ Palpate the area around the test site. If you feel swelling or edema, called *induration,* it should be measured and documented.

♦ Use a measuring device, preferably with concentric circles, marked in millimeters. The area is measured and documented in millimeters (mm). If a measuring device is included with the serum, use this. (*Rationale: It is important to obtain an accurate measurement of the induration/erythema area.*) Figure 50-3 illustrates measurement of induration/erythema.

♦ Observe for erythema. Assess the extent of the erythema. Redness without swelling is usually considered insignificant.

To evaluate the results of an *intradermal skin test:*

♦ Record the measurement of induration. (*Rationale: Exact measurements will enable evaluation of the extent and validity of the reaction.*) Findings used in interpretation of induration areas in intradermal skin tests are outlined in the accompanying box. The wheal may also have "pseudopods" (asymmetrical footlike outgrowths). In this case, draw a diagram of the pattern and indicate all measurements.

If there is an area of erythema, measure and document this separately from induration.

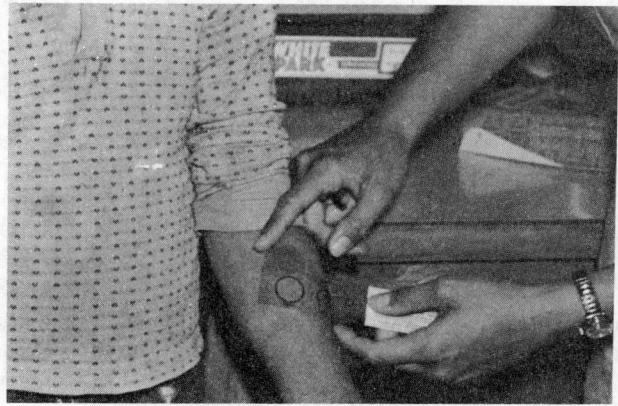

Figure 50-3. A measuring device used in determining size of induration. Courtesy of the American Lung Association

Interpretation of Induration Areas in Skin Tests

Intradermal Skin Test

0–4 mm: *not significant,* "negative"
5–9 mm: *inconclusive,* "doubtful" (another test may be performed)
10 mm +: *significant,* "positive"

Patch or Scratch Skin Test

2 mm or smaller: 0 ("negative")
Induration (including erythema): 3–5 mm: 1+
Induration and erythema 6–10 mm: 2+
Induration and erythema (round) 11–15 mm or more: 3+
Induration and erythema over 15 mm, *with pseudopods:* 4+

To evaluate the results of a *patch or scratch skin test:*

♦ Measure erythema *and* induration as for intradermal test.

The findings are interpreted on a scale from 0 to 4+. The box indicates interpretation of these findings.

In a person with *immunosuppression* a reaction of 4 to 10 mm induration may also be considered significant. In this person, referred to as *anergic,* the test is a "false negative." It *appears to be negative* because the person's body cannot respond to the antigen by producing antibodies. This does not mean that the person has not been exposed to the disease.

If a person is judged to be anergic, a two-step test may be done or controls used. Two-step tests or controls are routine practices in many health facilities. In some cases, antibodies are given. (Chapters 77 and 78 contain more discussion about immunity and immunosuppression.)

An elderly person may also be anergic. In this case, a false negative result is obtained because the immune system has lost the ability to respond to the antigen. Other tests (such as chest x-ray, sputum culture, or two-step test) are necessary to determine if the person is truly negative.

Assessment of the Musculoskeletal System

The examiner assesses the function of the muscles, bones, and joints; looks for full range of motion without pain in all joints; and observes for any lumps or nodules. Both sides of the body should be symmetrical. The person should be able to use any prescribed ambulation aids, such as a cane or walker, safely.

If the person has a cast, splint, or traction in place, special nursing assessments are made. The greatest danger in this case is pressure from the immobilization device. Chapter 70 describes this assessment in detail.

The accompanying box lists many components of the assessment of the musculoskeletal system, the head and neck, and the extremities.

Assessment of the Neurologic System

Components of assessment are outlined in the accompanying box. The most important aspects of the neurologic examination are general observations made during the course of the interview. Much can be determined simply by conversing with the patient. Adapt the assessment to the individual. As areas of abnormalities are identified, further in-depth assessment is warranted.

Keys to Nursing Assessment
The Musculoskeletal System

History

- History of previous injuries
- History of disorders in family members

Objective Assessment

- Range of motion in all joints
- Swelling in joints, abnormal lumps
- Posture and movement (both sides of body should be symmetrical)
- Gait, balance
- Amputations
- Redness, obvious deformities
- Use of ambulation aids or prostheses
- Comparison of laboratory tests with normals
- Reports of x-ray, ultrasound, MRI, or other diagnostic tests

Assessment with Cast, Splint, or Traction in Place

- Color, motion, sensitivity of distal part (signs of pressure)
- Severe pain, pressure, loss of function
- Ability to move fingers and toes
- Hemorrhage, drainage, signs of infection
- Condition of pin site

Subjective Assessment

- Pain, discomfort, muscle cramps
- Difficulty in moving, stiffness, limited range of motion
- Ability to perform activities of daily living

Assessment of the Head and Neck

History

- Regularity of professional dental care
- Daily dental hygiene; brushing, flossing
- History of frequent sore throats

Objective Assessment

- Presence of deviated nasal septum
- Color of mucous membranes, lips, mouth

- Condition of teeth, dental caries, missing teeth, malocclusion
- Use of dentures
- Presence of halitosis
- Bleeding or sore gums, evidence of gum disease, ulcerations
- Presence of lesions, scars, alopecia
- Presence of swollen lymph nodes, node tenderness, shape
- Shape of head, symmetry of face
- Neck problems (swelling, limited movement, pain)
- Distention of jugular veins
- Epistaxis (nosebleeds)

Subjective Assessment

- Complaints of sore throat, frequent runny nose, nasal stuffiness
- Difficulty in swallowing
- Halitosis, foul taste in mouth
- Voice changes
- Headache

Assessment of the Extremities

History

- Previous injuries

General Assessment

- Color, scars on limbs
- Condition of nails
- Venous distention in legs, hands, or arms
- Peripheral pulses in legs and arms
- Difference in temperature from right to left leg or arm
- Ability to move all joints
- Obvious deformities, contractures, amputations
- Use of prosthesis or ambulation aids
- Complaints of pain, discomfort, limited movement

When assessing for neurologic disorders, the reports of the family are particularly important. The patient may not be able to tell you exactly what is happening or the family's perception of the problem may be different from that of the patient. The nursing history includes any information that might be helpful in diagnosis.

Special Considerations in Children
Neurologic Assessment

Usually a child is more comfortable with a parent present. The parent may help you ask the questions or assist in other ways. The parent may also be able to answer some of the questions if the child is unable to do so.

Level of Consciousness and Mental Status

An individual's level of consciousness (LOC) can be determined by using an evaluation tool such as the *Glasgow coma scale*. This tool assesses eye, motor, and verbal response to obtain a numerical score from 3 to 15. A change in the score of 2 points or more is considered significant and should be reported and documented immediately. The tool is explained in Figure 50-4.

The examiner also assesses short- and long-term memory, speech, overall emotional status, judgment, and overall behavior. Is the patient acting appropriately?

Other Neurologic Assessments

Muscle Tone and Strength. When assessing muscle tone and strength, the examiner looks for abnormalities such as **spastic** (rigid) or **flaccid** (limp) extremities. Involuntary movements such as tremors or shaking are noted. Range of motion of all joints is checked. The strength of both arms or both legs is tested simultaneously. (*Rationale: Symmetric examination allows you to detect a difference in strength.*) When assessing hand grasps, for example, the examiner requests the person to squeeze both hands at the same time. To assess leg strength, have the person push both feet against each of the examiner's hands at the same time.

Balance, Coordination, and Protective Reflexes. The examiner can assess balance and coordination by observing whether the patient is able to sit on the edge of the bed or stand without support. A lack of balance and coordination is a safety concern.

If the person is able to stand, the *Romberg test* may be performed. This is done by having the person stand with feet together, arms extended, and eyes closed. If the patient must take a step or hang onto something to maintain balance, the test result is considered *positive*. The examiner monitors the person carefully so that injury does not occur during the test.

Keys to Nursing Assessment
The Nervous System

Nursing History

- History of mental health disorder
- History of chemical abuse; over-the-counter drug use
- Patient history of related disorders such as diabetes mellitus, stroke, human immunodeficiency virus infection, sexually transmitted diseases
- Family history of neurologic disorders, cardiovascular disorders, diabetes mellitus, degenerative disorders
- Recent injury, history of previous head injury
- History of exposure to toxins, poisons, drug overdose, industrial chemicals, animal bites
- Reports of family about patient's behavior and changes in behavior

General Assessment

- Body temperature measurement
- Level of consciousness, eye signs (PERRLA)
- Signs of increasing intracranial pressure
- Speech patterns, ability to move on command or follow instructions
- Overview of selected cranial nerve function
- Protective reflexes
- Muscle tone, strength, balance, coordination, mobility level, posture
- Hearing and vision screening
- Orientation to time and place
- Ability to concentrate
- Behavior, attitudes
- Involuntary movements, mannerisms, tics, tremors
- Comparison of laboratory test results with normal values
- Reports of tests

Subjective Assessment

- Presence of seizures, vertigo, tremors, tics, tingling, paralysis, weakness, numbness
- Headaches
- Dizziness, vertigo, syncope (fainting)
- Confusion, alertness
- Long- and short-term memory
- Excessive fatigue
- Abnormal or bizarre behaviors, appropriateness of speech

Gait may be observed for strength and balance. Findings should be the same on both sides of the body.

The examiner observes the presence or absence of protective reflexes. These include cough, gag, and blink. These protective reflexes are necessary to prevent injury. Absent cough and gag reflexes may result in choking and respiratory complications caused by aspiration of mucus or food.

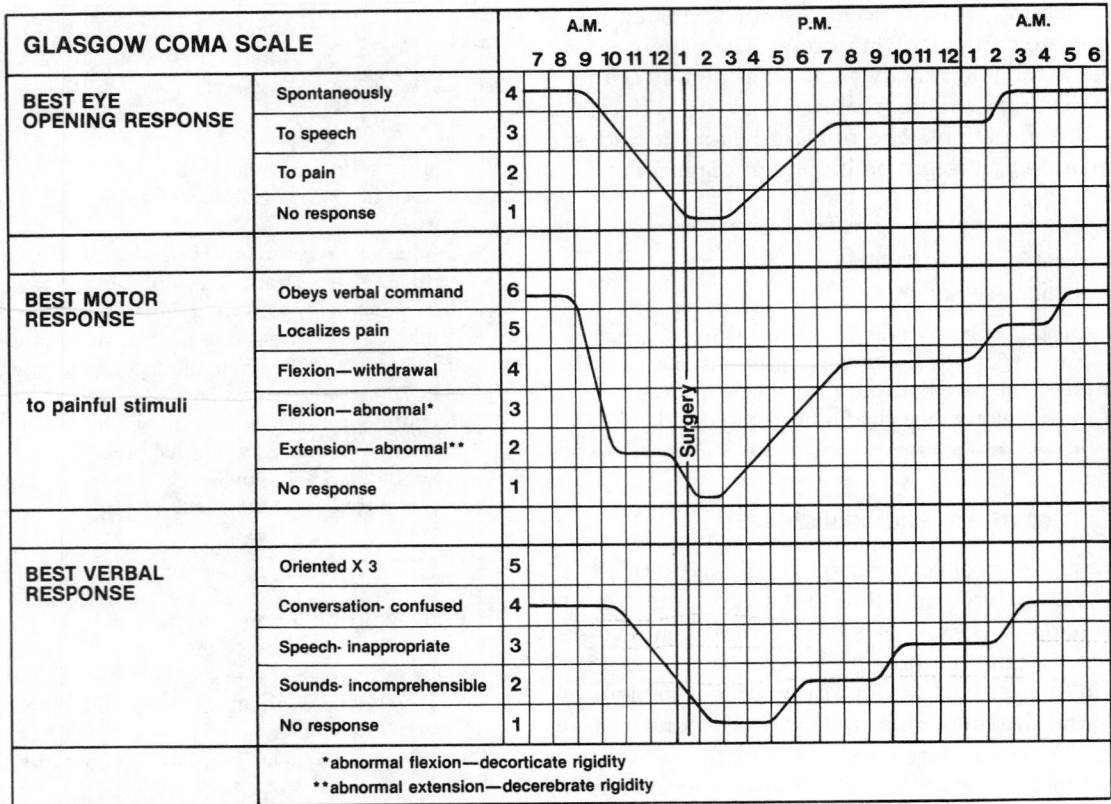

GLASGOW COMA SCALE			A.M. 7 8 9 10 11 12	P.M. 1 2 3 4 5 6 7 8 9 10 11 12	A.M. 1 2 3 4 5 6
BEST EYE OPENING RESPONSE	Spontaneously	4			
	To speech	3			
	To pain	2			
	No response	1			
BEST MOTOR RESPONSE	Obeys verbal command	6			
	Localizes pain	5			
	Flexion—withdrawal	4			
to painful stimuli	Flexion—abnormal*	3		Surgery	
	Extension—abnormal**	2			
	No response	1			
BEST VERBAL RESPONSE	Oriented X 3	5			
	Conversation- confused	4			
	Speech- inappropriate	3			
	Sounds- incomprehensible	2			
	No response	1			
	*abnormal flexion—decorticate rigidity **abnormal extension—decerebrate rigidity				

Figure 50-4. Glasgow coma scale for determining level of consciousness. How to score responses:

Scoring of eye opening: **4** = If the patient opens the eyes spontaneously when the nurse approaches; **3** = If the patient opens the eyes in response to speech (spoken or shouted); **2** = If the patient opens the eyes only in response to painful stimuli such as digital squeezing around nailbeds of fingers; **1** = If the patient does not open the eyes in response to painful stimuli.

Scoring of best motor response: **6** = If the patient can obey a simple command, such as, "Lift your left hand off the bed"; **5** = If the patient moves a limb to locate the painful stimuli applied to the head or trunk and attempts to remove the source; **4** = if the patient attempts to withdraw from the source of pain; **3** = If the patient flexes only the arms at the elbows and wrist in response to painful stimuli to the nailbeds (**decorticate rigidity**); **2** = if the patient extends the arms (straightens the elbows) in response to painful stimuli (**decerebrate rigidity**); **1** = if the patient has no motor response to pain on any limb.

Scoring of best verbal response: **5** = If the patient is oriented to time, place, and person; **4** = if the patient is able to converse, although not oriented to time, place, or person (eg, "Where am I?"); **3** = if the patient speaks only in words or phrases that make little or no sense (eg, "B-H, H-K."); **2** = if the patient responds with incomprehensible sounds such as groans; **1** = if the patient does not respond verbally at all.

Special Considerations in Aging
Neurologic Assessment

◆ If older people are hearing impaired, be sure they are wearing a hearing aid or can read your lips. Make sure they understand the questions or commands rather than assuming they are confused.

◆ Reassure older persons that you will not let them fall during the assessment. Older people may have a history of falling, may be unsteady on their feet, or may be fearful of falling.

Eye Signs. Cranial nerves III (oculomotor), IV (trochlear), and VI (abducens) are assessed with the pupil check (Fig. 50-5). Abnormal eye signs may also indicate increased intracranial pressure.

Eye signs are assessed as follows:

◆ The pupils of the eyes should be equal in size and round in appearance.

◆ Pupil reaction is checked by shining a small flashlight quickly into the eye. The pupil should contract immediately when light hits it and should quickly dilate when the light is removed. If the pu-

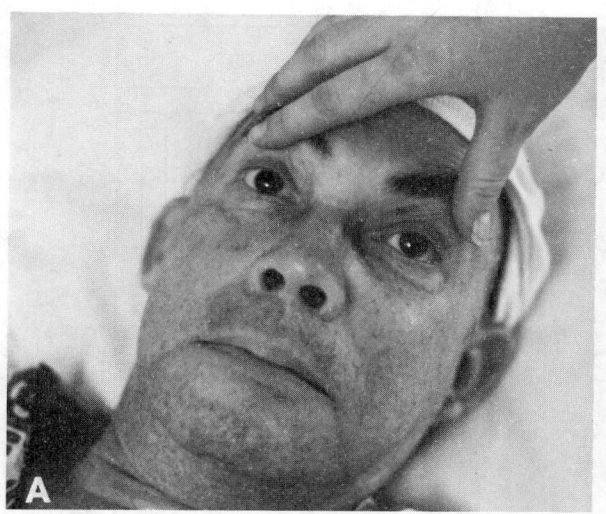
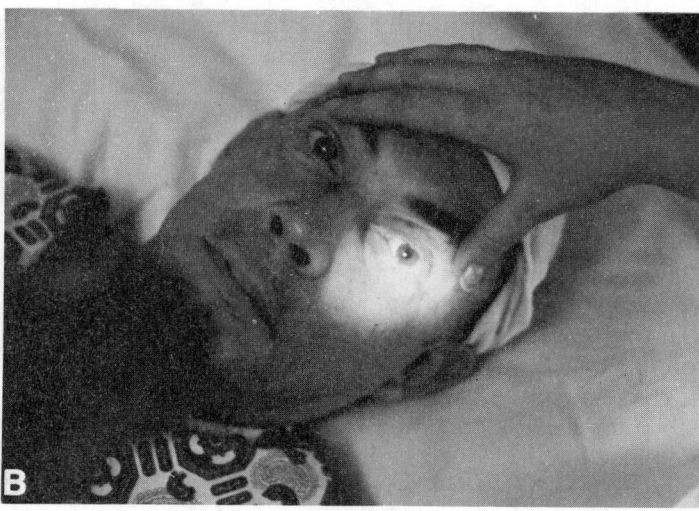

Figure 50-5. Assessment of eye signs is an important activity in nursing assessment and neurologic nursing. Pupils should be equal in size (PE), at about 2 to 6 cm. They should be round (R). The pupil of each eye should contract immediately when a light is shined directly into it—react to light (RL). When an object is held close and then farther away, the pupils should change size to indicate proper accommodation (A). The two eyes should move in a coordinated fashion when following a moving object (+C). These signs, when normal, can be abbreviated in the chart as PERRLA +C. **(A)** Illustration of the visual examination of the eyes; **(B)** illustration of checking the accommodation of the pupils.

pil changes size rapidly, this is considered "brisk." Slow pupil change is described as "sluggish."

◆ Accommodation of the eye is tested by having the patient look at a distant object and then at a near object (about 6 inches away). The size of the pupil should change if the eye is accommodating correctly.

◆ Documentation of the normal pupil check is called PERRLA and follows:
  ◆ PE pupils equal
  ◆ R round
  ◆ RL react to light
  ◆ A accommodation OK

◆ To check coordination between the eyes, have the patient watch your moving finger. The eyes should move together. Normal coordination can be added to the above documentation as follows:
  ◆ +C eyes coordinate with each other

Sensory Assessment. Assessment of pain, temperature, touch, and pressure are important aspects of the neurologic examination. All are senses that protect the human body from injury. If any of these are absent, the examiner must take steps to provide protection for the person. Absence of the sense of pressure, for example, places an individual at risk for developing pressure areas and skin breakdown. Absence of the sensation of temperature places an individual at risk for burns or frostbite.

Much of this assessment can be determined during the course of basic care. Observing the patient during a painful procedure or noticing the patient frequently change position in bed or wheelchair provides the nurse with information regarding pain and pressure sensation.

Cranial Nerve Function. The neurologist will perform the in-depth examination of cranial nerve function; however, the nurse can assist by monitoring certain aspects of the cranial nerves.

As described in the section on assessment of eye signs, the gross function of cranial nerves III, IV, and VI can be evaluated in that manner. In addition, cranial nerves V (trigeminal), VII (facial), XI (accessory), and XII (hypoglossal) are assessed by the following simple actions. Have the patient clench the teeth (cranial nerve V), stick out the tongue (XII), shrug the shoulders (XI), and smile and raise the eyebrows (VII). Cranial nerve I (olfactory) is assessed by having the patient identify familiar odors. Cranial nerve II (optic) is functioning if the patient can see. These simple checks, combined with the pupil checks, offer a quick screening of 9 of the 12 cranial nerves. (The functions of cranial nerves VIII—vestibulocochlear, IX—glossopharyngeal, and X—vagus are beyond the scope of this book.)

Any deviation from normal in any of the cranial nerves or in eye signs should be documented and brought to the attention of the physician for further evaluation. Many hospitals have a neurology documentation form on which eye signs, intracranial pressure (ICP), vital signs, level of consciousness (the Glasgow coma scale), extremity control and strength, and other pertinent data are all recorded for easy access.

Assessment of the Endocrine System

The endocrine system manufactures and distributes hormones throughout the body. These hormones regulate most of the body's processes and activities. Therefore, a disorder in the endocrine system can produce signs and symptoms in any organ or system of the body. Laboratory tests are an integral factor in the physician's identification of endocrine disorders. The accompanying box lists some of the components of the nursing assessment of endocrine function.

Assessment of the Sensory System

The sensory system provides information about the world around us and about the status of the internal body. The accompanying box outlines sensory assessment. The nurse may be involved in vision or hearing screening. If a disorder is suspected on this gross evaluation, the person is referred to a physician for follow-up. To a lesser degree, other senses can be assessed by the nurse. Assessment of special senses and protective reflexes was described briefly in the discussion of neurologic assessment.

Screening of Vision

Screening for Visual Acuity. The nurse may be asked to do initial visual assessment or screening in the school or physician's office. A Snellen eye chart may be used in assessment. This chart consists of letters of the alphabet, numbers, or the letter E placed in various positions, such as upside down or backward. For small children, a chart with pictures of familiar objects such as houses or trees may be used. The figures or letters on the Snellen chart are of different sizes and are placed in rows.

The line at which the patient can identify more than half of the figures correctly is recorded as the line of *visual acuity.* Visual acuity is expressed as a fraction and is based on a standard of normal vision. When a person stands 20 feet away from the chart, the line marked 20 should be able to be read. This means the person has 20/20 vision, which is considered normal. If the person can see at 20 feet only what should be seen at 100 feet, the vision is described as 20/100, and the person most likely is nearsighted, a condition called *myopia.* If the person can see at 20 feet what should be seen at 15 feet, the vision is 20/15 and the person is

most likely farsighted, a condition called *hyperopia.* The larger the denominator in the reading, the poorer the vision.

A person with a best corrected reading of 20/200 or worse in each eye is considered *legally blind.* This term does not mean the person is unable to see anything but, rather, may detect movement or see light and darkness.

If the person is unable to see the chart, the examiner's fingers are held up for counting. The distance at which a correct answer is given should be noted; for example, "counting fingers at 4 feet." With even less vision, the ability to see should be noted by the examiner's waving hand in front of the person's eyes. This would be noted as "detects movement at __ feet." When the person has very poor visual acuity, a bright light may be shone into the eye. A notation is made if the light is seen, "light perception."

Screening for Color Blindness. The *Ishihara plates* may be used for assessing color recognition. Instructions for use accompany the plates. Color blindness is an hereditary defect of the cones in the retina. It most often affects males and rarely affects African Americans. Most often, in color blindness, the person is unable to distinguish red and green hues or, less commonly, yellow and blue. There is no cure for color blindness, but the person should be made aware of limitations.

Visual Fields Assessment. Visual field assessment is done to determine central and peripheral vision loss.

Keys to Nursing Assessment
The Sensory System

Nursing History

◆ Last eye examination; last ear examination, hearing test
◆ History of glaucoma, cataracts, circulatory disorders, stroke
◆ History of allergies
◆ Previous eye or ear surgery
◆ History of acute or chronic infections, other disorders, trauma
◆ History of environmental exposure to chemicals, noise; use of protective eyewear or hearing protection
◆ Medication use; use of recreational drugs

Vision Screening

◆ Evidence of disorders, lesions, ptosis, discharge, redness, foreign objects, trauma
◆ Pupillary reaction to light; screening with ophthalmoscope
◆ Visual difficulties on routine screening (gross visual acuity), vision loss
◆ Screening for color blindness
◆ Screening for visual field deficits
◆ Assessment of extraocular muscles
◆ Use of glasses, contacts, eye prosthesis
◆ Assessment of related cranial nerve function

Hearing Screening

◆ Discharge, redness, masses, foreign objects, trauma
◆ Excessive ear wax
◆ Hearing difficulties on routine screening
◆ Use of hearing aid, communication ability
◆ Disorders of balance, vertigo
◆ Assessment of related cranial nerve function

Subjective Assessment

◆ Complaints of visual difficulties, photophobia (intolerance to light), eye pain
◆ Symptoms such as "flashers" or "floaters"
◆ Difficulty in hearing, frequent ear infections, drainage, tinnitus (ringing in the ears), vertigo, dizziness
◆ Use of eye or ear medications
◆ Ability to feel sensations in various parts of the body
◆ Ability to taste
◆ Ability to smell
◆ Neurologic status, level of consciousness

Central vision loss may be due to such problems as optic neuritis, inflammation of the optic nerve, central nervous system tumors, or age-related macular degeneration in the retina of the eye. Peripheral vision is the ability to see objects in the outer limits of the visual fields. Loss of peripheral vision suggests the possibility

of advanced glaucoma or hemianopsia (vision only in half of the visual field) due to stroke or tumor.

Peripheral vision can be estimated with the "confrontation" method, using finger counting or a light. The examiner and patient sit face to face and the patient covers one eye. During the test, the patient is asked to focus on an object straight ahead. The examiner brings an object from outside the patient's view into the expected field of vision. The object is brought into the field from each of four quadrants:

◆ Superior (from above the head)
◆ Inferior (from below the chin)
◆ Nasal (from the side of the occluded eye across the nose)
◆ Temporal (from the outside in)

The patient is instructed to indicate when the object is first seen. This information is carefully documented. The physician will follow up with further testing.

Extraocular Muscle Assessment. This examination assesses the functioning of the external muscles of the eyeball (extraocular). A complaint such as *diplopia* (double vision) may indicate a muscle disorder. Gross assessment of the extraocular muscles is done by asking the patient to follow the examiner's finger or a light source with both eyes simultaneously. The examiner traces a large H in the air. The eyes should have full and parallel range of motion (both eyes moving together) in all directions.

Screening for Hearing

The nurse often does a preliminary hearing screening of the patient. If any deficit is noted, the patient is followed up by the physician. It is important to determine the cause of any hearing loss because hearing loss may point to a more serious problem (such as a brain tumor).

The assessment of the patient with a hearing deficit begins with the history. Included in the assessment should be questions about:

◆ Recent and previous ear infections, history of ear tube placement, history of punctured eardrum
◆ Any medication use, particularly medications damaging to hearing (look up individual medications)
◆ Childhood illnesses
◆ Family health history of hearing disorders, hereditary hearing deficits
◆ Prolonged noise exposure
◆ Symptoms of eighth cranial nerve (auditory nerve) disorders (such as unilateral hearing loss—on one side only, sudden hearing loss, or hearing loss accompanied by vertigo, tinnitus, or ear fullness)

Tinnitus is a ringing, buzzing, or other sound heard in the ear. It is not caused by any identifiable stimulus but is found in several ear disorders, infection of the eustachian tube, trauma, drug toxicity, or tumors.

Visual Assessment. During the physical examination, the external ear is inspected for its shape, size, and lesions. The ear is palpated for pain and edema. Any redness, discharge, or foreign body is noted. The ear canal and tympanic membrane (ear drum) are examined with the otoscope (Fig. 50-6).

The **otoscope** is a lighted, bell-shaped instrument used in examining the external auditory meatus, the eardrum, and the middle ear through the translucent eardrum (tympanic membrane). The otoscope allows visualization of the area from which cerumen (wax) or a foreign object must be removed. The examiner can also learn much about the condition of the middle ear by looking at the tympanic membrane.

For hygienic purposes, the otoscope tip must be sterilized or discarded after each use. If a patient has an infected ear, the tip is changed before the other ear is examined.

Hearing Tests: Audiometry

Hearing tests indicate how well a person can hear and what type of hearing loss exists. Hearing loss is measured in *decibels* (db). A person is considered hard of hearing if the loss is from 35 to 65 db, and legally deaf if the loss is above 65 db. The legally hearing-impaired person does not necessarily live in a world of silence. Usually some sounds can be heard.

Gross Assessment of Hearing Acuity. A simple test involves measuring the distance at which a person can hear a watch tick or a pin drop.

Pure-Tone Audiometry. The audiometry test is accurate, reliable, and part of most school or industry health programs. Certain frequencies are important in everyday speech; this is known as the *speech range*. The audiometer makes it possible to test several children simultaneously; those who seem to have defective hearing on the initial screening test can then be tested again individually. A child who has a hearing loss should be referred to an otologist or other physician for evaluation.

Reflex Audiometry. Reflex audiometry is useful with very young children. A sound is presented; the child reacts by a reflex eye blink if he or she hears the sound.

Tuning Fork Tests. Several tests use a tuning fork to measure the degree and type of hearing loss. When air conduction hearing is tested, the tuning fork is held close to the ear meatus (opening). When bone conduction is tested, the tuning fork is touched to a bone of the skull.

In the *Weber test*, the tuning fork is placed on the midline of the scalp or on the forehead. The patient is asked to describe the tone in each ear. If the hearing is normal (or if the hearing loss is equal on both sides), the patient will hear the vibrations equally in both ears. If there is a conduction hearing loss, the vibration will be heard in the poorer (affected) ear. If the loss is sensorineural, the vibration will be heard only in the better (unaffected) ear.

In the *Rinne test*, air and bone conduction are compared. Normally, air conduction (sound transmission) lasts twice as long as bone conduction. If the patient hears better when the tuning fork touches the bone, a conductive hearing loss exists. If the person hears better when the tuning fork is held outside the auditory meatus, either a sensorineural loss or normal hearing is indicated.

Tympanometry (Acoustic Impedance Audiometry). This procedure can determine hearing acuity without the cooperation of the patient. The instruments are sealed in the external auditory canal. This procedure is used to determine fluid in the middle ear in children and to determine what type of lesion is causing a conductive hearing loss.

Electrophysiologic Audiometry. Because this type of testing does not require the cooperation of the subject,

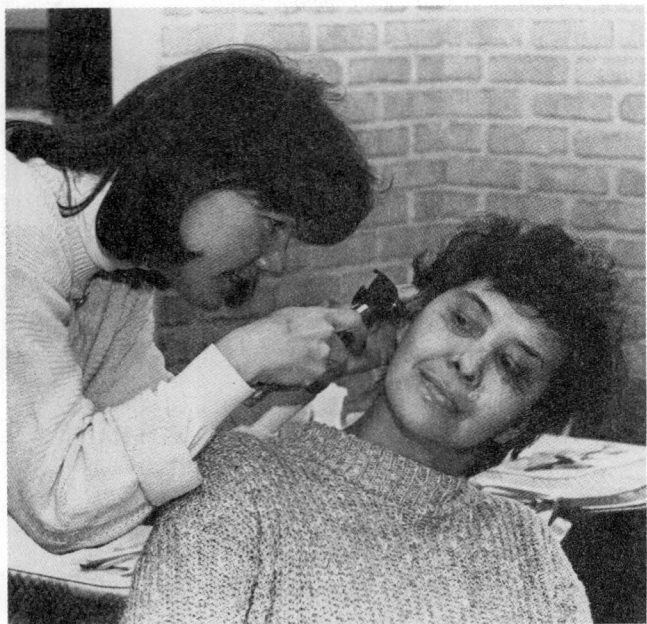

Figure 50-6. The nurse uses an otoscope to examine the ear of a patient. The eardrum and other structures of the outer ear can be visualized. (Photo courtesy of MCOSS Inc., Red Bank, NJ)

it is useful in testing small children. Two chief types of response are checked to see if the child hears the sound presented: the electrodermal reflex (EDR), which measures perspiration, and the electroencephalographic response (EER), which measures brain wave changes in response to sound. A computer is often used to decode and quantify the EER test results; this response is known as *evoked response audiometry*. It will detect abnormalities in the nerve pathways between the eighth cranial nerve and the brain stem.

Follow-up Audiometry. If some type of hearing loss is indicated on initial screening, an audiometry test by a specialist is conducted to determine the magnitude of the loss. Air conduction defects are measured by earphone, while bone conduction defects are measured by placing an oscillator on the mastoid process. If the results of the tests indicate that air and bone conduction losses are about equal, but the ratio of air conduction to bone conduction time is still about 2:1, a sensorineural loss is indicated.

Assessment of the Cardiovascular System

A complete cardiovascular assessment should begin on admission of the patient to the healthcare facility. The assessment includes both history and physical examination. The nursing assessment is concerned mainly with those issues that may interfere with the patient's ability to carry out activities of daily living (ADLs). The patient's weight and height are compared to determine obesity. Blood pressure and pulse are measured. The accompanying box lists other components of the cardiovascular nursing assessment.

The nurse should ask about the patient's health habits. Risk factors such as smoking and levels of exercise, rest, and nutrition are included in the questions. (Assessment for specific heart and blood vessel disorders is contained in Chapter 74.)

Inspection, palpation, and auscultation are used in the physical examination of the cardiovascular system. Certain symptoms, such as shortness of breath, may be observed while taking the patient's vital signs. Difficult breathing, edema, cyanosis, pain, fatigue, and leg ulcers are other possible indications of heart or blood vessel disorders.

Listening to Heart Sounds. The nurse listens to the patient's heart with a stethoscope. The nurse should be able to recognize deviations from normal. The normal heart sounds are heard as the valves open and close to let blood circulate. Signs of deviations from normal include:

Keys to Nursing Assessment
The Cardiovascular System

Nursing History

- Date of last ECG
- Previous transfusions of blood or blood products
- History of heart or blood vessel disorders
- History of blood dyscrasias
- History of related disorders (ie, hypertension, phlebitis, varicose veins, diabetes mellitus, atherosclerosis, kidney disorders)
- Smoking history (patient and family)
- Exercise level, nutritional status, stress level
- Medications taken, including aspirin (mild anticoagulant), blood pressure pills, over-the-counter medications

Objective Assessment

- Blood pressure measurement
- Pulse measurement: rate, volume, and regularity
- Measurement of peripheral pulses
- Blood return when skin pressed lightly (should be immediate); other circulation tests
- Auscultation of heart sounds
- Respiratory difficulties
- Presence of related disorders (leg ulcers, edema, cyanosis, varicose veins, evidence of hypovolemic shock, clubbed fingers)
- Comparison of laboratory test results with normal values
- Reports of diagnostic tests

Subjective Assessment

- Heart or chest pain/discomfort, palpitations, arrhythmias
- Symptoms such as dyspnea, shortness of breath, orthopnea
- General fatigue
- Vascular discomforts
- Easy bruising, petechiae, inability to stop bleeding, difficulty in healing wounds, frequent infections
- Leg pain or cramps, cold extremities, differences in temperature of right versus left leg/foot or hand, changes in skin appearance

---

- *Click or snap*: may be a symptom of a valvular disorder
- *Murmur*: may be caused by valvular damage
- *Friction rub*: pericardial surfaces (sounds like thumb and finger being rubbed together in front of the ear), may signal pericarditis, an inflammation of heart muscle
- *Cardiac tamponade*: muffled or faint heart sounds. Cardiac tamponade is the medical term for abnormal compression of the heart by excess fluid or blood in the pericardial sac.

If the nurse has any questions about heart sounds, this must be reported to the primary caretaker and carefully documented.

Assessment of the Immune System

Much of the assessment of the immune system involves obtaining an accurate nursing history and teaching the patient.

The examiner asks questions about risk factors for sexually transmitted diseases or potential immune disorders such as infection with the human immunodeficiency virus. Allergies also are assessed as part of the immune system. The accompanying box lists some of the components of nursing assessment of the immune system.

Assessment of the Respiratory System

A complete history is essential in assessing respiratory function and oxygen needs. The accompanying box lists components of nursing assessment of the respiratory system.

A penlight is used for visual inspection. With the patient sitting, look to see if the septum is greatly deviated and if the nose if symmetric. The nurse gently pushes up slightly on the tip of the nose and the nasal mucosa is inspected with the light for redness, bleeding, discharge, and any masses. A lighted *nasal speculum* may

---

Keys to Nursing Assessment
The Immune System

Nursing History

♦ History of high-risk sexual behavior
♦ Currency of immunizations and boosters
♦ History of drug abuse, especially IV
♦ History of "allergy shots", known allergies
♦ Recent injuries
♦ History of cancer, immune disorders, blood dyscrasias, allergies in family

General Assessment

♦ Frequent infections or illnesses
♦ Slow wound healing
♦ Dyspnea
♦ Joint pain, skin rash
♦ Visual disturbances
♦ Comparison of laboratory test results with normal values
♦ Results of physical examinations, skin tests, x-rays, or other diagnostic tests

---

Keys to Nursing Assessment
The Respiratory System

Nursing History

♦ History of asthma, allergies, orthopnea, emphysema, pneumonia, frequent upper respiratory infections
♦ History of chest trauma, previous open-chest surgery
♦ Previous skin tests done and results, any chest x-rays
♦ Regular use of supplemental oxygen, medications
♦ Smoking history (including family members)

Objective Assessment

♦ Visual observation of nose (symmetrical, presence of lesions), nasal mucosa (color, swelling, drainage, bleeding), septum (deviated or not)
♦ Visual observation of throat (redness, drainage, swelling); swollen neck glands
♦ Respiratory rate and character, observation of breathing patterns
♦ Chest symmetry, obvious deformity (such as barrel chest)
♦ Observation of sputum (amount—small, medium, large; consistency—thin, thick, tenacious, stringy; color—clear, describe other colors; odor—odorless, foul smelling—describe)
♦ Abnormal breathing movements or evidence of dyspnea, wheezing, bradypnea, tachypnea, hyperpnea, Cheyne-Stokes or Kussmaul's breathing, hyperventilation, use of accessory muscles, sternal retraction
♦ Signs/symptoms of hypoxia, cyanosis, air hunger, other symptoms
♦ Other signs/symptoms (hemoptysis, cough, etc)
♦ Lung/breathing sounds (normal, abnormal—crackles, rhonchi, wheeze)
♦ Oxygenation level, as measured by pulse oximeter or blood gas analysis
♦ Pulmonary function tests
♦ Ability to correctly use breathing aids such as inhaler, supplemental oxygen, incentive spirometer
♦ Comparison of laboratory test results with normal values
♦ Assessment of intradermal/skin tests for respiratory disorders
♦ Reports of diagnostic tests

Subjective Assessment

♦ Difficulty in breathing (dyspnea, orthopnea, shortness of breath)
♦ Nasal discharge, frequent nosebleeds, frequent colds
♦ Cough, hemoptysis (blood in sputum)
♦ "Sinus" headaches
♦ Chest pain, wheezing

be used for examination of the inner portion of the nares (nostrils).

Assessment of Cough

One of the most common respiratory symptoms is the cough. A cough is the contraction of muscles in the pharynx, as a result of irritation. The nurse assesses the cough for the following:

◆ Dry, loose, productive (producing material from the lungs), whooping or other unusual sound
◆ Frequency (occasional, frequent, prolonged spasms)
◆ Effect on the patient
◆ Presence of cyanosis during coughing (indicates obstruction of the air passages)

Assessment of Sputum

Sputum is material other than saliva that is expectorated from the mouth. It may be coughed up from the bronchi of the lungs or it may be a discharge caused by infection of the nasal-throat cavity. Discharge from infected sinuses may drain into the throat from the back of the nose.

The amount of sputum expectorated varies and should be documented as small, medium, or large. The amount can be estimated more accurately by filling an identical container with water to the same level as the sputum and then measuring the water.

Characteristics of sputum should be assessed. The *consistency* may be thin, watery, thick, stringy, **purulent** (containing pus) or **tenacious** (very sticky). The *color* may be clear, white, yellow, green, gray, black, or red. **Hemoptysis** refers to blood-tinged or bloody sputum. True hemoptysis is bright red and frothy, with air bubbles, indicating bleeding in the respiratory tract. (Conditions indicated by abnormal sputum are described in Chapter 79.) Normal sputum has no odor. If an odor is present, it must be described.

Assessment of Chest Movements

Both sides of the chest should move symmetrically when the patient breathes. If one side of the chest moves and the other does not, malfunction of one lung should be suspected.

Other abnormal breathing movements include abdominal breathing where only the abdomen moves; the chest does not. A person breathing in this manner usually is unaware of it. In infants, abdominal breathing indicates respiratory distress, whereas in adults this is rarely the case. If the sternum (breast bone) is drawn in on inspiration (*sternal retraction*), it is sign of respiratory distress, particularly in infants. Other signs of respiratory distress include distention of the veins of the neck, cyanosis, panic, and air hunger. For a discussion of these and other symptoms of *hypoxia* (lack of

oxygen) in the child, see Chapter 64; for adults, see Chapter 79.

Assessment of Breath Sounds

By listening to the sounds of breathing with a stethoscope, the nurse skilled in this assessment can determine whether they are normal. Normal breathing is not readily audible, whereas abnormal breathing sounds can be heard. Listen to each area of each lung, having the patient breathe deeply through the mouth. If abnormal sounds are heard, document the exact location.

Crackles and Rales. Crackles, also called rales (pronounced "rahls"), are a nonmusical sound usually heard on inspiration. They are categorized as coarse or fine. Crackles may or may not be cleared by coughing. *Coarse crackles* have a moist sound (gurgling); they sound like Velcro being pulled apart. They may also be called "moist rales." *Fine crackles* produce a sound similar to that heard when rubbing hair on your skin in front of the ear. The presence of crackles usually indicates congestion, caused by the presence of fluid or pus in the lung.

Rhonchi. Rhonchi can be heard on both inspiration and expiration but are more likely to be heard on expiration. Rhonchi consist of low-pitched, dry, rattling sounds in the throat or bronchus. Rhonchi are usually cleared by coughing.

Wheezes. Wheezing is a high-pitched musical whistling or squeaking sound. Wheezing usually indicates obstruction or closure of the bronchi and is often caused by conditions such as bronchial asthma or chronic obstructive pulmonary disease (COPD). Wheezing that accompanies a chest cold may be cleared by coughing. Asthmatic wheezing is usually not cleared by coughing.

Friction Rub. A friction rub is a grating sound caused by inflammation of the pleural surfaces. A friction rub sounds like the sound made when you rub your thumb and forefinger together next to your ear. The friction rub does not change with coughing. (It is important to differentiate between a cardiac [heart] friction rub and a pulmonary [lung] friction rub. They sound the same. The differentiation is made by the location in which each is heard.)

Assessment of the Digestive System

The nursing history is important in establishing the possibility of digestive disorders. What the patient tells you about bowel and nutritional habits is important information for the physician. One of the most significant signs of a digestive disorder is a *change in bowel habits*.

The nurse can also perform tests to determine occult blood in the stool and can auscultate to determine the presence or absence of bowel sounds. Components of the gastrointestinal nursing assessment are listed in the accompanying box.

Nursing Assessment of the Urinary System

The examiner asks about voiding habits or difficulties. This subjective information is vital in formulating both nursing and medical diagnoses. Significant symptoms include:

◆ Any change in voiding habits
◆ Polyuria (voiding excessive amounts of urine)
◆ Nocturia (excessive voiding at night)
◆ Dysuria (difficult or painful voiding)
◆ Frequency (excessively frequent voiding)
◆ Urgency (inability to wait to void)
◆ Hesitancy (inability to start the stream of urine)
◆ Urinary incontinence (loss of sphincter control), dribbling (drops of urine between voidings), enuresis (bed-wetting)
◆ Abnormal contents in urine—hematuria (blood), pyuria (pus), or malodorous (foul-smelling) urine

The examiner asks about frequency and severity of symptoms, as well as how long they have continued. Certain disorders in other body systems are significant when assessing urinary function. These and other elements of the nursing history, as well as other components of the urinary nursing assessment, are contained in the accompanying box.

Although there are many different types of urologic diseases and conditions, most patients with these disorders share many of the same symptoms: edema, dry and itchy skin, headache, nausea and vomiting, infection, inability to wait to void, frequent urination, pain and burning on voiding, incontinence, and irritability.

Physical Assessment

In addition to routine vital signs, inspection of the external urinary meatus is done. The examiner can detect external skin lesions, redness, or signs of irritation. In male patients, misalignment of the urethral meatus can be determined.

An *inguinal hernia* is the herniation of abdominal contents into the inguinal canal. This type of hernia accounts for about 75% of all hernias. Both men and women are checked for this condition, although it is much more common in men. Ask the patient to bear down or cough and palpate the inguinal area (groin) for bulging.

Keys to Nursing Assessment
The Digestive System

Nursing History

◆ Nutritional history, cultural dietary practices, appetite, changes in dietary patterns, sudden food intolerance
◆ Tobacco use, form used
◆ Alcohol use
◆ Recent weight gain or loss (unexplained)
◆ Patterns of bowel elimination (frequency, time of day, amount, size, character, consistency, shape, color, odor, floating)
◆ History of change in bowel elimination patterns
◆ Medications used (laxatives, stool softeners, antidiarrheals)
◆ Use of enemas
◆ History of digestive disorders (onset, frequency, causes, severity, symptoms, intervention used)
◆ Date of last rectal examination, colonoscopy, other tests

General Assessment

◆ (See "assessment of the head and neck" presented earlier in this chapter.)
◆ Tests for occult blood in stool, black stool (melena), observation of blood in stool or emesis, coffee-ground emesis
◆ Measurement of body weight compared to height
◆ Auscultation of bowel sounds (see Chapter 46)
◆ Assessment of abdominal masses, scars, or other abnormalities
◆ Signs such as jaundice
◆ Difficulty in chewing or swallowing
◆ Ability to safely purchase, prepare, and store foods
◆ Comparison of laboratory test results with normal values
◆ Reports of upper or lower GI x-rays, endoscopic procedures, ultrasound, CT scan, MRI, gastric analysis, guaiac of stool, or other diagnostic procedures

Other Assessment

◆ Presence of hemorrhoids, redness, rash or swelling in rectal area

Subjective Assessment

◆ Pain, difficult bowel movements, diarrhea, constipation, excessive gas, intolerance to specific foods
◆ Appetite and weight changes
◆ Weight loss programs
◆ Digestive discomforts (nausea, vomiting, pain, indigestion, heartburn, belching), hematemesis (vomiting of blood)
◆ Presence of blood in or on stool
◆ Use of enemas or laxatives
◆ High-risk behavior (bulimia, anorexia, bingeing, etc)
◆ Frequent mouth ulcers, canker sores
◆ Frequent halitosis

The experienced examiner also palpates the abdomen for tenderness or masses and the costovertebral junction for flank pain.

Assessment of the Urine

Assessments of urine include amount, color, clarity, and odor. Under normal conditions, urine is clear and described as yellow, straw colored, or amber, with an aromatic odor. It is also important to note if any blood, pus, or sediment is present. Aside from these specific factors, the overall intake and output record is important in assessing urinary disorders. The loss of the ability to concentrate and dilute the urine is one of the first signs of kidney disease; specific gravity of urine is the first screening test of urine dilution. If the urine output is excessive (greater than 1,500 mL/24 h), the patient is said to have *polyuria*; if the output is very small (100–500 mL/24 h), the patient is said to have *oliguria*; if there is no output (0–100 mL/24 h), the patient has *anuria*.

Several procedures used to assess urinary function may be performed by the nurse. These include tests such as the Bili-Labstix, which provides information about urinary tract and kidney status, carbohydrate metabolism, and liver and biliary tract status. It is a paper strip that, when dipped into urine, yields readings within 30 seconds. These readings include urine pH, sugar (glucose) content, as well as the presence of abnormal components such as protein, ketones, hemoglobin (blood), or bilirubin. Urine is also used for most pregnancy tests, which assess for the presence of the hormone human chorionic gonadotropin (HCG).

Assessment of the Reproductive System

Assessment of the reproductive system includes many of the same questions as are asked in urinary system assessment. This is particularly true for the male patient because the systems are so closely related. In addition, the nurse obtains a sexual history. Practices followed by the *patient's mother* during pregnancy have the potential to affect the patient's reproductive system throughout adult life (particularly the female patient).

The examiner examines the external reproductive organs. This includes inspection of the genitalia for lesions, erosions, rashes, scars, discoloration, and hair distribution. Varicosities are noted; breasts and testicles are palpated for lumps or other abnormalities.

Any unusual or questionable signs or symptoms must be reported to the physician and carefully documented. An overview of nursing assessment of the reproductive system is contained in the accompanying box.

Male Reproductive Organs. To inspect the glans penis of the uncircumcised male patient, retract the foreskin. There should be no buildup of smegma (oils and epithelial cells which can build up under the foreskin) if hygiene is good. (*Note:* Be sure to replace the foreskin after inspection, particularly in children or the neurologically impaired. If the foreskin remains retracted, the penis will swell. This becomes a medical emergency if it cannot be brought back over the glans. An emergency circumcision will need to be done to prevent necrosis of the head of the penis.)

Keys to Nursing Assessment
The Reproductive System

Nursing History

All Patients

◆ Mother's reproductive history; mother's use of drugs, smoking, alcohol, radiation exposure during pregnancy with this patient (especially women)
◆ Family history of reproductive disorder
◆ Sexual history, history of sexual dysfunction, painful intercourse
◆ History of high-risk behavior (multiple sexual partners, unprotected sex—heterosexual or homosexual, intravenous drug abuse)
◆ History of sterilization procedures
◆ History of any genital/reproductive surgery
◆ Methods of birth control used, satisfaction with method, previously used methods, and reasons for discontinuing

Female Patients

◆ Reproductive history (number of pregnancies, number of living children, type of delivery, abortions and type, inability to become pregnant), fetal blood Rh incompatibilities with children
◆ Menstrual history (age at onset—menarche, length of cycle, regularity, discomfort, last menstrual period [LMP], breakthrough bleeding, age at menopause)
◆ History of frequent vaginal or other reproductive tract infections

◆ History of sexually transmitted diseases or pelvic inflammatory disease (PID), treatment
◆ Date of last Pap test, mammogram, known breast conditions

Male Patients

◆ Male sterility
◆ Date of last testicular examination, prostate specific antigen (PSA) blood test

Objective Assessment

◆ Visual observation of external genitalia and breasts
◆ Penile or vaginal discharge, swelling, discoloration or lesions
◆ Swelling of scrotum, prostate enlargement, testicular masses
◆ Presence of urinary disorders in men
◆ Palpate anterior thigh for hernia
◆ Breast examination
◆ Comparison of laboratory test results with normal values
◆ Results of x-rays, mammography, or other diagnostic tests

Subjective Assessment

◆ Changes in breasts, results of breast self-examination
◆ Results of testicular self-examination
◆ Frequent infections, pain, other symptoms

Palpate the penis and scrotum for nodules, tenderness, and asymmetrical size or surface irregularities of the testes. Ask the patient if he has been performing regular testicular self-examination. Cancer of the prostate is distinguished from other prostate disorders by biopsy. Often this patient presents with obstructive symptoms—difficulty in voiding—and may have hematuria. On examination, the cancerous prostate often feels irregular and may have hard nodules. A PSA (prostate specific antigen) blood test also assists in diagnosis of prostate cancer.

Female Reproductive Organs. In the woman, observe for inflammation of the vaginal area or of Bartholin's glands. Age-related changes of the vagina or falling of the uterus (called prolapse) or other structures can be observed. The primary caregiver will assess vaginal and rectal tone and will perform a pelvic examination and Pap test.

The breasts are examined as for breast self-examination (see Chapter 84). The patient is asked about the regularity and results of her own breast self-examinations.

Keys for Review

Key Questions for Critical Thinking

1. Describe the difference in nursing responsibilities when assisting with the physical examination of the adult and of the child.
2. Describe the following positions and their uses: horizontal recumbent, dorsal recumbent, prone, Sims', Fowler's, knee–chest, dorsal lithotomy, and erect.
3. Describe the functions of the nurse when accompanying the physician on patient rounds.

Key Readings

Bates BA. Guide to Physical Examination and History Taking, Ed 6. Philadelphia, J.B. Lippincott, 1995

Beare PG, Meyers JL. Principles and Practice of Adult Health Nursing. St. Louis, C.V. Mosby, 1990

Berkow R (Ed). The Merck Manual of Diagnosis and Therapy, Ed 16. Rahway NJ, Merck & Co, 1992

Craven RF, Hirnle CJ. Fundamentals of Nursing: Human Health and Function. Philadelphia, J.B. Lippincott, 1992

Earnest VV. Clinical Skills in Nursing Practice, Ed 2. Philadelphia, J.B. Lippincott, 1993

Fischbach F. A Manual of Laboratory and Diagnostic Tests, Ed 3. Philadelphia, J.B. Lippincott, 1992

Kinney MR, Packa DR, Dunbar SB. AACN's Clinical Reference for Critical-Care Nursing, Ed 3. St. Louis, Mosby-Yearbook, 1993

Maas M, Buckwalter K, Hardy MA. Nursing Diagnoses and Interventions in the Elderly. Redwood City, CA, Addison-Wesley, 1991

O'Toole M (Ed). Miller-Keane Encyclopedia and Dictionary of Medicine, Nursing, and Allied Health, Ed 5. Philadelphia, W.B. Saunders, 1992

Scherer JC. Introductory Medical-Surgical Nursing, Ed 5. Philadelphia, J.B. Lippincott, 1991

Key Readings (continued)

Seidel HM, Ball JW, et al. Mosby's Guide to Physical Examination, Ed 2. St. Louis, Mosby-Yearbook, 1991

Smeltzer SC, Bare BG. Brunner and Suddarth's Textbook of Medical-Surgical Nursing, Ed. 7. Philadelphia, J.B. Lippincott, 1992

Smith AJ, Johnson JY. Nurses' Guide to Clinical Procedures. Philadelphia, J.B. Lippincott, 1990

Suddarth DS. The Lippincott Manual of Nursing Practice, Ed 5. Philadelphia, J.B. Lippincott, 1991

Taylor C, Lillis C, LeMone P. Fundamentals of Nursing: Art and Science of Nursing Care, Ed 2. Philadelphia, J.B. Lippincott, 1993

Enrichment Keys

Fuller J, Schaller-Ayers J. Health Assessment: A Nursing Approach, Ed 2. Philadelphia, J.B. Lippincott, 1994

"Assessing Patients" Section of Nurse's Photo-Library. Springhouse, PA, Springhouse, 1994.

Keys to Learning More

Chapter 53: patient assessments in the perioperative period

Chapter 54: surgical asepsis

Unit Twelve: maternal and child health and assessments

Unit Thirteen: pediatric nursing and assessments

Unit Fourteen: medical and surgical nursing and assessments of adults

Unit Fifteen: geriatric nursing and assessments of older adults

Chapter 87: nursing assessment in psychiatry

51 Infection Control Techniques

Keys for Learning

Learning Objectives

- Explain the chain of infection.
- List and discuss the major points involved in universal precautions.
- Describe how a patient's room might be set up when using barrier techniques.
- State the most important procedure in the prevention of disease spread in the hospital.
- Describe and demonstrate the use of appropriate personal protective equipment in infection control.
- Describe and demonstrate what to do before leaving a patient's room and precautions to take during medication administration, vital sign monitoring, and transport of a patient who is potentially infectious.
- Describe the components of protective (neutropenic/reverse) isolation.
- Differentiate between the use of protective isolation and the other types of isolation precautions.
- State general information in relation to infection control in pediatric units.

Key Terms

personal protective equipment   protective isolation

Keys to Understanding This Chapter

Chapter 5: basic needs of people including safety and freedom from disease; some patients must be protected from disease

Chapter 7: impact of communicable diseases on the community

Chapter 8: introduction to microorganisms

Chapter 15: skin and mucous membranes protect against disease

Chapter 21: concept of immunity

Chapter 30: medical asepsis and universal precautions

Chapter 45: personal hygiene

Chapter 46: assisting with elimination

Chapter 47: collection of specimens

Key Points

- Isolation procedures may vary among facilities. You should know the specific procedures in your facility.
- Infection is best controlled by prevention—breaking the links in the chain of infection.
- Universal precautions treat all blood and certain body fluids as if they are potentially infectious.
- Personal protective equipment helps prevent disease transmission.
- Before entering a patient's room, assess to determine personal protective equipment and other equipment needed.
- Body substance isolation expands on universal precautions by including body fluids such as urine, feces, and vomitus.
- Historically, various forms of isolation were recognized by the Centers for Disease Control and Prevention as effective toward prevention of disease transmission. These include category-specific and disease-specific isolation.
- Isolation is often frightening and misunderstood by patients and families.
- Handwashing is the most important means of preventing the spread of infection.
- Personal protective equipment should be discarded if it is a single-use item, becomes contaminated, or becomes ineffective due to damage.
- Isolation patients leave only for procedures that cannot be done at the bedside; those departments must be notified.

Key Topics Outline

Infection Control
  Universal Precautions
  Isolation
  Setting Up Patient's Room
Specific Procedures and Personal Protective Equipment
  Performing Nursing Procedures
Reverse (Protective/Neutropenic) Isolation

Rosdahl CB: Textbook of Basic Nursing, 6th ed. © 1995 J.B. Lippincott Company

The nurse must understand the basic principles related to the spread of disease before caring for patients. It is important for you to keep in mind the chain of infection, as discussed in Chapter 8. It is important to break this chain whenever possible. This is done by using careful infection control and barrier techniques.

Infection Control

Infection is best controlled by *prevention*. Several types of prevention methods are used in the healthcare facility. Medical asepsis, including good handwashing, disinfection, and sterilization, and prevention of nosocomial infections, were discussed in Chapter 30. Surgical asepsis is discussed in Chapter 54.

Three general techniques are used to prevent the spread of infection in the hospital:

◆ Universal precautions and body substance isolation
◆ Specific isolation techniques
◆ Protective isolation

Universal Precautions

The procedures of universal precautions have been carefully designed by the Centers for Disease Control and Prevention (CDC). This has been done in an effort to protect healthcare personnel and other patients from the spread of the human immunodeficiency virus (HIV), which is known to cause acquired immunodeficiency syndrome (AIDS), as well as disorders such as hepatitis B (HBV). Key points in universal precautions address the use of barrier techniques, including **personal protective equipment** (PPE). These are discussed in Chapter 30 and listed inside the cover of this book. The Occupational Safety and Health Administration (OSHA) enforces the use of universal precautions. OSHA regulations are discussed in Chapter 30.

Isolation

For some patients, such as those with communicable respiratory disorders (such as tuberculosis [TB]) or a disease that is resistant to medications, additional precautions must be taken. The patient must be placed in a room separate from other patients or isolated. Historically, various forms of isolation were recognized by the CDC as effective toward preventing disease transmission.

> **Key Concept**
> ◆ Specific procedures for an individual patient will often be prescribed, depending on the reasons for the precautions.
> ◆ Each hospital has established local protocols.

Traditional Isolation

Historically, there were two primary types of traditional isolation systems used in healthcare: category-specific isolation and disease-specific isolation. Some institutions may still follow these systems. However, because of OSHA regulations, universal precautions (discussed below) are mandatory for all patients.

Category-Specific Isolation. Specific categories of isolation (respiratory, contact, enteric, strict, or wound) are identified, using color-coded cards. This form of isolation is based on the patient's diagnosis. The cards are posted outside the patient's room and ask the visitor to check with the nurse before entering.

Disease-Specific Isolation. This type of isolation uses a single all-purpose sign. The nurse selects items on the card that are appropriate for the specific disease that causes the patient to be isolated.

Current Isolation Systems

Universal precautions and body substance isolation are two systems using barrier techniques, which have evolved recently in response to the prevention of blood-borne infections such as HIV and HBV. Chapter 30 discusses universal precautions in detail. (See also inside cover of this book.) Body substance isolation incorporates the same recommendations as universal precautions, but considers all body substances as potentially infectious, regardless of the patient's diagnosis. Body substance isolation advocates using barrier techniques whenever healthcare personnel have contact with moist body substances, mucous membranes, and nonintact skin. Body substance isolation eliminates the need for category-specific or disease-specific isolation systems except for certain airborne diseases, such as *Varicella* or pulmonary tuberculosis, that require special precautions, such as a private room with a sign on the door requesting visitors to check with the nurse before entering the room.

Key Concept

◆ Universal precautions—blood and certain body fluids from all patients regardless of their diagnosis are treated as infectious

◆ Body substance isolation—all body fluids treated as infectious

---

Setting Up a Patient's Room for Isolation

Patients may stay in their own rooms. The facilities for carrying out barrier techniques may not be the same in every hospital, but the principles are the same. Outside the patient's room or in a small room adjacent to the patient's room, supplies can be stored and a sink is available for handwashing.

Patient and Family Teaching

The first thing a nurse does when setting up the patient's room is to thoroughly explain the reasons for the barrier techniques to the patient and family. It is important for them to understand how easily disease organisms can be spread without special precautions. If they understand the preventive procedures that will be performed, they will usually cooperate. Explain that children are usually not allowed to visit a patient with a communicable disease because children are so susceptible to disease.

Barrier techniques may be frightening to patients. They may fear their disease and think people are afraid to come near them. The person may be lonely, missing the companionship of other patients and normal contacts with hospital personnel. The nursing staff should not avoid patients, even though it takes more effort to visit them. Try to plan your work so that you can stay in the room as long as possible at one time. Even when you are not going into the room, stop by the door and say hello.

Supplies and Equipment

The basic supplies and equipment for isolation include the following:

Inside the Room. The patient's room should be equipped with bedpan and urinal; wash basin and soap

dish; thermometer and holder (often a glass clinical thermometer is used); water pitcher and glass; emesis basin; toilet and facial tissues; toothbrush and dentifrice; and such personal items as shaving equipment, comb or brush, deodorant, shampoo, and cosmetics. (It may be necessary to dispose of these items when the patient is discharged). The patient should have a phone and television, if at all possible. You will also need some of the following: paper towels; plastic or paper bags to line the wastebasket for disposing of trash; washable blankets, pillows, and bedspreads, and impervious laundry bags, as well as the usual linens needed for a patient unit. It is ideal to have a sink with foot or knee controls and a linen bag and stand.

Outside the Room. Items to be placed outside the patient's room include a bedside stand or cabinet stocked with PPE, as required for that patient. You will also need clean laundry bags and large trash bags, biohazard bags and tape or tags for marking contaminated bags, and a sign for the door. The sign will depend on the infection control technique the hospital has adopted.

Nursing Alert

Before working in a pediatric unit a nurse should determine his or her immune status to communicable diseases of childhood. You may require immunization to prevent exposure and infection.

Specific Procedures and Personal Protective Equipment

Handwashing

Handwashing is basic to all nursing procedures. The CDC has stated that "proper handwashing before and after contact with each patient is the single most important means of preventing the spread of infection." (Review Chapter 30 for handwashing procedure.) Jewelry should not be worn when caring for patients because it may harbor microorganisms. It is difficult to disinfect adequately without special equipment and solutions.

General universal precautions are used when caring for patients. These include gloves and other PPE, as needed.

Key Concept

Each institution establishes its own policy about PPE to be used according to OSHA regulations.

Gloves

Gloves, which are used in all patient care when the patient's body substances are involved, protect the nurse from microorganisms that the patient may carry. The use of gloves also prevents the spread of organisms from one patient to another, to other hospital staff, or from hospital staff to patient. Disposable gloves are available in each patient unit and are used if there is anticipated contact with blood and body fluids or if the nurse has any break in the skin of the hands. Gloves used are discarded in the patient's room. The use of clean gloves is described in Chapter 30.

Eye Protection

Goggles, usually with side and forehead shields, are worn if there is any danger of the patient's body fluids splashing onto the nurse. Disposable goggles are to be made available in each patient's isolation unit. In some situations where extra protection is needed, such as in the operating room or morgue, full face shields are used. The specific situation dictates the type of eye protection to be used. The use of eye protection is described and illustrated in Chapter 30.

Gowns or Aprons

You wear a gown or protective apron to keep your clothing clean, in the instances when there is a potential for body substances to splash on your clothing. The accompanying box provides guidelines for using gowns.

Masks

When you are giving nursing care to patients with communicable diseases transmitted through the respiratory tract, it is necessary to protect yourself against airborne transmission. For example, if your patient has active pulmonary tuberculosis or is unable to control secretions, you will usually need to wear a mask to cover your nose and mouth. Each hospital establishes its own policy about the PPE to be used. Everyone coming in contact with the patient, including visitors, may wear a mask or the patient may be the only one to wear PPE if outside the room. Airborne diseases remain in the patient's room until it is disinfected; all visitors and staff should wear PPE.

The principle reason for wearing PPE is to keep organisms from entering or leaving the respiratory tract (yours or the patient's). In the operating room or nursery, masks protect the patient from possible infection by staff.

Masks are disposable to reduce the risk of cross-contamination. When you are not using the mask, dispose of it. A mask hanging around the nurse's neck is a menace, rather than a protection. The use of a mask is described in Chapter 30.

Nursing Skill Guidelines
Putting On and Removing Gown

- ◆ The inside of the gown is clean; the outside is contaminated.
- ◆ The gown must be long enough to cover your uniform or clothing completely; it must open down the back and must be full enough to overlap at the back. A tie around the waist keeps the gown in place.
- ◆ The neck of the gown is clean because you never touch that part with contaminated hands.
- ◆ If you have a long-sleeved uniform, roll the sleeves up above your elbows before you put the gown on.
- ◆ A supply of clean gowns is ready outside the patient's room to put on before you enter.
- ◆ After use, the gown is removed and disposed of inside out (contaminated side in). If disposable gowns are used, they are placed in the receptacle for contaminated material. If reusable gowns are used, they are placed in the linen hamper for laundering. Gowns are usually not hung in the room for reuse.
- ◆ After removing the gown, wash your hands thoroughly before you touch anything else.

Leaving a Patient's Room

Whenever you leave the room of a patient, you must take special care not to spread infection to other patients. Discard your gown and mask without contamination, and scrub your hands without spreading contamination to your upper arms. General information about this procedure is:

- ◆ General handwashing techniques are used. Special attention is paid to prevention of contamination.
- ◆ Always point your hands down when washing them. (Rationale: *This prevents contamination of your upper arms.*)
- ◆ Do not touch any part of the sink or the faucets. The ideal sink should have foot or knee controls, as well as a foot-controlled dispenser. (Rationale: *The sink is contaminated by organisms. A bar of soap spreads organisms.*)
- ◆ Paper towels must be used and thrown away in the designated container. (Rationale: *A common towel is contaminated and spreads organisms.*)
- ◆ Scrub your hands thoroughly at least twice, giving special attention to your nails. Do not wear rings.

Double Bagging. In some hospitals, refuse and linen are "double bagged" out of the patient's room. In other facilities, this procedure is no longer used because refuse and linen from all patients are considered contaminated and treated as such (per universal precautions).

The double-bag procedure is carried out by two nurses. The nurse inside the room is considered "contaminated" and the nurse outside is considered "clean." The contaminated nurse places patient items into a bag and closes the top. This entire bag, inside and out, is considered contaminated. The clean nurse, outside the room, folds the top of the clean bag down to make a collar or "cuff." The clean nurse keeps his or her hands outside this cuff.

The contaminated nurse touches only the *inside* of the clean bag; the clean nurse touches only the *outside* of the clean bag. The clean nurse folds over the top of the clean bag, seals it carefully and labels it, touching only the outside of the bag. Most materials are placed into prelabeled bags, so housekeeping and maintenance personnel will know what procedures to follow. Instruments and reusable items are double bagged and clearly labeled for sterilization. Glass or other breakable items must be identified as "glass-breakable." Even if the glass item is disposable, it should be labeled, because if it breaks, it may rip the bag and spread contamination or cut someone.

Nursing Alert

If a double-bagging procedure is not used, all discarded materials are considered contaminated.

Performing Nursing Procedures in Isolation

Administering Medications

Use universal precautions when you administer medications. Disposable materials are used and disposed of in the patient's room. The following nursing skills review pointers and add materials specific to patients in isolation.

♦ Unwrap medications before going into the room *(Rationale: This is difficult to do after you have put on your gloves.)*
♦ If you will need juice or applesauce to mix the medications, take them with you into the room. If a medication tray must be used, use a disposable one.
♦ Do not take medication cards into the patient's room.
♦ If you are not going to touch the patient, you may just wear a mask, if required. Do not touch the patient or anything in the room, and be sure to carefully scrub when out of the room.
♦ If you are giving an injection, gloves must be worn, as per body substance isolation precautions. Wear gown and mask, as required. Needles are placed into the sharps disposal container in the patient's room. As always, needles are not broken off, recapped, or detached from the syringe. "Safety syringes" are used in many facilities.

♦ Use disposable medication cups.
♦ Intravenous bags are used and discarded in the patient's room. In the rare case of an intravenous bottle, it must be labeled "glass" and placed into the appropriate container in the room.
♦ *All* materials are disposed of in the patient's room.

Sending a Specimen to the Laboratory

Before collecting a specimen, label the container. If you are sending a blood, urine, or other specimen to the laboratory, place it on a clean paper towel in the anteroom and carefully scrub when out of the room. Then, place the specimen into a zip-lock bag identified with the standard "biohazard" label. In some hospitals, a double-bagging procedure is used to take the specimen out of the room. Wash your hands again. Identify the specimen as biohazard; it is helpful if the laboratory personnel know of suspected organisms. As always, specimens should be taken to the laboratory as soon as possible. Remember to touch the request cards and the outside of the bag only with your clean hands, to protect the laboratory personnel.

Taking Vital Signs

Usually the equipment needed to take vital signs is kept in the patient's room and disinfected when the patient is discharged. These nursing skills describe some of the special procedures used in taking vital signs in an isolation room.

♦ Use the equipment in the room. You should not have to bring items in with you.
♦ Wear gloves and whatever other protective equipment is indicated.

Nursing Skill Guidelines
Caring for the Body After Death of a Person in Special Isolation

♦ The body is cared for as is any person who dies (discussed in Chapter 90).
♦ The body is wrapped while in the room and is usually placed in a plastic zippered bag.
♦ The body is transferred to a cart that has been draped with a clean bath blanket or sheet. The clean blanket is wrapped around the body by a clean person outside of the room.
♦ The room is decontaminated according to your facility's procedure.
♦ If you are the person who touched the body inside the room, you are considered contaminated and must wash your hands when leaving the room. Afterward, you may touch only the outside of the wrapping or shroud.
♦ Label the body properly. The pathologist treats all patients as if they have an infectious disease.

There will usually be a clock on the wall, so you will not need to use your watch. If you do need to bring your watch, place it on a paper towel and touch only the bottom of the towel with your contaminated hands or seal it in a Zip-Lock bag. Pick up your watch after you have scrubbed out of the room.

A glass clinical thermometer may be used and discarded when the patient is discharged. The blood pressure apparatus is usually on the wall. The cuff and stethoscope are disinfected when the patient is discharged.

Dishes and Meal Trays

Most hospitals treat all dietary items (dishes, trays, eating utensils) as potentially infectious, no matter where the patients are. Paper and disposable products may be used in isolation. Otherwise, appropriate precautions are used in handling all dietary trays and dishes.

Transporting the Patient to Other Departments

In rare cases, it may be necessary to transport the patient to another part of the hospital. The following nursing skills describe special precautions in transporting the isolated patient to other departments.

- Be sure you wear protective equipment, as needed.
- The patient must wear gown, gloves, or mask as indicated.
- If there is any drainage, make sure this is controlled and contained.
- The wheelchair or stretcher is draped with a clean sheet or bath blanket. The patient is wrapped in the clean material.
- If the patient is ambulatory, he or she should be escorted to the examination by a staff member.
- Notify the other department that the patient is on special isolation precautions, so personnel can take appropriate precautions.
- Carefully disinfect the wheelchair or stretcher after use.

Care of the Body After Death

If a patient dies, special precautions are taken to prevent the spread of infection. In many hospitals, these precautions are taken with all patients who die. The accompanying box describes care of the body after death.

Terminal Disinfection

Terminal disinfection refers to the care of a patient's unit and belongings after the illness is over. The process is the same whether the patient remains in the hospital, is discharged, or dies. The institution prescribes the method to be used, which should be sufficiently thorough to destroy the disease-causing organisms. Some organisms are more difficult to destroy than others. Also, some organisms can live up to 6 months on furniture and other surfaces.

Nursing Alert

Anything that touches the patient is contaminated and must be decontaminated or sterilized before it can be used for another patient. Stop to think before you do anything for the patient, or you might become contaminated and spread the disease. *One break in technique is all it takes to spread infection*! Remember, good handwashing is vital.

Special Considerations in Children
Nursing Procedures in Infection Control

- A higher percentage of pediatric admissions involve communicable illnesses than do adult admissions. Often the pediatric population is not immune to these diseases. If not contained, a hospital outbreak can result.
- Children are at greater risk of acquiring viral infections than adults.
- Young children may not be able to understand good handwashing and barrier precautions.
- Environmental surfaces must be kept as clean as possible because children may have physical and oral contact with them. Children may also put toys and other objects in their mouths. Some of the toys may be shared in the playroom.
- Barrier techniques are important to employees because they tend to have closer contact with pediatric patients than with adults by rocking, cuddling, and feeding.

General Procedures in Protective/Neutropenic Isolation

- Private room required.
- Healthcare workers and visitors may not enter if they have a cold, influenza, or other communicable disease.
- Anyone entering the room must wear a mask and practice strict handwashing before patient contact.
- The patient cannot receive fresh fruit, fresh vegetables, or flowers.
- Rectal temperatures, enemas, suppositories, intravenous and intramuscular injections, and other invasive procedures are avoided, if possible.
- The patient's temperature should be measured at least every 4 hours.
- If there is any reason to suspect an infection, a blood culture may be drawn.
- In some cases, special linens are used and hospital-laundered scrub suits are worn by staff. Hair covering is required in some units. Staff working in these units often wear lab coats if leaving the unit.
- Special air purification is used in some situations.

Protective (Reverse or Neutropenic) Isolation

Sometimes, it is the patient who must be protected from the outside environment. In such cases, the procedures are reversed: the microorganisms from other people are kept away from the patient. This is known as **protective isolation** or reverse or neutropenic isolation. This type of isolation attempts to prevent harmful microorganisms from coming into contact with the patient. General procedures for this type of isolation are given in the accompanying box.

Types of patients who might be placed in protective isolation are burn patients, immunocompromised (HIV, cancer chemotherapy) patients, patients following bone marrow transplnt, or patients with a low resistance from another cause (such as agammaglobulinemia).

Patients on protective isolation do not have a good immune response. Therefore they may become infected but not show classic signs and symptoms of infection. This occurs because they do not have enough white blood cells to create the normal inflammatory response.

Key Concept

◆ Barrier techniques prevent organisms from leaving the patient's room.
◆ Protective isolation prevents organisms from coming into contact with patients.

Keys for Review

Key Questions for Critical Thinking

1. Explain how barrier techniques relate to universal precautions.
2. Differentiate between techniques when the patient has a communicable disease and when the patient is to be protected.
3. Describe items needed to set up a patient's room for infection control. Discuss their use.
4. Describe the role of prevention in the control of disease spread.

Key Readings

Becker SI. "Learning About Infection Control" in "Controlling Infection" section of Nurse's PhotoLibrary. Springhouse, PA, Springhouse, 1993

Centers for Disease Control. Recommendations for Prevention of HIV Transmission in Health-Care Settings. MMWR 36(25), 1987

Craven RF, Hirnle CJ. Fundamentals of Nursing: Human Health and Function. Philadelphia, J.B. Lippincott, 1992

Key Readings (continued)

Earnest VV. Clinical Skills in Nursing Practice, Ed 2. Philadelphia, J.B. Lippincott, 1993

Hoeprich PD, Colin JM, Ronald AR. Infectious Diseases, Ed 5. Philadelphia, J.B. Lippincott, 1994

Smeltzer SC, Bare BG. Brunner and Suddarth's Textbook of Medical-Surgical Nursing, Ed 7. Philadelphia, J.B. Lippincott, 1992

Smith-Temple AJ, Johnson JY. Nurses' Guide to Clinical Procedures, Ed 2. Philadelphia, J.B. Lippincott, 1994

Taylor C, Lillis C, LeMone P. Fundamentals of Nursing: The Art and Science of Nursing Care, Ed 2. Philadelphia, J.B. Lippincott, 1993

Keys to Learning More

Chapter 54: use of surgical asepsis
Unit Twelve: assisting mothers and newborn babies
Unit Thirteen: pediatric nursing
Unit Fourteen: medical–surgical nursing

52 Patient Comfort and Pain Management

Learning Objectives

- Differentiate between acute and chronic pain.
- Describe pain locations.
- Identify major causes of pain.
- List and explain at least seven factors determining how people perceive pain.
- Describe the function of endorphins in pain management.
- Discuss measures used to intervene in the chronic pain syndrome.
- Differentiate between surgical and conservative treatment of chronic pain and describe forms of conservative treatment.

Key Terms

acute pain	endorphins	pain threshold
angina	gate control theory	pain tolerance
biofeedback	guided imagery	phantom pain
central pain	intractable pain	psychogenic
chronic pain	neuralgia	referred pain
deep pain	nociceptor	superficial pain

Keys to Understanding This Chapter

Chapter 5: basic human needs, which include comfort and safety

Chapter 14: organization of the body including pain receptors

Chapter 38: signs and symptoms

Chapter 39: transcultural considerations, which affect pain perception

Chapter 49: heat and cold application

Key Points

- Pain may be acute or chronic. If acute pain is not managed properly, it can develop into chronic pain.

Key Points (continued)

- Pain may be classified by location.
- Perception of pain is individual and depends on many factors.
- Both physical and psychological techniques are useful in pain management.
- The chronic pain syndrome greatly affects the life of the patient and the family.
- It is important to intervene in the cycle of chronic pain as early as possible.

Key Topics Outline

Encountering Pain
  Types of Pain
  Causes of Pain
  Factors in Pain Perception
Nursing Assessment
Pain Management
Chronic Pain Syndrome
  Intervention Into the Chronic Pain Cycle

Key Learning Activities

- Attend a headache seminar. Talk to people about their headaches. What therapeutic modalities do they use?
- Interview a person who has chronic pain. What has been helpful in pain management? What would this person recommend to other patients? How has the pain influenced the person's work, family activities, and relationships with others?
- Read more about the gate control theory of pain and pain management.

Pain is one of the most common reasons people contact a healthcare professional. It is also the chief reason people take medication. One of nursing's important interventions is to relieve pain and to make the patient comfortable. One of the considerations in all of the basic skills you learned in Unit Nine is to make the patient comfortable while you perform the required skills.

Encountering Pain

We all know what is meant by the term pain, but it is difficult to define. A noted pain theorist, Margot McCaffery says, "Pain is whatever the experiencing person says it is, existing whenever he says it does."[1] Pain is the body's way of signaling something is wrong.

Types of Pain

Acute pain is the sensation that results abruptly from an injury or disease. Usually it is short-lived. If the cause is not discovered or is not cared for properly, chronic pain may result. **Chronic pain** is pain that continues for a long period of time, sometimes for life. It is pain that continues beyond what would be expected to be a healing period for an acute pain. The patient often is depressed in relation to the pain.

Sometimes a definite objective cause cannot be documented. A group of associated symptoms surround chronic pain and the treatment must be aimed at alleviating these related symptoms. The treatment regimen for chronic pain differs from that for acute pain.

Intractable pain refers to chronic pain that is severe and constant or unrelenting. Usually nursing and medical procedures do not relieve this pain. The discussion of hospice nursing in Chapter 91 describes some means used to deal with intractable pain in terminally ill persons.

Location of Pain

Sometimes pain is categorized in relation to the area of the body where it originates.

Superficial pain originates in the skin or mucous membranes. The source usually can be located easily because there are many nerve endings in the affected structures. The patient often describes superficial pain as prickling, burning, or dull.

Deep pain originates in inner body structures. It may be manifested by vomiting, blood pressure changes, or weakness. The patient may have difficulty in pinpointing the exact location of deep pain. The patient often describes deep pain as aching, shooting, grinding, or cramping.

Central pain seems to originate within the brain itself, in the pain interpretation, and/or receiving centers.

Neuralgia is an intense burning sensation that follows a peripheral nerve. **Referred pain** is pain felt in a location different from the actual origin. **Phantom pain** occurs in amputations when the person feels pain in an area that has been amputated. **Angina** is pain connected with cardiac pathology.

Causes of Pain

Pain has several causes. Perhaps the most common is muscle tightness. You can test this theory by making a tight fist and holding it; after a few seconds, you begin to feel discomfort. This is caused by muscle spasms and by resulting decreased blood supply to that muscle. As oxygen supply to the muscle decreases, discomfort increases. This same sort of muscle tightness often occurs in pain. As pain increases, the body's natural response is to tighten muscles further. Fatigue, fear of the unknown, and lack of knowledge about management further tighten muscles and a cycle of pain can follow, as shown in Figure 52-1. This can develop into chronic pain.

Examples of other physical causes are disease, infection, trauma, cell growth or injury, lack of proper nutrition, metabolic factors, and temperature extremes. Chemical factors include toxins such as alcohol, drugs, cigarettes, and pollution in the air and water.

Pain may also be of **psychogenic** origin; that is, it originates in the mind and has no identifiable physical cause. Psychogenic pain can be as severe as pain from a physical cause. Most pain has both physical and psychogenic causes.

Factors in Pain Perception

The perception of pain is individualized. Pain is different in different people and at different times in the same person.

Nociceptors are sensory receptors of pain. They are free nerve endings in tissue; they respond to physiologic stimuli.

A person can stand pain up to the pain threshold (see Figure 52-1). **Pain threshold** is the point at which a stimulus is described as being painful. **Pain tolerance** denotes the point at which a person can no longer tolerate pain without analgesia.

Several factors influence patients' perceptions of pain or at least affect responses to pain. Some of these are:

---

1 McCaffery M. Cognition, Bodily Pain and Man–Environment Interactions. Los Angeles, University of California, 1968.

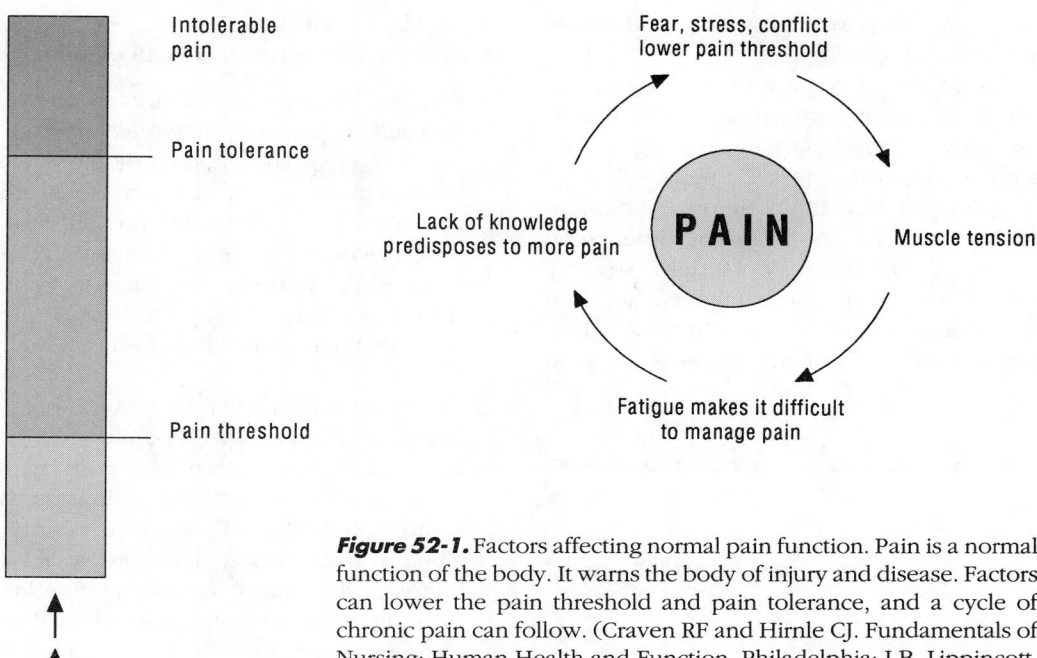

Figure 52-1. Factors affecting normal pain function. Pain is a normal function of the body. It warns the body of injury and disease. Factors can lower the pain threshold and pain tolerance, and a cycle of chronic pain can follow. (Craven RF and Hirnle CJ. Fundamentals of Nursing: Human Health and Function. Philadelphia: J.B. Lippincott, 1992.)

◆ *Cultural:* People with certain cultural backgrounds are conditioned to cry out when in pain; others are conditioned to be stoic.

◆ *Age:* Infants and young children feel pain but cannot verbalize pain. School-aged children and adolescents many times try to be brave and not give in to pain. Adults respond in varying ways. Older adults may not feel acute pain because of decreased sensations or perceptions.

◆ *History of pain:* The person who is chronically ill and has almost constant pain often learns to tolerate it. On the other hand, if a previous experience was very painful, a person may feel great pain when the experience is repeated. This is called *anticipatory pain.*

◆ *Anxiety:* Anxiety can actually cause physical pain. Tense muscles reinforce that pain.

◆ *Body image/self-image:* Feelings about oneself influences pain and pain reaction. The patient's personality may cause him or her to keep pain a secret.

◆ *Time of day:* Many people express greater pain at night. This might be caused by loneliness, boredom, overexertion, or actual increase in pain.

◆ *Suggestion:* Sometimes a person can be preconditioned to feel or not feel pain. For example, a woman told that childbirth is painful may have a great deal of discomfort; another woman may be preconditioned to have a more comfortable delivery.

◆ *Distraction:* If a person's attention can be diverted, he or she may not feel as much pain as would

otherwise be the case. Guided imagery is an example of a distraction technique.

◆ *Brain functioning:* In some cases, pain perception is distorted in the brain. It is possible to perceive pain when it seems that no cause exists (central pain) or to interrupt the perception of pain so that the patient is no longer bothered by the discomfort.

Nursing Assessment

Pain is *subjective;* that is, only the patient can describe it. Pain itself cannot be objectively observed by the nurse although some manifestations of pain can be observed. For example, the nurse can observe the patient crying, screaming, wringing the hands, or smoking excessively. However, the nurse does not know *why* the patient is doing these things unless told.

When the patient is admitted and during the hospital stay, it is important to determine as much as possible about pain. Questions asked about pain should include location, onset, duration, frequency, description, and what makes the pain better or worse. Any factors that seem to precipitate the pain must be identified.

Description of the intensity of pain includes *mild, slight,* or *moderate.* Duration of pain is described as *intermittent, spasmodic,* or *constant.* The quality of pain can be described as *boring, burning, constant, cramping, crushing, dull, excruciating, hammering, intermittent, knifelike, grinding, penetrating, piercing, pounding, radiating, sharp, shooting, spasmodic, stabbing, tearing, throbbing,* or *tingling.*

Associated characteristics of pain can be *visual disturbance, nausea and vomiting, fatigue and depression, anorexia, muscle spasms, anger and aggression, withdrawal,* and *regression.*[2]

Patients are often asked to rank their level of pain on a scale of 1 to 10. Their ranking from one time to the next gives you a more objective way of judging severity of the pain. Other assessment formats have also been developed for pain assessment. The accompanying box gives an overview of the nursing process in pain management.

Key Concept

If a patient feels pain, the pain is real.

Pain Management

It is preferable to use physical or psychological measures for pain relief rather than medication. These measures are determined by the physician. They may be given by a specially trained person and you may be asked to assist. Or you may give the treatment, such as application of heat and cold.

The Body's Natural Defenses Against Pain

The body has internal mechanisms that help control pain and its perception: endorphins and inhibition of pain transmission.

Naturally occurring analgesic substances called **endorphins** are produced by the body. These endorphins are produced by the brain and spinal cord. They are safe and occur naturally in the body as a result of exercise and certain other stimulation. They kill pain and elevate mood. Endorphin production is increased with acute pain but decreases or stops as pain becomes chronic. Some authorities believe that activities other than exercise, such as laughter, also increase endorphin production. It is also believed that intake of certain chemicals and foods, including caffeine, nicotine, alcohol, salt, and sugar decrease endorphin production.

Another theory, the **gate control theory**, says there is a gate control system in which there are fibers that close off pain sensations that would reach the brain if the gate were open.

---

[2] Craven RF, Hirnle CJ. Fundamentals of Nursing: Human Health and Function. Philadelphia, J.B. Lippincott, 1992.

Physical Techniques

Physical measures to control pain include:

◆ *Physical stimulus* (*cutaneous stimulation*): Gentle massage or pressure may relieve congestion or promote circulation and oxygenation, and thus relieve pain. Transcutaneous electrical stimulation is used to relieve low back pain (TENS unit).

◆ *Acupuncture:* This procedure involves insertion of tiny needles into specific "energy points" under the skin. It is used to treat pain. Heat or pressure (acupressure) may also be applied externally to these points.

◆ *Heat and cold:* The application of heat or cold may help to control localized pain.

◆ *Exercise:* Exercise can relieve pain by promoting circulation of the part, distracting the patient, and stimulating endorphin production.

◆ *Comfort measures:* A clean bed, a clean face and hands, restful music, or a semilighted room may promote relaxation and pain relief. Positional changes also help.

Psychological Techniques

Several psychological techniques can be helpful in controlling pain:

◆ *Distraction and diversion:* Activities such as visiting, games, television, or craft projects can divert the patient's attention.

◆ *Talking:* Sometimes the patient can relieve pain by verbalizing to the nurse about the pain.

◆ *Relief of anxiety:* The resolution of a personal problem may be all that is needed to relieve pain.

◆ *Deep relaxation:* Deep relaxation techniques can be effective in pain control. The procedure often involves *guided imagery.* For example, the patient controls a migraine headache with deep relaxation, followed by visualizing dilation of cranial blood vessels.

◆ *Hypnosis:* Hypnosis builds on deep relaxation but requires more focused attention and response to suggestions or commands. Suggestions made by the hypnotist focus attention away from pain and suggest its disappearance. Some patients are taught self-hypnosis to reinforce the suggestions.

◆ *Deep controlled breathing:* This technique has been used extensively in childbirth.

◆ *Group therapy:* Feelings can be verbalized and suggestions for pain control shared. The family may be involved in the group.

Medications

Some ointments and liniments relieve pain. They may contain a local anesthetic or may draw blood into the area to increase the temperature and improve circulation.

Overview of the Nursing Process
Pain Management

Assessment Priorities

The patient's description of the pain, pain experience: the pain's location, duration, quantity, quality, and chronology; aggravating factors; and phenomena associated with the pain

What meaning, if any, the pain has for the patient

The patient's coping strategies and their success or failure

Behavioral responses to pain (moving away from the stimuli; grimacing, moaning, crying; restlessness; protecting the painful area; withdrawal)

Physiologic responses (*sympathetic responses when pain is moderate and superficial:* increased blood pressure, pulse rate, and respirations; pupil dilatation; muscle tension and rigidity; pallor; increased adrenalin output and blood glucose; *parasympathetic responses when pain is severe and deep:* nausea and vomiting; fainting–unconsciousness; decreased blood pressure and pulse rate; rapid and irregular breathing)

Affective responses (exaggerated weeping and restlessness, withdrawal, stoicism, anxiety, depression, fear, anger, anorexia, fatigue, hopelessness, powerlessness)

Possible Nursing Diagnoses

Pain
  Chronic Pain
  Ineffective Individual Coping
  Knowledge Deficit (effective pain management program)
  Powerlessness
(*Note:* Initially, pain must be viewed as a symptom and its physical etiology pursued. Interventions for pain done prior to an accurate assessment may mask the true cause of the patient's pain, thus causing further suffering and possibly even death by allowing the progression of signs, symptoms, and the disease process.)

Planning

The nurse designs a plan of care with the patient and family to achieve the following general patient goals:

The patient describes a gradual reduction of pain using a scale of 0 (no pain) to 10 (pain as intense as it can get)

The patient demonstrates competent execution of a successful pain management program

Appropriate goals for the patient with chronic pain:

The patient verbalizes (demonstrates) the ability to control pain sufficiently to manage—enjoy everyday living

The patient's family relates feeling better able to cope with the patient's pain experience.

Implementation

Establish a supportive and trusting nurse–patient relationship.

Teach the function of pain and instill confidence that a successful pain management program can be developed.

Remove or alter the cause of pain (whenever possible) and alter factors that decrease pain tolerance.

Use appropriate noninvasive relief measures: distraction, imagery, relaxation, cutaneous stimulation (massage, application of heat or cold, vibration, pressure)

Administer the prescribed analgesic; if a patient-controlled-analgesia unit (PCA) is being used, instruct the patient about its use.

Assist with the use of other pain therapies as appropriate: acupuncture, biofeedback, neurosurgery, electrical nerve stimulation

Evalation

The adequacy of the plan of care is determined by evaluating the patient's achievement of the preceding goals. If the patient is unable to meet key goals, the plan must be modified. Key evaluative criteria include:

Patient experiences adequate relief.

Patient is satisfied with the pain management program.

Patient feels sufficiently comfortable to attend to the demands of everyday living.

Analgesics are often used for pain control. Medications may mask symptoms, so a serious disorder goes undetected. On the other hand, if the person truly is having pain, withholding an analgesic can intensify pain. If a needed analgesic is withheld for too long, it may be ineffective when given. Some patients are allowed to administer their own analgesia through a patient-controlled analgesia (PCA) pump.

Some medications used currently for chronic pain improve the patient's mood, thus assisting in muscle relaxation. When muscles are more relaxed, pain improves and endorphin production is often increased.

The preventive approach is often appropriate for the patient in whom pain can be predicted (eg, after surgery or before a painful treatment). If medication is given before pain occurs, the pain is often prevented, a smaller dose is usually needed, and side effects of the medication are usually prevented. It is possible, however, to become habituated to the use of an analgesic. The nurse should be alert to this. Addiction is not a problem when medications are given for a short time.

Chronic Pain Syndrome

Chronic pain can be destructive to a person's life-style and outlook. The patient's initial reaction is often one of frustration and anger, but it may become difficult to express this anger because family and friends become tired of hearing about it. The more anger the patient feels, the more difficult it is to express true feelings. The patient may even begin to feel that no one believes the pain is real.

If the person is not allowed to express feelings, anger is suppressed or turned inward and causes depression. Symptoms of depression can include extreme fatigue, inability to sleep, lack of interest in surroundings, lack of appetite or excessive appetite, guilt feelings, sexual impotence, and withdrawal from social activities. The depressed person suffers from lack of self-esteem and may feel worthless or a burden to others. Severe depression may contribute to suicide and chemical dependency.

As pain continues, the person withdraws and becomes inactive. This physical inactivity aggravates the situation because muscles and joints become stiff and begin to deteriorate and endorphin production stops.

Intervention Into the Chronic Pain Cycle

The chronic pain syndrome should be recognized as early as possible so aggressive steps can be taken toward treatment. Each factor makes pain worse and fortifies the cycle. Intervention is aimed at breaking this cycle. It is most effective to aim treatment at the symptoms surrounding the pain because it may not be possible to stop the pain itself. Therefore, treatment is aimed at raising the patient's self-esteem and dealing with anger, guilt, and frustration. Characteristics of the chronic pain syndrome and suggested nursing approaches are given in Table 52-1.

> **Key Concept**
>
> Patient care and patient teaching should aim at breaking the cycle of chronic pain as early as possible in the process.

Patient Teaching

An important factor in assisting the patient to deal with chronic pain is education. The patient needs to learn to recognize signs of and control of muscle tension. The patient must be taught the importance of activity and exercise and needs encouragement to continue the exercise schedule. Helping the family to deal with pain is important. The person must be encouraged to share feelings and the family needs assistance to know how best to support the patient. The accompanying box presents keys for teaching the patient and family.

Surgical Intervention

Surgery may be effective in alleviating pain. For example, in low back pain with a herniated disc as the causative agent, the disc may be removed.

Passive Conservative Treatment

Treatment modalities that do not involve surgery are called *conservative treatment*. These may be active or passive. Several forms of passive treatment may be

---

Table 52-1. The Chronic Pain Syndrome

Characteristics	*Suggested Approaches*
Loss of control	Gain control over one part of life at a time; set intermediate goals and target dates
Decreased self-esteem	Participate in support groups, affirmations
Decreased communication (family members don't want to hear about pain anymore)	Talk to others with chronic pain; limit talking about pain with family to a specified length of time each day.
Inappropriate life goals (only goal in life is to get rid of pain)	Try to control pain so that normal life can be resumed (try for longer period of time each day)
Change in relationships; lack of sexual activity; changed roles within family	Attend family and marriage therapy; financial counseling; explain to children why life is changed and what activities can continue; encourage family activities
Family and friends become angry over need to "take care" of patient, do patient's work	Participate in family therapy; vocational counseling; try to find "worthwhile" job within capabilities
Decreased activity	Find alternative activities, hobbies, entertainment; vocational counseling
Decreased endurance	Build up strength gradually; find activities that are possible (walking, swimming, low-impact exercise)

used. These modalities do not involve action on the part of the patient. Examples include physical therapy, whirlpool and heat treatments, passive range of motion (PROM), the continuous passive motion (CPM) machine, and traction.

Active Conservative Treatment

Active conservative treatment requires participation on the part of the patient. This type of treatment carries the most potential for lifetime pain management. Modalities include exercise, biofeedback, and guided imagery.

Exercise. Specific body parts are exercised actively by the patient. It is important to increase activity level gradually to build up flexibility of joints and strength of muscles. The patient needs to know what activities are allowed so further injury does not occur. The activities must be varied and enjoyable because exercise will be required on a permanent basis to prevent regression.

The exercise and activity program is built to increase endurance gradually. The patient needs to understand that some pain may occur as muscles are exercised; it is important to know how much pain is safe. Activity levels are increased a little each day, pushing just beyond the discomfort level. This also helps stimulate endorphin production, as well as to increase endurance and abilities.

Biofeedback. Because muscle tension often causes pain, it is important for the patient to learn how to control this tension. A **biofeedback** unit may be used for this purpose. This device will indicate when muscles are tense; the patient then learns how to reduce tension. Eventually, the patient will be able to recognize signs of muscle tension without the machine and will be able to take active measures to reduce stress.

The TENS Unit. Physical stimulation is provided by the transcutaneous electrical nerve stimulation (TENS) unit. The patient wears the device and controls electrical stimulation when there is pain. This gentle electrical shock covers pain, allowing the muscle to relax. The shock also stimulates production of endorphins. The implantation of an electrode along the spinal cord, which is activated by the patient, has been more effective than external stimulators.

Deep Relaxation and Guided Imagery. The patient is taught self-hypnosis or deep relaxation. Then a suggestion (**guided imagery**) is given that helps control pain. For example, the suggestion may be that pain occurring over a large area of the body is moving down and out of the body. In this way, a smaller area can be involved; the eventual goal is to eliminate the pain entirely. (This procedure is also used with cancer patients, visualizing their body's defense cells as large and strong and the cancer cells as small and weak.) Patients with chronic pain are helped to visualize themselves as important, valuable, and contributing members of society. They are also taught to picture themselves as powerful and able to conquer pain. In addition, they are helped to change their perception of the pain so it is not as troublesome.

Group Therapy

Group therapy has proved helpful. This gives the person an opportunity to express feelings and to talk about pain with other people who will understand. Members of the group can often offer suggestions as to how they handled the same situations and concerns. Some groups offer financial or vocational counseling.

Usually the family can benefit from a support group as well. They can learn how to deal with the patient's concerns and how to be most supportive. If pain continues for some time, they can learn to deal with their own feelings about the situation.

Stress Management

Pain is aggravated if the patient has a great deal of stress. There are many ways to deal with stress. The person with chronic pain must be assisted with these coping mechanisms; he or she will probably need to seek alternate activities because of the physical limitations of pain. If the person is taught to be more assertive, stress is often reduced. Other measures are physical activity, recreational activities, and a well-balanced diet.

Some therapists use a program similar to the 12 steps of Alcoholics Anonymous. The first is "I am powerless over this pain." This has proved effective in many cases.

Keys for Review

Key Questions for Critical Thinking

1. Describe the kinds of questions you would ask to determine if the patient has acute or chronic pain. To determine the location of pain?
2. Explain the body's defense against pain.
3. Chronic pain is difficult to treat. Discuss why this is so.
4. You work in a nursing home. Many of your residents have chronic pain. Describe your basic plans and rationale for conservative measurement of these residents.

Key Readings

Craven RF, Hirnle CJ. Fundamentals of Nursing: Human Health and Function. Philadelphia, J.B. Lippincott, 1992

NANDA Nursing Diagnoses: Definitions and Classifications 1992. Philadelphia, North American Nursing Diagnosis Association, 1992

O'Toole M (Ed). Miller-Keane Encyclopedia and Dictionary of Medicine, Nursing, and Allied Health, Ed 5. Philadelphia, W.B. Saunders, 1992

Smeltzer SC, Bare BG. Brunner and Suddarth's Textbook of Medical-Surgical Nursing, Ed 7. Philadelphia, J.B. Lippincott, 1992

Key Readings (continued)

Watt-Watson JH, Donovan MI. Pain Management: Nursing Perspective. St. Louis, Mosby-Yearbook, 1993

Enrichment Keys

Burckhardt CS. "Chronic Pain." Nursing Clinics of North America 25(4), pp. 863–870, December, 1990

Nolan MF. "Pain: The experience and its expression." Clinical Management 10(1):22–25, 1990

Slack J, Faut-Callahan M. "Pain management." Nursing Clinics of North America 26(2), pp. 463–476, June, 1991

Keys to Learning More

Chapter 53: pain related to surgery

Unit Eleven: medications

Unit Fourteen: adult medical-surgical care

Chapter 85: geriatrics

Chapter 89: rehabilitation and home care

Chapter 91: hospice care, where pain is a major issue

Unit *10* Surgical Intervention

53 The Person Who Has Surgery

Keys for Learning

Learning Objectives

- Discuss classifications for determining high-risk patients.
- List the main types of anesthetics and describe the stages of general anesthesia.
- Discuss the importance of patient teaching related to surgery.
- List all the important preoperative nursing steps.
- Correctly demonstrate the procedure for preoperative skin preparation.
- State the function of the recovery room and describe equipment found there.
- Describe the specific measures to be carried out when the patient returns from the recovery room.
- List the possible immediate postoperative complications and the measures to be taken by the nurse to alleviate them.
- State the nursing measures to be taken to alleviate postoperative pain, thirst, nausea, distention, and urinary retention.
- Outline procedures for turning-coughing-deep-breathing, huffing, and using the incentive spirometer.

Key Terms

anesthetist	evisceration	positive Homan's sign
anesthesiologist	intraoperative	postoperative
atelectasis	invasive	splinting
dehiscence	perioperative	thrombophlebitis
embolus	pneumonia	

Keys to Understanding This Chapter

Chapter 5: basic human needs the person must meet in the perioperative period, with the assistance of the healthcare team

Chapter 8: microbiology background to study sterile technique and prevention of infections during and immediately after surgery

Keys to Understanding This Chapter
(continued)

Unit Four: knowledge of normal anatomy and physiology to recognize deviations

Unit Five: nutrition and diet therapy, an important part of postoperative treatment

Chapter 32: sudden death and cardiopulmonary resuscitation sometimes needed in the immediate postoperative period

Unit Nine: nursing skills used in administering care to all patients

Key Points

- Use of narcotics can cause serious side effects. Watch carefully for these side effects, especially respiratory depression.
- Preoperative teaching is your first line of defense against postoperative complications. Teaching also helps to make the patient feel more at ease during this stressful time.
- Before giving any pre- or postoperative medication, always check for drug allergies.
- Early complications include hemorrhage, shock, hypoxia, and hypothermia. Be alert for early indications of these complications and respond to them quickly.
- Follow appropriate steps to alleviate the patient's postoperative discomforts. Try to anticipate the patient's needs based on your assessments.
- Pulmonary hygiene is extremely important in the prevention of later postoperative complications.
- Following the physician's orders for early postoperative mobility will also help to decrease the possibility of respiratory or circulatory complications.

Key Learning Activities

◆ Interview a respiratory therapist or anesthetist about types of equipment and medications used and why these change.
◆ Make arrangements to visit a same-day surgery unit. Note any differences in patient care and discharge teaching/planning than with the hospitalized surgical patient, and develop a care plan that reflects those differences.
◆ Set up a patient's room to receive the postoperative patient.

A common treatment of disease or disorder is surgical intervention. It is called *intervention* because the surgeon actually intervenes in the disease process by operating on the patient's body to repair, remove, or replace body tissues or organs. Surgery is considered an **invasive** process because an incision is made into the body or a part is removed.

Perioperative nursing includes routine assessments and nursing interventions in each of the phases of surgery and should focus on specific nursing care related to the particular surgery that is being performed.

Perioperative Care

The term **perioperative** refers to the total span of surgery, including before and after surgery. Surgical nursing is concerned with assisting with surgery or other mechanical interventions in the disease process or with the care of the patient before or after that intervention. The three phases of surgical nursing are:

◆ **Preoperative** nursing care: before surgery
◆ **Intraoperative** nursing care: in the operating room and the postanesthesia recovery room or postanesthesia care room
◆ **Postoperative** nursing care: after surgery

Factors in Surgery

Surgery is performed in several different types of medical facilities. If the surgery is extensive or if the patient is classified as high risk, the patient will be admitted to a hospital for surgery. Some patients present a higher than normal risk when undergoing surgery. The physician must assess the situation and weigh these risks against the level of urgency of the surgery. The risk factors may be outweighed by the necessity of the surgery. Table 53-1 classifies risk factors.

A less complex or less dangerous procedure may be performed in a walk-in or ambulatory center, often known as a Surgi-Center. In the Surgi-Center the patient enters, has the procedure performed, and goes home the same day. The ambulatory center may be part of a physician's clinic, may be free-standing, or may be a department of a hospital.

Nursing Considerations

A variety of nursing diagnoses may be established for the perioperative patient and family. Several examples follow:

◆ Fear
◆ Knowledge Deficit
◆ Anticipatory Grieving
◆ Body Image Disturbance
◆ Aspiration
◆ Ineffective Airway Clearance
◆ Pain
◆ High Risk for Altered Body Temperature
◆ Hypothermia
◆ Altered Tissue Perfusion (cerebral, peripheral)
◆ Fluid Volume Deficit
◆ Impaired Tissue Integrity

Table 53-1. Factors in Assessing the High-Risk Patient

Category	Risk Factor	Possible Complications
Weight	Obesity	Poor healing (less circulation in fat tissue)
		Hypostatic pneumonia (less activity)
		More difficult surgery (more fat tissues to dissect)
	Undernutrition, malnutrition	Poor healing (lack of nutrients)
		Skin breakdown (less padding over body prominences, lack of protein)
Status of hydration	Dehydration	Reduced circulation (lack of tissue fluid, electrolyte imbalance)
	Edema	Reduced circulation (retention of fluids, pressure within tissues)
Electrolyte balance	Imbalance	Many complications, depending on specific electrolyte
Age	Very young	Respiratory problems (poorly developed lungs)
		Existence of congenital conditions may cause various complications
	Very old	Poor healing (reduced circulation)
		Skin breakdown (friable skin, bony prominences, poor circulation)
		Confusion (may be caused by anesthesia or change in routine)
		Hypostatic pneumonia (lack of activity, poor lung tissue turgor)
		Dehydration or undernutrition (poor eating habits, confusion)
Use of chemicals	Smoking	Lung disorders (inflammation, increased mucous production, diseased lung tissue, chronic bronchitis, etc)
		Circulatory disorders, such as blood clots or poor circulation atherosclerosis, hypertension (nicotine constricts blood vessels)
		Cardiac disorders, such as atherosclerosis in heart vessels
		Digestive disorders, such as peptic ulcer
	Chemical abuse	Withdrawal symptoms (caused by removal of substance)
		Addiction (less resistance to dependency because of abuse)
		Lung disorders or circulatory disorders (general poor health and poor nutrition)
Use of certain precription drugs	Depends on specific drug	Bleeding disorders, fluid retention, confusion, and many other complications
Preexisting physical disorders	Depends on disorder	Poor circulation, slowed healing, tendency to clotting, pulse disorders, retention of fluids (heart disorders)
		Hypostatic pneumonia, poor oxygen exchange (lung disorders)
		Slowed healing, increased incidence of infections, insulin imbalances (diabetes)
		Inability to regulate blood sugar levels (diabetes mellitus)
		Allergic reactions to anesthesia or medications (allergies, asthma)
		Inability to control seizures (seizure disorders, epilepsy)
		Slowed healing, high incidence of infections (immune disorders, diabetes, cancer chemotherapy)
Psychological status	Excessive fear	Difficulty in understanding instructions, pulse disorders, cardiac arrest, difficulty in achieving anesthesia
	Intellectual impairment	Inability to understand instructions, lack of follow-through (psychiatric disorders, dementia, mental retardation)

◆ Impaired Skin Integrity
◆ Impaired Physical Mobility

Several nursing interventions are common to all surgical procedures:

◆ Provide emotional support to patient and family.
◆ Prepare patient physically for the surgery.
◆ Make sure all legal matters, such as signing a surgical permit, are carried out.
◆ Provide patient and family teaching.
◆ Provide routine preoperative and postoperative care.

The time available for each of these interventions depends in large part on where the surgery is performed and whether or not it is an emergency procedure. If the procedure is performed as an elective procedure and if the patient is a hospital inpatient, the preparation and teaching time may be considerably longer than if the patient is brought in by ambulance and operated on as an emergency. Levels of patient choice in surgery are the following:

◆ *Optional/Elective:* The condition is not life-threatening. The patient may choose whether or not to have surgery. (Examples are face lift, removal of nonmalignant birthmark, and tubal ligation for sterilization.)
◆ *Required/Nonelective:* The surgery is necessary at some time. The patient may have some choice as to *when* the procedure will be done. (Examples are hernia repair and replacement of hip joint.)
◆ *Urgent/Nonelective:* The surgery must be performed within a day or two to prevent further damage to the patient. (Examples are removal of malignancy and removal of severely diseased appendix or tonsils.)
◆ *Emergency:* The surgery must be performed immediately to save the patient's life. (Examples are tubal pregnancy, severe internal hemorrhage, and ruptured appendix.)

Anesthesia

A physician trained in anesthesiology is called an **anesthesiologist**, and a registered nurse trained in anesthesiology is called a nurse **anesthetist**. A visit from the anesthesiologist or anesthetist before the operation gives patients an opportunity to ask questions that may be troubling them. It is pleasant, too, for patients to recognize someone when they come to the operating room.

Types of Anesthetics. Anesthetics are divided into two main classes: general anesthetics, which suspend all bodily sensations; and local, regional, or spinal anesthetics, which create insensitivity of specific body parts without causing unconsciousness.

General anesthetics are administered intravenously, rectally, or by inhalation. Abdominal or chest surgery is usually performed with the patient under general anesthesia, as are some orthopedic and many genitourinary procedures.

The less anesthetic used, the safer it is for the patient; thus, *local anesthesia* is preferred whenever possible. A local anesthetic may be administered topically or by injection. Common procedures performed under local anesthesia include dental work, many types of plastic surgery or skin suturing, and some eye surgery. Much brain surgery is done using local anesthesia.

> **Key Concept**
> Patients receiving local anesthetic are often given some type of sedation also.

Anesthetics most often given by *inhalation* are halothane (Fluothane), nitrous oxide, and cyclopropane. The patient is usually prepared for *inhalation anesthesia* by an intravenous injection of thiopental sodium (Pentothal), etomidate (Amidate), fentanyl citrate with droperidol (Innovar), ketamine hydrochloride (Ketalar), or propofol (Diprivan). The patient falls asleep, after which he or she is intubated and maintained on an inhalation anesthetic. Pentothal or methohexital sodium (Brevital sodium) is sometimes given alone for minor procedures. A drug called midazolam HCl (Versed) is frequently used to induce sleepiness and relieve anxiety, as well as for "conscious sedation" in procedures such as endoscopy. It often causes amnesia regarding the procedure as well.

Stages of General Anesthesia.[1] If a slow-acting drug is used, the patient passes through recognizable stages of general anesthesia. As the patient "wakes up" from the anesthesia these stages are reversed. The stages are:

1. *Stage of analgesia/amnesia:* reflexes present, heart rate normal, slower rate and increased depth of respiration, normal blood pressure, some dilation of eyes with reaction to light.
2. *Stage of dreams and excitement:* active reflexes, increased heart rate, irregular breathing, increased blood pressure, pupils widely dilated and divergent.
3. *Stage of surgical anesthesia:* involves four planes with third and fourth plane best for surgery. Progressive loss of reflexes, decreased heart rate, progressively depressed respirations until apneic, nor-

[1] Adapted from Patrick MJ, et al. Medical-Surgical Nursing: Pathophysiological Concepts. Philadelphia, J.B. Lippincott, 1991, p. 376.

mal to decreased blood pressure, constricted pupils to slightly dilated and centrally fixed.

4. *Stage of toxic or extreme depression*: no reflexes, weak and thready heart rate, respiration completely flaccid, decreased blood pressure, widey dilated pupils. (Danger stage.)

Key Concept

The anesthetized patient is completely dependent on others; he or she cannot control the most basic body functions, including breathing. It is vital that this person be closely observed and monitored *at all times*.

The accompanying box describes nursing care guidelines for the patient receiving anesthetics.

Preoperative Nursing Care

You will be asked to assist the surgical nurse in the care of preoperative patients. It is important to carry out preoperative orders exactly; they affect the success of the operation. The orders concern the physical preparation of the patient, but as you carry them out, remember the patient's feelings and need for reassurance. Many patients are admitted the day of surgery and often will not arrive on your unit until after surgery. In emergency surgery the preoperative period may be short. To the extent possible, emotional support should be provided all patients. The organization of preoperative nursing care is outlined in the accompanying box.

Nursing Alert

Be sure the patient has signed the operative permit *before* any presedation medications are given. Otherwise, it is illegal and the next-of-kin will need to be called for permission to operate.

Preoperative Checklist

The healthcare facility will have a preoperative checklist for you to use in your care of the patient. All the items must be checked off before surgery is performed. Each facility has its own version of the checklist. The list may be shortened if ambulatory surgery is done or if the patient is to have a local anesthetic. The box entitled "Organizing Preoperative Nursing Care" defines the items included in the checklist. If you have any questions about the checklist, consult your team leader.

Nursing Skill Guidelines
Providing Care for the Anesthetized Patient*

◆ It is vital to check for allergies before any patient has surgery or before administering any postoperative drug.

◆ Any abnormal laboratory results pre- or postoperatively must be brought to the physician's attention immediately.

◆ Extreme apprehension following the administration of preoperative medication *must* be brought to the attention of the surgeon immediately.

◆ The use of spinal anesthetics requires that the patient be kept flat until the anesthetic has worn off, sometimes up to 12 hours. It is also important to observe urine output very carefully and to watch for bladder distention.

◆ Watch carefully for signs of respiratory distress following the use of neuromuscular blockers or any type of general anesthetic. Be cautious with the use of postoperative narcotics because of the patient's decreased respiratory drive from anesthesia.

◆ When narcotics are being used, naloxone (Narcan) should be kept at an easily accessible location to reverse the effect in cases of severe respiratory distress or suppression.

◆ Watch carefully for signs of circulatory depression following the using of neuromuscular blockers or any general anesthetic.

◆ Neuromuscular blockers may potentiate when used with other central nervous system depressants, including alcohol.

◆ When an epidural or spinal anesthetic is used, be sure to keep Narcan at an easily accessible location for reversal of untoward effects, watch for respiratory depression, and safeguard the injection site. The same principles apply when the patient is receiving postoperative medication via these routes.

◆ When using topical anesthetics, watch for skin irritations. The eye blink reflex may be retarded by the use of eye anesthetics, causing the eyes to become dry.

◆ Many new anesthetics that have a short duration are being used currently. Patients may arrive on your unit much more alert than they have in the past. They require pain medication sooner than they did with some other anesthetics. Always be watchful for adverse effects, even with short-acting medications.

Kathleen McCullough, Hennepin County Medical Center, Minneapolis.

Surgery may need to be canceled if preoperative care is not performed correctly or if the nurse does not check off items accurately. A preoperative goal is to have the patient in the best possible physical and emotional condition for surgery. A well prepared patient is much more

Nursing Skill Guidelines
Organizing Preoperative Nursing Care

◆ Check the chart and note the preoperative orders.
◆ See that the operation permit is signed. This must be witnessed. (Nursing students should not witness legal papers of any type.)
◆ Prepare the operative area, as ordered.
◆ Check the patient's medical history for any essential respiratory, cardiac, or other drugs taken routinely. Notify the physician of these medications. The patient may need to take these despite NPO status.
◆ See that all specimens and blood samples have been collected and sent to the laboratory.
◆ Note and attend to any change in diet, as ordered.
◆ Give a sedative, if ordered
◆ Withhold fluids and foods, as directed. Usually, the patient is NPO before surgery.
◆ Give preoperative instruction and provide emotional support to the patient and the family.

Before the Operation

◆ Record temperature, pulse, and respiration (TPR), and blood pressure (BP). Report immediately to the nurse in charge any marked deviation from normal so that it can be reported to the physician.
◆ Make sure the patient's weight is recorded on the chart. (This helps to determine drug dosages.)
◆ Help the patient with bath and other hygiene measures. The patient must remove all clothes before going to surgery and wear only a clean hospital gown.
◆ Remove any prosthesis. Remove wigs, contact lenses, false eyelashes, glasses, and false fingernails.
◆ Remove jewelry and valuables and put them in a safe or give them to the patient's family. Be sure that the patient's wedding band is included with these unless the patient does not wish to remove it and it is securely bound or taped to the hand. Carefully document what is done with the valuables.
◆ Help the patient put on elastic stockings, if ordered.
◆ Have the patient void immediately before going to the operating room (OR). If the patient is unable to void, inform the charge nurse and document this fact on the chart.

◆ Remove hairpins. Long hair should be pulled back and covered with a surgical cap or a cotton towel. (Hair should be washed the evening before surgery, if possible.)
◆ Remove complete or partial dentures and place them in a denture cup with clear water. Label the cup and put it in a safe place, such as the drawer of the bedside table.
◆ Remove makeup or nail polish. (The anesthetic observes the nailbeds and lips, along with the oximeter.)
◆ Be sure that all items on the preparation checklist have been accounted for and that the list is signed and attached to the chart. Items to be included are identification band; permit; prep and shave; enema; blood work; urinalysis; temperature/pulse/respiration and blood pressure; dentures removed; contact lenses or glasses removed; jewelry removed or secured; the patient voided or catheterized; hairpins, makeup, and nail polish removed; NPO. The chart will be taken to the OR with the patient. (This checklist is usually completed by 6 AM if the patient is first on the OR schedule.) Some procedures may be carried out the previous evening, especially if the patient is scheduled for early surgery. In many cases, a student nurse is not allowed to do the final sign-off of the chart. Learn the hospital's rules.
◆ Preoperative medications are given, as ordered, after all personal care items are completed. This will help to ensure safety for the patient (who should not be active after taking a sedative) and it will enhance the effects of the medications.
◆ Be sure the side rails are *up* and the bed is in *low* position after medicating the patient.
◆ Be sure all preoperative charting is up to date and signed before the patient goes to the operating room.
◆ When the patient leaves for surgery, begin to prepare the unit for the patient's return postoperatively.

Note: Some procedures may be done in the OR area if the patient comes in on the morning of surgery.

---

likely to have successful surgery and an uneventful course of recovery, leading to optimum rehabilitation.

Key Concept

There is a reason for each step in preoperative preparation. If you omit any steps, you are jeopardizing the patient. Many of these steps will be done by the patient at home when admission is the day of surgery.

Emotional Support of Patient and Family

If this is the patient's first experience with surgery, the patient may be apprehensive. Most people fear pain; some are concerned about losing consciousness; and others are afraid they will die. Some are fearful of cancer or of being disabled. If the patient has had an operation before, he or she may compare the previous experience to this one. If the previous experience was difficult, the patient may be very frightened.

The patient or family may wish to speak with a spiritual advisor or with the hospital chaplain. You might help to arrange this meeting. The patient and family also often wish to meet with the surgeon before surgery, and the anesthetist or anesthesiologist usually visits the patient before surgery.

A thoughtful nurse will explain to the patient's family that the patient will be taken to surgery 30 minutes to an hour before the surgical procedure is scheduled. The family should also know that after surgery, the patient will be taken to the recovery room, where he or she will be observed by specially trained personnel until vital signs are stable and full consciousness returns. If the family understands these procedures, they will be less upset by the length of time the patient is gone. The nurse should also inform the family where they may wait for news. The patient may be transferred to another unit after surgery; in that case, the family must know where the patient will be.

One of the most helpful means of preparing the patient and family is to explain what will happen during and after surgery. If the patient understands procedures he or she will be more relaxed and cooperative. The patient should have a chance to practice exercises and use equipment, such as the incentive spirometer, before surgery. Equipment can be frightening and should be explained to the patient and family.

The patient and family need to know what to expect when the patient returns from the operating suite. If there will be equipment such as tubes, intravenous lines, or suction, they should know about this beforehand. Explain the preparation for the operation to the patient as you go along, and tell the patient how each step helps both patient and surgeon.

Preoperative teaching should concentrate on several major points, as listed in the accompanying teaching box. Methods of effective instruction should be followed.

◆ Organize your teaching.
◆ Explain what you are going to do.
◆ Demonstrate the procedure.
◆ Supervise the patient's practice.
◆ Reinforce successful behavior.
◆ Review the procedure.

If there are any patient questions that you cannot answer or equipment you do not understand, be sure to ask someone for help. Your confidence in equipment use will instill confidence in the patient.

Assessments

Observation. The patient must be observed carefully during preparation for surgery. Record in the chart and report to the team leader at once any unusual reactions or observations.

Keys to Patient/Family Teaching
Preoperative Teaching

Patient teaching preoperatively must include:

◆ Anticipation of patient questions and having answers for them
◆ Reason for special equipment by bedside
◆ How to turn in bed without assistance
◆ Discomforts to be expected and how to alleviate them
◆ Splinting of the incisional area
◆ Deep breathing exercises
◆ How to use the incentive spirometer
◆ Exercises to be performed postoperatively
◆ Amount and kind of ambulation allowed or expected following surgery
◆ Description of operating room or recovery room. (Sometimes, especially in the case of children, a tour of these areas is helpful.)
◆ Wound care
◆ Nutrition

Physical Examination and Laboratory Tests. Before the surgical procedure, the patient is given a complete physical examination. Admission vital signs recorded on the patient's chart are used as *baseline data* for comparison during the physical examination, during the surgery itself, and immediately postoperatively. The patient's weight is recorded on the chart in pounds *and* kilograms because dosages of medications, including anesthetics, are calculated on the basis of the patient's weight.

Routine preoperative tests often include chest x-ray examination, complete blood count (CBC), and urinalysis (UA) before surgery. Other tests and examinations are performed as needed. An electrocardiogram (ECG) is usually obtained on all patients over age 40. Blood is drawn for a "type and crossmatch" if there is any possibility that a blood transfusion will be needed because of blood loss during surgery. A bleeding–clotting test, such as the prothrombin time, is often ordered. The nurse notifies the physician of routine medications taken by the patient. Information on allergic reactions is necessary.

Skin Preparation

Skin preparation is important in preparing a patient for surgery. Because the skin is normally oily and harbors a multitude of bacteria, it must be cleansed properly to prevent wound contamination. The patient may be required to shower with antibacterial soap before surgery.

The skin is most often prepared early on the morning of surgery, except in an emergency. The skin is cleansed with an anti-infective agent and the area is shaved because microorganisms adhere to hair. This is

Overview of the Nursing Process
Preoperative Nursing Care

Assessment Priorities

Nursing History

Patient's understanding of the proposed surgical procedure (clarify any misperceptions)

Past experiences with surgery

Fears (fear of the unknown, fear of pain or death, fear of changes in body image of self-concept)

Factors that increase surgical risk or the potential for postoperative complications: 1) **Past and present illnesses:** cardiovascular diseases, pulmonary disorders, renal and liver function alterations, metabolic disorders (especially diabetes); 2) **medications:** anticoagulants, diuretics, tranquilizers, adrenal steroids, antibiotics; 3) **life-style factors:** nutrition (history of malnutrition or obesity); use of alcohol, nicotine, or recreational drugs; activity level

Adequacy of coping patterns and support systems

Pertinent sociocultural factors (eg, health beliefs and practices, economic concerns, cultural considerations, such as language barrier problems)

Physical Examination

Vital signs the morning of surgery (report any significant deviation from normal)

Accurate height and weight (medications may be calculated on the basis of these data, especially for children)

General systems review, noting in particular any new cardiopulmonary developments that place the patient at high risk for surgery

Results of all preoperative diagnostic tests are to be recorded in the patient's record and if abnormal, reported.

Possible Nursing Diagnoses

Anxiety
Ineffective Coping
Decisional Conflict
Fear
Anticipatory Grieving
Knowledge Deficit
Powerlessness

Planning

The nurse designs a plan of care with the patient and family to achieve the following general patient goals. Prior to surgery the patient:

Demonstrates physical preparedness for surgery (absence of significant deviations from normal in the vital signs, no signs of infection)

Verbalizes any concerns or fears related to the surgery

Provides *informed* consent for the surgery

Correctly demonstrates how to turn, deep breathe, use equipment (such as the incentive spirometer), and perform splint incision (when appropriate)

Verbalizes understanding of postoperative pain management program

Verbalizes understanding of postoperative activity plan

Implementation

Nursing actions to meet the patient's psychological needs

Establish a supportive and trusting nurse–patient relationship

Develop and implement a teaching plan that 1) familiarizes the patient–family with what to expect on the day of surgery. 2) prepares the patient to participate in the pain management program, and 3) enables the patient to state the purpose of deep breathing and to demonstrate it, as well as incentive spirometry, leg exercises, and turning in bed.

Counsel the patient–family about helpful coping strategies and available resources. At the patient's request, invite a spiritual counselor to see the patient.

Nursing actions to meet the patient's physical needs

Maintain nutrition and hydration; if the patient is NPO (nothing by mouth) for 8 to 12 hours prior to surgery, ensure that the patient understands the reason for this restriction and remove all food and fluids from the bedside.

Evaluate the patient's bowel status and determine the need for an order for bowel elimination. If a Foley catheter is ordered prior to surgery, explain its use prior to insertion.

Carry out preoperative skin and hygiene orders.

Facilitate sleep and rest in the immediate preoperative period.

Remember that many patients are not admitted until the morning of surgery. The nurse must then *teach* the above preoperative care.

Evaluation

The adequacy of the plan of care is determined by evaluating the patient's achievement of the preceding goals. If the patient is unable to meet key goals, the plan must be modified. Key evaluative criteria are:

Patient's physical preparedness for surgery

Patient's mental preparedness for surgery

Patient's understanding of and ability to participate in care postoperatively

An uneventful course of recovery.

known as a "surgical prep" (Fig. 53-1). Some patients are asked to shower first, using antibacterial soap.

Some hospitals have "prep teams" who do all the surgical preparations (preps). However, you should be acquainted with the procedure and be able to perform it if required.

Nursing Skill
Preparing the Patient's Skin for Surgery

Supplies and Equipment

Disposable razors or complete disposable prep tray
Waxed paper bag or plastic bag
Bath blanket
Antibacterial soap such as pHisoHex
Acetone or nail polish remover
Anti-infective agent (Betadine, or agent as specified)
Waterproof pads, such as Chux
Scissors
Cotton-tipped applicators
Gloves
Clean patient gown

Procedure

1. Check the physician's orders. Determine exact area to be prepped and any special instructions. You will be prepping an area larger than the incisional site. *(Rationale: This will allow for proper draping of the patient without contamination caused by touching an unprepared area.)*
2. Wash your hands and don gloves. *(Rationale: Minimize the risk of infection because the skin will be broken. You also need to protect yourself.)*
3. Assemble the equipment and take it to the bedside.
4. Introduce yourself and explain the procedure to the patient. *(Rationale: Minimize the patient's anxiety.)*
5. Close the patient's door or pull the bed curtains. Use a bath blanket to cover the patient. *(Rationale: Provide privacy.)*
6. Set up tray, using warm water.
7. Place waterproof pads on the bed.
8. Expose the area to be prepped. You may prep a portion at a time if the area is extensive.
9. Assess the skin condition of the patient. Report any redness, rash, lesions, or breaks in the skin before beginning the prep. *(Rationale: The surgery may be postponed or special precautions taken if any of these conditions exist. There is a greater risk of infection if the skin is not intact before surgery.)*
10. Clip long hair at the site with scissors. *(Rationale: Prevent pulling with the razor.)*
11. Moisten gauze or sponge with warm water, and dampen the skin. Lather with shaving soap. Allow the hair to soak in the soap for 3 to 4 minutes. *(Rationale: This softens the hair.)*
12. Shave the area carefully with firm strokes of the disposable razor, held gently at a 45° angle (Fig. 53-1).

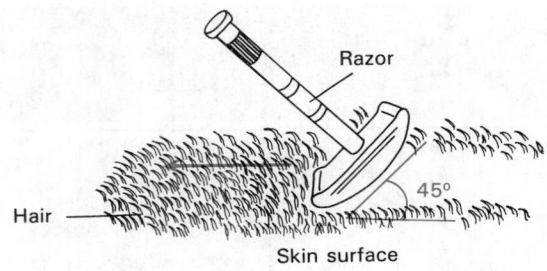

Figure 53-1. Shave in the direction of hair growth at a 45° angle.

13. Shave with the direction of hair growth. Avoid pressure on the razor, especially over bony prominences. *(Rationale: Avoid scratching or nicking the skin, which might open the area to infection.)*
14. If you do cut or nick the patient's skin, report it to your instructor or team leader immediately.
15. Rinse the razor frequently in clear water. Use a new razor if the razor becomes dull. Reapply soap solution as needed. Refill the basin with warm water as needed. *(Rationale: The hair must be kept moist.)*
16. Shave entire area, even if no hair is visible. *(Rationale: Ensure removal of fine hairs.)*
17. Rinse away excess soap and hair debris.
18. Scrub the area with an anti-infective soap (such as pHisoHex) for 10 minutes unless otherwise ordered. Scrub from the proposed surgical site outward to the periphery. Carefully scrub skin folds. Scrub the perianal or rectal area last. *(Rationale: Scrub from cleanest area outward.)*
19. Remove excess lather.
20. Cover the area with a thin film of anti-infective soap and allow to air dry, or pat dry with a sterile towel. If ordered, cover the site with a sterile towel or gauze.
21. Carefully inspect the skin at the completion of the scrub. Report any nicks or cuts immediately.
22. Cleanse the umbilicus with a cotton-tipped applicator. In some cases you may need to cleanse skin folds with an applicator as well. Use an orangewood stick for cleaning toenails and fingernails.
23. If surgery is to be performed on the hand or foot, clip nails. In some situations, as with a diabetic patient, a physician's order is required to clip the nails.
24. Remove nail polish, as ordered.
25. Make the patient comfortable. Be sure the call light is within reach. Instruct the patient as to the preservation of the scrub.
26. Wash your hands before leaving the room.
27. Discard all materials, according to your facility's protocols.
28. Wash your hands again after disposing of the supplies and equipment.
29. Report and document the time of the skin prep and the area prepared. Comment on the condition of the skin and reactions of the patient after the procedure was finished. Be sure to sign your name and title. *(Rationale: Documentation must be completed before the patient goes to the operating room.)*

Intestinal Preparation

Intestinal preparation will be in keeping with the physician's orders, the operation, the anesthetic, and the patient's condition. In many surgical procedures the intestinal tract should be as empty of feces as possible. The patient is usually given an enema to facilitate the surgery and to prevent intestinal distress. Be sure that the patient has expelled *all* of the enema. (An anesthetized patient may expel the remainder on the operating table.) The patient may also be asked to drink a polyethylene glycol-electrolyte solution, such as GoLYTELY, to cleanse the bowel. A large amount of GoLYTELY must be taken—as much as several quarts. The patient will need encouragement and positive reinforcement during this process.

Usually no food is given the morning of the operation and only a very small amount the night before, according to the individual requirements. (*Rationale: A patient is less likely to be nauseated or to vomit if the stomach is empty.*) If some vomiting does occur, aspiration into the lungs is less likely.

Key Concept

The patient may be asked to self-administer an enema at home. Usually sodium phosphate is used (Fleet phospho-soda). The patient may need instruction in the procedure or reassurance that he or she will be able to do the procedure.

Preoperative Medication

Three types of medications are used preoperatively: sedatives, narcotics, and drying agents. They are summarized in the accompanying key medications box.

Because the patient should have as much rest as possible before surgery, a *sedative* is usually ordered the evening before surgery. (It is usually a one-time order and is *not* PRN.) The sedative also helps to stabilize the blood pressure and pulse.

Key Medications
for Preoperative Care

◆ *Sedatives:* amobarbital sodium (Amytal), chloral hydrate (Noctec), ethchlorvynol (Placidyl), methotrimeprazine HCl (Nozinan), midazolam HCl (Versed), pentobarbital sodium (Nembutal Sodium), and secobarbital sodium (Seconal Sodium).
◆ *Narcotics:* alfentanil HCl (Alfenta), fentanyl citrate (Sublimaze), meperidine HCl (Demerol), morphine SO_4 (Morphine), and sufentanil citrate (Sufenta).
◆ *Drying agent:* atropine sulfate.

Nursing Considerations

◆ Observe for respiratory distress or bradypnea. These medications often are contraindicated in patients with severe respiratory disorder.
◆ Observe for inability to arouse patient, extreme lethargy or drowsiness, fatigue, oversedation.
◆ Observe for other central nervous system symptoms, such as dizziness, blurred vision, nightmares, ataxia.
◆ May potentiate action of oral anticoagulants and antihypertensive drugs.
◆ Elderly people or children may have opposite of desired reaction (paradoxical excitement).

On the morning of surgery, a preoperative *narcotic* is given to relax the patient and enhance the effects of anesthesia. It may be ordered for a specific time of day or "on call to OR." In the latter case, the medication is given when the operating room calls to have the patient transported to the operating room.

A *drying agent* is given to help inhibit body secretions so that less mucus is produced, and there is less likelihood of aspiration and atelectasis. Production of gastric and intestinal secretions is also reduced, so there is less abdominal distention postoperatively.

Key Concept

Before giving any preoperative medications, make sure the patient does not have any drug allergies and that the surgical permit has been signed and witnessed.

Before giving preoperative medications, explain to the patient the purpose of the drug and its probable effects. Once the narcotic has been given, explain to the patient that the side rails will be raised and that he or she must remain in bed and should request assistance to go to the bathroom. Explain to the family that the patient has been partially sedated and that, although they may stay in the room, they should not expect the patient to carry on a conversation. The patient should not smoke.

Key Concept

Be sure to offer the bedpan or urinal to the patient immediately before he or she is taken to the operating suite.

Transport of the Patient

If the patient is in the hospital preoperatively, the nurse should prepare the patient's room so the operating room staff can conveniently move the patient. Furniture should be moved so that the operating room cart can be put next to the bed, and all items should be taken off the bedside stand so they will not be knocked off. Make the patient as comfortable as possible. Make sure that the checklist on the chart is complete and signed; the chart will accompany the patient to the operating room where it will be given to the anesthetist or operating room nurse. Note on the front of the chart if the patient has any drug allergies or is taking cortisone, insulin, an anticonvulsant, or an anticoagulant. In most hospitals, a patient with allergies wears a special red name band, along with the regular one. Send a clean bath blanket with the patient.

Nursing Alert

To prevent errors, always be certain that the patient is properly identified before being taken to the operating room. *No* patient should be allowed to go to the operating room without an identification bracelet!

Intraoperative Nursing Care

Often the nursing student will observe in the operating room as a part of the student experience. This will not only give the nursing student a better idea of operating procedures, but will also help the student to understand the patient's feelings and apprehensions. Many graduate nurses are specially trained to work in the operating room or postanesthesia recovery room.

Nurses and surgical technologists assist the surgeons in the operating room. There are two basic categories of assistant, the *sterile assistants* and the *circulating assistants*. The *sterile nurse* (*scrub nurse*) is scrubbed, gowned, and gloved and functions within the sterile field. Duties include handing instruments to the surgeon, threading needles and cutting sutures, assisting with retraction and suction, and handling specimens.

The *circulating nurse* works outside the sterile field. Duties include opening packs and delivering supplies and instruments to the sterile team, delivering medications to the sterile nurse, labeling specimens, and keeping records during the surgical procedure; this person acts as a patient advocate by monitoring the patient and maintaining patient safety. In most cases the circulating nurse must be an RN.

Special Considerations in Aging
Perioperative Care

- ◆ Height and weight are used to calculate dosages of narcotics and anesthetics; the elderly are more susceptible to overdose.
- ◆ Baseline respiratory assessment is important because the elderly are more susceptible to aspiration pneumonia.
- ◆ Early mobility is important because they are more susceptible to disuse syndrome.
- ◆ Skin and body fat assessments are made because color, turgor, and temperature assessments are not always reliable.
- ◆ When moving and positioning, consider the patient's friable skin and fragile bones.
- ◆ Blood pressure and oxygen saturation are monitored because the elderly are more susceptible to hypertension or postural hypotension.
- ◆ Parenteral fluids may overload circulation because of decreased kidney function.
- ◆ Fluid and electrolyte balance changes more quickly.
- ◆ The elderly often have coexisting diseases.
- ◆ The patient should wear hearing aid and glasses if possible; be sure room is well-lighted.
- ◆ Patient may have poor peripheral vision; be careful not to startle.
- ◆ Patient may react differently to medications than expected; may have difficulty excreting medications.
- ◆ The elderly patient is more susceptible to postoperative urinary retention and constipation.
- ◆ The patient may be confused; teach in small "doses"; teach family.
- ◆ Offer to tape wedding ring in place.

Postoperative Nursing Care

The Recovery Room

Nearly all hospitals have a room or a suite set aside for the care of patients immediately after surgery. The room is variously called the recovery room (RR), postanesthesia recovery room (PAR), and postanesthesia care unit (PACU). In the RR the patient is carefully monitored until he or she is fairly recovered from the anesthesia.

Key Abbreviations and Acronyms for Perioperative Care

IV	Intravenous
NPO	Nothing by mouth
OR	Operating room
PACU	Postanesthesia care unit
PAR	Post anesthesia recovery
RR	Recovery room
TCDB	Turn, cough and deep breathe (hyperventilate)
TCH	Turn, cough, hyperventilate

This room is located next to the operating rooms so that physicians and nurses are quickly available when needed. Concentrating postoperative patients in a limited area makes it possible for one nurse to give close attention to two or three patients at the same time (Fig. 53-2).

In the RR are found all the articles that may be needed for care:

♦ *Breathing aids*: oxygen, suction equipment, nasal and oral airways, pulse oximeters, mechanical breathing bag or other resuscitation equipment, emergency equipment such as laryngoscopes, "trach" sets, endotracheal tubes

♦ *Circulatory aids*: blood pressure apparatus, stethoscope, intravenous solution, tourniquets, syringes and needles, cardiac monitors, cardiac arrest equipment, cardiac drugs and respiratory stimulants, and defibrillators

♦ *Drugs*: narcotics, sedatives, and drugs for emergency situations

♦ *Other supplies*: surgical dressings, sandbags, and various other items

Each patient unit has a recovery bed equipped with side rails, poles for intravenous medications, wheel brakes, and a chart rack. The bed can be moved easily and adjusted to elevate or lower the head or foot. The bedside stand holds tissues, emesis basin, tongue blades, face cloth, and towel. Each unit has outlets for piped-in oxygen, suction, and blood pressure apparatus.

> ### Key Concept
> In the case of ambulatory surgery, the patient may recover in a special reclining lounge chair.

Moving the Patient to the Recovery Room

When a patient is being moved to the RR, every effort is made to avoid unnecessary strain or possible injury and to accomplish the transfer as quickly as possible with the least exposure.

The anesthesiologist and circulating nurse go to the RR with the patient to make certain that the patient's condition is satisfactory.

The anesthetist or anesthesiologist is responsible for monitoring the patient's condition throughout the surgical procedure until that responsibility is transferred to the RR nurses. The anesthesia person reports the patient's condition to the nurse in charge and leaves postoperative orders and any special instructions required.

Occasionally, the nurse will be asked to care for the immediate postoperative patient in the patient unit. Before the patient arrives, the same equipment as would be found in the recovery room must be on hand.

Receiving the Patient in the Nursing Unit

When the patient is nearly awake, the RR staff should call the nursing station and report on the patient's condition, indicating what special equipment will be

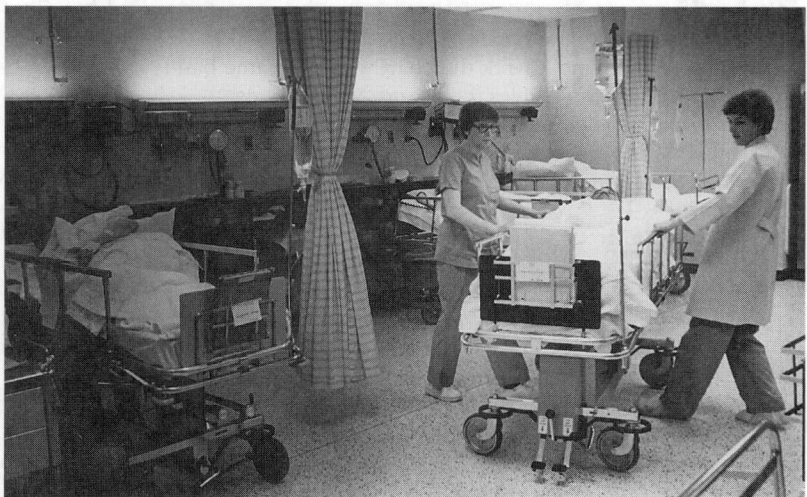

Figure 53-2. The recovery room is near the operating room, in case of emergency. Specially trained nurses assist and monitor patients until they are fully awake. Note the readily available wall suction, blood pressure, oxygen, and other equipment. (© Bistram Photography; photo courtesy of Unity Medical Center, Fridley, MN)

needed for the patient when he or she returns to the station. The nurse will then have time to prepare for the patient's arrival. The preparation of a room for a surgical patient includes opening the bed by pulling all the top linens to the foot or side of the bed (see Chapter 44). The furniture is arranged so that the patient can be easily transferred from the recovery room cart to the bed.

The nurse should also have on hand tissues, an emesis basin, a blood pressure cuff and stethoscope, rectal or tympanic thermometer, a frequent vital signs chart, an intravenous standard, and suction and oxygen equipment, if required.

When the patient arrives from the RR, the nurse should immediately check the vital signs to make sure they compare favorably with the readings obtained by the RR staff. A report will be brought from the recovery room with the patient. It is given by the RR nurse to the floor nurse.

When the patient is settled in bed, and after vital signs have been taken and all immediate orders carried out, the nurse should see that the patient's family is notified that the patient is back in the room. Although the family should not visit for long, they can help reassure the patient by spending a few minutes in the room.

Nursing Alert

No patient should be left alone until he or she has fully regained consciousness. Check the physician's orders and carry them out immediately.

Nursing Skill
Receiving the Patient From Recovery Room

Procedure

1. Carefully identify the patient. Check the name band with another nurse. Check the chart with the name band before the RR nurse gives the report. Wear gloves. *(Rationale: The patient is not fully conscious. It is important to make sure you have the correct patient. This patient has non-intact skin. You will be exposed to body substances.)*

2. Attach drainage apparatus, as ordered, for drainage from a cholecystostomy, catheters, or chest tubes before the RR nurse leaves. Attach gastric or other tubes to the appropriate suction device. *(Rationale: These items must be in proper working order. Chest tube suction must be operating properly **to maintain life.**)*

3. Keep the patient flat (often in Sims' position) until he or she wakes up (unless specifically ordered otherwise). Keep side rails up. *(Rationale: The semianesthetized patient could fall from bed.)*

4. Maintain an open airway. You can feel exhaled breath by holding your hand in front of the patient's nose. Just because the chest or abdomen is moving does not necessarily mean that the patient is breathing. Watch for any signs of respiratory distress. *(Rationale: Anesthesia and sedatives can upset respirations.)*

5. Carry out any order for immediate administration of drugs or oxygen. *(Rationale: This patient must be stabilized and made comfortable as soon as possible.)*

6. Assess patient for level of consciousness or ability to move extremities, in the case of spinal anesthesia. *(Rationale: This is part of your ongoing assessment and documentation.)*

7. Take vital signs as ordered. Blood pressure is usually taken often for the first hour and gradually less often, if it is stable. Be sure to watch for signs of shock, such as restlessness or panic. Check temperature every 2 to 4 hours. *(Rationale: The immediate postoperative period can be the most dangerous. Changing blood pressure and pulse are the first indicators of difficulty.)*

8. Inspect dressings; note signs of hemorrhage and any unusual amount of drainage. If necessary, reinforce but *do not change* dressings. Notify the team leader of unusual drainage. *(Rationale: The physician may wish to see the character of the drainage; the dressing may be weighed to determine exact blood loss. Removing the dressing might upset the suture line.)*

9. If vomiting occurs, turn the patient's head to the side. *(Rationale: This helps to empty the mouth, thus preventing aspiration.)* Use the emesis basin to catch the emesis. Check to see if antiemetics can be given. *(Rationale: The emesis basin is specially shaped to fit around the neck. Excessive vomiting should be prevented.)*

10. If the patient retches excessively, check to make sure the dressings and incisions are intact and suction equipment is operating properly. *(Rationale: The quick and violent movements of vomiting can interfere with the suture line. The stitches or staples can rip out. If vomiting occurs, it may mean the suction is not operating properly.)*

11. Measure emesis; note on the chart the time, amount, and nature of the emesis. Report it to the nurse in charge. Save the emesis if it appears unusual. *(Rationale: This is important information for the physician.)*

12. If the patient is receiving intravenous fluids or blood, check the rate of flow and the time for the next bag. Make sure that the needle is in the vein. Check intravenous site for swelling or redness. *(Rationale: It is important to maintain a patent [open] IV for adequate hydration and in case emergency medications must be given. Swelling or redness are signs of IV infiltration—see Chapter 57.)*

13. Discard gloves. Wash your hands. *(Rationale: You have been exposed to the patient's body substances.)*

14. Record intake and output. This includes any oral and intravenous fluids, as well as drainage, voiding, and emesis. *(Rationale: An accurate record of intake and output is necessary. The patient must be rehydrated.)*

15. Document all treatments and patient reactions. Be sure to include level of consciousness or returning sensation in extremities. *(Rationale: This provides continuity of care.)*

Immediate Postoperative Complications

The nurse should observe the patient immediately postoperatively for complications, including hemorrhage, shock, inadequate oxygen, and hypothermia.

Hemorrhage

Hemorrhage at the time of surgery causes shock and indicates the need for blood transfusions or other fluid replacement. Usually, the patient's blood is routinely typed and crossmatched before surgery so that compatible blood will be available. Prompt action is necessary because excessive bleeding could be rapidly fatal.

Secondary hemorrhage sometimes occurs after the patient returns from surgery; consequently, the wound dressing should be inspected frequently. If you note bleeding, report it. Be sure to look *under* the patient. (Blood may pool there.) However, concealed bleeding, also called occult or internal bleeding, is revealed mainly through the signs of shock.

Shock

The type of shock that is most dangerous after surgery is known as *circulatory or hypovolemic shock.* It is most frequently associated with severe hemorrhage. In severe hemorrhage the blood supply to peripheral blood vessels is reduced. Circulation becomes insufficient and the blood is unable to carry out its normal functions.

The nurse should be on constant alert for signs of shock, as listed in the accompanying box.

If shock occurs, the nurse provides the following care:

♦ Control hemorrhage (use direct pressure, if needed).
♦ Put the patient in the Trendelenburg position, unless contraindicated. Elevate the lower part of the body so that patient's feet are higher than the head (*unless the patient has had brain surgery or spinal anesthesia, in which case he or she should be kept flat*). (*Rationale: The Trendelenburg position helps drain blood out of the feet and legs, thus providing more blood for the brain.*)
♦ Supply heat sufficient to keep the body at a normal temperature. (*Rationale: The temperature can drop very quickly in shock.*)
♦ Give oxygen and drugs as ordered by the physician.
♦ Administer blood, plasma, or other parenteral fluids as ordered by the physician. (*Rationale: Restore fluid balance.*) *Parenteral* means by injection, rather than by way of the gastrointestinal tract. Electrolytes will probably be added to the intravenous line to restore electrolyte balance as well.

Signs of Shock

♦ Drop in blood pressure (systolic below 90 in adult means possible shock; below 80 means actual shock)
♦ Narrowed pulse pressure (the heart beats faster and less effectively)
♦ Restlessness and anxiety
♦ Extreme thirst
♦ Cold, moist, pale skin
♦ Drop in body temperature
♦ Increased pulse rate (rapid and weak or thready)
♦ Deep, rapid, gasping respirations (air hunger)
♦ Complaints of ringing in the ears and spots before the eyes
♦ Pallor or blueness (cyanosis) of the lips, nailbeds, gums and conjunctiva (dark-skilled persons also show pallor or blueness, or a dusky gray, as compared to their natural skin tone)

♦ The physician may order vasopressor drugs. (*Rationale: Increase blood pressure.*)

Hypoxia (Hypoxemia)

Anesthetics and preoperative medications sometimes depress respirations and interfere with oxygenation of the blood, causing a condition known as hypoxia. Mucus blocking the trachea or the bronchial passages also lowers the amount of oxygen entering the lungs. Oxygen and suction equipment should always be on hand for emergency use. Hypoxia is discussed in more detail in Chapters 79 and 80. Symptoms of hypoxia include dyspnea, rapid pulse, initial elevated blood pressure, and then cyanosis and lowered blood pressure, dizziness, and cyanosis.

Treatment for hypoxia includes administering oxygen and placing the patient in the Trendelenburg position (head lowered, feet elevated). Many patients today are monitored with the pulse oximeter. The physician orders the minimum acceptable oxygen concentration (usually about 95%). The following are nursing skills in applying and monitoring the pulse oximeter.

♦ Choose the sensor appropriate for the patient's size. (*Rationale: Inappropriate size may cause inaccurate results.*)
♦ Choose the appropriate location. The adhesive sensors and finger clip sensor for adults can be placed on the index, middle, or ring finger. All adhesive sensors can also be placed on a toe unless the patient has decreased circulation in the lower extremities. There is also a small earlobe clip for use on infants. The neonate adhesive sensor may also be placed on the foot.
♦ Before applying the sensor, use an alcohol wipe on

the site. (*Rationale: Make sure the site is clean and dry.*)

♦ Remove any fingernail polish or acrylic nails on the fingers to be used. (*Rationale: They could interfere with the reading.*)

♦ If you have any doubts about the site chosen, check the proximal pulse and capillary refill. Capillary refill is checked by pressing on the patient's skin. The normal color should return *immediately* when pressure is released. (*Rationale: Decreased circulation could skew oxygen saturation readings.*)

♦ Check the sensor's markings to make sure the light-emitting diode and photodetector are correctly aligned. They should be opposite each other. (*Rationale: If they are not aligned, the sensor will give an inaccurate reading.*)

♦ Attach the sensor to the patient cable and turn it on. You should have a digital read-out or lightbar to show your readings and alarm settings (Fig. 53-3). The type will depend on your facility's monitor.

♦ Always make sure the alarms are on before you leave the patient. The monitors come with preset limits. The limits can be changed per physician's order or your facility's policy. If you turn off the monitor, the alarm limits will default back to the original settings.

♦ The pulse oximeter will give audible and visual alarms. You can silence the audible alarm for 60 seconds at a time by pressing "audio alarm off." It will reset after 60 seconds.

♦ Move an adhesive sensor every 4 hours and clip type every 2 hours. Watch for signs of tissue breakdown or irritation from adhesives or clips. (*Rationale: Prevent tissue necrosis.*)

♦ In the patient's chart, document the oximeter readings and location of sensor. Notify your instructor or team leader of any changes in readings of over 5%.

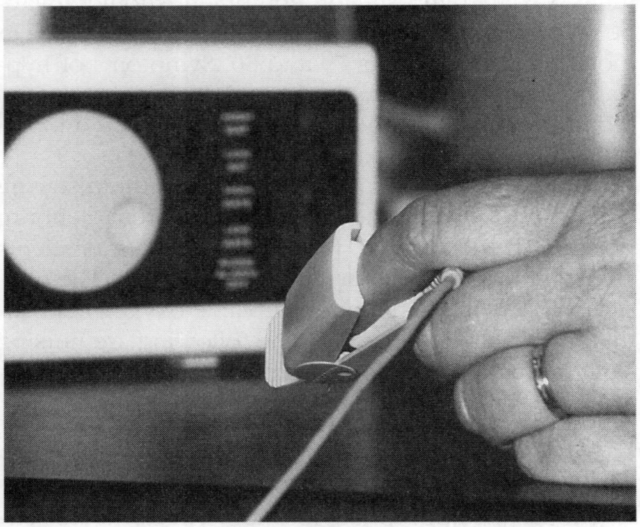

Hypothermia

Patients often complain of feeling cold after surgery. This can cause hypoxia and cardiac stress if severe enough. Significant signs and symptoms of hypothermia are:

♦ Temperature below 97.5°F (36.4°C) *rectally*
♦ Shivering and "goose flesh"
♦ Patient complaints of being extremely cold

Apply warmed blankets and give oxygen by means of a heated nebulizer. This raises core temperature.

Nursing Alert

Heated oxygen administration is contraindicated in patients who have had ear, nose, or throat surgery or who have chronic obstructive pulmonary disease.

Postoperative Discomforts

By the time the patient has returned from the recovery room to the ward or room, he or she is usually awake and fully aware of a number of discomforts. Medications used for postoperative complications are summarized in the accompanying medications box.

Pain. Pain usually is the first postoperative discomfort the patient will notice. The competent nurse is wise enough to know the value of sufficient medication to ease pain. If the patient receives medication early and subsequent doses are spaced properly, he or she will be kept relatively comfortable. Make sure the patient is conscious and vital signs are stable before giving pain medication so that respirations are not depressed and the patient is not put in unnecessary danger. Pain medications used are frequently narcotics similar to those given preoperatively, in addition to analgesics such as ibuprofen. Chapter 52 describes ways to assist a patient to manage pain.

Thirst. Thirst is present postoperatively, usually because of a decrease of fluids preoperatively, loss of fluids during surgery, anesthetic recovery, and dryness

Figure 53-3. The pulse oximeter measures oxygen levels in the patient's circulating blood. The oximeter shown here is applied to the finger with the sensing unit over the fingernail. The reading is shown as a digital readout on the machine shown in the background and is expressed as a *percentage of oxygen saturation.* Usually, the goal is to maintain patients at approximately 95% or better oxygen saturation. (Photo by Kimberly Malcolm)

Key Medications
for Postoperative Care

Postoperative Nausea

♦ benzqinamide HCl (Emete-con)
♦ cyclizine lactate (Marezine)—given preoperatively to prevent postoperative vomiting
♦ prochlorperazine (Compazine, Stemetil)—also given for postoperative nausea; available in injectable, syrup, rectal suppository and sustained-release tablet forms
♦ trimethobenzamide HCl (Tebamide, Tigan)—also given to prevent emesis—available in capsules, injectable and suppositories

Postoperative Constipation

♦ Various forms of docusate, a stool softener (Surfak, Kasof, Colace, Diocto, Regutol, Stulex)
♦ magnesium citrate (Citroma), magnesium hydroxide (Milk of Magnesia, MOM), magnesium sulfate (Epsom Salts)
♦ psyllium (Metamucil, Siblin)—chewable pieces, effervescent powder, granules, powder, wafers

Nursing Considerations: Antinausea Medications

♦ Allergy may cause anaphylaxis
♦ Side effects include drowsiness, dizziness, lethargy, dry mouth and respiratory passages, orthostatic hypotension, constipation
♦ May aggravate glaucoma

Nursing Considerations: Laxatives and Stool Softeners

♦ May stimulate gastrointestinal motility (avoid gastrointestinal bleeding, obstruction, perforation)
♦ Elderly patients may have extrapyramidal side effects (see Chapter 87) to any medication or may react oppositely (paradoxical reaction)

lation soon after an operation helps the patient to expel flatus. Small amounts of solid food also help.

Key Concept

If a patient is complaining of distention or "gas pains," do not give ice or allow the patient to take fluid through a drinking straw.

If discomfort increases and nursing measures do not bring relief, the physician usually orders one or more of the following: heat applied to the abdomen; insertion of a rectal tube; or intramuscular injections of neostigmine (Prostigmin), a drug that stimulates peristalsis. The nurse assesses the patient for the presence of bowel sounds on each shift. This is done by listening to the patient's abdomen with a stethoscope (see Chapter 46).

If intestinal paralysis persists, a serious complication known as *paralytic ileus* may develop. In that case, a nasogastric tube is inserted.

Nausea. If the patient complains of nausea, medication should be given to prevent emesis. Often these are given intramuscularly. See the accompanying box.

Urinary Retention. It is important to check voiding in the new postoperative patient because some patients have difficulty voiding. The nurse can aid the patient in voiding by assisting the patient to sit upright, pouring warm water over the vulva, placing the hands in warm water, and just running water so that the patient can hear it. If the patient has not voided within 8 to 12 hours of surgery, catheterization, as ordered, will bring relief. Intake and output should be recorded accurately for all new surgical patients.

caused by the drying agent (such as atropine). Most patients receive fluids intravenously during surgery and immediately postoperatively. This helps to prevent thirst, as does rinsing the mouth. Most physicians allow sips of water or ice chips in small amounts soon after surgery.

Distention. Temporary paralysis of intestinal peristalsis allows gas to accumulate in the intestine and causes distention. Normal peristalsis is disturbed by handling of the intestines during a surgical procedure, by anesthesia and drugs used during surgery, by the lack of solid food, and by restricted body movements. Accumulated gas (flatus) causes sharp pains that often are more distressing than the pain of the incision. Ambu-

Constipation. Disruption of the normal diet and the daily elimination schedule, pain medications, and inactivity may cause constipation. Usually, the routine postoperative orders will include a medication to prevent this complication. Nursing measures to help prevent constipation include encouraging fluid intake (particularly fruit juice), assisting the patient to sit up on the commode or bedpan, and promoting ambulation. Medications may help (see the box).

Restlessness and Sleeplessness. The patient may be restless and have difficulty sleeping. Every effort should be made to relieve these symptoms by ordinary nursing measures. Medications to promote sleep and relieve pain also play an important part.

Prevention of Later Postoperative Complications

Attention to preventive measures, improvements in medical practice, and early ambulation have all gone a long way toward eliminating the hazards that once accompanied an operation. Preoperative patient instruction is important in preventing postoperative complications.

Respiratory Complications

The principal respiratory complications following surgery are pneumonia and atelectasis. **Pneumonia** results from an infection of the lungs or from accumulated fluid. This can happen as a result of the inhibition of normal clearance mechanisms (such as coughing) caused by anesthesia. This is also called *hypostatic pneumonia*. **Atelectasis**, the collapse of a portion of the lung caused by plugs of mucus closing bronchi, causes acute and severe symptoms that may be aggravated by inactivity. Patients often are reluctant to cough or breathe deeply because of incisional pain. The patient may become somewhat cyanotic and respirations and pulse may become very rapid as he or she struggles to obtain oxygen. The nurse should assess lung sounds at least once per shift (see Chapter 50).

Exercises and Breathing Techniques. Respiratory complications can be reduced or eliminated by performing respiratory exercises or treatments such as deep breathing, coughing, chest percussion, and the incentive spirometer. Some of these exercises are explained in the accompanying box of guidelines. Ambulation if also encouraged.

Splinting or supporting the operative area with a pillow, folded bath towel, or blanket, during coughing exercises is an important part of postoperative care of patients after chest or abdominal surgery. Splinting is shown in Figure 53-4. The patient's willingness to cough can be greatly increased by the nurse who can gain the patient's confidence and who can make the procedure as comfortable as possible. The key is to explain the procedure in advance and gain the patient's cooperation and assistance. The turn, cough, and deep breathe procedure (TCDB), formerly called turn, cough, and hyperventilate (TCH) procedure, the huffing procedure, and the incentive spirometer procedure are in the box.

Deep breathing is aided by use of the incentive spirometer, which forces the patient to concentrate on inspirations and is less hazardous than TCH. It also gives the patient immediate feedback.

Incentive spirometers come in two types, flow-activated and volume-activated devices. The *flow-activated* incentive spirometer usually consists of one or more balls in a vertical tube. Because deep breaths (volume) are the objective, the length of time the patient suspends the ball at the top of the tube determines the depth of the breath. *Volume-activated* devices come in many shapes, but because they measure volume directly, they make it easier for the patient to understand when he or she has accomplished a deep breath. Figure 53-5 shows the incentive spirometer in use.

> ### Key Concept
> Any of the breathing exercises will be more effective if they can be taught and practiced preoperatively.

Circulatory Complications

Thrombophlebitis and emboli are two of the more serious circulatory complications that can develop after surgery. **Thrombophlebitis** is the formation of a blood clot in a vein. It is caused by *venous stasis* (the slowing or stopping of the return flow of venous blood as a result of increased clotting), lack of activity, increased pressure within vessels, and other factors. It most often develops in the calf of the leg.

If thrombophlebitis does occur, the following supportive measures may be ordered:

- ◆ Elevate the affected body part.
- ◆ See that the patient gets bed rest.
- ◆ Administer anticoagulants as directed.
- ◆ Avoid rubbing the body part.
- ◆ Apply warmth as directed.

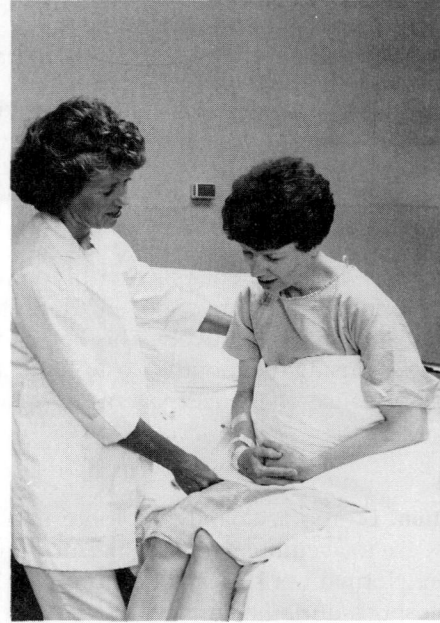

Figure 53-4. The abdominal or chest incision is splinted by holding a pillow or folded bath blanket and pulling it tightly against the incision. This helps to make coughing or deep breathing more comfortable and promotes better oxygenation.

Assisting the Patient With Postoperative Exercises

♦ The postoperative patient will be better able to perform these exercises if they were taught in the preoperative period.
♦ Wear gloves for these procedures
♦ Explain the procedures before assisting with them.
♦ Document all procedures and results.

Splinting an Incision

♦ The idea of the procedure is to relieve pressure on the abdominal suture line, and thus, to relieve pain.
♦ The patient should be braced while lying or sitting on the bed.
♦ A pillow, folded bath blanket, or large towel is used as a splint to distribute pressure evenly across an incision. The nurse can assist the patient to hold the splint for the first few postoperative days. The patient will be able to hold it after that.
♦ The pillow or bath blanket is grasped at the edges and stretched across the incision. The nurse can hold from behind.
♦ Pressure is applied by firmly pushing down on the splint (for the patient who is lying in bed) or by pulling the splint toward you from behind (when the patient is sitting). This should be done during the patient's cough.
♦ The nurse should anticipate the timing and strength of each cough. This can be done by counting aloud and by feeling the movement of the patient's breathing as the patient prepares to cough.

Turning, Coughing, and Deep Breathing (TCDB)

♦ Instruct the patient to take a deep breath and hold it for 2 to 5 seconds. (Rationale: This allows the air to reach the most severely deflated areas of the lung.)
♦ Instruct the patient to then do a strong double cough with the mouth open. (Rationale: This helps the patient mobilize and remove secretions.)
♦ Repeat this process several times each hour, especially for the first few days postoperatively and while the patient remains bedridden. At first, this must be done 24 hours a day.
♦ This process may be ordered to be done during times when the patient is awake, after the first few days postoperatively. (Rationale: The patient is now more active and the chance of respiratory complications is decreased; the patient needs uninterrupted rest.)

Huffing

♦ Instruct the patient to take a deep abdominal breath and then force it out in several short, quick breaths.
♦ The patient then takes a second, deeper breath and forces it out in short panting movements.
♦ The third breath is still deeper and is exhaled quickly in a strong "huff." The combination of these three breaths constitutes one huff. (Rationale: This series may help to loosen more secretions than just coughing.)

♦ This series is repeated as many times or for as long a time as is ordered.

Using the Incentive Spirometer

♦ Position the patient in the most upright position possible without discomfort. (Rationale: This allows better use of the diaphragm.) Figure 53-5 illustrates the use of the incentive spirometer.
♦ Explain the operation of the particular spirometer to the patient. Set a goal—number of seconds or a specific volume—to be attained. Mutually agree on the number of times and how often the procedure is to be done. Follow physician's orders.
♦ Have the patient cough to remove as much mucus as possible before the treatment.
♦ Instruct the patient to take slow, deep breaths and to hold the breath at the end of inspiration for 2 to 5 seconds. (Rationale: This allows the air to reach the most severely deflated areas of the lung.)
♦ The procedure should be repeated until the patient has achieved the goal or given his or her best effort at least 8 to 10 times. The nurse must take care to make certain that the patient does not repeat the process too rapidly. (Rationale: This may produce the unwanted effect of hyperventilation.)
♦ Coughing or huffing should be repeated at the end of the procedure. (Rationale: To clear the lungs as much as possible.)
♦ Be sure to wash your hands thoroughly following the procedure. (Rationale: To protect yourself and other patients.)

Leg Exercises

♦ Position the patient in a semi-Fowler's position.
♦ Bend the knee and raise the foot. Hold for a few seconds.
♦ Extend the leg and lower it to the bed.
♦ Do this five times with each leg. (Rationale: To help maintain muscle tone for ambulation and to decrease venous stasis.)
♦ Trace circles with the feet by bending them down, in toward each other, up and then out. Repeat this five times with each foot. (Rationale: To promote circulation and contribute to optimal respiratory exchange.)
♦ Position the patient in a side-lying position.
♦ Flex and extend the hip joint by using a bicycling motion. Repeat this five times on each side.
♦ Encourage the patient to exercise the legs as much as possible when in bed.

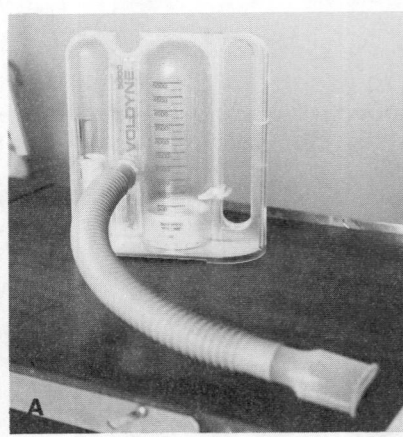 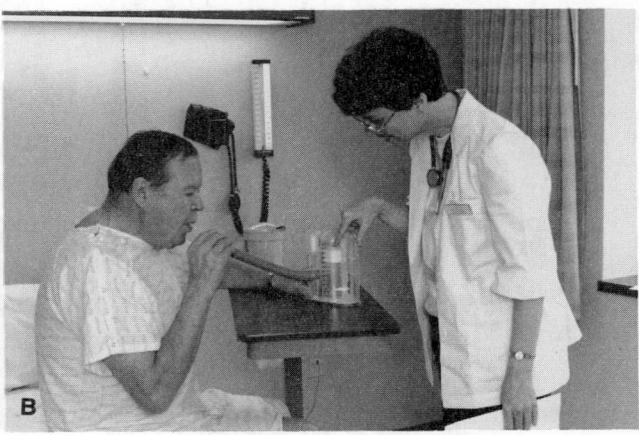

Figure 53-5. Incentive spirometers. **A:** Flow-directed incentive spirometer. **B:** Patient using incentive spirometer. Teach the patient how to use the device and to use it regularly. Immediate feedback regarding effectiveness is provided by the machine. (Source: Craven RF and Hirnle CJ. Fundamentals of Nursing: Human Health and Function. Philadelphia, J.B. Lippincott, 1992)

An **embolus** occurs when a piece of a clot or thrombus breaks off and enters the circulatory system, usually ending up in the lungs and causing such serious complications that death may follow. Symptoms of embolism depend on its location. Common symptoms include severe pain, nausea and vomiting, and severe shock. If the embolism is in an arm or leg, circulation distal to the embolus is often cut off, with related symptoms, such as numbness and absence of pulses. Gangrene, requiring amputation, may also result.

Avoiding Circulatory Disorders. One means of avoiding circulatory disorders is to apply elastic stockings, elastic roller bandages, or antiembolic stockings as ordered by the physician (see Chapter 48). Other nursing measures used to prevent circulatory disorders include leg exercises every 2 hours (see box), complete range of motion every shift, and ambulation as soon as possible after surgery.

Assessing for Thrombophlebitis. The nurse flexes the patient's foot up toward the knee (dorsiflexion) with the leg straight, as a means of evaluation for the presence of thrombophlebitis. If pain occurs behind the knee on dorsiflexion, this is known as a **positive Homan's sign** and must be reported immediately.

Complications of Bed Rest. Dangers of prolonged bed rest include respiratory and circulatory complications, development of pressure sores, generalized edema, contractures, osteoporosis, difficulty in weight bearing and balance, formation of renal calculi, scrotal edema, constipation, loss of appetite, and general mental depression and disorientation. Thus, the sooner the patient can move about after surgery, the better.

The patient will at first merely dangle the legs over the edge of the bed, then sit in a chair, and finally walk. Early ambulation, sometimes on the day of surgery, assists circulation, improves respiration, prevents lung congestion, and aids in voiding and bowel activity. It promotes better eating and sleeping patterns, encourages the patient to be more self-sufficient, and provides tangible evidence to the patient that he or she is making a quick recovery and that things are going well.

Ambulating and Positioning. Patients should be ambulated as soon as possible after most surgical procedures. The specific procedures for assisting the patient to dangle, to move from bed to chair, to walk, and to use crutches or a walker are described in Chapter 43.

Other Complications

Wound Infection. A temperature elevation occurring 2 or 3 days after surgery, severe pain, and redness and swelling around the incision are usually signs of a wound infection. Staphylococcal organisms persist widely; nurses must be ever vigilant to prevent infection from spreading. The nurse assesses the wound at least every 4 hours and documents the findings. Sterile technique and careful handwashing are important when changing dressings. The nurse also wears gloves and carefully disposes of all waste materials, according to universal precautions.

Treatment includes administration of antibiotics, increased fluids, rest, and an adequate diet to build up resistance. If necessary, the wound is drained. In some cases, the wound is cleaned or flushed with a solution (wound irrigation).

Wound Dehiscence. If the surgical incision separates or opens, this is referred to as **dehiscence**. Prompt action must be taken to prevent evisceration of abdominal contents.

Wound Evisceration. Evisceration is a serious complication of abdominal surgery. In this event, the edges of the wound separate and the abdominal organs protrude. Usually the patient will describe this sensation by saying "something gave." The condition is not common, but the nurse must be prepared to deal with it. The most a nurse can do is to cover the protruding organs with sterile gauze that have been wet with sterile normal saline and to lose no time in reporting the incident. The greatest dangers from evisceration are infection, rupture or strangulation of the intestine, and hemorrhage. Patients at risk for evisceration include persons whose wounds do not heal well, such as those with diabetes mellitus, elderly persons with friable (fragile) skin, people who are morbidly obese, and persons with invasive cancer of the abdomen.

Additional Supportive Measures

Providing Adequate Nutrition. The patient needs to have adequate food and fluids as soon as possible following surgery. Most people who have uncomplicated surgery can function adequately on intravenous therapy for a short time. The person should resume oral intake as quickly as possible. Usually, the patient will be started on a progressive diet. First a clear liquid diet is offered, then a full liquid diet, and finally a soft or general diet. Generally speaking, the sooner the patient can tolerate food, the sooner he or she will begin to recover in other ways.

Certain categories of patients require more extensive dietary therapy and should be evaluated by a dietitian, in cooperation with the physician. Special attention should be given to the person who is:

- Frail and elderly
- Obese
- Severely underweight
- Diabetic
- Suffering from a malabsorption disorder
- A victim of anorexia nervosa or bulimia
- Diagnosed as having a defect in digestion
- Running a high fever for any length of time
- A victim of severe trauma or amputation
- Suffering from a large infection
- Severely burned
- Experiencing drainage from any body orifice or wound
- Suffering from severe diarrhea
- Unable to resume oral intake within 8 to 10 days
- Vomiting for a period of time

To rebuild tissue after the trauma of surgery, the patient needs to take in nutrients in excess of normal body needs. *Protein* is particularly necessary to rebuild wounded or diseased tissue. (See also Chapter 28.)

Irrigating Wounds. Many patients have a wound that must be irrigated. The physician will issue a specific order as to the type of solution to be used, and the nursing procedure or protocol book identifies the procedure to be used. In some cases the irrigation will follow sterile procedures; in others, the procedure will be clean. One specific procedure for wound irrigation is contained in Chapter 54. Skills in managing drainage in wounds follow:

- In reporting and documenting the patient's condition, the nurse should note the amount, color, odor, and consistency of any drainage.
- Gloves are always worn when doing dressing changes. Gowns, masks, and face shields may need to be worn, depending on the potential for contamination of yourself or the wound.
- If the physician has ordered that the dressing is to be reinforced, the nurse is not to remove it to assess the incisional area, maintain the suture line.
- Any drainage noted should be outlined on the dressing with ink and dated, timed, and initialed. *(Rationale: Assist with monitoring the amount of drainage.)*
- Usually, dressings are reinforced and the physician notified of unusual drainage in the immediate postoperative period. Dressings should not be changed without a physician's order.
- Dressings and drainage tubes/devices should be disposed of according to the facility's policies for universal precautions and biohazardous waste.
- Drainage may be directly from the incision site, from a separate wound drain, a portable suction device, or any combination thereof.
- The patient's chart should inform the nurse if a packing is in place and indicate when and if it should be removed.
- The nurse should observe and document that the packing is in place and that the drainage is not excessive. Describe all drainage as to quantity and quality.

Changing Dressings. The nurse is often asked to assist with a dressing change. There is a difference between dressing reinforcement and dressing change. The nurse can reinforce a dressing without an order, but a dressing change is done under the direction of the physician or on the physician's order. Sterile dressings are changed using strict aseptic technique. The general principles of sterile technique are covered in Chapter 54.

Removing Sutures and Staples. The nurse may be asked to assist in removing sutures following surgery. Generally, this consists of having a disposable suture removal kit available. The physician may require other materials, including a bandage to apply following removal of the sutures. Sutures are readily removed. A sterile scissors is used to cut the suture and a sterile tweezer to pull the thread out. The physician pulls on the side next to the knot. The graduate nurse may be asked to remove sutures after uncomplicated surgical procedures.

Today many surgeons choose to close the skin with staples. Staples are inert, do not cause infection, and are quickly inserted. To remove staples, follow the manufacturer's instructions. Usually, a special staple remover is required. Chapter 54 describes sterile technique for suture and staple removal.

Providing Intravenous Therapy. Most patients come back from the operating room with an intravenous therapy (IV) infusion. Many types of intravenous solutions and several methods of administration are commonly used. These methods are discussed in Chapter 57 (in relationship to administration of medications).

It is important to know how to care for the patient who has an intravenous apparatus. Special procedures are to be followed when giving daily care, ambulating the patient, and positioning the patient. It is also important to recognize when the intravenous line has infiltrated and to know how to discontinue it safely. It is important to assess and monitor the infusion site every hour and to make sure the infusion is running. Most patients will have an intravenous pump/controller to maintain a consistent rate of flow. The patient's total intake and output is also recorded.

> **Key Concept**
>
> The patient who is having surgery needs not only physical preparation but also kind and gentle emotional support.

Keys for Review

Key Questions for Critical Thinking

1. Discuss the urgency of various types of surgery and where they might be performed.
2. Discuss inpatient teaching compared to teaching of an outpatient.
3. Describe the actions that are taken when the patient arrives in the nursing unit following surgery.
4. Develop a teaching plan for the patient who will need to use the incentive spirometer in the postoperative period.

Key Readings

Ball KA. "Laser technology" Symposium. The Nursing Clinics of North America 25(3), pp. 617–738, September 1990

Berkow R (Ed). The Merck Manual of Diagnosis and Therapy, Ed 16. Rahway, NJ, Merck & Co, 1992

Craven RF, Hirnle CJ. Fundamentals of Nursing: Human Health and Function. Philadelphia, J.B. Lippincott, 1992

Earnest VV. Clinical Skills in Nursing Practice, Ed 2. Philadelphia, J.B. Lippincott, 1993

NANDA Nursing Diagnoses: Definitions and Classifications 1992. Philadelphia, North American Nursing Diagnosis Association, 1992

Nursing '93 Drug Handbook. Springhouse, PA, Springhouse, 1993

O'Toole M (Ed). Miller-Keane Encyclopedia and Dictionary of Medicine, Nursing, and Allied Health, Ed 5. Philadelphia, W.B. Saunders, 1992

Key Readings (continued)

Smeltzer SC and Bare BG. Brunner and Suddarth's Textbook of Medical Surgical Nursing, Ed 7. Philadelphia, J.B. Lippincott, 1992

Taylor C, Lillis C, Lemone P. Fundamentals of Nursing: The Art and Science of Nursing Care, Ed 2. Philadelphia, J.B. Lippincott, 1993

Enrichment Keys

Clower GG. "My most humorous moment in nursing." NSNA Imprint 41(1), January 1994

Keys to Learning More

Chapter 54: surgical asepsis

Unit Eleven: medications and their administration

Chapter 61: indications for a cesarean delivery and pre- and postoperative nursing care

Unit Thirteen: treatments administered to children, including surgical intervention

Unit Fourteen: disorders of adults, many of which require surgery

Chapter 89: rehabilitation techniques sometimes necessary following surgery

Chapter 90: the person who is dying

54 Surgical Asepsis in Nursing Care

Keys for Learning

Learning Objectives

- List at least five examples of sterile areas and five examples of nonsterile areas of the body.
- Differentiate between medical and surgical asepsis and sterilization and disinfection.
- List nine guidelines to follow when using sterile technique.
- Open a sterile tray and a sterile package without contaminating them and hand sterile supplies to another nurse.
- Assist a physician with a dressing change and with the removal of stitches, skin clamps, or staples.
- Apply a wet-to-dry dressing or packing.
- Describe the procedures for female and male catheterization.
- Describe care of the patient with a urinary catheter and procedures performed.
- Describe the procedure for removal of an indwelling catheter.

Key Terms

autoclave	residual urine
catheterization	sterile
clean	sterilization
disinfection	surgical asepsis
medical asepsis	

Keys to Understanding This Chapter

Chapter 8: microbiology gives you a background to study sterile technique and prevention of infections

Chapter 25: anatomy of the male and female genitals; needed for catheterization

Chapter 30: medical asepsis, as differentiated from surgical asepsis

Unit Seven: components of the nursing process used in all of your nursing care and effective communication

Keys to Understanding This Chapter
(continued)

Unit Eight: effective communication and documentation

Chapter 50: physical examination and nursing assessment, information useful in assessing patients having sterile procedures

Unit Nine: basic nursing skills

Chapter 51: use of surgical mask

Chapter 53: person who has surgery

Key Points

- "Clean" applies to medical asepsis. It implies that all gross contamination is removed and that *many* microorganisms have been removed.
- "Sterile" means that the item is free of *all* microorganisms and spores.
- When a sterile item is touched by *anything* unsterile, it becomes contaminated and is no longer sterile. Discard an item if you contaminate it or if you are not sure whether it is contaminated.
- Catheterization is the procedure of inserting a flexible tube through the urethra into the bladder to remove urine. It is an aseptic procedure for which sterile equipment and techniques are required.
- Do not cut a catheter to remove it.
- Patient and family teaching is important, especially if the patient will be going home with a need to perform a sterile procedure or catheter care.

Key Topics Outline

Medical and Surgical Asepsis
Sterilization and Disinfection
Sterile Technique
  Equipment
  Wounds and Dressings
  Urinary Catheterization

While nurses perform any nursing procedure, they assess their patients. Nurses recognize the signs of pain, infection, poor tissue healing, poor circulation, excess drainage or bleeding, lowered blood pressure, shock, or pain. These are also considered when caring for patients who are having a dressing change, suture removal, urinary catheterization, or other sterile procedure.

Medical and Surgical Asepsis

As part of the prevention of disease spread it is essential that you understand the difference between "clean" and "sterile."

Clean implies that all gross contamination is removed and that *many* microorganisms have been removed. Mechanical cleansing and use of disinfectants are sufficient for that purpose. "Clean" is **medical asepsis**. **Sterile**, however, means that the item is free of *all* microorganisms and spores. (A spore is a resting stage of *some* microorganisms, resistant to environmental changes.) If an area is sterile, it must be kept free of all microorganisms, to prevent infection and disease. In these instances sterile technique, or **surgical asepsis** is used.

Many parts of the body are clean but not sterile. Examples are the skin, the mouth and digestive tract, and the upper respiratory tract. These areas are open to the outside and are impossible to keep sterile. Other parts of the body are sterile. Either they do not normally open to the outside (such as the abdominal cavity or the ovary) or they do not normally contain any microorganisms. Some of these areas (such as the urinary bladder) may be prone to infection, even though they are normally sterile.

Medical Asepsis or Clean Technique

The main concept in nursing related to medical asepsis is that of preventing the spread of the disease from one person to another, whether it be from patient to nurse, patient to patient, or nurse to patient. Medical asepsis is discussed in Chapter 30. Handwashing is one of the most important factors in medical asepsis; the skin cannot be sterilized, but it can be cleaned. *Isolation or infection control*, used when the patient has a communicable disorder, is a variation of medical asepsis and is discussed in Chapter 51. In some cases, *protective isolation* is used to protect the patient.

Surgical Asepsis or Sterile Technique

Surgical asepsis or sterile technique differs from medical asepsis in that in surgical asepsis all microorganisms are destroyed. *Sterile technique* means that no organisms will be carried to the patient. It destroys microorganisms *before* they can enter the body.

Sterile technique is followed for changing dressings, administering parenteral (outside the digestive tract) medications, and performing surgical and other procedures, such as urinary catheterization. Surgical asepsis is accomplished by first sterilizing articles and then avoiding any contact with unsterile articles. When a sterile article is touched by an unsterile article, it becomes contaminated—it is no longer sterile.

> **Key Concept**
> ◆ Sterile to sterile remains sterile. Sterile to clean becomes contaminated.
> ◆ Think before you touch anything.

Sterilization and Disinfection

Sterilization is the destruction of *all* microorganisms and spores, whereas **disinfection** destroys *most* pathogens but not necessarily their spores. Sterilization and disinfection are necessary in performing surgical and medical asepsis and in preventing the spread of harmful bacteria. Equipment used by a patient is sterilized or discarded. The discharged patient usually takes home the wash basin, mouth care utensils, and items such as the incentive spirometer, or the items are discarded. Occasionally, a piece of equipment is sterilized for reuse.

Sterilization is the process of exposing articles to heat or to chemical disinfectants long enough to kill all microorganisms and spores. Boiling for 10 minutes destroys most but not all organisms. Exposure for 15 minutes to steam under 18 pounds of pressure at a temperature of 257°F (125°C) will kill even the toughest ones; a pressure steam sterilizer is called an **autoclave**. Chemical disinfectants powerful enough to destroy germs or heat cannot be used on certain articles, such as plastic. Most plastic items are disposable.

Moist heat dulls the sharp cutting edges of some instruments; therefore, they are better sterilized by dry heat or chemicals. Gas sterilization using ethylene oxide (EO) and radiation are other methods. Most sharps, such as scalpels and suture removal scissors, are disposable. Needles used for injections are discarded.

The supplies used for surgical and other sterile procedures must be free of all organisms, both pathogenic and nonpathogenic. Anything that comes into contact with an open wound or break in the skin, that is introduced into a sterile body cavity, or that punctures the skin must be sterile. In most hospitals sterile supplies are prepared in a central supply room (CSR), also called central sterile supply (CSS), or are purchased in a sterile condition and disposed of after being used. Some items, such as surgical towels are packaged in cloth, paper, or plastic wraps, secured with a special type of masking tape, labeled, and sterilized.

Key Concept

- ◆ Sterilization is the destruction of all microorganisms and spores.
- ◆ Disinfection is the destruction of most pathogens but not spores.

Handling Sterile Supplies and Equipment

As previously stated, every movement in aseptic procedure is a link in the chain of asepsis; if you break one link by contaminating something, the chain is broken and you open the door to infection.

Key Concept

- ◆ Never touch sterile with unsterile articles.
- ◆ Discard an article if you contaminate it or if you are not sure whether it is contaminated. Do not risk using a contaminated one.

Sterile Technique

The accompanying box describes precautions to be taken to prevent contamination. The rest of this chapter discusses sterile technique.

Nursing Skill Guidelines
Using Sterile Technique

- ◆ Once you have put on sterile gloves and/or a gown, you cannot touch anything that isn't sterile.
- ◆ Reaching over a sterile field when you are not wearing sterile clothing contaminates the area.
- ◆ If a sterile wrapper becomes wet, the wrapper and its contents are no longer sterile.
- ◆ If your mask becomes wet, it no longer screens out microorganisms, and you must change to a new mask.
- ◆ If you are wearing sterile gloves to perform a sterile procedure, keep them in front of you, between your nipple line and waist. If they move above or below these areas, they are considered contaminated.
- ◆ Your back is not sterile, even though you are wearing a sterile gown.
- ◆ If you are not sure you have caused contamination, assume that you have. *If in doubt, consider the objects in question to be contaminated.*
- ◆ Skin cannot be rendered sterile; it can only be made clean.
- ◆ Parts of the body that are not exposed to the outside are considered sterile. This includes the abdominal cavity, the urinary bladder, and usually the uterus. The gastrointestinal tract is not sterile, because it is actually a tube within the body that opens to the outside at both ends. In addition, unsterile items (food) are introduced into the gastrointestinal tract daily.

In many nursing situations, you will be required to open a package and maintain the sterility of its contents. Nursing Procedure 54–1 is basic to many sterile procedures.

Hair Covering

In some cases, especially in the operating room, you will be asked to wear a cap or hood to cover your hair. Remember that none of your hair can be showing. If you have long hair, you will need to wear a special type of hood. If your hair is short, you can wear a surgical cap. A male nurse with a beard often wears a surgical hood to cover his entire face, except the eyes.

Surgical Mask

Specifics for donning a surgical mask are covered in Chapter 51. In strict sterile situations, such as the operating room or protective isolation, the mask is worn with the hair covering. The purpose of the mask is to form a barrier to stop the transmission of harmful microorganisms. In the operating room or during a sterile procedure, the mask keeps harmful organisms from your respiratory tract from spreading to the patient. In

Supplies and Equipment

Sterile supplies (as needed for procedure)
Waist-high table

Suggested Procedure and Rationale

1. Gather supplies. Check expiration date on sterile supplies.
   (Rationale: Organization facilitates performance of the skill. Outdated sterile package is considered contaminated.)
2. Wash hands.
   (Rationale: Handwashing prevents the spread of organisms.)
3. Explain procedure to patient.
   (Rationale: Providing information fosters patient cooperation.)
4. Prepare waist-high working area.
   (Rationale: Keeping sterile objects above waist level maintains sterility.)
5. Place sterile package on working area. Remove outer covering or plastic wrap if one is present.
   (Rationale: Outer covering protects sterile contents.)
6. Grasp edge of outermost flap and open away from you toward the back of the table.
   (Rationale: Opening top flap away from nurse prevents reaching over a sterile field and contaminating it.)

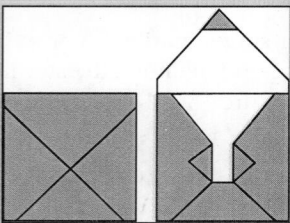

Step 6   Opening top flap away from nurse.

7. Fold each side flap down toward table. Holding the underside of the wrapper, snap the side and lay flat on table.
   (Rationale: This will help to keep the wrapping from curling back onto its original position.)

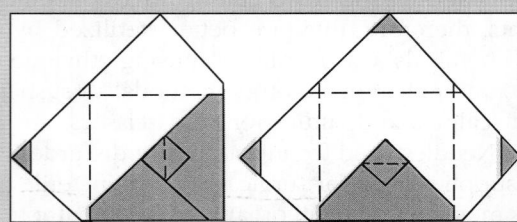

Step 7   Folding side flap down.

8. Grasp tip of near flap and open back toward you. Pull flap downward from underneath and snap into place.
   (Rationale: Flaps are unfolded and sterile field is prepared.)

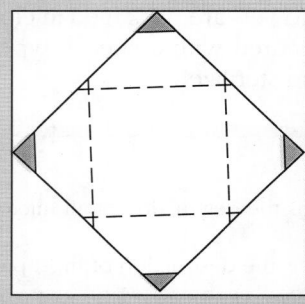

Step 8   Opening near flap toward nurse.

9. Drop any additional sterile items onto sterile field.
   (Rationale: Sterile item touching sterile item maintains surgical asepsis.)

---

the case of the infectious patient, the mask protects you from the patient's harmful organisms.

Sterile Gown

The sterile gown is worn in the operating room, in protective isolation, and sometimes in the delivery room. You can touch with your hands only the parts of the sterile gown that will touch your body after the gown is in place. Therefore, touch only the inside of the gown with your hands or body. Someone will tie the strings for you; the back of the gown is considered contaminated, even though it was sterile when you put it on. Any part of the gown below the level of your waist and above the nipple level is also considered contaminated. Be careful when you are wearing a sterile gown not to touch anything that is not sterile.

Your instructors will give you specific instructions in how to put on a gown and gloves without contaminating yourself or anything else in the sterile area.

Sterile Gloves

For some procedures you will need to put on sterile gloves. Remember that once you have the gloves on, you cannot touch anything unsterile without contaminating your gloves. Therefore, you must make all your preparations before you put on your gloves.

> ### Key Concept
>
> Whenever the cover on a sterile tray, or a gown, mask, dressing, drape, or other cloth/paper item becomes wet, it is considered *contaminated.*

A method of gloving, called *open gloving,* is described in Nursing Procedure 54–2. A procedure called *closed gloving* is often done when a sterile gown is also being used. That procedure is beyond the scope of this book.

Wounds and Dressings

The type of wound and its condition will determine the type of dressing to be used and the frequency of dressing changes. Sometimes the physician orders the type and time for dressing changes, but some nurses make those decisions also. Check what your facility's procedure is.

Changing a Sterile Dressing

Dressings are changed so that the nurse may evaluate wound healing and so that a dry dressing will be applied. Wounds heal better in a dry environment. The steps in changing a sterile dressing are given in Nursing Procedure 54–3.

Applying a Wet-to-Dry Dressing or Packing

A dry dressing promotes healing. The following skill is used in applying a wet-to-dry dressing or packing.

◆ Gather the following supplies and equipment: clean gloves, sterile gloves, biohazard disposal bag, waterproof bed pad, sterile dressings or packing or disposable dressing kit, medication or solution as ordered, sterile cup(s), tape or Montgomery straps, draping materials, and sterile forceps or cotton-tipped applicators.

◆ Follow the steps in Procedure 54–3 to remove old dressing or packing. (*Rationale: Dressing removal debrides wound and prepares it for healing.*)

◆ Set up area. Place sterile cup on bedside table close to patient.

◆ When opening multiuse bottles, set bottle cap upside down so inside of cap does not touch anything. (*Rationale: The inside of bottle caps must remain sterile for the next use.*)

◆ With label toward palm of hand, pour off a small amount of solution into a trash receptacle. (*Rationale: The outside of the bottle is contaminated. The label must be kept dry so it is readable and doesn't fall off.*)

◆ Pour ordered solution into cup. Use two cups if a different solution is needed for cleaning wound.

◆ Open sterile packages and place materials on sterile field. (*Rationale: You must maintain sterile technique. This necessitates setting up materials before donning sterile gloves.*)

◆ If sterile container of solution is provided in your dressing kit, it is not prepoured.

◆ Put on sterile gloves as directed in Nursing Procedure 54–2 and set up sterile supplies.

◆ Carefully saturate a gauze pad or packing strip of size or amount needed to fill the wound cavity. Gently squeeze out excess moisture so it is damp but not dripping unless ordered otherwise.

◆ Gently pack gauze or packing into wound bed. Use a sterile cotton-tipped applicator or forceps to tuck dressing into cavity or under skin surfaces. (*Rationale: Wet-to-dry dressings are used to provide a mild debridement of wound bed. Complete coverage of wound bed ensures entire wound is debrided when dressing is removed.*)

◆ Cover wet dressing with dry sterile dressing, as ordered.

◆ Complete sterile dressing change as listed in Nursing Procedure 54–3.

◆ Properly dispose of gloves and wash hands.

◆ Document procedure, results, appearance of wound and drainage, and how patient tolerated the procedure.

Removing Stitches, Skin Clamps, or Staples

Sutures (stitches) and skin clamps may be removed at the time of the dressing change. A suture removal kit is used and discarded after use. If you are asked to remove stitches, you must first have instruction. Use sterile technique. Skin clamps and staples are removed according to the manufacturer's recommendations. Follow the procedures used in your hospital.

Irrigating Sterile Wounds

The physician may order a sterile wound irrigation. This is done to remove debris from an open wound following injury or surgery that has been complicated by infection. Heat or medications may also be applied using this method. The three major types of wound irrigation are:

◆ *Manual irrigation* with a hand-held syringe that can be sterile or clean

◆ *Continuous wound irrigation* with an infusion-type setup

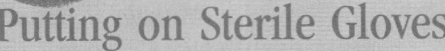

Putting on Sterile Gloves

Supplies and Equipment

Sterile gloves (appropriate size)

Procedure

1. Wash hands.
   (Rationale: Handwashing prevents the spread of organisms.)
2. Open the outer glove package carefully following Procedure 54-1 on clean, dry, flat surface at waist level or higher.
   (Rationale: A clean, dry surface that is waist level or higher protects the sterile gloves from contamination.)
3. If there is an inner package, open it in the same way, keeping sterile gloves on inside surface with cuffs toward nurse.
   (Rationale: Gloves remain sterile and ready to apply.)

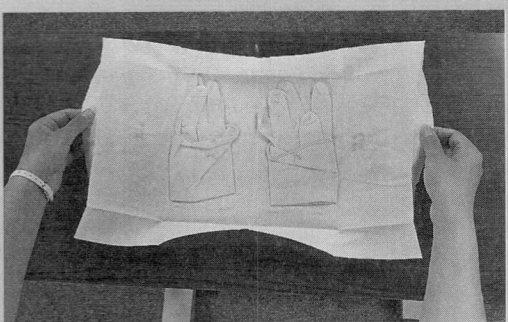

Step 3   Opening the inner glove package

4. Use nondominant hand to grasp *inside* upper surface of cuff of glove for dominant hand. Lift glove up and clear of wrapper.
   (Rationale: Inner surface of glove can be touched by clean hand. Outer surface will remain sterile.)

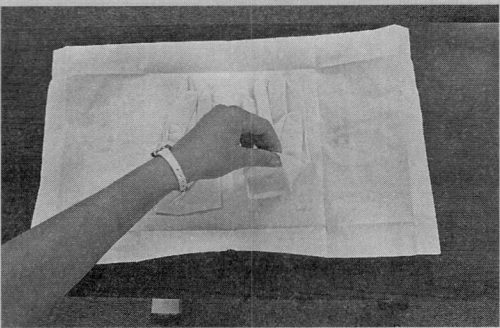

Step 4   Grasping the cuff and lifting the glove

5. Insert dominant hand into glove, placing thumb and fingers in proper openings. Leave the cuff in place.
   (Rationale: Attempts to unfold glove cuff may result in contamination of glove.)

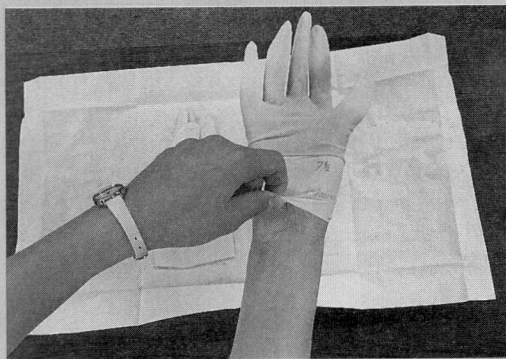

Step 5   Inserting dominant hand into the glove

6. Slip fingers of sterile gloved hand *under (inside) cuff* of remaining glove while keeping thumb pointed outward. Lift glove up and clear of wrapper.
   (Rationale: Sterile gloved hand is protected by cuff as unsterile hand is inserted.) Keep thumb out of the way.

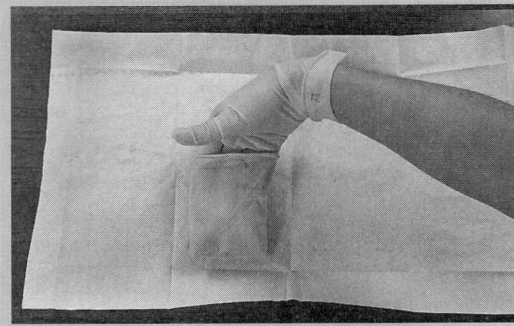

Step 6   Slipping sterile gloved fingers under sterile cuff

(continued)

7. (a) Insert nondominant hand into glove. (b) Adjust gloves and snap cuffs into place. Avoid touching inside glove and wrist areas.
   (Rationale: Gloves remain sterile when touching other sterile areas.)

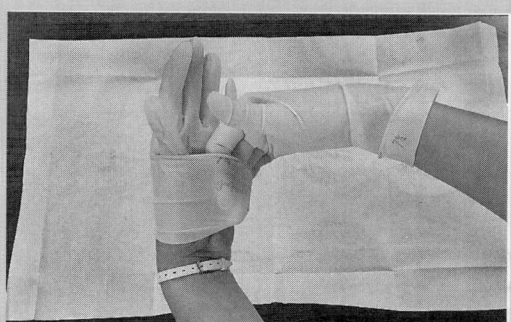

Step 7a   Inserting nondominant hand into glove

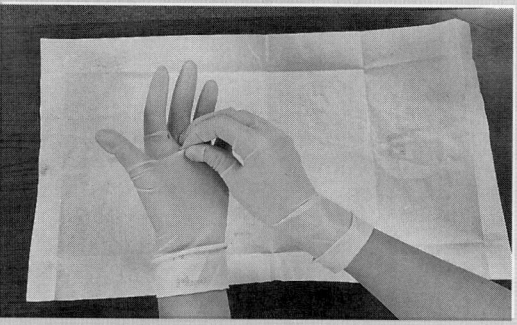

Step 7b   Adjusting gloves, touching only sterile areas (Photos © B. Proud.)

8. Keep sterile gloved hands above waist level. Make sure not to touch your clothes.
   (Rationale: Holding hands above waist level helps keep them within sight and prevents accidental contamination.)

♦ *Intermittent irrigation* alone or combined with gentle suction, such as a Hemovac

The nurse will be responsible for performing the manual irrigation and for monitoring and emptying the continuous or intermittent irrigation, usually after the tubes have been inserted by the physician.

Manual Sterile Irrigation. The skills for manual sterile irrigation are discussed here.

Nursing Skill

Performing Sterile Wound Irrigation

Supplies and Equipment

Disposable sterile irrigation pack
Irrigation solution, as ordered
Biohazardous waste bag
Clean gloves
Waterproof bed pad
Eye goggles or face guard
New dressings, as ordered
Clean basin or irrigating pouch

Procedure

1. Carefully wash your hands. *(Rationale: Washing hands prevents contamination.)*
2. Check physician's orders and carefully gather all equipment and supplies. *(Rationale: Physician's orders may have changed. Once a wound is exposed, the procedure should be completed as quickly as possible.)*
3. Close the door and pull the curtains. Cover with a bath blanket. *(Rationale: Protect the patient's privacy and prevent chilling.)*
4. Introduce yourself and explain the procedure. *(Rationale: The comfort level is higher in a patient who understands the procedure.)*
5. Put on clean gloves and eye shield or face guard. *(Rationale: The nurse's hands are protected by the gloves. If material splashes, the nurse's face and eyes must be protected.)*
6. Position the patient so the solution will run from the upper end of the wound downward. Place the waterproof pad and clean basin or irrigating pouch under the area to be irrigated. *(Rationale: The bed pad protects the bed linens. The clean basin or pouch will catch the irrigating solution.)*
7. Drape the patient using a bath blanket. Expose the patient as little as possible.
8. Remove old dressing and discard as described in Nursing Procedure 54–3. Discard gloves. Wash hands again.
9. After washing hands, open irrigation tray, using sterile technique. Carefully pour solution with the label facing the palm into irrigation bottle. *(Rationale: Outside of bottle is no longer sterile. Solution must be poured before you don gloves. Spilled solution will cause contamination and would make label unreadable.)* If the bottle has been opened previously, pour off a small amount of solution.
10. Place bottle close to patient on overbed table. Make sure to date and initial the bottle after opening. Include patient's name. *(Rationale: The solution will be used for one patient only. It must be clearly identified and kept handy.)*

(Text continues on page 647)

Changing a Sterile Dressing

Supplies and Equipment

Clean gloves
Plastic biohazard bag
ABD pads
Sterile saline or water
Bath blanket
Sterile gloves

Sterile dressings, as ordered
Tape or Montgomery straps
Waterproof pads
Forceps from sterile suture removal set (optional)

Procedure

1. Explain procedure to patient.
   (Rationale: Providing information fosters patient cooperation.)
2. Gather supplies after checking physician's order for dressing change.
   (Rationale: Organization facilitates performance of the skill. Checking physician's order clarifies type of dressing ordered, presence of drains, and schedule for dressing change.)
3. Wash hands.
   (Rationale: Handwashing prevents the spread of organisms.)
4. Close the door or pull the bed curtains. Assist patient to comfortable position. Expose only the area to be redressed using bath blanket if necessary. Place waterproof pad under patient to protect the bed.
   (Rationale: This protects the patient's privacy and prevents chilling.)
5. Prepare plastic bag as receptacle for soiled dressings. Fold back cuff and place within reach of working area.
   (Rationale: Plastic bag prevents transmission of organisms from soiled dressing.)

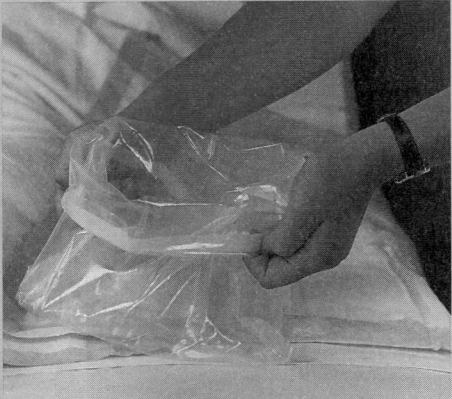

Step 5   Preparing a bag for the soiled dressings

6. Put on clean gloves. Untie Montgomery straps or gently loosen tape. Remove soiled dressing, being careful not to tear the wound or dislodge any drains. Use sterile saline to moisten dressing if it is sticking to wound. Lift soiled side of dressing away from patient's view.
   (Rationale: Gloves act as a barrier. Dressing must be removed cautiously to maintain integrity of sutures and prevent discomfort for the patient. The sight of drainage or blood may upset the patient.)
7. Assess amount, color, odor, and consistency of drainage. Observe wound and surrounding tissue.
   (Rationale: Assessment provides indication of presence of infection.)
8. Removal gloves and place in plastic bag
   (Rationale: Gloves are contaminated with wound drainage.)

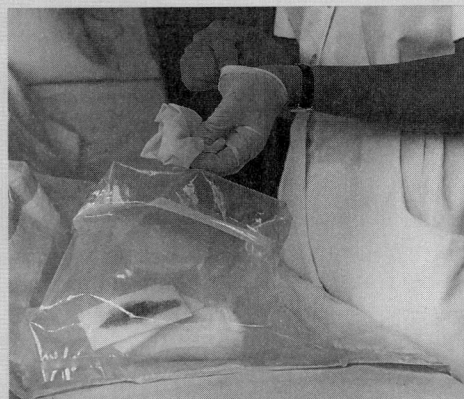

Step 8   Removing soiled gloves (Photos © B. Proud.)

9. Open sterile dressings on bedside table. Uncap sterile saline or other solution ordered by physician to cleanse wound.
   (Rationale: Organization of sterile supplies ensures that supplies needed are present and placed in order of use.)
10. Put on sterile gloves.
    (Rationale: Sterile gloves maintain surgical asepsis.)
11. Moisten sterile dressings and cleanse wound, if ordered, moving from top to bottom or from center of wound outward (forceps may be used for this). Use a new swab or gauze pad for each cleansing motion.
    (Rationale: Cleansing from clean to dirty prevents introducing organisms into the wound.)

(continued)

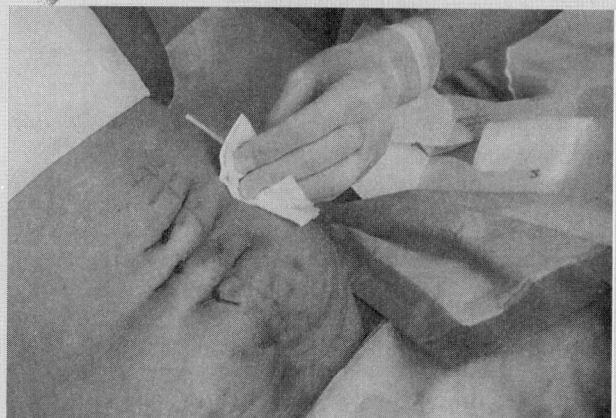

Step 11　Cleansing the wound

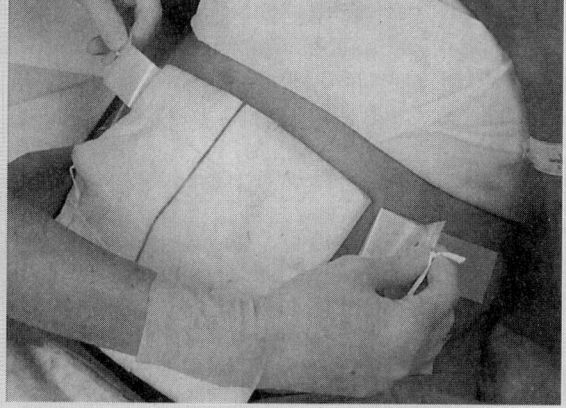

Step 14　Applying Montgomery straps

12. If necessary, use gauze pad to dry wound using same motion.
    (Rationale: Moisture provides a medium for organisms to grow and multiply.)
13. Apply layer of dry sterile dressings over incision and wound area. Pad with additional dressings. Cover with sterile ABD pad, if required.
    (Rationale: Inner layer of dressing acts as a wick. Additional dressings and outer pad absorb drainage and protect the wound.)
14. Remove gloves and place in disposal bag. Apply tape or tie Montgomery straps.
    (Rationale: Tape is easier to apply when gloves have been removed, but it can also be put on with gloves. If there is any question, use gloves.)

15. Reposition and cover patient. Handle only *outside* of bag, keeping your hands inside the cuff, and carefully closing it. Dispose of bag with used supplies according to agency policy.
    (Rationale: Proper disposal prevents transmission of organisms.)
16. Wash hands.
    (Rationale: Handwashing prevents the spread of organisms.)
17. Document wound care and all assessments.
    (Rationale: Documentation provides coordination of care.)

11. Open sterile dressing tray if one is to be used.
12. Put on sterile gloves.
13. Prepare inside of irrigation tray and dressing tray. Place irrigation syringe into bottle. Open packs of dressings and prepare other items. *(Rationale: It is important to keep the materials sterile.)*
14. Carefully assess the amount and character of drainage and size and condition of wound and surrounding tissue. *(Rationale: This information must be reported and documented.)*
15. Draw up solution into the syringe.
16. Explain following steps as you proceed. *(Rationale: The patient or family may need to continue the treatment after discharge.)*
17. Hold syringe just above top end of wound and force fluid into the wound slowly and continuously (Fig. 54–1.) Use enough force to flush out debris but do not squirt or splash fluid. Irrigate all portions of wound. Do not force solution into wound pockets. Continue irrigating until solution draining from bottom end of wound is clear. *(Rationale: These procedures ensure that you will remove debris and infectious products but not damage the wound.)*

18. Using sterile 4 × 4s, gently pat dry the edges of the wound (unless the wound is to have a wet-to-dry dressing, then dry only surrounding skin). Work from cleanest to most contaminated areas. *(Rationale: This helps to prevent further contamination by removing culture medium for microorganisms. The dressings will remain dry for a longer period of time, and contamination is not spread.)*
19. Apply sterile dressings as ordered.
20. Make the patient comfortable.
21. Teach the patient to observe for excess drainage or severe pain. Teach any other pertinent observations. *(Rationale: The patient's observation may alert the staff to problems and result in quick action.)*
22. Discard all materials, remove gloves, and wash hands carefully. *(Rationale: These procedures help to prevent contamination.)*
23. Document and report the treatment and your observation of the wound. *(Rationale: Pertinent observations may assist the team in further patient care planning.)*

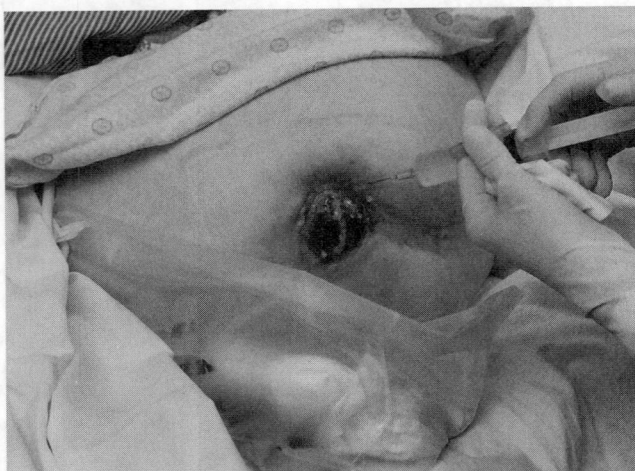

Figure 54-1. Sterile wound irrigation is carried out with a large syringe and the solution prescribed by the physician. Often, there is no needle on the syringe. The solution is sprayed into the wound, flushing out debris, including pus, dead tissue, and blood. Note that the irrigation is directed from the top, allowing it to drain into the self-adhesive drainage pouch below. The syringe and drainage pouch are then discarded and the wound redressed. (Photo courtesy of 3M Health Care)

Intermittent or Continuous Irrigation. Intermittent or continuous wound irrigation follows the same principles. However, catheters are placed into the wound and the solution is dispensed using a setup similar to that of an intravenous apparatus. Drainage is by gravity. This device is often used following prostate surgery (TURP).

If suction is to be used, a device such as a Hemovac is often installed. This device is emptied and negative pressure is reestablished by squeezing the container. Smaller amounts of drainage can be removed with a Hemovac. This device is often used following breast or neck surgery. Use of the portable wound suction pump follows.

◆ Introduce yourself and assist patient to a comfortable position. Wash your hands. Wear gloves.
◆ Explain procedure, using this time as an instruction period for patient and family if this procedure is to be continued at home. (*Rationale: Discharge teaching is begun as soon as possible to facilitate a smooth transition to the home. Teaching helps decrease anxiety.*)
◆ Open emptying port or plug. Hold suction device over collection container and tip it so drainage empties from port. Remember to use a sterile container if you are collecting a specimen for culture. Make sure suction device is empty. Measure drainage. (*Rationale: This patient is usually on intake and output. Drainage is considered output.*)
◆ Wipe plug and outside of emptying port with alco-

hol wipe. (*Rationale: All actions are aimed at decreasing transfer of microorganisms and the chance of wound infection.*)
◆ Reestablish suction by squeezing device flat and then securing plug into the port (Fig. 54–2). (*Rationale: This creates a gentle vacuum.*)
◆ Check patency of suction at least once a shift. It must be checked often even if there is large amount of drainage or sudden change in amount of drainage. (*Rationale: It is vital to maintain suction to ensure healing of wound.*)
◆ Place device as close to site as possible. For mobile patients, attach tabbed piece of tape around the tubing and secure with a pin to patient's gown. Be careful not to puncture the tube. Be sure there is no tension on the tubing. Instruct patient to be careful not to pull on tubing. (*Rationale: These steps minimize tension and prevent trauma on wound and insertion site.*)
◆ Dispose of drainage and gloves, wash hands, and make patient comfortable.
◆ Carefully document and report amount and character of drainage and of surrounding skin, as well as any other observations.

Urinary Catheterization

The bladder is the reservoir for urine, and when 200 to 250 mL has collected there, the urge to void (urinate) occurs. If the bladder cannot be emptied normally, it becomes distended as urine collects, and urine may dribble from the urethral opening. A distended bladder is also prone to infection and can cause chronic kidney disorders.

Catheterization is the procedure of inserting a tube called a catheter through the urethra into the bladder to remove urine. It is an aseptic procedure for which sterile equipment (usually disposable) is required.

Catheterization is most commonly used to relieve urinary retention when the patient is temporarily unable to void, to remove urine remaining in the bladder (**residual urine**) when voiding only partly empties it, and to prevent urine from touching sutures in the perineum.

At one time catheterization was considered necessary to obtain an uncontaminated specimen of urine. However, many physicians now recommend "midstream urine collection" and "clean catch." The need for catheterization following surgery has also diminished as early ambulation for surgical patients has increased.

It is not considered safe to remove more than 750 to 1,000 mL of urine from the bladder at any one time. If the flow of urine seems undiminished after this quantity has been withdrawn, clamp or remove the catheter and report it to the charge nurse so the physician can be

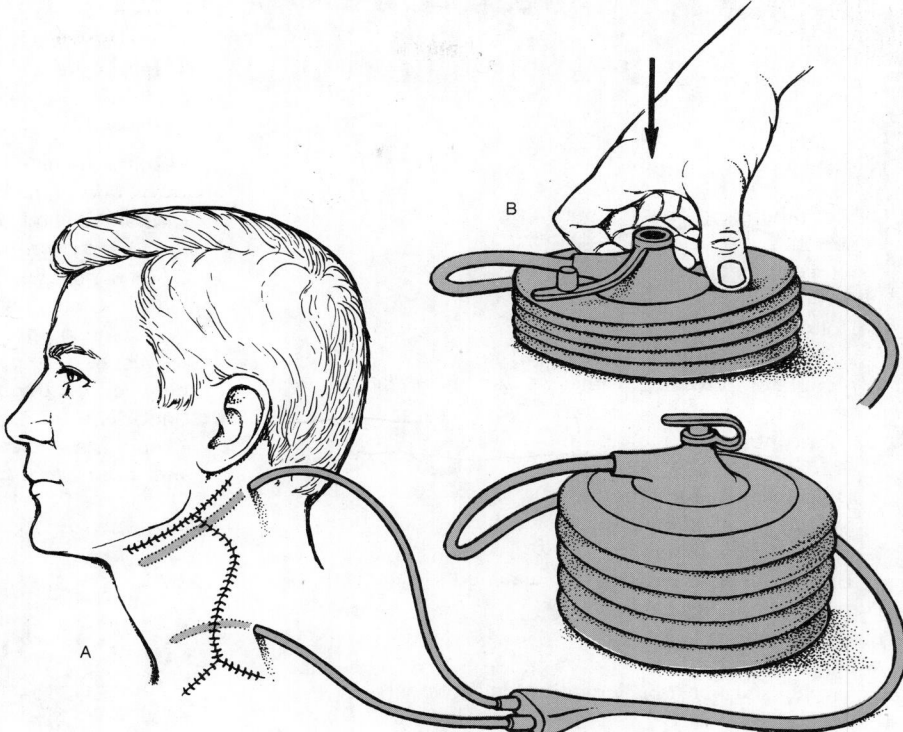

Figure 54-2. (A) Two perforated catheters are draining the incisional area following a radical neck dissection. By means of a Y tube, drainage is drawn into a portable wound-suction receptacle. When full, open top plug of receptacle and empty. **(B)** To reestablish negative pressure, compress receptacle as indicated and replace plug; suction drainage will resume. (Brunner L, Suddarth DS: The Lippincott Manual of Nursing Practice, Ed 4. Philadelphia, J.B. Lippincott, 1986:120)

notified. (*Rationale: If a patient is admitted with a greatly distended bladder, it is considered safer to relieve the distention gradually to prevent bladder damage and possible shock.*)

> **Nursing Alert**
>
> Some patients are sensitive or allergic to latex and may have an allergic reaction to the catheter.

Types of Catheters

The catheters most commonly used are made of latex or plastic, although metal catheters are used occasionally by physicians. Catheters should be discarded after they have been removed. (It is difficult to sterilize a catheter adequately.) Every type of catheter has a rounded tip, to prevent injury to the meatus or the urethra. Catheters are graded in French (Fr) sizes, the same as rectal tubes. Sizes 14 Fr, and 16 Fr are suitable for the female patient; 20 Fr and 22 Fr are usually used for the male patient. The larger catheter is used for the man because it is stiffer and will be easier to push the distance of the male urethra. The 8 Fr and 10 Fr catheters are used for children because they are smaller.

The Retention (Indwelling) Catheter. The retention catheter provides temporary or permanent drainage of urine. It may be necessary for an incontinent or unresponsive

patient, following bladder injury or surgery, in cancer of the bladder, or in bladder infection. The Foley catheter is a "balloon-tip" catheter and is perhaps the most commonly used retention catheter. The Foley catheter has a tube inside the catheter opening into a small balloon above the opening in the tip that provides the outlet for the urine. After the Foley catheter is inserted, the balloon is inflated with sterile water or saline through a small projecting tube near the outer end of the catheter, which is capped with a plug. Balloon sizes vary. Most hold 5 to 30 mL of fluid. A prefilled syringe usually is used to inject the solution into the balloon through this plug. The prefilled syringe usually contains 2 to 3 mL more than that stated balloon size, allowing for balloon inflation as well as the length of tubing used to fill the balloon.

When the syringe is withdrawn, the tube stays plugged. No other plug or clamp is needed. The inflated balloon keeps the catheter from slipping out of the bladder.

Catheterizing the Female Patient

Many situations require the placement of a urinary catheter. These include cesarean delivery, bladder or vaginal repair, and cancer of the bladder. Urinary disorders are discussed in Chapter 82. Nursing Procedure 54–4 summarizes steps in catheterizing the female patient.

The Lateral Position for Female Catheterization. In some cases it is preferable to have the woman in a side-lying

(Text continues on page 652)

Catheterizing the Female Patient

Supplies and Equipment

Sterile catheterization tray containing the following sterile
supplies:
Gloves
Basin
Cotton balls
Antiseptic solution
Straight or indwelling catheter (size appropriate for pa-
tient).
Lubricant
Forceps
Drapes (plain and fenestrated)
Syringe prefilled with water or saline
Specimen container
Urine collection bag (may be attached to catheter)
Flashlight or additional lamp
Plastic biohazard bag
Waterproof pad
Velcro leg strap or nonallergenic tape (optional)
Bath blanket
Clean gloves, soap, water, washcloth, and towel

Procedure

1. Explain procedure to patient.
   (*Rationale: Providing information fosters patient
   cooperation.*)
2. Gather supplies after checking physician's order for
   catheterization.
   (*Rationale: Organization facilitates performance of
   the skill. Checking the physician's order clarifies insertion of a straight or indwelling catheter.*)
3. Wash hands.
   (*Rationale: Handwashing prevents the spread of
   organisms.*)
4. Close the door or pull the bed curtain. Adjust bed to
   a comfortable working height. If right handed, preferred position is on the patient's right side.
   (*Rationale: Bed at proper height and appropriate position prevents back strain. Closing curtain or door
   protects the patient's privacy.*)
5. Assist patient into a supine position with feet spread
   apart and knees flexed. Use bath blanket to drape
   patient.
   (*Rationale: Dorsal recumbent position allows visualization of the urinary meatus. Bath blanket provides
   warmth and privacy.*)
6. Put on clean gloves. Wash perineal area with soap.
   Rinse and dry. Remove gloves and wash hands
   again.
   (*Rationale: Area is cleansed prior to introducing
   catheter into meatus.*)

7. Ensure adequate lighting. Position a lamp at the foot
   of the bed or another nurse may hold a flashlight.
   (*Rationale: Good lighting improves visualization of
   the urinary meatus.*)
8. Open the sterile catheterization tray on bedside table.
   Put on sterile gloves. Pick up sterile drape and shake
   open. Grasp upper corners and fold back over sterile
   gloves. Ask the patient to lift buttocks. Place drape
   between her thighs with the upper edge under the
   buttocks.
   (*Rationale: Protecting the gloves with the drape
   maintains sterility while positioning the drape.*)

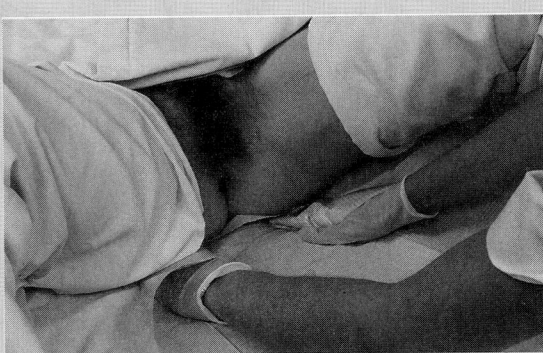

Step 8   Placing the drape while protecting sterile gloved hands

9. Set up equipment on tray:
   a. Open package with antiseptic and pour over cot-
      ton balls.
   b. Remove plastic covering from catheter. For in-
      dwelling catheter, attach prefilled syringe to bal-
      loon inflation port and inflate balloon with appro-
      priate amount of fluid. After balloon inflates,
      aspirate fluid back into syringe, leaving the sy-
      ringe connected to the port and the balloon flat.
   c. Open lubricant and lubricate tip (1–2 inches) of
      catheter. The catheter tip may be left inside the
      sterile lubricant package until needed.
   d. Unscrew the cap from the specimen container if
      one is needed.
      (*Rationale: Preparation of supplies ensures that
      all equipment is present. Inflating the catheter
      balloon before use checks for leaks or a nonfunc-
      tioning balloon. Lubrication of the catheter in-
      creases comfort.*)

(continued)

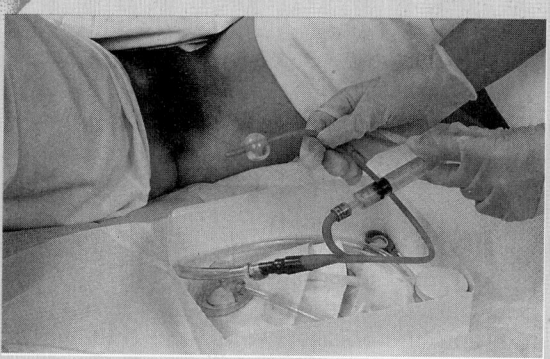

Step 9 Testing the balloon on an indwelling catheter

10. Move catheterization tray with equipment onto sterile drape between patient's thighs.
    (Rationale: All supplies are easily available, decreasing likelihood of reaching and contaminating equipment.)

11. Using nondominant hand, separate and gently spread the labia minora to expose the urinary meatus. Keep this hand in position.
    (Rationale: The nondominant hand is now considered contaminated. Spreading the labia allows easier cleansing and visibility.)

12. With sterile dominant hand, use forceps to pick up cotton ball and cleanse both labial folds and then the meatus. Use one cotton ball for each stroke, moving from top to bottom or front to back, and discard each used swipe in plastic bag. Cleanse meatus last.
    (Rationale: Moving from clean to dirty lessens the chance of introducing organisms into the bladder.)

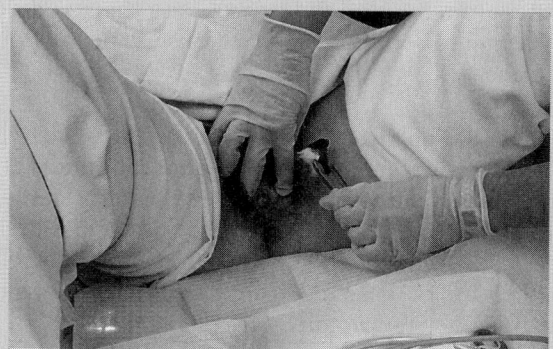

Step 12 Cleansing from front to back

13. Pick up catheter approximately 3 inches from the tip with sterile dominant hand. Place drainage end in basin. If catheter is indwelling, it may already be attached to drainage tubing.
    (Rationale: Sterile setup will not be contaminated by draining urine.)

14. Ask the patient to breathe deeply and slowly through her mouth. Insert the catheter gently into the meatus advancing it 2 to 3 inches until urine begins to drain. (See Figure 25-4 for location of meatus.) If catheter is to be indwelling, advance it another 1 to 2 inches. Never force insertion of the catheter if resistance is felt. Move nondominant hand to hold catheter in place. Collect urine specimen if one is ordered.
    (Rationale: Asking the patient to focus on breathing relaxes the sphincter and the catheter meets less resistance on entering the meatus. Forcing the advancement of the catheter may injure the meatus or mucous membranes.)

15. If catheter is not to be indwelling, remove it after urine has drained. For indwelling catheter, inject fluid to inflate balloon. Pull gently on catheter to check that it is secure.
    (Rationale: Balloon holds catheter in place in the bladder.)

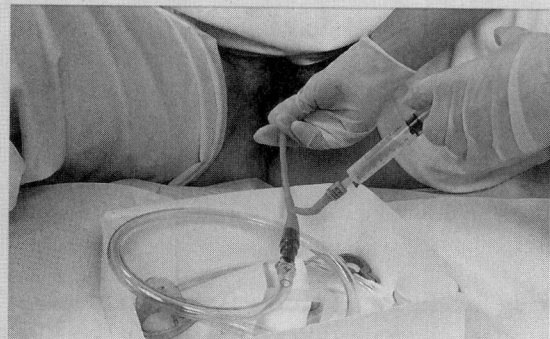

Step 15 Injecting sterile water to inflate the balloon

16. Use leg strap or tape to anchor tubing from indwelling catheter. Position drainage bag below the level of the bladder. Catheter should pass *over* leg.
    (Rationale: Properly positioned tubing decreases tension on the catheter. Drainage bag below bladder level uses gravity to promote the flow or urine and decreases risk of urinary stasis.)

17. Dry patient's perineal area if necessary. Remove gloves. Reposition and cover the patient. Lower the bed. Remove equipment.
    (Rationale: These measures ensure patient comfort and security.)

18. Dispose of equipment according to agency policy. Dispose of gloves.
    (Rationale: Proper disposal prevents transmission of organisms.)

19. Wash hands.
    (Rationale: Handwashing prevents the spread of organisms.)

20. Document size and type of catheter inserted and patient's response. Record amount of urine obtained, appearance, and collection of specimen if one was obtained.
    (Rationale: Documentation provides coordination of care.)

position for catheterization, rather than supine. The side-lying position does not expose the patient as much, it is more comfortable because the legs can be relaxed, and it is the only position possible for the patient who has had back surgery or who has contractures of the legs. When the patient is relaxed, insertion of the catheter is easier. The side-lying position also makes it easier to maintain sterile technique because only one labium needs to be held in position. Because the nurse does not have to reach over the patient's leg, the nurse is less likely to contaminate the catheter.

The patient lies on her side with her knees drawn up to her chest. If the nurse is right handed, the patient should lie on her left side, and vice versa. The patient's buttocks should be near the side of the bed where the nurse is standing, and the patient's shoulders should be near the other side of the bed. Stand behind the patient, near her buttocks. Follow the same sterile technique and general procedure as for the back-lying position.

Catheterizing the Male Patient

It is more difficult to catheterize a male patient because the urethra in the man is longer and more curved than that in a woman. Sometimes, in addition, an enlarged prostate gland constricts or obstructs the urethra. Previous infection in the urethra can also cause strictures. Nursing Procedure 54–5 describes male catheterization.

Caring for the Patient After Catheterization

After the catheterization of any patient, be sure the patient is comfortable and that the signal cord is within reach.

Be sure that the balloon is inflated or that another device is available to hold the catheter in place and that the catheter tubing is secured externally to avoid pulling and discomfort. To avoid pulling, hypoallergenic tape should be used to hold the catheter to the abdomen in the man and to the thigh in the woman. The patient may feel the urge to void due because of presence of the catheter in the urethra. Explain this to the patient.

In both men and women the tubing should extend straight down from the bed level to the bag ("straight drainage"). Extra tubing may be placed on the bed with the patient, so movement is possible. (*Rationale: Loops hanging down can promote urinary stasis and infection.*) If an indwelling catheter is left in place, attach the drainage apparatus to the bed, maintaining its sterility. Chapter 46 describes the care of the patient with a catheter in more detail.

Emptying the Urinary Drainage Bag. The nurse will be asked to empty the drainage bag, using sterile technique. Skills used in emptying urinary drainage bag follow.

◆ Carefully pull the drain tube located on the bottom of the bag out of its storage pocket, without touching it below the level of the clamp. Hold it over a container and release the clamp, making sure that the drain tube does not touch anything. (*Rationale: You avoid touching the lower part or the inside of the drain tube because pathogenic organisms can travel up the system and cause a bladder infection.*)

◆ When the urine has drained out, clamp the tube, wipe the tip with an alcohol wipe, and carefully replace it into the storage pocket. Be sure the clamp is far enough up the tube to allow most of the tube to fit into the pocket. (*Rationale: These procedures help to maintain the sterility of the catheter's closed drainage system.*)

◆ Most patients with indwelling catheters are on intake and output (I&O). Therefore, you collect the urine in a graduated container and measure it before disposing of it in the toilet. Rinse the graduate with cool water. Specific gravity may be ordered. It is important to observe the color, odor, and other characteristics of the urine. (*Rationale: The nurse's observations are important to the healthcare team when they evaluate the patient's response.*)

◆ If the patient will be going home with an indwelling catheter, teach the person what you are doing as you do it. You may ask the patient to do a return demonstration after you have demonstrated the procedure. (*Rationale: Patient teaching and documentation are important components of the nursing care plan.*)

◆ Properly dispose of your gloves and wash your hands.

◆ Record output on the appropriate sheet and document and report any special observations about the urine.

Collecting Specimens for Culture. The nurse may be ordered to collect specimens of urine for culture. In this case it is again important to observe careful sterile technique, and the drainage system usually remains closed. Wear clean gloves to protect yourself. The specimen for culture is collected using a sterile syringe and a small-gauge (approximately #25) needle. In some cases, a needleless system is used. The catheter is clamped just below the aspiration port and a very small amount of urine is allowed to collect (wear gloves). The port is cleansed with alcohol and allowed to dry and the specimen is drawn up into the syringe. The catheter is unclamped as quickly as possible, to avoid damage to the urethra or bladder. Urine specimens are not collected from the drainage bag. (*Rationale: There is a much greater chance of contamination in the bag than exists further up the catheter. In addition, it is not*

(Text continues on page 655)

Catheterizing the Male Patient

Supplies and Equipment

Same as for "Catheterizing the Female Patient"

Procedure

1. Follow steps 1 through 4 for female catheterization in Nursing Procedure 54-4.
2. Assist the patient to lie on his back with legs slightly apart. Position the drape or bath blanket so only the penis is uncovered.
   (Rationale: This prevents chilling and protects the patient's privacy.)
3. Put on clean gloves. Wash perineal area with soap. Rinse and dry. Remove gloves and wash hands again.
   (Rationale: Area is cleansed prior to introducing the catheter into meatus.)
4. Open the sterile catheterization tray on bedside table. Put on sterile gloves. Pick up sterile drape, shake open, and lay on patient's thighs. Place opening of fenestrated drape over penis.
   (Rationale: Using the drape provides a sterile field.)
5. Set up equipment on tray (same as step 9, Nursing Procedure 54-4). Catheter tip for male catheterization should be lubricated 5 to 7 inches.
   (Rationale: The longer male urethra necessitates lubricating a longer portion of the catheter.)
6. Move catheterization tray onto the sterile drape.
   (Rationale: All supplies are easily available, decreasing likelihood of reaching and contaminating equipment.)
7. Use nondominant hand to grasp penis. If patient is uncircumcised, retract foreskin before cleansing. With forceps, pick up cotton ball and cleanse from meatus outward in a circular motion. Repeat three times using each cotton ball only once.
   (Rationale: Moving from clean to dirty lessens the chance of introducing organisms into the bladder.)

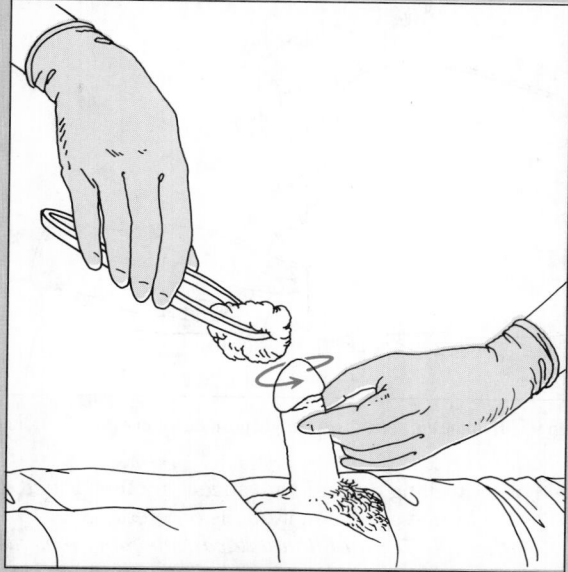

Step 7   Cleansing the penis

8. Pick up catheter approximately 3 inches from the tip with dominant hand. Place drainage end in basin. If catheter is indwelling, it may already be attached to drainage tubing.
   (Rationale: Sterile setup will not be contaminated by draining urine.)
9. Lift the penis to an upright perpendicular position. Gently pressing the end of the penis from two sides may help to open the meatus. Ask the patient to bear down as if voiding. Insert the catheter gently into the meatus advancing it 7 to 9 inches or until urine begins to drain. If resistance is encountered when passing the catheter, rotate the catheter slightly or withdraw it rather than forcing it.
   (Rationale: Holding the penis upright straightens the urethral canal. Rotating the catheter helps ease the catheter past the prostate gland.)

(continued)

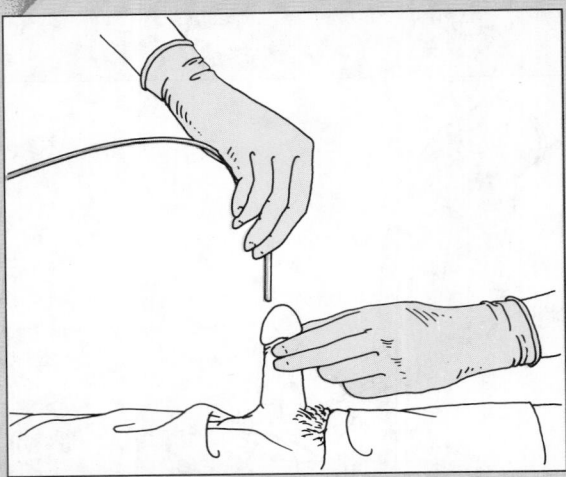

Step 9 Holding the penis in an upright position for inserting the catheter

10. For indwelling catheter, advance it another 1 inch. Collect urine specimen if one is ordered.
    (Rationale: The additional advancement of the catheter ensures that balloon will be inflated in the bladder rather than in the urethral canal.)
11. Follow steps 15 through 20 in Nursing Procedure 54-4 for female catheterization. Exceptions for the male patient include:
    a. Tape or secure the catheter to the lower abdomen or upper thigh allowing some slack in the tubing.

b. Return the foreskin to its original position in the uncircumcised man.
    (Rationale: Securing the catheter to the lower abdomen may reduce urethral pressure at the angle of the penis and scrotum. Returning the foreskin to its original position prevents impaired circulation and pressure on the urethra.)

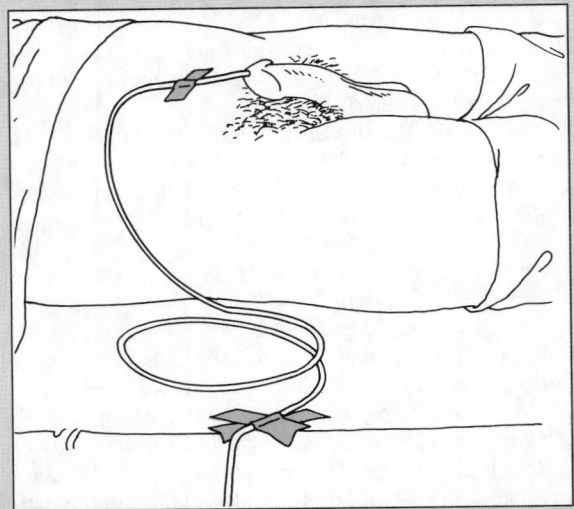

Step 11b Securing the catheter to the lower abdomen

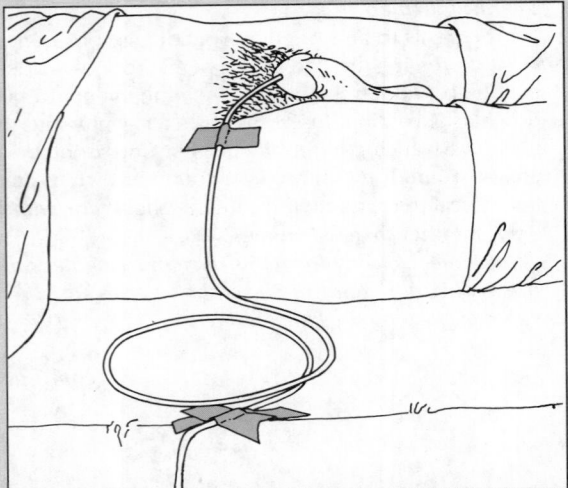

Step 11a Securing the catheter to the upper thigh

known when the urine drained into the large bag.) See also Chapter 47 for information on specimen collection and handling.

> **Key Concept**
>
> It is vital to prevent infection when working with urinary catheter or drainage systems.

Irrigating the Urinary Catheter. The purpose of irrigating the catheter is to cleanse the lumen of the catheter tubing, thus promoting patency of the tube. A physician's order is required before the procedure is performed. The physician will also order the type and amount of solution to be used. The following nursing skill describes irrigating the urinary catheter.

Nursing Skill
Irrigating the Urinary Catheter

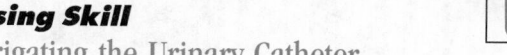

Supplies and Equipment

Clean gloves
Sterile gloves
Waterproof pad
Irrigating solution
Sterile irrigating syringe
Alcohol wipe

Procedure

1. Wash your hands. Assemble equipment and supplies.
2. Explain to the patient what you are going to do and why. Close the door or pull the bed curtains. *(Rationale: These actions decrease the patient's anxiety and provide privacy.)*
3. Don clean gloves.
4. Access catheter/tubing connection. Place waterproof pad under connection.
5. Set up sterile irrigating field (see Nursing Procedure 54–1).

6. Disconnect catheter from tubing and place a sterile cap on tubing to protect it. Do not allow tubing to fall on floor. *(Rationale: All actions decrease the possibility of contamination of tubing.)*
7. Discard gloves, and wash hands. Don sterile gloves.
8. Draw up 30 mL of irrigation solution (or other ordered amount).
9. Insert the syringe into tip of catheter and slowly inject solution. Solution should be room temperature, unless otherwise ordered. *(Rationale: This decreases the possibility of bladder spasms.)*
10. Remove syringe and allow solution to drain out by gravity.
11. Repeat these steps until solution drains freely. Do not continue if no solution returns from catheter. Report this to your instructor or team leader. *(Rationale: This prevents overdistention of the bladder and ensures adequate irrigation of bladder.)*
12. Cleanse end of catheter with alcohol wipe and remove cap from tubing. Cleanse end of tubing also. *(Rationale: Decrease possibility of contamination.)*
13. Reconnect tubing to catheter. Make sure urine is draining.
14. Dispose of waste and remove gloves.
15. Wash your hands.
16. Settle patient in a comfortable position.
17. Chart the time the procedure, amount of irrigation solution used and the amount returned, results, and how the patient tolerated the procedure.
18. *Note:* If you are instilling a medication, place a clamp on the catheter after you inject the solution. Return after the designated time and unclamp catheter. *(Rationale: This prevents the solution from running out of the bladder.)*

Removing the Foley Catheter. The removal of the indwelling catheter is a simple procedure. The nurse is careful to prevent trauma to the urethra and tries to make the patient as comfortable as possible. Actions in removing the Foley catheter are given in Nursing Procedure 54–6.

Removing the Foley Catheter

Supplies and Equipment

Gloves

Waterproof pad

Syringe (size is determined by volume of fluid used to inflate balloon)

Soap, water, washcloth, and towel

Procedure

1. Explain procedure to patient.
   (Rationale: Providing information fosters patient cooperation.)
2. Gather supplies after checking physician's order for removal of catheter.
   (Rationale: Organization facilitates performance of the skill.)
3. Wash hands before putting on gloves.
   (Rationale: Handwashing prevents the spread of organisms. Gloves act as a barrier.)
4. Close the door or pull the bed curtains. Adjust bed to a comfortable working height. Place waterproof pad between patient's thighs.
   (Rationale: Closing curtain or door protects the patient's privacy. Bed at proper height prevents back strain. The waterproof pad prevents soiling the bed linen.)
5. Attach hub of syringe to inflation port or insert needleless hub. Deflate the balloon by completely aspirating all the fluid.
   (Rationale: Balloon must be completely deflated so as not to traumatize urethra on removal.)

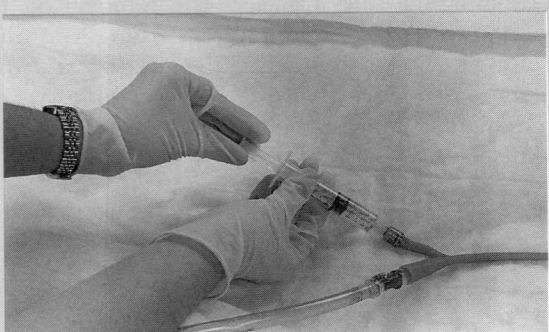

Step 5 Deflating the balloon

6. Pull the catheter out gently and slowly.
   (Rationale: This eases the catheter through the urethra.)
7. Wrap catheter in waterproof pad. Remove catheter, drainage bag, and equipment from bedside, disposing according to agency policy. Measure urine in drainage bag and record on I&O form.
   (Rationale: Proper disposal prevents transmission of organisms. Urine measurement provides accurate record of output.)

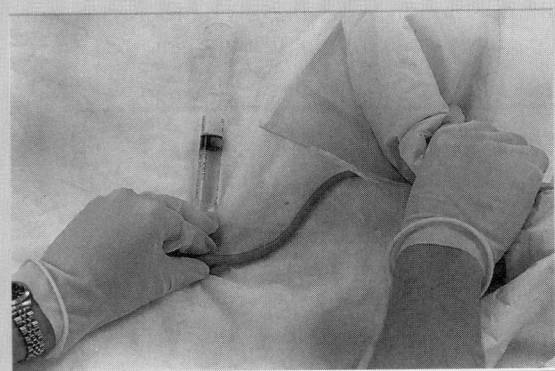

Step 7 Wrapping the catheter in a waterproof pad (Photos © B. Proud.)

8. Assist patient to cleanse and dry perineal area. Return to position of comfort.
   (Rationale: These measures ensure patient comfort.)
9. Remove gloves and wash hands.
   (Rationale: Handwashing prevents the transmission of organisms.)
10. Document removal of catheter on appropriate form.
    (Rationale: Documentation provides coordination of care.)

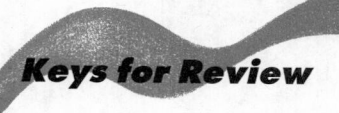

Keys for Review

Key Questions for Critical Thinking

1. Describe the difference between medical and surgical asepsis. Give examples of when each is used.
2. List nine guidelines to follow when using sterile technique. Describe rationale for each.
3. Describe when you would wear a hair covering, surgical mask, sterile gown, and sterile gloves. At what point in procedures would you don and remove them?
4. Describe the differences between female and male catheterization. Describe your explanation of the procedures to a woman and man.
5. Patient teaching is important. Describe key points in teaching a patient going home with an indwelling catheter.

Key Readings

Berkow R (Ed). The Merck Manual of Diagnosis and Therapy, Ed 16. Rahway, NJ, Merck & Co, 1992

Cooper DM. "'Wound Healing" Symposium. The Nursing Clinics of North America 25(1), pp. 163-277, March 1990

Craven RF, Hirnle CJ. Fundamentals of Nursing: Human Health and Function. Philadelphia, J.B. Lippincott, 1992

Earnest VV. Clinical Skills in Nursing Practice, Ed 2. Philadelphia, J.B. Lippincott, 1993

NANDA Nursing Diagnoses: Definitions and Classifications 1992. Philadelphia, North American Nursing Diagnosis Association, 1992

O'Toole M (Ed). Miller-Keane Encyclopedia and Dictionary of Medicine, Nursing, and Allied Health, Ed. 5. Philadelphia, W.B. Saunders, 1992

Key Readings (continued)

Smeltzer SC, Bare BG. Brunner and Suddarth's Textbook of Medical Surgical Nursing, Ed 7. Philadelphia, J.B. Lippincott, 1992

Smith-Temple AJ, Johnson JY. Nurses' Guide to Clinical Procedures, Ed 2. Philadelphia, J.B. Lippincott, 1994

Taylor C, Lillis C, LeMone P. Fundamentals of Nursing: The Art and Science of Nursing Care, Ed 2. Philadelphia, J.B. Lippincott, 1993

Enrichment Keys

Korniewicz D, Kirwin M, Larson E. "Do your gloves fit the task?" American Journal of Nursing 91(6):38-40, 1991

Larson E. "Handwashing: It's essential—even when you use gloves." American Journal of Nursing 89:934-939, 1989

Keys to Learning More

Unit Eleven: medication administration, parenteral medications administered using sterile technique

Unit Twelve: sterile procedures used in obstetrics

Unit Thirteen: treatments administered to children, including sterile procedures

Unit Fourteen: disorders of adults, many of which require surgical asepsis

Unit *11* Pharmacology and Administration of Medications

55 Introduction to Pharmacology and Mathematics

Learning Objectives

- Define the key terms in this chapter.
- Describe how the nurse is expected to account for narcotics and controlled drugs.
- Describe how to use drug reference books.
- Describe routes of administration of drugs and give an example of each.
- Describe at least three forms in which a drug may be available.
- Describe the necessary parts of a medication order.
- Identify the various measurement systems.
- Convert between different measurement systems.
- Use the metric system in calculating medication dosages.
- Demonstrate the use of ratio and proportion to calculate dosages of medications.

Key Terms

agonist	medication
ampule	official name
antagonist	pharmacology
caplet	potentiating
capsule	registered pharmacist
chemical name	synergistic
diluent	tablet
enteric-coated	trade name
generic name	transdermal
household measurement	vial

Keys to Understanding This Chapter

Chapter 4: legal implications must be considered when giving medication

Chapter 5: meeting basic needs sometimes requires medications for assistance

Keys to Understanding This Chapter
(continued)

Unit Four: understanding basic normal anatomy and physiology helps to recognize unwanted medication side effects

Unit Seven: administration of prescribed medications requires knowledge of phases of nursing process

Chapter 52: pain is sometimes relieved by medication

Chapter 53: the person who has surgery receives various medications

Key Points

- Medications are substances that modify body functions. They are used to prevent disease, aid in diagnosis and treatment of disease, or restore and maintain function of body tissues.
- Many laws, rules, and regulations concern the prescription, storage, and administration of drugs.
- The patient has the right to know what drugs are being given and to request the generic form of a drug.
- The patient may also refuse to take medications, unless there is a court order.
- The administration of medications is an activity which must be taken very seriously to prevent errors.
- Nurses have a responsibility to know how and where to look up information on drugs with which they are not familiar.
- A medication error can have serious consequences on a patient's condition and can cause death.
- Drugs are available in many forms.
- The nurse must understand how to calculate a drug dosage in case a drug is provided in a different dosage than the prescription. Ratios, proportions, and fractions are used.

Rosdahl CB: Textbook of Basic Nursing, 6th ed. © 1995 J.B. Lippincott Company

Key Learning Activities

◆ Interview a pharmacist in the community or in a hospital. What is the person's educational background? What are the person's major duties? What suggestions would the pharmacist have for better cooperation between nurses and the pharmacy department (in a hospital)?
◆ Practice doing conversions from the apothecary to metric system.
◆ Take a math placement test to determine if you need further review before administering medications.

A **medication** is a substance other than food that modifies body functions. Medications are used to prevent disease, aid in the diagnosis and treatment of disease, and restore or maintain functions in body tissues. **Pharmacology** is the study of chemicals and their effect on the body. A **registered pharmacist** (RPh) is a person licensed to prepare and dispense drugs.

Patients may feel apprehensive about medicines. Fear that an injection will hurt, that a medication will have an offensive taste, or that a capsule will stick in the throat may increase anxiety. Patients may think they are being made subjects for experimentation or that nothing will help them. They may simply be tired of taking medications.

Most patients want to know what a medication is and why it is being given. It is reassuring to be told what is being done. "I've brought you something for your cough," or "to relieve your pain," or "to help you sleep."

Key Concept

An important part of nursing practice is teaching patients about their medications and documenting that teaching.

Legal Aspects

Federal Drug Standards

Standards of strength and purity of drugs are essential to protect the public from the dangers of misuse or adulteration (adding of impure or inferior substances).

The Food, Drug, and Cosmetic Act empowers the Food and Drug Administration (FDA) to enforce drug standards. The publication that defines standards for the approval of drugs is called *The United States Pharmacopeia and the National Formulary* (USP[NF]). The USP and NF are now published as single volumes. They are revised every 5 years and supplements are published frequently to keep the information current.

Control of Narcotics and Schedule Drugs

In 1970, Congress passed the Comprehensive Drug Abuse Prevention and Control Act, commonly referred to as the "Controlled Substance Act." The Drug Enforcement Agency (DEA) was organized to enforce this act. The act regulates manufacturing, distributing, and dispensing drugs that are to be controlled. There are five classifications or "schedules" of controlled substances. The degree of control depends on these classifications (see the accompanying box).

The medications in schedules II, III, IV, and some others must always be kept in a double-locked drawer or cupboard. There are special forms in each healthcare facility that are used for recording the usage of these controlled substances. The forms verify the patient's name, dosage of the drug, time of administration, name of the person who prescribed the medication, and name and signature of the person who gave it. Keys to the narcotic cupboard or drawer are always carried by a nurse who is on duty.

Counting Narcotics and Schedule Drugs. The drugs are counted by two nurses at the beginning of each shift: the nurse going off duty and the nurse coming on duty.

Controlled Substances

Controlled Substances (Schedule Drugs) are classified on the following basis:

- *Schedule I* (C–I): high abuse potential, no accepted medical use (examples: heroin, LSD, mescaline)
- *Schedule II* (C–II): high abuse potential, severe dependence liability (examples: narcotics, barbiturates, amphetamines; includes drugs such as codeine, morphine, secobarbital)
- *Schedule III* (C–III): less abuse potential, moderate dependence liability (examples: nonbarbiturate sedatives, some narcotics in limited doses; includes drugs such as paregoric tincture or seconal suppositories)
- *Schedule IV* (C–IV): still less abuse potential, limited dependence (examples: some sedatives and antianxiety agents, nonnarcotic analgesics; includes drugs such as chloral hydrate, diazepam [Valium], phenobarbital)
- *Schedule V* (C–V): limited abuse potential (examples: small amounts of narcotics used as antitussives [cough medicines] or antidiarrheals, codeine cough syrup). Some of these medications may be kept in an unlocked area.

The count must agree or a search is undertaken to find any missing drug.

The nurse who is carrying the narcotic keys has a responsibility to keep track of them and to make sure that they are turned over to the next nurse in charge. As a student, you should return the keys to the charge nurse immediately after giving a narcotic. (Be sure you have signed out the drug.) In most nursing programs, students are not allowed to give narcotics or schedule medications without direct supervision. In many facilities nursing students are not permitted to handle the narcotics store.

Patients' Rights

Patients have the right to know what drugs are being given to them, why, and what the possible side effects might be. They have the right to refuse to take drugs unless a court order gives the physician the right to force medications. They also have the right to request generic drugs rather than brand name drugs. (Generic drugs are often less expensive.)

Nursing Considerations

As a nurse, you have an important responsibility to each patient to be knowledgeable about all drugs given. There is no excuse for administering a drug without first knowing the appropriate dosage and possible adverse effects. You should become familiar with some of the standard reference books, so you can always practice safely. Even if you are not giving drugs, you should be familiar with the drugs your patients are receiving. It is important that you know the possible actions of drugs so you can observe and report their effects intelligently. This knowledge should be applied every time a medication is given. This is not as difficult as it seems because the science of pharmacology has given us detailed information about the actions of a vast number of drugs. The information helps you to recognize both favorable and unfavorable effects. It also reminds you that drugs affect people as individuals.

> **Key Concept**
>
> It is up to you, as a nurse, to know as much as possible about the drugs you give. If a patient has an undesirable reaction from a drug and you do not recognize this reaction and take the appropriate action, you are at fault for a medication error, as much as if you had given the wrong drug.

When a patient is admitted to a healthcare facility, the assessment includes a detailed drug history. The history enables the physician to decide which drugs are both safe and effective for treating this patient. It is vital to determine if the patient has any allergies before giving drugs.

Drug References. The hospital formulary is prepared by and used in hospital pharmacies. Updated annually, the formulary lists the drugs available in that hospital pharmacy and provides information about the hospital's policies on the dispensing of drugs.

The *United States Dispensatory* (*USD*) discusses both official (the name identified in the USP[NF]) and unofficial drugs.

Key Abbreviations and Acronyms for Pharmacologic Care

DEA	Drug Enforcement Agency
OTC	Over-the-counter
RPh	Registered pharmacist
TO	Telephone order
VO	Verbal order
PDR	Physician's Desk Reference
USD	United States Dispensatory
USP(NF)	United States Pharmacopeia and National Formulary

The *Physician's Desk Reference (PDR)* is a recognized source of information on drugs. A new edition is published every year with more frequent updates. The *PDR* consists of seven sections: manufacturers' index, product name index, product classification index, generic and chemical name index, product identification section, product information section, and diagnostic product information. It also includes a list of poison control centers and a guide to the management of drug overdose. In the *PDR*, you can find information about therapeutic doses of drugs, side effects, expected therapeutic effects, and other special information.

Facts and Comparisons is used in many pharmacies. This book lists drugs under the following classifications: nutritional products, blood modifiers, hormones, diuretics and cardiovascular drugs, autonomic drugs, central nervous system drugs, gastrointestinal (GI) drugs, anti-infectives, and biologicals. This book is updated monthly and provides the most current drug information available.

Many other drug reference books are available.

Drug Preparations and Actions

Drug preparations are available for oral, topical, inhalant, and injectable administration; these are called *routes of administration*. They are discussed further in Chapter 57. Drug classifications are discussed in Chapter 56.

Names of Drugs

The rapid increase in the number of drugs and the variety of names often given the same drug are confusing. The **chemical name** describes the chemical composition of the drug. The **generic name** is often similar to the chemical name and is assigned by the first manufacturer of the drug. The generic name is simpler than the chemical name and may be used in any country by any manufacturer. The **official name** is the name identified in the USP(NF). The **trade name** (proprietary or brand name) is the copyrighted name assigned by the drug company making the drug and is followed by the symbol ®. If more than one company makes the same drug, it will have the same generic name but may have several different trade names. For this reason many physicians order drugs using only the generic name. Examples of these names for one drug are given in the accompanying box.

Many drugs are listed on the medication Kardex or on the package under both the generic name and the trade name. If this is not the case, you will need to look up the drug that was prescribed, if the order uses one form of the name and the package is labeled with another. You need to *make sure* you are giving the correct

Drug Names

The following presents an example of the different drug names for the drug ibuprofen.

Chemical name: 2-(4-isobutylphenyl) propinoic acid
Generic name: ibuprofen
Official name: ibuprofen
Brand names: Motrin, Amersol (available in Canada), Rufen, Advil (OTC), Nuprin (OTC)

drug. (Many reference books list drugs under both the trade name and the generic name. It is often easier to look up a drug under the generic name.)

Drug Actions

The form of a drug, its properties, and the desired effect determine the method of administration. A drug that produces a desired response is called an **agonist.** A drug that has an opposing effect (one drug acts against the other) is called an **antagonist.** There may be a **synergistic,** or **potentiating,** effect (one drug enhances the effect of the other). In potentiation or synergism, the combined action of the two drugs is greater than the sum of the two when given separately.

The nurse must be aware not only of the desired actions of various drugs but also undesired reactions as well. The nurse must be on the alert constantly for *adverse reactions* and *side effects* to be able to report and document them carefully.

Nursing Alert

Be aware of the patient who develops an allergy to medications. Watch for a rash, difficulty breathing, or other symptoms of anaphylaxis. Be aware that a rash may not develop immediately; a rash may not be apparent until the patient has been taking the medication for many days.

Drug Forms

Drugs are prepared in forms suitable for the various methods of administration. These forms are liquids, solids, semisolids, metered-dose inhalants, transdermal, and continuous-release medications.

Liquids. Liquids are administered *orally, parenterally,* or *topically.* Parenteral administration routes include *intramuscular, subcutaneous, intradermal,* and *intravenous* injection. Oral administration of liquids is most often used in pediatrics, psychiatry, or geriatrics. Topical use of liquids includes instillations and irrigations, usually of the eye or ear. Lotions may also be used topically. A *tincture* is another form of a liquid drug; it contains alcohol.

Ampules are sealed glass receptacles that usually contain one dose of a liquid drug.

Vials are rubber-stoppered glass receptacles containing one or several doses of a drug in either liquid or powder form. Powders must be reconstituted in sterile water or sterile normal saline for injection, as specified by the manufacturer. The water or saline is the **diluent**; it dilutes the powder.

Disposable syringes containing single doses of a drug for injection are also widely used. One type of disposable syringe such as a Tubex contains one dose of a drug in a cartridge unit, with an attached sterile needle that fits into a metal or plastic holder. The cartridge is discarded after use.

Solids. Solid drugs are given by mouth in the form of tablets or capsules. A **tablet** is a compressed, spherical form of a drug; tablets may be **enteric-coated** (a coating that does not dissolve until the tablet reaches the intestine), or they may be plain. A **caplet** is a tablet in the shape of a capsule, to make it easier to swallow. A **capsule** is a drug in powdered or pellet form that has been enclosed in a soluble cylindrical gelatin-like capsule. The reason for using a capsule may be that the drug has a disagreeable taste or that the coating may delay the action of the drug. Tablets, caplets, and capsules can be made to release the medication at one time or they may be time-released medications (released over a period of time).

> **Nursing Alert**
>
> Be sure to check before crushing a tablet, caplet, or capsule. Time-released medications should not be crushed.

A *powder* is another form of a solid drug; a powder is most often mixed with a liquid for oral administration. It may also be applied topically or inhaled.

A *pill* technically is absolutely round, although in common usage, tablets are sometimes called "pills" as well.

Semisolids. Drugs in semisolid form are usually given as vaginal, urethral, or rectal suppositories. They are solid when inserted and melt at body temperature. Other semisolid drugs are ointments and pastes; these are generally used for topical application.

Inhalers. Oral or nasal *inhalers* deliver the drug topically to the area of desired effect. These inhalers are metered and discharge a constant amount of the drug with each actuation. The advantage of this type of delivery is the reduction of systemic effects to the rest of the body. This is especially important when using steroids or sympathomimetics.

Transdermal Medications. Transdermal (through the skin) preparations have a similar advantage. In these delivery systems, the drug is incorporated into a resin in a patch and placed on the skin. It will deliver a controlled amount of the drug through the skin into the blood over a period of time (usually 12–24 hours). The drug is continually absorbed through the skin while the patch is intact. Drugs that are used transdermally bypass the GI tract. Thus, drugs that would be destroyed by the digestive system can be given by this means. In most cases a smaller amount of the drug is needed for the same desired effect as oral preparations.

How Drugs Are Prescribed

Drug Dosage

The *dose* is the amount of a drug given as treatment. The *minimal dose* is the smallest amount necessary for a therapeutic effect. The *therapeutic dose* is the amount required to obtain the desired effect in a particular patient, or in most patients. The *maximal dose* is the largest amount that can be given safely. The *toxic dose* is an amount that causes symptoms of outright poisoning. The *lethal dose* is an amount that will cause death.

In prescribing the dosage of any drug, the physician considers the following individual differences:

Age. Children are more sensitive to drugs than adults and can tolerate less of a drug because of their smaller size. The effects of drugs on elderly people may differ from the effects on younger adults. Body changes, particularly in the liver or kidneys, can lead to the accumulation of drug, which can lead to serious adverse reactions and symptoms of overdose. Older people may also have a *paradoxical* (opposite) response to any drug.

Gender. Some drugs are more soluble in fat, others in water. Because women usually have more body fat and men more body fluid, the effects of medications are different in men and women. In addition, many drugs given to the mother may be harmful to an unborn fetus or to a nursing infant.

Weight. Dosage is often prescribed in relation to a patient's weight, especially when a specific concentration of the drug in the blood is desired. Larger doses are required in heavier persons. (To calculate the dosage for certain drugs the patient's weight is recorded in kilograms.)

Patient's Condition. The nature of a disease and its severity may make a difference in the dosage. More of a drug is required to quiet a highly disturbed patient or to control severe pain than is required to treat less extreme agitation or less severe pain. Renal and hepatic function may make a difference in the amount of drug required.

Patient's Disposition and Psychological State. A highly nervous person requires less of a stimulant and more of a depressant drug. The opposite is true of a less anxious or more stoic patient.

Method of Administration. The speed with which a drug enters the circulation may affect the dosage. This, in turn, depends on how the drug is given. Intravenous and intramuscular methods are more rapid-acting than the oral method. Drugs administered rectally are absorbed more slowly than drugs administered either orally or by injection.

Distribution. Some drugs are distributed evenly throughout the body and reach all cells; others appear only in certain body fluids or tissues. For example, one antibiotic may enter the spinal fluid, but another may never reach it.

Environment. The temperature may influence the speed of absorption; heat causes faster absorption and cold may decrease absorption because it decreases metabolic rate and circulation.

Time of Administration. Time of day is a factor in drug administration. For example, if a sleep medication is given in the morning, the person will probably not go to sleep. If medications are given at mealtime, they are usually absorbed more slowly. A diuretic is best administered in the morning so frequent urination does not interrupt sleep.

Elimination. Normally, a drug remains in the body long enough to do its work and is eliminated by the excretory organs, in the urine, feces, breath, or perspiration. Some drugs leave the body in their original form, whereas others have been made inactive by chemical changes that have occurred in their structure. If these processes are slow, the effect of the drug may be too prolonged; if they are too rapid, the drug may be excreted before it can do its work effectively. If the drug cannot be eliminated because of kidney or liver dysfunction, toxic levels of the drug may accumulate in the blood. Furthermore, chemical changes also may result in the formation of substances that are harmful if the body is unable to dispose of them rapidly enough.

Prescriptions

Some drug preparations can be purchased without a prescription and are known as *over-the-counter* (OTC) drugs. Federal law requires a prescription for any drug that is not considered safe to use without a physician's supervision. Many prescriptions cannot be refilled without the written or telephoned authorization of the physician. Prescriptions cannot be refilled more than one year after the date they are written.

A prescription (medication order) is a written formula for preparing and giving a drug preparation. Physicians (MD), osteopaths (DO), dentists (DDS and DMD), nurse practitioners (NP), midwives (CNM), and veterinarians (DVM) are the only persons licensed to write prescriptions for drugs. *The nurse may give a drug preparation only on an order from one of these people.* In the hospital, the orders are written in a special form in the patient's chart.

The physician writes the prescription, but the *pharmacist* is the only person qualified and licensed to make up drug preparations. In a hospital, the prescription is sent to the hospital pharmacy; otherwise, it is prepared by a local pharmacist. Every hospital has its own procedure for handling orders for prescribed drugs.

The prescription (medication order) has several parts (Table 55-1). Abbreviations commonly used in medication orders are listed in Table 37-2.

Verbal Orders

Sometimes orders are given verbally by physicians, such as in an emergency or on the telephone. Most hospitals allow only the registered nurse to accept verbal orders. However, in extended care facilities and nursing homes, licensed practical nurses *may* be allowed to take verbal medication orders. Most facilities require that verbal orders be signed by the physician within 24 hours.

The nurse who has taken a verbal order sees that such an order is written in the proper place, identified as a verbal order (VO) or a telephone order (TO), and later signed by the physician. This is important because a written order protects the physician, the patient, and the nurse. It is a permanent record that cannot be disputed and is always available for reference.

The nurse is responsible for carrying out an order as it is written: the nurse is *never* permitted to make even the slightest change. If you have any reason to question an order, or if you do not understand or cannot read an order, you must consult the charge nurse, team leader, or physician before proceeding.

Table 55-1. Parts of a Prescription

Part	Procedure/Rationale
Patient's *full* name	To avoid confusion with another patient with same surname; patient's room number or medical record number may be included
Date/time of day	Tells when order is to be started; may tell when order is to be discontinued; prescription must be rewritten if drug is to be continued
Name of drug	Generic name preferred to trade name; sometimes both are used
Dosage/amount of drug	Stated in measurement system used by hospital; may also be expressed as number of capsules or tablets or in fluid volume
Time/frequency of dose	The hospital nursing service usually determines the schedule for drug routines; the physician may give less definite directions. (For example, certain drugs must be given before meals, whereas others must be given with or after meals for maximum effect. It is important to differentiate between a drug to be given every 6 hours and one to be given 4 times a day.)
Method/route	It is usually understood that the oral method is to be used if no other method is specified, although oral (PO) should be specified. Otherwise, the physician specifies the method, especially if the drug can be given in more than one way.
Physician's signature	Essential for legal reasons or if there is some question about the order; an unsigned order may mean the physician had not finished writing it or that it was not written by a physician.

Key Concept

The nursing student *never* takes verbal or telephone orders for medications.

Systems of Measurement

Drugs are measured by both dry and liquid methods. Two systems are used for measuring drugs, the *metric system* and the *apothecaries' system*. In addition, there

Table 55-2. Systems of Measurement

System	Unit	Abbreviations/Symbols
Metric	milligram	mg
	gram	g, gm
	cubic centimeter	cc*
	liter	L
	milliliter	mL
	kilogram	kg
	microgram	mcg or μg
Apothecaries'	grain	gr
	minim	m, min, ɱ
	dram	dr, ℨ
	ounce	oz, ℥
	pint	pt
	quart	qt
Household	drop	gtt
	teaspoon	t, tsp
	tablespoon	T, tbsp

* 1 cc = approximately 1 mL.

is the system of **household measurement** that is used in cooking. The units of measurement with their corresponding abbreviations are given in Table 55-2. These are measures that you will use to measure medicines, solutions used in nursing treatments, and fluids taken in and excreted by the patient. All hospitals do not use the same system. Nurses must understand all of the measuring systems and know the equivalents to convert from one system to another. Drugs must be measured in the same terms as those in the drug order.

You may also be asked to administer a drug in *units*, such as insulin for diabetes or penicillin for an infection. You will also hear the term *units* used in connection with recommended dietary allowances of vitamins. It is important to know that some drugs are prescribed by the amount to be given, rather than by the specific dosage. For example, multivitamins are prescribed by the number of tablets, and milk of magnesia is prescribed by the volume of fluid.

Nursing Alert

Administering drugs is one of the most important functions you will have as a nurse. Take your responsibility seriously. A medication error can cause a patient's death.

The Metric System

The metric system is the most widely used measurement system in the world. It is often used in medicine. The U.S. monetary system is based on the metric system. The metric system is based on a decimal system in which measurements are in increments of 10. Length, weight, and volume are all measured in this manner.

Length is measured in meters; volume in liters; weight in grams. Greek and Latin prefixes are used to describe various increments of these basic units. For example:

◆ deci- (divide by 10; 1/10)
◆ centi- (divide by 100; 1/100)
◆ milli- (divide by 1,000; 1/1,000)
◆ micro- (divide by 1,000,000; 1/1 millionth)
◆ deca- (multiply by 10; × 10)
◆ hecto- (multiply by 100; × 100)
◆ kilo- (multiply by 1,000; × 1,000)

In addition to medication administration, nurses use the metric system in other aspects of care. For example, amounts of oral fluid intake and urinary output are measured in milliliters (mL), and newborns are weighed in grams (g) and measured in centimeters (cm). When measuring the size of an incision or ulcer, you often measure in centimeters. The dilation of the cervix during delivery is always stated in centimeters.

Metric Conversions by Moving the Decimal Point. Metric conversions are made by moving the decimal point. When you move the decimal point to the *right*, you will get a *larger number* and a *smaller unit of measure*. For example: 1.0 gram = 1,000.0 mg. The decimal point was moved to the right. One gram is equivalent to 1,000 milligrams

When you move the decimal point to the *left*, you get a *smaller number* and a *larger unit of measure*. For example: 1,000.0 g = 1.0 kg. The decimal point was moved to the left. One kilogram is equivalent to 1,000 grams.

Hint: To get a *smaller unit of measure*, move the decimal point to the *right*; you will get a larger number

To get a *larger unit of measure*, move the decimal point to the *left*; you will get a smaller number. The accompanying box gives you examples of metric measures and equivalents.

Household Measurement

Household measurement is widely used in the home. It uses terminology with which most people are familiar. This system is often used to measure medications given at home, for example, tablespoon and teaspoon. It is necessary to know the conversions between the metric and household systems when teaching patients and their families. The physician usually orders the medication in the metric system, but the patient only has household measurement tools at home. For example:

5 mL = 1 teaspoonful (approx.)
15 mL = 1 tablespoonful (approx.)

Metric Measures and Equivalents

Weight is measured in grams:

1 kilogram (kg) = 1000 grams (g) (=2.2 pounds)
1 milligram (mg) = 0.001 (1/1000) gram
1 milligram (mg) = 1000 micrograms (mcg)
1 microgram (mcg) = 0.000001 gram (1/1,000,000 or 1/1 millionth of a gram) = 0.001 milligram
454 grams = 1 pound

Volume is measured in liters:

1 liter (L) = 1000 milliliters (mL)
1 milliliter (mL) = 0.001 liter (L)

Length is measured in meters:

1 meter (M) = 100 centimeters (cm) = 1000 millimeters (mm)
1 centimeter (cm) = 0.01 meter (M) or 1/100 meter
1 millimeter (mm) = 0.001 meter or 1/1000 meter
2.54 cm = 1 inch

Note: Volume is sometimes expressed in terms of cubic centimeters (cc); the proper designation is milliliter (mL). (1 mL = approximately 1 cc).

The Apothecary System

This system is an ancient system and is seldom used, although many products still are expressed with this system and some physicians still use it. For example:

5 grains (of aspirin) = 325 mg (approx.)
½ grain (codeine) = 30 mg (approx.)
1 grain = 60 mg (approx.)

Conversion From One System to Another

Conversion from one system of measurement to another can be done by using simple mathematics. Table 55-3 identifies systems of measurement and their equivalent relationships. The term equivalent does not mean exact or equal. There is some discrepancy because of the inaccuracy of the apothecary system. For example, the original grain was defined as the weight of a grain of wheat.

Dosage Calculation

Most medications are ordered and supplied in the metric system. At times, however, liquid and oral medications may be ordered in apothecary or household measure. If a medication is ordered in one unit of measure and supplied in another unit of measure, the nurse must calculate the amount of medication needed in the measurement system in which it is ordered.

Dosage calculations are an important responsibility. If the calculated dosage seems unusual or if the nurse

Table 55-3. Systems of Measurements in Their Equivalent Relationships

	Metric	*Apothecaries'*	*Household*
Dry measures	1 g	15 gr	¼ tsp
	28–30 g	1 oz	
	60–65 mg	1 gr	
Liquid measures	1 mL	15 m	15 drops
	5 mL	1 fl dr	1 tsp
	15 mL	3 fl dr	1 tbsp
	30 mL	1 fl oz	
	500 mL	1 pt (approx.)	2 measuring cups
	1000 mL (1 L)	1 qt (approx.)	4 measuring cups

has any doubts about the accuracy of the calculation (eg, the calculated dose seems too large or too small), he or she should ask another nurse or pharmacist to check the calculation. The calculation of medications with important or toxic side effects should always be double-checked by another nurse. (Examples include insulin and digitalis preparations.)

Ratio and Proportion

Ratios and proportions are frequently used to calculate medication dosages. A ratio is the relationship of one quantity to another. A ratio may be written as a fraction or separated by a colon, for example, 2/3 or 2:3. When two ratios are set equal to each other, they are said to be *in proportion* to each other. A true proportion consists of two ratios separated by an equals sign (=) or a double colon (::). This indicates that the two ratios are equal.

For example:

$$\tfrac{2}{3} = \tfrac{6}{9}$$

or

$$2{:}3{::}6{:}9$$

or

2 is to 3 as 6 is to 9

This is a valuable relationship. When written with the colon, the first and last numbers are referred to as the *extremes* and the second and third (middle) numbers as the *means*.

$$2{:}3 \quad :: \quad 6{:}9$$

means
extremes

There are three rules that apply when using ratios.

Rules of Ratios

◆ The product of the means equals the product of the extremes. The *product* is the answer you get

when you multiply. Therefore, $2 \times 9 = 18$ (product of the extremes) and $3 \times 6 = 18$ (product of the means).

◆ The product of the means divided by one extreme yields the other extreme. Therefore, $3 \times 6 = 18$ and $18 \div 2 = 9$.

◆ The product of the extremes divided by one mean yields the other mean. Therefore, $2 \times 9 = 18$ and $18 \div 6 = 3$.

THEREFORE, when 3 of the 4 factors of a ratio are known, the missing factor can be found, using simple mathematics.

Dosage Calculations Using Ratios

Ratio and proportion is probably the most commonly used method of calculating dosages.

To use the ratio and proportion method, the numbers to be multiplied must be in the same unit of measurement. Therefore, you must convert if this is not true.

#1. EXAMPLE: The prescription is 1 mg Haldol IM (intramuscularly) and the medication is available in an ampule with a strength of 5 mg/1 mL. How many mL should be given?

SOLUTION: Set up a ratio.

Known factors:

medication available = 5 mg (strength)	<u>Factor 1</u>
in 1 mL (per volume)	<u>Factor 2</u>
prescribed dosage = 1 mg	<u>Factor 3</u>
volume (mL) needed to give = X mL	<u>Unknown factor</u>

◆ (Product of means, divided by one extreme, equals other extreme.)

Set up units in the same position on each side.

5 mg is to 1 mL as 1 mg is to X mL

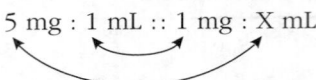

Remember: Units of conversion must cancel properly.

Cross-multiply:

$$1 \times 1 = 1 \div 5 = \frac{1}{5} = \frac{2}{10} = 0.2 \text{ mL}$$

(You need to convert to tenths so you can measure in a syringe.)

You would measure up 0.2 (2/10) mL in your syringe.

You can also calculate tenths by dividing the numerator (top number) by the denominator (bottom number) (See the section on fractions later in this chapter.)

$$\frac{1 \text{ (numerator)}}{5 \text{ (denominator)}} \quad \frac{1}{5} = 5\overline{)1.0}^{0.2} = \frac{2}{10} \text{ or } 0.2 \text{ mL}$$
$$\underline{1\,0}$$

#2. EXAMPLE: The prescription of Penicillin G (oral tablets) is 375 mg. Tablets are supplied in 250 mg scored tablets (able to be divided in half). How many tablets do you give?

Set up a ratio:

250 mg is to 1 tablet as 375 mg is to X tablets
250 mg : 1 tablet :: 375 mg : X tablet

Multiply means:
375 mg × 1 tablet = 375 mg tablets
and 375 mg tablet ÷ 250 mg = X tablets
Therefore, X = 1.5 tablets
You would give 1½ tablets

$$\begin{array}{r} 1.5 \\ 250\overline{)375.0} \\ \underline{250\,0} \\ 125\,0 \\ \underline{125\,0} \end{array}$$

You would need to split one of the scored tablets in half. (You cannot divide tablets except where they are scored.)

Occasionally, tablets are scored so they can be divided into halves *or* fourths.

#3. EXAMPLE: The prescription is 75 mg Trazodone. The medication is provided in 150 mg scored tablets. How many tablet(s) are needed?

SOLUTION: Set up a ratio:

150 mg is to 1 tablet as 75 mg is to X tablets
150 mg : 1 tablet :: 75 mg : X tablet

Multiply means:
75 mg × 1 tablet = 75 mg tablets
and 75 mg tablet ÷ 150 mg = X tablets
Therefore, X = 0.5 tablets
You would give 0.5 tablet (½ tablet)

$$\begin{array}{r} 0.5 \\ 150\overline{)75.0} \\ \underline{75\,0} \end{array}$$

Note: If the dosage for tablets does not come out exactly, the prescribed dosage *cannot* be given.

#4. EXAMPLE: You are administering a tube feeding. The patient is supposed to receive 75 mL/h. The bag contains 500 mL. How many hours will this feeding bag last?

Set up a ratio:

75 mL : 1 hour :: 500 mL : X hours

Multiply means:
1 hour × 500 mL = 500 mL hr
and 500 mL hr ÷ 75 mL = X hrs.
Therefore, X = 6.66 . . . = 6⅔ hours

$$\begin{array}{r} 6.66\ldots \\ 75\overline{)500.00} \\ \underline{450} \\ 500 \\ \underline{450} \\ 500 \\ \underline{450} \end{array}$$

The bag will last 6 hours and 40 minutes.

Fractions

Fractions can be either *common fractions* or *decimal fractions*.

Common Fractions. A *fraction* is a portion or piece of a whole that indicates division of that whole into equal parts. Common fractions have a numerator (the top number) and a denominator (the bottom number). For example:

$$\frac{3}{4} \quad \frac{\text{numerator}}{\text{denominator}}$$

¾ can be pictured as: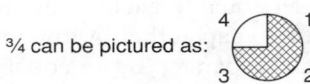

The numerator refers to a *part* of the whole and is the top number. The denominator refers to the *total number of parts* and is the number on the bottom.

To multiply fractions:

$$\frac{2}{3} \times \frac{3}{4}$$

1. Multiply the numerators to get the new numerator.

$$\frac{2}{3} \times \frac{3}{4} = \frac{6}{}$$

2. Multiply the denominators to get the new denominator.

$$\frac{2}{3} \times \frac{3}{4} = \frac{6}{12}$$

3. Reduce the fraction to its lowest terms. (Divide both numbers by 6.)

$$\frac{6}{12} = \frac{1}{2}$$

To divide fractions:

$$\frac{3}{4} \div \frac{2}{3}$$

1. Write the problem.

$$\tfrac{3}{4} \div \tfrac{2}{3}$$

2. Invert the divisor.

$$\tfrac{3}{4} \div (\tfrac{3}{2})$$

3. Multiply the numerators and denominators.

$$\tfrac{3}{4} \times \tfrac{3}{2} = \tfrac{9}{8}$$

4. Reduce the fraction to its lowest terms.

$$\tfrac{9}{8} = 1\tfrac{1}{8}$$

Decimal Fractions. Decimal fractions are fractions in which 10 is always the denominator. The 10 is sometimes omitted when fractions are written and a decimal point is inserted in the numerator (as many places from the last number on the right as there are ciphers [zeros] of 10 in the denominator). Therefore, $1/10 = 0.1$ and $1/100 = 0.01$.

3/4 can also be written as a decimal by converting it to tenths, or in this case, hundredths. 4 goes into 100, 25 times and 25 times 3 is 75. Therefore, $3/4 = 75/100$ths or 0.75.

$$\frac{3}{4} = \frac{X}{100} \quad \overset{\text{cross-multiply}}{4\,X = 300} \quad X = 4\overline{)300} \quad X = 75$$
$$\frac{28}{}$$
$$\frac{20}{20}$$

Replace X with 75: $\dfrac{75}{100} = 0.75$

Dosage Calculations Using the Formula Method

When the prescribed or desired dosage is different from what is available or "what you have," a dosage calculation is necessary to determine the quantity of drug to give. Use ratio and proportion to solve dosage calculations.

The formula method can be used when calculating dosages in the *same system* and the *same units of measurement*. The following formula can be used to calculate the amount of medication needed.

$$\frac{\text{Desired amount or prescribed amount (D)}}{\text{Available dosage (what's on hand) (A)}} \times \text{Quantity (eg, 1 pill or 1 tablet or 5 mL)} = \chi$$

Desired amount divided by Available dosage × Quantity = amount to give

---

#1. EXAMPLE: The prescribed dose is $1\tfrac{1}{4}$ mg digoxin and the medication is supplied as $\tfrac{1}{2}$ mg tablets.

Desired amount $1\tfrac{1}{4}$ mg   (or $\tfrac{5}{4}$)
Available dosage $\tfrac{1}{2}$ mg
in what Quantity   1 tablet

Set up the problem $\dfrac{D}{A} \times Q = X \qquad \dfrac{5/4}{1/2} \times 1 \text{ tablet} = X$

Because this calculation is in fractions, follow the rules for working with fractions (see the section on fractions earlier in this chapter).

1. Write the problem.

$$\tfrac{5}{4} \div \tfrac{1}{2} \times 1 \text{ tablet} = \chi$$

2. Invert the divisor.

$$\tfrac{5}{4} \div (\tfrac{2}{1}) \times 1 \text{ tablet} = \chi$$

3. Multiply the numerators and denominators.

$$\tfrac{5}{4} \times \tfrac{2}{1} \times 1 \text{ tablet} = \chi$$

$$\tfrac{10}{4} \times 1 \text{ tablet} = \chi$$

4. Reduce the fraction to its lowest terms.

$\tfrac{10}{4}$ tablet $= 2\tfrac{2}{4} = 2\tfrac{1}{2}$ tablets. You would give $2\tfrac{1}{2}$ tablets.

#2. EXAMPLE: The prescribed dose is 1/400 gr of a medication. The tablets provided are 1/200 gr per scored tablet.

◆ Desired amount: 1/400 gr
◆ Available dosage: 1/200 gr
◆ In what Quantity: 1 tablet

Set up the problem.

$$\frac{D}{A} \times Q = \chi \qquad \frac{\tfrac{1}{400}\ \text{gr}}{\tfrac{1}{200}\ \text{gr}} \times 1 \text{ tablet} = \chi$$

Use the rules for calculating fractions.

1. Write the problem.

$$1/400 \div 1/200 \times 1 \text{ tablet} = \chi$$

2. Invert the divisor.

$$1/400 \div (\tfrac{200}{1}) \times 1 \text{ tablet} = \chi$$

3. Multiply the numerators and the denominators.

$$\frac{1}{400} \times \frac{200}{1} \times 1 \text{ tablet} = \chi$$

$$\frac{200}{400} \times 1 \text{ tablet} = \chi$$

4. Reduce the fraction to its lowest terms.

$$\frac{200}{400} \text{ tablet} = \frac{1}{2} \text{ tablet}$$

Because the tablets are scored, the nurse can give $\frac{1}{2}$ tablet. (Remember that some tablets cannot be broken in half.)

Key Concept

In a fraction, a larger denominator denotes smaller pieces. Therefore, $\frac{1}{400}$ is only half as much as $\frac{1}{200}$.)

Significant Figures

This term refers to figures which have practical meaning. For example, a dosage prescribed is 1.325 mL. When measured with a syringe containing markings of 1.3 mL, 1.4 mL, and 1.5 mL, the last two numbers (the "25") cannot be measured. Therefore, the dosage that can be measured is 1.3 mL and 1.3 mL is the significant figure. (The amount given is 1.3 mL because this amount is closer to the prescribed dosage than 1.4 mL.)

Percentages

The term *percentage* refers to the number per hundred. Therefore, 20% equals 20 per hundred. Percent has no specific units of measure. It is actually a ratio. To con-

vert from percentage to a fraction, the percent number becomes the numerator and 100 is always the denominator.

EXAMPLE: 20% = 20/100

a. To convert a fraction to a percent, put the fraction in the format that has 100 as the denominator; then multiply by the number required so the denominator equals 100. Thus, the numerator becomes percentage.

EXAMPLE #1:

$$\frac{4}{10} = \frac{40}{100} = 40\% \text{ (multiply both sides by 10)}$$

EXAMPLE #2:

$$\frac{9}{20} = \frac{X}{100} \qquad \overset{\text{cross multiply}}{20X = 900} \qquad X = 20\overline{)900} = 45$$

$$\begin{array}{r} 80 \\ \hline 100 \\ 100 \\ \hline 0 \end{array}$$

Replace x with 45: $\frac{9}{20} = \frac{45}{100} = 45\%$

(20 goes into 100 5 times; $9 \times 5 = 45$)

b. You can also determine the percentage of any fraction by dividing the numerator by the denominator.

$$20\overline{)9.00} = 0.45 \qquad 0.45 = \frac{45}{100} = \underline{45\%}$$
$$\begin{array}{r} 0.45 \\ 80 \\ \hline 100 \\ 100 \end{array}$$

Key Concept

Be sure to use reference books or tables if you have any questions about dosage conversions. It is a good idea to have another nurse double-check your calculations until you are confident in doing them.

Keys for Review

Key Questions for Critical Thinking

1. Describe schedule drugs and discuss the role of the nurse in storing and accounting for these types of drugs.
2. Discuss how you would proceed if you thought a drug order was erroneous.
3. Describe the actions of an agonist and an antagonist drug and provide examples of each.

Key Readings

Alfaro-LeFevre R. Drug Handbook: A Nursing Process Approach. Reading, CA, Addison-Wesley, 1992

Batasini PH. Pharmacological Calculations for Nurses: A Worktext, Ed 2. Albany, NY, Delmar Publishers, 1991

Boyer MJ. Math for Nurses: A Pocket Guide to Dosage Calculation and Drug Preparation, Ed 3. Philadelphia, J.B. Lippincott, 1994

Clayton B, Stock Y. Basic Pharmacology for Nurses, Ed 10. St. Louis, Mosby-Yearbook, 1992

Craven RF, Hirnle CJ. Fundamentals of Nursing: Human Health and Function. Philadelphia, J.B. Lippincott, 1992

Dunlop K. Mathematics for Health Occupations. Albany, NY, Delmar Publishers, 1991

Henke G. Med-Math: Dosage Calculation, Preparation, and Administration, Ed 2. Philadelphia, J.B. Lippincott, 1995

Pikar G. Dosage Calculation, Ed 3. Albany, NY, Delmar Publishers, 1991

Key Readings *(continued)*

Scherer J. Introductory Clinical Pharmacology, Ed 4. Philadelphia, J.B. Lippincott, 1992

Swonger A, Matejski M. Nursing Pharmacology: An Integrated Approach to Drug Therapy and Nursing, Ed 2. Philadelphia, J.B. Lippincott, 1991

Taylor C, Lillis C, Lemone, P. Fundamentals of Nursing: The Art and Science of Nursing Care, Ed 3. Philadelphia, J.B. Lippincott, 1993

Keys to Learning More

Chapter 56: classifications of medications and their medical uses

Chapter 57: administration of medications

Unit Twelve: many medications are used in childbirth; many are dangerous in pregnancy

Unit Thirteen: pediatric disorders and administration of medications to children

Unit Fourteen: adult disorders, many of which require medications

Unit Fifteen: special considerations in giving medications to older adults

Chapter 87: psychiatric medications and serious side effects, such as tardive dyskinesia

Chapter 88: substance abuse, including drug abuse

Unit Seventeen: death, dying, and hospice nursing, where special medications are often required

56 Classification of Medications

Keys for Learning

Learning Objectives

♦ Describe the most common antibiotics.
♦ Discuss development of resistance by pathogens to antibiotics.
♦ List and describe three classifications of antineoplastics, the types of dermatologic agents, and common analgesics and barbiturates.
♦ Define the term digitalizing dose.
♦ Describe types of digitalis preparations and the dangers of overdose.
♦ Describe three drugs used to control blood pressure and two types of drugs that control the viscosity of the blood.
♦ Demonstrate the ability to use reference books related to medications.
♦ Describe the side effects of steroid use over an extended period of time.
♦ Discuss the nursing assessment required when a patient is receiving medications.
♦ Describe the most common side effects of narcotics and antibiotics.

Key Terms

antiarrhythmic	bronchodilator	productive
antibiotic	cathartic	sedative
anticonvulsant	depressant	seizure
antihypertensive	hemostatic	stimulant
antitussive	hypnotic	vasoconstrictor
bactericidal	nonproductive	vasodilator
bacteriostatic	potentiation	

Keys to Understanding This Chapter

Chapter 4: legal aspects of drug production and administration
Chapter 8: types of organisms; categories
Chapter 39: ethnic and religious background when assessing response to medications

Keys to Understanding This Chapter
(continued)

Chapter 50: nursing assessment skills helpful in evaluating patients' responses to medications
Chapter 52: medications are often used for pain
Chapter 53: surgical patients receive medications and anesthesia
Chapter 55: introduction to pharmacology and math

Key Points

♦ It is important for nurses to know basic classifications and uses of drugs.
♦ Always use a current reference book to look up medication-related questions.
♦ It is the nurse's responsibility to know expected and unexpected effects of drugs being administered.
♦ Administration of medications is a great responsibility. Incorrect medication administration may cause further damage or even death.
♦ New drugs are developed and released each year. The Federal government has the responsibility for research as to safety of drugs.

Key Topics Outline

Anti-infective Drugs
    Antibiotics
Dermatologic Agents
Drugs That Affect the Central Nervous System
    Analgesics
    Narcotic Analgesics
    Nonnarcotic Analgesics and Anti-inflammatory Drugs
    Hypnotics and Sedatives
    Anticonvulsants
    Psychotropic Drugs
    Autonomic Drugs
Drugs That Affect the Endocrine System
Drugs That Affect the Eye
Cardiovascular Drugs

Rosdahl CB: Textbook of Basic Nursing, 6th ed. © 1995 J.B. Lippincott Company

Key Learning Activities

◆ Interview a pharmacist and tour the pharmacy. How many different medications are stocked there? How do they determine which to have on hand? What information do they require from a patient before dispensing a medication? What are most of the over-the-counter medications used for?

◆ Look at package inserts from at least three prescription drugs. What type of information is included? Do all package inserts have the same information? Report back to the class.

◆ Look in your medicine cabinet at home. What kinds of prescription medications do you have? What kinds of over-the-counter medications do you have? What are the dates on the bottles or packages? What condition were they prescribed for?

New drugs are constantly being tested for approval by the Food and Drug Administration (FDA) and are regularly appearing on the market. Some older drugs may be replaced by newer, more effective ones. Others may be removed from the approved list because their continued use has been shown to have dangerous effects on health.

This chapter is presented as a reference for the major classifications of drugs and their actions. (All drug tables are at the end of the chapter for convenience.) It is not intended to be a total listing of all the drugs available. As you study this chapter, keep in mind that individual drugs are prescribed for *individual patients.*

Nursing Alert

Dosages given in all tables in this book are based on the usual adult dose. (An adult is considered to be someone ages 20 to 60.) There may be variations, based on the judgment of the physician. Smaller doses are usually prescribed for children. *If in doubt about the dose of any drug, look it up!*

Anti-infective Drugs

Antibiotics

An **antibiotic** is a chemical compound that is used to treat bacterial infections. It is a product of living cells and is either produced naturally by living cells (such as bacteria, yeasts, or molds) or semisynthetically (by cells in the laboratory). Although antibiotics are produced by living cells, the term "antibiotic" is commonly used to mean any drug that acts as an antimicrobial agent. Antibiotics are classified as *broad-spectrum* if they are effective against many organisms, and specific, or *narrow-spectrum* if they are effective against only a few microorganisms. Antibiotics may be **bacteriostatic** (retard the growth of bacteria) or **bactericidal** (kill bacteria).

Antibiotic-Resistant Organisms. A microorganism may not be sensitive to the action of a particular antibiotic. If an antibiotic is used indiscriminately, especially for minor ailments, it may eventually become ineffective. Sometimes the antibiotic destroys those microorganisms that are sensitive to it; the population of harmful microorganisms that is not sensitive to the antibiotic then has an opportunity to multiply to a dangerous level. Another possibility is the occurrence of a mutation, a change in the microorganism that renders it able to withstand the antibiotic. We then say that the microorganism is *resistant* to the drug (eg, penicillin-resistant staphylococcus).

Effectiveness. Several factors are important for an antibiotic to be effective. It should be a stable substance, not destroyed by tissue enzymes; it should not be inhibited by the presence of serum, pus, or blood or be eliminated too rapidly by the kidneys. The selected antibiotic should be soluble in water and diffuse readily into body tissue. Ideally, the antibiotic will not sensitize the patient and cause an allergic reaction nor should it kill the normal and useful bacteria (normal flora) that reside in the human body. Furthermore, it should be well absorbed from the gastrointestinal (GI) tract, if given orally. Finally, it should not be antagonistic to other antibiotics. The best antibiotic is one that has most of these characteristics (see the accompanying box).

Not all antibiotics are equally effective. The physician must sometimes use a less effective drug because of the patient's reactions or because of a specific disease organism.

Selecting the Appropriate Antibiotic. Physicians often take a sample of the wound or infected area. A *culture* is grown in the laboratory and *sensitivity tests* are done on the culture to identify the antibiotic that is most appropriate to inhibit the growth of that particular organism. Cultures may be done of blood, sputum, pus or wound drainage, urine, or mucous membrane discharge. This is known as a *culture and sensitivity* (C&S) test. The culture specimen must be sent to the laboratory immediately after it is obtained to ensure the accuracy of the test results. Once antibiotic therapy is started, the C&S will not be accurate.

At the present time, the penicillins, erythromycins, cephalosporins, aminoglycosides, and tetracyclines are the most effective and most widely used antibiotics. In some infections, any one of several antibiotics will be effective, whereas in others, only one specific antibiotic will be of value. Sometimes, a combination of antibiotics is required to control an infection. Sometimes, antibiotics are used with other drugs to improve their effectiveness. Antibiotics from many classifications are listed in Table 56-1 at the end of the chapter.

Penicillins

Penicillin inhibits the growth of susceptible bacteria and is bactericidal when there is a sufficiently high concentration of the drug in the body. Penicillin is excreted rapidly in the urine and is remarkably free of toxic effects.

Penicillin is most effective against gram-positive organisms, such as streptococci, staphylococci, and pneumococci. It is also active against some gram-negative organisms, such as gonococci and meningococci, and against the organism that causes syphilis. It is not effective against the tubercle bacillus or in viral infections or typhoid fever. Therefore, penicillin is a fairly narrow-spectrum antibiotic.

Administration. Penicillin can be given by several routes. The intramuscular (IM) route is most often used with the slower-acting penicillins. The intravenous (IV) route is used in severe infections when a high blood level of the drug is desired. The oral route is the easiest way to administer penicillin and is usually effective for all but the most severe infections. Gastric secretions destroy some of the drug, so the oral dose is often larger than the parenteral dose.

Side Effects or Adverse Reactions. Penicillin has few side effects, even in large doses, except for the person who is sensitive or allergic to it. (Penicillin sensitivity occurs in about 5% of North Americans.) In some cases, penicillin causes a comparatively mild allergic reaction, such as hives or a rash. In the more common penicillin reactions, the symptoms may be delayed from 5 to 14 days after administration. In severe cases, a penicillin allergy may cause immediate *anaphylaxis*. These immediate, severe reactions occur in 4 to 15 people out of 100,000 and can cause death.

Patients with a history of any allergy or of a previous reaction to any drug should have a sensitivity test before receiving penicillin. A mild allergic reaction is usually treated with an antihistamine such as Benadryl. In severe reactions, epinephrine, aminophylline, or oxygen may be required.

Preparations. Penicillin is available in liquid, tablet, and parenteral forms. The dosage is measured in units or milligrams and will vary with individual needs and with the type of penicillin used.

Nursing Alert

Penicillins share cross-allergenicity. Therefore, if a patient is allergic to one penicillin, caution should be used when giving another. There is also a slight cross-allergenicity to cephalosporins.

Cephalosporins

The cephalosporins are derivatives of a substance called cephalosporin-C and are structurally related to the penicillins. If proper conditions exist, the cephalosporins are usually bactericidal. These drugs are produced semisynthetically and have a broad spectrum of action.

Cephalosporins are active against gram-positive cocci, including staphylococci resistant to penicillin G, and gram-negative bacteria, including *Escherichia coli*, *Proteus mirabilis*, and *Klebsiella* species. This group of drugs is used frequently in mixed infections and in patients allergic to the penicillins. There is a 10% chance of a person also being allergic to a cephalosporin when allergic to penicillin. Both oral and injectable forms are available. The cephalosporins have become the most widely used drugs in the hospital setting. Examples are given in Table 56-1.

Guidelines for the Use of Antibiotics

- ◆ Certain antibiotics are widely used because they are effective against many organisms.
- ◆ Other antibiotics may be used because they are effective against organisms that are resistant to the commonly used antibiotics.
- ◆ Certain antibiotics are used because an individual is sensitive to the commonly used ones.
- ◆ The dosage prescribed depends on the severity of the illness and the susceptibility of the organism to the drug.
- ◆ The side effects of antibiotics vary. Some have very few or mild side effects; others may cause reactions, and sometimes even permanent damage. It is important to recognize the adverse reactions and be alert in observing and reporting them.
- ◆ The antibiotic of choice in any infection is that which has been proven effective against the identified microorganisms and which has the lowest potential for side effects. A drug that is more potent than necessary should *not* be used.
- ◆ A culture and sensitivity (C & S) test should be done *before* administration of any antibiotic. After an antibiotic is started, the culture will not be accurate.

Tetracyclines

The tetracyclines are broad-spectrum antibiotics effective against a wide variety of organisms. They are usually administered orally because they are very painful when given by injection; they are available, however, for intramuscular or intravenous use.

Oral absorption is decreased by the presence of food and some dairy products, especially milk, in the stomach. For this reason, tetracyclines should be given on an empty stomach (1 hour before or 2 hours after a meal), and no food should be eaten for 1 hour after they are given. The absorption of tetracyclines is also influenced by the presence of calcium, magnesium, and aluminum in the stomach. Therefore, the patient is not given antacids such as Gelusil, Maalox, or Milk of Magnesia with tetracycline and should limit dairy products. (Bicarbonate of soda may be used for patients who have acid indigestion.) Iron has also been shown to inhibit the absorption of tetracyclines.

Side Effects or Adverse Reactions. The tetracyclines have relatively few side effects; nausea, vomiting, and diarrhea are the most common. Intestinal infection is possible because tetracyclines also kill microorganisms that normally live in the digestive tract. Photosensitization (sensitivity to light), especially to sunlight, may develop. In children, discoloration of the teeth is possible.

Allergic reactions are possible with tetracyclines. Symptoms include a skin rash, burning eyes, and vaginal or anal itching.

Tetracyclines are contraindicated in pregnant women and in persons with liver damage. Examples are also listed in Table 56-1.

> ### Nursing Alert
> The symptoms of a serious reaction to tetracyclines include diarrhea with liquid feces and shreds of intestinal lining. Although rare, this can be fatal, especially in children or elderly people. Therefore, *any* diarrhea in a patient receiving a tetracycline must be reported *at once*.

Aminoglycosides

Aminoglycosides are potent bactericidal antibiotics. They are active against many aerobic gram-negative organisms and some aerobic gram-positive organisms. They are most often used parenterally (by injection) because they are not systemically absorbed after oral administration in patients with intact GI mucosa.

Aminoglycosides can cause serious adverse reactions and toxicity and a patient who is receiving an aminoglycoside must be carefully monitored. Aminoglycosides are often combined with other antibacterial drugs for use in serious infections. Table 56-1 provides examples of commonly used aminoglycosides.

Erythromycins

Erythromycin is a bacteriostatic agent that is active against some gram-negative cocci and bacilli. (Other gram-negative organisms and viruses, yeasts, and fungi are resistant to this drug.) It is a highly effective drug when used against susceptible organisms. Many derivatives of the original drug are used. It is most often used for streptococcal infections in patients who are allergic to penicillin.

Erythromycin drugs are administered most frequently by mouth but can cause GI distress. Erythromycin should be given 1 hour before or 2 hours after a meal. Table 56-1 lists erythromycin, the most commonly used form of these drugs.

Sulfonamides and Other Urinary Antiseptics

Sulfonamides (commonly called sulfa drugs) are widely used as antimicrobial agents, chiefly because of their low cost and effectiveness in treating common bacterial infections. They are *bacteriostatic* agents, permitting normal body processes to eradicate infection. The use of sulfonamides is usually indicated only in the following conditions: chancroid, trachoma, toxoplasmosis, urinary tract infections, and as an alternative to penicillin in rheumatic fever if the patient is allergic to penicillin. Sulfonamides are also used to treat some common sexually transmitted diseases (STDs). Sulfonamides are not tolerated well by certain ethnic groups.

Common Sulfonamides. Several sulfa drugs are described in Table 56-1, along with other anti-infective agents. *Sulfisoxazole* (Gantrisin) is often the drug of choice for urinary tract infections. This drug is seldom given to infants less than 2 months of age and must be used carefully in pregnant women. Infant doses are based on body weight. (Sulfisoxazole should not be used to treat the group A β-hemolytic streptococcus, which causes "strep sore throat," because it does not prevent sequelae, such as rheumatic fever.)

Sulfisoxazole is available in tablet form; for children, it is available in pediatric suspension. An injectable form is also available but should be used only when the patient cannot take oral medications. The long-acting form of sulfisoxazole is acetyl sulfisoxazole.

Nursing Considerations. It is a nursing responsibility to encourage fluid intake with sulfonamides, unless contraindicated. Adequate fluid intake must be maintained to prevent *crystalluria*, the excretion of crystals in the urine, which causes kidney irritation. Kidney stone formation is also a complication of inadequate fluid intake.

Other Urinary Antiseptics. *Nitrofurantoin* (Macrodantin, Furadantin) is effective against a wide range of gram-negative and gram-positive organisms. It should always be administered with milk or food to minimize gastric irritation.

Other Antibiotics and Anti-infective Drugs

The antibiotics previously discussed are the most effective and the most widely used. Other antibiotics and antibiotic-like compounds are also available. Some are used when the causative organism has shown resistance to the more popular antibiotics; others are used in patients who show allergies to the more popular drugs.

The drugs in Table 56-1 are not all derived from living organisms such as mold or algae and so some of those listed technically are not antibiotics. However, they have antimicrobial actions and are commonly referred to collectively as antibiotics.

Dermatologic Agents

Absorption of medication from the skin is poor and uncertain. It is affected by the condition of the sweat glands and pores that penetrate the epidermis from the deeper subcutaneous tissue and by the adequacy of the blood supply to the area. Absorption is increased if the skin is macerated (softened), either by water or by perspiration. Chapter 68 describes many disorders of the skin, the related nursing care, and specific methods of administering drugs in dermatologic conditions.

Drugs applied to the skin or into body openings, for example the ear, eye, or rectum, are called *topical agents*. Dermatologic agents are medications applied to the skin to treat local skin conditions. Types of dermatologic agents include soothing agents, antiseptics, anesthetics, corticosteroids, antifungals, and pediculocides (see Table 56-2 at the end of the chapter.) It is impossible to sterilize the skin, but sufficient washing will remove most bacteria and loose epithelium. Strong antiseptics can cause more harm than good by causing an irritation that breaks down the skin's natural resistance to bacteria.

Transdermal medications are topical agents designed to be absorbed through the skin for systemic effects. They are prepared in a medication patch form or a gel form. The medication patches are made using special membranes that allow medication to be slowly absorbed. A patch should be removed and the skin washed thoroughly before another patch is applied. Sites should be rotated. Nitroglycerin and scopolamine transdermal patches are in common use.

Drugs that Affect the Central Nervous System

The nervous system affects many body processes. When its functions are disturbed, certain drugs will increase or decrease the activity of the nerve centers in the brain or in the nerve pathways. **Stimulants** help to speed up certain mental and physical processes; **depressants** slow them down.

Many drugs have a stimulating effect on the central nervous system (CNS), but only a few are medically valuable for this purpose. In the past, stimulants were used in diet pills, but they were found to be dangerous. The most valuable stimulants are drugs that stimulate the respiratory centers in the brain; these drugs are usually used to counteract the toxic effects of depressant drugs, such as overdoses of barbiturates. Other than to counteract overdose, stimulant drugs are not commonly prescribed today.

Drugs that depress the activities of the CNS include analgesics that relieve pain, hypnotics and sedatives that bring rest and sleep, and general anesthetics that cause loss of consciousness. In addition to discussing these depressants, we will also consider some of the drugs known as selective depressants, which are used for the symptomatic treatment of various conditions.

Table 56-3 at the end of this chapter describes many of the drugs that have an effect on the CNS.

Analgesics

The analgesic drugs relieve pain but do not cause unconsciousness. Patients receiving analgesics may go to sleep because they are more comfortable, but the drug itself does not induce sleep; (narcotics may promote sleep, particularly in an overdose). Aspirin and acetaminophen (Tylenol) are commonly used over-the-counter (OTC) analgesics.

Narcotic Analgesics

Narcotic analgesics are called opiates because they are naturally occurring or synthetic agents that are opium derivatives or act like opium derivatives. Opium is the hardened, dried juice of a poppy plant. The most widely used opium alkaloids in drug therapy are *morphine* and *codeine*, which affect mainly the CNS. The most commonly used narcotic analgesic is *meperidine hydrochloride* (Demerol). It is described later in this section as a morphine substitute (see also Table 56-3).

Nursing Alert

It is important to monitor the patient's pulse, respiration, and blood pressure when narcotics are being given. The first sign of narcotic overdose is often *respiratory depression* (lowered respiratory rate).

All drugs produced from opium or opium derivatives are habit forming and are subject to the narcotic regulations of the Harrison Narcotic Act, which was amended by the Controlled Substances Act of 1970 (see Chapter 55).

Morphine (Morphine Sulfate, MS)

The most important function of morphine is its ability to relieve severe pain (such as in heart attack [MI]) and thus bring rest and sleep. It also relieves fear and anxiety and promotes a feeling of well-being. It is helpful in slowing peristalsis in such conditions as diarrhea, peritonitis, and stomach and bowel surgery. It can also relieve apprehension before anesthesia.

Side Effects or Adverse Reactions. Morphine depresses respiration, and severe morphine poisoning may cause respiratory failure and death. It contracts the pupils of the eyes and may cause nausea and vomiting. In toxic amounts, it lowers blood pressure and slows heart rate. Because it slows peristalsis, it may cause constipation. Allergic reactions to morphine occur fairly frequently.

Morphine is not recommended to relieve pain when a milder drug will do as well. This is especially true of pain in prolonged illness because habit formation (chemical dependency) is almost sure to occur. Exceptions are such painful conditions as inoperable or terminal cancer when recovery is impossible and morphine is the patient's only source of comfort and relief. Morphine is more effective if it is given *before* pain becomes extreme. Nurses sometimes mistakenly withhold a dose of morphine for as long as possible for fear of encouraging chemical dependency. There is little or no danger of habit formation when morphine is given for a short time to relieve severe pain. Many morphine-type analgesics are used after surgery.

Poisoning. Opium or morphine poisoning is usually the result of attempted suicide. The significant early symptoms of poisoning are *slow respirations* (less than 12/min), *deep sleep*, and *constricted pupils*. Emergency treatment involves the use of narcotic antagonists, such as naloxone (Narcan), which counteracts the action of morphine. If breathing decreases dangerously, the nurse must maintain an airway, begin mouth-to-mouth or breathing bag resuscitation, and call for assistance. It may be necessary to insert an endotracheal tube and administer supplemental oxygen.

Hydromorphone Hydrochloride

Hydromorphone hydrochloride (Dilaudid) is prepared from morphine and has about five times the analgesic effect of morphine, but this effect does not last as long. The effect is prolonged if the drug is given by suppository. It causes very little drowsiness, nausea, or vomiting but does depress respiration. It is an addictive drug.

Codeine

Codeine is a derivative of morphine, but its action is milder. It is especially effective in relieving cough, but it also relieves minor irritations and mild to moderate pain. It has a less depressing effect on the CNS than morphine and is less habit forming. It is also less constipating. Codeine is a common ingredient in cough mixtures.

Other Narcotic Analgesics

Other narcotic pain relievers are effective and have fewer unfavorable side effects than morphine. These drugs are often used as substitutes for morphine (see Table 56-3).

Meperidine hydrochloride (Demerol), used instead of morphine to relieve pain that is not severe, acts quickly, but its effect is not prolonged. It is often used before anesthesia or immediately postoperatively and is less likely than morphine to cause nausea and vomiting. A normal dose has few ill effects on respiratory or heart action; it is often given to obstetric patients in combination with other drugs. Possible side effects of Demerol include dizziness, nausea and vomiting, headache, and fainting; toxic amounts of this drug may cause dilated pupils, mental confusion, seizures, respiratory depression, and even death. Demerol is definitely habit forming, perhaps more so than morphine.

Methadone hydrochloride (Dolophine) is much like morphine in that it is an effective pain reliever and has similar lasting effects. It is slightly more effective than morphine in relieving chronic pain and is effective for cough. It may cause nausea and vomiting, itching, constipation, and respiratory depression and may be habit forming. It is sometimes used to assist a person in withdrawal from morphine or heroin.

Percodan, a combination of aspirin and oxycodone, is used to treat moderate pain. Side effects are similar to those of other narcotics. Onset of action occurs in 10 to 15 minutes, with a duration of 3 to 6 hours.

Fentanyl (Sublimaze) is a narcotic analgesic used as premedication for induction of anesthesia, maintenance of anesthesia, and as needed postoperatively. It has short duration of action so the dosage can be readjusted, often every 1 to 2 hours. It is also available in a transdermal patch (Duragesic). The patch delivers the drug over a 72-hour period; it is used most often for terminal cancer patients who cannot ingest oral forms of narcotic analgesics.

> **Nursing Alert**
>
> All narcotics, synthetic narcotics, and many barbiturates have potential for habituation or addiction. The patient should receive only medications that are absolutely necessary and should be weaned from any drug as soon as possible.

Accounting for Narcotics

An important role for nurses in many institutions is the safekeeping of narcotics and other controlled substances. The procedures for narcotic record-keeping are presented in Chapter 55.

Nonnarcotic Analgesics and Anti-inflammatory Drugs

The nonnarcotic analgesics are chemically related to morphine but are not classified as narcotics. They are less potent than the narcotic group and have less addiction potential (see Table 56-3).

Antipyretic analgesics are drugs that have the ability both to relieve pain and to reduce fever.

Salicylates

The salicylates, aspirin being the most common, are derived from salicylic acid. They are most effective in relieving pain in joints and muscles and reducing fever by increasing heat elimination from the body. Normal doses of salicylates do not affect respiration or circulation. Salicylates do not cause sleep and are not habit forming. If taken with sufficient liquid, salicylates are readily absorbed from the stomach and duodenum. It is important to increase intake of water while taking salicylates to facilitate excretion by the kidneys. (These drugs sometimes give the urine a brownish green color.) Salicylates will reduce the symptoms of a cold or influenza but will not cure it. They are specifically effective in relieving the pain or discomfort of headache, neuralgia, rheumatoid arthritis, rheumatic fever, and dysmenorrhea.

Side Effects or Adverse Reactions. The salicylates have remarkably few toxic side effects, but if used extensively for every minor discomfort, they can cause mild poisoning, with such symptoms as dizziness, ringing in the ears, hearing and vision disturbances, nausea and vomiting, heartburn, and diarrhea. Buffered tablets are believed to be less likely to cause GI disturbances than plain salicylates. Aspirin must be used cautiously; it is capable of impeding blood coagulation and thereby promoting hemorrhage. Therefore, aspirin is contraindicated in patients taking coumadin. Some physicians prescribe daily aspirin to help prevent heart attacks.

Salicylic acid is too irritating to be taken orally but is often used in ointments and other preparations. (Corn removers contain salicylic acid.)

Salicylates should not be used in children or teenagers to treat chickenpox or flu symptoms because of the danger of developing Reye's syndrome, a rare but serious disease.

Preparations. *Acetylsalicylic acid,* ASA, (aspirin) is a bitter drug available in tablets (plain or enteric-coated), capsules, or rectal suppositories. Flavored chewable tablets are available for children and should be kept out of the child's reach because they may be mistaken for candy. (Non–aspirin-containing drugs, such as Tylenol, are usually recommended for children.) Aspirin is often combined with other drugs and used as a more potent analgesic.

Nonsalicylate Analgesics

All nonsalicylate analgesics can cause gastric irritation. They are contraindicated in patients with history of peptic ulcer, gastritis, or ulcerative colitis. To lessen gastric irritation, these drugs should always be given with milk, food, or antacids. If severe GI symptoms persist, the drug must be discontinued. Some nonsalicylate analgesics are as follows:

Acetaminophen (Tylenol, Datril) has the same analgesic and antipyretic properties as aspirin, but with fewer side effects; Tylenol is often prescribed for people allergic to salicylates and is commonly used for infants and children. It has few GI side effects. Acetaminophen is less effective as an anti-inflammatory and is less useful than aspirin for treating arthritis and other inflammations.

Phenylbutazone (Butazolidin) relieves pain and inflammation of rheumatoid arthritis and other inflammatory diseases, but because of a high incidence of adverse effects, it is recommended only for those who do not respond or who are allergic to other drugs. It should be given with meals or milk to reduce gastric upset.

Nonsteroidal Anti-inflammatory Drugs

Nonsteroidal anti-inflammatory drugs (NSAIDs) are used primarily to treat inflammation but also have analgesic and antipyretic (fever-reducing) activity. NSAIDs, a large class of drugs, are used to treat mild to moderate pain. Most NSAIDs can cause gastric upset and should be given with food. They should *not be given* with salicylates or anticoagulants (because of the danger of bleeding) or with certain psychiatric medications, especially lithium (because renal clearance is reduced and toxicity may occur). For the same reason, a person receiving cyclosporine to prevent organ transplant rejection also should not receive NSAIDs.

Ibuprofen (Motrin, Advil, Midol-200, Nuprin, Rufen) is a potent anti-inflammatory agent used to relieve mild to moderate pain and to relieve symptoms of rheumatoid arthritis. Ibuprofen is available without prescription in a 200-mg strength. Ibuprofen is indicated for minor aches and pains, fever reduction, and dysmenorrhea. It is often recommended to control fever in infants and small children. (At this time, the children's form requires a prescription.)

Indomethacin (Indocin) is chemically unrelated to other drugs in this class. It is effective in treating arthritis, bursitis, and other joint diseases. It should always be given with meals or milk.

Hypnotics and Sedatives

Sleeplessness is not always caused by pain; a hospital patient may be disturbed by unfamiliar noises, lack of privacy, personal worries, or minor discomforts. A nurse can correct many of these irritations without drugs, but sometimes the physician orders drugs to ensure adequate rest and sleep. A **hypnotic** is given at bedtime and produces sleep rather quickly. A **sedative** is given in divided doses throughout the day and has a relaxing effect, so the patient naturally sleeps better at night (see Table 56-3). The tranquilizing drugs have effects similar to sedatives. Because of the possible dangers of overdose, many barbiturates, which are hypnotics, and sedatives are counted in many institutions in the same way narcotics are counted.

Barbiturates (Hypnotics)

The ideal hypnotic acts quickly, brings a natural sleep without "hangover," is not habit forming, and does not have harmful effects on the body. The search for this kind of drug has given us hundreds of barbiturates, but only a few approximate these requirements.

Barbiturates produce sleep, quiet restless and nervous patients, and prevent and control seizures. Often they are used before anesthesia or for obstetric sedation.

Barbiturates are easily absorbed and can be given orally or by injection. Preparations are available for many types of action: ultrashort, short, intermediate, and long.

Side Effects or Adverse Reactions. The patient may have "hangover" reactions; he or she may be depressed and listless or emotionally disturbed. Sometimes, a barbiturate causes skin rash or urticaria (hives) or can precipitate an asthmatic attack. It may cause restlessness and unpleasant dreams or confusion. Elderly patients, especially, are likely to become confused and need careful watching if they get up for the bathroom at night.

Severe barbiturate poisoning causes deep sleep or stupor; the patient becomes comatose, with slow or rapid shallow breathing and a weak rapid pulse. This may lead to death from respiratory failure.

Slow poisoning from barbiturates may also occur, with such symptoms as mental confusion and depression, loss of memory and incoherent speech, weight loss, GI upset, and anemia. Judgment is impaired so it is unsafe for the person to drive a car or use machinery.

Indiscriminate use of barbiturates is frequent. Addiction may occur if large doses are taken over a long period of time. People sometimes use barbiturates for suicide attempts, so they must be carefully prescribed.

Other Hypnotics

In addition to barbiturates, many other drugs are used as hypnotics (see Table 56-3). *Chloral hydrate* (Noctec) is the oldest of the hypnotics and is still used extensively today. It is often given to older patients because of its relative safety. Its chief disadvantage is gastric irritation and its unpleasant taste; gelcap forms are now available. *Flurazepam* (Dalmane) is useful in most sleep disorders; it is chemically related to *diazepam* (Valium). *Paraldehyde* is not used as often today as it once was although it may be useful in detoxification from alcohol. A newer drug, *estazolam* (ProSom) is quite safe and effective. It should not be used with alcohol. It may be metabolized more quickly in a smoker and more slowly if the person is taking oral contraceptives and certain other drugs. It should *not* be used during pregnancy. Another relatively new drug, triazolam (Halcion), has been blamed for adverse effects and is no longer extensively used.

Anticonvulsants

Seizures (convulsions) are signs of brain disorders associated with changes in the brain's electrical activity. **Anticonvulsants** are CNS depressants that help to prevent or control different types of seizures, which vary from mild to severe.

The most widely used anticonvulsant is *phenytoin* (Dilantin). It is available in tablet, capsule, suspension, and injectable forms. The incidence of adverse reactions with phenytoin is quite high, and almost all patients on this drug are to some extent adversely affected. The most common side effects are nervousness, hyperplasia of the gums, skin rash, and excess growth of facial hair.

Other commonly used anticonvulsants include *clonazepam* (Klonopin, Rivotril), *primidone* (Mysoline), *carbamazepine* (Tegretol), *mephobarbital* (Mebaral), *phenobarbital* (Barbita, Luminal Ovoids, Solfoton), *ethosuximide* (Zarontin), and *valproic acid, valproate sodium* (Depakene, Depakote). In emergency situations, magnesium sulfate ($MgSO_4$) may be used.

The dosage of these drugs is usually adjusted to the individual patient, with gradually increasing dosages administered until the desired blood level is attained or until seizures are under control. Many of these drugs require periodic dosage adjustment with chronic use.

Psychotropic Drugs

The two major groups of psychotropic drugs are *tranquilizers* and *antidepressants* (see Table 56-3). These drugs are used primarily in mental health and chemical dependency units of the hospital, but they may be used for any patient.

Tranquilizers

A *tranquilizer* effects a change toward tranquility in the behavioral state of an individual. Tranquilizers are not a substitute for an understanding nurse, but they do help the healthcare team find reasons for disturbed behavior. They have a direct effect on the patient's level of anxiety, and they reduce hyperactivity without impairing consciousness. Tranquilizers are commonly classified as either major or minor agents. Major tranquilizers affect more severe symptoms, whereas minor tranquilizers treat milder conditions.

Tranquilizers are not without risk. Common unfavorable reactions associated with many of them are skin rash and urticaria or itching. Sometimes chills and fever develop, with edema, double vision, and diarrhea. Large doses may cause coma and a marked fall in blood pressure. Furthermore, these drugs are potentiated when combined with alcohol. (**Potentiation** means that the effect of the combination is greater than the sum of the effects of each drug used alone.)

A patient can become mentally and physically dependent on tranquilizers. Severe withdrawal symptoms can follow abrupt discontinuance. These symptoms occur most often in patients who have used the drug for some time.

Major Tranquilizers. *Chlorpromazine* (Thorazine) is a member of the phenothiazine group. It is the most important and widely used major tranquilizer. It relieves overactive behavior; with the aid of chlorpromazine, many patients whose behavior made it necessary to confine them to mental institutions are now able to live at home. It does not cure mental and emotional disorders, but changes patients' behavior to make it more acceptable and manageable. Chlorpromazine is available in oral tablets or in injectable form for more rapid response. Thorazine may cause drowsiness and sleep (which may be desirable in some instances), mouth dryness, nausea, vomiting, sensitivity to light, and dermatitis. Toxic effects, such as trembling, drooling, muscular rigidity, jaundice, sore throat, and anemia, are warnings to consult the physician immediately. Dosage is based on the severity of the symptoms. A serious side effect, *tardive dyskinesia*, can result when using any psychotropic medication (see Chapter 87). Extrapyramidal side effects can also occur.

Haloperidol (Haldol) is a tranquilizer whose precise mode of action is still being investigated. It has been used effectively for controlling moderate to severe agitation and hallucinations. Extrapyramidal side effects (such as Parkinson-like symptoms) occur frequently, but sedative effects are less of a problem than with phenothiazines. The oral form is available in tablets or a liquid concentrate. The IM form is also available in a *decanoate,* which is long-acting. These injections are helpful in management of psychiatric patients who tend to be noncompliant, because an injection is only needed every 2–4 weeks.

Minor Tranquilizers. *Meprobamate* (Miltown, Equanil) is a calming drug that relieves anxiety and tension (thus relieving insomnia), decreases irritability, and promotes a feeling of well-being and relaxation.

Chlordiazepoxide (Librium) is a versatile drug that relieves anxiety and tension and is used to ease alcohol withdrawal symptoms. Given intramuscularly, it should be administered deep intramuscularly and injected slowly; intravenous administration is not recommended but may be done in an emergency.

Diazepam (Valium) is a drug that is valuable for relief of tension and anxiety. It is also a useful adjunct in the relief of skeletal muscle spasms, in acute alcohol withdrawal, in status epilepticus, and as premedication for anesthesia. It can be addicting.

Hydroxyzine pamoate (Vistaril, Atarax) was formerly used to relieve anxiety; it may also potentiate the effects of narcotics and barbiturates, increasing the effects of these drugs. It may be used to relieve nausea or pruritus and is sometimes used to aid sleep.

Antidepressants

Antidepressants alleviate depression; they have brought about a significant change in the treatment of various disruptions in mental health. Symptoms characterizing clinical depression are the expression of feelings of worthlessness, inadequacy, hopelessness, and guilt. Persons with such symptoms may have suicidal tendencies. Drugs used to treat depression provide relief of these symptoms but do not treat the underlying causes of depression.

Types of Antidepressants.

- ◆ Cyclic antidepressants, including *amitriptyline HCl* (Elavil, Endep), *imipramine HCl* (Tofranil), and *nortriptyline* (Pamelor).
- ◆ Monoamine oxidase inhibitors (MAO inhibitors), including *tranylcypromine sulfate* (Parnate) and *phenelzine sulfate* (Nardil).
- ◆ Serotonin uptake inhibitors such as *fluoxetine* (Prozac) and *sertraline HCl* (Zoloft) are new antidepressants.

Nursing Alert

Patients taking MAO inhibitors must be warned against eating foods with high tyramine content (such as some ripened cheeses, beef or chicken liver, meats prepared with tenderizer, beer, and raisins). Other prohibited foods include wine, chocolate, ripe bananas, and herring. These people also cannot use certain OTC agents, such as cold and hay fever products that contain sympathomimetic amines (drugs that mimic the sympathetic nervous system). The sympathomimetic amines can produce hypertensive crises in patients taking MAO inhibitors.

Antidepressants are effective in the treatment of endogenous depression (that which is ongoing and from within the person). Antidepressants generally take from 2 to 4 weeks to begin showing an effect.

Cyclics frequently have *anticholinergic* effects (such as dry mouth) and may cause *tardive dyskinesia* (impairment of voluntary movements). Tardive dyskinesia is a serious side effect and is a potent factor in the refusal of patients to take their medications. Once they have experienced this side effect, they are often afraid it will occur again. Tardive dyskinesia is discussed in detail in Chapter 87.

Imipramine hydrochloride (Tofranil) is an effective agent used to treat most types of depression; maximal benefit is not achieved for 1 to 2 weeks. Imipramine is also used in children for bedwetting (enuresis).

Amitriptyline hydrochloride (Elavil) produces antidepressant and mild tranquilizing effects. It is also commonly used for neuralgias.

Desipramine hydrochloride (Norpramin) is chemically related to imipramine and has the same pharmacologic properties; enteric-coated tablets are color-coded according to dosage.

Fluoxetine (Prozac) is used to treat depression and has been used experimentally to treat obesity. (Patients taking Prozac often lose weight.)

Lithium. *Lithium* is used in the treatment of the manic phase of bipolar (manic–depressive) illness. This drug reduces or prevents symptoms of motor hyperactivity, decreased need for sleep, and flight of ideas or grandiosity. Few side effects occur when blood levels are kept within normal limits. The patient on lithium should maintain adequate salt and fluid intake because lithium has a strong relationship to sodium and can cause toxicity if the patient is dehydrated, is receiving diuretics, or if the sodium level in the body is low. Lithium can cause renal (kidney) damage; NSAIDs should not be taken.

Autonomic Drugs

We do not consciously control the activities of the autonomic nervous system. Its responses are influenced by hormones and other chemicals and occur more or less automatically. Certain drugs, however, affect these responses, and some of these drugs are actually prepared from natural hormones. Two important hormones of the autonomic nervous system are epinephrine and norepinephrine, produced by the adrenal glands. These hormones may also be manufactured synthetically and administered as drugs.

Epinephrine

Epinephrine, Adrenaline, constricts blood vessels when applied to mucous membranes or wounds or when injected into tissues. It has no effect on unbroken skin. Because digestive enzymes destroy it, it is not given by mouth.

Epinephrine speeds up the heart rate, raises blood pressure, constricts surface blood vessels, and relaxes smooth muscles in the respiratory tract, causing bronchodilation. It is the most valuable drug for relief of acute attacks of bronchial asthma. It is especially useful in treating allergic reactions, such as anaphylaxis, serum reactions, hay fever, and urticaria. It is a powerful heart stimulant, but it must be used with great care so it does not seriously interfere with the heartbeat. As a last resort, when the heart has stopped beating, epinephrine injected directly into the heart muscle or into nearby veins has been known to restore heart action.

Nervous patients and those with hypertension or exophthalmic goiter who take this drug may become more nervous and develop tremor, anxiety, headache, difficulty in breathing, and stomach pain. More dangerous symptoms, resulting from large doses or intravenous administration, are dilatation of the heart, edema of the lungs, and cerebral vascular accident (CVA; stroke). Epinephrine is unsafe for patients with heart disease or hyperthyroidism or for those who are emotionally unstable.

Norepinephrine

Norepinephrine (levarterenol; Levophed) constricts blood vessels in most vascular beds. Levarterenol bitartrate is used to maintain blood pressure in hypotensive states resulting from such conditions as hemorrhage, trauma, and myocardial infarction.

In elderly people, excessive levarterenol may raise blood pressure to dangerous levels and cause CVAs. Like epinephrine, it can interfere with the heartbeat and must be used with caution.

Key points in administration of norepinephrine are frequent monitoring of blood pressure (arterial monitoring is best), giving the drug in a dilute intravenous solution, and being watchful about infiltration of the solution because infiltration may cause sloughing of tissue.

Drugs That Affect the Endocrine System

Many hormones are given to reduce the symptoms of particular hormone deficiencies. In addition to various sex hormones, the thyroid hormone may be administered. In many cases of overproduction of a hormone, the offending endocrine gland must be totally or partially removed.

The conditions caused by overproduction and underproduction of various hormones are discussed in Chapter 72. Specific hormone preparations are discussed in relation to each condition.

Insulin, produced in the pancreas and necessary for proper absorption and storage of glucose (sugar), is administered parenterally to help control diabetes mellitus. Oral hypoglycemic agents are available that increase the production or effectiveness of available insulin. These drugs are discussed in Chapter 72 in connection with diabetes mellitus, and many of them are presented in Table 56-4 at the end of this chapter.

Steroids are hormones. They include hormones produced by the adrenal glands (adrenocortical hormones). The most common adrenal cortical hormone is *cortisone*, which is an anti-inflammatory agent. It is used on a long-term basis in some situations, if other medications are not effective, although it may have serious side effects (see accompanying box). Cortisone must not be stopped abruptly because the body decreases its production of this hormone when it is given as a medication. If the patient abruptly stops the medication, the body will not have enough and a steroid crisis can develop.

Side Effects of Steroid Administration

The person receiving steroids on a long-term basis often suffers side effects. The patient and family must be able to recognize and deal with them:

- ◆ Cushingoid symptoms, including:
  - ◆ Swelling between the shoulder blades ("buffalo hump")
  - ◆ Swollen face ("moon face")
  - ◆ Increased appetite; abdominal distention; weight gain
  - ◆ Ecchymoses (hemorrhaging in the skin or mucous membranes)
  - ◆ Hirsuitism (increased body hair)
  - ◆ Aggravation of adolescent acne
  - ◆ Hypertension (high blood pressure)
  - ◆ General weakness
- ◆ Bone marrow toxicity; possible osteoporosis
- ◆ Masked infection
- ◆ Increased susceptibility to infections
- ◆ Development of peptic ulcers and gastrointestinal bleeding
- ◆ Suppression of growth
- ◆ Aggravation of diabetes mellitus
- ◆ Increased intracranial pressure, with projectile vomiting, severe headaches, diplopia, and/or seizures
- ◆ Cataracts
- ◆ Thrombophlebitis and/or embolism

Additional Points Related to Steroid Therapy

- ◆ To prevent a steroid crisis, the patient is weaned from steroids when treatment is completed. The patient should be cautioned not to suddenly stop taking the drug.
- ◆ Antacids are given with the steroid to prevent gastrointestinal upset or ulcers.
- ◆ The patient should have a mirror, so that the gradual progress of the side effects can be observed and they do not come as a shock.
- ◆ Counseling may be helpful for a child and/or parents and for adult patients.
- ◆ The patient needs to be reassured that the side effects are not harmful and will disappear when the drug is discontinued.
- ◆ Severe complications can occur if a child on steroids gets chickenpox or if an adult gets shingles. If this does occur, immediate medical care is necessary.

Drugs That Affect the Eye

Drugs may be used to treat eye infections and irritations, to dilate or constrict the pupil, to prevent or relieve pain, or to reduce pressure within the eye. Some of these drugs produce their effects by acting on the autonomic nervous system to relax and contract smooth muscle; others act directly on eye tissue. Make sure *only* solutions marked "for ophthalmic use" are used in the eyes.

Drugs that dilate the pupil are called *mydriatics*; those that constrict the pupil are called *miotics*.

Local anesthetics are used to prevent pain during eye examinations or operations. (They should not be used routinely in irritated or painful eyes because they would mask symptoms while allowing an injury to or irritation of the cornea to continue unchecked.) *Proparacaine* (Ophthaine) and *tetracaine* are commonly used in surgery.

Eye infections may be treated with antibiotics or sulfonamides specific for the causative organism. Examples of commonly used anti-infective agents are *gentamicin sulfate* (Garamycin) and *sulfacetamide* (Sulamyd). Most are available in solution or ointment form.

Drugs Used in Treating Glaucoma

Glaucoma is caused by abnormally high production or decreased absorption of fluid (aqueous humor) in the eye, resulting in increased intraocular (within the eyeball) pressure. Some drugs used to reduce production of this fluid by topical (local) application are *carbachol* (Carbacel) and *pilocarpine* HCl (Pilocel, Pilocar). These drugs are effective against chronic glaucoma. *Isofluorophate* (Floropryl), *physostigmine* (Eserine Sulfate, Isopto Eserine), and *echothiophate iodide* (Phospholine Iodide) are anticholinesterase drugs and are used when other drugs have not been effective.

Oral medications can also enter the systemic circulation and slow production of intraocular fluid.

Cardiovascular Drugs

Cardiovascular drugs are used for their effect on the action of the heart itself or for dilating or constricting blood vessels. They are used to remedy failures in heart action or circulation that would interfere with the body's supply of oxygen and nutrients and removal of waste products. When the heart loses its efficiency as a pump, the circulation fails. Disease or degenerating changes in the heart itself or in blood vessels can impair the heart's efficiency. Chapter 74 discusses these conditions in detail.

Certain drugs make the heart beat faster, whereas others slow it down but strengthen its force. This lat-ter type of drug is sometimes needed when the heart has been forced to beat faster than normal to make up for the weakness of its beat. In such instances there is danger of the heart becoming exhausted from overwork.

Cardiotonics

Cardiotonics are heart stimulants. See Table 56-5 at the end of this chapter. Atropine in large doses strengthens the heartbeat. Caffeine is a fast-acting stimulant that makes the heartbeat strong and rapid. Epinephrine is a powerful emergency stimulant for the circulation.

Digitalis

Digitalis is a widely used cardiotonic. It makes the heart beat slower and stronger, giving the heart time to rest between beats. This improves circulation and reduces edema in the lungs and abdomen, thus making breathing easier.

Dosages of digitalis vary according to individual needs. The dose that produces the desired optimum benefit for the patient, the *digitalizing dose*, is divided over a period from 1 to 2 days. This dose, slightly reduced, is the amount the patient will receive thereafter, the *maintenance dose*. Many patients who need digitalis must take it for the rest of their lives. Injectable forms of digitalis are used for rapid *digitalization*.

> **Nursing Alert**
>
> It is vital for the nurse to differentiate between an order for *digitoxin* and one for *digoxin* (two different digitalis preparations), because the names are similar, but the dosages are very different. A medication error in this instance could kill a patient!

Signs of Overdose. A patient who is receiving digitalis needs close medical and nursing observation because an overdose can dangerously lower the heart rate. Accuracy is especially important in giving this drug because it is potent; a tiny difference in amount can be dangerous.

Other symptoms of digitalis disturbance include nausea and vomiting, headache, diarrhea, and sometimes drowsiness and blurred or yellow vision. A record of the patient's intake and output of fluids is usually kept, and the patient is watched for signs of edema and breathing difficulty.

Digoxin (Lanoxin) is the most popular oral form of digitalis. There is a generic form available, but it is rarely used because of inconsistencies used in the binding agent that result in many adverse effects.

Nursing Alert

When giving any digitalis derivative, always count the apical pulse for 1 *full minute* before giving each dose. If the pulse is lower than 60 beats per minute (bpm) or if there is a change in rhythm, withhold the dose and immediately report these conditions to the team leader. (In some nursing homes, radial pulses are allowed because it is difficult to take apical pulse when the person is up and dressed. If there is any doubt about a radial pulse, it must be double-checked apically.)

Antiarrhythmics

Antiarrhythmics make the heart less active and decrease the heart rate. Some types of heart disease affect the rhythm of the heartbeat, causing the heart to quiver, without rest, between beats (fibrillation). This affects circulation and may lead to congestive heart failure. Some drugs steady heart rate by increasing the rest period, which changes a rapid, irregular pulse to one that is slow and regular (see Table 56-5).

Quinidine is used to treat atrial arrhythmias and to treat or prevent congestive heart failure; the difference between digitalis and quinidine is that digitalis stimulates more power in heart muscle, whereas quinidine restrains erratic heart muscle activity, causing slower, more regular action. This drug is available as quinidine sulfate.

Procainamide hydrochloride (Pronestyl) is more effective for ventricular than atrial arrhythmias. It is less toxic than quinidine and its effects last longer.

Verapamil hydrochloride (Calan) is the only calcium channel blocker approved for cardiac arrhythmias. It also has antianginal and antihypertensive effects (helps to reduce angina and high blood pressure).

Lidocaine is used to treat life-threatening ventricular arrhythmias. It is only available in intravenous or intramuscular forms. It can only be used with constant electrocardiographic monitoring. It is usually used only until the patient is stabilized on oral medications.

Drugs That Affect the Blood Vessels

Some drugs affect the circulatory system by constricting (**vasoconstrictors**) or dilating (**vasodilators**) blood vessels. The vasoconstrictors raise blood pressure; the vasodilators lower it. They produce their effects indirectly by action on the nervous system or directly by action on muscle cells in the blood vessels.

Vasoconstrictors

The vasoconstrictors (hypertensive agents) are used to control superficial hemorrhage, raise blood pressure, and relieve nasal congestion (see Table 56-5).

Levarterenol bitartrate (Levophed) is used to raise blood pressure after surgery, hemorrhage, or shock. It is given intravenously in a solution of dextrose or saline.

Metaraminol bitartrate (Aramine) is used to raise or maintain blood pressure in an emergency. It is given intramuscularly, subcutaneously, or intravenously, depending on the desired speed of reaction.

Ephedrine, in small doses, stimulates the heart and raises blood pressure; larger doses depress heart action.

Phenylephrine hydrochloride (Neo-Synephrine) relieves congestion in mucous membranes. It is also used to treat some types of shock; it raises and stabilizes blood pressure. Neo-Synephrine is sometimes used to treat allergic reactions or to dilate the pupil of the eye for examination or treatment. It is available in ophthalmic solution, as a decongestant nasal spray, and for injection.

Vasodilators

Drugs that dilate blood vessels (hypotensive agents) are used to treat peripheral blood vessel disease, coronary artery disease, and hypertension (see Table 56-5). Some vasodilators, the nitrates in particular, have been used for many years, especially in acute attacks of angina pectoris or to prevent such an attack. In these instances, they relieve angina pain caused by spasm (constriction) of coronary blood vessels.

Nitrates. People who are subject to angina attacks usually carry nitrates with them to use in an emergency.

Nitroglycerin, NG, acts quickly in 2 or 3 minutes when a tablet is placed under the tongue (*sublingual*); it is rapidly absorbed by mucous membranes, and the effects last for about 30 minutes. Once a bottle is opened, the tablets are good for only 6 months. Nitroglycerin is also available in long-acting capsules (Nitro-Bid) or as transdermal patches. The patches deliver the medication over 24 hours (Nitro-Dur, Transderm-Nitro). Nitroglycerin tablets should *always* be kept in the original glass container (which is usually brown) and should be protected from exposure to light. The patient should be alerted to the fact that the tablet may "fizzle" under the tongue.

Nursing Alert

Nitroglycerin should not be used in patients who have recently had a myocardial infarction (MI) or who have severe asthma, closed-angle glaucoma, or postural hypotension.

Amyl nitrite comes in glass ampules (pearls) covered with a thin coating so it can be crushed easily and inhaled; it is used for the prevention of or treatment for fainting (syncope). It has a strong and rather disagreeable odor. Two or three inhalations are a safe limit; more may cause overdosage. The nurse should know what to do for a person who takes an overdose. The patient may feel dizzy and faint from a sudden lowering of blood pressure and may have headaches. Large doses of these drugs exaggerate these symptoms and make the face and neck flushed and the pulse weak and rapid. In nitrate poisoning, the patient should be treated for shock. The head should be lowered and oxygen administered if the person is cyanotic (see Chapters 31 and 80).

Other Vasodilators. *Isoxuprine* (Vasodilan) is a vasodilator used in cerebral and peripheral vascular insufficiency. It is often used in pregnancy to stop contractions in premature labor, although it does not have FDA approval for this use.

Ethyl alcohol (ethanol) dilates blood vessels in the skin and is used for this purpose in some diseases of peripheral vessels, such as Raynaud's disease.

Hydralazine hydrochloride (Apresoline) reduces blood pressure and helps to control hypertension through peripheral vasodilation. Treatment begins with small doses; dosage is then adjusted to obtain the desired effect. Apresoline often causes unpleasant side effects, such as headache, palpitation, depression, and nausea and vomiting; more serious symptoms include chills, fever, pain in the heart region, and edema of the legs and feet.

Prazosin (Minipress) acts by reducing peripheral vascular resistance. The first dose is usually given at bedtime to decrease *syncope* (fainting or lightheadedness). Postural hypotension is another side effect of this drug.

Drugs That Reduce Blood Pressure

Drugs that reduce blood pressure are called **antihypertensives**. Some, the vasodilators, are described above.

Diuretics

Diuretics are drugs used to increase the amount of urine excreted by the kidneys, decreasing the volume of fluid circulating in the body, and thereby lowering blood pressure. Indications for diuretic use are edema, hypertension, congestive heart failure, and toxemia of pregnancy (preeclampsia/eclampsia). One side effect of diuretic use is excessive excretion of potassium (K+). Thus, potassium levels must be monitored in patients who are taking diuretics; supplemental potassium often is given.

Hydrochlorothiazide (Hydrodiuril) and *furosemide* (Lasix) are examples of potassium-wasting diuretics. *Spironolactone* (Aldactone) and *triamterene/hydroch-* lorothiazide(Dyazide) are examples of potassium-sparing diuretics. (The latter do not cause as much potassium excretion as do other drugs in this class.)

β Blockers

β Blockers (beta blockers) are commonly used as first line therapy for treatment of hypertension. They act directly on the heart to decrease heart rate by depressing atrioventricular node conduction and decreasing the strength of myocardial contraction; thereby, they decrease blood pressure. *Propranolol* (Inderal), *atenolol* (Tenormin), and *metoprolol* (Lopressor) are a few β blockers used to treat hypertension. Propranolol is also used to treat angina and cardiac arrhythmias and to prevent migraine headaches and stage fright.

Calcium Channel Blockers

Calcium channel blockers inhibit movement of calcium ions across the cell membrane, thereby depressing the mechanical contraction of myocardial and smooth muscle. Depression of impulse formation (automaticity) and conduction velocity in the heart also occurs. *Diltiazem hydrochloride* (Cardizem), *nifedipine* (Procardia), and *verapamil* (Calan) are used to treat hypertension and angina. Verapamil is also used to treat arryhthmias. (All of these antihypertensive drugs are listed in Table 56-5.)

Angiotensin-Converting Enzyme Inhibitors

Angiotensin-converting enzyme (ACE) inhibitors are drugs that reduce peripheral vascular resistance in the hypertensive patient by blocking the activation of angiotensin, a powerful vasoconstrictor, without decreasing cardiac output. ACE inhibitors are often used alone or in combination with thiazide diuretics. ACE inhibitors are becoming one of the most widely prescribed antihypertensives. Examples are *captopril* (Capoten), *enalapril* (Vasotec), and *lisinopril* (Prinivil, Zestril).

Miscellaneous Agents

Guanethidine sulfate (Ismelin) is a powerful drug, the effect of which is more noticeable when the patient is sitting or standing up. Orthostatic blood pressure must be taken and recorded regularly. Patients may feel weak and dizzy when they move about; it is especially important to safeguard elderly patients who may get up during the night.

Methyldopa (Aldomet) reduces blood pressure by lowering peripheral vascular resistance.

Pargyline hydrochloride (Eutonyl) is used for moderate to severe hypertension. (Eutonyl is an MAO inhibitor; therefore, patients using Eutonyl must be cautioned against eating certain foods, as described previously.)

Diazoxide (Hyperstat) is used in severe hypertensive crises.

Many of the vasodilators are also used alone, or in combination, to treat high blood pressure.

Drugs That Affect the Blood

Blood is composed of plasma, red cells, white cells, and platelets. Red cells are made up mainly of a substance called hemoglobin, which contains iron. Hemoglobin has the important job of carrying oxygen to every body cell. Normally, an adequate diet provides the essentials needed to form blood (iron, vitamin C, parts of the vitamin B complex, and animal protein). Drugs sometimes are needed to treat disturbances of the blood, such as anemia (decreased oxygen delivered to the blood because of a lack of or abnormal red blood cells) or leukemia, and to affect blood clotting.

Iron

Iron is an essential part of hemoglobin; it is distributed throughout body cells and is stored in blood-forming organs. Actually, the body needs only small amounts of iron from diet because it salvages iron from worn-out blood cells and uses it again. However, women up to and through menopause need up to four times as much iron as men. Iron deficiency causes anemia and is usually due to a massive hemorrhage or prolonged slow bleeding.

Many iron preparations are available. Iron is usually given by mouth, but preparations such as *iron dextran* (Imferon) are given by injection if the oral route is not feasible. Injection should be done by the "Z-track" method to prevent permanent skin discoloration (see Chapter 57).

Many oral iron preparations irritate the stomach, which is why they are given after meals or with food. Solutions containing iron should be taken through a straw because they stain the teeth, and the metallic taste is unpleasant. Iron usually causes very dark stools. Slow-release products are available and cause less stomach irritation.

Iron taken over a prolonged period may cause loss of appetite, nausea and vomiting, headaches, stomach pain, diarrhea, or constipation. Large doses can cause poisoning, especially in children.

Vitamins

Folic acid is indicated in patients with megaloblastic anemias or anemias associated with pregnancy, infancy, or childhood. It is often given routinely during detoxification from alcohol. Folic acid stimulates production of red and white blood cells in megaloblastic anemia. It is required to maintain normal erythropoiesis and nucleoprotein synthesis. Recent studies show that if taken before and during pregnancy, it may decrease the incidence of birth defects, especially spina bifida.

Vitamin B$_{12}$ (cyancobalamin) is necessary for the manufacture of red blood cells. It is not absorbed to any great extent orally, particularly in people with a deficiency of intrinsic factor, which is produced in the stomach and aids in the absorption of vitamin B$_{12}$ in the intestine. People with a lack of vitamin B$_{12}$ will develop pernicious anemia. Intramuscular injections of vitamin B$_{12}$ will arrest the disease. The dosage is measured in *micrograms* (abbreviated μg or mcg), and the amount given depends on the seriousness of the patient's need. Vitamin B$_{12}$ usually has no undesirable side effects.

Nursing Alert

It is possible to take too many vitamins. Symptoms of overdose depend on the specific vitamin, but they can lead to serious disorders and even death.

Coagulants

Drugs that promote blood clotting are called **hemostatics** or *coagulants*. When blood plasma lacks elements that cause blood to clot, certain drug preparations can be used to make up this deficiency.

Absorbable gelatin sponge (Gelfoam) is a form of gelatin used to stop capillary bleeding. It can be left in a surgical wound, where it will be completely absorbed.

Oxidized cellulose (Oxycel) comes in the form of a treated cotton or gauze pack that is absorbable and can be applied to check hemorrhage.

Vitamin K is necessary to make prothrombin, the substance that starts the formation of a blood clot. It is found in many foods, but sometimes the intestine is unable to absorb it. It may be given to patients who have a prothrombin deficiency, as in jaundice, or to newborns. (Most newborns receive an injection of vitamin K in the delivery room as a precautionary measure.) Available preparations are in forms that can be given by mouth, or by intramuscular or intravenous injection. Vitamin K is given *deep intramuscularly* because it tends to irritate tissues. The dosage is usually based on body weight. Subsequent doses of vitamin K are given, based on the patient's prothrombin time. (See Chapters 75 and 76 and the next section of this chapter for precautions in anticoagulant therapy.)

Anticoagulants

Anticoagulants, drugs to prevent abnormal clotting of blood, are important because clots in major blood vessels (coronary occlusion and CVAs) are one of the chief causes of death in the United States.

A combination of chemicals is used to prevent coagulation of blood collected for transfusions.

Heparin is useful in preventing postoperative thrombosis and embolism. If a patient is receiving heparin, the nurse should watch for bleeding from the wound or for blood in the urine (hematuria); these symptoms should be reported at once. Heparin is given by subcutaneous or intravenous injection. (Protamine sulfate is given intravenously to counteract an adverse action of heparin.) Heparin also may be used in a "heparin-lock" to keep a vein open for repeated intravenous injections.

Warfarin (Coumadin), a coumarin derivative, prevents venous thrombosis and pulmonary embolism, thrombophlebitis (inflammation of a vein), and blood clots. It is available in tablets; doses vary according to the patient's needs. There are few side effects, but overdosage can cause hemorrhage; nosebleed, bleeding into the skin, or blood in the urine should be reported. (The antidote for overdose of coumarin derivatives is vitamin K.)

> ### Nursing Alert
>
> Patients receiving any anticoagulant (and some coagulants) should have regular *prothrombin time* ("pro-time") or *clotting time* evaluations (such as the Lee-White evaluation) to make sure they are not becoming "overheparinized," or susceptible to hemorrhage. If the blood clotting time becomes too long, the anticoagulant dose must be decreased. The "sliding-scale" anticoagulant dose is based on the outcome of a daily clotting time.

Blood Products

Whole Blood, Blood Plasma, and Blood Proteins

Whole Blood. Whole blood is indicated primarily for a combination of rapid loss of both red cells and plasma, such as in massive hemorrhage. A transfusion of whole blood quickly increases the number of red blood cells, restoring blood volume and thus raising blood pressure. It may save a patient's life when survival depends on quick action. The blood given must be compatible with the patient's own blood group. For most transfusions, packed red cells are preferred because they provide only the blood component needed. (The administration of packed red cells also prevents circulatory overload.)

Blood Plasma. Blood plasma is the fluid part of blood that has been separated from the blood cells. It is frequently used to prepare products such as albumin, plasma protein fraction (PPF), immune globulin, and antihemophilic factor preparations. (Because of the risk of blood incompatibilities and disease transmission, nonplasma solutions are preferred for rapid fluid replacement.)

Plasma proteins are constituents of blood plasma that can be separated from plasma. Plasma proteins are obtained from pooled plasma and are heat treated to reduce the risk of hepatitis and human immunodeficiency virus (HIV) transmission. Plasma proteins do not contain clotting factors. *Albumin* is a plasma protein that has the same effect as plasma in treating shock, and it can be administered in smaller amounts. *Immune serum globulin* (γ globulin; gamma globulin) is also a plasma protein and is given to help the patient ward off a specific infection. Immune serum globulins can be administered intramuscularly.

Fibrinogen, a component of blood plasma, can be applied locally to stimulate blood clotting. Other plasma preparations include *normal human serum albumin* (used in treating shock) and *antihemophilic factor* preparations (a temporary aid to the person with hemophilia).

Platelets. Platelets can be removed from a fresh unit of blood. They are administered to patients who have inadequate platelet production, those undergoing intensive cancer chemotherapy, and those receiving large amounts of stored bank blood. Platelets may also be administered to patients with aplastic anemia and leukemia.

Administration of Blood Products. All blood products require special filters for administration. A thorough knowledge of blood or blood product administration is necessary. All intravenous solutions other than normal, or isotonic, saline (0.9% saline) cause *destruction* of red blood cells or other deleterious effects to the blood product (see Chapter 75).

Antineoplastic Drugs

As malignant diseases become more treatable, chemical agents have become increasingly important. True cures of malignant tumors are brought about by early surgery and radiation, and, in some cases, by drug therapy (chemotherapy). In some cases, antineoplastic ("against cancer") drugs are used as a palliative measure in tumors that are no longer curable by surgery, or for cancers such as leukemia, which spread throughout the body. The antineoplastic drugs can be divided into several large groups based on their probable mode of action. Chapter 76 discusses administration of antineoplastic drugs in more detail, as well as side effects and related nursing care.

Alkylating Agents. Alkylating agents inhibit cell division and thus prevent multiplication of malignant cells. However, they are often toxic to any cells that are rapidly multiplying such as those in the gastrointestinal

(GI) tract and bone marrow. Alkylating preparations include *mechlorethamine* HCl (nitrogen mustard), *cyclophosphamide* (Cytoxan), and *cisplatin* (Platinol).

Antimetabolites. Antimetabolites are compounds whose chemical structure is similar to substances normally used by cells for growth. These artificial relatives of essential substances are toxic to rapidly growing cells. Preparations include *methotrexate*, MTX (Amethopterin) and *fluorouracil*, 5-FU.

Hormones. It is believed that hormones slow the growth of tumors by making the environment less favorable for the tumor. For example, some mammary cancers are slowed by administration of androgenic (male) hormones. Hormone preparations include *testosterone, fluoxymesterone* (Halotestin), *diethylstilbestrol* (DES), as well as *tamoxifen* (Nolvadex), which is an antiestrogen hormone that competes for estrogen-binding sites and is used to treat breast cancer.

Drugs Used in Treating Allergies

The antihistamines are most effective in relieving the uncomfortable symptoms of hay fever and other allergic reactions. These drugs are not curative but do bring temporary relief. Their benefits are short lived, and they are merely adjuncts to more specific treatment. Many of these specific treatments and related nursing activities are described in Chapter 77.

The most common side effect of antihistamines is drowsiness, which may progress to deep sleep. There may also be mouth and throat dryness, uncertain muscular coordination, and muscular weakness.

Diphenhydramine (Benadryl) is an antihistamine that is available in oral and injectable form. It is more sedative than other antihistamines and is sometimes used solely as a sleep aid, particularly when psychotropic drugs are being given. In this way, medication side effects are prevented while sleep is promoted. *Chlorpheniramine* (Chlor-Trimeton) is slower acting but has fewer side effects than other antihistamines. Combinations of antihistamines and decongestants (Actifed, Dimetapp) are useful in treating sinusitis, rhinitis, nasal stuffiness, and postnasal drip. *Terfenadine* (Seldane) and *astemizole* (Hismanal) cause less drowsiness than other antihistamines.

Drugs That Affect the Respiratory System

Drugs That Act on the Respiratory Center

Oxygen and *carbon dioxide* are the two respiratory gases administered in the treatment of hypoventilation and hypoxia and are considered drugs when used in this way. Oxygen promotes adequate oxygenation of cells and thereby protects cell integrity. Carbon dioxide stimulates the respiratory center to increase the rate and depth of respiration.

Drugs are available that stimulate the depth and rate of respiration; however, the importance of mechanical or physiologic stimulation must not be ignored. (Indeed, the latter is generally superior to the use of drugs.) Respiratory depression caused by drug overdose is the most common indication for chemical agents; *doxapram HCl* (Dopram) is the most widely used chemical respiratory stimulant.

Drugs That Act on the Cough Center (Antitussives)

Coughing is a protective reflex to clear the respiratory tract of foreign bodies or secretions. A cough is **productive** when secretions are removed and **nonproductive** when it is dry and irritating. Treatment of cough is secondary to the treatment of the underlying disorder. Medications used to relieve cough include narcotic and nonnarcotic antitussives and expectorants. See Table 56-6 at the end of the chapter.

Narcotics. Narcotics, such as morphine and codeine, are effective **antitussives** (cough suppressants), but their use is limited because of their undesirable side effects and potential for habituation. Codeine is available in cough syrups.

Nonnarcotics. Nonnarcotic antitussives are widely used but are not as effective as narcotic agents. An example is *dextromethorphan* (which is contained in many OTC cough and cold preparations), such as Benylin, Delsym, Contac, and Robitussin.

Expectorants. *Expectorants* are drugs that increase secretion of mucus in the bronchi and help to expel sputum. Expectorants are taken with water, which helps increase the flow of mucus that protects the mucous membrane from irritation. Some expectorants may cause skin eruption, frontal sinus pain, or coryza (nasal discharge) if they are used for a long period of time. They have a metallic taste, and most patients find them unpleasant to take.

Bronchodilators

Drugs that cause relaxation of the smooth muscle of the bronchial tree are referred to as **bronchodilators** (see Table 56-6). This relaxation allows the diameter of the bronchioles and alveolar sacs to increase, and thus increases air exchange. These agents can also decrease respiratory tract congestion through vasoconstriction and reduction of mucous membrane swelling. Most drugs in this group are administered by oral aerosolization or inhalation to decrease systemic side effects of the drug. Treatment times are extremely variable and depend on patient response time. Oral agents, such as *terbutaline* (Bricanyl), *albuterol* (Proventil), or *theophylline* (Aminophylline), must be present in sufficient blood levels to provide adequate bronchodilator action.

Antihistamines and Decongestants

Antihistamines act by preventing the action of histamine produced in the body. These drugs have been used for various types of allergies and anaphylactic reactions (see Table 56-6). Antihistamines have their greatest effect on nasal allergies, particularly hay fever. Much difference of opinion exists as to the usefulness of these drugs in treating the common cold. They treat symptoms only and do not provide long-term relief or protect against reactions. They should be regarded as accessory agents to more specific treatment. Indiscriminate use may be harmful; people taking antihistamines may become drowsy while operating dangerous machinery or driving a car. As stated before, newer agents, such as *terfenadine* (Seldane) and *astemizole* (Hismanil), do not cross the blood–brain barrier; thus, they cause less drowsiness than other antihistamines.

Antihistamines are also contraindicated in patients with diabetes mellitus, without specific advice of the physician. They also should *not* be used by people with narrow-angle glaucoma.

Decongestants are often used orally or in nasal sprays or nose drops. They tend to dry up nasal secretions and thus reduce congestion in the nose and sinus tracts. Nasal decongestants should not be used for more than 3 days because of rebound congestion. Oral decongestants, such as *pseudoephedrine* (Sudafed), are contraindicated in patients with hypertension, without advice of a physician.

Drugs That Affect the Gastrointestinal System

Drugs affect the GI tract in numerous ways. They cleanse the mouth, stimulate peristalsis, relieve vomiting, and correct enzyme deficiencies and excess acidity.

Drugs That Affect the Mouth (Mouthwashes)

Oral hygiene is more effective in mouth care although some drugs are mildly helpful. Mouthwashes are not very potent germ killers because they cannot be used in strong concentrations without harming tissues. They are useful as disinfectants and in removing mucus from the mouth and throat. A 1% sodium bicarbonate (baking soda) solution ($\frac{1}{2}$ teaspoonful in a glassful of water) is a useful mouthwash for removing mucus. A 0.9% solution of sodium chloride (table salt) is *normal saline* and is as effective as any commercial preparation.

Hydrogen peroxide (H_2O_2), mixed half and half with water, may be used for mouth care in the unconscious patient or for the patient who must breathe through the mouth. Rinse with clear water after using peroxide to remove the taste.

Stannous fluoride is recognized as having beneficial effects in preventing tooth decay. It is found in many dentifrices. The American Dental Association has recommended the fluoridation of drinking water as a method for reducing dental decay. A 2% solution of sodium fluoride applied to children's teeth has also been found to be effective in preventing dental caries.

Drugs That Affect the Stomach

Certain drugs are used to control the excessive production of stomach acids; to aid digestion; to relieve distention from gas; and to prevent, control, or induce vomiting.

Antacids

Antacids are used to treat common upset stomach. See Table 56-7 at the end of the chapter. They are also used for peptic ulcers to reduce and control stomach acidity, giving the ulcer a chance to heal. A widely used home remedy antacid is sodium bicarbonate. The habit of taking this substance to avoid too much acid in the stomach can interfere with the body's electrolyte balance and cause systemic alkalosis. It can also cause acid rebound and can be a complication in cardiac distress. Other antacids are often preferred because they are not as readily absorbed and are not as apt to cause alkalosis. In very large doses, however, they may severely upset the acid–base balance of the body.

Some of the most commonly used antacids are *magnesium-aluminum hydroxide* (Maalox), *magnesium-aluminum hydroxide with simethicone* (Gelusil), and *aluminum hydroxide gel* (Amphojel). Liquids are generally more effective than tablet forms.

Histamine H_2 Antagonists

Histamine H_2 antagonists are drugs that inhibit gastric secretions that are mediated by histamine. They are indicated in the treatment of ulcers, gastric reflux, and hypersecretory conditions. Results are usually seen immediately, but complete healing can take up to 6 weeks or more. *Cimetidine* (Tagamet) and *ranitidine* (Zantac) are examples of H_2 antagonists.

Antiflatulents

Antiflatulents are drugs used to treat the symptoms of gas pressure in the digestive tract. *Charcoal* and *simethicone* (Mylicon) are antiflatulents that are used alone or in combination with each other.

Emetics

Emetics are agents given to induce vomiting. Their use has been replaced by gastric lavage (washing out the stomach) in many cases. Occasionally, emetics are used as a first aid measure when prompt evacuation of the stomach is needed, as is the case when certain poisons have been ingested.

Ipecac syrup is used only for the conscious patient because of the danger of aspiration. It is important to recover the dose of ipecac given, by emesis or lavage, because an unrecovered dose may exert toxic effects on the heart. The usual dosage is 15 mL, with another dose in 30 minutes if no results are observed. In the case of poisoning, contact the Poison Control Center before giving ipecac. (Some caustic substances cause more problems when emesis is produced. Chapter 31 describes emergency care in poisoning.)

Antiemetics

Antiemetics are given to produce symptomatic relief from nausea and vomiting (see Table 56-7). Numerous preparations have been used, but effective treatment usually depends on removal of the cause. Nondisease causes of nausea and vomiting may be emotional stress, motion sickness, pregnancy, or the effects of drugs or other treatments. When vomiting is caused by these conditions, CNS depressants, antihistamines, or tranquilizers may serve as antiemetics. Phenobarbital, a depressant, is occasionally used as an antiemetic. (A drug that was formerly used for nausea in pregnancy, Bendectin, has been *removed* from the market.)

Antispasmodics

The ideal antispasmodic agent should reduce secretion in the stomach and slow GI motility. A large number of drugs have been synthesized to capture this effect, but a great number of them have serious side effects. Generally, a drug that slows the stomach also causes blurred vision, dry mouth, and rapid heartbeat. The drugs listed in Table 56-7 are those that show the greatest antispasmodic activity with relatively fewer side effects than other drugs in this class.

Drugs That Affect the Intestine

Cathartics

Cathartics (laxatives) are drugs administered to induce defecation (see Table 56-7). A healthy person who eats a normal diet, gives attention to the impulse to defecate, drinks adequate fluids, and exercises sufficiently generally does not need a laxative. However, people who must lie in bed in one position, those receiving drugs such as morphine, codeine, or certain psychotropics, and those who have impaired muscle tone that affects the colon are likely to be constipated. Constipation is also associated with mental disorders, anemia,

and severe headache, and often occurs following administration of barium.

Elderly patients who have been taking cathartics for constipation most of their adult lives may need to continue this practice when in the hospital. Roughage in the diet is not a practical alternative to laxatives if the person is unable to chew. Furthermore, elderly people, like everyone else, are not likely to take kindly to the idea of changing lifetime habits. A mild cathartic taken regularly as prescribed by the physician is not likely to be harmful. Cathartics are contraindicated in cases of abdominal pain and after certain surgical procedures.

Cathartics are classified according to mode of action, as follows: bulk-producing agents, irritants, lubricants, saline cathartics, osmotic agents, and fecal softeners.

Bulk-Producing Cathartics. Bulk-producing laxatives stimulate peristalsis by increasing the stool's bulk and thereby modifying its consistency. The mechanism by which bulk-producing cathartics work is based on a normal stimulus, and therefore these laxatives are among the least harmful to the body. However, bulk-producing substances can cause fecal obstruction and impaction. Therefore, it is important to give them with adequate fluids and observe the patient for any untoward symptoms. Examples of bulk laxatives are *psyllium hydrophilic muciloid* (Metamucil and Konsyl).

Irritant Cathartics. Irritant cathartics irritate the large intestine, causing increased activity and bowel evacuation. Examples are *cascara sagrada* and *castor oil.*

Lubricant Cathartics. Liquid petrolatum, or *mineral oil,* is a lubricant used to soften feces. It is given to prevent straining with a bowel movement after rectal operations or for chronic constipation in inactive persons, such as elderly people. Mineral oil taken orally interferes with absorption of fat-soluble vitamins, A, D, E, and K. Therefore, some physicians do not prescribe it. It should be given between meals or at bedtime to avoid interfering with food absorption.

Saline Cathartics. Saline cathartics are soluble salts that are only slightly absorbed from the GI tract. Given with large amounts of water, they increase bulk in the intestine and cause distention. The distended colon stimulates smooth muscle contraction, followed by a thorough, quite rapid emptying of the bowel. Examples are *Milk of Magnesia* (M.O.M.), *magnesium citrate, magnesium sulfate,* and *Fleet's Phospho-Soda;* these drugs are usually given once a day at bedtime, as needed (PRN), or as a bowel prep before surgery or exams.

Osmotic Agents. In some cases, such as preparation for bowel surgery or examination, total emptying of the bowel is required. One such agent, *polyethylene glycol* *electrolyte solution* (Colyte, GoLYTELY) is not absorbed, so does not result in electrolyte imbalance. The patient is required to drink the solution over a period of 3 hours (a total of 4 L solution).

Fecal Softeners. Fecal softening agents are believed to act like a detergent by helping to permit water and fatty material to mix with fecal contents. They cause stools to become moist and bulky. These agents have a wide margin of safety and few undesirable side effects. Examples are *dioctyl potassium sulfosuccinate*—docusate potassium (Dialose, Kasof); *dioctyl sodium sulfosuccinate,* docusate sodium (D-S-S, Colace, Disonate); and *dioctyl calcium sulfosuccinate*—docusate calcium (Surfak, Pro-Cal-Sof). Liquid forms and powdered forms should be mixed with fruit juice to mask the taste.

Antidiarrheals

Diarrhea is a symptom of a disorder of the bowel associated with rapid passage of intestinal contents, fluid stools, and cramps. Diarrhea may produce serious consequences such as dehydration and loss of electrolytes, vitamins, and calories. Because diarrhea is thought to be a defense mechanism of the bowel, it often should not be stopped until its cause has been determined.

An antidiarrheal agent is a medication given to slow peristalsis and stop diarrhea, while allowing normal bowel movements (see Table 56-7). Examples of antidiarrheals are *diphenoxylate hydrochloride in combination with atropine* (Lomotil), *paregoric,* and *loperamide* (Imodium). Lomotil reduces intestinal motility and increases intestinal tone. It must not be given to children under the age of 2 years. It is used by travelers to combat cramping that often accompanies a change in food or a bacterial gastritis common in some countries. Paregoric is a derivative of morphine used to decrease the motility of the gut. Loperamide (Imodium) is now available without prescription and is as effective as Lomotil with greater safety.

Drugs That Affect the Urinary Tract

Diuretics

Diuretics are drugs that eliminate water and salts from the body by increasing the flow of urine. Because diuretics cause the elimination of both water and salts, the use of certain diuretics (for example, furosemide [Lasix] and hydrochlorothiazide [Hydrodiuril]) can also result in the loss of potassium. Patients taking these diuretics often also take a potassium supplement or increase potassium in their diet (eg, bananas and orange juice). See Table 56-8 at the end of the chapter.

When the flow of urine is inadequate, water and salts accumulate in the tissues and cause edema. An increased flow of urine usually reduces edema. Water acts as a diuretic, although it is not a drug, because if taken in increased amounts, water stimulates a reflex increase in fluid loss.

Many diuretics also reduce blood pressure, which can result in postural hypotension when the patient first begins taking the drug.

Xanthine Diuretics. The xanthine diuretics include caffeine and theophylline. These drugs are used rarely today as diuretics because they are inferior to thiazides and other diuretics.

Thiazide Diuretics. The thiazide diuretics are synthetic drugs chemically related to sulfonamides. The development of these agents marked a major breakthrough in the search for a potent oral diuretic. All thiazides are equally effective as diuretics although dosage and duration of action may vary. The thiazides have many advantages over other diuretics: ease of administration (oral), low cost, effectiveness over long periods, low toxicity, and few side effects. Examples include *bendroflumethiazide* (Naturetin), *chlorothiazide* (Diuril), and *hydrochlorothiazide* (Hydrodiuril, Dyazide).

Other Diuretics. *Furosemide* (Lasix) and bumetanide (Bumex) are effective, potent, rapidly acting diuretics; because of their potency, close medical supervision is required to monitor fluid and electrolyte balance. Supplemental potassium (K) is often prescribed when Lasix or Bumex is given. These are called "loop" diuretics because they inhibit reabsorption of sodium and chloride in the loop of Henle in the kidney.

Ethacrynic acid (Edecrin) is a potent diuretic with a short duration of action. Its use has largely been replaced by furosemide and bumetanide. Patients unresponsive to other diuretics usually respond to Edecrin.

Spironolactone (Aldactone) promotes diuresis and helps counteract the loss of potassium. It is effective in promoting diuresis in patients resistant to more common diuretics.

Triamterene (Dyrenium) potentiates (increases the action of) other diuretics. It causes increased elimination of sodium but does not cause a loss of potassium. For this reason, it is prescribed in the combined form with hydrochlorothiazide that is marketed under the brand name Dyazide.

Drugs That Affect the Muscle Tone of the Urinary Bladder

Bladder difficulties can result in a frequent desire to empty the bladder or an inability to empty it. In either case, the problem is one of poor muscle tone. *Neostig-*

mine methylsulfate (Prostigmin) and *bethanechol chloride* (Urecholine) improve muscle tone in the bladder, and L-*hyoscyamine sulfate* (Levsin) elixir relaxes bladder muscle. *Oxybutynin* (Ditropan) is an antispasmodic used to treat patients with bladder instability (eg, urgency, frequency, or urinary leakage).

Urinary Antiseptics and Antispasmodics

Urinary antiseptics exert antibacterial activity in the urinary tract with little or no systemic effect. The organisms that most commonly infect the urinary tract are the gram-negative bacilli, as well as some strains of streptococci and staphylococci. A number of antibiotics and sulfonamides inhibit growth of these organisms in the urinary tract; the one selected for use is generally determined by a laboratory culture of a urine specimen. Sulfonamides commonly used include *sulfisoxazole* (Gantrisin) and *sulfamethoxazole* (Gantanol). Several antibiotics covered earlier in this chapter are also effective against urinary tract infections.

Phenazopyridine (Pyridium) is a drug used primarily for its analgesic effect on the urinary mucosa. It relieves the symptoms of urgency and frequency of urination. Phenazopyridine is often used in combination with sulfa drugs. It colors urine bright orange.

Drugs That Affect the Reproductive System

Male Sex Hormones (Androgens)

Androgens are essential for the development and maintenance of male sex characteristics (see Table 56-4). Both sexes produce male and female hormones, but their effects are antagonistic to each other. Androgens are administered to men whose bodies do not produce a high enough level of these hormones. Androgens may also be administered to female patients to reduce the rate of spread of a cancer in the reproductive tract.

Drugs That Affect the Uterus

The uterus is a highly muscular organ with great ability to expand and contract. Drugs that act on the uterus are used either to increase or decrease uterine motility (muscular activity).

Drugs That Increase Uterine Motility

Oxytocins increase uterine contraction and may be used to induce or assist labor. The most commonly used are alkaloids of ergot and an extract of the posterior pituitary gland, oxytocin. Patients receiving these drugs during labor must be watched closely, with frequent

checks of blood pressure and monitoring of fetal status. Prolonged contractions of the uterus can diminish blood and oxygen supply to the fetus, and may promote rupture of the uterus.

Ergot Alkaloids. Preparations of ergot are used to promote contraction of the uterus back to its normal size after childbirth; these drugs also constrict the smaller blood vessels and thereby prevent postpartum hemorrhage. *Ergovine maleate* (Ergotrate) is given subcutaneously or intramuscularly immediately after delivery. Tablets for oral administration are also available.

Possible side effects of ergot-type drugs are nausea and vomiting, dizziness, headache, diarrhea, and abdominal cramps. These effects are most likely to occur after large doses of the drug, such as in a self-induced abortion. Severe poisoning may cause gangrene or blindness.

Methylergonovine Maleate. *Methylergonovine maleate* (Methergine) resembles Ergotrate in its action but is more powerful, has more prolonged effects, and is less likely to raise blood pressure.

Oxytocin. In addition to its use to induce labor, oxytocin may be given during childbirth to increase uterine contractions at the time of delivery if normal contractions fail to expel the fetus or placenta. Oxytocin is also used to contract the uterus and to reduce hemorrhage after the placenta is presented. This drug is usually administered by slow intravenous drip in dextrose 5% in water (D_5W).

Drugs That Decrease Uterine Motility

Many times, it is desirable to inhibit uterine contractions, for example, when premature labor threatens or when contractions are rapid and irregular. Drugs to relieve these conditions include certain CNS depressants and antispasmodics. Morphine or *meperidine* (Demerol), especially when combined with *promethazine* (Phenergan), tends to decrease uterine motility. An intravenous infusion of 10% alcohol in 5% dextrose has been used in premature labor, as has intravenous *diazepam* (Valium). *Magnesium sulfate* has a potent depressant effect on all muscular tissue and effectively relaxes the uterus when it is contracting abnormally. Magnesium sulfate is also used to treat the seizures of eclampsia (formerly known as toxemia of pregnancy) because of its CNS depressant properties. *Isoxsuprine* (Vasodilan) and *terbutaline* (Brethine) are used in oral form to treat premature labor although they are not FDA-approved for this use.

Ovarian Hormones

The ovaries secrete two important hormones that affect the activity of the sex glands (see Table 56-4 at the end of this chapter). One is follicular hormone and the other is luteal hormone.

Estrogen. Estrogens are responsible for development of sex organs and secondary sex characteristics, such as growth of breasts, distribution of hair, texture of the skin, and the maintenance of these all through life. When estrogen deficiency occurs, as in menopause, replacement therapy may be prescribed. Estrogen agents are also used for functional uterine bleeding, for failure of ovary development, to suppress lactation in postpartum patients, and to prevent osteoporosis in postmenopausal women. In some cases, men with cancers of male reproductive organs are given these drugs as a palliative (not curative) measure.

The side effects of estrogens include nausea and vomiting, diarrhea, dizziness, and skin rash. When these symptoms appear, they are usually mild and disappear with adjustment in dosage, use of another estrogen, or a change in method of administration.

Progesterone. Progesterone is secreted by the corpus luteum and influences uterine and ovarian conditions during pregnancy. It prepares the lining of the uterus for implantation of the ovum and for nourishment of the embryo. It suppresses ovulation during pregnancy and reduces the irritability of uterine muscle to prevent premature labor or spontaneous abortion. Progesterone may be of use in dysmenorrhea, menorrhagia, metrorrhagia, or threatened spontaneous abortion. Side effects are few, but some patients complain of headache, dizziness, and fever. Allergic reactions are also possible.

Drugs Used in Family Planning

Contraceptives are hormonal preparations used to limit the number of pregnancies (to control fertility). There are many contraceptive preparations; because oral contraceptives change so often, the nurse should consult a current drug reference for information. Other hormonal preparations are used to enhance fertility in women who have had difficulty conceiving. Chapter 63 describes and lists drugs commonly used to limit or enhance fertility.

Drugs Used in Treating Sexually Transmitted Diseases

Antibiotics are used to treat the STDs, syphilis and gonorrhea. Many other STDs can also be successfully treated with antibiotics, although some, such as her-pesvirus, are resistant to treatment. Chapter 63 describes STDs and their treatment.

Zidovudine (ZDU, Retrovir) is used to treat HIV infections and the complex of disorders related to acquired immunodeficiency syndrome. (See Chapter 78.)

Serums and Vaccines

Serums (sera) and vaccines for preventing or treating disease are discussed in Chapter 77 along with antigen and antibody reactions. Chapter 64 provides a discussion of immunization programs for children.

Immune Serums (Sera)

There are two types of immune sera: natural sera and antitoxins. Natural human sera are obtained from patients who have recovered from a disease and still have immune bodies in their blood. Examples are immune serum globulin (gamma globulin) and pertussis immune globulin. Antitoxic sera are produced in the bodies of animals that have been actively immunized by a specific toxin. They are given to neutralize toxins produced in human beings by certain diseases. Examples are diphtheria, tetanus, and gas gangrene antitoxins. The latter are needed when the patient has contracted a disease against which he or she has no antibodies.

Vaccines

Vaccines are preparations of disease organisms, live or attenuated (weakened), that cause the body to produce immunity to infectious disease. It may take several weeks for immunity to develop. Sometimes, if an effective human serum is available, a dose of the serum may be given before a vaccine to ensure immediate protection. This might be done when there is danger of immediate infection. Vaccines are available to treat many diseases that formerly afflicted much of the world's population.

Toxoids

A toxoid is a toxin modified so that it is nontoxic but still capable of stimulating the body to build immunity to a disease. Diphtheria toxoid and tetanus toxoid are the most widely used of this group and may be given separately or in combination. Triple antigens (diphtheria and tetanus toxoids and pertussis vaccine, known as DTP; and measles, mumps, and rubella vaccine, or MMR) are used for immunizing children.

Tests for Immunity

To determine if a person has been exposed to certain disease organisms, a tiny amount of the specific toxin is injected subdermally (under the skin) or intradermally (within the layers of the skin) on the forearm. If antitoxins to that disease are present in the person's blood, a reddened area (*erythema*) and swelling (*in-*

duration) will appear around the point of injection (see Chapter 50). The most common test of this type is the tuberculin test for tuberculosis. Purified protein derivative (PPD) is used for this test. A positive reaction does not necessarily mean that the person has an active case of tuberculosis, but it may indicate that he or she has been exposed to it. Several chapters including 50, 64, 77, and 79 describe the use of tuberculin tests in detail.

Key Concept

A person can be allergic to *any drug at any time*. The nurse must always be watchful for signs of anaphylactic shock or other signs of milder allergy. In some cases, the physician gives a small sample of the drug to test the person's reaction before prescribing it.

Keys for Review

Key Questions for Critical Thinking

1. Discuss the many actions of diuretics and describe the physiology of how they work.
2. Many drugs can affect the blood vessels. Describe the different effects that drugs have on blood vessels and relate those effects to the physiology of blood pressure.
3. You have to give a patient a drug with which you are not familiar. Describe how you would proceed with gathering all the information you need to give the drug safely.

Key Readings

Alfaro-LeFevre R. Drug Handbook: A Nursing Process Approach. Redding, CA, Addison-Wesley, 1992

Clayton B, Stock Y. Basic Pharmacology for Nurses, Ed 10. St. Louis, Mosby-Yearbook, 1992

Malseed R. Pharmacology: Drug Therapy and Nursing Considerations, Ed 3. Philadelphia, J.B. Lippincott, 1990

Nursing '94 Drug Handbook. Springhouse, PA, Springhouse, 1994

Physician's Desk Reference. Oradell, NJ, Medical Economics Co, published yearly with quarterly updates

Scherer J. Introductory Clinical Pharmacology, Ed 4. Philadelphia, J.B. Lippincott, 1991

Key Readings (continued)

Sewester S. Facts and Comparisons Drug Information. Philadelphia, J.B. Lippincott, updated monthly

Spratto G, et al. RN Magazine's Nurse's Drug Reference '95. Albany, NY, Delmar Publishers, 1995

Swonger A, Matejski M. Nursing Pharmacology: An Integrated Approach to Drug Therapy and Nursing, Ed 2. Philadelphia, J.B. Lippincott, 1991

Enrichment Keys

UDL Laboratories. Generic-Brand Comparison Handbook. UDL Laboratories Inc. Rockford, IL, 1991 (available to nursing students)

Keys To Learning More

Chapter 57: medication administration

Unit Twelve: medications as used in obstetrics

Unit Thirteen: pediatric medication administration

Unit Fourteen: medications as part of treatment for major adult disorders

Unit Fifteen: older persons and medication use

Chapter 87: medications in psychiatry

Chapter 88: chemical abuse and its treatment

Unit Seventeen: medication use in the dying patient

Chapter 92: transcription of medication orders

Table 56-1. Anti-infective Drugs

Name of Drug*	Usual Adult Dose	Notes
Penicillins		
Amoxicillin (Amoxil, Polymox)	Oral only: 250–500 mg q8h	Extended spectrum
Ampicillin (Polycillin, Omnipen)	Oral, IM, IV: 250–500 mg to 1 g q6h	Effective against several strains of bacteria; used as initial therapy for meningitis (until results of cultures are completed). Ampicillin with probenecid (Polycillin, Principen) used in gonorrhea.
Carbenicillin (Geopen, Pyopen)	Oral: 2–5 g q4–6h	Antipseudomonas activity; smaller dose in urinary tract infections
Cloxacillin (Tegopen)	Oral only: 250–500 mg q6h	Antistaphylococcus activity
Dicloxacillin	Oral only: 250–500 mg	Best absorbed of the oral antistaphylococcus medications
Methicillin (Staphcillin)	IM, IV: 1 g q4h to q6h	Antistaphylococcus activity
Nafcillin (Nafcil, Unipen)	Oral: 250–500 mg q4–6h Oral, IM, IV: 500 mg to 1 g q4–6h	Treatment of penicillin-resistant organisms; especially staphylococcus
Oxacillin (Prostaphlin, Bactocil)	Oral: 500 mg q4–6h By injection: 1 g q4–6h	Used for penicillin-resistant organisms, especially staphylococcus
Penicillin G, aqueous	Oral, IM, IV: 5 million to 20 million U/d, in divided doses	Oral form used for mild to moderate infections with penicillin-sensitive organisms; parenteral route used in severe infections
Penicillin VK (Penicillin V Potassium, V-Cillin-K, Pen-Vee K)	Oral only: 250–500 mg q6h	Mild to moderate bacterial infections
Piperacillin (Pipracil)	IM, IV: 3–4 g q4–6h	Extended spectrum; antipseudomonas activity; mixed infections
Ticarcillin (Ticar)	Parenteral only: 2–4 g q4–6h	Antipseudomonas; bacterial septicemia
Procaine penicillin G, aqueous (APPG, Crysticillin, Wycillin)	IM only: 600,000–4,800,000 U/d, in divided doses	Long-acting: moderate to severe infections
Cephalosporins		
Cefaclor (Ceclor)	Oral only: 250 mg q8h or 375 mg q12h	Most often used for organisms resistant to ampicillin, specific for otitis media
Cefadroxil (Duricef)	Oral: 1 g daily, in single or divided doses	Skin infections; tonsillitis caused by a β-hemolytic streptococcus (can cause renal impairment)
Cefamandole naftate (Mandol)	Parenteral only: 500 mg to 1 g q4–8h	Pneumonia; skin infections (can build up pressure in bottle due to CO_2 formation)
Cefazolin (Ancef, Kefzol)	Parenteral only: 500 mg to 1 g q6–8h (dose up to 12 g used in life-threatening infection)	Extended duration of action; used to treat wide range of infections, including septicemia
Cefoperazone (Cefobid)	IM, IV: 1–2 g q12h	Extended duration; antipseudomonas activity (may cause liver or kidney side effects)
Cefotaxime (Claforan)	Parenteral only: 1 g q6–8h	Extended spectrum
Cefoxitin (Mefoxin)	Oral: 1 g q6–8h	Better gram-negative and anaerobic activity
Cefuroxime sodium (Ceftin)	Oral: 125–500 mg q12h	Preoperative preparation, sinus infections
Cefuroxime sodium (Zinacef)	IM, IV: 750 mg to 1.5 g q8h	Broad spectrum
Cephlexin (Keflex)	Oral: 250–500 mg q6h	Skin infections: in children, used for otitis media
Cephalothin sodium (Keflin)	IV, deep IM: 1–2 g q4–6h	Severe infections; added to dialysis solution to prevent infections
Cephradine (Velosef)	Oral: 250–500 mg q6h IM, IV: 1 g q6–8h	Skin and respiratory infections (dose increased in lobar pneumonia); not affected by food

(continued)

Table 56-1 (continued)

Name of Drug*	Usual Adult Dose	Notes
Moxalactam disodium (Moxam)	Parenteral only: 1–2 g q8h	Extended spectrum; skin infections and uncomplicated pneumonia
Tetracyclines		
Doxycycline (Vibramycin)	100–200 mg daily	Oral and IV forms available; long duration of action; can cause photosensitivity
Minocycline (Minocin)	Oral: 50–100 mg q12h IV: 100–200 mg q12h	Broad spectrum, including acne; carriers of meningococci; in gonorrheal infections (oral: may take with food or milk)
Tetracycline (Sumycin, Achromycin)	Oral: 250 mg q6h IV: 250–500 mg q12h	Use in children may discolor teeth Not used during pregnancy May cause photosensitivity
Aminoglycosides		
Amikacin (Amikin)	IM, IV: 500 mg 2–3 times daily	Treatment of gram-negative infections, including pseudomonas and bacterial septicemia (nephrotoxic, ototoxic)†
Gentamicin (Garamycin)	Ophthalmic: drops/ointments IM and IV: 3–5 mg/kg/d (in divided doses)	Eye infections Nephrotoxic and ototoxic; reserved for serious gram-negative infections
Neomycin	Topical use as 1% solution or ointment; possible oral use as bowel prep	Toxicity with continued systemic use
Streptomycin	IM: 1–2 g q12h	When given IM, used to treat *Mycobacterium tuberculosis*
Tobramycin (Nebcin)	IM and IV: 3–5 mg/kg/d in divided doses	Similar to gentamicin in all aspects
Erythromycins		
Erythromycin (Erythrocin, E-Mycin, Ilosone)	Oral: 250–500 mg q6h IV: 500 mg to 1 g q6h	Oral forms can cause GI distress
Sulfonamides and Urinary Antiseptics		
Co-trimoxazole (trimethoprim and sulfamethoxazole) (Septra, Bactrim)	Oral: 1 double-strength tablet q12 h May also be given IV	A combination of two sulfa drugs for urinary tract infection and otitis media in children
Nitrofurantoin (Macrodantin, Furadantin)	Oral: 50–100 mg q6h	Oral use only; must be taken with food or milk; urinary antiseptic
Norfloxin (Noroxin)	Oral: 400 mg b.i.d.	Urinary tract infections
Sulfamethoxazole (Gantanol)	Oral: 2 g initially, then 1 g b.i.d.	Urinary tract infections
Sulfasalazine (Azulfidine)	Oral: 500 mg q.i.d.	Ulcerative colitis, oligospermia (lack of sperm cells) and infertility in men (withdrawal of drug reverses effect)
Sulfisoxazole (Gantrisin)	Oral: 4 g initially, then 1–2 g q.i.d.	A sulfa drug; must be given with plenty of water to avoid formation of urinary crystals
Antifungals		
Amphotericin B (Fungizone)	IV: 0.25–1 mg/kg/d	Parenteral antifungal agent; test dose required because of possible anaphylaxis
Fluconazol (Diflucan)	Oral: 200–400 mg/d initially, then 100–200 mg/d IV: 50–400 mg initially, then as per chart, based on creatinine clearance	Broad-spectrum antifungal
Ketoconazole (Nizoral)	Topical: 2% cream, once daily Oral: 200–400 mg daily	Antifungal
Miconazole (Monistat)	IV: 200–3600 mg/d in divided doses Vaginal: OTC	Severe systemic fungal infections, for vaginal yeast infection Intrathecal for fungal meningitis

(continued)

Table 56-1 (continued)

Name of Drug*	Usual Adult Dose	Notes
Nystatin (Mycostatin, Nilstat)	Oral: 5 mL q.i.d. in suspension Oral: 500,000–1,000,000 U t.i.d. Topical: apply b.i.d. or t.i.d.	Antifungal agent
Antivirals		
Acyclovir (Zovirax)	Oral: 200–800 mg 5 times/d IV: 5 mg/kg q8h Topical: Apply q3h × 7 d	Used for herpes simplex virus types I and II and shingles
Amantadine (Symmetrel)	Oral: 100 mg b.i.d.	Antiviral: influenza type A virus, respiratory tract infections
Zidovudine (AZT, Retrovir)	Oral: 200 mg q4h	Treatment of HIV infections (AIDS, advanced ARC); adjust dose PRN for hemotologic changes
Other Antibiotics and Anti-infectives		
Chloramphenicol (Chlormycetin)	Oral: 250 mg–1 g q6h	Very broad spectrum; can be toxic to bone marrow
Chloroquine phosphate (Aralen)	Oral, IV: 300 mg/d (base dose)	Antimalarial
Clindamycin (Cleocin)	150–600 mg q6–8h Vaginal: qHS × 7	Available in topical, oral, and injectable forms; effective against gram-positive infections
Ciprofloxacin (Cipro)	Oral: 250–750 mg q12h	Fairly wide spectrum, used for urinary tract infections
Isoniazid (INH)	Oral: Up to 300 mg daily	Treatment of tuberculosis (take with food)
Mebendazole (Vermox)	Oral: 100 mg one-time dose	Treatment of roundworm, pinworm, whipworm
Metronidazole (Flagyl)	IV: 500 mg q6h Oral: 250 mg t.i.d. for 7 d or 2 g as one-time dose	Treat anaerobes; treat trichomoniasis
Polymyxin B (Aerosporin)	IM, IV, intrathecal‡: 5,000–25,000 U/kg/d	Acute infections, especially pseudomonas; urinary tract, meninges, blood stream (extremely nephrotoxic)
Quinine sulfate	Oral: 650 mg q8h	Antimalarial, low doses for night leg cramps
Rifampin (Rifadin)	Oral: 300–600 mg once daily	Treatment of tuberculosis (discolors urine); for prophylactic use after Haemophilus influenza meningitis exposure
Vancomycin (Vancocin)	Oral: 500 mg–2 g/d in divided doses IV: 500 mg q6h	Used for resistant staph infections in penicillin-allergic patients

* A trade name appears in parentheses following the generic name of the drug.

† Nephrotoxic, damaging to kidney cells; ototoxic, damaging to eighth cranial nerve, causing hearing and balance disorders.

‡ Intrathecal, injection through the sheath (theca) of the spinal cord into the subarachnoid space.

Table 56-2. Dermatologic Agents

Type	Examples*
Soothing Agents	
Emollient preparations	*Glycerin:* in pure form, tends to dry skin; if mixed with rosewater, has a moisturizing effect
	Lanolin: used as ointment base; purified fat of sheeps' wool with water
	Urea: 2–40% promotes hydration and removal of excess keratin in dry skin
	Vitamin A & D ointment
	Zinc oxide ointment: 15% zinc oxide in simple ointment base
Lotions and solution preparations	*Burrow's solution:* aluminum acetate used for its astringent (drying) properties; used for poison ivy, insect bites, *etc.*
	Calamine lotion: used for dermatitis (itching, inflamed skin) caused by poison ivy, insect bites, or prickly heat
Anesthetics	
Benzocaine, lidocaine, cocaine	Sprays, lotions, or creams used for pruritus (itching) and pain due to wounds, minor burns, prickly heat, chickenpox, insect bites, sunburn
Antiseptics	*Benzalkonium chloride (Zephiran):* detergent type of agent; germicidal for a number of pathogens; activity reduced by soap solutions; most effective in 1:750 solution
	Chlorhexidine gluconate (Hibiclens): antimicrobial activity against a wide range of microorganisms; used as a surgical scrub and cleanser for preoperative bathing and wound cleansing
	Iodine: generally in alcohol solution (tincture) in concentration up to 7%
	Povidone-iodine (Betadine): stable compound slowly releases iodine; relatively nonirritating; contains 1% available iodine
	Thimerosal (Methiolate): organic mercury compound, used on abraded skin, concentration of 1:1000; available also as tincture (with alcohol)
Antifungals	*Gentian violet:* external application in solution of 1% of the dye; stains clothing
	Nystatin (Mycostatin): antibiotic; used for fungal infections of skin and mucous membranes; commonly used as vaginal suppository
	Tolnaftate (Tinactin): 1% concentration in a cream or solution to treat infections caused by *Trichophyton,* the organisms of athlete's foot
	Chlotrimazole (Lotrimin): antifungal used topically for athlete's foot and diaper rash; used vaginally for yeast infection; both forms available OTC
Corticosteroids	Betamethasone diproprionate (*Diprosone*): available in varying strengths and emollient bases; used for anti-inflammatory, antipruritic, and antiproliferative actions (avoid contact with eyes; apply sparingly)
	Desoximetasone (Topicort): available as cream, gel, or ointment (used cautiously in viral diseases; may macerate skin if covered with occlusive dressing)
	Hydrocortisone (Acticort, Bactine HC, Cortef, Hytone, Synacort, Unicort): aerosol, cream, gel, lotion, ointment, topical solution, rectal foam (used for dermatitis, may be used on face, groin, axillae, and under breasts; clean area before application; avoid eyes; use as directed)
Pediculocides (Kill lice)	*Lindane (Kwell):* available as lotion, ointment, or shampoo (keep away from eyes and mouth; potential for CNS toxicity in infants and children)
	Permethrin (Nix): shampoo (combing of nits [eggs of lice] not required); will prevent reinfection up to 2 wks; available OTC; no CNS toxicity if used as directed

* A trade name appears in parentheses following the generic name of a drug.

Table 56-3. Central Nervous System Drugs

Name of Drug*	Usual Adult Dose	Notes
Narcotic Agonist Analgesics		
Codeine	Oral or IM: 30–60 mg q4h PRN	Usually given in combination with aspirin (Empirin #3) or acetaminophen (Tylenol #3)
Fetanyl (Sublimaze, Duragesic)	Topical: 25–300 mcg/72 h IV: 1–30 mcg/kg	Dosage depends on use (induction of anesthesia, maintenance of anesthesia vs pain maintenance)
Hydromorphone (Dilaudid)	Oral or IM: 2–4 mg q4–6h	Shorter duration of action than morphine
Levorphanol (Levo-Dromoran)	IM: 2 mg q4h	For relief of moderate to severe pain
Meperidine (Demerol)	IM or oral: 50–100 mg q3–4h	Does not have antitussive (cough suppressant) effect of other narcotics
Methadone (Dolophine)	IM and oral: 2.5–10 mg q6–12h	Longer duration of activity; used as narcotic replacement to facilitate withdrawal
Morphine	Oral, IV, or IM: 10–15 mg q4h	Used to treat severe pain (eg, heart attack)
Nalbuphine HCl (Nubain)	IV, IM, subQ: 10 mg/70 kg	Synthetic narcotic agonist/antagonist; potent but with low potential for habituation and for respiratory depression
Oxycodone (Percodan, Percocet)	Oral: 5 mg q4h	Often combined with aspirin (Percodan) or with acetaminophen (Percocet)
Pentazocine (Talwin)	Oral: 50 mg q3–4h IM, IV, subQ: 30–60 mg q3–4h	Talwin may cause dependence. Oral form (Talwin NX) contains 50 mg pentazocine and 0.5 mg naloxone (Narcan). If injected as unintended use, naloxone will block effect
Propoxyphene HCl (Darvon†)	Oral: 65 mg q4h	In combination with aspirin or acetaminophen, produces greater pain relief (Darvon compound); potentiated by alcohol
Narcotic Antagonists		
Naloxone (Narcan)	IV: 0.4–2 mg q2–3min	Used as antidote in narcotic overdose; it prevents or reverses effects of opioids
Nonnarcotic Analgesics and Anti-inflammatory Drugs¶		
Acetaminophen (Tylenol, Datril)	Oral: 300–650 mg q4–6h	Analgesic and fever reducer; used in aspirin-allergic patients and children
Acetylsalicylic acid, ASA, aspirin	Oral or rectal; 81–650 mg (⁷⁄₄–10 grains) q4–6h	May cause GI distress in high doses; mild anticoagulant. Low dose (81 mg) used to prevent stroke and to prevent reinfarction following MI
Auranofin (Ridaura)	Oral: 6 mg daily	Used in arthritis (contains 29% gold)
Diclofenac (Voltaren)	25–75 mg b.i.d.	NSAID, used in arthritis and ankylosing spondylitis
Ibuprofen (Motrin, Advil, Nuprin, Rufen)	Oral: 200–800 mg q6–8h	Given with meals or milk if GI distress occurs. Available OTC in 200-mg strength and sometimes used for fever in children; NSAID
Indomethacin (Indocin)	Oral: 25–50 mg 3 or 4 times daily	Most commonly used in arthritis; gastric distress common; NSAID
Naproxen (Naprosyn, Anaprox)	Oral: 250–750 mg b.i.d.	Longer acting drug used for arthritis; NSAID
Phenylbutazone (Butazolidin)	Oral: 100 mg q.i.d.	For short-term use in arthritis (if used for longer time, may cause aplastic anemia and/or agranulocytosis); NSAID
Piroxicam (Feldene)	Oral: 20 mg once daily	Single daily dose in rheumatoid arthritis; NSAID
Sulindac (Clinoril)	Oral: 150–200 mg b.i.d.	For acute and long-term use in arthritis; NSAID
Hypnotic, Sedative, and Antianxiety Drugs		
Barbiturates		
Amobarbital (Amytal)	Oral: 65–200 mg h.s.	Hypnotic; intermediate duration of action
Pentobarbital (Nembutal)	Oral: 100 mg h.s.	Short-acting hypnotic; may be used as preanesthetic
Phenobarbital (Luminal)	Oral: 30–120 mg 2–3 times daily	Long-acting sedative; used principally as an anticonvulsant
Secobarbital (Seconal)	Oral: 100 mg h.s.	Short-acting hypnotic and pre-anesthesia sedative, used occasionally in pregnancy

(continued)

Table 56-3 *(continued)*

Name of Drug*	Usual Adult Dose	Notes
Benzodiazepines		
Alprazolam (Xanax)	Oral: 0.25–2 mg t.i.d.	Intermediate acting; 2-mg dose used to treat panic attacks
Chlordiazepoxide (Librium)	Oral: 10–25 mg 3–4 times daily IM: given deep IM	Long-acting drug to treat anxiety and alcohol withdrawal
Diazepam (Valium)	Oral: 2–10 mg up to q.i.d. IV: 5–10 mg PRN	Used to treat seizures, muscle spasm, anxiety; IV form for status epilepticus; used in alcohol detoxification
Flurazepam (Dalmane)	Oral: 15–30 mg h.s.	Hypnotic only; use dose of 15 mg in elderly
Lorazepam (Ativan)	Oral: 0.5–6 mg/d, in divided doses IM: Usual dose is 1–2 mg	Intermediate acting; sublingual administration absorbed faster than oral IM most often used to control dangerous behavior
Oxazepam (Serax)	Oral: 10–15 mg 3–4 times daily	Short-acting drug for anxiety and alcohol withdrawal
Triazolam (Halcion)	Oral: 0.125–0.5 mg h.s.	Shortest-acting hypnotic in this class; may have dangerous side effects
Miscellaneous		
Buspirone (BuSpar)	Oral: 5–20 mg t.i.d.	Management of anxiety disorders; not related chemically to benzodiazepines, barbiturates, or other sedative hypnotics; less sedative effects than benzodiazepines.
Chloral hydrate (Noctec)	Oral: 500 mg h.s. Rectal: 500 mg-1g h.s.	Oldest of currently used hypnotics; bitter taste; gel caps and suppositories available
Meprobamate (Equanil, Miltown)	Oral: 400 mg 3–4 times daily	Antianxiety and sedative with muscle-relaxing properties
Psychotherapeutic Drugs		
Antipsychotic Drugs		
Chlorpromazine (Thorazine)	Oral: 25–200 mg q.i.d. IM: 10–100 mg q4–6h	Higher doses may be used initially and then tapered down
Clozapine (Clozaril)	Oral: 25 mg b.i.d.; gradually titrated upward	Used to treat severely ill schizophrenics who do not respond to other drugs. Can cause severe blood dyscrasia; patient must have weekly WBC. Patient must be registered with government program.
Fluphenazine HCl (Prolixin)	Oral: 0.5–5 mg b.i.d. IM: $\frac{1}{3}$–$\frac{1}{2}$ oral dose (decanoate available)	Used to treat psychotic disorders. Can cause blood dyscrasias.
Haloperidol (Haldol)	Oral: 0.5–10 mg 2–3 times daily IM: 2–5 mg q4–8h (decanoate available)	Low sedative properties, high extrapyramidal effects (tics and abnormal involuntary movements); higher doses may be used
Lithium carbonate (Lithonate, Lithotabs)	Oral: 300–600 mg daily (dose based on blood levels and clinial response)	Treatment of manic phase of bipolar illness; (Maintain salt and fluid intake; lithium toxicity symptoms are diarrhea, vomiting, and muscle weakness); avoid NSAIDs
Perphenazine (Trilafon)	Oral: 4–16 mg q.i.d. IM: 5 mg q6h	IM form used as an antiemetic
Thioridazine (Mellaril)	Oral: 50–100 mg t.i.d.	Higher doses may be used
Thiothixene (Navane)	Oral: 2–10 mg t.i.d.	Side effects similar to Haldol, Mellaril, and Trilafon
Trifluoperazine (Stelazine)	Oral: 1–5 mg t.i.d.	IM injection available to control acute symptoms
Antidepressants‡		
Amitriptyline (Elavil, Endep)	Oral: 50–100 mg daily IM use also	Total daily dose may be given at bedtime to reduce sedative side effects (tricyclic).
Bupropion HCl (Wellbutrin)	Oral: 100 mg b.i.d.–150 mg t.i.d.	Used to treat depression. Contraindicated in seizure disorders.
Desipramine (Norpramin, Pertofrane)	Oral: 50–200 mg daily	Fewer anticholinergic and sedative effects than other drugs of this class (tricyclic)
Doxepin (Sinequan, Adapin)	Oral: 75–150 mg daily	Once daily dose at bedtime is most effective (tricyclic)

(continued)

Table 56-3 (continued)

Name of Drug*	Usual Adult Dose	Notes
Fluoxetine (Prozac)	Oral: 10–20 mg b.i.d.	Not related to tricyclics or other antidepressants (may cause drowsiness)
Imipramine (Tofranil)	Oral: 75–100 mg daily	Mild anticholinergic and sedative effects (tricyclic)
Maprotiline (Ludiomil)	Oral: 75–150 mg daily	Also relieves anxiety associated with depression (tricyclic)
Tranylcypromine sulfate (Parnate)	Oral: 10–20 mg daily	Monoamine oxidase (MAO) inhibitor (avoid tyramine-containing foods; eg, beer, cheese, beef); do NOT use with tricyclics.
Trazodone (Desyrel)	Oral: 150–400 mg daily	Effects noted earlier than those of other drugs in this class May be used also to aid sleep in depressed pt. Few serious side effects
Other CNS Drugs		
Carbemazepine (Tegretol)	Oral: 800–1200 mg daily	Used in mixed seizures, generalized tonic–clonic seizures, and treatment of pain associated with trigeminal neuralgia
Carbidopa/levodopa (Sinemet: contains 10 mg carbidopa and 100 mg levodopa)	Oral: 10/100 to 25/250 t.i.d. Sinemet CR (sustained release): 50/200	Antiparkinsonism agent. May cause hemolytic anemia, cardiac arrythmias. Contraindicated in glaucoma, melanoma; may interact with antihypertensives.
Cyclobenzaprine (Flexeril)	Oral: 10 mg t.i.d.	Centrally acting muscle relaxant; structurally related to tricyclics (may cause drowsiness and dry mouth)
Dantrolene sodium (Dantrium)	Oral: 25–100 mg 2–4 times daily IV: 2.5 mg/kg 1½ h prior to anesthesia	Skeletal muscle relaxant used for cerebral palsy, multiple sclerosis; also used for malignant hyperthermia
Dextroamphetamine (Dexedrine)	Oral: 10 mg daily	Used in adults for narcolepsy (a sleep disorder) Used in children for attention deficit hyperactive disorder (ADHD)
Diethylpropion	Oral: 25 mg t.i.d. or 75 mg sustained-release daily	Used for weight loss
Methocarbanol (Robaxin)	Oral: 500–700 mg q4h IM, IV: up to 2–3 g daily	Centrally acting muscle relaxant (may cause drowsiness)
Methylphenidate (Ritalin)	Oral: 20–30 mg/d in divided doses	Adults: narcolepsy Children: ADHD
Phenytoin (Dilantin)	Oral: 300–400 mg/d IV, IM: variable dosages	Anticonvulsant for generalized tonic–clonic and psychomotor seizures (gingival hyperplasia is frequent side effect)
Primidone (Mysoline)	Oral: 250 mg 3–4 times daily	Treatment of generalized tonic–clonic, psychomotor or focal seizures
Sumatriptan (Imitrex)	SubQ: 6 mg; may repeat in 1 h (limit 12 mg/d)	Treatment of severe migraine headaches; available by prescription (prefilled syringes) for home administration

* A trade name appears in parentheses following the generic name of the drug.

† There are several forms of Darvon in common use today. The nurse should consult a specific drug reference before administering any of these preparations because the names are similar but the therapeutic effects are different.

¶ NSAIDs are contraindicated when patients are taking any drug which may cause kidney damage, such as Lithium.

‡ The tricyclics, such as amitriptyline, imipramine, and doxepin can cause very annoying and severe side effects, including tardive dyskinesia (see Chapter 87).

CR, controlled release

Table 56-4. Drugs Affecting the Endocrine System

Name of Drug*	Route of Administration	Clinical Use and Notes
Sex Hormones#		
Estrogens		
Conjugated estrogens (Premarin)	Oral: 0.3–2.5 mg daily Topical (vaginal): @ h.s.	Replacement therapy, osteoporosis
Estrone (Theelin)	IM only: 0.5–2 mg weekly	Replacement therapy, prostatic cancer
Estradiol transdermal (Estraderm)	Topical patch: 0.05–0.1 mg/24 h	Replacement therapy in menopause; low dose with fewer side effects because of transdermal administration (Patch changed 2×/wk.)
Ethinyl estradiol (Estinyl)	Oral: 0.02–1.5 mg/d	Replacement therapy, prostatic and breast cancer
Progestins		
Levonorgestrel (Norplant)	Implant: 36 mg/implant—dose is 6 implants, in fan shape	Implant is effective for up to 5 y for contraception
Progesterone	IM only: 125–375 mg/d Suppository: 25–400 mg	Amenorrhea, functional uterine bleeding (unlabeled use) (Unlabeled use): used for premenstrual syndrome, premature labor, and to improve fertility, in combination with clomiphene (Clomid)
Medroxyprogesterone (Provera)	Oral: 2.5–10 mg daily, often given on cyclic basis	Amenorrhea; given after menopause with premarin as a prophylaxis for cervical cancer
Norethindrone (Norlutin)	Oral: 2.5–25 mg daily	Amenorrhea, endometriosis
Androgens		
Testosterone	IM only: 25–100 mg	Eunuchoidism§, impotence due to androgen deficiency, breast cancer, (give deep IM in gluteal muscle)
Testosterone enanthate (Delatestryl)	IM only: 50–400 mg q2–4 wk	As above, and oligospermia
Methyltestosterone (Oreton Methyl, Metandren)	Oral, buccal: 10–40 mg/d	As above and postpartum breast engorgement (Buccal administ. provides 2× androgenic activity as oral tablets.)
Anabolic Steroids**		
Nandrolone decanoate (Deca-Durabolin)	IM only: 50–200 mg/wk	Management of anemia associated with renal insufficiency
Oxandrolone (Oxandrin)	Oral: 2–5 mg b.i.d.-q.i.d.	To promote weight gain; for osteoporosis
Thydroid Hormones		
Natural		
Desiccated thyroid	Oral: 32–195 mg daily	Impure mixture of thyroid hormones; dose is started low and increased to most effective level.
Thyroglobulin (Proloid)	Oral: 32–200 mg daily	Hypothyroidism replacement therapy; contains T_3 and T_4
Synthetic		
Levothyroxine (Synthroid, Levothroid)	Oral: 88–100 mcg (μg) daily‡	Pure form of T_4 hormone; IV form available
Liothyronine (Cytomel)	Oral: 25–100 mcg (μg) daily‡	Pure form of T_3; short duration of action permits rapid dose adjustment.
Liotrix (Euthroid, Thyrolar)	Oral: dosed in equivalents to thyroid	A fixed ratio (4:1) of T_4 and T_3
Antithyroid Agents		
Methimazole (Tapazole)	Oral: 5 mg 1–3 times daily	Initial dose is higher; used for hyperthyroidism; inhibits synthesis of thyroid hormones.
Propylthiouracil, PTU, (Propyl-Thyracil, available in Canada)	Oral: 100–150 mg daily	Initial dose is higher; doses should be divided equally every 8 h

(continued)

Table 56-4 *(continued)*

Name of Drug*	Route of Administration	Clinical Use and Notes
Adrenal Gland Drugs†		
Betamethasone (Celestone, Valisone)	Oral: 0.6–7.2 mg daily	Anti-inflammatory agent
	Injection: 1–9 mg daily	
	Topical: 0.025–0.1%	
Cortisone (Cortone)	Oral: 25–300 mg daily	Naturally occurring anti-inflammtory agent
	Injection: 20–240 mg daily	
Dexamethasone (Decadron, Hexadrol)	Oral: 0.75–9 mg/d	Anti-inflammatory agent; Cushing syndrome depression test
	Injection: 20–100 mg/wk	
	Topical, aerosol: 0.1–0.4%	
	Ophthalmic: 0.05%	
Methylprednisolone (SoluMedrol, Medrol)	Oral: 4–48 mg/d	Anti-inflammatory agent; high-dose therapy used IV in treatment of shock or anaphylaxis, oral form available in 6-day Dospak
	IV: 10–40 mg initially, may repeat q4–6h	
Hydrocortisone (Solu-Cortef)	Oral: 20–240 mg/d	Naturally occurring antiinflammatory agent
	IM: 15–240 mg/d	
	Topical: 0.5–2.5%	
Prednisolone (Delta-Cortef)	Oral: 5–60 mg/d	Anti-inflammatory agent, not given IV
	IM: 4–60 mg/d	
	Ophthalmic: 1%	
Prednisone	Oral: 5–60 mg/d	Anti-inflammatory agent; most widely used oral agent
Triamcinolone (Artistocort, Kenalog)	Oral: 4–60 mg/d	Anti-inflammatory agent
	Injection: 5–40 mg/d	
	Topical: 0.1%	
Drugs Affecting Glucose Metabolism		
Insulins††		
Regular	SubQ, IV, IM: (100 U/mL; also in *concentrated* form, 500 U/mL)	Onset: $\frac{1}{2}$–1 h
		Peak: 2–5 h
		Duration: 6–8 h
		Rapid acting (only insulin that can safely be given IV)
Semilente (prompt-acting insulin zinc suspension)	SubQ, IM: (100 U/mL)	Onset: $\frac{1}{2}$–1$\frac{1}{2}$ h
		Peak: 5–10 h
		Duration: 12–16 h
		Rapid acting
NPH (Isophane insulin suspension)	SubQ, IM: (100 U/mL)	Onset: 1–1$\frac{1}{2}$ h
		Peak: 8–12 h
		Duration: 24 h
		Most widely used insulin
Lente (70/30) (Insulin zinc: contains 70% extended + 30% prompt insulin in suspension)	SubQ, IM: (100 U/mL)	Onset: 1–2$\frac{1}{2}$ h
		Peak: 7–15 h
		Duration: 24 h
		Intermediate duration
Protamine zinc, PZI (Contains protamine zinc + iletin)	SubQ, IM: (100 U/mL)	Onset: 4–8 h
		Peak: 14–20 h
		Duration: up to 36 h
		Long duration

(continued)

Table 56-4 (continued)

Name of Drug*	Route of Administration	Clinical Use and Notes
Ultralente (Extended insulin zinc suspension)	SubQ, IM: (100 U/mL)	Onset: 4–8 h Peak: 10–30 h Duration: over 36 h Longest duration
Oral Antidiabetic Agents		
Acetohexamide (Dymelor)	Oral: 250–500 mg daily	Oral drugs are not a substitute for insulin Doses in excess of 1500 mg/d are not recommended
Chlorpropamide (Diabinese)	Oral: 100–250 mg/d	Longest duration of oral agents
Glipizide (Glucatrol)	Oral: 5–30 mg/d	May be given in divided dose; give 30 min before meals
Glyburide (Micronase, DiaBeta)	Oral: 1.25–20 mg daily	Second-generation oral antidiabetic agent
Tolazamide (Tolinase)	Oral: up to 500 mg/d as required	Doses greater than 1 g/d are not recommended

* A trade name appears in parentheses following the generic name of the drug.
″ Medications used for fertility control are described in Chapter 63.
† Doses of these drugs can vary widely, (Dosages of insulin are given in units.)
‡ This dosage is given in micrograms (μg or mcg); a microgram is one thousandth of a milligram.
** Anabolic steroids can be very dangerous when used for body building; physician's supervision is required. They are illegal for athletes.
†† Dosages of insulin are based on blood sugar levels and are individual to each patient. Only the suspension of 100 U/mL is available in the United States, except for emergency use. *Human Insulin Note:* Human insulin is derived from recombinant DNA synthesis and has fewer adverse immunogenic responses associated with its use. It is available as Lente, Regular, NPH, and ultralente.
§ Eunuchoidism is failure of a male to develop male sex characteristics.

Table 56-5. Cardiovascular System Drugs

Name of Drug*	Usual Adult Dose	Notes
Cardiotonics		
Digitoxin (Crystodigin)	Oral: maintenance dose of 0.05–0.2 mg daily	Excreted very slowly from the body
Digoxin (Lanoxin)	Oral or IV: maintenance dose of 0.125–0.25 mg daily	Low potassium levels increase toxicity of digitalis drugs
Antiarrhythmics		
Bretylium (Bretylol)	IV: 5–10 mg/kg, q15–q30 min; may use up to 30 mg/kg (may be repeated)	Give slowly in nonemergency situations.
Disopyramide (Norpace)	Oral: 200–300 mg initially; then 100–150 mg q6h	Depresses contractility of heart
Lidocaine (Xylocaine)	IV: 50–100 mg initially, then drip at 1–5 mg/min (may be repeated in emergency)	Acts primarily on ventricles; increased toxicity with reduced hepatic function
Procainamide (Pronestyl, Procan)	Oral: 250–500 mg q4h (IV for emergency)	Half-life is 4 h; adverse effects include arthritis-like symptoms
Propranolol (Inderal)	Oral: 10–80 mg b.i.d. to q.i.d. Long acting: 80–160 mg/d IV: 1 mg/min up to 10 mg	Decreases conduction, contractility, and automaticity of heart
Quinidine sulfate	Oral and IM: 200–400 mg q.i.d.	Similar in action to procainamide; GI distress is common
Verapamil HCl (Calan, Isoptin)	Oral: 240–320 mg/d in divided doses IV: 0.075–0.15 mg/kg	Calcium channel blocker; depresses phase 4 of depolarizaton of heart
Vasoconstrictors and Sympathomimetics†		
Dobutamine (Dobutrex)	2.5–10 mcg (μg)/kg/min‡	Less increase in heart rate and cardiac arrhythmias than with other drugs
Dopamine (Intropin)	IV: 2–5 mcg (μg)/kg/min (higher doses in emergency)‡	Increases cardiac output and renal blood flow
Epinephrine (Adrenalin, HCl)	IM or SubQ: 0.5 mL of 1:1000 solution IV: used in cardiac arrest	Used in anaphylaxis (severe allergic reaction) and as hemostat (to stop bleeding)
Isoproterenol (Isuprel)	IV: 1–10 mcg (μg)/min‡	Stimulates cardiac contractility; increases heart rate and cardiac output
Levarterenol, norephinephrine (Levophed)	IV: 2–4 mcg (μg)/min‡	Restores blood pressure in acute hypotensive states
Metaraminol (Aramine)	IV: 2–5 mg direct IV to maintain BP at desired level	Increases BP but heart rate is usually decreased; may be used as infusion titrate
Vasodilators and Antiangina Agents		
Amyl nitrite	Inhalation: up to 0.3 mL	Relieves acute angina; excessive side effects limit use; may be abused
Cyclandelate (Cyclospasmol)	Oral: 200–400 mg b.i.d. to q.i.d.	Acts directly on smooth muscle to relax blood vessels
Isosorbide dinitrate (Isordil, Sorbitrate)	Oral: 5–30 mg q.i.d. Sublingual: 2.5–10 mg q.i.d.	Prophylactic use in angina pectoris
Minoxidil** (Lonifen)	Oral: 5–40 mg daily in single dose	Direct-acting vasodilator (major side effect is unusual hair growth)
Nitroglycerine (Nitrostat)	Sublingual (most common route): 0.15–0.6 mg PRN for chest pain	Drug of choice in angina; rapid action, short duration
Nitroglycerin ointment (Nitro-Bid, Nitrol)	Topical: 1-inch spread, usually over chest area; q6h	Prophylactic use; excess dose may cause headache
Nitroglycerin transdermal (Nitro-Dur, Transderm Nitro)	Topical: 0.1–0.6 mg/h	Apply transdermal patch once daily; alternate application sites
Nylidrin (Arlidin)	Oral: 3–12 mg 3–4 times daily	Side effects include dizziness, tachycardia, hypotension

(continued)

Table 56-5 (continued)

Name of Drug*	Usual Adult Dose	Notes
Papaverine (Pavabid)	Oral: 100–300 mg 3–5 times/d IV, IM: 30–120 mg q3h	Relaxes all smooth muscle (contraindicated in AV heart block)
Verapamil (Calan)	Oral: 80–120 mg t.i.d.	Used for vasopastic and unstable angina at rest
Antihypertensives		
Atenolol (Tenormin)	Oral: 25–100 mg once daily	May be used alone or with diuretics; acts mostly on the heart
Captopril (Capoten)	Oral: 12.5–50 mg 2–3 times/d (take 1 h before meals)	ACE inhibitor; combined with thiazide diuretics to lower blood pressure. Also used for heart failure.
Clonidine (Catapres)	Oral: 0.1–0.4 mg b.i.d. Transdermal patch: sustained release over 7 d	Sedative effects minimized by bedtime administration
Enalapril (Vasotec)	Oral: 2.5–40 mg, single or in 2 divided doses IV: 0.625–1.25 mg q6h	ACE inhibitor; used for heart failure and hypertension
Labetalol (Normodyne)	Oral: 50–300 mg b.i.d. IV: 200–400 mg b.i.d.	Action is both to lower peripheral resistance and directly on the heart as β (beta) blocker.
Methyldopa (Aldomet)	Oral and IV: initial 250 mg b.i.d.; may increase to 500 mg q.i.d.	Drowsiness may occur during first days of therapy; with prolonged use, patietns can develop positive Coombs' test (indicative of blood disorder)
Metoprolol (Lopressor)	Oral: 50–100 mg daily or b.i.d.	Acts mostly on the heart; β blocker without the side effects of bronchospasm
Nadolol (Corgard)	Oral: 40–80 mg once daily	β blocker; contraindicated in patients with asthma or bronchospasm
Nitropruside sodium (Nitropress)	IV only: 30 mcg (μg)/kg/min‡	Used in hypertensive crisis— for immediate lowering of BP; and in cyanide toxicity with overdose
Prazosin (Minipress)	Oral: initial 1 mg 2–3 times daily; may increase to 2–5 mg t.i.d.	Acts by reducing peripheral vascular resistance (possible postural hypotension and syncope with first dose; give first dose at bedtime)
Propranolol (Inderal)	Oral: 40–240 mg b.i.d.	Also used to treat arrhythmia, angina, migraine and stage fright; not indicated for asthmatics because it can cause bronchospasm (β blocker)
Reserpine (Serpasil)	Oral: 0.1–0.25 mg daily	Originally an antipsychotic drug; causes much sedation; causes less decrease in heart rate than other drugs
Verapamil (Calan)	Oral: 80 mg t.i.d.	Calcium channel blocker (effects observed in first week)

* A trade name appears in parentheses following the generic name of the drug.

† These drugs "mimic" the action of the sympathetic nervous system; they are used to raise blood pressure.

‡ This dosage is given in micrograms (μg); a microgram is one thousandth of a milligram.

** Minoxidil is also available in 2% topical solution to treat baldness, called Rogaine.

Table 56-6. Respiratory System Drugs

Name of Drug*	Usual Adult Dose	Notes
Antitussives (control cough)		
Benzonatate (Tessalon)	Oral: 100 mg t.i.d.	Anesthetizes receptors in respiratory tract to reduce cough reflex
Codeine	Oral: 10–20 mg q4–6h	A narcotic, generally combined with other products in cough syrup
Dextromethorphan, DM (Delsym, DM Cough, Robidex, Sucrets, Contac)	Oral: 10–30 mg q4–8h	Available in many OTC syrups; said to be as effective as codeine for cough
Diphenhydramine (Benylin, Benadryl)	Oral: 25–50 mg q4h	An antihistamine with antitussive properties, causes drowsiness
Hydrocodone (Hycodan, Hycomine)	Oral: 5–10 mg q6–8h	Schedule III narcotic; depresses cough reflex center in medulla
Expectorants		
Potassium iodide, saturated solution (SSKI)	Oral: 300–600 mg 3–4 times daily	Decreases viscosity of mucous by increasing respiratory secretions
Guaifenesin (Robitussin)	Oral: 100–400 mg q4–6h	Widely used but some doubt as to clinical efficacy; thins mucous
Iodinated glycerol (Organidin)	Oral: 60 mg q.i.d.	Similar to potassium iodide
Bronchodilators		
Albuterol (Proventil, Ventolin)	By inhalation: 2 puffs q4–6h	Most selective bronchodilator available
Aminophylline (Aminophyllin)	Oral: 200–250 mg q6–8h IV: maintenance dose of 0.9 mg/kg/h	Dose affected by age, heptic and cardiac status, and smoking history
Epinephrine HCl (Adrenalin)	SubQ: 0.2–0.5 mg q2h for acute asthma attack	Short duration; side effects include CNS stimulation and heart palpitations.
Epinephrine bitartrate (Primatene, Medihaler-Epi)	By inhalation: 1 puff PRN to releive acute bronchospasm	For temporary use only
Isoetharine (Bronkosol)	By inhalation: 0.25–1 mL of 1% solution diluted with saline	Rapid onset of action but relatively short duration
Isoproterenol (Isuprel, Medihaler-Iso)	By inhalation: 1 or 2 puffs repeated q4h as needed	Excessive use may lead to loss of effectiveness (rebound congestion)
Metaproterenol (Metaprel, Alupent)	By inhlation: 2–3 puffs as needed; not to exceed 12/d Oral: 10–20 mg 3–4 times daily	Rapid-acting agent when taken by inhalation route
Terbutaline (Brethine, Bricanyl)	Inhalation: 2 puffs q4–6h Oral: 2.5–5 mg q6h SubQ: 0.25 mg once; repeat in 15–30 min	Not recommended in children under 12; oral form sometimes used to stop contractions in premature labor
Theophylline (Theo-Dur, Slo-Phyllin, Bronkodyl, Theon, Theobid)	Oral: initially 3–5 mg/kg q6h, then 100–200 mg q6h	GI upset, headache, dizziness, nervousness are most common side effects of oral administration; effectiveness decreased by cigarette smoking

(continued)

Table 56-6 (continued)

Name of Drug*	Usual Adult Dose	Notes
Antihistamines		
Astemizole (Hismanal)	Oral: 10 mg daily	Once-a-day dose; not recommended for use in children
Chlorpheniramine (Chlortrimeton)	Oral: 4 mg q4–6h	Available OTC
Cyproheptadine (Periactin)	Oral: 4 mg q8h	Additional indications include urticaria and appetite stimulation.
Diphenhydramine (Benadryl)	Oral: 25–50 mg q6–8h	Sedative effects quite pronounced; also indicated for motion sickness and as sleep aid.
Promethazine (Phenergan)	IM: 25–50 mg; repeat in 2–4 h	Marked sedative action; also used for postoperative nausea and vomiting.
Terfenadine (Seldane)	Oral: 60 mg b.i.d.	Causes less drowsiness than chlorpheniramine. Contraindicated when taking erythromycin, and in patients with hepatic dysfunction
Triprolidine (Actidil)	Oral: 2.5 mg 3–4 times daily	Most commonly used combined with pseudoephedrine (Actifed) or ketoconazole (Nizoral)
Corticosteroids		
Beclomethasone diproprionate (Vanceril, Beclovent)	By oral inhalation: 2 puffs 3–4 times daily	Fewer side effects than systemic steroids
		Always use 5 min after bronchodilator (not for acute attacks—for preventive use only)
Flunisolide (Nasalide)	By nasal inhalation: 2 sprays in each nostril b.i.d.	For treatment of seasonal or perennial rhinitis
Triamcinolone acetonide (Azmacort)	By oral inhalation: 2 puffs 3–4 times daily	Same as beclomethasone
Decongestants		
Ephedrine	Oral: 25–50 mg q4–6h	CNS stimulation may be a side effect; rebound congestion often reported; primarily used as a bronchodilator.
Phenylephrine HCl (Neo-Synephrine HCl)	Topical: spray or drops in nostrils q3–4h	Oral form also available in many OTC cold preparations
Pseudoephedrine (Sudafed, Novafed, Afrinol)	Oral: 30–60 mg 3–4 times daily	Avoid in patients with hypertension.
Oxymetazoline (Afrin)	Topical: drops or spray in nostrils b.i.d.	Longer duration and less rebound congestion than other nasal solutions
Miscellaneous Products		
Cromolyn sodium (Intal)	Capsule for inhalation: 20 mg q.i.d. Solution for nebulization: 20 mg q.i.d. Aerosol spray oral: 2 sprays q.i.d. Aerosol spray nasal: 1 spray each nostril, 3–6 times/d	Drug is antiasthmatic, antiallergic, and mast cell stabilizer. Used for prophylactic management of bronchial asthma (not for acute attacks).

* The trade name appears in parntheses following the generic name of the drug.

Table 56-7. Gastrointestinal System Drugs

Name of Drug*	Usual Adut Dose	Notes
Antacids		
Aluminum hydroxide (Amphojel, Alternagel)	Oral: 600 mg 3–6 times daily, between meals and at bedtime	May have constipating effect; may impair absorption of certain drugs; OTC
Aluminum-magnesium hydroxide (Aludrox, Maalox, Gelusil, Mylanta)	Oral: 15–30 mL 3–6 times daily, between meals and at bedtime	Combination products tend to be less constipating, with equal acid-reducing ability; OTC
Calcium carbonate (Titralac, Tums)	Oral: 0.5–2 g as needed	High dose may cause hypercalcemia; may reduce absorption of tetracycline antibiotics, OTC.
Dihydroxy aluminum sodium carbonate (Rolaids)	Oral: 1 or 2 tablets as required	Routine high doses may induce constipation, OTC.
Antiemetics		
Benzquinamide (Emete-Con)	IM: 50 mg initially; repeat in 1 h and every 3–4 h PRN	For nausea and vomiting associated with anesthesia and surgery
Dimenhydrinate (Dramamine)	Oral: 50–100 mg q4–6h IM: 50 mg q4–6h PRN	An antihistamine; for nausea, vertigo, and motion sickness; OTC
Meclizine (Antivert, Bonine)	Oral: 25–10 mg daily in divided doses	Prevention and treatment of nausea and vomiting associated with motion sickness; treatment of Meniere's Disease
Metoclopramide (Reglan)	Oral: 10 mg q.i.d. IV: 1–2 mg/kg, repeated every 2–3 h × 4	GI stimulant with antiemetic properties; primarily used with cancer chemotherapy
Prochlorperazine (Compazine)	Oral: 5–10 mg 3–4 times daily IM: 5–10 mg, repeated in 4–6 h Rectal: 25 mg every 4–6 h	For postoperative nausea and vomiting; also used after chemotherapy or radiation cancer therapy
Scopolamine (Transderm-Scop)	1 patch every 72 h	Topical patch provides sustained release over 72 hours. Used for motion sickness and to relieve spasticity; used preoperatively to reduce secretions.
Thiethylperazine (Torecan)	IM, oral or rectal: 10–30 mg daily in divided doses	Actions and side-effects similar to Compazine; acts directly on vomiting center
Trimethobenzamide (Tigan)	Oral: 250 mg 3–4 times daily IM: 200 mg 3–4 times daily Rectal: 200 mg 3–4 times daily	As with most antiemetics, less effective by oral route than by injection
Antispasmodics		
Belladonna alkaloids	Oral: 1 tablet 3–4 times daily	Usually combined with phenobarbital (Donnatal)
Dicyclomine (Bentyl)	Oral: 10–20 mg 3–4 times daily IM: 20 mg q4–6h	Probably effective for hypermotility of bowel
Glycopyrrolate (Robinul)	Oral: 1 mg b.i.d. or t.i.d.	Used in peptic ulcer therapy; also used to reduce secretions during anesthsia
Propantheline (Pro-Banthine)	Oral: 15 mg q.i.d. (before meals and h.s.)	Used in peptic ulcer therapy, possesses antisecretory as well as antipasmodic capabilities
Laxatives (Cathartics)		
Bisacodyl (Dulcolax)	Oral: 10–15 mg Rectal: 10 mg	Must be swallowed whole, not chewed; not to be taken within 1 h of antacids
Castor oil (Neoloid)	Oral: 15–60 mL	Irritant laxative generally used as prep prior to bowel x-rays
Docusate (Colace, Surfak, Doxinate)	Oral: 50–250 mg	Fecal softener; take with full glass of water; higher doses required for initial therapy
Glycerin	Rectal: 1 suppository; retain for 15 min	Hyperosmolar agent (to cause a bowel movement)

(continued)

Table 56-7 (continued)

Name of Drug*	Usual Adult Dose	Notes
Magnesium hydroxide (Milk of Magnesia, M.O.M.)	Oral: 15–30 mL PRN	Saline laxative with onset of action in ½–3 h
Magnesium sulfate, Epsom salt	Oral: 15 g dissolved in water	Saline laxatives that attracts and retains fluid in colon and initiates perstalsis
Methylcellulose (Methocel, Cologel, Citrucel)	Oral: 0.5–2 g t.i.d.	Bulk-producing laxative to be taken with full glass of water
Mineral oil, MO	Oral: 15–30 mL	Lubricates intestinal mucosa, softens stool and thus promotes its passage
Phenolphthalein (Ex-Lax, Correctol)	Oral: 1–2 tablets at bedtime	Stimulant laxative with onset in 6–10 h
Polyethylene glycol electrolyte solution (Colyte, GoLYTELY)	4 L solution, 240 mL every 10 min	Used for bowel cleansing prior to GI examination
Psyllium (Metamucil, Hydrocil)	Oral: 1 teaspoon 1–3 times/d	Bulk laxative; considered to be the safest laxative; onset about 12–24 h
Sodium phosphates (Fleet Phospho-soda)	Oral liquid: 20–30 mL in glass of water Enema: 60–135 mL as enema	Used as bowel prep (much less volume to drink than GoLYTELY) and for fecal impaction. Not used in abdominal pain or appendicitis; contraindicated in cardiac disorders.

Antidiarrheals

Bismuth subsalicylate (Pepto-Bismol)	Oral: 30 mL every ½–1 h up to 8 doses/d	Used for "traveler's diarrhea"; may cause black, tarry stools
Diphenoxylate with atropine (Lomotil)	Oral: 2.5–5 mg q.i.d.; may reduce dosage when controlled	Related to meperidine and therefore subject to drug abuse; used for "traveler's diarrhea"
Kaolin-pectin mixture (Kaopectate)	Oral: 60–120 mL after each loose stool	For symptomatic treatment of diarrhea; absorbs excess fluid and reduces intestinal inflammation
Loperamide (Imodium)	Oral: initially 4 mg, then 2 mg after each loose stool up to 16 mg/d	Clinical improvement should be noted within 48 h
Paregoric	Oral: 5–10 mL up to q.i.d.	An opium derivative; sometimes combined with kaolin and pectin.

Miscellaneous Gastrointestinal Drugs

Bethanechol (Urecholine)	Oral: 10–50 mg b.i.d. to q.i.d.	Stimulates gastric motility; usually used to stimulate atonic bladder
Chenodiol (Chenix)	Oral: 500–750 mg b.i.d.	Used to dissolve gallstones; indicated only in patients considered poor surgical risks
Cimetidine (Tagamet)	Oral: 200–400 mg b.i.d. to q.i.d.; or 800 mg h.s. IM, IV: 300 mg q6–8h	Inhibits secretion of gastric acid; indicated in treatment of ulcers
Dexpanthenol (Ilopan)	IM, IV: 250–500 mg repeat at 2 h, then q6h	Indicated in prevention and treatment of adynamic postoperative ileus
Metoclopramide (Reglan)	Oral: 10 mg, 30 min before meals IV: 2 mg/kg, then reduce	Used to treat delayed gastric emptying; IV form used for nausea prevention with cancer chemotherapy
Omperazole (Prilosec)	Oral: 20–40 mg once daily	Given once daily for 4–6 wk; not recommended for more than 6 mo of therapy
Rantidine (Zantac)	Oral: 150 mg b.i.d., 300 mg h.s.	Similar in almost all respects to Cimetidine; longer acting, so is given only twice daily
Simethicone (Mylicon)	Oral: 40–80 mg q.i.d., after meals and at bedtime	A defoaming agent used to relieve excess gas in GI tract; may be combined with antacids; should be chewed
Sucralfate (Carafate)	Oral: 1 q.i.d., before meals and at bedtime	Used in treatment of ulcers; forms a protective barrier at ulcer site to protect against acid

* A trade name appears in parentheses following the generic name of the drug.

Table 56-8. Urinary System Drugs

Name of Drug*	Usual Adult Dose	Notes
Bumetanide (Bumex)	Oral: 0.5–2.0 mg daily IM, IV: 0.5–1 mg given over 2–3 h Do not exceed 10 mg/d	Action similar to furosemide, much smaller doses needed
Chlorothiazide (Diuril)	Oral: 500 mg 1–2 times daily	First thiazide diuretic; increases potassium excretion
Chlorthalidone (Hygroton)	Oral: 25–100 mg daily	Long duration of action (up to 72 h)
Ethacrynic acid (Edecrin)	Oral: 25–100 mg once daily IV: 50–100 mg	More potent than thiazide group; can cause ototoxicity†
Furosemide (Lasix)	Oral: 20–80 mg daily IV: 20–40 mg initially; increase in 20-mg increments	Concomitant administration (at the same time) with gentamicin may increase ototoxicity
Hydrochlorothiazide (Oretic, Hydrodiuril)	Oral: 25–100 mg daily	Usual initial drug for hypertension treatment
Mannitol	IV: 50–200 g/24 h	Osmotic diuretic; rapidly excreted
Mercaptomerin (Thiomerin)	IM, subQ: 25–250 mg daily	This drug has largely been replaced by other diuretics
Spironolactone (Aldactone)	Oral: 25–200 mg daily	Administered combined with hydrochlorothiazide (Aldactazide); potassium-sparing diuretic
Triamterene (Dyrenium)	Oral: 50–100 mg b.i.d.	Administered combined with hydrochlorothiazide (Dyazide)
Trichlormethazide (Naqua, Metahydrin)	Oral: 2–4 mg daily	Similar in action to hydrochlorothiazide and chlorthalidone

* A trade name appears in parentheses following the generic name of the drug.

† Ototoxicity: damaging to eighth cranial nerve, causing hearing and balance disorders.

57 Administration of Medications

![wave graphic]

Keys for Learning

Learning Objectives

◆ Differentiate between local and systemic effects of drugs.
◆ List six routes of administration; state the relative rates of absorption, effectiveness, and safety of each.
◆ Describe and demonstrate the steps to be taken before medications are given.
◆ Describe how to administer and record a STAT medication, a PRN medication, and an HS medication.
◆ Describe how to sign out and administer narcotics.
◆ State the five rights in giving drugs and the importance of each.
◆ State the steps to be followed when a medication error occurs; when a patient refuses a medication; when a medication is to be "wasted."
◆ Describe and demonstrate correct methods for the various types of injections.
◆ Demonstrate use of different types of syringes and related safety precautions.
◆ Describe the use of total parenteral nutrition and state nursing precautions.
◆ Describe the use of the infusion pump, piggyback administration, and heparin lock.

Key Terms

buccal	intradermal	parenteral
enteral	intramedullary	phlebitis
hub	intramuscular	subcutaneous
hyperalimentation	intravenous infusion	sublingual
induration	lumen	transdermal
infiltration		transfusion

Keys to Understanding This Chapter

Chapter 4: legal and ethical aspects of nursing
Unit Four: normal body structure and function
Chapter 30: medical asepsis and universal precautions
Unit Seven: nursing process

Keys to Understanding This Chapter
(continued)

Chapter 37: documentation and reporting
Chapter 42: vital signs
Chapter 49: heat and cold application, sometimes used rather than medications
Chapter 52: patient comfort and pain management
Chapter 54: surgical asepsis, used for parenteral administration
Chapter 55: mathematics and pharmacology
Chapter 56: classification of medications

Key Points

◆ Administration of medications is perhaps the single most dangerous function of the nurse. The rules of safe administration are essential and must be followed precisely.
◆ Be familiar with the medications you administer. Use drug references for any questions regarding the medication.
◆ Follow the five "rights" of medication administration faithfully.
◆ Follow through with complete and timely documentation of medication administration.
◆ Always follow universal precautions as they apply to the administration of medications.
◆ Monitor intravenous infusions and sites carefully.

Key Topics Outline

Preparing to Administer Medications
Times of Administration
Safety in Administering Medications
Routes of Administration
Enteral Administration
 Administering Oral Medications
 Feeding Tube Administration

Rosdahl CB: Textbook of Basic Nursing, 6th ed. © 1995 J.B. Lippincott Company

Key Learning Activities

◆ Read two or three different nursing journal articles or helpful hint columns on administration of medications. Try to find material on more than one route of administration. Begin a notebook of helpful information.

Key Learning Activities (continued)

◆ In clinical, while reading your patient's chart, observe the doctor's medication orders and compare them with the medication administration record. Note that many medications can look like something similar and that doses can be used in different units of measure than what may be available. This information can be added to your notebook of helpful hints.
◆ Practice using the reference books available in your school or clinical facility. Quiz each other about medications.

Key Nursing Procedures

Probably the single most dangerous function of the nurse is the administration of medications. All the rules of safe administration must be followed. It is also important to know the desired and undesirable side effects of drugs so you can carefully observe and document patient reactions.

Preparing to Administer Medications

Some of the abbreviations and acronyms with which you need to be familiar are listed in the accompanying box.

Storage of Medications

In most healthcare facilities, a special unit in each patient area is provided for storing medications. It is equipped with cupboards, a sink, running water, and work space. This unit should not be accessible to the public or to patients.

Some hospitals and many nursing homes store medications in locked movable carts. Medications for each patient are stored in individual drawers of the cart; this helps prevent patients from receiving the wrong medications.

Medications should be arranged in an orderly fashion. Some require refrigeration or brown bottles to preserve their chemical properties. Every drug should be clearly labeled. *If a label is illegible, send the container back to the pharmacy.* *Never* label or relabel a drug yourself, and *never* change containers or bottles.

Key Abbreviations and Acronyms for Medication Administration

DRF	Drip rate factor
HS	Hour of sleep
IM	Intramuscular
IV	Intravenous
IVPB	IV piggyback
MAR	Medication administration record
NG	Nasogastric
PICC	Percutaneous intravenous central catheter
PRN	As needed
R	Rectal
S	Sublingual
STAT	Immediately
SubQ	Subcutaneous
TD	Transdermal
TPN	Total parenteral nutrition
V	Vaginal

All narcotics and other controlled substances are kept double-locked in the medication room or in a "med" cart. They must be signed out as they are given and accounted for at the end of each shift. If, as a graduate, you are asked to administer these medications, you will be taught to follow the specific procedures of the facility where you work. Nursing students are sometimes allowed to give narcotic drugs and other controlled substances, under the supervision of the clinical

Nursing Skill Guidelines
Setting Up Medications

◆ Always give your undivided attention to setting up and administering medications. *(Rationale: A medication error could cause serious injury or death.)*

◆ Check the medication order with the MAR, or the patient's Kardex. Make certain that the MAR and physician's orders are identical. If medication cards are used, they must match the order *exactly*.

◆ Always read the medication label three times: (1) when you take it from the shelf or drawer; (2) before you remove the medicine from the container; and (3) before you put back or discard the container. *Never* give a medication from an unlabeled container or if you cannot read the label. Make sure the label on the container checks *exactly* with the MAR or the medication card.

◆ Be completely familiar with abbreviations, as well as generic versus trade names. Use extreme caution with drugs that have similar names.

◆ Check the medicine to make sure it is not spoiled or outdated. *(Rationale: It may lose its effectiveness or it may become toxic.)*

◆ If unit dose medications are used, it is a good idea not to open the package until you are ready to give the medication. *(Rationale: This provides a double-check. If the patient refuses, the med won't be wasted. Patients can be sure they are getting the correct med.)*

◆ If unit dose is not used, measure the dose with appropriate equipment. Hold the measure at eye level with your thumbnail on the line of the desired amount when measuring liquids. Pour liquid medications from the unlabeled side of the bottle. *(Rationale: This avoids soiling the label. A soiled label may be unreadable.)* The meniscus (lower part of the curve at the surface of the contained liquid) should be at the indicated level.

◆ If unit dose medications are not available, shake the required number of tablets or capsules into the cap of the container. Small paper cups (souffle cups) are usually provided for passing meds. Never handle medications with your fingers. *(Rationale: If you shake out too many, you can put them back if you have not touched them. Once medications have been handled, they are contaminated. They cannot be used or returned to the container.)*

◆ Administer each medication as you prepare it. *(Rationale: To avoid medication errors.)*

◆ *Never* give a drug that someone else has prepared. *(Rationale: You take responsibility for all medications you give.)*

◆ Do not leave medications at the patient's bedside.

---

instructor. See Chapter 55 for further information on schedule drugs.

Checking the Medication Record

Various systems are used to keep medication records. A card system may be used in some facilities, most often long-term care facilities. In many institutions, the order is copied (transcribed) onto the patient's medication administration record (MAR) or medication Kardex. Some facilities are using computerized patient records, which include medication records.

Whatever system is used, the medication record most often includes the patient's name, the drug name, the dosage, the route of administration, and the times the medication is to be given. Sometimes, the *trade* name and the *generic* name are stated on the record. The nurse is responsible for checking that the transcription of the medication order is correct by comparing it with the physician's original order.

Setting Up Medications

Routines vary slightly from one healthcare facility to another, but safety rules are the same everywhere. It must be remembered that rules have been established to protect the patient and to protect hospital personnel

from mistakes that could have serious results. The accompanying box lists guidelines for setting up medications.

Nursing Alert

Patients may be allergic to medications, as well as to foods. Some patients are allergic to latex, including gloves, catheters, tourniquets, balloons, and rubber bands. Always double-check for *any* allergies before giving medications or performing any procedures.

Unit Dose Systems

Many pharmaceutical companies supply tablet, capsule, liquid, and injectable forms of various drugs in individual prepackaged containers. These packages are usually marked with both the generic and trade name of the drug, as well as the dose contained in the package. Because each dose is packaged separately, it is often referred to as a *unit dose system*. The unit dose method provides greater safety when administering drugs than does a *stock* drug supply (large quantities of medications kept on the nursing unit) because the name and dose of the drug are on each dose, unit, or package of the drug. In the hospital pharmacy, before the drug is sent up to the nursing station, the unit dose package is labeled with the patient's name. The unopened package may be taken directly to the patient with one dose at a time. (Some facilities put only one day's medication supply in the med cart drawer at a time.)

The nurse takes the MAR or medication card along when administering medications. Do *not* remove the medication from the package until you are at the patient's bedside. This provides an additional safety check for the nurse and the patient. If the patient is paranoid, they can watch you open the package or they can open it themselves, under your supervision. It also prevents waste if, for some reason, the medication is not given.

Other Medication Systems

Some hospitals use a computer system to handle drug dispensing. The nurse keypunches the coded orders, which are electronically relayed to the pharmacy. The pharmacy may also be automated for handling routine drugs. Unit dose medicines may be dispensed to the nursing station by means of a conveyor, pneumatic tube system, or courier.

Times of Administration

STAT. If a medication is ordered *stat*, it is to be given *immediately*. Check the order, write the medication order on the medication Kardex, and set up and administer the medication as soon as possible. Be sure to chart stat medications *as soon as they are given* (not before), so there will be no duplication. (In some facilities, "given," your initials, and the time are written next to the order, so the physician knows the STAT order was followed.) When using the medication card system, the card should be torn almost in half as soon as the medication has been given and charted. Keep this card for later reference when reporting off at change of shift. Mark the med order off on the Kardex (as given). Tell the team leader that you are giving a stat medication.

PRN. If the patient asks for a PRN (as needed or on request) medication, be sure to give it as soon as possible. You must check the chart to be sure that the correct time period has elapsed since the last dose of the PRN medication. It is also important to check the dose last given because some orders are written with a dose range, rather than with a specific dose. If there is any chance of duplication, check before giving the medication. Be sure to chart and report *immediately after* giving a PRN medication.

It is important to assess the patient's need for PRN medication. It is unwise to give PRN drugs, particularly narcotics, unless they are needed. However, drugs should not be denied to the patient who really needs

them. Keep in mind that patients may experience pain and other symptoms in a variety of ways. If in doubt, check with your team leader.

Hour of Sleep (HS). Bedtime medications, such as sleeping pills and laxatives, are often ordered PRN. If so, ask the patient whether he or she needs a sleep medication or a laxative, and set up the medication if the person requests it. Chart it immediately *after* administering it.

Safety in Administering Medications

The accompanying box provides guidelines for safety in medication administration. The "five rights" and proper disposal and charting of errors and refusals are also safety factors.

The Five "Rights"

The Right Patient. Be sure that you give each medication to the right patient. Check the name on the MAR and unit dose package (if one is being used) with the patient's identification band. (Never give a medication to a patient who does not have an identification band; the bed tag is *not* sufficient identification.) Ask the patient's name, if the patient is conscious and oriented. The patient must *state* his or her name, and not just answer "yes" or "no" to a question such as "Are you Mr. Winter?"

Stay with the patient until oral medication is swallowed. If left alone with a medication, the patient may dispose of it or hoard it. For an elderly or confused patient, it may be necessary to check the mouth to make sure the medication was swallowed. In some cases, liquid medications are ordered, to make sure it is taken.

The Right Medication and the Right Dose. Double-check the medication card (if used), and the unit dose package (MAR if used) to make sure you are giving the correct medication and the dose that was ordered. (*Never* give a medication that someone else has prepared. If a mistake occurs, you will be held responsible.) Check each label three times.

Pay attention when a patient questions the correctness of a medication. If a patient has been getting a red tablet or capsule and is offered a white one instead, it will not be surprising if he or she suspects a mistake. Recheck the order, the label, and the MAR. If a patient reports an allergy to a medication, check again before giving the medication.

The Right Time. Check the time for giving a drug with the MAR. Follow the routine of the hospital as to intervals or routine times when medications are given. You must know which types of medications are usually

Nursing Skill Guidelines
Safety in Administering Medications

◆ Do not place different types of drugs together in a cup unless each is in a unit/dose package. *(Rationale: The patient might not take one medication, and you would not be able to identify for certain which drug was left in the cup.)*

◆ *Never* leave a medicine tray, package, or cup within reach of patients or visitors. If you must leave the room, take the medication with you. Lock it up if necessary. Lock the medication cart each time you leave it. *(Rationale: The medications may be taken by the wrong person or not taken.)*

◆ Healthcare facilities have established times for medication administration. If medications are not given within the time limits set by the facility, this constitutes a *medication error.*

◆ Always chart medications as soon as you have given them. *Never* chart a medication before you give it. Record the time, name of the drug, and dose. Add your initials so the physician will know who gave the drug. *(Rationale: The medication record is a legal document; it is used regularly in planning patient care. It must be accurate.)* Sign your full name and status (LPN, RN, student) at the bottom of the medication Kardex or MAR, so it is known who gave medications during that shift.

◆ Record and *report immediately* any unusual patient reaction, an unfavorable change in the patient's condition, refusal to take medicine, or inability to take all of it.

◆ If you find that you have forgotten to give a medication, you must report this promptly. This is a *medication error.*

◆ Discard an unused or open dose of a medication; never return it to a stock container. Medications should be disposed of according to the policy of the individual healthcare facility. You must have a witness cosign with you if you discard a narcotic.

◆ If a patient refuses a medication, chart the medication as you normally would, then circle the time and write "Ref" next to it. The same procedure is followed for any other reason a scheduled medication is not given on time—circle the time and indicate a reason ("emesis," "on pass," "PT," etc.).

◆ Check *very carefully* for drug allergies. Check the MAR, the chart for allergies, and the physician's orders. Ask the patient if he or she is allergic before giving any drug. Note any allergies on the front of the chart and apply a special red "allergy" identification band to the patient.

The Five "Rights" of Giving Drugs

◆ Select the *right patient.*
◆ Select the *right medication.*
◆ Give the *right dose.*
◆ Give the medication at the *right time.*
◆ Give the medication by the *right route.*

given four times a day during waking hours or every 6 hours around the clock. You must also know whether a medication is to be given before or between meals or with food or milk.

You must give a drug within 30 minutes either way of the time for which it is ordered. Any deviation from these limits constitutes a *medication error.* Be sure you know the abbreviations for times, such as "t.i.d." (three times a day) and "b.i.d." (twice a day). Ask if you are not sure.

The Right Route. Check the physician's orders and the MAR to verify the route by which the medication should be given. *Remember:* Some drugs can cause death if given by the wrong route. You should know the correct route for certain medications.

Medication Errors and Refusals

Occasionally, a medication error may occur. This must be reported *at once* to prevent danger to the patient. In some cases, immediate emergency action must be taken to prevent undesirable complications or death. Medication errors include giving the wrong medication, giving a medication at the wrong time or in the wrong dose, giving a medication by the wrong route, or administering a medication to the wrong patient. This is why the five "rights" are so important. If you have any doubt about a medication, ask before giving it, to prevent an error. On the other hand, if you think you might have made an error, do not hesitate to report it at once. Do not think of yourself at this time, but think instead about the patient and the dangers to health and life. Report the medication error according to your facility protocol.

Use correct procedure in disposing of a medication that the patient refuses to take. Method of disposal varies according to facility policy. Be sure to note on the chart or medication record that the medication was refused and why.

If a drug is set up, opened, and not given, it should be disposed of, according to the facility protocol. In the case of a schedule narcotic, another nurse must witness the disposal and cosign the drug sheet. (If a drug package is unopened, it may be returned to the medication drawer or cupboard.)

Nursing Alert

Documentation: If medication is *not* given, in most facilities the nurse must indicate this by circling time and adding initials; for example, (0800) CR. The reason for holding it is then charted in the nurses notes. If the reason can be indicated on the medication administration record or Medex (for example, (0800) Ref CR or (0800) NPO CR), it need not be documented in the nurses notes.[1]

---

[1] "Drug Administration" packet, Anoka Technical College, Anoka, MN.

Charting of Medications

An important part of the administration of medications is charting or documentation. This record tells other members of the nursing and medical staff which medications the patient received and documents how the patient reacted to them. A comprehensive discussion of charting in general and of charting of medications is presented in Chapter 37. In many facilities, the drug order and documentation of administration of drugs are both on the MAR. Many hospitals record all meds and treatments using *military time* (the 24-hour clock).

Medication Teaching

An important component of medication administration is teaching the patient. The patient should know:

♦ What medications are being given
♦ Why he or she is taking the medication
♦ The dosage
♦ The expected effects
♦ Possible undesirable side effects
♦ How long the medication will be needed

The patient should be able to verbalize this information back to you. The patient should be able to demonstrate special procedures (such as administration of insulin). All teaching *must* be documented. (If it is not well documented, it is considered not to have been done.) This is an important component of the nursing care plan and is required by JCAHO. There may be printed information available about medications for patient use.

Routes of Administration

Table 57-1 shows routes of administration of drugs.

Local and Systemic Effects

Drugs can have many effects on the body. A *therapeutic effect* is the desired effect of a medication. It will produce the result for which the medication was given. An *adverse effect* or *side effect* is a response that is not intended or desired. Some adverse effects are minor and can be ignored; others are potentially harmful. Medication *toxicity* is an undesired effect a medication has on body tissues that is most often harmful and must be treated. It results from a buildup of the medication in the blood, internal ingestion of a medication intended for external use, or an overdose of the medication.

The method chosen to administer a drug depends on the nature of the drug and the desired effect. There may be a *local effect* at the site where the drug is applied. Local effects may be attained by applying drugs to the skin or mucous membranes (topical application).

Antiseptics such as alcohol on a laceration or scratch or soothing drugs such as a lotion applied directly to a rash are examples of drugs used for a local effect. Drug preparations are applied to the mucous membranes of the eye, mouth, nose, throat, and genitourinary tract by swabbing, spraying, instillation, or irrigation; they are inserted into the vagina and rectum in the form of suppositories. Drug-saturated packs can be inserted into body cavities.

In a *systemic effect*, the drug is absorbed into the circulation and carried to body cells. There are several methods for introducing drugs into the circulation and obtaining systemic effects; the choice depends on the nature and the amount of the drug to be given, the speed of its action, and the patient's condition. These methods of administration include oral ingestion, intramuscular injection, intravenous infusion, sublingual, rectal, and inhalation. Transdermal patches are drug patches which may be applied to the skin; they are absorbed systemically and yield a desired drug level over time. Speed of absorption depends on the route; intracardiac (directly into the heart) is the fastest, followed by intravenous (into a vein), inhalation, intramuscular, subcutaneous, oral, rectal, and transdermal.

Enteral Administration

Enteral administration is given through the digestive tract. This can include oral, sublingual, buccal, feeding tube, or rectal administration.

Administering Oral Medications

More medications are given by mouth than any other way. Liquid medications may be given full strength or diluted with water, milk, or fruit juice, depending on the drug. Some substances do not mix well. You must check to see what the appropriate solvent would be. Small amounts of liquids, measured in minims, must be diluted or most of the medication will be left in the medication cup.

The patient swallows the drug when it is administered orally, whether as liquid, capsule, tablet, or pill. The oral route is convenient and economical but has drawbacks. Some drugs have an unpleasant taste or odor; others injure the teeth or irritate the lining of the stomach. Patients who are nauseated or vomiting cannot take drugs by mouth. Digestive enzymes destroy the effectiveness of certain drugs. In some instances, patients may be uncooperative and refuse to swallow the medication. Furthermore, there is the danger of an unresponsive patient aspirating a medication into the lungs. Patients should be told if a solid medication is to be chewed or swallowed whole. Nursing skills used in

Table 57-1. Routes for Administering Drugs

Route	How Drug Administered	Term Used to Describe Route
Given by mouth (to be swallowed)	Patient swallows drug	Oral administration (PO)
Applied to mucous membranes	Inserting drug into	
	Vagina	Vaginal administration (V)
	Rectum	Rectal administration (R, PR)
	Placing drug under tongue	Sublingual administration (SL)
	Place drug between cheek and gum	Buccal administration
	Placing drug into direct contact with mucous membrane	Instillation (such as eye)
	Flushing mucous membrane with drug in solution	Irrigation (as in urinary bladder or eye)
	Instilled into eye	Eye drops, ointment
	Instilled into ear	Ear drops
Given via respiratory tract	Having patient inhale drug	Nasal inhalation
	Using nasal spray	Aerosolized administration
	Giving nose drops	Note gtts
Given by suppository	Inserting suppository into	
	Rectum	Rectal administration (R)
	Vagina	Vaginal administration (V)
Given through the skin	Placing drug patch or ointment on skin	Transdermal administration (TD)
	Rubbing drug into skin	Inunction (topical administration)
Given by feeding tube	Drug is instilled through feeding tube into stomach or intestine	Types of tubes:
		Nasogastric (NG)
		Gastrostomy (GT)
		Jejunostomy (JT)
Given by injection	Injecting drug into	Injection
	Subcutaneous tissue	Subcutaneous injection (SubQ)
	Muscle tissue	Intramuscular injection (IM)
	Corium (under epidermis)	Intradermal injection
	Vein	Intravenous injection (IV)
	Artery	Intra-arterial injection
	Heart tissue	Intracardiac injection
	Peritoneal cavity	Intraperitoneal injection
	Spinal canal	Intraspinal injection
	Bone	Intraosseous injection
	Subarachnoid space	Intrathecal injection
	Bone marrow cavity	Intramedullary injection
	Large vein (such as subclavian)	Total parenteral nutrition (TPN)

Adapted from Taylor C, Lillis C, LeMone P: Fundamentals of Nursing: The Art and Science of Nursing Care, Ed 2. Philadelphia, J.B. Lippincott, 1993.

oral administration of medications are given in Nursing Procedure 57-1.

Sublingual Administration. A **sublingual** (SL) drug is placed under the patient's tongue, where it dissolves and is absorbed. The patient must be able to understand instructions to keep the drug under the tongue and not chew or swallow it. The patient should not drink anything until the drug is absorbed.

Buccal Administration. Buccal refers to the cheek or mouth. Buccal administration involves placing the medi-

cation between the cheek and gum. These skills are summarized in the nursing skill box. Actions will depend on patients ability to self-administer the medication. If the patient requires assistance, the nurse must wear gloves.

Rectal Administration. The rectal method consists of the instillation of a liquid or insertion of a suppository drug preparation into the rectum. It is used if a patient is vomiting or has had oral surgery, if the taste of a drug is offensive, or if the action of the digestive enzymes would interfere with its effectiveness. It can also be

(Text continues on page 722)

Supplies and Equipment

Medication Kardex, cards, or computer record
Medication cart
Disposable medication cups
Water or juice
Straws (optional)
Mortar and pestle or pill crusher or tablet cutter (optional)

Procedure

1. Wash hands.
   (Rationale: Handwashing prevents the spread of organisms.)
2. Gather equipment. Use medication Kardex, cards, or computer record to verify medication order. Check any inconsistency with physician or pharmacist.
   (Rationale: Organization facilitates performance of the skill and reduces the chance of a medication error.)
3. Prepare one patient's medication at a time.
   (Rationale: This lessens the chance for a medication error.)
4. Unlock medication cart or drawer.
   (Rationale: Keeping medication setup locked provides security if the area is unattended.)
5. Proceed from top to bottom of medication Kardex or computer record when preparing medications.
   (Rationale: This ensures that a medication order will not be missed for a specific time.)
6. Select correct medication from drawer or shelf. Compare label to medication order on Kardex, card, or computer record. Complete any necessary calculations:
   a. Pour pill from a multidose bottle into the container lid and transfer the correct amount to a medication cup.

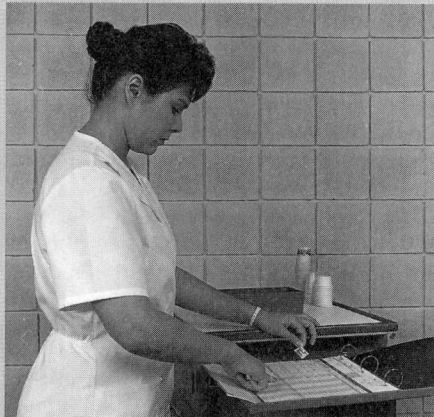

Step 6   Comparing a unit-dose medication to the order on the Kardex

b. Leave unit dose medications in wrapper and place in medication cup.

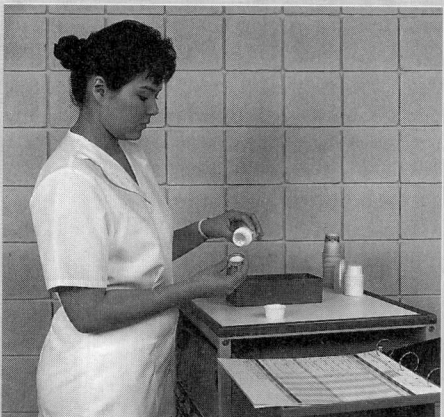

Step 6a   Pouring a pill from a multi-dose vial

c. Measure liquid medication by holding the medicine cup at eye level and reading the level at the bottom of the meniscus. Pour from the bottle with the label uppermost and wipe neck with a paper towel if necessary. Sometimes calibrated droppers are provided.

(Rationale: Comparing medication to written order is a medication check to prevent an error. Pouring medication into the lid eliminates handling the drug. Unit dose wrappers keep medication clean and safe. Holding a cup at eye level to pour a liquid gives the most accurate measurement. Pouring away from the label and wiping the lip of a bottle helps keeps the label legible.)

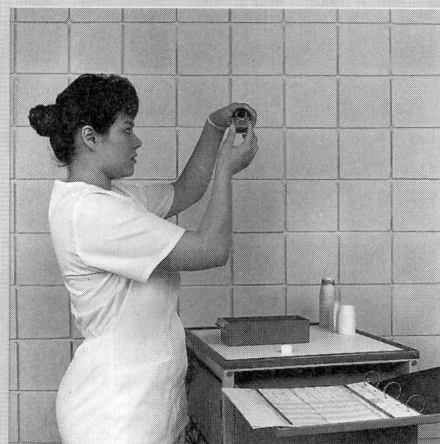

Step 6c   Measuring liquid medication

(continued)

7. Recheck each medication with written record. *(Rationale: This is the second medication check to ensure preparation of the correct dose.)*
8. When all medications have been prepared, compare each one again to the medication order. *(Rationale: All medications should be checked three times to prevent errors.)*
9. Crush pills if patient is unable to swallow them:
   a. Place pill in paper soufflé cup in mortar or pill crusher. Cover pill with another paper soufflé cup placed inside the first one. Crush pill until it is in powder form.

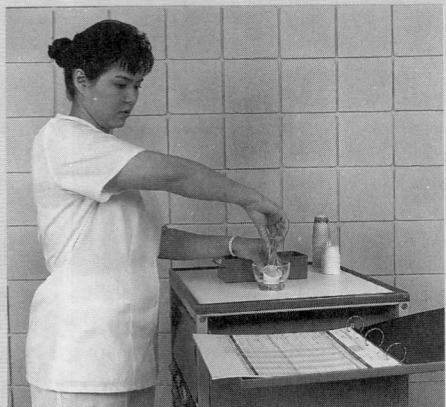

Step 9a Preparing to crush a pill

   b. Do not crush time-release capsules or enteric-coated tablets.
   c. Dissolve in water or juice or mix with apple sauce to mask the taste.
   (Rationale: Crushed medication is easier to swallow. Enteric-coated tablets that are crushed may irritate the mucosal lining of the stomach. Opening and crushing the contents of a time-release capsule may interfere with its absorption.)
   d. Cut tablets at score mark only. *(Rationale: This ensures accuracy.)*
10. Take medication to patient once it is prepared. Medication should be given as close to the ordered time as possible.
   (Rationale: Agency policy usually considers 30 minutes before or after the ordered time as an acceptable variation.)

11. Identify the patient before giving the medications:
   a. Check the name on the identification bracelet.

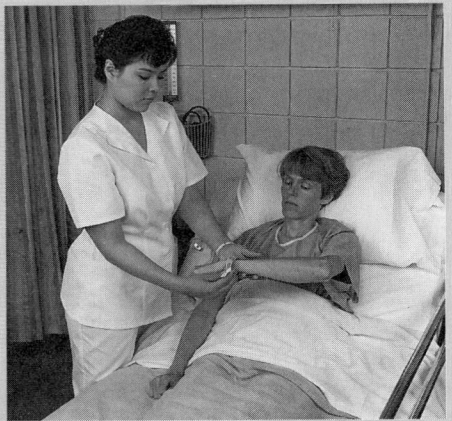

Step 11a Checking the patient's identification bracelet

   b. Ask the patient his or her name.
   c. Ask a staff member to identify the patient.
   (Rationale: Medication may be administered to the wrong patient if identity is not established. Checking the identification bracelet is the most reliable method.)
12. Complete necessary assessments before giving medications.
   (Rationale: Nurse's responsibility includes checking that the patient is not allergic to the drug. Additional checks include assessment of blood pressure, apical pulse rate, or respiratory rate depending on the action of the medication.)
13. Assist the patient to a comfortable position.
   (Rationale: Sitting as upright as possible makes it easier to swallow medication and less likely to cause aspiration of fluids.)
14. Administer the medication:
   a. Offer water or fluids to take with medication. Be aware of any fluid restrictions if they exist.
   b. Ask patient how he or she prefers to take the medication (ie, one at a time, all at once, from the cup or their hand).
   c. Open unit dose medication packages and give medication to patient.
   d. Review the name and purpose of the medication.
   e. Discard any medication that falls on the floor.
   f. Mix powder medications with fluids at the bedside.

(continued)

g. Record fluid intake on intake and output form. *(Rationale: Patient preference determines method of taking medication and involves patient in the administration process. Medication that falls on the floor is considered contaminated. Powdered forms of drugs may thicken when mixed with fluid and should be given immediately. Recording fluid intake with medication maintains accurate documentation.)*

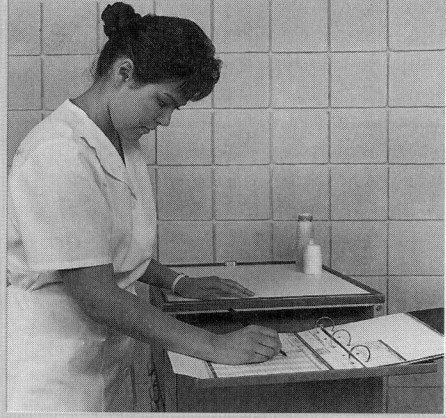

Step 17a   Documenting administration (Photos © B. Proud.)

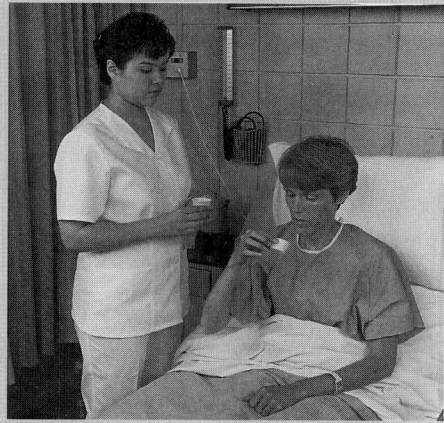

Step 14   Administering the medication

15. Remain with the patient until all medication has been taken. Check the patient's mouth, if needed. *(Rationale: The nurse's signature on the medical record indicates that the patient has taken the medication. It is unsafe to leave medication at the bedside.)*
16. Wash hands. *(Rationale: Handwashing prevents the spread of organisms.)*
17. Record medication administration on the appropriate form:
    a. Sign after drugs have been given.

b. If a medication was refused, record this according to agency policy on the medication record.
c. Document vital signs or particular nursing assessments according to agency format (ie, apical pulse, blood pressure reading).
d. Sign in narcotic book for controlled substances when they are removed from locked area. *(Rationale: Documentation provides coordination of care and verifies reason medications were omitted and specific nursing assessments needed to safely administer medication. Federal law regulates special documentation for narcotics or other dangerous drugs.)*
18. Check on the patient within 30 minutes after giving medication. This is particularly important following pain medication or any PRN (as needed) med. *(Rationale: This verifies response to the medication and, particularly, relief of pain after an analgesic.)*

Nursing Skill

Administering Sublingual or Buccal Medications

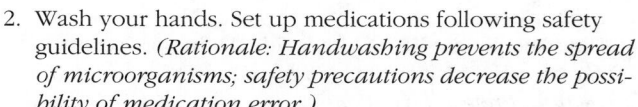

Supplies and Equipment

Medication Kardex, cards, or computer record
Medication
Disposable cups
Gloves, if needed

Procedure

1. Gather equipment and check the medication order against the original physicians order. *(Rationale: The right medication must be given to the right patient.)*

2. Wash your hands. Set up medications following safety guidelines. *(Rationale: Handwashing prevents the spread of microorganisms; safety precautions decrease the possibility of medication error.)*
3. Instruct the patient to place and keep the medication under the tongue, if sublingual, or between the cheek and gum, if buccal.
4. If assistance is required, don gloves. *(Rationale: This protects you and the patient.)*
5. Place medication in proper position.
6. Instruct the patient to keep the medication in place until it is dissolved. Tell the patient not to chew the medication. *(Rationale: Allowing the medication to dissolve allows the medication to be absorbed properly.)*
7. Tell the patient not to put anything in the mouth until the medication is completely absorbed. *(Rationale: This will ensure that the correct dose is absorbed.)*

8. Teach the patient the effects and side effects of the medication and to notify you if any symptoms are experienced. (*Rationale: Potential problems will be identified and addressed.*)
9. Record the medication given (note SL for sublingual) and any significant responses, per your facility's protocol.

---

used in an unresponsive patient or a small child. The major drawback is that the patient may not be able to retain the entire amount of the drug, and, if part of it is expelled, there is no way of knowing how much has been retained. Absorption is also very slow. Drug preparations administered rectally are usually given in small amounts.

If "half a suppository" is ordered, it must be cut in half lengthwise. Check with the pharmacy first to make sure this is safe. (*Rationale: Cutting this way*

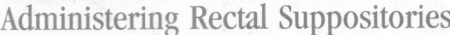

Nursing Skill
Administering Rectal Suppositories

Supplies and Equipment

Medication Kardex, cards, or computer record
Medication
Gloves

Procedure

1. Gather equipment and check the medication order against the original physician's order. (*Rationale: The right medication must be given to the right person.*)
2. Wash hands. Set up medication following safety guidelines. Suppositories usually are kept refrigerated until they are used. Wear gloves. (*Rationale: Handwashing prevents the spread of microorganisms; refrigeration prevents suppositories from melting.*)
3. Explain to the patient what you are going to do and why. (*Rationale: This will decrease the patient's level of anxiety and make the patient relax more so medication can be administered.*)
4. Have the patient lie on either side. Drape properly. (*Rationale: This position will provide easy access to the rectum. Protect the patient's privacy.*)
5. Insert the suppository at least 2 to 4 inches (2 inches for children, 4 inches for adults) and direct it against the rectal wall. (*Rationale: This places the suppository past the rectal sphincters and maximizes absorption.*)
6. Instruct the patient *not to expel* the suppository. The patient should maintain this position a minimum of 5 to 10 minutes; usually 30 to 45 minutes. (*Rationale: Having the patient retain the suppository will allow the medication to work effectively.*)
7. Dispose of your gloves and wash your hands.
8. Record the medication given (note R for rectal) and the patient's response.

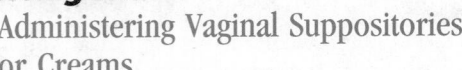

Nursing Skill
Administering Vaginal Suppositories or Creams

Supplies and Equipment

Medication Kardex, cards, or computer record
Medication
Gloves

Procedure

1. Gather equipment and check the medication order against the physician's original order. (*Rationale: Right medication must be given to the right patient.*)
2. Wash hands. Set up medication following safety guidelines. Suppositories are usually kept refrigerated until they are used. (*Rationale: Handwashing prevents the spread of microorganisms; refrigeration prevents suppositories from melting.*)
3. Explain to the patient what you are going to do and why. (*Rationale: This will decrease the patient's level of anxiety and provide patient teaching about the prescribed medication and its expected effects.*)
4. Wear gloves. (*Rationale: Gloves will protect against accidental exposure to blood or body fluids.*)
5. Position the patient comfortably on her back or side so you can see the vaginal orifice. Drape properly. Cleanse the perineum.
6. Insert the suppository at least 2 inches (4.5 cm) into the vagina. (*Rationale: You must clear the external vaginal muscles or the suppository will be expelled.*)
7. Instruct the patient to remain lying down for about 20 minutes. (*Rationale: Having the patient remain in that position will maximize medication absorption.*)
8. If administering a cream, lubricate the applicator, insert it gently to full length and then remove it, as the plunger is depressed. (*Rationale: Instilling the cream as the applicator is removed will ensure that the medication is properly distributed.*)
9. Offer the patient a sanitary pad. (*Rationale: A sanitary pad will collect excess drainage and protect the patient and the bed from drainage.*)
10. Dispose of gloves and wash your hands.
11. Record the medication given (note V for vaginal) and the patient's response.

---

maintains its "bullet" shape and the correct dosage of medicine.)

Vaginal Administration. Although the vagina is not part of the digestive tract, vaginal suppositories are given in a similar manner as rectal suppositories.

Feeding Tube Administration

Some medications must be administered through the patient's feeding tube (see Nursing Procedure 28-1). Medications will need to be in a liquid form or be dissolved in a liquid (after crushing a pill or opening a capsule). Coated or time-release medications cannot be crushed or exposed to stomach acids or they may become ineffective. Only medications specified as *enteral* may be given via feeding tubes.

Nursing Skill
Giving Medications via a Feeding Tube

Supplies and Equipment

Medication Kardex, cards, or computer record
Medication
Fluids, as needed
Mortar and pestle or pill crusher
Gloves
Large syringe
Stethoscope

Procedure

1. Check medication order. If more than one medication is to be given, make sure they are compatible.
2. Check with the pharmacist if you are not sure of restrictions related to the medications.
3. Wash your hands. Set up medication following safety guidelines. (*Rationale: Handwashing prevents the spread of microorganisms. Safety precautions will decrease the possibility of medication error.*)
4. Gather needed equipment. Wear gloves. (*Rationale: Gloves protect both you and the patient.*)
5. Explain to the patient what you are going to do and why, as appropriate for that patient. (*Rationale: Explanations decrease the patient's anxiety.*)
6. Position the patient with the head elevated about 30°, if possible. (*Rationale: An elevated head decreases the risk of aspiration.*)
7. Check placement of the tube and aspirate for residual stomach contents if ordered (see Nursing Procedure 28-1).

   ◆ If the patient has a button-type gastrostomy tube (GT), do not aspirate (this may damage the antireflux valve). Also do not aspirate if the patient has a jejunal tube (JT).

   ◆ If there is a high residual or gastric contents are unusual in any way, hold the medication and contact your team leader.

   ◆ If 50 mL or more of undigested formula is aspirated in adults or 10 mL or more in infants, check with the team leader before medication administration.

8. After aspirating, pinch or clamp tubing and remove the syringe.
9. Remove plunger from the syringe and reconnect the syringe to the tube.
10. Be sure that medication is dissolved or well mixed, especially if medication was crushed. (*Rationale: Some medications may adhere to the feeding tube, causing the tube to become clogged.*)
11. Release the clamp and pour the medication into the syringe.
12. If the medication does not flow down the tube, insert the plunger and give a slight pressure to start the flow. (*Rationale: Sometimes this action will start the flow.*)
13. Remove the plunger and watch to see if the medication flows.
14. If medications do not flow, repeat the step.
15. When all the medication has gone in the tube, flush the tube with ordered fluid or about 15 to 30 mL water. This amount may vary depending on the size of the patient and any fluid restrictions. Be sure to add this free water to the tube feeding intake sheet. (*Rationale: These fluids help dissolve food or medication in tube. Accuracy in recording intake is important.*)
16. Clamp the tube and remove the syringe.
17. Reconnect the feeding or replace the tubing plug.
18. Keep the head of the bed elevated for at least 30 minutes after medication administration. (*Rationale: This decreases the possibility of aspiration.*)
19. Be sure the patient is positioned comfortably.
20. Dispose of waste appropriately and wash your hands.
21. Document medication given and patient response. Report any unusual findings.

Parenteral Administration

Parenteral administration includes any method of administering a drug other than through the digestive tract. Drugs may be absorbed via the mucous membranes of the eyes or the respiratory tract; they may be absorbed through the skin.

The term *parenteral* is most commonly used to denote drugs that are injected by needle into body fluids or tissues. These medications must be soluble, absorbable, and sterile.

Eye (Ophthalmic) Administration

In many eye disorders, medications are instilled or administered directly into the eye. These include liquid medications, ointments, and medication-impregnated discs that resemble contact lenses.

Administering Eye Drops. Eye drops are instilled for various reasons: to contract or dilate the pupil, to treat an infection, to provide lubrication, or to produce a local effect such as anesthesia. It is often the nurse's responsibility not only to carry out the procedure, but also to instruct others in it. The bottle of eye drops is discarded when the eye drops are discontinued. The accompanying nursing skill describes how to administer eye drops.

Nursing Skill
Administering Eye Drops

Supplies and Equipment

Medication Kardex, cards, or computer record
Medication, with dropper
Gloves, if needed
Goggles, if needed
Clean cotton balls
Disposable tissues

Procedure

1. Check the medication order against the physician's original order. *(Rationale: The right medication must be given to the right patient.)*
2. Wash your hands carefully. If drops are to be placed in both eyes, wash your *hands before and after treating each eye. (Rationale: Handwashing deters the spread of microorganisms.)*
3. Wear gloves (and sometimes, goggles). *(Rationale: This will avoid exposure to body fluids.)*
4. Wipe the eyelids and lashes clean with a cotton ball, using a different cotton ball for each eye. Wipe from inner to outer corners (canthi). *(Rationale: This action prevents the spread of infection from one eye to the other.)*
5. Have the patient lie down or sit with head tilted backward. *(Rationale: This will help facilitate instillation and dispersion of medication.)*
6. Provide patient with a tissue. *(Rationale: There may be an overflow of medication or tears.)*
7. Check the label on the bottle; do not instill any medication in the eye unless it is labeled *ophthalmic. (Rationale: A medication error could endanger the patient's vision.)*
8. Gently retract the lower eyelid with the thumb and a finger or with two fingers. *(Rationale: This exposes the lower conjunctival sac.)*
9. Rest the hand in which you are holding the squeeze-bottle or tube against the patient's forehead if necessary. *(Rationale: This steadies the hand.)* (Fig. 57-1).
10. Ask the patient to look up, and instill the prescribed number of drops into the center of the everted (turned outward) lower lid (the conjunctival surface). *(Rationale: Instilling the drops into the conjunctival sac will avoid having drops fall directly into the cornea and possibly injuring it.)*
11. Press on the inner canthus of the eye when instilling eye drops. *(Rationale: This prevents the solution from draining into the tear duct and minimizes the risk of systemic effects.)* This is particularly important in glaucoma.
12. Instruct the patient to close the eyelids and apply gentle pressure for 1 minute. *(Rationale: This allows distribution of medication.)*
13. Wipe off any excess with a cotton ball.
14. Repeat for other eye, if ordered, using a fresh cotton ball and washing hands.
15. Dispose of gloves and wash your hands after procedure. Document the procedure.

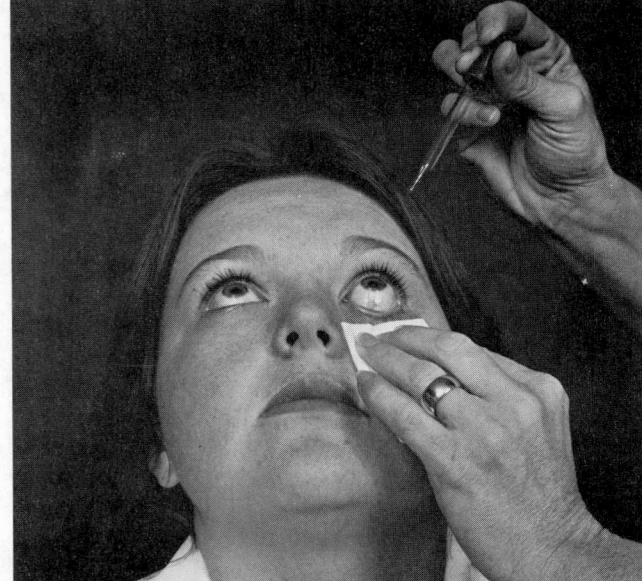

Figure 57-1. The nurse exposes the lower conjunction of the eye where he or she will place eyedrops by having the patient look up and by applying pressure downward with two fingers over the bony prominence of the cheek. The thumb may be used for applying pressure downward if it is more convenient for the nurse. In many cases, gloves are worn when giving eyedrops.

Administering Eye Ointments. Eye ointments are usually applied to both eyes, even though only one eye is affected. Great care is required not to spread infection from one eye to the other. For this reason a separate tube is reserved and labeled for each eye. Nursing skills include the following:

◆ Follow the first 9 steps above.
◆ Before administration, wipe the tube with another cotton ball and discard a small amount of ointment. *(Rationale: This maintains sterility of the ointment.)*
◆ Apply the ointment inside the lower lid, in a thin line, from inner to outer canthus. The eyeball itself is not touched with the tube. *(Rationale: This helps to avoid irritating the cornea.)*
◆ Ask the patient to blink a few times. *(Rationale: This will disperse the medication.)*
◆ If medication is to be instilled into the other eye, wash your hands in between.
◆ Gel-type medications are often given at bedtime. *(Rationale: They blur the vision.)*
◆ Use a cotton ball or tissue to wipe away any excess.
◆ Dispose of gloves and wash your hands.
◆ Document the procedure, noting the patient's reactions.

Key Concept

An infection in one eye can easily spread to the other eye.

The Ocusert System. This system has been developed for persons who need continuous eye medication. It is simple and easy to use. The drug (pilocarpine HCl) is placed in a tiny oval disc that resembles a small soft contact lens. Each Ocusert system contains enough medication to last 1 week. The drug is released continuously, so there is no danger of patients forgetting to use eye drops, and it is being delivered while patients are sleeping, as well as during the day. This type of drug delivery system is also called *releasing-system insert.* Once patients become accustomed to placing the system into the eye, they will probably find it simple and convenient to use.

Guidelines for using the Ocusert system include:

- Wash your hands and put on gloves.
- Read the manufacturer's instructions for specific guidelines.
- Place the Ocusert-Pilo system in the eye, positioning it under the lower or upper eyelid. It is not visible when in place. The medication will be released slowly and without interruption.
- Replace the system weekly.
- Instruct the patient that if the system falls out, it should be rinsed in cool tap water and repositioned.
- Do not use the system if it looks deformed or damaged.

Administering Ear Drops

Medications are given by instillation from a squeeze bottle or a dropper.

To better visualize the ear canal and help ensure that medication and treatments provide the greatest benefit, the auditory canal should be properly positioned. Gently pull the auricle up, back, and slightly outward for the adult. *Never* introduce an irrigating tip or applicator into the ear past the point where you can see—you might damage the eardrum. To straighten the ear canal of a child, pull down and backward on the earlobe (Fig. 57-2).

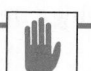

Nursing Skill
Administering Ear Drops

Supplies and Equipment

Medication Kardex, cards, or computer record
Medication, with dropper
Gloves, if needed
Disposable tissues
Cotton balls and normal saline, if needed

Procedure

1. Check the medication order against the original physician's order. (*Rationale: The right medication must be given to the right patient.*)
2. Take the medication out of the refrigerator 15 to 30 minutes before administration. It must be as close to body temperature as possible. (*Rationale: The eardrum is very sensitive. Medication not at room temperature can cause pain or nausea or both. A hot solution can cause permanent damage.*)
3. Wash your hands. Don gloves if there is discharge from the ears. (*Rationale: Both actions deter the spread of microorganisms.*)
4. Have the patient lie on the side with the affected ear upward. (*Rationale: This position aids medication drainage into the ear.*)
5. Explain to the patient what you are going to do. (*Rationale: The patient is more cooperative if he or she understands the procedure.*)
6. Remove excess drainage with a dry wipe. If the drainage has dried, use cotton balls soaked with normal saline solution. (*Rationale: Drainage can interfere with effectiveness of medication.*)
7. Draw up the amount of solution needed in the dropper. (*Rationale: Unused solution should not be returned to the bottle; it is contaminated.*)
8. Straighten the ear canal as shown in Figure 57-2. (*Rationale: This action will allow better visualization of the ear canal.*)
9. Rest your other hand containing the dropper on the patient's head. (*Rationale: This position steadies your hand.*)
10. Hold the tip above the auditory canal and allow drops to fall on the side of the canal. (*Rationale: The patient will feel discomfort if the drops fall directly on the tympanic membrane.*)
11. Instruct the patient to remain in that position for 5 to 10 minutes. (*Rationale: This allows medication to run into the ear canal for maximum effectiveness.*) You may wish to place a small cotton pledget in the ear canal. (*Rationale: This catches the drainage.*)
12. If the procedure is ordered for the other ear, be sure to allow 10 minutes between instillations. Wash your hands after the first instillation and use separate marked bottles for each ear. (*Rationale: Using separate equipment will prevent cross-contamination and reinfection. The time is needed for the first ear to receive the medication.*)
13. Replace equipment, keeping each patient's ear medication separate. (*Rationale: This will prevent cross-contamination.*)
14. Dispose of gloves, and wash your hands. (*Rationale: This prevents spread of microorganisms.*)
15. Document procedure. Be sure to note any significant patient reaction.

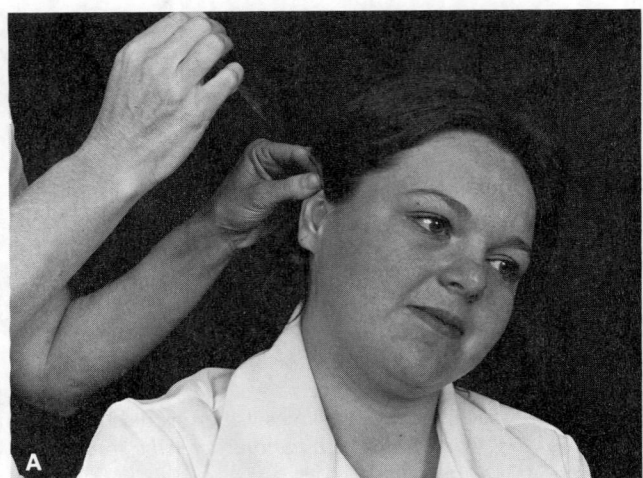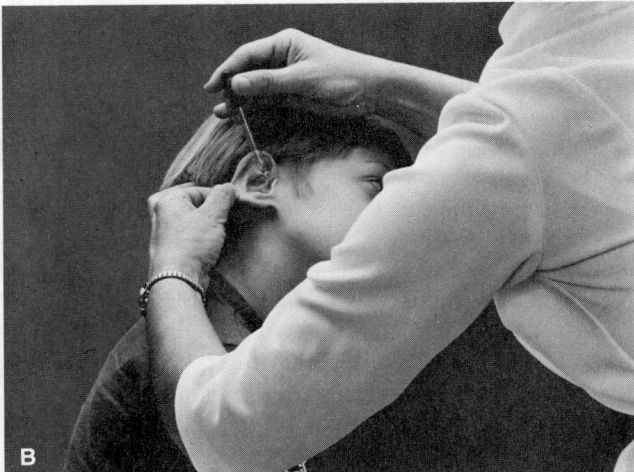

Figure 57-2. **(A)** The nurse pulls the pinna of the ear up and back to straighten the ear canal in adult patients. He or she then places eardrops on the side of the canal. Disposable gloves should be worn if drainage is present. **(B)** The nurse pulls the pinna of the ear down and back to straighten the auditory canal in children. He or she then places the eardrops on the side of the canal. Disposable gloves should be worn if drainage is present.

Nasal Medications and Respiratory Administration

Inhalation or Aerosolized Administration. Drugs that can be vaporized may be given through the respiratory tract. The drug is rapidly absorbed and quickly effective. Nebulizers that produce a fine mist are used for inhalation. The finer the mist, the farther it will travel into the respiratory tract when inhaled. This is important in an emergency, as in administration of oxygen or bronchodilators.

Inhalers are hand-held devices. They are also called *metered-dose nebulizers*. These devices work by having increased pressure inside the unit, which, when pumped by the patient delivers a preset amount of drug in a mist form through a chamber into the patient's oropharyngeal area. It is then inhaled into the lungs. The order is written as the number of "puffs" to be given. Inhalers are available in a variety of shapes and sizes. Extenders and chambers are also available to increase the volume of medication.

Nebulizers work on the basis of compressed air or oxygen forcing medication through tubing to a mouthpiece or mask as a mist that the patient inhales. A variety of styles are available (see Chapter 80). The order is written as to the volume (mL) of medication to be placed into the chamber. The treatment is usually continued until the medication is gone.

These methods require some level of coordination and may be difficult for a child or confused adult to use. Nursing skill guidelines are given in the accompanying box.

Teach the patient when he or she is breathing comfortably; the patient must be able to concentrate. Teach the use, effects, and side effects of the medication. Be careful to note if the patient should perform mouth care after the treatment. (*Rationale: Some medications can adversely affect taste if left in contact with the mucous membranes.*) Observe the patient carefully to ensure correct use.

Special Considerations in Children
Aerosol and Inhalation Therapy

To ensure that the young child receives an accurate dose, a mask may be used or the mouthpiece held close to the nose and mouth so the child inhales the medication with normal respiration. Restraint in a highchair or being held by an adult may be necessary.

Nose Drops. When used properly, nose drops provide an effective nasal treatment, and they are often administered in the hospital. The order usually calls for a specific number of drops (gtts) in each nostril.

Some people use nose drops far too often. As a result, the medications lose their effectiveness and eventually cause swelling of the turbinates (the condition they are supposed to prevent). This is called a *rebound effect* (rebound congestion). Many nose drop preparations are sold over the counter without a prescription, and their prolonged use can be damaging. People with hypertension should *never* use nose drops. The drug contained in nose drops can increase the blood pressure, even in a nonhypertensive person. Nursing skills for administering nasal drops or sprays follow:

◆ Check the medication order against the physician's original order. (*Rationale: The right medication must be given to the right patient.*)

Nursing Skill Guidelines
Administering Aerosolized Medications

◆ Check the medication order against the physician's original order. (*Rationale: The right medication must be given to the right patient.*)

◆ Wash your hands. Wear gloves. Set up medication following safety guidelines. (*Rationale: These steps prevent contamination and decrease the possibility of medication error.*)

◆ Teach the patient how to use his or her particular device.

Inhaler

◆ The inhaler should be shaken well immediately prior to use. (*Rationale: Shaking aerosolizes the fine particles.*)

◆ Spray once into the air. (*Rationale: This fills the mouthpiece.*)

◆ Instruct the patient to take a deep breath and exhale completely through the nose. Then the person grips the mouthpiece with the lips, pushes down on the bottle, and inhales as slowly and deeply as possible through the mouth. (*Rationale: The procedure is designed to allow the medication to come in contact with the lungs for a maximum amount of time.*)

◆ Have the person hold their breath for about 10 seconds and then exhale slowly with pursed lips.

◆ Repeat for each "puff" ordered, waiting 5 minutes or as prescribed between puffs. (*Rationale: This achieves maximum benefit.*)

Nebulizer

◆ Fill the nebulizer cup with the ordered amount of medication. Turn on the oxygen or air at the prescribed liter flow. (*Rationale: Make sure the required amount of medication is given.*)

◆ Instruct the patient to close the lips around the mouthpiece and breathe through the mouth. (If a mask is used, the patient may breathe normally.)

◆ Instruct the patient to continue the treatment until he or she can no longer see a mist on exhalation from the opposite end of the mouthpiece or vent holes in the mask. (*Rationale: This ensures that the entire dose is inhaled.*)

◆ The nebulizer cup and mouthpiece should be cleansed with warm soapy water, rinsed, and dried after each use. Follow your facility's protocols for frequency of changing the tubing and cup for each patient. (*Rationale: Guidelines decrease the possibility of introducing microorganisms into the respiratory tract.*)

General Considerations

◆ Avoid treatments immediately before or after meals. (*Rationale: You want to decrease vomiting or appetite suppression, especially with medications that cause the patient to cough or expectorate or are done in conjunction with percussion/bronchial drainage.*)

◆ If the patient is to continue treatments at home, be sure he or she has a complete understanding of the medication and has demonstrated the ability to do the treatment. (*Rationale: Once home, the patient may not have a resource for teaching. This could result in incorrect dosing or inability to use or maintain equipment.*)

◆ Wash your hands and discard gloves. (*Rationale: This decreases the possibility of contamination.*)

◆ Document procedure and patient's response. Document any teaching done and the patient's ability to follow the teaching.

◆ Wash your hands. Prepare medication following safety guidelines. (*Rationale: Handwashing prevents the spread of microorganisms. Safety precautions decrease possibility of medication error.*)

◆ If using a *spray*, the patient should be sitting up with the head tilted back. The tip of the bottle is placed just inside the nares aimed toward the midline of the nose. Squeeze the bottle while the patient inhales. Instruct the patient to maintain this position for approximately 5 minutes. (*Rationale: This position will allow the medication to maintain contact with the nasal mucosa. Leaning forward may allow the medication to run out the nares.*)

◆ Teach the patient that decongestant sprays can cause increased heart rate and blood pressure and rebound nasal congestion. (*Rationale: Frequent use can stimulate the sympathetic nervous system.*)

◆ If instilling *drops*, position the patient in the same way. Insert the dropper just inside the nares and instill the prescribed number of drops in each nares as ordered. Elevate the nares slightly by pressing with the thumb. Try not to touch the nares with the dropper. (*Rationale: This will decrease contamination of the dropper and decrease the possibility of the patient sneezing.*)

◆ Instruct the patient to maintain the head position for up to 5 minutes. (*Rationale: To increase contact with the medication.*)

◆ Wash your hands. (*Rationale: Handwashing prevents the spread of microorganisms and decreases contamination.*)

◆ Record medication given and the patient's response.

Transdermal Administration

Some drugs are available in **transdermal** patches. That means their effects are passed through the skin. These drugs yield systemic effects. The patches should be placed on clean, hairless parts of the body, typically on the trunk, unless otherwise indicated by the physician. The patches should be changed when ordered by the physician. Some patches need to be changed daily and some weekly, depending on the drug.

Nursing skills in administering transdermal medications are:

◆ Check the order against the physician's original order. (*Rationale: The right medication must be given to the right patient.*)
◆ Wash your hands. Prepare medication for administration following safety guidelines.
◆ Teach the patient the use, effects, and side effects of the medication.
◆ Make sure the application site is clean, dry, and free of hair. Transdermal patches should be applied to the upper trunk of the body whenever possible and sites should be rotated. (*Rationale: Cleanliness of the site and placement of the patch will affect the absorption rate of the medication. Other parts of the body will have different circulation and will affect the rate of absorption, as will placing a new patch on the old site.*) Some medications may require that the old patch be left in place for 30 minutes following application of a new patch (so that a constant level of medication is maintained). Some patients may have difficulty tolerating the adhesive used to apply the patch and altering the sites allows the skin a chance to recover.

◆ Note carefully the location of the current patch before removing it. Be sure to cleanse the skin carefully. (*Rationale: This prevents inaccurate dosing and decreases the potential for skin breakdown or irritation.*)
◆ Place the new patch, applying firm pressure to the edges. Instruct the patient to notify you of any side effects immediately. Check on the patient after 30 minutes. (*Rationale: Applying pressure to the edges ensures an adequate seal with the patient's skin.*)
◆ Wash your hands thoroughly. (*Rationale: Washing your hands will prevent any medication from being absorbed into your skin.*)
◆ Record the medication given and the patient's response. Record TD for transdermal administration on the medication record.

Administration by Injection

Injection is a method of introducing liquid drugs into the tissue through a needle. The injection may be intradermal, subcutaneous, intramuscular, or intravenous. When an intravenous route is used, the method is usually known as an *infusion.* (Other routes such as intracardiac, intramedullary, intrathecal, intraosseous, and intraperitoneal are used only by physicians or specially trained nurses.) The parenteral routes commonly used by nurses are presented in detail following the information on general principles and preparation of medication.

General Principles

Injections are given in various ways, but the basics discussed here apply to every method. Sterile equipment is a must in giving injections to avoid introducing harmful organisms into the tissues or bloodstream.

A drug may be administered by injection for the following reasons:

◆ The drug is most effective when given by this route or is unavailable in any other route.
◆ The desired action is needed quickly.
◆ It is necessary to ascertain the accuracy of the dose of drug injected or retained.
◆ The patient is nauseated or vomiting.
◆ The patient's mental or physical condition renders him or her unable to swallow oral medication.
◆ The drug cannot be absorbed by way of the digestive system.

Injected drugs are absorbed faster than those administered orally, and they are absorbed even more quickly as the routes move from the tissues to the bloodstream. The faster method is generally the intravenous one, with the exception of intracardiac injection (directly into the heart), which is used in emergencies and administered by a physician.

An injection may be momentarily painful when the needle pierces the skin because pain receptors are located there. Deeper insertion of the needle does not mean greater pain. Injecting the solution fairly slowly distributes it more evenly in the tissues and prevents painful pressure. The needle should be inserted and removed *quickly*, however. Gently massaging the area after the needle is withdrawn speeds absorption and helps relieve discomfort.

The nurse should not be afraid to give an injection, but it is important to realize that possible dangers *do* exist. The injection may enter a blood vessel, in which case the drug could be absorbed too rapidly and cause damage. Paralysis or nerve damage, as well as scar formation, necrosis, and sloughing of the tissues, embolism, and abscess or cyst formation may also result.

Syringes

Measurements are stamped on the barrel of the syringe (Fig. 57-3). Milliliters are subdivided into tenths. A subcutaneous or intramuscular injection is usually given with a 2- to 3-mL syringe. Special syringes are used for tuberculin and other intradermal skin tests and for insulin injections.

Syringes are disposable. In one type, the entire unit is discarded after one use. In another type, the medication is premeasured in a disposable cartridge–needle unit that is clamped in a nondisposable holder. Disposable systems are used to prevent cross-contamination. Do not touch the inside or the tip of the barrel or the shaft of the needle. (*Rationale: Touching any of these areas could contaminate the injection setup and could cause an infection in the patient.*)

Needleless systems are available for use with an IV setup. This syringe has a plastic tip which can be inserted into a special port.

The *safety syringe* is becoming more popular. It has a plastic sheath which is pulled down after a medication is drawn up, to protect the needle. After the injection has been given, this sheath is pulled out and twisted and locked into place. This precludes recapping needles and prevents needlesticks to nurses and other personnel.

Insulin Syringes. Insulin, a drug used to control diabetes mellitus, must be given subcutaneously; it cannot be given by mouth because digestive enzymes destroy it. The physician prescribes the dosage, according to the needs of the patient, and adjusts it if necessary.

Insulin syringes are marked in *units* on the sides of the barrel. Insulin syringes are disposable to prevent the possibility of cross-contamination. The methods of administering insulin are presented in Chapter 72. *Note:*

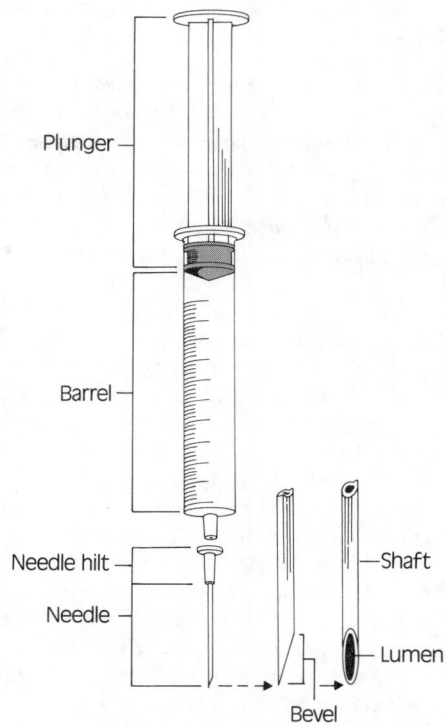

Figure 57-3. Parts of a needle and syringe.

No other type of syringe can be used to give insulin. (Units are *not* equivalent to mL.)

Tuberculin Syringes. Minims and milliliters may be identified on tuberculin syringes. These syringes have a very small diameter and are marked in fine gradations up to 1 mL. They are always clearly marked in tenths and may be graduated in hundredths of a milliliter.

The Needle

Needles are made of stainless steel and are disposable. The needle is hollow (the **lumen**); the part attached to the syringe is called the **hub** or hilt (see Figure 57-3). The needle has a sharp point and a beveled (slanted) edge, so that it can be inserted easily and with minimum discomfort to the patient. Always inspect a needle before giving an injection to be sure that the point is perfect; a dull or damaged needle should never be used. Be sure the needle is firmly attached to the syringe.

The length and gauge of the needle chosen depend on the type of medication given, the route, the site of injection, and the patient's weight. Needle lengths vary from $\frac{1}{2}$ inch to 5 inches. The gauge (diameter) of the needle varies from #14 to #28. The larger the gauge number, the smaller the diameter. For example, a tuberculin test is given with a short, fine needle about $\frac{1}{2}$

Nursing Alert

- *Universal precautions* dictate that needles *not* be recapped after use. This helps to prevent a needle stick to the nurse. Diseases such as acquired immunodeficiency syndrome and hepatitis B are spread by contaminated body fluids, such as blood.
- Be careful when placing needles in the "sharps" container and when carrying a used syringe/needle.
- Dispose of used syringe/needles *immediately*. Most hospitals have a sharps disposal container in each room. Otherwise, there are containers on the medication and treatment carts.
- Any finger stick is potentially dangerous to the nurse and must be reported *immediately*.
- If a needle must be recapped, place the cap on a level surface and "scoop" it up with the needle. Do not touch the cap while this is being done.
- Small styrofoam-filled boxes are also available. Stick the needle into the styrofoam to prevent accidental finger sticks while transporting the equipment back to a sharps disposal container. (This method is used in areas such as psychiatry and for occasional injections in home care.)
- There are new devices available for recapping needles that will prevent needle sticks, such Gard Recapper®. These devices allow the nurse to uncap and recap the needle without danger. The safety syringe, using a plastic sheath, has been previously described.

to ³⁄₄ inches (1.1–1.65 cm) long, 25 gauge. An intramuscular injection is given with a larger needle, about 1¹⁄₂ to 2 inches (3.3–4.4 cm) long. The gauge depends on the viscosity (thickness) of the medication (20–22 gauge is usual). The length depends on the patient's size. The administration of blood requires a larger gauge needle.

Preparing Medications for Administration by Injection

Drugs that are given by injection are packaged in many ways. Some are dispensed as powders because they would deteriorate in a solution. They are diluted, immediately before use, with the solution (sterile water or normal saline) suggested by the manufacturer. If the drug will remain stable in a solution, it is dispensed in an ampule, a vial, or a prefilled syringe. There are single dose ampules and single and multidose vials.

An *ampule* is a glass container that holds a single dose of medication. Because there is no way to prevent contamination of an open ampule, any unused medication must be discarded. A *vial* is a glass container with

a self-sealing stopper. Because of this self-sealing stopper, vials can contain more than one dose of a medication. Procedure 57-2 shows how to draw up medication from an ampule and from a vial.

A *prefilled syringe* provides a single dose of medication and is prepared by the manufacturer of the medication or by the pharmacy. If all the medication in the syringe is not needed, the excess amount can be discarded into the sink or toilet by pushing the plunger until the quantity needed is correct (the syringe will have a scale marked on the barrel). Tubex and Carpuject are two common types of prefilled syringes.

The Intradermal Injection

An **intradermal** injection is a shallow injection, just beneath the epidermis (Fig. 57-4). These injections are usually performed for diagnostic purposes. A tubercu-

(Text continues on page 733)

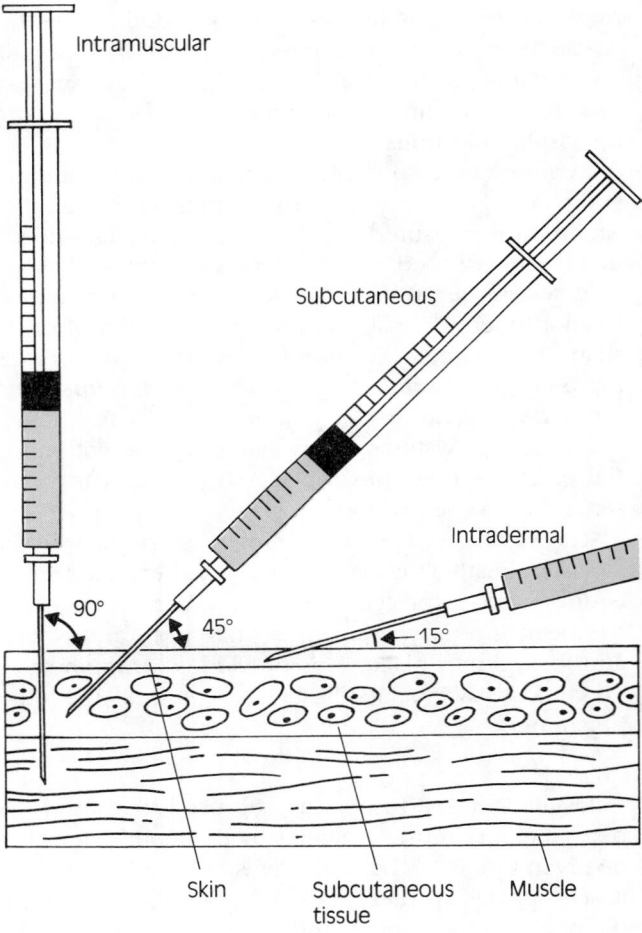

Figure 57-4. Comparison of the angles of insertion for intramuscular, subcutaneous, and intradermal injections. A SubQ may be given at a 90° angle if a short needle is used or if the person is heavy.

Drawing Up Medication From an Ampule or Vial

Supplies and Equipment

Syringe and needle
Alcohol swab or gauze pad
Ampule or vial of medication
Medication card, Kardex, or computer record
Filter needle (optional)

Procedure

1. Wash hands.
   (Rationale: Handwashing prevents the spread of organisms.)
2. Gather equipment. Use medication Kardex, cards, or computer record to verify medication order. Check any inconsistency with physician or pharmacist.
   (Rationale: Organization facilitates performance of the skill and reduces the chance of medication error.)
3. Unlock medication cart or drawer. Check expiration date on medication.
   (Rationale: Keeping medication setup locked provides security if the area is unattended. Outdated medication may be ineffective.)

Ampule

4. Hold ampule upright. Use finger to tap on stem of ampule or hold ampule by the stem and rotate hand in a circular motion.
   (Rationale: All medication in the ampule should be in the lower part prior to snapping off the stem.)

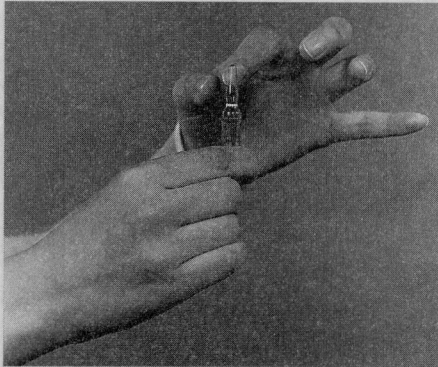

Step 4   Tapping the stem of an ampule

5. Grasp the stem with alcohol swab or gauze pad.
   (Rationale: Pad protects the nurse's finger from glass particles when stem is removed.)

6. Snap off neck of ampule away from your hands and face.
   (Rationale: Snapping off the ampule stem away from the face protects the nurse's face from small glass particles.)

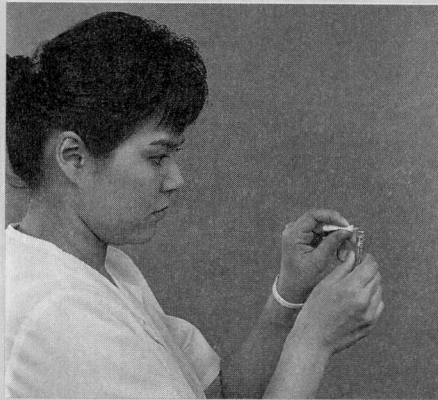

Step 6   Snapping off the neck of an ampule

7. Remove cap and insert needle into ampule. Certain agencies may recommend use of a filter needle. Withdraw the medication. Avoid touching rim of ampule with needle and injecting any air into ampule. Use one of the following methods:
   a. Keeping ampule *upright* on a flat surface, insert needle into solution and aspirate medication into syringe.

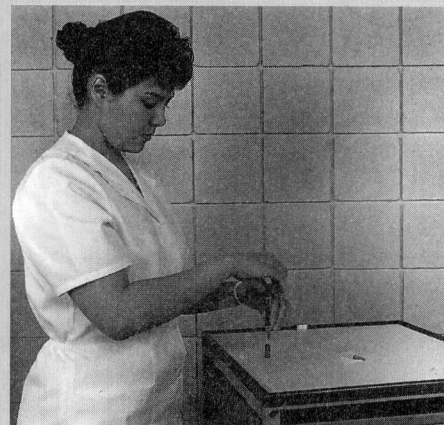

Step 7a   Keeping an ampule upright when withdrawing medication

(continued)

b. *Invert* the ampule, insert needle into the solution and aspirate medication into syringe.
(Rationale: Keeping the needle in the solution prevents aspiration of air. Touching the sterile needle against the ampule rim contaminates the needle. There is no need to inject air into ampule because contents are not under pressure.)

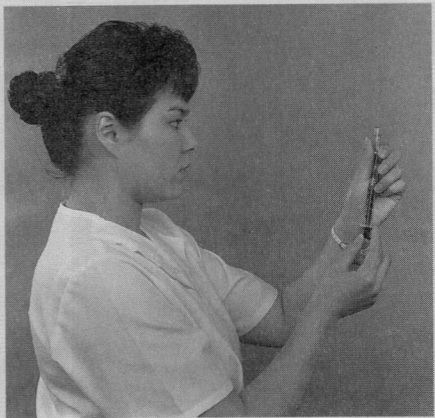

Step 7b   Inverting an ampule to withdraw medication

8. Remove needle from solution in ampule. Hold needle upright and discard any air that has been withdrawn into syringe. Discard any excess medication into plastic cup or sink.
(Rationale: Checking amount of medication withdrawn from ampule ensures that correct dose is administered.)
9. Change needle if necessary, recap the needle, or pull the safety sheath over the needle. *Do not* lock the safety sheath.
(Rationale: Cap maintains sterility of needle.)
10. Discard used ampule in sharps container.
(Rationale: Proper disposal prevents accidental injury.)

Vial

11. Remove metal or plastic cover from vial and cleanse the rubber port with alcohol swab.
(Rationale: Cap and cleansing with alcohol swab decrease the possibility of introducing contaminants into the vial.)

12. Remove needle cap and add amount of air to syringe equal to amount of medication that will be withdrawn from vial. Some agencies may recommend the use of a filter needle.
(Rationale: Injecting an equal amount of air prevents buildup of negative pressure in the vial.)
13. Insert needle through center of rubber stopper and inject air into vial keeping the needle above the solution.
(Rationale: Air should be injected into air space rather than bubbled through solution so accurate dose is withdrawn into syringe.)

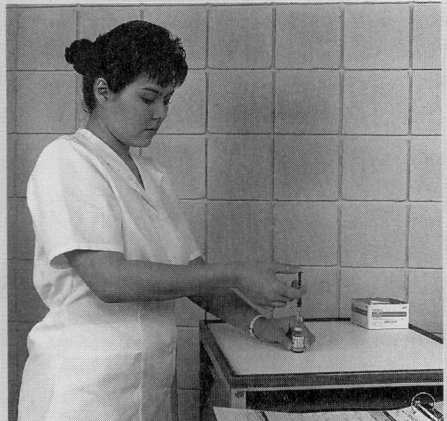

Step 13   Adding air to the vial

14. Invert the vial. Steady vial and syringe in nondominant hand at eye level. Brace little finger against plunger.
(Rationale: Holding vial and syringe securely prevents contamination of the medication. The plunger is held in case negative pressure already exists in the vial. This could force the plunger out.)
15. Move needle into solution.
(Rationale: Medication rather than air will be aspirated.)
16. Use dominant hand to pull back on plunger of syringe. Withdraw accurate dose into syringe. Remove needle from vial.
(Rationale: Positive pressure in vial promotes easy aspiration of fluid into syringe.)

(continued)

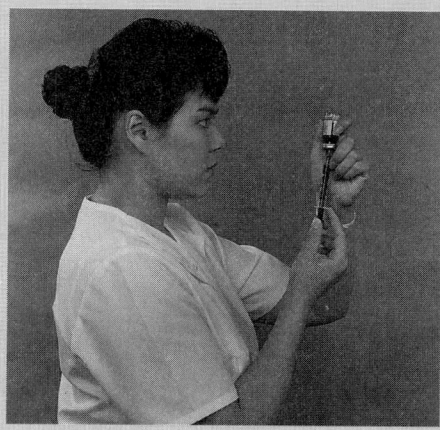

Step 16 Withdrawing medication from a vial (Photos © B. Proud.)

17. Hold needle upright and recheck syringe contents for presence of air. Tap barrel of syringe to move air bubbles upward prior to expelling them. Reinsert needle into solution if it is necessary to withdraw any additional medication.
    (Rationale: Removing air bubbles ensures that accurate amount of medication was withdrawn.)
18. Change needle if necessary, recap the needle, or pull safety sheath over needle. Do not lock.
    (Rationale: Cap maintains sterility of needle.)
19. Discard used single dose vial or store multidose vial according to agency policy.
    (Rationale: Proper disposal prevents transmission of organisms.)
20. Wash hands.
    (Rationale: Handwashing prevents the spread of organisms.)
21. Always wear gloves when administering injections.
    (Rationale: This protects yourself.)

lin syringe with a 25- to 26-gauge needle is used. Preparation of the patient and the substance to be injected is the same as for other injections. The inner aspect of the lower arm is a common site for intradermal injections.

If the test is given to determine sensitivity (such as the purified protein derivative [PPD] test), the injection site is checked at 48 hours and 72 hours. The evaluation of the injection site is based on *induration* (a hardness) and, to a lesser extent, on *erythema* (redness). The evaluation procedure is described in Chapter 50. Controls may be given, along with the desired test material (such as tuberculin). *(Rationale: This ensures the person is producing antibodies.)*

Nursing Skill
Giving an Intradermal Injection

Supplies and Equipment

Medication
Medication card, Kardex, or computer record
Sterile syringe and needle
Alcohol swab
Disposable gloves

Procedure

1. Check the medication order against the physician's original order. *(Rationale: The right medication must be given to the right patient.)*
2. Wash your hands. Wear gloves. Set up medication following safety guidelines. *(Rationale: This prevents contamination and decreases the possibility of medication error. Gloves are worn because the patient's skin will be pierced.)*
3. Explain to the patient what you are going to do and why. *(Rationale: This decreases the patient's anxiety and helps increase the patient's cooperation.)* Teach the medication's use, effects, and side effects to the patient.
4. Choose an injection site on the inner aspect of the forearm that is not heavily pigmented or covered with hair and cleanse the site with an alcohol pad in a circular motion from the center outward. Allow the alcohol to dry. *(Rationale: Hair or discoloration may interfere with assessment of the site after injection. Cleansing in this manner decreases microorganisms on the skin and prevents dragging contaminants from a dirty surface to a clean one.)*
5. Uncap the needle (usually a ¼- to ½-inch, 26- or 27-gauge needle) and use your nondominant hand to pull the skin over the injection site slightly taut. *(Rationale: Firmer skin makes it easier to access intradermal tissue.)*
6. Place the needle, bevel up, at a 15° angle (almost flat with the skin) and insert it just until the bevel is no longer visible (see Figure 57-4). *(Rationale: To access the intradermal, but not subcutaneous, tissue.)*
7. Slowly inject the medication (usually 0.25 mL or less). Watch for a blister or *wheal* to form. *(Rationale: This indicates that the medication is correctly placed. Intradermal sites can tolerate only small amounts of medication.)*

8. Withdraw the needle quickly and at the same angle at which it was inserted. *(Rationale: This minimizes damage to the tissues.)*

9. Do not massage the site. *(Rationale: This could displace the medication and give false readings to a test.)*

10. Discard the needle and syringe in a sharps container. Lock the safety sheath in place. Do not recap the needle. *(Rationale: This decreases the possibility of injury from a needle stick or infection.)*

11. Properly dispose of gloves and wash your hands.

12. Record the medication given, the site, and the patient's response. Note when test results should be assessed in the chart and on the Kardex. Occasionally, the site is circled with pen. Follow your facility's protocol for this. *(Rationale: Test results can be false if not read at the appropriate time. Marking the site can allow careful observation of the correct area, especially if controls are used.)*

The Subcutaneous Injection

In **subcutaneous** injection, a small amount of a drug is injected into the subcutaneous tissue (*hypodermically*—under the skin). This method is used to give drugs that are soluble and nonirritating, such as insulin. A subcutaneous injection ("SubQ") is given in an area where bones and blood vessels are not near the surface, commonly the upper part of the arms and the thighs. For the occasional subcutaneous injection, the arm is the most convenient site. If a patient is having injections regularly, a different location is chosen each time; for example, use the right arm, then the left arm, then the right thigh, then the left thigh. The abdomen is also an area frequently used for injections; the back may also be used. Try to find a spot in each area that has not been used for at least 1 inch in all directions.

Recommendations as to angle of administration and length of needle vary. The nurse must assess the patient's body mass and use judgment for each patient. An undernourished or emaciated patient has less subcutaneous tissue than a stouter person; a $\frac{1}{2}$-inch needle is used. The solution is usually injected at a 45° angle, but it may be necessary to increase this angle slightly (see Figure 57-4). In a very heavy person, a 90° angle is used (usually with a $\frac{5}{8}$- to 1-inch needle, because a short needle may not reach the subcutaneous tissue). Using a needle that is too long can cause damage by hitting a bone or a nerve; a 25-gauge needle is commonly used. Actions in giving a subcutaneous injection are given in Nursing Procedure 57-3.

The Intramuscular Injection

In **intramuscular** (IM) injection, a drug is injected into the muscle beneath the subcutaneous tissue. This method is used when giving irritating drugs or large amounts of a drug because deep muscle tissue has fewer nerve fibers. Also, larger doses can be given intramuscularly. Absorption of the drug is faster because muscle tissue has a great number of blood vessels. The injection is given in much the same way as a subcutaneous injection, except that a longer needle is used and the drug is injected into muscles, instead of into tissues directly beneath the skin (see Figure 57-4). Most often a $1\frac{1}{2}$- to 2-inch, 20- to 22-gauge needle is used depending on the type of medication.

Intramuscular injections are more difficult and dangerous to give than subcutaneous injections for several reasons. The needle must penetrate thick muscles. If the drug is injected into subcutaneous tissues, it is not absorbed quickly and may cause pain and serious irritation. The possibility of striking bones, large nerves, and blood vessels is greater when a longer, larger needle is used. Paralysis or nerve damage can result from injecting in an incorrect site. Nursing Procedure 57-4 outlines steps in giving an intramuscular injection.

Injection Sites

Intramuscular injections are usually given in the thick gluteal muscles of the buttocks, although small injections may be given in the side of the thigh in the vastus lateralis muscle (part of the quadriceps femoris) or in the outer part of the upper arm in the deltoid muscle. These sites are shown in Figure 57-5.

The Dorsogluteal Site. The dorsogluteal (posterior gluteal) site is not used for infants less than 18 months old or small children because they may not have enough muscle mass. It is commonly used for intramuscular injections in adults. However, keep in mind that debilitated adults may also lack enough muscle mass to use this site. The thick layer of fat in some people may make it difficult to assess muscle tissue.

The way to locate this site is to draw an imaginary line, after palpating, from the posterior iliac spine to the greater trochanter of the femur. The injection should be given above and lateral to this line (see Figure 57-5**A**). Ideally, the patient should be lying prone with toes pointed inward; this reduces discomfort from the injection by forcing the gluteal muscles to relax.

The Ventrogluteal Site. The preferred site for injection in the hip area is the ventrogluteal (side gluteal) site; it is recommended for adults and for children who have been ambulating for more than 2 years. The location of your hand differs, depending on whether the patient is lying on the back, abdomen, or side. The right hand is used for the left hip and vice versa.

(Text continues on page 737)

Giving a Subcutaneous Injection

Supplies and Equipment

Medication
Sterile syringe (1–3 mL) with 25–27-gauge needle (1/2 or
   5/8 inch in length)
Gloves
Alcohol swabs
Medication card, Kardex, or computer record

Procedure

1. Wash hands.
    *(Rationale: Handwashing prevents the spread of
    organisms.)*
2. Gather equipment. Use medication Kardex, cards, or
    computer record to verify medication order. Check
    any inconsistency with physician or
    pharmacist.
    *(Rationale: Organization facilitates performance of
    the skill and reduces the chance of medication
    error.)*
3. Prepare medication. If necessary, withdraw from am-
    pule or vial according to Nursing Procedure 57-2.
    *(Rationale: Preparation of medication before enter-
    ing patient's room facilitates administration.)*
4. Add air to syringe according to agency policy.
    *(Rationale: For a heparin injection, 0.1 mL of air is
    generally recommended to clear the medication from
    the needle.)*
5. Explain procedure to patient.
    *(Rationale: Providing information fosters patient
    cooperation.)*
6. Identify the patient before giving the medication. Re-
    fer to step 11, Nursing Procedure 57-1.
    *(Rationale: Medication may be administered to the
    wrong patient if identity is not established.)*
7. Put on gloves. Close the door or pull the bed
    curtains.
    *(Rationale: Gloves act as a barrier. Closing curtain
    or door protects the patient's privacy.)*
8. Assist patient to a comfortable position. Select appro-
    priate site using anatomic landmarks.
    *(Rationale: Correct identification of site decreases the
    risk of injury.)*
9. Cleanse the skin with an alcohol swab. Start at site
    and move outward with a circular motion. Allow area
    to dry. Place alcohol swab on a clean, nearby
    surface.
    *(Rationale: Cleansing injection site with antiseptic
    prepares the site for the injection.)*

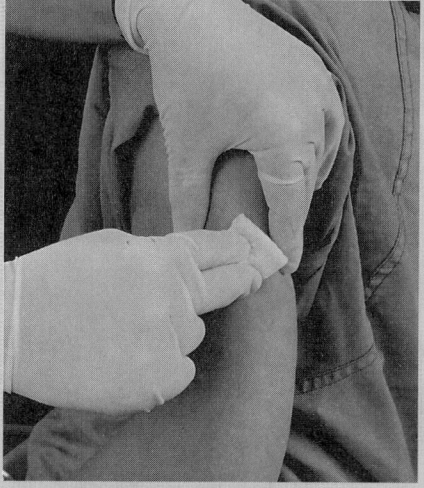

Step 9   Cleansing the site

10. Remove needle cap or retract sheath. Use nondomi-
    nant hand to gently bunch or spread tissue at injec-
    tion site.
    *(Rationale: Size of patient determines method of
    preparation of site. Skin that is spread taut facilitates
    needle entry. Bunching the area, if patient has excess
    tissue, may be necessary to ensure that needle is
    placed in subcutaneous tissue.)*

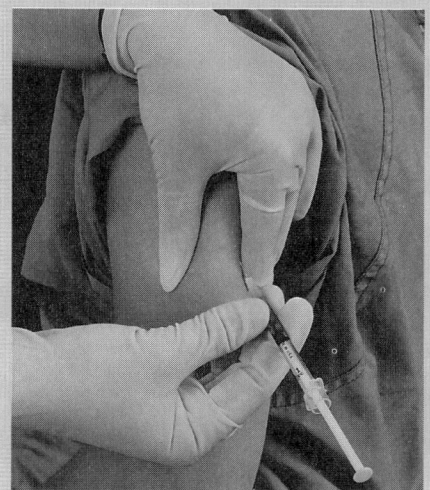

Step 10   Bunching tissue at the injection site

(continued)

11. Hold syringe in dominant hand like a pencil or dart.
    (Rationale: This position prevents accidental loss of medication while inserting needle.)
12. Insert needle quickly at correct angle. Usual rule is 45° for 5/8 inch needle or 90° for 1/2 inch needle. Check agency policy.
    (Rationale: Quick entry of needle is less painful. Correct angle delivers medication to subcutaneous tissue.)

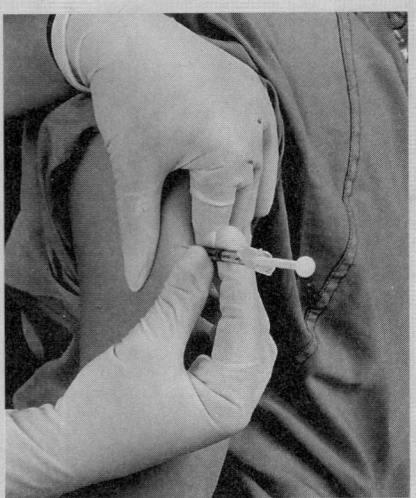

Step 12 Preparing to insert the needle (90-degree angle for a 1/2-inch needle)

13. Release skin and move nondominant hand to steady lower end of syringe.
    (Rationale: This prevents movement of the syringe, which can be painful for the patient.)
14. Aspirate for a blood return by pulling back on plunger with dominant hand. If blood enters syringe, needle should be removed and a new injection prepared. Aspiration is usually contraindicated for a heparin injection.
    (Rationale: A blood return indicates intravenous placement of needle. Medication becomes contaminated by blood and must be redrawn. Heparin is usually not aspirated because of its anticoagulant activity.)

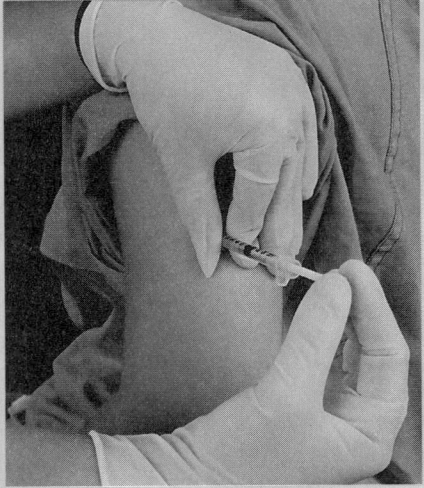

Step 14 Aspirating for blood

15. If no blood appears, inject the medication at a slow and steady rate.
    (Rationale: Rapid injection may be painful for the patient.)

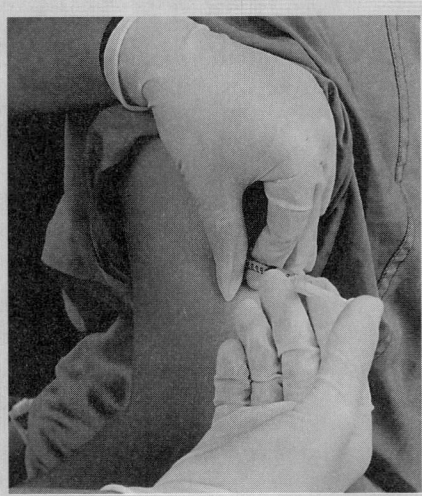

Step 15 Injecting the medication (Photos © B. Proud.)

16. Remove needle quickly at the same angle it was inserted.
    (Rationale: Slow withdrawal of needle may be uncomfortable for the patient.)

(continued)

17. Massage the site gently with alcohol swab unless contraindicated for specific medication.
(Rationale: Massaging the site promotes absorption of the medication and increases patient comfort. Heparin site is not massaged because of anticoagulant action of medication.)
18. Do not recap needle. Place uncapped needle and syringe in appropriate container. If using safety syringe, pull sheath over the needle, and twist until it locks into place.
(Rationale: Most accidental needle sticks occur while recapping needle. Proper disposal prevents injury.)

19. Assist patient to return to position of comfort. Remove gloves and wash hands.
(Rationale: Handwashing prevents the spread of organisms.)
20. Record medication administration on the appropriate form. Indicate subcutaneous site that was used.
(Rationale: Documentation provides coordination of care. Rotation of sites prevents injury to subcutaneous tissue.)
21. Check on patient response to medication within appropriate period of time.
(Rationale: Drugs administered parenterally have a more rapid response.)

In the procedure, the index finger is placed on the patient's iliac spine and the middle finger is moved down to form a V with the index finger. The middle finger is slipped to a point just below the crest of the ileum. The palm of the hand rests on the patient's hip. The triangle between index and middle finger is the injection site (see Figure 57-5**B**).

The ventrogluteal site is recommended because it is a safer and less painful location for injection than the dorsogluteal site. The fat layer is thinner in this area, while the gluteal muscle is thicker, even in very thin patients. One disadvantage is that the patient can see what is going on; to avoid this, the patient can be on the back, the side, or the abdomen for this injection.

Alternative Sites. Other sites that may be used for intramuscular injections are shown in Figure 57-5. They include the *vastus lateralis* (lateral thigh) and *deltoid* (upper arm). Another site in the thigh is rectus femoris (anterior thigh). Sites in the thigh are often chosen when injecting babies and small children. Many clients find the rectus femoris site uncomfortable and it is most often used in adults only when other sites are contraindicated. However, it is convenient in self-injection. The abdomen is also used for self-injection.

The *vastus lateralis* is a thick muscle that is being used more frequently for intramuscular injections. It is a desirable site for infants and children whose gluteal muscles are poorly developed. There is little risk of injury with this site because there are no large nerves or arteries surrounding the site. It is located on the anterolateral aspect of the thigh. It is identified by dividing the thigh into thirds both horizontally and vertically. The injection is given in the *outer middle third.*

The *deltoid* muscle can be used for intramuscular injections, but should be used only for small amounts of liquid. There is also a risk of radial artery and nerve damage with this site. Children under 18 months old should not receive injections in this site because of poor muscle development. It is located on the lateral aspect of the upper arm, 1 to 2 inches below the shoulder joint (acromium). Hepatitis B vaccine and tetanus toxoid are examples of medications given in the deltoid site.

Table 57-2 presents further guidelines on choosing sites.

The Z-Track Method

Certain drugs, such as iron preparations, are irritating to the skin and must be injected deeply. They are given *intramuscularly*. The Z-track or zig-zag method keeps the solution from leaking onto the skin. First, pull the skin to one side and insert the needle. After ascertaining that the needle is not in a blood vessel, inject the medication. Wait a few seconds and remove the needle. Allow the skin to return to its original position as you remove the needle. As the tissues slide past each other, the needle track is closed. A Z-track injection site is *not* massaged (Fig. 57-6).

Nursing Alert

Any intramuscular injection must be given into *healthy* muscle tissue for proper absorption to occur. If a patient requires intramuscular injections frequently, the sites should be rotated, and a notation of the site used each time should be made on the patient's chart. The rotation of injection sites is particularly important in the diabetic patient.

Giving an Intramuscular Injection

Supplies and Equipment

Medication
Sterile syringe (1–3 mL) with appropriate needle:
   Adult: 21–23-gauge needle, 1–1.5 inch in length
   Child: 25–27-gauge needle, 0.5–1 inch in length
Gloves
Alcohol swab
Medication card, Kardex, or computer record

Procedure

1. Wash hands.
   (Rationale: Handwashing prevents the spread of organisms.)
2. Gather equipment. Use medication Kardex, cards, or computer record to verify medication order. Check any inconsistency with physician or pharmacist.
   (Rationale: Organization facilitates performance of the skill and reduces the chance of medication error.)
3. Prepare medication. If necessary, withdraw from ampule or vial according to Nursing Procedure 57-2.
   (Rationale: Preparation of medication before entering patient's room facilitates administration.)
4. Add 0.2 mL air to syringe according to agency policy.
   (Rationale: Air in syringe clears medication from needle and helps keep drug in muscle tissue.)
5. Explain procedure to patient.
   (Rationale: Providing information fosters patient cooperation.)
6. Identify the patient before giving the medication. Refer to step 11, Nursing Procedure 57-1.
   (Rationale: Medication may be administered to the wrong patient if identity is not established.)
7. Put on gloves. Close the door or pull the bed curtains.
   (Rationale: Gloves act as a barrier. Closing curtain or door protects the patient's privacy.)
8. Assist patient to a comfortable position. Select appropriate site using anatomic landmarks.
   (Rationale: Correct identification of site decreases the risk of injury.)

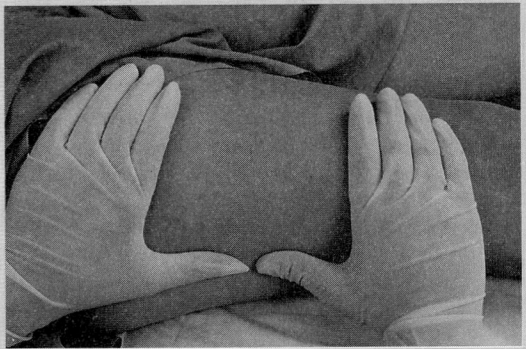

Step 8   Selecting the appropriate site using anatomic landmarks

9. Cleanse the skin with an alcohol swab. Start at site and move outward with a circular motion. Allow area to dry. Place alcohol swab on a clean, nearby surface or hold between fingers of non-dominant hand.
   (Rationale: Cleansing injection site with antiseptic prepares the site for the injection.)
10. Remove needle cap. Use nondominant hand to spread tissue at injection site.
    (Rationale: Skin that is spread taut facilitates needle entry.)
11. Hold syringe in dominant hand like a pencil or dart.
    (Rationale: This position keeps finger off plunger, preventing accidental loss of medication while inserting needle.)
12. Insert needle quickly at a 90° angle.
    (Rationale: Insertion is less painful and enters muscle tissue.)

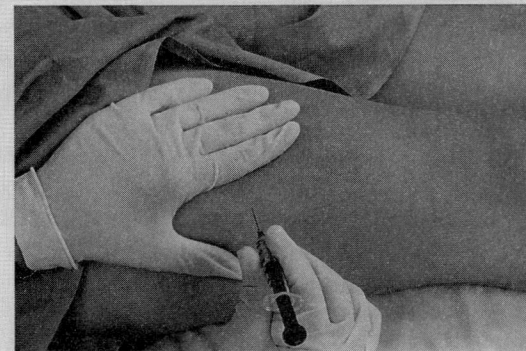

Step 12   Inserting the needle

(continued)

13. Release skin and move nondominant hand to steady lower end of syringe.
    (*Rationale: This prevents movement of the syringe, which can be painful for the patient.*)

14. Aspirate for a blood return by pulling back on plunger with dominant hand. If blood enters syringe, needle should be removed and a new injection prepared.
    (*Rationale: A blood return indicates intravenous placement of needle. Medication becomes contaminated by blood and must be redrawn.*)

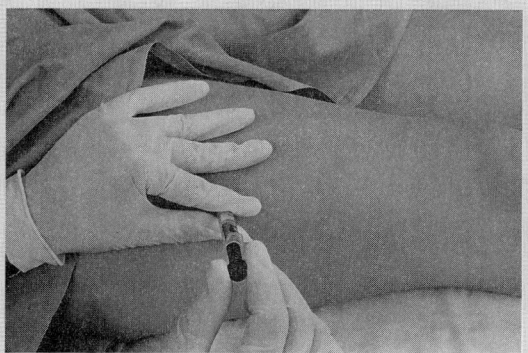

Step 14 Aspirating for blood

15. If no blood appears, inject the medication at a slow and steady rate.
    (*Rationale: Rapid injection may be painful for the patient.*)

16. Use nondominant hand to spread skin around needle entry site. Remove the needle quickly at the same angle it was inserted.
    (*Rationale: Slow withdrawal of needle may be uncomfortable for the patient. Taut skin provides for easier removal of needle.*)

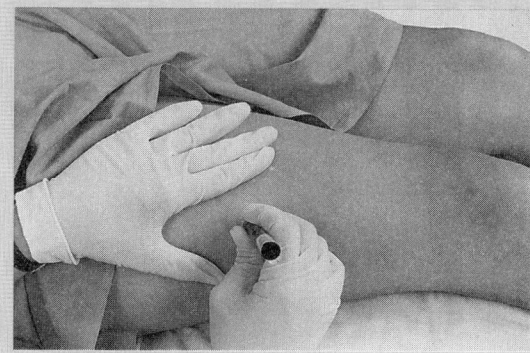

Step 16 Spreading the skin when removing the needle (Photos © B. Proud.)

17. Massage the site gently with alcohol swab.
    (*Rationale: Massaging the site promotes absorption of the medication and increases patient comfort.*)

18. Do not recap needle. Place uncapped needle and syringe in appropriate container. Use safety syringe, if available.
    (*Rationale: Most accidental needle sticks occur while recapping needle. Proper disposal prevents injury.*)

19. Assist patient to return to position of comfort. Remove gloves and wash hands.
    (*Rationale: Handwashing prevents the spread of organisms.*)

20. Record medication administration on the appropriate form. Indicate intramuscular site that was used.
    (*Rationale: Documentation provides coordination of care. Rotation of sites prevents injury to muscle tissue.*)

21. Check on patient response to medication within appropriate period of time.
    (*Rationale: Drugs administered parenterally have a more rapid response.*)

Intravenous Injection and Infusion. A drug may be injected *intravenously*, directly into a vein (given intravenously [IV]), to obtain the needed effect quickly or when it is impossible to inject the drug into other tissues. A large quantity of solution is given by *infusion*, that is, the solution flows into the patient's vein with the aid of gravity or an infusion pump. The starting of an intravenous injection (*venipuncture*) requires technical skill and usually must be done by a physician or registered nurse. Intravenous infusion is commonly given for dehydration and excessive loss of blood, to dilute poisons in the blood and other body fluids, or to provide electrolytes, drugs, and nutrients. If blood is given, this method is called a **transfusion**. Drugs are *not* added to a blood transfusion. The technique of administering blood is described briefly in Chapter 75. A special type of intravenous infusion called total parenteral nutrition (TPN) is discussed in the next section.

Intracardiac Injection. In extreme emergencies, such as a cardiac arrest, the physician may inject a drug directly into the left ventricle of the heart. The heart then pumps the drug into the body with its next contraction or compression.

Intrathecal or Intraspinal Injection. A physician may elect to administer a medication by direct injection into

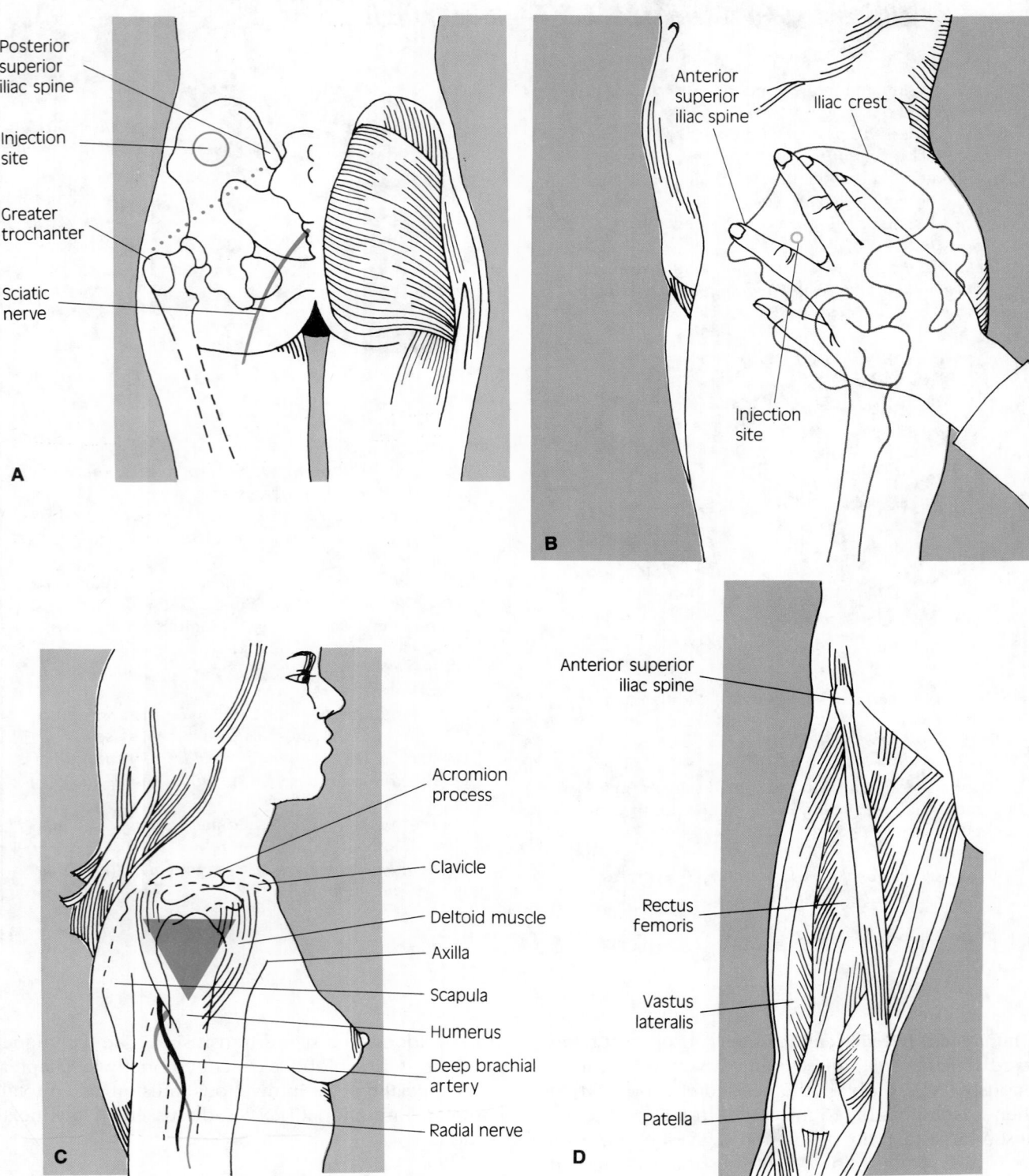

Figure 57-5. Intramuscular injection sites. **(A)** Dorsogluteal site: lateral and slightly superior to midpoint of a line drawn from trochanter to posterior superior iliac spine. **(B)** Ventrogluteal site: located by placing palm on greater trochanter and index finger toward anterior superior iliac spine. Middle finger is then spread posteriorly away from index finger as far as possible. The injection is made in the middle of the triangle formed by the fingers. **(C)** Deltoid site: located by palpating the lower edge of the acromion process. At the midpoint, in line with axilla on lateral aspect of upper arm, triangle is formed. **(D)** Vastus lateralis site: identified by dividing thigh into thirds horizontally and vertically. Injection is given in outer middle third.

Table 57-2. Choosing Sites for Intramuscular Injections

Site	Age Group	Amount of Solution per Injection
Deltoid (Upper arm)	Children 18 mos to 15 y	0.5 mL
	Children over 15 y and adults	0.5–2.0 mL
Rectus femoris (Anterior thigh)	Infants and toddlers	0.5–1.0 mL
	Preschoolers	up to 1.5 mL
Ventrogluteal (Side hip)	Toddlers over 3 y	1.0 mL
	Preschoolers	up to 1.5 mL
	School-age children	up to 2.0 mL
	Older children and adults	up to 2.5 mL
Dorsogluteal (Back of hip)	Children less than 3 y	up to 1.0 mL
	Children 3–6 y	up to 1.5 mL
	6–15 y	up to 2.0 mL
	15 y and older	2.0–4.0 mL
Vastus lateralis (Side thigh)	Children older than 15 y	up to 2.0 mL
	Adults	up to 5.0 mL

the spinal canal to maximize the specific effect of the drug on the central nervous system or to give spinal anesthetic. This technique is basically the same as that for the lumbar puncture. Nurses do not administer drugs intraspinally, unless they are trained as Registered Nurse Anesthetists and are directly supervised by an anesthesiologist.

Parenteral Therapy

Injection of fluids is known as parenteral therapy, and the various methods of injecting large quantities of fluid into the body are called *infusions*. During, after, and many times before a surgical procedure, the patient may experience a loss of fluids and electrolytes through bleeding, vomiting, excessive perspiration (diaphoresis), or drainage. When the loss is severe and is not replaced by fluids taken orally, fluids and electrolytes must be replaced parenterally.

Methods

Several routes are available for the injection of parenteral fluids: intravenous, intramuscular, subcutaneous, and **intramedullary** (into the bone marrow cavity). The commonly used method for substantial amounts of

fluid is **intravenous infusion** (IV); In intravenous infusion, the solution drips into a vein at a rate ordered by the physician (usually in drops per minute or milliliters [mL] per hour). The safest way to regulate an infusion is with an electronic infusion pump or controller. A Microdrip setup may also be used.

Total parenteral nutrition (TPN), the administration of all nutrients parenterally (also called total parenteral alimentation, TPA, or hyperalimentation), involves the use of a large central venous catheter. The other methods mentioned above (intramuscular, subcutaneous, intramedullary) cannot be used for large amounts of fluids or for TPN.

Intravenous Infusion

Intravenous infusion is widely used. You will not be responsible for starting an infusion, but you should know how to care for a patient who is having this treatment. Usually, a plastic catheter is inserted into a vein. Attached to it is a length of tubing connected to a plastic bag containing the prescribed solution. A clamp on the tubing regulates the flow of fluid. In many hospitals, an electronic infusion pump is used to regulate the drip rate of the intravenous infusion. In some situations when the fluid is being infused into an arm vein, the arm may be immobilized. This is less common with a catheter than with a needle in the vein.

Many facilities are using "needleless" systems. The type of system and its components vary depending on the facility and brand choice. All types aim to decrease the risk of injury from needle sticks, either by sheathing

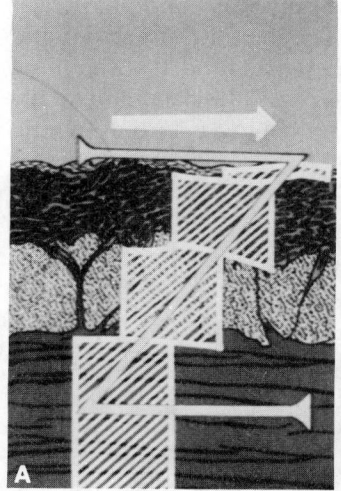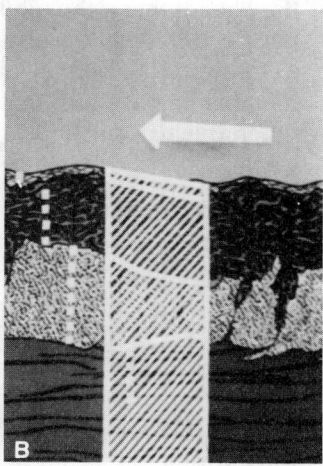

Figure 57-6. Z-track injection. **(A)** The tissue is tensed laterally at the injection site before the needle is inserted. This pulls the skin, subcutaneous tissue, and fat planes into a Z-formation. **(B)** After injection, tissues are released while the needle is withdrawn. As each tissue plane slides by the other, the tract is sealed.

the needle or by using plastic connectors and access devices. Needleless systems vary by manufacturer and you must follow your facility's protocol for use of the system.

Needleless systems may require special syringes and tubing. Also used are safety syringes, a sheath-type system that encloses the needle in a plastic housing. Both systems are intended to decrease the possibility of injury from needle sticks. Always dispose of used needleless systems following your facility's protocol for sharps and biohazardous waste.

Infusion Pumps and Controllers

Electronic infusion devices can control the amount of intravenous fluid to be infused. They automatically regulate the flow and alert the nurse through an alarm system when air is in the tubing, when the bag or bottle is empty, and when the flow is obstructed.

Infusion pumps are the most accurate of these devices. They use positive pressure to deliver the prescribed volume of fluid. *Infusion controllers* use gravity and the height of the intravenous container in relation to the location of the intravenous site to maintain a precise flow rate. The *pump* regulates flow by volume; the *controller* senses the number of drops infusing.

Setting up and programming an infusion pump is different for each brand of pump. Setting up a controller is much less difficult. Before using a pump or controller, proper instruction is needed. The first few times a nurse works with a pump or controller, another nurse should double-check the setup to make sure it is correct. In addition, safety features are built into each machine to avoid erroneous programming.

When using an infusion pump or controller, teach the patient that if the tubing becomes obstructed or the bag becomes empty, an alarm will sound. It is important to forewarn the person; otherwise, the patient or family member might think that something is terribly wrong when the alarm sounds.

Microdrip Setup

The microdrip setup allows the solution to be administered in very small drops so that the amount given is carefully regulated. The microdrip has a drip rate factor (DRF) of 60 drops per milliliter (mL) of fluid. This is in comparison to common systems, which have a DRF of 15 drops/mL or 10 drops/mL. The nurse is responsible for knowing the DRF of the system in use. Check the information packed with the tubing before using it.

The microdrip setup has many advantages over conventional gravity set-ups. Because it delivers the fluid in small drops, it can be used in situations where careful regulation is necessary, for example, in children and older adults, or in patients with heart disease where an overload of fluid would be especially dangerous.

Infusion Rate

If an infusion pump or controller is not used, the size of the catheter, the height of the solution bag or bottle, and the position of insertion site all influence the rate of infusion. A catheter with a larger diameter will allow the solution to flow faster. The higher the bottle or bag, the faster the infusion will flow. Appropriate guidelines are given in the accompanying box.

If the insertion site allows a great deal of patient movement, the solution can flow alternately faster or slower depending on the position of the insertion site, for example, when a patient has an insertion site in the lower arm that can be freely movable. If the insertion site allows the catheter to become kinked, the solution will flow more slowly. In some instances, immobilization of the insertion site is desirable to allow a regulated flow. An arm board can be attached to the lower arm, for example, that will keep the insertion site stable but will not restrict arm movement completely.

A slower rate of infusion is usually necessary for an older person, a small child, a patient with kidney or heart disease, or a patient with a head injury. A rapid rate of infusion may cause circulatory overload (or increased intracranial pressure) in these patients. However, a faster rate of infusion is usually desirable for a person who has lost body fluids, as for example, from diarrhea or vomiting, or for a patient who cannot eat for a short period, as for example, immediately after surgery.

Every effort should be made to make the patient receiving an infusion as comfortable as possible.

Nursing Skill Guidelines
Calculation of IV Infusion Rate

◆ If you are not using an intravenous controller, you need to calculate infusion rates. The formula is:

$$\frac{\text{Flow Rate}}{\text{(drops/min)}} = \frac{\text{mL solution}}{\text{hours to administer}}$$
$$\times \frac{\text{DRF (drops per mL)}}{60 \ \text{(min/h)}}$$

◆ OR: Divide mL/hour (ordered) by 60 = mL/min. and multiply by DRF (drops/mL) = drops per minute.

◆ The *drip rate factor* (DRF) varies with the tubing used. This is stated on the box. Most common DRFs are 15 drops/mL or 10 drops/mL. The Microdrip has a standard of 60 drops/mL.

◆ After the drip rate is determined, the intravenous bag is taped and labeled for each hour to double-check your calculations. Frequent checking of the taped information is needed to keep the infusion on time.

When the infusion is completed, the catheter is withdrawn from the vein and pressure is applied with a gauze pad over the puncture site for a short time to prevent oozing of blood. The nurse should wear gloves for the procedure to maintain universal precautions and avoid exposure to blood. A bandage is then applied to the site.

Intravenous Solutions

The most commonly used intravenous solutions are dextrose in water (5% solution in sterile water, called D_5W), 5% dextrose in 0.25% normal saline ($D_5\frac{1}{4}NS$), and 5% dextrose in 0.45% normal saline ($D_5\frac{1}{2}NS$). Also used is a solution of 5% dextrose in normal saline (D_5NS), and normal saline solution (NS, 0.9% NaCl). Normal saline is the *only* solution to be used in conjunction with a blood transfusion. Ringer's solution and Ringer's lactate may be used in the operating room or emergency department. The physician is responsible for ordering the exact type of intravenous solution and the rate at which it is to be given. It is the nurse's responsibility to check the solution to be used with the physician's order. If drugs or electrolytes are to be added, this is usually done by the pharmacy.

Intravenous Drugs

Many drugs, including antibiotics, electrolytes, and vitamins, are commonly added to an intravenous infusion. Most hospital pharmacies add the drugs ordered by the physician to the intravenous solution. Medications may be added to intravenous solutions in a laminar flow hood, which reduces the risk of contamination. Because of the growing number of drugs administered intravenously and the dangers of drug incompatibilities, having the pharmacy personnel prepare the solutions reduces the chances of dangerous drug or electrolyte combinations and of errors in mixing medications. If nurses are going to add medications to infusions, in-service instruction is needed.

Piggyback Administration of Drugs. Frequently, medications are given intermittently through the intravenous infusion. You may hear this practice referred to as "IV piggybacks" or abbreviated as IVPB. The ordered medication is diluted into a predetermined amount of compatible solution in a separate infusion bottle or bag. This is usually done by the pharmacy. It is then connected with special tubing and a needle or needleless setup to the primary infusion system and administered over a period of 20 to 30 minutes or as ordered (Fig. 57-7).

Intravenous tubing is often set up so that the piggyback can be added and the flow begun and when the piggyback is completed, the system automatically switches back to the main solution bag. (It is not necessary to open or close clamps to divert the flow; the relative pressures of the solution in the bags will change the flow from the empty piggyback bag to the main bag.) If this type of setup is not available, the nurse will need to watch. When the drug is completely infused, close the clamp on that tube and *switch* back to the main infusion.

Nursing Considerations

The patient who is receiving intravenous therapy must be monitored for adverse reactions to the infusion (see the accompanying box). The following are nursing skill guidelines for monitoring the patient who is receiving intravenous therapy.

◆ Watch for adverse reactions. One such problem is **infiltration**, in which the IV solution is infusing into tissues instead of the vein (see box).
◆ Make at least hourly checks of the rate, the tubing connections, amount and type of solution present.

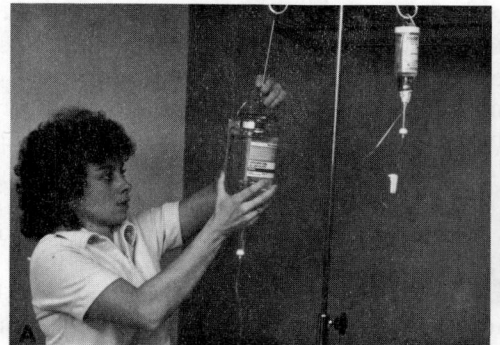
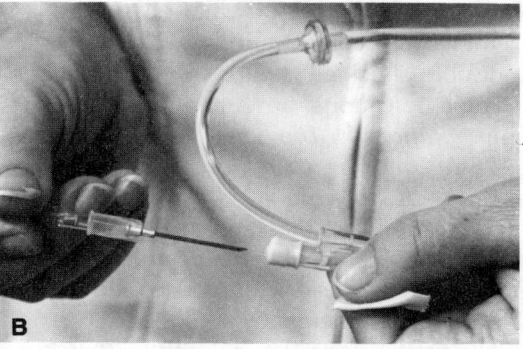

Figure 57-7. Preparing for piggyback infusion. **(A)** The medication in the small container on the side will infuse before the solution in the lower container. **(B)** A needle is used to connect the secondary tubing with the primary tubing.

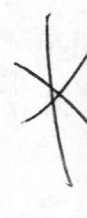

Nursing Alert

Watch for adverse reactions in intravenous therapy
- Infiltration
  - Area feels cold and hard to the touch
  - Pain and burning sensation at the site
  - Blood does not return in the tubing when the bag is lowered below the level of the patient
  - Edema
  - White, raised area on the arm
  - Flow rate may or may not be slow
- Fluid overload
  - Increased pulse rate
  - Dyspnea
  - Increased blood pressure
  - Engorged neck veins
- Inflammation or **phlebitis**
  - Redness and warmth along the vein
  - Pain or burning sensation at the site
  - Slow flow rate
  - Tenderness
  - Edema of the vein above the insertion site
  - Hardened feel to the vein
- Infection
  - Fever
  - Chills
  - Redness, swelling, or discharge at the insertion site
  - Malaise

If you see any of these signs, discontinue the intravenous infusion as soon as possible and notify the physician; for infiltration, apply moist, warm packs to the area.

If using an electronic infusion device (pump or controller), check that all settings are correct.
- Safeguard the site and be aware of tubing and pump during transfers, ambulation, or other activities. If a pump is not being used, remember that the system works on the principle of gravity. If the bag of solution is too low, blood will flow up the tubing and may cause complications.
- Be sure to double-check all clamps when changing tubing, adding medications, or removing the line from a pump. *(Rationale: The patient may inadvertently receive an overdose of medication or fluid that could be life-threatening.)*
- Always check to make sure that medications, solutions, or additives are compatible before adding anything to the solution. Nurses usually do not add to IV solutions, except in an emergency or in the ICU.
- Protect the site from getting wet or soiled. *(Rationale: This reduces the risk of infection.)*
- If the patient will be off the unit for tests or procedures unaccompanied, be sure there is adequate

solution to be infused while the patient will be away. *(Rationale: Do not depend on the personnel in another department to do this because they may not have the training to maintain the infusion.)*

The Heparin Lock

Many patients have a heparin lock ("hep lock") in place. A heparin lock is an intravenous catheter that is inserted into a vein and left in place. A sterile plug is attached to the end of the catheter, through which medications can be given. About 2 mL of the drug heparin or normal saline is instilled into the apparatus about every 8 hours to prevent clotting at the insertion site. With a heparin lock in place, a new venipuncture does not need to be done each time an intravenous medication is to be given. The heparin lock also removes the necessity for a continuously running intravenous line when that therapy is no longer needed. Many times, patients are sent home with a heparin lock.

Hospital protocol is carefully followed for a heparin lock. The physician prescribes the medication and dose. In some hospitals, a "heparin lock kit" is available, which contains prefilled syringes, two containing normal saline and one containing a dilute heparin solution. An example of a protocol for giving a medication by heparin lock is outlined in Nursing Procedure 57-5.

Total Parenteral Nutrition

Total parenteral nutrition (TPN), or total parenteral alimentation (TPA), was formerly known as *hyperalimentation*. TPN is a method by which large quantities of fluids and nutrients are administered to a patient. By this means, the desired levels of carbohydrates, proteins, fats, vitamins, minerals, water, and electrolytes can be provided. The infusion of TPN requires an intravenous line in a large blood vessel, such as the subclavian vein (called a *central line*). Insertion of a central line is performed by a physician, under aseptic conditions. The insertion site must also be kept sterile and is cared for as described in the agency protocol. (Hospital LPNs usually do not work with central lines.) The nutritive solution is concentrated and could cause irritation, clots, or swelling if given into a smaller vessel. The high concentration of dextrose also provides an excellent medium for bacterial growth.

Nursing Considerations. The nurse must observe certain precautions in caring for the patient who is receiving TPN. Aseptic technique must be followed during changes of bottles, tubing, filters, or dressings. Because the catheter is in a major blood vessel, infection would spread rapidly throughout the body. Dressings at the insertion site must be kept clean to prevent bacteremia (presence of bacteria in the blood). Vital

Administering Medication by Heparin Lock

Supplies and Equipment

Medication
Medication card, Kardex, or computer record
Alcohol swabs
Gloves
Watch with second hand

For Flush

Saline vial
Heparin flush solution
Syringes (2–3) with 21–25-gauge needle

For Bolus Injection

Syringe with 21–25-gauge needle or needleless equipment

For Intermittent Infusion

IV bag or bottle with 50–100 mL solution
IV tubing
Tape
21–23-gauge needle or needleless equipment
IV pole
IV pump (optional)

Procedure

1. Wash hands.
   (Rationale: Handwashing prevents the spread of organisms.)
2. Gather equipment. Use medication Kardex, cards, or computer record to verify medication order. Check any inconsistency with physician or pharmacist.
   (Rationale: Organization facilitates performance of the skill and reduces the chance of medication error.)
3. Unlock medication cart or drawer. Check expiration date on medication.
   (Rationale: Keeping medication setup locked provides security if the area is unattended. Outdated medication may be ineffective.)

For Bolus Injection

4. Prepare medication. If necessary, withdraw from ampule or vial according to Nursing Procedure 57-2.
   (Rationale: Preparation of medication before entering patient's room facilitates administration.)
5. Explain procedure to patient.
   (Rationale: Providing information fosters patient cooperation.)
6. Identify the patient before giving the medication. Refer to step 11, Nursing Procedure 57-1.
   (Rationale: Medication may be administered to the wrong patient if identity is not established.)

7. Put on gloves.
   (Rationale: Gloves act as a barrier.)
8. Cleanse heparin lock port with alcohol swab.
   (Rationale: Antiseptic removes surface contaminant and decreases potential for introducing microorganisms into the system.)

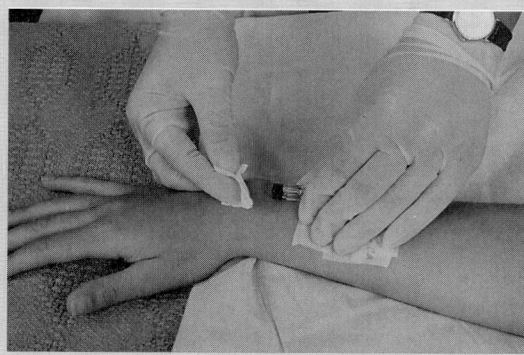

Step 8   Cleansing the port with an alcohol swab

9. Steady heparin lock with nondominant hand. Insert needle of syringe containing 1 mL saline into center of port. Aspirate for possible blood return. Flush lock with saline. Remove needle and discard syringe in sharps container without recapping it.
   (Rationale: Saline clears tubing of any heparin flush or previous medication. Blood return on aspiration generally indicates that catheter is positioned in vein although blood return does not always occur. Most accidental sticks occur when recapping a needle. Proper disposal prevents injury.)

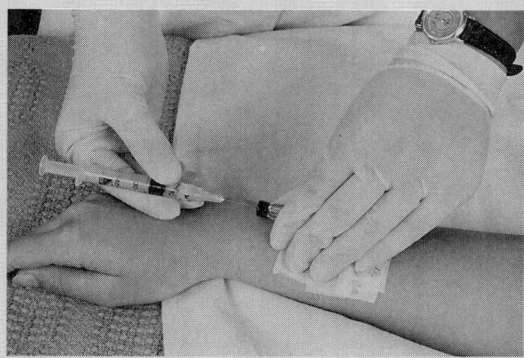

Step 9   Inserting the syringe with the saline flush

(continued)

10. Cleanse port again with alcohol swab. Insert needle of syringe containing medication. Inject medication slowly according to prescribed rate, using watch with second hand. Withdraw the syringe and dispose of properly.
    (Rationale: Rapid injection of medication can lead to speed shock.)

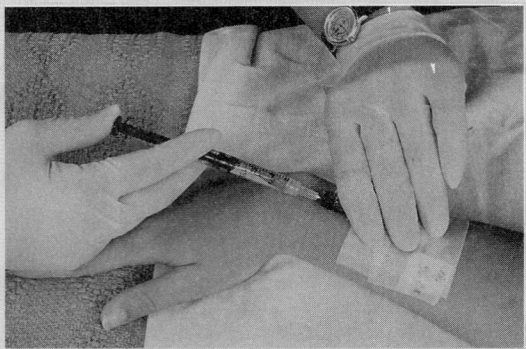

Step 10 Timing the administration of IV medication

11. Cleanse port with alcohol swab. Flush lock with 1 mL heparin flush followed by 1 mL saline, or according to agency policy. Some agencies recommend only a saline flush to clear the lock.
    (Rationale: Flush clears the lock of medication and keeps it patent.)

For Intermittent Infusion

12. Use premixed solution in bag. Connect tubing and add needle or needleless component. Prime tubing with solution.
    (Rationale: Preparation of medication before entering patient's room facilitates administration.)
13. Follow steps 5–9 for bolus injection through heparin lock.)

14. Cleanse port again with alcohol swab. Insert needle or needleless component attached to IV setup into port. Attach to IV infusion pump or calculate flow rate and regulate drip according to prescribed delivery time. Clamp the tubing and withdraw the needle when all solution has been infused. Follow agency policy regarding disposal of equipment.
    (Rationale: Rapid injection of medication can lead to speed shock.)

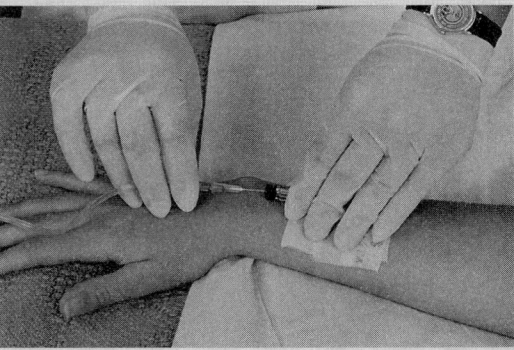

Step 14 Connecting an intermittent infusion set-up to a heparin lock
(Photos © B. Proud.)

15. Repeat step 11 for bolus injection through heparin lock. *(Rationale: Ensures that all medication has been given.)*
16. Remove gloves and wash hands.
    (Rationale: Handwashing prevents the spread of organisms.)
17. Record IV medication administration on the appropriate form and heparin and/or saline flush. Record fluid volume in bag (often 50 mL) on intake and output record.
    (Rationale: Documentation provides coordination of care.)
18. Check on patient response to medication within appropriate period of time.
    (Rationale: Drugs administered parenterally have a more rapid response.)

signs must be checked frequently for evidence of a developing infection. Guidelines are given in the accompanying box.

The catheter must be taped securely at the insertion site to prevent it from being dislodged. All connections must be secure. Put a piece of tape on each connection; then bridge with another piece of tape for safety. Fold over each end of each piece of tape, to facilitate removal. Transparent dressings over the catheter inser-

tion site facilitate observation of the site. This dressing is usually left in place unless it is soiled. Your facility may use "click-lock" or Luer-Lok syringes and tubings to help ensure the connections are secure. This will ensure that no air can enter the tubing; an air embolism would be a serious or fatal complication.

Because TPN solutions contain a high concentration of glucose, a patient's blood is usually tested for glucose several times a day. Excess glucose usually indicates that

Nursing Skill Guidelines
Caring for the Patient With an Intravenous or TPN Line

◆ Check the insertion site for redness, swelling, or tenderness at least every 8 hours. *Document* that the site has been checked and document the condition of the site.

◆ Run TPN through a filter in the tubing; do *not* run lipids (fats) through the filter.

◆ If there is any difficulty, report it at once. The physician may order the intravenous line or TPN to be discontinued or to be irrigated.

◆ Change intravenous dressings every 72 hours (unless the hospital or nursing home has a policy otherwise). Change the dressing if it becomes wet or contaminated with drainage.

◆ Change intravenous tubing every 72 hours or as per agency protocol. Mark it so others will know when it was last changed.

◆ Wear gloves when changing dressings or tubing.

◆ The fewer times the nurses handle dressings, the lower the risk of infection.

◆ There are two types of dressings; gauze and transparent. Some hospitals use both types, based on the insertion site of the intravenous line.

---

the body is unable to use all of the available carbohydrates. The rate of infusion for TPN must be constant to prevent episodes of hypoglycemia or hyperglycemia. Most hospitals use an electronic infusion pump to regulate the rate of infusion. Intake and output of fluid must be measured accurately and the patient must be weighed daily; all of these must be recorded accurately.

Most hospitals follow a special protocol for the care of the patient receiving TPN. Be sure to follow the nursing procedures in your facility.

Long-Term Infusion

The Hickman catheter is a type of *intravascular* (within the blood vessel) device, which in inserted into the superior vena cava. The Hickman catheter is used for patients who will need an intravenous or TPN infusion for a long time. The advantage of the Hickman is its lower risk of infection or infiltration because of its deeper placement.

A similar device is the *implantable* device, such as the Infusaport or Portacath. This catheter is placed in the superior vena cava. However, it has a port just below the skin surface in the subcutaneous tissue, where medications are infused. This device is often used for cancer chemotherapy. (Administration of chemotherapy is discussed in Chapter 76.)

Another type of catheter is the percutaneous intravenous central catheter (PICC). This type of catheter is inserted at the antecubital site and threaded up the vein to a large central vein. The length is determined by measuring the patient's arm to the central location; it may be well over a foot in length. These lines can remain in place for weeks or months with similar advantages to the Hickman catheter. However, it does restrict the use of the arm because excessive use can cause outward migration of the line or irritation at the insertion site.

Nursing Alert

◆ The administration of blood is called a *transfusion.*

◆ Blood and drugs are *not* administrated together.

◆ Drugs are *never* to be added to a blood transfusion.

Administering Drugs to Children

Chapter 64 discusses medication administration to children. Keep in mind that a child can tolerate only a fraction of the adult dosage of a drug; therefore, drug overdoses and drug errors are more apt to occur in children. Because a child is also more likely to be allergic to drugs, the nurse should be watchful for any untoward reaction.

The nurse may be required to calculate pediatric doses because most medications are packaged in adult doses. In-house pharmacies may not provide premeasured pediatric doses. Pediatric doses are usually calculated based on body surface area, using the child's height and weight, as applied to the "West Nomogram." Generally, these calculations are made by the physician, but you should be able to determine if the dose is correct. The most common way for pediatric drugs to be ordered is milligrams of medication per kilogram of body weight (mg/kg). Review a copy of your facility's protocol before administering any medications to children.

Unit *12* Maternal and Newborn Nursing

three types of cells will ultimately form the fetus and its adjoining structures.

Amniotic Fluid. Other cells in this cavity eventually form a fluid-filled sac (the **amnion**) in which the embryo floats. The fluid in the amnion (*amniotic fluid*) has the following functions:

♦ It helps cushion the fetus against injury.
♦ It regulates temperature.
♦ It allows free fetal movement.

An excess of amniotic fluid (>2,000 mL) is called **hydramnios**; over 5000 mL is usually called *polyhydramnios.* These may be an indication of fetal abnormalities. A test called an *amniocentesis* may be done to determine fetal abnormalities or fetal lung maturity. It involves obtaining a sample of amniotic fluid from the pregnant woman by puncturing the abdomen. Because of the risks involved, an amniocentesis is not done merely to determine the sex of the fetus, although the sex of the fetus is revealed by the procedure.

Sex Chromosomes. The sex is determined by the father's sperm at the time of fertilization. A female ovum carries only one type of chromosome to determine sex; it is called X. A male sperm cell may carry either an X or Y sex chromosome. If the ovum is fertilized by a sperm cell carrying a Y chromosome, the fetus will be a boy (XY); if the sperm cell carries an X chromosome, the fetus will be a girl (XX).

Fetal Circulation

In utero, the fetus is attached to the placenta by the umbilical cord, which consists of two arteries and one large vein twisted about each other (Fig. 58-1). Circulation in the fetus differs from circulation in the newborn. The fetus secures oxygen and food from the woman's blood, instead of using its own lungs and digestive system; however, because the fetal and the maternal blood are in separate capillaries and do not mix, there must be a place where the interchange of gases, food, and wastes can take place. This occurs in the *placenta*. Fetal capillaries in the placenta are surrounded by maternal capillaries, and the exchanges take place across the capillary membranes. In this way, the woman's blood supplies food and carries off wastes from the fetus. The placenta will be expelled from the uterus following the birth of the newborn; in this context, it is called the *afterbirth.*

Deoxygenated blood from the fetus is returned to the placenta through the two umbilical arteries. The oxygenated blood is returned to the fetus from the placenta by a single vessel, the umbilical vein. This is another *exception* to the classification that all arteries carry oxygenated (bright red) blood, and all veins carry deoxygenated (dark red) blood. These three vessels are intertwined and make up the *umbilical cord,* which is approximately 20 inches (51 cm) long. The cord is protected by a soft, jellylike substance called *Wharton's jelly* and enters the fetus' body approximately in the middle of the abdomen at the *umbilicus (navel).* Some of the oxygenated blood from the umbilical vein passes through the fetal liver, while the majority enters the inferior vena cava through the ductus venosis, a structure unique to fetal circulation. From the inferior vena cava, the blood flows into the right atrium.

Because the lungs are not functioning yet, the bulk of blood is shunted to the left atrium of the heart. This shunt occurs through another fetal structure, the *foramen ovale.* The foramen ovale is an opening between the right and left atria, and it permits the majority of blood to bypass the right ventricle. A small portion of blood passes from the right atrium to the right ventricle and makes its way into the pulmonary artery. It is then shunted through the ductus arteriosus, a connection between the pulmonary artery and aorta that allows shunting of blood around the fetal lungs.

Normally, with the newborn's first few respirations, the lungs are expanded, because the pressure within the thorax is altered. The foramen ovale closes, and the ductus arteriosus and ductus venosus shrivel up and become fibrous ligaments. A congenital heart defect in a child occurs if these events do not take place. These defects and their treatment are discussed in Chapters 62 and 65.

Fetal Vulnerability. The fetus is vulnerable to a number of potentially harmful influences that could result in *congenital* (present at birth) defects. The basic embryonic structure is determined by genes, so a defective gene may be responsible for certain congenital defects. Environmental factors also can cause congenital anomalies. These environmental factors are discussed later in this chapter.

Fetal Development

Normal fetal growth and development follow a definite and predictable pattern. For example, growth and development, before and after birth, follows the *cephalocaudal* (head to toe) principle. Each fetus grows at its own rate, however. The *average rates* of fetal development are described and illustrated in the accompanying box. The typical 9-calendar-month pregnancy is divided into 3-month segments, referred to as **trimesters.**

Birth Weight. The newborn's heredity and the mother's nutritional status have some influence on the neonate's weight at birth. A newborn weighing 10 lb (4,540 g) or more is often difficult to deliver. However, the

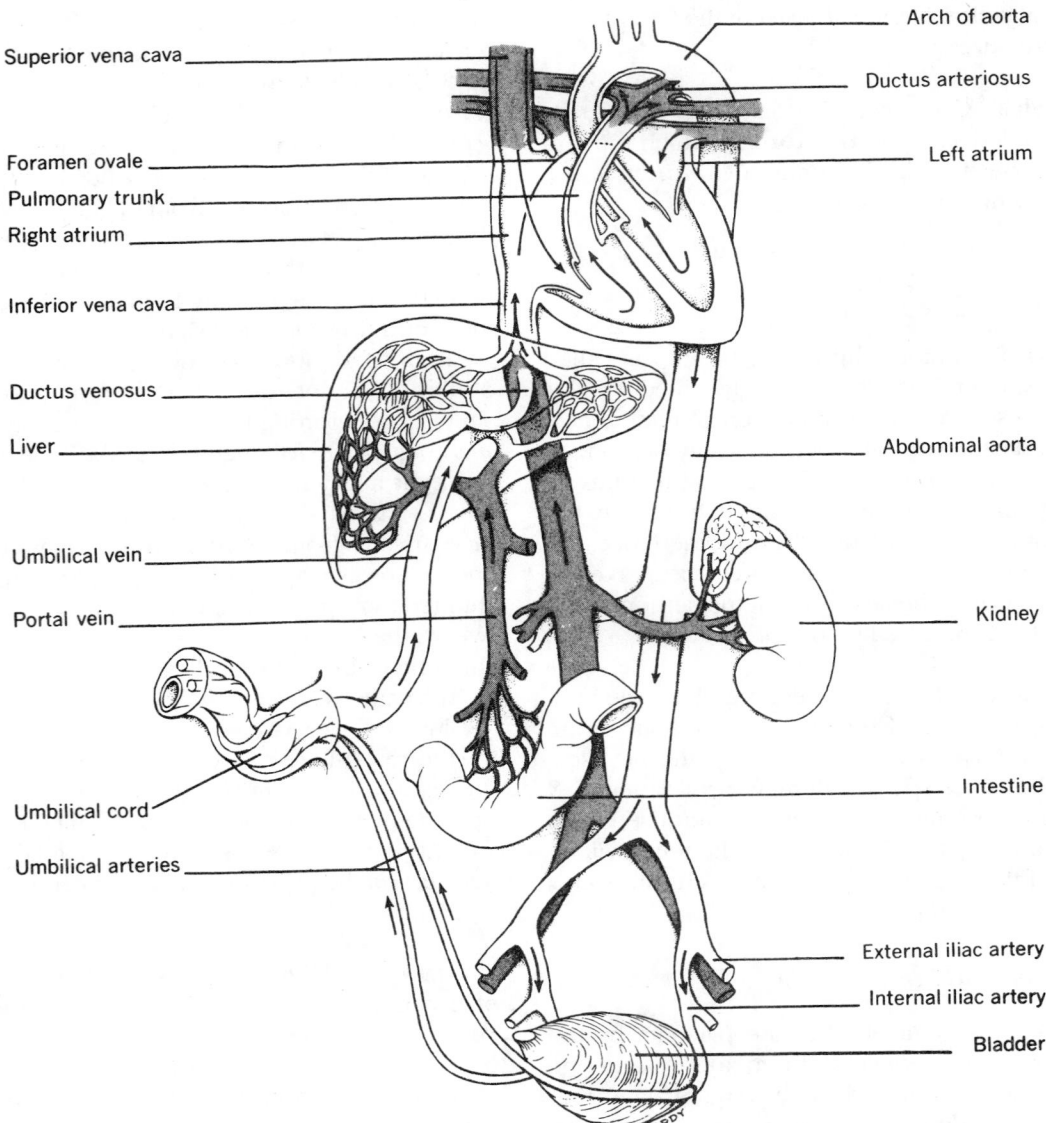

Figure 58-1. Diagram of fetal circulation shortly before birth; the course of blood is indicated by arrows. The baby's blood travels through the blood vessels in the umbilical cord to and from the placenta, where exchanges of gases (oxygen and carbon dioxide) and digestive products (nutrients and wastes) take place. Here is an exception to the rule of veins and arteries: The fetal umbilical arteries carry deoxygenated blood, and the umbilical vein carries oxygenated blood.

smaller the child at birth, the less likely the chances are of survival. A newborn weighing less than 2⅕ lb (1,000 g) is considered immature. With today's neonatal intensive care units, however, chances for survival of very small newborns are improving. Birth weight problems are discussed in Chapter 62.

Multiple Births. In some cases, more than one fetus is the product of a single pregnancy. This is known as a multiple birth. The most common multiple birth is that of twins (occurring in approximately 1 in 100 births).

Other less common multiple births include triplets (three babies), quadruplets (four babies), quintuplets (five babies), and so on. With the use of fertility drugs, multiple births with more than two babies occur more often than in the past.

Multiple births can be identical or fraternal. *Identical* twins develop from a single ovum, fertilized by a single sperm cell. This single fertilized ovum splits after fertilization, developing into two or more babies instead of one. Identical twins must be the same sex, and there is usually one shared placenta.

Fraternal twins develop from two ova, each of which is fertilized by a separate sperm cell. There are two placentas. Fraternal twins may look alike or may look different from each other. In some cases, blood tests are the only way to be sure if twins are identical or fraternal. Twins of the opposite sex are always fraternal.

Signs and Symptoms of Pregnancy

The signs and symptoms of pregnancy are customarily divided into three categories: presumptive, probable, and positive (Table 58-1).

Presumptive symptoms appear early and may be noted only by the patient (subjective). For this reason, they are often referred to as *symptoms*. While pregnancy may be presumed, these symptoms may indicate other conditions as well. Probable signs and symptoms also appear early in pregnancy but are more objective. Often, the probable signs can be observed by medical personnel and by the patient herself. While probable signs are more definite than the presumptive symptoms, they still are not absolute. Positive signs are definite proof of an existing pregnancy.

Presumptive Symptoms of Pregnancy

Presumptive symptoms of pregnancy involve body changes, largely as a result of changes in hormone levels.

Amenorrhea. Absence of menstruation is often one of the first indications of pregnancy, but a missed menstrual period does not always signify conception.

Morning Sickness. Nausea may begin soon after the first missed menstrual period and usually disappears by the third month of pregnancy. Approximately 50% of all pregnant women experience some nausea or vomiting. Although it is called morning sickness because it occurs most commonly at this time, this nausea or vomiting may occur any time during the day. If this condition lasts beyond the fourth month, is excessive (**hyperemesis gravidarum**), or affects the general health of the woman, it is considered a complication of pregnancy. This will be discussed in Chapter 61.

Frequent Urination. When the enlarging uterus presses against the urinary bladder, it may cause the woman to feel the need to urinate more frequently. As the uterus rises into the abdominal cavity, the pressure is relieved, and the condition usually subsides until quite late in the pregnancy.

Changes in the Breasts. Many of the breast changes that occur in pregnancy are similar to those that are present during the normal menstrual cycle, just before the menstrual flow begins. They include enlargement, heaviness, tingling, throbbing, or tenderness. As the preg-

Average Fetal Development

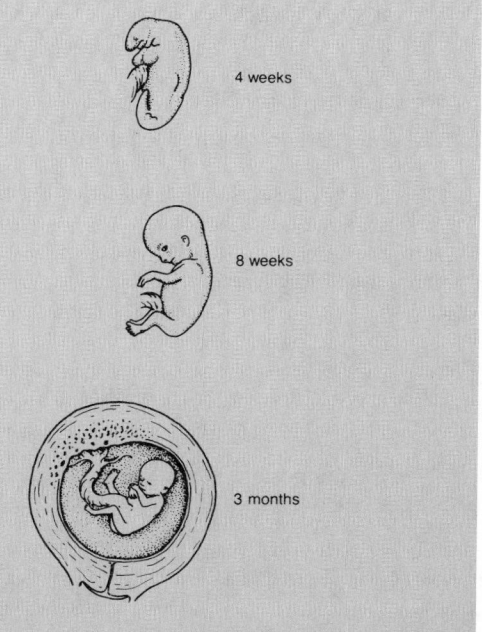

First Lunar Month

The fetus is 0.75 to 1 cm in length.
Trophoblasts embed in decidua.
Chorionic villi form.
Foundations for nervous system, genitourinary system, skin, bones, and lungs form.
Buds of arms and legs begin to form.
Rudiments of eyes, ears, and nose appear.

4 weeks

Second Lunar Month

The fetus is 2.5 to 5 cm in length and weighs 4 g.
Fetus is markedly bent.
Head is disproportionately large, due to brain development.
Sex differentiation begins.
Centers of bone begin to ossify.

8 weeks

Third Lunar Month

The fetus is 7 to 9 cm in length and weighs 28 g.
Fingers and toes are distinct.
Placenta is complete.
Fetal circulation is complete.

3 months

(continued)

Average Fetal Development (continued)

Fourth Lunar Month

The fetus is 10 to 17 cm in length and weighs 55 to 120 g.
Sex is differentiated.
Rudimentary kidneys secrete urine.
Heart beat is present.
Nasal septum and palate close.

Fifth Lunar Month

The fetus is 25 cm in length and weighs 223 g.
Lanugo covers entire body.
Fetal movements are felt by mother.
Heart sounds are perceptible by auscultation

Sixth Lunar Month

The fetus is 28 to 35 cm in length and weighs 680 g.
Skin appears wrinkled.
Vernix caseosa appears.
Eyebrows and fingernails develop.

Seventh Lunar Month

The fetus is 36 to 38 cm in length and weighs 1200 g.
Skin is red.
Pupillary membrane disappears from eyes.
The fetus has an excellent chance of survival if born now.

Eighth Lunar Month

The fetus is 38 to 42 cm in length and weighs 2.7 kg.
Fetus is viable.
Eyelids can open and close.
Fingerprints are set.
Vigorous fetal movement occurs.

Ninth Lunar Month

The fetus is 43 to 49 cm in length and weighs 1,900 to
2,700 g.
Face and body have a loose wrinkled appearance because
of subcutaneous fat deposit.
Lanugo disappears.
Amniotic fluid decreases.

Tenth Lunar Month

The fetus is 48 to 52 cm in length and weighs about
3,000 g.
Skin is smooth.
Eyes are uniformly slate colored.
Bones of skull are ossified and nearly together at sutures.

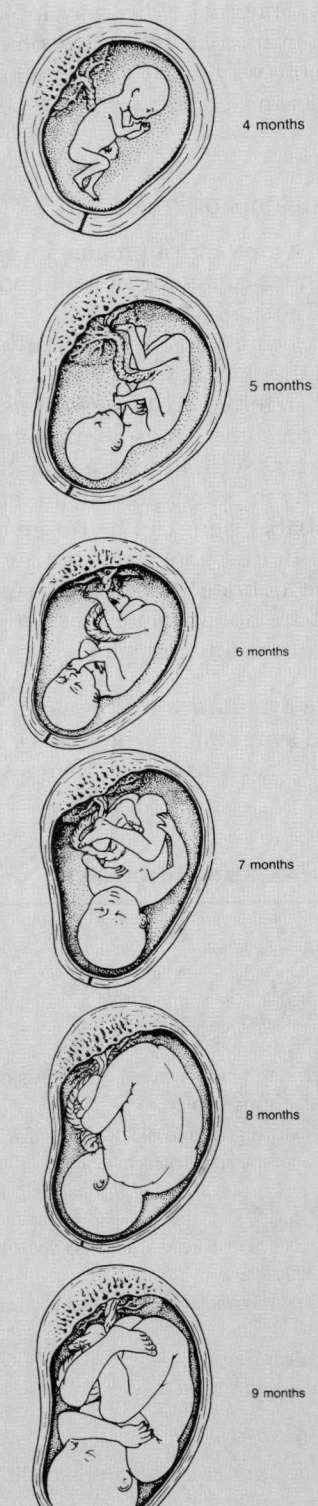

4 months

5 months

6 months

7 months

8 months

9 months

Table 58-1. Signs and Symptoms of Pregnancy

	Presumptive Symptoms	***Probable Signs and Symptoms***	***Positive Signs***
1–4 wk	Amenorrhea Nausea (ends by 12th wk) Frequent urination (absent in second trimester, recurs in third trimester) Fatigue	Basal body temperature elevation Positive urine pregnancy test RIA test positive	Ultrasound can diagnose pregnancy at 4 wk
6–8 wk		Chadwick's sign Goodell's sign Hegar's sign Softening and flexion of uterine fundus	
About 10–12 wk		Uterus at level of symphysis pubis	Fetal heart tones (FHT) heard faintly Ultrasound can measure FHT
18–20 wk	Quickening	Ballotement	FHT heard distinctly
20–24 wk		Uterus at umbilicus	Fetal movement felt by examiner
Other	Breast changes Chloasma Linea nigra	Enlargement of abdomen	

nancy progresses, the areolar tissues and the nipples enlarge and darken.

Fatigue. During the early months of pregnancy, the woman may experience drowsiness and a tendency to tire easily. She may find that she requires more rest and sleep than usual.

Pigmentation Changes. Skin changes occur as a result of pregnancy. In addition to changes in the breasts, a suntanned, bronzed masking may appear across the face of dark-haired women and is known as **chloasma** or *melasma* (chloasma gravidarum), or the "mask of pregnancy." A definite pigmentation of the abdomen often appears as a dark line extending from the umbilicus to the pubis and is known as the **linea nigra.**

Key Abbreviations Used in Pregnancy

BBT	Basal body temperature
EDD	Estimated date of delivery
FHT	Fetal heart tones
G (I, II, III)	Gravida (number of pregnancies)
HCG	Human chorionic gonadotropin
LMP	Last menstrual period
PIH	Pregnancy-induced hypertension
RIA	Radioimmunoassay

These changes in skin color are a result of alterations in hormonal levels.

Quickening. The first movements of the fetus felt by the expectant woman are called **quickening.** This is first experienced toward the end of the fifth lunar month (18th–20th week) of gestation. It is described as a light, "fluttery" sensation. This "feeling of life" is not a positive sign of pregnancy, because it cannot be corroborated objectively by anyone other than the woman and because it can be simulated by movement of gas within the colon.

Probable Signs of Pregnancy

The probable signs are more objective and are more likely to be observed by a physician or midwife during examination. They are more certain than the presumptive signs of pregnancy.

Basal Body Temperature Elevation. Elevation of basal body temperature is one of the earliest signs of pregnancy. However, to be accurate, the temperature must have been taken and recorded before pregnancy occurred so that comparisons can be made.

Positive Urine Pregnancy Tests. Most pregnancy tests are based on the fact that the hormone human chorionic gonadotropin (HCG) is secreted by the chorionic villi of the placenta. This hormone can be detected in small amounts in the urine and the blood of a pregnant woman by about the 15th day of pregnancy. Urine tests are available for home use and offer quick results with 90% to 95% accuracy.

Positive Radioimmunoassay (RAI). This is a blood test that is performed in the laboratory and is completed in approximately 1 hour. It is fairly reliable and can determine pregnancy approximately 8 days after conception.

Cervical Changes. At 6 to 8 weeks' gestation, a marked softening of the cervix takes place. This is known as *Goodell's sign.* (Before pregnancy, the cervix feels like the tip of the nose; during pregnancy, it feels like the earlobe.)

Uterine Changes. At 6 to 8 weeks' gestation, the lower uterine segment (between the body of the uterus and the cervix) softens. This softening is called *Hegar's sign.* There is also a softening of the fundus of the uterus at about 6 to 7 weeks' gestation and a flexion of the fundus at about 7 to 8 weeks' gestation. Enlargement of the uterus also is an important aid to the diagnosis of pregnancy. It occurs steadily throughout the pregnancy. The uterus rises above the symphysis pubis by 12 weeks' gestation and reaches the umbilicus by the 20th to the 24th week.

Vaginal Changes. Increased blood supply to the vaginal area during pregnancy results in a visible color change of the mucous membrane. The tissue develops a dark violet hue and is known as *Chadwick's sign.* This generally occurs in about the sixth week of gestation.

Ballottement. Gentle tapping of the abdomen of the pregnant woman will cause the fetus to "bounce" in the amniotic fluid. This rebound reaction can be felt by the examiner. **Ballottement** appears at approximately 16 to 18 weeks' gestation when the fetus is small compared with the quantity of amniotic fluid.

Enlargement of the Abdomen. As the uterus increases in size, the abdomen is forced outward. As the abdomen enlarges, the posture and gait of the woman is altered as well.

Positive Signs of Pregnancy

When the following signs are present, there is an unquestionable diagnosis of pregnancy.

Fetal Heart Beat. The fetal heart beat (*fetal heart tones*) can be detected by using either Doppler ultrasound or a special stethoscope called a fetoscope. Fetal heart tones can be heard faintly by a skilled examiner as early as 11 to 12 weeks' gestation. They can be heard more distinctly by the 18th to 20th week of gestation. Normal fetal heart rates range from 120 to 160 beats per minute.

When assessing the fetal heart rate, the examiner must be aware of two other audible sounds to avoid confusion. The *funic souffle* is a swishing sound produced by the pulsation of blood as it is propelled through the umbilical cord. Its rate is the same as the *fetal* heart rate. The *uterine souffle* is a swishing sound produced by the maternal blood as it flows through the large vessels of the uterus. Its rate is the same as the *woman's* heart rate. (Thus, the examiner feels the woman's radial pulse at the same time as he or she assesses the fetal heart rate.)

Ultrasonography Examination. The most common instrument used to evaluate fetal heart tones, fetal size, and estimated due date is the *Doppler ultrasound.* The Doppler converts ultrasonic frequencies (high-frequency sound waves) into audible frequencies or onto a video monitor. It can diagnose pregnancy as early as the fourth week of gestation and allows fetal heart rates to be heard by the 11th week of gestation. The ultrasound is safe, painless, and relatively inexpensive.

Fetal Movement Felt by Examiner. An examiner or nurse may be able to feel fetal movement by about the fourth or fifth month of pregnancy. At first the movements are felt faintly, but as the fetus grows and muscle strength increases, the movements become stronger. It is important to differentiate these fetal movements from other movements within the woman's body.

Prenatal and Antepartal Care

Prenatal refers to the period between conception and the birth of the newborn, while **antepartal** refers to the period between conception and the onset of labor. Theoretically, antepartal would be the correct term for the discussion in this chapter. The two are often used interchangeably, and because prenatal still seems to have wide usage, it is retained here.

The goal of good prenatal care is the maximum physical and mental fitness of the woman with the reward of an uncomplicated delivery and a healthy mother and newborn. Because the public has become so aware of the value of prenatal care, a woman often seeks care as soon as she suspects that she is pregnant. In recent years, emphasis has been placed on premarital and prepregnancy examination to encourage positive maternal and child health.

Consulting a Practitioner

The practitioner begins to care for the woman by taking a complete history of the woman and her partner to learn about their past illnesses and whether there is a familial susceptibility to certain diseases, such as Tay-Sachs, diabetes, and sickle cell anemia, which can affect the pregnancy. The practitioner is interested in learning whether a multiple pregnancy has occurred in either family. He or she must know of any difficulties experienced by the woman during previous pregnancies or deliveries. The obstetric history of the woman's mother also may be significant. The medical and obstetric history provides an accurate record of the patient's past and present health and gives the birth attendant pertinent data.

The First Visit

The partner should be encouraged to go with the woman on her first visit to the practitioner. It is helpful for him to be present at subsequent visits too so that he can hear firsthand what the practitioner says. Parenthood is a partnership in which both partners have an equal interest. Also, the woman might be encouraged to carry out her program if the father understands it.

The practitioner performs a complete physical examination of the woman, which includes the following:

◆ Head-to-toe assessment, including the gums, teeth, thyroid gland, heart, lungs, breasts, and all body systems
◆ Blood and urine tests, including blood type, Rh factor, and human immunodeficiency virus status
◆ Blood pressure and weight
◆ A pelvic examination, including a Pap test and a test for gonorrhea and syphilis
◆ Purified protein derivative test for tuberculosis
◆ Rubella titer to determine susceptibility to German measles

The practitioner examines the pelvic organs for signs of pregnancy and to take measurements. Pelvic measurements are needed to determine whether the bony passageway is wide enough for the newborn; this is especially important in a first pregnancy. The woman's blood type and Rh factor are determined. If the woman is Rh negative, she should receive RhoGAM at 28 weeks' gestation and following any invasive procedure (ie, amniocentesis) to prevent Rh isoimmunization.

A rubella titer is done to determine the woman's level of immunity to rubella (German measles). If she is not immune, she is not vaccinated during pregnancy because the rubella vaccine is live and can have a teratogenic effect on the fetus. This condition is discussed further in Chapters 61 and 62.

The urine is examined for albumin, sugar, and the presence of bacteria.

The practitioner advises the expectant woman about her diet and other health habits. She is told what she should observe about herself between visits and what she must report immediately (see the accompanying box).

Determining the Estimated Date of Delivery

It is desirable for the woman who thinks she is pregnant to consult a physician after one menstrual period has been missed. Many women do not keep an accurate rec-

---

Keys to Patient/Family Teaching
Danger Signs in Pregnancy to Report

◆ Excessive or irritating vaginal discharge
◆ Rupture of amniotic membrane
◆ Vaginal bleeding
◆ Swelling of extremities or face
◆ Dyspnea
◆ Blurred vision or spots before the eyes
◆ Dizziness or fainting
◆ Headaches
◆ Decrease in urine output
◆ Burning with urination
◆ Persistent vomiting
◆ Abdominal pain or severe back pain
◆ Chills
◆ Fever
◆ Chest pain
◆ Altered fetal movement
◆ Epigastric pain
◆ Lower abdominal pressure

---

ord of menstrual periods and often do not resume normal periods after discontinuing birth control pills. In these cases, the physician determines the estimated date of delivery (EDD), also called the estimated date of confinement (EDC), based on objective physical evidence.

A full-term pregnancy is (in theory) 280 days after the last menstrual period or 266 days after fertilization. The 280 days equal 40 weeks or 10 lunar (9 calendar) months; the 266 days equal about 9 calendar months. The duration of pregnancy is estimated by the practitioner using the first day of the last normal menstrual period.

Commonly used methods for determining EDD are:

◆ Nägele's rule: Count back 3 months from the first day of the last menstrual period and add 7 days. This method is quite accurate if the woman's menstrual cycle is regular.
◆ Measure the fetus using ultrasound.

The actual duration of pregnancy varies greatly, and one should remember that the EDD is an *estimated* due date. Only about 4% of women deliver on their estimated due date.

Routine Examinations

The pregnant woman will want to know the routine for her return visits to the birth attendant or midwife. Usually, the practitioner sees the expectant woman every 4 weeks up to 32 weeks' gestation, then every 2 weeks until the 36th week, then every week until delivery. If necessary, she will be seen more often. The practitioner will ask for a first-morning specimen of urine each time to check for the presence of protein, glucose, blood, and ketones; check her blood pressure and weight, and measure the fundal height to determine if the size is appropriate for gestational age.

Albumin in the urine may indicate pregnancy-induced hypertension a condition characterized by hypertension, edema, and proteinuria. In approximately the fourth month, an ultrasound is often done. Any other procedure will be determined by the patient's condition; a specific treatment given to one pregnant woman may not be necessary for another (see accompanying box).

Pregnancy is a normal process for which a woman's body is built. To help adjust to pregnancy, she must have the right food, enough rest, and adequate recreation and exercise. Generally, the woman can continue doing most things she did regularly before she became pregnant.

Nutritional Needs

Studies show that an newborn's chances for good health are greater with a reasonably high birth weight. The nutritional requirements of a pregnant woman are different from those of a nonpregnant woman. The woman's caloric needs increase during pregnancy because she has to meet energy requirements for fetal, placental, and maternal tissue development. Quality of diet, rather than quantity, is stressed however, and the pattern of weight gain is more important than the amount of weight gained.

The woman's daily food requirements are those of the food guide pyramid (see Chapter 26). In addition to the basic food guide pyramid, she should make the following adjustments to her diet:

- Increase caloric intake by approximately 300 calories daily.
- Increase calcium intake before the last half of the pregnancy; calcium is essential to the development of the fetus' bones and teeth and for blood clotting. Milk intake should be increased to 3 to 4 cups daily.
- Maintain iron intake; it is essential in the production of hemoglobin. Iron is stored by the fetus to be used after birth, because breast milk contains little iron. Most physicians order an iron supplement during pregnancy because of its importance in the diet.
- Folic acid (folate), a B vitamin, is given to help prevent congenital defects, most notably spina bifida. Four hundred mg daily is recommended; 200 mg from food and 200 mg as a supplemental vitamin.
- Increase intake of most vitamins. Many physicians prescribe supplemental vitamins during pregnancy.
- Increase protein intake; protein is essential for building and repair of all body tissues and aids in the production of milk for the nursing mother.
- Avoid empty calories. (This includes alcohol, sugared soda drinks and other sweets, and salty foods.)

Routine Screening Tests During Pregnancy

At 15 to 20 weeks, a triple screen test is recommended. This test measures the maternal serum levels of alpha-fetoprotein, estriol, and human chorionic gonadotropin. Abnormal levels of these substances may indicate the presence of abnormalities, such as neural tube defects or chromosomal disorders.

At 26 to 28 weeks, all patients should be screened for abnormal carbohydrate metabolism to rule out gestational diabetes. If there is a strong history of diabetes, large infants, glycosuria, or unexplained fetal deaths, the test should be performed at 12 to 13 weeks' gestation.

- Use iodized salt; it promotes proper functioning of the thyroid gland.
- Include a wide variety of foods. Especially during the first few months of pregnancy if the woman is experiencing nausea, a variety of foods will encourage proper nutrition.
- Do not take laxatives or enemas unless the physician specifically orders them. Stool softeners (such as docusate sodium—Colace) are ordered more often than laxatives. Fiber is essential to prevent and treat constipation.
- Increase fluid intake to 8 to 10 glasses per day to assist in kidney and bowel function. Water is the preferred fluid.

Table 26-1 also lists amounts of specific nutrients needed by the pregnant woman, in comparison to other women.

The nurse working with an antepartal woman should keep in mind her general health, age, cultural and religious backgrounds, likes and dislikes, food allergies or sensitization, and socioeconomic status. These factors will affect her diet and the pattern of weight gain. Dietary counseling should begin at the first visit and continue throughout all follow-up visits.

Weight Gain. Obstetricians advise a gain of approximately 25 to 30 lb above normal weight, depending on age, prepregnancy weight, and general health. Weight should increase gradually from the sixth week after conception to the end of the full term. (The suggested rate of weight gain over the three trimesters is 3–5 lb during the first trimester and 1 lb per week during the second and third trimesters.)

Appetite. Changes in the woman's body during the early part of pregnancy may interfere with her appetite, so attention must be given to supplying her with proteins, vitamins, and iron throughout pregnancy.

Many pregnant women find that they are extremely hungry after the first few weeks of pregnancy. They should monitor what they eat and be careful not to fill up on empty calories. Rich foods, highly spiced foods, and fried foods are not desirable. In the latter months, several small meals taken daily, rather than three large ones, will probably help the woman feel better, because she will not have as much space in her abdomen for a distended stomach.

Pica. Pica is an abnormal craving for nonfood items during pregnancy, such as clay, dirt, or corn starch. If left untreated, pica can lead to serious nutritional and other physical disorders.

General Health Practices

Elimination. It is preferable for the woman to have a daily bowel movement, although not all women normally do so. A woman who has a tendency toward constipation may have increased difficulties during pregnancy due to decreased peristalsis. Plenty of water, fruits and vegetables, and moderate exercise encourage regular elimination.

Skin and Hair. The oil and sweat glands are more active than usual during pregnancy, so a daily warm (not hot) bath or shower is important. There is no proof that a tub bath is harmful at any time during pregnancy. Of course, the woman must be careful not to slip or fall in the tub or the shower. During the last few weeks of pregnancy, the woman should not take a tub bath if she is home alone. She may have difficulty getting out of the tub and may need assistance.

The hair may be oilier than usual; frequent shampooing will probably be needed. A permanent or hair dye may be safely used during pregnancy.

Teeth. Good oral hygiene should be practiced during pregnancy. The woman who eats a balanced diet and sees her dentist regularly does not need to worry about tooth damage during pregnancy. Necessary dental work should be done, and sources of infection should be treated. Many dentists do not want to perform oral surgery, such as root canal, during pregnancy, unless it is an emergency.

The diet should include good sources of calcium, such as milk and cheese. Some women experience an increase in salivation, called *ptyalism,* during pregnancy. Although this is irritating to the woman, it does not cause tooth decay or gum irritation.

Breasts.* Except for the use of a supportive bra, no elaborate breast care is needed prior to breast-feeding.

Studies show that complicated prenatal nipple preparation rarely makes a difference in successful breast-feeding. A woman who is considering breast-feeding may decide against it if presented with a list of nipple exercises and special creams and ointments she is required to purchase. Women who plan to breast-feed should bathe as usual and use minimal or little soap on the nipples. Nipples should be gently patted dry. The nipple secretes its own natural moisturizer, which should not be removed with soap or other chemicals. Alcohol, tincture of benzoin, and lanolin ointments also should be avoided. (These substances may damage the areola and nipple and have not been shown to be effective in preventing sore and cracked nipples. Lanolin is also a common allergen and may contain insecticide residuals and DDT.)

Wearing a nursing bra with the flaps down, and exposing the nipples to air and sunshine may help to condition the nipples. Harsh treatment of the nipples prenatally may cause sore and cracked nipples and should be avoided. Nipple exercises and stimulation should not be done, especially in the third trimester when they can cause uterine contractions and premature labor. Flat nipples should be treated with breast shields worn in the last trimester and after delivery between feedings. Inverted nipples are rare and can be treated with a nipple shield.

Rest. The pregnant woman tires more easily, and should have enough rest to prevent fatigue. It is better to prevent fatigue than to have to recover from overfatigue. The woman knows how much rest she ordinarily requires, and she should plan to have more if she needs it. Going to bed earlier, getting up later, or taking an afternoon nap may help. Short daytime periods of rest will be beneficial if the woman really relaxes. Pregnant women are able to carry on normal household activities without harm if they avoid heavy work and get additional rest.

Later in pregnancy, postural discomforts may make sleeping difficult. Simple measures, such as additional pillows at the back or a pillow supporting the weight of the abdomen or the top arm while the woman lies on her side, will usually relieve these minor problems.

During the last months of pregnancy, the woman should rest on her *left* side for at least 1 hour in the morning and afternoon. (*Rationale: This position relieves fetal pressure on the renal veins, helps the kidneys excrete fluid, and increases flow of oxygenated blood to the fetus.*) It is also advisable for the woman not to sleep on her back. (*Rationale: The weight of the uterus can interfere with the circulation in the aorta and the vena cava, thus depriving woman and fetus of oxygen.*)

Exercise. Exercise improves circulation, appetite, and digestion; it also aids elimination and helps the woman

---

* Courtesy of Gwendelyn Combs-Marshall, Nutri Source.

sleep better. The woman's customary exercises may be safely continued. Swimming in a pool can be beneficial; however, swimming in lake water in later stages of pregnancy is not advised because of the danger of infection. Specific prenatal exercises are a part of childbirth education. Walking in fresh air is excellent exercise. Whatever the exercise, it should not be fatiguing. Exercising should be daily, rather than sporadic.

Posture. Because the weight of the pregnant uterus is concentrated in front, the woman tends to lean or tilt backward to maintain her balance. This posture is beneficial to those who ordinarily have poor posture. However, the change in body alignment causes a strain on back and leg muscles. This factor, plus the natural softening of the pelvic joints, causes many of the pains of the back, legs, and feet, which are common in late pregnancy. Rib strain and swelling of the ankles and the feet also are common. Some women find it helpful to wear a special maternity girdle, which lifts the abdomen up and in, while holding the back flat. However, the examiner should be consulted about the advisability of wearing a girdle.

Sexual Relations. Sexual intercourse during pregnancy is not harmful as long as it is not unduly uncomfortable and no high risk factors are present (ie, placenta previa). Sexual intercourse is often physically difficult and awkward late in the pregnancy. Pregnancy diminishes sexual desire in some women, while increasing it in others. Mutual understanding by the pregnant woman and her sexual partner will eliminate misunderstandings.

Clothing. By about the third month, the woman will discover that her clothing is becoming tight, and she will need to obtain maternity or looser clothing. Modern maternity clothing is attractive, fashionable, comfortable, and nonconstricting. Queen-size pantyhose can substitute for maternity panty hose. Garters, constrictive knee socks, and knee-high pantyhose must *not* be used, because they restrict blood flow. Comfortable shoes should be worn; flat heels are less awkward and provide a better base of support. The woman will probably have difficulty tying shoelaces or fastening buckles late in the pregnancy.

The woman should wear a wide-strapped bra that supports the breasts without causing pressure on the nipples. An underwire bra is usually more comfortable for the woman with heavy breasts. A good nursing bra is essential after delivery if the woman plans to nurse. The woman should purchase two or three bras of the chest size she usually wears but with a larger cup size.

Travel. Most women who drive continue to do so during pregnancy, at least until the last months when driving may become uncomfortable (fetus, woman, and steering wheel cannot occupy the same space at the same time). The woman must be sure to buckle her seat belt *under* her enlarging abdomen. The shoulder strap should be used and may be placed to the side of the abdomen. It is particularly important to use seat belts during pregnancy to protect the woman and fetus. A car with air bags provides added protection.

Long trips are exhausting for anyone, but because families in the United States are so much on the move, it frequently becomes necessary for the pregnant woman to travel. Travel by air or train is recommended for long, tiring trips. If the woman is to travel by car, she should plan to stop at least every 2 hours to go to the bathroom, stretch, relax, and walk around. This helps to prevent pooling of the blood in the lower extremities. The pregnant woman should not fly in a small plane that is not pressurized, because the lower atmospheric pressure decreases oxygen to the fetus.

It is a good idea for the expectant woman to consult her obstetrician about travel plans, because there are special conditions and times during pregnancy that may make traveling unwise. It is also unwise to take a long trip away from home when the woman is close to term.

Employment. Many employed women continue to work during pregnancy; this is permissible if the expectant woman's and the fetus' health are not endangered. The law states that in most situations, a maternity leave of absence, without loss of seniority, must be granted to a woman who requests one. Ruled out during pregnancy are jobs that involve heavy lifting, operating dangerous machines, continuous standing, or working with toxic substances. Radiation also should be avoided.

Teratogenic Factors

A **teratogen** is an environmental agent or factor that causes defects in the fetus. Most teratogenic effects occur in the first trimester of pregnancy, often before the woman knows that she is pregnant. These events occur after fertilization and are *not* genetic, although they are congenital (present at birth). Some examples of teratogens include the following.

Diseases. Fetal damage caused by rubella and complications caused by maternal herpesvirus will be discussed in Chapter 62. To avoid another dangerous infection, *toxoplasmosis,* the pregnant woman should not handle cat litter and should cook meat well, especially poultry. She should wash her hands carefully after handling raw meat and wash all raw fruits and vegetables thoroughly before eating them. Gloves should be worn while gardening or cleaning. Immunization with a live virus (ie, rubella) should be avoided, because this may cross the placental barrier and cause fetal infection.

Medications. The accepted practice is for the pregnant woman not to take any medications unless they are absolutely necessary and are ordered by the obstetrician. Prescribed medications should be taken in the smallest effective dose and should be discontinued as soon as possible. The safety of any drug in pregnancy is unpredictable.

Even commonly used medications can cause problems in the fetus. For example, aspirin, a mild anticoagulant, can cause a prothrombin problem in the fetus. Medications such as nose drops, diet pills, diuretics, and cold remedies also can cause serious difficulties.

Some medications cause defects that show up many years later in the child. Diethylstilbestrol (DES), previously taken in pregnancy to prevent miscarriage, has been linked to later cervical cancer in girls and infertility in boys born to women who took DES. Antineoplastic drugs (used to treat cancer) are particularly teratogenic, as are many types of hormones (see accompanying box).

Drug Abuse. Street or recreational drugs, such as amphetamines and stimulants, can cause difficulties for the fetus. Addicting drugs, such as cocaine and heroin, can cause congenital addiction and abnormalities in the newborn. Other drugs are either known or suspected teratogens. Substance abuse and chemical dependency will be discussed further in Chapter 88. Some of the effects of drugs and alcohol on pregnancy and the fetus are discussed in Chapters 61 and 62.

> **Nursing Alert**
>
> If you suspect any type of drug abuse in a pregnant woman, report it to the physician immediately, so steps can be taken to protect the fetus as much as possible.

Nicotine and Caffeine. The use of tobacco, which contains nicotine, and caffeine-containing beverages and foods also can be harmful. Items containing caffeine include coffee, some teas, most cola drinks, some other soft drinks, and chocolate (in candy or as a drink). As one of the methylxanthines, caffeine is believed by some to contribute to *mastitis,* an inflammation and swelling of breast tissue in the woman, and is irritating to the fetus. Caffeine crosses the placenta.

Nicotine can cause premature birth or death of the neonate because it decreases the amount of oxygen available to the fetus. Smoking seems to have the most harmful effects on the fetus during the last 6 months of pregnancy; smokers tend to have smaller babies.

Alcohol. The woman is urged not to use alcohol while she is pregnant. A serious disorder, *fetal alcohol syn-*

Categories of Drug Safety in Pregnancy

The Food and Drug Administration has rated drugs as to their relative safety during pregnancy.

Category A—Human studies fail to demonstrate fetal risks.

Category B—Animal studies fail to demonstrate fetal risks.

Category C—Animal studies have demonstrated fetal risks; no controlled human studies are available.

Category D—Human fetal risk exists, but life-threatening situation may outweigh the risks.

Category X—Proven fetal risks exist; drug is contraindicated in women who are or may become pregnant.

N.R.—Not rated.

Drug handbooks usually identify the pregnancy risk for each drug.

Drugs are particularly dangerous to the fetus in the first and third trimesters of pregnancy. In the first trimester, the fetus is being formed and is particularly sensitive to teratogens. The third trimester is dangerous, because when the neonate is born, the mother's circulatory system is no longer available to help metabolize or excrete drugs, and the newborn's immature circulatory and excretory systems must take over.

drome, can occur (see Chapter 62). A daily consumption of as little as 1 to 3 oz of alcohol during the first trimester of pregnancy can be harmful to the fetus.

Other Teratogens. Other teratogens include maternal dietary deficiencies. Food, air, and water pollutants also may play a role. Radiation is particularly dangerous. The specific negative effects of many of these teratogenic factors are discussed in Chapter 62.

Minor Discomforts of Pregnancy

Even in normal pregnancies, many common complaints appear—the so-called minor discomforts of pregnancy. These disorders are minor, not in the sense that they do not cause true discomfort, but because they are not serious and do not threaten the life of the fetus or the woman. Some discomforts are so common that they are called symptoms of pregnancy.

Morning Sickness. Morning sickness is the most common symptom and discomfort of early pregnancy. It is believed to be the result of a general reduction in stimuli to the smooth muscles of the stomach and intestine, accompanied by diminished gastric motility. The symptoms may be caused by physiologic changes, such as hormonal and metabolic changes. Many women experience morning sickness before they have any idea that they are pregnant.

The nausea, with or without vomiting, may occur at any time of the day. In a small percentage of women, it persists throughout the day. It usually starts early in the first trimester and subsides by the time the woman enters her second trimester. Frequent small meals and dry carbohydrate foods (such as air-popped popcorn or soda crackers) taken before arising may be helpful. The pregnant woman also might try limiting her fluid intake and lying in bed for 20 to 30 minutes in the morning, taking liquids and solids at separate times, avoiding greasy foods and those with strong flavors and odors, and resting after meals. It also is helpful to drink carbonated, noncaffeinated, beverages.

> ### Key Concept
>
> Hyperemesis gravidarum is a serious condition characterized by uncontrollable nausea and persistent vomiting, leading to dehydration if unchecked.

Nausea can often be relieved if the person lies on the *right side*. This position shifts the stomach contents away from the cardiac sphincter and into the lower part of the stomach, thus relieving the pressure on the sphincter.

Heartburn. Heartburn or *pyrosis* is a burning sensation felt in the throat and esophagus, caused by a decrease in motility of the stomach or an incompetent cardiac sphincter. This permits the stomach contents to "back up" into the esophagus, creating the irritation of the esophagus. The heart is not involved; the name refers to pain in the area of the heart. To relieve the discomfort of pyrosis, the woman should eat small frequent meals; avoid overeating; chew food thoroughly; eliminate rich, spicy, or fried foods; and avoid lying down after meals. Low-sodium antacids may be ordered but should not be taken without an order from the physician. The woman should be instructed to avoid home remedies, such as baking soda.

Gingivitis. Spongy, swollen, or bleeding gums may develop. This may be caused by increased congestion of blood due to hormonal influences or by a deficiency of vitamin C in the diet. The condition improves with good oral hygiene and an increase in fruits containing ascorbic acid (vitamin C). An astringent mouthwash may be comforting. A hard bristle toothbrush should be avoided, because it can irritate the tender gums.

Shortness of Breath. Dyspnea or shortness of breath is caused by the pressure of the fetus on the diaphragm. It is usually troublesome only in the latter weeks of pregnancy and is relieved as the fetus settles into the pelvic cavity (*lightening*) or by delivery. It is aggravated when the woman lies down; she will rest and sleep much more comfortably if she is supported and elevated by pillows at her back.

Leg Cramps. Cramps in the calf of the leg can be painful. The general belief is that they are caused by an excessive accumulation of phosphorus or by a decrease in calcium in the body. Cramps also can be related to fatigue, chilling, and muscle tension. Calcium lactate or calcium gluconate, taken before meals, or vitamin B will usually provide relief and prevent recurrence of the cramps. The woman also can try forcing her toes upward and exerting pressure on the knee to straighten her leg. She can try elevating her legs, applying heat, and avoiding fatigue. She should have her birth attendant examine her to rule out thrombophlebitis.

Varicose Veins. Varicose veins may develop in the later months of pregnancy, usually in the legs and sometimes in the groin, vulva, or rectum (hemorrhoids). The tendency to develop varicosities is hereditary, and the increased intra-abdominal pressure from the enlarged uterus as well as prolonged standing hasten their development. The patient should not wear garters or tight clothing that would interfere with circulation, and she should avoid being on her feet for any length of time. When the pregnant woman must be on her feet, she should move around, rather than standing in one spot for long periods of time. Elevating her legs in bed several times daily will help drain the blood. She also can apply elastic bandages or stockings in the morning and avoid crossing her legs at the knees. Nylon elastic and support stockings are attractive and might make her more comfortable.

Varicose veins in the vulva area may be decreased by lying down several times a day with the buttocks elevated on pillows.

Any time the woman experiences painful veins or edema in her legs, she should notify her practitioner; he or she can initiate measures to prevent deep or superficial thrombophlebitis (see Chapter 74).

Edema. Toward the end of pregnancy, fluids collect in the body, especially in the feet and legs, partly because of added pressure of the uterus on the blood vessels. Elevating the legs will usually give some relief. Edema will be relieved by having the patient rest and sleep on her left side. Less salt in the diet is recommended, because salt tends to hold fluids in the body. Generalized edema may be a symptom of *pregnancy-induced hypertension*. If this situation occurs, the physician must be notified at once.

Vaginal Discharge. In addition to the natural increase in secretions from the vaginal and the cervical glands during pregnancy, certain infectious organisms, such as *Trichomonas vaginalis,* or an eroded cervix may be the cause of vaginal discharge. Usually the practitioner prescribes medicated tablets, creams, or suppositories.

Routine douching is not recommended during pregnancy. An unclean douche tip can introduce bacteria into the birth canal or uterus. Moreover, if the solution is too hot or the pressure too great, it can cause premature rupture of the amniotic sac. The physician might prescribe a medicated vaginal douche if the woman is not too close to delivery. Women in general, but particularly pregnant women, should wear cotton panties because they are more absorbent and allow air to circulate. They should refrain from using bubble bath or bath oils. All women should be taught to wipe from front to back after going to the bathroom. These measures help prevent vaginal and bladder infections. It is important to promote comfort and cleanliness by bathing daily.

Constipation. Constipation and flatulence (gas) are not unusual in pregnancy. They are thought to be caused by decreased peristalsis. Increased fiber in the diet, exercise, and adequate fluid intake may solve the problem. Occasionally, the physician orders a mild stool softener. Less often, a mild laxative may be ordered.

Nursing Alert

The woman must be cautioned not to take any drugs without a physician's order. Particularly dangerous are laxatives, diuretics, stimulants, depressants, or hormones.

Hemorrhoids. The veins in the rectum sometimes become congested (varicosed) and may be very painful. This condition is usually a result of constipation and straining to evacuate the bowels and uterine pressure interfering with the flow of venous blood. Regular bowel habits will help prevent hemorrhoids. If this condition develops, ice or witch hazel compresses (Tucks) or sitz baths will bring relief. The physician may prescribe suppositories, analgesic ointments, or anesthetic sprays.

Other Discomforts. Faintness or dizziness, nosebleeds, and heartburn also cause discomfort during pregnancy.

A condition called *supine hypotensive syndrome* may occur in the late stages. When the woman is lying on her back, the weight of the uterus exerts pressure on the large abdominal blood vessels; this causes her blood pressure to fall, and she feels faint. Also, uterine blood flow may be diminished. Lying on her *left side* should bring relief. The woman should be instructed to avoid the supine position, not to stand up too quickly or for too long, and to avoid fatigue.

Backaches are caused by postural changes and softening of the pelvic joints. The woman should be taught to use proper body mechanics and avoid lifting heavy loads; she should not wear high-heeled shoes.

Miscellaneous Concerns

Stretch Marks. Some pregnant women develop reddish or white lines on the thighs, breasts, and abdomen. These are called *striae gravidarum,* or stretch marks, and are caused by the stretching and rupture of internal tissues. Vitamin E oil or cocoa butter may help keep these marks less noticeable, but they will not prevent them.

Preparing for Parenthood

Many fears about delivery can be allayed by patient education. If the woman knows what will happen and what to expect, she is less likely to be apprehensive. An understanding nurse can help her verbalize and work out her concerns. A prenatal class for the woman and her partner or close friend is recommended.

Pregnancy and Parenthood
The ideal family-centered care begins with preparation for parenthood. Contemporary social influences have encouraged the recognition that an understanding and affectionate father contributes tremendously to a successful pregnancy and that this good start helps to shape a stable and happy family life.

Prenatal Classes
Prenatal classes are held for the father and mother together. The woman may bring a friend or relative instead. Information is presented in such a way as to minimize fear. The anatomy and physiology of childbearing is presented; the parents learn the process of labor and delivery. The expectant woman is taught exercises that help to develop general muscle tone while strengthening and controlling the particular muscles used in labor and delivery. Special emphasis is placed on breathing techniques. The partner is trained to coach the woman in these exercises. Also covered are postpartum care and the psychological tasks of pregnancy involving the woman and her partner. A tour of the hospital's maternity department is included to familiarize the parents with the area. Parents can often choose between a birthing room or the delivery room.

Most birth attendants feel that this instruction is valuable. It is recognized that fear aggravates pain in any situation; therefore, education to minimize fear is desirable. The patients are more relaxed and cooperative, and labor time is often shortened. In addition, prenatal classes provide an opportunity for expectant parents to meet other couples with whom they can discuss mutual concerns. The accompanying box presents an overview of the nursing process as it relates to normal pregnancy.

❖ *Overview of the Nursing Process*
Normal Pregnancy

Assessment Guidelines

Nursing History

Medical history of both parents
Genetic history of both parents
Ethnic background of both parents
Feelings about the pregnancy (reproductive choice)
Woman's obstetric history
Pertinent lifestyle factors:
> Nutrition, balance between activity and rest, sexual activity, teratogenic factors (exposure to diseases; use of prescription, OTC, and "recreational" drugs; ingestion of alcohol, nicotine, and caffeine)

Presence of discomforts common to pregnancy:
> Morning sickness, shortness of breath, leg cramps, constipation, hemorrhoids, vaginal discharge, gingivitis, edema, varicose veins, stretch marks

Recognition of danger signs in pregnancy and ability to state appropriate response
Preparedness for labor and delivery experience
Preparedness for parenting
Effect of pregnancy on self-concept
Adequacy of coping skills and resources
Superstitions and fears

Physical Examination

Assist the primary practitioner with the assessment and documentation of a complete physical examination that includes a pelvic examination
After the first prenatal visit:
> Vital signs and weight
> Urine test for sugar and albumin
> Examination of the abdomen
> Presence of edema
> Fetal heart rate

Ultrasound (if indicated)

Possible Nursing Diagnoses

Activity Intolerance
Anxiety
Body Image Disturbance
Ineffective Breathing Pattern
Decisional Conflict
Constipation
Ineffective/Disabling Family Coping
Diversional Activity Deficit
Altered Family Processes
Fatigue
Fear
Fluid Volume Excess

Knowledge Deficit (specify)
Altered nutrition (Less or More than Body Requirements)
High Risk for Altered Parenting
Altered Role Performance
Self-Care Deficit
Self-Esteem Disturbance
Altered Sexuality Patterns
Sleep Pattern Disturbance
Urinary Incontinence, stress

Planning

The nurse designs a plan of care with the woman and family to achieve the following general goals:
Throughout the pregnancy, the woman's weight gain (overall nutritional status) and general lifestyle patterns support fetal growth and development
The woman reports she feels able to cope with the physical and emotional changes accompanying pregnancy.
The woman and her partner correctly demonstrate breathing and other relaxation techniques for labor.
The woman describes and uses appropriate strategies for dealing with any of the discomforts of pregnancy.
The long-term goal is the uncomplicated delivery of a healthy newborn without maternal harm.

Implementation

If they request advice and circumstances are appropriate, counsel the couple about reproductive choices.
Develop and implement a teaching plan that corrects any knowledge deficiencies about conception, fetal growth and development, general health practices for the woman, and the labor and delivery experience.
Teach the woman strategies for dealing with any of the discomforts of pregnancy that present, such as morning sickness or leg cramps.
Refer the woman to prenatal classes.

Evaluation

The adequacy of the plan of care is determined by evaluating the woman and her family's achievement of the above goals. If the woman is unable to meet key goals, the plan must be modified. The basic evaluative criteria follow:

Maximum physical and mental health of woman throughout pregnancy
Uncomplicated delivery
Healthy mother and newborn after delivery

Natural Childbirth

Natural childbirth is a broad term used for management of labor. It has gained popularity in the United States because of women's desire to be alert and in control during the birth experience and able to bond with the newborn immediately after birth. Its methods are based on careful prenatal education, support by the father and those in attendance during the labor and birth, and application of controlled breathing and voluntary muscle relaxation.

Nurses working in the labor and delivery areas must understand the various breathing and relaxing techniques so that they can be helpful to their patients.

Doctors and nurses are making an effort to provide more homelike *birthing rooms* in hospitals. Some hospitals are designed to allow the woman to labor, deliver, and recover all in the same room. Many hospitals encourage partners and other family members to remain with women through labor and participate in the birthing. In some hospitals, the partner not only coaches the woman through labor, but cuts the cord, bathes the newborn, and stays with the mother and neonate. Such participation will help to bond the family unit.

Concerns and Superstitions

It is natural for a pregnant woman to be concerned about delivery and about the condition of her child. However, most pregnancies and newborns are normal.

If the woman is gravely worried, the nurse should inform the practitioner, who can discuss the matter with the woman. It is not possible to assure every woman that she will have a perfectly normal child, because there are many conditions that cannot be predicted. This situation is particularly challenging if the woman has previously given birth to a physically or mentally impaired child.

Many superstitions surround pregnancy. The one that comes to mind most often is the belief that the woman can mark her fetus or influence its mind if she sees something unpleasant or ugly. This is *impossible,* because there is no direct connection between the nervous systems of the woman and fetus. The woman also cannot tie knots in the umbilical cord by stretching her arms; the fetus may turn in the uterus and cause a knot, but the woman has nothing to do with it. Also, a hopeful woman's special interest in art and music cannot have any effect on her unborn fetus.

> **Key Concept**
>
> Most pregnancies are normal, and most babies born are normal.

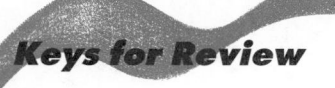

Keys for Review

Key Questions for Critical Thinking

1. Compare fetal and newborn circulation. Describe the functions of the umbilical vein and arteries, ductus venosus, foramen ovale, and ductus arteriosus.
2. Describe the difference between presumptive, probable, and positive signs and symptoms of pregnancy. Discuss at least three examples of each.
3. Using Nägele's rule, calculate a patient's EDD if the woman reports that the first day of her last menstrual period was October 5.
4. List at least six danger signs the woman should report immediately. Describe why they are urgent and dangerous.
5. List at least six minor discomforts of pregnancy. Describe medical treatment for each. Plan appropriate patient teaching for each.

Key Readings

Auvenshine M, Enriquez M. Comprehensive Maternity Nursing: Perinatal and Women's Health, Ed 2. Boston, Jones and Bartlett, 1990

Berckow R (Ed). Merck Manual of Diagnosis and Therapy, Ed 16. Rahway, NJ, Merck Research Laboratories, 1992

Dumas L (Ed). "Women's Health." Nursing Clinics of North America 27(4), 821-993, December, 1992

MacLaren A. Nurses' Clinical guide to Maternity Care. Springhouse, PA, Springhouse, 1992

May KA, Mahlmeister LR. Maternal and Neonatal Nursing: Family-Centered Care, Ed 3. Philadelphia, J.B. Lippincott, 1994

Miller-Keane Encyclopedia and Dictionary of Medicine, Nursing and Allied Health, Ed 5. Philadelphia, W.B. Saunders, 1992

Key Readings *(continued)*

Pillitteri A. Maternal-Newborn Nursing: Care of the Growing Family, Ed 2. Boston, Little Brown, 1985

Reeder SJ, Martin LL, Koniak D. Maternity Nursing: Family, Newborn, and Women's Health Care, Ed 17. Philadelphia, J.B. Lippincott, 1992

Sherwen L, Scoloveno M, Weingerten C. Nursing Care of the Childbearing Family. Norwalk, CT, Appleton & Lange, 1991

Keys to Learning More

Chapter 59: the family during normal labor, delivery, and the postpartal period

Chapter 60: care of the normal neonate

Chapter 61: complications related to childbirth

Chapter 62: disorders of the neonate

Chapter 63: sexuality, infertility, and fertility control

Chapter 90: care of a patient who is dying, including caring for a family whose newborn dies

59 Normal Labor, Delivery, and Postpartum Care

Keys for Learning

Learning Objectives

- Define the key terms in this chapter.
- Describe signs of approaching labor.
- Describe the differences between true and false labor.
- Describe fetal monitoring; differentiate between internal and external monitoring, and state the role of the nurse.
- Describe the normal maternal changes during labor and delivery. Describe postpartum nursing care.
- Describe nursing care during each stage of labor.

Key Terms

after-pains	engorgement	lightening
amniotomy	episiotomy	lochia
colostrum	intrapartum	os
crowning	involution	postpartum
dilation	labor	show
effacement	lactation	

Keys to Understanding This Chapter

Unit Five: nutritional needs, including the woman immediately after delivery and while she is nursing

Unit Four: normal human anatomy and physiology, information used as a baseline for determining deviations from normal during labor and delivery

Unit Seven: nursing process used to assist in performing all nursing care during labor and delivery

Chapter 54: sterile technique, which is used in the labor and delivery rooms and in some aspects of postnatal care

Unit Eleven: medications and their administration, including those used in labor and delivery

Key Points

- The onset of true labor may be difficult to recognize, even for the multigravida.

Key Points (continued)

- During labor, the nurse is responsible for frequent assessments to keep the birth attendant or midwife informed of progress or deviations from normal.
- Episiotomies or lacerations may occur, even with the "normal" labor and delivery process.
- The fourth stage of labor is a critical time for the mother and her newborn. The major concern during this time is preventing maternal hemorrhage (and maintaining the newborn's respiratory and cardiac function).

Key Topics Outline

Labor
  Signs of Approaching Labor
  Onset of Active Labor
Stages of Labor
First Stage
  Station, Lie, Position and Presentation
  Nursing Care During the First Stage
  Fetal Monitoring
Second Stage
  Nursing Care During the Second Stage
Third Stage
  Nursing Care During the Third Stage
Fourth Stage
  Nursing Care During the Fourth Stage
Postpartum Care
  Postpartum Changes
  Assisting the New Mother
  Breast Care
  Perineal Care
  Diet
  Minor Discomforts
Postpartum Examination and Discharge
  Discharge
  Six-Week Check-Up

The childbearing family has many needs throughout the various stages of labor. These special needs can be met only by a skillful, knowledgeable, compassionate, and caring nurse. Using the nursing process as a systematic approach can provide comprehensive nursing care. A maternal care nurse is in an ideal position to promote family participation and to focus on the critical needs of each family member.

Although the parents have looked forward to delivery, they may be apprehensive. The nurse provides encouragement and support and helps the woman meet her basic needs.

Careful observations are made after delivery. The nurse must carry out tasks to prevent the development of complications and to promote rapid healing of tissue. The nurse also functions as a teacher to provide knowledge the mother needs for self-care and neonatal care.

Labor

Labor is a series of processes by which the uterus contracts and expels the fetus. No one is certain what causes labor to begin, but approximately 38 weeks after fertilization (40th week), the fetus is ready to be born. **Intrapartum** is the period of time in which labor and delivery take place.

Signs of Approaching Labor

Several signs and symptoms indicate that true labor is approaching.

Lightening. Lightening is the settling of the fetus lower into the pelvis. Lay people often say, "the baby has dropped." It normally occurs 2 to 3 weeks before the onset of labor in primigravidas. If the patient is a multigravida, this may not occur until labor begins. While lightening allows the pregnant woman to breathe more easily, she will notice an increase in pelvic pressure and urinary frequency.

Braxton-Hicks Contractions. During pregnancy, the muscles of the uterus prepare for labor and delivery by tightening and relaxing at intervals. These contractions, called Braxton-Hicks contractions, are usually painless, short, and irregular. As labor approaches, they may become stronger and somewhat regular. These *false labor* contractions may sometimes be mistaken for true labor. False labor may be experienced from the 38th week of pregnancy onward. The woman may obtain some relief by walking or lying down.

Energy Spurt. Some women experience a spurt of energy just prior to the beginning of labor and take on an excessive number of household chores.

Bloody Show. During pregnancy, the cervix is sealed by a plug of mucus. Just prior to labor, the cervix opens slightly and this mucus plug is dislodged. At the same time, some of the capillaries of the cervix rupture, staining the sticky mucus a pinkish color. This is called the **show** or *bloody show* and indicates that labor is about to begin.

True Versus False Labor

It is often difficult for the woman to distinguish between true and false labor contractions. They are described in Table 59-1.

False labor contractions are generally confined to the lower abdominal area, they are mostly irregular, and their intensity does not substantially increase with time. While false labor may be annoying, the contractions come and go from time to time, and the discomfort can be relieved by ambulating. In false labor, there is *no change* in the dilation of the cervix on examination, and there is no bloody show.

True labor, on the other hand, is characterized by involuntary rhythmic and productive contractions of the uterine muscles. These contractions occur at fairly regular intervals, starting at about 20 to 30 minutes apart and lessening to about 2 to 3 minutes apart. The contractions of true labor usually last about 30 seconds at

Table 59-1. Description of Contractions in True and False Labor

True Labor	False Labor
Regular, rhythmic	Irregular
Increase in duration, frequency, and intensity	Do not increase much in duration, frequency, and intensity
Increase with ambulating	Decrease with ambulating
Start in back, radiate to abdomen	Primarily located in lower abdomen
Dilate and efface cervix	No cervical changes
"Show" usually present	"Show" not present

first and then last longer as labor progresses. The interval between the contractions of true labor gradually decreases, while the intensity increases. The bloody show usually appears during this time. Usually, the true labor contraction feels like low back pain that moves gradually around to the abdomen. These contractions help to dilate and efface the soft cervix.

Onset of Active Labor

The following are two common signs of active labor:

- ◆ Regular contractions
- ◆ Rupture of the membranes

Whenever one or both of these signs are present, it is time for the woman to notify her birth attendant or midwife and go to the hospital if directed to do so.

Contractions

Contractions of the uterine muscles bring about the birth of the fetus. These contractions are *involuntary*; therefore, the woman cannot hurry, slow, lengthen, or shorten them. There are three phases to a contraction:

- ◆ *Increment.* Contractions are building or increasing in strength.
- ◆ *Acme.* The contraction has reached its peak in strength.
- ◆ *Decrement.* The contraction is decreasing in strength.

Other terminology related to contractions includes the following:

- ◆ *Intensity.* Total strength or severity from onset to acme
- ◆ *Duration.* Length of time from the beginning of a contraction to the end of that contraction

- ◆ *Frequency.* Length of time from the onset of one contraction to the onset of the next contraction

In the past, contractions were referred to as "labor pains." It is important not to reinforce the idea of pain. "Labor contractions" is the preferred term. The nurse may tell the woman she may feel some "discomfort."

A contraction lasting 2 minutes or longer is called a *tetanic* or *tonic* contraction and should be reported immediately. The duration of contractions increases from 30 seconds to between 60 and 90 seconds near full dilation of the cervix.

The time between contractions is called the *relaxation time* and is equally important. If the relaxation time is short or absent, the fetus may suffer from lack of oxygen, and the woman may become extremely tired.

The *intensity* of contractions (mild, moderate, or strong) is also estimated. The woman may be asked to classify the intensity on a scale from 1 to 10. This helps to quantify a subjective symptom (discomfort). The nurse's documentation of observations of contractions should include their frequency, duration, intensity, and the length of the relaxation time as well as the patient's reactions and statements (Fig. 59-1).

Nursing Alert

Report immediately any contraction that lasts 2 *minutes* or longer. This is a tetanic or tonic contraction. Complications of a tetanic contraction include *uterine rupture,* which is immediately life-threatening, and fetal distress.

Rupture of the Membranes

The fetus lies in a membranous sac filled with amniotic fluid (commonly called the *bag of waters*). By the 40th week of the cycle, the amniotic fluid volume has reached approximately 1,000 mL or 1 quart. Prior to delivery, the membrane must break. This may occur

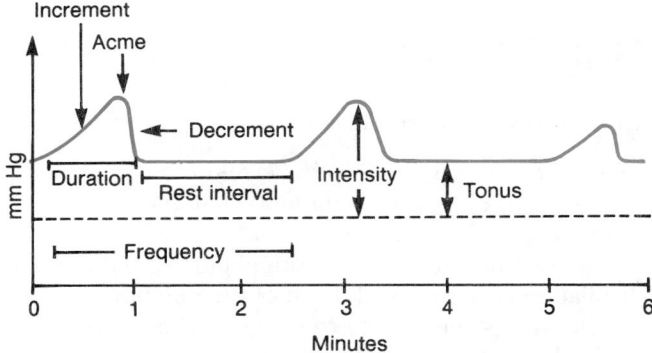

Figure 59-1. Changes in intrauterine pressure, as indicated by fetal monitor, during contractions. Note the indications of duration, intensity, frequency, and rest.

Key Abbreviations and Acronyms for Labor and Delivery

AROM	Artificial rupture of membranes
L&D	Labor and delivery
LOA	Left occiput anterior (position)
1st PPD	First postpartum day
PROM	Premature rupture of membranes
ROA	Right occiput anterior
SROM	Spontaneous rupture of membranes
SVE	Sterile vaginal examination

early in labor or just prior to delivery. The membrane may break with a sudden gush or a gentle trickle. If the membranes break without medical intervention, this is termed *spontaneous rupture of membranes* (SROM). This occurs in almost 25% of births.

The birth attendant may artificially rupture the membranes (AROM). An **amniotomy** is performed using a special hook. Performed under sterile conditions, this procedure often causes true labor to begin or speeds up the labor process.

The Nitrazine Test. A simple test determines if the amniotic sac has ruptured. A strip of nitrazine paper is placed against the vaginal wall and compared to a color standard. The normal pH of the vagina is 5.0 (acidic); the pH of the amniotic fluid is 7.0 to 7.5 (neutral to slightly alkaline). If the paper turns blue, it is probably amniotic fluid, indicating the amniotic sac has ruptured. If the test or urine strip remains yellow, it is probably in contact with vaginal secretions.

Nursing Assessment. When the bag of waters ruptures in the hospital, the time, method of rupture (spontaneous or artificial), and color of fluid are recorded by the nurse.

Stages of Labor

Labor is divided into four stages:

- The first stage (*dilation*) begins with onset of true labor and ends with complete dilation of the cervix.
- The second stage (*expulsion*) begins with complete dilation and ends with birth of the newborn.
- The third stage (*placental*) begins with delivery of the newborn and ends with delivery of placenta.
- The fourth stage (*recovery*) begins after delivery of the placenta and ends when the patient's condition is stable, usually about 1 hour later.

First Stage

In the first stage of labor, the uterine muscles contract to supply pressure to stretch and dilate the cervix. This stage normally lasts from 8 to 18 hours for the primigravida and 1 to 14 hours for the multigravida, and it is accompanied by the breaking of the bag of waters.

Cervical Changes

Two distinct changes take place in the cervix during the first stage of labor: dilation and effacement.

In **dilation,** the cervical **os** (mouth or opening), normally held closed by a circular muscle, begins to open. Dilation is measured in centimeters, from 1 to 10 cm. *Complete* dilation, 10 cm (about 3.9 inches), is necessary to allow the fetus to be expelled from the uterus.

Effacement refers to the thinning of the cervix. The cervix, normally long and thick, shortens or thins as a result of contractions. This thinning (or pulling back) is measured in percentages. The higher the percentage, the thinner or shorter the cervix (100% is considered *complete* effacement). Medical personnel are able to estimate the amount of dilation and effacement by feeling the cervix during a rectal or sterile vaginal examination.

> **Key Concept**
>
> When dilation is 10 cm and effacement is 100%, the woman is said to be "complete."

Phases

The first stage of labor is divided into three phases, which are detailed in Table 59-2.

Station, Lie, Position, and Presentation

Station. Station means the degree of descent of the fetal head (or presenting part) in the birth canal. Stations of the presenting part are measured in relation to the level of the ischial spines of the woman's pelvis. At station zero, the fetal head is said to be *engaged;* that is, the widest part of the presenting part of the fetus is at the midpelvis. The other stations are measured 1 to 5 cm above or below station zero (Fig. 59-2).

Lie. Lie denotes the position of the fetus' spinal cord (the "long part") in relation to that of the woman. The normal lie of the fetus is *longitudinal* and denotes that the fetus' spine is parallel to the woman's spine. If the head is the presenting part, the longitudinal lie promotes a normal delivery. In a *transverse* lie, the fetus is lying crosswise in the uterus and cannot be delivered in that position.

Table 59-2. First Stage of Labor

Phase	Frequency of Contractions	Duration of Contractions	Character and intensity of Contractions	Cervical Dilation	Mother's Behavior
Latent	5–20 min	30–50 sec	Irregular, mild	0–4 cm	Follows directions, excited, talkative
Active	2–4 min	45–60 sec	Regular, moderate to strong	4–8 cm	Serious, apprehensive
Transitional	2–3 min	60–90 sec	Regular, very strong	8–10 cm	Difficulty following directions Frustrated, irritable

Position. Position refers to the relationship between some designated referral point on the presenting part of the fetus to the woman's pelvis. For example, if the top (crown) of the fetal head is presenting, the *occiput* (head) is the designated point. The occiput may be in the woman's right or left anterior, right or left posterior, or right or left transverse pelvic opening (Fig. 59-3). In a frank breech presentation, the sacrum is the designated point; the sacrum may be in any part of the woman's pelvic area. These positions are often designated by the obstetric personnel and in the charts by initials. See examples of three positions in Figure 59-3. Other positions are possible; some of them make delivery difficult or dangerous.

Presentation. Presentation means the presenting part of the fetus, or the part of the fetus that first enters the birth canal. The usual presenting part is the head; this is called the *cephalic* or *vertex* presentation. When the buttocks or a foot is the presenting part, it is known as a breech presentation. Complicated labor often occurs when parts of the body other than the fetus' head present (see Chapter 61)

Nursing Care During the First Stage

Admission

Hospital procedures for the admission of women in labor vary little. The nurse asks about the expected date of delivery or expected date of confinement. If the newborn is preterm, special precautions are taken, and special equipment is readied. The nurse also asks how close the contractions are and how long they last, whether the patient has noticed any bleeding, and whether the bag of waters has ruptured. The anesthesiologist or anesthetist will want to know when the patient last ate.

Routine admission procedures include temperature, pulse, and respiration; blood pressure; and urine testing for sugar and albumin.

The birth attendant may examine the woman's heart, lungs, and abdomen and listen to the fetus' heartbeat. In most hospitals, an external fetal monitor is applied to the woman's abdomen to obtain a baseline fetal heart rate tracing. A sterile vaginal examination is often performed to determine how far labor has progressed.

Any bright red bleeding must be reported at once. A patient who is bleeding should never be examined vaginally until placenta previa is ruled out by ultrasound. The nurse must remember to keep both parents informed of the labor progress and to observe closely at all times for any signs of fetal distress. The accompanying box lists danger signs in labor. The nurse *must* report any of these to the physician *immediately.*

> **Nursing Alert**
>
> Be sure to ask the woman on admission about allergies to povidone-iodine (Betadine), lidocaine (Xylocaine), or any other drugs.

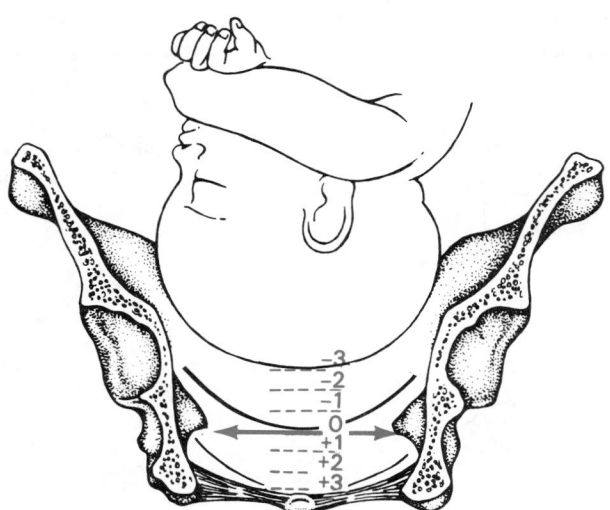

Figure 59-2. Stations of the fetal head. This diagram shows the relationship of the fetal head to the pelvic bones, specifically the ischial spines, during the labor and delivery process. Station zero (0) represents the level of the ischial spines.

Nursing Assessment to Monitor Labor Status

Uterine Contractions. Uterine contractions are one means of assessing the patient's progress. If the pregnancy is full term, the fundus of the uterus (where the strongest muscular contractions can be felt), is located just above the umbilicus. The nurse's hand should rest there lightly to best evaluate uterine contractions. As the uterus contracts, the abdomen becomes hard and rigid. The uterus then relaxes, as indicated by the softening of the muscle fibers. Uterine contractions also can be assessed using external and internal devices (monitors or ultrasound).

Sterile Vaginal Examination. The progress of labor also is assessed by a sterile vaginal examination (SVE), which is usually performed by the birth attendant, midwife, physician or registered nurse. In addition to the degree of cervical dilation and effacement, the examiner is able to determine the presenting part, station, size of the pelvic outlet, and status of the membranes.

The nursing student assists by ensuring that the patient is draped properly. Students should not be asked to perform vaginal examinations. If, as a graduate, a nurse is asked to perform vaginal examinations, the hospital must provide inservice instruction in the procedure.

Emotional and Physical Support

Nursing support during the first stage of labor is directed toward making the woman as comfortable as possible and encouraging her to rest.

Observation and Monitoring of Voiding. One of the nurse's important duties is to be sure that the patient's bladder is empty. A full bladder prevents the fetus' head from descending into the pelvis and thereby slows the progress of labor. It may be necessary to catheterize the patient.

Vital Signs. Carefully observe the physical state of the woman during labor and delivery. Record vital signs at

Danger Signs in Labor

◆ Sharp, unremitting pain
◆ Prolonged contractions or failure of the uterus to relax (rigid uterus after a contraction)
◆ Change in character of the fetal heart beat; abnormal deceleration pattern on fetal monitor
◆ Bleeding
◆ Extreme maternal exhaustion
◆ Cessation of labor after it has begun
◆ Hypotension or increased pulse rate of the mother
◆ Prolapse of the umbilical cord
◆ Irregular fetal heartbeat
◆ Passage of meconium-stained amniotic fluid when fetus is in vertex position
◆ Exaggerated movement of the fetus
◆ A pH value below 7.2 of fetal blood drawn from scalp veins (indicating fetal acidosis)

regular intervals. Each hospital has specific routines, which should be followed carefully.

Comfort Measures. Labor is exactly what it says: hard work. The nurse should stay with the woman and do everything possible to help her relax and rest between contractions. The nurse can sponge the woman's face and hands occasionally, rub her back, offer her a sip of water or ice chips from time to time, change her gown if it becomes damp, and see that the air in the room is fresh. The father or support person should be encouraged to become involved in these comfort measures. The father needs support from the nurse also.

The woman might prefer to have the head of the bed up during the first part of labor. If she does lie flat, however, she should lie on her *left side* (rather than on her back). This will help prevent hypotension, which

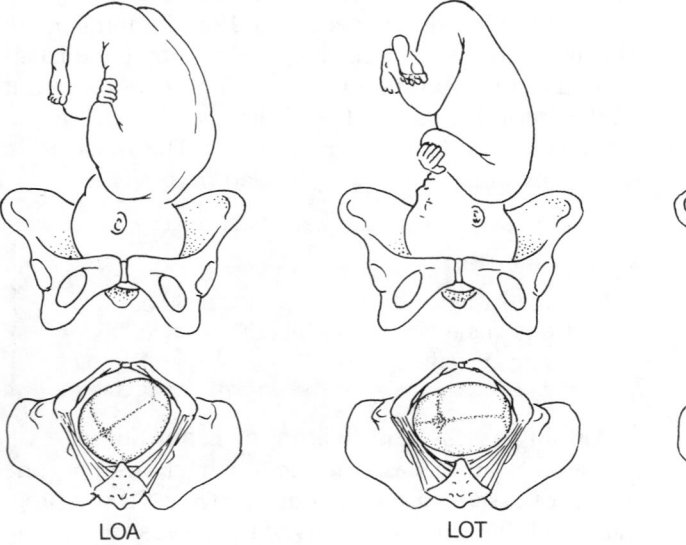
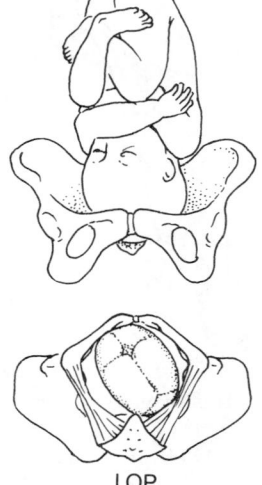

LOA   LOT   LOP

Figure 59-3. Examples of fetal positions. (LOA) Left occiput anterior (as seen from the front and from below), (LOT) Left occiput transverse. (LOP) Left occiput posterior.

results from compression of her aorta and vena cava by the weight of the uterus falling backward against the spine. She may be permitted to ambulate if the bag of waters is intact.

The woman should be encouraged to breathe slowly and deeply. She should be encouraged to use any techniques learned in prenatal class to relax her muscles. She may need to be coached by the father and nurses to do so.

Food and Fluids. Water and clear fluids are usually allowed during the very early stages of labor. (Solid or liquid foods may cause the woman to vomit, particularly if she is to have a general anesthetic.) In a prolonged labor, intravenous solutions may be given to maintain caloric and fluid intake and to lessen exhaustion and dehydration.

Relief of Discomfort

If the woman desires, she may be given some medication to make her more comfortable and to relax her. The type of drug may vary with the locale, the physician, and the condition of the patient. Analgesics reduce the discomforts of labor; sedatives promote rest; and tranquilizers relax the patient. Sometimes a combination of two drugs is administered.

Nursing Alert

Medications may slow labor if given too early or may cause the newborn to be lethargic if given too late. The woman often makes the decision for the use of medication during labor, after consulting her physician.

Many patients receive some form of anesthesia during labor and delivery. General anesthesia is rarely used because the patient receiving this type of anesthesia is asleep when the newborn arrives. Babies born this way may not breathe spontaneously and may be difficult to awaken. General anesthesia is generally used in emergency situations only (ie, emergency cesarean delivery) due to the possibility of newborn depression. (In most cesarean deliveries, general anesthesia is not given until *after* the baby is delivered.)

Epidural Block. One of the most common methods of anesthesia today is *epidural* anesthesia, also called the *lumbar epidural block*. In epidural anesthesia, a small catheter is inserted into the epidural space within the spinal column. The catheter is taped into place, and a test dose of the anesthetic drug is given. If there are no undesired side effects, the drug can be carefully administered either intermittently or continuously using a pump through the catheter during labor and delivery.

Most women receive relief of pain within 20 minutes with this method of anesthesia. An anesthesiologist should monitor the administration of this type of anesthesia, because serious side effects (ie, maternal hypotension) can occur.

The woman receiving epidural anesthesia during labor should be positioned on her side, with her head slightly raised. If she lies on her back, a small firm pillow should be placed under her right hip so that the uterus is tilted to the left. This will help prevent the compression of the woman's aorta and vena cava.

Nursing Alert

If the woman receiving anesthesia or analgesia complains of any of the following, report it *immediately*:

◆ Inability to move the legs
◆ Numbness in the legs
◆ Ringing in the ears
◆ Dizziness
◆ A metallic taste

or

◆ If the woman has hypotension or seizures

These are serious side effects of anesthesia and can be fatal to the woman and/or fetus.

Other Local Anesthetics. Other anesthetics can be injected into the spinal canal (saddle block), the caudal space (caudal block), or the pudendal nerve (pudendal block). Sometimes the local anesthetic is injected around the cervix (cervical block). Although the patient is awake during delivery, sensation is lost in the site anesthetized.

The following anesthetic agents can be used:

◆ Tetracaine hydrochloride (Pontocaine)
◆ Dibucain hydrochloride (Nupercainal)

Each type of anesthesia has distinct advantages. The patient's needs and wishes and the availability of medications dictate the form used. Many women see labor as a natural function and desire to deliver with little or no medication.

Fetal Monitoring

Continuous electronic monitoring of the fetal heart during labor is routine in many hospitals. The purpose of the fetal monitor is to record the rate and quality of the fetal heartbeat during a uterine contraction and when the uterus is relaxed. It can give an *early warning of fetal distress,* so corrective measures can be started immediately. An electronic fetal monitor is always used in the following situations:

◆ If the fetus seems to be in distress
◆ If the delivery is being induced

◆ If the woman has a chronic disorder
◆ If there is a complication of pregnancy

The normal fetal heart rate is 120 to 160 beats per minute.

External (Indirect) Monitoring

External monitoring is most commonly used. External monitoring is based on the Dopper effect. High-frequency ultrasound waves directed to the fetal heart bounce back to a transducer on the woman's abdomen. The receiver amplifies the fetal heart sounds. The signal is converted to audio (sound) and simultaneously printed out on electrocardiograph paper. In addition, a pressure-sensitive device, called a tocodynomometer, is used to monitor contractions. Placed directly over the fundus, the device transfers an electrical impulse to the monitor, creating a readout.

The relationship between the fetal heartbeat and uterine contractions can be studied because they are printed out simultaneously.

Internal (Direct) Monitoring

If the external monitor's printout signals a fetal or maternal problem, an internal, or direct, monitor is used because it is more accurate. An electrode, such as the scalp clip or spiral, is passed through the dilated cervix and attached directly to the presenting part of the fetus. The internal monitor can provide more precise information including the fetal electrocardiogram. The external sensor may still be used to measure the intensity and length of uterine contractions, or a catheter (intrauterine pressure catheter) may be inserted into the uterus. The catheter can then directly measure the uterine contractions according to the pressure placed on it (see Figure 59-1).

Key Concept

The most important factor in fetal monitoring is the *relationship* between the fetal heart rate and the contractions.

Evaluation of Fetal Monitor Information

The nursing student or licensed practical nurse is not usually responsible for fetal monitoring but should understand the basic theory and terminology. *The team leader must be notified if any signs of fetal distress appear on the fetal monitor.* Accelerations are transient increases of the fetal heart rate of 15 or more beats per minute. Any acceleration of 60 or more beats per minute is considered a complication. The fetus may be in danger.

Decelerations (slowing) of the fetal heart rate are categorized according to when they occur in relation to a contraction. For example, an *early deceleration* begins early in the contraction, hits its low point at the peak of the contraction, and returns to baseline at the end of the contraction. Early decelerations are due to vagal nerve stimulation resulting from pressure on the fetal head and are considered a *normal* response of the fetus to labor. They should "mirror" the pattern of the contraction.

Decreased variability, *little to no fluctuation in the fetal heart rate, is a danger sign* and may indicate an abnormality in the fetal nervous system or maternal use of central nervous system depressants.

Nursing Alert

Variable decelerations occur anytime during and after contractions. This usually indicates umbilical cord compression; it can usually be altered by changing the woman's position or by giving her oxygen.

Late decelerations begin late in the contraction, and the fetal heart rate recovery occurs after the contraction is over. It is related to placental insufficiency and is a significant sign of fetal distress.

The fetal heart rate should not fall below 100 BPM.

Second Stage

The second stage of labor begins with the complete effacement and dilation of the cervix and ends with the expulsion of the neonate. It usually lasts about 1 hour for a primipara. The second stage of labor for a multipara usually lasts about 25 minutes but can take up to 1 hour.

During this stage, abdominal muscles and the diaphragm join the uterine muscles to push the newborn out. The woman may say she feels "pushing pains" or a "bearing down" feeling. The rectum dilates, the perineum bulges, and the top of the fetus' head (**crowning**) appears (Fig. 59-4A).

Coaching the Woman. In this stage, the woman is able to help deliver the newborn. She takes a deep breath and holds it, and then pushes with each contraction. If she relaxes too, she can work better when the next contraction comes. The nurse or the coach encourages the woman to push only *with* contractions and to rest in between.

If a woman tells you the baby is coming, *believe her,* get assistance immediately, and check for crowning. If a delivery occurs suddenly without advance warning and preparation, it is called a *precipitous delivery.* A patient may "precipitate" in the labor room bed if her claim that the birth is imminent is ignored.

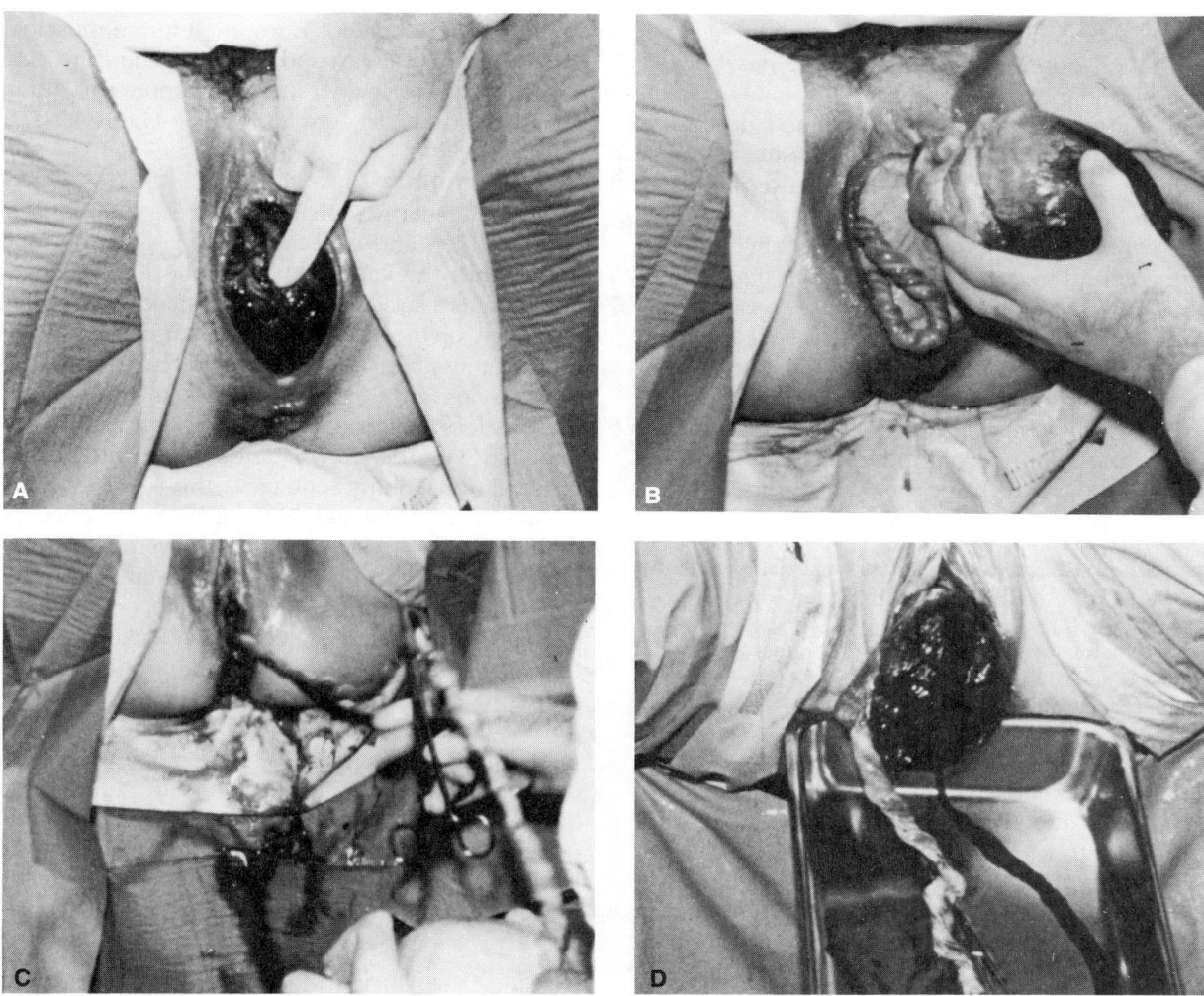

Figure 59-4. Second and third stages of labor. **(A)** "Crowning" of the fetal head. Note the bulging of the perineum and the dilation of the anal sphincter. **(B)** The head is normally born face down. After the head is born, the baby turns, and one shoulder at a time is delivered, as shown here. Notice the twisted umbilical cord. From the time the shoulders are born until delivery of the entire infant is usually only a split second. **(C)** The cord is quickly clamped in at least two places to prevent hemorrhage of mother or baby. **(D)** The third (placental) stage of labor begins with the birth of the baby and ends with the delivery of the placenta.

Episiotomy. Often the birth attendant makes an incision in the perineum, called an **episiotomy,** which enlarges the vaginal opening and allows the fetus to be delivered more easily. It helps to preserve the structure and strength of the perineal muscles and prevents a jagged laceration or a tear extending to the anus, which would be difficult to repair and could leave permanent damage.

End of Second Stage. The expulsion of the neonate in a normal presentation involves the birth of the head, face downward, and immediate rotation to the side (see Figure 59-4*B*). The shoulders are born, one at a time, and the rest of the newborn follows quickly. The cord

is clamped in two places (see Figure 59-4*C*) and cut between the clamps at this time. This completes the second stage of labor.

Nursing Care During the Second Stage

Often the practical or registered nurse will assist in the delivery or birthing room. If you are assigned to assist the woman, you most likely will stand at her head, instructing her on how to breathe and when to push and informing her of what is going on. If you are assisting the birth attendant, you may be responsible for passing equipment, medication, and other items. If you are caring for the newborn, you will need to make sure that he or she is breathing and is kept warm. You also will perform other routine procedures for the newborn, as described in Chapter 60.

Aseptic conditions must be maintained during delivery. The nurse wears a clean scrub suit, a cap to cover the hair, and a mask. The father also is dressed appropriately.

If the patient is going to deliver in a delivery room, she is transferred to the delivery room on her bed and moves over to the delivery table with the assistance of the circulating nurse. The table, which is split across the middle, is opened (broken), and the buttocks are positioned at the break in the table. The feet are placed in stirrups. Perineal preparation is done to cleanse the skin and remove secretions from the genitalia. (Shaving is rarely done today.) In some cases, a birthing chair is used.

Key Concept

Many women choose to deliver in a birthing room. The family stays in the same room for labor, delivery, and the postpartum period.

Clearing the Newborn's Airway. After the head is delivered, the birth attendant or midwife will suction the nose and mouth of the neonate with a bulb syringe. The birth attendant checks for a nuchal cord and removes it from the newborn's neck. The anterior shoulder is delivered and then the posterior shoulder and the remainder of the body. The neonate cries out, and the lungs expand. The nurse notes the time of delivery for the legal records. This entire portion of the delivery often takes only a few seconds.

Clamping the Cord. When the cord stops pulsating, two Kelly clamps are applied, and the cord is cut between them by the birth attendant or father (see Figure 59-4*C*). An umbilical clamp is applied, and the nurse must make certain it is attached securely.

Receiving the Newborn from the Birth Attendant. Once the newborn is stable, he or she may be held for a short time by the mother or father. However, the nurse is responsible for its care. The newborn must be kept warm, yet parents should have time to hold and bond with the neonate. Overhead warmers allow the nurse and father to observe the newborn. The nurse determines and records the Apgar score (see Table 60-1).

Third Stage

The third stage of labor extends from the time the newborn is expelled until the placenta and membranes are expelled. The placenta is attached to the uterine wall, but after the neonate is born, the uterine muscles contract to shear it away and expel it. The third stage of labor can take anywhere from 1 minute to 1 hour, but it usually takes 5 to 10 minutes (see Figure 59-4*D*).

Delivery of the Placenta

The placenta is delivered after the uterus rises into the abdomen and becomes globular. As the placenta moves into the vagina, the umbilical cord lengthens, and there is a sudden trickle or gush of blood. The birth attendant or the nurse keeps a hand firmly over the empty uterus until it feels firm and hard, indicating that the muscles and the blood vessels are contracted, and there is less danger of hemorrhage. If the placenta is expelled with the shiny side out, it is called *Schultze's* presentation ("Shiny Schultze"); this is the fetal side and occurs in approximately 80% of births. If it is expelled with the dull side out, it is called *Duncan's* presentation ("Dirty Duncan"); this is the maternal side, which is rough and irregular.

Following the delivery of the placenta, it may be necessary to administer an oxytocic medication to assist the uterus to contract, thereby minimizing bleeding. The birth attendant examines the expelled placenta and membranes to determine if it is intact. (Retained placental fragments are a major cause of hemorrhage following delivery.) The birth attendant also examines the cervix, vagina, and perineum and then sutures the episiotomy. Blood loss during a normal delivery is approximately 300 mL.

Nursing Care During the Third Stage

The third stage is relatively short. After the delivery of the newborn in the second stage, the placenta is delivered in the third stage. It is a *dangerous period* for the mother because of the possibility of hemorrhage.

Delivery of the Placenta

The uterus may rise in the abdomen, causing the placenta to separate from the uterine wall. The placenta is delivered with a little blood following it. The open vessels at the placental side bleed until the uterus contracts.

The nurse records the following information about the delivery of the *placenta:*

♦ Exact time the placenta was delivered
♦ Whether it was delivered spontaneously or removed manually
♦ Which side of the placenta presented

The nurse may be instructed to administer oxytocics or gently massage the fundus to minimize blood loss.

After the birth attendant has examined the cervix and vagina and sutured the episiotomy, the nurse cleanses the perineum and removes the mother's legs from the stirrups, if stirrups were used.

Charting the Delivery

- Complete information about the type of delivery and procedures used
- Sex and condition of the baby at birth (include Apgar score)
- Time of birth
- Time at which the placenta was expelled
- Condition of the fundus
- Any medication administered
- If an episiotomy was done
- Condition and vital signs of the mother

Nursing Alert

Bring the mother's legs down from the stirrups *slowly* and *together*. This helps to avoid further trauma and discomfort.

Change the mother's gown, apply perineal pads, cover her with a warm blanket, and transfer her to the recovery room if that is the hospital's policy. Otherwise, the mother recovers in the room where she delivered.

Before the mother leaves the delivery or birthing room, the nurse completes the documentation. The accompanying box lists information for the chart.

Fourth Stage

Some hospitals identify a fourth stage of labor: recovery. *Recovery* includes the first hour following the expulsion of the placenta. In this hour, the mother's body

Charting for the Postpartum Patient

Assessment of the fundus:

- Firmness (*consistency*)—firm, boggy (and result of massage)
- At center or deviated (*location*)
- Height (*position*)

Height of the fundus. One possible way of documenting fundal position is shown below:

2/U = 2 finger widths over umbilicus
1/U = 1 finger width over umbilicus
 UU = fundus at level of umbilicus
U/1 = 1 finger width below umbilicus
U/2 = 2 finger widths below umbilicus

Lochia:

- Rubra, serosa, alba (*character*)
- Excessive, moderate, scant (*amount*)
- Odor

begins the process of **involution,** when her reproductive organs resume their normal size. Total involution takes about 6 weeks. The mother must be observed closely for signs of hemorrhage, urinary retention, hypotension, and undesirable side effects from anesthesia. The recovery period is discussed later in this chapter.

Nursing Care During the Fourth Stage

The first hour after delivery is the fourth stage of labor. Following delivery, the mother might feel chilled and shake uncontrollably. This may be in response to a cool room, sudden hormonal shifts, or the sudden change in intra-abdominal pressure after the fetus and placenta are expelled.

Key Concept

Be sure the mother has several warm blankets available if she needs them. Many hospitals have a recovery room where the mother and newborn are taken after delivery and where the mother and father can fondle and care for their newborn during the first hours. Sometimes the mother recovers in the same birthing room where she delivered. In some hospitals, the neonate is first taken to the nursery for initial admission examination, and then the newborn is returned to the recovery room. Other hospitals admit the newborn when the mother arrives in the postpartum area.

Immediately following delivery, the mother experiences extreme fatigue, close to exhaustion, just as she would after any extremely vigorous physical activity or hard work. At the same time, she is relieved and excited. She is interested in seeing and holding her newborn and having a visit with the father. The bonding between parents and newborn should be encouraged *immediately.* The nurse must allow time for the family to be together as soon as possible.

The mother is observed closely for several hours after delivery for signs of complications. Charting for the postpartum patient is listed in the accompanying box. In addition, vital signs and maternal complaints are documented.

Nursing Assessment

Vital Signs. The mother's blood pressure and pulse are checked every 15 minutes for the first 1 or 2 hours or until stable; they are then checked every half hour for 1 hour or longer. The routine varies according to hospital policy. Usually after the first 12 hours, vital signs are checked every 4 hours for 12 hours and then every 8 hours if there are no difficulties.

Fundus and Perineum. When vital signs are taken, the fundus of the uterus and perineum also are checked. The reason for keeping a close check on the fundus is to see that it remains firm and contracted. If it becomes soft and boggy, the nurse cups a hand around the fundus and massages it gently until it regains firmness.

Patient Participation in Care

The woman is encouraged to massage her own fundus at regular intervals. If this measure is not sufficient, the physician may order an intravenous or intramuscular oxytocic drug to be administered. Oxytocic drugs are ergonovine maleate, egometrine maleate (Egotrate Maleate), and oxytocin (Pitocin). *Oxytocics* promote uterine contraction and help prevent hemorrhage.

A rising fundus may indicate uterine hemorrhage. If this does not respond to massage, it should be reported immediately. A fundus located to the right of the midline often indicates a full bladder. Having the mother void will usually return the fundus to its earlier location. If this does not occur, notify the team leader.

The perineum is checked to make sure the stitches are intact and there is no excessive bleeding and for edema or bruising.

Lochia. Lochia is the vaginal discharge that occurs following delivery. It consists of blood and the broken down lining of the uterus. Immediately following delivery, it is bloody and should be moderate in amount.

Large obstetric sanitary pads are worn for the first few days after delivery. Wearing gloves, the nurse checks lochia during the immediate postpartum period. The nurse assesses the amount, character, and color of the lochia. Normal lochia changes are described in the next section.

The amount is described as scant, moderate, or large; it should have a fleshy, never a foul, odor.

Voiding. Observe and record the mother's first voidings after delivery. Failure to void may indicate swelling or injury to the urinary system. If the mother feels the urge to void but is unable to do so or if the fundus shifts to one side, this should be reported. If the mother is not able to void within 6 to 8 hours after delivery, catheterization may be necessary.

Encourage Food and Fluids

The mother may be thirsty and hungry after delivery. She should be encouraged to drink fluids to replace those lost in labor and delivery. After tolerating liquids, she can gradually add solid foods.

Putting the Newborn to Breast

If the mother plans to breast-feed, she should be encouraged to put the newborn to her breast in the delivery or recovery room. The neonate usually is alert at this time, and the stimulation of the breast encourages the secretion of endogenous (within the mother's body) oxytocin.

Patient Teaching

Patient teaching begins early because mothers are discharged a short time after delivering. The mother receives instruction in breast care, perineal care, fundus observation, care of the stitches, fluid intake, voiding, ambulation, engorgement, and involution. She must know danger signs. A mirror is used to check stitches. She observes lochia changes. She also is taught how to care for her baby.

Transfer out of the Recovery Room

The mother remains in the recovery room or is closely observed in the birthing room long enough to ensure that her condition is satisfactory, usually 1 to 2 hours. When the mother's condition is stable, she is transferred to her postpartum room if she delivered elsewhere.

Complete information about the delivery and other procedures must be recorded on the woman's chart before she is moved. Check the charting from the delivery room and the recovery room to make sure that the chart is *complete.* Documentation is transferred with the mother.

Postpartum Care

Postpartum refers to the period following delivery, usually about 6 weeks long, during which the reproductive organs return to their normal nonpregnant state (involution). The general care of the postpartum patient is similar to that of other patients. Observe the woman's overall state, her appetite, her activity, and how well she sleeps and rests. Note temperature, pulse, respiration, and blood pressure. The special needs of the postpartum patient must be met, and observations must be made. An overview of the nursing process during postpartum care accompanies this discussion.

Each day the patient must be *assessed* to make certain she is progressing satisfactorily and to detect early signs of complications. To prepare the patient for the assessment, the nurse asks the patient to empty her bladder and assists her in lying flat in bed. Universal precautions should always be followed when there is possible contact with body secretions.

Postpartum Changes

The process by which reproductive organs return to their nonpregnant state is called **involution.** To provide competent nursing care to the postpartum patient,

Overview of the Nursing Process
Postpartum Care

Assessment Priorities

Immediate Postpartum Care

Blood pressure and pulse q15 min × 1–2 h or until stable, then q30 min × 1 h; then q4h × 12 h or as ordered

Fundus of the uterus, lochia, and stitches (if present) are checked at the same time as the BP and pulse

Any signs of hemorrhage (Check the perineal pad, and be alert to the possible pooling of blood under the patient.)

First voidings

Bonding with infant

General Postpartum Care

After the first 12 h, vital signs are checked q4 h × 12 h and then q8h

Breasts, fundus of the uterus, lochia, and stitches (if present), and legs (for signs of thrombosis) are checked at least once every shift

Voidings and bowel elimination

Adequacy of self-care behaviors: breast care, perineal care, response to discomforts

Quality of maternal-newborn bonding and family dynamics

Adequacy of parenting skills

Knowledge of what to expect after discharge

Possible Nursing Diagnoses

Impaired Adjustment
Anxiety
Body Image Disturbance
Ineffective Breast-Feeding
Decisional Conflict (specify)
Constipation
Ineffective Individual Coping
Altered Family Processes
Anticipatory Grieving
High Risk for Infection
Knowledge Deficit (specify)
Pain
High Risk for Altered Parenting
Personal Identity Disturbance
Altered Role Performance
Self-Care Deficit
Self-Esteem Disturbance
Altered Peripheral Tissue Perfusion
High Risk for Fluid Volume Deficit

Planning

The nurse designs a plan of care with the mother and family to achieve the following goals:

Mother's body demonstrates beginning return to normal, nonpregnant state: (1) fundus remains firm and contracted and moves downward; (2) lochia progresses on schedule from lochia rubra to lochia alba.

In the breast-feeding mother, (1) the breasts begin to produce milk by the third or fourth day; (2) the breasts are not engorged.

Breast engorgement in the non-nursing mother does not last more than 2 or 3 days.

Mother demonstrates correct perineal care.

Incision (episiotomy or cesarean incision, if present) appears to be healing.

Elimination patterns, urinary and bowel, return to normal, prepregnant state.

Whenever observed, parent(s) demonstrates (1) adequate bonding with infant and (2) competence in parent-newborn interactions.

Parent(s) demonstrate adequate parenting skills: holding newborn, bathing, dressing, feeding.

Mother repeats discharge instructions.

Implementation

Immediate Postpartum Care

Facilitate parent-newborn bonding.

Answer any questions the parent(s) has about the delivery experience, condition of neonate, or other matters.

Use warm blankets if requested to keep the mother warm.

If the fundus if soft and spongy, cup a hand around the fundus, and massage it gently until it becomes firm and contracted.

Use a cold pack or compresses (Tucks) for episiotomy pain if indicated.

Report immediately any sign of hemorrhage.

Report delayed voiding (note whether fundus is displaced from midline).

Give a cleansing bath; use this opportunity to explain breast care, perineal care, care of stitches, and to provide instruction about fluid intake, voiding, ambulation, engorgement, and involution.

(continued)

Overview of the Nursing Process
Postpartum Care *(continued)*

General Postpartum Care

Reinforce teaching about the details of self-care initiated during the initial cleansing bath.

Allow the mother to talk about her labor and delivery experience.

Be sensitive to the mother's fluctuating needs to be cared for and to regain her independence.

Teach the nursing mother and non-nursing mother how to care for the breasts.

Be sensitive to the patient's comfort needs; use positioning, ambulation, massages, compresses, and analgesia as necessary to relieve discomforts and pain (*Caution:* Never rub or massage a patient's sore calf; evaluate for thrombosis.)

Observe the mother and newborn during the neonate's feeding times, and offer suggestions as necessary.

Teach parenting skills.

If indicated, role model healthy interactions with the newborn, and demonstrate neonate care skills.

Begin discharge teaching as soon as possible; if indicated refer the mother and family to the public health nurse for follow-up care.

Evaluation

The adequacy of the plan of care is determined by evaluating the mother or family's achievement of the above goals. If key goals are not met, the plan must be modified. The basic evaluative criteria follow:

Return of uterus to normal size, incision(s) heals, no infection

Maximum physical and mental health of mother

Satisfactory bonding and parenting skills.

---

the nurse must understand the physiologic changes that occur following childbirth.

Uterus

Immediately after delivery, the uterus weighs approximately 2 lb (900 g) and is about the size of a grapefruit. It can be felt at the level of or slightly below the umbilicus. After delivery, it begins to return to its normal position and size. When this process is complete, the uterus will weigh about 2 oz (50 g) and will be low, at or near the center of the pelvic cavity.

Uterine Fundus. The fundus is palpated regularly to make sure it is contracted. It should be positioned midline and feel firm to the touch. If the uterus is deviated to the side, the nurse should be suspicious of a distended bladder. Increased bladder size will prevent the uterus from constricting, thus causing the uterus to relax. The uterus should contract after the patient voids. (A contracted uterus should *not* be massaged.)

A soft or boggy uterus indicates relaxation of the muscles and is a *danger sign*. A boggy fundus must be massaged to encourage muscle contraction. The nurse cups a hand around the fundus of the uterus (at about the level of the umbilicus) and rotates the hand gently. The second hand is placed over the symphysis pubis to stabilize the uterus. This massage is continued until a firm mass is felt. Be sure to teach this process to the mother, and document this teaching.

The *height* of the fundus is an indication of the progress of involution. By palpating the abdomen, the nurse can locate the fundus and then measure its height

in relation to the umbilicus. Normal involution occurs when the fundus descends one finger width each day. A full bladder and other complications interfere with this process. The fundal height is recorded as indicated earlier in this chapter.

Lochia

The flow of lochia continues for 3 to 4 weeks with the following changes occurring:

◆ For the first 2 days, lochia is bright red, mostly blood, and is called *lochia rubra*. It should smell like blood; a foul odor points to infection.

◆ After the bleeding diminishes, the color of the discharge changes to pink or brown tinged; the lochia is now called *lochia serosa* for approximately the next 7 days.

◆ By the 10th day, the lochia is yellow or white, has decreased greatly in amount, and is called *lochia alba*.

The amount of lochia flow after delivery should be about the same as a menses. It should not contain large clots, and it should change color as described. The nurse records the amount, color, and any other characteristics that may be significant. It is important to teach the mother the normal sequence of lochia change, because she will probably go home the first or second postpartum day.

Cervix and Vagina

The cervix is soft and edematous following delivery. It constricts and firms during the postpartum period. The vagina, too, regains muscle tone, and lacerations and episiotomies heal. The vagina and vulva lose the congested, purplish color and return to the prepregnant pinkish hue.

Stitches and the Perineum

The patient turns on her side to facilitate a better view of the perineal area. If the patient had an episiotomy, the nurse examines the stitches to detect inflammation, redness, and the healing process and to make certain the stitches are intact. A flashlight may be needed.

The perineal area also is inspected for hematomas, ecchymosis, and edema. Hemorrhoids are noted so that measures to alleviate them can be initiated.

If the patient is unable to ambulate, perineal care may be administered. A fresh perineal pad is applied, usually to the panties, and the panties pulled straight up. If tabbed pads are used, the front is attached first.

Abdominal Wall and Weight Loss

The abdominal wall often remains soft and flabby for several weeks following childbirth, due to the extensive stretching of the tissue and loss of muscle tone. By approximately 6 weeks after delivery, the muscle tone is regained. The mother begins an exercise program gradually as the birth attendant or certified nurse midwife recommends.

How quickly a mother regains her figure depends on the amount of weight she gained prenatally, the amount of weight she lost during the delivery, the amount of exercise she has after delivery, her diet and eating pattern, and whether she is breast-feeding. Body weight decreases approximately 12 to 15 lb (5440–6800 g) at delivery and about 5 lb (2270 g) during the next few days, due to loss of excess body fluid.

Breasts

Changes in the breasts following childbirth prepare for the nourishment of the newborn. During the last half of pregnancy and the first day postpartum, colostrum is produced. **Colostrum** is a thin yellowish secretion that provides vitamins and immune bodies to protect the newborn against some infections. On about the second or third day postpartum, the breasts begin to secrete milk.

Each time a newborn is put to breast, milk is secreted. **Lactation,** the production of milk, is due to the release of the hormones prolactin and oxytocin. As the newborn sucks the nipple, a reflex reaction occurs whereby the posterior pituitary gland releases oxytocin, which causes the milk-producing cells to produce milk and move it to the milk ducts (see Chapters 19 and 25). The oxytocic hormone also results in uterine contractions, and mothers often verbalize that they experience abdominal cramping while breast-feeding. The entire process is commonly known as the "let-down reflex;" the milk is said to "let down" or "come in." If the mother does not plan to nurse her neonate, bromocriptine mesylate (Parlodel) may be given to prevent breast engorgement.

The nurse examines the nipples to determine that they are in good condition and observes for cracking, caking, dryness, or bleeding. If the mother is breast-feeding, the nurse observes whether the nipple protrudes sufficiently for adequate nursing. The breasts are palpated gently to determine if they are soft, firm, or engorged. The breasts are normally soft until about the third day, when milk production occurs.

Engorgement. Engorgement is defined as congestion of the breast, due to increased blood supply in the lymphatic and venous systems. This results in full, hard, and painful breasts.

The nursing mother's engorgement is relieved by the following:

◆ Wearing a supportive bra
◆ Frequent breast-feeding
◆ Applying warm packs to the breast for 15 minutes prior to nursing. An alternative is to stand in the shower with warm water spraying on the breast for 15 minutes prior to nursing.

The non-nursing mother's engorgement is relieved by the following:

◆ Wearing a supportive bra
◆ Avoiding excessive fluid intake
◆ Placing cold packs on her breasts three to four times a day
◆ Avoiding stimulation (ie, hot shower spray)
◆ Medications, as prescribed

Engorgement in the nursing and non-nursing mother generally subsides in 24 to 48 hours.

Bladder

During pregnancy and labor, there has been an added strain on the urinary system. The abdominal muscles may be weakened. In addition, there is often bruising and swelling of the urethra and general loss of muscle tone. During the puerperium, there is an increased demand on the kidneys and bladder as the mother's fluid balance is restored. Because of these factors, new mothers may have difficulty voiding. Common difficulties include voiding in small amounts, residual urine, dysuria, or urinary retention.

The bladder may be palpated for a rounded bulge in the suprapubic region. This indicates distention. By questioning the patient regarding voiding, the nurse can gain information related to urinary symptoms.

Constipation and Hemorrhoids

The mother may be constipated for 1 to 2 weeks following delivery because the abdominal muscles have been stretched, and the intestine has been inactive. Diet, adequate fluids, and activity help to regulate this condition.

Many physicians routinely order stool softeners (ie, docusate sodium [Colace]) or mild laxatives until good bowel function is reestablished. A suppository or small enema may be needed if the laxative is not effective. (The new mother should never take an enema without a specific physician's order.)

If hemorrhoids have bothered the mother during pregnancy, they may still cause discomfort. Ice packs, witch hazel pads (Tucks), suppositories, creams, ointments, or sitz baths may be necessary.

Legs

The patient's legs are exposed, and she is asked to straighten her legs on the surface of the bed and to flex her feet toward her face. Pain on flexion of the feet indicates a *positive Homan's sign* and suggests thrombophlebitis.

Assisting the New Mother

Bathing. When the mother is ambulating and stable, she is permitted to take a shower. The nurse will need to assist her the first time, assembling supplies and instructing her on the procedure. The nursing mother should be instructed to avoid using soap on the nipples. *(Rationale: Soap will cause the nipples to dry and crack.)* A cesarean birth mother will often receive a bed bath the first day after childbirth.

Activity and Rest. The newly delivered mother needs a combination of rest and activity. In most hospitals, the mother is up within 4 hours after a normal delivery. *(Rationale: This helps to prevent respiratory and circulatory complications.)*

The new mother should be encouraged to nap during the day, and in some cases, visitors may need to be restricted. Analgesics may facilitate her ability to rest.

Ambulation. The nurse assists the new mother in her initial ambulations. She should be encouraged to first sit on the edge of the bed and take deep breaths. When she gets up at first, she should move slowly. The nurse or father should remain with her the first few times the mother gets out of bed or until she feels totally stable.

Sometimes the patient experiences an increase in lochia while ambulating; this may alarm her. The nurse monitors the flow and assures the patient that the increase is likely to be due to gravity when arising. The nurse explains that the increased lochia helps to drain

the uterus and helps it to return to its normal position and size.

A Public Health Nursing referral may be done.

Breast Care

Breast care differs, depending on whether the mother is bottle feeding or breast-feeding.

The Non-nursing Mother

The mother who does not wish to nurse her newborn may receive medication to prevent lactation. She should wear a bra that gives firm support. She may have fluids "ad lib" for the first 24 hours after delivery, but after this time, fluids are often restricted. Ice packs can be applied to reduce discomfort.

The Nursing Mother

Nursing the newborn is beneficial for the following reasons:

◆ Breast milk is readily available and convenient.
◆ Milk is the correct temperature.
◆ Milk contains antibodies.
◆ Nursing helps in the bonding process.
◆ Nursing speeds the involution process.
◆ Breast milk is less likely to cause allergic reactions and other neonatal difficulties.
◆ Nursing mothers may have a lower incidence of later developing breast cancer.
◆ Breast milk is cheaper than formula.

Most mothers can nurse their babies unless there are complications, such as severely retracted nipples, infections, or breast malformations. The first requirement for breast-feeding is a good supply of milk; milk production is influenced by emotional status, diet, fluid intake, and rest. The mother who is happy, wants to nurse the neonate, and is not worried or overtired has excellent chances for having a good milk supply. An adequate diet based on the food guide pyramid and ample fluids are essential. Intake of dairy products may be increased. Supplemental vitamins are often prescribed while breast-feeding. (See Chapter 26 for dietary modifications in the nursing mother.) Breast care for the mother who is nursing her newborn varies among hospitals. The goal is to simplify procedures while avoiding infection.

In some hospitals, the mother cleans her nipples before each feeding; this is not the case in other hospitals. *(Rationale: Breast milk contains lactic acid, which acts as a natural cleanser for the nipples.)* Infant feeding is discussed in Chapter 60.

Expression of Milk. *Expression of milk* means artificial emptying of the breasts. This may be used when a preterm newborn must be fed in the newborn intensive care unit or for the convenience of a working mother.

An electric breast pump offers the best method for expressing milk, because the suction is steady and controlled. Milk also can be expressed by hand. Milk that is to be used later should be collected in a sterile bottle and refrigerated. Refrigerated milk should be used within 48 hours. Breast milk can be kept in a home freezer for 1 month or in a frozen food locker for 6 months.

Perineal Care

Perineal care provides comfort and cleanliness and prevents odor and infection. Whether or not she has an episiotomy, the woman should be encouraged to use a peri bottle (a flexible plastic bottle containing clear, warm water). In addition to promoting healing, the peri bottle helps keep the perineum infection-free. Initial perineal care is done by the nurse with the patient in bed on a bedpan. When the patient is ambulatory, she attends to herself. Methods vary, but the purpose is the same: to avoid contamination from fecal material.

Teaching the Mother Perineal Care

Perineal care must always be given after the patient voids or has a bowel movement. The mother is taught to wash her hands and change the perineal pad every 2 to 3 hours during the day. The pad she is wearing is removed carefully and placed in a paper bag for later disposal.

After voiding or a bowel movement, the mother cleanses herself from front to back with tissues, using fresh tissues for each stroke and discarding them in the toilet. Tepid water is sprayed from the peri bottle on the perineum; tissues are used to pat dry from front to back, on each side, and then in the middle. It is important that undue pressure be avoided if the stitches of the episiotomy have not yet dissolved. The mother should pat the stitches dry, not wipe them. Without touching the inner surface of the perineal pad, she fastens the tab of the sanitary belt or attaches the sticky part of the pad to her panties from front to back so it will not slip forward.

> **Nursing Alert**
>
> The perineal pad is always moved from clean to dirty. Thus, when a soiled pad is removed, the panties are pulled straight down. If a sanitary belt is used, the pad is unhooked from the front first. When a clean pad is applied, it is hooked on the front first. This helps to prevent infection.

Relief of Discomfort

A soothing analgesic ointment or spray is applied as ordered. Witch hazel (Tucks) pads may be used. Sitz baths are encouraged for the mother who has stitches. Frequent sitz baths (four times a day) will increase the mother's comfort and promote healing of the episiotomy. Oral analgesics and warm or cold compresses may relieve discomfort. Squeezing the buttocks together before sitting down helps provide a cushion.

Diet

The new mother should have a nutritious, well-balanced diet. If she is nursing, extra quantities of milk and other liquids may be added.

Minor Discomforts

After-pains. For the first few days after delivery, the mother may have painful cramps as the uterine muscles contract. These are called **after-pains** and are more likely to occur in multigravidas. Breast-feeding stimulates uterine contractions, and therefore often brings on the cramping. An analgesic may be ordered as needed for these pains. Heat application is sometimes ordered.

> **Key Concept**
>
> The intensity of after-pains seems to be related to the presence or absence of dysmenorrhea in this mother.

Postpartum Examination and Discharge

Discharge

The birth attendant checks the patient before discharging her from the hospital. She is told to return for a follow-up examination at the end of 6 weeks, and she is usually advised not to have sexual intercourse or to use vaginal douches until then.

Routine discharge procedures are followed when mother and newborn leave the hospital, and specific obstetric procedures also are performed. The mother should be informed that menstruation will resume in 6 to 8 weeks if she does not nurse her neonate. If she does nurse, menstruation is usually delayed for 4 to 5 months or until she stops nursing.

Although ovulation does not usually occur during the nursing period, prolonging this period is no guarantee that pregnancy will not occur; many nursing mothers do become pregnant. *The new mother should be made aware that it is possible for her to become pregnant before the first normal menstrual period, because ovulation occurs before menstruation.*

Patient teaching on all aspects of postpartum and newborn care and documentation of this teaching are vital. The new mother must know when to call the physician or midwife for assistance.

Six-Week Checkup

The practitioner examines mother and neonate approximately 6 weeks after delivery. The purpose of this examination includes making sure that the mother's uterus has returned to normal size, that her episiotomy has healed, and that no infection is present. The examiner will advise the mother at that time regarding resumption of activities.

Keys for Review

Key Question for Critical Thinking

1. A pregnant woman is complaining of back pain, regular contractions which are getting stronger, and "some blood" on her underwear. Determine whether this is true or false labor and why. Describe the directions the woman should be given.
2. Differentiate between duration and frequency of contractions.
3. List the four stages of labor, describe each, and describe nursing care that takes place.
4. Differentiate between the maternal and fetal side of the placenta.
5. Describe the greatest danger to the mother during the immediate postpartum period. Describe what actions the nurse takes to prevent it and actions the nurse takes as it develops.

Key Readings

Auvenshine M, Enriquez M. Comprehensive Maternity Nursing: Perinatal and Women's Health, Ed 2. Boston, Jones and Bartlett, 1990
Jaffe MS, Melson KA. Maternal-Infant Health Care Plans. Springhouse, PA, Springhouse, 1989
Ladewig L, London M, Olds S. Essentials of Maternal-Newborn Nursing, Ed 2. Redwood City, CA, Addison-Wesley, 1990

Key Readings (continued)

MacLaren A. Nurses' Clinical guide to Maternity Care. Springhouse, PA, Springhouse, 1992
May KA, Mahlmeister LR. Maternal and Neonatal Nursing: Family-Centered Care, Ed 3. Philadelphia, J.B. Lippincott, 1994
Pillitteri A. Maternal and Child Health Nursing: Care of the Childbearing and Childrearing Family, Ed 2. Philadelphia, J.B. Lippincott, 1995
Reeder SJ, Martin LL, Koniak D. Maternity Nursing: Family, Newborn and Women's Health Care, Ed 17. Philadelphia, J.B. Lippincott, 1992
Sherwen L, Scoloveno M, Weingerten C. Nursing Care of the Childbearing Family. Norwalk, CT, Appleton & Lange, 1991

Keys to Learning More

Chapter 60: care of the normal neonate
Chapter 61: complications related to childbirth
Chapter 62: disorders of the neonate
Chapter 63: fertility control
Chapter 90: care of a patient who is dying, which applies when caring for a mother whose newborn dies

60 Care of the Normal Neonate

Keys for Learning

Learning Objectives

- Describe the Apgar scale.
- Describe assessments made routinely on the newborn.
- Identify causes of neonatal heat loss and ways to prevent cold stress.
- Describe identification of the neonate and reasons for careful identification.
- Describe characteristics of the normal neonate.
- State normal vital signs of the neonate.
- Demonstrate the steps involved in bathing and weighing the neonate, the routine daily care, and care of a circumcision.
- State characteristics of the normal neonate's stools.
- State the nurse's responsibilities in assisting the nursing mother and the bottle-fed newborn.
- Demonstrate burping (bubbling) the neonate.

Key Terms

acrocyanosis	desquamate	neonate
Apgar score	fontanels	phenylketonuria
bonding	galactosemia	phimosis
caput succedaneum	imperforate	pseudomenstruation
circumcised	lanugo	smegma
cephalhematoma	meconium	vernix caseosa

Keys to Understanding This Chapter

Chapter 5: basic needs of all people

Chapter 9: characteristics and activities of the normal neonate and infant used as a baseline for assessing deviations from normal in the delivery room and nursery

Unit Five: nutritional needs of all people, including the neonate

Unit Seven: nursing process used in performing all nursing care for the neonate

Unit Eight: documentation

Chapter 54: sterile technique, which is used in some aspects of neonatal care

Unit Eleven: basics of medication administration

Key Points

- Accurate assessment of the neonate requires information from prenatal through postnatal periods.
- Maintaining adequate ventilation includes ensuring a patent airway and proper body temperature.
- Teaching is a major role for the nurse and involves parents at all phases of the nursing process.
- The newborn has social and physical needs.

Key Topics Outline

Initial Care of the Newborn
  Maintaining the Airway
  Other Assessments
  Cord Care
Newborn Care in the Delivery Room
  Warmth
  Identification
  Protection Against Disease
  Bonding
Characteristics of the Normal Newborn
  Body Size
  The Head and Body
  Skin
  Movement and Activities
  Influences of Maternal Hormones
Admission to the Newborn Nursery
  Protection for the Newborn
  Admission Procedures
  Examination by the Birth Attendant
  Neonatal Laboratory Screening
Daily Care of the Newborn
  Nursing Assessment
  Other Daily Care
Infant Feeding
  Breast-feeding
  Bottle Feeding
Bubbling the Newborn
  Supplements
Discharge of the Mother and Newborn

The care the newborn receives in the first several months of life will be closely related to normal or abnormal growth and development as a healthy infant. Nurses are in a unique role to act as teachers to parents and to act as an advocate for the newborn.

The normal newborn is born with the reflexes and body systems needed to live outside the uterus. However, assistance is needed to meet daily needs. The nurse assists the **neonate** (the term used for a child in the first 4 weeks of life) and teaches the new parents to care for their newborn.

Initial Care of the Newborn

Maintaining the Airway

As soon as the neonate is born, the birth attendant removes secretions from the newborn's respiratory tract manually or with a small, soft-bulb syringe. In some instances the birth attendant or midwife holds the newborn's head down so that gravity can assist in removing secretions. At this point, the neonate takes its first breath and makes its first sounds.

The newborn's skin has a bluish or dusky tinge at first, but as soon as oxygen enters the circulating blood in quantity, the skin of the white newborn turns lighter and assumes a natural tone. The African American newborn may remain slightly darker. Sometimes if the mother has been medicated recently or has had a long-lasting anesthetic, the newborn does not breathe at once and must be stimulated.

Modifications in the Respiratory and Circulatory Systems. Many changes occur in the newborn's respiratory system at birth. The lungs must expand and fill with air on the first inspiration. This is why it is so important that the newborn's airway be clear when the first breath is taken. Excess secretions in the neonate's airway can cause aspiration pneumonia or death.

At birth, some of the circulatory structures shown in Figure 58-1 must close to allow blood to flow to the heart, lungs, and liver. If these circulatory changes do not occur spontaneously, the newborn will not have adequate oxygenation.

Assessment: Apgar Score

The **Apgar score** was named for the physician who developed the scale. It provides a quick way of assessing the physical condition of the newborn and of determining whether he or she needs assistance or resuscitation.

The Apgar scale is used to measure the degree of depression or lack of it that the newborn exhibits (Table 60-1). The newborn is evaluated at 1 minute and 5 minutes after birth. A number from 0 to 2 is given on each sign of the Apgar scoring chart, and all the numbers are totaled. Both the 1-minute and the 5-minute Apgar scores are recorded on the newborn's chart.

◆ If the total score is 10, the newborn is in the best possible condition.
◆ If the score is 5 or more, the newborn usually does not need resuscitation.
◆ If the score is under 5, the newborn is in danger.
◆ If the score is 3 or less, the newborn usually needs emergency resuscitation.

Resuscitation of the Newborn

If following tactile stimulation breathing does not begin, the respiratory center is probably depressed, and *emergency action must be taken*.

The newborn must be resuscitated immediately; permanent brain damage can occur if the neonate is without oxygen for more than 4 minutes. When respiratory difficulties develop in the delivery room, the birth attendant or anesthesiologist assists the neonate, but the nurse may be the person to initiate resuscitation in the newborn nursery. Nursing skills used in resuscitation follow.

◆ Gloves are often worn.
◆ The purpose of resuscitation is to establish an airway, provide oxygen to the lungs, and stimulate the newborn to breathe.
◆ The neonate is positioned in a supine position. (*Rationale: The supine position facilitates drainage and counteracts shock.*)
◆ The neck is maintained in a neutral position. (*Rationale: Hyperextension can cut off the airway.*)
◆ Gentle suction is provided. If a bulb syringe is used, the bulb is compressed before insertion. The mouth is suctioned before the nose. (*Rationale: Suctioning the nose first may trigger a reflex gasp-*

Overview of the Nursing Process
Care of the Normal Neonate

Assessment Priorities

Immediate Assessment

Apgar (heart rate, respiratory effort, muscle tone, reflexes, color)

Newborn's weight and length (on arrival in the newborn nursery)

Complete physical examination on admission to newborn nursery

Continuing Assessment

Rate and type of respirations (note if the neonate is crying or sleeping while the rate is taken), skin color, apical pulse, blood pressure and temperature (initial rectal temperature to ensure patency of rectum); vital signs are recorded q4h for the first 24 h or oftener

Signs of respiratory distress: retractions of the lower chest and xiphoid process, dilation of the nostrils, or expiratory grunts

Dextrose stix checks (check agency parameters)

Daily weight

Cord condition

Voiding and stools

Skin color for signs of jaundice or cyanosis

Sleep—activity patterns

Bonding

Adequacy of parenting behaviors

Any signs of difficulty or abnormalities (be alert to whining or sharp, high-pitched cries)

Possible Nursing Diagnoses

Ineffective Airway Clearance

High Risk for Aspiration

High risk for Altered Body Temperature

Ineffective Breast-Feeding

Ineffective Breathing Pattern

Ineffective Family Coping

Altered Family Processes

Impaired Gas Exchange

Altered Growth and Development

High Risk for Altered Body Temperature

High Risk for Infection

Altered Nutrition, Less than Body Requirements

High Risk for Altered Parenting

Planning

The nurse designs a plan of care with the family to achieve the following general patient goals:

The newborn's feeding and daily weight reflect normal growth and development

Whenever observed, the vital signs fall within the normal newborn range

The neonate demonstrates no signs of respiratory distress, infection, or other disease processes

The parents demonstrate (1) comfort in holding and interacting with the newborn and (2) adequate parenting skills

Implementation

Immediate Care in the Delivery Room

Suction: Keep the nose and mouth clear of secretions.

Ensure warmth.

Administer silver nitrate or antibiotic ointment solution to the neonate's eyes and vitamin K as ordered.

Place identification bands on newborn and mother.

Take the neonate's footprints and the mother's thumb print.

Complete the delivery information on the chart before the neonate leaves the delivery room.

Continuing Care

Follow the hospital's procedures for the initial cleansing and daily bathing of the newborn.

Cleanse the cord three times daily with alcohol or other solution per hospital policy.

Facilitate the mother's breast or bottle feedings.

Reposition the newborn from side to side; sleeping on the stomach or back is discouraged.

Role-model healthy parenting behaviors for the parent(s) if indicated.

Teach the parent(s) parenting skills.

Refer the mother to appropriate support groups (eg, mothers of twins, breast-feeding group).

Refer the family to a public health nurse if this is necessary.

Instruct the mother about follow-up care for the newborn during discharge.

Evaluation

The adequacy of the plan of care is determined by evaluating the newborn and family's achievement of the proceding goals. If key goals are unable to be met, the plan must be modified. The basic evaluative criteria are:

Healthy newborn at discharge.

Parents comfortable with parenting skills and roles (siblings prepared to welcome a new family member)

Table 60-1. The Apgar Scoring Chart

Sign	0	1	2
Heart rate	Absent	Slow (less than 100)	Over 100
Respiratory effort	Absent	Slow, irregular	Good, crying
Muscle tone	Flaccid	Some flexion of extremities	Active motion
Reflexes, irritability	No response	Weak cry or grimace	Vigorous cry
Color	Blue, pale	Body pink, extremities blue	Completely pink

ing motion, which can lead to aspiration of material [meconium or mucus] in the mouth.)

◆ Occasionally a newborn needs to be intubated in the delivery room. This is usually done by anesthesia personnel.

◆ Oxygen is provided by mask or anesthesia bag. It is important that the mask be of the proper size to seal over the newborn's mouth and nose.

◆ Physical stimulation, such as rubbing the newborn's chest and feet, may help breathing.

◆ Medication may be necessary to stimulate the newborn to breathe on its own.

◆ The neonate usually takes nothing by mouth (NPO) until respiratory status is stabilized. *(Rationale: This prevents aspiration.)*

◆ The newborn may be given antibiotics if extensive resuscitation has been done. *(Rationale: This will prevent infections because the newborn has been exposed to potential microorganisms.)*

Continuing Assessment of Respiratory Status

For several hours after birth, the nurse continues to assess the newborn's respiratory status. Respiratory status is considered normal if there are synchronized movements of the diaphragm and abdominal muscles. The chest should expand as a whole.

Signs of Respiratory Distress in the Newborn*

◆ *Retractions* of the lower chest and of the xiphoid process.
◆ *Retractions* of the upper chest
◆ *Opposition movements* of the upper and lower chest
◆ Nasal flaring
◆ *Expiratory grunts*
◆ Tachypnea

Additional information about respiratory status can be gained by observation of skin color, color of nailbeds and oral mucosa, pulse rate, level of activity, and character of cry.

* Figure 62-2 illustrates these abnormal movements.

Signs of respiratory distress are outlined in the accompanying box. Any of these signs must be reported immediately to the physician. (See Figure 62-2.)

The nurse also assesses the general condition of the neonate and evaluates respiratory status by skin color, rate of respiration, and general activity. Neonates are obligatory nose breathers at a rate of 30 to 60 breaths per minute. (They have great difficulty breathing through the mouth.)

Other Assessments

The birth attendant will perform an examination to determine obvious physical defects in the neonate. Patency of the nose and esophagus can be determined by passing a number 5 to 8 French suction catheter through the nares.

As part of the routine assessment, the nurse documents the following on the chart:

◆ Rate of respirations (note if crying or sleeping)
◆ Type of respirations (note abnormal symptoms, such as retraction, dilation of nares, expiratory grunts, and unusual crying sounds)
◆ Pulse
◆ Blood pressure
◆ Temperature
◆ Weight (daily)

These assessments are made several times a day for the first day of life and then on a daily basis. If complications are suspected, assessments are made more often.

Cord Care

The stump of the cord begins to shrivel and darken soon after birth. The clamp often is removed after 24 hours, as long as no bleeding is evident. *(Rationale: This prevents tension on the drying stump.)* Triple Dye may be applied to the cut cord and around the umbilicus (*periumbilical* area) to prevent infection. One application of Triple Dye is usually sufficient, although some physicians order this to be done daily.

Because fetal circulation was maintained through the umbilical cord, it is possible for the neonate to hemorrhage in a very short time through the cord. Therefore, the clamps or ties must be secure, until they can be safely removed. The nurse caring for the newborn must assess the cord for bleeding at frequent intervals during the first few hours of life.

Newborn Care in the Delivery Room

Warmth

When a neonate is born, he or she is exposed to a drastic change in temperature. As heat loss occurs and because the newborn's temperature control center is not completely developed, he or she is susceptible to *cold stress*. In this situation, the newborn's body is more apt to experience respiratory distress syndrome, acidosis, apnea, or increased respiratory rate. It is important, therefore, to maintain the body temperature of the neonate.

The neonate is wrapped in a warmed blanket immediately after delivery to protect from drafts and chills. Sometimes a cap is placed on the newborn's head. *(Rationale: More heat is lost through the head than through any other part of the body.)* The newborn may be placed on the mother's abdomen or into an isolette or newborn warmer.

Nursing skills used to prevent neonatal heat loss are the following:

- ◆ Transport the newborn in an isolette.
- ◆ Delay the first bath until the temperature has been stable at 98.6°F (37°C).
- ◆ Give the newborn a bath under a radiant heater.
- ◆ Don't wash off all vernix initially.
- ◆ Cover work table and scales so they are not cold.
- ◆ Organize work so that the neonate is uncovered for a minimum amount of time.
- ◆ Keep the newborn away from outside walls.
- ◆ Keep the newborn wrapped in a warm blanket.
- ◆ Make sure there are no drafts in the room.
- ◆ Keep portholes closed on an incubator.
- ◆ Heat any oxygen or humidified air given.
- ◆ Tell the mother not to unwrap her newborn immediately after birth.
- ◆ Keep a hat on the neonate's head.

Nursing Alert

If the newborn's body temperature is below 96°F (35.5°C), a newborn warmer or isolette is needed.

Identification

It is important to identify each newborn properly following birth. Before the neonate leaves the delivery room, he or she is given an identification band. A name band or bracelet is applied to the mother's wrist, and two are applied to the neonate—one to the ankle and one to the wrist. These bands have identical numbers and information regarding name, birth date and time, birth attendant's name, and sex of neonate. (If the newborn has a common last name, the full name of the mother is included.)

Each time the neonate is brought into the mother's room, the identification bands are double-checked. At discharge, one of the newborn's identification bands is removed and placed on the chart, which the mother signs.

Key Concept

Many precautions are taken in newborn nurseries to prevent the kidnapping or mixing up of newborns.

Newborn Footprint. A second identification is the footprint of the newborn and the thumbprint of the mother. These prints are taken before either the mother or neonate leaves the delivery room and are part of the permanent chart.

Nursing Skill
Footprinting the Newborn

Supplies and Equipment

Two infant footprinters or inked pad
Tissues or "baby wipes"
Prescribed solution
Lotion

Procedure

1. Wash your hands.
2. Remove the vernix from the bottom of the newborn's feet before it dries. *(Rationale: Dried vernix is more difficult to remove, and vernix obscures the footprint.)*
3. Cleanse the newborn's foot gently with the solution specified by the hospital.
4. Hold the neonate's ankle between your thumb and middle finger, placing your index finger behind the toes.
5. Keeping the newborn's knees flexed and legs close to the body, gently touch the inked footprinter to the foot. Place the heel on the chart and "walk" the foot over the chart with a heel-to-toe motion.
6. Remove the excess ink from the neonate's foot with lotion, and dispose of the footprinter. *(Rationale: An individual footprinter is usually used for each foot.)*
7. Follow the same procedure for the other foot.
8. Press the mother's right thumb on the inked pad and then press on the record, gently rocking from one side to the other. This must be done *before* mother *or* baby leaves the delivery room.
9. Wash your hands thoroughly and document the procedure.

Other Identifying Information. The chart also includes information about the neonate's sex, hour of birth, condition, and type of delivery. Any identifying marks, care of the eyes, and mother's Rh status are documented. The chart *must* be made out before the newborn leaves the delivery room.

The nurse must be especially careful if the newborn has a common name. In all cases, the mother's full name and the date and time of the neonate's birth are of critical importance and should be carefully documented on the chart.

The Birth Certificate. A certificate of the newborn's birth is completed and signed by the birth attendant or midwife who delivered the newborn as soon as possible after birth. The birth certificate is filed with the State Department of Vital Statistics. It is best to choose a name for the neonate *before* the birth certificate is filed; this precludes later confusion.

Protection Against Disease

Eye Prophylaxis. To protect a newborn from ophthalmia neonatorum, a severe eye infection (often caused by the gonorrhea organism), a 1% solution of silver nitrate ($AgNO_3$) or an antibiotic solution or ointment (such as erythromycin) is instilled in the newborn's eyes immediately after delivery. This is required throughout the United States for all newborns.

Key Concept

Eye prophylaxis is delayed until parents and newborn have had a few minutes to look at each other.

Vitamin K. Because of a lack of intestinal bacterial flora, the newborn is not able to produce an adequate amount of vitamin K, which is important for production of certain coagulation factors by the liver. Thus, an intramuscular injection of vitamin K is usually administered during the first hour after birth. This must be documented and reported to the nursery nurse.

Other Precautions. The newborn may need specific treatment in the presence of maternal infection or if the mother is a habitual substance abuser.

Bonding

Bonding is the promotion of attachment between parents and newborn. Birth is traumatic for the neonate: He or she leaves a dark environment for a bright one, a warm environment for a cold one, and a relatively quiet, secure home for a complex, noisy world. The newborn needs to feel secure, loved, and comfortable during the first hours of life. Such a feeling is promoted when the parents hold, caress, soothe, touch, and speak to the newborn. A mother who has chosen to breast-feed should be encouraged to do so immediately. Father and siblings also can hold the neonate soon after birth.

Characteristics of the Normal Newborn

The first 24 hours of life are critical for the neonate. The nurse must be aware of the characteristics of the normal newborn so that accurate assessments can be performed.

Body Size

The weight of the normal newborn ranges from 5.5 to 10 lb (about 2500–4540 g), with girls usually weighing less than boys. The neonate loses weight (usually 5%–10%) during the first few days after birth and then begins to gain. The length of the normal newborn ranges from 18 to 22 inches (about 45.75–56 cm) with boys usually approximately 0.5 inch longer than girls.

The Head and Body

The newborn has a large head, averaging 13 to 14 inches (33–35.5 cm) in circumference. It is supported by a short neck and a chest somewhat smaller than the head (10–12 inches [25.5–30.5 cm] in circumference). The newborn has a large, protruding abdomen.

The newborn's head may be shaped irregularly, depending on the type of delivery. If the newborn was delivered breech or by cesarean delivery, the head is usually round, but if the neonate was delivered vaginally the head may be *molded* (elongated) because of the overlap of skull bones during the birth process. This molding is temporary.

Caput succedaneum is an accumulation of fluid within the scalp of the newborn, which causes it to be puffy and edematous. It is caused by pressure to the head during delivery and disappears within a few days. **Cephalhematoma** is an accumulation of blood between the bones of the skull and the periosteum (the membrane that covers the skull). It is not drained because of the danger of infection. The neonate's appearance may upset the parents, but they should be reassured that the fluids will eventually be absorbed.

Fontanels. Fontanels are soft spots in the newborn's skull. Two major fontanels can be felt. The soft spots are formed by the junction of the individual skull bones.

(These bones do not fuse completely before birth, to facilitate delivery.) The *anterior fontanel* is above the forehead, is diamond shaped, and closes between the ages of 12 and 18 months. The *posterior fontanel* is located on the crown of the head (near the back of the head or occiput), is smaller and more triangular, and closes by the third month of life.

Eyes. The newborn's eyes appear blue or gray at birth. The neonate may appear cross-eyed, because he or she is unable to focus the eyes. The newborn usually has eyelashes and eyebrows at birth. The eyelids may appear red and edematous because of the irritation of the silver nitrate or erythromycin. The neonate keeps his or her eyes closed most of the time, because they are still sensitive to bright lights. During the first several weeks of life, the neonate is unable to produce tears, because the lacrimal glands are not yet functioning.

Skin

The skin of a white newborn is pink or red soon after birth. The skin of African American and other nonwhite neonates may appear pink or tan, with some pigment changes occurring within hours or days of delivery. The newborn typically has a small face, flat nose and ears, and receding chin. If forceps have been used for delivery, small bruises may appear on the face or head.

The nose and cheeks may have pinhead-sized white spots, caused by obstructed oil and sweat glands. These are called *milia.* Sometimes white or grayish-colored bumps are found on the hard and soft palate of the mouth. These are known as *Epstein's pearls.*

Various types of birthmarks may occur. Some disappear early in life; others are permanent. One type, which often appears on the eyelid or forehead of the newborn, is known as *stork bite.* The skin of some neonates is sensitive, so red, hive-appearing, raised lesions known as *erythema toxicum,* or newborn rash, may occur.

Petechiae, which are small purplish dots on the skin, may be present, because of the pressure caused by labor. The buttocks, lower back, or upper legs of non-white babies often have dark blue areas of discoloration, called *mongolian spots.*

Veins may be seen. Fine, downy hair, called **lanugo,** may be found on the face, shoulders, and back. The skin also may be covered with a white, thick, cheesy material, the **vernix caseosa,** which is composed of epithelioid cells and secretions from sebaceous glands. It protects the skin from the amniotic fluid in utero. It is especially noticeable in the hair and skin creases.

Because of slowed peripheral circulation, the extremities of the newborn often appear cyanotic; this condition is called **acrocyanosis**. This cyanosis is exaggerated when the newborn is exposed to cold. Generalized cyanosis or pallor must be reported. It could indicate a heart defect.

Movement and Activities

Maturity. The birth attendant observes posture, various flexibility tests and reflexes, and specific physical characteristics to determine neuromuscular and physical maturity of the newborn; if the neonate's scores are too low, he or she is treated as premature.

Behavior. The typical newborn sleeps approximately 20 hours a day. He or she awakens easily and cries when hungry or uncomfortable. The arms and legs move freely and symmetrically. The extremities are often flexed. The newborn is unable to support the weight of the head.

Reflexes. Certain reflexes are present at birth, even though the nervous system of the newborn is immature. These reflexes indicate the adequacy of neurologic functioning in the neonate; their presence or absence indicates abnormalities:

- The *rooting reflex* is elicited when the newborn is stroked on the lip or cheek. The normal neonate reacts by turning the head toward the direction of the stimulus.
- The *sucking reflex* is demonstrated as the newborn grasps the nipple with the lips. Sucking should be automatic.
- The *gag reflex* is stimulated when the back of the throat is touched by an object. This is a protection against choking.
- The *grasp reflex* is evidenced by a tight grasp of a finger placed into the newborn's hand. This reflex disappears as the newborn grows older.
- The *Moro* or *startle reflex* is caused by a sudden noise or jarring of the crib. This reaction causes the newborn to throw the arms out and draw the legs up.
- The *tonic neck reflex* is a postural reflex. When the neonate is lying on the back and turns the head to one side, the leg and arm of the corresponding side extend, and those of the opposite side flex.
- The *Babinski reflex* occurs when the sole of the foot is scraped from heel to toe. The big toe fans out and hyperextends.
- Other normal reflexes include *stepping, crawling, blinking, sneezing,* and *coughing.*

Senses. The neonate can see shades of light and darkness following birth and blinks in response to bright lights but is unable to focus the eyes.

The newborn is able to hear after delivery, as evidenced by reactions to loud noises. Parents are encouraged to talk in a soothing voice.

Touch is well developed in the neonate; he or she responds to discomfort, such as pain and wetness.

The senses of smell and taste are present soon after delivery, although less is known about them. Newborns are known to increase sucking when glucose water is offered. Research has shown that newborns at 1 week of life are able to distinguish their mother's milk by smelling their mother's breast pads.

Influences of Maternal Hormones

The newborn of either sex may have swollen breasts because of the presence of maternal hormones. The labia of the female newborn may appear edematous, and a small amount of mucous bloody discharge may be expelled from the vagina. This is known as **pseudomenstruation.** The scrotum of the male neonate may appear large, and a testicle should be palpable in each sac.

Admission to the Newborn Nursery

When the newborn is transferred from the delivery room to the newborn nursery, the nursery nurse must be given certain information:

♦ Length of first and second stages of labor
♦ Time of rupture of the membranes
♦ Type of delivery and any difficulties
♦ Analgesics and anesthetics that were used in delivery
♦ Condition of the newborn at delivery
♦ The newborn's Apgar score
♦ Whether infant resuscitation as needed
♦ Whether vitamin K was given
♦ Whether eye prophylaxis was performed

Protection for the Newborn

The techniques used by the nursery personnel isolate each newborn from direct contact with other babies. All people working in the nursery (and the father or coach) follow a specific handwashing and scrub technique. Nursery personnel usually wear hospital scrub suits and the father wears a gown over his clothes. People with an infectious disease are not allowed in the obstetric area.

Each newborn is placed in a separate crib or warmer equipped with a firm, waterproof mattress. The crib has clear sides, so the neonate can be observed at all times. If the newborn's temperature is not yet stabilized, the isolette or newborn warmer is used.

Each newborn has its own equipment and supplies. *Equipment is never shared.* The nursery is well lighted and heated to approximately 75°F. The nursery is *never* left unattended, and newborns are within sight at all times.

> **Nursing Alert**
>
> Bulb syringes are kept at each newborn's cribside. *(Rationale: The nurse must be alert to possible choking. The bulb syringe is used to suction the neonate if needed.)*

Nursery Infections. A hospital nursery can be a hazardous place for a newborn if an infection is present. Epidemics of a skin infection (such as impetigo) and staphylococcal infections may occur. A fatal type of neonatal diarrhea is a particular danger. Some hospitals have two nurseries; one is used while the other is being disinfected. Babies with identified infections are isolated from well babies, and in a questionable case, the newborn is kept isolated.

Admission Procedures

Nursing Assessment

The nurse assesses the newborn on admission. It is important to note the physical characteristics, including the appearance of the newborn, behavior, and reflexes. The nurse observes the cord and makes certain that the clamp is securely attached. The number of vessels in the umbilical cord are counted. Normally, there should be three—two arteries and one vein. If only two vessels are observed, there is a strong possibility of congenital defects in the newborn.

Weight and Length. The newborn is weighed immediately after arriving in the newborn nursery. The weight is recorded on the chart in grams and converted to pounds for the mother's benefit.

The easiest way to measure the neonate is to stretch him or her out full length in the bassinet. Place a small mark on the sheet at the bottom of the feet and at the crown of the head, and measure between the marks.

The nurse also measures and records head circumference and chest circumference. The head usually measures 1 or 2 inches (2.54–5 cm) more than the chest. These measurements are often recorded in centimeters. The procedure for measuring head circumference is discussed in Chapter 64.

Vital Signs. Respiration, pulse, and temperature are taken and recorded every hour or two immediately after birth and then every 4 hours for the first 24 hours. The initial temperature is taken rectally to establish patency of the rectum. The tympanic or axillary routes are used for subsequent temperatures.

Elimination. The passage of stool and urine—including the amount, color, and consistency—is recorded. If the newborn does not void within 24 hours after birth, the birth attendant will determine the patency of the urethra. Any deviation from normal should be charted and reported to the physician.

Cleansing

Procedures for the initial cleansing of the neonate differ among hospitals. Sometimes the father is allowed to cleanse the newborn in the delivery room, or a staff member may merely wipe off the blood and some of the vernix. In some facilities a complete body bath and shampoo are done once the neonate is stable and the body temperature is within normal limits. Care is taken to prevent the newborn from being chilled during any bathing procedure.

Examination by the Birth Attendant

Within 24 hours of birth, the newborn must be examined thoroughly by the birth attendant. The birth attendant reviews the chart, including the labor and delivery record and the prenatal record. When examining the newborn, the birth attendant evaluates the circulatory, respiratory, digestive, and neurologic systems thoroughly. The birth attendant also observes the reproductive, urinary, musculoskeletal, and endocrine systems carefully. The nurse's assessments and charting during the first few hours are important to the birth attendant's examination.

Neonatal Laboratory Screening

When the neonate is a few hours old, hemoglobin and hematocrit tests are often ordered. Because of increased blood volume, the hemoglobin is normally 15 to 18 g/100 mL of blood. The normal hematocrit for the newborn is 45% to 60%. It is important to rule out anemia. In most cases, the heel-stick method is used to obtain peripheral blood for examination in the neonate. This may be a nursing function in your facility.

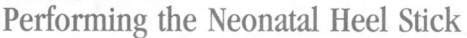

Nursing Skill
Performing the Neonatal Heel Stick

Supplies and Equipment

Warm, moist pack
Gloves
Alcohol wipe
Sterile gauze or cotton ball
Sterile lancet
Capillary tubes or PKU cards
Pen and labels

Procedure

1. Warm the heel for at least 5 minutes, using a warm, moist pack. *(Rationale: This helps to dilate the capillaries and arterioles and will enhance blood flow.)*

2. Wash hands and don gloves. *(Rationale: Universal Precautions require gloves in procedures involving blood.)*

3. Cleanse the heel with alcohol. Dry with sterile gauze or a cotton ball. *(Rationale: It is important to prevent infection. The presence of alcohol might alter the results of the test.)*

4. Firmly restrain the foot with your free hand.

5. Using a sterile lancet, puncture the skin on the *side of the sole of the heel.* The puncture must be deep enough to obtain free blood flow but not so deep as to touch the bone (approximately 2–2.4 mm). *(Rationale: A serious complication is necrotizing osteochondritis, an inflammation of the bone. The skin on the side of the heel is thinner, to facilitate blood flow and the puncture. This location also is believed to cause less pain.)*

6. Discard the first drop of blood. *(Rationale: This could contain contaminants from the skin.)*

7. Collect blood according to hospital protocol. If capillary tubes are used, avoid getting any air bubbles into the tube. In some cases, materials are added to the sample; usually the tube is plugged. If phenylketonuria cards are used, be sure the blood covers the entire circle. Label the sample carefully—the laboratory needs to know that it is a heel-stick sample. It may need to be placed on ice for transport to the laboratory. *(Rationale: Protocols must be followed exactly to maintain accuracy of the tests.)*

8. Tests should be done immediately. Do not expose the sample to air. Do not allow the blood to clot. *(Rationale: These actions can cause changes in the pH, CO_2 or lactic acid levels.)*

9. Apply pressure to the site with a sterile gauze square or cotton ball. Make sure bleeding has stopped. Apply a bandage.

10. Comfort the newborn.

The physician may order a Dextrostix test, which helps to monitor the blood glucose level of the neonate. A small sample of blood is obtained from a heel stick and tested with a reagent strip. The blood glucose level testing procedure is described in Chapter 72.

Most states in the United States require testing for specific diseases in the newborn. A test is done to rule out **phenylketonuria,** an inherited disorder caused by the body's inability to digest protein normally. Tests are made for **galactosemia,** a hereditary disease. Phenylketonuria and galactosemia are discussed in Chapters 62 and 65. Tests of thyroid function also can rule out *hypothyroidism,* also known as cretinism (see Chapter 72). This disorder has a much better prognosis if it is treated before the age of 3 months.

The newborn's urine may be tested for drugs, such as cocaine or marijuana. If these are present, this indicates maternal substance abuse. Care of the neonate born to the substance-abusing mother is discussed in Chapter 62.

A test for G6PD deficiency may be done, especially in babies of African, Asian, and Mediterranean origin.

Daily Care of the Newborn

Routine care of the newborn requires meeting the basic needs of food, cleanliness, comfort, and safety. It also requires careful nursing assessment for signs of abnormalities or problems.

Nursing Assessment

Vital Signs

Respiration and Pulse. Respiration is taken first, then pulse. *(Rationale: Respirations and pulse increase when the neonate is disturbed. Values are not accurate if the newborn is moving or crying.)* Chart whether the neonate was sleeping, awake, or crying when pulse and respiration were taken.

Respirations are counted for 60 seconds. The newborn breathes through the nose, and the nurse will observe the abdomen rise and fall with each breath. Respirations should be quiet and may be irregular. The normal respiratory rate ranges from 30 to 60 respirations per minute when the newborn is at rest. (Signs of respiratory distress are described earlier in this chapter.)

The pulse is taken apically for 60 seconds. The pulse is rapid and may be irregular; the normal range is 120 to 160 beats per minute. Warm the stethoscope in your hand before taking the pulse.

Temperature. Most newborn nurseries use the tympanic temperature probe to measure the temperature of neonates after the initial rectal temperature. The tympanic temperature probe may be set to convert to the rectal temperature equivalent. The tympanic method is considered the safest method and is fast and accurate. The tympanic probe is inserted into the neonate's ear, while the head is held steady. It will record within a few seconds.

If the tympanic method is not to be used, rectal or axillary temperatures may be ordered. The normal neonate's rectal temperature is between 98°F and 99°F (36.7°C and 37.1°C). To measure the temperature rectally, gently insert the temperature probe approximately 0.5 inch (1.3 cm). Hold the newborn's feet with one hand and the probe with the other hand. Place a dry diaper over the neonate so that you will not get wet if he or she voids while the temperature is being taken. Keep the probe in place until the instrument beeps. Hold the probe at all times. (Many hospitals do not do routine rectal temperatures because of injury potential.)

Blood Pressure. Blood pressure usually is low, ranging from 50 to 80 mm Hg systolic and 30 to 50 mm Hg diastolic. Follow hospital protocol for location to be used (usually the leg). The smallest size cuff is used.

Daily Weight. The neonate is weighed once a day. Bath time is an excellent time to do this. Nursing skills in weighing a neonate follow:

Nursing Skill
Weighing the Neonate

Supplies and Equipment

Towel
Transfer paper
Clean diaper
Infant scale

Procedure

1. Wash your hands before the procedure. This scale is cleaned between uses. *(Rationale: This prevents spread of infection.)*
2. Pad the scale with a towel. *(Rationale: This prevents excess heat loss in the neonate and prevents startling the infant.)* Deduct the weight of the towel. *(Rationale: To ensure accuracy.)*
3. Remove all of the newborn's clothes. Place a transfer paper on the scale, and weigh the newborn as quickly as possible. *(Rationale: Minimizes exposure and discomfort.)*
4. Keep your hand above the neonate at all times (Fig. 60-1). *(Rationale: This protects the neonate from falling.)* Never leave the newborn unattended.
5. Dress the newborn. Use a clean diaper. Place the newborn back in the crib. Discard the transfer paper. *(Rationale: The diaper was contaminated. Make sure the baby is safe before cleaning up the area.)*
6. Wash your hands. *(Rationale: This prevents cross-contamination.)*
7. Record the weight in grams on the chart. *(Rationale: Grams are used for consistency and to promote greater accuracy.)* Convert to pounds for the mother's information.

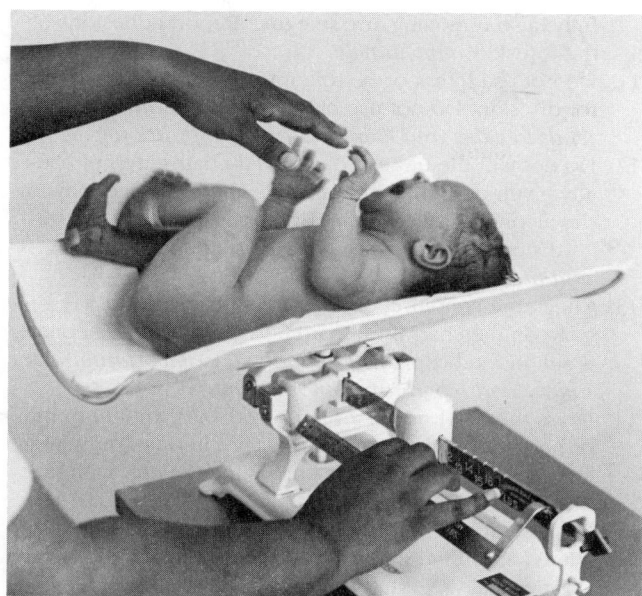

Figure 60-1. Weighing the newborn. A clean transfer paper is placed on the scale. The baby is weighed undressed. The nurse keeps one hand over the neonate at all times to prevent falls.

Eyes, Nose, and Ears

Redness, swelling, or discharge should be reported and recorded on the chart; the physician will prescribe the necessary treatment.

Elimination

Urination. The newborn often voids immediately after birth. Nursing assessment is important to make sure the neonate voids, usually within 4 to 8 hours after delivery. At first the urine is concentrated and may be pink (caused by *urates*). After the first 2 or 3 days, the neonate voids 5 to 12 times daily.

Nursing Alert

If the newborn does not void within the first 18 to 24 hours after birth, the physician must be notified. *(Rationale: This may be a sign of imperforate urethra, a ureteral blockage, anuria, or other disorder.)*

Stools. The first stool is a gray or black puttylike mass of matter, called the *meconium plug.* During the first days, the stools are dark green, sticky, and tarry. This indicates the presence of **meconium,** a waste product formed in the newborn's intestine in the latter months of pregnancy.

Later, the stool changes to greenish-yellow (*transitional stool*) and then to yellow. The stools of breast-fed babies range from pale green to golden yellow, are

smooth, and pasty or "seedy." A neonate fed a formula of cow's milk has a brighter yellow and more formed stool. The stools smell like sour milk; breast-fed stools have less odor. The newborn normally has several stools a day, fewer if breast-fed.

Nursing Alert

If the newborn does not pass a meconium stool within 24 hours, the physician must be notified. *(Rationale: This may be a sign of **imperforate** anus [closed anus] or inspissated meconium [hardened stool], causing a bowel obstruction. These conditions usually must be surgically corrected immediately.)*

Cord Care

Observe carefully for redness, drainage, or any other sign of infection. *(Rationale: The cord is an excellent portal of entry for infection until it is healed.)* Many hospital protocols include daily application of alcohol to reduce infection and speed the drying process.

Daily care assessments of the neonate are summarized in the accompanying box.

Other Daily Care

Maintaining Body Temperature

The neonate's temperature control center is immature, so the temperature may be elevated if the room is too warm. Alternatively, the neonate's body temperature may need to be supported by external means for the first few days of life, especially if the room is cool. Caps, additional clothing, and extra blankets promote warmth.

Skin Care

The skin of the neonate dries the first few days after birth, and cracks may appear in the folds; it also may **desquamate** (peel) in large or small flakes. The skin of the newborn is usually reddish and wrinkled, although it should become smooth and of a color typical of its race within 2 weeks. If any *jaundice* appears, especially in the first 24 hours after birth, it should be reported at once.

The newborn's skin is sensitive. To prevent irritation, his or her buttocks should be thoroughly cleaned following a bowel movement. If any rash or irritation occurs, it should be reported. *(Rationale: This could be a source of infection.)*

Cleansing the Newborn

Hospital routines for bathing neonates vary. The normal routine is to give a sponge bath every day with water and a soft wipe or to use a mild germicidal soap. It is essential to prevent chilling or overtiring.

Nursing Skill
Cleansing the Neonate

Supplies and Equipment

Stethoscope
Temperature probe
Baby wipes, soft cloth, or prescribed materials
Baby soap
Cotton balls
Antiseptic for cord stump
Clean clothes and diaper
Clean crib linens
Trash bag
Cleanser for buttocks
Fine comb or brush
Pan of warm water
Watch or clock with second hand

Procedure

1. Wash your hands thoroughly before beginning the procedure. Individual equipment and a modified isolation technique are used. *(Rationale: It is vital to prevent the spread of infection among newborns, because their defense mechanisms are immature.)*
2. Assemble equipment needed. *(Rationale: Once you begin, you cannot leave the neonate.)*
3. Take respiration, pulse, and temperature *first* if ordered. Then undress the newborn and take the weight *before* giving the bath.
4. Keep the neonate warm and secure. Be sure to support the newborn during the procedure so that he or she does not become frightened. *(Rationale: The first few days of a newborn's life may play a part in shaping attitudes toward the general environment; therefore, it is important that he or she feels safe and secure.)*
5. Assess the neonate as you bathe him or her. Note skin color, blemishes or rash, abnormal jerking or twitching, bleeding or abnormal discharge, and congenital abnormalities.
6. Begin the bath by wiping the eyes, stroking from the inner corner to the outer corner. A clean area of the wipe is used for each eye. Wipe the rest of the neonate's face, including the ears.
7. Moisten the hair; rinse and dry it. Gently comb or brush it, even if the baby has minimal hair.
8. Wash the newborn's body with clear water, working from the head down. Soap is used sparingly, if at all. *(Rationale: It tends to dry the skin.)* Give special attention to the folds of the skin.
9. Cleanse the genital area last, assessing for signs of rash or irritation. Cotton balls or baby wipes can be used to cleanse the perineal area from front to back. Cleanse the vulva carefully, removing all **smegma** (excess secretions and dead skin cells). If pins are used, close them when you remove them, and keep them out of the newborn's reach. *(Rationale: These are all safety precautions.)*
10. Care for a circumcision as prescribed. Observe for any unusual swelling or bleeding. Cleanse the penis care-

fully, also removing any smegma. Report adhesions of the foreskin *immediately*.
11. Do not use lotion or petroleum jelly unless prescribed for dry skin. Do not use baby powder. *(Rationale: It tends to cake, and there is a risk of aspiration.)*
12. Do not wet the unhealed cord. Tub baths are not usually given until the cord falls off. The physician may order alcohol, Triple Dye, or antibiotic ointment for the cord stump. *(Rationale: These help speed the healing and prevent infection.)*
13. Check the condition of the cord at least once a day. Note on the chart if the cord falls off while the neonate is still in the hospital. *(Rationale: It is important to document and report any abnormalities.)*
14. Dress the newborn in a diaper and shirt, and wrap him or her in a blanket. Hold him or her in one arm while changing the linen on the crib. Wipe the crib with the prescribed antiseptic.
15. Discard all trash properly.
16. Make sure the newborn is in a comfortable and safe position.
17. Wash your hands.
18. Document all observations.

Key Concept

Any abnormal sign or symptom must be reported at once. A newborn's condition can change quickly.

Parent Teaching

Many hospitals provide demonstration baths with newborn manikins for new mothers; demonstrations are often given by a nursing student. Later, the mother is expected to perform the procedure for the nurse to show she has fully understood.

The neonate usually does not receive a tub bath until he or she is about 2 weeks old. The cord must fall off before a tub bath is given. However, the demonstration is given during prenatal class or while the mother is in the hospital. Document all teaching. The skills for giving a neonatal tub bath follow.

Nursing Skill
Giving a Tub Bath

Supplies and Equipment

Baby bath tub
Bath thermometer
2 wash cloths
Towels
Baby soap
Clean clothes and diaper
Skin care materials, as prescribed

Procedure

1. Wash your hands before you start the procedure.
2. Have all the equipment ready and conveniently placed before you start. *(Rationale: You should not leave the neonate once you begin the procedure.)*
3. Be sure that the room is warm enough and that the newborn is protected from drafts. Check the temperature of the water carefully; it should be warm, not hot (98°F, or 37°C, is the usual maximum temperature). *(Rationale: Babies chill or burn easily.)*
4. Carefully support the neonate's head and body with a moderately firm grip when you put him or her in the tub.
5. Use a soft wash cloth and towel and a minimum of soap.
6. Rinse all the soap off; dry the skin folds well.
7. Assess for skin irritation or abnormalities.
8. Clean and care for the equipment, and replenish used supplies.
9. Wash your hands.
10. Document the procedure, noting any unusual symptoms.

Care of the Penis

In male babies, the foreskin (prepuce) covers the glans penis or extends beyond it. The opening may be very small, a condition known as **phimosis.** A secretion called smegma may collect beneath the foreskin, and drops of urine also may remain, causing irritation. If circumcision is not performed, the physician may order that the foreskin be stretched and retracted over the glans penis for cleaning once every day. This must be done gently and carefully. Replace the foreskin immediately; a tight foreskin will cause edema and pain.

Circumcision. Some male newborns may be **circumcised** (part or all of the foreskin is removed). Ritual circumcision is performed on all Jewish male babies. If the baby has been circumcised, he must be kept clean and assessed for bleeding, swelling, and voiding. A sterile petrolatum dressing may be applied after each voiding for 24 to 48 hours to keep the diaper from sticking. Circumcision is usually performed shortly before the newborn leaves the hospital or after discharge; for this reason, the mother should be instructed in the care required, and the teaching should be documented.

Nutrition

Birth attendants differ in their procedures for feeding newborns. Many mothers who breast-feed are allowed to do so in the delivery room. Other birth attendants prefer that the newborn remain NPO for 3 to 4 hours after birth. The first feeding usually consists of sterile water and is often given by the nurse. If all is normal, the mother gives the newborn as many other feedings as she wishes; if the mother is tired, the nurses may feed the neonate.

If the baby takes too much food, takes it too fast, or is not properly burped (bubbled), the food may be regurgitated. (This is simply an overflow and should not be thought of as vomiting.) Food remaining in the esophagus may cause hiccups, which can usually be stopped with sips of water.

Many physicians order vitamin supplements for the newborn, especially the breast-fed baby, who might not be receiving the benefits of the vitamins and iron present in most prepared formulas.

> ### Nursing Alert
> A healthy baby is eager for food; however, if he or she refuses to nurse or to take the bottle, spits up or vomits, or has an unusual amount of discomfort from gas, the physician should be notified. Sometimes, a simple change in formula will relieve these digestive symptoms. If this is not effective, however, these symptoms may indicate a congenital digestive malformation or disorder.

Sleep

Except when being fed, the newborn sleeps most of the time, although not deeply. The baby will awaken and cry when hungry or uncomfortable. Most authorities recommend that the baby sleep on the side and be repositioned from side to side. Many physicians suggest that the baby not be placed on the stomach until he or she can raise the head. Research in the area of sudden infant death syndrome (SIDS) suggests a higher incidence of SIDS when the newborn is positioned prone. Although positioning the newborn on its back has been discouraged in the past, SIDS research is dispelling past fears of choking. A pillow is not used because of the danger of suffocation.

Holding the Newborn

It is important that the newborn feel secure at all times. Babies are usually dressed in shirts and diapers and then wrapped securely in a receiving blanket. This allows the neonate to have much the same position and feeling of security that was experienced in the uterus. When the newborn is lifted, the head, neck, and buttocks must be supported. The baby should be held close to the nurse's body to provide security. The "football" hold is a convenient method of holding a newborn, because it provides the nurse with a free hand so that additional tasks can be performed (Fig. 60-2).

The Baby's Responses

The newborn baby cries and tightens the muscles in response to sudden loud sounds, changes in position, the feel of something cold touching the skin, or any

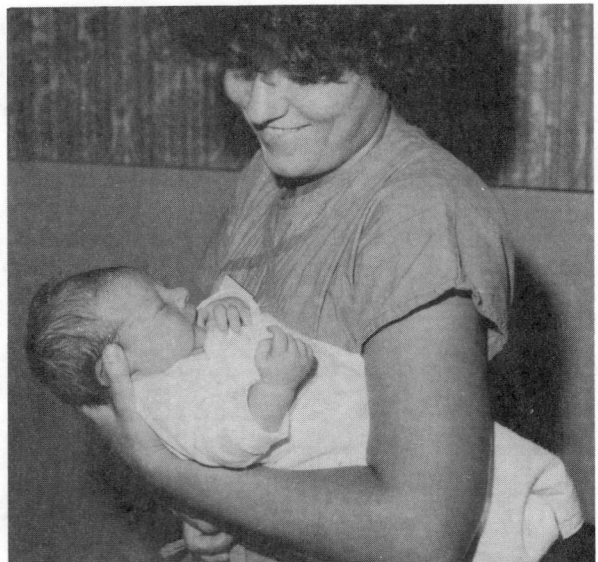

Figure 60-2. Football hold for carrying the newborn.

interference with movements. The baby relaxes if held and rocked and patted lightly.

Crying is the only way a baby can ask for help. He or she cries if hungry, wet, uncomfortable, disturbed, or sick. The cry of the healthy newborn is lusty. The baby who gets more care usually cries less.

Hunger cries are healthy, demanding cries, and the newborn may put fingers in the mouth as an additional sign of hunger. After being fed, the baby is quiet unless he or she has swallowed air from the bottle and needs to bubble.

Infant Feeding

Newborns are usually fed "on demand," or approximately every 3 to 4 hours. An important nursing skill is the proper method of bringing the neonate to the mother.

Nursing Skill
Bringing the Neonate to the Mother

Procedure

1. Wash your hands.
2. Dress the neonate warmly.
3. Weigh the breast-fed baby.
4. Carry the baby carefully. The football hold is often used.
5. Instruct the mother to wash her hands. (*Rationale: This prevents infection of the neonate.*)
6. Compare the wrist band of the mother with that of the baby. (*Rationale: You must ensure the right baby is with the right mother.*)
7. Provide privacy for the mother and her newborn.

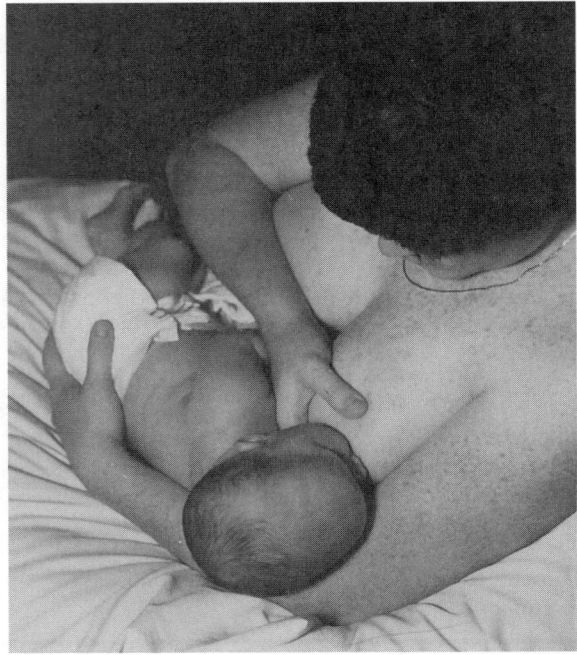

Figure 60-3. Position for breast-feeding. (Used with permission of Chele Marmet and the Lactation Institute, 16430 Ventura Blvd., Encino, CA 91436.)

8. Assist the mother into a comfortable position (Fig. 60-3). (*Rationale: She will be in the same position for about 20 minutes.*)
9. Show the mother how to hold and bubble the neonate. Have her demonstrate in return. (*Rationale: This is for safety.*)
10. When the feeding is finished, check with the mother on how the baby fed, or determine the amount of formula missing from the bottle. Check if baby was bubbled.
11. Weigh the breast-fed infant.
12. Make sure the baby is clean and dry before placing him or her in the crib. Follow hospital procedure for placement in the crib. (*Rationale: Positioning is aimed at preventing aspiration.*)
13. Wash your hands.
14. Document on the baby's chart, including how much breast milk/formula was taken, and any other pertinent observations.

Breast-Feeding*

More than 50% of newborns are breast-fed today. Advantages of breast-feeding for the baby include the following:

◆ Decreased incidence of allergies
◆ Nutritionally superior

* Most of the information in this section is from Gwendelyn Combs-Marshall, Certified Lactation Educator, Nutri Source.

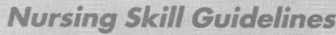

- Economical
- Readily available
- Promotes transfer of maternal antibodies
- Enhances maternal-newborn bonding
- Possibility of higher IQs†

Breast-feeding also is beneficial to the mother. It speeds involution of the uterus, promotes neonate bonding, and delays ovulation. Many researchers believe nursing also reduces the risk of breast cancer. No matter what the nurse's personal feelings or beliefs about breast-feeding, as a healthcare professional, it is important to promote and facilitate breast-feeding because it is undeniably an excellent healthy choice for the newborn and mother.

First Feedings. The mother will often nurse her newborn immediately after birth and again within 4 hours. If the mother does not ask to nurse, the birth attendant or nurse may suggest it. The delivery room staff should cooperate if the mother agrees. Most modern delivery tables are wide enough to accommodate nursing. Thermal heat or a radiant warmer may be used to heat the nursing couple if the room is cool or if the mother is shivering from strenuous labor or from medication. Breast-fed neonates usually should not get supplementary water or bottles in the nursery; this helps to avoid nipple confusion and encourage nursing at the breast. Nursing skills in helping to position the mother and neonate for breast-feeding are given in the accompanying guidelines box.

Many women feel a slight tingling sensation when they begin to nurse. This is the "let-down" reflex when the sucking action of the newborn triggers the brain to release milk from the alveolus to the baby. Many "let downs" occur during a single nursing session. The let-down reflex can be impaired when the mother is stressed, cold, or in pain. Alcohol also can inhibit milk flow.

> **Nursing Alert**
>
> Stay with the mother the first time the baby goes to breast to show her what to do.

Feeding Schedule. All babies should be fed on demand, that is, when they are hungry. Babies are all different, and their nursing patterns will vary. During the fist few days, the baby gets colostrum, which is rich in disease-fighting immunities and nutrients. Although the mother's milk is not in yet, it is important for the new-

---

Nursing Skill Guidelines
Positioning and Assisting with Breast-feeding

- Proper positioning during breast-feeding is important. The mother and newborn should be comfortable. The cradle or football holds are most commonly used, or the mother can lie on her side. *(Rationale: Proper positioning helps the newborn receive the milk easily. It also helps to minimize nipple soreness, plugged ducts, and mastitis.)*
- *The arm supports the newborn.* The mother is supported with pillows, and she uses one arm to support the newborn. If she uses the cradle hold, the back of the newborn's head should be in the crook of her arm, and her hand should hold the newborn's bottom or thigh. The proper positioning in the cradle hold is given in Figure 60-3.
- *The other hand supports the breast.* The mother's hand opposite the nursing breast should be used to support the breast. The mother should place her hand below her breast on her rib cage. She should use as many fingers as necessary to support her breast without covering any of her nipple. Her thumb should be placed *above* her nipple. This grasp is called the C-hold or palmar grasp. *(Rationale: This will ensure proper positioning and prevent nipple soreness.)*
- The neonate's body should be turned toward the mother's body so that they are tummy to tummy.
- *Tickle the neonate's bottom lip or corner of mouth.* Stroke the newborn's bottom lip with the nipple to trigger the rooting reflex. This will coax the neonate to open his or her mouth. Wait until the mouth is open wide. *(Rationale: If it is not, the neonate will grasp on the tip of the nipple and cause soreness for mother.)*
- *Pull the neonate in close.* As soon as the mouth is open wide, move the newborn quickly to the breast so that the nipple goes past the gums and well into the mouth. The newborn should have the whole areola in his or her mouth, not just the nipple. (The areola is the darkened area surrounding the nipple.) The mother's arm should support the newborn, and the newborn's nose and chin should touch the breast. If the nose is covered, the mother gently presses her breast near the neonate's nose so he or she can breathe easily.
- To stop nursing, place a finger between the baby's mouth and the areola to break suction.
- If pain is felt while nursing, break suction and begin again. *(Rationale: Pain in not a normal part of breast-feeding.)*
- Both breasts are offered at each feeding, alternating the starting side. *(Rationale: Each breast should be emptied regularly.)*

---

† Lucas A, Marley R, et al. "Breast milk and subsequent intelligence quotients in children born preterm." Lancet 339:261-264, 1991

born to nurse often. This will help to condition the nipples for nursing and stimulate milk production. Frequent nursing also will prevent engorgement and related complications. Milk production is stimulated by the neonate's sucking; the more sucking, the more milk will be produced. It is not uncommon for newborns to be too sleepy to nurse. Sleepy babies can often be aroused by a diaper change, being undressed, or a sponge bath. It is normal for newborns to fall asleep while nursing.

When the mother's milk "comes in," by the third or fourth day, a breast-feeding baby may nurse 8 to 12 times a day. The breast from which the baby nursed last during the previous feeding should be offered first because it may not have been emptied completely. It is often easy to tell which breast to offer because it feels fuller than the other. The baby should nurse about 10 minutes on one breast before being offered the second breast. It is often best to let the baby signal when to switch breasts to get the right balance of calories. When the baby first begins nursing, he or she gets *foremilk,* which is relatively low in fat. *Hindmilk* appears at the end of the feeding and is higher in fat and calories.

Many women seem concerned about their milk supply after a few weeks because their breasts feel softer. This is normal and is due to the body's adjustment to the neonate's needs. Often, a baby who has settled into a nice feeding pattern will begin to nurse more often. This baby is probably experiencing a growth spurt. Although the mother may not have enough milk the first day, her body will quickly adapt, and her milk supply will increase. During the early days and months, many babies will suck for pleasure, which is often called *non-nutritive sucking.* When a baby is actually nursing you will hear a "suck-suck-swallow" pattern. There will be no swallow during non-nutritive sucking.

Elimination. Signs that the newborn is receiving adequate nutrition are at least six to eight wet diapers and one to two stools per day. Once the baby has passed the meconium (within 24–48 hours), the baby's stool will be loose and unformed and range in color from pea soup to yellow to tan. The stool will appear seedy and will have little odor. By 6 weeks of age, most breast-feeding babies have one or two bowel movements a day. This is because breast milk is so well absorbed.

Common Problems During Breast-Feeding

Sore and Cracked Nipples. Sore nipples are most often caused by improper positioning of the neonate at the breast. In the early days of nursing, a baby with a vigorous suck may cause nipple discomfort. Sore nipples caused by an enthusiastic baby should subside as the nipples get conditioned to nursing. Treatment of sore nipples includes swabbing the affected nipple with

Medications and the Nursing Mother*

Many drugs pass into breast milk from the mother. Not all drugs pass in the same concentrations; it depends on fat solubility, water solubility, and other factors. Drugs taken by the mother that are *particularly dangerous* to the nursing neonate follow:

◆ Anticancer drugs (chemotherapy)
◆ Radioactive substances (such as those used for diagnostic tests)
◆ Lithium (used to treat psychiatric disorders)
◆ Chloramphenicol (Chloromycetin, Chloroptic)
◆ Phenylbutazone (Butazolidin)
◆ Atropine (used to dilate pupils of the eyes, to dry secretions before surgery, and in other situations)
◆ Thiouracil
◆ Iodides
◆ Mercurials

* *Merck Manual of Diagnosis and Therapy, Ed 16. Rahway, NJ, Merck Inc, 1992.*

breast milk and allowing it to dry there. Dry heat, such as a 60-watt lamp held 18 inches from the breast, or use of a warm (not hot) hair dryer after nursing will help ease symptoms. Routine use of nipple ointments should be discouraged. Soap should not be used on the breasts. (*Rationale: It is drying, and this would promote cracking of the nipples.*)

Engorgement. Engorgement is the extreme fullness of the areola or breast. Some engorgement is normal. The best treatment is prevention by frequent nursing. If engorgement is already present, have the mother use warm heat before nursing and then manually express some milk. This allows the neonate to get a proper grasp on the nipple and prevents further pain for the mother. Massage also helps to soften the engorged breast to allow for easier hand expression or nursing. A good fitting nonwaterproof cotton bra is essential. (*Rationale: Waterproof bras hold in moisture, which can cause irritation or maceration of the nipples. The breasts should be firmly supported.*) The most important treatment is to nurse frequently, even around the clock.

Plugged Ducts. Plugged ducts or tender lumps in the breasts of an otherwise healthy lactating woman, are usually caused by incomplete emptying of the breasts. The treatment is to continue nursing. Massaging the area and applying heat prior to nursing will help to ensure complete emptying of the breast. Nursing on the opposite breast first will allow the affected breast to "let down," easing nursing on the affected side. Proper positioning of the newborn and changing the neonate's position also may help. The mother's bra should be checked for proper fit.

Mastitis. If an organism is present, such as *Staphylococcus aureus* or *Escherichia coli,* and the mother's resistance to disease is lowered because of stress or illness, mastitis can result. Mastitis is a systemic breast infection that must be treated with antibiotics. For a discussion and treatment of mastitis, see Chapter 61.

Maternal Diet for Breast-Feeding

A well-nourished mother ensures an adequate and nutritious milk supply for her newborn and protects her own health. On the other hand, a poorly nourished mother or one who is restricting her calories may not produce enough breast milk. It is recommended that the nursing mother receive about 500 calories a day above her non-nursing caloric intake. Adequate fluids also are important for milk production. See the food guide pyramid and Table 26-1 in Chapter 26 for specific food types and amounts suggested for the nursing mother.

The nursing mother need not restrict her intake of favorite foods just because she is nursing, although a few foods may cause concern. *Alcohol* does appear in the breast milk, and large quantities in the maternal diet have been shown to inhibit the let-down reflex. Babies of heavy alcohol drinkers nurse less often and for shorter periods. However, small amounts of alcohol tend to ease the let-down reflex and relax the mother. *Caffeine* also is transferred to breast milk. A moderate intake is fine; however, if the baby appears wakeful, restless, or irritable, the mother may want to cut down on her caffeine intake.

Cow's milk has inconclusively been linked to colic in newborns. If the baby is colicky, the mother may want to eliminate fluid milk from her diet for 2 weeks to see if it makes a difference. Colic usually worsens if a breast-fed baby is switched to human milk substitute. *Strongly flavored foods* may cause temporary colic in some neonates. Colic usually lasts approximately 24 hours. Common offenders are onions, garlic, beans, and rhubarb.

Many medications are passed from mother to infant via breast milk, as briefly introduced in the accompanying box. The nursing mother should consult her baby's pediatrician before taking any drugs.

Key Concept

The nursing mother should be encouraged to avoid stringent weight loss diets, which may adversely affect the quantity and quality of her breast milk.

Infant Nutrition

The nutritional needs of infants are best met by breast milk or human milk substitute for the first 4 to 6 months of life. Early introduction of solids may increase the risk of allergy and has no advantages over human milk or its substitute. See Chapter 64 for a complete discussion of infant nutrition.

Nursing Alert

Your hands and the mother's hands must be washed before putting the newborn to breast or giving the bottle. *(Rationale: This maintains cleanliness and helps to prevent infections.)*

Bottle Feeding

If the mother does not want to nurse her baby, her feelings should be respected. Research has provided satisfactory formulas for replacing breast milk. Breastfeeding may not be desirable when the mother has a chronic disease, if the nipples are severely inverted, or if the baby has certain abnormalities. In the event of a premature baby and in some other situations, the mother may express her milk and it may be bottle-fed to the baby.

A variety of formulas is available; each product available has its own advantages. The physician orders the formula according to the newborn's need.

During the first week of feeding, most babies increase their intake from 1 to 3 oz per feeding, with a total intake of 12 to 15 oz in 24 hours. This amount increases to approxmately 20 oz in 24 hours by the end of the second week. Intake increases rapidly thereafter. By the third week, many babies will drop an evening or a night feeding and sleep longer without hunger.

The mother's hands are washed before she is handed the baby, and care is used in keeping the nipple clean. The rate of flow from the nipple should be checked, to make certain that it is a constant drip. Nipple openings are made either with a "cross" cut or with holes. If the openings are not large enough, the holes can be enlarged by putting a red-hot needle through them. If the opening is too large, the baby may tend to choke.

While the baby is eating, the bottle should be tilted so that milk is in the neck of the bottle at all times or so the plastic liner folds in on itself, to keep the baby from swallowing air. The baby should be bubbled at intervals during the feeding.

Feeding does not just provide food for the baby; it also gives the baby a sense of security and of being loved. *Always hold the baby* and cuddle him or her during the feeding. Hold the bottle-fed baby exactly as you do the breast-fed baby, and encourage the mother to do the same. To prevent aspiration of milk and to promote bonding, *do not prop the bottle.* A propped bottle may also contribute to ear infections because the milk can flow through the eustachian tube.

Preparing the Formula. Because bacteria thrive in milk, care is exercised when preparing the newborn's formula. Most mothers use either a premixed formula or a formula that is simply mixed with water. If the formula is purchased in small, disposable bottles, the bottles are already sterilized. When using disposable bottles, the mother must be sure that the plastic bag is securely fastened into the holder and that the baby cannot pull the end of the bag through the side of the holder while feeding. Also, bottles usually do not need to be disinfected if an automatic dishwasher is used. Formula is usually given at room temperature.

Key Concept

The major problem in formulas is overdiluting or underdiluting the formula while mixing. The mother must be taught to *measure carefully,* so the baby is receiving a consistent and accurate formula at each feeding.

Bubbling the Baby. Newborns must be properly bubbled (burped) during and after each feeding to prevent regurgitation of food and possible aspiration into the lungs. *This must be done whether the baby is breast-fed or bottle fed.* The breast-fed baby should be bubbled between breasts; the bottle-fed baby should be bubbled after every 0.5 to 1 oz of fluid for the first day or so. All babies should be bubbled after a feeding. The time between bubblings gradually increases, but the mother must be sure that the baby is not retaining any gas in the stomach at the end of the feeding.

There are several correct ways to hold the baby during bubbling, but in all cases, the baby must be held so that gas in the stomach is expelled without causing regurgitation. The baby may be held upright on the knee or held upright against the shoulder. *Gently* pat or rub the baby's back. Alternatively, the baby can be placed prone over the knees and his or her back can be gently rubbed.

Nursing Alert

Some cases of SIDS, or "crib death," may be caused by regurgitated food or fluid that has collected in the respiratory passages. Therefore, the nurse should stress the importance of proper bubbling.

Supplements

The physician may suggest that vitamin concentrates be added to feedings when the newborn is 2 to 3 weeks old. Milk contains the other essential nutrients for the first 6 months of life, although iron is often given to prevent iron-deficiency anemia.

Discharge of the Mother and Newborn

Prior to discharge, the birth attendant examines the neonate thoroughly. All birth records must be completed. The mother must be instructed regarding care of the newborn. She also is notified when the newborn must return to the birth attendant's office for an examination.

Sometimes the family requires or requests a Public Health or Home Care referral. If this is done, a visiting nurse will contact the new parents once they arrive home.

Nursing Alert

Before any mother or new baby is discharged, the identification bands must be verified. The mother's ID band and the newborn's ID band are compared. The mother signs the chart, indicating she has received the correct baby.

Keys for Review

Key Questions for Critical Thinking

1. Describe the importance of the Apgar score immediately following birth. Describe steps to be taken to maintain the newborn's airway.
2. Describe the importance of identification in the delivery room. Describe activities that maintain an accurate identification following birth.

Key Questions for Critical Thinking
(continued)

3. Describe daily care of the neonate and why each activity is important.
4. Develop a teaching plan for an adolescent mother regarding bathing and holding the newborn. Develop a teaching plan for the mother of a circumcised neonate.

Key Readings

Auvenshine M, Enriquez M. Comprehensive Maternity Nursing: Perinatal and Women's Health, Ed 2. Boston, Jones and Bartlett, 1990

Ingalls AJ, Salerno MC. Maternal and Child Health Nursing, Ed 7. St. Louis, C.V. Mosby, 1990

Jackson DB, Saunders RB. Child Health Nursing: A Comprehensive Approach to the Care of Children and their Families. Philadelphia, J.B. Lippincott, 1993

Kenner C. Nurses' Clinical Guide to Neonatal Care. Springhouse, PA, Springhouse, 1992

Lawrence RA. Breastfeeding: A Guide for the Medical Professional, Ed 3. St. Louis, C.V. Mosby, 1989

MacLaren A. Nurses' Clinical Guide to Maternity Care. Springhouse, PA, Springhouse, 1992

May KA, Mahlmeister LR. Maternal and Neonatal Nursing: Family-Centered Care, Ed 3. Philadelphia, J.B. Lippincott, 1994

Mohrbacher N, Stock J. The Breastfeeding Answer Book. Franklin Park, IL, La Leche League, 1991

Pillitteri A. Maternal and Child Health Nursing: Care of the Childbearing and Childrearing Family, Ed 2. Philadelphia, J.B. Lippincott, 1995

Key Readings (continued)

Reeder SJ, Martin LL, Koniak D. Maternity Nursing: Family, Newborn and Women's Health Care, Ed 17. Philadelphia, J.B. Lippincott, 1992

Sherwen L, Scoloveno M, Weingerten C. Nursing Care of the Childbearing Family. Norwalk, CT, Appleton & Lange, 1991

Enrichment Keys

Castiglia PT, Harbin RE. Child Health Care: Process and Practice. Philadelphia, J.B. Lippincott, 1992

Keys to Learning More

Chapter 61: complications related to childbirth
Chapter 62: disorders of the neonate and related nursing care
Chapter 63: fertility control
Chapter 64: care of infants and young children

61 Complications Related to Pregnancy and Childbirth

Keys for Learning

Learning Objectives

- ◆ Describe five complications of pregnancy and the treatment of each.
- ◆ Discuss care of the pregnant diabetic woman.
- ◆ Describe special needs of the adolescent mother and the family whose newborn has died.
- ◆ Describe tests of fetal maturity and related nursing care.
- ◆ Describe nursing care in emergency delivery and in postpartum hemorrhage.
- ◆ Define premature and precipitate labor, premature rupture of membranes, placenta previa, abruptio placentae, prolapsed cord, polyhydramnios, retained placenta, and uterine rupture. Describe nursing care for each of the above.
- ◆ Discuss nursing care in labor that has been induced.
- ◆ Describe indications and preoperative and postoperative nursing care in cesarean delivery. Describe special care needed by the cesarean neonate.

Key Terms

abortion	hyperemesis gravidarum
abruptio placentae	mastitis
amniocentesis	placenta previa
choriocarcinoma	polyhydramnios
cystitis	preeclampsia
dystocia	pregnancy-induced hypertension
eclampsia	psychosis
ectopic	puerperal
forceps	thrombophlebitis
hematoma	version
hydramnios	

Keys to Understanding This Chapter

Chapter 5: basic needs, some of which may be threatened during a complicated pregnancy and childbirth

Unit Four: normal human anatomy and physiology, used as a baseline for determining deviations from normal during complicated pregnancy and childbirth

Unit Seven: nursing process used in performing all nursing care, especially during a complicated pregnancy or childbirth

Unit Nine: nursing skills needed in patient care, including during a difficult pregnancy or childbirth

Chapter 53: skills needed to care for a person who has surgery, such as cesarean section

Chapter 54: sterile technique, which is used in the delivery room and in many aspects of care of the woman with complications

Unit Eleven: medications, many of which are used in complicated pregnancy and delivery

Key Points

- ◆ Many spontaneous abortions occur for unknown reasons. However, fetal maldevelopment and certain maternal factors account for other cases. The type of spontaneous abortion dictates the medical and nursing management.
- ◆ Ectopic pregnancy is a significant cause of maternal morbidity and mortality.
- ◆ Existing medical disorders, such as diabetes mellitus, cardiac disorders, and chemical dependency, will complicate pregnancy and require special care.
- ◆ Premature separation of the placenta and placenta previa are differentiated by the type of bleeding, uterine tonicity, and the presence or absence of pain.
- ◆ Dystocia is active labor which does not result in effective dilation or effacement of the cervix.

Rosdahl CB: Textbook of Basic Nursing, 6th ed. © 1995 J.B. Lippincott Company

Although pregnancy, labor, and delivery are considered normal physiologic processes, complications may arise at any time and may have serious consequences for the woman or her fetus. The terms *high risk* or *at risk* are used when psychological or physiologic factors could significantly increase the chances of mortality or morbidity of the woman or fetus. Early prenatal care helps identify these problems so that interventions can begin.

Complications related to childbirth have a physical and an emotional impact. The woman faces many hazards to her own physical well-being and is concerned about her fetus. For example, prolonged and difficult labor is physically and emotionally draining. This fatigue can interfere with the initial bonding between mother and newborn. During any time of crisis related to complicated childbirth, the family deserves the best possible medical and nursing care. This includes technical, physical, and emotional nursing care.

Complications of Pregnancy

Interrupted Pregnancy

Abortion

Abortion describes the termination of any pregnancy before the fetus is *viable*, that is, before it is able to survive outside the uterus. Abortion remains a controversial issue. Certain religions declare abortions to be contrary to natural law. Roman Catholic hospitals, for example, may not permit them. A nurse or physician may refuse to participate in an induced abortion based on religious or moral grounds.

Abortion is considered the most risky and least acceptable method of family planning or birth control. Contraceptives should be encouraged instead.

Classifications. Two major categories of abortion follow:

Key Abbreviations and Acronyms for Complex Pregnancies and Labor and Delivery

CPD	Cephalopelvic disproportion
D&C	Dilation and curettage
FAT	Fetal activity test
FBP	Fetal biophysical profile
HELLP	Hemolysis, elevated liver enzymes, low platelet count
NST	Nonstress test
OCT	Oxytocic challenge test
PIH	Pregnancy-induced hypertension
PROM	Premature rupture of membranes

◆ *Spontaneous* (without intervention; by natural causes), often called "miscarriage" by lay people
◆ *Induced* (with the aid of mechanical or medical agents)

Authorities estimate that approximately 10% to 20% of all pregnancies end in spontaneous abortion. Abnormalities or defects in the fetus are the most frequent causes of spontaneous abortion. Maternal alcohol use and cigarette smoking contribute to small or abnormal fetal development. Other causes of abortion include maternal disorders, trauma (such as a motor vehicle accident), dietary factors, and abnormalities of pregnancy.

A *threatened abortion* exists any time bleeding or cramping occurs in the first 20 weeks of pregnancy without major cervical dilation. Many birth attendants will not take extreme measures to save such a pregnancy, because a spontaneous abortion is often nature's way of disposing of a malformed fetus. However, if bleeding is slight, hormones or muscle relaxants may be given, and the patient is put to bed with her feet elevated for 48 to 72 hours. If bleeding stops, she may undertake limited activities. If true uterine contractions occur, the prognosis is more guarded.

An *inevitable abortion* is one in which the loss of the products of conception cannot be prevented. It is characterized by increased cramping, increased blood loss, and progressive dilation of the cervix.

An *incomplete abortion* is one is which some of the products of conception are expelled, but some are retained in the uterus. Extensive bleeding may occur. In this case, a dilatation and curettage (D&C) of the uterus is often performed.

A *complete abortion* is one in which all the products of pregnancy (placenta and fetus) are expelled, the uterus is contracting toward normal size, and the cervix is closed. The same care is given that would routinely follow a delivery. The patient should be observed closely for signs of hemorrhage; her blood pressure checked to see that it remains stable; changes in skin color noted and reported, especially pallor or cyanosis; and the pulse checked (a weak, rapid pulse is a sign of shock). The birth attendant checks to make sure the uterus is contracted. The number of perineal pads used and the amount of bleeding also should be documented.

A *missed abortion* is one in which the fetus has died but remains in the uterus. If the fetus is not expelled spontaneously within 1 month, the pregnancy will be terminated and a D & C done.

Septic abortion is the term given when the contents of the uterus become infected before, during, or after an abortion. *Septic (endotoxic) shock* may occur and may cause maternal death.

Habitual abortion means that a woman spontaneously loses several successive pregnancies. In such a case, the birth attendant usually makes every possible effort to save the pregnancy. Attempts are made to determine the cause of the repeated abortions and to correct the situation if possible. Sometimes surgery is performed.

A *criminal* or *illegal* abortion is the intervention in pregnancy without medical or legal justification. Abortion is not legal in all situations or in all places. Because an illegal abortion is normally carried out in an unsterile environment by nonmedical people, the risks to the pregnant woman are great. Major risks include hemorrhage and infection.

A *therapeutic abortion* is the legal termination of pregnancy under the direction of a physician. Induced abortion, before the 16th to the 20th week of gestation, is legal in most parts of the United States and in many other countries and may be done for medical or personal reasons. (In the latter case, the term "therapeutic" is often not used).

Medical reasons for therapeutic abortion include severe maternal cardiac disease, severe renal or hypertensive disorder, or a fetus with a high probability of congenital anomaly. In some maternal psychiatric disorders or family crises, abortion is performed as an elective procedure. Certain congenital disorders, which can be determined by amniocentesis at about the 14th week of gestation, are an indication for abortion to avoid the birth of a severely impaired neonate. If the woman has rubella (German measles) during pregnancy, especially during the first trimester, the likelihood of fetal defects is strong, and an abortion may be performed (see Chapter 67).

A new drug called dinoprostone (Prostin E$_2$) may be used to abort a pregnancy after the first trimester, or to treat an incomplete abortion, a dead fetus, or a benign hydatidiform mole.

Complications of Abortion. When the placenta separates from the uterus, large blood vessels are exposed, and this can lead to severe infection or hemorrhage. During the time when abortions were performed illegally and often under unsanitary conditions, sepsis was a common concern. Untreated, postabortion sepsis can be fatal; sterility (inability to conceive) is another common result. Thus, it is vital to maintain sterile conditions and to remove all the products of conception from the uterus.

If the aborting woman is Rh-negative and the father is Rh-positive, immune globulin (RhoGAM) should be given as a precautionary measure. Even a pregnancy of short duration could be enough to cause the Rh-negative woman's body to build up anti-Rh antibodies. These antibodies could cause difficulty in future Rh-positive pregnancies.

Premature Dilation of the Cervix

Some habitual abortions are the result of premature dilation of the cervix. This situation is also called "incompetent cervix." This is an unfortunate name, because it implies that the woman is deficient or has done something wrong; this can threaten the woman's self-esteem. Premature dilation of the cervix simply means that the cervix muscle is not able to support a pregnancy. Causes of this condition include cervical infections, such as chlamydia; cervical or vaginal cancer; previous cervical biopsies or conizations; and prior multiple D&Cs. The cervical weakness may be congenital; one cause of this is maternal exposure to diethylstilbestrol in utero.

In the case of premature dilation of the cervix, by about the fifth or sixth month of gestation, the weight of the fetus is enough to force the cervix to dilate, causing spontaneous abortion. Minor surgical procedures are used in the pregnant woman with an incompetent cervix. A nonabsorbable suture or band of fascia is placed around the cervix. This is called a *cervical cerclage* (Shirodkar or McDonald technique). This suture or fascia holds the cervix closed during the pregnancy; when the woman begins labor, the suture is removed.

Ectopic Pregnancy

The word **ectopic** means outside; therefore, an ectopic pregnancy is one that remains outside the uterus (Fig. 61-1). The most common ectopic pregnancy is a *tubal pregnancy*, one that occurs in the uterine or ovarian tube. In some cases, an abdominal or ovarian pregnancy is encountered, but this is rare.

Factors predisposing to ectopic pregnancy are tubal occlusion, an intrauterine contraceptive device, tumors, pelvic infections, endocrine imbalance, or abnormal tubal development. The symptoms of an ectopic pregnancy begin with spotting or bleeding 2 or 3 weeks after a missed menstrual period. Often there is accompanying pain, which may be quite severe. A tubal pregnancy always requires surgical removal of part or all of the affected tube to prevent rupture of the ovarian tube, a dangerous complication. An untreated ectopic pregnancy can be fatal in a short time.

Hydatidiform Mole

In hydatidiform mole, the embryo dies in utero, but the chorionic villi degenerate, forming grapelike clusters of vesicles. At first, the pregnancy appears normal, but then the uterus enlarges more rapidly than usual. The woman has episodes of spotting and bleeding and brownish red discharge; "tapioca-like" vesicles may be discharged. Preeclampsia symptoms may be noted, and the woman typically has symptoms of severe nausea and malaise. The mole can become very large.

Once the diagnosis is certain, the uterus is usually emptied by an induced abortion, followed approximately 48 hours later by a careful dilation of the cervix and curettage of the uterus (D&C).

The amount and character of bleeding should be documented and the expelled tissue saved and sent for pathologic examination. Aseptic technique is used in all cases to avoid infections. Because the experience is frightening, the parents need a great deal of emotional support.

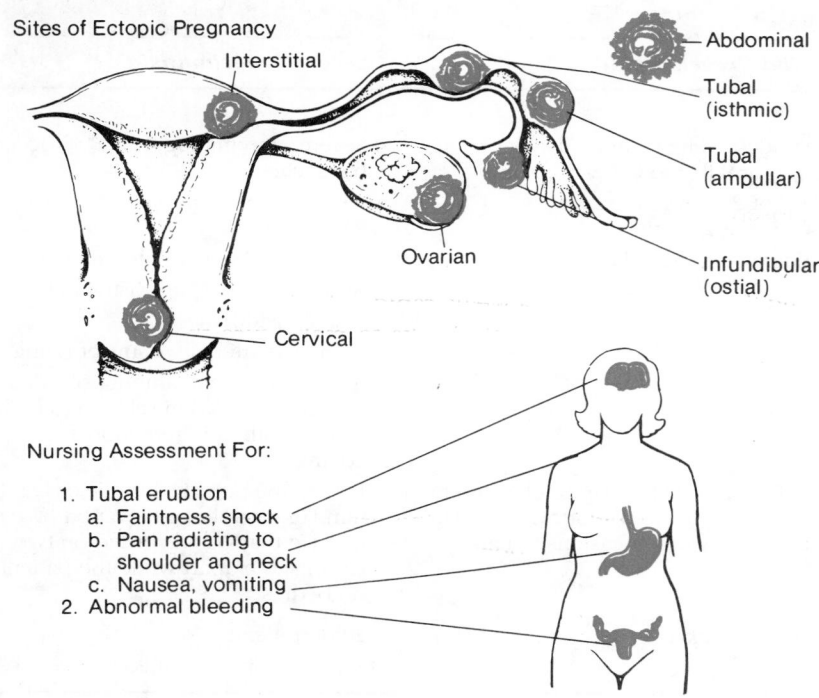

Sites of Ectopic Pregnancy

Interstitial

Abdominal

Tubal (isthmic)

Tubal (ampullar)

Ovarian

Infundibular (ostial)

Cervical

Nursing Assessment For:

1. Tubal eruption
   a. Faintness, shock
   b. Pain radiating to shoulder and neck
   c. Nausea, vomiting
2. Abnormal bleeding

Figure 61-1. Ectopic pregnancy.

Follow-up after delivery of a hydatidiform mole is essential. A human chorionic gonadotropin titer must be done; the titer ratio should fall after delivery. If the titer remains high or rises, this often indicates a situation known as metastatic mole, which is treated with chemotherapy and may be rapidly fatal. In addition, the mole—benign in itself—may be the forerunner of a malignant tumor known as **choriocarcinoma.**

Maternal Disorders Caused by Pregnancy

Hyperemesis Gravidarum

Hyperemesis gravidarum, pernicious vomiting, is more severe than simple morning sickness. The cause is unknown; however, various theories suggest causes ranging from toxins in the woman's bloodstream to a possible hormonal imbalance or an emotional condition. For example, women whose established reaction pattern to stress involves gastrointestinal disturbances often react in the same way to pregnancy.

Simple morning sickness usually begins at the second to fourth week and ends at approximately the 12th week of gestation, although it may continue throughout the pregnancy. Persistent vomiting to the point of excessive weight loss, dehydration, severe loss of appetite, and acetone in the urine are the symptoms of hyperemesis gravidarum. The woman also may have excessive salivation (*ptyalism*), epigastric and rib discomfort, constipation or diarrhea, nutritional anemia, and electrolyte imbalances. Few drugs can be used without potential harm to the fetus.

The woman may receive intravenous (IV) glucose and water with electrolytes, antiemetics, and sedatives. In the more severe stages, severe headache, mental aberrations, delirium, coma, jaundice, and cyanosis may occur; in rare cases, death may occur. In rare instances, an abortion may be necessary to save the woman's life.

Pregnancy-Induced Hypertension

Hypertensive disorders of pregnancy are characterized by one or more of the following signs: hypertension, edema, proteinuria, and in severe cases, seizures and coma. **Pregnancy-induced hypertension** (PIH) may occur during pregnancy, labor, delivery, or the postpartum period. It is a major cause of maternal death, stillbirth, and death in newborns yearly.

The exact cause of PIH is unknown, but the symptoms result from a vasoconstriction and vasospasm of blood vessels throughout the body. The central nervous system, kidneys, or liver may be affected. Decreased blood flow to the placenta and uterus may endanger the fetus.

Prompt treatment of hypertensive disorders—controlling symptoms as much as possible and allowing labor to start normally or initiating it when the safety of the woman and the fetus permits—seems best.

PIH is divided into *preeclampsia* and *eclampsia*, depending on the symptoms. Table 61-1 describes the signs and symptoms of preeclampsia and eclampsia.

Preeclampsia. The patient who was previously progressing normally but develops one or more hyperten-

Table 61-1. Signs and Symptoms of Preeclampsia and Eclampsia

Mild Preeclampsia	Severe Preeclampsia	Eclampsia
		Symptoms of severe preeclampsia PLUS: Rapid pulse
Sudden weight gain: 2 lb/wk (0.9 kg) or 6 or 8 lb/mo (2.72–3.63 kg)	Severe, unremitting frontal or occipital headache	
1+ or 2+ proteinurea (<5 g in 24° urine)	3+ or 4+ proteinuria (≥5 grams in 24° urine)	
Edema—fingers, face, legs, feet	Nausea and persistent vomiting	
	Abdominal pain, epigastric pain	
	Visual disturbances	
	Localized arterial spasms of retina	
	Abnormally small amount of urine secretion (oliguria) in relation to fluid intake; with fluid retention and edema	
B/P ≥ 140/90 mm Hg or elevated by ≥30 mm Hg systolic or ≥15 mm Hg distolic on two occasions 6 h apart	B/P ≥ 160 mm Hg systolic or ≥110 mm Hg diastolic or elevation of ≥30 mm Hg diastolic recorded on two occasions, 6 h apart while the patient is on bedrest	Very high blood pressure (over 170/110; systolic can be above 200)
		Maximum urine albumin level with scanty urine output
		Fever
Hyperreflexia	Hyperreflexia Weight gain, as in mild preeclampsia	Seizures, coma

sive or other symptoms, usually after the 20th week of gestation, has **preeclampsia.** It develops in approximately 5% of pregnancies, most often in primigravidas and women with a history of high blood pressure or vascular disorders. Although the symptoms most often allow the physician to intercept and treat it early, it can occur explosively, perhaps the day after the examination. An expectant woman should be instructed to report these symptoms to her birth attendant immediately.

It is also possible to predict preeclampsia by a test in which the patient's blood pressure is measured while she is lying on her back and again while she lies on her left side. This is referred to as the "roll-over test." It is used more often in the examiner's office than in the hospital. If the diastolic blood pressure is 20 mm Hg higher (or greater) when she is lying on her back, preeclampsia is likely. She will be advised to rest on her left side as much as possible. This woman is usually seen by her birth attendant every 2 days during her entire pregnancy.

Mild preeclampsia may be treated at home with sedation or tranquilizers and a regular diet (with salted foods omitted in some cases). Resting in a lateral position (particularly on the left side) aids in placental circulation. The woman is encouraged to rest most of the time; she should avoid climbing stairs.

Medical Management and Nursing Considerations. Patients with *severe preeclampsia* symptoms, identified in Table 61-1, are admitted to the hospital. Weight, intake, and output are checked daily. Output must be at least 30 mL/h. The patient may have an indwelling catheter. Vital signs are taken at least every 2 hours; the fetal monitor is used to assess the status of the fetus. A low-fat, high-protein diet may be used, or the woman may take nothing by mouth and have an IV, such as Ringer's solution. The urine is checked for albumin at least twice daily. External stimuli are reduced as much as possible. See the sample nursing care plan for an adolescent with PIH.

The patient and her family need to understand that the following precautions are necessary.

♦ Visiting is restricted.
♦ The room is kept quiet and fairly dark.
♦ Sedatives are given.
♦ Padded side rails are up at all times for safety.
♦ The woman is on bed rest.
♦ She should lie on her left side as much as possible. *(Rationale: This helps to facilitate renal circulation in the woman and placental circulation in the fetus.)*
♦ A preeclampsia tray is kept at the bedside.
♦ All intake and output is measured.
♦ Vital signs are taken often; weight is taken daily.
♦ Level of consciousness and reflexes are checked often.

♦ Blood will be drawn periodically.
♦ The fetus will be monitored.

The drug of choice in the treatment and prevention of severe preeclampsia is magnesium sulfate (MgSO$_4$) given intravenously or intramuscularly. This is a potent anticonvulsant drug that acts by slowing neuromuscular conduction and depressing central nervous system irritability, thus reducing muscle excitability and hyperreflexia. While the vasodilating effects of MgSo$_4$ will lower the blood pressure slightly, this action is only transient. The main reason for administering MgSO$_4$ is to prevent seizures, not lower blood pressure.

Because of its effects on the central nervous system, respirations and deep tendon reflexes must be assessed frequently while the patient is receiving the drug. The nurse must observe and report any changes. Urinary output also must be monitored because oliguria can result from excessively high levels of magnesium sulfate in the bloodstream.

If MgSO$_4$ does not control seizures, diazepam (Valium) may be used. Furosemide (Lasix) may be needed to stimulate urine output. Potassium (K$^+$) often is given with Lasix.

Calcium gluconate (Kalcinate) is a specific antidote for magnesium sulfate and is used if toxicity occurs. It is kept at the bedside of the patient at all times while she is receiving magnesium sulfate.

An IV is usually kept running to administer fluids and to keep the vein open in case emergency drugs must be given. Electrolytes are replaced intravenously, as needs are determined by blood tests. If the blood pressure remains dangerously elevated, additional medications (ie, labetalol HCl [Normodyne, Trandate]) may be ordered. However, it is important not to reduce the woman's blood pressure too much or too fast, because this would cause *anoxia* in the fetus. Blood pressure is usually maintained above 130/80.

Nursing Alert

If the woman's blood pressure spontaneously drops quickly, this may be an indication of maternal hemorrhage.

When the patient at or near term is stabilized, the fetus will usually be delivered. *Induction* (causing the fetus to be born, usually with medications) will be done if the cervix is ripe. If it is not ripe, cesarean delivery is done. If the fetus is not mature enough to survive, the pregnancy may be sustained for a short time. If the woman's condition worsens, the baby will usually be sacrificed to save the woman's life.

Angela Barr is a single, white 16-year-old, gravida 2 (para 0, abortion 1) in the 30th week of her pregnancy. She presented to the emergency department (E.D.) with a BP of 190/110 and complaints of persistent headache (3 days) and blurred vision. She had one prenatal clinic visit prior to presentation without follow-up. She is malnourished and reports a high-carbohydrate (low-protein) diet. She was admitted to the prenatal unit with the diagnosis of severe preeclampsia (pregnancy-induced hypertension [PIH]) for evaluation and to prevent eclampsia. The long-term maternal goal is survival with minimal morbidity; eclampsia is one of the three leading causes of maternal death in North America. The long-term fetal goal is to be as mature as possible at birth without significant post-delivery complications. Two top-priortiy nursing diagnoses developed for Miss Barr follow.

Nursing Diagnosis *High Risk for Injury: Eclampsia Related to Diet and Lack of Prenatal Care as Evidenced by BP (190/110), Headache, Blurred Vision*

Goal 1: Patient verbalizes serious nature of PIH syndrome and possible harmful consequences for mother and fetus.

Goal 2: Patient demonstrates complete recovery from PIH.

Goal 3: Healthy infant is delivered.

Nursing Actions (assess/do/teach)	Rationale	Evaluative Statement
1. Assess the patient's understanding of preeclampsia and the necessity of treatment; explain how she can best participate in the plan of care.	Compliance is enhanced when the patient values the plan of care.	6/25, Goal 1 not met; cannot understand why "the big-to-do"; wants to go home. Revision: Continue intensive one-on-one counseling.
2. Careful monitoring: a. BP q5–30 min until stable, then q2–4h during acute period; TPR and level of consciousness at least q4h b. Signs of hyperreflexia or hyporeflexia c. Serum electrolytes, urine protein, hematocrit, and plasma or urinary estriols d. Daily weights, signs of edema (check sacrum while on bedrest) e. 24-hour fluid intake and hourly urine output f. Level of consciousness, check reflexes; signs of hyperactivity, seizures, coma, or cyanosis g. Fetal heart rate; beginning signs of labor	The patient's status can change rapidly in a life-threatening manner.	
3. Keep on bed rest in left side-lying position in a quiet room with dimmed lighting and emergency supplies available. Restrict visitors.	This position facilitates blood flow to the fetus; light and noise may spark convulsions.	
4. High-carbohydrate, low-fat, and moderate-protein diet with moderate sodium	Diet is essential to medical regimen and fetal development.	
5. Sedatives, antihypertensives, and anticonvulsants to be readily available; IV in place and kept open	These may be needed in an emergency.	

(continued)

Nursing Diagnosis: *Ineffective Individual Coping Related to Multiple Stressors (Pregnancy, Youth, Illness, and Uncertain Future) and Lack of Resources as Evidenced by Refusal to Deal With Present Situation and Denial of Its Gravity ("What's so Hard About Having a Baby?")*

Goal: When acute preeclampsia period is resolved, patient (1) verbalizes feelings about pregnancy and (2) identifies personal and community resources that will enable her to support herself and the baby.

Nursing Actions (assess/do/teach)	Rationale	Evaluative Statement
1. Continue to asses the patient's grasp of her current situation and the appropriateness of her response; correct any misconceptions about the realities of parenting.	Denial is a common defense mechanism; appropriate in the short term but must be replaced by careful planning prior to discharge.	3/24 Goal partially met; patient is beginning to talk about what she will need to do to be prepared to care for the baby and herself at home.
2. Explore the patient's personal and external resources; reinforce coping strategies that worked in the past; make referrals as necessary.	The patient's self-esteem and adequacy as a parent will depend on the support she is able to mobilize.	

Nursing Alert

The HELLP syndrome is a major complication of preeclampsia:

♦ *H*emolysis
♦ *E*levated *l*iver enzymes
♦ *L*ow *p*latelet count
♦ Eclampsia

Eclampsia. Few women progress to the serious stage called eclampsia, although if preeclampsia is left untreated, this progression most likely will occur. **Eclampsia** is one of the most severe complications of pregnancy. It is characterized by generalized tonic-clonic seizures, a very rapid pulse, and a very high blood pressure (see Table 61-1). It develops in 1/200 women with preeclampsia.

After a seizure, the patient may regain consciousness within a few minutes, or she may remain in a coma for several hours or days. Seizures may recur in either instance. Even when a patient awakens after seizures, she may be confused. The treatment for eclampsia is basically the same as that for severe preeclampsia, with delivery performed as soon as possible.

If seizures continue, the coma deepens. The "slushy" respirations characteristic of lung edema are audible, and the prognosis is now poor. The primary causes of maternal death due to hypertension are circulatory collapse, cerebral hemorrhage, and renal failure. A major complication is abruptio placentae with maternal hemorrhage. Following delivery, the patient who had PIH must continue to be monitored. If the elevated blood pressure continues for more than 42 days after delivery, she is diagnosed with chronic hypertension. A 6-week checkup should include extensive evaluation of the patient's blood pressure, complete blood count, blood urea nitrogen, urinalysis, and creatinine.

A mild sedative, such as phenobarbital, may be used as a precaution after delivery.

Existing Medical Disorders Complicating Pregnancy

Diabetes Mellitus

Diabetes mellitus is an endocrine disorder in which the pancreas fails to produce sufficient insulin for proper use of glucose. This condition is discussed in detail in Chapter 72. A diabetic woman needs special care and monitoring during pregnancy, because insulin requirements may fluctuate. Even when the diabetes is monitored carefully, the pregnant woman and her developing fetus are at risk.

Potential problems during pregnancy include fetal death, *macrosomia* (oversized fetus), a fetus with a respiratory disorder, difficult labor, preeclampsia or eclampsia, polyhydramnios, and congenital malformations.

Diabetes tends to be more difficult to control durin[g] pregnancy. The patient may become *hyperglyc*[emic] with resulting acidosis or diabetic coma. She become *hypoglycemic*, with resulting hypoxia in the fetus. The non–insulin-dependent diabetic woman may need to have insulin injections during pregnancy. Depending on the condition of the woman and fetus, diabetic women may be delivered early (36th to 38th week of gestation) by induction or cesarean delivery.

The diabetic woman and her family are taught blood glucose testing, adjustments to make, and signs for which to watch. Family teaching is important because the woman may not be able to recognize signs soon enough or may not be able to take actions in time. The accompanying box lists subjects for patient teaching.

Diabetic women should be under the care of an internist and an obstetrician during pregnancy. Frequent prenatal visits are essential. Careful fetal monitoring is necessary during labor, and the newborn must be assessed carefully. Generally these newborns are treated as premature neonates.

Nursing Alert

Reactions to too little or too much insulin are a danger to the woman, especially during labor and immediately after delivery. The woman's body reacts to the trauma of birth, and the glucose level is easily upset.

Gestational Diabetes. Approximately 3% of pregnant women will develop carbohydrate intolerance for the first time during pregnancy. Thus, all women are screened at 26 to 28 weeks' gestation with a 1-hour glucose test. While some women can be managed by diet alone, others will require insulin. The majority of women will return to prepregnancy glucose levels following delivery.

Cardiac Disorders

Pregnancy places additional strain on the heart. The greatest danger occurs during the last trimester of pregnancy and during labor and delivery. The cardiac patient in labor should be assessed for dyspnea, chest pain, and pulmonary edema.

During pregnancy, the woman with a cardiac condition should get plenty of rest and avoid activities that result in shortness of breath. She should maintain a diet that will prevent excessive weight gain and water retention. This usually means that sodium (salt) is restricted. The prognosis depends on the woman's age and the severity and type of heart disease.

Women with cardiac disorders can often successfully deliver their babies. The current belief is that it is safer for the woman to undergo a normal delivery than have an abortion, which was sometimes done in the past. The extra strain of a cesarean delivery is also avoided, if possible. However, she may be induced and delivered early to prevent a difficult labor.

Keys to Patient/Family Teaching
The Pregnant Woman With Diabetes

Patient and family teaching of the pregnant woman with diabetes includes the following:

♦ Method for self-testing blood for glucose several times a day
♦ Insulin and diet adjustments based on glucose level
♦ Method of insulin injections if the woman has not used insulin previously
♦ Signs of hyperglycemia and hypoglycemia
♦ Actions to take if hyperglycemia or hypoglycemia occur
♦ Signs and symptoms of beginning preeclampsia

Chemical Dependency

The addicted pregnant woman is often malnourished and fails to seek prenatal care. Drug use may account for a stillborn child, spontaneous abortion, abruptio placentae, and numerous congenital defects. Some of these conditions, as they relate to the newborn, are discussed in more detail in Chapter 62.

Disorders Affecting the Fetus

Infection

Maternal infections can damage the fetus. For instance, a severe respiratory disease, such as viral pneumonia, can cause fetal anoxia. If the woman contracts rubella early in pregnancy, fetal malformation is a strong possibility. (Congenital rubella syndrome is discussed later in this chapter.) If the woman's rubella titer is low (below 1:10), this means she does not have antibodies to fight rubella. If this woman is exposed to rubella, gamma globulin may be given. An abortion also may be done. After the pregnancy, the mother is immunized for rubella, after making sure she is not pregnant again.

Sexually transmitted disease in the woman is often transmitted to the fetus. Syphilis, gonorrhea, herpesvirus II, and acquired immunodeficieny syndrome are all transmitted by way of the maternal-fetal circulation. These conditions in the newborn are discussed in Chapters 62 and 65.

Rh Sensitization. Rh sensitization occurs less frequently than in the past because it can be prevented in the majority of cases. In Rh sensitization, some of the Rh-positive red blood cells from the fetus cross the placental barrier and enter the maternal circulation. Because the Rh-positive cells become antigens in the Rh-negative woman, they stimulate the formation of antibodies within the woman's circulatory system. These antibodies return to the fetus, destroying the fetal red blood cells. An Rh-negative woman who has produced these antibodies is said to be sensitized. The neonate in this situation is born with a condition known as *erythroblastosis fetalis.*

The sensitization of the woman in erythroblastosis fetalis usually occurs at or near the first delivery, so the antibodies do not always affect the fetus being carried at that time. However, in subsequent pregnancies with Rh-positive fetuses, the already sensitized woman usually produces large numbers of antibodies. Some neonates are born only mildly affected, whereas others are severely affected. Efforts to save the fetus may include intrauterine transfusion if the pregnancy is less than 32 weeks' duration or early delivery at 34 to 38 weeks.

Erythroblastosis fetalis can be prevented by administering anti-D gamma globulin (RhoGAM) to the Rh-negative woman. This drug should be administered during pregnancy and 72 hours following the birth of an Rh-positive neonate and following an *abortion.* RhoGAM prevents the woman's body from building up anti–Rh-positive antibodies. Erythroblastosis fetalis is thus prevented, even in Rh-positive fetuses. The availability of RhoGAM has made this disorder rare in the United States.

> **Nursing Alert**
>
> *Each* time an Rh-negative woman delivers or aborts, RhoGAM must be administered again.

ABO Incompatibility. ABO incompatibility can arise if the woman's blood type is A and the fetus' is B or AB; if the mother is B and the fetus is A or AB; and if the mother is O and the fetus is A, B, or AB (see Chapter 75).

ABO incompatibility is not detectable before birth. It can occur in a first pregnancy and does not increase in severity with subsequent pregnancies. It is usually clinically milder than Rh factor incompatibility. The problem is indicated by jaundice in the neonate within the first 36 hours; phototherapy (treatment with a special light) is often useful in treating the jaundice.

Placental and Amniotic Disorders

Placenta Previa

Placenta previa is a condition that occurs when the placenta has implanted in the lower segment of the uterus, rather than in the upper wall (Fig. 61-2). *Low implantation* is the attachment of the placenta at the opening or border of the cervical os but not covering it. If the placenta partially obliterates the cervical os, it is a *partial placenta previa.* If the placenta totally covers the cervical os, it is called *total placenta previa.*

Predisposing factors are numerous and include closely spaced pregnancies, abnormalities in uterine structure, late fertilization, and old cesarean scars. Painless vaginal bleeding during the later months of pregnancy is the primary symptom and is due to the separation of the placenta from the uterine wall.

> **Nursing Alert**
>
> Placenta previa is an emergency that may require immediate cesarean delivery. Signs of shock or a rising uterus, which may become very hard without contractions, must be reported immediately. (The blood may be trapped inside the uterus.)

If undetected before labor begins, placenta previa will result in hemorrhage, because the cervical dilation causes increased tearing of the placental tissue. The severity of hemorrhage in relation to the progress of labor determines the method of delivery to be used: In total placenta previa, cesarean delivery is performed; in partial placenta previa, the amount of cervical involvement dictates the method of delivery, although caesarean delivery is usually done if the previa covers more than 30% of the cervical os when the cervix is fully dilated. A patient may be hospitalized several times before hemorrhaging becomes severe enough to warrant cesarean birth.

Other potential complications of placenta previa are loss of uterine muscle tone, uterine rupture, retention of placental tissue, and air embolism, a serious complication caused by exposure of uterine sinuses and blood vessels to the air. The fetus is at considerable risk, and fetal shock and maternal or fetal death are possible.

Diagnosis and Management. If vaginal bleeding occurs, the patient should be hospitalized *immediately* and placed on bed rest. The nurse should anticipate the need for fetal monitoring, IV and blood administration, possible cesarean delivery, vaginal packing, and emergency infant resuscitation.

Diagnosis is most often obtained by ultrasonography (Doppler ultrasound), which can usually identify the exact location of the placenta. In some situations, x-rays may be used (including *placentography* to visualize the placenta).

If the fetus is diagnosed as *viable,* a sterile vaginal examination may be done (by the physician only) in the operating room. The operating room is prepared with a double setup to allow for an emergency cesarean delivery if this becomes necessary.

If the woman is bleeding and a vaginal delivery is planned, an *amniotomy* (rupture of the amniotic sac) is performed. An oxytocin induction may be started. If bleeding continues or labor does not begin quickly and progress rapidly, a cesarean delivery is done.

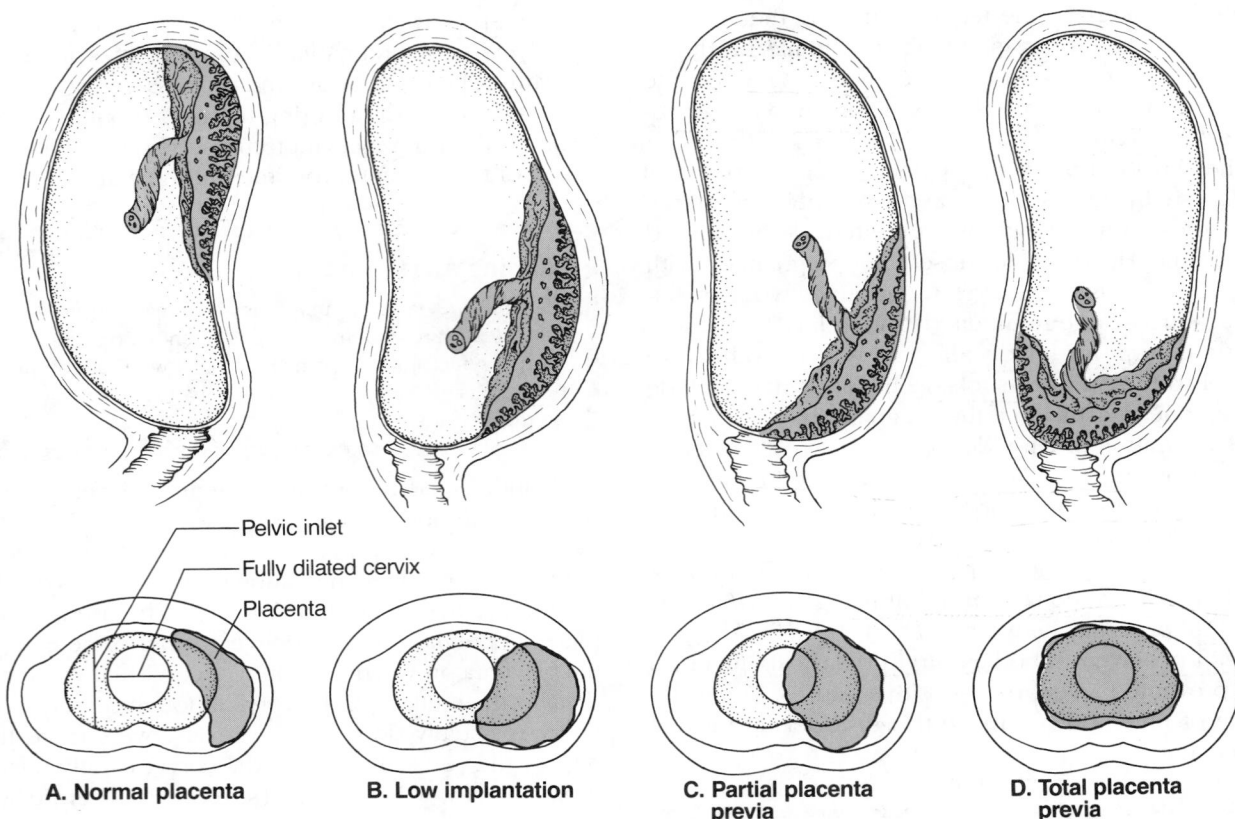

Pelvic inlet
Fully dilated cervix
Placenta

A. Normal placenta   **B. Low implantation**   **C. Partial placenta previa**   **D. Total placenta previa**

Figure 61-2. Placenta previa. **(A)** Normal placenta. **(B)** Low implantation. **(C)** Partial placenta previa. **(D)** Total placenta previa. (Redrawn from Benson RC. Handbook of Obstetrics and Gynecology, Ed 6. Los Altos, CA, Lange Medical Publications, 1977.)

Modern surgical methods and the use of blood transfusions have greatly reduced maternal mortality, although placenta previa is still considered serious. The prognosis for the neonate depends on the effect of maternal hemorrhage on fetal circulation and oxygenation.

Maternal Postpartal Assessment. The mother must be assessed carefully for hemorrhage following a placenta previa delivery. If the bleeding continues to be severe, an emergency hysterectomy may be done.

Abruptio Placentae

Abruptio placentae (abrupt separation) of the normally implanted placenta from the uterine wall is a grave complication of later pregnancy (Fig. 61-3). It usually develops after the 20th week of gestation, and it often occurs without labor.

Some of the predisposing factors of the separation are pressure on the vena cava by the enlarging uterus (associated with hypertension), preeclampsia, poor placental circulation, substance abuse (ie, cocaine), grand multiparity, and women who have had numerous abortions or stillbirths. Physical trauma, such as a motor vehicle accident, also can cause immediate placental separation. The extent of the separation determines the amount of danger to the fetus. Abruptio placentae is a common cause of stillbirth.

Abruptio placentae can occur during active labor, giving rise to fetal distress. The bleeding that results from the separation may be apparent or hidden. If bleeding is externally visible, it is often dark. The uterus becomes tender and rigid, and symptoms of maternal shock may occur. Fetal movement may increase or decrease. If the woman experiences extreme pain or the uterine fundus rises, it may indicate that there is bleeding and pooling behind the placenta (retroplacental hemorrhage).

Other possible maternal complications include bleeding into the uterine muscle, precipitous labor (fast and uncontrolled), loss of uterine tone, and oliguria leading to acute renal failure. Maternal death may occur. Dangers to the fetus include anemia, anoxia, and death.

Management. The treatment of abruptio placentae depends on the severity of the separation. The diagnosis and vaginal examination are carried out under a double setup by a physician, because if abruptio pla-

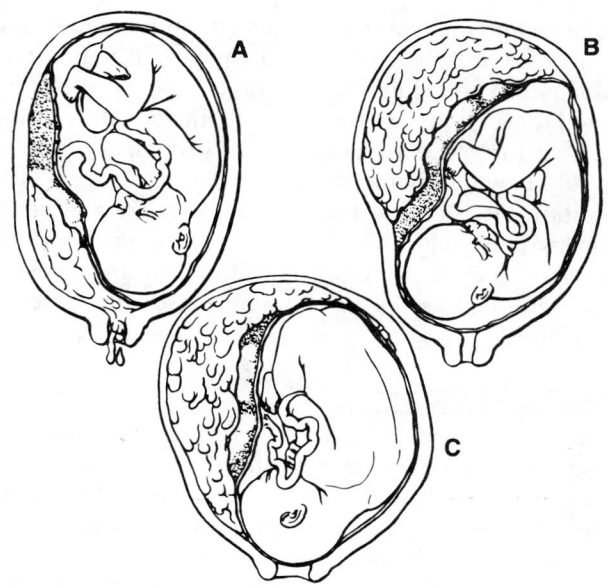

Figure 61-3. Premature separation and abruptio placentae. **(A)** Separation is low and incomplete; vaginal hemorrhage is evident. **(B)** Separation is high, causing fundus of uterus to rise. Fetus is in grave danger. External hemorrhage is not present, but amniotic fluid is port-wine color. **(C)** Complete abruption with fetus in grave danger. External hemorrhage is prevented because fetus' head is in cervical os.

centae cannot be differentiated from placenta previa without a vaginal examination, cesarean delivery must be anticipated.

The fetus must be continuously monitored so that a cesarean delivery can be done if necessary. The upper limit of the fundus is identified and marked on the woman's abdomen with a felt tip pen. The fundus is then observed for changes or movement upward. If it moves upward, blood may be collecting within the uterus; this is a dangerous situation, usually calling for immediate cesarean delivery.

Before a cesarean birth, lost maternal blood must be replaced. During this time, maternal and fetal vital signs must be monitored constantly.

The fetus will be delivered vaginally if the cervix is ripe, if induction causes productive contractions, and if there is no fetal distress. However, if the woman's blood pressure drops or the fetus experiences anoxia, cesarean delivery will be done immediately. In a few cases, a hysterectomy may need to be done to control the bleeding. (A cesarean delivery, followed immediately by a hysterectomy is known as a Porro's section.)

With modern treatment, abruptio placentae is rarely fatal to the woman. However, the outlook for the newborn's survival depends on the severity of the separation and the degree to which his or her oxygen supply has been affected.

> **Key Concept**
>
> Any bleeding in pregnancy or labor is a serious sign.

Polyhydramnios

In **polyhydramnios** (or **hydramnios**) there is an excessive amount of amniotic fluid (more than 2,000 mL; more than 5000 mL in polyhydramnios). Seen in approximately 10% of pregnant diabetics, it also accompanies fetal anomalies, such as spina bifida and anencephaly. The woman's abdomen is excessively large, producing dyspnea and difficulty with movement. The skin is stretched tightly, and excessive stretch marks (striae gravidarum) may be present. Uterine muscles also have been stretched, which may lead to ineffective contractions (dystocia) and failure of the muscles to contract following childbirth.

Prolonged Pregnancy

A pregnancy continuing beyond 42 weeks is known as prolonged (postdate) pregnancy. In this case, the obstetrician may induce labor or do a cesarean delivery. The condition of the fetus is a determining factor. If there is any indication of fetal distress, a cesarean delivery is most likely done. Risks to be considered include placental insufficiency, in which the placenta deteriorates and uteroplacental circulation is compromised.

Other Considerations

Multiple Pregnancy. A multiple pregnancy is one in which more than one fetus is developing in the uterus at the same time. Twin pregnancy is the most common type, although triplets, quadruplets, and other multiples may develop. If a multiple pregnancy is suspected, ultrasound is diagnostic. Labor is not ordinarily more difficult than in a normal pregnancy, although preterm and precipitate (sudden, progressing faster than normal) deliveries are relatively common.

Adolescent Pregnancy. More than 1.2 million adolescent women in the United States become pregnant each year, representing nearly 20% of births. Pregnancy in a girl younger than age 16 places a particular strain on her body; this adolescent is undergoing not only the normal changes of adolescence, but also those needed to sustain a pregnancy. Iron requirements are high for both adolescence and pregnancy, and anemia may result. The young woman may need special dietary instructions or vitamin supplements.

Adolescent pregnancy complications often involve preeclampsia, eclampsia, and spontaneous abortion.

Babies are often preterm and small for their gestational age at birth. Perinatal mortality is increased, and neonates often develop slowly. Pregnant adolescents are at high risk for infections and sexually transmitted diseases.

Prenatal classes are offered through the local public health department or the hospital. The patient should attend to understand her nutritional needs and the process of pregnancy.

The school-age girl should be given information about continuing her education. By law, public school education must be made available to pregnant teenagers. Counseling services should be offered, because the girl may be afraid to go to her parents for help. The Salvation Army, her local church group or clergy member, Planned Parenthood of America, the local social service agency, and the family physician may provide further aid. Financial assistance also may be available.

Pregnancy in the Older Woman. The woman older than 40 years encounters more risks than the woman between 16 and 40 years of age. Bodily changes in preparation for menopause may have begun. The older woman who is having her first child has an increased incidence of complications in pregnancy, such as ectopic pregnancy, gestational diabetes, and hypertensive disorders, in addition to problems during labor and delivery, such as hypertonic or hypotonic dystocia and hemorrhage. She also has a greater-than-normal chance of having a mentally disturbed or malformed child. The older mother who is a grand multipara may be more likely to have a precipitate delivery, a placenta previa, hydramnios, hypotonic dystocia, or a hemorrhage because of an atonic uterus.

Pregnancy in the Divorced or Widowed Woman. The woman who has recently been separated by death or divorce from her husband has special emotional needs. The nurse can respond to these needs and remain with the woman as much as possible during labor and delivery. A relative often acts as the labor "coach."

Assessing Fetal Status

Various tests are used to assess fetal status or fetal maturity. The most commonly used include amniocentesis, ultrasonic scanning, the oxytocic challenge test (OCT), and the nonstress test (NST).

Amniocentesis
Amniocentesis is the insertion of a needle through the maternal abdominal wall into the amniotic sac and the withdrawal of amniotic fluid. This invasive test can be performed in the examiner's office or on an outpatient basis. Amniocentesis should always be preceded by an ultrasound scan to determine the location of the placenta and the fetal parts. The examiner confirms the fetal position by palpation and cleanses the area and anesthetizes the skin site. A long, sterile needle is inserted through the abdominal wall, through the uterine wall, and into the amniotic sac. Approximately 20 mL of fluid is withdrawn. The needle is removed, and the insertion site is covered with a bandage. There is some risk involved with amniocentesis. Placental and fetal damage, premature labor, or abortion may result, although these risks are minimized by the use of ultrasound.

Information Provided. Amniocentesis tests for fetal abnormalities or establishes fetal maturity. For example, diagnosis can be made of some types of intellectual impairment, such as Down syndrome and Tay-Sach's disease; inherited disorders, such as muscular dystrophy and cystic fibrosis; and some fetal abnormalities, such as spina bifida. Amniocentesis is frequently used to determine the status of an Rh-positive fetus in an Rh-negative woman. An amniocentesis may be ordered when the birth attendant suspects intrauterine growth retardation or when exact determination of fetal maturity or sex is essential.

Nursing Considerations. The patient is instructed to empty her bladder before the test (to prevent bladder rupture). The woman's vital signs are monitored during the test and for at least 1 hour afterward. Fetal heart tones (FHTs) are monitored to ensure the fetus is not in distress; the external fetal monitor is most often used. The woman is instructed to notify the birth attendant if she has any difficulties after returning home. This includes *any* bleeding or cramping.

Ultrasonic Scanning
An ultrasound scan uses high-frequency sound waves to produce a picture of intrauterine activity. The graphic recording of this picture is called a sonogram. From this image, the examiner can learn a great deal about the developing fetus.

A transducer, placed on the skin of the abdomen, passes sound waves into the fetus. Because of various densities of body tissues (such as bones and muscles), the waves are echoed back to the transducer at different rates. The echo is transformed by computer into an image on a monitor.

Information Provided. Ultrasound can determine gestational age, fetal head size, location of the placenta, and some fetal anomalies. Multiple pregnancies can be identified. In some cases, the sex of the fetus also can be determined. Ultrasound also is used in conjunction with tests such as amniocentesis. The woman is often allowed to watch the fetus move and the heart beat.

She is often given a print and/or videotape of the ultrasound to take home.

Nursing Considerations. The nurse explains to the woman that a *full bladder* is necessary for the test so that the fetal parts will be moved up into the abdomen. This allows for better visualization of the fetus. The patient will be asked to drink large amounts of liquids and will not be allowed to empty her bladder. This test takes 20 minutes, and there are no known harmful effects on the woman or fetus. This is a noninvasive test.

Oxytocic Challenge Test

The OCT, also known as the *stress test,* is a way to evaluate the response of the fetal heart to contractions. It provides information as to how well the placenta is supplying oxygen to the fetus. Therefore, it is particularly useful in detecting fetuses who are beginning to experience difficulty because of inadequate placental circulation.

Although the OCT is not dangerous in itself, it may stimulate labor. Thus, it is generally performed in the labor and delivery area of the hospital, rather than in the clinic setting.

Uterine contractions can be initiated by nipple stimulation, but most often are initiated by IV oxytocin. An IV administration of oxytocin by infusion pump is begun. Its rate of administration is increased until three contractions are produced in 10 minutes. The reaction of the fetal heart is determined using the fetal monitor. If, toward the end of a contraction, the fetal heart rate decreases (late deceleration), uteroplacental insufficiency is indicated, which may lead to death of the fetus. An OCT is classified as positive when there are persistent late decelerations with more than 50% of the contractions. A decision is made about continuing the pregnancy or performing a cesarean delivery.

Nonstress Test (NST)

The NST provides information on the fetal heart rate in response to fetal activity. The healthy fetus is active in utero, and the fetal heart rate will normally increase as the fetus moves in the uterus. To perform the NST, an external fetal monitor is strapped to the woman's abdomen, and she is asked to press a button each time she feels the fetus move. This monitoring process is carried out for approximately 40 minutes.

An NST is classified as reactive when there are at least two episodes of fetal heart rate accelerations of 15 beats per minute lasting at least 15 seconds within a continuous 10-minute period. A reactive test shows that the fetal heart rate increases with every fetal movement and that the fetus is doing well.

A nonreactive test shows that the fetal heart rate did not increase with activity and that the fetus may thus be suffering from lack of oxygen. The fetus may fail to

be active during the course of the test. Methods are then used to stimulate the fetus. These include palpating or shaking the uterus, making loud noises, or stimulating the woman's nipples.

Fetal Biophysical Profile (FBP)

The biophysical profile combines an NST with ultrasonic assessment of the fetus. Using ultrasound, the examiner evaluates fetal breathing movements, fetal tone, fetal body movements, and amniotic fluid volume. Each of the five components, including the nonstress test, are scored as 0 (abnormal) to 2 (normal).

Complications of Labor and Delivery

Approximately 85% of all deliveries are considered normal; 15% are considered complicated. One of the nurse's duties in the labor and delivery area is to assess for possible complications. The lives of two people are at stake.

Premature Rupture of Membranes

In 10% to 12% of all pregnancies, the bag of waters ruptures, but the patient does not go into labor for several days or weeks. Several complications may arise:

◆ Premature labor
◆ Intrauterine infection (the fetus is particularly susceptible to infections)
◆ Malpresentations and prolapsed cords during labor

If the bag of waters breaks with a sudden gush, the diagnosis is obvious, but if there is a slow trickling of amniotic fluid, it is more difficult to diagnose. Nitrazine tests may be used.

The woman should be admitted to the hospital when premature rupture of the membranes occurs. The woman and fetus are then assessed. Ultrasound and amniocentesis will determine fetal maturity, and labor is induced if the fetus is sufficiently mature.

Premature Labor

Labor that occurs before the 37th week of gestation is premature, but it often produces a viable (live) newborn. However, because prematurity is a leading cause of infant mortality, the birth attendant often attempts to postpone delivery until the fetus is more mature.

The patient is placed on bed rest. Tocolytic agents, such as those listed in the accompanying box, may be given to stop the contractions if there is no fetal distress, if the membranes are intact, and if the patient is dilated less than 4 cm. Medications are usually given intravenously until contractions cease, after which they may

Key Medications
to Stop Labor (Tocolytic agents)

- Ritodrine HCl (Yutopar)
- Terbutaline sulfate (Brethine, Bricanyl)
- Magnesium sulfate
- Indomethacin (Indocin)
- Nifedipine (Procardia)
- Dexamethasone (Decadron)

Nursing Considerations

- Side effects of these drugs include dizziness, headache, tremor, and GI symptoms
- Side effects of ritodrine include maternal hypotension and pulmonary edema and maternal or fetal tachycardia
- Dexamethasone may be given to speed maturation of fetal lungs
- Indomethacin also may be given to the premature infant after birth to close a patent ductus arteriosus

be administered orally. The woman and fetus must be followed closely for the remainder of the pregnancy.

Precipitate Labor and Delivery

A precipitate labor is one that is brief (shorter than 3 hours) and in which contractions are usually severe. It most often occurs in induced labor or multiparity. A precipitate delivery may be so rapid that the woman cannot be taken to the delivery room or prepared for delivery; the physician or midwife is not always present.

The nurse should stay with the patient, put the signal light on for help, remain composed, and assist the patient as much as possible until help arrives. The principles of asepsis should be applied as the situation allows. Delivery should never be prevented in any way. The nurse should simply assist with the birth and make sure that the newborn is breathing adequately.

Because of the force and speed of labor, possible trauma can occur to the mother and newborn. Dangers to the mother include perineal laceration, hemorrhage, infection, and uterine rupture; to the newborn, anoxia, subdural hematoma, and fractures. The neonate who is born outside the delivery room is isolated to make sure he or she does not carry infection to the other neonates.

Uterine Rupture

A ruptured uterus is one of the most serious complications of labor; fortunately, it is rare. Predisposing factors include a previous cesarean delivery or any uterine scar. Severe tonic labor contractions in which there is no period of relaxation, dystocia, cephalopelvic dispro-

portion, or injudicious use of drugs, such as oxytocin to stimulate uterine contractions, also may give rise to rupture.

When a rupture is threatened, the patient complains of continuous and intense pain, and a Bandl's ring may be noted (thickened upper uterine segment and a thin, distended lower segment). The patient appears apprehensive and restless. Contractions are tonic, pulse is rapid, and urination is frequent. If the threat of rupture occurs before delivery, the fetus is usually in great distress, as shown by irregular or absent FHTs.

Constant fetal monitoring is vital. The patient with a rupture may need an emergency cesarean delivery, followed by an immediate hysterectomy. This is needed to save the mother's life; the newborn's life may or may not be saved.

Symptoms of rupture are a sharp, tearing pain followed by a sudden cessation of pain. The patient is anxious and shows signs of shock and hypotension; her pulse is rapid and weak. (She is hemorrhaging internally.) Emergency measures must be used to treat for shock and hemorrhage. The patient is prepared at once for an emergency Porro's cesarean section (delivery of the baby and immediate removal of the uterus—hysterectomy).

Dystocia

Dystocia, difficult or abnormal labor, is active labor that does not result in effective dilation or effacement of the cervix. Therefore, the labor is long but does not progress. Dystocia may be related to fetal factors, uterine or passageway abnormalities, or faulty uterine contractions. Dystocia not only exhausts the woman, but also predisposes her and her fetus to possible danger and even death.

Uterine Inertia

Uterine inertia (dysfunctional uterus) refers to insufficient, uncoordinated contractions that do not produce effective dilation. It is also called *hypotonic dystocia*. Causes include emotional stress, a thick and rigid cervix, and excessive or premature use of analgesic medications. Uterine inertia occurs most often in primigravidas. However, it also is identified in some grand multiparas who have weak muscle tone in the uterus. Other women may suffer from uterine inertia if they have an overdistended uterus because of an extremely large fetus, a multiple pregnancy, or hydramnios.

Nursing care includes early recognition and prompt notification of the physician; assessment of cervical dilation, if any; accurate evaluation of pain; assessment with the fetal monitor of fetal heart rate as related to the pattern of contractions; and positive emotional support and reassurance for the parents. The nurse must anticipate and be prepared to assist with medical treatments, such as IV fluids or efforts to stop the ineffective labor with medications such as morphine. Sleep and rest enables the uterus to achieve a normal pattern when labor resumes. Other treatment may include IV infusion of oxytocin or a cesarean delivery.

Dystocia Caused by the Fetus

Sometimes the size of the fetus as compared with that of the woman's pelvis or the position or presentation causes dystocia.

Cephalopelvic Disproportion. Cephalopelvic disproportion means that the presenting part, usually the fetal head, is too large to pass through the woman's pelvis. This may be related to maternal diabetes (which often results in large babies), heredity, or maternal nutrition. Caesarean delivery should be anticipated; however, some birth attendants use cesarean birth as a last resort.

Abnormal Fetal Positions and Presentations. Normally, a baby is born in a vertex position (head first). However, if an abnormal fetal position is assumed within the uterus, labor is difficult, and vaginal delivery may be impossible. Depending on the position of the head, difficulties may still occur. For example, if the face is the presenting part, vaginal delivery is often impossible, because this angle causes a cephalopelvic disproportion. The abnormal position also may cause a hand, foot, or buttocks to present. Ultrasonography can identify fetal position, as can the location of FHTs. A cesarean delivery may be done in abnormal position or presentation.

Posterior. The most common abnormal fetal position is an *occiput posterior presentation* (toward the woman's back), designated right (ROP) or left (LOP). Delivery can be difficult or impossible, because the fetal neck is overflexed, the face is uppermost, and the head diameter is too large to pass through the birth canal. This presentation can occur if the maternal pelvic floor is relaxed. The woman typically complains of a continuous low backache, and FHTs are heard on the woman's flank (side).

Medical management may include manual rotation of the fetus (**version**) before engagement, delivery assisted by forceps, or cesarean delivery. The nurse helps the patient do pelvic rocking exercises. Emotional support should be given, and the woman's lower back should be massaged. (Pelvic rocking is done while lying flat in bed. The abdomen is rocked from top to bottom, alternating back and forth. First, the backbone is pressed against the bed and the hips are rocked away from the bed, while the vaginal muscles are tightened. The buttocks are then pressed into the mattress, while the small of the back is lifted.)

Transverse. The *transverse lie* usually results in a *shoulder presentation*. The fetus lies crosswise, so there is

risk of a prolapsed cord or descent of the fetus' arm if the membranes rupture. Management may include version, but a cesarean delivery will most likely be done.

Face-Brow. In a *face-brow presentation* (occipitomental), the fetus' head is unfavorably positioned for delivery. Predisposing factors include a transverse lie, multiparity, polyhydramnios, and a low-lying placenta. The woman may deliver spontaneously if flexion of the fetus' neck occurs. The patient should be reassured, and the nurse should anticipate medical measures, such as version or cesarean delivery if the fetal position cannot be altered.

Breech. Breech presentation occurs in 3% of all deliveries. In a *complete* breech, the buttocks presents with the knees bent and the feet next to the buttocks. A *footling* breech is one in which one or both feet present (single footling or double footling). In a *frank* breech, the buttocks presents with the legs extended straight up (the legs and feet are entwined around the face). Predisposing factors are placenta previa, cephalopelvic disproportion, multiple pregnancy, small fetus, tumors, and polyhydramnios. If the mother has had a previous breech, a subsequent breech is more likely.

Fetal mortality is higher in breech deliveries than in any other kind of delivery. The risks to the woman include laceration and hemorrhage; to the fetus, the risks include birth injuries and fetal anoxia, which may be caused by early rupture of the bag of waters and by cord prolapse. Also, the head is delivered last, so asphyxia can occur; the head cannot undergo normal molding and may be caught in the birth canal.

Medical measures may include diagnostic ultrasound and fetal maturity studies, the use of forceps for the aftercoming head, or cesarean delivery. Nursing care is the same as for any laboring patient. The nurse should anticipate that FHTs will be located at or above the umbilicus, and meconium-stained amniotic fluid may be present. The nurse also should prepare for infant resuscitation if a spontaneous delivery occurs.

Cord Problems

Prolapsed Cord

In a prolapsed cord, the fetal umbilical cord precedes the baby. The cord may protrude from the cervix or may drop as low as the vulva. An occult (hidden) prolapse is difficult to determine because the cord is compressed between the fetus and the uterine wall. A prolapsed cord is a serious complication, because as the fetus' head descends, it may press the cord against the hard structures in the woman's pelvis, cutting off fetal circulation. This condition usually requires an emergency cesarean delivery.

A prolapsed cord can result from any factor that interferes with the engagement or adaptation of the presenting part to the pelvis, such as multiple pregnancy, a transverse lie, an abnormal presentation (such as a footling), hydramnios, or a high presenting part when the membranes suddenly rupture.

Sometimes this condition is detected early by electronic fetal monitoring. The birth attendant or nurse must insert a sterile gloved hand into the vagina to hold the fetal presenting part away from the cord so that the fetal circulation is not cut off while the woman is being prepared for an emergency cesarean delivery. If the cord has prolapsed outside the vagina, it is covered with sterile towels, moistened with warm, sterile normal saline. This prevents drying and caking of the cord and fetal blood. The woman should be placed in the Trendelenburg or knee-chest position as ordered. Fetal monitoring is essential. The nurse should notify the physician at once and must be prepared for resuscitation of a depressed neonate. A postoperative complication may be maternal puerperal infection.

Cord Around Fetal Neck (Nuchal Cord)

As the fetus moves within the uterus, the umbilical cord may become wrapped around the neck. If this condition is discovered before labor, cesarean delivery may be done. If it is not discovered until the woman is in labor, the cord may have become so tightly wrapped around the neck that the fetus is not able to receive oxygen. In this case, the birth attendant may use forceps to speed delivery, and the cord will be cut immediately. If there is a loose nuchal cord, the birth attendant may be able to slip it over the fetus' head.

Intrapartum Hemorrhage

Adherent Placenta

When the placenta fails to separate or to be expelled within 20 to 45 minutes after delivery or when parts of the placenta remain in the uterus, there is danger to the mother. This condition is called *adherent placenta* or *retained placenta*. The tissue must be removed soon after delivery so that an infection or hemorrhage does not develop.

There are three types of adherent placenta. *Placenta accreta*, the most common, is characterized by abnormal adherence of the placenta to the uterine muscle. In this condition, the deciduous membrane normally found between the placenta and the uterine wall is absent. *Placenta increta* penetrates the uterine wall. In *placentae percreta*, the uterine wall is invaded down to the serosal layer. The more extensive the penetration, the more danger there is to the woman and fetus.

In addition to physical factors, predisposing factors to intrapartum hemorrhage include precipitate delivery, administration of oxytocin too soon after delivery, and mismanagement of the third stage of labor.

The birth attendant may need to remove the placenta manually and may do a postpartum curettage of the uterus. Vigorous attempts at removal may lead to hemorrhage, shock, or rupture of the uterus. If the uterus is ruptured or if bleeding is not controllable, a hysterectomy must be performed to save the mother's life.

The nurse should carefully assess the mother immediately postpartum for signs of hemorrhage or shock. Anticipate the need for anesthesia, and have long, sterile gloves (version gloves) ready for the birth attendant.

Other Considerations

Induction of Labor

The birth attendant may induce, or start, labor before the woman begins naturally. Labor is induced only in certain instances, because it is not without risk. Reasons for induction include the possibility of fetal death without labor, worsening signs of pregnancy-induced hypertension, a large or post-term fetus, and maternal diabetes mellitus. The birth attendant must determine if the birth canal is large enough before inducing labor. If a cephalopelvic disproportion exists (the fetal head is larger than the pelvic inlet), induction can be fatal. Fetal maturity also must be evaluated to make sure that the fetus can survive outside the uterus.

Nursing Considerations. Nursing assessment is important during induction. The fetus is carefully monitored for fetal distress. The woman's blood pressure and pulse should be taken every 10 to 15 minutes during an IV or suppository induction, and at least every ½ hour following the rupture of the bag of waters. Any sign of maternal or fetal distress is an emergency situation and *must be reported to the physician immediately*. The nurse provides physical and emotional support to the woman and her partner during induction.

Induction with Drugs. Drugs are administered parenterally or orally to induce labor. An oxytocic is the most commonly used drug, although prostaglandin vaginal suppositories may be administered. The accompanying key medications box provides nursing considerations.

Amniotomy. Labor also can be induced by *amniotomy*, which means rupturing the amniotic membranes with a special hook. This procedure is performed by the physician under sterile conditions, at times assisted by the nurse. Labor usually follows quickly. The nurse should chart the time of the amniotomy, the color and approximate amount of fluid, and the effects on the woman. If labor does not begin spontaneously after amniotomy, induction with medications will usually follow. The woman must be watched for signs of uterine infection if delivery does not occur within 24 hours.

Key Medications
for Induction of Labor

◆ Oxytocin (Pitocin, Syntocinon)

Nursing Considerations

◆ Oxytocin is given IV, using a piggyback setup with a solution of normal saline or D5W (5% dextrose in water) to keep the vein open.
◆ The drip rate is adjusted for optimum rate, character of contractions, and optimum relaxation time between contractions.
◆ The infusion pump must be used to ensure an accurate measurement and delivery of the drug.
◆ A fetal monitor must be used to make sure the fetus is not in danger.

Emergency Delivery

Sometimes there is not enough time for the woman to get to the hospital for delivery. In this case, police officers, rescue personnel, or nurses may be asked to assist at emergency childbirth.

Nursing Considerations. Delivery should *never* be prevented; this can cause great damage to the woman and the fetus. The birth attendant should remain calm and deliver the baby as safely as possible. The best aseptic technique must be followed.

Usually there are few complications in a precipitous delivery. Important interventions in the care of the newborn include ensuring respirations and proper body temperature. It is not advisable to cut the cord unless the services of the birth attendant will not be available. However, the cord should be *double-tied* once the newborn is breathing or the placenta is delivered to prevent maternal hemorrhage. The neonate and placenta should be kept together if a birth attendant or hospital's services are anticipated. Putting the neonate to breast immediately helps the uterus to contract and prevents maternal hemorrhage. The mother will be examined for retained placental tissue, lacerations, and other complications once she receives medical assistance. Nursing skill guidelines in emergency delivery are listed in the accompanying box.

Lacerations. During a precipitous or emergency delivery, a laceration or tear into the perineal tissue and anus may occur. Lacerations are classified in several categories: The first degree involves the perineal skin and vaginal mucous membranes; the second degree involves muscles of the perineal body; the third degree involves the anal sphincter; and the fourth degree extends to the anal canal. All are repaired by sutures while the woman is still on the delivery table or in the emer-gency department. Cervical tears also are repaired to prevent hemorrhage.

Operative Obstetrics

Sometimes it becomes necessary to assist the woman with the delivery of the baby. The most common means to do so are version, forceps delivery, vacuum extraction, episiotomy, and cesarean birth. Episiotomy is discussed in Chapter 59.

Version

Version is used to turn the fetus to a more desirable presentation. In *external version*, the patient lies on her back with her knees flexed, and the birth attendant maneuvers the fetus through the uterine wall to a more favorable presentation. In *internal version*, the fetus is turned with the birth attendant's sterile gloved hand inside the uterus. Because the cervix must be dilated to perform the internal version, the fetus is generally delivered at the same time. The nurse must have long, sterile version gloves available for the birth attendant.

Forceps Delivery

Sometimes the birth is assisted with **forceps**, which are double-bladed, curved instruments that fit around the fetus' head. Their purpose is to increase traction and assist in rotating the fetus during delivery. Maternal in-

Nursing Skill Guidelines
Assisting in an Emergency Delivery

◆ Provide as much privacy as possible for the woman.
◆ Wear gloves, if available.
◆ Do not attempt to prevent delivery.
◆ Follow aseptic technique as closely as possible. (Remember that newspapers are quite clean.)
◆ Make sure the membranes have ruptured.
◆ Make sure the newborn's airway is clear before he or she takes the first breath.
◆ Initiate respiration in the newborn.
◆ Keep the neonate warm.
◆ Tie off the umbilical cord in two places.
◆ Do not cut the umbilical cord.
◆ Have the mother hold the newborn and put it to breast.
◆ Get medical assistance as soon as possible.
◆ Make sure the mother's uterus contracts after delivery of the newborn and placenta.
◆ Write down the time of birth of the neonate and the placenta. Write down the mother's name and address.
◆ Keep the mother warm.
◆ Reassure the mother.

dications for forceps delivery include exhaustion, heart disease, and prolonged labor. Fetal indications include fetal distress (as indicated by an irregular heartbeat, FHT below 100, or a late deceleration pattern on the fetal monitor) and a prolapsed umbilical cord.

Forceps deliveries are classified according to the *station* of the presenting part; that is, the position of the fetal head in relation to the ischial spines (see Figure 59-2). *Midforceps* delivery is used when the head is at the ischial spines (engaged), and the station is zero. The most commonly used forceps procedure is the *low forceps*, in which the fetal head is on the perineal floor (+2 station). Before forceps are applied by the practitioner, the FHTs are checked (preferably with the fetal monitor), a sterile vaginal examination is done to determine whether dilation and effacement are complete, and the membranes are ruptured. The patient is usually catheterized prior to the sterile vaginal examination if forceps delivery is anticipated.

Nursing Considerations. The nurse is responsible for documenting the time of delivery and use of forceps and observing the newborn. If there are any marks or injuries from the forceps, the nurse must document them on the newborn's chart. The mother's physical status, vital signs, and emotional reactions also are documented.

Vacuum Extraction

An alternative to forceps delivery is vacuum extraction, whereby a round, metal cup is placed on the fetal head. Suction is created by a special pump to secure the cup to the presenting part (the fetal head), and traction is exerted to ease the fetus gently out of the uterus. The patient must be fully dilated before the vacuum extractor can be used. The nurse will need to document the procedure and observe the newborn and the mother.

Cesarean Delivery

A cesarean delivery is a surgical procedure used to deliver the baby through an incision in the abdomen and the uterus. Any complication of labor may be an indication for performing cesarean delivery. In some instances, the woman may have an elective cesarean birth. If the mother has had previous cesarean births, the physician may prefer to do another to avoid the risk of a ruptured uterus. The high number of cesarean births in the United States is controversial.

Preoperative Care. Cesarean delivery may be scheduled in advance or may be an emergency procedure. A cesarean delivery is not usually done if the fetus is dead.

The nurse should prepare the parents for the procedure. The parents are concerned about the woman's safety, the fetus' safety, and the mother's recovery, not only from childbirth, but also from major surgery. A complete explanation is given to the father or coach. Many hospitals allow fathers in the operating room during cesarean delivery, because they can support the woman during this procedure, just as they can during vaginal delivery.

Preoperative care in abdominal surgery is discussed in Chapter 53. However, the woman does not receive narcotics or strong sedatives, because the fetus' respiration could easily become depressed. The nurse assesses for symptoms of fetal distress or unusual discomfort the woman might experience.

Generally, the woman is given an epidural or spinal anesthetic. In many cases, the woman is not anesthetized further, so the fetus will not be anesthetized. In some cases, local anesthesia is used until the fetus is delivered; the woman then receives general anesthesia for the remainder of the procedure. The woman should be forewarned that she will be awake for at least the first part of the procedure.

Preparing the Operating Room. The operating room must be prepared for abdominal surgery and for care of a newborn. An isolette or *incubator* and resuscitation and suction equipment are required. Surgical nurses and a special nurse to care for the newborn are present at the delivery.

Postoperative Care. The mother is given routine postoperative care. Vital signs should be assessed, lochia and nipples observed, and the fundus checked. Fundal assessment may be difficult because of the abdominal dressing, but it is important to do so; this mother can hemorrhage, as can any postpartum patient. Intake and output are recorded for 24 to 48 hours. IV fluids are usually continued for 24 hours after surgery. Diet is advanced as tolerated. Perineal care is administered, and oxytocic drugs are administered as ordered. Early ambulation and breathing exercises are important. The patient usually goes home on the third or fourth postoperative day.

Newborn Care. The newborn's respiratory status for the first few days of life must be assessed carefully, because he or she is more likely to experience respiratory distress than a neonate born vaginally. During a vaginal delivery, approximately 40% of the fluid in the fetal lungs is squeezed out when the fetal chest is compressed while passing through the birth canal. A newborn delivered by cesarean birth does not experience this compression and may experience respiratory distress due to retained fluids. This infant also has not had the stimulation of the birth experience.

Complications of the Postpartum Period

If undetected and untreated, a postpartal or **puerperal** (occurring following the birth of a baby) complication can become so severe that the mother may require re-hospitalization within days of discharge. Therefore, the postpartum assessment provides valuable information in detecting problems. Postpartum complications include circulatory disturbances, infectious processes, and emotional disorders.

Circulatory Disturbances

Hematoma

Bleeding into the subcutaneous tissue in the perineal area is called a postpartum **hematoma**. The hematoma may be caused by a precipitous delivery, prolonged pressure during labor and delivery, large varicosities in the pelvic area, or a vein that has been cut or pricked during episiotomy or its repair.

The patient experiences symptoms of severe pain in the perineal area, especially after a bowel movement or if the bladder becomes overly distended.

The perineal area should be assessed for discoloration and swelling. Cold compresses or a medicated pad, such as Tucks (containing witch hazel), may be used; sometimes compresses soaked in a magnesium sulfate solution are used. Sitz baths may be soothing. Analgesics are often given to relieve discomfort. The patient may be returned to the delivery room for incision and ligation of a blood vessel. Small hematomas will be absorbed without treatment.

Postpartum Hemorrhage

Average blood loss during a normal delivery is approximately 300 mL; any loss of more than 500 mL within 24 hours is considered a hemorrhage. A postpartal hemorrhage is classified as early if it occurs within 24 hours after delivery. A late hemorrhage may occur from 2 days to 6 weeks following delivery.

Postpartum hemorrhage is usually caused by uterine atony (lack of muscle tone), which prevents the uterine muscle from contracting and closing the venous sinuses. Other causes are retention of a fragment of placental tissue (which prevents the blood vessels from contracting) and tears or breaks in the reproductive tract as a result of delivery. Symptoms include steady or gushing external vaginal bleeding. The uterus is usually located high and feels boggy. The mother's pulse is often rapid, and the blood pressure drops in relation to the severity of the hemorrhage.

Nursing Considerations. The patient's life may depend on prompt nursing care. The area over the uterus should be grasped, cupping it with both hands. While supporting the lower part of the uterus with one hand, the other hand is used to massage gently but firmly. If the uterus cannot be located because it is boggy, the lower abdomen should be massaged until the uterus contracts. The woman is placed into the Trendelenburg position, and her vital signs are monitored. The physician is notified, and IV oxytocin infusion is anticipated.

If the cause of the bleeding appears to be a laceration or retained placental tissue, the patient will usually be prepared for a sterile vaginal examination and treatment. If the blood loss is extensive, she will probably require a blood transfusion.

Nursing Alert

Postpartum hemorrhage may occur quickly. Take action and report if any of the following occurs:

◆ Copious vaginal bleeding
◆ Boggy uterus (*massage first* and then report)
◆ Uterus high in the abdomen
◆ Signs of maternal shock

Thrombophlebitis

Thrombophlebitis involves a clot in a blood vessel, with resultant inflammation. In a new mother, thrombophlebitis typically occurs in the femoral vessels in the leg. Early ambulation has greatly lessened the occurrence of thrombophlebitis in new mothers.

Symptoms include swelling, slight elevation of temperature, pain, and redness or whiteness in the affected area. A positive Homan's sign occurs (calf pain on flexion of the foot). The symptoms most often develop in the second postpartal week and may persist for weeks or months.

Treatment consists of bed rest with elevation of the affected part, local application of heat, analgesics, antiembolism stockings, and anticoagulants. After the acute stage has passed, the patient may have to wear a support stocking for some time.

Nursing Alert

Carefully assess the woman with thrombophlebitis. If the clot breaks away, it can enter the circulation as an *embolism* and become fatal.

Infectious Processes or Puerperal Infection

Puerperal infection is an infection in any part of the reproductive tract after childbirth. It was the major cause of maternal deaths before asepsis was practiced. Predisposing conditions include the presence of injured tissues or retained pieces of placenta and lowered maternal resistance. The infection may be mild or severe, local or general; however, like any infection, it is preventable or treatable.

Staphylococcus and *Streptococcus* are common organisms causing puerperal infection. Because these organisms can be carried by hospital personnel, those who work in the labor room wear caps, clean or sterile suits or gowns, and gloves. In the delivery room, aseptic technique is practiced, and masks are worn. The father also wears hospital garb in the delivery room or during the birth in the birthing room. Hands are washed prior to and after all examinations. The patient's articles, such as peri pads, must be handled in an aseptic manner, and the mother must be taught proper perineal care. Personnel with upper respiratory or gastrointestinal symptoms should not be in contact with the patient.

Fever with a possible chill is the outstanding symptom of puerperal infection. Infection is suspected if the patient's temperature is elevated to 100.4°F (38°C) orally on any two successive days during the first 10 days postpartum. A tender, high uterus; headache; general malaise; and dark-colored, foul-smelling lochia are other symptoms of infection. The episiotomy suture line may appear infected. The nurse must assess the characteristics of the lochia, the height of the fundus, and the appearance of the perineum.

The infected mother may be isolated or moved to another floor. The newborn may be isolated and is not brought to the mother for feeding. Antibiotics are administered. Fluids are encouraged, and the bed is placed in Fowler's position to promote drainage of lochia.

Cystitis

Cystitis, an inflammation of the bladder, is caused by a microorganism. It occurs frequently following childbirth because of urinary retention, residual urine, and trauma to the bladder and urethra during delivery. When urine remains in the bladder, it becomes a breeding place for bacteria.

Symptoms of cystitis include frequency and urgency of urination, pain and burning on urination, hematuria, low abdominal pain, fever, and malaise. Once a urine specimen is obtained, antibiotics are administered. Fluids are encouraged.

Mastitis*

Mastitis is an infection of the breast most commonly caused by *Staphylococcus aureus*, *Escherichia coli*, and rarely *Streptococcus*. This organism usually enters the

body through cracked or fissured nipples. The highest incidence occurs in the second or third week postpartum. Symptoms of mastitis include localized tenderness, redness, heat, fever, malaise, and sometimes nausea and vomiting. Mastitis should be treated immediately to avoid abscess and chronic mastitis, which may last for up to 4 months and require extensive antibiotic therapy.

Predisposing conditions to mastitis are plugged milk ducts, poor drainage of ducts and alveolus, the presence of an organism, stress and fatigue, and tight-fitting clothing. Treatment of mastitis includes local massage, moist heat, antibiotic therapy, rest, and frequent nursing. The woman requires teaching related to self-care. The accompanying box lists teaching subjects.

Postpartum Blues and Postpartum Psychosis

Approximately 50% to 80% of all women experience a mild depression, called *postpartum blues*, 3 to 10 days after delivery. These blues appear to be a normal hormonal reaction. It usually resolves itself if the woman has a good support system. If symptoms last longer than 2 weeks, however, a postpartum **psychosis** can be suspected. This condition rarely occurs in women with no previous psychiatric history.

Assessment by the nurse during the early postpartum period is helpful in diagnosing and intervening with these patients. Such patients may be suicidal or homicidal. Hospitalization and child-protective services may be needed. Prognosis, with appropriate medications, is usually good, but the condition may recur following subsequent deliveries.

Keys for Patient/Family Teaching
Prevention of Complications of Mastitis

Patient teaching related to prevention of complications of mastitis includes the following:

- ◆ The mother continues to nurse the newborn on both breasts, beginning with the unaffected breast to ease let-down reflex on the other side.
- ◆ Bed rest is mandatory. The newborn can be taken to bed with her for frequent nursing.
- ◆ The mother must follow antibiotic therapy regimen for at least 10 days.
- ◆ Hot packs are used on the breast for comfort.
- ◆ The mother should drink plenty of fluids.
- ◆ Mild analgesics, such as acetaminophen, can be used for pain relief.
- ◆ The mother should wear a well-fitting support bra.
- ◆ Document all teaching.

Information adapted from Lawrence RA. Breastfeeding: A Guide for the Medical Professional, Ed 3. St. Lous, C.V. Mosby, 1989.

---

* Courtesy of Gwendelyn Combs-Marshall, Certified Lactation Educator.

When the Newborn Dies

Occasionally, in spite of excellent prenatal care, a fetus or newborn dies. This is a difficult time for the parents. The nurse must be as supportive as possible and give the parents a chance to vent their feelings. A visit by the hospital chaplain or social worker may be appreciated; the nurse can ask if the family wishes to have someone called. In many hospitals, the mother is moved from the obstetrics unit so that she will not hear crying babies or see happy parents. The nurse should be familiar with hospital policy and should respect the parents' wishes. Allow the mother to hold the child and take photos if she wishes. The family also may choose to donate tissues to help other people. The family should be given the opportunity to have a funeral or have the hospital cremate the body. Referral to an organization such as "The Compassionate Friends" is often helpful.

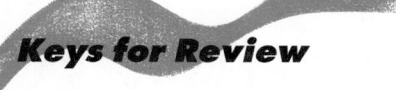

Keys for Review

Key Questions for Critical Thinking

1. Discuss the relationship of substance abuse to pregnancy. Discuss possible maternal, fetal, and neonatal effects.
2. Differentiate between placenta previa and abruptio placentae and describe symptoms of each. Describe related nursing care.
3. Describe steps taken in emergency delivery. Describe the rationale for each step.
4. Place yourself in the position of a woman who has just been told she must have an emergency cesarean birth because of complications. Describe your feelings. Discuss what information you want and the nursing care you would like to receive.

Key Readings

Auvenshine M, Enriquez M. Comprehensive Maternity Nursing: Perinatal and Women's Health, Ed 2. Boston, Jones and Bartlett, 1990

Berckow R (Ed). Merck Manual of Diagnosis and Therapy, Ed 16. Rahway, NJ, Merck Research Laboratories, 1992

MacLaren A. Nurses' Clinical Guide to Maternity Care. Springhouse, PA, Springhouse, 1992

May KA, Mahlmeister LR. Maternal and Neonatal Nursing: Family-Centered Care, Ed 3. Philadelphia, J.B. Lippincott, 1994

Key Readings (continued)

Pillitteri A. Maternal and Child Health Nursing: Care of the Childbearing and Childrearing Family, Ed 2. Philadelphia, J.B. Lippincott, 1995

Reeder SJ, Martin LL, Koniak D. Maternity Nursing: Family, Newborn and Women's Health Care, Ed 17. Philadelphia, J.B. Lippincott, 1992

Sherwen L, Scoloveno M, Weingerten C. Nursing Care of the Childbearing Family. Norwalk, CT, Appleton & Lange, 1991

Keys to Learning More

Chapter 62: neonatal disorders
Chapter 63: fertility control
Chapter 84: female reproductive disorders
Chapter 90: death and dying, helpful information when caring for a mother whose fetus or newborn dies

Key Resources

The Compassionate Friends, Inc.
"A self-help organization offering friendship and understanding to bereaved parents and siblings"
National Office
P.O. Box 3696
Oak Brook, IL 60522-3696
(708) 990-0010
(708) 990-0246 (FAX)

62 Disorders of the Neonate

Keys for Learning

Learning Objectives

- Define the term high-risk neonate.
- Describe the classification of neonates according to size and gestational age.
- Define characteristics and nursing care specific to the premature neonate.
- Describe the medical problems related to the large-for-gestational-age newborn.
- Describe various injuries that may occur during the birth process.
- Describe common disorders of each body system of the neonate, listing symptoms and treatment measures.
- Describe fetal effects resulting from sexually transmitted diseases and other infectious conditions.
- Describe neonatal effects of drug and alcohol use during pregnancy.

Key Terms

anencephaly	microcephaly
atelectasis	phenylketonuria
congenital	phototherapy
cytomegalovirus	physiologic jaundice
epispadias	pyloric stenosis
esophageal atresia	respiratory distress syndrome
genetic	spina bifida
galactosemia	teratogenic
hydrocephalus	thrush
hypospadias	toxoplasmosis

Keys to Understanding This Chapter

Chapter 9: basis for recognizing deviations from normal development in the neonate

Unit Four: basis for recognizing deviations from normal body structure or function

Chapter 32: sudden death and cardiopulmonary resuscitation

Keys to Understanding This Chapter
(continued)

Unit Seven: nursing process

Unit Eight: communication

Unit Nine: nursing skills in patient care, including the neonate with complications

Chapter 54: sterile technique, which is used in many aspects of neonatal care

Unit Eleven: basics of medication administration

Chapter 60: care of the normal neonate

Key Points

- Being able to identify risk situations affecting mother and newborn is of vital importance when planning adequate care.
- High-risk newborns have special problems caused by immaturity, alterations in structure or functioning of systems, and metabolic imbalances.
- Parents need assistance to accept the newborn with special needs and the care he or she will require.
- The alert nurse is invaluable to the survival of the infant in respiratory distress.
- Nursing skills in assisting to interpret data, make decisions, and provide therapy are crucial to the compromised infant's survival.
- The nurse is commonly the first to observe the signs of drug dependence in the newborn.

Key Topics Outline

The High-Risk Neonate
    Classification of High-Risk Neonates
    Nursing Considerations in the Premature Neonate
    Potential Complications in High Risk Neonates
Hemolytic Conditions
Birth Injuries
Congenital Disorders
    Musculoskeletal Disorders
    Nervous System Disorders

Rosdahl CB: Textbook of Basic Nursing, 6th ed. © 1995 J.B. Lippincott Company

At birth the newborn takes on the functions of breathing, eating, digesting, eliminating, and stabilizing body temperature. If problems develop with any of these vital functions, the newborn will often have difficulty surviving. The newborn with a complication is considered *high risk* or *compromised.* Due to advanced technology and improved medical and nursing care, high-risk neonates have an ever-increasing chance of survival.

The nurse may be the first to recognize disorders in the newborn. Through accurate assessments, the nurse is often able to detect abnormalities and report them promptly. Difficulties can often be alleviated or corrected if treatment is begun promptly.

The High-Risk Neonate

The mother, her family, and the high-risk neonate are highly vulnerable. Protecting the newborn by maintaining a warm environment, adequate oxygen, and safety is a priority for nursing care. The newborn's basic needs of oxygen, nutrition, fluid, and elimination must be monitored and met carefully. The survival and well-being of the neonate depend on the collaborative efforts of the medical and nursing team. The nurse also must remember that the newborn belongs to a family that has many other needs.

Parents are shocked when told about a defect in their newborn. At such times, the nurse usually is present to provide support. Parents need to verbalize their fears, hopes, and disappointments. Sometimes they need to have more knowledge so that they can make decisions relative to the treatment of the disorder. Most of all, parents want a caring nurse—one who will listen.

Baptism. If the neonate's condition is poor and the family is Christian, the newborn may be baptized according to the parents' wishes. Anyone can perform a baptism in an emergency. However, if clergy or a hospital chaplain is available, this person should perform the baptism. If the parents wish to have a nurse baptize their newborn or the products of conception into the Christian faith, water is poured over the head or other skin surface and the following words are spoken: "I baptize you in the name of the Father, of the Son, and of the Holy Spirit [Holy Ghost]." The parents and priest or minister should be made aware that the baptism has taken place. A record of the procedure is inserted on the mother's chart. Two witnesses should be present whenever possible, and their names should be documented on the chart.

Classification of High-Risk Neonates

Newborns may be classified by their size and gestational ages, as defined in the accompanying box. Neurologic assessments are done on all neonates to determine maturity. Useful abbreviations and acronyms are listed in a second box.

Small-for-Gestational Age Neonate

Small-for-gestational age (SGA) newborns are at risk; mortality is greater than 10%. Causes of SGA include the following:

◆ Maternal conditions (ie, pregnancy-induced hypertension, cardiac and renal disease, and diabetes mellitus)
◆ Poor maternal nutrition
◆ Intrauterine infections
◆ Maternal substance abuse, including alcohol
◆ Maternal cigarette smoking
◆ Congenital malformations
◆ Twins and other multiple births
◆ Fetal and placental abnormalities

The characteristics of the SGA newborn include an abnormally large head in relation to the body; loose,

Classification of Neonates

Based on Size

♦ *Appropriate for gestational age* (AGA): refers to a neonate whose growth is within normal limits

♦ *Small for gestational age* (SGA): refers to a newborn whose birth weight is below the 10th percentile expected for that gestational age

♦ *Large for gestational age* (LGA): refers to a newborn who is larger than 90% of the babies born at that gestational age

♦ *Low birth weight* (LBW): weighs less than 5.5 lb (approximately 2,500 g)

♦ *Very low birth weight* (VLBW): weighs between 500 and 1,499 g (approximately 1–3.5 lbs)

♦ *Immature:* weighs less than 1000 g (2.2 lb)

♦ Based on Gestational Age

♦ *Preterm:* born prior to the 37th completed week of gestation (before 295 days, counting from the first day of the last normal menstrual period); accounts for 6% to 8% of all births in the United States

♦ *Term:* born between the 38th and 42nd weeks of gestation

♦ *Posterm:* born after the 42nd week of gestation

dry skin; sparse or absent hair; wide skull sutures caused by inadequate bone growth; and diminished muscle and fatty tissue. Specific problems faced by the SGA neonate include hypothermia, hypoglycemia, respiratory distress, prolonged infantile apnea or SIDS, and delayed neurologic development.

Large-for-Gestational Age Neonate

Large-for-gestational age (LGA) newborns are those whose birth weights exceed the 90th percentile of newborns of the same gestational age.

LGA newborns are born most often to diabetic mothers. Although the newborn is large and appears fat, it is not necessarily healthy. Elevated blood glucose levels in the woman increase the glucose available to the fetus. This stimulates additional insulin production by the fetal pancreas. The problem arises when the fetus is delivered and the supply of excess glucose is terminated. This newborn quickly uses all available carbohydrates and may develop hypoglycemia. Other problems facing the LGA neonate include birth injury (ie, fractured clavicle, skull fracture, and brachial nerve palsy), as well as respiratory disorders.

Post-term Neonate

The fetus who remains in the uterus beyond 42 weeks of gestation is called post-term. Such a newborn is not necessarily in better condition than the full-term newborn. The post-term neonate often has respiratory or nutritional problems because the placenta is unable to provide adequately for the fetus after the normal time of gestation. As a result, the post-term newborn may be SGA. The post-term neonate has long fingernails and hair; has dry, parched skin; lacks vernix caseosa; and looks wrinkled and old at birth. He or she may have swallowed meconium or aspirated it into the lungs.

Preterm Neonate

Neonates classified as preterm are those born prior to 37 weeks' gestation. Despite advances in the early identification and treatment of preterm labor, preterm deliveries affect approximately 10% of all births in the United States. Causes of preterm delivery include the following:

♦ Poor prenatal care
♦ Maternal age extremes (ie, younger than 19 or older than 35)
♦ Low socioeconomic status
♦ Poor maternal nutrition
♦ Chronic disorders (ie, hypertension, diabetes, renal disorders)
♦ Antepartum trauma or infection
♦ Uterine anomalies
♦ Premature cervical dilation

The preterm infant appears thin, with minimal subcutaneous fat; lanugo on the face, back, arms, and legs; skin is transparent; breast tissue is barely palpable; testes may be undescended: breathing is irregular and weak; body temperature is frequently subnormal; and the cry is weak. Neurologic assessments reflect an immature central nervous system as demonstrated by diminished or absent reflexes.

Nursing Considerations in the Premature Neonate

To conserve the small neonate's energy, he or she is handled as little as possible (see the sample nursing care plan for the premature neonate). Usually, a bath is

Key Abbreviations and Acronyms for Neonatal Disorders

AGA	Appropriate for gestational age
FAS	Fetal alcohol syndrome
HIV	Human immunodeficiency virus
LBW	Low birth weight
LGA	Large for gestational age
NEC	Necrotizing enterocolitis
PIA	Prolonged infantile apnea
PKU	Phenylketonuria
PT	Preterm
RDS	Respiratory distress syndrome
SIDS	Sudden infant death syndrome
SGA	Small for gestational age
VLBW	Very low birth weight

Baby boy LeFevre was born at 34 weeks' gestation, weighing 2,250 g, with Apgar scores of 4 and 6. He is preterm but appropriate for gestational age (PT AGA). Nursing priorities for Baby LeFevre include thermoregulation, respiration, and nutrition. Three priority nursing diagnoses from his plan of care follow.

Nursing Diagnosis: *Ineffective Thermoregulation Related to Large Body Surface Area (Increased Radiant and Conductive Heat Losses) and Reduced Brown Fat Stores as Evidenced by Temperature Swings Below 97.4°F and Above 98.8°F*

Goal 1: Infant's temperature remains within acceptable range for his weight.

Goal 2: Whenever observed, infant shows no signs of problems associated with cold stress (increased oxygen consumption; increased glucose consumption with associated hypoglycemia, poor weight gain, acidosis, and decreased surfactant production) or overheating (increased insensible water loss through the skin, increased oxygen consumption, apnea, and burns).

Nursing Actions (assess/do/teach)	Rationale	Evaluative Statement
1. After the initial rectal reading, take an axillary temperature q30 min until stabilized in the range of 97.4°–98.8°F (36.4–37°C); continue to monitor temperature and weight gain frequently.	This ensures temperature stability and assesses for cold stress and hyperthermia. Cold stress can decrease weight gain.	1. 5/20, Goal 1 met; temperature remains within acceptable range.
2. Dry the preterm newborn immediately, place under radiant heat, keep a hat on his head, wrap in warm blankets, or place in warm incubator (incubator air temperature for first 24 hours, 33.3°C ± 0.7); maintain a neutral thermal environment.	This decreases radiant and conductive heat losses.	2. 5/20, Goal 2 met; no signs of cold stress or overheating.
3. Even after the initial stabilization, all care and treatment must include the prevention of heat loss; keep away from windows, cold walls, drafts.	These actions decrease radiant and conductive heat losses.	
4. Monitor the newborn's daily weight.	Cold stress can decrease the speed of weight gain.	4. 5/25, Goal 2 being met. Daily weight beginning to increase.

Nursing Diagnosis: *Ineffective Breathing Pattern Related to Immature Lungs and Decreased Surfactant Production as Evidenced by Progressive Difficulty in Breathing and Substernal Retractions Noted 45 Minutes After Birth*

Goal 1: Whenever observed, the infant's respirations fall within the normal range; blood gases are within normal limits.

Goal 2: The infant demonstrates no signs of respiratory distress (xiphoid retractions, nares dilatation, expiratory grunt, tachypnea, cyanosis, hypoxemia, acidosis).

(continued)

Nursing Actions (assess/do/teach)	Rationale	Evaluative Statement
1. Frequent monitoring and close observation of breath sounds, respiratory rate, skin color, mucous membrane color, and any sign of respiratory distress; observation of oximeter readings	The newborn's status can change rapidly; the newborn's response to therapy is assessed.	1. 5/20, Goal 1 met; respirations within normal limits
2. General supportive measures: minimal handling, neutral thermal environment, adequate caloric intake and hydration; oral feedings contraindicated with marked increase in respiratory rate	Oxygen use is conserved. Danger of aspiration is increased.	2. 5/20, Goal 2 met; no signs of respiratory distress
3. Oxygen therapy 40%–50% through plastic hood, as ordered	Apply just enough pressure to open and keep open most of the alveoli; this maintains PO_2 at satisfactory level. Suctioning helps keep the airway patent.	
4. Careful suctioning as needed, based on assessment.		

Nursing Diagnosis: *Altered Nutrition, Less than Body Requirements Related to Small Stomach Capacity With High Caloric Requirement and Fatigue with Sucking*

Goal 1: Infant demonstrates consistent weight gain (approximately 20–30 g/d)

Nursing Actions (assess/do/teach)	Rationale	Evaluative Statement
1. After the first sterile H_2O feedings, initiate nipple feedings of expressed breast milk; before initiating nipple feedings, observe for any signs of stress, tachypnea, respiratory distress, or hypothermia that increase the risk of aspiration; during feedings observe for signs of difficulty with feeding (tachypnea, cyanosis, bradycardia, lethargy, and uncoordinated suck and swallow reflexes).	This causes less severe lung tissue reaction to H_2O, should aspiration occur.	5/24, Goal partially met; weight gain of 15–20 g most days.
2. Two-hour feedings until the infant tolerates 15 mL at each feeding; 3-hour feedings until infant tolerates 30 mL, then 4-hour feedings; feed in semisitting position and bubble gently after each 0.5–1 oz. Position on right side of abdomen after feeding.	The preterm newborn's stomach capacity is small. This position prevents aspiration.	
3. Assess tolerance of feedings: check for abdominal distension, gastric residuals, emesis.	You want to prevent development of necrotizing enterocolitis (NEC).	
4. Gavage feed infant, as needed.	Gavage feeding helps to conserve energy; decrease oxygen consumption, and decrease risk of aspiration.	

not given immediately. It is difficult to control the temperature of the premature infant; thus, he or she must be kept warm. The bed is warmed, a stockinette cap is worn, and the temperature is taken often. Oxygen is supplied if necessary. Figure 62-1 illustrates care provided for a premature neonate in the neonatal intensive care unit.

Isolette Care. The isolette simulates the environment within the uterus as closely as possible. The isolette is transparent, so the neonate can be seen at all times. An even level of temperature, humidity, and oxygen is maintained. The isolette is covered by a hood, and nurses give care through portholes.

Feeding. Feeding varies. In some instances, no food is given for 36 hours, because digestion is an additional burden on the newborn's body. In other instances, formula or expressed breast milk is given using a nipple or a nasogastric tube (gavage feeding). Formula is prescribed in small amounts on a 2- to 3-hour schedule, to avoid distending the small stomach or adding to respiratory distress.

Elimination. Because the premature newborn's kidneys are not fully developed, he or she may have difficulty eliminating wastes. Accurate output is determined by weighing the diaper before and after the infant urinates. The diaper's weight difference in grams is approximately equal to the amount of milliliters voided.

Protection Against Infection. Good handwashing, the first defense against infection, must be performed by all who come in contact with the infant. Because premature neonates are susceptible to infections, they are isolated and attended by nursery personnel who are

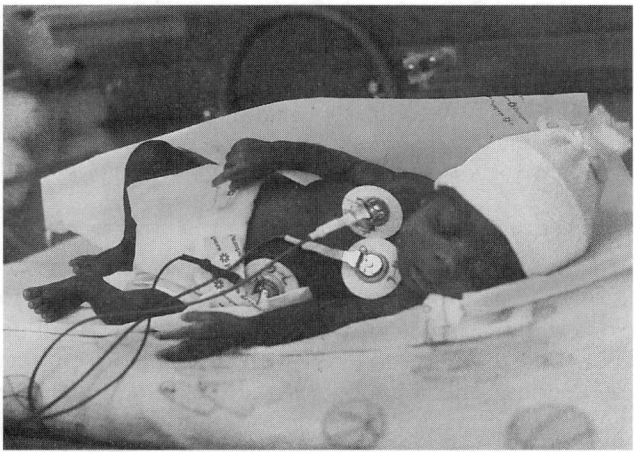

Figure 62-1. A neonate in the neonatal intensive care unit. Note the electrodes for constant monitoring and the cap on the neonate's head to maintain body heat.

trained to follow special aseptic techniques. Generally, the premature neonate is not dressed so that the nurse can observe breathing. Their contacts with other people are limited as much as possible. However, the mother and father, taught to wear a gown and gloves, are encouraged to touch and hold the neonate, if the newborn's condition permits, to promote bonding.

Assessments. The premature neonate is assessed carefully. Observations include color (pink, cyanotic, jaundiced); respirations (normal/abnormal: rate, retractions, expiratory grunt, nasal flaring); pulse (rate, strength, regularity); amount, frequency, and description of stools and voidings; general appearance; weight; and activity level. Any abnormal symptoms must be reported. If the newborn is having difficulties, monitors will be attached, and care will be given in the neonatal intensive care unit.

Respiratory Status. Figure 62-2 illustrates the measures for determining respiratory status. This assessment is particularly important in premature newborns.

Respiratory distress syndrome (RDS) is a leading cause of death in premature newborns. In RDS, the lungs cannot expand normally and thus do not get enough air for proper oxygenation. The cause is unknown, although there are several theories. A deficiency in a substance called _pulmonary surfactant_ exists, resulting in incomplete expansion of the lungs. **Atelactasis,** partial or complete collapse of a lung, is common.

The infant with RDS demonstrates dyspnea and cyanosis. The respiration rate increases, and the nares flare. The chest muscles retract during inspiration, and this is accompanied by tachycardia and an expiratory grunt. If the condition cannot be corrected, it is usually fatal, but if the infant survives the first few days of life, recovery is usually complete.

RDS is treated by administering oxygen in an atmosphere of high humidity and sometimes by using a mechanical ventilator. The newborn is fed by gavage or through a central line (total parenteral nutrition) to prevent aspiration into the lungs. Usually antibiotics are given.

Retrolental fibroplasia often led to blindness in premature newborns in the past. It occurs when a concentration of oxygen over 40% is given for a prolonged time. Excessive concentrations of oxygen must be avoided, and the premature neonate's blood Po_2 level (oxygen level) must be carefully monitored by the respiratory care staff.

Potential Complications in High-Risk Neonates

Meconium or Amniotic Fluid Aspiration

In the hypoxic fetus, the anal sphincter relaxes, allowing meconium to pass into the amniotic fluid. Meconium aspiration can occur at birth. If the first breath

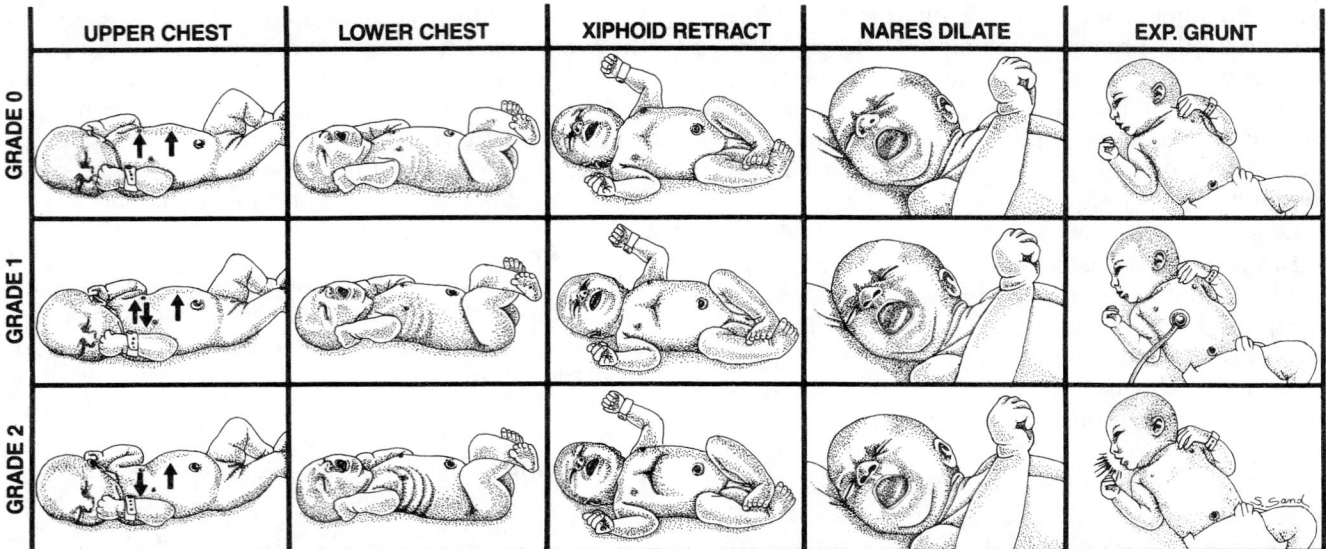

Figure 62-2. The Silverman-Andersen index of neonatal respiratory distress. Observation of retractions. An index of respiratory distress is determined by grading each of five arbitrary criteria. Grade 0 indicates no difficulty; grade 1 indicates moderate difficulty; and grade 2 indicates maximum respiratory difficulty. The retraction score is the sum of these values; a total score of 0 indicates no dyspnea, whereas a total score of 10 denotes maximal respiratory distress.

is taken prior to suctioning, the neonate may aspirate meconium an amniotic fluid into the lungs.

Any aspirated fluid can lead to atelectasis, pneumonia, and other pulmonary problems. An aspiration bulb is kept at the cribside for the purpose of clearing respiratory passages. Treatment is supportive. Oxygen is given, fluids are encouraged, and temperature is regulated. Antibiotics may be given.

Cyanosis

If the newborn does not establish initial breathing, he or she turns blue or dusky, a condition known as cyanosis.

Respiratory difficulty may be due to a prolapsed cord during delivery (a condition in which the cord becomes compressed between the fetus' head and the woman's pelvis), a congenital heart defect, faulty respiratory apparatus, a birth injury to the brain, a congenital defect in the brain stem, medications, or even the analgesic or anesthetic the mother was given.

Treatment is initiated promptly for newborns who do not breathe as soon as they are born. First, it must be determined whether the air passages are clear of obstructive substances, such as amniotic fluid and mucus. Soft catheters, bulb syringes, and mechanical suction machines are used to remove this material. The newborn's head is lowered to facilitate postural drainage. The back is rubbed to stimulate respiration. If the infant fails to respond, additional resuscitation measures (ie, mechanical ventilation) are begun.

Physiologic Jaundice

In many newborns, the bilirubin level is elevated (*hyperbilirubinemia*), causing **physiologic jaundice.** This results from the inability of the newborn's immature liver to handle bilirubin, a byproduct of red blood cell breakdown. This excess bilirubin appears in the bloodstream, causing the skin to appear yellow. A heel-stick blood test (see Chapter 60) may be ordered to determine the degree of hyperbilirubinemia. If the level is sufficiently high, phototherapy will be initiated.

Nursing Alert

Physiologic jaundice usually appears about the third day of life. Jaundice that appears immediately after birth should be reported, because this is more likely to indicate hemolytic disease, such as erythroblastosis fetalis.

The use of fluorescent lights to alleviate jaundice is known as **phototherapy.** To provide maximum skin exposure, the newborn is naked except for a small diaper. The eyes are covered with dressings to protect the retinas. The newborn is then placed under the lights. The newborn's temperature must be monitored carefully to prevent hypothermia or hyperthermia. Generally the infant is placed on a 3-hour feeding schedule. *(Rationale: Frequent feedings help to speed the excretion of bilirubin.)* The urine and stool may be green. The neonate is removed from the lights for feeding, checking vital signs, and bonding.

Vomiting, Diarrhea, and Dehydration

Newborn vomiting may be a symptom of a congenital defect (ie, esophageal atresia), birth injury (ie, intracranial hemorrhage), or infectious process. There is a distinct difference between vomiting and the normal spitting up of the newborn.

Diarrhea is most commonly caused by bacteria, although it also may be caused by an incompatible formula or an allergy. In diarrhea of the newborn, the stool is formless, greenish-yellow, and has a foul smell. Evidence of severe diarrhea requires that the infant be isolated *immediately* to prevent possible infection of other infants. Stool cultures must be obtained. Dehydration can occur very quickly.

The greatest concern in newborn vomiting or diarrhea is *dehydration,* which, if unchecked, leads to an electrolyte imbalance. Dehydration develops quickly in the small infant, because he or she has so little reserve fluid. Treatment must be started immediately, or the newborn may die. Intravenous fluids are given, along with humidified oxygen; lost electrolytes must be replaced.

Necrotizing Enterocolitis

Necrotizing enterocolitis is a serious disorder causing varying amounts of the bowel wall to necrose (die). It is more common in premature babies, especially if the membranes ruptured early or if the newborn suffered anoxia; bottle-fed babies are more susceptible. Symptoms include lethargy, abdominal distention, hypothermia, apnea, and irritability. The bowel is rested by using a nasogastric tube and suction, parenteral fluids and total parenteral nutrition, and antibiotics. X-rays are taken frequently to evaluate progress.

Hypoglycemia

All infants have the potential for decreased blood sugar soon after birth. However, there is a greater susceptibility in LGA newborns of diabetic mothers, newborns with erythroblastosis fetalis (discussed in the next section), and newborns with heart disease or galactosemia. Hypoglycemia occurs when the blood glucose level reads below 40 mg/100 mL with a Dextrostix or 30 mg/100 mL when blood glucose is determined in the laboratory. (These determined critical values may vary between hospitals.)

Signs of hypoglycemia normally relate to the central nervous system. These include tremors, irritability, jitteriness, high-pitched or weak cry, and eye rolling. There may be observable changes in vital signs (such as apnea and tachycardia). The newborn may be cyanotic or pale, eat poorly, and have seizures. Treatment consists of a carefully calculated infusion of 10% to 15% glucose, decreasing the amount as the neonate can tolerate oral feedings. The infant must be assessed carefully for changing status.

Hemolytic Conditions

Hemolytic conditions often result from an Rh or ABO blood incompatibility. In both, the mother builds up antibodies against antigens from her own fetus.

Erythroblastosis Fetalis. *Erythroblastosis fetalis* can occur when an Rh-negative mother gives birth to an Rh-positive neonate, resulting in an Rh incompatibility that causes the woman's antibodies to destroy the fetus' red blood cells. This condition is uncommon today, because it can be prevented if Rh-negative women are given RhoGAM following any invasive procedure (ie, amniocentesis), after any abortion, at 28 weeks' gestation, and following delivery of an Rh-positive neonate. Some cases are still seen in women who do not have prenatal care or who have had a previously untreated abortion.

An intrauterine transfusion to the fetus may be given prior to birth. Phototherapy is used in milder cases after birth. If this does not help, a series of *exchange transfusions* probably will be given. As the infant grows older, he or she will produce red blood cells independently, and the condition will be outgrown.

ABO Incompatibility. ABO incompatibility occurs when the mother has O-type blood and the neonate has A, B, or AB type or when the mother is group A or B, with a newborn of the opposite blood group. The disease usually is mild and is characterized by jaundice and an enlarged spleen. Treatment usually consists of phototherapy.

Birth Injuries

Various injuries may occur during the birth process. Some of these are serious, but most can be corrected.

Fractures. One of the most common birth injuries is a fractured clavicle. Signs and symptoms of a fractured clavicle include asymmetrical Moro reflex and crying when the affected arm is moved. Fractures rarely are complicated and usually heal without difficulties.

Intracranial Hemorrhage. Intracranial hemorrhage can be a dangerous birth injury. Seen primarily in the preterm infant, additional causes include difficult delivery, precipitate labor and delivery, or prolonged labor. Seizures, respiratory distress, cyanosis, a shrill cry, and muscle weakness are symptoms. The prognosis varies with the extent of the injury and treatment. To prevent hemorrhage, vitamin K is given intramuscularly to every newborn soon after delivery. Treatment is similar to that in an adult.

The newborn with intracranial hemorrhage is positioned with the head of the bed slightly elevated. Oxygen, vitamin K, antibiotics, anticonvulsive medications, and sedatives are administered. Feeding is by gavage tube. Complications that may result include cerebral hemorrhage, cerebral palsy, hydrocephaly, and mental retardation.

Brachial Plexus Injury. Brachial plexus injury results from trauma to the brachial plexus during a difficult delivery (ie, shoulder dystocia). One example of brachial plexus injury is Erb-Duchenne paralysis, which results from trauma to the fifth and sixth cranial nerve. The infant is unable to elevate the affected arm, which lies limply at the side. Grasp reflex is present. Lower plexus injury results in symptoms in the hand and forearm, with the grasp reflex absent. Treatment of both includes range-of-motion exercises and possible splinting. Prognosis depends on the degree of nerve damage.

Facial Paralysis. Facial paralysis (Bell's palsy) occurs when the facial nerve is injured, usually as a result of forceps delivery. If the nerve tissue is damaged, paralysis may be permanent. Usually only one side is affected, and the eyelid and mouth may droop on that side. The infant's sucking mechanism may be impaired, requiring special feeding. The infant also may need saline irrigation or patching of the eye to retain moisture. Plastic surgery is sometimes effective in improving appearance. Fortunately, most cases of facial and brachial paralysis are temporary.

Congenital Disorders

Disorders of the neonate may involve any body system and some involve several systems. Disorders of the neonate may be broken into the following types:

◆ **Congenital:** abnormalities that exist at birth (may be genetic or acquired)
◆ **Genetic:** hereditary in origin
◆ **Teratogenic:** anything that causes severe abnormalities in the fetus (eg, maternal illness, medications, environmental toxins, vaccinations, or inoculations); acquired disorders

More information on most of the following disorders is given in Chapters 65, 66, and 67.

Musculoskeletal Disorders

Talipes (Clubfoot). In clubfoot, one or both feet turn out of the normal position. The condition occurs more often in males. Early diagnosis and treatment usually yield an excellent prognosis. Exercise, corrective shoes, braces, casts, and surgery also may be used.

Congenital Dislocated Hip. Congenital dislocated hip occurs more frequently in females and is believed to be caused by faulty embryonic development of the hip joint. The head of the femur fails to be situated firmly in the acetabulum. Early treatment is necessary to prevent permanent damage.

The first sign of this condition may be a limitation of abduction on the affected side when the thigh is flexed (Ortolani's sign). The affected femur is shorter than the unaffected femur; the skin folds of the thigh and buttocks are asymmetric, and a slight click may be heard with abduction of the hip. Diagnosis is usually confirmed with x-ray studies.

Treatment usually consists of stabilizing the head of the femur into the acetabulum and holding it there for a period of time. This may be accomplished by using a "triple" diaper, providing bulk in the groin region to force the leg into abduction or with thick foam pads or splints. In extreme cases, a cast may be needed. (See Chapter 65.)

Polydactylism and Syndactylism. The presence of extra fingers and toes is called polydactylism. Often the extra digit will hang limp, boneless. In this case, a suture is tied tightly around the appendage, and the digit will fall off. Occasionally surgery is necessary. *Syndactylism* is the fusing together of two or more digits. Separation of the digits may be possible by surgery.

Nervous System Disorders

Hydrocephalus. Hydrocephalus is caused by an overabundance of cerebrospinal fluid in the ventricles of the brain and untreated, results in an enlarged head. The newborn also may exhibit bulging fontanels and nervous irritability. Hydrocephalus is treated by surgically inserting shunts that drain the ventricles. (See Chapter 65.)

Spina Bifida. Spina bifida is a congenital anomaly in which the vertebral spaces fail to close, allowing a herniation of the spinal contents into a sac. If the meninges covering the spinal cord herniate through the vertebral space, they are called a meningocele. If spinal cord nerve fibers and meninges herniate, it is referred to as a myelomeningocele. Surgery may correct the problem; the prognosis depends on the extent of the deformity. Folic acid (folate) taken during pregnancy has been proven to greatly reduce the incidence and severity of spina bifida.

Down Syndrome. Down (Down's) syndrome, also called trisomy 21, is often identified in the newborn nursery by typical physical features, although final diagnosis can be made only by chromosomal analysis. Physical and mental manifestations may range from mild to severe. One deep crease runs horizontally across the hands. Eyes are slanted, and the tongue is large and protruding. The infant is flaccid. There is usually accompanying mental retardation and heart defects; cataracts and gastrointestinal disorders may be present. (See Chapter 67.)

Anencephaly and Microcephaly. The child with **anencephaly** has an absence of part or all of the brain. The skull is flat, and the newborn will live for only a short time, if at all. A child with **microcephaly** has an abnormally small head. The child may or may not live, depending on the extent of deformity. Because the brain does not develop as normal, there is almost always some mental retardation.

Cardiovascular Disorders

Several congenital heart and blood vessel defects are seen in newborns. Some of these are illustrated in Chapter 65. Cardiovascular defects include the following:

- *Patent ductus arteriosus,* in which the ductus arteriosus fails to close at birth
- *Atrial and ventricular septal defects,* which are abnormal openings between the respective chambers of the heart
- *Tetralogy of Fallot,* in which four major heart defects occur simultaneously
- *Coarctation of the aorta,* which is a narrowing of the aorta as it leaves the heart

One of the characteristic features of many congenital heart disorders is cyanosis, which becomes more pronounced when the newborn cries. The birth attendant and nurse must assess carefully for heart murmurs. Other signs may be respiratory difficulty, easy tiring, and abnormal vital signs. The newborn will be treated symptomatically. Medications, such as cardiotonics, may be ordered; surgical repair may be necessary.

Respiratory Disorders

Choanal Atresia. Choanal atresia occurs when the nostrils are closed at the entrance to the throat so that air cannot pass through. Neonates are obligatory nose breathers; thus, the atresia must be surgically corrected quickly to open the nostrils.

Gastrointestinal Disorders

Cleft Lip and Palate. A *cleft lip,* which occurs in approximately 1 in 600 births, is a vertical opening in the upper lip, which may appear as a notch in the lip or may extend upward into the nose. When the palate is split, the condition is known as *cleft palate;* this condition occurs less frequently than cleft lip. Cleft lip or cleft palate can be one sided (unilateral) or two sided (bilateral). Clefts also are classified as complete or incomplete.

Cleft lip and palate cause difficulty with feeding if the newborn is not able to suck effectively. In addition, milk that goes into the mouth may be expelled through the nose. Special nipple and feeding devices assist in feedings. (See Chapter 65.)

Esophageal Atresia. In **esophageal atresia,** the upper end of the esophagus ends in a blind pouch, making it impossible for the newborn to obtain food. Surgery must be performed quickly. The baby sometimes is maintained on total parenteral nutrition until surgery.

Tracheoesophageal Fistula. When esophageal atresia is accompanied by a tracheal fistula, the situation is much more life-threatening. Because food or mucus is channeled from the esophagus directly into the lungs, this condition must be corrected immediately, or the child will aspirate and suffocate. Emergency surgery is performed immediately with no feedings given prior to surgery.

Pyloric Stenosis. Pyloric stenosis is a congenital anomaly in which there is an increase in the size of the musculature at the junction of the stomach and small intestine. This causes the pyloric opening to be constricted, preventing food from passing through. The newborn initially vomits a milky substance. Later the vomiting becomes projectile. The neonate is fussy and hungry, loses weight, and becomes dehydrated. Surgical correction is necessary.

Imperforate Anus. In an *imperforate anus,* the rectum ends in a blind pouch, causing an obstruction to the normal passage of feces that must be corrected immediately. Imperforate anus is suspected if the neonate does not pass a stool within 24 hours of delivery, or if the nurse has difficulty obtaining a rectal temperature.

Phenylketonuria. Phenylketonuria (PKU) is a genetic defect that renders the infant incapable of metabolizing certain amino acids, which are spilled into the blood and tissues in the form of *phenylalanine.* No cure exists for this disease, but it can be controlled with a special diet. Treatment is initiated as soon as possible after birth. Untreated, PKU results in mental impairment, behavior problems, or retardation and other abnormalities. All neonates are tested for PKU prior to discharge from the hospital and at the 6-week checkup (See Chapter 65).

Galactosemia. Galactosemia is a genetic disorder in which the newborn is incapable of metabolizing galactose; thus, galactose builds up in the body and causes vomiting, diarrhea, jaundice, and mental retardation. Early diagnosis and dietary management can help prevent mental retardation.

Genitourinary Disorders

Exstrophy of the Bladder. In bladder exstrophy, the abdominal wall fails to develop, and the interior of the bladder lies exposed. Infection is a common problem, and surgery is necessary.

Hypospadias and Epispadias. When the urethra opens on the bottom side of the penis, the newborn has **hypospadias.** This condition causes problems later in toilet training, because the child is unable to direct the urinary stream. Surgical repair involves the use of the foreskin, so circumcision should *not* be done on this newborn. Less common is **epispadias,** in which the meatus is located on the upper side of the penis.

Infections

Maternal Infections

Infections present in the woman during pregnancy or delivery can have an adverse effect on the fetus.

Sexually Transmitted Diseases
The nurse must be nonjudgmental when dealing with cases of sexually transmitted diseases. Chapter 63 discusses individual diseases.

Syphilis. In most states, the law requires that pregnant women be tested for syphilis. If the test is positive, prompt treatment with penicillin early in pregnancy will prevent harmful effects on the neonate. Untreated syphilis can lead to premature labor and delivery, congenital infection, anomalies, and stillbirth.

Signs of syphilis in the newborn are general skin eruptions of rose spots, blebs on the soles and palms, *snuffles* (a catarrhal discharge from the nasal mucous membrane), a hoarse cry, cracks and ulcerations around the anus and mouth, and a positive blood test. The affected newborn is isolated and treated with antibiotics.

Gonorrhea. If the organism causing gonorrhea gets into the eyes of the infant during delivery, it causes a bilateral conjunctivitis, which, if untreated, can lead to blindness (*ophthalmia neonatorum*). The prophylactic installation of silver nitrate or antibiotic ointment into the eyes soon after birth will prevent this condition. This is done in all states. Once the infant has contracted the disease, large doses of antibiotics are given. The infant is isolated to prevent spread to other infants.

Herpesvirus II. Herpesvirus II can complicate a pregnancy and can be dangerous to the newborn. If the virus becomes active prior to the 20th week of gestation, a spontaneous abortion or stillbirth may occur. Active virus later in pregnancy may cause premature labor or local infection of the eyes, skin, or mucous membranes.

If a woman is known to be infected with herpesvirus and is near term, a cesarean delivery is usually done, unless the amniotic fluid is considered contaminated. In this case, the infant probably is already infected. After delivery, the neonate is isolated to prevent transmission of the virus to others in the newborn nursery.

Acquired Immunodeficiency Syndrome. The human immunodeficiency virus (HIV) which causes acquired immunodeficiency syndrome (AIDS) can be transmitted through the placenta or during delivery. The fetus with congenital AIDS may be stillborn; the living neonate may have a guarded prognosis. However, although nearly all infants born to HIV-infected mothers test positive for the HIV *antibody*, recent research has revealed that only about 1 in 4 of these infants test positive for the HIV *antigen*. It is now believed that only the antigen-positive neonates will go on to develop full-blown AIDS and that the other ¾ will have a normal life span. Immediate and continued treatment with drugs may be recommended for antigen-positive infants. Chapter 78 discusses AIDS and its treatment.

> **Nursing Alert**
>
> Infections can be transmitted to nursing personnel. Therefore, universal precautions are followed in the care of all mothers and newborns.

Other Maternal Infections
Rubella (German Measles). The virus of rubella (German measles, 3-day measles) can be dangerous in pregnancy but has no permanent ill effects on the mother. However, it causes defects in the fetus, known as *congenital rubella syndrome*. Common defects in this newborn are cataract, deafness, congenital

heart defects, cardiac disease, and mental retardation. (German measles is referred to as *rubeola* in French and Spanish.)

Toxoplasmosis. The protozoan responsible for **toxoplasmosis** is found in animal (cat) feces and in rare or uncooked meat. Although the pregnant woman may be asymptomatic, possible neonatal effects include stillbirth, premature delivery, microcephaly, hydrocephaly, seizures, and mental retardation.

Thrush. Thrush is a yeast infection, in which milklike spots form in the newborn's mouth. It is transmitted to the newborn during delivery if the mother has a *monilial* infection. It also can be spread by infected hospital personnel or family members failing to use proper aseptic technique. The infected infant is isolated and treated with antifungal medications, or a gentian violet solution is applied to the affected mouth area. It is important to wipe the neonate's mouth with a gauze sponge after each feeding, because lactose (the sugar in milk) promotes the growth of *Candida albicans,* the causative organism.

Cytomegalovirus. Cytomegalovirus, which belongs to the herpesvirus group, can be transmitted by an asymptomatic woman to the fetus through the placenta or through contact during delivery. Possible effects on the neonate include SGA, microcephaly, hydrocephaly, and mental retardation.

Other Infections

Other infections may be transmitted in the nursery if aseptic measures are not used. One of the most common infections is *bronchopneumonia,* which is dangerous because the neonate is not strong enough to cough up secretions and may choke. Postural drainage along with the proper concentration of oxygen and humidity aids breathing. Antibiotics and suctioning may be required.

Impetigo contagiosa is a skin infection usually caused by *Staphylococcus* or a *Streptococcus.* With the development of antibiotic-resistant strains of staphylococcal organisms, the infection rate in staphylococcal infections has risen. It is dangerous to have an outbreak of "staph" in the newborn nursery, because it is so difficult to control. Therefore, isolation procedures must be followed.

The Chemically Dependent Neonate

All drugs, including alcohol and nicotine, can adversely affect a fetus. Crack-addicted babies are becoming a serious problem in the United States. The newborn of a chemically dependent mother also will most likely be dependent, because the drugs have reached the fetus by placental exchange. As a result, the dependent neonate will have withdrawal symptoms after birth. Chemically dependent neonates are more likely to be preterm, premature, or of low birth weight and are more likely to have intellectual impairment. Spontaneous abortions, abruptio placentae, and stillbirths also are more common in chemically dependent women.

Fetal Alcohol Syndrome

Maternal use of alcohol is a major factor in contributing to physical defects in the fetus. The result is a condition called fetal alcohol syndrome (FAS). Possible neonatal effects of FAS include growth deficiency, microcephaly, facial abnormalities, cardiac anomalies, and mental retardation. The degree of defect present seems to be related to the level of alcohol intake; however, it is not known precisely what level of intake will not affect the newborn. Research has shown that as little as 1 ounce a day can adversely affect the fetus.

Nursing Alert

Because a safe level of alcohol intake during pregnancy has not been established, pregnant women should be advised to avoid alcohol completely.

Cocaine Exposure and Neonatal Effects

Cocaine-dependent newborns often experience a significant withdrawal syndrome, which can last 2 to 3 weeks. Newborns experiencing withdrawal from cocaine or crack may demonstrate the following signs and symptoms:

◆ Irritability
◆ Marked jitteriness
◆ Rapid changes in mood
◆ Lethargy
◆ Hypersensitivity to noise and external stimuli
◆ Poor feeding
◆ Irregular sleep patterns
◆ Tachypnea
◆ Tachycardia
◆ Diarrhea
◆ Diminished interactive behavior

These neonates may have experienced small strokes (cerebrovascular accidents) in utero due to sudden changes in the woman's blood pressure. Also, prenatal exposure to cocaine has been implicated as a cause of sudden infant death syndrome in infancy.

Key Concept

The addicted newborn is *hypersensitive*. Most affected are the central nervous and gastrointestinal systems. Keys to handling an addicted neonate follow:

◆ Provide eye contact.
◆ Touch the neonate.
◆ Rock *up and down* (***not*** side-to-side—this makes the newborn more hyperactive).

Heroin and Neonatal Effects

Signs and symptoms of heroin withdrawal include the following:

◆ Jitteriness
◆ Hyperactivity
◆ Shrill, persistent cry
◆ Frequent sneezing or yawning
◆ Increased tendon reflexes
◆ Decreased Moro reflex
◆ Irregular sleep patterns

Treatment of the Chemically Dependent Neonate

Approximately 50% of neonates born to addicted mothers will experience withdrawal symptoms serious enough to require treatment.

Care of these neonates is based on the type and extent of withdrawal symptoms and focuses on ensuring adequate respiration, nutrition, and temperature. Environmental stimuli must be kept to a minimum; sedation may be necessary.

Key medications for the heroin-addicted newborn are listed in the accompanying box.

Maternal Marijuana Use and the Newborn

Marijuana is thought to be one of the most abused drugs in the United States today, with an estimated 20 million users. It crosses the placenta. Used during pregnancy, it may cause shortened gestation or a precipitate labor of less than 3 hours. There is evidence to suggest a higher incidence of meconium staining and aspiration. No increased incidence of congenital complications or effects on the growth and physical parameters is specific to marijuana use alone. When used with alcohol, decreased birth weight and increased risk for FAS are expected. Much more research is needed for long-term follow-up studies on these newborns.

Key Concept

Nursing assessments of the neonate are important in diagnosis and treatment. Careful initial assessments are vital to the newborn's future, because mother and neonate go home so soon after birth.

Key Medications
for the Heroin-Addicted Infant

◆ Phenobarbital (Luminal)
◆ Camphorated tincture of opium (paregoric)
◆ Diazepam (Valium)

These drugs may be used singly or in combination.

Keys for Review

Key Questions for Critical Thinking

1. Describe the care of the premature newborn in an isolette.
2. Differentiate between physiologic jaundice and the hemolytic jaundice that occurs in blood group incompatibility. Describe nursing care and management for both.
3. You have a 2-day-old SGA newborn in your care who has just developed diarrhea. Describe your actions. Explain why diarrhea is dangerous to this newborn and to other newborns in the neonatal intensive care unit.

Key Questions for Critical Thinking
(continued)

4. A newborn of a cocaine-addicted mother has just arrived in your neonatal intensive care unit. Describe what you expect to see in the newborn and how you will handle each of these problems.

Key Readings

Auvenshine M, Enriquez M. Comprehensive Maternity Nursing: Perinatal and Women's Health, Ed 2. Boston, Jones and Bartlett, 1990

Cloherty JP, Stark A. Manual of Neonatal Intensive Care, Ed 3. Boston, Little, Brown, 1991

Kenner C. Nurses' Clinical Guide to Neonatal Care. Springhouse, PA, Springhouse, 1992

Marks MG. Broadribb's Introductory Pediatric Nursing, Ed 4. Philadelphia, J.B. Lippincott, 1994

Perez-Woods R, Malloy MD. "Positioning and skin care of the low-birth-weight neonate." NAACOG's Clinical Issues in Perinatal Nursing and Women's Health Nursing 3(1): 97-113, 1992

Peters H, Theorell CJ. "Fetal and neonatal effects of maternal cocaine use." Journal of Obstetric, Gynecologic, and Neonatal Nursing 20: 121-126, 1991

Sherwen L, Scoloveno M, Weingerten C. Nursing Care of the Childbearing Family. Norwalk, CT, Appleton & Lange, 1991

Enrichment Keys

Alfonso D, Hurst I, et al. "Stressors reported by mothers of hospitalized premature infants." Neonatal Network 11(6): 63-70, 1992

Bass L. "What do parents need when their infant is a patient in the NICU?" Neonatal Network 10(4):25-33, 1991

Enrichment Keys (continued)

Blanche S, Mayaux MJ, Rouzious C, Teglas JP. Relation of the course of HIV infection in children to the severity of the disease in their mothers at delivery. N Eng J Med 330(5):308–312, 1994

Ladden MG, Damato E. "Parenting and supportive programs." NAACOG's Clinical Issues in Perinatal and Women's Health Nursing 3(1):174-187, 1992

LeBlanc M. "Thermoregulation: Incubators, radiant warmers, artificial skins, and body hoods." Clinics in Perinatology 18(3):403-421, 1991

May KA, Mahlmeister LR. Maternal and Neonatal Nursing: Family-Centered Care, Ed 3. Philadelphia, J.B. Lippincott, 1994

Roncoli M, Medoff-Cooper B. "Thermoregulation in low-birth-weight infants." NAACOG's Clinical Issues in Perinatal and Women's Health Nursing 3(1):25-33, 1992

Keys To Learning More

Chapter 63: fertility control

Unit Twelve: nursing care of children

Chapter 88: chemical dependency and the substance-abusing parent

Chapter 90: care of a patient who is dying, which applies when caring for a mother whose newborn dies

63 Sexuality, Fertility, and Sexually Transmitted Diseases

Learning Objectives

- Describe individual differences in sexual orientation.
- Discuss sexual dysfunction from occasional difficulties to consistent disruption of basic needs.
- Compare advantages and disadvantages of various types of contraceptives.
- Describe methods of determining a woman's fertile period.
- Describe common sexually transmitted diseases and their treatment.

Key Terms

asexual	orgasm
bisexual	pediculosis pubis
contraceptive	priapism
dyspareunia	sexuality
gay	sexually transmitted diseases
heterosexual	sterility
homosexual	tubal ligation
infertility	vaginismus
impotence	vasectomy
lesbian	

Keys to Understanding This Chapter

Chapter 4: legal and ethical aspects of nursing. Ethics are considered in working with people who have a sexual orientation or sexual practices different from yours.

Chapter 5: basic needs, including sexuality and sexual expression

Chapter 7: community health; laws must be followed in reporting cases of infectious diseases, including some sexually transmitted diseases and acquired immunodeficiency syndrome (AIDS).

Chapter 8: microbiology, a basis for studying infections of the genital tract

Keys to Understanding This Chapter
(continued)

Chapter 25: normal anatomy and physiology of the male and female reproductive systems

Unit Seven: nursing process used to assist in performing all nursing care

Chapter 54: sterile technique used in some aspects of caring for patients with sexually transmitted diseases

Unit Eleven: medications and their administration

Chapter 61: complications of pregnancy, including those caused by maternal infections

Chapter 62: disorders of the neonate, many of which result from maternal sexually transmitted diseases

Key Points

- Human sexuality involves the whole body, mind, and spirit and is core to the personality of the individual.
- Sexual assault is a crime of violence. Victims need support, encouragement, and treatment to aid them in dealing with the aftermath.
- Sexual dysfunction is a male's or female's inability to enjoy or engage in sexual activity for any reason.
- Infertility can be caused by male or female factors.
- Birth control is an important task for individuals at various stages of their fertile years. Counseling in this area must be bias free and geared to the needs and preferences of the individual.
- Sexually transmitted diseases have the potential of not only causing sterility, but also, as in AIDS, death.

Key Topics Outline

Human Sexuality
    Sexual Orientation
    Sexual Assault
    Sexual Dysfunction

Rosdahl CB: Textbook of Basic Nursing, 6th ed. © 1995 J.B. Lippincott Company

Key Learning Activities

◆ Visit a rape crisis intervention center, and listen to telephone calls and counseling. Ask counselors questions regarding sexual assault and what happens to victims and offenders.
◆ Visit a Planned Parenthood or similar clinic to discover what information is provided.
◆ Observe Norplant being inserted. Interview the patient to determine why she selected this method of contraception.

Sexuality, fertility, and potential for disease are some of the most basic needs and fears that rule the individual. They have affected humans since the beginning of time. This chapter briefly discusses these topics.

Human Sexuality

Sexuality is the way in which individuals physically, mentally, emotionally, and socially experience and express themselves as sexual beings. It involves much more than sexual contact. It begins at birth and is a vital part of an individual's makeup and personality. It includes anatomy, learned or adopted behaviors, attitudes, feelings, and relationships with all other humans. The nurse must be sensitive to these core human feelings and needs to deliver care in a nonjudgmental manner, in both verbal and nonverbal interactions.

Sexual Orientation

Individuals have an inherent or acquired tendency to be attracted emotionally and physically to people of one gender or the other or both. One's orientation may be heterosexual, homosexual, bisexual, or asexual.

Individuals who are attracted to the opposite sex are said to be **heterosexual**, while those attracted to the same sex are **homosexual**. Men who are sexually attracted to other men are generally referred to as **gay**. Women who are sexually attracted to women often prefer to be called **lesbians**. Individuals who are attracted to both sexes are **bisexual**. People who are not particularly attracted to either sex are considered **asexual**.

Partly because of the AIDS crisis in the United States (discussed in Chapter 78), people are speaking more candidly about homosexuality.

> **Key Concept**
>
> All people, no matter what their sexual orientation, should be taught methods of safer sex (ie, monogamous relationship, use of condoms) if they engage in sexual activity.

Sexual Assault

Rape is a violent crime. Heightened awareness of its implications has resulted in more sensitive treatment of the victim. The victim, whether female or male, should be encouraged to seek treatment immediately following a sexual assault. A person who has been raped should *not* shower, bathe, or douche before being examined. The nurse will need to assist the physician with the pelvic examination and provide emotional support to the rape victim. The police should be notified; usually a female officer will wish to interview the female victim. Although men also are victims of sexual assault, they tend to be less likely to come forward.

Careful and factual documentation is essential in making up the patient chart. Hospitals have protocols that must be followed (ie, handling of victim's clothes and other pieces of evidence). This ensures that the victims' rights are protected and that the appropriate information is available for legal purposes. This chart will often be used in court.

Crisis intervention centers, rape centers, and special telephone services are available to provide emergency advice and counseling. In some centers, group therapy sessions are held for the victims, which aim to help the person regain emotional health. Sexual abuse of children is discussed in Chapter 65.

Many times victims of rape want to put the experience behind them as quickly as possible and refuse to seek help or leave treatment early. Many of these people later experience flashbacks and other symptoms of post-traumatic stress disorder (PTSD). They should be encouraged to seek help at that time.

Sexual Dysfunction

Sexual dysfunction is caused by a variety of physical or psychological factors and can be perceived as frustrating or incapacitating to the individual. Sexual dysfunction is the inability to enjoy or engage in sexual activity. The person may be reluctant to seek help due to difficulty in speaking about such a personal problem with a stranger.

Male Sexual Dysfunction

The most common sexual dysfunction in males is **impotence**, the inability to achieve or sustain an erection. This condition also is referred to as *sexual arousal disorder* or *erectile dysfunction*. Medical causes include sexually transmitted diseases (STDs); chronic disorders; open-heart surgery; surgery for prostate disorders; hormonal disorders (such as diabetes mellitus); medications; chemicals, such as tobacco, alcohol, and cocaine; some types of neurologic damage; and certain degenerative disorders. Of greater importance, however, are psychological factors. An occasional episode of impotence is not uncommon and should not be cause for alarm. It is the *continued* inability to perform sexually that merits careful investigation. If no physical cause can be found, psychological counseling of both partners is often in order. Extreme tension, feelings of guilt or inadequacy, obesity, and exhaustion can be factors.

Treatment. In addition to counseling, several treatment options are available. Any medications the patient uses must be analyzed. According to clinical indications (if the patient can tolerate the absence of the drugs) and after consulting the patient's primary physician, drugs that affect sexual function should be reduced or discontinued.

Next, any basic *endocrine abnormality* should be treated. Occasionally, hormone levels can be normalized by intramuscular injection of a long-acting testosterone; in some cases, oral testosterone is used.

Drug-induced erection is another method of treatment. By chemically stimulating the nerves in the penis, an erection may be caused by oral medication (such as yohimbine). Another method involves the injection of a medication (papaverine) alone or in combination with other drugs (ie, phentolamine or prostaglandin E_1) directly into penile tissue. These drugs will dilate the blood vessels of the penis, allowing them to fill normally with blood, which results in an erection. A possible complication is **priapism**, continued erection accompanied by pain.

Finally, two *surgical options* are available. The first is the placement of a penile implant. There are many different implants: the semirigid rod, mechanical devices, the self-contained prosthesis, and the inflatable prosthesis. Each device has its own advantages and disadvantages. The semirigid rod is the easiest device to implant, yet is the least natural. The inflatable prosthesis mimics a natural erection best, yet it is the most expensive. The other surgical procedure is the penile revascularization. Only recently has this type of surgery not been considered experimental. Only approximately 5% of all impotent men are candidates for penile vascular surgery. Such surgery involves the reconstruction of arterial blood supply or the removal of veins that drain blood from the penis too rapidly.

Female Sexual Dysfunction

Sexual function in the female is a complicated and sometimes misunderstood process, which involves much more than **orgasm** (the culmination of sexual excitement). Up to 30% of normal females do not experience orgasm with intercourse. The sexual response cycle is divided into appetite, excitement, orgasm, and resolution. Inhibitions can occur at any or all of these phases.

Medical causes include **dyspareunia** (painful intercourse), **vaginismus** (involuntary contraction of vaginal outlet muscles, which prevents penetration by penis), hormonal imbalances, and chronic disorders (ie, diabetes). Women experiencing sexual dysfunction should be referred for medical and psychological counseling.

Infertility

Infertility affects approximately 15% of all couples and refers to the inability to conceive and produce live babies after adequate sexual exposure. **Sterility** is the absolute inability to procreate (eg, absence of live sperm or non-producing ovaries). Approximately 50% of infertility is due to combined male and female factors.

Male Infertility. Approximately 35% of infertility is due to male factors. Infertility in the man may be due to undescended testicles, orchitis after mumps, irradiation of the testes, untreated STD, obesity, internal adhesions, glandular disturbances, infection, impotence, or emotional tension. Although 1 mL of semen contains literally millions of sperm cells, the number of normal active spermatozoa may be comparatively small, and this decreases the chances of fertilization.

Key Abbreviations and Acronyms for Reproduction and Sexually Transmitted Disease

AI	Artificial insemination
AIDS	Acquired immunodeficiency syndrome
BBT	Basal body temperature
CMV	Cytomegalovirus
DES	Diethylstilbestrol
HIV	Human immunodeficiency virus
HPV	Humanpapillomavirus
HSV	Herpes simplex virus
IUD	Intrauterine device
IVF	In vitro fertilization
NGU	Nongonococcal urethritis
NGC	Nongonococcal cervicitis
PID	Pelvic inflammatory disease
PTSD	Post-traumatic stress disorder
RPR	Rapid plasma reagin
STD	Sexually transmitted disease
VDRL	Venereal disease research laboratory

Female Infertility. Approximately 35% of infertility is due to female factors. There are many reasons for female infertility. First, the ovum may not mature or be released properly. The sperm and the egg may fail to unite. The fertilized egg may not implant in the uterus. The causes of these situations may be hormonal, anatomic, or psychological. The woman may have a displaced uterus, obstructed ovarian tubes, cervical or vaginal infection (such as endometriosis), ovarian cysts, scar tissue from pelvic inflammatory disease (PID), or a fibroid tumor. Irradiation may have permanently damaged all of the ova. (All ova ever produced are present in the ovaries of the female at birth; any damage to the ova at any time will probably cause permanent inability to bear normal children.)

Diagnosing Causes

If desired conception has not taken place after 1 year of regular, unprotected intercourse, a physician should be consulted. Couples in their middle to late 30s may wish to consult a specialist earlier if there is any reason to suspect a problem. The physician will check the general health of both partners and order tests of the semen and of vaginal and cervical secretions.

A procedure to inflate the fallopian tubes with carbon dioxide (*Rubin's test*) may be done to determine patency (openness) of the tubes. An x-ray study may take place (*hysterosalpingogram*). Sometimes a light curettage (scraping) of the uterus is performed to determine whether the lining of the uterus is undergoing the normal changes necessary to receive a fertilized ovum. The charting of basal body temperature for 3 to 4 months will determine if and when the female is ovulating. Ovulation must occur for pregnancy to take place. The ova may be studied to determine if they are maturing properly.

Treatment

A woman can determine when she ovulates due to an abrupt fall and then a rise in body temperature. In a healthy woman, sexual intercourse at the time of ovulation often results in pregnancy. The woman takes her oral temperature before arising each day and records it on a chart. At the time of ovulation, temperature should be slightly elevated. Cervical mucus also changes in appearance and consistency when ovulation occurs. The woman correlates it with temperature increase as an indicator of ovulation. Chapter 25 describes and illustrates the menstrual cycle. Chapter 58 describes normal pregnancy.

Artificial insemination may be used to enhance the chance of conception. In this process, male sperm (the husband's or a donor's) is artificially implanted into the woman's cervix. Fertility drugs may be ordered, but these have a tendency to cause multiple pregnancies. (This is believed to be related to these potent drugs resulting in the release of more than one egg.)

Modern technology now offers a vast number of choices for couples experiencing infertility. Artificial insemination is used if the husband's sperm count is too low or if the woman's body interferes with sperm motility.

In vitro fertilization (IVF) is the fertilization of the woman's or donor's egg outside of the woman's body. The resulting fertilized ovum (zygote) is then inserted into the uterus. IVF is used if physical factors in the woman interfere with normal motility of the sperm, if the sperm count is low, or if the woman is not producing viable eggs (ova).

These procedures have raised many moral, ethical, and legal dilemmas. There have been many court battles regarding IVF, sperm banks, surrogate motherhood, and ownership of frozen sperm or frozen fertilized ova. The couple should receive competent counseling prior to undergoing any of these procedures.

Fertility Control

Many methods of birth control are available. Any method should be safe, effective, and inexpensive; have minimal side effects; and be easy to obtain and use. There is no ideal method for everyone; there are advantages and disadvantages to each. The individual using a particular method of **contraception** must be comfortable with it and committed to using it correctly

Ling Chan is a 20-year-old, Southeast Asian, newly married, new mother. Two days after delivering a healthy baby boy, she asks the nurse for information about contraception. "This first baby wasn't really planned . . . and I'm not sure we can handle more than one child for a while . . . at least not until we both get ourselves settled. I don't know much about the different methods of contraception, and I'm not sure which would be best for us."

Nursing Diagnosis: *Knowledge Deficit: Fertility control related to inexperience, as evidenced by questions*

Goal 1: Mrs. Chan correctly describes the action, effectiveness, preparation, administration, side effects, complications, and risk factors associated with the common contraceptive methods.

Goal 2: Mrs. Chan selects a contraceptive method that she believes will suit her needs and for which she is not at high risk of serious complications.

Nursing Actions (assess/do/teach)	Rationale	Evaluative Statement
1. Because the patient has requested this information and is highly motivated to learn, begin by assessing what she already knows and correct any misperceptions (eg, some women believe they cannot get pregnant while they are breast-feeding); ask the patient if she would like her partner to be present for the teaching session.	Teaching should be tailored to the individual needs of the person or couple.	3/8 Goal 1 met; patient correctly described the major methods of contraception. 3/8 Goal 2 partially met; both Ling and her husband wish to use the pill. Ling's history (smokes 1 pack per day and family history of diabetes and heart attack; mother died at age 45) places her at high risk for serious complications; Ling understands these risks and is able to verbalize danger signs.
2. Using charts and printed materials (or actual devices) instruct about the action, efficacy, preparation and administration, side effects, complications, and risks of the natural and artificial methods of contraception.	All the facts are provided that the person or couple need to make an informed choice.	
Once the patient states a preference for a particular method, carefully assess her level of risk for developing complications and explain these. Once she has selected a method, instruct her about the early danger signs of complications and what she should do if they occur.	The risk of serious complications should be minimized.	

to attain optimum effectiveness. This requires careful communication between nurse and patient to ensure that the best method for this individual has been recommended. The accompanying nursing care plan shows how the nursing process is used for sharing fertility information. Table 63-1 compares several methods of fertility control.

Methods of birth control are effective only if the individuals who use them do so correctly. To be sure the method chosen is the best for that individual, the following should be considered:

- Lifestyle
  - Age and sexual activity

Table 63-1. Methods of Fertility Control and their Relative Effectiveness*

Method	Pregnancy Rate	Drug Contained/ Brand Name	Action	Comments
No protection	85%–90%			
Subcutaneous implant	Less than 1%	Levonorgestrel (Norplant System)	Hormonal	Effective up to 5 y
Injections	Less than 1%	Medroxyprogesterone acetate (Depo-Provera)	Hormonal	Given every month
Oral contraceptives	1%–3%	Usually combined—estrogen (such as estradiol, estriol) and progesterone Brand names include the following: *Monophasic* (taken for 20–21 days): Demulen, Levlen, Ovral, Nordette, Ov-con-35, Brevicon, Loestrin, *Biphasic* (one color taken for 10 days, next color for 11 days): Nelova 10/11, Ortho-Novum 10/11 *Triphasic* (sequence specified by manufacturer): Tri-Levlen, Triphasil, Tri-Norinyl, Ortho-Novum 7/7/7	Hormonal Simulates pregnancy and depresses ovulation	One pill daily (21 days of medication, 7 days without) in various patterns
"Morning-after" pill	1%	Estrogen/progestin combined (Ovral)	Hormonal	Emergency only
Intrauterine devices	2%–5%	Progestasert ParaGuard, TU-380A	Prevents implantation in uterus	Can remain in place for 4 years
Chemical barriers	5%–25%	Spermacidal douches, suppositories, and so forth	Kill or immobilize sperm	Most effective if used with mechanical barrier Must remain in place for several hours after intercourse
Mechanical barriers	10%–15%	Male condoms used alone Condoms (male and female), cervical cap, diaphragm	Block sperm from fertilizing egg	Most effective when combined with chemical barrier Must remain in place in female for several hours after intercourse
	5%–25%	Collagen sponge with spermicide		
	5%–20%	Diaphragm with spermicide		
	2%–10%	Condom with spermicide		
Natural family planning (rhythm method)	11%–30%	None	Planned intercourse to coincide with woman's infertile time	Requires mutual cooperation Woman's cycle must be regular
Withdrawal (coitus interruptus)	25% when used with extreme care; usual pregnancy rate higher	None	Withdrawal before ejaculation	Requires mutual cooperation Pre-ejaculation fluid may contain sperm
Female sterilization	Less than 0.5%	Tubal ligation	Blocks path of egg (ovum)	
Male sterilization	Less than 0.15%	Vasectomy	Blocks path of sperm	

* Percentages in this table are estimated using a number of sources.

- ◆ Number of partners
- ◆ Need or desire for spontaneity
- ◆ Level of maturity
- ◆ Understanding of personal health
- ◆ Comfort with touching own body
- ◆ Religious and cultural beliefs
- ◆ Effectiveness
  - ◆ Reaction to unplanned pregnancy
  - ◆ Plans for future pregnancy
  - ◆ Ability to take or use contraceptives as prescribed
- ◆ Risk
  - ◆ Patient or partner's health history
  - ◆ History of STDs

Hormonal Methods

Norplant

Norplant is a relatively new contraceptive method that is gaining in popularity due to the length of protection (5 years) and the ease of use. The system involves implantation of six rubberlike capsules on the undersurface of the woman's upper arm during the first 7 days after onset of menses. The capsules contain a synthetic hormone called levonorgestrel, which helps prevent ovulation. Effective within 24 hours of insertion, Norplant can be inserted immediately after childbirth or abortion; 6 weeks after birth if the mother is breast-feeding. It is entirely reversible with fertility returning in approximately 3 months.

The following are possible side effects:

- ◆ Abnormal menstruation: excessive bleeding, spotting, irregular periods, missed periods
- ◆ Weight gain
- ◆ Headache
- ◆ Acne
- ◆ Decreased effectiveness if the woman weighs 70 kg (154 lb) or more, or if one of the implants falls out
- ◆ May aggravate preexisting depression
- ◆ May aggravate diabetes mellitus or hyperlipidemia
- ◆ Visual changes

The following are contraindications:

- ◆ Acute liver disease or jaundice
- ◆ Pregnancy
- ◆ Thromboembolic disease
- ◆ Severe visual impairment

Anyone using this method needs to be under a physician's care.

Medroxyprogesterone Acetate (Depo-Provera)

Medroxyprogesterone acetate (Depo-Provera) is a hormone that is administered by injection every 3 months. It is an extremely effective synthetic hormone similar to progesterone. Recently approved by the Food and Drug Administration, medroxyprogesterone works by preventing ovulation. Return of fertility can take anywhere from 3 to 18 months.

Possible side effects of medroxyprogesterone include the following:

- ◆ Irregular or absent menstrual bleeding
- ◆ Weight gain
- ◆ Headaches
- ◆ Nervousness
- ◆ Decreased libido
- ◆ Breast tenderness or excessive enlargement
- ◆ Pulmonary embolism
- ◆ May aggravate diabetes mellitus, kidney disease, seizure disorders, cardiac disorders, and mental illness

Contraindications include the following:

- ◆ Pregnancy
- ◆ Cancer of breast or reproductive organs
- ◆ Previous stroke
- ◆ History of liver disease
- ◆ History of blood clots in legs

Use of this method requires the care of a physician.

Birth Control Pills

Birth control pills, also referred to as oral contraceptives, are widely used in the United States and Canada. The woman takes one pill every day for 21 or 28 days, starting at the end of the menstrual period. The 21-day supply requires the individual to stop taking the pill for 7 days before resuming a new pack. The 28-day supply provides seven nonhormonal pills; thus, there is no interruption in the woman's pattern of taking a pill daily. The most popular pill contains a synthetic progesterone and an estrogen, which simulates pregnancy; hence, the woman does not ovulate and cannot become pregnant. The pills must be taken as prescribed to ensure effectiveness.

Possible side effects include the following:

- ◆ Weight gain
- ◆ Headache
- ◆ Nausea

Some side effects can be relieved with minor changes in the type of pill.

Prolonged exposure to estrogen can increase risks for some women, for example, changes in the blood vessels of the retina of diabetics. Vision could be impaired.

Contraindications include the following:

- ◆ High blood pressure
- ◆ Heart defects
- ◆ Blood disorders (drug promotes clotting)
- ◆ Women over age 40
- ◆ Heavy smokers
- ◆ Obesity

"Morning-After" Pill

The *morning-after* pill contains diethylstilbestrol (DES). It has been approved in the United States for *emergency use only* (such as rape or incest) and is taken no later than 24 hours after intercourse. DES prevents implantation of a fertilized egg by interfering with the production of progesterone. DES has been shown to cause cervical cancer in the daughters of some women who received it during pregnancy to prevent spontaneous abortion.

Intrauterine Devices

The intrauterine device (IUD) is inserted into the uterus by a physician. Two brands of IUDs are available in the United States; Progestasert and ParaGuard. Progestasert is a T-shaped device that releases a small amount of progesterone daily. ParaGuard also is a T-shaped device made of copper that can be left in place for up to 4 years. Their function is to prevent the fertilized ovum from implanting in the uterus. Factors in IUD insertion are listed in the accompanying box.

Risks of IUDs include the following:

◆ Increased risk of PID if woman has many partners
◆ Ectopic pregnancy

The physician may decide not to insert an IUD in any of the following situations:

◆ Recent STD or other pelvic infection. The IUD also may become a site for infection, which can cause scarring and later infertility.
◆ Possible pregnancy (insertion of the IUD may cause abortion). The IUD may be inserted during the menstrual period as a safeguard.
◆ Abnormally heavy menstrual flow, spotting between periods, or copious vaginal discharge
◆ Severe menstrual cramps
◆ Anemia, a bleeding disorder, or fainting spells
◆ Severely displaced or flexed uterus or another gynecologic problem
◆ Diabetes, circulatory problems, or atherosclerosis

The greatest danger is uterine or cervical perforation, although these situations occur rarely.

The IUD offers continuous protection without the woman participating actively. It is highly effective, and the non-medicated IUD avoids the problem of possible harmful hormonal effects.

> ### Nursing Alert
>
> If a woman becomes pregnant with an IUD in place, the device is usually removed by 7 weeks' gestation to avoid spontaneous abortion, ectopic pregnancy, septic abortion, or premature labor.

IUD Insertion and Use

If you are asked to assist with the insertion of an IUD or Progestasert device, keep these points in mind:

◆ The physician makes sure the patient is not pregnant.
◆ The patient should have a Pap test and tests for sexually transmitted diseases before having any device inserted.
◆ Sterile aseptic technique is used for insertion.
◆ The patient may feel a sharp pain when the IUD is inserted.
◆ The patient may have cramps for a few days, but these should not continue.
◆ Menstrual flow may be heavier or last longer than normal after the IUD has been inserted.
◆ The device may be expelled within the first few months. (If the woman does not expel it within 2 to 3 months, it will probably remain in place.)
◆ The woman should check monthly to make sure that the IUD is in place. (Slender threads attached to the device can be felt protruding from the cervix.) She should have a yearly Pap test and pelvic examination to assure there is no irritation from the IUD.
◆ The ParaGuard IUD is effective for 4 years.

Barrier Methods

Chemical Barriers

Spermicidal creams, vaginal foams, jellies, suppositories, and tablets offer contraceptive protection to the woman. The foams are most effective when used with a diaphragm.

Mechanical Barriers

A man can use a condom, a rubber sheath applied to an erect penis before sexual intercourse. Condoms also are used as protection against HIV and STDs. A female condom has been introduced recently. The latex condom is attached to a flexible ring, which is inserted like a diaphragm. The condom protrudes from the vagina, providing protection for the external genitalia as well.

Mechanical devices for the woman include the cervical cap and the diaphragm. They must be fitted by the physician and must be inserted each time prior to intercourse. Mechanical devices are more effective when used in combination with spermicidal foam, gel, or cream.

The collagen sponge absorbs the ejaculate in its collagen strands and keeps the sperm away from the cervix. It is about the size of a tampon. It is wet with tap water and inserted. Like the diaphragm, it should be left in place for *6 hours following intercourse.* Some research has connected the use of sponges with toxic shock syndrome.

A mechanical barrier must be used faithfully or it is not effective. Some people object to the use of such devices, saying they are not spontaneous.

Natural Family Planning

For many people and for various reasons, mechanical or chemical fertility control is not acceptable. For them, *natural family planning* may be a viable, although often less effective, way of preventing pregnancy. These methods offer no protection against sexually transmitted diseases.

Rhythm Method

The rhythm method involves limiting sexual intercourse to the time of the female menstrual cycle in which the woman is most likely infertile. This method is reliable only in women who ovulate regularly and know when they are fertile. This can be determined through disciplined monitoring of the basal body temperature each morning before rising. The temperature drops, then rises during ovulation. Usually this is accompanied by an increase in vaginal mucus. The woman is generally considered fertile during the 2 days before and 2 days after ovulation.

Withdrawal

Coitus interruptus is one of the oldest forms of fertility control. It involves a need for tremendous awareness and disciplined control on the part of the man and woman. The man must be aware of the approach of his climax and withdraw prior to it. This method is controversial and risky because most men release small amounts of pre-ejaculatory fluid, which could contain semen. Anyone using this method must be prepared for unplanned pregnancy. It is included in family planning counseling because many young people are embarrassed to seek other means and may use it as their first form of birth control. Although it is not ideal, it is preferable to nothing at all.

Induced Abortion

Abortion (the interruption of an established pregnancy) is discussed in Chapter 61. It is a controversial means of family planning and is not encouraged as a primary means of controlling pregnancy.

Sterilization

Because several permanent sterilization procedures are possible, the partners usually make the decision together concerning which method they will use.

Vasectomy

The man may have a **vasectomy**, in which the vas deferens is ligated and sometimes partially removed. This procedure is relatively easy and painless and may be done in the physician's office under local anesthesia. There are only two small scrotal incisions, and the postoperative course is usually uneventful. Recently, efforts have been made to reanastomose the ligated vas, that is, to reverse vasectomies with some success. However, the man who chooses to have a vasectomy should anticipate that he will remain sterile because the revision procedures often are not successful. The man should understand that he will *not* be impotent, just sterile.

Postoperative Care. The only postoperative complication of a vasectomy may be scrotal tenderness, swelling, or impotence for 1 to 2 days. Infection may occur but usually is mild. Sitz baths, ice packs, and analgesics are usually all that are needed to relieve postoperative discomforts. It is important for the man to have regular sperm counts following a vasectomy. In rare cases, the sperm find an alternate pathway, and the man is then no longer sterile.

The patient must be told that it may take up to 6 weeks after a vasectomy for the semen to be totally sperm free, because semen is stored in the body. A sperm count is usually done 6 weeks to 2 months postoperatively. If the sperm count is zero, the vasectomy was most likely successful. Patient teaching includes reminding the patient to use birth control measures until the sperm count remains at zero for 6 weeks. However, a sperm count should be done again after 6 months and then yearly to assess the continuing effectiveness of the surgery.

The emotional aspects are often of more concern than the physical ones. The man should feel confident in his decision to have a vasectomy. Talking with other men who have had a vasectomy may reassure him that he will not lose his sexual potency or drive.

Tubal Ligation

Tubal ligation is the most common and effective procedure for permanent sterilization in women. It is usually done in a same-day surgery center or immediately following a vaginal delivery. It is easier to perform following childbirth because the uterine/ovarian tubes are more accessible.

The easiest and most convenient way to do a tubal ligation is through an endoscope (laparoscopic tubal ligation). Performed under epidural, spinal, or general anesthesia, this minor operation is often referred to as the "Band-Aid tubal." Each uterine tube is usually ligated (tied off), cut, and a portion removed. Only one stitch is necessary in one or two incisions, and it is absorbable, so the woman does not need to return to the surgeon for stitch removal.

Postoperative Care. Mild postoperative discomfort may result from manipulation of the ovaries (cramping) or from the abdominal distention with carbon dioxide for better visualization (shoulder pain). The patient can expect to leave the hospital as soon as she has recovered from the anesthesia. Someone should be available to drive her home after surgery. There may be a slight vaginal discharge or spotting for a few days postoperatively.

Tubal ligation may be performed at the time of other abdominal surgery through an abdominal incision; all or part of the uterine tube may be removed. It also may be done vaginally. Normal menstrual periods and libido should resume after tubal ligation.

Sexually Transmitted Diseases

Sexually transmitted diseases (STDs) are contracted through sexual intercourse or other sexual contact with an infected person, and their signs are frequently seen in the urogenital tract. STDs are the fastest growing and most prevalent communicable disease in the United States today.

The increased incidence cannot be attributed to one cause. Sociologically, in the last 2 or 3 decades, there has been a great deal of freedom in sexual and lifestyle choices. The popularity of certain birth control methods also is a factor in the spread of STDs. For example, the use of IUDs and oral or implanted contraceptives do not protect couples from HIV or other STDs. A barrier method, such as a condom, *must* be used for safer sex, even if another fertility control measure is used.

Key Concept

There is no "totally safe sex." Use of a condom provides *safer sex.*

The most widespread STDs are *gonorrhea* and *chlamydia.* Genital herpesvirus and condyloma (genital warts) are becoming more common. Syphilis also is becoming more prevalent among some populations. The disease most in the news today is HIV, which causes AIDS and which is often spread sexually. HIV and AIDS are discussed in Chapter 78.

We became complacent in the past because penicillin was effective in killing the organisms that caused syphilis and gonorrhea. Tetracycline was effective against chlamydia. However, antibiotic-resistant organisms (especially gonococcus) have emerged, and penicillin-resistant gonorrhea is increasing, particularly among young people. In addition, no specific antibiotic or other treatment has been found at this writing that will prevent or cure the HIV infection, AIDS, or her-

pesvirus II. A person also may have more than one STD at the same time, which makes treatment more difficult.

Gonorrhea

Gonorrhea is due to infection by gonococcus (*Neisseria gonorrhoeae*) and is the most widespread venereal disease (probably because of its shorter incubation period). Certain strains are becoming penicillin resistant.

Gonorrhea attacks the genital tract in men and women and can spread to other parts of the body. It can be difficult to diagnose and treat because it is frequently associated with other STDs (ie, syphilis).

Signs and Symptoms. The symptoms of gonorrhea may appear anywhere from 3 days to 2 weeks after sexual contact with an infected person. Usually the first symptom is pain and a burning sensation when urinating, followed by a yellowish, purulent discharge. This infection also is the cause of reproductive tract symptoms in both sexes. Prostatitis or an infection of the seminal vesicles and sterility may develop. Without treatment, the disease progresses to the epididymis.

Approximately 50% of women are asymptomatic. Clinical findings in women include cervical tenderness, dyspareunia, purulent anal discharge, dysuria, and a yellow-green purulent vaginal discharge. Sterility may result when strictures form in the uterine tubes. Douching, sexual intercourse, and menstruation may spread the infection to the ovary and cause abscess.

In men and women, the oral and anal structures may be involved. If the organisms enter the bloodstream, arthritis, heart disease, liver damage, or central nervous system damage may occur. Before antibiotics were known, many patients with gonorrhea became arthritic. Antibiotics or silver nitrate is instilled into the eyes of newborns to prevent blindness that can be caused by maternal gonorrhea. Meningitis, peritonitis, PID (pelvic inflammatory disease), sterility, or a fatal endocarditis (inflammation of heart tissue) are other possible consequences.

Diagnostic Tests. A smear of the discharge is cultured and examined microscopically. Some physicians advocate obtaining throat cultures, because the organisms can be spread to other areas of the body.

Key Concept

A serologic test for syphilis (Venereal Disease Research Laboratory [VDRL] or rapid plasma reagin [RPR]) should be done at the same time as the gonococcus smear. The causative organism of syphilis can be transmitted as a "passenger" on the gonorrhea organism.

Medical Treatment. Treatment of choice for gonorrhea is one intramuscular injection of ceftriaxone sodium (Rocephin) plus a 7-day course of doxycycline. (If the woman is pregnant, erythromycin is substituted for the doxycycline.) All sexual partners also must be treated simultaneously to prevent reinfection. All cases of gonorrhea must be reported to public health authorities.

If treatment is delayed, the disease is spread to other parts of the body (ie, joints, tendons, meninges). While the infection is active, careful and frequent handwashing is a must. Universal Precautions are used. The *patient* also should be taught to wear gloves when coming into contact with his or her own body secretions. Precautions to avoid touching the eyes are especially important, because the eye is particularly susceptible to gonorrheal infection.

With an advanced infection, the patient needs bed rest and may require sitz baths and massive doses of intravenous antibiotics. The patient is not considered disease free until cultures have been negative for at least 7 days without antibiotics.

Nursing Alert

Having gonorrhea once does not confer immunity; the person is particularly subject to *reinfection*. It is important to trace and treat all contacts at the same time to avoid reinfection ("ping-pong infection"). Reinfection by an asymptomatic carrier is common.

Syphilis

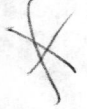

Syphilis is a destructive disease that can cause consequences throughout the body. It is known as "the great imitator" because its symptoms resemble those of many other diseases. There has been a marked increase in syphilis in recent years. The spirochete (*Treponema pallidum*) thrives in moisture and lives for a short time outside the human body. Contact with a syphilitic lesion by kissing or by sexual intercourse transmits the spirochetes to the mucous membranes. It also can enter through cuts or breaks in the skin. Pregnant women may abort or transmit syphilis to their unborn infants, causing deformities.

After entering the body, the spirochetes immediately multiply, gain access to the bloodstream, and in 10 days to 3 months, the first syphilitic lesion (primary lesion, or chancre) appears.

Key Concept

The incidence of syphilis is increasing, particularly in young people.

Diagnostic Tests. Syphilitic infection can be detected by certain blood tests, such as the fluorescent treponemal antibody absorption (FTA-ABS), treponema pallidum immobilization test, or a smear taken from a syphilitic lesion. The VDRL and RPR are common tests that are reliable, inexpensive, and easy to perform. The original blood test for syphilis (1906) was called the Wassermann and is sometimes used. Tests for syphilis and gonorrhea are always done as part of prenatal care. Some states also require premarital blood tests for these disorders.

The VDRL or RPR is not conclusive until at least 2 weeks after infection. However, the VDRL is able to identify three-fourths of the syphilis cases 6 weeks after infection, and virtually all cases of secondary syphilis. False-positives may occur in heroin addicts or in people who have recently had measles, infectious hepatitis, infectious mononucleosis, chickenpox, rheumatoid arthritis, or systemic lupus erythematosus.

Stages of Syphilis

Primary Stage. The primary lesion, the chancre, may appear on the penis, inside the vagina, on the nipple, or in a crack at the side of the mouth. This is *not* to be confused with herpes simplex, or the canker sore. The chancre is deep, painless, hard, and oval-shaped with serous drainage. It contains millions of spirochetes, but in 2 to 6 weeks, this lesion will disappear spontaneously, whether the patient has received treatment or not. Sometimes, enlarged lymph nodes also appear. Blood tests are usually positive during the primary stage. Large doses of penicillin, given intramuscularly, are usually curative.

Secondary Stage. Approximately 2 to 4 weeks after the initial infection, the secondary stage begins; it may last 2 to 6 weeks. A macular copper-colored rash appears on the soles of the feet and palms of the hands. Serologic tests (ie, VDRL, RPR, FTA-ABS) would also be positive at this stage. Wartlike spots may develop on the mucous membranes or around the anus. These spots are extremely infectious. Patches of the patient's hair may come out, and he or she may have a fever, headache, or sore throat. The person may have none of these symptoms and may feel normal and well. This stage also *ends spontaneously*. During the first and second stages of syphilis, the patient is highly infectious, even though there may be no symptoms. This is the main reason for the spread of the disease. The patient believes that he or she is cured, or the patient decides he or she did not really have syphilis. Secondary syphilis also may be cured by large doses of penicillin.

Latent Stage. This stage may last anywhere from several years to several decades. The only indication of the disease is a positive serologic test, although the test may also be negative in later stages.

The final stage of the disease involves major body organs (ie, heart, nervous system, liver, bones, and eyes). The person is now less contagious to others but may be critically ill. Eventually, the overt damage of the tertiary stage is seen. The patient may have a heart attack, valvular heart disease, severe brain damage (paresis), meningitis, severe bone or liver disease, or blindness.

Another manifestation of syphilis at this stage is tabes dorsalis (locomotor ataxia), in which the nervous system is involved. It is accompanied by a sharp, burning pain in the legs; they feel numb, and then cold or warm. The patient seems not to know where his or her legs are and cannot walk without watching them closely. The gait is jerky, and the patient cannot find his or her way in the dark. Joint function is lost. Intramuscular benzathine penicillin G is an effective treatment of syphilis at any stage.

Key Concept

Although treatment can destroy the syphilis organisms at any stage of the disease, drugs cannot reverse any damage already present. *Damage is irreversible.*

Herpes Genitalis and Herpesvirus II

Herpesvirus genitalis is a viral infection that is sexually transmitted. Referred to as genital herpes or HSV (herpes simplex virus), it is widespread in the United States, where it is the second most common STD, particularly among young people. Genital herpes may be found in conjunction with another STD and is most common in people who have multiple sexual partners, making it difficult to trace. It is more common in women than men.

The organism causing the condition is *Herpesvirus hominis,* type II. (*Herpesvirus hominis* type I causes common canker sores in the mouth and "cold blisters.") Herpesvirus type I is mainly associated with nongenital lesions but sometimes does involve the genital tract. *Herpesvirus type II* causes almost entirely genital lesions (blisters). There is a close association between genital herpes and cervical or prostate cancer. Any woman who has had herpesvirus II should have a Pap test at least every 6 months to rule out cervical cancer. Men who have had a herpes infection should have a rectal examination and a PSA test yearly for prostatic cancer. There also seems to be some association between genital herpes and diseases such as Hodgkin's disease and lymphosarcoma, so the patient also must have a complete physical examination on a regular basis.

Special Considerations Related to Herpesvirus II

Predisposing and Precipitating Factors to the Herpesvirus Infection

- Multiple sexual partners or excessive sexual activity
- Anxiety or fatigue
- Vaginal or labial irritation
- Sunburn
- Wearing tight clothes, especially synthetics or a wet bathing suit
- Fever
- Certain time of menstrual cycle
- Taking birth control pills
- Hormonal imbalance

Other Considerations

- Closely associated with cervical cancer
- Closely associated with prostatic cancer
- Closely associated with Hodgkin's disease and lymphosarcoma
- Great danger to the newborn if mother has herpesvirus
- Disease is very contagious at certain times.
- The virus can penetrate a condom.

Babies delivered vaginally may become infected; therefore, if the mother has active lesions, the baby is usually delivered by cesarean delivery. It is vitally important to the welfare of the baby that the mother reveal her infection.

There is no cure for genital herpes, but the condition requires effective management to prevent possible complications. The initial lesion will heal without treatment, although the condition usually is recurrent. Two-thirds of people who have an initial outbreak will have a recurrence. The infection is communicable only when the lesion is present and during the immediate *prodromal* period (just before the onset of symptoms).

Key Concept

The recurrence of herpes symptoms often coincides with the menstrual cycle in the woman or during times of stress.

Signs and Symptoms. The initial lesion resembles a fever blister or the common canker sore. In *women,* the lesions begin on the external genital labia approximately 6 days after exposure and can spread and become painful; they may be painless if they spread into the vagina. The lesion often looks like a pimple surrounded by a reddened area; it then progresses to a papule, a vesicle, and finally a crust. (This sequence lasts from 1–3 weeks.) Systemic symptoms, such as headache, general malaise, fever, and node tenderness, often exist at the same time as the occurrence of the initial lesion. Other symptoms of a primary infection in women include dysuria (painful voiding), vaginal discharge, perineal discomfort, and dyspareunia (painful sexual intercourse). The lesions may be extremely painful. However, approximately 10% of all people infected are not aware of it.

In the *male*, the major symptom is a painful lesion, usually on the penis, which may be mistaken for the chancre of syphilis. The uncircumcised man may carry the herpesvirus in the smegma, a secretion that collects under the foreskin.

Secondary infections usually are localized, causing a painful lesion. Precipitating factors include anxiety, fatigue, excessive sexual activity, excessive vaginal or labial irritation, sunburn, tight clothes (especially synthetics), and fever; recurrence also seems to be related to hormonal imbalance and to the menstrual cycle. Birth control pills increase the possibility of infection, because they alter the vaginal secretions so that the virus grows faster and is more easily transmitted.

Diagnostic Tests. Screening should be done at the same time as screening for syphilis and gonorrhea. Cultures should be done on any suspicious lesion. Diagnosis is possible only when the lesion is present. Only viral cultures can differentiate herpesvirus I from herpesvirus II. It is believed that the virus buries itself, perhaps in the central nervous system, between outbreaks and is not observable.

Key Concept

Diagnosis of herpes simplex virus type II is possible *only* when a lesion is present.

Medical Treatment. Because herpesvirus II is not curable, the patient needs emotional support. Treatment is mostly symptomatic and is directed at reducing discomfort and preventing secondary infection. Oral analgesics, such as aspirin, may be given to reduce systemic discomfort. Sitz baths may relieve discomfort but do not have any effect on the course of the disease. Cleanliness and dryness are essential to promote healing. Cotton underwear is useful. The woman may need to be catheterized, although extreme caution must be used to avoid spreading the infection into the bladder. Acyclovir (Zovirax) ointment has shown promise in treating herpes outbreaks. Topical ointments, such as dexpanthenol (Panthoderm), may help to relieve discomfort.

Sexual contact should be avoided by the patient, especially if lesions or any symptoms are present. If her-

pes is present in the vagina or on the cervix in the woman or on the penis in the man, a condom offers no protection, because viruses are small enough to penetrate the condom. If the patient has an oral lesion, he or she must be counseled to use only his or her own toothbrush. The person should not share food or engage in kissing. The patient must be taught meticulous handwashing to prevent spread of the lesions to another part of the body. Universal Precautions must always be followed.

Chlamydia

Chlamydia trachomatis infection is the most common STD in the United States. Approximately 50% of affected individuals are asymptomatic; thus, chlamydia is called the "silent STD." Chlamydia infections are twice as common as gonorrhea, but because the chlamydial infection does not have to be reported by law, the statistical findings are not certain. Chlamydial infections account for approximately half of the nongonococcal urethritis in men and the nongonococcal cervicitis in women. It causes at least two-thirds of the acute epididymitis in young men and can lead to sterility in men and women. Chlamydia is a common cause of PID—approximately one-half of all cases—and is linked to cervical dysplasia and abacterial cystitis (urethral syndrome) in women. In infants, it is linked to nongonococcal ophthalmia neonatorum and neonatal pneumonia (see the accompanying box).

The symptoms of chlamydial infections in men include painful urination and a watery discharge from the penis. Women may have vulvar itching and burning, grayish-white vaginal discharge, dysuria, and spotting between menstrual periods. Nonpregnant patients are generally treated with oral tetracycline or doxycycline for 7 days; pregnant women are prescribed erythro-

---

Chlamydial Infections

Chlamydial infections are believed to be related to many other conditions, including the following:

◆ Pelvic inflammatory disease—causes about half of cases
◆ Female infertility (due to scars in uterine tubes)
◆ Male infertility (due to epididymitis)
◆ Stillbirths
◆ Premature births
◆ Newborn infections (such as conjunctivitis)
◆ Infant pneumonia, as long as 6 weeks after birth
◆ Ectopic pregnancy
◆ Urethritis and cystitis in men and women
◆ Cervical dysplasia and cervicitis (possible precursors to cervical cancer)

mycin. A condom must be used, and both sexual partners must be treated simultaneously to avoid ping-pong reinfection.

Genital Warts

Technically called *condyloma acuminatum*, genital warts are caused by the human papillomavirus (HPV). The HPV is spread sexually, and the lesions may not appear for up to 6 months after exposure. The presence of a positive Pap test in a sexually active female is often the first sign that the HPV is present. A specific test, the Virapap, can indicate certain strains of HPV. Precancerous or cancerous changes also may be seen on the cervix.

The genital warts are pinkish, cauliflower-shaped growths appearing on and around the genital structures and the anus. When acetic acid (vinegar) is applied, the lesions turn white. Additional clinical signs include pruritus (itching), dyspareunia (painful intercourse), and chronic vaginal discharge. The greatest danger in an HPV infection is the *predisposition to cervical cancer.* (There are approximately 50 strains of the HPV; approximately 10 of these strains are directly related to the later incidence of cancer, particularly of the cervix.)

Predisposing factors for genital warts include the following:

♦ Sexual intercourse at a young age
♦ Frequent sexual intercourse
♦ Multiple sexual partners
♦ Cigarette smoking
♦ The presence of other STDs

Medical Treatment. Follow-up is necessary as soon as the Pap test is positive and particularly if the virus is discovered. Lesions must be actively treated as soon as possible to reduce the possibility of cancer. The most common treatment is weekly external application of podophyllin 10% to 25% in benzoin tincture (Pod-Ben-25). The drug is caustic, and the treatment is sometimes painful. This drug cannot be used if the wart or surrounding tissue is irritated or inflamed. It also cannot be used in a diabetic, if the person has poor circulation, or during pregnancy.

If topical medications are not effective, carbon dioxide, laser therapy, cryosurgery (application of extreme cold), or cautery treatments may be performed. In severe cases, more extensive surgery may be needed.

It is important to *treat both sexual partners simultaneously* to prevent retransmittal of the disease. Treatment assists in bringing the virus under control but does not necessarily cure the person.

Prevention. The best prevention of venereal warts is abstinence from sexual activity. Because this is not prac-

tical, the patient is advised to use a condom for intercourse; the application of spermicidal creams also seems to be helpful in controlling the spread of the virus.

Other Sexually Transmitted Diseases

There are other diseases that are usually spread by sexual contact. Unfortunately, many people do not know about them, so they do not seek medical advice when there are symptoms.

Chancroid. *Chancroid* is caused by *Haemophilus ducreyi.* The first symptom is a soft sore, different from the hard chancre of syphilis. Symptoms occur most often in men, but women may be carriers. Chancroid is almost always spread by sexual contact, especially in hot, humid climates. The lesions appear in the genital area 3 to 5 days after contact and develop into irregular ulcers, surrounded by edema and erythema. They bleed easily when touched. The infection often spreads to the inguinal lymph nodes. This disease is most common in tropical countries, as are *granuloma inguinale* and *lymphogranuloma venereum.* They are all treated with antibiotic therapy.

Cytomegalovirus. Cytomegalovirus (CMV), a member of the herpes family, is transmitted by any close contact (ie, intercourse, kissing, breast-feeding). Although individuals with CMV are typically asymptomatic, possible clinical findings include upper respiratory symptoms, fatigue, retinitis, and pneumonia. Treatment includes symptomatic relief (ie, bed rest, acetaminophen); there is no specific treatment or vaccine for CMV. Immunocompromised individuals (such as persons with AIDS or who are undergoing cancer chemotherapy) may be given immunotherapy and an antiviral agent to control symptoms.

Trichomoniasis. *Trichomoniasis* is caused by the *Trichomonas vaginalis* organism and is usually spread by sexual intercourse. "Trich" is sometimes called a "dirty" infection, because it produces foul-smelling discharge. It is treated with metronidazole (Flagyl) and is discussed further in Chapter 84.

Pubic Lice (Crabs)

Pubic lice or **pediculosis pubis** are tiny parasites that attach themselves to pubic hair follicles and cause intense itching. The condition of having lice (commonly called crabs) is known as pediculosis. It can be spread by sexual contact, infested bed linens, and clothing or close physical contact.

Diagnosis is based on viewing the lice or their eggs (*nits*) attached to the hair follicles. Treatment consists of applying a drug such as lindane (Kwell) or pyrethrins

(Barc, Pyrinyl, RID) to the affected area and thoroughly cleaning all clothing and personal articles. Because Kwell is contraindicated during pregnancy, alternate medications (ie, Eurax) must be ordered if the woman is or suspects she is pregnant. The lice die within 24 hours after being separated from the body, but the nits can live for approximately 2 weeks. A repeat treatment is needed at that time. Sexual partners must be simultaneously treated, and household members must be carefully monitored.

HIV Infection and Acquired Immunodeficiency Syndrome

This disease was first described in 1980 and exists throughout the world in slightly different forms. The people who have the highest incidence in the United States are male homosexuals, intravenous drug abusers and their sexual partners, Haitian immigrants to the United States, infants of affected mothers, and more recently, heterosexuals. The causative agent is present in the blood, and some cases have been recorded as a result of blood transfusions before routine testing of donor blood was done. Today testing is available for blood, which has made transfusions much safer. In keeping with body substance isolation, nurses wear gloves when coming in contact with any body fluids to protect themselves against the possibility that their patient might be human immunodeficiency virus (HIV)-positive, have AIDS, hepatitis, or any other communicable disease.

The causative organism, HIV, has been identified. Research continues into the possibility of a cure or vaccine. The disorder is mentioned in this chapter because the greatest avenue of spreading continues to be sexual contact. The Surgeon General has recommended the use of condoms for *safer sex*, although it is known that condom use does not absolutely prevent the spread of AIDS or HIV. Because HIV primarily affects the immune system, it is considered in detail in Chapter 78.

Keys for Review

Key Questions for Critical Thinking

1. Describe human sexuality and how is it expressed.
2. Discuss factors in sexual dysfunction and describe treatment used for each. Discuss psychological problems and interventions the nurse can use for these problems.
3. Describe factors that influence fertility and infertility. Discuss various kinds of counseling or teaching used for each.
4. Discuss ways in which the transmission of STDs can be prevented. Describe ways you personally can prevent transmission.

Key Readings

Andrist LC. AWHONN's Clinical Issues in Perinatal and Women's Health Nursing: Women's Issues in Women's Health Care Nursing. Vol 4, No 2. Philadelphia, J.B. Lippincott, 1993

"Choice of contraceptives." The Medical Letter on Drugs and Therapeutics, New Rochelle, NY, Medical Letter Inc. 34(885):111-114, December 11, 1992

"Depo-Provera contraceptive injection." Upjohn 3-17, November 1992

Duleba AJ, et al. "Prognostic factors in assessment and management of male infertility." Human Reproduction 7(10):1388-1393, 1992

Herbst AL, et al. Comprehensive Gynecology, Ed 2, St. Louis, Mosby-Yearbook, 1992

Key Readings (continued)

Kresch AJ, et al. A Guide to Managing Endometriosis. Krames Communications, 1991

Lethbridge DJ. "Coitus interruptus: considerations as a method of birth control." Journal of Obstetric, Gynecologic, and Neonatal Nursing 29(1), January/February, 1991

Martinez AR, et al. "The reliability, acceptability and applications of basal body temperature (BBT) records in the diagnosis and treatment of infertility." European Journal of Obstetrics and Gynecology and Reproductive Biology 47:121-127, 1992

Morley JE. "Mangement of impotence." PostGraduate Medicine 93(3), February 15, 1993

Reeder SJ, Martin LL, Koniak D. Maternity Nursing: Family, Newborn, and Women's Health Care, Ed 17. Philadelphia, J.B. Lippincott, 1992

Scheifele S. Tubal Sterilization: Making an Informed Choice. Krames Communications, 1990

Smeltzer SG and Bare BG. Brunner and Suddarth's Medical-Surgical Nursing, Ed 7. Philadelphia, J.B. Lippincott, 1992

Keys to Learning More

Chapter 78: autoimmune disorders, including HIV infection and full-blown AIDS

Chapter 83: male reproductive disorders

Chapter 84: female reproductive disorders

Unit *13* Assisting the Young Person Who Has a Dysfunction

64 Fundamentals of Pediatric Nursing

Keys for Learning

Learning Objectives

♦ Explain the importance of obtaining immunizations, and recognize at what ages these are administered.
♦ List safety guidelines for the hospitalized child.
♦ Recognize and explain the three phases of adjustment experienced by the hospitalized child.
♦ Identify appropriate sites and methods used to obtain vital signs in different age groups.
♦ Describe the procedure for obtaining a urine specimen from an infant or very young child.
♦ List the signs of respiratory distress. Describe oxygen administration to a child.
♦ Explain the role of play as related to the hospitalized child.
♦ List key points in pediatric medication administration.
♦ Discuss general preoperative and postoperative care of the pediatric patient.

Key Terms

immunization   pediatrics
pediatrician

Keys to Understanding This Chapter

Chapter 5: basic needs of all people, including children
Unit Three: normal growth and development knowledge helps in recognizing deviations
Unit Four: body structure and function for recognizing deviations
Unit Five: nutrition and diet therapy
Unit Six: pediatric safety and first aid
Unit Seven: nursing process used in the care of all patients
Unit Eight: communication skills necessary for the care of children and relating to parents
Unit Nine: basic nursing skills adapted slightly for children
Chapter 50: physical examination and nursing assessment

Keys to Understanding This Chapter
(continued)

Chapter 54: sterile technique
Unit Eleven: administration of medications
Chapter 62: neonatal disorders

Key Points

♦ Basic care in pediatrics is the same as for adults, but some procedures may need to be modified.
♦ Pediatrics requires knowledge of normal growth and development; these milestones help determine developmental delays.
♦ Children may need assistance to meet basic needs simply because of age.
♦ Teaching of parents or caregivers is vital; most pediatric care is done at home.
♦ Very young children are susceptible to many communicable diseases.
♦ Maintenance of pediatric safety is vital.
♦ Vital signs vary according to size and age.
♦ The respiratory tract of children is small and susceptible to infection.
♦ Play is children's work and their means of communication.
♦ Administration of medications to children involves precise calculation; it is usually based on body weight in kg.

Key Topics Outline

Health Maintenance
    Infant Care
    Toddler Care
    Preschooler Care
The Hospital Experience
Basic Pediatric Nursing Procedures
    Admitting the Child to the Hospital
    Assisting With the Physical Examination

Rosdahl CB: Textbook of Basic Nursing, 6th ed. © 1995 J.B. Lippincott Company

Key Learning Activities

◆ Create a therapeutic play project for use in the hospital setting. How could it be altered to apply to different age groups?
◆ Visit a day care center. Compare normal child growth and development with that of children who are ill.
◆ Plan a parent education topic. Use an illness or disease, normal growth and development, or safety issue. What information should be emphasized? How would you present the material?

Pediatrics is the area of care dealing with children. The area of nursing care is called pediatric nursing. The medical specialist in this field is called a **pediatrician.** The in-hospital care of children has greatly decreased, and many children are seen as outpatients or receive care from parents in the home. Prevention, prompt attention to illness, new drugs, and home care are factors in pediatrics and continued health for children.

The nurse will encounter ill and physically or mentally challenged children in settings other than the hospital. This may be in school, a physician's office, or a day surgery center. The fundamentals of pediatric nursing apply no matter where you encounter the child. The next chapter in this unit discusses infants, toddlers, and preschoolers. Well care of neonates is discussed in Chapter 60, and the school-age child, adolescent, and young adult are discussed in Chapter 66. Pediatric nursing procedures in this chapter can for the most part be used or adapted across the board. Many of the skills in Unit Nine are applicable or adaptable to pediatric nursing. Abbreviations in child care, and especially immunizations, are listed in the accompanying box.

> **Key Concept**
>
> Basic principles of safety and child care apply to both well and ill children.

Health Maintenance

Health maintenance or *health supervision* of the growing child involves such activities as regular physical examinations; completion of required immunizations;

Abbreviations Used in Pediatric Nursing

BRAT	Bananas, rice, applesauce, toast
DDST	Denver Developmental Screening Test
DT	Diphtheria and tetanus toxoids
DTP	Diphtheria and tetanus toxoids and pertussis vaccine
e-IPV	Enhanced-potency inactivated poliovirus vaccine
HBV	Hepatitis-B vaccine
Hib	*Haemophilus influenzae* type-B conjugate vaccine
MMR	Measles, mumps, and rubella viruses in a combined vaccine
OFC	Occipital-frontal circumference
OPV	(Live) oral poliovirus vaccine

health, safety, and nutrition education; and parental counseling. These are covered in routine trips to a primary caregiver. Even the well child is seen in the caregiver's office for neonatal checkups, 6-month checkups, and immunizations, as well as preschool and athletic physicals. The child also may come in with a presenting physical complaint.

Nursing in a well-child clinic or pediatrician's office offers a prime opportunity for parent teaching regarding normal growth and development and routine child care and safety. Some of the items discussed in parent teaching are listed in the accompanying box. The pediatric nurse must be well versed in the care of children of all groups to identify deviations from normal growth and development. Specific information is obtained during each visit according to the age of the infant or child.

This may include vital signs, height and weight, occipital-frontal circumference (OFC) of the head, abdominal girth, or limb measurements. The height and weight are often plotted on a growth chart that allows comparison with other American children of the same age. This helps in identifying a child who may have an abnormality related to physical growth.

The Denver Developmental Screening Test is a tool used to identify developmental delays in infants, toddlers, and preschoolers. If a delay is identified or suspected, a more detailed evaluation of the child may be performed.

Key Concept

Growth grids and charts using white, middle-class American children as a norm pose a problem for children from other cultures or whose parents are very small. For example, Southeast Asian people tend to be smaller than many other children born in the United States. This must be taken into consideration when discussing "norms" with parents.

Physical Examination

The primary caregiver will complete a physical examination. This is a point of reference in evaluating future illnesses. Many examiners use a head-to-toe checklist. The sequence of this type of examination is listed in a box in Chapter 50. Some assessments may follow the body systems (similar to the organization of this book). In this way, a pattern is established, and nothing is overlooked. When an abnormality exists, it is noted and described in detail on the child's chart.

Immunization

Immunization makes it possible to provide temporary or permanent protection against certain diseases. Early immunization is important to protect small children. Immunization should be given only to children who are not experiencing signs and symptoms of illnesses.

The laws in most states now require that children have five diphtheria, tetanus, pertussis immunizations and four oral polio vaccine immunizations before starting kindergarten. Records of immunizations must be presented to the school. Refer to Table 64-1 for the recommended immunization schedule for many of the diseases described in the text.

Key Concept

If a family cannot afford immunizations, they usually can receive them at no cost or a reduced fee at their local health department.

Keys to Family Teaching
Family Teaching for the Parent of a Young Child Includes the Following:

Infant
♦ Proper diet and feeding techniques
♦ Teething
♦ Feeding routine, colic, and spitting up
♦ Need to suck: pacifiers
♦ Positioning and sleep habits
♦ Diaper rash
♦ Bathing and bathing safety
♦ Urinary and bowel habits
♦ Crib safety
♦ Use of a car restraint or device
♦ Accident prevention: suffocation, drowning, poisoning, and falling
♦ Beginning dental care: wipe the infant's gums with a damp cloth to remove excess food

Toddler
♦ Dental care: dental visits
♦ Weaning from the bottle
♦ Diet and solid food
♦ Behavior patterns: separation anxiety, negativism, and temper tantrums
♦ Discipline and limit setting
♦ Poison prevention
♦ Toilet training

Preschooler
♦ Eating habits: dawdling over food, "picky" eaters
♦ Night waking, bedtime fears, and nightmares
♦ Development of a positive self-concept and body image
♦ Aggressive behavior and sibling rivalry
♦ Preparation for school
♦ Thumb sucking; dental care
♦ Care for common childhood diseases

Tuberculin testing varies from state to state. One test is recommended during the first 2 years of life or before admission to school. Some states require another test during the school years. Additional testing is indicated if tuberculosis exists within a given population. The means of performing and interpreting the tuberculin test is discussed in Chapters 50 and 57.

Infant Care

Infancy is considered to be the first year of life. Infant health supervision includes parent teaching, assessment of developmental milestones, growth assessment, and immunizations. Much of the examination will center around discussion with the parent and anticipatory

Table 64-1. Recommended Schedule for Active Immunization of Normal Infants and Children

Recommended Age	Vaccine(s)	Comments
At birth (before hospital discharge)	HBV*	(see footnote)
2 mo	DTP,† OPV,** Hib,ˣ HBV	Can be initiated earlier in areas of high endemicity
4 mo	DTP, OPV, Hib, HBV	2-mo interval desired for OPV to avoid interference
6 mo	DTP, (OPV), Hib	OPV optional for areas where polio might be imported (eg, some areas of southwest United States)
12–15 mo	Hib, HBV	
15 mo	MMR,‡ PPD˅	MMR and PPD recommended at same time
18 mo	DTP, OPV	Consider as part of primary series—DTP essential
4–6 y	DTP, OPV	Up to seventh birthday
12 y	MMR	
14–16 y	TD§	Repeat every 10 y for lifetime

* HBV—Hepatitis B virus vaccine. (Infants of HBV positive mothers and those in high-incidence areas should follow schedule above; others may begin series at 1–2 mo and may receive third injection as late as 18 mo.)

† DTP—Diphtheria and tetanus toxoids with pertussis vaccine.

** OPV—Oral, attenuated poliovirus vaccine, contains poliovirus types 1, 2, and 3 (e-IPV [enhanced potency-inactivated poliomyelitis vaccine] may be used in children who are HIV+ or who have frequent exposure.) Note: Many states require that the child have had 5 DTP before starting school; 4 oral polio vaccine also required before school.

‡ MMR—Live measles, mumps, and rubella viruses in a combined vaccine. Some states specify MMR at 1 year of age; however, 15 mo is more common. (MMR should *not* be given before 1 year of age.)

§ TD—Adult tetanus toxoid (full dose) and diphtheria toxoid (reduced dose) in combination.

ˣ Hib—*Haemophilus influenzae* type b conjugate vaccine.

˅ PPD—Purified protein derivative (test for previous exposure to tuberculosis)

Report of the Committee on Infectious Diseases, American Academy of Pediatrics, Ed 19. 1982; update by MN Department of Health, Immunology & Epidemiology section, March, 1993.

teaching. Important subjects to include in teaching about infancy were listed in the box at the beginning of this chapter.

General observations include the following:

◆ How the parent holds the infant
◆ If the infant "cuddles" to the parent
◆ General cleanliness
◆ The infant's response to painful procedures
◆ Appearance of health or illness; normal weight or excessive thinness

Specific observations include the following:

◆ Equal, active movement of all extremities
◆ General activity level
◆ Alertness of the infant
◆ Skin color, warmth, and texture
◆ Tone and pitch of the infant's cry
◆ General respiratory status

Toddler Care

Toddlerhood is considered from 1 to 3 years. As the child progresses through toddlerhood, independence and autonomy become important. Well-child assessments include the following:

◆ The age of weaning from the bottle to a cup

◆ The age at which toilet training was started and completed
◆ Language development
◆ Play patterns and activities
◆ Sleep patterns

Behavior patterns and related problems and discipline used at home should be discussed. Discussion regarding dental care is appropriate during the toddler visits, and parents should be encouraged to begin dental checkups as early as 12 months of age.

Assessment necessitates a strong focus on safety, because children at this age are very mobile but lack the judgment to protect themselves.

Also observe parent–toddler interaction. Subjects to include in teaching are listed in the box at the beginning of this chapter.

Preschooler Care

The child is a preschooler from 3 through 5 years. The physical examination for the 3- to 5-year-old focuses on the child's readiness for school. Height and weight are again plotted on the growth grid and compared with those of other American children. A systems checklist is used to evaluate the child's physical condition. Attention also focuses on sleep patterns, safety, and relationships with peers, siblings, and parents.

Evaluation of the child's speech, hearing, and vision is of prime importance in preschool years. Each must be within normal limits to ensure an individual's readiness to learn. It also is important to determine if the child's developmental age is commensurate with chronologic age. Because an adequate attention span is an essential prerequisite for learning, the child's ability to pay attention and focus on a task should be assessed. Gross and fine motor control should be evaluated. These problems are evaluated earlier, but they become a special focus in the preschool examination. Subjects to include in teaching are listed in the box at the beginning of this chapter.

The Hospital Experience

Many pediatric procedures are completed in the same-day surgery area of the hospital. Examples of these procedures include circumcision, insertion of polyethylene tubes, detailed dental work, hernia repairs, and cystoscopy. The child having major surgery will almost always be admitted to the hospital on the morning of surgery.

Most of the preparation for surgery will be done at home before admission. Because patients are discharged from same-day surgery to home, postoperative teaching must be emphasized, and parents must be thoroughly instructed in care of the child at home. Documentation of teaching and instruction given to parents is essential.

Hospitalization can be traumatic and disturbing. Often children do not understand what is happening or why they are being taken away from their home. Illness also threatens body image.

Even before children are 1 year old, they become frightened of strangers and are aware of their mother's absence. From this age through 5 years, the child often exhibits severe anxiety if separated from home and family. Even 6- and 7-year-olds continue to experience fear of separation when they are ill. As a rule, older children are able to understand the need for hospitalization. Nursing skills for calming infants, toddlers, and preschoolers are given in the accompanying box.

Very young children have concrete thought processes and often misinterpret what is being said. (Statements in parentheses give an example of what the child might be thinking.) The following statements give examples of what should be *avoided*:

◆ "I am going to take your blood pressure." (Where are you taking it?) Say something like, "I am going to find out how strong your heart is beating right now."
◆ "I am going to give you a shot." (Are you going to shoot me with a gun?) Say something like, "I am going to give you some medicine in an injection."

◆ "You are on a BRAT diet. (Am I a brat?) You might say, "You are on a special diet so you don't have cramps in your stomach."

Keep sentences short; phrase statements so the child knows *what to do*, not what to avoid. (For example, if you say, "*Don't* run into the street," the child may only hear "run into the street.") Tell children that nurses work at night too. Otherwise, they may worry that no one will be there and that they will be alone.

Family-Centered Care

Most hospitals make an effort to meet the security needs of the child as part of a family unit. Parents are encouraged to remain with their child during the hospital stay and should be encouraged to participate in their child's care. If they are not able to remain with the child, the parents should assure the child they will return and relate the time of their return so the child will be able to understand ("before lunch" "after Daddy gets off from work"). Parents and children are relieved of great anxiety in this way.

Parents react in various ways, depending on the seriousness of the child's illness and the immediate threat to the child's life, the life situation of the parents, the ego resources of the parents, the parents' former experiences with illness and hospitalization, the parents' individual style of coping with stress, and the parents' beliefs and values.

> **Key Concept**
>
> The pediatric nurse cares not just for the sick child, but for the entire family as well.

Preparation for Hospitalization

One goal of nursing care should be to assist the child to adjust to the reality of hospitalization as much as possible and to understand that strangers are trying to help. One way to help children overcome fear is to prepare them for the experience at their level of comprehension. They should be told what to expect, so they do not feel they are being punished or abandoned by being placed in the hospital. If possible, they should be given a hospital tour prior to admission (Fig. 64-1). It helps if they help pack for the trip to the hospital.

Stages of Adjustment

Before accepting the situation, most children, particularly those up to age 3 or 4 years, go through three phrases of adjustment before accepting hospitalization: protest, despair, and denial. Each phase extends into the next.

In the *protest* phase, the child's need for the mother is conscious and sorrowful. The child cries and rejects

Nursing Skill Guidelines
Calming Children for Assessments and Procedures

General Guidelines

- Explain procedures at the child's level of understanding.
- Explain procedure to the parent.
- Don't tell the child that it won't hurt, if it will.
- If at all possible, do not perform painful procedures in the child's bed. Use examination or treatment room. The child's bed should be a "safe place."
- If you promise that you will stay with the child throughout the procedure, keep your promise.
- Give an analgesic before the procedure is started if possible.
- Try not to restrain the child any more than is absolutely necessary.
- Don't tell the child not to cry. Crying is a normal response to pain. It is not necessary to further embarrass the child.
- After the procedure, explain any undesired effects that the child or parents should watch for, and tell him or her to call you if they develop.
- If possible, tell the parents and the child the result of the procedure or test.
- Stop in from time to time to make sure the patient's condition is stable and to reassure him or her that you care.
- Document unusual reactions. It would also be a good idea to note on the Kardex any measures that help to make a repeated procedure less disagreeable for a specific child.

Infants

- Change diaper before treatment
- Feed before treatment, unless this might cause nausea
- Offer a pacifier
- Interact with the infant before performing procedure
- Position the infant in the accustomed sleeping position if possible
- Release the thumb for sucking if possible

- Softly sing repetitious songs
- If singing doesn't work, try whistling (some babies will pause in crying long enough to go to sleep)
- Rub the back and arms in a constant rhythm
- Distract infant with a toy, book, or picture
- If the infant has a history of respiratory difficulties, place the child on the stomach and vigorously pat on the back. (Some children associate back pounding with ease of breathing.)
- Hold children in your arms

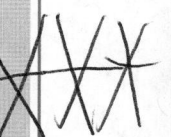

Toddlers

- Let the child play with equipment before doing procedure.
- Explain procedure in relation to toddler's senses, using simple words and short sentences.
- Encourage parents to participate by supporting and comforting the child when possible.
- Allow the child to hold a security object during procedure.
- Distract rather than restrain whenever possible.
- Praise the child for being "helpful."
- Allow child to cry without feeling like a baby.
- Allow child to hold equipment or help whenever possible.
- Allow child to play with equipment after procedure.

Preschoolers

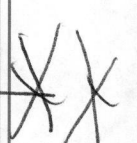

- Prepare preschooler for sensations to be experienced in simple words.
- Use dolls or puppets to explain procedures.
- Allow preschooler to play with the teaching aids.
- Assure the preschooler of privacy.
- Encourage preschooler to talk about the procedure; clarify any misunderstandings or questions.
- Encourage preschooler to help in a reasonable way with procedure.
- Verbally praise preschooler and reward in some way (eg, stickers, stars).

Adapted in part from Jackson DB, Saunders RB. Child Health Nursing: A Comprehensive Approach to the Care of Children and their Families. Philadelphia, J.B. Lippincott, 1993.

---

hospital staff because he or she is distressed and afraid; the child wants his or her parent or other caregiver.

In the *despair* stage, the child becomes inactive and sad. Usual comfort measures, such as thumb sucking and clutching a blanket, become prominent. He or she still watches constantly for the parent but is quiet and withdrawn.

The *denial* phase has been interpreted as a sign that the child is protecting himself or herself from anxiety by rejecting the parent. In truth, the need for him or her is more intense than ever.

The goal is to reach a stage of *acceptance* or adjustment.

The Child From Another Culture

The child and parents from a culture different from that of most of the patients or nurses in the hospital may be confused and frightened. It is especially frightening and difficult for a child who does not understand

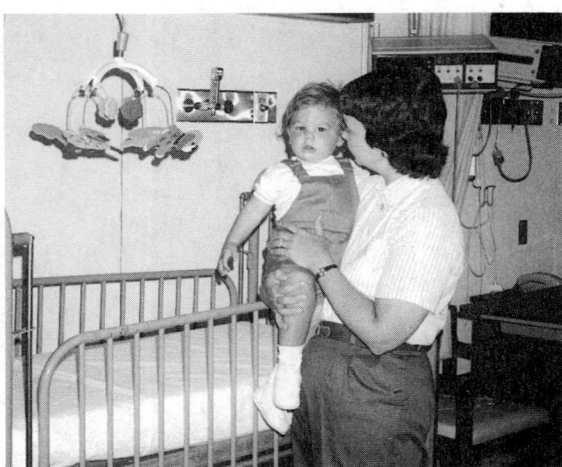

Figure 64-1. Before hospital admission, the parent accompanies the child on a tour of the hospital facilities. The cribs, lights, and equipment can be shown and explained to the child. (Jackson DB and Saunders RB. Child Health Nursing: A Comprehensive Approach to the Care of Children and Their Families. Philadelphia: J.B. Lippincott, 1993)

the language spoken in the hospital. It is helpful if parents are able to translate for their child and if they are allowed to be with the child as much as possible. Try to communicate with the child, and help him or her feel comfortable and relaxed. Pictures of common items can be made available so the child can communicate needs and feel less isolated.

> **Key Concept**
>
> A smile is a universal language.

Basic Pediatric Nursing Procedures

Admitting the Child to the Hospital

The admission of the child to the hospital is similar to admission of the adult, except that the nurse must be aware of the needs of *the parents and the child*. Try to make the patient as comfortable and secure as possible; you need to earn the child's confidence and elicit cooperation. Often if the child sees his or her parents accept and trust you, he or she will be more willing to accept you as a caregiver.

The parents are asked about special needs of the child, likes and dislikes, allergies, and special vocabulary, especially for items such as using the "potty." Include the child in this information gathering as much as possible by directing questions to him or her also. The child should be introduced to roommates. A play-

room can be a nonthreatening environment for the child, parents, and nursing staff to get to know each other.

Assisting With the Physical Examination

The equipment is the same as that for an adult, except in some cases it is smaller. Most important in this examination is the child's cooperation. If the child is too young or too ill to understand how to cooperate, you will have to restrain him or her for parts of the examination. (Restraint can frighten the child more than the examination, so do your best to get a child to cooperate without restraint.)

> **Key Concept**
>
> Much of the admission can be performed while the child sits on the parent's lap.

Making Up the Crib

The crib is prepared for the child's arrival. The mattress is usually covered with a waterproof material. The linens usually include a mattress pad, contour bottom sheet, sometimes a draw sheet, and a blanket. Where possible, use a fitted or contour sheet for the bottom of the crib so it stays in place. The crib can be made up with a bath blanket instead of a top sheet. A pillow is not used for the small child because of the danger of suffocation. Youth beds for older children are made up the same way as adult beds.

Assessing on Admission

The nurse observes the child very carefully for any sign of a rash, abrasion, discharge, or alteration in level of consciousness. Note complaints of pain or other symptoms in the same manner as for an adult patient. If you have reason to think the child has been battered or abused in any way, report it to your charge nurse—this is a legal responsibility.

Vital Signs

Vital signs are obtained and documented on admission. Table 64-2 lists normal ranges of vital signs for various ages.

Respiration. Respirations are taken before other vital signs, because an accurate respiratory rate cannot be obtained if the child is crying. If a respiratory rate cannot be obtained because of the child's crying, the nurse should observe for signs of respiratory distress, such as skin color or pallor and breath sounds. (Figure

Table 64-2. Average Vital Signs for Children

Age	Average Pulse (bpm)*	Average† Respiration	Systolic** Blood Pressure‡	Diastolic** Blood Pressure‡
Infant	100–160	30–60	74–100	50–70
Toddler	80–110	20–40	80–112	50–80
Preschooler	70–110	22–34	82–110	50–80
School-Age	65–110§	18–30	84–120	54–80
Adolescent	60–90	12–16	94–140	62–88

Temperature reanges are the same as for an adult.
* bpm = beats per minute.
§ girls = 5 bpm higher.
‡ Boys' blood pressure is slightly higher.
† Hazinski MF. Nursing Care of the Critically Ill Child, Ed 2. St. Louis, C.V. Mosby, 1992.
** Skale N. Manual of Pediatric Nursing Procedures. Philadelphia, J.B. Lippincott, 1992.

62-2 describes and illustrates signs of respiratory distress such as xiphoid retraction, nares dilation, and expiratory grunt.) Appropriate documentation should be made on the patient's chart.

Pulse. If the child is older than 2 years, the pulse may be taken radially; if younger than 2 years, the pulse is taken apically. The pulse is initially counted for 1 full minute. (If the child's vital signs have been stable and the child is not in respiratory distress, pulse may be counted for 30 seconds and multiplied by two.) The size of the bell or diaphragm of the stethoscope is smaller for an infant than for an adult.

Temperature. An oral temperature is taken on the older child. A rectal or tympanic temperature is taken if the child is younger than 6 years or is disoriented, unconscious, or in severe respiratory distress. In many hospitals rectal temperatures are preferred for infants older than 1 month.

Rectal temperatures should not be taken if the child has had rectal surgery. Tympanic temperatures should not be taken if the child has had ear surgery or has ventilating tubes or infection. The axillary method is used only if other methods are not possible. Regardless of the method used, the nurse should remain with the patient to ensure patient safety. The nurse should hold the temperature probe in place for the required time.

Blood Pressure. A smaller blood pressure cuff is used for a child; when choosing a cuff, measure the width of the cuff against the width of the arm. The cuff should cover approximately two-thirds of the upper arm. The *bladder* of the cuff should be long enough to encircle the arm without overlapping. Be sure to use the *same size* cuff each time. Cuff size will vary with age and size of patient.

The most important concept is the blood pressure or temperature *trend*. Determine whether it is going up or down.

Nursing Alert

If blood pressure is taken on the thigh in an infant (birth to 1 year), record the thigh pressure.

In children older than 1 year, thigh pressure is approximately 20 mm Hg *higher* than arm pressure.

If the radial artery (wrist) must be used, radial blood pressure is 10 mm Hg *lower* than that of the brachial artery.

Weight and Height. All children are weighed on admission. The small child is weighed on an infant or child scale. The infant or small child is weighed in grams. Often, this weight is converted to pounds for the mother's benefit (454 g = 1 lb). Weight in grams allows accurate dosage calculating for administration of medication, particularly intravenous (IV) fluid administration. To maintain medical asepsis, a paper must be placed on the scale before the child is weighed. The scale must be disinfected after the procedure. While the child is being weighed, the nurse keeps one hand just above the child to make sure he or she does not fall. After the child is weighed, the paper is discarded and the weight documented. To maintain medical asepsis, the nurse's hands should be washed before and after weighing. Body substance precautions should be used if the child has diarrhea, nausea, or observable open lesions. Any deviations in weight must be reported immediately. These procedures help to assess edema or dehydration. The infant is measured with a paper tape measure. One way to do this is to mark the length of the child head to toe on the bed and then measure between the marks rather than trying to measure a moving baby. Standing heights are recorded for the older child.

The following skills are used when weighing an infant. (Step-by-step procedure is in Chapter 60.)

◆ Weigh at the same time each day, preferably before feeding or as ordered by the primary caregiver.
◆ Balance the scale carefully before obtaining the weight.
◆ Weigh without clothes or diaper.
◆ Note additional equipment being weighed (eg, IV, arm board, brace cast).

Head Circumference

The OFC of the head is measured in children up to 2½ years of age and in any child with a questionable head size. This measurement is compared with a chart of normal sizes to determine any abnormality.

Nursing Skill
Measuring Occipital-Frontal Circumference

Supplies and Equipment

Disposable paper tape measure

Suggested Procedure and Rationale

1. Wash your hands.
2. Gather necessary equipment
3. Explain to the parent and child (if appropriate) what you are going to do and why.
4. Place the tape measure over the most prominent part of the occiput and around the forehead, just above the supraorbital ridges (eyebrows).
5. Make sure the infant's head is held in a stable position.
6. Tighten the tape so the reading is accurate.
7. Read the measurement over the forehead. Discard the tape and wash your hands.
8. Record and document the measurement.
9. Compare it with previous measurements. You also may compare it with a table of normal measurements for that age.
10. Notify your instructor of any significant deviations from normal or previously obtained measurements.

Key Concept

OFC reflects intracranial volume pressure. It can be a significant measurement. Factors that affect head circumference include brain development, intracranial pressure, hydrocephalus, brain tumor, and some congenital defects, such as microcephaly.

Chest Circumference

The chest circumference is measured and compared with the OFC. Normally the neonate's head is larger than the chest. The chest and head measurement are approximately equal at 1 to 2 years of age. The chest then begins to become larger than the head. By age 5, the chest is about 2 to 3 inches (5–7⅔ cm) larger than the head.

Other Measurements

Other measurements include abdominal circumference, extremity length, and extremity circumference. Be sure to note where on the extremity a circumference measurement was taken.

Nursing Alert

A disposable paper tape measure should be used when measuring infant length or OFC. *(Rationale: Cloth tape measure may stretch and alter measurement findings. Disposable tape measures also prevent cross-contamination.)*

Daily Assessment and Documentation

The pediatric nurse must be observant and note all information about the child, including normal behavior and reactions, abnormal symptoms, and unfavorable signs.

Because children often cannot tell the nurse how they feel, whether or not they have voided or had a bowel movement, or how much they have eaten, the nurse must be responsible for recording this information.

Diet. Observe how much the child eats and drinks throughout the day. Intake and output for a child does not just mean fluid intake and output; it also means food intake and all types of output. Accuracy is important, because it is easy for the small child to become dehydrated. The nurse also should note if an infant spits up formula or if the young child does not want to eat. Many hospitals have special pediatric menus to cater to the likes of the child. It is not unusual to see items such as pizza, soup, corn dogs, hamburgers, and ice cream on the special menu.

Nursing Alert

Illness and separation from family and home can alter the child's appetite greatly. Also, be aware of candy in the child's bedside stand. Eating candy can decrease appetite for regular meals.

Output. Assess number, color, and consistency of stools and any emesis, voiding, or other drainage. Diapers should be weighed to obtain an accurate assessment of urine output.

General Appearance. Note the child's activity level, skin color and warmth, comfort level, cry (lusty or weak), responsiveness to environment, and general respiratory status.

Parents' Comments. Note statements made by parents about the child's condition. Because the parent is more familiar with the child's normal activity and appearance, they may notice signs the nurse has missed.

Physical Signs. Be on the lookout for signs, such as seizures, changes in vital signs, cough, congestion, wheezing, nasal discharge, rash, or any other irregularity.

Visitors. Note whether the parents are at the bedside or if they visit frequently. If the parents do not visit, this could indicate a family problem. The nurse also should observe and report interaction between parents and child.

Discharging a Child

Children are discharged from the hospital in much the same way as adults, except they are taken home by their parents, who are responsible for follow-up care. Be sure the child has been properly discharged by the physician and has appointment slips, medication prescriptions, and physician's orders. The parents must be taught follow-up care, and this teaching *must be documented.* The child should be carried or taken to the car by wheelchair or wagon. The nurse or attendant must accompany the child and parents to the entrance of the hospital. Most states require children be placed in a car seat or restraining safety device when traveling in a car. Some hospitals make car seats available to parents who are unable to afford one by the time of discharge.

Meeting Basic Needs

Assisting With Safety

The nurse is legally responsible for the safety of the child while in his or her care. The accompanying nursing skill guidelines outline safety care.

Preventing the Spread of Disease

The hospitalized infant needs to be protected from contagious illness that may spread from other infants. The nurse and family of the child younger than 2 years are usually asked to wear gowns when handling a child with a contagious disease to prevent the spread of infection.

In many hospitals, nurses use disposable gowns. If reusable gowns are used, a nurse's gown is hung at the bedside of each child and is used whenever that child is handled. This gown should be changed at least once each shift and more often if needed. Because the inside of the gown is considered clean and the outside contaminated, the gown is hung right side out. The nurse scrubs before putting the gown on and scrubs thoroughly after removing it. Gloves are worn if the nurse will come into contact with any body fluids or substances, including stools, emesis, urine, or blood.

Using Pediatric Safety Devices

Special measures should be taken to prevent accidents or injuries from falls. Even if a small child sleeps in a regular bed at home, he or she is usually put in a crib in the hospital. This is done not only to control the child, but also to take into account the likelihood of regression. Sometimes it is necessary to enforce bedrest by applying a patient safety device called a restraint. Small children also should be restrained whenever in a high chair or wheelchair or whenever they are up unattended. The safety device, however, should not be substituted for good nursing observation (Fig. 64-2).

A physician's order is usually required for application of any restraint device. Restraints must be released and reapplied every 1 to 2 hours and the skin and circulation checked every hour. These safety measures must be documented. There are legal responsibilities related to restraints. Guidelines for restraints are given in the accompanying box.

Assisting With Nutrient Intake

At mealtime, the children may be out of bed in high chairs or seated at a small table. The parents are encouraged to help feed the child, because most children will eat better for the parents. All small children must be restrained when up, and all food and fluid consumed or eaten as intake must be recorded after meals. Children must *always* be supervised when eating.

Encouraging Fluids. It is often difficult to get children to take fluids, because they do not understand the reasons for drinking when not thirsty. Ask parents about the child's favorite liquids. Small amounts offered frequently are usually taken better. Ask parents to help. Aside from actual fluids, acceptable fluid substitutes are ice pops, ice cream, gelatin, soda, and fruit drinks.

Nursing Skill Guidelines
Providing Pediatric Safety in the Hospital

◆ Wash your hands before and after giving patient care. Follow Universal Precautions or Body Substance Precautions. (*Rationale: Pediatric nursing often involves contact with body fluids. Following these guidelines will help protect yourself, other staff, patients, and visitors from contamination or exposure to biohazardous substances.*)

◆ Make sure side rails on beds and cribs are up at all times. Beds should always be in the lowest position unless the nurse is performing specific procedures. (*Rationale: This prevents injuries from falls.*)

◆ Adequately support children when you are carrying or transferring them. Always support the head and neck, and watch the position of extremities carefully. (*Rationale: Correct positioning decreases the possibility of injury and gives the child a sense of security.*)

◆ Supervise ambulatory children.

◆ Be aware of policies specific to the unit for fire, severe weather, external alerts, and so forth. (*Rationale: Children will need more attention and assistance than adults in emergency situations.*)

◆ Keep children away from electrical equipment, cords, and outlets. Keep them away from heat sources (ie, radiators, lamps, heat vents). If using heat therapy, check temperature and closely monitor the skin. (*Rationale: A child's skin is more sensitive to heat and more easily burned than an adult's.*)

◆ Never leave a child younger than 10 years alone in any amount of water. Check frequently on older children. (*Rationale: This prevents accidental drowning. Drowning can occur in small amounts of water.*)

◆ Use safety restraints when transporting a child. Never leave a child unattended. Always use the provided safety devices when a child is in a high chair.

◆ Use disposable diapers unless the child is sensitive to them. (*Rationale: Pins are not required, and they are disposable and therefore safer.*)

◆ If safety pins must be used, keep them closed whenever they are removed. Do not leave pins lying out, because they are easily swallowed. Put your fingers between the child's skin and the pin when applying a pin. (*Rationale: This prevents choking or injuries to yourself, the child, other staff, or visitors.*)

◆ Check all toys for small removable or broken pieces. (*Rationale: Small pieces can be swallowed or aspirated.*)

◆ Supervise children when they are using pens, pencils, or scissors. (*Rationale: Sharp objects can cut the child.*)

◆ Use only toys that can be disinfected. Remind parents that if a toy cannot be disinfected, it may need to be thrown away.

◆ Disinfect toys on a regular basis (always between use by different children or if dirty or contaminated). (*Rationale: Disinfection will decrease the possibility of contamination from microorganisms.*)

◆ Do not allow latex balloons to be used; mylar is acceptable. (*Rationale: Latex balloons can pop, and the pieces can be aspirated; mylar balloons will not pop.*)

◆ Be alert for any broken equipment, furniture, or glass items. (*Rationale: This will prevent accidental injuries.*)

◆ When taking temperatures, assess the child's ability to cooperate. (*Rationale: If the child is uncooperative, the thermometer could break, or the reading could be inaccurate.*)

◆ Check the graphic sheet to see which route has been used for temperatures. Occasionally the physician will order a specific route.

◆ Always stay with a child while taking his or her temperature.

◆ Hold thermometers in place in most cases.

◆ Supervise children when they are out of their room. They should never be in the medication room, diet kitchen, or utility room. (*Rationale: This will decrease the risk of injury.*)

◆ Never prop a bottle to prevent choking and ear infections.

◆ Never leave a young child unattended when eating.

◆ Cut food into small bites.

◆ Avoid giving foods that are slippery and hard to chew.

◆ Teach parents good safety practices, and make sure they understand why you are using safety precautions. (*Rationale: They will be more receptive to safety practices if they understand reasons. Teaching helps decrease home accidents.*)

Gavage Feeding. Sometimes the child will be fed through a gastrostomy "button." These are usually used for children, because they are less bulky and less uncomfortable than an external tube. A syringe or tube feeding bag is attached to an adapter and primed with the tube feeding. The adapter is then attached to the button and the tube feeding administered. A bolus tube feeding is usually administered over 30 minutes, using only gravity. In some cases, a pump, such as the Kangaroo, is used.

Administering Parenteral Fluids. Because approximately 80% of a small child's weight is water, the child becomes dehydrated more easily than the adult. If he or she has diarrhea, a high fever, or difficulty excreting wastes, the fluid and electrolyte balance of the body may be upset, and fluids and electrolytes must be administered parenterally to maintain homeostasis.

Too much fluid is dangerous for a child, so an infusion pump is usually used to control the exact amount of fluid the child receives. This device delivers fluids at

- Explain to parent and child what you are doing and why. Be sure restraint is not seen as punishment. *(Rationale: Teaching helps decrease fears and prepares parents before seeing the child in a restraint.)*

Commonly Used Restraints

Bubble Tops—Made of clear plastic and attached to the top of the crib

- Be sure it is firmly attached to the crib. *(Rationale: This prevents it from falling and injuring the patient.)*
- Be sure it is the correct size for the crib. *(Rationale: This prevents the child from being able to climb out around it or getting his or her head stuck.)*
- Use for any child who may be able to climb or jump over the sides of the crib.

Jacket—A smaller version of that used for adults; can be used in cribs, highchairs, beds, or wheelchairs

- Apply jacket over clothing or patient gown. *(Rationale: You want to decrease skin irritation.)*
- If a child restraint jacket is used, the straps come out on each side after the jacket is applied. They usually cross in front and tie in back. *(Rationale: This prevents getting caught in straps and choking or strangling.)*
- Tie straps to back of chair or frame of bed or crib. Tie to movable part of bed. Do not tie straps to side rails. *(Rationale: It is important to be able to raise bed or lower side rails without tightening or loosening restraints. A restraint tied in the wrong place can interfere with use of equipment or strangle the child.)*
- Check circulation every 1 to 2 hours, and allow child to exercise. *(Rationale: These activities prevent skin breakdown, promote circulation, maintain muscle function, and decrease possibility of respiratory complications.)*
- Document and report any evidence of skin irritation.

Clove Hitch or Commercial Wrist Device—A Kerlix bandage or stockinette applied in a figure-eight knot or a manufactured device used to retain one or more extremities

- Apply padding under the restraint.
- Tie a knot so the device cannot become too tight.
- Check extremity every hour for circulation and signs of skin breakdown.
- Remove restraints every 2 hours, and allow child to exercise the extremity.

Armboards—Used to protect IV sites

- Pad with washcloth or small towel, and fasten with tape. *(Rationale: Washcloth will absorb perspiration and is more comfortable. Also, it can be changed and washed if soiled.)*
- Secure armboard to patient's extremity after the IV is placed and secured. *(Rationale: If the board must be removed, the IV site remains secured.)*
- Check circulation every hour.

- Loosen or reapply tape as needed.
- Document circulation checks.

Less Commonly Used Restraints

Mummy Restraint—Used to restrain the entire body with a small blanket. Only the head is exposed.

Crib Net—A net placed over the top of the crib and secured to the bed frame to keep child from climbing or jumping out of the crib.

Papoose Board—A plastic frame onto which the child can be strapped in almost any position. It is commonly used when infants are circumcised. It is uncomfortable and should be used only for brief procedures, such as starting an IV.

Glove—Prevents child from scratching or pulling on tubes.

Sleeve Restraint—Tongue blades are inserted into a sleeve with long pockets and ties. The child's arm is slid into the sleeve and the straps tied under the opposite arm. Used to keep a child from bending his or her arm and pulling on tubes or other devices or disrupting a facial suture line.

Documentation

Devices often are documented by a checklist. This list allows the nurse to state specific patient reactions and the number of times the safety devices were applied and removed.

Knots Used For Restraints

"Quick-Release" Knot

Wind the strap of the restraint twice around the wheelchair post or bed frame. Make a loop by folding the remainder of the strap in half. Slip the middle of this loop under the part wrapped around the wheelchair post, and tighten. You now have "half a bow." If the patient pulls on the strap from the patient end, the knot will tighten. However, when you pull on the free end, it will release easily. The free end must be out of reach of the child. This knot is safer than a traditional knot, because it can be released quickly in an emergency.

"Hold-Fast" Bow

To tie a bow that will not come untied spontaneously, wrap the second end all the way around before pulling through the loop to make the second half of the bow. The knot will come untied when you pull on the free end just like any other bow knot but will not easily come untied. This knot is handy for shoelaces and restraints that are tied to each other. This must be kept out of reach of the child.

> **Nursing Alert**
>
> - Make sure straps are not too long. *(Rationale: The child might become caught or might strangle.)*
> - Make sure restraints are not too tight. *(Rationale: The circulation may be impaired.)*

✓ every 30 minute and remove every 2 hours

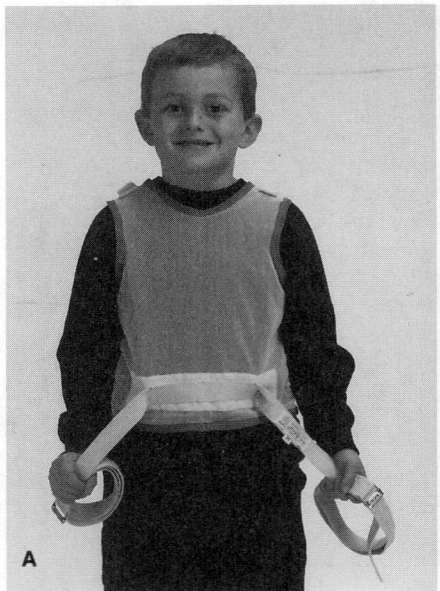 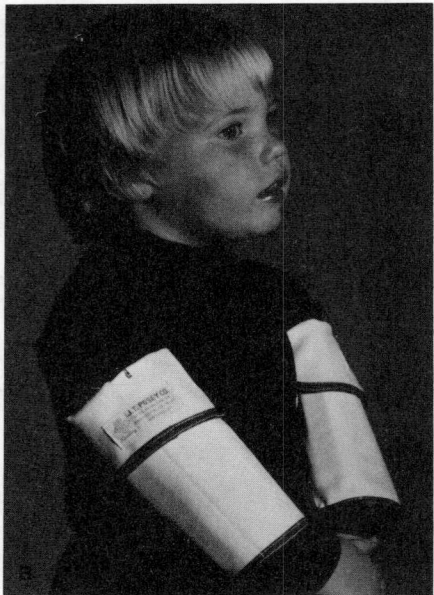 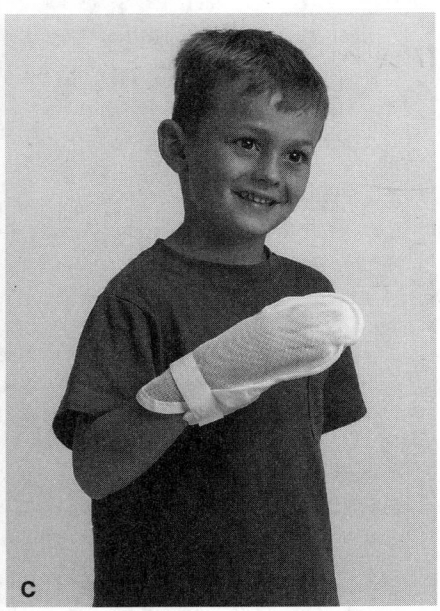

Figure 64-2. Examples of pediatric restraints. **A:** Jacket; **B:** Elbow or sleeve; **C:** Glove or mitt. Product photos provided by the Posey Company, Arcadia, CA.

a precise, preselected rate. An alarm is activated if the IV is not infusing properly, the rate is altered, or the bag is empty.

The child may need to be restrained to prevent pulling on the tube. The IV may be administered into the arm, neck veins in the older child, or scalp or neck veins in the infant or toddler.

Children with recurring long-term problems often have a Hickman or Broviac catheter for administration of fluids. This allows for prompt access for blood specimens, for the infusion of IVs, chemotherapy, or antibiotics, or for total parenteral nutrition therapy.

The child receiving long-term cancer chemotherapy or other IV medications may have a central line. These include Hickman, Broviac, jugular, and percutaneous intravenous central catheter (PICC) lines. The following nursing skills are used when assisting the child with a long-term IV catheter or central line:

◆ Monitor for signs and symptoms of infection at the site. This is the most common complication of this type of therapy. (Signs of infection include redness, pain, and elevated white blood count or temperature.) Observable signs and symptoms should be documented with notes made of laboratory findings that may indicate infection.

◆ Dressings should be changed every 24 hours if gauze dressing is used and every 72 hours if a transparent dressing (such as Tegaderm) is used. The dressing should be changed any time it becomes wet or loose. Use sterile technique to change dressings. (See Chapter 54.)

◆ Carefully monitor the IV catheter and tubing for any tears or leaks.

◆ Secure connections carefully. Children are more apt to pull on catheters and tubing. Use Luer-lok or click-lock connectors or tape connections securely.

◆ Use restraint devices as necessary to keep child from pulling on IVs.

◆ Monitor the site for signs of infiltration (hardness, white area, severe pain).

◆ Teach parents to care for the IV if the child will be discharged with it in place. Allow them to practice with equipment while the child is in the hospital.

◆ After the IV has been removed, monitor the site carefully for hemorrhage.

Assisting With Elimination

Bladder Elimination

Disposable diapers are used to promote cleanliness unless the child is allergic or has a bad diaper rash. In this case cloth diapers are used and are covered with disposable diapers.

Pediatric Urine Collection. Because the small child cannot void on command, the pediatric urine bag is used to collect a urine specimen. The bag is disposable and has an adhesive neck applied to the infant's skin. The nursing skill for pediatric urine collection follows.

Nursing Skill
Collecting Urine in a Urine Collector

Supplies and Equipment

Urine collector of appropriate size and type
Water for cleansing
Washcloth
Gloves

Procedure

1. Offer fluids half an hour before applying the collector bag.
2. Wash your hands.
3. Employ body substance precautions. Gather needed supplies.
4. Explain to parents what you are going to do and why. *(Rationale: Many procedures are unfamiliar and frightening to parents and child. Teaching helps decrease fears and increase cooperation.)*
5. Position the child on his or her back with legs apart and knees bent (frog-leg position). You may need the assistance of another adult to position the child properly so you can accurately apply the collector.
6. Gently cleanse and dry perineal area. You may use plain water and a wash cloth to cleanse the labia or penis. Remove any powder or lotion. *(Rationale: Clean, dry skin is necessary for the adhesive to stick.)*
7. Peel backing off adhesive surface and apply bag to perineum. With females, it is easiest to seal it from the bottom up to the pubis; do the opposite with males. Be sure the skin is smoothed during application, by gently pulling on the skin as needed.
8. With males, place the penis in the bag and apply the bag to the pubis and scrotum (Fig. 64-3). Be sure the foreskin is in its normal position in an uncircumcised male before applying the bag. *(Rationale: Keeping the skin smooth helps form a tighter seal and prevents leaking of the specimen.)*
9. Cover the bag with a loose-fitting diaper or underpants. *(Rationale: This discourages the child from pulling on the bag. Tight-fitting diapers or pants may dislodge the bag or cause the seal to burst after the child has voided.)*
10. Offer fluids after the bag is applied. *(Rationale: This encourages voiding.)*
11. Check the bag every 15 to 30 minutes to see if the child has voided.
12. After the child has voided, gently remove the bag as soon as possible. *(Rationale: This prevents loss of the specimen and makes the child more comfortable.)*
13. Cleanse the perineum.
14. Apply a clean diaper or underpants.
15. Place the urine in a specimen cup through the emptying port provided on the outside of the bag.
16. Discard waste appropriately. Discard gloves.
17. Wash your hands.
18. Send specimen to the lab following your facility's policy.
19. Document that the specimen was obtained. Note the amount and characteristics of the urine and how the child tolerated the procedure.

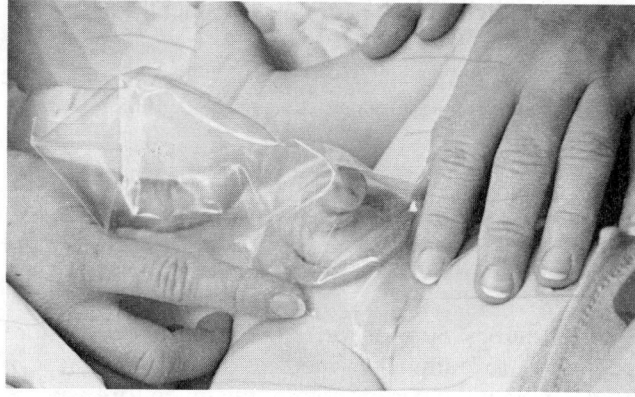

Figure 64-3. Disposable urine collection devices are available for infants and small children who have not yet achieved voluntary bladder control. Gloves are usually worn. (Jackson DB and Saunders RB. Child Health Nursing: A Comprehensive Approach to the Care of Children and Their Families. Philadelphia: J.B. Lippincott, 1993)

Catheterization. A child is not catherized unless absolutely necessary, because the procedure can cause distress, and delicate structures can be damaged. Catheterization also can introduce bacteria into the bladder, causing a urinary tract infection.

If catheterization is necessary, the small child usually has to be restrained during the procedure; the most common means of restraint is the papoose board. It is helpful to have another nurse assist with the procedure. The child can be restrained in this manner for the absolute minimum length of time only!

After insertion, the catheter must be securely taped to prevent the child from pulling it out. A small child may need to be restrained. Special perineal care must be given.

Bowel Elimination

Enemas are generally discouraged for infants. They are given to children in the same way as adults, although a smaller quantity of solution is used. For a tap water enema, a *maximum* of 300 mL is used for an infant; a maximum of 500 mL for a child from age 1 to 12. Disposable pediatric enemas are available in measured amounts and are much safer than the enema bag. The temperature of the solution must not exceed 105°F (40.6°C); 101°F (38.3°C) is more desirable. Disposable enemas are usually given at room temperature. For a small child, a rubber-tipped bulb syringe also may be used. Be careful not to use too much pressure when instilling the fluid.

Sometimes, the child will not be able to retain the solution. In this case, several folds of toilet tissue or a piece of soft foam rubber may be held around the tube to help the child hold the solution. The thickness of disposable diapers usually makes a bedpan unnecessary. You may need to restrain a small child or ask for assistance.

> **Nursing Alert**
>
> A tap water enema can be particularly dangerous to a small child, because it can cause electrolyte changes and/or a fluid shift.

Suppositories. Suppositories are often needed, more frequently to administer medication than to cause a bowel movement. Drugs commonly given this way are Tylenol and anticonvulsive or antinausea drugs. The nurse must explain the procedure to the child and urge the child not to expel the suppository. The nurse should insert the suppository and hold it in place by gently pressing on the anal sphincter from the outside until the child no longer feels the urge to expel it. The nurse should use a clean glove when inserting a suppository. The suppository should be lubricated with water soluble lubricant before insertion unless it has a slippery or greasy consistency.

Diarrhea. When young children have diarrhea, the main dangers are dehydration and spread of disease. Because the small child becomes dehydrated very quickly as a result of diarrhea, quick preventive measures must be taken. Nurses must carefully follow Universal Body Substance Precautions (see Chapter 51) when a child has diarrhea.

Assisting With Daily Cleanliness

Infant Bath. The infant is usually given a tub bath in a small bedside tub. Be sure to bring all equipment needed when the bath is started, because the child cannot be left alone after the bath is begun. The child is weighed before the bath and covered with a bath blanket or as hospital policy requires. The specific procedure for an infant bath is presented in Chapter 60.

The eyes are cleansed first with clear water from inner canthus to outer canthus; the rest of the face is then washed. (A separate cotton ball is used for each eye.) The outer ear canals are not probed. The hair is shampooed as necessary—daily if there are signs of cradle cap (a collection of oily secretions on the head).

Place the infant into the tub, or use the washcloth. Sometimes, a mild soap is used; other times, the bath is given with clear water. Perineal and genital care are given.

After the bath, the infant is dressed, and hair is combed. Fingernails and toenails are cleaned. Many hospitals do not allow nails to be trimmed without a specific physician's order. Oil or lotion may be applied

to irritated areas. Assess for signs of diaper rash or any other unusual signs, and report them to the charge nurse.

Oral Hygiene. The infant is given oral hygiene by wiping the gums with a damp wash cloth or gauze pad after each feeding. Pediatric dentists now encourage this type of oral hygiene for all infants.

By age 3, the child should be able to brush the teeth with adult supervision. By age 8, the child should be independent in brushing or flossing, with occasional checking by the nurse.* You may need to teach these procedures to the child.

The nurse must assist with brushing the teeth. All children should be encouraged to rinse often with water. If the child is mature enough to rinse the mouth and spit the solution out, a well-diluted mouthwash can be used.

Meeting Oxygen Needs

The primary cause of cardiopulmonary arrests in pediatrics is respiratory in origin. A newborn without cardiac anomaly has a heart that has been designed to last a lifetime. Small children have respiratory tracts that are anatomically different from adults. This, in addition to an immature immune system, places infants and young children at high risk for respiratory problems.

The pediatric nurse must be skilled at assessing respiratory status in infants and young children. The pediatric patient is not able to tell you he or she is having difficulty breathing. The child's status can change quickly, and early signs can be difficult to see.

> **Nursing Alert**
>
> Change in respiratory rate of an acutely ill child is significant. An infant with a rapid respiratory rate expends a great deal of energy. When the respiratory rate becomes too slow, it may be an indication that the infant is becoming too tired. This is an infant who is at high risk for respiratory arrest.

The nurse must be alert for restlessness, apprehension, and panic, because these may indicate respiratory problems. Darkening of skin color, particularly around the nose and mouth, called *circumoral cyanosis*, is a significant sign of poor oxygenation. An infant with an expiratory grunt requires immediate attention, because this is a late sign of respiratory distress (see Figure 62-2).

* Dental Health Advisor, Whittle Communications LP, 1993.

The following are signs of pediatric respiratory distress:

◆ Restlessness, apprehension, panic
◆ Tachycardia
◆ Tachypnea
◆ Nasal flaring
◆ Wheezing
◆ Stridor
◆ Change in color
◆ Expiratory grunt
◆ Retractions (substernal, subcostal, intercostal, suprasternal)
◆ Respiratory rate and character (gasping, shallow, labored)

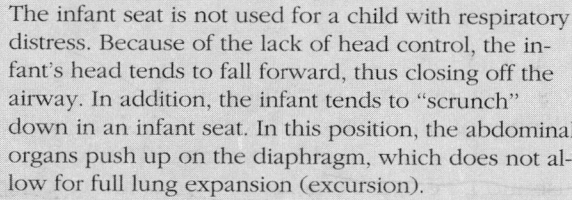

Nursing Alert

The infant seat is not used for a child with respiratory distress. Because of the lack of head control, the infant's head tends to fall forward, thus closing off the airway. In addition, the infant tends to "scrunch" down in an infant seat. In this position, the abdominal organs push up on the diaphragm, which does not allow for full lung expansion (excursion).

Administering Oxygen

Preterm or premature newborns are placed in an isolette. The newborn isolette provides oxygen and warmth. The unit has a built-in humidifier to provide moisture.

It is difficult to administer oxygen to the small child by nasal catheter or face mask because of the child's limited ability to understand and cooperate. If only humidity is needed, an oxygen mask may be used. It is placed *near* the child, as a "blow-by" set up.

Mist Tent. The child with a respiratory condition may be placed in a *mist tent*, which provides oxygen and humidity to liquefy secretions and aid breathing (Fig. 64-4). These devices may be used to administer humidity only, humidity and oxygen, or medications.

A bath blanket is placed on top of the bed linens to absorb moisture so the child will be kept warm and dry. The tent should be flushed with oxygen or air *before* the child is placed in it. The plastic tent is tucked securely around the crib mattress and is sealed with a folded bath blanket if the bottom edge does not reach the foot of the bed. The reservoir is filled with distilled water. The nurse is responsible for documenting the procedure and for documenting its effects and any signs of dyspnea, cyanosis, or other difficulties. Linens should be changed often.

Skills in caring for the child in a mist tent follow:

◆ Allow the child to explore a tent before being

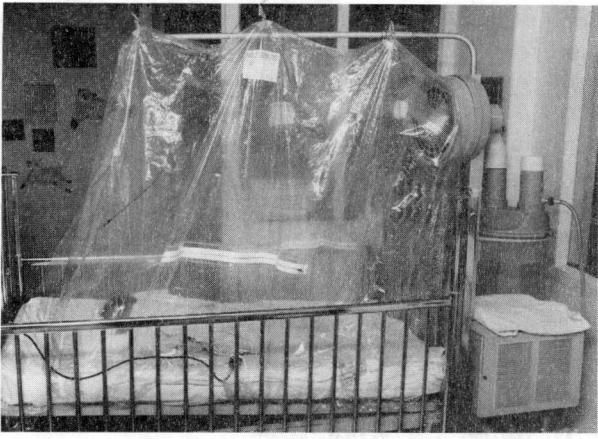

Figure 64-4. The mist tent supplies humidity and oxygen. (Jackson DB and Saunders RB. Child Health Nursing: A Comprehensive Approach to the Care of Children and Their Families. Philadelphia: J.B. Lippincott, 1993)

placed in it. Explain to the parents and child why and how the tent is used to reduce fear, thus reducing oxygen need.
◆ Wash your hands. Gather the necessary equipment
◆ Place the child in the tent after it is set up and turned on. Be sure to tuck it in securely.
◆ If the child will not stay in the tent, a jacket or other type of restraint may be needed. If a restraint is used, check the child's skin for signs of breakdown at least every 2 hours.
◆ Perform a thorough respiratory assessment every 1 to 2 hours or more often if necessary.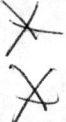
◆ Observe the child for shivering, lethargy, decreased temperature, or irritability. Change the child's pajamas and bed linens frequently as they become damp.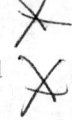
◆ Monitor the child for intake and output and signs or symptoms of dehydration.
◆ Provide diversional activities; use toys that are safe in an oxygenated environment and can be cleaned.
◆ Teach parents how to interact with the child, and encourage them to spend time with the child.
◆ Provide small feedings with frequent rest periods.
◆ Document respiratory assessment data and patient tolerance of the tent. Also document any teaching and the parent's response.

To provide a clean environment, mist tents are discarded after use. Tents are used for as short a time as possible, because they are difficult to keep germ free and are restrictive for the child.

Oxyhood. The oxyhood is a plastic box that fits over a small child's head. Oxygen can be administered in any concentration by means of a blender, which controls the amount of oxygen that mixes with room air and then enters the hood. The oxygen must be humidified to prevent damage to respiratory mucosa. *The flow rate must be high enough so carbon dioxide is flushed out of the hood.* The advantage of the oxyhood is that it maintains a constant concentration of oxygen, because the patient is in a high-flow atmosphere. Nursing skills in administering oxygen to an infant through the oxyhood follow.

Nursing Skill

Administering Oxygen Through an Oxyhood

Supplies and Equipment

Oxygen hood (or other device)
Regulator
Oxygen source

Suggested Procedure and Rationale

1. Wash your hands before and after giving care.
2. Collect needed equipment. Be sure you have the correct size hood.
3. Explain to the parents what you are going to do and why.
4. Set up equipment. Most facilities have wall outlets for oxygen.
5. Attach flow regulator to the oxygen.
6. Connect tubing to the port on the hood and to the flow regulator.
7. Turn the flow meter to the ordered rate to flush the hood.
8. Place the hood over the head and neck of the infant (Fig. 64-5).
9. Monitor the infant for respiratory distress and respiratory status frequently to ensure oxygen level is sufficient.
10. Notify your team leader or instructor of any significant changes or signs of respiratory distress.
11. Document the time oxygen was started, rate of flow, and assessments of the infant.

Intermittent Positive Pressure Breathing. Another method of administering oxygen in combination with medication is intermittent positive pressure breathing (IPPB). This device is used almost exclusively with cystic fibrosis and is described further in Chapter 80.

Nursing Alert

It is dangerous to administer oxygen to an infant in high concentrations over a long period of time. The greatest danger is that of *retrolental fibroplasia*, an eye disorder that can cause blindness.

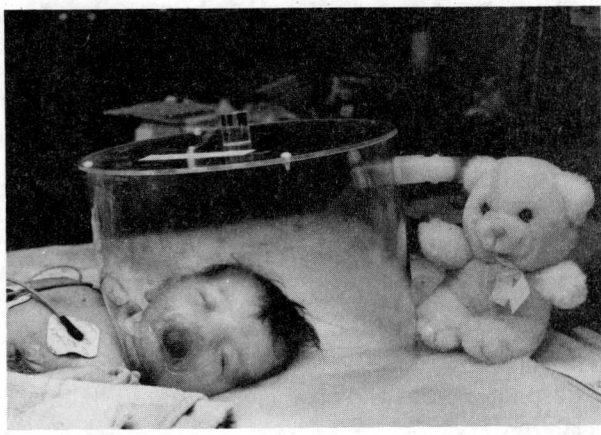

Figure 64-5. The oxyhood is placed over the head and neck of the infant. (Jackson DB and Saunders RB. Child Health Nursing: A Comprehensive Approach to the Care of Children and Their Families. Philadelphia: J.B. Lippincott, 1993)

Resuscitation

Resuscitation of the pediatric patient poses a special challenge for all healthcare personnel. The pediatric nurse also must be skilled in emergency medication administration. Pediatric emergency drugs are calculated according to a child's body weight. Pediatric units have a specialized emergency cart, known as a crash cart or code blue cart, which is stocked with medication and equipment of various sizes. Those caring for children in an emergency situation must be familiar with the sizes and use of this equipment.

Nurses caring for children should receive training each year in pediatric basic life support. Ventilation and chest compressions must be done with the utmost care to prevent further complications (see Chapter 32).

Meeting Diversional and Recreational Needs

Play is an important part of a child's growth and development. It is especially important to give children something to do while in the hospital. Children of all ages love to read or to be read to. They all need to be talked with and included in conversation. Children have a great need to have someone listen to them.

Play is therapeutic, because physical activity helps the child to strengthen muscles and improve coordination. Play is also important in the social development of a child and can be an emotional outlet for the hospitalized child who is under the stress of strange surroundings and painful procedures. Play also can help children to learn more about the world. The nurse can use play to teach children and to prepare them for certain clinical procedures. For example, the nurse and patient can play-act deep breathing or taking medications.

Many children regress to a previous stage of psychosocial development when they are frightened, ill, or injured. By observing children at play, the nurse can learn a great deal about their physical and mental status.

Many hospitals that specialize in pediatrics have a "child-life" department that addresses diversional and medical play therapy.

Advanced Pediatric Procedures

The nurse performs other procedures or assists the physician in procedures. The nurse also assists and comforts the child during painful procedures. A nursing skill guidelines box for calming children appears at the beginning of this chapter. These methods are helpful in calming the child undergoing a painful procedure.

Assisting With Diagnostic Procedures

Venipuncture. If a blood sample from a very young child is to be taken from the jugular vein, the nurse will assist the physician by holding the child. The child is restrained with the head extended over the edge of the table, and the table edge should be padded. The child must be held perfectly still. After the procedure, any signs of swelling or bleeding around the puncture site should be noted.

The preferred site for venipuncture is the femoral area. When this site is used, the nurse stands at the child's head and holds the child on the back with legs spread apart (frog-leg position). The child must be held securely while the physician does the procedure. The nurse can easily talk to the child when he or she is in this position.

Heel Stick Blood Samples. Blood may be obtained from an infant by heel stick. A disposable heel warmer may be applied first to increase blood supply to the area. A sterile lancet is used to obtain the sample after cleansing the area with an alcohol sponge. This procedure is detailed in Chapter 60.

Lumbar Puncture. When lumbar puncture is done, the infant or child is held with the back curved while the legs are restrained with a sheet (Fig. 64-6). The general lumbar puncture procedure is described in Chapter 71.

Therapeutic Procedures

Managing Fever

Fever in a child does not always indicate serious illness; teething or recent immunization can be the cause. Because fever is one way the body fights pathogens, it may be better to let a low-grade fever run its course than to give antipyretic medications.

If the oral temperature is below 102°F (38.8°C), use the following guidelines:

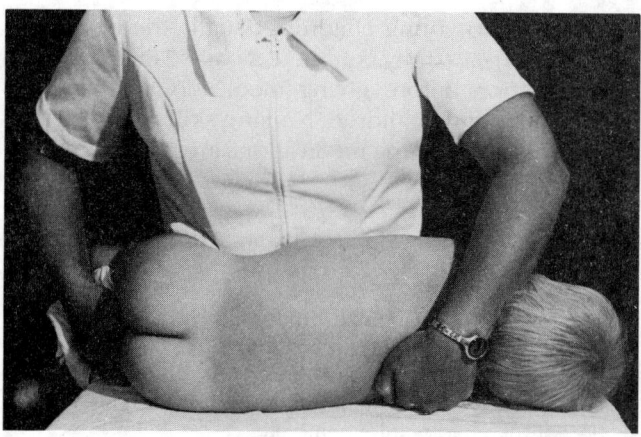

Figure 64-6. Position for lumbar puncture. While the child lies on the side with the back curved, the nurse holds the child's head and shoulders with one hand and arm and holds the legs (wrapped together with a sheet) with the other hand and arm. This position allows the nurse to talk to the child, give comfort, and answer questions. The nurse also can see what the physician is doing.

◆ Keep the child quiet.
◆ Do not overdress the child; use minimum clothes for comfort.
◆ Encourage fluids.
◆ Generally do not use antipyretics.

If the temperature is between 102°F and 104°F (38.8°C–40°C), use the preceding measures and the following:

◆ Call the physician; antipyretics may not be ordered.
◆ Put the child to bed.

If the oral temperature is over 104°F (40°C), use all the preceding measures and the following:

◆ Give nonaspirin fever-reducing medication. *Do not give aspirin* because of the danger of Reye's syndrome.
◆ Sponge with lukewarm water until further instructions are received from the physician.

Giving a Therapeutic Sponge Bath to a Child. Children who do not respond to routine fever treatment may respond to a tepid sponge bath. *Alcohol and ice are not used. (Rationale: They lead to hypothermia, and alcohol fumes are irritating.)*

Generally, the temperature of the water should be 85°F and 95°F (29.4°C–35°C). This procedure is used infrequently, because a cooling blanket is more efficient. Follow the procedure for giving an adult a tepid sponge bath in Chapter 49, keeping in mind the previous points.

Administering Medications. Nursing students or new graduates may or may not be allowed to administer medications to young children. Usually the new graduate must successfully complete a course in medication administration before giving medications to any patients, particularly children. Nursing skill guidelines for administering pediatric medications are given in the accompanying box.

Nursing Alert

The nurse must recognize children's medication dosages, whether or not that particular nurse is giving medications. The nurse also must know the side effects of each drug being administered so that observation of the child will be complete.

The Child Having Surgery

Although many preoperative and postoperative procedures are the same for adults and children, there are certain differences.

♦ The child often cannot verbalize discomfort or symptoms he or she may be experiencing. Therefore, it is your responsibility to watch for any untoward signs.

♦ A child cannot be assessed in the same manner as an adult, because the lungs are smaller, respiration is more rapid, the heart is smaller and beats faster, and the urine volume and amount of blood in the body are less. Therefore, a small deviation from normal is more important than in an adult.

♦ The child will need less analgesia after surgery to control pain because of smaller body size and faster absorption time.

♦ Rapid rate of metabolism and growth increases the healing ability of tissues.

♦ Substances are excreted from the body faster in a child; drugs may wear off sooner.

♦ The child can become dehydrated very quickly.

♦ Electrolytes are not as stable in a child.

♦ The high metabolic rate in infants and small children dictates a high caloric intake.

♦ The child lacks the physical resources available to adults. Thus, the child's general condition can change rapidly.

Consider the child's parents and their emotional needs. If parents are included in the child's preoperative and postoperative care, everyone will be more comfortable and cooperative. Teaching is vital (see p. 624).

The nurse in the operating room must remember that children will be more cooperative if they hear familiar voices and see familiar faces. Thus, a visit from the nurse or anesthesiologist before the operation helps to relieve anxiety. The child's waiting period should be as short as possible after arriving in the operating room.

Preoperative Care

Many hospitals have a "preop party" for children who are to have surgery. The children have an opportunity to tour the hospital and to meet the nurses before surgery. If the child is to go directly to the operating room on the morning of surgery, it is important to try to alleviate fear of the unknown.

The same principles prevail for care of children who undergo surgery as for adult patients. General preoperative and postoperative care (see Chapter 53) should be reviewed. Following are some additional guidelines.

♦ Because most preoperative preparation will be done at home by the parents, they need careful instructions. The parents should be involved as much as possible in preparation for surgery. They may come to the hospital with the child and stay during the history of the physical examination. Often the parents accompany the child to the door of the operating room.

♦ The medical history and physical examination are obtained by the physician; the practical nurse or nursing student may do a part of the nursing history. Be sure to include the parents when obtaining the nursing history.

♦ General laboratory work is done. Blood type and crossmatch are done if necessary. Dehydration, shock, and electrolyte imbalance are often dangerous and more likely to occur in a child. Blood is not given unless it is absolutely necessary.

♦ The operative permit is signed by the parents or guardian because the child is not of legal age. (The nursing student should not witness the operative permit.)

♦ The operative procedure is explained to the parents and child as simply and frankly as possible; explain the postanesthesia recovery room (PAR), wake up, IV, early ambulation, turning and deep breathing, forcing fluids, and getting up to go the bathroom.

♦ The parents are taught any care they will have to provide when they take the child home.

♦ If any special equipment, such as nasogastric suction, chest tubes, or catheters will be in place, explain the need for them and how they are used.

♦ Tell parents where they can wait during surgery so the physician will know where to find them.

♦ Carefully document all preoperative procedures and teaching.

Evening Preoperative Preparation. The child may go to the clinic or hospital the day before surgery for needed

Nursing Skill Guidelines
Administering Medications to Children

- Never give a child a choice of whether or not to take medicine. Do not say, "It's time for your pill, okay?"
- The child should be given choices whenever possible, for example, the type of juice or placement of a band aid.
- Never surprise or sneak up on a child or give an injection while the child is asleep. This will traumatize a child and may cause nightmares or difficulty sleeping.
- Tell the child that it is okay to cry.
- Following administration of an injection, do not tell the child he or she has been "good." Use the term "brave."
- Keep explanations simple and brief.
- Do not lie to the child. For example, do not tell the child that an injection will not hurt.
- Be positive, firm, and kind.
- Do not prolong completion of your task.
- There is seldom a "standard" dose of medication for the pediatric patient. Most doses are calculated based on the patient's weight in grams or kilograms.
- Accuracy in administration is vital. Liquids are usually the best method of measurement because smaller doses can be measured and because you can be sure it is swallowed.
- Because of smaller size and higher rate of metabolism, children absorb and excrete medication more quickly than adults. Watch closely for adverse side effects.
- Catheter-tip syringes are usually used for administering liquids to infants. Use the smallest syringe possible to administer medicine to ensure accuracy of measurement. Infants also may be given liquid medications through a nipple.
- Pills may be crushed or capsules emptied and contents placed in applesauce or pudding or dissolved in ice cream, juice, or formula. Because some medications cannot be mixed with certain types of foods, check a drug reference before using this technique. If adding a medication to any of these items, use only a small amount of the solute. Do not add a medication to an entire bottle of formula or cup of juice. *The child may not completely finish it and consequently not receive the prescribed dose of medication.*
- It is recommended to use the anterior thigh for giving IM injections to children younger than 3 years. *(Rationale: Their other muscles are not well enough developed.)* The deltoid site may be used if no other alternative is available and if there is sufficient muscle mass.
- Do not describe medicine as any type of candy. *(Rationale: This could lead to accidental overdose or poisoning.)*
- Use verbal and nonverbal communication to assess pain. Even young children can use a simplified pain scale such as a smiling or non-smiling face to describe their pain level.
- Be sure to monitor respiration when giving narcotics. *(Rationale: Children are particularly susceptible to respiratory depression.)*
- Always check the child's identification band before giving a medication. Do not ask the child. *(Rationale: Children may not be able to tell you their name, may tell you another name, or answer to any name asked of them.)*
- Be sure to explain to young children that medicine is not a punishment for being "bad" or refusing to cooperate. Use simple terms to explain why they are receiving medication.
- If the child is to receive an IV medication, be sure to explain that after the initial insertion, they will not be getting another "poke" with each dose.

Nursing Alert
Children may be more likely than adults to experience a paradoxical reaction to medication (a reaction *opposite* to that expected).

blood work and x-rays. The child returns home and is admitted in the morning. The parents will perform preoperative procedures as they have been taught. The child will probably need to take nothing by mouth (NPO) after midnight.

An admission questionnaire is sent home with the parent. This form is to be completed and returned to the hospital when the child is admitted. The admitting nurse reviews this questionnaire with the parents to make sure it is accurate and understandable. Make sure an operative permit has been signed. Reports of all blood work and preoperative x-rays must be on the chart.

Nursing Assessments on Preoperative Admission. When the child comes to the hospital on the morning of surgery, the nurse must assess for and document any signs of upper respiratory infection (URI), such as fever, cough, or runny nose. This is absolutely vital. An upper respiratory infection would make respiratory complications more likely and probably cause surgery to be delayed until the infection is cleared. A child is more likely to have a URI than an adult. Also be sure to chart the presence of an open wound, rash, or other unusual conditions.

Preoperative Preparations the Morning of Surgery. On the morning of the operation, the child is asked to void, and temperature, pulse, respiration, and blood pressure are recorded. Preoperative medications are given, and any hairpins or jewelry are removed. The child should be wearing hospital pajamas, and must be wearing an identification band. Ordered surgical preparation should be done, and the nurse should check to see that all laboratory reports are on the chart and that blood work is done. Everything, including toys, is taken out of the bed. If the patient is going to be taken to the operating room in the crib, the sheets are changed. The child is kept NPO. It is an important safety factor to remind the child and parents to limit activity after preoperative medication is given. The child may rest in bed or be held by the parent, but if he or she has to go to the bathroom, help must be provided. When everything is done, the nurse should sign the chart. Emotional support should be given to the parents and the child. The parents might wish to consult with the hospital chaplain.

Postoperative Care

The nurse should prepare the room to receive the patient. (Review Chapter 53 for general postoperative care.) Arrange the room so the cart from the recovery room can be moved in easily. The room should have available an IV stand, emesis basin, tissues, blood pressure apparatus, drainage equipment as needed, and any other supplies needed for the particular patient. In most hospitals, a postoperative checklist is provided on which vital signs are documented. The nurse also is responsible for assessing the patient carefully, documenting and reporting accurately, and notifying the parents when the child has returned to the pediatric unit. The nurse observes the following guidelines:

♦ When the child returns from surgery, check vital signs, according to hospital routine and physician's orders. Children's vital signs may change quickly.

♦ Monitor flow of IV, or program the controller; monitor fluid intake and output.

♦ Check positioning; the side or abdomen position is best (to prevent aspiration).

♦ Turning, coughing, and deep breathing are important, especially for an older child. Younger children do not seem to have as much difficulty with postoperative respiratory complications. (Be sure to support the incisional site with a bath blanket or pillow while encouraging the child to deep breathe.)

♦ Encourage the older child to move the toes, ankles, and legs if permitted to prevent thrombophlebitis.

♦ Reorient the child to the room—explain the IV, oxygen, suction and drainage tubes, and dressings to child and parents.

♦ Inspect the operative site for discharge or bleeding; note equipment in use, such as a Foley catheter, suction drainage, bottles, casts, or traction. Be sure everything is connected and operating properly.

♦ Check color, motion, and sensitivity of toes or fingers if a cast is in place. Reattach weights to traction as ordered.

♦ A child usually recovers from anesthesia much more quickly than an adult. However, considerate care and close observation are essential.

♦ Check for voiding; take a positive approach, and follow the physician's postoperative orders. Many times a child can be up on the afternoon of surgery. (Remember, the oral intake may be diminished, but the child has probably had 500—1,000 mL of IV fluid.) Saying "I am going to help you to the bathroom" is a much better approach than forcing or coercing the child.

♦ Fluids are given according to physician's orders. Usually about 1 hour after returning from PAR, sips of water or ice chips can be given. Check for return of peristalsis (flatus, bowel movement). If bowel sounds are not present, consult the charge nurse before giving fluids or ice, to prevent gas pains.

♦ Refresh the child when permitted; wash the face and hands, and change the gown and bed linens.

♦ Set goals for the child. Encourage walking; use medications as needed for discomfort. Early ambulation prevents complications.

♦ The young patient often recovers from surgery quickly. Many patients are discharged the afternoon of surgery or the next day. Parents must be taught specific postoperative procedures and observations for the patient's safety and the parents' security. Carefully document all teaching.

Keys for Review

Key Questions for Critical Thinking

1. Describe the importance of teaching parents about the care of their children.
2. Describe immunization, the diseases each prevents, and recommended ages for each.
3. Describe safety measures needed and rationale in caring for the hospitalized child.
4. Describe the parameters of restraints, including when and why they are used, types of restraints, and legal ramifications.

Key Readings

Castiglia PT, Harbin RE. Child Health Care: Process and Practice. Philadelphia, J.B. Lippincott, 1992

Mazinski MF. Nursing Care of the Critically Ill Child, Ed 2. St. Louis, Mosby-Yearbook, 1992

Jackson DB, Saunders RB. Child Health Nursing: A Comprehensive Approach to the Care of Children and Their Families. Philadelphia, J.B. Lippincott, 1993

Murray R, Zentner J. Nursing Assessment and Health Promotion Strategies Through the Life Span. East Norwalk, CT, Appleton & Lange, 1993

O'Toole M. (Ed). Miller-Keane Encyclopedia and Dictionary of Medicine, Nursing and Allied Health, Ed 5. Philadelphia, W.B. Saunders, 1992

Key Readings (continued)

Pomar PJ (Ed). Nurses and Family Health Promotion; Concepts, Assessment, Intervention. Philadelphia, W.B. Saunders, 1992

Skale N. Manual of Pediatric Nursing Procedures. Philadelphia, J.B. Lippincott, 1992

Whaley LF. Nursing Care of Infants and Children, Ed 4. St. Louis, Mosby-Yearbook, 1991

Enrichment Keys

Culture and chronic illness: raising children with disabling conditions in a culturally diverse world. Pediatrics 91 (Suppl. 5, part 2): 1023–1081, 1993

Keys to Learning More

Chapter 65: nursing care of the infant, toddler, and preschool-age child.

Chapter 66: nursing care of the older child

Chapter 67: nursing care of the child with special needs

Unit Thirteen: disorders of adults, including similar disorders and treatment to that for children

Chapter 80: techniques in oxygen administration

Chapter 89: rehabilitation techniques for adults and children

Chapter 90: death and dying, including children

65 Care of the Infant, Toddler, or Preschooler

Learning Objectives

- Discuss common childhood communicable diseases.
- Describe types of trauma in children, including treatment, prevention, and parent education.
- State the nurse's responsibility regarding reporting of suspected abuse.
- Discuss common musculoskeletal and nervous system disorders.
- Discuss the care of a child with a cleft lip or palate, including feeding and safety measures.
- Discuss anemia.
- Discuss common respiratory tract disorders.
- Discuss dehydration and fluid and electrolyte imbalances in children.
- Describe celiac disease and its nursing care.
- List common urinary and reproductive disorders; discuss symptoms, diagnosis, and treatment.

Key Terms

bronchiolitis	intussusception	roseola
cryptorchidism	leukemia	rubella
encephalitis	marasmus	rubeola
encopresis	meningitis	spina bifida
enuresis	meningomyelocele	tetanus
hermaphroditism	rickets	torticollis
hydrocele		

Keys to Understanding This Chapter

Chapter 5: basic needs of all people, incuding children

Unit Three: understanding normal growth and development to help recognize deviations

Unit Four: normal body structure and function

Keys to Understanding This Chapter
(continued)

Unit Five: information about special diets

Unit Six: safety and first aid

Unit Nine: basic nursing skills adapted slightly for children

Chapter 50: physical examination and nursing assessment

Chapter 53: the child who has surgery

Unit Eleven: administraton of medications

Chapter 64: needs of the hospitalized child

Key Points

- Many childhood communicable diseases can be prevented through immunization.
- Trauma is the number-one cause of death in children.
- The young child depends on others to meet basic needs. When these needs are not met, it is considered child neglect.
- Sudden infant death syndrome is sudden, unexplained death of a seemingly healthy child.
- Meningomyelocele is the most serious form of spina bifida; it may cause paralysis or other disorders.
- Lack of supervision exists in more than 90% of all near-drowning events.
- Parents of a child born with facial defects need emotional support and encouragement.
- Reye's syndrome is decreasing as parents learn about the hazards of aspirin use in children.
- Gastrointestinal illness places the young child at high risk for fluid and electrolyte imbalance or dehydration.
- Structural defects of the heart result in abnormal shunting of oxygenated and deoxygenated blood.

Key Learning Activities

◆ Visit a pediatric immunization clinic. Observe parent teaching. Inquire about cost, scheduling, and populations at risk of not receiving immunizations.
◆ Develop a poster showing safety tips. Include the topic of prevention regarding poisoning, drowning, suffocation, and burns.
◆ Interview three pediatric nurses. Ask them to describe their most memorable patient. What was the child's illness? Why do they remember this patient? How do they feel about the patient's outcome?

In Chapter 64 you learned that caring for the hospitalized child requires knowledge of normal growth and development. You also learned that children's vital signs differ from those of an adult. Normal curiosity of children and their inability to make safe decisions places them at risk for a variety of injuries. Congenital physical defects are responsible for a number of health-related disorders, requiring support of the child and family.

Many diagnostic, x-ray, and laboratory procedures are similar for children and adults. If you want to review a procedure, consult the index for its location in this book. The accompanying box will help you understand some of the abbreviations and acronyms in this chapter.

Communicable Diseases

The most common diseases in children are the communicable ones—those transmitted from one person to another. Children with common communicable diseases are cared for at home unless there are complications. If the disease is especially contagious, the child may be placed in isolation (see Chapter 51).

It is impossible to keep people from being exposed to contagious diseases. Children are often most infectious to others before symptoms appear. This period between the time the child is exposed and the time required for the disease to develop is called the *incubation period*.

The goal of communicable disease management is control. The child is admitted to the hospital only if he or she requires hospital treatment, and precautions must be taken to prevent the spread of the disease to other children. Nursing and medical management involves controlling the avenues of the spread of infection.

Diphtheria

Diphtheria begins with a sore throat, fever, and often generalized aching and malaise. Inflammation of the throat (the disease also may appear in the nose, larynx, or trachea) is followed by formation of a dirty gray membrane that is closely adherent and cannot be removed witout causing bleeding. The causative bacillus produces a poison that can weaken the cardiac muscle. The patient is very ill and must be observed closely. The mortality rate is between 5% and 10%, although the disease is rare today because it can easily be prevented by immunization. People who have no symptoms of diphtheria may be carriers. They are treated prophylactically with antibiotics.

Tetanus

Tetanus is a highly fatal disease caused by an anaerobic organism (one that cannot live in the presence of oxygen). It is characterized by convulsive contractions of all voluntary muscles. Tetanus is preventable by the administration of the tetanus *toxoid* that causes the body to build up antibodies. In the event of an injury, such as a cut or puncture wound, tetanus *antitoxin* is given immediately to provide ready antibodies. Chapter 21 introduces the concept of immunity.

Whooping Cough (Pertussis)

Whooping cough is caused by a bacillus. Infants do not receive immunity to it from their mothers. so even very young infants are susceptible. However, whooping cough is easily prevented by immunization (diphtheria, tetanus, pertussis). Parents must make sure their child is immunized. People have become complacent. There are indications that pertussis is becoming more common in the United States.

Whooping cough occurs rarely in people who are 10 years of age and older. The inoculation period is from 7 to 14 days. The symptoms begin with bronchitis and a slight elevation in temperature. The cough steadily grows worse, leading to paroxysms of coughing, characterized by a "whooping" sound. The child may cough so hard that he or she vomits or becomes dyspneic. The first stage lasts about 1 week; the severe coughing stage lasts from 2 to 3 weeks. It takes about another 2 or 3 weeks for the cough to disappear, but whooping cough can last for several months. The most serious complication is bronchopneumonia.

The child is kept isolated throughout the whooping period. Antibiotics and other medications are given. Close supervision is needed because of respiratory difficulties and nutritional problems.

Measles (Rubeola)

Rubeola (common measles, red measles, 7-day measles) is caused by a virus found in the nose, mouth, throat, and eyes and in their discharges. It is highly communicable and may not be recognized in its early stage as the symptoms often resemble cold symptoms. The incubation period is from 10 to 14 days. Measles begins with a slight temperature rise, a runny nose, and watering eyes. About the second or third day, bluish white pinpoint spots with a red rim (*Koplik's spots*) appear in the mouth. Small dark red areas appear on the head and spread throughout the body. These red areas grow larger and group together, giving the skin a blotchy appearance. The respiratory symptoms increase. The patient sneezes frequently, the eyes are sore, and the discharge becomes purulent; light hurts the eyes (*photophobia*); the throat is sore, and the patient has a hacking cough. The rash, which may last for up to 10 days, is greatest about the fourth day. During the second week, the skin begins to flake off in tiny powderlike flakes (*desquamation*) for 5 to 10 days. The patient itches all over and must be discouraged from scratching.

Measles is rarely fatal, but the complications can be serious. The infection may spread to the middle ear (*otitis media*). Pneumonia is a common development, and encephalitis (brain inflammation) develops occasionally and may cause death. Measles is most hazardous to the very young child; however, one episode seems to confer immunity. It is important that all children be immunized because of the seriousness of complications. Outbreaks of measles occur periodically because immunizations are not kept up to date.

Gamma globulin confers temporary immunity if given within a few days after exposure. If gamma globulin is given later but before symptoms appear, the attack will be mild; however, it has no effect if administered after the disease develops.

Mumps

Mumps, also called *epidemic parotitis*, is a viral disease that affects the salivary glands, especially the parotid. Children younger than 2 years and adults seldom contract mumps. However, if they do, the aftereffects can be serious, including sterility in the male. For this reason, children should be protected by administration of the mumps vaccine at approximately 15 months of age.

Close contact is required for mumps to be transmitted. The incubation period is from 2 to 3 weeks. The first sign is usually a swelling of the parotid gland, on one side or both. Sometimes, the child has a low-grade fever, headache, and general malaise before the swelling appears. The swollen gland is painful, and opening the mouth and eating are uncomfortable. The swelling begins to disappear by the second or third day and is usually gone by the 10th day. The disease is considered communicable until the patient's swelling disappears. Complications are infrequent in the child.

German Measles (Rubella)

German measles (rubella) is caused by a virus but is mild and lasts only a short time. However, German measles can cause serious congenital malformations if contracted by a pregnant woman. All children should be immunized, not only for their own protection, but for that of pregnant women with whom they may come in contact. (*Note:* "Rubella" refers to *German measles* in French and Spanish.)

The symptoms of rubella are similar to those of rubeola but are not nearly as severe; spots do not appear on the oral mucous membrane. Sometimes the facial rash is the first noticeable sign of infection. Another symptom often seen is the swelling of the lymph nodes in the occipital region (behind the ears and at the back of the neck). The rash spreads quickly and disappears just as rapidly. Although complications in the child are rare, they can be serious. One attack or one immunization should confer lifelong immunity.

The immunization measles, mumps, rubella (MMR) is given to protect against this group of diseases.

Measles Encephalitis

Measles **encephalitis** is inflammation of the brain. It is a dangerous complication of measles. It has been called "sleeping sickness." Approximately 1 in every 1,000 cases of measles becomes encephalitis, and the ensuing brain damage may be permanent. The disease can be fatal, especially for younger children; therefore, every child should be vaccinated against measles.

Chickenpox (Varicella)

Chickenpox is caused by the same virus that causes herpes zoster (shingles), a condition in adults. Chickenpox usually begins with a slight, sometimes unnoticeable, fever. A rash appears on the face and trunk and then develops into blisters surrounded by a red ring. The eruptions proceed from *papules* (red, elevated skin areas), to *vesicles* (blisterlike elevations filled with serous fluid), to *pustules* (filled with lymph or pus), and finally to a flat crust that falls off in 1 to 3 weeks. The child is usually isolated for 10 to 12 days or until dry crusts have formed, after which the disease is not as communicable. Aspirin should not be given, because of the danger of developing Reye's syndrome, which is discussed later in this chapter.

The chickenpox virus is found in the nose and throat, in the blisters, and in the crusts. The incubation period is from 14 to 16 days.

Serious complications are rare, and the most likely is infection due to scratching the blisters, which can leave scars or "pock marks." Ordinarily, the only child for whom chickenpox is very dangerous is the newborn or the child on steroid therapy. An immunization for chickenpox is being tested in some areas. The administration of acyclovir (Zovirax) is helpful in reducing symptoms.

Roseola

Roseola is a benign disease of infants. A high fever lasting a few days is followed by a rash when the temperature falls. It is believed to be caused by a virus but is not as communicable as many other diseases. The child may experience febrile seizures, but other complications are rare. One attack seems to confer lifelong immunity.

Poliomyelitis

Polyiomyelitis is a contagious viral disease that attacks the central nervous system and can cause temporary or permanent paralysis and weakness (in approximately 50% of patients). Vaccines have all but eliminated the disease in the United States, yet the spread of poliomyelitis is increasing in some parts of the world. The Sabin oral vaccine is used most often. All children should be immunized.

> **Key Concept**
>
> Parents should be taught the importance of immunizations.

Reye's Syndrome

Reye's syndrome is an acute and potentially fatal disease of childhood. The etiology of the disease is unknown; however, in most cases it follows a viral illness. It also has been related to the use of aspirin during a viral illness.

Characteristics of the disease include fever, impaired liver function, and severely impaired level of consciousness. Elevated blood ammonia levels also are present.

Public education regarding the dangers of aspirin use for sick children has drastically reduced the incidence of this disease, and early diagnosis and aggressive medical intervention have greatly improved the prognosis.

Streptococcal Infections

Scarlet Fever

Scarlet fever, also known as *scarlatina*, is caused by streptococci. The symptoms of scarlet fever develop after an incubation period of 1 to 7 days and include the appearance of a generalized flush or redness, caused by a rash of pinpoint red spots crowded together (macular rash). Flaking of the skin (desquamation) follows. The tongue becomes coated with a white substance, which later clears. The most common complications are ear infections and nephritis, arthritis, cardiac problems, and pneumonia. The most serious complication is rheumatic fever. If treated promptly, however, the prognosis is good. The patient must be kept on bed rest until symptoms disappear, and antibiotics are given.

Streptococcal Sore Throat

"Strep throat" is caused by the group A β-hemolytic (beta-hemolytic) *Streptococcus*. It is common in young children. The most serious complication is rheumatic fever and rheumatic heart disease; nephritis also can follow strep throat. Strep throat is treated with large doses of antibiotics, most often penicillin. To prevent complications, treatment must be started as soon as possible. White patches on the tonsils could be due to strep. Elevated temperature that does not fall after acetaminophen (children's Anacin, Datril, Panadol, Tylenol) is given also points to strep. If the patient complains of a "lump" in the throat rather than a sore throat

Key Abbreviations and Acronyms Used in Pediatric Nursing

ALL	Acute lymphocytic leukemia
AML	Acute myelogenous leukemia
BRAT	Bananas, rice, applesauce, toast diet
FTT	Failure to thrive
HUS	Hemolytic uremic syndrome
ITP	Idiopathic thrombocytopenia purpura
JRA	Juvenile rheumatoid arthritis
LTB	Laryngotracheobronchitis
ORS	Oral rehydration solution
PDA	Patent ductus arteriosus
PIA	Prolonged infantile apnea
PKU	Phenylketonuria
RSV	Respiratory syncytial virus
SBE	Subacute bacterial endocarditis
SIDS	Sudden infant death syndrome
T&A	Tonsillectomy and adnoidectomy
URI	Upper respiratory infection
UTI	Urinary tract infection

and feels "sick all over," it is likely that he or she has strep. A child who has a history of strep throat should be seen by a physician, who will do a culture immediately; it is the only way to differentiate strep throat from a simple sore throat.

> ### Key Concept
>
> Specimens must be obtained for culture and sensitivity prior to beginning treatment with antibiotics. Culture specimens obtained after administration of antibiotics will be inaccurate.

Rheumatic Fever

Rheumatic fever is also caused by the group A β-hemolytic *Streptococcus.* This disease is a killer and a crippler. Rheumatic fever remains one of the leading causes of death among children and is a leading cause of heart disease in people younger than age 50. It most often develops in children between 5 and 15 years of age. One attack does not guarantee immunity; on the contrary, it increases susceptibility to further attacks.

Rheumatic fever belongs to a group of diseases called *collagen diseases*, which are diseases of connective tissues. Rheumatic fever usually follows a streptococcal infection, such as scarlet fever or strep throat. It is believed to result from continued streptococcal infections, in which the patient becomes sensitive to the organism or develops a type of allergic response.

Therefore, prompt treatment of streptococcal infections greatly reduces the risk of rheumatic fever.

Signs and Symptoms. The symptoms of rheumatic fever vary in degree from mild to severe; the child may complain of symptoms that are not always associated with the disease. Loss of weight and appetite, fatigue and irritability, aches, pains, and tenderness in the extremities may be signs. However, symptoms may be more clear-cut. The fever may begin suddenly, especially after a cold or sore throat, and is highest in the evening. The most significant symptom of rheumatic fever is *polyarthritis*, in which the shoulders, elbows, wrists, or knees swell and become excruciatingly painful. The pain travels from one joint to another and may affect several joints at the same time. The pain usually lasts for a few days to a week in each joint, then subsides gradually. Fortunately, the arthritis of rheumatic fever does not cause joint deformities, and the joints are usually normal after the attack.

Signs to watch for include jerky, uncontrolled movements of the face, neck, arm, and leg muscles (Sydenham's chorea); small nodules under the skin over the elbows, ankles, legs, knuckles, and at the back of the head; and frequent nosebleeds.

A common and serious complication of rheumatic fever is *rheumatic carditis*, or rheumatic heart disease, in which lesions of the valves impair the efficiency of the valves and thus increase the heart's workload. The symptoms may be mild or so severe that cardiac failure occurs.

Medical Treatment. When rheumatic fever does occur, most cases are treated at home. When severe instances of carditis or heart failure occur, hospitalization is necessary.

The course of the disease depends primarily on whether the heart is involved and if so, to what degree. Recovery time is directly affected by the degree of carditis. The active phase of rheumatic fever usually lasts from 1 to 4 months, but one outbreak is likely to be followed by others. The key to treating rheumatic fever is to prevent permanent heart damage. Complete bed rest is ordered. It is fairly easy to keep a child inactive when the disease is acute because he or she is so sick. However, aggressive patient teaching is needed during convalescence when it is harder to regulate activity.

Antipyretics, such as acetaminophen, are given for several purposes: relief of pain, reduction of fever, and increased prevention of heart damage because of their anti-inflammatory properties. Aspirin may be ordered, because it is also a mild anticoagulant and thus aids circulation. However, other drugs are safer because of the danger of Reye's syndrome associated with aspirin. Cortisone reduces inflammation but is prescribed only if absolutely necessary because of associated adverse reactions.

An antibiotic (usually penicillin) is administered; if the patient is allergic to penicillin, another antibiotic is given. Because recurrence is probable, some physicians prescribe a small daily dose of penicillin for life. There is growing controversy about the benefits of continued prophylactic penicillin therapy for long periods; many physicians now recommend that patients be "weaned" gradually. However, if there is any sign of a strep throat, prophylactic therapy must be resumed immediately after a physician has been consulted.

The American Heart Association has classified heart disorders and the activities that can be safely undertaken for each, and these are listed in the accompanying box. The physician will designate the classification for individual children.

The outcome of this disease depends on the extent of heart damage, with the valves being the most common sites of damage. It is possible, although difficult, to repair or replace heart valves. Neither the chorea nor the arthritis is likely to have serious consequences. The carditis may be fatal, or recovery may be complete. Most children recover and lead normal lives.

Diagnostic Tests

- White blood count (WBC) and erythrocyte sedimentation rate (ESR, commonly known as "sed rate") are elevated.
- C-reactive protein is positive.
- Cardiac enzymes, such as the serum glutamic-oxaloacetic transaminase (SGOT), may be increased if severe carditis is present. This test is more commonly called the AST (aspartate aminotransferase) today.
- Antistreptolysin-O (ASO) titer is elevated.

Parasitic Infestations

Parasites live in or on the body of another living thing. Common parasites that infest humans include bacteria, protozoa, fungi, insects, and worms. Parasitic infestations are grouped according to the body system they affect.

Intestinal parasites infest the gastrointestinal (GI) tract at some point in their life cycle. Fecal contamination, uncooked flesh of animals or fish, and infected plants or water are often the source of infection. These parasites thrive where human excrement is not hygienically disposed of, where food is inadequately cooked, and where poverty and human overcrowding exist. The nurse will often see an order for a stool specimen for ova and parasites (O&P). The ova (eggs) and the parasites (worms) are examined. When handling a stool specimen, gloves are always worn, and care sould be taken not to contaminate oneself. Medications used in parasite infestations are summarized in the accompanying box.

Restriction of Activity in Heart Disorders*

Class I: Patients can take part in any activity; children can go to school and do anything that other children do.

Class II: Patients are allowed ordinary activities but not strenuous ones; children can go to school but must not take part in competitive sports, such as races, football, basketball, or tennis.

Class III: Patients must be moderate about ordinary activity and must avoid strenuous ones; children can go to school but should be given extra time for such activities as climbing stairs.

Class IV: Patients definitely must limit even ordinary activities; children must learn not to run, should never be allowed to become overtired, and should have definite rest periods.

Class V: Patients should have complete rest; children may be allowed to sit up in a chair or may have to stay in bed.

* American Heart Association.

Pinworms. Pinworms are one of the most common infestations in children. The eggs are ingested and mature in the cecum. The hatched worms lay ova in anal and perineal folds, which causes local itching. The child will scratch, especially around the anus; may grind the teeth while sleeping; and is often tired, anorectic, and irritable. The worms may be seen in the anal region or on stool.

The cellophane tape test is used to obtain and identify pinworms. Tape is wound around the end of a tongue blade with the sticky side out. After spreading the child's buttocks, the tape is pressed against the anus. The tape is transferred to a microscope slide and examined for eggs. The early morning hours are the most favorable for finding pinworms.

Giardiasis. *Giardia intestinalis* or *Giardia lamblia* is another protozoan that can cause illness in children or adults. Drinking stream water and careless disposal of human excrement by campers and backpackers into rivers, lakes, and streams provide the opportunity for infestation. Day care centers have the greatest prevalence of *Giardia*. Young children may have the disease but most often carry the protozoa without symptoms. Their caretakers often are the ones who become ill. The key to transmission is survival of the *Giardia* cysts, even with what is thought to be adequate cleaning and handwashing.

Symptoms of giardiasis include diarrhea, flatulence (gas), belching, nausea, fatigue, cramps, vomiting, and anorexia. However, people under stress or with immune deficiencies may be sicker and often have less resistance to the disorder.

Key Medications

for Parasites

◆ Some of the medications are effective against more than one parasite.
◆ *Tapeworms*—quinicrine HCl (Atrabrine), niclosamide (Niclocide)
◆ *Roundworms*—piperazine (Antepar, Bryrel, Entacyl in Canada)
◆ *Hookworms*—tetrachloroethylene
◆ *Pinworms*—mebendazole (Vermox), pyrantel pamoate (Antiminth)
◆ *Lice*—lindane (Kwell, Scabene)
◆ *Scabies*—crotamiton (Eurax) or lindane (Kwell).

Nursing Considerations: Anthelmintics

◆ Patients should use good personal hygiene and careful handwashing and avoid food preparation during treatment. All family members should be treated simultaneously.
◆ The patient with a seizure disorder, kidney malfunction, severe malnutrition, or anemia must be observed carefully and may not be able to use these medications.
◆ Side effects include dizziness, drowsiness, headache, seizures, diarrhea, nausea, and vomiting.
◆ A potential side effect of piperazine is hemolytic anemia.

Nursing Considerations: Lindane

◆ Treatment for lice includes careful washing and cleaning of all household items and clothing. Entire family may need simultaneous treatment.
◆ Observe for skin irritation
◆ Do not apply to open lesions, rash, or to face, eyes, mucous membranes or urethral meatus.
◆ Avoid inhaling the fumes. Also, the medication is extremely dangerous if swallowed.
◆ Itching may continue for a few days after treatment and may require antipruritic medication.
◆ CNS toxicity is a potential side effect and is more likely in infants, small children, and the aging.
◆ Treatment, especially for lice, may need to be repeated.

Tapeworms. Tapeworms are detected by the discovery of ova in stool. The child complains of dizziness, abdominal pain, or diarrhea. Medications are usually effective in eradicating the worms.

Flukes. Flukes are found in polluted drinking or swimming water. Specific drugs are usually effective.

Roundworms. Roundworms (ascaris species) are most common in warm climates where living conditions are not clean. They are transmitted in feces used as fertilizer. The larvae burrow into the intestine and enter the bloodstream and then migrate to the lungs, liver, or heart. Finally, they return to the intestine and grow to maturity. The infection may not be suspected until a worm is passed in stool or is vomited. Symptoms that also must be treated include diarrhea and intestinal obstruction, sometimes with intestinal rupture.

Hookworms. Hookworms are a type of roundworm. Most often they enter the host through bare feet. They then circulate through the bloodstream into the lungs, where they migrate to the mouth and throat and are swallowed. These worms destroy red blood cells, thus causing anemia. The abdomen may become distended. Blood or hookworm ova may be found in stool. Iron tablets or blood transfusions may be needed to treat anemia.

Pediculosis. Lice also can infest the child. This condition is called pediculosis and is discussed in Chapter 68.

Skin Disorders

Nevi

A nevus (plural, *nevi*) is an abnormal mark on the skin; it can be congenital or acquired and pigmented or vascular. Some types are called "birth marks." There are three major types of nevi: *intradermal* (common moles), *junctional* (flat or raised at the junction of the dermis and epidermis), and *active junctional* (most likely to develop into melanoma).

Pigmented nevi (*birthmarks* or *moles*) are either simple brown spots or dark hairy spots composed of cells containing melanin. Although normally harmless, the nevi must be closely watched, because they can develop into malignant melanomas. Pigmented nevi are removed if there is any chance that they are malignant and sometimes for cosmetic reasons. *Vascular nevi* (*angioma*) are called *hemangiomas* (overgrowth of blood vessels) or *lymphangiomas* (of lymph vessels). *Capillary hemangioma* (*port-wine stain, nevus flammeus*) is a red or purple lesion that usually does not fade. There is no known treatment. *Immature hemangioma* (*strawberry mark, nevus vasculosus*) usually regresses and disappears, so treatment is usually not necessary. A *cavernous hemangioma* is a raised, red lesion that does not regress.

Mongolian spots are irregular dark blue-green areas, generally found on the lower back. They are almost always present in Asian infants and are frequent in Mediterranean and African people but are rare in white people. They usually disappear by about the age of 5 or 6 years.

Rash

Many small babies have a rash of unknown cause. Their skin is very delicate and easily irritated. If no cause can be determined, the rash should be treated symptomatically. Exposure to air generally relieves the rash and other symptoms, such as itching. The physician may order an ointment or lotion.

Eczema

Eczema is a severe dermatitis characterized by remissions and exacerbations. It seems to be familial. Infantile eczema is often severe and accompanied by much discomfort from itching, burning, and oozing or crusting. The mildest form is called *cradle cap*. It appears to be worse in the winter. It may be due to an allergy, although the parents often do not know the cause. Eczema can occur anywhere on the body.

Symptoms and Treatment. The baby with severe eczema is miserable; he or she cries and wants to scratch constantly. It is a good idea for the nurse to spend a lot of time with this baby, because when the baby is alone, he or she will have to be restrained to prevent scratching. The scratching could lead to severe excoriation, infection, future scarring, or a dangerous complication called *eczema herpeticum* (eczema complicated by herpesvirus).

One effective restraint is the elbow restraint, also used in connection with cleft lip repair. The child's hands must be tied down to prevent him or her from scratching the face. It is a good idea to restrain a child in a rocking chair so that he or she can move but cannot scratch.

Dermatitis packs or therapeutic baths often relieve itching. Sometimes antibiotic or cortisone ointments are applied.

The diet should be adjusted to eliminate identified allergy-producing substances. Dietary adjustments often include soybean formulas. Gradually, foods are added to the diet at the rate of one new food per week (called an *elimination* diet).

Musculoskeletal and Orthopedic Disorders

Orthopedic nursing is discussed in Chapter 70. Before caring for a child in a cast or in traction, it is vital to review specific related procedures.

Congenital Hip Dysplasia and Dislocation

One or both hips may not be properly located in the ball and socket joints; the head of the femur may be displaced, or the acetabulum may not develop properly. This is known as *dysplasia*, and it causes hip dis-

location. If the disorder is unilateral (on one side only), the buttock on the affected side will have an additional crease, and the child's two knees will not be level when lying on the back with hips and knees flexed and the soles of the feet flat on the bed (the Allis' sign). The knee on the affected side is lower. X-ray studies are diagnostic. This condition is more frequent in females, is uncommon among African Americans, and occurs most often on one side only.

If untreated, the dislocation will cause deformity in later life, characterized by a shorter leg and limited abduction on the affected side. Later, the patient will walk with a limp and have lordosis (concave curvature of the lumbar spine) and a protruding abdomen.

Medical Treatment. If dysplasia is diagnosed before dislocation occurs, the condition can be treated medically. (Most affected infants have dysplasia without dislocation). This disorder is usually discovered when the child is in the newborn nursery or at the 6-week checkup.

To treat dysplasia, the child is placed in a *splint brace* or a similar cast to maintain the hips in an abducted position for 3 or 4 months. The small infant may be corrected with the use of triple or quadruple diapers, which keep the hips abducted. These measures keep the head of the femur within the acetabulum.

If the hip has been dislocated, it must be repositioned and maintained in that position. If ligaments or muscles have been torn, a spica (body) cast may be worn for 6 to 9 months. Sometimes, traction is necessary first.

When the child has been walking for several years, skeletal traction may be used to try to abduct the hips gradually. If this is unsuccessful, surgical repair is needed. If closed reduction under general anesthesia and casting are unsuccessful, an open reduction (through an incision) is performed. A *tenotomy* (transection of a tendon) also may be necessary. If the child has not been treated and is older than 6 years, the prognosis for prolonged maintenance of the repair is poor.

Nursing Considerations. The child should be handled carefully but should be picked up to encourage normal social development. The pillow splint or cast must be protected from soiling and wetting.

Normal rules for cast care apply (see Chapter 70). The nurse should watch for any signs of irritation or pressure. The child should be turned often, exercised if possible, and taken to the play room and to meals.

The parents should be instructed in the child's care. It is helpful to obtain a hospital bed with a Balkan or Bradford frame and trapeze so the child can move about in bed.

Clubfoot (Talipes)

The term *clubfoot* describes a foot that is twisted or bent out of shape as a result of hereditary factors or an abnormal position in utero. It occurs more commonly in males and more often in multiple births than in single births. Unilateral clubfoot is slightly more common than bilateral clubfoot.

Medical Treatment. Treatment includes casting or splinting to correct one deformity at a time. Surgery may be necessary for older children or for those with severe defects. The type of surgery performed depends on the specific defect. In young children, usually the soft tissues only need to be repositioned, because bones are not yet calcified. In older children, however, the bones may need to be repositioned.

The usual procedures and precautions for observing and caring for a child in a cast are observed (Fig. 65-1). The parents are taught how to care for the child and what symptoms and complications to look for. A great deal of patience is required, because the child may be in a splint or cast for several years.

Torticollis

Torticollis, also called *wryneck*, may be congenital or acquired. The congenital type is caused by failure of the sternocleidomastoid muscle to lengthen as the child grows. It must be corrected, or curvature of the upper spine and abnormal elevation of the shoulders will result.

Treatment includes passive or active exercises, surgical correction, or casting. The child must be examined periodically until after puberty to make sure there is no recurrence.

Osteogenesis Imperfecta

Osteogenesis, called "brittle bones," may be congenital or acquired. It is a skeletal deformity due to abnormal calcification and mineralization of bone.

Symptoms and Treatment. Symptoms include easily fractured bones and poor posture or body alignment. If the child is born with the disorder, the prognosis is poor. Parents should be instructed in proper handling techniques to decrease their fear of harming their infant or child. The older the person is when symptoms appear, the better the prognosis.

Treatment is aimed at preventing deformities. Traction or immobilization may be used. Parents should be encouraged to emphasize normal development of their child. Advise the parent that development of fine motor skills and avoidance of strenuous activity will prevent some fractures. The parents must learn how to recognize fracture and how to splint correctly. Fostering independence and responsibility during physical activity also is important.

Juvenile Rheumatoid Arthritis

Juvenile rheumatoid arthritis (JRA) is a generalized systemic disease of the entire musculoskeletal system. It can lead to deformities, such as contractures, and impaired movement of body parts. The cause is unknown. Several research theories have linked JRA to infection or to an abnormal immune response. Girls are more likely to be affected than boys.

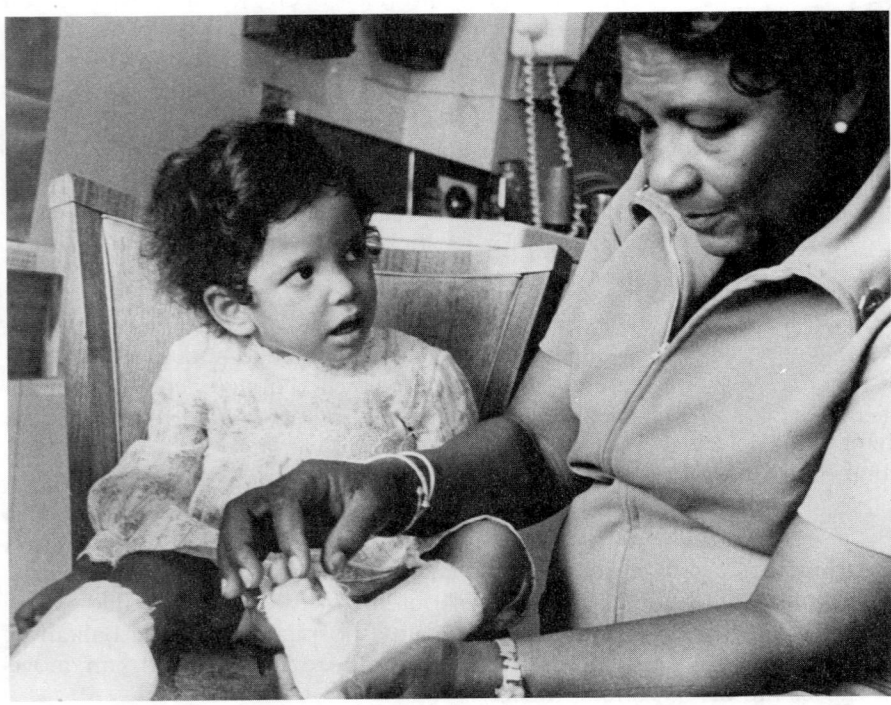

Figure 65-1. This child has had casts applied to treat bilateral clubbed feet. The nurse is checking the circulation in her foot by observing the toes for color, motion, sensitivity, and temperature. (Courtesy of Visiting Nurse Service of New York.)

Symptoms and Treatment. Many of the characteristic symptoms of arthritis are present, such as painful joint movement and subcutaneous nodules. The child's growth may be arrested; malformation may occur as a result of uneven maturation of bones or joints. Some drugs, such as acetaminophen and nonsteroidal anti-inflammatory drugs, help to relieve the symptoms.

Many children experience a spontaneous remission with no recurrence. Only about 20% continue to be affected as adults. Nursing care during the acute phase includes exercising the limbs, helping the child with activities of daily living, and sometimes applying heat in the form of a hot bath, packs, or whirlpool treatments.

All aspects of therapy must involve the child and parents. Counseling may be necessary, because parents often experience guilt and anxiety. Social development and helping the child to develop a positive attitude toward school also are important.

Rickets

Rickets is a skeletal condition caused by a vitamin D deficiency that prevents bones from metabolizing calcium properly. Rickets is rare in the United States because of the use of vitamin D-fortified milk.

The child with rickets does not walk or crawl at the normal age and may be small for his or her age. The bones may be lumpy; because they are weak, weight bearing bends the bones, which causes characteristic bowed legs or knock-knees. X-rays show abnormal calcification. Treatment involves administration of vitamin D and physical therapy to prevent deformity or to correct existing deformities.

Trauma

Children are susceptible to injury from falling, choking, drowning, poisoning, and burns or from being caught in a moving object. Parents must constantly be alert to prevent accidents, yet because the young child is constantly on the move, it is difficult to watch him or her every moment. As a result, trauma is the number-one cause of death in children.

Fractures

Although children's bones are not as brittle as those of adults, children receive more accidental blows and injuries and consequently suffer many fractures. Falls are frequent among children with nervous system disorders, because their balance and coordination are impaired. Some fractures also are due to abuse by parents or guardians. Treatment of fractures includes casts and traction. When a child is in a cast or traction, the nurse checks circulation by assessing skin color, sensitivity, and temperature; motion; and pulse (see Chapter 70).

Fractures most commonly seen in children are those involving the radius, ulna, and clavicle.

Burns

Burns are discussed at the end of Chapter 68. Most of the information there also applies to burns in children, but it must be adapted to the younger child.

The chief nursing problems in treating burns are combating shock, alleviating pain, and restoring fluid and electrolyte balance. Secondary problems include prevention of infection and reconstruction or repair of damage. Children who have been severely burned are best cared for in a specialized burn unit. The treatment is long-term. In addition, the child and the parents need understanding and emotional support.

The extent of burns is determined on a percentage basis. Because the child's body surface differs in proportion from the adult's, a different method of determining the extent of the burn must be used. Remember that the infant's head is large in proportion to the body to get a better idea of the percentages of burn.

- *The newborn:* The head is 17% of the entire body surface; each arm, 8%; each leg, 13%; the front or back, 20%; and genitals, 1%.
- *The 3 year-old:* The head is 15%, each arm, 8%; each leg, 14%; the front or back, 20%; and genitals, 1%.
- *The 6-year old:* The head is 11%, each arm, 8%; each leg, 16%; front or back, 20%; and genitals, 1%.
- *Over age 12:* The "rule of nines" applies (see box in Chapter 68): the head is 9%; each arm, 9%; each leg, 18%; front or back, 18%; and genitals, 1%.

Burns may be *first, second, third,* or *fourth* degree (see box in Chapter 68). Burns also may be classified as *partial thickness* or *full thickness,* relating to the type of grafting that may be needed. Refer to Chapter 68 for nursing care of burns. Chapter 31 describes emergency first aid.

Poisoning

Poisonous substances are found in most households. The inquisitive toddler, who puts anything and everything into the mouth, can easily ingest one or more of these substances. Cleaning compounds are a major problem, because they are usually under the sink or on the floor of the bathroom closet and are easily accessible to toddlers.

A common type of poisoning in children is aspirin poisoning. Drug companies have attempted to alleviate the problem by installing safety caps on bottles. One of the difficulties encountered with medications manufactured for children relates to the appearance of these drugs. They are packaged attractively, taste good, and are in "fun" shapes. As a result, many small children mistake medications for candy.

Poisonous house plants and cigarette butts also should be kept out of reach. Cigarette butts may be *poisonous* if eaten. Lead poisoning (plumbism) results from inhaling or eating leaded substances. It is discussed in Chapter 66. The family must be taught poison prevention measures. A list of teaching subjects is given in the accompanying box.

Medical Treatment. In the event of poisoning, it is important to call the local *poison control center* immediately; its specially trained personnel can determine the best treatment for the particular poison. The poison control center number should be taped on each phone in the home. In most larger U.S. cities, dialing 911 also will provide immediate access to emergency assistance. The poison control staff will tell you if vomiting should be indicated or not.

Physicians recommend that *syrup of ipecac* be kept in every household, especially if children are present. Syrup of ipecac is an *emetic*; it causes vomiting within a short time. (It is important to know that vomiting should *not* be induced if a caustic substance, such as ammonia, has been ingested because the poison would burn again while being vomited.) The usual dose of syrup of ipecac for the toddler is 15 mL; this dose should be decreased for the younger child (the crawler). (All doses given *must* be recovered.)

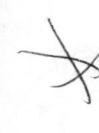

Activated charcoal is used to absorb poisons. If emesis is to be induced, this must be done before activated charcoal is administered. Charcoal is not mixed with food or given with any other drugs, because it will absorb these substances. The dose is approximately 5 to 10 times the amount of poison ingested.

Emergency Treatment. When the child is brought to the hospital, specific procedures are performed. Sometimes the stomach is washed out (gastric lavage), usually with normal saline, in an effort to remove as much of the poison as possible. This procedure must be done quickly to keep as much of the harmful substance from being absorbed into the bloodstream as possible. If a caustic substance, such as lye or kerosene, has been swallowed, vomiting is not induced, because the poison will burn as much on the way up as it did when swallowed. If it has been several hours since the drug was ingested, the stomach is not lavaged, because most of the substance probably will have been absorbed already. In this case, the symptoms are treated.

Nursing Considerations. The nurse may be asked to assist with gastric lavage. In most hospital emergency rooms, the needed equipment is packaged as a gavage set. A suction machine and ordered drugs and solutions are required. The nurse assists the physician with the

---

Keys to Patient/Family Teaching
Prevention of Poisoning

Patient and family teaching related to poison prevention includes the following:

◆ Poisonous chemicals should be labeled with warning labels and stored in cabinets with locks on the doors.
◆ Medications and poisonous materials should be kept in original containers, never in a soda bottle or similar inviting container.
◆ Childproof caps should be used whenever possible.
◆ Children should be taught the dangers of these materials and to stay away from such poisonous materials.
◆ Edibles and nonedibles should not be in the same cabinets.
◆ Children should not be left alone when there are poisonous materials nearby.
◆ Medicines and vitamins should never be treated as candy. Medicines resembling candy, animals, and people should not be bought.
◆ Read labels carefully when using products. Heed precautions. Do not give medicines in the dark.
◆ Dispose of poisonous materials and medicines carefully. Destroy medicines by flushing in toilet and washing down in sink rather than throwing in trash.
◆ Keep ashtrays with cigarette butts and ashes away from children.
◆ Do not have poisonous plants in the house or in the yard.
◆ The local Poison Control Center's phone number should be kept by all phones in the house.
◆ Keep syrup of ipecac and activated charcoal in the house.
◆ Poisoning can take place while visiting in the homes of friends and relatives. Watch children carefully when visiting.
◆ If suspected poisoning occurs, remain calm as you dial emergency and give information to the operators.

---

procedure, documenting all pertinent information and procedures performed and giving support to the child and family. The nurse also must be ready to assist in suctioning (to prevent aspiration), administering oxygen and resuscitation, catheterizing, inserting an intravenous catheter or nasogastric tube, drawing blood samples, or performing x-rays or electrocardiograms (ECGs).

After lavage, the child is generally kept for 1 or 2 hours before being discharged, unless much of the poison was absorbed into the bloodstream. In this case, the child is admitted to the hospital overnight for observation. The nursing care then involves assessing the child for any change in level of consciousness (LOC) and for signs of dizziness, nausea, vomiting, unusual behavior, extreme drowsiness, or excitement. Sometimes irreversible physical or mental changes occur. Surgery must be performed occasionally to correct the physical damage caused by ingested caustic substances. The patient may have renal failure and may require dialysis.

When the child is released from the hospital, the parents must be instructed to watch for unfavorable symptoms and must be advised to return the child to the emergency room if they occur.

Foreign Objects

Small objects should be kept out of reach of young children as much as possible. Children should be taught never to put anything into a body opening. Again, parents must be constantly alert, keeping dangerous objects away from children.

Aspiration or Swallowing of Foreign Objects. A child will often swallow or aspirate a small object. If it is not sharp and has entered the intestinal tract and seems to be moving through the intestine, it will generally pass through. Nursing care would then involve close observation of stools to ascertain that the object has been excreted; x-rays may be needed.

If an object is aspirated into the lungs, it may be coughed out. If not, bronchoscopy or lung surgery may be necessary to remove the object, because it could cause an infection if allowed to remain in the lungs. Aspiration of an object also could cause suffocation. See Chapter 32 for emergency removal of a foreign object from the throat. Family teaching regarding choking appears in the accompanying box.

A Foreign Object in the Eye. Many times a child will get a cinder, eyelash, or other object in the eye and irritate it further by scratching or rubbing. Sometimes surgery is necessary to remove the object if ordinary first-aid measures are not effective.

Objects in the Nose or Ears. Many times children put small objects, such as buttons or peanuts, into their ears or nose and then cannot remove them. A child who has inserted an object into the nose will often have halitosis (bad breath). Because a serious infection can result, the object must be removed by the physician.

Objects in the Rectum or Vagina. Objects in the rectum or vagina must be removed carefully by a physician to prevent damage to the tissues.

Keys to Patient/Family Teaching
Prevention of Choking

Patient and family teaching related to prevention of choking includes the following:

- Food eaten by children should be cut into small pieces.
- Children should be taught to chew slowly and thoroughly and to avoid laughing or talking while they are eating.
- Only foods appropriate for the child's age should be served. Avoid nuts, popcorn, chewing gum, hard candies, and so forth before age 4 years.
- Children should not walk, run, play, or cry with food or foreign objects in their mouth.
- Small objects, such as coins, beads, and marbles should be kept from children until school age.
- Small household and carpentry items, such as pins, buttons, toothpicks, thumbtacks, screws and nails, and so forth, should be put away carefully after use. If they are being used and children are in the vicinity, the child should be watched carefully.

Lacerations, Puncture Wounds, Abrasions, and Crushing Injuries

Many children come into the emergency room with cuts and punctures from knives, forks, pencils, or other sharp objects found in the home. The obvious preventive measure is to keep such objects out of the child's reach.

The child also may sustain a crushing injury from being caught in a car door or under a heavy piece of furniture or from being hit by a moving bicycle or car. Serious injuries also can occur in electric car windows or garage doors. Bruises and abrasions can result from a fall from a tricycle, a wagon, or playground equipment.

Many such injuries are not serious enough to warrant the child's admission to the hospital. Lacerations are sutured, antiseptics and dressings are applied, and x-rays are taken if needed to determine whether a fracture was sustained. Usually a tetanus booster is given. Puncture wounds in particular are watched for signs of infection and are kept open as much as possible so that they can drain and heal from the inside. The parents may be instructed to soak the wound periodically to facilitate drainage.

Injuries Caused by Animals. A dog bite can be very serious. Children should be warned *never* to annoy a dog that is eating (even their own family dog) or pet any unfamiliar dog. Frequently, the face is bitten, and plastic or reconstructive surgery may be required. It should be determined if the dog has received rabies immunization; if not, the the dog must be isolated and watched for signs of rabies or distemper. If the dog becomes ill or cannot be found, the child must be given prophylactic rabies injections; a tetanus booster also should be given. Very few cases have documented survival of humans infected with rabies.

The most dangerous complication of a cat scratch is infection. As in the case of dog bites, the cat must be watched for signs of rabies.

Wild animals also bite people, particularly if trapped or frightened. They are often carriers of rabies or other diseases.

Suffocation

Suffocation in children may be caused by a number of circumstances, including a foreign object being aspirated or a child being smothered by a plastic bag or a pillow. Very young children should not be given pillows until they are able to turn themselves over freely.

Suffocation can result if a small infant who has an upper respiratory infection cannot cough up the mucus plugging the bronchi. Humidity usually helps to loosen secretions so that the baby can cough them up. Infants are "nose breathers" and have not yet learned mouth breathing. For this reason, a bulb syringe should be available to assist in keeping the nasal airway clear of mucous accumulation.

A child also can suffocate if he or she becomes trapped in a discarded refrigerator. Children seeking treats from large freezers have been known to fall into the freezer and be unable to rescue themselves. Any of these situations could be rapidly fatal if the door closes and the child is trapped inside. State laws generally call for doors to be removed from all discarded refrigerators or for the refrigerator to be turned tightly against a wall.

Drowning and Near-Drowning

In approximately 90% of all drowning incidents, adult supervision is lacking. The areas in which drownings occur are age related. Infants are subject to drowning in bathtubs, toilets, or containers of standing water, such as a dog dish or pail. The highest incidence of drowning for the preschooler occurs in swimming pools. Adolescents more commonly have drowning experiences in rivers and lakes. A drowning can take place in any body of water. The outcome of the event depends on the length of time the child has been submerged and the water temperature.

Near-drowning is defined as "survival for at least 24 hours following submersion in a body of fluid." When submersion begins, the child gasps, chokes, and swallows water. In almost all cases, the airway spasms and closes off (laryngospasm), preventing water from entering the lungs. If the child is rescued at this point, it is referred to as *dry drowning,* because no water entered the lungs. If the child remains in the water, car-

diopulmonary arrest occurs, and the airway relaxes, allowing water to enter the lungs. This is known as *wet drowning.* It is important to note whether the child was found floating in the water or found at the bottom of the pool. A child experiencing a dry drowning will float because of the air still trapped in the lungs. When the lungs fill with water, the child's body sinks.

A child who has a near-drowning in cold water will experience the diving reflex. The diving reflex occurs when the face is exposed to cold water. Blood is diverted from the periphery of the body to the heart and brain, preserving vital functions. Because of this reflex and a slowed metabolic rate, individuals may be resuscitated, even after prolonged periods of submersion in cold water.

The most common complication of near-drowning is aspiration pneumonia. This may occur when the child vomits and then aspirates or who aspirates the submersion fluid. Children who have been submerged in contaminated water are at greater risk for respiratory infection.

Key Concept

The two most effective ways of preventing near-drowning are adequate adult supervision at all times and water safety training.

Sudden Infant Death Syndrome

Sudden infant death syndrome (SIDS) is the sudden, unexplained death of a seemingly healthy infant. This diagnosis can only be made following postmortem examination. SIDS is diagnosed when no cause of death can be identified. A condition called prolonged infantile apnea (PIA) is defined as cessation of breathing for at least 20 seconds, or for a shorter time, with accompanying bradycardia, cyanosis, and/or pallor. When this condition is discovered (a "near miss"), an apnea monitor can be used to prevent SIDS.

Although the etiology of SIDS is unknown, one theory suggests that an abnormality in brain steam function results in faulty respirations. Incomplete bubbling after feeding has also been blamed.

In addition, to experiencing profound shock and grief, parents of SIDS infants often feel overwhelming guilt. Nurses must be particularly sensitive to this tragic situation and offer support and compassion. Parents should be provided with information regarding support groups such as The Compassionate Friends and the SIDS Foundation (addresses at the end of this chapter).

Some children at high risk are placed on an apnea monitor until about 1 year of age. Nursing skills in apnea monitoring follow. The nurse can also teach parents how to use the monitor.

Nursing Skill
Using the Apnea Monitor

Supplies and Equipment

Apnea monitor with electrodes
Material to cleanse skin

Suggested Procedure and Rationale

1. Wash your hands.
2. Gather equipment.
3. Explain to the parents what your are going to do and why. *(Rationale: Teaching helps decrease parents' anxiety and gives them a better understanding of procedures.)*
4. Prepare infant's skin by making sure it is clean and dry. *(Rationale: If skin is clean and dry, electrodes will make better contact and will stick better. There will be less chance of skin breakdown.)*
5. Apply electrodes (either to the infant or to the electrode belt, depending on type of monitor used.)
   a. The electrode belt should be placed at the nipple line.
   b. Skin electrodes are usually best placed between nipple and armpit and may be repositioned somewhat. *(Rationale: Proper placement of electrodes ensures accurate readings on the monitor. Moving the electrodes helps prevent skin breakdown.)*
6. Insert lead wires. The white lead wire inserts on the right side (mnemonic: white = right). The black inserts on the left. There may be additional color-coded lead wires depending on system used.
7. Insert the corresponding lead wire into the cable and, insert the cable into the monitor. The cable is usually color coded to match lead wires.
8. Attach the belt to the infant. The belt should be snug, but you should be able to insert two fingers under it. *(Rationale: Ensure accurate readings without causing respiratory compromise or skin breakdown.)*
9. Make sure the monitor is plugged in, the cable attached, and the alarms properly set.
10. Turn the monitor on. Indicator lights should be on.
11. Settle the infant comfortably, or allow parents to hold and comfort their infant. *(Rationale: Comforting the infant helps decrease respiratory distress and makes him or her feel safer.)*
12. If monitor alarms:
    a. Check the infant immediately!
    b. Check the infant's breathing and color. If the infant is pink but not breathing, wait until the 10th beep before stimulating. If the infant is not pink, start stimulation *immediately. (Rationale: The infant may resume breathing without intervention. The alarm may be mechanical in origin, and the infant may not require any stimulation.)* Believe your observations of the infant before believing the monitor.
13. Use this stimulation sequence: Gently touch; gently shake; strong shake; start CPR! *(Rationale: Use as little intervention as necessary to get the infant to resume breathing.)* After the problem is resolved, the alarm will stop.
14. Press reset button to turn off alarm indicator. *(Rationale:*

The alarm will stop when the problem is resolved, but the alarm needs to be reset.)
15. Document and report any alarms and nursing responses. Document the infant's condition. Always note alarm settings when starting and ending any contact with the infant and at least every hour in between. *(Rationale: Monitor alarms can be altered by other staff or visitors on purpose or by accident. Check them frequently to ensure they are set correctly.)*

Child Abuse

Abuse of children is a widespread, socially significant problem. Hundreds of children die each year as a result of abuse, and hundreds more are temporarily or permanently injured.

Child abuse can take several forms, including neglect, physical abuse, and sexual abuse. The nurse who suspects that a child has been abused is obligated by law to report it to the nursing supervisor or physician or the authorities. Signals of child abuse are listed in the box.

Key Concept

A sudden change of behavior in a child of any age is a clue that abuse may be occurring.

Neglect

Child neglect can be divided into emotional and physical. An emotionally neglected child is one who has been deprived of love, affection, and attention from the parent or adult caregiver. Physical neglect is described as a lack of basic physical needs, such as food, water, clothing, and adequate medical care.

The neglected child may appear disheveled, unclean, and malnourished and may show evidence of untreated dental problems. An emotionally neglected child may demonstrate self-destructive behaviors or be passive and withdrawn. The child also may have difficulty sleeping or nightmares, and may exhibit signs of depression and suicidal tendencies.

Physical Abuse

The term physical abuse has not been clearly defined in a universally accepted manner. Most often it refers to a situation in which a child has been physically harmed, and injury has occurred. The injury is inflicted intentionally and can vary from minor bruising to death. The *shaken baby syndrome* is an example of physical abuse in which an adult holds an infant by the shoulders and violently shakes the baby. This usually occurs when the adult becomes frustrated after attempts to quiet a crying infant. The immature development of the infant neck

Keys to Nursing Assessment
Detecting Child Abuse

Signals: Common Perpetrators of Child Abuse

- Parents who have suffered abuse, neglect, or rejection in their past
- Parents who have histories of being dependent and now demonstrate dependency on others
- Parents who have one or more of the following personality traits: hostility, a tendency to blame others, punitiveness, low self-esteem, or a tendency to act impulsively
- Parents caring for out-of-wedlock, unwanted, or foster children
- Parents who are young and immature
- Parents in troubled marital relationships that include excessive demands from spouse, rejection or abuse by spouse, unmet needs
- Parents who use drugs excessively
- Parents who expect children to meet their needs and expectations and are overcritical and do not see the child in a positive light
- Parents who use extreme discipline measures
- Parents who indicate a loss of control in disciplining, such as slapping, shaking, and hitting the child
- Parents overwhelmed by the emotional and physical needs and demands of their children
- Parents who are unable to cope with daily activities, which can lead to irritability and low frustration level
- Parents who seldom touch or look at their child, who react with impatience, or who ignore their child's crying

Signals: Possible Abuse of School-Age Children

- The child lies about injury.
- The child exhibits behavior problems.
- The child sometimes expects abusive behavior, as if it is the only kind of attention they receive; therefore, child acts in a way that invites abuse.
- The child becomes a lawbreaker

- The child often uses and eventually abuses drugs and alcohol, especially starting at an early age.
- Frequent truancy
- Self-injurious behavior, suicidal thoughts or attempts
- Promiscuous sexual behavior

The younger child often admits to abuse because he or she is unaware that beating is an unacceptable behavior. The older child may attribute an injury to an improbable cause—possibly lying for fear of parental retaliation.

Signals: Possible Abuse of Young Children

- Injuries at various stages of healing (could not have happened at same time)
- Sophisticated sexual knowledge in a young child
- Agreement with parents on illogical cause of injury
- Burns, lacerations, or serious bruises without appearance of accident; unexplained fractures; chunks of hair missing
- Parental labeling of child as "different" or "bad"
- Attempts at staying away from home
- Attempts to hide abuse scars with clothing
- Frequent injuries
- Extreme fear of adults; fear of being touched
- Appearance of neglect: dirty, unkempt, extremely thin, lethargic
- Stomach problems, colitis, rectal/vaginal bleeding, frequent headaches

Signals of Child Neglect

- Abandonment of child by parent
- Inadequate medical, dental care; inadequate hygiene, clothing, supply or quality of food, lack of sleep
- Unmet physical or mental problems
- Inadequate heat or repair of home
- Isolation of family from usual social contacts
- Excessive demands of child (expected to do all the housework or accept total care of younger sibling)
- Child left without custodial care or supervision

---

muscles and lack of head control, along with violent shaking, results in cerebral trauma or hemorrhage. Death or serious intellectual impairment can ensue.

Evidence of physical abuse can take several forms. Unexplained bruises in various stages of healing or numerous unexplained fractures that have healed in a child may indicate physical abuse.

> **Key Concept**
>
> Accidental brain injury can occur when a child is thrown into the air and caught. Parents should be cautioned about the dangers of this type of play.

Sexual Abuse

Sexual abuse of a child ranges from exposure and fondling to anal or vaginal intercourse, incest, and rape. The typical pattern is one of secrecy. The person abuses the child, sometimes as early as 1 year of age, and as the child grows older, the abuser tells the child to keep it a secret. By the time the child is old enough to realize that what is happening is not normal, he or she is too ashamed and afraid to reveal the truth. The child's reaction is one of guilt and fear. In many cases, the entire situation is repressed, only to surface as flashbacks, nightmares and/or self-injurious behavior years later.

Many schools have programs to teach young children about sexual abuse and incest. These programs demonstrate "right touch, wrong touch" and help the child to say "no" and to seek help. The child is taught not to go with strangers and to report any incidents to someone in authority.

Child pornography has become a growing concern. Sadly, hundreds of children disappear each year, many of whom are forced into pornography ("kiddie porn"). Satanic cults also subject children to many types of abuse, sexual and physical.

Sexual abuse is difficult to identify and harder to prove. Some of the indications that a child may be sexually abused follow:

◆ A sudden change in behavior
◆ Symptoms of abdominal pain, gastric distress, or headaches
◆ Signs of emotional disturbance
◆ Avoidance of touching or physical contact
◆ Vaginal or rectal bleeding or lesions

Nursing Considerations. Often the first response of the nurse to abuse of a child is anger. Be objective. Be aware of possible personal problems of the suspected abuser, such as low self-esteem, rejection, and isolation. Include objective explanations, and be consistent in your approach. Suspected abusers are often in an environment that is *out of control*, and their only way of coping is to abuse their child.

Key Concept

If you *suspect* child abuse, you must, by law, report it immediately. A nurse who does not do so is committing a crime. Those reporting suspected abusers are legally protected against recourse.

Parent Anonymous groups throughout the country assist abusers in breaking the cycle. Support groups provide ongoing help to abusers who have completed counseling programs and need day-to-day assistance in pursuing a nonabusive lifestyle.

Your role as a nurse is important. You can be the key to reporting and dealing with the problem:

◆ *Believe the child.* If a child confides in you, always assume that the child is telling the truth.
◆ *Observe the child's reactions.* Look not only for marks and bruises, but also for reactions. The child who draws away when touched or who is autistic should be considered a victim of abuse until proven otherwise. The child sometimes attempts to protect the abuser and will make excuses for "accidents."
◆ *Document your observations.* Carefully observe the signs of abuse. Be objective. Identify and document every observation to the last detail. Measure bruises and abrasions, and take photographs.

◆ *Teach the child.* The child needs to learn what activities are inappropriate and what to do if someone tries to exploit him or her.

The accompanying sample nursing care plan addresses a nurse's concern about a child who appears to be abused.

Failure to Thrive

Inadequate physical growth is termed *failure to thrive* (FTT). This may involve only weight, or it may involve weight and height. Characteristic developmental symptoms include developmental retardation, retarded motor development, inadequate social response, and delayed language development. The child is withdrawn and apathetic, does not relate to the environment, and does not cry. The child shows "flat affect" (no response to external stimulation).

If the cause of FTT is *physical*, the child appears small for age on the growth grids. Such children do not appear "abnormal." Undernourished infants are passive and withdrawn; developmental lags are experienced early in life. If the cause is related to the *social or home situation*, the child often appears to have a "starved" look. He or she has spindly arms and legs, a "pot belly," and an unnaturally old appearance. Mothers of FTT infants are often unaware of the amount of food the infant needs or is taking and do not understand the nutritional needs of the child, thus causing a physical difficulty. The parents should not be blamed, but family counseling and parenting skill education are often needed.

FTT may be caused by a physiologic problem, such as cystic fibrosis, celiac disease, gastroenteritis, parasites, or diabetes mellitus. More commonly, FTT has a social rather than a congenital physical cause.

Nursing Considerations. A developmental history should be taken of FTT children. Look at the parents' reactions to the pregnancy. Questions to ask include, "What is the 24-hour feeding pattern?" For additional assessment factors, refer to the accompanying box.

The infant who is diagnosed as FTT is often hospitalized from 10 days to 2 weeks. The child is fed on demand, at least every 2 to 3 hours. If the weight gain is appropriate, FTT is definitely diagnosed. If the child does not gain weight, physiologic reasons must be sought. A physical examination is essential, including a complete blood workup.

The caretaker (mother or father) should be with the infant, to provide care and spend as much time as possible with the infant. Tender, loving care and stimulation are essential. Hold the child, and rock and cuddle him or her. The caretaker also must be educated to look for positive signs from the child (smile, responsiveness).

Accurate recordings of intake and output (I&O) are essential. Be sure to follow the feeding schedule. In an

Freddie Meers is a 4-year-old white boy admitted to the pediatric unit from the emergency department in severe respiratory distress with hypoxemia, retention of carbon dioxide, and respiratory acidosis. He is well known to the nurse admitting him because this is his fourth admission for asthma; his first admission was when he was 30 months old. During the assessment, the nurse notices bruises on the back and torso in several stages of healing and what appears to be a cigarette burn on the buttock. The child is too ill to provide any history, and when questioned about the bruises, the mother states that "'Freddie is clumsy and falls frequently." In the past this nurse was concerned about Freddie's extreme fear of adults and exaggerated eagerness to please his parents. Although stabilizing the child medically is the nurse's first priority, the nurse also resolves to report Freddie as a suspected case of child abuse. Included on the plan of care are the following diagnoses.

Nursing Diagnosis: *Altered Parenting Related to Unmet Social/Emotional/Maturational needs of the Parents and Multiple Family Stressors as Evidenced by the Child's Physical and Psychological Trauma and the Parent's Inattention to the Child's Needs*

Goal: Parents verbalize the need for professional assistance to resolve personal problems and develop parenting skills.

Long-Term Goal: Parents actively participate in individual or group counseling until effective parenting skills are developed and consistently used.

Nursing Actions (assess/do/teach)	Rationale	Evaluative Statement
1. Assess the parent's potential to abuse: history of abuse as a child, unrealistic expectations of children (role reversal), lack of knowledge of parenting skills, social isolation, and lack of resources to deal with multiple life stresses.	Abusive parents were often abused as children. Parents may direct their anger and frustration toward the helpless child.	8/1, Goal not met; parents continue to deny there is a problem. *Revision:* Continue to work one on one with mother.
2. Attempt to establish a supportive relationship with one or both parents; talk about how difficult it can be to raise children (while not condoning abuse), and take advantage of any opportunities that present to act as a role model for positive interactions with the child and to teach parenting skills. Recommend that the parents voluntarily seek professional counseling.	Abusing parents have rarely learned to trust others and may feel defensive about their deficiencies.	8/5, Goal partially met. Mother agrees to meet with counselor after speaking to child protection worker and learning alternatives.
3. Avoid the tendency to become a substitute parent for the child to the exclusion of the child's natural parents.	This only intensifies the parent's feelings of inadequacy, worthlessness, and isolation.	
4. Report the case to the Child Protective Services.	All states have mandatory laws for reporting child maltreatment.	
5. Initiate discharge planning as soon as the legal disposition for placement has been decided (temporary foster home placement or return to parents).	This will ensure continuity of care.	
6. Reassure the child that he is safe in the hospital.		

(continued)

Nursing Diagnosis: *Altered Growth and Development Related to Inadequate Caretaking as Evidence by Listlessness and Decreased Responses*

Goal 1: Child demonstrates interest in everyday activities and positive affective responses.

Goal 2. Child begins to demonstrate healthy self-esteem behaviors.

Nursing Actions (assess/do/teach)	Rationale	Evaluative Statement
1. Continue to assess the child's ability to trust his environment and to participate in everyday activities.	Meeting the child's anxiety needs are fundamental to care.	1. 8/1, Goal 1 partially met; child is beginning to enjoy playing with other children and responds positively to primary nurse.
2. Provide a consistent caregiver to demonstrate acceptance of and affection for the child while at the same time attempting to modify negative behavior; implement a program of attention based on play, group interaction with other children, and quiet time with the child.	Acceptance is critical to the child's development, as are consistent behavior standards.	2. 8/1, Goal 2 partially met; child is still "trying too hard" to be accepted; displays an exaggerated fear of rejection; occasional disruptive behavior.
3. Accept temporary regression in the child.	This is a necessary mechanism to cope with the present crisis.	
4. Praise the child's abilities (realistically).	This will promote his self-esteem	

Familial Causes

- Early separation of mother from infant, which leads to inappropriate bonding
- Major depression of parent early in child's life
- Major crisis in family, which takes time away from family life
- Serious illness of the infant, which leads to an inability to form a strong familial bonding
- Parents who are isolated or have marital problems; single parents
- Very young parents and parents with minimal parenting skills
- Serious illness/death of parent or sibling

Infant-Related Causes

- Prematurity, illness, congenital malformation, malabsorption disorders
- Reduced responsiveness and interaction with others in environment
- Dislike of cuddling, slow social development (eg, doesn't smile), difficulty in feeding

older child, accurate food and fluid intake must be recorded.

Neurologic Disorders

Encephalocele

If the bones of the skull do not close correctly, a portion of the brain may protrude through the opening. This condition is known as *encephalocele*. The amount of damage in the functioning of the child depends on the size and location of the encephalocele and on the presence or absence of strangulation or rupture of parts of the brain. The chief danger in this condition is possible rupture of the meningeal sac, leading almost inevitably to meningitis or encephalitis. The defect can be surgically corrected but sometimes is delayed until the child is 1 year old. Until surgery is performed, meticulous nursing care is necessary to prevent damage or infection.

Spina Bifida

Spina bifida is a malformation of the spine, usually the lower spine, in which a part of the vertebral or spinal column is open or missing. The condition may be asymptomatic or may cause severe paralysis, depending on how large the opening is and whether the meninges or spinal cord herniate through the opening. Prenatal amniocentesis can detect this disorder; elective abortion may be done. Genetic counseling may be indicated. Folic acid (folate) taken during pregnancy helps to prevent spina bifida. The three forms of this disorder are spina bifida occulta, meningocele, and meningomyelocele.

Spinal bifida occulta is an opening in the vertebral column with no apparent symptoms. It is discovered only if an x-ray is taken for an unrelated reason or if an investigation is done because a dimple is present over the backbone. A small tuft of hair or port wine stain is sometimes present in the vertebral area. Although this condition may cause problems when the child undergoes a growth spurt during puberty, it generally does not cause difficulty. It may be corrected by surgery if necessary.

Meningocele occurs when one of the meninges (the spinal cord covering) protrudes or herniates through an opening in the vertebral column (Fig. 65-2**B**). The patient with a meningocele may have no disability. On the other hand, there may be muscle weakness, difficulty with bowel and bladder control, and rarely paralysis. Corrrective surgery is needed. Generally, the child will lead a normal life after surgery.

Meningomyelocele or *myelomeningocele* (see Figure 65-2**C**) is the most serious form of spina bifida. The meninges and part of the spinal cord protrude through an opening. The child has a visible lesion on the back. This patient is most often paralyzed and may have bladder and bowel control problems. Serious possible complications include **meningitis** (inflammation of the meninges covering the spinal cord), encephalitis, and hydrocephalus (see next section). The nurse must handle the defect with great care to avoid spinal cord damage. Surgery is needed to prevent infection and to preserve as much nerve function as possible. Surgery is often done very soon after birth.

Nursing Considerations. A nursing goal in treating any of these children is to prevent further damage. The most common problem is loss of sensation in the legs, so the nurse must be sure to protect the child against possible leg injury. Careful examination also is necessary to assess for pressure areas and tight clothing, which can be irritating and cause skin breakdown or lack of sufficient circulation to a part. Good skin care must be given, and diapers must be changed immediately after voiding and defecating.

The nurse assists in preoperative and postoperative surgical management. Precautions should be taken to protect the child from infection in the area of the defect. Another common site for infection is the bladder, because the child is often catheterized. The child can be

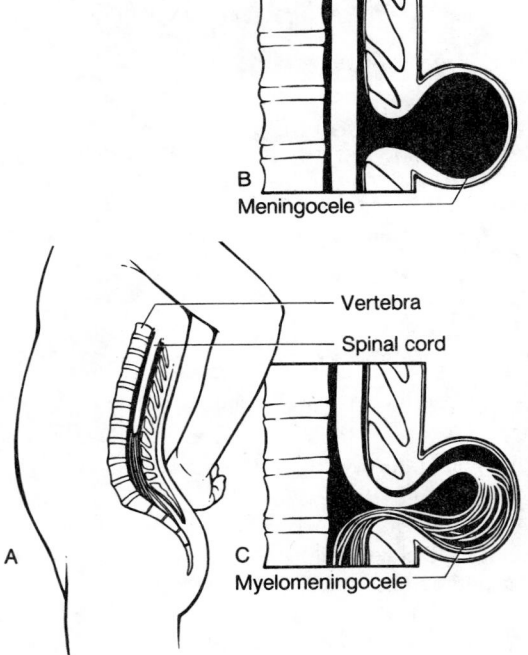

Figure 65-2. Cross-section of a normal spine **(A)** compared with a meningocele **(B)** and a myelomeningocele **(C)**. (May KM, Mahlmeister LR. Maternal and Neonatal Nursing: Family-Centered Care, 3rd ed. Philadelphia: J.B. Lippincott, 1994)

predisposed to infection if the catheter is not properly managed. If kidney damage or other urinary system damage occurs, a urinary tract diversion may be required.

The nurse must pay special attention to positioning, because it is important to prevent musculoskeletal deformities. The nurse also assists the child in range-of-motion exercises (passive or active). The child is usually seen by a physical therapist. Sometimes orthopedic surgery must be performed to correct deformities. The nurse also is important in providing psychological support to the parents and the child.

Nursing Alert

For some reason, children with spina bifida tend to be extremely sensitive to latex. The nurse must make sure they do not come in contact with items such as tourniquets, catheters, rubber bands, gloves, balloons, or various tubes made of latex.

Hydrocephalus

The brain and spinal cord are enclosed in spinal fluid, which circulates constantly. If this circulation is disrupted, fluid collects and causes swelling of the head and brain damage. This is called *hydrocephalus*. This disorder often develops because the brain or spinal cord is not properly developed or because of a spinal cord defect, such as spina bifida. It also can occur as a complication of meningitis, head injury, or cranial hemorrhage.

The symptoms of hydrocephalus include progressive enlargement in the circumference of the head. The sutures between the cranial bones open because of increased accumulation of fluid. Brain tissue atrophies progressively as pressure in the cranial cavity increases. The nurse should be alert to the possibility of seizure activity. The child cannot control voluntary muscle movements and may die of respiratory complications, malnutrition, or infection. Diagnosis of hydrocephalus is made on the basis of lumbar puncture, computed tomography (CT) scan, positron-emission tomography (PET) scan, or magnetic resonance imaging (MRI). Sometimes the CT scan is enhanced by the injection of an intravenous (IV) dye, iohexol (Omnipaque). (Chapter 50 lists precautions in dye use.) An electroencephalogram (EEG) also may be done.

Treatment is to insert a shunt or bypass surgically, which will allow the fluid to circulate around the defect or blockage. This procedure should be performed as soon as possible after birth, because brain damage that occurs is irreversible.

Nursing Considerations. Preoperatively, the child is given nursing care to prevent skin breakdown, and precautions are taken to prevent infection. The child is turned frequently from side to side to prevent aspiration and pressure sores. It is especially important to prevent pressure areas on the enlarged, fragile head.

Gavage feedings or total parenteral nutrition may be given to prevent malnutrition, because this child often has difficulty eating. Feed the child carefully and slowly. Place the child's head, neck, and shoulders on a pillow to distribute the pressure exerted on the infant's head evenly while holding the infant.

The child's head is carefully assessed. Assess the fontanels for tension or fullness; measure and record occipital-frontal head circumference daily (see Chapter 64). It also is important to keep the head clean and dry.

Postoperatively, the child is assessed for signs of shock or hemorrhage; the incisional area is assessed for leakage of spinal fluid. Vital signs are taken according to hospital routine or as directed by the physician. The child is positioned on the side away from the operative side to prevent pressure and damage to the shunt valve. I&O must be recorded accurately to determine if the child is retaining fluids. Usually, hyperalimentation is given.

Because shunts are not always effective, the nurse must observe carefully for any signs of increasing intracranial pressure, such as bulging fontanels, changes in eye appearance, or LOC (level of consciousness). Another frequent complication is infection. Report any

sign of infection immediately. If the shunt is performed before brain damage occurs and if it is successful, the child will be able to lead a normal life.

The parents need to know major developmental milestones of all children to identify any problems their child may have after discharge. They should be encouraged to prepare goals for their child that are appropriate to ability and potential. Focusing on the child's *strengths* is very important. Referral to special education programs may be necessary.

Key Concept

Head measurements (OFC and other measurements, as ordered) are an important aspect of nursing care in hydrocephalus. An increase in head size indicates increasing fluid in the brain. For this reason, the circumference of the head is measured at the same place on the head each time. Mark the head with ink or indicate on a drawing exactly where the measurements are to be taken. In this way, each nurse will measure in the same location, and the measurements can be compared accurately. Document these measurements carefully.

Microcephaly

The microcephalic child has a very small brain. The head tends to be small, and the child is intellectually impaired to a degree determined by the size of the brain. This condition is congenital. No cure is known, and the child is treated symptomatically.

Craniostenosis

Craniostenosis occurs when the fontanels close before they should; the child's skull is too small to allow for normal brain development. If one suture closes and others remain open, malformations can occur.

Craniostenosis must be treated surgically as soon as possible to prevent brain damage. The surgery, which consists of opening the suture lines by craniotomy, is usually successful, although it may need to be repeated. If surgery is done soon enough, the brain usually develops normally.

Febrile Seizures

Febrile seizures are convulsions that may occur in children usually between the ages of 6 months and 3 to 5 years. The etiology of this seizure type is unknown. It is often related to an acute illness in which the body temperature rises above 101.8°F. The seizure most often occurs when the fever is rising. It is unknown why some children experience febrile seizures and others do not; however, there is some evidence that heredity may play a role.

Treatment of febrile seizures is aimed at controlling fever with acetaminophen, tepid sponges, or other measures. Medications also may include lorazepam (Ativan) or phenobarbital. There is controversy about whether long-term antiepileptic drug therapy should be instituted, because febrile seizures are usually benign. Other factors that help determine the appropriateness of long-term drug therapy include EEG findings, age at which the first seizure occurred, recurrences of seizures, and seizure type (tonic-clonic versus other types). Chapter 71 contains a discussion of seizure disorders.

Breath-Holding Spells

A breath-holding spell is an episode during which a child holds his or her breath and becomes unconscious; it usually follows a period of intense crying. The child will often exhibit seizurelike activity of the extremities. It is important to note that this is *not* a true seizure disorder.

A typical breath-holding episode may occur following a fall in which the child hits the head. The child begins to cry violently and holds the breath on exhalation. This results in a period of unconsciousness, with some myoclonic (muscle-jerking) type movements. This activity mimics a seizure and can be frightening for parents. The child then begins to breathe spontaneously and recovers within seconds. Other injuries and tantrums may result in breath-holding episodes. These episodes are benign and are usually outgrown by the age of 5 years.

Disorders of the Eyes, Nose, and Mouth

Strabismus

Strabismus, commonly known as "crossed eyes," is an inability to move the eyes together. Although strabismus is usually congenital, it may develop as a result of a childhood disease. The normal newborn is cross-eyed because control of the eye muscles has not yet developed; therefore, correction may not be advisable until the child is older.

There are two chief classifications of strabismus: *paralytic strabismus* (the muscles of one eye are underactive) and *concomitant strabismus* (both eyes move, but the deviation of the affected eye is always the same). Other terms associated with strabismus are *convergent* (both eyes looking toward the center), *divergent* (both eyes looking outward), and *vertical* (the affected eye [or eyes] moves only on a vertical plane).

Concomitant strabismus may always involve the same eye (*monocular*), both eyes alternately (*alternating*), or both eyes (*binocular*). The person uses the unaffected eye at any particular time. If one eye is used all the time, the other eye does not participate in vision, and the resulting double vision (*diplopia*) causes the unused eye to weaken. In *alternate strabismus*, each eye is dominant at various times and monocular weakness is not as likely to occur. In *latent strabismus*, the muscle imbalance is overcome with great effort, so the child complains of eye strain, headache, and diplopia.

Medical Treatment. The unaffected eye is patched to stimulate the unused eye; corrective eyeglasses (which can be prescribed as early as 1 year of age) are ordered; eye exercises and miotic drugs are prescribed (to contract the pupils of the eyes); and surgical intervention may be done. Treatment begins early to prevent further damage and to improve the child's appearance.

The affected muscles are corrected surgically to match the unaffected muscles. Sometimes a computer is used to more accurately calculate the correction.

Nursing Considerations. Often elbow restraints are all that is needed to protect the eyes, and the child can be up and about soon after surgery. Many children have *photophobia*, which is sensitivity to light; sunglasses may help. If the child is to be on bed rest or is to have the eyes covered following surgery, he or she should be prepared for this preoperatively. To avoid frightening the child whose eyes are covered, you must speak before you touch the child.

Rarely is the strabismus patient hospitalized; this is outpatient surgery. Thus, the parents must be taught preoperative and postoperative care.

Errors of Refraction and Ptosis of the Eyelids

A small child's eye muscles are not developed enough to permit normal accommodation of the pupils. However, because other factors also may be involved, the child should be examined regularly after 3 years or earlier if symptoms appear. Red, puffy, and watering eyes or frequent rubbing of the eyes may indicate difficulty in seeing. The child also may complain of dizziness, headache, or double vision. It is important to determine whether visual difficulties arise from an error of refraction, which can usually be corrected by eyeglasses, or from another problem, such as a brain tumor.

Ptosis, or drooping eyelids, is usually congenital. In most cases, it is corrected by surgery.

Epistaxis

Epistaxis, or nosebleed, is common in children. Foreign objects pushed into the nose, systemic disorders, trauma, and allergy can be causes. Bleeding can usually be stopped by applying pressure or cold compresses across the bridge of the nose. The nose may need to be packed by the physician to stop hemorrhage. The child's blood volume is lower than that of an adult, so a nosebleed is potentially dangerous. Also blood may be swallowed. Any symptoms, such as vomiting "coffee-ground" material, should be reported. Cautery or application of a substance such as silver nitrate ($AgNO_3$) is used to control epistaxis if it occurs frequently.

Nursing Alert

If a child with nosebleed also has a head injury, *do not* stop bleeding without specific physician's orders. *(Rationale: Holding blood inside the nasal cavity can increase intracranial pressure.)*

Cleft Lip and Cleft Palate

Cleft lip and cleft palate are deformities that commonly occur together at birth. They result from failure of the upper lip and palate to close completely during the second and third months of gestation (Fig. 65-3). Each of these defects also may occur separately. Cleft lip is more common in males; cleft palate is more common in females. Evidence also indicates that there is a slight tendency for familial occurrence.

Cleft palate appears as an opening in the roof of the mouth that leads into the nose. The cleft lip may be no more than a notch in the upper lip or may extend up into the nostril on one or both sides. The cleft in the lip may be complete or incomplete and may be complicated by other factors, such as a lip muscle separated by the cleft, skin that is thinner than normal, missing hair follicles and sweat glands, a flattened nostril on the affected side, and a missing part of the jaw and teeth. Mental retardation is *not related* to cleft lip or cleft palate.

Surgical Treatment. Surgical repair of cleft lip is called a *cheiloplasty.* The cleft is sutured, generally when the child is quite young. Very little preoperative preparation is needed with a young infant. The goal of surgery is to restore function to the lip and to improve the child's appearance.

A skin graft or revision of the scar may be necessary later. The scar is quite prominent immediately after the operation but usually becomes unnoticeable as the child grows older. The male may grow a moustache to cover the scar.

Immediate postoperative care is directed toward maintaining the airway, preventing shock or hemorrhage, using proper feeding techniques, and preventing injury to the suture line. Sometimes a Logan bow (curved metal bar) is placed over a repaired cleft lip to

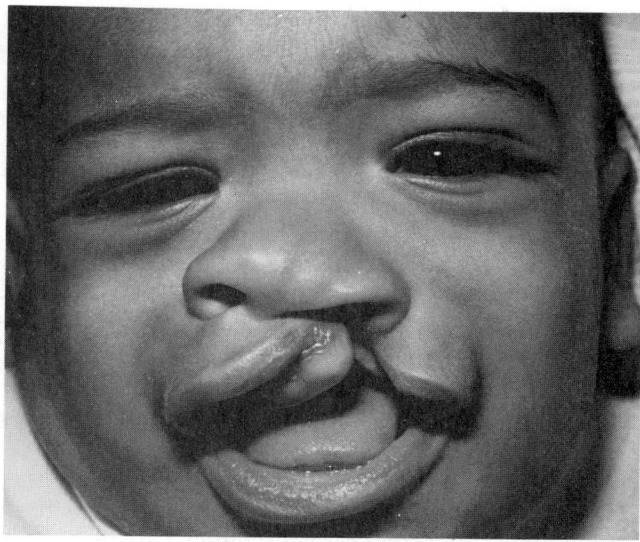

Figure 65-3. Unilateral cleft lip and palate. (Krause CJ. et al. Aesthetic facial surgery. Philadelphia, J.B. Lippincott, 1991.)

decrease tension on the suture line. Often these children need to have ventilating tubes (polyethylene [PE] tubes) inserted in the tympanic membrane to reduce the incidence of frequent ear infection. A restraint device often is needed to keep the child from rubbing the suture line.

Surgical repair of a cleft palate is called a *palatoplasty.* It is done when the child is 2 to 6 years old. The goals of this surgery are to restore normal speech, avoid damage to the suture line of the lip, and close the palate as much as possible. The palate may be repaired surgically by placement of a graft or with the use of a dental prosthesis, which is either attached to the teeth or provides replacement for the missing teeth and part of the jaw. The prosthesis aids speech by closing the hole between mouth and nose. Surgical repair of the palate is usually done in one procedure, but it may be carried out in several stages if the cleft is severe.

Dental surgery is often necessary to rebuild missing gums and replace missing teeth. The prosthetic palate may include prosthetic teeth. The mouth must be kept very clean as a protection against tooth decay and infection. Consistent dental care is needed.

Rhinoplasty, which is repair of the nose, is at times necessary; however, this is usually not done until the person is an adolescent.

Speech Therapy. Defective speech is one challenge faced by the child with a cleft palate. A cleft lip alone generally does not present speech problems.

The child will not be able to produce some speech sounds until the palate is repaired. The parents and nurse should speak clearly to the child and listen carefully to what the child is saying. The speech therapist can give guidelines about appropriate exercises.

Speech aids to prevent air flow between the nose and mouth are useful. These aids are attached to a palate prosthesis and extend back into the throat. The speech aid does not move as the uvula would move in normal speech. Instead, the child is trained to make the throat move to produce sounds and learn to speak. The child may be fitted for the aid as soon as he or she has enough teeth to anchor the prosthesis. The prosthesis is made of soft plastic and is removed and cleaned after eating. It is changed approximately every 2 years to fit the child's growing mouth. Sometimes the surgeon uses a prosthetic palate until the child is older and then does surgical palate repair.

Nursing Considerations. Nursing care begins at birth and involves the actual care and family teaching.

Feeding the Child. Part of the soft palate is missing in cleft palate, and the uvula is almost always absent, as is a part of the hard palate. As a result, the mouth and throat are not separated from the nose. Thus, if the baby is fed by usual methods, milk is regurgitated through the nose. If he or she also has a cleft lip, sucking is not normal.

Some babies can be fed by using a soft nipple with large holes. The baby is held upright so that milk is not drawn into the nose. Occasionally a special flattened nipple (duckbill nipple) or a cleft palate nipple with a flap to cover the hole in the palate is used. In other cases, a special feeder is used. Figure 65-4 illustrates one type of feeder.

The following are recommendations for feeding these infants:

- Feed slowly in small amounts, and bubble frequently.
- Feed some clear water last.
- Hold the infant upright.
- Clean the mouth and cleft carefully after each feeding.
- Dilute solids and spoonfeed.
- In extreme cases, gavage feeding may be necessary until part of the palate is covered.
- Prevent aspiration.

Providing Oral Hygiene. Oral hygiene is essential. A small infant may be given sterile water after feeding; the older child may be encouraged to use mouthwash and to brush the teeth often.

Preventing Infections. Because the pathway is open between the mouth and nose, pressure in the eustachian tubes is not equalized by swallowing. Infections develop easily and may cause partial hearing loss. Parents should be instructed in ways to prevent ear infections in their child. The child should be protected from colds and upper respiratory infections.

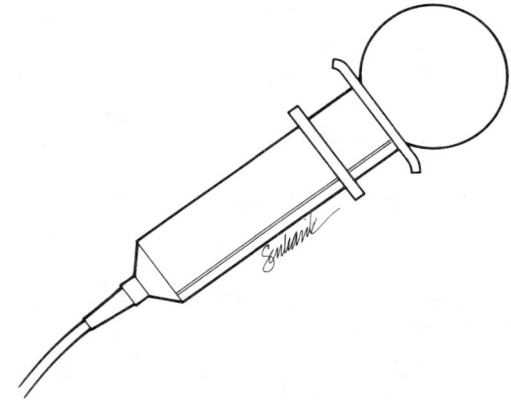

Figure 65-4. A Brecht feeder allows formula to pass directly to the neonate's posterior oropharynx. (May KM, Mahlmeister LR. Maternal and Neonatal Nursing: Family-Centered Care, 3rd ed. Philadelphia: J.B. Lippincott, 1994)

Addressing Emotional Aspects. How the child adjusts to a cleft lip or palate depends largely on how parents and other people react to the deformity. It is a difficult situation for parents. Parents often have preconceived ideas as to what their baby may look like, and the child with cleft lip or palate may not meet that expectation. Group discussion with other parents who have faced the same problem provides support. Parents can learn to help their child deal with teasing. (Chapter 67 contains a discussion of emotional aspects of children who are physically challenged.)

Providing Postoperative Care. Nursing care is aimed at preventing strain on the suture line and preventing deformities or complications. Nursing skill guidelines in postoperative care are given in the accompanying box.

Baby Bottle Syndrome

If bottle feeding continues after the child has teeth or if the bottle is used as a pacifier, a deformity called *baby bottle syndrome* (nursing bottle mouth) can occur. Baby bottle syndrome is caused by the contents of the bottle continually coming in contact with the teeth for prolonged periods of time, resulting in numerous dental caries. This condition most frequently occurs in children between 18 and 36 months of age. It is important for the nurse to teach parents how to prevent this condition. Subjects to be taught are listed in the accompanying box.

Tonsillitis

Tonsillitis, an inflammation of the tonsils, is caused by *Streptococcus* or *Staphylococcus* organisms. Symptoms include a sore, reddened throat, with swelling and sometimes pustules on the tonsils. Swallowing is difficult, and the patient's WBC and temperature are elevated. A throat culture is done to determine the offend-

Nursing Skill Guidelines
Providing Postoperative Care in Cheiloplasty and Palatoplasty

Care Specific to Cheiloplasty (Cleft Lip Repair)

◆ Apply tongue blade or other arm restraints. *(Reason: This will prevent child from bending the elbows to touch suture line.)*

◆ Position child on the back or side but not the abdomen. *(Reason: This prevents child from rubbing the surgical site on the bed.)*

◆ Cleanse suture line after each feeding and as necessary with prescribed solution. *(Reason: This promotes healing and prevents undue scarring.)*

◆ Try to prevent unnecessary crying. *(Reason: This will avoid pull on suture line.)*

◆ Provide quiet diversion whenever possible.

◆ Give glucose water first, then formula, as per physician's orders. Feed child with Brecht nipple, preemie nipple, medicine dropper, syringe, or small spoon, depending on extent of repair, age of child, and physician's order. *(Reason: This prevents injury to surgical site, while providing adequate nutrition and medications.)*

◆ Give child water after formula. *(Reason: Clear away any mucus that has formed, and promote healing of the site.)*

◆ Unless ordered by physician, do not use straws. *(Reason: Use of straw may put pressure on surgical site from the sucking motion.)*

Care Specific to Palatoplasty (Cleft Palate Repair)

◆ Provide nursing care similar to cleft lip repair *except:*

◆ Place child on abdomen or side, not on the back. *(Reason: This will decrease choking and danger of aspiration.)*

◆ Keep mouth clean and free from irritation. *(Reason: The suture line is inside the mouth. Cleanliness helps promote healing.)*

◆ If child is old enough to understand, tell him or her not to rub the site with the tongue. *(Reason: This will help maintain integrity of suture line and promote healing.)*

◆ The child may be NPO for the first 24–48 hours after surgery. The diet is then advanced to liquids. This may be necessary for 10–14 days postoperatively. After liquids are tolerated and the physician's order is received, the diet may be advanced to soft solids. Be sure the child does not have potato chips, popcorn, candy, or other hard or scratchy foods. Teach parents about diet restrictions. *(Reason: Some foods may damage suture line.)*

◆ Discourage sucking and blowing. Do not feed child with nipple or straw; fluids are best taken from a cup. *(Reason: Sucking can cause strain on suture line; blowing can force fluids into eustachian tube.)*

◆ Do not use food with extremes in temperatures. *(Reason: The child may not have sensation in the roof of the mouth and extremely hot or cold foods could cause injury.)*

◆ Feed child from the side of a spoon. Do not insert spoon into mouth. *(Reason: The spoon could damage the suture line.)*

◆ Be sure to do parent teaching about patient care and diet restrictions before discharge. *(Reason: The parents will be providing care after discharge. Teaching them in the hospital provides a comfortable setting in which to practice.)*

◆ Encourage parents to visit often.

Keys to Patient/Family Teaching
Prevention of Baby Bottle Syndrome

Family teaching to prevent baby bottle syndrome includes the following:

◆ Infants should not take a bottle to bed or fall asleep with a bottle. Never prop a bottle.

◆ The infant's mouth should be cleaned or teeth brushed after feeding.

◆ Infants should be weaned to a cup by 1 year of age.

◆ Children should not be allowed to walk around with a bottle.

◆ Begin regular dental checkups after tooth eruption.

◆ Give juice in a cup as early as possible.

◆ Keep pacifiers clean.

ing organism, and drug sensitivity tests are run to determine the treatment of choice.

Key Concept

Because the tonsils are so close to the eustachian tube, tonsillitis can easily spread to the middle ear and cause otitis media. Infants and toddlers are most often affected, because their eustachian tube is short and straight and does not drain well.

Medical and Surgical Treatment. The patient is kept in a high-humidity environment, and large doses of antibiotics are given. If the child has difficulty swallowing, a soft diet may be offered. Fluids are encouraged, and acetaminophen (Tylenol) is given to lower temperature and relieve discomfort.

If the child has had numerous streptococcal infections in a short time, removal of the tonsils (*tonsillectomy*) may be indicated, although this is controversial. Tonsillectomy also may be done in the case of a recurring peritonsillar (around the tonsil) abscess. Usually, tonsillectomy is not done following a single episode of tonsillitis. Removal of the tonsils and adenoids is called a *tonsillectomy* and *adenoidectomy* (T&A).

Nursing Considerations. Most T&A surgery is performed in same-day surgery centers. Before surgery, the child must be free of upper respiratory infections. Accurate assessment is necessary on admission.

The parents are instructed in preoperative care that is to be given at home: Routine preparation includes giving the child nothing by mouth after midnight. The nurse is often asked to give preoperative instructions. When the child arrives at the facility, the nurse completes preoperative care. Preoperative medication is not usually given to young children.

Postoperative nursing care is directed at preventing hemorrhage, the most common complication. The nurse must observe the child for spitting up of a great deal of bloody sputum or vomiting of "coffee-ground" material. Blood may be swallowed, so some vomiting of dark blood is not unusual. Bloody sputum or vomiting must be assessed (see box). The nurse should position the child on the side or abdomen or with the head of the bed elevated to prevent aspiration.

Fluids should be encouraged after the child is awake and fully responding. Clear fluids are best; milk tends to form a film in the throat. Usually ice pops, soda pop, fruit drinks, gelatins, and sherbet are used and are well accepted by children.

> **Nursing Alert**
>
> Red juices and frozen pops should be avoided for the postoperative T&A patient. Emesis of red juice may be difficult to differentiate from bloody emesis.

Many physicians write a "diet as tolerated" order. A special pediatric diet is often available, so the child can help choose which foods and liquids are most appealing. The child should not drink fluids through a straw. Normal drinking and swallowing promote healing. (Sucking also can dislodge clots or stitches and lead to hemorrhage.) Gum chewing also may be encouraged if supervised carefully; chewing gum promotes the flow of saliva, which is soothing and encourages healing. Use pain medications as needed so that the child can drink more comfortably and rest better. An elevated temperature postoperatively may indicate *dehydration* and the need to force fluids. This elevation also may point to infection, although it is not common.

> **Keys to Nursing Assessment**
> **Signs of Oral–Nasal Hemorrhage**
>
> ◆ Frequent swallowing
> ◆ Bright red blood or partially digested blood in the emesis ("coffee ground" emesis)
> ◆ Vital signs; watch for the usual signs of shock— lowered blood pressure, increased pulse, panic, pallor, cyanosis
> ◆ Nausea or vomiting
> ◆ Assess amount, frequency, color, and consistency of emesis

The patient is usually discharged the day of or the day after surgery. Sometimes an antibiotic prescription may be given as prevention against infection. Home care instructions should be explained to the parents, including signs of hemorrhage and respiratory distress. The child should continue with high fluid intake and soft foods. He or she should play quietly and rest in bed much of the time for approximately 1 week before returning to school or other normal activities.

Sensory System Disorders

Otitis Media

Otitis media is a middle-ear infection resulting from fluid accumulation. It is the most common bacterial infection of early childhood. Seventy to 80% of all children have at least one episode of otitis media.

It may be defined as *acute* if its onset is rapid and short, *subacute* if fluid involvement lasts between 3 weeks and 3 months, and *chronic* if it lasts longer than 3 months. Complications include hearing loss, scarred or ruptured tympanic membrane, inner ear infection, mastoiditis, or meningitis.

Dysfunction of the eustachian tube, which causes accumulation of fluid, may be caused by bacterial infections, viral nasopharyngitis, enlargement of lymphoid tissue in the nasopharynx area, tumors, foreign bodies, allergies, and other physiologic factors in the infant. "Propping" of a baby's bottle also may allow fluid to flow through the eustachian tube and cause otitis media.

Pain may or may not be present. In an infant, this may be expressed by pulling or scratching the ear and being irritable. Older children will complain of pain. Signs of infection, swollen glands, and loss of appetite, sometimes with vomiting, are other symptoms.

Definite diagnosis is made when a bulging tympanic membrane is seen on otoscopic examination. Landmarks of the bony prominences are obscured. If the eardrum ruptures, there may be bleeding or purulent (containing pus) drainage.

The most serious complication of otitis media is loss of hearing, which may be permanent. In many children, the hearing loss may go undetected until they enter school. Other rare complications include mastoiditis (inflammation of the mastoid process), chronic otitis media, and occasionally encephalitis or meningitis.

Medical and Surgical Treatment. Treatment of otitis media involves restoring the normal function of the eustachian tube and maintaining or improving hearing. A PE tube is inserted as a temporary or permanent accessory eustachian tube, allowing drainage of the accumulated fluid in the middle ear and equalization of pressure on each side of the eardrum. Hearing is restored after placement of PE tubes. The patient with a PE tube must not get water into the ears when swimming or taking a shower.

PE tubes (ventilating tubes) are placed by a physician called an *otolaryngologist* (an ear, nose, and throat specialist) as an outpatient procedure. PE tubes allow the pressure within the ear to equalize with atmospheric pressure. They also promote drying of the middle ear cavity.

Antihistamines and decongestants may be administered, and warm, moist packs are applied. Acetaminophen for fever and (if the patient is older than 6 years) codeine for pain may be prescribed. Antibiotics are prescribed. After 10 days, the child's ears are inspected by the physician or nurse practitioner. If the tympanic membrane remains reddened or if other symptoms persist, another course of antibiotic therapy may be indicated.

Surgical procedures in otitis media and its complications are *tympanoplasty* (reconstruction of the middle ear, either with the placement of a homograft transplant of the structure or with a prosthesis) and *myringoplasty* (reconstruction of the eardrum, usually with a graft of temporalis fascia).

Cardiovascular Disorders

Disorders of the cardiovascular system can be a result of congenital heart defects, hemorrhage, fluid and electrolyte imbalance, neurologic disorders, respiratory illnesses, or ingestion of poisons. These can quickly result in congestive heart failure and shock in the infant or small child.

Heart Defects

Some children are born with a structural abnormality of the heart. This is called congenital cardiac anomaly. Various types of heart defects may occur. Some of these defects are associated with other disorders, such as Down syndrome or fetal alcohol syndrome. An infant with a significant defect will show evidence of congestive heart failure or poor oxygen tissue perfusion. This is the result of abnormal shunting of blood between the chambers of the heart.

The infant with a heart defect may show signs of cyanosis, depending on the origin of the condition. Other symptoms may include dyspnea, coughing or choking, pulse rate over 200, heart murmurs, failure to gain weight, difficulty in feeding, listlessness, and a general sickly appearance. The child should be observed for symptoms of respiratory distress and change in pulse rate and rhythm.

> **Key Concept**
>
> Some congenital heart anomalies cause *cyanosis*. Others do not and are called *acyanotic*.

The older child often has poor physical development, low tolerance to physical activity, clubbing of fingers and toes, cyanosis in certain cases, elevated blood pressure and pulse rate, and possibly an enlarged heart. Frequently the child may need to squat or sit to facilitate breathing, especially on exertion. Cyanosis is more difficult to determine in dark-skinned patients. No matter what the skin tone, in cyanosis a definite duskiness is present in the skin, lips, and nailbeds.

Definite diagnosis is made by auscultation (listening for heart sounds), x-ray studies, ECG, careful physical examination, and a complete history. At times, cardiac catheterization and angiocardiography may be done. However, because these procedures carry some risk, they are not done unless necessary.

Several nursing diagnoses are commonly seen in children with congenital heart defects:

◆ Impaired Gas Exchange related to impaired circulation
◆ Fluid Volume Excess related to decreased kidney perfusion
◆ Ineffective Family Coping related to life-threatening diagnosis
◆ Altered Nutrition, Less than Body Requirements related to fatigue
◆ Altered Growth and Development related to inadequate nutritional intake

Ventricular Septal Defects. Ventricular septal defects are the most frequent congenital anomaly of the circulatory system (Fig. 65-5). There is an abnormal opening between the left and right ventricles. This defect is usually acyanotic because the greater pressure in the left ventricle causes a shunt from left to right, so the blood

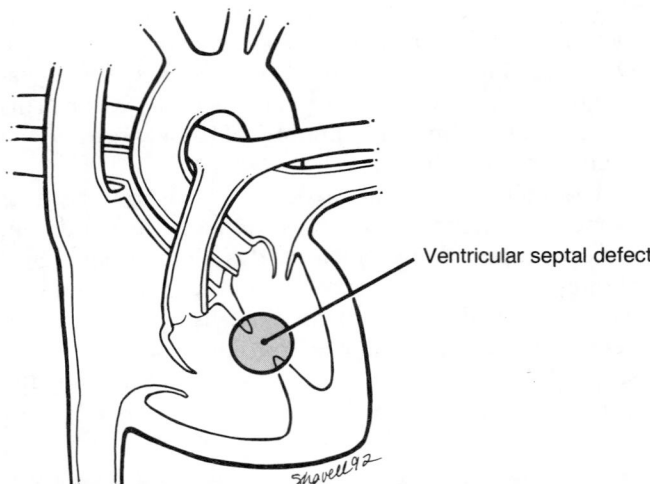

Figure 65-5. In a ventricular septal defect, there is a hole in the wall of the septum that separates the left ventricle from the right ventricle. Normally, the deoxygenated blood flows through the superior vena cava and inferior vena cava into the right atrium, right ventricle, and pulmonary artery. In a ventricular septal defect, some of the oxygen-rich blood from the left ventricle flows through the defect and recirculates through the lungs. (Jackson DB and Saunders RB. Child Health Nursing: A Comprehensive Approach to the Care of Children and Their Families. Philadelphia: J.B. Lippincott, 1993)

pumped to the body is oxygenated. If pulmonary hypertension exists, the shunt may go the other way, and the patient will be cyanotic. These defects can usually be corrected in open-heart surgery by placing a patch (usually of Teflon) into the opening. If the opening is small and there is no pulmonary hypertension, the child may be asymptomatic. Surgery may be unnecessary or may be postponed until the child is older. In some cases, an "umbrella" occluder may be placed via catheter and surgery avoided or postponed.

Atrial Septal Defects. An atrial septal defect is an abnormal opening between the right and left atria. The majority of these defects occur in the area of the foramen ovale (Fig. 65-6). Those lower in the septum are more likely to involve the mitral and tricuspid valves and the septum. Usually, the shunt is from left to right, so the patient is acyanotic. These defects are closed surgically or with an occluder unless there is severe pulmonary hypertension. If the valves are involved, the operation is much more complicated and may include valve replacement.

Patent Ductus Arteriosus (PDA). The ductus arteriosus is a vessel between the aorta and the pulmonary artery that normally closes before birth or very soon after. (This ductus allows the prenatal circulation to bypass the lungs.) When it remains open (patent), it is called

patent ductus arteriosus (Fig. 65-7). When the left ventricle pumps blood into the aorta, which should go to the body, some of that oxygenated blood is returned to the pulmonary circulation via the patent ductus, because of the higher pressure in the aorta. This increases the pressure in the lungs, as well as the volume of (oxygenated) blood. The heart must work harder and the child lacks oxygen in body cells.

The ductus may be closed with a foam plug or an umbrella occluder placed via cardiac catheterization. If these measures do not work, surgical ligation and severing of the ductus correct this defect. This closed-heart procedure was one of the first surgical procedures performed. It is usually done even if the patient does not show symptoms because of the danger of subacute bacterial endocarditis (SBE).

Transposition of the Great Vessels. In transposition, the aorta and the pulmonary artery are reversed, so each connects to the wrong side of the heart. If no shunts or septal defects exist, the child will die early because of lack of sufficient oxygenation to the cells of the body because only unoxygenated blood is circulated systemically. Surgical correction is not always successful but should be attempted.

Tetralogy of Fallot. Tetralogy of Fallot is a combination of four major defects: *pulmonary stenosis* (narrowing of the pulmonary artery), which leads to pulmonary hypertension; *ventricular septal defect, overriding aorta,*

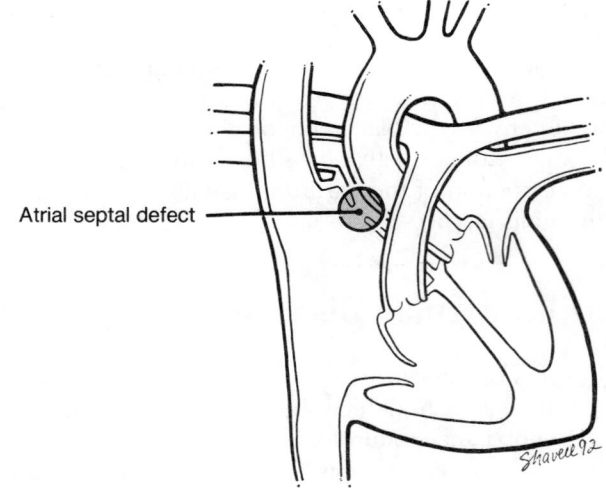

Figure 65-6. In an atrial septal defect, there is an abnormal communication between the right atrium and left atrium, allowing blood to be shunted from left to right through the atrial septum. This hole is usually in the area of the foramen ovale, which normally closes at birth. (Jackson DB and Saunders RB. Child Health Nursing: A Comprehensive Approach to the Care of Children and Their Families. Philadelphia: J.B. Lippincott, 1993)

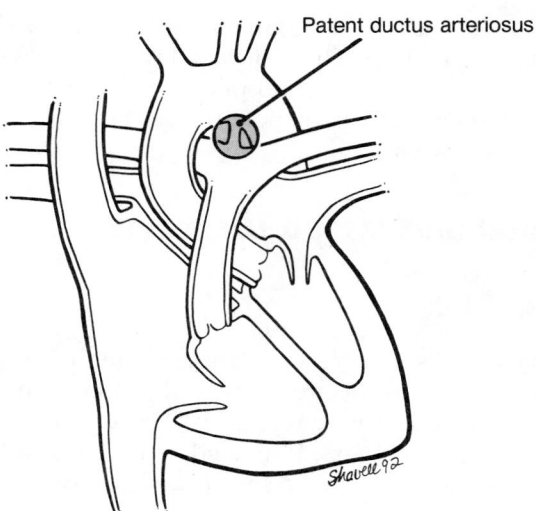

Figure 65-7. In patent ductus arteriosus, a connection (shown in the circle) exists between the aorta and pulmonary artery. This ductus should close at birth, but remains open (patent). Pressure is higher in the aorta than the pulmonary artery, and blood flows from the aorta through the patent ductus arteriosus into the pulmonary artery. This means there is an excess volume of blood flowing through the lungs and a lack of oxygenated blood to the body. (Jackson DB and Saunders RB. Child Health Nursing: A Comprehensive Approach to the Care of Children and Their Families. Philadelphia: J.B. Lippincott, 1993)

also called dextroposition of the aorta (the aorta receives venous and oxygenated blood); and *right ventricular hypertrophy.* The right ventricle is enlarged because the heart must pump harder to compensate for the unoxygenated blood and to pump blood into the lungs.

The patient with a severe defect in any of these areas is cyanotic and shows other symptoms, such as squatting to breathe, convex fingernails, and clubbed fingers. Often this child does not survive beyond 2 years of age. If the child survives, surgical procedures may correct some of the defects, depending on their severity. The corrective surgery is complicated and is usually deferred until the child is at least 6 years old. Palliative surgery may be performed earlier to provide an artificial patent ductus arteriosus by means of a shunt. This operation (the original "blue-baby" operation) increases blood flow to the lungs and reduces cyanosis and dyspnea.

Pulmonary Stenosis. Pulmonary stenosis is the narrowing of the right ventricular overflow tract (Fig. 65-8), which decreases blood flow into the lungs. On rare occasions, pulmonary stenosis also involves a narrowing (stenosis) of the pulmonary artery. If symptoms are present, the valve is surgically corrected (*commissurotomy*). Closed- or open-heart surgery may be indi-

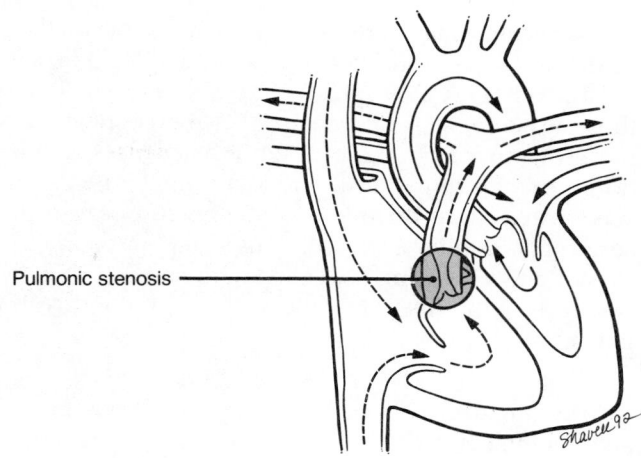

Figure 65-8. In pulmonary stenosis, the right ventricular outflow tract narrows. (Jackson DB and Saunders RB. Child Health Nursing: A Comprehensive Approach to the Care of Children and Their Families. Philadelphia: J.B. Lippincott, 1993)

cated, and the valve may be replaced with an artificial valve. If the pulmonary artery is greatly stenosed, a vessel graft may be done.

Aortic Stenosis. In aortic stenosis, an aortic valve malfunction causes the heart to work harder to pump blood to the body. The treatment is similar to that for pulmonary stenosis.

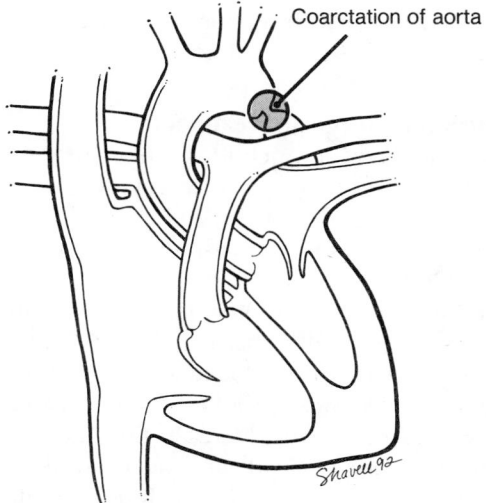

Figure 65-9. In coarctation of the aorta, there is an abnormal narrowing (shown in the circle) of the aorta that causes an obstruction to the blood flow from the left side of the heart. Because of this narrowing, the pressure in the aorta and left ventricle increases. To help carry blood through the narrowing, blood vessels around it and the left ventricle enlarge. (Jackson DB and Saunders RB. Child Health Nursing: A Comprehensive Approach to the Care of Children and Their Families. Philadelphia: J.B. Lippincott, 1993)

Coarctation of the Aorta. In coarctation (constriction) of the aorta, the aorta narrows, and the blood flow is obstructed (Fig. 65-9). The symptoms are similar to those of aortic stenosis, except that the coarctation is usually further from the heart and thus causes circulation problems in the arms and head. In children, conservative medical treatment is attempted because the surgical procedure is difficult. Surgical correction consists of either excising the coarctation and suturing the two ends of the vessel together or using a blood vessel graft.

Tricuspid Atresia. Tricuspid atresia is the absence of an opening between the right atrium and the right ventricle, which decreases pulmonary circulation because the only routes by which the blood can get to the lungs are through a ventricular septal defect, a patent ductus, or the bronchial vessels. This restriction leads to pulmonary hypertension. The child will die soon after birth unless corrective surgery is performed. Because oxygenated blood mixes with unoxygenated blood, the child is cyanotic.

Anomalous Venous Return. In anomalous venous return, pulmonary veins empty into the right half of the heart instead of the left half, bringing oxygenated blood to the wrong side of the heart. If all the pulmonary vessels empty in this way, there must be an accompanying septal defect or the child will die. If some of the vessels empty on the wrong side of the heart, the child will be cyanotic, and surgical correction will be necessary. This child usually suffers from pulmonary hypertension.

Medical and Surgical Treatment

Generally, the older a child is when surgery is performed, the better the prognosis. However, if a child is exhibiting symptoms of heart failure, pulmonary hypertension, or severe cyanosis, surgery must be performed earlier.

Sometimes, palliative surgery is performed early, and corrective surgery is attempted when the child is older. In some cases activity is reduced to lessen strain on the heart, and medications are administered to strengthen the activity of the heart, decrease fluid accumulation and workload of the heart, and decrease the chance of infection. Medications may include digitalis compounds, diuretics, and antibotics. Some children regularly receive oxygen. The child is brought to the best possible physical and mental condition before surgery is carried out.

In some cases of open-heart surgery, it is necessary to bypass the heart circulation by means of a heart-lung pump (pump oxygenator). Heart action is temporarily stopped. Closed-heart surgery is much safer, although any open-chest surgery is serious.

Surgery may be done under *hypothermic* (reduced body temperature, which slows all body processes) or *hyperbaric* (increased atmospheric pressure, which enables the blood to carry more oxygen) conditions.

Blood and Lymph Disorders

Kawasaki Disease

Kawasaki disease (mucocutaneous lymph node syndrome) is a disorder resulting in inflammation of the blood vessels (vasculitis), which occurs in children younger than 5 years. Untreated, children with Kawasaki disease may develop severe cardiac problems. The cause of this disease is unknown.

Symptoms of Kawasaki disease include the following:

◆ Prolonged fever of 5 days or more
◆ Red and infected eyes
◆ "Strawberry tongue" and cracked, dry lips and oral mucous membranes
◆ Edema of hands and feet: reddened and peeling soles and palms
◆ Rash, particularly in perineal area
◆ Swollen lymph nodes

Diagnosis of Kawasaki disease is based on assessment of the previously listed symptoms. Blood work may reveal increased ESR, anemia, and abnormal urinalysis.

Medical treatment includes administration of acetaminophen and gamma globulin. Nursing care is supportive and should include frequent oral care, skin care, and cardiac monitoring.

Anemias

Anemia is a condition of an abnormally low number of red blood cells, low content of hemoglobin, or a defect in red cell function. Anemia also may be caused by a combination of these factors. There are many types of anemia; the most frequent childhood type is iron-deficiency anemia (see Chapter 75). Many doctors recommend an iron-fortified formula for all babies in an effort to prevent this condition. Some anemias respond to vitamins and iron. The child and family must be taught to follow a nutritious diet, with emphasis on eating meat or other complete proteins, vegetables, and fruits. Some anemias are seen when bottle feeding continues for too long, and the child does not get other needed foods. Anemia also can result from hemorrhage, hemolytic disease, malabsorption of vitamin B_{12}, and hereditary factors.

Sickle Cell Anemia

Sickle cell anemia is hereditary and is seen primarily in people of African descent. It is a recessive trait, so only a *small percentage of people show any symptoms.* It is characterized by red blood cells that become abnormally shaped like a "sickle" when hypoxia occurs. The sickle shape of the cells allows for clumping, and capillaries are closed by clumps of blood cells. Because the blood cannot circulate properly and carry oxygen to the cells of the body, anemia results. People with a severe active form of the disease will probably not live past 40 years of age.

In addition to anemia, the person with active sickle cell disease, called *sicklemia,* shows symptoms of jaundice, ulcerated areas around the ankles, and nausea and vomiting. Hemiplegia or other symptoms of cerebral vascular insufficiency may be present.

The treatment is symptomatic. Blood transfusions are given to relieve painful episodes and increase the hemoglobin level. The patient with severe sickle cell anemia should avoid high altitudes and, when traveling by air, should fly only in a pressurized cabin. (Chapter 75 discusses this condition in more detail.)

Purpura

Idiopathic thrombocytopenic purpura (ITP) is the most common acquired bleeding disorder of childhood. The acute form is seen most often in children between the ages of 3 and 7 years. Symptoms include easy bruising, often without an obvious cause, petechiae (tiny internal hemorrhages) on the mucous membranes, frequent nose bleeds, and bleeding into the bladder or GI tract. Symptoms appear suddenly, and the child may look as though he or she has been physically beaten.

The disease is seldom fatal in children. In most cases symptoms run an acute course and then clear, with recovery within 6 weeks. The greatest risk is intracranial hemorrhage (less than 5% of cases). Sometimes the cause of the disease cannot be identified, although an affected mother can transmit it to her fetus.

Nursing Considerations. Nursing care involves close observation for hemorrhage, avoidance of injury, and bed rest. The patient is not given intramuscular injections because of danger of hematoma formation. Rectal temperatures or enemas are not recommended because of the possiblity of trauma to the mucous membranes. Transfusions of platelets are of limited benefit. The patient may receive steroids. In extreme cases, a splenectomy, which is surgical removal of the spleen, is performed.

Keep the side rails up and pad them. A soft tooth brush should be used to brush teeth to avoid injury to the gums. Urinary catheterization should be avoided, because of the danger of hemorrhage and infection. Invasive procedures, such as venipuncture, should be *avoided* if at all possible for the same reasons. If venipuncture must be done, to prevent hemorrhage, pressure should be exerted on the puncture site for *at least 20 minutes* after inserting the needle.

Hemophilia

Hemophilia is a hereditary bleeding disorder in which there is a deficiency in one of the factors necessary for blood clotting. Internal and external hemorrhage can occur with even a minor injury. Bleeding into joints, most commonly the knee, ankle, and elbow, results in severe pain. Death can occur as a result of hemorrhage.

Nursing Considerations. The nurse should try to prevent injury to the child by gentle handling and should use measures to try to stop hemorrhage. Tympanic temperatures are taken to reduce the risk of hemorrhage. Periodic transfusions of blood products may be required.

In the past, many children with hemophilia died at an early age; today, however, because of improved management, many reach adulthood and middle age.

The family must be taught to recognize the symptoms of bleeding, to get medical assistance immediately when needed, and to protect the child from injury without being overprotective.

Leukemia

Leukemia is a group of associated disorders characterized by malignancies in the bone marrow and lymphatic system. It is classified into two major types, depending on the specific cell involved: *acute lymphocytic (lymphoid) leukemia* (ALL) and *acute myelogenous leukemia* (AML). ALL is sometimes called lymphatic, lymphoblastic, stem-cell, or blast-cell leukemia.

With today's improved antileukemic drugs and intensive treatment, a remission rate of 85% to 95% can be induced in ALL; many of these children will be cured. The survival rate for AML is not as high, although about 75% of these children will experience at least one remission. These statistics are in sharp contrast to those of only a few years ago. Factors relating to prognosis include type of cell involved (*histologic type*; ALL has a better prognosis), *age at onset* (the child between 2 and 8 years of age has a better prognosis), *initial white blood count* (a low white blood count has a better prognosis), the child's *sex* (females have a better prognosis), and specifically in AML, length of *time needed* to achieve remission (rapid remission usually means a better prognosis).

ALL is the most common form of the disease seen in children and is more common in males and in children younger than 5 years old. Normal bone marrow is replaced by primitive cells incapable of manufacturing red blood cells. The excessive number of WBCs also can destroy normal red blood cells. The patient is severely anemic and bleeds readily. Death from hemorrhage is a possibility because of insufficient platelets. Because white cells are defective, the child is highly susceptible to infection, and this, rather than the leukemia itself, may be the cause of death. The untreated child generally does not live longer than 4 to 6 months after the onset of ALL.

AML accounts for 10% to 20% of childhood leukemias. AML also is called granulocytic, myelocytic, monocytic, myelogenous, monoblastic, or monomyeloblastic leukemia. AML carries a less favorable prognosis than ALL.

A diagnosis is made on the basis of medical history, which often indicates sudden illness with general malaise, high fever, joint pains, bleeding from body orifices, and enlargement of the liver, spleen, and lymph nodes. The child is pale and lethargic and bruises easily. Instead, the child may become ill gradually, with increasing weakness and pallor. The white blood count is usually elevated, with characteristic abnormal cells. The patient is anemic, with a hemoglobin as low as 4g to 8g. Positive diagnosis can be made by bone marrow and lymph node biopsies.

Medical and Surgical Treatment. *Chemotherapy.* Generally, the child is managed by chemotherapy. Drugs are now given in higher doses and for longer periods than formerly to prevent relapse. Remissions are not uncommon. The length of survival seems to be directly related to the length of remission and to how soon the remission occurs after therapy is begun.

Antineoplastic (anticancer) drugs must be carefully administered. Many drugs are given IV through a central line. Oral drugs are sometimes used, alone or in combination with IV therapy. Key medications are listed in the accompanying box.

Side effects and adverse reactions of chemotherapy include alopecia (loss of hair), bleeding, oliguria (low urine volume), retention of fluids, edema, anorexia (loss of appetite), nausea and vomiting, rashes and skin lesions, severe headache, fluctuations in body temperature, and tissue necrosis around the injection site. Inflammation and ulceration of the GI tract may occur, with ulcerated sores in the mouth often the first symptom. Chapter 76 describes cancer treatment in detail. Check the child's mouth each day with a flashlight to make sure there are no ulcerations, reddened areas, or white patches. Any unusual symptoms should be reported immediately.

Platelet Therapy. Platelet apheresis is a process through which platelets only are removed from a donor's blood. The amount removed is equivalent to that which would be collected from 6 to 10 U of whole blood. (A well

person can safely donate platelets up to twice a week for short periods of time.) The platelets are then transfused into the leukemic child. It is hoped that platelet therapy will forestall death by hemorrhage until a chemotherapeutic cure is found.

> ### Key Concept
> The only known food that helps to build platelets is fresh parsley. Encourage the parents to feed the child parsley daily.

X-Ray Therapy. X-ray therapy may be a part of the regimen; however, it can cause vomiting, diarrhea, severe electrolyte imbalance, and rapid dehydration in children.

Combination Chemotherapy and Radiation. In some cases, chemotherapeutic agents and radiation are combined for maximum effectiveness. This may be hard on the patient and may reduce the antibody levels to the point at which infections occur. The patient may be kept in the hospital in protective isolation during this treatment and during bone marrow transplant (see Chapter 51).

Bone Marrow Transplant. If the child does not improve with other treatments, a bone marrow transplant may be done. The donor marrow usually is removed from the pelvic bones. Donor marrow must match the recipient; family members are most likely to match. A bone marrow transplant may be considered a last resort, but up to 70% of children survive more than 2 years after transplantation.

Bone marrow is transplanted through an IV infusion, similar to a blood transfusion. The transplanted marrow naturally grafts itself within the patient's bones, replacing diseased marrow and making new blood cells.

Nursing Considerations. Treat the symptoms, and make the child as comfortable as possible, encouraging the child to be as active as the disease will permit. Institute means to prevent infection or injury. Rectal temperatures are *not* taken, because of the danger of injury. A cough or any other symptom of an upper respiratory infection must be reported immediately. *Any* infection can result in generalized septicemia and can cause death. Nursing care of patients receiving chemotherapy, radiation, and blood tranfusions is discussed in Chapters 75 and 76.

The child and family need skilled emotional support. Help the parents accept the course of the disease; *always* offer hope of remission. The sick child is a part of a family unit and should be involved in family life and childhood friendships as much as possible.

Nursing Alert

The child undergoing treatment for leukemia usually has very low immunity to disease; the greatest danger is infection. It is important to protect this patient through excellent nursing technique.

Cancer

Malignant lymphoma (Hodgkin's disease), lymphosarcoma, and other sarcomas, such as osteogenic sarcoma, are not uncommon in children. The prognosis may be poor because malignancies in children often progress quickly and may not be detected at an early stage. The most common cancers in children are those of the brain, kidney, adrenal glands, bones, and structures of the central nervous system.

Any brain tumor is serious because the increase in size puts undue pressure on the brain, and this can cause brain damage. Very young children are less likely to have malignant tumors than older people. In children, the most common brain tumors are *gliomas* of the cerebellum, the brain stem, or the optic nerve; *pinealomas*, tumors of the pituitary; and *congenital* brain tumors. They are most likely to be fast growing, and may be inoperable. However, whenever possible, immediate surgery and follow-up radiation or chemotherapy are required to prevent further complications.

Aside from the physical effects of childhood cancer, the emotional effects may require even more nursing

assistance. The nurse also needs to provide emotional support to the family.

Respiratory Tract Disorders

Sample nursing diagnoses seen in respiratory illness are the following:

◆ Ineffective Airway Clearance related to excessive mucus production, ineffective cough, or swollen airway
◆ Impaired Gas Exchange related to narrowed airway
◆ Fear related to breathlessness
◆ Fatigue related to increased effort of respirations

Upper Respiratory Infection

Upper respirtory tract infections are common in children and in adults. They may be caused by a virus or by bacteria. Respiratory distress symptoms are illustrated in Figure 62-2.

Usually there is a high temperature; dyspnea with thick, tenacious sputum and mucus; and edema of the throat. If there is no cough, the patient will find it difficult to get rid of secretions. The child is often kept at home unless there are complications.

The general treatment includes antibiotics, humidity, oxygen, rest, and occasionally a tracheostomy. A small child may be put in a mist tent, or a humidifier may be used. The child with a contagious disease is kept in his or her room, and only adults may visit. Gowns should be worn by nurses and visitors.

Pneumonia

Pneumonia, an inflammation of the lung, usually with consolidation and drainage, is common in children and adults. It may initially be an infectious disease, may be secondary to another disease, or may result from aspiration. The physician differentiates pneumonia from other upper respiratory infections by means of a chest x-ray. It is usually treated with antibiotics, bed rest, and fluids (see Chapter 79).

When administering antibiotics for any reason, parents must understand that it is imperative for the child to take the *entire* antibiotic prescription. If the child stops taking the prescription before all the medicine is taken, the organism may not be killed and may return. Resistant strains of pathogens also can develop in this way.

Croup

The symptoms of laryngotracheobronchitis (LTB) known as *croup*, are laryngeal spasm, dyspnea, and increased mucus production. The child also has a harsh, seal-like cough; the chest rattles when the child breathes. He or she may be cyanotic. The child usually has a high fever; a rapid pulse; cold, clammy skin; and a flushed face.

The patient is placed in a mist tent humidifying device. Oxygen may be given to assist respirations. Expectorants are often given to loosen secretions and to assist the child in coughing up the mucus. An older child may be propped up on pillows to make breathing easier.

The nurse must observe the child's respiratory condition. If distress is severe (severe *croup epiglottis*), a tracheostomy may be required.

Acetaminophen to reduce temperature and sedatives to relieve anxiety are given when the patient's respiratory status has been assessed; fluids are forced. If the patient cannot take fluids orally, IV fluids are given. Clear liquids, ice pops, gelatin, and other fluids should be offered frequently.

Asthma

Asthma is the most common major allergic disorder in children (1%–2% incidence). Breathing difficulties occur because of bronchial spasms, obstructive edema, thick secretions, and panic. Wheezing, particularly when exhaling; rapid and shallow breathing; and a severe cough are symptoms of asthma.

Treatment is symptomatic. Allergy tests, followed by specific desensitization may be recommended. Inhalant drugs and nebulization treatments are used frequently to assist the school-age child to tolerate activity (such as physical education classes) better. Use of the medications prevents respiratory distress or treats it promptly. Many school-age children routinely have measured dose inhalers at home and school to assist in their ongoing care plan for asthma.

Nursing Alert

Status asthmaticus, which can be fatal, is a condition that exists when the acute episode cannot be relieved by medications. Treatment includes administration of IV fluids and drugs, such as aminophylline, and anti-inflammatory agents.

Bronchiolitis

Bronchiolitis is a viral respiratory infection resulting in inflammation of the bronchioles. It is seen most often in children younger than 2 years and tends to be a seasonal illness, occurring in winter and early spring.

The illness begins with symptoms of a cold, which gradually become worse. Chest x-rays reveal "air trapping" in the lungs. The illness usually resolves within 10 days. A severe case of bronchiolitis may require hospitalization and treatment with IV fluids and oxygen administered by mist tent (see Chapter 64).

Respiratory Syncytial Virus. Respiratory syncytial virus (RSV) is believed to be the cause of more than half the cases of bronchiolitis. RSV bronchiolitis is particularly prevalent in infants and toddlers and is easily transmitted by direct and indirect contact. The child with RSV is usually placed on contact isolation. All people caring for the child must observe strict handwashing procedures and wear disposable goggles.

Diagnosis of RSV is based on symptoms and a positive nasal culture smear. Treatment may include the use of an antiviral agent called ribavirin. This is administered by mist tent or face mask. Nursing skills for administering ribavirin therapy follow:

- Wash your hands.
- Gather equipment and medication.
- Explain to parent (and child if old enough) what you are going to do and why. (Rationale: *This will decrease anxiety and promote cooperation.*)
- Perform thorough respiratory assessment before beginning and at least every 2 to 4 hours. Refer to Figure 62-2. (Rationale: *Respiratory infections can cause decreased air exchange. Thorough assessment of patient's respiratory status can determine impending airway obstruction and assure prompt treatment.*)
- Ribavirin may be administered using Oxyhood or tent or ventilator for intubated patients.
- It is usually given for 3 to 5 days, for 12 to 20 hours a day.
- 20 mg ribavirin per 1 mL water is placed in a small-particle generator (nebulizer) connected to Oxyhood or tent. (Rationale: *Ribavirin must be administered as a mist to be effective.*)
- If patient is intubated, antibacterial filters must be added to the circuit of the ventilator tubing; filters must be changed every 24 hours. This should be performed only by well-trained therapists, physicians, and nurses. (Rationale: *Precipitation of drug in ventilator tubing around expiratory valve could obstruct the valve, resulting in high positive-end expiratory pressure.*)
- Dispose of waste appropriately, and wash your hands. (Rationale: *This will prevent spread of mircoorganisms.*)
- Document procedure, medication given, and patient response. Include respiratory assessment data. Report any signs and symptoms of respiratory distress.

Nursing Alert

Pregnant women should avoid contact with the child receiving ribavirin.

Gastrointestinal Disorders

The student should review the information on abdominal surgery on children in Chapter 64 as well as Chapter 53 before caring for a child undergoing any surgery discussed in this section. Sample nursing diagnoses seen in GI disorders are the following:

- ◆ Fluid Volume Deficit related to excessive fluid loss from frequent diarrhea
- ◆ Altered Nutrition: Less than Body Requirements related to excessive vomiting
- ◆ High Risk for Impaired Skin Integrity related to exposure of skin to frequent loose stools
- ◆ Altered Growth and Development related to inadequate intake or absorption of nutrients

Pyloric Stenosis

In pyloric stenosis, also called *congenital hypertrophic pyloric stenosis*, the pyloric sphincter is thickened, narrowing the canal through which food passes from the stomach to the intestine. It is seen more commonly in males than females. The stenosis may be so extensive that the obstruction is complete; the pylorus then closes, and food cannot pass into the intestine. As a result, food is regurgitated into the esophagus, causing severe vomiting. Vomiting is the most common symptom of pyloric stenosis.

An infant usually does not show signs of pyloric stenosis until he or she is a few weeks to 2 months old. The symptoms include projectile vomiting, loss of weight, hunger, irritability, and dehydration. Often, constipation and oliguria (decreased urine formation) are associated. Diagnosis is made on the basis of an upper GI x-ray examination.

Medical and Surgical Treatment. The treatment of choice for pyloric stenosis is surgery (*pyloromyotomy*). However, if the child is a poor surgical risk for other reasons and if the stenosis is not life-threatening, medical means of treatment may be used. These include sedation, antispasmodic drugs, and thickened feedings. Medical means of treatment also are used in developing countries where surgery is not available.

Nursing Considerations. Before surgery, fluids are given intravenously to correct fluid and electrolyte imbalance due to vomiting. (Electrolyte studies identify the type of solution to administer intravenously). An accurate record of I&O is vital, as is clear notation of the amount and type of vomitus.

Postoperatively, precautions are taken to prevent aspiration or other respiratory distress. The baby is positioned on the side, with the head slightly elevated. Care is scheduled so a bath is given before feeding. Glucose water or plain water feedings are usually started 2 to 3 hours after surgery; the child is bubbled frequently. The amount fed is increased when the child is able to retain more. The diet progresses from glucose water to half-strength formula to full-strength formula. Recovery is usually uneventful.

Chalasia

A newborn may vomit because the cardiac sphincter is not functioning properly. This condition is called chalasia. As a result, food is regurgitated into the esophagus. If dehydration or malnutrition do not occur, there is usually no treatment, because this condition often resolves itself. If caused by a hiatal hernia or an abnormally short esophagus, surgery may be necessary. An upper GI x-ray is diagnostic.

Meckel's Diverticulum

Meckel's diverticulum is a congenital disorder in which a small portion of the ileum ends in a blind pouch just before its junction with the colon. The symptoms include the passage of bloody or tarry stools. There is no pain unless the diverticulum is inflamed. Treatment consists of removing the pouch surgically. Complications are rare. Preoperative and postoperative care is routine.

Hernia

A *hernia* is protrusion of part of an organ through an abnormal opening. In children, a congenital defect is most often the cause of hernia. There are several types of hernias.

Diaphragmatic hernia, which occurs rarely, is a condition in which a portion of the intestine protrudes through the diaphragm.

With an *umbilical hernia*, a portion of the intestine protrudes through a weak umbilical ring, producing a bulge beneath the navel. Because this condition usually disappears by the time the child is 3 or 4 years old, surgery is not usually needed. Strangulation is rare, with surgery necessary only if the protruding part is large or other congenital defects are present.

In an *indirect inguinal hernia* (most frequent in males), the intestine protrudes through the round ligament into the inguinal area and may descend into the scrotal sac. Surgery is required if strangulation develops. In the female, inguinal hernia may involve the ovary or the uterus, and immediate surgery is needed to prevent damage to these structures.

A *direct inguinal hernia* protrudes through the weakest part of the abdominal wall. Because the peritoneum overlying the protruding abdominal contents is transparent, the contents can be visualized, and all or part of the abdominal contents may be seen. Should the hernia rupture, severe hemorrhage, peritonitis, a generalized septicemia, or strangulation could occur. Surgery is usually performed early in life.

The treatment of choice for many hernias is surgery. The specific procedure varies with the condition. Preoperative and postoperative care is routine. Often hernia repair is completed in the 1-day surgery suite and may be done by laparascope.

Diarrhea

Diarrhea is a sudden increase in frequency of loose and watery stools. It is most often caused by infectious organisms in the GI tract. Stress, prolonged temperature elevation, and spoiled food are other causes. Also, certain antibiotics can alter the bacteria normally present in the intestine, and this will result in an increase in number of stools.

Diarrhea can be *very dangerous* in the small child. The smaller he or she is, the greater the possibility of fluid and electrolyte imbalance and dehydration. Severe diarrhea can be fatal in an infant.

Medical Treatment. Milder forms of diarrhea can be treated at home. Oral rehydration solutions (ORS), such as Lytren and Pedialyte are given to the child with diarrhea. Several ORSs are available in different flavors, which older children find more palatable. Diet eventually progresses to bananas, rice, applesauce, and toast (BRAT) and clear liquids, such as gelatin and clear broth.

In *severe diarrhea*, stools are frequent and forceful, green or yellow liquid. The child is lethargic and irritable. Skin turgor is poor, the eyes and anterior fontanels are sunken, and the pulse is weak and rapid, indicating dehydration. Oliguria also develops.

Hospitalization is often necessary to replace water loss and restore fluid and electrolyte balance. Electrolyte studies determine what IV solution is necessary, a chest x-ray determines if there is a complicating respiratory condition, and a stool culture identifies the causative organism. The child is placed on enteric isolation to prevent spread of organisms to other patients (see Chapter 51).

Nursing Considerations. The nurse wears gloves and gown when caring for the child with diarrhea.

In *severe diarrhea*, continuous IV therapy is necessary to rest the GI tract and replace body fluids. Because restraints may be necessary during IV infusion, comforting the child is important, and make sure to release restraints periodically so he or she can change position at will. The nurse must maintain accurate I&O records and must describe carefully the amount and character of all stools. No food or fluids are given by mouth for 24 to 48 hours to rest the GI tract. Petrolatum soothes dry lips.

Good skin care is essential, because the buttocks can become sore and irritated. Thorough, gentle cleansing from the front of the perineal area to the back is necessary each time the diaper is changed. The buttocks are exposed to air as much as possible. Sitz baths in clear tepid water and nonprescription ointments help ease discomfort.

When the number of stools has diminished, clear liquids are gradually begun. Each hospital has its own routine, or the physician may specify which fluids are allowed. Oral electrolyte solutions, such as Pedialyte, are often given. The dosage is based on the child's weight and is ordered by the physician. Milk is avoided; it tends to aggravate diarrhea. As the child is able to retain fluids without an increase in number of liquid stools, the variety and quantity of fluids are increased (such as carbonated beverages). Depending on the physician, either half-strength skim milk or a soybean formula is given. The next step is gradual introduction of antidiarrheal solid foods. Fruits should be scraped or peeled, and foods such as ripe bananas, applesauce, and puffed or popped rice cereal are given (BRAT diet). Cottage cheese and yogurt may be offered in place of meat, although they must be given carefully because they may aggravate diarrhea. Following this regimen, the child gradually resumes a normal diet.

When electrolyte balance is attained, diarrhea has subsided, and the child is taking fluids and antidiarrheal solids, the parents are instructed in diet, and the child is discharged.

Lactose Intolerance

If a child has frequent attacks of diarrhea, the problem may be lactose intolerance, which is an inherited disorder characterized by an inability to metabolize lactose in milk and milk products. It is more common in African Americans than in whites; about 85% of African Americans have this disorder. It is also common in Asians in the United States. The lactose-intolerant person cannot drink milk or eat dairy products; not only are dairy products not properly absorbed and metabolized, but their presence also interferes with absorption of other food substances. If the problem is not recognized and treated, the child may die from malnutrition.

Symptoms include vomiting, listlessness, and FTT. These symptoms usually appear 1 to 2 weeks after birth and are most common in bottle-fed babies. The child is switched to a meat-base or Nutramigen formula. The diet must be supervised for years before changes can be made. This person may never be able to drink milk but may become able to tolerate cheese and yogurt.

Intestinal Obstruction

Intestinal obstruction may be a consequence of poor peristalsis, a neoplasm, an ingested foreign object, or a stricture. The person is nauseated and vomits, but vomiting does not provide relief, nor does food or a laxative. There may be severe pain. Symptoms vary according to the location of the obstruction and whether it is partial or complete. A newborn may be obstructed simply because of underdeveloped muscles (atonic colon).

Medical measures may provide relief; surgery is performed if symptoms do not disappear. If the obstruction is complete, immediate surgery must be performed to prevent internal rupture and peritonitis or gangrene. The general preoperative and postoperative care is similar to any other GI surgery. Nasogastric suction, antispasmodic drugs, and analgesics may be indicated.

Intussusception

Intussusception is the telescoping of one part of bowel into another. It is usually caused by hyperactive peristalsis in one part of the bowel and hypoactivity in the other part. One danger is that blood supply may be cut off, causing gangrene. This condition is most common in infants, yet usually the infant has been doing well. A definite diagnosis is based on the findings of a lower GI x-ray. The procedure itself often reduces the intussusception; if this is not the case, surgery is needed to prevent complications. Preoperative and postoperative care is routine, and the healthy child seldom has complications.

Colic

Colic is not serious; it is more troublesome to parents than to the infant. It is more common in infants who are very small at birth or who are born early but are large for gestational age. There are frequent episodes of crying, and the infant doubles up as though in great pain. The symptoms seem to be worse in the evening. Many doctors believe that a nervous mother is more likely to have a colicky baby. Current research points to a possible physical cause of colic.

Treatment consists of feeding the baby slowly and using bottles with disposable, collapsible inner bags to reduce the amount of air the infant swallows. The formula is usually switched to one with a soybean base. In any event, the baby almost always outgrows the condition by the time he or she is 3 or 4 months of age. Parents also may be encouraged to give the infant a pacifier to encourage more sucking. Soothing the infant through touch, rocking, and a gentle voice also are recommended. The parents should be encouraged to get a babysitter or a relative to assist. The parents of a baby with colic need a break from the constant crying of the baby; counseling may be indicated to prevent child abuse.

Metabolic Disorders and Nutritional Deficiencies

Marasmus

Marasmus more correctly describes a general FTT. It seems to be related to such conditions as kwashiorkor (protein deficiency), rickets (vitamin D deficiency), and scurvy (vitamin C deficiency). Causes of marasmus might be a general systemic disease, an absorptional problem, or neglect or abuse.

Symptoms of marasmus are edema, lowered blood volume, and blood pressure, lowered body temperature, and a general appearance of ill health. The child's abdomen protrudes, the eyes are sunken, and he or she is generally weak and listless. Physical growth lags behind that of normal children the same age. The child usually continues to eat well. Mental development may or may not be slowed.

Nursing Considerations. Nursing care involves restoration of hydration and nutrition, maintenance of body temperature, and general tender loving care. The child usually responds well to treatment.

Many parents are not knowledgeable about diets and parenting. An important part of nursing care in such cases is to teach parents about nutrition and general aspects of child care, including bathing and shampooing. The importance of affection and recreation should be included in teaching. Parents must especially be taught feeding routines: how to give first solids, how to hold the baby, how to keep air out of the neck of the bottle, and how to bubble the baby. These teaching factors are discussed earlier in this chapter.

Biliary Atresia

One cause of malnutrition may be biliary atresia, a defect in the bile ducts that prevents bile from escaping from the liver. The lack of bile causes defective digestion and elimination. In some cases, surgery must be performed to relieve the obstruction.

Celiac Disease

The most common malabsorption syndrome in children is celiac disease, which is a chronic intestinal disorder of infants and young children. It involves inflammation of the small bowel and malabsorption of nutrients. Celiac disease is thought to be congenital, although its effects may not be apparent for several months or years. Usually, however, the condition shows up within 6 months after birth.

The basic defect in this disease is an inability to absorb carbohydrates, particularly wheat, oats, barley, and rye protein. (These grains contain *glutens*, a tough, elastic substance.) When a child with celiac disease eats grains containing glutens, the glutens are excreted virtually unchanged in the stools, which are fatty and float. Undernutrition results from lack of carbohydrate. Remission usually occurs when gluten-containing foods are omitted from the diet. Breast-feeding seems to postpone the appearance of symptoms.

Celiac disease is characterized by enormous, floating fatty stools, anorexia (refusal to eat and lack of appetite); undernutrition and FTT; distended abdomen and wasted buttocks; excessive flatus; and arrested growth (Fig. 65-10). Diagnosis is verified by a jejunal biopsy and clinical improvement of the child when placed on a gluten-free diet. More than one child in a family may have the disorder, indicating a familial tendency. The disorder may vary in degree from mild to severe. The more severe form of the disorder is discussed here.

Medical Treatment. Treatment of celiac disease includes strict adherence to a gluten-free diet (see Chapter 28). The person is not allowed any cereal grains, such as wheat, barley, rye, and oats, and is not allowed any malt. This includes malted milk and beer. The child also is not allowed lactose, which is the sugar contained in milk and dairy products. This diet must continue in some form for life. However, after the growth spurt of adolescence, a small amount of gluten-containing foods may be introduced. If any difficulty occurs, they must be removed again.

Celiac Crisis

During the first 2 years of life, an affected child often has the symptoms of large watery stools, vomiting, and a distended abdomen. Prior to this, the same child will have had irregular weight gain and periods of occasional vomiting, but a celiac crisis is sudden and more severe.

In celiac crisis, the child is dehydrated, and the fluid and electrolyte balance is severely disturbed. The child is treated symptomatically on an emergency basis. IV fluids are administered. Corticosteroids may be helpful during celiac crisis.

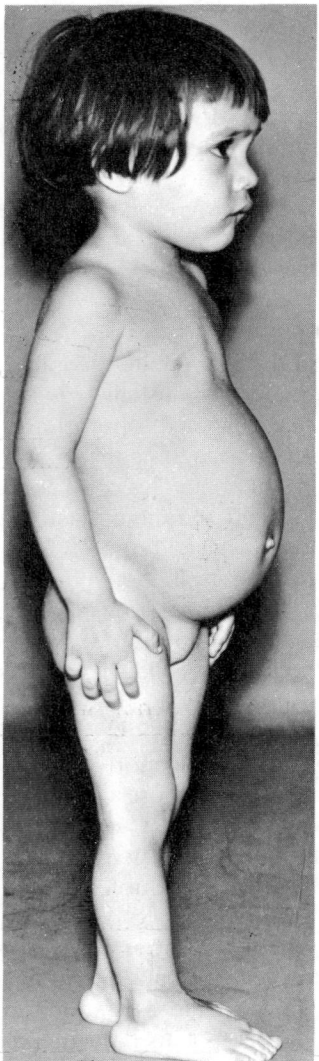

Figure 65-10. Celiac disease, showing protuberant abdomen.

> ### Key Concept
>
> It is necessary to differentiate celiac disease from cystic fibrosis of the pancreas. The symptoms are similar in early stages, but treatment is different.

Cystic Fibrosis

Cystic fibrosis of the pancreas (mucoviscidosis) is a chronic and incurable condition. It is the most common lethal genetic disease in white people. It affects the pancreas, respiratory system, and in adult males, reproductive organs. It is rare in African American and Asian people. Many children with cystic fibrosis eventually die from complications; however, with active treatment, children live past adolescence fairly often. In cystic fibrosis, mucus-producing glands secrete mucus in ab-

normally large quantities. These viscid secretions collect in the lungs, pancreas, and liver, disrupting normal functions of these organs.

Symptoms and Diagnosis. The first manifestation is a malabsorption syndrome with celiac symptoms, followed by respiratory or cardiac manifestations. The stools are thick and sticky and have a strong odor. Although a good appetite is apparent, the child will not gain weight. He or she looks emaciated and has a large abdomen. This acquired malnutrition is due to an inability to absorb fat-soluble vitamins.

Diagnosis is made on the basis of stool specimens and pulmonary function testing, with specific diagnosis made on the basis of a sweat test to determine the sodium chloride content of sweat. If the sodium chloride content is too high, it indicates a positive diagnosis if other symptoms are also present.

Medical Treatment. The patient is treated with massive doses of antibiotics to prevent infection. Drugs such as *pancreatin* (Dizymes, Pancreatin) and pancrelipase (Cotazyme, Creon, VioKase) seem to be useful in counteracting pancreatic insufficiency. Dietary control is aimed at increasing vitamin intake and correcting respiratory symptoms. The high-calorie, high-protein diet includes supplementary vitamins, because nutritional problems are present in 80% of cases. Pancreatic extract is given, as is salt in hot weather. Active exercise, such as swimming, running, or biking, seems to be helpful.

A major goal in management is maintenance of a patent airway. The patient receives frequent intermittent positive pressure breathing (IPPB) treatments and ambitious chest physiotherapy with careful pummeling of each lobe of the lungs to prevent pulmonary obstruction and infection. The goal of IPPB is to assist the patient to breathe more deeply and to loosen secretions. The mechanical device forces room air or oxygen-rich air into the airway. Thus, the patient's lungs are expanded more completely, and respiratory disorders can be treated or prevented. Chapter 80 describes various means of oxygen administration and therapy in more detail.

The patient should sleep in a humidity tent so propylene glycol or another agent can be inhaled. Exercises can be taught to incease lung capacity, and these will help the patient cough up secretions. The patient and family are instructed in postural drainage. The small child may need suctioning. Bronchodilators and iodides help thin secretions. Immunity to all contagious diseases of childhood must be maintained, especially those affecting the respiratory tract directly. Gamma globulin given on a regular basis is not recommended but may be given if the child becomes ill or is exposed to a respiratory infection.

Phenylketonuria

Phenylketonuria (PKU) is a hereditary metabolic disorder. If untreated, PKU causes severe retardation that begins during the first year of life. PKU is detected by a blood test, which is done after delivery and is required by law in most states. However, because babies are discharged from the hospital so soon after delivery, the test *must be repeated at the 6-week checkup.* (The blood test is not accurate until after the infant has had several feedings of formula or breast milk.) If PKU is present, siblings also should be tested. People with PKU are most often blue eyed and blond and have sensitive skin.

Treatment must start as soon as possible. Existing damage is irreversible, but treatment prevents further damage. A special substitute formula is used in place of the usual milk in the diet. Phenylalanine-containing foods are avoided; these include most breads, eggs, meat, milk, cheese, and legumes or nuts. Artificial sweeteners containing phenylalanine, such as Nutra-sweet, are omitted. Low-protein natural foods, such as fruits, vegetables, and certain cereals, are allowed. These dietary restrictions usually continue for life.

As the PKU child reaches school age, learning difficulties may develop. Most regional PKU clinics recommend yearly psychological and intellectual evaluation. Many PKU children are eligible for learning disability services in school. Communication between school, family, and physician is essential. Strict adherence to dietary limitations is strongly encouraged.

Megacolon

In megacolon, also known as *Hirschsprung's disease* or aganglionic megacolon, the colon lacks parasympathetic nerve supply. Because of lack of peristalsis, the abdomen becomes abnormally large. If a large segment of colon is affected, palliative treatment may be all that is possible. In 90% of children with Hirschsprung's disease, the aganglionic area is in the rectosigmoid segment of the bowel. Surgical treatment may be effective if the damaged or malfunctioning portion of colon can be removed.

Symptoms and Diagnosis. Symptoms are caused by accumulation of feces in the bowel and include diarrhea or constipation, nausea, and vomiting. The abdomen becomes distended, and bowel movements are not normal, resulting in malnutrition. Usually the effects of Hirschsprung's disease appear shortly after birth. The newborn fails to pass meconium within 24 to 48 hours. There may be signs of obstruction, such as bile-stained or fecal vomiting, abdominal distention, irritability, feeding problems, FTT, or dehydration. The older child exhibits intractable constipation that usually requires laxatives and saline enemas. Surgery is usually required eventually.

Diagnosis is made on the basis of medical history, x-ray studies, barium enema, and palpation of the distended abdomen. A proctoscopy usually reveals an empty rectum and lower colon, and biopsy of the rectal wall usually indicates an absence of nerve fibers.

Medical and Surgical Treatment. Corrective surgery is delayed if possible until the infant is about 1 year old and better able to withstand the procedure. During this time, it is important to prevent constipation. Small saline enemas, stool softeners, and digital removal of fecal impactions are used. Sometimes colonic irrigations are done; they are similar to an enema except that a larger tube is used and is passed up into the descending colon. Drugs that act on the parasympathetic and sympathetic nervous systems may be given to improve peristalsis. Surgery often involves a temporary colostom

> **Key Concept**
>
> Watch for abdominal distention, temperature spikes, and irritability following surgery for Hirschsprung's disease. These are signs of possible anastomotic leaks.

Nursing Considerations. Preoperative preparation includes saline enemas to evacuate the colon. Accurate records of the quantity of solution are kept. The return solution should be clear of fecal particles. Antibiotics are administered as a bowel preparation.

Postoperative care involves keeping the wound clean and dry. The wound must be completely healed before a rectal temperature probe or suppository can be used. Tympanic temperatures are usually taken. The child will have a first liquid bowel movement approximately 3 to 4 days after surgery. Because bladder trauma can occur from extensive surgical manipulation, the urine is assessed for blood.

Clear oral feedings are begun when active bowel sounds are present. The diet is increased as tolerated. When the child is discharged from the hospital, parents are instructed to watch closely for foods that increase the number of stools and to avoid them. The parents need assurance that the child will eventually achieve sphincter control and be able to eat a normal diet. Complete continence may take several years to attain, however. Because the child with Hirschsprung's disease is hospitalized for surgery so early in life, parental emotional bonding may be difficult to establish. It is important to encourage the parents to participate in their child's care as much as possible in the hospital.

Urinary and Reproductive Disorders

Exstrophy of the Bladder

Exstrophy of the bladder, more common in males, occurs when the two sides of the lower abdomen fail to grow together, and the bladder is exposed. This condition is treated by positioning the child on the side or back and keeping the bladder area as clean and dry as possible. Sometimes the exposed bladder is kept moist with ointments or saline packs. Surgery is usually not performed until the child is about 3 or 4 years old, at which time the bladder is usually removed and urine diverted into the colon. Urinary diversion and care of the patient with a urinary disorder are described in Chapter 82.

Hermaphroditism

Hermaphroditism is a condition in which the individual exhibits both male and female characteristics. If any doubt arises about an infant's sex, studies are performed immediately. The buccal mucosa or skin structure is microscopically examined for a female or male chromosomal pattern. Hormonal and anatomic studies also may be done. Normal social and emotional development demands that the sex be established as soon after birth as possible. Depending on the physical problem, treatment may be surgical to revise or remove structures or medical to provide appropriate hormones.

Hypospadias and Epispadias

In *hypospadias*, the urinary meatus is located on the bottom of the penis; in *epispadias*, the meatus is located on top of the penis. These conditions can usually be surgically corrected and are not life-threatening. Minor hypospadias is quite common and usually requires no correction. If surgery is required, it is almost always done in two stages. Circumcision is contraindicated prior to surgical correction of this displacement of the urinary meatus because the foreskin may be used for surgical correction of the condition.

Preoperative nursing care is the same as in any surgery; the surgery is not done if an upper respiratory infection is present. The parents and child must be prepared intellectually and emotionally for surgery. Postoperative care includes the following:

◆ Wear gloves.
◆ The penis is usually wrapped in petrolatum gauze to prevent swelling, pain, and bleeding.
◆ A urinary or suprapubic catheter is placed during surgery; the patient is placed on the back or side, and restraints may be necessary.
◆ Assess urinary output often. Empty drainage at change of shift; record color and amount of urine.
◆ Check catheter for kinks; be sure it is connected to straight drainage and that the collecting bag is below level of bladder.
◆ Assess periodically for any swelling or bleeding.
◆ A bed cradle may be used to prevent pressure on surgical site.
◆ Keep the child's hands busy with diversional activities to prevent him from disturbing the dressings or catheter.

Polycystic Kidney

Polycystic kidney is characterized by cysts or tumors on the kidney. If the condition is bilateral, treatment is not usually effective.

Cryptorchidism

Cryptorchidism is an *undescended testicle*. It is discussed in detail in Chapter 83. It is common at birth but usually corrects itself spontaneously. If not, surgical treatment, an *orchiopexy*, is performed in early childhood to prevent sterility. Because undescended testes are often associated with hernia and hydrocele, surgical repairs are usually completed together. If an undescended testicle is found in an older child, surgery must *not* be postponed. A delay could result in sterility, because sperm cannot tolerate the heat inside the body.

Nursing Considerations. The child is admitted the day of surgery. Parents are instructed in preoperative preparation. The nurse assesses the patient to make sure that no symptoms of upper respiratory infection exist; if they are present, surgery will probably be postponed.

Postoperatively, if bowel sounds return and the child takes and retains fluids, voids, and ambulates properly, discharge to home care can be as early as 24 hours after surgery. The patient may return from surgery with an abdominal dressing, as a result of accompanying hernia repair. The dressing must be assessed often for drainage. The parents must be taught what to look for if the child is going home soon after surgery. (*Remember:* The nurse always wears gloves when handling dressings.)

Enuresis

Enuresis is the inability of the child to control the bladder, especially at night. More commonly, it is known as bed-wetting. It is more common in males than females. A complete urologic workup is necessary to discover if there is a physical cause. If the cause is physical, such as severe infection, bladder trauma, diabetes mellitus, small bladder capacity, meatal stenosis, or bladder spasm, it can often be treated. The child may not empty the bladder completely with voiding, or he or she may be an exceptionally sound sleeper.

If no physical cause can be found, a possible underlying emotional problem should be investigated. Family stress or problems with school can be associated with enuresis. It is important for parents not to shame or criticize the child for bed-wetting. If the condition persists into grade school, low dosages of an antidepressant, such as imipramine hydrochloride (Tofranil) have sometimes been used to promote continence. Counseling can sometimes assist the child and family.

Encopresis

Encopresis is incontinence of feces without physical cause. Many children with encopresis experienced coercive toilet training by their parents. Usually, symptoms begin with stool withholding late in infancy.

Treatment is geared to improving family relationships and understanding personality patterns. Nursing support, coupled with a nonjudgmental, nonpunishing parental approach, is fundamental to the therapeutic plan. Inpatient psychotherapy may be needed. Oil retention enemas and mineral oil are usually prescribed. Regular bowel habits should be established. Increased dietary bulk also is recommended.

Hydrocele

A **hydrocele** is an accumulation of serous fluid within the scrotal sac, causing the scrotum to become very large and painful. If the fluid is not reabsorbed spontaneously, excision and drainage may be necessary. A hydrocele is often associated with a hernia.

Hemolytic Uremic Syndrome

Hemolytic uremic syndrome (HUS) is a rare, acute condition occurring in children, usually between the ages of 6 months and 3 years. Three conditions occur with this illness: renal failure, hemolytic anemia, and thrombocytopenia.

Although the exact etiology is not known, HUS is thought to be caused by a virus. The disease usually follows an episode of diarrhea and vomiting or, less commonly, an upper respiratory infection. The inner lining of the arterioles surrounding the glomerulus of the kidneys becomes swollen and clogged with platelets and fibrin. As red blood cells move through these arterioles, they become damaged and are removed by the spleen. This results in hemolytic anemia. The child appears pale, bruised, and hypertensive, with diminished or absent urine output.

Treatment includes management of hypertension, dialysis and blood transfusions, and nutritional support.

Urinary Obstruction

Urinary obstruction can occur as a result of a neoplasm (cancer), calculi (stones), or severe infection. It is important to relieve the obstruction to prevent complications, such as hydronephrosis. Catheterization or antibiotics can be effective; otherwise, surgery is performed.

Pyelonephritis

Pyelonephritis (pyelitis) is a potentially dangerous kidney inflammation. (See Chapter 82 for a detailed discussion.) It is a bacterial infection that can migrate to the kidneys by way of the bloodstream, or it may be a complication of cystitis (inflammation of the urinary bladder). Because the urinary tract has a mucous membrane, cystitis can often lead to pyelonephritis and urinary tract infection. The short urethra of females makes them more prone to the infectious process. The accompanying box describes patient teaching to help prevent urinary tract infections in females.

Symptoms of pyelitis include dysuria (painful voiding) with frequency and urgency, fever, chills, and headache. Low back pain also may be present. There may be abdominal tenderness and pain. Culture and sensitivity tests are done to determine the causative organism so that appropriate antibiotics can be prescribed.

Pyelonephritis is curable in most cases; if not treated, it can lead to serious complications.

Acute Glomerlonephritis

Acute glomerlonephritis is also called acute post-streptococcal glomerulonephritis. This inflammation is the most common form of nephritis found in young children between the ages of 5 and 10 years. It is the result of an immunologic reaction to infection elsewhere in the body, most often to streptococci. Damage to the glomeruli of the kidney may cause urine output to decrease or cease.

The initial and main symptom is smoky urine or hematuria. The eyes may be puffy, and blood pressure is elevated. A throat culture may reveal group A β-hemolytic *Streptococcus*. Kidney enlargement also may be present.

Blood tests show mildly to moderately elevated blood urea nitrogen and creatinine. The urine shows the presence of red blood cells (microscopic or gross hematuria) and elevated WBCs. The urine values, including abnormal protein, indicate impaired renal function. There may be an elevated ASO (antistreptolysin-O) titer.

The patient is kept on bed rest during the acute phase. Activity is permitted as the hematuria clears and blood pressure returns to normal. The child is kept in a room away from children with upper respiratory infections. The diet is high in calories and low in sodium, protein, and potassium. Fluids may be restricted. Daily weights are taken to determine if the child is accumulating fluid in the tissues. Temperature, pulse, and respiration and blood pressure are important. Antibiotics and cortisone may be prescribed, although the use of these steroids is controversial.

In most cases, recovery is complete. In a few cases, chronic nephritis may develop, and the patient may need to be maintained on dialysis.

Chronic Glomerulonephritis

Chronic glomerulonephritis may be a complication of acute nephritis or may occur without preceding illness. The symptoms are unpredictable, and kidney damage usually is progressive. It can lead to hypertension, proteinuria, hematuria, and uremia.

The disease tends to progress in three stages. The first stage is the *latent stage*, with few outward symptoms. Albumin appears in the urine, and the patient may be anemic. No special treatment is needed at this time. In the second stage, *edema*, fluid is retained. Treatment includes a high-protein, low-salt diet. Steroid use is controversial; they are sometimes prescribed but are not used widely, as was the practice in the past. In the *stage of uremia*, the third stage, the kidneys begin to fail. No medical treatment is available for this stage. The patient may be maintained by dialysis until a suitable donor for a kidney transplant can be found. These patients are often excellent candidates for a kidney transplant.

Components of nursing care include the following:

- ◆ Accurate assessment of vital signs, I&O, and daily weights
- ◆ Daily assessment of renal function; observation for signs of fluid, electrolyte, and acid–base imbalance.
- ◆ Low-sodium, high-calorie diet, with adequate protein
- ◆ Good skin care (because of pruritus—itching and edema)
- ◆ Good oral hygiene, with care taken not to damage fragile gums
- ◆ Instructions to parents to have child take medications as ordered, to have child take diuretics in the morning so that sleep is not disrupted, to report symptoms of urinary tract infections, and to avoid contact with people with upper respiratory infections
- ◆ Explanation to child and parents about side effects of steroids if they are to be given (see Chapter 56)

Nephrotic Syndrome

In nephrotic syndrome, the kidney degenerates. It occurs most often in children between $1\frac{1}{2}$ and 5 years of age. Nephrotic syndrome is characterized by generalized edema and the presence of protein or blood in the urine. Urine output is scanty, and blood pressure is elevated. The abdomen is distended; the child is uncomfortable. He or she does not eat, because fluid in the abdomen and chest causes discomfort. The child is susceptible to other infections.

Palliative measures are symptomatic. Edema is reduced by administering corticosteroids and by limiting fluids and salt intake. The side effects of steroids are described in Chapter 56. Diuretics are used to reduce edema. The nurse should encourage the child to eat. The child should be protected from exposure to infections. Careful skin care is needed, and the child must be assisted to move about in bed. If the child is having difficulty breathing, he or she may be more comfortable sitting up.

The child is very ill and needs expert nursing care, emotional support, and kindness. Although steroids may induce a remission, the disease is not often curable. Nursing care is similar to that in chronic glomerulonephritis and includes checking weight at the same time each day, on the same scale, with the child wearing the same amount of clothing. Temperature, pulse, and respiration; blood pressure; and I&O are checked regularly. A low-sodium, high-protein diet appropriate for the child's age and limited fluids are given.

Renal Failure

Renal failure is a serious condition and usually must be treated by dialysis or kidney transplant. It may be caused by poisoning, chronic nephritis, or severe anaphylactic reactions.

Wilms' Tumor

Wilms' tumor, called *nephroblastoma*, is a malignant adenosarcoma of the kidney, most common in the 3- to 4-year-old child. It is one of the more common neoplasms of childhood, usually affecting one kidney only.

In most cases, there are no symptoms until the tumor is far advanced. Microscopic hematuria may be present but usually not until late in the course of the disease.

Diagnosis is made on the basis of palpation of the abdominal mass, x-ray studies, and biopsy during a laparotomy (surgical exploration of the abdomen).

Treatment for Wilms' tumor depends on "staging." There are five stages of the tumor's progress, which are shown in the accompanying box.

Staging in the Progress of Wilms' Tumor

Stage I	The tumor is well encapsulated and is limited to the kidney. it is totally removed by surgery.
Stage II	The tumor extends into the abdominal cavity. Often it can be totally removed.
Stage III	The tumor extends into the abdominal cavity to such an extent that it cannot be removed entirely.
Stage IV	The tumor has metastasized to distant sites (eg, lungs, liver, bone, brain).
Stage V	There is bilateral kidney metastasis.

Surgical removal, when done, is followed by irradiation to the site of the tumor and to both sides of the spine. Chemotherapy is often used.

Whenever a child is to have surgery, the parents and child should be prepared. If the child is old enough to understand, dolls, puppets, and drawings can be used to explain placement of tubes and to play out fears.

Nursing Alert

In Wilms' tumor, the abdomen is *never* unnecessarily palpated preoperatively. The tumor could rupture and disseminate. Extreme caution should be used when handling this child at all times.

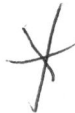

Keys for Review

Key Questions for Critical Thinking

1. Explain actions you would take in developing rapport with a child with a skin disorder and his or her parents.
2. You are teaching a parents' group about the number-one cause of death in children. Discuss how it is preventable. Describe your main teaching points.
3. You are working in an emergency room when a parent brings a 2-year-old child in for poisoning. Discuss questions you would ask. Describe protocol you would follow.
4. Describe the difference between drowning and near-drowning. Describe how you would teach a parent to prevent drowning.
5. Describe the differences and similarities in types of child abuse. Describe factors for each that would make you suspect abuse. Discuss actions you should take if you suspect child abuse.

Key Readings

Berkow R (Ed). The Merck Manual of Diagnosis and Therapy, Ed 16. Rahway, NJ, Merck & Co, 1992

Castiglia PT, Harbin RE. Child Health Care: Process and Practice. Philadelphia, J.B. Lippincott, 1992

Hazinski MF. Nursing Care of the Critically Ill Child, Ed 2. St Louis, Mosby-Yearbook, 1992

Jackson DB, Saunders RB. Child Health Nursing: A Comprehensive Approach to the Care of Children and their Families. Philadelphia, J.B. Lippincott, 1993

Murray R, Zentner J. Nursing Assessment and Health Promotion Strategies Through the Life Span. East Norwalk, CT, Appleton & Lange, 1993

NANDA Nursing Diagnoses: Definitions and Classifications 1992. Philadelphia, NANDA, 1992

Nursing '93 Drug Handbook. Springhouse, PA, Springhouse, 1993

Key Readings *(continued)*

O'Toole M. (Ed). Miller-Keane Encyclopedia & Dictionary of Medicine, Nursing & Allied Health, Ed 5. Philadelphia, W.B. Saunders, 1992

Pomar PJ (Ed). Nurses & Family Health Promotion: Concepts, Assessment, Intervention. Philadelphia, W.B. Saunders, 1992

Skale N. Manual of Pediatric Nursing Procedures. Philadelphia, J.B. Lippincott, 1992

Whaley LF. Nursing Care of Infants and Children, Ed 4. St. Louis, Mosby-Yearbook, 1991

Wong DL. Essentials of Pediatric Nursing, Ed 4. St. Louis, Mosby-Yearbook, 1993

Keys to Learning More

Chapter 66: disorders of older children

Chapter 67: children with special needs

Chapter 68: skin disorders, including burns

Chapter 70: care of patient in traction or cast

Chapter 71: seizure disorders

Chapter 72: endocrine disorders, including diabetes mellitus

Chapter 74: cardiovascular disorders

Chapter 75: blood and lymph disorders

Chapter 76: cancer

Chapter 77: allergies

Keys to Learning More *(continued)*

Chapter 79: respiratory disorders

Chapter 80: oxygen administration

Chapter 81: digestive disorders

Chapter 89: rehabilitation techniques for adults and children

Chapter 90: death and dying

Key Resources

American Sudden Infant Death Syndrome Institute
    275 Carpenter Drive
    Suite 100
    Atlanta, GA 30328

Sudden Infant Death Syndrome Clearing house
    8201 Greensboro Drive
    Suite 600
    McLean, VA 22102

National Sudden Infant Death Syndrome Foundation
    10500 Little Patuxent Parkway
    Suite 420
    Columbia, MD 21044

The Compassionate Friends, Inc. (A nationwide support group for bereaved parents and siblings)
    P.O. Box 3696
    Oak Brook, IL 60522-3696
    (708) 990-0010; (708) 990-0246 (FAX)

66 Care of the School-Age Child or Adolescent

Learning Objectives

- ◆ Discuss general principles of nursing care for the school-age child or adolescent.
- ◆ Describe symptoms of infectious mononucleosis.
- ◆ Identify skin disorders common in the school-age child and adolescent.
- ◆ Describe three postural defects and their treatment.
- ◆ Name three types of bone tumors found in the child.
- ◆ Identify symptoms of chronic ulcerative colitis, and describe treatment.
- ◆ Describe anorexia nervosa, bulimia, and obesity.
- ◆ Discuss clinical depression in the adolescent.
- ◆ Identify warning signs of suicide.

Key Terms

acne	insomnia	orthodontia
anorexia nervosa	kyphosis	scoliosis
bulimia	lordosis	sebum
cataplexy	malocclusion	somnambulism
dermabrasion	mittelschmerz	somniloquism
dysmenorrhea	narcolepsy	
hypersomnia		

Keys to Understanding This Chapter

Unit Three: normal growth and development

Unit Four: normal body structure and function

Unit Five: dietary information

Unit Six: safety and first aid

Unit Nine: basic nursing skills

Chapter 50: physical examination and nursing assessment

Unit Ten: surgery and surgical asepsis

Unit Eleven: medication administration

Chapter 63: sexually transmitted diseases

Keys to Understanding This Chapter
(continued)

Chapter 64: basics of pediatric nursing

Chapter 65: care of the infant and young child

Key Points

- ◆ Hormonal changes occurring in the older child result in certain disorders, including acne vulgaris, menstrual difficulties, and emotional disorders.
- ◆ Young people in this age group place high importance on physical appearance and peer acceptance. This impacts on adjustment to many illnesses and disorders.
- ◆ The most important aspect of treatment of Legg-Calvé-Perthes disease is maintaining the affected extremity as nonweight bearing.
- ◆ Anorexia nervosa and bulimia, although related to nutrition, are psychological disorders requiring long-term treatment.
- ◆ The suicidal child most often has depression and feelings of hopelessness and despair. This child may "cry out" with gestures and words.

Key Topics Outline

Health Maintenance
  School-Age Child Care
  Adolescent Care
Infectious Diseases
Parasitic Infestations
Skin Disorders
Musculoskeletal Disorders
Endocrine Disorders
  Diabetes Mellitus
Sensory System Disorders
Gastrointestinal Disorders
  Inflammatory Bowel Disease

Key Learning Activities

♦ Design a poster outlining distinguishing characteristics of various skin disorders. Include pictures or drawings.
♦ Create a survey identifying things that make people sad or happy. Survey your friends and classmates. Discuss the difference between feeling sad and having clinical depression.

Pediatric nursing continues with the study of the school-age child and young adult. Some physical conditions are more common in this age group.

Health Maintenance

A head to toe or checklist format may be used for school-age and adolescent health maintenance examinations. These examinations are often required before participation in athletics or extracurricular activities. There also may be a physical complaint or a referral from the school nurse.

School-Age Child Care

The school-age child's height and weight should continue to be plotted on the growth grid to establish a comparison with other American children of the same age. Emphasis should be on successful completion of school work and relationships with peers, siblings, and parents. Nutrition, elimination, and sleep patterns should be evaluated. The child needs a measles, mumps, rubella (MMR) booster at age 12.

Adolescent Care

Health supervision issues for the adolescent should focus on puberty and a smooth transition to young adulthood. The adolescent requires an update of the diphtheria tetanus (DT) immunization.

Special Concerns

The adolescent is capable of expressing individual concerns. Thus, it is important to talk separately to the parents and adolescent. The adolescent's privacy must be respected. A tactful approach encompasses everything from draping to detailed explanations of procedures to be performed. The adolescent may present with such problems as acne vulgaris, menarche and menstruation dysfunction, inadequate nutrition, sexually transmitted diseases, suicidal ideation, or chemical

abuse. The transition from childhood to adolescence can be difficult. Many adolescents benefit from professional counseling.

The Hospitalized Adolescent

Adolescents need certain accommodations to preserve their self-respect and identity. They do not belong either on the pediatric ward or the adult ward; a special unit should be provided for them. When this is not possible, the roommate should be the same sex and approximately the same age.

Relationships with peers should be maintained. Friends should be allowed to visit, but their activity should be regulated so that they do not overtire the patient. A telephone should be available for use by the hospitalized adolescent. (Set a "curfew" for its use.)

Illness or injury can be a serious threat to self-image. Many young people worry about damage to their bodies or about death. Because they are likely to be acutely aware of emerging sexuality, their modesty must be respected. The young person is striving for independence, so the nurse should attempt to include the patient in care as much as possible.

Key Concept

The hospitalized adolescent may be too embarrassed to ask questions. A bulletin board or brochure rack well stocked with informational pamphlets about adolescent concerns is one way to communicate with the adolescent.

Infectious Diseases

Acute Infectious Mononucleosis

Mononucleosis is a self-limiting disease characterized by flulike symptoms. It is caused by the Epstein-Barr virus. The mode of transmission is not completely known; however, it is believed that it is spread by oral secretions or droplets. At one time it was known as the "kissing disease."

The symptoms of mononucleosis initially appear as flulike: headache, low-grade fever, anorexia, and fatigue. This typically develops into a sore throat, swollen cervical lymph nodes, and an elevated temperature. An enlarged spleen, rash, and tonsillitis also may accompany this illness.

Medical Treatment. The treatment for mononucleosis is symptomatic. It is important for the adolescent to get plenty of rest. Treatment of fever and occasionally antibiotics for sore throat or tonsillitis are important. Fluids should be encouraged.

Streptococcal Infections and Rheumatic Fever

Streptococcal infections and rheumatic fever are mentioned here because they are frequently seen in school-age children and adolescents. The importance of proper bed rest and the correct medication regimen must be stressed. Rheumatic fever is not as common as streptococcal infections because of public awareness of the need to treat "strep" infections (see Chapter 65).

Lyme Disease

Lyme disease, also called Lyme arthritis, is a tick-borne illness that has become prominent in some parts of the United States in the last decade. Anyone who spends time outdoors or near wooded areas populated with deer and certain other animals is at risk. The disease is transmitted by a spiral-shaped bacterium (spirochete). Spirochetes are passed to a human or an animal by the bite of a deer tick, which is less than half the size of the common wood tick (approximately the size of a printed period).

Signs and Symptoms. In approximately 30% of humans, there is a distinct ring-shaped rash; as it fades, there is central clearing with red edges. The person also has flulike symptoms. These people are easily diagnosed and treated with antibiotics. Generally, they have no further problems. However, in a majority of people, there is no rash. In these people, the spirochetes travel through the blood, settle in the tissue, and begin to multiply. There are no immediate symptoms. Weeks after the bite, the person may begin to complain of angina, chronic fatigue, headaches, facial palsy, limb numbness, heart arrhythmias, or intellectual impairment. Many months, or even years, later, chronic symptoms, such as pain (caused by nerve degeneration), loss of muscle function, and even psychiatric disturbances, may develop. The most characteristic symptom is an arthritis that resembles rheumatoid arthritis. Because of the diversity of symptoms, Lyme disease has been called the "great imitator." Polymerase chain reaction is a relatively new laboratory test that can identify specific spirochetes. This, along with other general blood tests, aids in the diagnosis of Lyme disease.

Lyme disease can still be treated with antibiotics after the later symptoms develop, but diagnosis and treatment are much more difficult. The symptoms are often treated as individual entities with no thought of Lyme disease as the cause because there was no rash.

Prevention. Preventive measures should be taken by people who cannot avoid potentially infested areas. Areas of greatest concentration are the Pacific coast, upper Midwest, and Northeast coastal states. People who spent time in the outdoors should be taught preventive measures. See the accompanying box for patient teaching.

Nursing Alert

In the pregnant woman, Lyme disease can cause miscarriage, stillbirth, or fetal abnormalities.

LaCrosse Encephalitis

This disorder can affect children and is carried by the Tree Hole mosquito. It is most common in the upper midwest and northeast. The virus causes symptoms ranging from mild headaches and flu-like symptoms to mental confusion and seizures. It may cause permanent CNS damage and, rarely, death. The source of most

---

Keys to Patient/Family Teaching
Prevention of Lyme Disease

Patient and family teaching for prevention of Lyme disease includes the following measures when outdoors, particularly in the woods:

- Long sleeves and long pants should be worn with cuffs tucked into socks.
- Light-colored clothing makes it easier to see ticks. Skin and clothing should be checked frequently for ticks.
- Brush clothing off before entering house.
- Insect repellents containing DEET or permathrin are used.
- Walk on paved or cleaned areas rather than in the woods.
- After leaving infected areas, the body is checked for ticks. Use a mirror or have someone help.
- If a tick is attached, grasp it at its head with tweezers and pull it out with steady pressure.
- Grass and weeds should be kept short around the home.
- Use tick and flea collars on pets; brush pets often.

Tree Hole mosquitos is within the child's own yard or immediate neighborhood. Removal of breeding spots that hold water controls the insect.

Parasitic Infestations

Pediculosis

Pediculosis means infestation by lice on the head, body, or pubic area. It is on the rise; many cases are being reported in schools. Signs and symptoms include severe itching and the presence of small, dark bugs and lighter eggs (nits) attached to hair shafts. Chapter 68 describes the treatment in detail.

> **Key Concept**
>
> The nurse should be aware of the stigma of uncleanliness that is attached to the presence of lice. The affected child and parents need emotional support, reassurance, and vigorous instruction.

Scabies

Scabies is caused by a mite, which burrows under the skin. Although this condition is usually seen in adults, children also can be infected. This condition is discussed in Chapter 68.

Skin Disorders

Acne Vulgaris

A skin eruption called acne vulgaris, or simply **acne**, is common in adolescents and young adults. It is characterized by blackheads, pimples, cysts, nodules, and scarring and is most commonly seen on the face, back, chest, and upper arms. Acne usually is first seen during puberty and is slightly more common in boys than girls. Research indicates that hormonal changes during puberty accompanied by oversecretion of **sebum** are the underlying causes of acne. Diet plays no significant role in the development or progression of acne; however, a well-balanced nutritional diet is recommended for the purpose of good overall health. Some individuals may be sensitive to certain foods, in which case those foods are avoided. Stress seems to cause an increase in flare-ups of acne.

Acne can leave permanent scars on the face. It often has an emotional effect, because it usually occurs when a young person is agonizingly conscious of personal appearance and peer group approval.

Medical and Surgical Treatment. Treatment includes topical and systemic medications.

Dermabrasion, a surgical means of smoothing the skin, may be considered only after active acne has ceased. This procedure is used to minimize scarring. Key medications are listed in the accompanying box.

Nursing Considerations. The nurse must recognize that physical appearance is very important to the adolescent. Personal hygiene should be reviewed to prevent infection. Good general health and diet are included in the management of acne vulgaris. Instructions regarding medications and skin care regimen are essential. Teaching subjects are summarized in the accompanying box.

Impetigo Contagiosa

Impetigo contagiosa is an infection that can be caused by staphylococci or mixed bacteria. The reddened vesicles break open and leave a sticky yellow crust, usually on the face and hands (Fig. 66-1). Impetigo is highly contagious, and precautions should be taken to isolate the patient and equipment to prevent the spread of infection.

Key Medications
for Acne Vulgaris

Topical Agents

- benzoyl peroxide (Desquam, Fostex, Oxy-10, Clearasil)—antibacterial agent
- retinoic acid, tretinoin (Retin-A)
- tetracycline cream
- erythromycin cream

Systemic Agents

- tetracycline (such as Panmycin Achromycin)
- isotretinoin (Accutane)—careful monitoring by physician needed because of serious side effects; used only when other agents not effective

Nursing Considerations—Topical Agents

- When combined with other agents, may cause excessive drying of skin
- Avoid application to mucous membranes or eyes; avoid inflamed skin or sunburned skin
- Use with caution if fair-skinned; use with caution in eczema or other skin conditions
- May cause bleaching of hair or clothing

Nursing Considerations: Tetracycline

- Take 1 hour before or 2 hours after any food, especially milk, dairy products, or meat.
- May interact negatively with iron, lithium, and oral contraceptives
- Do not use with renal (kidney) or hepatic (liver) dysfunction; drink plenty of water

The crusts are removed with soap and water. Oral systemic antibiotics are usually used.

Nursing Considerations. Nursing care is aimed at preventing the spread of infection. Good handwashing is essential. Towels and linens for the infected child should be kept separate from others. The child should be discouraged from scratching or touching infected sites.

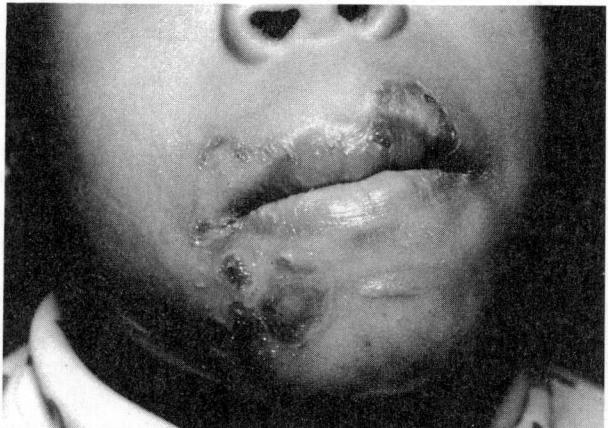

Figure 66-1. Impetigo. Nonbullous impetigo. Moist expanding perioral crusts with minimal surrounding erythema characteristic of streptococcal infection of the skin. (Courtesy of Bernard A. Cohen, M.D.)

Athlete's Foot (Tinea Pedis)

Athlete's foot, also called *tinea pedis,* is a fungus infection that attacks the skin between the toes. Watery blisters form in moist weepy spots that burn and itch. It is common among school-age children and young people. The organism responsible for infection (often *Candida albicans*) grows in dark, damp places and is found on floors of public baths and showers.

Commercial preparations are available for treating athlete's foot. If the infection does not respond to these preparations, a dermatologist should be consulted. Medications used in athlete's foot are Pedi-Dri foot powder, undecylenate acid and zinc undecylenate (Desenex powder, ointment, solution, or cream), tolnaftate (Tinactin), or Lysol solution. Young people will find teaching about athlete's foot helpful (see box).

Musculoskeletal Disorders

Trauma

Because the school-age child and adolescent are usually very active, they are subject to many kinds of injuries. The nurse will see many fractures, burns, and other forms of trauma in this age group. Consult the index for discussions of these conditions.

Postural Defects

Postural defects are the most common musculoskeletal problems occurring during early school years and adolescence. Common postural defects occurring during puberty or adolescence include lordosis, kyphosis, and scoliosis (Fig. 66-2).

Lordosis is an exaggerated curvature of the lumbar spine in which the pelvis tips forward. It may occur as a result of a disease process, or it may be idiopathic. It may be associated with obesity, in which excess abdominal weight throws off the center of gravity. It is also associated with hip dislocations or contractures and is accompanied by pain.

Kyphosis is an abnormal curvature of the thoracic spine that results in a "hunchback" appearance. It can

result from diseases, such as tuberculosis, compression fractures, or arthritis, or it can be caused by poor posture. When kyphosis is caused by poor posture, it is often accompanied by lordosis, giving the child the appearance of swayback.

Scoliosis is a side curvature, resulting in an S-shaped appearance of the spine. There are two types of scoliosis: functional and structural. Functional scoliosis is the result of poor posture. Structural scoliosis is rare and is due to defects in spinal muscles or bones. It is the most common of the postural defects and is seen more frequently in girls.

Diagnosis. *Diagnosis* is made by observation and radiography (x-ray). Postural defects, especially scoliosis, are often discovered by the child's pediatrician or during school screenings. The examination is simple and takes relatively little time. The child faces the screener, stands straight with feet 2 to 3 inches apart. The examiner looks at the symmetry of the upper torso. The student is then instructed to place the chin on the chest, place the hands together, and bend over, allowing the hands to hang freely. The screener looks for any asymmetry, such as unequal shoulder height, elbow levels, or height of the hips. The child is also observed for abnormal curvature of the spine. If curvature is present, a scoliometer (leveling device), is used to detect the degree of curvature. Referral and treatment are based on the degree of curvature.

Medical and Surgical Treatment. Treatment of postural defects depends on the cause and degree of defect. If the cause of the defect is functional, the child may benefit from counseling. Nagging or harassing the child to stand or sit up straight usually does not help. Many traction devices and braces are used in the treatment of postural defects. Certain exercises also may help in mild cases. The Milwaukee brace is a commonly used device that extends from the chin to the hips and is specially fitted to the child. It is regularly adjusted as the child grows.

A somewhat more controversial method of treatment is the use of electrical stimulation. Electrodes are attached to the muscles of the back at night. It is thought that electrical stimulation of the muscles helps correct the curvature by increasing muscle tone.

Surgical intervention may be necessary to correct a postural defect. In these instances intervention includes application of a device to the spinal column to force realignment of the spine. The child usually undergoes spinal traction prior to the surgery. One of the most well-known spinal devices is the Harrington rod, which is actually secured to the vertebral bones.

Following surgery, the child may require a cast or brace for immobilization. Surgery is only done following more conservative treatment of the defect.

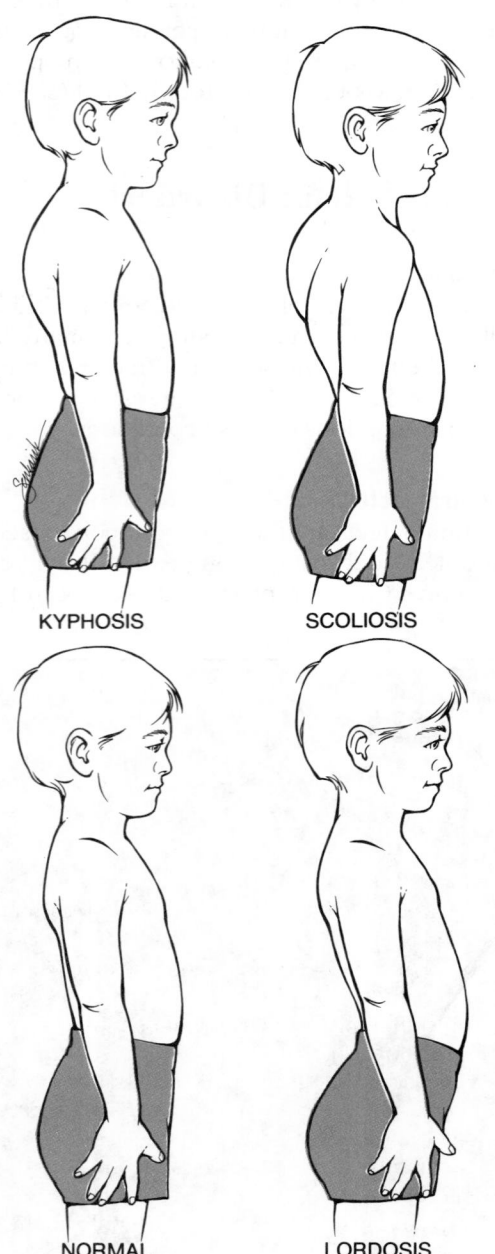

Figure 66-2. Profiles of children with normal and abnormal spinal curves.

Nursing Diagnosis. Some of the nursing diagnoses that will be seen on a nursing care plan are the following:

- Impaired Physical Mobility related to presence of brace, traction, or casts
- High Risk for Injury related to restricted movements
- High Risk for Impaired Skin Integrity related to presence of brace
- Body Image Disturbance related to chronic skeletal deformity or use of body brace

The nurse helps clarify the individualized goals of care for the patient and family. Plans are made to return to activities of daily living as much as possible. The nurse helps strengthen the adolescent's body image and helps the family support a positive image.

> **Key Concept**
>
> Because scoliosis most often affects adolescent girls and the treatment involves limitations and much distress, emotional support is of great importance.

Legg-Calvé-Perthes Disease

This disease occurs as a result of a lack of blood supply to the hip joint, which causes necrosis of the joint. It has several other names, among them coxa plana, slipped femoral epiphysis, Legg's disease, Legg-Calvé disease, and Legg-Calvé-Waldenström disease. It occurs in children between the ages of 2 and 12 years and is more common in boys and in white people. It may be caused by an injury or another disease process; it is also associated with low birth weight. Both hips may be affected; however, more frequently only one hip is affected. The disorder most often clears spontaneously, but treatment is necessary to prevent subsequent hip deformities. Stages of the disease are given in Table 66-1.

Medical Treatment. Treatment initially focuses on reducing inflammation by placing the child on bed rest. Traction may be used when muscle lengthening is necessary. Eventually an abductor brace or leg casts are applied. The goal of treatment is to maintain the head of the femur in the acetabulum. Abduction of the lower extremities is accomplished with the use of a variety of appliances, such as abductor braces, splints, or casts. A light-weight abductor brace allows the child to maintain almost normal activity. The most important aspect of treatment is to maintain the non–weight-bearing status of the child. The prognosis of Legg-Perthes disease depends on compliance with non-weight bearing on the affected extremity.

Surgical Treatment. Various types of nails or pins are used to secure the trochanter to the head of the femur.

Table 66-1. Stages of Legg-Calvé-Perthes Disease

Stage	Description	Duration
Stage I	Interruption of circulation to hip joint, resulting in necrosis of femoral head	Approximately 1–3 weeks; may last up to 1 year
Stage II	Depositing of new connective tissue because of new blood supply	6 months to 1 year; child may have definite, constant limp; also may have severe pain, aggravated by activity and relieved by rest
Stage IIIa	Granulation of new bone replaces connective tissue	1–2 years
Stage IIIb	Regeneration and completion of bone growth; shape of joint fixed	2–3 years (depending on whether medical or surgical treatment used)

If this surgery is done, the child only has a few months of non-weight-bearing. Surgery is usually reserved for children over age 6 who have a relatively severe femoral head deformity.

Dental Malocclusion

Malocclusion refers to faulty positioning of the teeth, which results in improper alignment of the jaws and teeth. In addition to being difficult to clean, malocclusion may cause facial deformities and difficulty eating and chewing. The correction of tooth positioning and jaw deformities is called **orthodontia**. Generally, orthodontic care should begin when the permanent teeth begin to erupt, between the ages of 8 and 12 years. Sometimes treatment is delayed until the child is older, depending on the severity of the problem.

Malignant Bone Tumors

Malignant tumors are not as common in children as they are in adults. However, tumors tend to grow faster in children than adults. General nursing care of the patient with cancer is discussed in Chapter 76.

Osteogenic sarcoma is a type of cancerous bone tumor, often seen in males between the ages of 10 and 30 years. The diaphysis of the long bones is frequently involved, and other bones may be involved as well. The cancer metastasizes by way of the circulatory system, often to the lungs first. Treatment may involve amputation of the affected extremity, along with radiation and chemotherapy. Aggressive treatment can reduce the mortality rate of this cancer.

Ewing's sarcoma is a bone malignancy that arises from the bone marrow and affects the long and flat bones. It is more commonly seen in males between the ages of 10 and 20 years. Radiation is used as treatment. The prognosis is guarded.

Parosteal sarcoma is less deadly than osteogenic sarcoma. It arises from the bone surface rather than the interior of the bone.

Endocrine Disorders

Diabetes Mellitus

Young insulin-dependent diabetics should be encouraged to test their blood for glucose, self-admininister their injections as soon as possible, and lead a normal, independent life (Fig. 66-3).

There are few dietary and exercise restrictions, and the diabetic can learn to regulate insulin intake according to diet and activity.

The young diabetic may be more "*brittle*" or difficult to control than the adult. Diabetes counseling must emphasize regulation of diet and insulin administration to reflect physical activity. Diabetes is discussed in detail in Chapter 72.

Sensory System Disorders

Retinitis Pigmentosa

Retinitis pigmentosa (RP) is characterized by a slowly progressive, bilateral retinal degeneration that often results in blindness. Adolescents are more likely to be affected than other people.

Generally, night blindness is the first symptom. The person is often myopic (near-sighted) as well. As the disease progresses, the visual field constricts, causing tunnel vision. The physician can often see a characteristic dark pigmentation in the retina, which is known as a *bone spicule*. Other ocular defects can occur, including cataracts, glaucoma, or blind spots. *Macular degeneration* occurs; when the macula is invaded, the person becomes blind. (This condition is often associated with hearing disorders.)

The patient should wear dark glasses in the bright sun to avoid further irritation of the eyes and to enhance remaining vision. The person may not be able to drive a car at night because of night blindness. Refer this person for counseling. The National Retinitis Pigmentosa Foundation provides literature and information about the disorder. Retinitis pigmentosa is a hereditary disease; therefore, genetic counseling is also important.

Juvenile Glaucoma

Glaucoma refers to abnormally high intraocular pressure, resulting in eye damage and decreased vision. It may be caused by trauma, hemorrhage into the eye, tumor, inflammatory eye diseases, or developmental

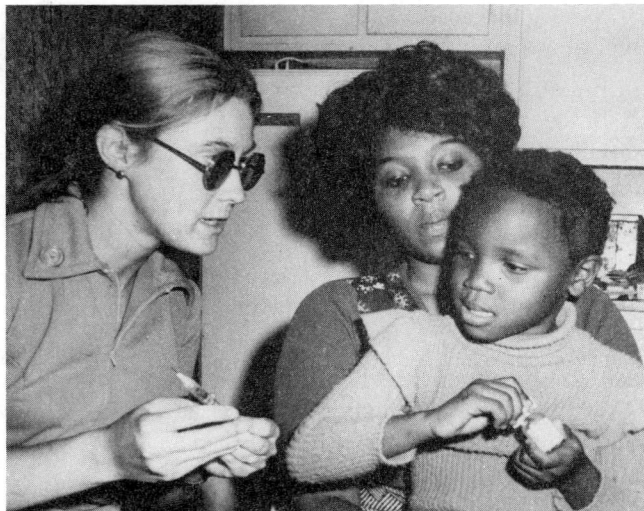

Figure 66-3. The nurse is instructing this young insulin-dependent diabetic patient and the child's mother in the proper technique of insulin administration. (Courtesy of Visiting Nurse Service of New York.)

abnormalities in the infant and young child. Early symptoms in the pediatric patient include frequent tearing, photophobia (sensitivity to light), and cloudiness of the cornea.

Surgery is performed as early as possible to prevent damage to vision. Medications to control intraocular pressure also are used. (See Chapter 73.)

Gastrointestinal Disorders

Inflammatory Bowel Disease

Inflammatory bowel disease (IBD) is a chronic gastrointestinal disorder. The two most common types of inflammatory bowel disease are Crohn's disease and chronic ulcerative colitis. Refer to Chapter 81 for information regarding Crohn's disease.

Chronic Ulcerative Colitis

Chronic ulcerative colitis (CUC) is a relatively common disorder of adolescents and young adults, which results in inflammation of the colon and rectum. One of the most pronounced symptoms of CUC is severe diarrhea. This may be accompanied by weight loss, anorexia, and delays in growth. A delay in the appearance of secondary sex characteristics also may be evident if the disease occurs before puberty. The distal colon shows evidence of ulceration, inflammation, and bleeding, which eventually may result in scarring of the gastrointestinal mucosa. An autoimmune component is believed to be associated with this illness, because it is often accompanied by arthritis, chronic hepatitis, and autoimmune anemia and because it responds to steroid treatment.

Medical and Surgical Treatment. One of the most important methods of treating CUC is administration of steroids. The difficulty with this is that many side effects are associated with steroid administration, some of which may cause further delay in growth (see Chapter 56). A colectomy, which removes the portion of the bowel that is diseased, results in care of symptoms. This is done only after conservative treatment has failed.

Appendicitis

Appendicitis occurs most frequently during adolescence. Appendectomy, a relatively simple surgery, is performed. Generally the young person recovers without difficulty. Occasionally, the appendix ruptures prior to surgery, exposing the peritoneum to gastrointestinal bacteria. In these cases, the child receives antibiotics, usually intravenously, to treat or prevent peritonitis. Nursing care for the postappendectomy patient is discussed in Chapter 81.

Disorders of the Reproductive System

Many disorders affect the reproductive system of the older child and adolescent. Many are related to hormonal changes.

Menstrual Difficulties

Difficulties with menstruation include delayed menarche (onset of menstruation), discomfort, and altered patterns. Pain occurring with ovulation is referred to as **mittelschmerz**. **Dysmenorrhea**, painful menstruation, is a common problem while regular periods are being established. There are two types of dysmenorrhea. When no pelvic disease is present, it is referred to as *primary* dysmenorrhea. When organic pelvic disease is present, it is called *secondary* dysmenorrhea.

Treatment of dysmenorrhea is symptomatic, unless an underlying physical cause can be identified. Analgesics, such as acetaminophen and ibuprofen, help reduce discomfort and inflammation.

Abnormal Sexual Development

Precocious and retarded sexual development may occur.

Defects in anatomic structure also can occur. If possible, these are corrected when the child is very young. These conditions are particularly distressing to the young person, because peer pressure is so significant at this stage of development. The nurse must consider the emotional aspects of this condition. Patients should be referred to the appropriate specialist.

Sexually Transmitted Diseases

Most sexually transmitted diseases (STD) in the United States occur in people younger than 25 years. The nurse should urge young people who think they might have an STD to see a physician. Physicians must, by law, treat STDs without reporting this fact to the patient's parents. There also are many free public clinics that provide tests and treatment for STDs.

Certain STDs are more prevalent in adolescents and young adults. These include syphilis, gonorrhea, genital herpesvirus, and genital warts. The incidence of many of these disorders is increasing, even with the massive amount of public education about safer sex and condom use. Many of these disorders have grave implications for young people because they render them unable to bear children; the HIV virus can cause AIDS, which usually is fatal. Chapter 63 describes these and other STDs, fertility control, and other issues related to sexuality.

Emotional and Psychological Disorders

Adolescents have several difficult developmental tasks that must be achieved before they can be considered adults. In some cases, the stress becomes overwhelming, and the young person develops emotional disorders. In addition to psychological factors, some of the following may involve physical factors.

Sleep Disorders

Narcolepsy

Narcolepsy is a brief attack of irresistible sleep, which is often precipitated by an alteration in the young person's emotional status. This can be traced to a conflict situation. Nighttime sleep is basically normal. However, an earlier appearance of rapid eye movement (REM) sleep is often reported. REM designates the type of sleep, most often occurring toward morning when a person dreams.

There is often conflict over competition or an expression of unacceptable aggression in this person. Boys are more likely to be affected than girls. There is no significant relationship between narcolepsy and seizure disorders, although a seizure disorder must be ruled out. Hallucinations may occur just as the person is falling asleep *(hypnagogic hallucinations)*. Another symptom is *sleep paralysis*. Narcolepsy may be accompanied by **cataplexy** which is an attack of muscular weakness and lack of muscle tone.

Hypersomnia

Hypersomnia is an uncontrollable urge to sleep, which is characterized by *lengthy* periods of sleep (12–18 hours). Hypersomnia must be differentiated from absence seizures. There may be a physiologic cause, such as brain damage or another physical illness. The disorder may be a manifestation of a psychological problem. The person sleeps to "escape the world."

Nightmares and Somnambulism

Nightmares and sonambulism (sleep walking) also are common childhood occurrences and are usually outgrown. The common nightmare frightens the child, but he or she can be comforted by the parent and will go back to sleep. The child often can tell all about the nightmare in graphic detail the next morning.

Somnambulism, which is sleep walking, usually occurs during the later stages of non-REM sleep. There is no recall of the episode when the child awakens. The sleep walking episode can last from several minutes to a half hour or longer. Sleep walking is more common in boys than in girls and is more common if the person is fatigued, under stress, or has taken a hypnotic or sedative medication. Trauma, central nervous system infections, or seizure disorders may be predisposing factors. Most commonly, however, somnambulism is related to anxiety. Often the child sleep walks once or twice and never does it again.

The major concern with sleep walking is physical protection. Do not threaten or abruptly awaken a sleep walker, but observe safety measures to avoid injury.

Night Terrors or Terror Disorder

Night terrors or terror disorder (pavor nocturnus), not to be confused with simple nightmares, almost always occurs in children, not in adults. It is not common. The child awakens screaming and is panicky. Such a child cannot be consoled and may be incoherent. After the terror has passed, the child usually cannot recall what caused it. The condition is usually outgrown. If blood is seen on the pillow after a child has a nightmare, the possibility of a psychomotor seizure disorder must be considered. A sleep study (polysomnogram) can differentiate these sleep disorders from seizure disorders.

Somniloquism

Sleep talking is called **somniloquism** and is common in young people. It may or may not be associated with sleep walking. The person often can carry on a logical conversation but will not remember it the next morning.

Insomnia

Insomnia is difficulty in falling asleep. It may be caused by *hyperkinesis* (hyperactivity) or may be a symptom of an emotional problem.

Eating Disorders

Food and eating behaviors change as the child develops. They can take on new meanings in adolescence as a result of family stress or peer pressure. A few of the nursing diagnoses that will be seen on a nursing care plan for a patient with an eating disorder are the following:

◆ Altered Nutrition: Less than Body Requirements related to self-induced vomiting, excessive use of laxatives
◆ High Risk for Fluid Volume Deficit related to inadequate oral intake, vomiting, laxative abuse
◆ Body Image Disturbance related to distorted perception of body weight
◆ Self-Esteem Disturbance related to denial of eating disorder
◆ Constipation related to inadequate diet, laxative abuse
◆ Ineffective Individual Coping related to altered family dynamics, changes in role expectations

Of prime importance in the care of a person with an eating disorder is the teaching factor. The patient needs to understand bodily functions and the need for nourishment to sustain the body and its functions. To have the patient comply with teaching, the nurse must develop a strong rapport with the patient. This is not an easy task.

Anorexia Nervosa

Anorexia nervosa is a disorder most commonly seen in white, upper middle class, female adolescents. It is characterized by extreme weight loss with no underlying causative physical disorder. The adolescent with anorexia nervosa does not have a loss of appetite but refuses to eat. There is an obsession with food and with not eating food. The adolescent usually focuses on preparing, talking about, and purchasing food but refuses to eat. Hunger is extreme and always present. The obsession is directed toward being thin. The adolescent has a distorted image of her own body and continues to see herself as overweight, even after becoming dangerously thin. This is a long-term psychological problem, which involves complex family relationships. Signs and symptoms of anorexia nervosa are listed in the accompanying box.

Complications can be life-threatening and include lowered blood pressure, bradycardia, hypokalemia, and congestive heart failure. Severe malnutrition must be treated before long-term counseling can begin. Most severe cases require hospitalization.

Bulimia

Bulimia, known as *gorge–purge syndrome,* is an eating disorder characterized by binge eating. It is more common in older adolescents and young women. Typ-

Signs and Symptoms of Anorexia Nervosa

- ◆ Extreme weight loss
- ◆ Menstrual irregularities
- ◆ Unexplained amenorrhea
- ◆ Weakness
- ◆ Fatigue
- ◆ Light-headedness
- ◆ Constipation
- ◆ Low blood pressure
- ◆ Bradycardia (slow pulse)
- ◆ Hypokalemia (potassium deficiency)
- ◆ Thinning hair
- ◆ Distorted body image
- ◆ Excessive exercising
- ◆ Low body temperature
- ◆ Dry skin
- ◆ Congestive heart failure

ically, the individual eats large amounts of food, usually in secret. Following this binge, an attempt is made to purge the system of food by self-induced vomiting or using laxatives and diuretics. Recurrent vomiting can cause dental caries by stomach hydrochloric acid, electrolyte imbalances, and even death. The individual has feelings of guilt and depression during periods of binging. Long-term counseling is necessary to overcome this illness.

Obesity

Obesity is the result of regular high consumption of calories, particularly from fats, resulting in excess accumulation of fatty tissue. It is classified as being in excess of 15% of optimum weight. The child who is obese is most often less active than the leaner child. A hereditary factor is related to obesity. Obesity is rarely caused by slow thyroid function.

There is a major psychological impact to the child who is obese. Making and keeping friends is difficult, and socialization and self-esteem are greatly affected. Treatment consists of diet and exercise with medical supervision, behavior modification, and counseling. Chapter 26 describes eating patterns and suggestions for healthy diets for children of all ages.

Enuresis and Encopresis

Enuresis (bed wetting) and *encopresis* (involuntary bowel movement with no physical cause) that continue into the school years require a physician's intervention. The cause is often emotional. Counseling or psychiatric

assistance, in combination with drugs, usually corrects the problem. Sometimes, a meatal stenosis needs to be surgically corrected. Encopresis most often requires intensive psychotherapy. In any event, the parent should not shame or belittle the child, because such parental attacks may cause lasting psychological damage.

Behavioral Problems

Although behavioral problems in childhood may have a physical basis, more often the cause is an inability to establish healthy relationships with others. Emotional problems may be manifested by withdrawn or destructive behavior or by bizarre speech. A child in need of professional assistance may be identified by inability to control impulses or behavior, behavior very different from others in the same age group, absence of friends, difficulty in learning even through he or she tests well, persistent physical symptoms that seem to have no physical basis, and specific deviant behaviors.

Many psychiatric units in large hospitals deal exclusively with young people. Keeping children in a unit separate from the adult unit is beneficial.

The Chronic Lawbreaker

One way a youngster indicates that he or she is having problems is by defying the law. Many police forces employ specialists or counselors to assist young people who are "asking for help" by being in constant trouble with the law. The most effective means of dealing with the problem is through family counseling.

Refusal to Go to School

Another problem facing parents of school-age children is refusal to go to school, or *school phobia*. This often occurs after a summer vacation or a brief illness. A change in school or neighborhood, a new sibling, divorce, or a family member's death may precipitate school avoidance.

The child (usually 5–10 years old) who has school phobia suffers from a fear of leaving his or her parents. The child "plays sick" and is so tense that he or she may actually become ill; in other instances, the child asks to stay home because of very minor physical complaints. If the child is allowed to stay home, the symptoms diminish immediately, only to recur the next morning. If the case is severe, the child may refuse to leave the house for any reason. This situation is often recognized by the school nurse, because the young person spends a great deal of time in the nurse's office once they get to school. (School phobia in an adolescent is often evidence of a more serious problem.)

Keys for Review

Key Questions for Critical Thinking

1. Describe the effect of hormonal changes on the adolescent female and male.
2. You work in an area where Lyme disease is prevalent. Describe the advice you would give your adolescent patients and rationale for this advice.
3. Describe similarities and differences between anorexia nervosa and bulimia. Describe nutritional factors involved. Describe psychological factors.

Key Readings

Behrman RE. Nelson's Textbook of Pediatrics, Ed 14. Philadelphia, W.B. Saunders, 1992

Castiglia PT, Harbin RE. Child Health Care: Process and Practice. Philadelphia, J.B. Lippincott, 1992

Hazinski MF. Nursing Care of the Critically Ill Child, Ed 2 St. Louis, Mosby-Yearbook, 1992

Jacksom DB, Saunders RB. Child Health Nursing: A Comprehensive Approach to the Care of Children and Their Families. Philadelphia, J.B. Lippincott, 1993

Murray R, Zentner J. Nursing Assessment and Health Promotion Strategies Through the Life Span. East Norwalk, CT, Appleton & Lange, 1993

O'Toole M. (Ed) Miller-Keane Encyclopedia and Dictionary of Medicine, Nursing and Allied Health, Ed 5. Philadelphia, W.B. Saunders, 1992

Pomar PJ (Ed). Nurses and Family Health Promotion: Concepts, Assessment, Intervention. Philadelphia, W.B. Saunders, 1992

Skale N. Manual of Pediatric Nursing Procedures, Philadelphia, J.B. Lippincott, 1992

Whaley LF. Nursing Care of Infants and Children, Ed 4. St. Louis, Mosby-Yerbook, 1991

Enrichment Keys

Health risk behaviors among adolescents who do and do not attend school—United States, 1992. MMWR 1994:43:129–132

Keys to Learning More

Chapter 67: children and adolescents with special needs

Unit Fourteen: physical disorders in adults, many of them experienced by children and adolescents

Chapter 68: skin disorders

Chapter 70: cast and traction care

Keys to Learning More (continued)

Chapter 71: seizure disorders

Chapter 72: endocrine disorders, including diabetes mellitus

Chapter 73: disorders of hearing and vision

Chapter 74: cardiovascular disorders

Chapter 75: blood and lymph disorders

Chapter 76: cancer

Chapter 77: allergic disorders

Chapter 78: immune disorders

Chapter 79: respiratory disorders

Chapter 80: oxygen therapy

Chapter 81: digestive disorders

Chapter 83: male reproductive disorders

Chapter 84: female reproductive disorders

Chapter 87: psychiatric nursing

Chapter 88: substance abuse

Chapter 90: death and dying

Key Resources

American Anorexia/Bulimia Association Inc.
133 Cedar Lane
Teaneck, NJ 07666

Juvenille Diabetes Foundation International
432 Park Avenue
New York, NY 10016

National Safety Council
444 N Michigan Avenue
Chicago, IL 60611
1-800-621-7619

National Scoliosis Foundation
93 Concord Avenue, PO Box 547
Belmont, MA 02178

Retinitis Pigmentosa Foundation Fighting Blindness
1401 Mount Royal Avenue
4th Floor
Baltimore, MD 21217-4245
410-225-9400

Scoliosis Association
PO Box 51353
Raleigh, NC 27609
919-846-2639

67 The Child or Adolescent With Special Needs

Keys for Learning

Learning Objectives

- Define attention deficit-hyperactivity disorder, and discuss the characteristic behaviors.
- Differentiate between genetic and acquired congenital disorders.
- Describe and compare major features of Down syndrome and fragile-X syndrome.
- Discuss the symptoms and treatment of chronic lead poisoning.
- Differentiate between cerebral palsy and Duchenne muscular dystrophy, and describe the treatment for each.
- Discuss how impairment of vision, hearing, or speech affects growth and development of children.
- Discuss the overall impact on the family who has a child with special needs.

Key Terms

amniocentesis	chromosomes	pica
ataxia	congenital	plumbism
autism	echolalia	teratogens
chelation	genetic	schizophrenic

Keys to Understanding This Chapter

Chapter 5: basic needs of all people

Chapter 7: community health agencies, many of which assist children with special needs

Unit Three: knowledge of normal growth and development assists in recognizing deviations

Unit Four: normal body structure and function, also basic to recognizing deviations

Unit Seven: nursing process skills used in the care of all patients

Unit Eight: communication skills used in care of all patients

Keys to Understanding This Chapter
(continued)

Unit Nine: basic nursing skills used in caring for children and adolescents

Chapter 50: physical examination and nursing assessment

Chapter 61: complications of childbirth

Chapter 62: disorders of the neonate

Chapter 64: basic pediatric nursing

Chapter 65: care of the infant, toddler, and preschooler

Chapter 66: care of the school child and adolescent

Key Points

- A genetic disorder is a physical or mental abnormality occurring because of an abnormal gene.
- Parents of a special needs child will often grieve over the loss of the expected "perfect child."
- A common finding in children with learning disabilities is low self-esteem.
- Exposure to alcohol or drugs during fetal development can result in physical or mental neonatal abnormalities.
- Duchenne muscular dystrophy is one of the most common muscle disorders in children.
- Substance abuse occurs most often in families with a difficulty (divorce, abuse, chronic alcoholism, financial problems). Often the substance abuser has low self-esteem and uses drugs to escape reality.

Key Topics Outline

Learning Disabilities
  Specific Learning Disabilities
  Attention Deficit Hyperactivity Disorder
Autism

Key Learning Activities

◆ Design a poster or presentation for your classmates about the effects (health hazards, potential outcomes) of maternal exposure to alcohol, narcotics, or infections during pregnancy.

◆ Visit a special education classroom. Describe the atmosphere (stimulation, handicap access, safety, student seating, teacher–student interactions, methods of communication, and socialization).

◆ Discuss long-term care of child with special needs, including costs, foster care, legal issues, education, and family needs.

The process of growing and maturing may be difficult, even under the best of circumstances. Life offers many challenges daily to all children during maturation. The child with a special need such as a long-term physical or emotional disorder and the family face not only ordinary day-to-day challenges, but additional ones as well. The entire family and all aspects of daily life are affected when a child has special needs or a chronic illness or is dying.

Nurses can assist the child and family by providing support and education. Families can be referred to a wide variety of support groups. Providing families with accurate information regarding the situation is essential.

Families experiencing any grieving process require support and acceptance of their feelings.

Key Concept

Parents with a physically or mentally challenged child go through a grieving process. This grieving occurs because of the loss of the "perfect child" that was expected during pregnancy. Grieving may occur intermittently throughout their lives, as their child reaches or fails to reach major milestones of growth and development. Grieving does not mean that the parents do not love their child. Support and understanding help parents cope with this challenge.

Key Abbreviations and Acronyms for Special Needs of the Pediatric Patient

ADHD	Attention deficit-hyperactivity disorder
CP	Cerebral palsy
FAS	Fetal alcohol syndrome
II	Intellectual impairment
IQ	Intelligence quotient
SLD	Specific learning disabilities
WISC-R	Weschler Intelligence Scale (for children)—Revised
MD	Muscular dystrophy
DMD	Duchenne muscular dystrophy

Learning Disabilities

A learning disability is a disorder in one or more of the processes involved in understanding or using language. There are many types of learning disabilities. They can be related to specific aspects of learning, such as memory, attention span, processing, or sequencing of information. A learning disability affects not only school performance, but all aspects of a child's life. Education must be individualized for the child with special needs.

Specific Learning Disabilities

Specific learning disabilities (SLD) are educational concerns. Most authorities believe that 10% to 20% of school-age children have some SLD. Although a learning disability may occur along with various other handicaps, such as sensory impairment or low IQ, they are *not* the result of these conditions. Children of normal intellectual functioning also can have difficulty with a specific aspect of learning.

There are many types of learning disabilities. SLD can include such disorders as inability to calculate or draw, and *dysphasia* (an impairment of speech). These disorders are evidenced by difficulty with speaking, writing, listening, talking, spelling, or calculating. *Dyslexia* is one of the most common disorders in which the person has difficulty with reading, spelling, or writing words. Often the child reverses letters or numbers.

Nursing Considerations. Nurses assisting children with learning disabilities must understand the specific type of disability and set achievable goals. The child with a problem listening and understanding must be given only one or two instructions at a time; these must be reinforced periodically. Children with listening deficits benefit from visual reminders; a tape recorder can be helpful for reinforcing information for the child with visual processing difficulties. Help and encouragement are important for the child to achieve progress. Keep in mind that patient teaching will need to be adjusted to account for the SLD.

Key Concept

It is easy to become frustrated when a child does not follow instructions. This child may continue to play with intravenous pumps or other equipment after repeated requests not to do so. This may be a behavioral problem or may be a learning disorder. The nurse must be patient and sensitive and offer praise and positive reinforcement (many children with SLD have low self-esteem). Manipulate the hospital environment to reduce unnecessary stimulation.

Attention Deficit-Hyperactivity Disorder

Attention deficit hyperactivity disorder (ADHD), also called minimal brain dysfunction and attention deficit disorder with hyperactivity (ADDH), involves a learning disability and a behavioral disorder. The child with ADHD has difficulties related to attention span and is extremely distractable. The child also is impulsive, disruptive, and hyperactive. The child may show poor eye–hand coordination; abnormalities may be seen on EEG. The manifestations of the disorder usually appear in most situations whether at home or elsewhere.

According to the American Psychiatric Association, the onset of the disorder is before the age of 4 years in approximately half of the cases and is six to nine times more common in boys.

For a child to be diagnosed with ADHD, at least 8 of the 14 criteria established by the American Psychiatric Association must be present for at least 6 months (see accompanying box). Diagnosis of ADHD is made only after other medical and psychiatric disorders are ruled out.

A child suspected of having ADHD undergoes a multidisciplinary evaluation, which includes speech and language, psychological, medical, and educational testing. A thorough neurologic evaluation and feedback from teachers and parents are essential.

The cause of this disorder is controversial; studies are continuing. A "disturbance of the neurotransmitters" (chemicals) in the brain has been speculated, but research has not identified any specific abnormality.

Nursing Considerations. Many problems are associated with ADHD. These include low self-esteem, poor social interaction, immaturity, and learning disabilities. The nurse working with the child with ADHD must understand that although strong emotional problems may develop, it is *not* classified as an emotional disorder. Treatment must be addressed from a multidisciplinary

---

Diagnostic and Statistical Manual of the American Psychiatric Association: Criteria for ADHD

1. Often fidgets with hands or feet or squirms in seat (in adolescents, this may be limited to subjective feelings of restlessness)
2. Has difficulty remaining seated
3. Is easily distracted
4. Has difficulty awaiting turn in group situations
5. Often blurts out answers before questions have been completed
6. Has difficulty following instructions
7. Has difficulty sustaining attention
8. Often shifts from one uncompleted activity to another
9. Has difficulty playing quietly
10. Often talks excessively
11. Often interrupts or intrudes on others
12. Often does not seem to listen
13. Often loses things necessary for tasks
14. Frequently engages in dangerous actions without considering the consequences

The child must have eight or more of these for a 6-month period to be diagnosed ADHD.

approach. A behavioral therapist may set up a behavior modification program. The school system must address any difficulties with learning and socialization, and the physician is involved with monitoring medication and the child's overall physical health. The nurse teaches the parents to minimize environmental stimuli, use consistent discipline, set limits, and focus on positive behaviors.

Although stimulant medications have proven to "work miracles" for some children, they are only part of the total behavioral, educational, and psychological approach to helping the child.

The current drug of choice is methylphenidate hydrochloride (Ritalin), a central nervous system stimulant that affects mental rather than motor activities. Side effects include decreased growth rate, increased heart rate and blood pressure, and sleep disturbances. Pemoline (Cylert) and other cerebral stimulants also may be used. Side effects are similar.

Antidepressants are the second drugs of choice. They are less likely to cause sleep disturbances, are not associated with growth retardation, and have a decreased risk of dependence.

Key Concept

The American Disabilities Act states that all children are entitled to free and appropriate education from the age of 3 to 21 years. This education is to be provided in the least restrictive environment.

Tourette Syndrome. Tourette Syndrome is an organic CNS disorder with an unknown cause, although there is a chemical neurotransmitter abnormality. This child exhibits tics (facial and motor movements, and vocal tics). About ¼ of these children show symptoms such as compulsive swearing. The child's behavior may deteriorate after trauma. Although these children are often of normal intelligence, they often have SLD and also show ADHD symptoms. Medications such as acetaminophen help with muscle spasm discomfort. Stimulants such as methylphenidate HCl (Ritalin), combined with haloperidol (Haldol) may help control behavior. A specific medication is pimozide (Orap) which blocks dopamine receptors in the brain. Many of these children improve as they near adulthood.

Autism

Autism is a severe developmental disorder characterized by intellectual, social, and communication deficits. Autism is not actually a disease but a syndrome of specific behaviors that may vary widely, thus making it difficult to diagnose. The cause of autism is unknown; however, statistics show that more boys are affected than girls.

The autistic child typically demonstrates a profound lack of social interaction with others. The child does not respond to verbal stimulation and does not like to cuddle or be touched. A bizarre attachment to mechanical objects may occur. Repetitive or ritualistic behaviors (eg, rocking, head banging, clicking of teeth, turning the head back and forth) are commonly seen in children with autism. Impaired verbal and nonverbal communication, temper tantrums, and self-destructive behavior also may be evident. **Echolalia** (repetition of words said by others) is one form of language impairment that may be seen. These children are believed to be preoccupied within themselves, perhaps having fixed delusions and hallucinations. They may become very upset or assaultive when interrupted.

Autism is most often associated with some degree of mental or cognitive impairment. Some autistic children are profoundly mentally impaired. Others may have superior intelligence in a particular area, such as math, art, or music (a savant). Other children have a photographic memory.

There is no known cure for autism; the prognosis varies widely. Psychiatric symptoms occur in approximately half of autistic children during adolescence. Intervention requires professionals with expertise in speech and language and behavior control. Education is a lifelong process.

Nursing Considerations. Nursing interventions include emphasizing the positive and focusing on the skills the child has. The nurse teaches parents to give the child immediate feedback and to continue social interaction with the child using short sentences and simple commands. Parents need to be concerned about safety but should maintain normal daily routines.

Genetic Disorders

Genetics is the study of heredity. Within the nucleus of almost every human cell are 23 pairs of **chromosomes**. Each chromosome contains hundreds of genes, placed in specific locations on the chromosome. Each gene (the unit of heredity) is responsible for a specific human characteristic (eg, hair color, size of nose, eye color). The correct position, shape, and alignment of genes results in a normal, healthy child. Any abnormality, of even a single gene, can have profound physical or mental consequences.

Genetic Versus Congenital Disorders

A **genetic** disorder is a physical or mental abnormality resulting from a defect in genetic structure. This defective gene can be familial (the parent has the defective gene and passes it on to the offspring), or it can occur with no apparent cause. A genetic disorder is in-born and is present at birth but may not be apparent.

Congenital simply means "present at birth"; it may or may not be genetic. A congenital defect or disorder can result from a defective gene; it is then genetic. A congenital disorder also can be the result of maternal factors or conditions during pregnancy or childbirth (acquired disorder).

> ### Key Concept
>
> Some congenital and genetic disorders are not identified until the child fails to achieve certain normal milestones of development.

Diagnosis

Some genetic disorders can be diagnosed immediately by identifying physical characteristics or by laboratory studies. Others demonstrate signs and symptoms gradually over time. Many disorders can be detected prenatally with **amniocentesis**, although this test carries a certain risk to the fetus. If the parents choose to maintain the pregnancy, they can prepare themselves for the disability and how to deal with it. Parents also may choose to abort a defective fetus.

Chromosomal studies are performed when a genetic disorder is suspected. A blood sample is taken, and if a chromosomal problem is suspected, further studies may be recommended.

Genetic Counseling

Genetic Counseling is provided to people seeking information about possibilities of genetic disorders in the family. A professional genetic counselor specializes in identifying genetic profiles (of individuals and families). During counseling, an extensive health history is taken. This includes chronic health problems, miscarriages, birth defects, and causes of death of other family members. The counselor also inquires about employment, ethnic background, and exposure to toxins. A family tree (profile) is designed; this indicates the probability of genetic disorders. Counseling includes education regarding genetics, how disorders are inherited, and individual risks of genetic disorders. The genetic counselor does not make decisions for people about family planning. Information and options are provided, and the couple makes their own decision. The genetic counselor's role is one of support and information.

Genetic counseling is a form of preventive health-care with the goal of preventing genetic defects. The nurse should encourage couples or individuals at risk for transmitting genetic disorders to seek genetic counseling before pregnancy. The genetic counselor helps them to make educated, informed decisions. Informa-tion on genetic counseling can be obtained from the National Foundation of the March of Dimes.

> ### Key Concept
>
> Genetic counseling is particularly indicated for an adult who has a known genetic disorder.

Intellectual Impairment

The intellectually impaired individual demonstrates below average intellectual abilities, accompanied by difficulty with independent functioning. These people also have been described as mentally retarded, mentally disabled, or intellectually challenged. The severity of the handicap or disability is determined in large part by scores achieved on standard intelligence tests. Tests such as the Wechsler Intelligence Scale for Children-Revised and Stanford Binet are used to determine degrees of intellectual impairment. Although actual intelligence quotient (IQ) scores obtained should not be used to determine a child's abilities, the scores usually must be reported so that the child can qualify for special education assistance in public schools. (Remember that these IQ tests were normed using middle-class, English-speaking people and may not be universally appropriate.)

Causes of cognitive impairment are many and varied. Chromosomal defects account for some. In addition, prenatal exposure to infections, drugs, and chemicals or maternal malnutrition play a role. Neonates who are premature, are small for gestational age, and have cranial defects or trauma are at great risk for cognitive impairment. The etiology is unknown in many cases.

Levels of Functioning

The child who is *borderline* intellectually impaired is most often able to function independently with special education assistance. Developmental delays are common, but many of these children achieve most of the milestones of normal child development.

The majority of cognitively impaired children fall into the category of *mild impairment.* Most of these children qualify for full-time special education. However, those who are higher functioning may develop reading skills at a fifth- or sixth-grade level. The *moderately* cognitively impaired child is unable to function independently and achieves a maximum mental age of 3 to 7 years. Training focuses on self-care activities (activities of daily living), and the child will eventually require assisted-care living arrangements.

The child who is *severely* mentally disabled requires a great deal of assistance with activities of daily living but can conform to daily routines and repetitive activities. Language development is minimal.

The *profoundly* mentally handicapped child will require complete assistance with all aspects of daily life. Some of these children may eventually be toilet trained; however, many are not. Verbalization is extremely limited.

Although the use of IQ scores for purposes other than agency placement and funding is discouraged, the following categories are generally accepted. These IQ categories are according to the American Association on Mental Retardation.

◆ Borderline: 83 to 68
◆ Mild: 67 to 52
◆ Moderate: 51 to 36
◆ Severe: 35 to 20
◆ Profound: below 19 (not able to test)

Special Considerations in Aging

Aging people who are mentally handicapped present special problems. They are often left without primary caregivers when their parents die or become disabled. It may be a difficult adjustment for this individual to enter an assisted-living situation when they are middle-aged or older.

Association for Retarded Citizens

The Association for Retarded Citizens in each county assists intellectually impaired people and their families. This association provides support groups, supplies and literature, education, advocacy in housing, employment, and referrals for group homes, respite care, and medical care.

Genetic Intellectual Impairment

Down Syndrome

Down syndrome (also called Down's syndrome), a developmental disorder, results from a chromosomal abnormality. This abnormality in the chromosomes results in varying degrees of intellectual impairment; it occurs in 1 in 50 to 900 births, depending on the type. The incidence of Down syndrome increases in older mothers, particularly in those older than 35 years.

There are three main types of Down syndrome. In 95% of all cases, there is an extra chromosome on the 21st pair of chromosomes. This is known as *trisomy 21*. The two other, much less common types are *translocation* and mosaicism. *Translocation* (3%–4% of cases) is a genetic abnormality passed from parent to child and is not associated with advanced maternal age. *Mosaicism* (1% of cases) is rare and is not genetic; it occurs because some cells have 46 chromosomes, and others have 47.

Characteristics. Down syndrome is most often diagnosed at birth by recognizable physical characteristics. Although this is a primary means of identifying Down syndrome, chromosomal studies confirm the diagnosis. Typical characteristics of Down syndrome include a small, flat nose and upward, outward slanting eyes. (For this reason, the disorder was called "Mongolism" in the past.) Other characteristic features include white dots on the iris of the eyes (Brushfield's spots); short, sparse eyelashes; small, low-set ears; and downward-curved mouth with protruding tongue. These children usually have short, square hands with an abnormal crease straight across the palm (simian line). They also have short, stubby feet, with a wide space between the big toe and the rest of the toes and a transverse crease across the sole of the foot. The muscles are flabby, and joints can easily be hyperextended without causing pain to the child.

Related Disorders. Many physical disorders are associated with Down syndrome. Congenital cardiac defects occur in approximately 35% of Down syndrome infants. There is an increased incidence of leukemia and severe respiratory illness, thyroid disorders, megacolon, and hypotonic abdominal muscles. Puberty may be delayed.

Nursing Considerations. Nursing interventions for the child with Down syndrome must focus on prevention of complications from related disorders and education and support for the family. A sample nursing care plan gives examples of nursing care of a child with Down syndrome. Early intervention by medical and educational professionals is essential in attaining optimal health and level of function.

Education enables a child with Down syndrome to have a fuller life and to feel pride in accomplishments. Children with Down syndrome, however, need a great deal of repetition to foster learning. Speech development may be slower than motor development. Stammering can occur in a child under stress. A decrease in relative IQ scores occurs with age because of the abstract thinking that is required at a higher mental age.

Fragile X Syndrome

Fragile X syndrome is an inherited genetic abnormality of the X chromosome; it results in cognitive impairment and distinctive physical features. Intellectual impairment ranges from SLDs to profound mental handicaps. Up to 1 in 1,000 children may be affected.

Characteristics. The child with fragile X syndrome typically has a large head, long face, and large chin. Eyes may be wide set, and ears are large and often protruding. The child typically has a broad nose, high palate, large testicles, and large hands. There is a noted speech

Joey Baker is a 12-year-old white boy with the admitting diagnosis of appendicitis and Down syndrome. He has had acute abdominal pain with vomiting and loss of appetite for 2 days. He has had an appendectomy. His mother and older sibling stayed with him throughout the night. His mother reports that he is able to function at the level of a 4- or 5-year-old but needs constant supervision and direction. Two nursing diagnoses from the plan of care follow. The diagnosis "anxiety" was developed on admission. The diagnosis "High Risk for altered growth and development" was suggested by the mother's consistently overprotective behaviors.

Nursing Diagnosis: *Anxiety Related to New Experience of Pain and Hospitalization as Evidenced by Withdrawal and Uncustomary Lack of Responsiveness*

Goal: Patient will feel sufficiently secure and safe to cooperate with the plan of care and treatment regimen. (Patient will trust the nurse.)

Nursing Actions (assess/do/teach)	Rationale	Evaluative Statement
1. Determine the child's usual pattern of daily activities, and duplicate this as closely as possible; if family members wish to participate in care, facilitate this; recommend that the family provide familiar comfort items, such as own pajamas or favorite toy.	Changes in routine are especially threatening to the mentally handicapped child.	6/6, Goal partially met; Pt beginning to trust nurse sufficiently to take medicine, allow assessment of incision.
2. Assess the child's reaction to illness and hospitalization; common fears of children are separation, loss of control, bodily injury and harm; plan interventions that minimize these stresses, and help the child to feel safe in the strange hospital environment; explain all procedures simply in a manner the child can understand—enlist the parent's help as necessary.	The child with Down syndrome poses a special challenge to the nurse, who bases care on the child's unique responses to the stress of illness; entering into the mind and experience of the child offers the best guarantee that the experience of hospitalization will be positive for the child.	

(continued)

delay; stuttering may be present. Heart murmur, caused by mitral value prolapse, may be present. Table 67-1 on page 943 compares fragile X to Down syndrome.

Learning is affected, not only by lower IQ, but also by shortened attention span and hyperactivity. The child also may exhibit autistic-type behaviors and temper tantrums.

Nursing Considerations. There is no cure for fragile X. Early interventions is essential to maximize the child's potential. Many of the nursing interventions for Down syndrome are appropriate for this child as well. The nursing interventions for the child with mental retardation remain the same regardless of the etiology. The child will benefit from speech and occupational therapy. Special education assistance is most helpful. Because fragile X syndrome is inherited, genetic counseling is recommended for all family members.

Other Genetic Disorders

Neurofibromatosus is characterized by "café-au-lait" spots and benign skin tumors. The child has neurologic, cognitive, and speech impairment. ADHD and seizures are common.

Tay-Sachs is an inborn error of metabolism, primarily affecting Ashkenazi Jews. At about 1 year of age, the

Nursing Actions (assess/do/teach)	Rationale	Evaluative Statement
3. Accept that the mentally handicapped child may revert to the coping strategies of a younger child: physical resistance, aggression, negativism, and regression; assist the family to understand these behaviors if they present.	Most children cope with the stress of illness by regressing to a more dependent and secure level of functioning.	
4. Be especially sensitive to any pain the child is experiencing, because it may be difficult for the child to communicate his comfort needs; offer analgesics and other comfort measures as appropriate.	Physicians and nurses tend to underestimate the existence of pain in children.	

Nursing Diagnosis: *High Risk for Altered Growth and Development Related to Mother's Overprotection as Evidenced by Excessively Protective and Permissive Maternal Behaviors and Dependence of Child on Mother*

Goal: Mother verbalizes the importance of the child developing self-control, independence, initiative, and self-esteem.

Nursing Actions (assess/do/teach)	Rationale	Evaluative Statement
1. Understanding that the stress of hospitalization is affecting the mother and child, assess the mother's overall adjustment to the child's handicap; stages of adjustment are overprotection, rejection, denial, gradual acceptance.	"Benevolent overreaction" is a common early response to a handicapped child; but the child's development is contingent on the parent's ability to accept and work with the handicap realistically.	6/6, Goal not met; mother very defensive about her parenting and rejects any discussion of Joey's need to develop more independence and self-control. *Revision:* Continue to work with both parents, and refer for counseling or support group if appropriate.
2. Affirm the positive parenting behaviors the mother exhibits, and talk about the difficulties of raising a handicapped child; counsel that overprotection is a common parental reaction but one that results in a vicious cycle of overprotective, permissive parent and dependent, demanding child; teach parenting strategies that promote the child's self-control, independence, initiative, and self-esteem; refer for professional counseling if necessary.	Overprotection in a parent is usually resistant to change once firmly established; professional counseling may be needed.	

Table 67-1. Comparison of Characteristics of Down Syndrome and Fragile X Syndrome

Down Syndrome	Fragile X Syndrome
Head—round, small, and short	Head—abnormally large
Face—flattened profile	Face—long; large, protruding jaw
Ears—small, low-set	Ears—large, protruding
Eyes—upward, outward slant; epicanthal folds; Brushfield's spots	Eyes—wide set; epicanthal folds
Nose—small; depressed nasal bridge	Nose—flattened nasal bridge
Hands—short, square; Simian creases	Hands—Simian creases
Mouth—high-arched palate; protruding tongue; mouth curved downward	Mouth—high-arched palate
Behavioral—low-normal intelligence to severely mentally handicapped; language delay	Behavioral—mild to profoundly mentally handicapped; short attention span, hyperactivity; temper tantrums; autistic-like behaviors; speech delay

child becomes hypotonic and loses vision. Death usually occurs before age 4. A blood test is available to determine carriers.

Gaucher disease also affects Ashkenazi Jews and involves the CNS. These children rarely live beyond age 5.

Torsion dystonia, in the dominant form, involves the population at large. It involves the CNS and although intelligence remains normal, many physical and developmental difficulties occur.

Congenitally Acquired Disorders

Prenatal exposure to **teratogens** can cause abnormal development in an embryo or fetus. Alcohol, drugs, maternal diseases, and toxic substances are teratogens and can cause a wide range of fetal abnormalities. In addition, trauma or anoxia during the birthing process or a problem during fetal development, such as maternal German measles, can cause fetal disorders. Maternal malnutrition during fetal development and low birth weight are important contributing causes of intellectual impairment. Disorders of the neonate and related symptoms are discussed in Chapter 62. (Chapter 88 addresses the general topic of substance abuse.) These conditions are congenital but *not* genetic; they are acquired. Many of these conditions cause difficulties for the child during infancy and beyond.

Fetal Alcohol Syndrome

Fetal alcohol syndrome (FAS) is the result of maternal alcohol consumption, perhaps as little as one ounce per day. The majority of infants with FAS have growth retardation and developmental delays in addition to below-normal mental functioning. These infants tend to be extremely irritable. As the child becomes older, a shortened attention span and hyperactivity become evident. Other features include microcephaly (small head); eye and ear defects, which include septal defects and tetralogy of Fallot; impairment of fine motor movement; and memory deficits. There is no cure for FAS. Early identification and intervention are necessary to maximize the child's potential and prevent further complications. Public education regarding the dangers of consuming *any alcohol* during pregnancy is the key to prevention.

Narcotic-Exposed Neonate

The long-term outcome of the neonate exposed to maternal narcotic use is not completely known. First, the newborn must withdraw from the narcotic. In addition, these children may have cognitive impairment, behavioral disorders, learning disabilities, and ADHD. Some of these difficulties also may be the result of a dysfunctional home environment, in which the mother may be continuing her drug use. In addition, mothers who use drugs regularly are often malnourished and frequently exposed to infections during pregnancy. The narcotic-exposed newborn faces long-term social, physical, emotional, and mental challenges.

Key Concept

Substance abuse is one of the most common causes of cognitive impairment and physical disabilities in children. Behavioral and psychosocial problems may result.

Infants Exposed to Maternal Infections

Many maternal infections have a critical effect on the fetus, with resulting long-term consequences. Fetal exposure to chickenpox or toxoplasmosis can result in mental retardation and microcephaly; toxoplasmosis also can cause deafness or cognitive impairment. Maternal herpesvirus can cause seizures and paralysis in the newborn. The outcome of prenatal exposure to rubella (German measles) includes disabilities and visual impairment.

Acquired Immunodeficiency Syndrome in Children

The majority of children who are human immunodeficiency virus (HIV)-positive or who have acquired immunodeficiency syndrome (AIDS) are infected prenatally by their HIV-positive mothers. However, recent research has shown that while a very high percentage of babies born to HIV-positive mothers test positive for the HIV *antibody*, only about 1 in 4 test positive for the *antigen*. Therefore, many of these infants will live a normal life span and most likely will not go on to develop full-blown AIDS.

A small percentage of children, usually adolescents or older children, have become infected with the virus through sexual contact or intravenous drug use. These children usually develop the AIDS-related complex of disorders.

Signs and Symptoms. One of the differences between children with HIV-related infections and adults is that prior to 1 year of age, the infant's immune system is immature. An infant is less able to fight off the opportunistic infections associated with AIDS, which results in quicker disease progression in those who are antigen-positive. Approximately half of these infants develop *Pneumocystis carinii pneumonia*. (Diseases such as Kaposi's sarcoma and tuberculosis, although common in adults with AIDS, are uncommon in children.) An infant with AIDS usually has delayed growth and presents as a typical failure to thrive baby. Most of these infants also have enlarged livers; many develop lymphoid interstitial pneumonia. These infants and children have a greater incidence of bacterial sepsis and neurologic involvement than the adult.

Treatment. Zidovudine (Retrovir) continues to be the primary treatment for pediatric AIDS. Antibiotics and gamma globulin are used to treat opportunistic infections. Common childhood illnesses, such as chickenpox, measles, otitis media, and upper respiratory infections, can be deadly to the infant or child with AIDS. Immunizations and isolation from other sick children are critical; a simple case of otitis media can quickly develop into meningitis in this child.

Other Considerations. Other factors complicate the care of the pediatric AIDS patients. The mother may be too ill to care for the child; if no other family members are available, foster care may be necessary. Keeping the child isolated from sick siblings at home is difficult, as is providing the child with adequate nutrition when the budget is limited.

Environmentally Acquired Defects

An environmentally acquired defect occurs as a result of an event in the child's environment, including trauma, ingestion of poisons, and infections. These can cause permanent brain damage and mental impairment; they are usually not reversible.

Chronic Lead Poisoning (Plumbism)

Lead is toxic to the human body. It is a substance that is found almost everywhere: in water, old paint, contaminated dust, and dirt. One of the most common causes of lead poisoning, also called **plumbism**, in children is through ingestion of leaded paint chips. A federal law prohibiting the use of lead in paints has reduced the number of lead poisoning cases. However, children living in older homes, usually in inner cities, remain at risk. Many times, older homes in deteriorating neighborhoods need repair; they may have chipped paint. Inquisitive and hungry children may eat paint chips. (Eating nonfood items is called **pica**.)

Nursing Alert

Lead is contained in items other than paint: newspaper print, unwashed fruits and vegetables, old toys and eating utensils, old pipes and plumbing, soil containing lead from old chipped paint, sand and dirt on playgrounds, and air pollution from unleaded gasoline. If the dust from scraped, leaded paint is inhaled, it can have just as deleterious an effect as if the paint were eaten. The buildup of lead can take place gradually.

Signs and Symptoms. Early symptoms of lead poisoning are so general that they can be easily missed or attributed to other childhood illnesses. Signs and symptoms of lead poisoning include the following:

◆ Hyperirritability
◆ Anorexia, nausea, and vomiting
◆ Abdominal pain
◆ Headache
◆ Fatigue, decreased play
◆ Intermittent vomiting (lead colic)

◆ Anemia, pallor
◆ Constipation
◆ Behavior changes
◆ In more severe cases, weakness, clumsiness
◆ Impaired level of consciousness and mental abilities
◆ Seizures
◆ Coma
◆ Encephalopathy (brain degeneration)

The most severe complication of lead poisoning is *lead encephalopathy*. This may result in a number of central nervous system disorders, including seizures, cerebral palsy, cognitive impairment, and attention deficit disorder. Untreated encephalopathy usually results in severe brain damage and death.

Treatment. The child first must be removed from the lead source. If the case is mild, the child is treated symptomatically. Anemia is treated with diet and iron supplements; seizures are treated with antiseizure medications.

Chelation is the administration of a drug that combines with lead to draw the lead out of the body. The drug of choice for chelation is edetate calcium disodium (calcium disodium versenate, calcium EDTA), given IV, and dimercaprol (BAL in oil), given deep IM. Recently approved by the Food and Drug Administration, 2,3-dimercaptosuccinic acid (DMSA) has the advantage of oral administration.

Long-term residual effects of plumbism include intellectual impairment, learning disabilities, or seizures. These require a multidisciplinary approach involving schools, social services, and the healthcare system. Early recognition of symptoms helps alleviate long-term consequences of chronic lead poisoning.

> **Key Concept**
>
> The most effective means of treating plumbism is through public education and prevention.

Neuromuscular Long-Term Disorders

Cerebral Palsy

Cerebral palsy (CP) is a general term used to describe movement disorders in children and may be accompanied by intellectual and learning deficits. Unlike other movement disorders, CP is not a progressive disorder. However, it is the most common permanent physical disability of childhood.

There are many known causes of CP, all of which are based on asphyxia and ischemia of the brain. Prenatal causes include maternal infection, excess radiation, fetal anoxia, pregnancy-induced hypertension, maternal diabetes, abnormal placental attachment, and malnutrition. Other causes include birth trauma, brain infections (eg, meningitis), encephalitis, head trauma, prolonged anoxia during childbirth or in very early infancy, brain tumor, and cerebral hemorrhage or clot.

Classifications. There are three major types of CP, although mixed forms also occur. The majority of children have *spastic cerebral palsy* (approximately 70%). Symptoms include hypertension, deep-tendon reflexes, and increased stretch reflexes. There is rapid alteration of muscle contraction and relaxation, muscle weakness, underdevelopment of affected extremities, and a tendency to develop contractures. The child with spastic CP walks on the toes with a scissorlike gait, crossing one foot in front of the other.

The child with *dyskinetic cerebral palsy* characteristically has abnormal involuntary movements, such as grimacing and sharp jerks. These movements disappear during sleep and increase with stress. The child has difficulty with speech, caused by involuntary facial movements. (Formerly called athetoid CP, this type affects approximately 20% of children with CP.)

Ataxic cerebral palsy results in incoordination and imbalance. There is nystagmus (rapid, repeated movements of the eyeball), muscle weakness, tremor, and lack of leg movement during infancy. When the child begins to walk, the feet are held far apart, causing a wide gait. The child with ataxic CP is unable to make fine or sudden movements.

Diagnosis. CP is diagnosed by symptoms demonstrated during infancy. Certain critical observations can direct the healthcare practitioner to look closely for other symptoms. The infant who has difficulty sucking or has arm or leg tremors with voluntary movement should be worked up for CP. The infant who crosses the legs when lifted from behind rather than pulling them up is also of concern. Other signs include difficulty in diapering because the legs are hard to separate and use of the arms and hands, but not the legs.

Treatment. Disabilities associated with CP are permanent; treatment is aimed at preventing complications and maximizing the child's potential. Helping the child learn self-care activities is a continuing goal. Improving communication through speech therapy and appropriate educational assistance is important. Physical and occupational therapy help maintain muscle strength and assist with adaptive measures. Braces or splints may aid in ambulation. Orthopedic surgery is sometimes us to correct severe contractures. The child who ha zures is often maintained on antiepileptic dru

Duchenne Muscular Dystrophy

Duchenne muscular dystrophy (Duchenne-Landouzy dystrophy) is the most common degenerative muscular disorder of children. Approximately half of all cases are inherited X-linked genetic disorders affecting only male offspring. A lack of protein product (dystrophin) in the muscles results in progressive muscle wasting.

Signs and Symptoms. Symptoms begin to appear around age 3 years. Prior to this, there may be noticeable developmental delay. The child's gait appears as a waddle. A positive Gowers' sign occurs. (The child needs to use the upper extremity muscles to compensate for weak hip muscles by pushing to an upright position using the hands to "climb up" the legs to a standing position. The child starts at the ankles and alternating hands, gradually pushes to an upright position, using the legs as the "climbing pole.") Figure 67-1 illustrates Gowers' sign. The child also may walk on the toes, fall frequently, and have difficulty hopping or running. These children often develop lordosis because of the unusual gait.

Delayed intellectual development and borderline IQ may be present. Gradual atrophy of the muscles occurs; by 11 to 12 years, the child is unable to walk. Contracture deformities can occur, especially of the hips and knees. Deterioration of respiratory muscles results in cardiac problems and respiratory failure.

Duchenne muscular dystrophy is diagnosed by the presence of symptoms, electromyogram, muscle biopsy, and elevated enzyme levels (aspartate aminotransferase—ALT [formerly SGOT], and creatine phosphokinase-CPK).

Treatment. There is no cure or treatment for Duchenne muscular dystrophy. The goal is to maintain physical function as long as possible. This disease is devastating, and emotional support must be provided for the child and family.

Mental Illness

Childhood Depression

Depression in children and adolescents can be difficult to identify. Many adolescents are moody and withdrawn, and it can be difficult to differentiate this from clinical depression. Younger children have a more difficult time expressing themselves and their feelings, and depression can go unnoticed.

Typical symptoms of depression include isolation and sadness, withdrawal from friends and family, fatigue and decrease in activity level, decrease in appetite, and a change in sleep patterns. Sleep pattern changes may be excessive sleep or an inability to sleep. School grades may decline, and the child may miss school for various reasons. The child may make statements that reflect low self-esteem. The key clue is a *marked change* in behavior.

Causes of depression vary. Some depression is related to chemical imbalances in the brain. Other cases are situational and occur in response to a traumatic event, such as the death of a family member or pet or the breakup of a relationship. Children with low self-esteem or those overwhelmed with a stressful situation are more prone to depression. Depression also can occur in children with a chronic illness or disability.

Treatment. The first step in treating children with depression is identifying the symptoms. Although it is difficult to recognize depression in children, the nurse should understand that all behavior is meaningful. Characteristics of depression should be investigated thoroughly to prevent further complications or suicide. Psychotherapy and counseling are necessary and may be provided on an outpatient basis. More serious cases of depression may require hospitalization. Family counseling is always helpful; antidepressant medications may be necessary.

Suicide

Suicide rates are on the rise; the age of the children is declining. Adolescent suicide is the third leading cause of death in 15- to 19-year-olds. Girls attempt suicide more often than boys, but boys succeed more often.

Many situations are associated with suicide and suicide attempt. Family problems may be involved. For example, financial difficulties, divorce, separation, or alcoholism can be factors related to suicide. For example, an adolescent who is experiencing the physical and emotional changes typical of the age group has minimal coping skills with which to deal with family-related stressors. A family under stress adds to that with which the adolescent must cope. A sample nursing care plan for an adolescent girl who has attempted suicide

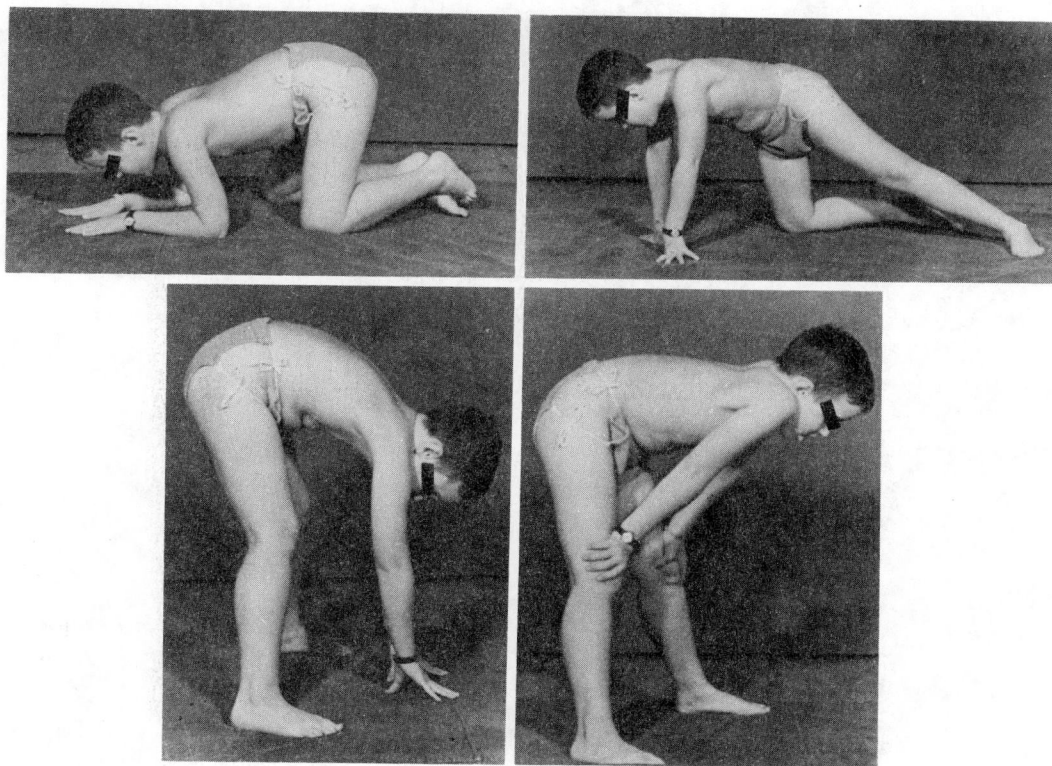

Figure 67-1. Gowers' sign in muscular dystrophy. A series of maneuvers is necessary to achieve an upright posture because of pelvic and trunk weakness. The child has to climb up his legs when rising from the floor. (Morrisey R.T. (ed.) Lovell and Winter's Pediatric Orthopaedics, 3rd ed. Vol. I. Philadelphia, J. B. Lippincott, 1990)

is provided. Depression, substance abuse, and low self-esteem are risk factors for suicide. Children with conduct disorders also are at risk.

Signs and Symptoms. Suicide ideation are thoughts or ideas of suicide that often involve a plan. This usually precedes an attempt at suicide and may be verbalized by the adolescent. A suicide gesture is a half-hearted attempt at inflicting personal injury. The injury is not intended to cause death. Suicide gesture and suicide ideation are a means of crying out for help. Ignoring these symptoms of despair can result in the death of an adolescent. Both are key warning signs and should not be ignored.

Other key warning signals include morbid discussion and preoccupation with death, giving away important personal belongings, and a sudden cheerfulness following a somber, withdrawn, depressed period. This sudden cheerfulness may be an indication that the adolescent has made a decision to commit suicide and is relieved that the decision has been made. It is a warning sign that can be easily missed. The accompanying box lists nursing assessments to be made in suicidal adolescents.

Treatment. All attempts or verbalization of suicide should be taken seriously and the child seen by a professional immediately. Intensive and long-term psychological counseling is essential. Children with severe depression and suicidal thoughts may have to be hospitalized and closely monitored until therapy is in place and suicide is no longer an immediate threat. (See Chapter 87.)

The nurse may want to use a no-suicide contract with the child in which the child agrees not to attempt suicide for a specified period of time and will contact help immediately if he or she feels suicidal. Children are usually very conscientious about wanting to "keep their word," and a no-suicide contact can be effective in certain situations.

Childhood Schizophrenia

The **schizophrenic** person loses contact with reality, sometimes as a result of a sudden severe emotional experience or sometimes as a result of an inability to adjust to the environment. Familial tendencies have been noted. Some of these children are helped by play therapy, behavior modification, and drug therapy. However, schizophrenia is often chronic. The person

An Adolescent Hospitalized for Attempted Suicide

Sherri Locke is a 15-year-old high school sophomore hospitalized after ingesting a "handful of my mom's Valium." Her mom reports that Sherri has a 2-year history of attention-getting behaviors: rebellious dress and personal conduct, truancy and failing grades at school, choice of rough dating partners, disregard for curfew. "I hardly recognize her anymore as my daughter." Sherri states she's sorry her suicide didn't work. "I wanted my parents to be sorry after I was dead . . . now they'll just be mad." Sherri's parents divorced 3 years ago.

Nursing Diagnosis: *High Risk for Self-Directed Violence Related to Desire to Punish Parents and Low Self-Esteem as Evidenced by Suicide Attempt*

Goal 1: Sherri displays no self-directed violence.

Goal 2: Sherri describes a positive plan of action to use in times of crisis similar to the one that prompted her suicide attempt.

Nursing Actions (assess/do/teach)	Rationale	Evaluative Statement
1. As soon as her medical condition is stabilized, evaluate the extent of her emotional pain, establish a direction for therapy, and assess the likelihood of a repeated suicide attempt; never discount the gravity of a suicide attempt by dismissing it as "merely" a bid for attention; factors to consider in evaluating the gravity of a suicide attempt: social set, intent, method, history, stress, mental status, support.	Prevention of a repeat occurrence is the first concern; early recognition, management, and prevention are priorities of care.	1/2; Goal 1 met; no new suicidal behaviors 1/2; Goal 2 not met; Sherri is unwilling to talk about the future and to discuss new coping strategies; *Revision:* Continue counseling.
2. Ensure that the environment is safe and free from any potentially harmful objects; make clear to the adolescent that her life is valued and that she will be protected from doing herself harm.	Relief of depression may signal that the adolescent now has the energy to execute a death wish. Structure and security are critical during the crisis period.	
3. Establish a supportive and caring nurse–patient relationship.	The adolescent needs to know that someone cares.	
4. Make referrals for counseling postdischarge—ideally, the whole family will engage in counseling; explore the adequacy of the patient's coping strategies; provide her with a "hotline" crisis number.	The adolescent's suicide may be symptomatic of a dysfunctional family. Swift and efficient crisis intervention may be life-saving in the future.	

must learn how to manage his or her life with the disorder.

Signs and Symptoms. The following are characteristics of childhood schizophrenia:

♦ Young people can develop schizophrenia as early as 5 or 6 years.

♦ The child has many characteristics of the autistic child, such as lack of speech, ritualistic behavior, and intolerance of change.

♦ Personality and cognitive development are affected.

♦ The child often "hears voices" (auditory hallucinations).

♦ The child has impaired interpersonal relationships.

♦ The child is often out of touch with reality, has a

Danger Signals for Suicide Prevention

- Lack of involvement in school activities
- No close friends
- Inability to communicate with parents
- Extreme anxiety, tenseness, abrupt changes in behavior, withdrawal, and sadness
- Change in eating pattern
- Change in sleeping pattern
- Sudden giving away of prized or valuable possessions
- Actual suicide threats, a suicide note, overuse of drugs, constant talk of death, talk of willingness to die or being ready for death, talk of being worthless or no good, talk of death as a release from pressure and pain
- Self-injurious behaviors, such as cutting or scratching oneself, self-inflicted cigarette burns, etc.
- Very dangerous and life-threatening activities, such as playing "Russian roulette" with a gun or "chicken" with a car
- Deep, lingering depression with loss of energy and desire
- Sudden relief of acute, long-term depression without treatment. This may mean that the person has made the actual decision to commit suicide or now has the energy to go through with it
- Depression, feelings of hopelessness, feelings of helplessness, low self-esteem, loneliness and isolation, impulsiveness, ambivalence
- Withdrawal from friends and family
- Unusual neglect of personal appearance, radical personality change
- Any suicide gesture

When any of the preceding danger signs are noticed, seek skilled, professional help immediately

distorted sense of what is real, or does not know where he or she is or what day it is.
- The child has an inappropriate affect (eg, laughs at a sad event).
- Other symptoms include delusions, paranoia, and aggression toward others.

There are many theories as to the cause of childhood schizophrenia. These include biochemical and organic causes, inadequate parent–child relationships, childhood sexual abuse, ritualistic abuse, and if the parents' mental health has been less than adequate, an increased tendency for children to develop psychoses.

Treatment. Treatment centers on modifying the child's behavior to cope with reality and organize thoughts. Medications are often helpful in controlling symptoms; however, they also may have the opposite effect in chil-

dren. Because behavior is so difficult for all involved, intensive and long-term treatment often is required. Home care with respite care, medical assistance, and social service assistance is preferred. The child must be monitored to ensure medication compliance.

Substance Abuse in Children and Adolescents

The transition from childhood to adolescence can be one of confusion and turmoil. Any change in family structure adds additional stress to the developmental tasks of the emerging adolescent. The use of chemicals to alter the consciousness is seen as a way of dealing with stress, raising faltering self-esteem, and being accepted by peers. Any chemical has the potential for abuse. Signals of substance abuse are given in the accompanying box. Effects of chronic drug use on the body systems are illustrated in Figure 67-2.

The most commonly used drug is alcohol. Other drugs used by young people include marijuana, lysergic acid diethylamide (LSD), amphetamines, barbiturates, narcotic analgesics, and occasionally heroin. Cocaine offers the user a euphoric "high" and can be inhaled as a powder, smoked in free-base form, or smoked in a water pipe ("crack cocaine").

Inexpensive household cleaners, hair spray, or paint in aerosol cans can be inhaled (huffing). This practice is extremely dangerous because it is toxic to the central nervous system. The user may lose consciousness and may have seizures. Also inhaled are fumes from glue, markers, and correction fluid.

Methamphetamine (crank, meth, crystal) is an inexpensively made drug that produces a longer, more intense high than cocaine. LSD, once a popular hallucinogenic drug of the 1960s, is being used again today.

Prevention. One of the major ways to prevent substance abuse is by public education. In addition, the young person must feel that he or she is worthwhile; the nurse can aid in building self-esteem. Treatment depends on the extent of the abuse, the age at which abuse began, and whether physical dependence exists. Support groups, individual counseling, and family counseling can be beneficial. Chapter 88 describes substance abuse and detoxification.

Key Concept

Probably the most important factor in breaking the cycle of chemical abuse is building a positive self-esteem in children. Because children cannot be prevented from having access to drugs, all nurses and parents can do is teach them to enjoy life without chemical abuse and to have positive self-esteem to resist peer pressure.

Children of Alcoholics

Generally, programs for children of alcoholics are begun as early as possible, preferably at age 2 or 3 years. Experts believe that the repeating cyclic pattern of chemical dependency in families can be broken by counseling and group therapy for these young children. Therapy is aimed at building self-esteem, building a personal identity apart from the alcoholic, assisting the family and child to set limits for behavior, establishing consistency, encouraging healthy interaction between the child and other children and adults, encouraging the child to trust others and be open and honest in relationships, and learning to differentiate between healthy touching and abusive touching.*

Sensory Disorders

The child with a sensory disorder poses a special challenge for the nurse. Altered senses have a major impact on growth and development, academic performance, development of socialization skills, and communication.

Visual Impairment

The most frequent causes of visual impairment include prenatal cataracts caused by heredity or maternal rubella, optic nerve atrophy, and retrolental fibroplasia resulting from oxygen toxicity.

Other causes of visual impairment include refractory errors, strabismus, and trauma (see Chapter 65 for a discussion of these causes). The visually impaired child is more dependent on others to learn socialization skills with other children. They lack visual cues and imitation, resulting in socialization delays. For an older child, special education intervention assists the child academically, along with audio tapes and instruction in the use of Braille reading.

The nurse teaches parents to remove limitations in the surrounding environment and to assist the child to achieve independent function.

If the child has partial sight, clocks with large numbers, calendars with large letters, and books with large print may decrease frustration. Non-sighted children should be encouraged to participate in activities with their peers, such as music, guided skiing, swimming, etc. If an infant has a visual impairment, the parents should encourage exploration while ensuring safety.

Hearing Impairment

Hearing impairment can result from prenatal exposure to cytomegalovirus, herpes, rubella, or syphilis. Meningitis, chronic ear infections, Down syndrome, exposure to loud noises, and certain medications also may cause damage to hearing. Studies have examined the effects of exposure to sound inside an isolette or oxyhood. Manifestations of hearing impairment in a child includes such behavior as avoiding social interaction,

---

* Courtesy of Children Are People, Inc., St. Paul, MN; used with permission.

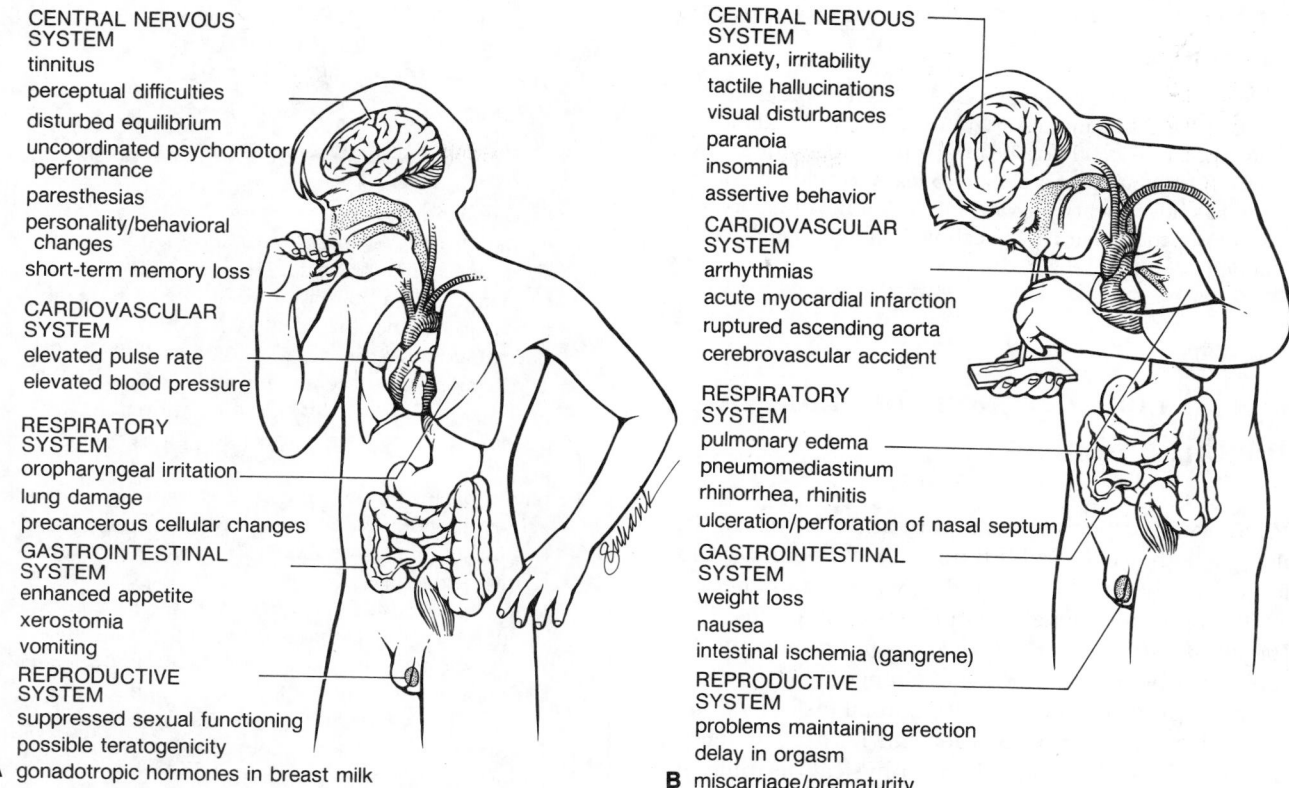

CENTRAL NERVOUS SYSTEM
tinnitus
perceptual difficulties
disturbed equilibrium
uncoordinated psychomotor performance
paresthesias
personality/behavioral changes
short-term memory loss
CARDIOVASCULAR SYSTEM
elevated pulse rate
elevated blood pressure
RESPIRATORY SYSTEM
oropharyngeal irritation
lung damage
precancerous cellular changes
GASTROINTESTINAL SYSTEM
enhanced appetite
xerostomia
vomiting
REPRODUCTIVE SYSTEM
suppressed sexual functioning
possible teratogenicity
A gonadotropic hormones in breast milk

CENTRAL NERVOUS SYSTEM
anxiety, irritability
tactile hallucinations
visual disturbances
paranoia
insomnia
assertive behavior
CARDIOVASCULAR SYSTEM
arrhythmias
acute myocardial infarction
ruptured ascending aorta
cerebrovascular accident
RESPIRATORY SYSTEM
pulmonary edema
pneumomediastinum
rhinorrhea, rhinitis
ulceration/perforation of nasal septum
GASTROINTESTINAL SYSTEM
weight loss
nausea
intestinal ischemia (gangrene)
REPRODUCTIVE SYSTEM
problems maintaining erection
delay in orgasm
B miscarriage/prematurity

Figure 67-2. Effects of chronic substance abuse on the body. **A,** Effects of chronic marijuana use. Psychic and perceptual effects may vary widely. Chronic use may result in psychologic dependence, but physical dependence is rare. **B,** Effects of chronic cocaine use. Repeated use can lead to an overwhelming psychologic dependence, which is characterized by extreme involvement in procuring and using the drug daily. There is also a true physical dependence. Data from Malseed R. Pharmacology: Drug Therapy and Nursing Considerations, Ed 3. Philadelphia, J. B. Lippincott, 1990

playing alone, acting timid, not learning to talk, and displaying poor socialization skills.

Nursing Considerations. One of the major problems a child with impaired hearing faces relates to speech development. Communication and safety are major issues facing the hearing-impaired child. Promotion of communication is critical. Speech therapy and the use of sign language are important interventions, as is the use of hearing aids, if appropriate, and lip reading. Assistance with socialization in school is essential; classmates must be taught to relate to the child and that this child is not intellectually impaired.

Speech Impairment

Impairment of speech can result from a hearing deficit or from muscular disorders (eg, Tourette syndrome, brain dysfunction) or from cleft lip or palate. Speech also can be influenced by environmental and emotional factors. Disorders in articulation are related to the ability to produce the correct sound. An example is the child who speaks with a lisp (pronounces "th" instead of "s"). A dysfluency is an interruption in the natural flow of speaking. This includes the child who stutters, although stuttering is normal in preschool children. (At this age, the child's ability to understand is more developed than vocabulary and command of the language.) When stuttering is present in the school-age child, it requires evaluation.

Some children benefit from speech therapy. Others require surgical intervention or orthodontics. Evaluation by an ear, nose, and throat specialist or neurologist also may be appropriate, depending on the specific circumstances. Hearing is tested, and referral to a psychologist or counselor is indicated for the child with an emotionally related speech disorder. A computer is beneficial to many children, especially if they are unable to communicate verbally.

Key Concept

A common cause of aphasia or a speech disorder in children is a hearing disorder. A professional audiologist should test a child's hearing if there is any question. It is difficult for a person to learn to talk if he or she has never heard anyone speak. If a hearing person loses their hearing, speech will often be maintained or can be regained.

Special Considerations in Pediatric Rehabilitation

When a young person has a permanent physical disability, whether caused by trauma or congenital condition, he or she must adjust to this, while simultaneously achieving normal developmental tasks of adolescence. *The physically challenged person is not abnormal.* The person simply has additional challenges.

Accomplishments of developmental tasks *without* a physical or emotional disorder can be a challenge to the child or adolescent. When a physical disability intervenes, these tasks provide additional challenges. Guidelines in general nursing skills in caring for the child or adolescent with special needs are outlined in the accompanying box. Behavior modifications, feeding training, and speech development follow.

Behavior Modification

Behavior modification involves positive reinforcement, which encourages the child to repeat desired behavior. Skills may need to be repeated many times before they are learned. If the child is intellectually impaired, the task should be made as simple as possible. Give praise when the task is done correctly; do not use punishment.

Usually the mentally impaired person is unable to generalize from one situation to the next, so you must teach each specific skill, task, or behavior. The person needs a routine and needs to do things the same way each time. There are specific techniques for teaching dressing skills, feeding skills, toilet training, and other activities of daily living. Teaching should take place in a quiet place, with few distractions. The place should be neat and kept in the same order at all times. Patience is the most important factor in training the person with intellectual impairment.

Feeding Training

Some children with severe learning disabilities and intellectual impairment have great difficulty eating. It will take great patience to feed them and to teach them

Nursing Skill Guidelines
Working With a Child or Adolescent With Special Needs

- Emphasize the positive; stress what the person can do. Reinforce success; praise the person for each accomplishment, no matter how small.
- Encourage the person to be as independent as possible. Encourage self-care. Help the person by showing how to do things. Reinforce by repeating instructions and return demonstrations.
- Encourage development of positive self-esteem. The person lacks role models with similar disabilities, making it more difficult to develop a positive self-image. Encourage participation in support groups.
- Find a balance between the need for assistance and achieving independence in activities of daily living (ADLs). Parents may need to be encouraged not to be overprotective.
- Emphasize "normalcy." Encourage the person to do all the "normal" things others do, for instance, music, sports, academic success. Encourage participation in many activities for a well-rounded life. Often the person can do more than others believe.
- Encourage normal social contacts. The person should participate in peer activities.
- Encourage regular school attendance when possible. Schools are obligated to provide assistance as needed. Encourage parents to discuss the person's problem and limitations with teachers, the school nurse, counselors, or others in close contact with the child or adolescent.
- Offer emotional support. The person will get discouraged. Listen to his or her problems. Let him or her express himself or herself.
- Observe for depression. A physical or emotional disorder may threaten future plans, resulting in depression.
- Consider the person's family. Involve them in planning and activities. Especially try to involve other siblings who might feel neglected.

to eat. See the accompanying box for helpful points when training the intellectually impaired person to eat.

Speech Development

Speech development is often difficult. Nurses and parents must be patient and encourage the child to say each word as slowly and clearly as possible. Do not use baby talk. Encourage the child to listen, and even if he or she cannot answer, be sure to talk to the child. Tell the child what you are doing, and try to anticipate questions. Read to the child, and encourage him or her to look at the pictures. The child may be able to communicate by using an electric typewriter or computer.

Nursing Skill Guidelines
Feeding the Intellectually Impaired Child

◆ Ensure correct positioning, preferably in a sitting position. *(Rationale: This position helps to close the larynx against the epiglottis.)* Flex the head slightly. You may need to use a pediatric safety device.
◆ Teach the child to suck by massaging the cheeks or by using a special nipple. A nipple or bottle is appropriate for the infant and young toddler; as the child becomes older, there is a need for age-appropriate behavior, and a cup or glass should be used. A straw may be helpful. Encourage blowing too. *(Rationale: These actions build up muscles used in speech.)*
◆ Assist the person to learn to drink from a cup by using sucking movements.
◆ Teach or remind the child to chew. If necessary, manipulate the jaw up and down.
◆ Remind the child to swallow. *(Rationale: This prevents aspiration.)*
◆ Place food on the side of the mouth, not in the center. Do not rush. *(Rationale: You want to prevent choking.)*
◆ Encourage the child to use the lips to remove the food from the spoon, to bite off pieces of food, to move food around in the mouth with the tongue. *(Rationale: These exercises also prepare the muscles for speech.)*
◆ Keep the eating atmosphere pleasant. If possible, have several people eat together. Provide role models.
◆ Allow the person to do as much self-feeding as possible. Keep the table neat and clean.

Key Concept

◆ Encourage the young person with a disability to participate in educational, social, and recreational activities.
◆ Working with people with long-term disorders and their families offers you the opportunity to use all your technical skills and interpersonal nursing skills.
◆ Keep the lines of communication open by developing active listening skills. Observe verbal and nonverbal cues for potential problems.

Long-Term Care

Children with long-term disabilities or degenerative disorders might be in the hospital for an extended time or be readmitted often. These children need special nursing care and attention.

A basic sense of trust must be established between the child and nurse. Ideally, the child should have the same nurse. This child needs to learn self-care as soon as possible and reinforce this as often as possible. The long-term patient can sometimes be given responsibilities on the unit to increase feelings of self-worth and usefulness.

The Family. Plan the child's care carefully according to the physician's orders. Consider age, sex, developmental level, home environment, medical problems, and prognosis. Do not forget that the hospitalized child is still a member of the family. Be considerate of parents, siblings, and other relatives. Also, be aware that long-term hospitalization drains the family's emotional well-being and finances. The child must have a sense of security; having basic needs met is important. Allow the child to do as much for himself or herself as possible, and assist with other needs without embarrassing the child.

Involving the Patient in Care. Long-term hospitalization usually means treatments and diagnostic tests that can lead to physical discomfort and apprehension in the child. Make an effort to minimize this by allowing parent and child to talk about their fears. Answer questions simply and truthfully. Focus on what the child can do during a painful procedure. Explain treatments just before they are done, rather than too far in advance so that the child's imagination does not run wild.

Allow the child to maintain social contacts with friends, classmates, and relatives as much as possible. It is easy for a child with a long-term illness to become overly dependent.

Keeping Up With School. If the child is of school age, educational needs are included in the care plan. A teacher is provided by the school district. Nursing staff should provide sufficient time and a quiet room for the teacher and student. School helps maintain normalcy in the child's life.

Community Resources. Use social service agencies in the community to help meet the long-term patient's educational, medical, recreational, and financial needs. A public health nursing referral is helpful. Voluntary associations have a special interest in various disorders; often it is helpful for the patient and parents to talk with other families who have faced the same situation.

Key Concept

Respite care should be provided so that the parents or other care givers of a severely disabled child can get occasional rest and a break.

The Child With a Poor Prognosis

It can be difficult for a nurse to work with a child who has a terminal illness. The nurse must deal with personal feelings and emotions before dealing with those of the patient and family.

The nurse should offer emotional support to the child and to the parents. You can be most helpful by listening and offering understanding support and kindness. They may not want to talk; they may just want to know you are there if they need you.

The Child Who is Dying

The child who is dying has special fears and concerns. Most people are afraid of separation (or "going away"). Children might fear medical procedures or mutilation; they sometimes feel that death is punishment for something they have done. Most children, like adults, fear pain. The child's greatest fear is that of being alone. Someone should be there at all times. Listen to the child and answer the child's questions as honestly as possible. Help the child to verbalize feelings. Treat any symptoms, and keep the child as comfortable as possible.

What to Tell the Child. Whether or not to tell the child that the prognosis is poor is controversial. Most experts agree that the older child probably knows anyway, because he or she can sense changes in the attitudes of others. Advocates of this view feel that the child might have a distorted idea of the situation. It is usually better to explain the facts so that the child can verbalize feelings and fears and deal with them. The child who has not been told that he or she is dying will have to deal with feelings alone, because most often he or she knows by the way people act. This makes it much more difficult for the child than it would be if feelings could be shared. What the child is told also depends in large part on how the parents are dealing with the situation.

The terminally ill child should be allowed to participate in whatever ward activities can be physically tolerated and should be allowed to do as much self-care as possible.

The Parents

Parents of a dying child might deny that their child is dying or strike out at members of the nursing team without meaning what they say. You can be helpful to parents by letting them be involved in the child's care. Tell them the truth. Encourage them to share their feelings and frustrations. *Always* refer to their child by name—before and after death.

The nurse must realize that parents are deeply upset and shattered. The most common reactions of parents are denial, guilt, anxiety, and acceptance, in that order. They should be given privacy and the opportunity to mourn. Most parents will benefit greatly from referral to a grief support group, such as "The Compassionate Friends," or to a hospice program. It is not unprofessional for the nurse to let the parents know that nurses feel their loss too. The nurse should be able to handle the death of a child with empathy, reverence, gentleness, and genuine nursing skill (see Chapter 90).

Key Concept

The physician may ask the parents of a fatally injured child if they wish to donate the child's tissues or organs for transplant to another person. This is a difficult decision, and parents need a great deal of emotional support from the nurse and representatives of the donor network. Donation of organs or tissues often helps parents to cope better later.

Keys for Review

Key Questions for Critical Thinking

1. Discuss the difference between congenitally acquired disorders and environmentally acquired disorders.
2. Describe and discuss the various forms of intellectual impairment.
3. Discuss how visual, hearing, and speech impairment affect growth and development, and describe appropriate nursing interventions.

Key Questions for Critical Thinking
(continued)

4. Discuss long-term care of the child with special needs, including cost, family needs, foster care, legal issues, and education.

Key Readings

American Psychiatric Association. Diagnostic and Statistical Manual of Mental Disorders, Ed 4-revised. Washington, DC, American Psychiatric Association, 1994

Barkely R. Attention Deficit Hyperactive Disorders. New York, Guilford Press, 1990

Behrman RE. Nelson's Textbook of Pediatrics, Ed 14. Philadelphia, W.B. Saunders, 1992

Castiglia PT, Harbin RE. Child Health Care: Process and Practice. Philadelphia, J.B. Lippincott, 1992

Hazinski MF. Nursing Care of the Terminally Ill Child, Ed 2. St. Louis, Mosby-Yearbook, 1992

Jackson DB, Saunders RB. Child Health Nursing: A Comprehensive Approach to the Care of Children and Their Families. Philadelphia, J.B. Lippincott, 1993

Murray R, Zetner J. Nursing Assessment and Health Promotion Strategies Through the Life Span. East Norwalk, CT, Appleton & Lange, 1993

Pomar PJ (Ed). Nurses and Family Health Promotion: Concepts, Assessment, Intervention. Philadelphia, W.B. Saunders, 1992

Thomas CL (Ed). Taber's Cyclopedic Medical Dictionary, Ed 17. Philadelphia, F.A. Davis, 1993

Wong DL. Essentials of Pediatric Nursing, Ed 4. St. Louis, Mosby-Yearbook, 1993

Enrichment Keys

Gaffren DA. The Seasons of Grief: Helping Children Grow Through Loss. New York, Plume, 1988

Romond J. Children Facing Grief. St Meinrad, IN, Abbey Press, 1989

Keys to Learning More

Chapter 70: musculoskeletal disorders, many seen in children

Chapter 71: neurologic disorders, including seizures and spinal cord injuries

Chapter 72: endocrine disorders, many seen in children

Chapter 73: sensory disorders, many seen in children

Keys To Learning More (continued)

Chapter 78: HIV infection, a more detailed discussion of a disease that affects children

Chapter 87: psychiatric nursing

Chapter 88: substance abuse

Chapter 89: rehabilitation techniques used in adults and children

Chapter 90: death and dying

Key Resources

American Speech-Language-Hearing Association
10801 Rockville Pike, Department AP
Rockville, MD 20852
301-897-5700

The Compassionate Friends, Inc.
P.O. Box 3696
Oak Brook, IL 60522-3696
708-990-1100
708-990-0246 (FAX)

March of Dimes Birth Defects Foundation
1275 Mamaroneck Ave
White Plains, NY 10605

Muscular Dystrophy Association
3561 E. Sunrise Ave
Tucson, AZ 85718
602-529-2000

National Association for Retarded Citizens
2501 Ave J
Arlington, TX 76011

National Easter Seal Society
2023 W Ogden Av
Chicago, IL 60612
312-726-6200

Office for Handicapped Individuals
Department of Education
Room 3106, Switzer Bldg
400 Maryland Ave SW
Washington, DC 20202
202-245-0080

United Cerebral Palsy Association
1522 K St NW
Washington, DC 20005
800-872-5827

Unit *14* Assisting the Adult With a Physical Dysfunction

68 Skin Disorders

Keys for Learning

Learning Objectives

- Define terms related to dermatology.
- Describe types of skin grafts and related nursing care.
- Describe measures to assist the patient with pruritus.
- Describe and demonstrate skills required to apply dermatologic dressings and give therapeutic baths.
- Discuss common skin disorders, their treatment, and nursing care.
- Discuss measures used to eliminate parasites, particularly lice.
- State stages of recovery in burns, and describe emergency, continuing, and rehabilitative nursing care.
- Describe three malignant and three nonmalignant tumors of the skin.
- Demonstrate the ability to give safe and competent nursing care to people with dermatologic disorders.

Key Terms

allograft	dermatitis	impetigo
angioedema	eczema	psoriasis
autograft	eschar	scabies
carbuncle	folliculitis	urticaria
condylomata acuminata	furuncle	vitiligo
contractures	heterograft	warts
debridement	homograft	xenograft

Keys to Understanding This Chapter

Chapter 15: the integumentary system
Chapter 16: fluid and electrolyte balance
Chapter 28: diet therapy and special diets
Chapter 30: medical asepsis
Chapter 45: personal hygiene and skin care
Chapter 48: bandages and binders
Chapter 49: heat and cold application
Chapter 50: physical examination
Chapter 54: surgical asepsis

Key Points

- The skin protects the body in various ways: it prevents microorganisms from entering the body; keeps the body from losing too much fluid; and helps prevent injury to fragile organs.
- Body substance precautions must be used when caring for patients with skin problems. Patients often have open, draining wounds.
- The skin may be exposed to a variety of allergies and infections
- Extent of burns is determined by a variety of means. Depth and percentage of burns are significant.

Key Topics Outline

Anatomy and Physiology Review
Diagnostic Tests
Medical and Surgical Treatments
    Common Medical Treatments
    Common Surgical Treatments
Nursing Process
    Data Collection
    Nursing Diagnosis
    Planning and Implementation
    Evaluation
Allergies
Chronic Skin Disorders
Infections
    Bacterial Skin Infections
Infestations by Parasites
Sebaceous Gland Disorders
    Burn Trauma
    Burn Prevention
    Immediate Care
    Stabilized Hospital Care
    Rehabilitation
Neoplasms
    Nonmalignant Tumors
    Skin Cancer

Key Learning Activities

- Review the Universal Precautions manual in your institution. Study Body Substance Precautions.
- Visit a burn unit. Observe assessments and nursing care.

Dermatology is the study of diseases of the skin; a *dermatologist* is the physician who specializes in this field. The nurse specializing in care of people with a skin disorder is called a *dermatologic nurse.* In addition to specializing in the field of dermatology, nurses see skin problems in many other patients for which they care. For instance, the infant may have a rash or the older person may have problems with itching. Some systemic disorders include skin manifestations. These conditions are discussed with the system that is primarily involved in the condition.

The nurse should be familiar with general terms used in documentation to describe skin disorders. In addition to key terms at the beginning of this chapter, the accompanying box gives additional terms used in dermatology.

Anatomy and Physiology Review

The skin as a system includes epithelial and connective tissue, nerves, and sweat and oil glands (see Chapter 15). It is composed of two layers: the epidermis, or outermost layer, and the dermis, which lies underneath. The dermis is usually called the "true skin." Nerve endings in this layer provide a variety of sensations. Cells located in the dermis give the skin elasticity, allowing it to stretch.

The skin protects the body in many ways: It helps prevent microorganisms or foreign substances from entering the body; it helps prevent injury to fragile organs; and it keeps the body from losing too much fluid.

Diagnostic Tests

Because so many skin disorders are manifestations of disorders in other body systems, diagnostic tests are covered in other sections of this book. If a systemic disorder has skin manifestations, the systemic disorder is first diagnosed and then the symptoms appearing in the skin are treated. Some diagnostic tests used to determine the origin of a skin disorder are skin tests for allergies; laboratory tests for blood dyscrasias, such as leukemia or lupus erythematosus; blood glucose and other tests for diabetes mellitus; and surgical biopsy to determine skin cancer. Direct observation is often the diagnostic tool used first to determine disorders of the integumentary system (skin).

Medical and Surgical Treatments

Common Medical Treatments

Skin disorders make people uncomfortable. Treatment is aimed at making the patient comfortable and treating systemic problems. Medications used in pru-

Key Terminology for Skin Disorders

Crusts	The dried residue of exudate
Dermatitis	Inflammation of the skin
Desquamation	The process of flaking or shedding
Excoriation	A scraped area
Fissure	A crack or cleft in the skin
Macules	Flat, discolored spots on the skin (such as freckles)
Papules	Solid elevations of the skin (such as warts) that do not contain fluid
Pruritus	Itching
Purpura	Discoloration of the skin due to the presence of blood in the tissue outside of the blood vessels (such as an ecchymosis, petechiae, or hematoma)
Pustules	Vesicles that contain pus
Scales	Thin flakes of skin
Ulcer	An open area produced by sloughing of necrotic (dead) inflammatory tissue
Vesicle	An elevation that contains clear or serous fluid
Wheals	Localized areas of edema (such as hives). Wheals may or may not itch.

ritus (itching) are listed in the box. The physician may order moist dressings or packs or therapeutic baths. These are discussed in the Nursing Process section in this chapter.

Removal of Exudate, Crust, or Eschar

The physician will generally remove loose skin, crusts, or denuded tissue. This process is called **débridement. Eschar**, the slough following a burn, is also removed. Débridement is a sterile procedure. It is often carried out at the same time moist packs are changed. The nurse is frequently asked to assist. The nurse should receive full instructions on how the procedure is to be done, because each patient is treated differently. Débridement and escharotomy are discussed in more detail in the Burns section at the end of this chapter.

Common Surgical Treatments

Although skin disorders make patients uncomfortable, one of the most damaging effects of a skin disorder is disfigurement.

Key Medications
for Pruritus

Antihistamines

- clemastine fumarate (Tavist)
- dexchlorpheniramine maleate (Dexchlor, Polargen)
- diphenhydramine HCL (Benadryl)
- trimeprazine tartrate (Temaril)

Tranquilizers

- hydroxyzine HCl and pamoate (Atarax, Vistaril)

Nursing Considerations

- These medications often cause drowsiness. Warn the patient not to drive or work around machinery.
- Potentiated by alcohol and other sedating drugs.
- Dry mouth is a common side effect. Encourage the patient to drink juices and other fluids, not just water. Sucking on hard candy or ice chips or chewing sugarless gum is helpful.
- Other side effects include stomach distress, diarrhea or constipation (administer medication with milk or food), and urinary frequency or retention.
- A life-threatening blood disorder, agranulocytosis, may be caused by clemastine fumarate and trimeprazine tartrate.
- Antihistamines are usually contraindicated in patients with asthma.
- Antihistamines should be discontinued 4 days before allergy skin tests, to preserve test accuracy.
- Advise the patient to use a sunscreen.
- Use with caution in elderly patients.

Plastic Surgery

Plastic surgery is one way to reverse these effects. Plastic surgery may be performed for cosmetic effects, to repair congenital defects, or to repair results of accidents. This is also called *reconstructive surgery.*

Skin and Tissue Grafts

Skin grafts are used to cover areas of skin lost through wounds, burns, or infections. A graft is a transplant of skin. The patient's own skin may be used, or cadaver skin is frequently used. (In this case the donated skin helps to seal the wound while new skin forms underneath.) Grafting is a painstaking procedure that may be done in stages. These procedures may be done over many months, depending on the size and numbers of areas to be covered and the success of each surgical procedure.

There are two major types of grafts, as illustrated in Figure 68-1. One type is called a *free graft.* This means that skin has been completely removed from its original site and grafted onto the recipient site (see Figure 68-1**A**). The other type is *pedicle graft.* In this type of graft,

one end of the graft remains attached to the donor site so that it can continue to receive nourishment until new circulation is established. The other end is attached to the recipient site of the same person's body. In some situations, the patient must assume an unnatural position until the graft begins to grow in the new site, at which time the graft can be separated from the donor site. This type of graft is used when a large area of skin is to be replaced, such as an ear, part of a hand or foot, or a large part of the face or tissue (see Figure 68-1**B**). Other types of grafts are named in relation to the donor.

Nursing Considerations. Every plastic surgeon has a preferred method of caring for the surgical area. They all require scrupulous attention to aseptic technique, protection of the grafts, keeping a new graft immobilized, and preventing infection at the donor site. Postoperatively, the surgical site may be swollen and bruised. The nurse prepares the patient by explaining preoperatively what is to be expected.

An important part of nursing care in reconstructive surgery stresses emotional support. The patient is often self-conscious about appearance and may want to stay away from others. He or she should be visited frequently and given emotional support and reassurance.

❖ Nursing Process

Data Collection

The nurse carefully observes and assesses the skin condition of all patients. Chapter 50 describes nursing assessment of the skin, hair, and nails. This assessment establishes a baseline for future comparisons, and the nurse should report any changes that occur in these assessments. The nurse assesses skin color (compared with the person's usual color) and skin texture and turgor. Skin lesions are noted. Common skin lesions are illustrated in Figure 68-2. These terms are defined in a box at the beginning of this chapter and are used throughout the chapter. Whether the skin is intact also is noted. In addition, subjective symptoms, such as itching, are important.

The nurse observes the patient's emotional response to the skin disorder or disease by answering the following questions. Is the patient so disabled by pain or itching that he or she needs assistance or encouragement to meet daily needs? Is the disorder so disfiguring that it affects social activities or self-esteem? Is the patient anxious or fearful of the outcome? Is the situation life-threatening?

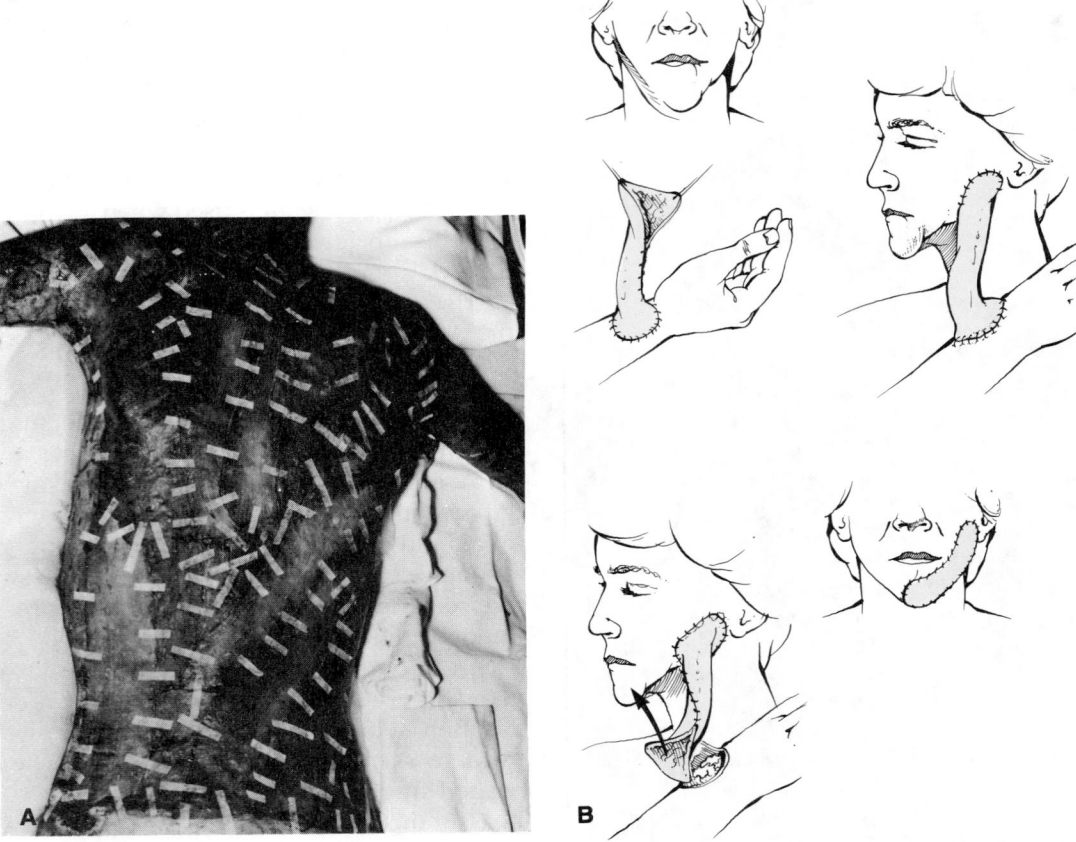

Figure 68-1. **(A)** Multiple skin grafts have been applied to this patient's back following a severe burn. Notice that tape is used instead of suturing. Tape is easier to apply, more likely to hold, and more comfortable for the patient. This patient recovered from his injuries and has normal movement of his extremities. (Photo courtesy 3M Health Care.) **(B)** Pedicle graft. 1. Cheek deformity. 2. Tube flap attached to carrier site. 3. Flap to recipient site. 4 and 5. Carrier end is detached and tube flap is opened and inset.

Nursing Diagnosis

Based on data collection, a number of nursing diagnoses may be established. The following are just a few that may be seen on nursing care plans for the patient with a skin disorder:

♦ High Risk for Infection related to laceration, rash, skin lesions, skin cancer, burn trauma
♦ Fluid Volume Excess related to edema
♦ Fluid Volume Deficit related to burn trauma
♦ Ineffective Breathing Pattern related to pain
♦ Impaired Social Interaction related to disfigurement
♦ Sexual Dysfunction related to pruritus, pain, skin lesions
♦ Ineffective Individual Coping related to chronic condition
♦ Body Image Disturbance related to skin lesions, disfigurement, pruritus, pain

Nursing Alert

Use Body Substance Precautions when caring for patients with skin problems. Such patients often have open, draining, or weeping wounds. Wear gloves whenever coming into contact with any body fluids or drainage; wear eye goggles if there is any possibility of splashing.

Planning and Implementation

The patient and nurse plan together for effective care to meet patient needs based on the nursing diagnosis. The nurse provides preoperative and postoperative care for the patient undergoing plastic surgery or skin grafting. In the patient with severe burns, the nurse may assist in débridement of dead tissue or eschar or in life-sustaining treatments. The patient with a skin disorder

Keys to Patient/Family Teaching
Pruritus

Patient and family teaching for the patient with pruritus includes the following:

- ◆ Cotton clothing should be worn. Irritating materials should be kept away from body.
- ◆ New clothes should be washed before wearing.
- ◆ Clothes should be rinsed in clear water. Fabric softeners, starch, and antistatic chemicals should not be used.
- ◆ Only cool or lukewarm baths should be taken. Soothing baths or localized skin preparations may be used as ordered.
- ◆ Lotion may be used on dry skin if physician allows.
- ◆ Nonallergenic makeup can be used.
- ◆ Skin testing can be done to determine allergens. Eliminate allergens if possible.
- ◆ Medications should be taken as prescribed.
- ◆ Activities that cause body to become overheated should be avoided.
- ◆ Fingernails should be kept short. Cotton gloves can be worn and the hands covered with cotton socks at night.
- ◆ Slap rather than scratch the itching area. Slapping will provide the same stimulation as scratching without continued irritation.
- ◆ The person who cannot exercise should sit in a rocking chair to provide exercise without further skin irritation.
- ◆ Relaxation audiotapes may be used to assist in falling asleep.

also may require assistance in meeting daily self-care needs, dealing with itching or pain, and working through the emotional aspects of having a disfiguring or chronic disorder. The nurse teaches the patient about the disorder and necessary treatments. A nursing care plan is developed to meet patient needs. A sample nursing care plan for a patient with burns is provided later in the chapter.

Assisting the Patient who Has Pruritus

Pruritus is often a symptom of a skin disease but also may arise from disorders in other systems of the body. Examples are liver disorders, cancer, diabetes mellitus, or thyroid disturbances. Dryness of the skin causes pruritus, particularly in elderly patients. The main problem in dealing with pruritus is that the patient is almost irresistibly compelled to scratch. This may lead to breaks in the skin, which can become infected and can cause scars.

Telling the patient not to scratch probably will be futile. Try to divert the patient's attention with other activities. Oral tranquilizers, antihistamines, or topical corticosteroids are sometimes ordered. These medications and related nursing considerations are listed in a box earlier in the chapter. Patient education about the proper use of medications following discharge may be necessary.

Hypnosis is often helpful in severe cases. Be sure to document patient reactions, noting which measures are effective. The patient will appreciate your advice on how to deal with itching. The guidelines in the accompanying patient teaching box may be helpful.

Giving Therapeutic Baths

A special therapeutic bath cleanses the patient's body; soothes the skin; relieves itching; helps remove dead skin, eschar, or crusts; and offers a way of applying medication to the entire body at one time. Therapeutic baths also provide an opportunity to apply warmth to the body so physical therapy and range-of-motion exercises can be performed more comfortably.

The therapeutic bath is given in a bathtub that is disinfected before and after the bath or in a whirlpool tank. The whirlpool bath is shown in Figure 68-3. The nurse follows the physician's orders regarding the substance to be used, the length of time the patient is to be in the bath, and other treatments to be carried out at the same time. (The hospital will specify how the tub is to be cleaned; colloids and oils used in these baths are often difficult to remove.)

Agents used in the bath often include oatmeal or other cereals, starch, or baking soda. Detergents and antipruritic preparations may be ordered. Soap is not used because of its drying effect. Medicated bath oil is used instead. Use tepid water (not hotter than 100°F or 30°C); a very hot bath aggravates pruritus. The tub will be very slippery, particularly if oil is used. Protect the patient from falling.

Care should be taken to pat the skin dry after the therapeutic bath; avoid rubbing. Rubbing increases irritation. Nonirritating linens should be used, and special laundering procedures are followed to remove all soap.

Soiled linen is placed in a labeled laundry bag and sent to the laundry. Clean laundry is obtained from central supply in labeled "allergy packs."

Applying Moist Dressings

Moist packs are applied to reduce swelling and weeping in acute dermatitis, to soften and remove exudate and crusts, and to relieve pruritus and discomfort. These dressings may be clean or sterile, depending on whether skin is intact. The dressing may be open or closed. A *closed dressing* is covered with plastic or a firm material. The *open dressing* is not covered because

Primary Lesions

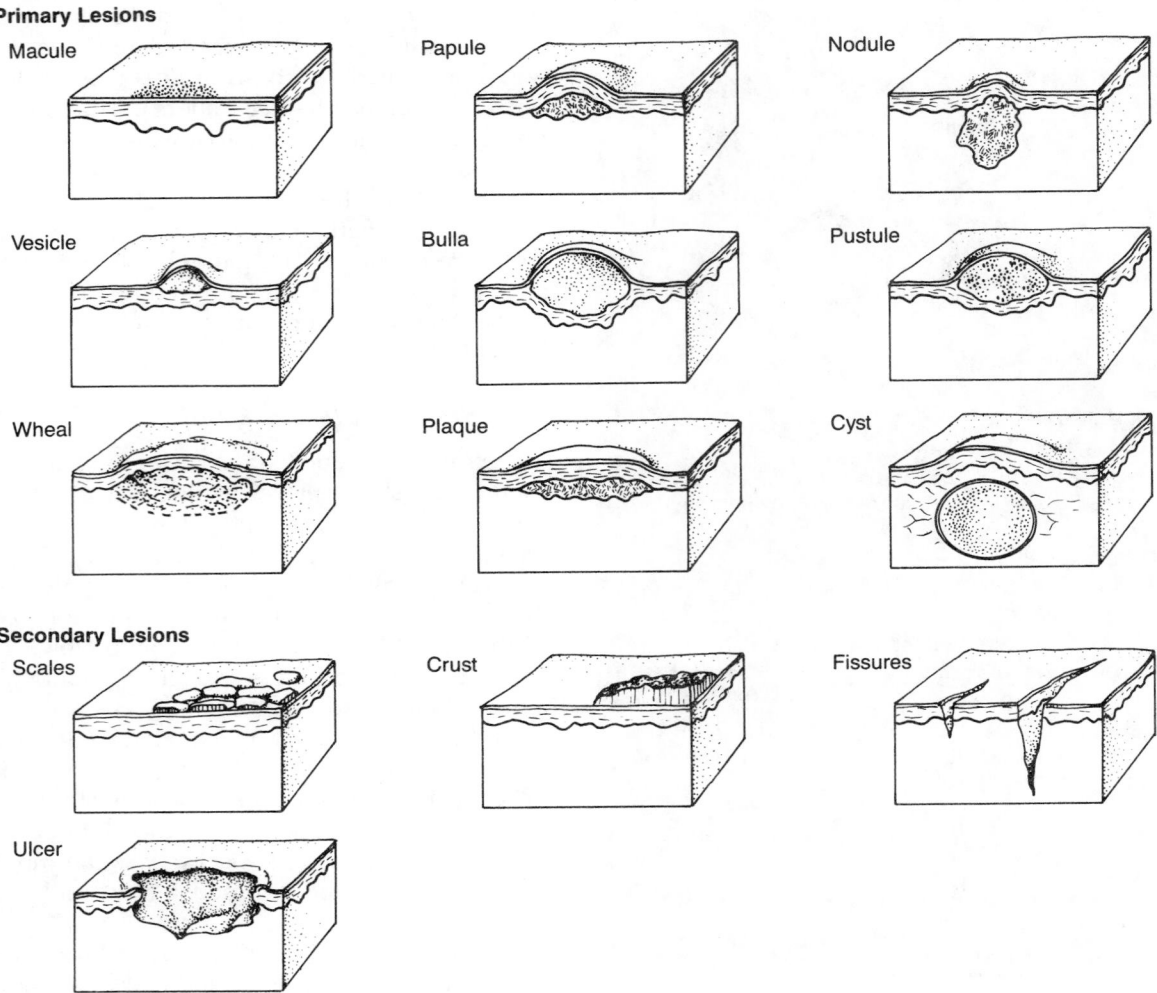

Figure 68-2. Common types of skin lesions. (Smeltzer SC, Bare BG. Brunner and Suddarth's Textbook of Medical-Surgical Nursing, ed 7. Philadelphia: J.B. Lippincott, 1992)

of the danger of tissue necrosis caused by lack of oxygen. Because the dressing is open, the fluid will evaporate rapidly and will require frequent changing or resoaking. The basic procedure for applying moist packs is discussed in Chapter 49.

Many solutions can be used on moist dressings, and the physician will specify which is to be used. Generally, the pharmacy will mix the solution and send it to the nursing unit. The procedure should be explained to the patient.

The pack is soaked in the solution and applied, semidripping, to the affected area. The packs are kept wet, as ordered. It is essential that moist packs be changed or resaturated at least every 2 hours. Protect the bed, the rest of the patient's body, and your own body from the solution.

A bed cradle should be available if packs are to be applied to the legs or trunk. Blankets should be provided so the patient will not become chilled.

Document the procedure and your observations when packs are removed. Used dressings are considered contaminated.

Maintaining Fluid and Electrolyte Balance

Fluid and electrolyte balance and general nutrition may be difficult to maintain because of developing exudates or because of serum lost due to inflammation or burns. The nurse should encourage fluid intake and encourage the patient to eat. Generally, a high-calorie, high-protein diet is given.

Considering Food Allergies

Skin disorders can be caused or become aggravated by food allergies. The patient may know what the offending foods are, or skin tests may be used to determine this. Chapter 77 discusses allergies in detail. Check to

Prevention of Burns

Family teaching regarding prevention of burns includes the following:

◆ The very young and very old are more likely to have accidents. Special preventive measures must be considered for these people.
◆ Portable heaters should be placed where there is no danger of falling over them or brushing against them. They should not stand near curtains, bed-spreads, or furniture that can catch fire easily from heat or flames. Use the type that will shut off automatically if the heater is tipped over.
◆ Candles should not be used for heat or light. They should not burn when no one is in the room.
◆ Place electrical appliances where no one will trip over them. Nothing should be used that has a frayed cord. Multiple outlet plugs should not be used. Cords should not run under rugs.
◆ Nothing should be stuck into an appliance that is plugged in (eg, a fork in a toaster).
◆ A qualified electrician should do work in the home.
◆ Children should be taught not to touch hot stoves and radiators. Handles of pans on the stove should be turned inward. Matches must be placed in a safe place out of the reach of children. Hot liquids should be kept out of the reach of infants and toddlers.
◆ People who are cooking indoors or out must be aware of loose clothing or flowing sleeves that could catch fire.
◆ Instructions should be followed carefully for heating pads and other equipment.
◆ The family should be aware of overhead wires in the yard or neighborhood. Wires should not be touched with metal ladders. Children should not climb up to them or fly kites in the vicinity. Any wire found disconnected or on the ground must be checked by an expert, particularly following a storm.
◆ There should be smoke alarms throughout the house; batteries must be checked regularly.
◆ Care must be taken with electrical appliances around water. Special lights and equipment are needed for swimming pool areas and for outdoor decorating.
◆ Overexposure to the sun or to the rays of a tanning bed are dangerous.
◆ Safety goggles should be worn when working with chemicals. Avoid inhaling chemical fumes in enclosed places. This is true of household cleaners.
◆ Have routine practice fire drills so family members know what to do in case of a fire. Develop a system where people will meet after a fire so the family will know if everyone is out of the house.
◆ Places of employment and schools should have routine fire drills. If this is not the case, insist on them.

see if the patient is on a restricted diet, and check the tray.

Providing Emotional Support

There may be a relationship between skin problems and emotional difficulties—skin eruptions may be the manifestation of underlying psychological problems. Furthermore, the itching that accompanies many skin disorders gives rise to emotional distress and physical discomfort. Itching is often more irritating than pain and more difficult to control.

Chronic skin problems can become an emotional challenge. Often the same disorder flares up at intervals throughout the patient's life, and the person must be assisted to cope. Group therapy may be helpful.

The patient's outward physical appearance may be unattractive. This person needs acceptance and support, probably more than many other patients. Allow the patient to express feelings, and provide companionship.

The use of touch can be therapeutic. The patient with a skin condition may be touched with bare hands, unless the person is contagious or has an open or draining lesion. Therapeutic touch can be effective with gloved hands as well.

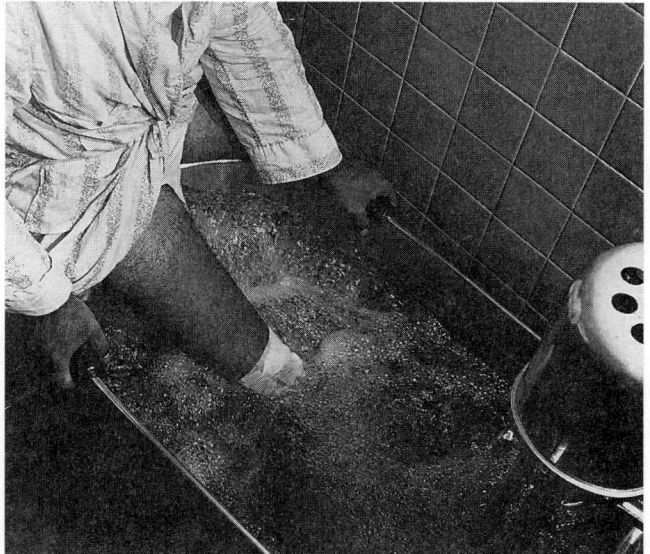

Figure 68-3. The whirlpool bath is often used in dermatologic nursing. The warm, circulating water can loosen crusts or eschar; it can clean a draining wound; and it is usually soothing to the patient. Severe pruritus may be treated in this way; oil is sometimes added to the water for its soothing effect. Whirlpool tubs come in sizes to fit the arm or leg (shown here) or in a large butterfly-shaped model that will accomodate the entire body. The large model might be used in a burn; in this way, much dead tissue could be removed from the burn without touching the patient. (Photo courtesy of 3M Health Care.)

Evaluation

Routinely, the nurse, patient, and family evaluate outcomes of care. Have short-term goals been met? Are long-term goals still realistic? What rehabilitation, home nursing, or other community services are needed? Planning for further care takes into consideration the patient's prognosis, complications, and patient responses to care given.

Allergies

Urticaria

Urticaria, commonly called *hives,* is characterized by the sudden appearance of edematous, raised pink areas called wheals that itch and burn. They may disappear as quickly as they came or may remain for several days. In most instances, acute urticaria is an allergic reaction to a foreign protein, such as an insect bite.

Contact allergens, such as face powder, can cause an urticaria that is known as *contact dermatitis.* The most common contact allergens are soaps, nickel jewelry or other products, perfumes, dyes, plants such as poison ivy, rubber, and insecticides. Stress and anxiety are thought to be important aggravating factors.

Urticaria of more than 6 weeks' duration is known as *chronic urticaria.* The exact cause of this disorder remains unknown in 80% to 90% of people. The person with an unexplained rash also should be examined for the possibility of Lyme disease.

Edema associated with urticaria is only a temporary annoyance, unless it involves extensive vital areas. If it becomes **angioedema,** which is gross swelling of the lips and tissues around the eyes, or edema of the larynx, which makes breathing difficult, death can occur.

Mild reactions can be treated with cool or ice water compresses or tepid baths with colloidal oatmeal or baking soda dissolved in the water. Antipruritic lotions, such as calamine lotion, may help. Antihistamines, such as astemizole (Hismanal) and azatadine maleate (Optimine), are often used for chronic urticaria. In severe cases, epinephrine may be administered. Chapter 77 discusses specific nursing care of the patient who has an allergy.

Nursing Alert

Angioedema associated with urticaria can become life-threatening. Look for the following:

◆ Extreme swelling of the lips
◆ Swelling around the eyes
◆ Dyspnea (difficult breathing)

Chronic Skin Disorders

Vitiligo

Vitiligo is a disorder in which areas of the skin are completely lacking in melanin pigmentation. Pigment cells (melanocytes) cannot be detected in the depigmented areas. The cause of vitiligo is unknown. No effective remedy is known, although the use of certain drugs, such as methoxsalen (Oxsoralen), followed by exposure to sunlight or ultraviolet light, offers temporary relief. The treatment is prolonged and time consuming and must take place under a physician's supervision. Cosmetics designed to cover birthmarks offer a practical solution to vitiligo.

Dermatitis or Eczema

Dermatitis means inflammation of the skin. The term eczema is often used interchangeably with atopic dermatitis. **Eczema** appears as small vesicles on reddened and pruritic skin. Sometimes the vesicles burst and ooze, after which crusts form. Persistent irritation and scratching make the skin leathery and thick. Eczema may be found in the folds of the elbows, the knees, and on the face, neck, wrists, and hands.

Eczema may spread to involve other areas. It may disappear completely for months or sometimes years but may recur at any time.

Eczema has a definite relationship to heredity, allergy, and emotional stress. Sometimes a family history will indicate the presence of an allergy, such as hay fever or asthma. Children who have eczema often develop these conditions later. There also may be an autoimmune component. As a person grows older, emotional factors seem to aggravate the eczema.

Treatment consists of applying moisturizing creams, corticosteroid ointments, wet dressings, or starch baths for inflamed skin. Antihistamines are used to relieve the itching, and tranquilizers are sometimes used to relieve the tension or anxiety that contribute to the condition. Childhood eczema is discussed in Chapter 65.

Psoriasis

Psoriasis most commonly affects young adults, people of early middle age, and men more often than women. The cause is unknown, although it is sometimes attributed to heredity or a metabolic disorder. Some researchers believe that it may be a systemic immune disorder. The course of psoriasis is unpredictable. In most patients, the disease remains localized. In some, however, its severity is incompatible with a productive life. Spontaneous clearing is rare, but unexplained exacerbation (flare-ups) or improvement is common. Stress and anxiety frequently precede flare-ups of the disease.

Signs and Symptoms. The hallmark of psoriasis is red patches covered with silvery scales that are constantly shed (Fig. 68-4). These patches appear mainly on the extensor surfaces of the elbows and knees, on the scalp, and on the lower back. The nails may begin to loosen at the beginning of the fingertips (*onycholysis*).

Medical Treatment. Treatment of psoriasis is generally not totally successful. The main objective of treatment is to reduce scaling and itching. Wet dressings may be used or lubricating ointments may be applied and covered. Ointments containing coal tar, anthracin, salicylic acid, or corticosteroids may be prescribed. Ultraviolet light treatments or exposure to the sun may be useful, with careful supervision by a physician. An intensive treatment of tar preparations and ultraviolet light is used in hospitalized patients. Methotrexate (Mexate) and oral retinoids (synthetic derivatives of vitamin A) are useful in patients with severe, extensive psoriasis. They require close supervision. A fairly new treatment is called *photochemotherapy.* It combines a photosensitizing agent (psoralen) with ultraviolet light.

Infections

Warts

Warts (verrucae) are small, flesh-colored, brown or yellow papules caused by a virus known as the *human papillomavirus.* Most warts are not painful, with the exception of the plantar wart on the sole of the foot, which grows inward due to the pressure of body weight.

Common warts are found most often on the hands, especially of children, or on other sites often subjected to trauma, but they may grow anywhere on the skin. *Filiform* warts are slender, soft, thin, fingerlike growths seen primarily on the face and neck. *Plantar* or *palmar* warts are firm, elevated or flat lesions occurring on the soles and palms.

Condylomata acuminata, or venereal warts, are warts that grow in warm, moist areas of the body. They often develop in areas that rub together, such as skin folds.

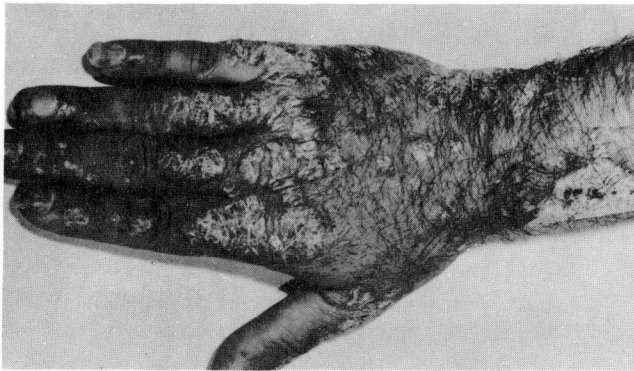

Figure 68-4. Severe psoriasis of the hand.

They may develop in clusters. These warts are frequently found on the foreskin and penis, particularly in uncircumcised men. They also can develop on vaginal and labial mucosa and in the urethral meatus and perianal (around the anus) area. **Condylomata acuminata** lesions are becoming more common in young people (see Chapter 63).

Medical Treatment. Common warts and filiform warts are best treated by destruction with electrodesiccation and curettage. Electrodesiccation involves treatment with short, high-frequency electric sparks, while curettage involves scraping or suctioning. Warts also are treated by the application of liquid nitrogen or by the use of keratolytic agents. In keratolytic treatment, salicylic acid and lactic acid are applied in the form of a solution or tape.

Bacterial Skin Infections

Impetigo and folliculitis are the primary bacterial infections of the skin. **Impetigo** is most commonly caused by streptococcal or staphylococcal bacteria and is contagious among infants and young children. Impetigo appears as vesicles that ooze and develop a golden yellow crust. The infections should be treated with systemic antibiotics, for example, penicillin. Lesions may be soaked with warm tap water to remove crusts and promote drying.

Folliculitis is a staphylococcal infection starting around the hair follicle. Lesions consist of superficial or deep pustules or follicular nodules. The face is a common site for deep folliculitis. Superficial folliculitis may respond to aggressive topical hygiene with antibacterial soaps and the use of topical antibiotics. Folliculitis on the male beard can be difficult to treat and may require the use of systemic antibiotics. Men with particularly curly facial hair have more difficulty because the hairs easily become ingrown.

Folliculitis may lead to the production of a furuncle, also called a *boil.* A **furuncle** starts as a firm, red, tender nodule. After a few days, the furuncle may discharge pus and finally a core. Furuncles are found most frequently in areas of hair-bearing skin that are subject to friction and moisture, especially the face, scalp, buttocks, and axillae. *Furunculosis* is the term for recurrent boils. Furunculosis develops in patients who are unable to be permanently rid of the *Staphylococcus* organism. There is no evidence that these patients harbor a particular strain of *Staphylococcus* or have any deficiency in their host defense mechanism.

A **carbuncle** is composed of several interconnecting boils in a cluster. They usually drain at multiple sites and are commonly found on the back of the neck, the back, and the thighs.

It is dangerous to pick or squeeze a boil, because this may spread infection to the surrounding tissue and possibly to the bloodstream. Special precautions should be taken with boils on the face, because the skin area drains directly into the cranial venous sinuses.

Medical Treatment. Treatment of boils consists of applying warm, wet dressings or soaks to localize the infection at one spot. Larger boils should be carefully incised and drained by a physician after they come to a point. After boils are drained, only topical antibiotics are needed. Furuncles or carbuncles associated with surrounding cellulitis or those associated with fever or located on the upper lip, nose, cheek, or forehead may ·be treated with oral antibiotics that are active against *Staphylococcus.* A culture and sensitivity test should be done before treatment to determine the most effective antibiotic.

Infestations by Parasites

Parasites live on another organism and take something from that organism. Scabies, lice, and bedbugs are parasites.

Scabies
Scabies are caused by a mite (*Sarcoptes scabiei*) burrowing under the outer layer of skin. One month or more after the mites enter the body, the skin begins to itch, especially when heavily covered. Red spots with a row of blackish dots $1/8$- to $1/2$-inch long with tiny vesicles and depressions appear, especially between the fingers. Other sites of involvement may include the wrist, antecubital fossa (front of the elbow), points of the elbow, nipples, umbilicus, lower abdomen, genitalia, and gluteal cleft (between the buttocks).

Scabies are acquired principally through close personal contact but may be transmitted through clothing, linens, or towels. Because the parasites get into bed clothing and personal garments, special precautions are necessary to keep scabies from spreading. All family members should be treated or examined for evidence of the condition simultaneously. The usual recommended treatment is a bath to open infected spots, followed by an application of a prescribed medication, such as crotamiton (Eurax) or lindane (Kwell) lotion to the entire body. The infected person must wear clean clothing and use clean bed linens and does not remove the medication for 8 to 12 hours.

Lice
Two types of lice (called pediculosis) infest humans: the lice that inhabit the head or body (*Pediculus humanus*) and crab lice (*Phthirus pubis*), which inhabit the genital region. They are very difficult to eradicate, because their eggs, called *nits,* can live for a long time on clothes or bedding or in overstuffed furniture. Symptoms include extreme pruritus (itching) and the presence of nits (eggs). The disease is most common in children. Outbreaks are fairly common in schools and day-care centers.

Preparations containing lindane (gamma benzene hexachloride), such as Kwell, Gamma Benzene, or Scabene, are highly effective if applied directly to the affected area, allowed to remain for 12 to 24 hours, and then completely removed with soap and water. Kwell is also available as a shampoo. The treatment usually needs to be repeated. The first treatment should kill most of the live lice. The second treatment kills the lice that hatch after the first treatment. After each treatment, inspect the patient; treated nits are expected to remain. It is important to look for live bugs. (All must be killed to prevent reinfestation.)

Nursing Considerations. It is important to treat everyone in the family and close contacts at the same time. Clean all linens and clothes in hot water; expose them to hot air in a clothes dryer. Items that cannot be washed should be dry cleaned and stored in plastic bags. For the child in school, check locker mates. Usually, if more than two cases of lice occur in a school class, the entire class must be checked. Children should be taught not to share combs or hats.

Key Concept
The nurse should be aware of the stigma of uncleanliness that is attached to the presence of lice. A child with lice and the parents need emotional support.

Bedbugs
The bedbug lives in clothing or bedding and is quite difficult to eradicate. Spraying all crevices in furniture, walls, and floors with an insecticide usually eliminates the insect. The bedbug usually bites the legs and feet, causing itching and burning. Lotions containing menthol or phenol or 0.5% hydrocortisone are applied to the bitten areas.

Nursing Alert
The nurse admitting a person who has been living on the streets or in shelters should be particularly alert for the presence of parasites, such as lice or bedbugs. It is important to treat the infected person immediately, to prevent transmission to others.

Sebaceous Gland Disorders

Sebaceous Cysts

When a sebaceous gland, which secretes oils, becomes plugged, a small, hard nodule forms. Called *cysts*, these hard nodules are not treated unless they become large and annoying, in which case they are drained or excised surgically.

Seborrheic Dermatitis, Seborrhea, and Dandruff

Seborrheic dermatitis and dandruff are conditions that cause scaling, primarily of the scalp, that is often associated with itching. *Seborrheic dermatitis* is an inflammatory condition that, in addition to erupting on the scalp, often occurs in areas of the body that have a large concentration of sebaceous glands, such as the eyebrows, eyelids, ears, axillae, groin, and skin under the ears and the breasts. It is characterized by yellowish, greasy scaling of the skin. An excessive sebaceous discharge that forms large scales or cheeselike plugs on the body is known as *seborrhea*. (*Seborrhea sicca* is a dry, scaly seborrheic dermatitis.) Dry flakes on the scalp (desquamation) are called *dandruff*.

Medical Treatment. Frequent shampoos are the mainstay of treatment, as advised by the physician. Some shampoos for treatment of the condition contain selenium sulfide suspension (Selsun Blue); others contain coal tar. Tincture of green soap or some other cleansing solution also may be used. In some cases, lotions or solutions containing corticosteroids are prescribed. These products are used sparingly once or twice daily according to the physician's directions.

If the seborrheic dermatitis is in a location other than the scalp, corticosteroid creams or ointments are prescribed. A low-fat diet, exercise, sunlight, reduction of stress, and rest also help, although there is no known cure.

Burn Trauma

Burns are traumatic injuries caused by thermal, electric, chemical, or radiation agents. A burn destroys cells by damaging the protein in them.

Burn Prevention

Children and adults need to be warned about the danger of burns, how to prevent, and what to do if they occur. This is especially true of occupants if their house is burning; they need a designated spot to meet. Keys to family teaching regarding burn prevention are given in the box on page 963.

Severity of Burns

Severity of injury from burns is related to depth, extent, age, parts of body burned, medical history with concurrent disorders, and amount of respiratory injury from smoke inhalation. Assessments are made during initial care in the hospital and frequently during the course of burn care.

Inhalation injuries are suspected if the burn patient was in a closed area with the fire and smoke. Singed nasal hairs, burns of the face, and soot-stained sputum are clear indications of smoke inhalation. The patient also may be hoarse or have a cough.

Burns are classified by three or four degrees of damage according to the depth of the burn and the amount of grafting likely to be needed. The accompanying box illustrates and summarizes the depth and four degrees of damage. These assessments are made after gentle cleansing of the burn area. Assessments are documented on the healthcare facility's form. An example of such a form for estimating percentage of body burned is given in the box.

Some institutions use the "rule of nines" for estimating percentage of body burned. It is similar to the figures in the box, but the body is divided into multiplications of nine. For instance, one arm is equal to 9%, and the entire back is equal to 18%. (See comparisons between child and adult described in Chapter 65.)

Special Considerations in Children
Burns

A superficial burn is critical if it covers two-thirds or more of the body of an infant.

Patients younger than 5 years have difficulty recovering from burns because their thin skin receives deeper burns, and they have incomplete immune systems and become dehydrated easily.

Recovery and Complications

There are four stages of problems and recovery. Each has its own effects on symptoms, assessment, medical therapy, and nursing care.

In *neurogenic shock*, fear and pain are most severe. A drop in blood pressure may cause death, especially in the very young or elderly.

In *fluid-loss shock*, systemic effects are most severe. Fluid is lost, blood volume drops, blood becomes thicker, and circulation is less efficient. Hematocrit reading and urine volume and specific gravity must be watched closely, as well as daily weights.

During *slough and infection*, eschar, which is the dead tissue, is separated from the live tissue, and an open wound is left. The wound often becomes infected, and antibiotics are administered.

Degree of Damage

First degree (superficial, partial thickness): characterized by red skin; usually not dangerous

Second degree (deep, partial thickness): characterized by destruction of outer layer of skin and formation of blisters; heals usually without grafting

Third degree (partial to full thickness): characterized by destruction of epidermis and dermis, with possible destruction of fat and muscles; emergency situation requiring immediate hospitalization and treatment; skin grafting necessary

Fourth degree (total full thickness): characterized by destruction of bone tissue; seen in nuclear radiation and explosions; very often fatal unless burn area is small

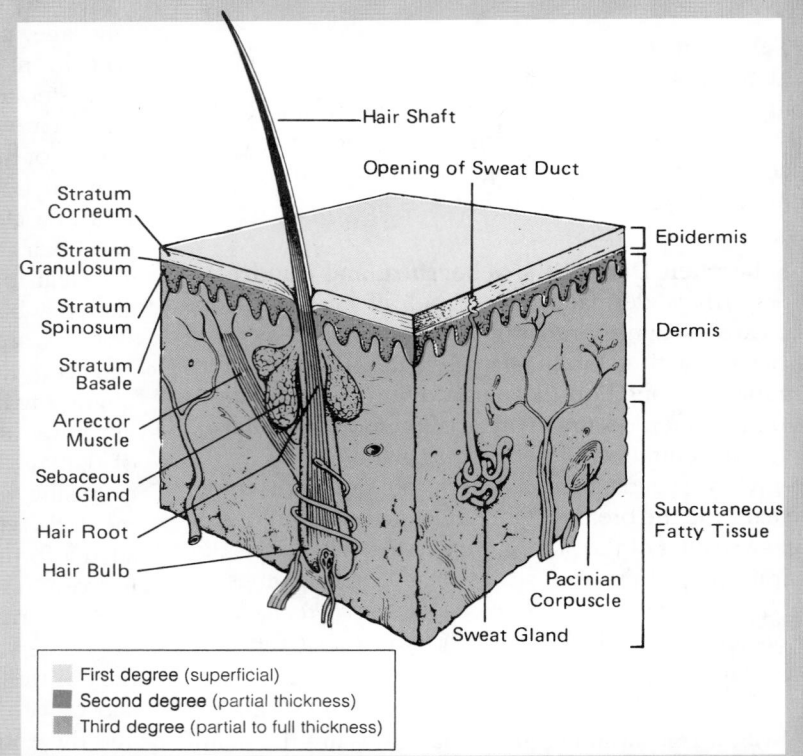

☐ First degree (superficial)
■ Second degree (partial thickness)
■ Third degree (partial to full thickness)

Sample Burn Evaluation Chart for Estimating Percentage of Body Surface Burned (indicated by shading). (Courtesy of Crozier-Chester Medical Center, Philadelphia, PA)

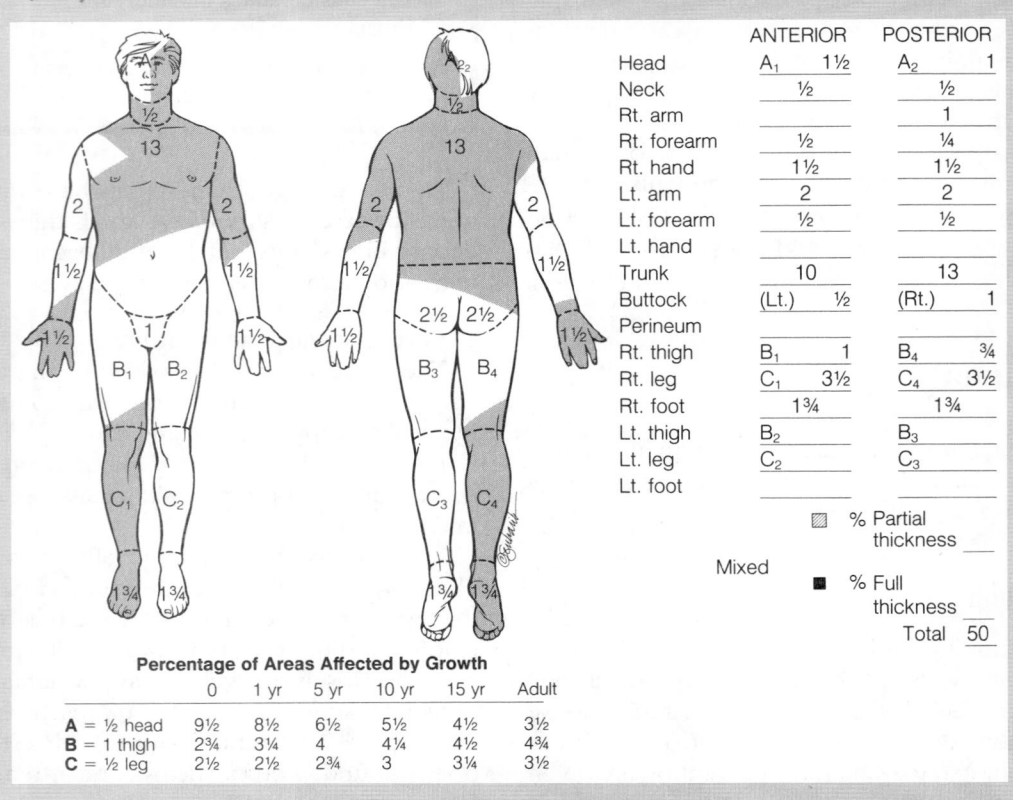

	ANTERIOR		POSTERIOR	
Head	A_1	1½	A_2	1
Neck		½		½
Rt. arm				1
Rt. forearm		½		¼
Rt. hand		1½		1½
Lt. arm		2		2
Lt. forearm		½		½
Lt. hand				
Trunk		10		13
Buttock	(Lt.)	½	(Rt.)	1
Perineum				
Rt. thigh	B_1	1	B_4	¾
Rt. leg	C_1	3½	C_4	3½
Rt. foot		1¾		1¾
Lt. thigh	B_2		B_3	
Lt. leg	C_2		C_3	
Lt. foot				

Mixed ▨ % Partial thickness ___

■ % Full thickness ___

Total 50

Percentage of Areas Affected by Growth

	0	1 yr	5 yr	10 yr	15 yr	Adult
A = ½ head	9½	8½	6½	5½	4½	3½
B = 1 thigh	2¾	3¼	4	4¼	4½	4¾
C = ½ leg	2½	2½	2¾	3	3¼	3½

Sample Nursing Care Plan
A Person With Burns

Mr. Lionel DeStephano, a 76-year-old male was admitted to the Regional Burn Center with second-degree burns extending over 10% of the right side of his body, involving his upper thigh and lower abdomen. One nursing diagnosis for Mr. DeStephano's plan of care follows.

Nursing Diagnosis: *Fluid Volume Deficit Related to Increased Capillary Permeability in Area of the Burn as Evidenced by Weeping and Wound Edema, Altered Vital Signs, Decreased Urinary Output, and Decreased Serum Potassium*

Goal: 8/6/95, Patient will achieve improved fluid and electrolyte balance.

Nursing Actions (assess/do/teach)	Rationale	Evaluative Statement
1. Monitor sensorium, vital signs, arterial blood gases, and electrolytes, noting and documenting trends.		Goal met; 8/6, patient is maintaining fluid output of approximately 50–70 mL/h; has stable vital signs and blood values within normal limits
2. Maintain accurate intake and output records; measure urine output hourly.	Less than 30–50 mL could indicate decreased renal flow.	
3. Titrate fluids and replace electrolytes as prescribed.	This will maintain homeostasis and decrease potential for renal problems.	
4. Weigh patient daily.		
5. Position patient to increase venous return, and administer oxygen as indicated.	This action helps maintain tissue perfusion.	
6. Be alert to signs of fluid overload.	After the acute phase, the fluid starts to reenter the vascular system from the tissues.	
7. Monitor IV fluid replacement.		

During the *repair* stage, healing begins in the burned area, and the general body condition improves. Skin grafting is begun. Blood may be given, and the patient is placed on a high-calorie, high-protein diet.

Complications. Various complications can occur following a burn. These include infection, general gastrointestinal disturbances, hypostatic pneumonia, kidney failure, anemia, skin ulcers, and contractures.

Impaired circulation or difficulty in moving or breathing may occur as eschar begins to tighten. An *escharotomy* (incision into eschar) may be needed to relieve the difficulties.

Multiple ulcers in the stomach and duodenum may develop approximately 1 week after the injury. These are called Curling's ulcers and are believed to be the result of stress. Cimetidine (Tagamet) helps prevent this condition. The first symptom of Curling's ulcers often is bleeding, as evidenced by bloody sputum or emesis or by tarry stools.

Contractures are abnormal shortening of muscles and other resulting deformities. They are the most serious long-term complications of burns.

Because the patient often must be immobilized for some time, special care should be taken to provide passive or active range-of-motion exercises as soon as possible. The patient is often reluctant to move because of pain or fear of pain. Therefore, it is important for the nurse to encourage the patient to exercise and explain why. If the burn is near a joint, contractures are more likely to form and may need to be released surgically. If medication prescribed as needed (PRN) is given before exercises, pain is reduced.

The Multidisciplinary Approach

Physical Therapy. The patient is often taken to the physical therapy department for whirlpool treatment and exercises. The whirlpool serves several purposes: It helps clean the body and often assists in removing eschar; it can serve to apply external medication; it gives warmth, so the patient can exercise with less pain; and it helps stimulate viable (live) tissue. When the whirlpool treatment is completed, the physical therapist exercises the patient's extremities.

Occupational Therapy. The seriously burned patient is usually in the hospital or rehabilitation center for some time and needs to be occupied with diversional activity. He or she also may need counseling or job retraining after release from the hospital and help in learning how to manage household activities. These services can be provided through occupational therapy or referral to vocational counseling.

Social Service. Because of the long-term nature of a severe burn, the patient may need assistance in arranging for care of his or her family during hospitalization and the rehabilitation period. Financial aid may be needed as well.

Immediate Care

The best first-aid for a burn is immediate application of cold packs or cold water. First-aid is discussed in Chapter 31.

> **Nursing Alert**
>
> Under no circumstances should ointments or salves be applied to an extensive burn; removing them causes further unnecessary discomfort, and their presence makes it difficult for the physician to determine the extent of the burn. They may also introduce pathogens into the wound.

All personnel working with a burn patient should use aseptic techniques when preparing the room and providing supplies. When the patient arrives in the hospital, the clothes are carefully removed, taking care not to cause further damage to the burn site. The patient may be placed on sterile sheets if the burn is severe. Personnel should show concern and give encouragement to the patient who is fearful, probably in pain, and may feel a sense of loss. Body systems are assessed immediately.

Vital Signs. Height, weight, and vital signs are recorded. Because the burn patient is subject to shock, vital signs should be taken often. The patient is often on a cardiac monitor. The nurse also should be alert to any change, such as tachycardia, which may indicate a worsening condition or a rise in temperature, indicating dehydration or the beginning of an infection.

Respiratory Status. It is important that respiratory status be carefully monitored, because the patient probably has inhaled smoke and may have sustained burns of the lungs. Smoke inhalation is often the cause of death in the patient who is not noticeably burned externally. The nurse should assess the rate and depth of respirations. It is particularly important to observe the patient when burns are in the head and neck area.

> **Nursing Alert**
>
> The presence of a cough should be reported immediately. The amount and character of any sputum should be noted. Black or gray sputum indicates smoke inhalation.

Oxygen therapy should be initiated. Because of possible respiratory complications, an endotracheal tube should be kept at the patient's bedside and a tracheostomy done if necessary. The nurse should begin immediate measures to prevent hypostatic pneumonia. Blood gases and pH are measured frequently to determine respiratory status and general body status. Respiratory therapy is prescribed.

Fluid and Electrolyte Balance. The patient loses body fluids constantly from open wounds. It is essential to replace fluids to maintain the circulatory volume, thus preventing the collapse of blood vessels, which could result in serious or fatal shock. The patient usually will receive intravenous fluids and plasma. The nurse must be sure that intake and output are recorded accurately. A central line is often in place, and the patient receives total parenteral nutrition (TPN).

The patient often has a nasogastric tube to suction. The partial thromboplastin time (PTT) and the gastric secretions are monitored to determine electrolyte levels. A drug such as cimetidine (Tagamet) may be given to reduce gastric secretions. A sample nursing care plan for a burn patient with fluid volume deficit accompanies the text.

Renal Function. Urine output must be monitored, because commonly renal function slows or stops after the body has undergone such a severe shock. The urinary output is measured at least hourly for the first few days, with attention paid to its specific gravity. A very high or a very low urine output is significant. Also, a very high urine-specific gravity should be noted (very concentrated urine). If the output is too low (less than 30 mL/h), dialysis may be needed. Acidosis also is a frequent complication.

Prevention of Infection. The patient may be placed in protective isolation to prevent pathogens from reaching him or her. The patient is highly susceptible to infection, because resistance is low, and there are many open areas on the body. (See Chapter 51 for a discussion of protective isolation.) The patient is given intravenous antibiotics. Antibacterial body packs or other topical medications may be applied.

Pain Management. The patient with a first- or second-degree burn is in a great deal of pain. The patient with a third-degree burn, which is deeper and more severe, is not in as much pain because nerve endings have been destroyed. Because morphine is often given to relieve pain, the nurse must be alert for symptoms of respiratory depression. Because the period of recovery is prolonged, less addicting drugs will be ordered as soon as the pain is better tolerated.

Prevention of Further Skin Breakdown. The patient is often placed in a special fluidized bed to prevent pressure areas and eliminate unnecessary handling and moving.

Stabilized Hospital Care

Dressings
Several types of solutions and substances are used as dressings, including gauze impregnated with an antibiotic or drug and moist packs soaked in a substance such as silver nitrate. Sterile dressings may be used.

Types of Dressings. Two types of dressings are used. Open dressings are continuously applied wet dressings.

Closed dressings are not often used; however, in some cases, they reduce the patient's pain and anxiety. Nursing skills in applying burn dressings follow:

◆ Explain the procedure to the patient.
◆ Give PRN medication approximately $\frac{1}{2}$ hour before a dressing change. This relaxes the patient. The dressings may be loosened by moistening them with warmed, sterile, normal saline if ordered.
◆ Wear goggles and gloves when changing dressings.
◆ Assess the condition of the burn; extra dry indicates dehydration; wet, soupy, and strong odor indicates infection; redness and swelling at the edge of the wound indicates cellulitis; and clean, pink, and shiny is a healthy sign.
◆ All dressings and packs are contaminated when removed from the body and should be disposed of accordingly.

In some cases the patient wears a tight occlusive dressing, face mask, or pressure dressing. The pressure may be applied to a specific burn area, such as an arm, or the patient may wear a full body pressure suit. This helps to prevent the development of keloid (scar) tissue. These devices are often used.

Topical Agents. The application of topical agents to the burned area is currently the widest used therapy.

Mafenide acetate (Sulfamylon) is an effective bacteriostatic cream used against many gram-negative and gram-positive bacteria. This cream is applied in a thick layer to the entire burned area with a sterile, gloved hand. The area is then usually allowed to remain open to the air. Disadvantages of this treatment include the patient experiencing burning pain following application and the possibility of the patient developing metabolic acidosis.

Silver sulfadiazine (Silvadene) is a bacteriocidal cream used against many gram-negative and gram-positive bacteria. It may be applied in a thin layer to the burned area with a sterile, gloved hand. A common protocol specifies that the wound then be covered with Vaseline-coated Adaptic, followed by sterile dressings. The entire dressing can be held in place with a Kling or a Kerlix, which is wrapped around the torso or the limb. (Some gram-negative bacilli are resistant to the effects of Silvadene. If this occurs, Silvadene is used in conjunction with other antimicrobial agents.)

Povidone (Betadine) covers a broad spectrum of microbicidal action. It is applied as a cream, usually three times a day. It is nonirritating and nonsensitizing.

Silver nitrate is still prescribed today by some physicians, although it is not used as often as it once was. Silver nitrate (0.5%) solution is applied to gauze dressings that are placed on the burn areas. The dressings are kept moist by using a bulb syringe to apply the solution. It is often thought that the bacteriocidal action of silver nitrate on burn areas is so effective that cross-contamination does not result; thus, protective isolation technique is not usually necessary.

Nursing Alert

Silver nitrate will blacken anything with which it comes into contact. Therefore, take measures to protect your uniform and hands. Linen to be used in this treatment is identified, to prevent staining of excess linens. Care also must be taken to prevent permanent staining of the walls and floors of the patient's room. The patient's visitors need to be cautioned about the staining as well.

Other Treatments

Débridement. The skin and other dead tissue that is burned and charred is known as eschar. It is usually thick, dry, and black or dark brown. Eschar must be débrided (removed) to expose the viable (living) tissue. In this way, grafting can be successfully performed.

The packs and external medications assist in loosening and softening the eschar, although the whirlpool is more commonly used because it is the most comfortable method for the patient. Physicians are now using laser scalpels for excision (removal) of eschar. This method causes minimal blood loss and less pain than previously used methods.

Nursing Alert

Offer the patient a PRN pain medication approximately ½ hour before any painful procedure, such as débridement, is to be done.

Electrolyte Balance. Electrolytes are lost through leakage from the wounds and because of impaired kidney function. The laboratory does daily determinations of blood and gastric pH and electrolytes, and the physician prescribes appropriate replacement therapy.

Dietary Management. Good nutrition to rebuild injured tissues is vital to the burn patient, who needs as many as 6,000 calories daily. The diet should be high calorie and high protein and is usually supplemented by vitamin preparations. The patient must be urged to eat. Tube feedings or total parenteral nutrition (TPN) may be used. (The cimetidine or other drug ordered earlier to prevent excess acid formation in the stomach may be continued.) Extra between-meal protein supplements, such as Resource or Resource Instant Crystals, also may be needed. Accurate recording of food intake is often ordered; it is the nurse's responsibility to record exactly what the patient eats and any significant observations (such as refusal to eat, choking, difficulty in swallowing, or vomiting). Daily weights usually are ordered.

Bowel Function. Often, stool softeners such as docusate Na (colace) are given to avoid straining. Record all bowel movements (time, amount, consistency, and other characteristics).

Rehabilitation

Reconstructive or Cosmetic Surgery

Skin Grafting. Skin grafting replaces tissue that cannot heal by itself because of extensive damage. It also is done for cosmetic reasons to limit the amount of scarring. If the patient has enough intact, undamaged skin, an autograft is done. An **autograft** is a graft using the person's own skin. When healing begins and the eschar is completely removed, the plastic surgeon cuts paper-thin slices of skin from an unaffected part of the patient's body and places these grafts on the affected area.

If the patient's own skin cannot be used, cadaver skin graft or skin from another person (**homograft** or **allograft**) may be used. Immunosuppressive medications may be given to prevent rejection of the foreign skin. In many cases, the foreign skin is allowed to be rejected but is in place long enough to allow new tissue growth underneath.

In some severe burns, especially in areas such as the hands, which are prone to contractures, pigskin (a **heterograft** or **xenograft**) is grafted in place. The patient's body will reject the pigskin in approximately 1 week, but before this occurs, the pigskin will aid in retention of body fluids, protect the open wound from infections, and promote healing.

Skin grafts are delicate; care should be taken not to disturb them so they can attach to the live tissue underneath and grow. Assess the graft and report if it seems to be detaching. It is important to follow the protocol of your hospital for the care of the *graft site* and the *donor site*.

Emotional Aspects. There are many emotional aspects to be considered in burns. The burn patient may become demanding, expecting much attention in later stages of care because so much attention is given immediately after the injury. The patient must be allowed to express feelings. At the same time, the patient needs honesty, understanding, and firmness. The patient should participate in developing a realistic nursing care plan. Family members also should participate. If the patient is in isolation, there is the added element of loneliness. Because there is often a realistic concern about appearance, the nurse can be most helpful by listening and encouraging the patient to become involved in a support group.

There is a danger of overdependence or addiction to pain-relieving drugs. Nursing measures should be used to promote patient comfort and reduce drug use to the minimum (see Chapter 52).

Prognosis

Although the course of treatment is long and arduous, current techniques help the person return to optimum functioning. Most patients are able to live productive lives.

Special Considerations in Aging

Burns

Older people may not realize they are being burned; they may be paralyzed or confused, or they may not be able to feel the burn.

Patients older than 60 years have difficulty recovering from burns because they have very thin skin and usually receive deeper burns. Also, the immune systems of adults older than 60 are often compromised.

Older patients with cardiovascular disease may not be able to withstand the additional trauma of a burn.

Neoplasms

Nonmalignant Tumors

There are many nonmalignant tumors of the skin, including warts, cysts, angiomas, keloids, and nevi (see Figure 68-2).

Moles

Moles, or pigmented nevi, are usually benign, although they may become cancerous, especially if they are very dark, hairy, and elevated. A biopsy should be performed if a mole has these characteristics.

Angiomas

Angiomas, or birthmarks, are vascular tumors of the skin, with involvement of underlying tissues and blood vessels. Some angiomas, such as the "port wine" angioma, are difficult to remove or if very large, inoperable. Other "strawberry" angiomas tend to involute (regress or disappear) spontaneously. Most angiomas, however, are neither very noticeable nor very dangerous.

Keloids

Keloids are benign tumors that develop from scars. Plastic surgery, for cosmetic reasons, may be performed to hide these scars.

Skin Cancer

Skin cancer is the most common form of cancer and the most curable. Because the lesion is visible, the patient usually seeks early treatment. The most common types

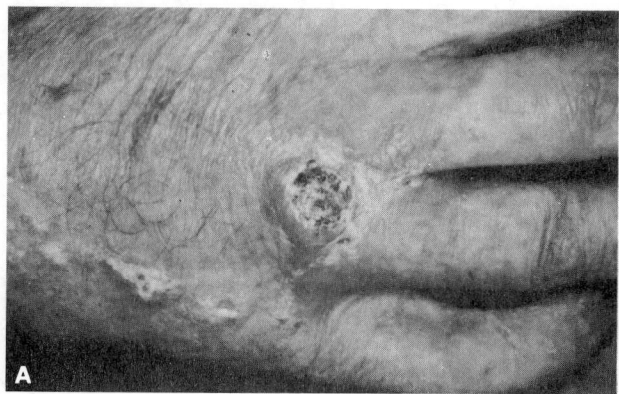
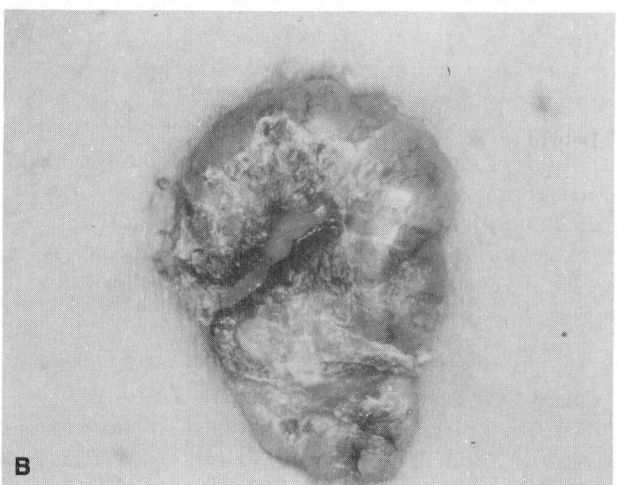
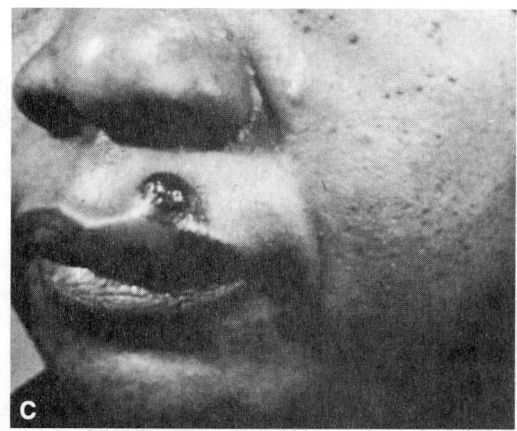

Figure 68-5. Skin cancers. **(A)** Squamous cell carcinoma. **(B)** Basal cell carcinoma. **(C)** Melanoma. (A and B, courtesy of Mervyn L. Elgart, M.D.; **C,** courtesy of Medichrome, Clay-Adams, Inc., New York.)

are *squamous cell carcinoma, basal cell carcinoma,* and *malignant melanoma* (Fig. 68-5).

Exposure to the sun is the leading cause of skin cancer. Light-haired, fair-skinned, light-eyed people are at high risk for skin cancer. Also at high risk are individuals who are prone to sunburn or who do not tan. People older than 40 years are more susceptible than younger people. Smoking also seems to increase susceptibility.

Observation and early investigation of changes in a mole and of new growths is vital; a deeply pigmented mole should be checked. A physician must be consulted when any changes in a wart or mole occur, including such factors as size, shape, color, flaking, bleeding, sudden elevation, hair growth, or sudden itching or burning.

Patient teaching is of utmost importance in controlling skin cancer. All people, especially those at risk, should be taught preventive measures (see box).

Treatment. Most forms of skin cancer are treated by curettage (scraping) or electrodesiccation (removal with intermittent electric sparks). Wide excision (surgery) may be necessary. Radiation therapy may be used for older patients or for those for whom excision is not practical or possible. Mohs' chemosurgery is sometimes performed. In this process, tissue is first fixed with zinc chloride and the cancer is then removed, in layers, under local anesthesia. If serial excisions are removed for biopsy, this is simply called Mohs' surgery.

Basal Cell Carcinoma

Basal cell carcinoma appears as a small, fleshy bump or nodule and usually is found in areas that are repeatedly exposed to the sun or other ultraviolet light. It is the most common skin cancer in white people. This cancer is very slow growing and does not metastasize. However, it may extend below the skin to the bone and cause considerable local damage.

Squamous Cell Carcinoma

Squamous cell carcinoma may appear as nodules or as red scaly patches. Squamous cell carcinoma is the second most common skin cancer found in white people. It is typically found on the rim of the ear, face, lips, and mouth. This cancer increases in size, developing into a large mass; the cancer may metastasize. The cure rate for squamous cell carcinoma is 95% with early treatment.

Malignant Melanoma

Malignant melanoma is the most virulent of all skin cancers but is almost always curable in its early stages. Melanoma may suddenly appear without warning, but it also may begin in or near a mole or other dark spot on the skin. It has a strong tendency to metastasize, and once colonies of melanoma cells reach vital internal organs, the disease becomes much more difficult to treat.

Mycosis Fungoides

This condition is a chronic, malignant skin neoplasm. Lymph nodes and internal organs are involved, and large, painful, ulcerating lesions develop on the skin. It is fatal. Treatment with nitrogen mustard (Mustargen) is palliative. This patient needs expert nursing care for the pain, itching, and disfigurement of the disorder.

Key Concept

Many dermatologic disorders are stressful. The nurse can be most helpful by providing a safe, comfortable, and supportive environment for the patient.

Keys for Review

Key Questions for Critical Thinking

1. You have assisted in the admission of a patient and have just identified the presence of lice. Describe what nursing care is needed. Describe what you will say to the patient and to his or her family.
2. A patient reminds you that he or she has many allergies and "very sensitive skin." Write a plan of care for this patient, addressing the necessary nursing interventions.
3. Discuss why angioedema is considered life threatening. Describe its signs and symptoms. Discuss what care you would give a person with these symptoms.

Key Questions for Critical Thinking

(continued)

4. Identify the body systems affected in the severe burn patient. Identify how each body system is affected. Discuss what care you would give a person with these symptoms.

Key Readings

Berkow R (Ed). The Merck Manual of Diagnosis and Therapy, Ed 16. Rahway, NJ, Merck & Co, 1992

Key Readings (continued)

Craven RF, Hirnle CJ. Fundamentals of Nursing: Human Health and Function. Philadelphia, J.B. Lippincott, 1992

Dyer C, Roberts D. "Thermal Trauma." Nursing Clinics of North America 25(1), March 1990

Earnest VV. Clinical Skills in Nursing Practice, Ed 2. Philadelphia, J.B. Lippincott, 1993

Fischbach F. A Manual of Laboratory and Diagnostic Tests, Ed 3. Philadelphia, J.B. Lippincott, 1992

NANDA Nursing Diagnoses: Definitions and Classifications 1992. Philadelphia, NANDA, 1992

Nursing 93 Drug Handbook. Springhouse, PA, Springhouse, 1993

O'Toole M (Ed). Miller-Keane Encyclopedia and Dictionary of Medicine, Nursing, and Allied Health, Ed 5. Philadelphia, W.B. Saunders, 1992

Smeltzer SC, Bare BG. Brunner and Suddarth's Textbook of Medical-Surgical Nursing, Ed 7. Philadelphia, J.B. Lippincott, 1992

Smith AJ, Johnson JY. Nurses' Guide to Clinical Procedures. Philadelphia, J.B. Lippincott, 1990

Taylor C, Lillis C, LeMone P. Fundamentals of Nursing: Art and Science of Nursing Care, Ed 2. Philadelphia, J.B. Lippincott, 1993

Keys to Learning More

Chapter 69: disorders in fluid and electrolyte balance

Chapter 75: blood and lymph disorders

Chapter 76: cancer

Chapter 77: allergic disorders

Chapter 78: human immunodeficiency virus, acquired immunodeficiency syndrome, and autoimmune disorders

Chapter 89: rehabilitation and home care nursing

Key Resources

American Burn Association
    Shriner's Burn Institute
    University of Cincinnati
    202 Goodman Street
    Cincinnati, OH 45219
    513-751-3900

National Institute of Arthritis and Musculoskeletal and Skin Diseases
    National Institutes of Health
    Bethesda, MD 20892
    301-496-4000

National Psoriasis Foundation
    6443 SW Beaverton Hwy, Suite 210
    Portland, OR 97221
    503-297-1545

69 Disorders in Fluid and Electrolyte Balance

Keys for Learning

Learning Objectives

- Define homeostasis.
- Differentiate between overhydration and dehydration, and describe related nursing care.
- Define edema, and state its causes.
- Define skin turgor; describe how it is evaluated.
- Describe four primary acid–base disturbances.
- Differentiate between alkalosis and acidosis, and outline nursing care for each.

Key Terms

edema

fluid volume deficit

fluid volume excess

metabolic acidosis

metabolic alkalosis

Keys to Understanding This Chapter

Chapter 14: organization of the body

Chapter 16: fluid and electrolyte balance

Chapter 24: the urinary system

Chapter 28: diet therapy

Chapter 38: signs and symptoms of illness or injury

Chapter 46: elimination

Chapter 50: physical examination and nursing assessment, including fluid and electrolyte balance

Chapter 53: surgical intervention

Chapter 57: administration of medications

Chapter 68: skin disorders

Key Points

- Fluid and electrolyte disturbances are possible in anyone but are particularly common in ill and hospitalized patients, including those undergoing surgical and diagnostic procedures. The risk of serious disturbances increases in patients at the extremes of the age spectrum.
- All nursing care should include assessment of the level of hydration and observation for dehydration.

Key Points (continued)

- Edema is a symptom of many disorders. Edematous skin is very friable and prone to breakdown. Good skin care is imperative, as is patient positioning.
- Measurement of intake and output is a valid key in the assessment of fluid balance.
- Respiratory acidosis, if not corrected, could lead to the need for mechanical ventilation.
- A simple treatment for respiratory alkalosis, usually caused by hyperventilation, can be to have patients breathe into a bag, replacing needed CO_2 in the body.

Key Topics Outline

Anatomy and Physiology Review

Diagnostic Tests
  Laboratory Tests

Medical Treatments

Nursing Process
  Data Collection
  Nursing Diagnosis
  Planning and Implementation
  Evaluation

Maintenance of Water Balance

Maintenance of Electrolyte Balance

Maintenance of Acid–Base Balance

Key Learning Activities

- List alternatives for a patient who needs to take more fluids but does not like water or who drinks too much plain water.
- Locate your facility's list of measurements or conversions for household containers, such as a styrofoam cup, ice cream container, drinking glass, or soup bowl.
- Make a chart of ways to determine fluid volume excess and deficit. Locate pictures if possible.

Rosdahl CB: Textbook of Basic Nursing, 6th ed. © 1995 J.B. Lippincott Company

A normal balance between the body's fluids and electrolytes and a normal acid–base balance must exist for a person to be healthy. We call this balance between the fluids, electrolytes, and acids and bases in the body *homeostasis*. It is a dynamic process by which the body constantly adjusts to internal and external stimuli. Disorders in body systems can positively or negatively influence homeostasis.

Anatomy and Physiology Review

The body constantly uses mechanisms called *feedback* to maintain balance. The nervous and endocrine systems are most intimately involved in this feedback. The digestive, urinary, respiratory, and integumentary systems also are involved in making changes in response to feedback.

Water is the primary body fluid and is vital to life. It comprises 50% to 75% of the human body. Variations depend on the person's age, muscle mass, and sex. Body fluids (blood, lymph, tissue fluid) are located in two compartments. They are *intracellular* (fluid within cells) and *extracellular* (fluid outside of cell walls). Extracellular fluid includes *intravascular* fluid or plasma (fluid within the vascular system) and *interstitial* fluid (fluid in which tissue cells are bathed). *Total body water* refers to the total amount of water in the body expressed as a percentage of body weight. Body fluids are constantly moving between compartments by specialized mechanisms called passive transport (osmosis, diffusion, filtration) and carrier-mediated transport (facilitated diffusion, active transport, endocytosis, exocytosis). Electrolytes are vital links in the transport of fluids across cell membranes.

The nurse monitors the patient for actual or potential threats to fluid and electrolyte balance. Much of nursing is directed toward assessing and maintaining homeostasis. Any disorder, disease, or injury can disrupt homeostasis.

Key Concepts

Fluid and electrolyte disturbances are possible in anyone but are particularly common in ill and hospitalized patients, including those undergoing surgical and diagnostic procedures.

The risk of serious disturbances in fluid and electrolyte balance increases in patients at the extremes of the age spectrum and in those who have preexisting or chronic illnesses.

Diagnostic Tests

Laboratory Tests

Many laboratory tests are aimed at evaluating the fluid–electrolyte or acid–base balance of the body. Blood tests include liver function studies, blood pH, blood gas evaluations, and measurement of specific blood electrolyte levels. Urine and other body fluids are studied for composition and abnormal components. In some cases, urine is collected for 24 hours so an entire day's output can be studied.

Medical Treatments

Oral and Intravenous Administration of Fluids and Electrolytes

Once an imbalance is determined, fluids, electrolytes, and other substances can be administered to the patient. Some of these substances, such as potassium, can be administered orally. However, some electrolytes either cannot be absorbed when taken orally or would not be absorbed quickly enough. In this case, intravenous (IV) administration of electrolytes is often the treatment of choice. An IV is started and specific electrolytes are added to the infusion, or a bolus (one-time large dose) of a particular electrolyte may be administered in extreme cases. Blood levels are monitored, and the dosage to be given is adjusted accordingly. Administration of IV fluids is discussed in Chapter 57.

❖ *Nursing Process*

Data Collection

The nurse must carefully observe and assess all patients for potential disorders in fluid or electrolyte balance. Chapter 50 describes the physical examination and nursing assessment, including fluid and electrolyte balance. This assessment establishes a baseline for future comparison and determines the presence of suspected complications. The nurse should report any changes in this baseline level.

When assessing the patient's fluid and electrolyte balance, the nurse makes judgements about factors such as the appearance and turgor of the patient's skin, the volume and specific gravity of urine, the relative balance between intake and output, and comparisons of daily weights. The accompanying box lists some of the components of nursing assessment. Chapter 50 offers a more detailed discussion.

Nursing Diagnosis

Based on data collection, the following nursing diagnoses may be established for the person with a disorder in fluid or electrolyte balance:

♦ Altered Urinary Elimination related to urinary retention or excessive urinary output
♦ Urinary Retention related to excess blood level of sodium
♦ Fluid Volume Excess related to electrolyte imbalance (as evidenced by edema, pulmonary edema, hypertension, ascites [fluid in the abdominal cavity], sodium retention)
♦ Fluid Volume Deficit related to electrolyte imbalance (as evidenced by hypotension, hyperthermia, rapid weight loss, dry skin, poor skin turgor, concentrated urine)
♦ Impaired Tissue Integrity related to edema, poor skin turgor, and dehydration
♦ Impaired Physical Mobility related to edema

Planning and Implementation

The patient, nurse, and healthcare team plan together for effective care to meet patient needs. The patient with a fluid or electrolyte imbalance may require assistance in meeting daily needs, maintaining a balance between intake and output, and understanding more about the disorder, its prognosis, and its treatment. The patient must follow the prescribed regimen to resolve the imbalance. A nursing care plan is developed to meet these needs.

Teaching the Patient and Family

The nurse can teach the patient and family a great deal about fluid and electrolyte problems, especially if the person will be cared for in the home. The patient should be included as much as possible in planning the diet and dietary restrictions and in the time and amount of food and fluids to be consumed. If the person understands the rationale for special diets or limitations, he or she is more likely to comply. The same is true for the person who will do the shopping and food preparation in the home. Some of the subjects to be included in patient and family teaching are summarized in the accompanying box.

Positioning and Edema

Edema, which is the abnormal accumulation of fluid in interstitial spaces, usually accompanies fluid volume excess disorders. Edema, its assessment, and illustrations are discussed in Chapter 50 and later in this chapter.

Edematous areas should be handled carefully. Edematous skin is friable and prone to skin breakdown, sloughing, and ulceration. The person's position should be changed frequently. The patient is positioned for maximum comfort. Elevation of an edematous body part, usually the feet and ankles, helps the area drain.

Assessing Daily Fluid Balance

Accurate intake and output records are kept. Intake and output of fluids should be roughly equal. If they differ greatly, the patient's level of hydration should be evaluated. Urine specific gravity and daily weights are checked. Skin turgor is evaluated by lifting a fold of skin between your thumb and forefinger (see Chapter 50). The extremities are assessed for edema. Intravenous fluid administration is monitored to prevent circulatory overload. Breathing is assessed to detect the serious complication of pulmonary edema. Drainage is assessed. The patient is weighed daily to detect rapid unexplained weight loss or gain.

Administering Medications

Medications are administered as ordered with observation of results and side effects. Diuretic drugs and electrolytes may be given. Urinary output should increase shortly after diuretics are begun.

Assisting With Mouth and Skin Care

The patient with fluid volume deficit should be given good mouth and skin care. These actions should be taken at least every 2 hours. Skin and mucous membranes are prone to breakdown, cracking, and infections.

Evaluation

Periodically, the nurse, patient, family, and other members of the healthcare team evaluate the outcomes of care. Have short-term goals been met? Are long-term goals still realistic? Planning for further nursing care takes into consideration the patient's prognosis and any complications and the patient's response to care given.

Maintenance of Water Balance

The correct amount of water (hydration) must be maintained in all areas of the body: within tissues, around tissues, and in circulation fluids (blood, plasma, lymph). If this balance is upset, several problems can occur, including fluid volume excess and fluid volume deficit.

The Person With Fluid Volume Excess

Fluid volume excess is excessive retention of water and sodium in the extracellular fluid. Overhydration refers specifically to excess water in the extracellular spaces. The following are possible causes of fluid volume excess:

♦ Increased fluid intake (as in too rapid administration of IV fluids containing sodium)
♦ Decreased urine output (as in kidney or liver disorders)
♦ Physical disorders (such as congestive heart failure or cardiac insufficiency that results in a decreased ability of the heart to pump effectively)
♦ Excess ingestion of sodium (for example, from sodium-containing medications)

Nursing care in fluid volume excess includes the daily assessments discussed previously, administration and observation of diuretics, and often a sodium-restricted diet.

The Person Who Has Edema

Edema is a symptom of many disorders, including the following:

♦ Congestive heart failure, thrombophlebitis, and cirrhosis of the liver, all of which increase venous pressure and cause faulty reabsorption of water and electrolytes
♦ Low protein levels, which cause fluid to be drawn out of the blood vessels and into the tissue spaces
♦ Poor lymphatic drainage, which reduces osmotic pressure
♦ Sodium retention due to a kidney disorder that causes extra sodium to be reabsorbed rather than excreted. The increased sodium causes water to be drawn out of the circulation and into the tissues.
♦ Inflammation, which dilates the arteries and increases the permeability of the capillary walls

Dependent edema occurs in an area that hangs down (in a dependent position). It is common in the feet and ankles. *Pitting edema* occurs when a dent remains for some time after edematous tissue over a bone is pressed with a finger (see Figure 50-1). *Pulmonary edema* is an accumulation of fluid in the lungs. It is a symptom of various heart and blood vessel disorders, nephrosis, cirrhosis of the liver, and IV therapy that is administered too fast.

The Person Who Has Fluid Volume Deficit

Fluid volume deficit is a deficiency of water and electrolytes in the extracellular space. Dehydration refers to a decreased volume of water, but this does not occur without electrolyte changes. The following are possible causes of fluid volume deficit:

♦ Inadequate fluid intake and starvation
♦ Loss of body fluids, for example from excessive sweating, diarrhea, vomiting, excessive urine output, excessive drainage, gastrointestinal suction
♦ Prolonged fever
♦ Inability of the body to conserve and reuse water by concentrating the urine

Fluid replacement therapy or hyperalimentation may be needed in this patient. The nurse monitors these procedures. Chapter 57 has a complete discussion of IV fluid therapy. Oral intake of fluids is encouraged unless the patient is nauseated; this is the easiest and safest way to restore proper hydration.

Key Concept

Fluid volume deficit can occur in may disorders. Assessment of the level of hydration and observations for fluid volume deficit should be a part of all nursing care.

Table 69-1. Electrolyte Functions and Imbalances

Electrolyte	Functions	Disorders	Comments
Potassium (K)	Major electrolyte in intracellular fluid Controls cellular osmotic pressure Activates enzymes Regulates acid–base balance Maintains nerve and muscle function Influences kidney function Influences sugar uptake	*Excess:* hyperkalemia *Deficiency:* hypokalemia (weakness, tachycardia, nausea) may cause medications not to be absorbed. May aggravate mental disorders. May be life-threatening.	Potassium cannot be stored; it must be taken daily. (Renal patients must be careful with salt substitutes; they are high in potassium.) Potassium may be required when certain diuretics, such as Lasix, are given. (Some diuretics are "potassium-sparing.")
Sodium (Na)	Major electrolyte in extracellular fluid Influences distribution of water Maintains acid–base balance Maintains nerve function	*Excess:* hypernatremia *Deficiency:* hyponatremia	May cause water retention and hypertension
Calcium (Ca)	Major component of bones and teeth Affects permeability of cell membranes Role in blood coagulation and maintenance of heartbeat Affects nerve function	*Excess:* hypercalcemia (lethargy, muscle weakness) *Deficiency:* hypocalcemia (neuromuscular irritability)	Hypocalcemia is rare. Special care is needed when patient with hypocalcemia is taking digitalis.
Magnesium (Mg)	Thought to be needed in activation of enzymes Aids some neuromuscular functions	*Excess:* hypermagnesemia *Deficiency:* hypomagnesemia (tetany, low blood pressure, seizures, psychotic symptoms)	Hypermagnesemia is rare. Specific antidote for magnesium intoxication (from overtreating fluid volume deficit)— calcium gluconate Hypomagnesemia often coexists with low calcium and low potassium.
Chloride (C)	Key role in acid–base balance Maintains water balance	*Excess:* hyperchloremia (metabolic acidosis) *Deficiency:* hypochloremia (metabolic alkalosis)	Hypochloremia usually associated with deficit of sodium and potassium
Phosphorus (P) and phosphate (PO$_4$)	Component of bone Involved in most metabolic processes	*Excess:* hyperphosphatemia *Deficiency:* hypophosphatemia	No observed response to hyperphosphatemia

Maintenance of Electrolyte Balance

There is a delicate balance between the fluids and electrolytes of the body. For the body to function properly in all aspects, the electrolytes within the body also must be properly balanced. In electrolyte imbalances (either too much or too little of an electrolyte; Table 69-1), serious consequences occur in body functioning.

Maintenance of Acid–Base Balance

Acid–base balance must be maintained for body functions to be carried out adequately. The body's cellular activity requires an alkaline medium. Extracellular body fluids are normally maintained at a pH of approximately 7.4; intracellular fluids have a slightly lower pH. Alterations of even a few tenths can be incompatible with

Causes and Symptoms of Acidosis and Alkalosis

Metabolic acidosis	Causes could be diabetes mellitus, diarrhea, nausea and vomiting, kidney failure, aspirin overdose, anorexia, bulimia, excessive dieting, shock, Addison's disease, renal disease, ileostomy, or duodenal fistula.	Metabolic alkalosis	Causes could be nasogastric tube, too much bicarbonate, vomiting, therapy with strong diuretics, steroid therapy, gastrointestinal fistula, starvation, bulimia.
Respiratory acidosis	Causes could be sedative overdose, pneumonia, emphysema, or asthma.	Respiratory alkalosis	Causes could be hysteria and hyperventilation, high fever, aspirin poisoning.
Symptoms	Hypoventilation: shallow respiration; disorientation; headache; warm, dry skin; drowsiness; nausea and vomiting; diarrhea; fruity-smelling breath; acidic blood; acidic urine; CNS depression; stupor; seizures; lethargy and coma.	Symptoms	Hyperventilation; deep and rapid breathing; CNS symptoms; muscle twitching, tetany, and tremors; dizziness; nausea and vomiting; diarrhea; alkaline urine and blood pH; irritability; restlessness; seizures; ECG changes; coma.

cellular activity. Imbalances in pH can result in acidosis or alkalosis.

Metabolic Acidosis

A deficit in bicarbonate ions or an excess in hydrogen ions causes a condition called **metabolic acidosis**. This means that the blood is more acidic than it should be. Causes and symptoms are listed in the accompanying box.

A condition called *respiratory acidosis* is characterized by an increase in carbon dioxide in the blood. It may occur in pneumonia, emphysema, asthma, and after administration of large doses of certain drugs (barbiturates, narcotic analgesics). Symptoms and treatment are similar to those of metabolic acidosis (see box).

The nurse administers IV infusions as ordered. Treatment of choice is bicarbonate or lactated Ringer's solution. Monitor laboratory values. Careful assessment is vital; the acidosis may become worse, or the patient may become *alkalotic* as an overreaction to the treatment. Assess the level of consciousness. The patient can lose consciousness if acidosis worsens. Assess the character of respiration. If the respiratory rate or character changes, the person can be compensating for the condition, or the situation may be worsening. The physician must be notified of respiratory changes so he or she can evaluate the patient's condition. This situation should be evaluated by the physician. Assist respirations, elevate the head of the bed, and administer oxygen; a mechanical ventilator may be needed. Assess urine pH.

Metabolic Alkalosis

Metabolic alkalosis is caused by an excess of bicarbonate (the blood is more basic than normal). See the box for causes and symptoms.

A condition called *respiratory alkalosis* is a deficit of carbonic acid and an oversupply of oxygen. This situation is usually caused by hyperventilation. Symptoms are similar to those of metabolic alkalosis. Treatment is directed at reducing the cause of the hyperventilation. A simple treatment is to have patients breathe into a bag so that they will rebreathe their own CO_2 and thus replace the CO_2 needed in the body.

The nurse administers IV solutions as ordered. Treatment of choice is sodium chloride or potassium chloride. Monitor laboratory values. Careful assessment is vital. Make sure the alkalosis does not worsen or reverse and become acidosis. Tingling in the fingers and toes and muscle twitching are ominous signs.

Special Considerations in Aging
Fluid and Electrolyte Balance

- ◆ The elderly client has decreased renal and respiratory function.
- ◆ Many medications affect renal and cardiac function and fluid balance.
- ◆ Routine procedures, such as a laxative prior to colon x-rays, may induce serious volume deficit.
- ◆ Alteration in fluid and electrolyte balance has the potential to produce profound changes in the elderly, with a rapid onset of signs and symptoms.
- ◆ Signs and symptoms of fluid and electrolyte disturbances may be subtle or atypical, such as confusion.
- ◆ Skin turgor is less valid, due to decreased elasticity of skin.
- ◆ Elderly people may deliberately restrict fluid intake to avoid embarrassing incontinence.
- ◆ The nurse may need to intervene to deal with incontinence.

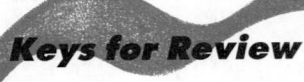

Keys for Review

Key Questions For Critical Thinking

1. Define homeostasis. Describe how fluid and electrolyte balance or imbalance affect it.
2. Describe the necessity of assessing hydration in *all* patients.
3. Explain the role of potassium in fluid balance.
4. List special considerations of the elderly client with regard to skin turgor. Discuss why the elderly patient may deliberately restrict fluids.

Key Readings

Berkow R (Ed). The Merck Manual of Diagnosis and Therapy, Ed 16. Rahway, NJ, Merck & Co, 1992

Kozier B, Erb G, et al. Techniques in Clinical Nursing, Ed 4. Redwood City, CA, Addison-Wesley, 1993

Metheny N. Fluid and Electrolyte Balance: Nursing Considerations, Ed 2. Philadelphia, J.B. Lippincott, 1992

NANDA Nursing Diagnoses: Definitions and Classifications 1992. Philadelphia, North American Nursing Diagnosis Association, 1992

Nursing '94 Drug Handbook. Springhouse, PA, Springhouse, 1994

O'Toole M (Ed). Miller-Keane Encyclopedia and Dictionary of Medicine, Nursing, and Allied Health, Ed 5. Philadelphia, W.B. Saunders, 1992

Smeltzer SC, Bare BG. Brunner and Suddarth's Textbook of Medical-Surgical Nursing, Ed 7. Philadelphia, J.B. Lippincott, 1992

Key Readings (continued)

Taylor C, Lillis C, LeMone P. Fundamentals of Nursing: The Art and Science of Nursing Care, Ed 2. Philadelphia, J.B. Lippincott, 1993

Enrichment Keys

Chambers JK. "Common Fluid and electrolyte disorders." Symposium in Nursing Clinics of North America 22(4), pp. 749–872, December, 1987

Jackson DB, Saunders RB. Child Health Nursing: A Comprehensive Approach to the Care of Children and their Families. Philadelphia, J.B. Lippincott, 1993

Keys to Learning More

Chapter 72: endocrine disorders
Chapter 74: cardiovascular disorders
Chapter 75: blood and lymph disorders
Chapter 76: cancer
Chapter 79: respiratory disorders
Chapter 81: digestive disorders
Chapter 82: urinary disorders
Chapter 91: hospice nursing

70 Musculoskeletal Disorders

Keys for Learning

Learning Objectives

- Describe how musculoskeletal disorders are diagnosed.
- Describe preventive nursing care of the orthopedic patient, including positioning, mobility, skin care, neurovascular assessment, and prevention of deformities.
- Describe types and purposes of casts and their application. Describe nursing care of the patient with a cast, splint, or traction.
- Differentiate between skeletal traction and skin traction and describe devices used.
- Define compartment syndrome, fat embolism, and other orthopedic complications with symptoms, treatment, and nursing care.
- Describe common bone and joint diseases and trauma.
- Describe symptoms, treatment, and nursing care for a fractured hip.
- Describe intervertebral disk disease, its symptoms, and forms of treatment.
- Describe types of amputation and related nursing care.
- Differentiate between rheumatoid and osteoarthritis; describe symptoms, treatment, and nursing care.

Key Terms

ankylosis	osteomyelitis
arthritis	osteoporosis
arthroplasty	rickets
arthroscopy	scleroderma
bursitis	sequestration
compartment syndrome	sprain
dislocation	strain
fracture	synovectomy
myelogram	tenosynovitis
orthopedics	traction

Keys to Understanding This Chapter

Chapter 17: musculoskeletal system

Chapter 31: first aid

Chapter 43: body mechanics and positioning, canes, walkers, wheelchairs, crutches

Chapter 45: personal hygiene and skin care

Chapter 50: physical examination and nursing assessment

Chapter 52: patient comfort and pain management

Unit Ten: surgical intervention

Unit Eleven: pharmacology and medication administration

Chapter 67: degenerative disorders, child with special needs

Unit Thirteen: children and young people with dysfunctions, including musculoskeletal disorders

Key Points

- Careful nursing assessments and knowledge of potential neurovascular complications are essential in orthopedic nursing.
- The orthopedic nurse needs to be aware of and try to prevent complications caused by decreased mobility of orthopedic patients.
- There are many different methods of treating orthopedic injuries including: casts, splints, internal fixation, external fixation, traction, and surgeries such as arthroscopy, total joint replacement, or lumbar decompression.
- Early treatment of orthopedic complications is necessary to prevent further injury to the area involved.
- The several types of musculoskeletal injuries, such as sprains, strains, dislocations, and fractures, require different forms of treatment.
- Treatment of musculoskeletal disorders and diseases can include drug therapy, exercise, surgery, physical therapy, diet, or resting the affected part.

Key Learning Activities

◆ Interview a person who has had a cast. What is the person's reaction? What helped to achieve maximum comfort?
◆ Interview a person who has been in traction. What are the reactions? What helped to achieve maximum comfort?

The specialty of medicine that treats diseases and injuries of bones, joints, and muscles is called **orthopedics** (ortho). The surgeon who specializes in this area of medicine is an *orthopedist*. Orthopedic nursing involves preventing further complications for the patient. Complications are discussed later in the chapter.

Anatomy and Physiology Review

The musculoskeletal system is composed of the bones of the skeleton and the muscles. The skeleton is divided into the *axial* skeleton (skull, vertebral column, rib cage) and the *appendicular* skeleton (extremities, pelvic girdle). There are three major types of muscle tissue: *cardiac* (heart), *smooth* (involuntary), and *skeletal* (voluntary, striated).

In Chapter 17, you learned that the skeletal system supports the soft tissues of the body, and the bones and joints act as levers, facilitating movement when muscles contract. The skeletal system also protects underlying organs and is responsible for producing many blood cells. Bones have the chemical ability to store minerals, especially calcium and phosphorus, for later use.

Diagnostic Tests

The nurse is usually responsible for preparing the patient for physical examinations and radiographic tests and procedures. This involves discussing the preparation, the actual procedure, and postprocedure activities with the patient; carrying out physical preparation; and documenting all aspects of care. Some of these procedures are discussed further in Chapter 71.

Laboratory Tests

Several laboratory tests are available to assess bone and muscle conditions. For example, the erythrocyte sedimentation rate (ESR), red blood cell (RBC) count, complete blood cell (CBC) count, rheumatoid factor level, and the blood levels of calcium and phosphorus indicate musculoskeletal condition.

X-ray Evaluations

Before any x-ray procedure is done, it must be determined if the patient is pregnant. If so, precautions are taken. Before a radiopaque dye is given, the presence of allergies must be assessed and ruled out. (See Chapter 50 for precautions when dyes are used.)

Radiography is by far the most common method used to assess the general state of bones. An x-ray is a means of visualizing bones and other internal structures to determine if there is any deviation from normal.

Arthrogram. An arthrogram is an x-ray of a joint (such as a knee or shoulder). After a radiopaque or radiolucent substance has been injected, a sequence of x-rays is taken.

Myelogram. The **myelogram** is an x-ray examination of the spinal cord and vertebral canal after a contrast medium has been introduced into the spinal subarachnoid space. This is a particularly valuable diagnostic procedure when the spinal cord is believed to be compressed, as in herniated intervertebral disk or a tumor encroaching on the spinal subarachnoid space.

Computed Tomography. Computed tomography (CT) scanning provides a three-dimensional radiographic view of the body part being scanned. The scan is noninvasive and painless. The amount of radiation received by the patient is equivalent to a conventional chest x-ray. The scanner takes a series of cross-sectional pictures of the body part in minute "slices" across the coronal plane. The image is recorded on a detector. A computer calculates the amount of radiation absorbed by various body tissues and produces a printout. The computer is able to detect differences in radiation absorption and differences in density of tissues that are too subtle to be seen on a conventional x-ray.

Other Diagnostic Tests

Magnetic Resonance Imaging. In magnetic resonance imaging (MRI), a powerful magnetic field enables the MRI scanning machine to produce detailed images of internal organs without use of potentially dangerous ionizing radiation or x-rays. Signals are produced by use of a magnetic field and radiofrequencies. Measurable signals are produced and these are translated into visual images by a computer. Three-dimensional imaging of any portion of the body is possible using MRI. MRI is much safer and less expensive than invasive procedures such as biopsy, surgery, or use of radioactive isotopes or dyes. Therefore, it is becoming the examination of choice in many cases. The precautions and nursing care of the patient who is to have an MRI are presented in Chapter 71.

Gallium (Ga^{67}) Scan: Bone Scan (Scintiscan, Scintillation Scan). This test is used to detect tumors and other pathology. A radioisotope is injected intravenously; the patient must lie quietly while the scanning is done. This scan cannot differentiate between malignant disease, inflammation, or other pathology.

Electromyogram. The electromyogram is a test of electrical conductivity, similar to the electrocardiogram or the electroencephalogram. It measures the electrical impulses within the muscles (myo = muscle). The physician can determine whether or not the muscles are responding normally to a stimulus.

Medical and Surgical Treatments

Common Medical Treatments

Fractures of bones are common. A splint is often used to immobilize a fracture temporarily, but the most com-

Key Abbreviations and Acronyms for Musculoskeletal Function

AEA	Above elbow amputation
AKA	Above knee amputation
AROM	Active range of motion
BEA	Below elbow amputation
BKA	Below knee amputation
CMS	Color, motion, sensitivity (circulation, mobility, sensation)
CPM	Continuous passive motion
CT	Computed tomography
DJD	Degenerative joint disease
DVT	Deep vein thrombosis
IVD	Intervertebral disk
MRI	Magnetic resonance imaging
ORIF	Open reduction, internal fixation
PROM	Passive range of motion
RA	Rheumatoid arthritis
ROM	Range of motion
PERRLA	Pupils equal, round, and reactive to light and accomodation
SLE	Systemic lupus erythematosus
THA	Total hip arthroplasty
TKA	Total knee arthroplasty
TLSO	Thoracolumbar sacroorthosis
TMJ	Temporomandibular joint

mon method of immobilizing a fracture after initial first aid treatment is a cast. The cast remains in place until the bone ends have joined together.

Many hospitals have a special cast and splint room. In larger hospitals, specialized technicians work in this area. If you are asked to assist, the physician will specify the cast or splint material desired and will direct its application.

Often, the patient is given an analgesic, narcotic, or anesthetic before cast application. Medication is less frequently given for application of a splint. If a general anesthetic is used, the immobilizing device is applied in the operating room or day surgery center and routine preoperative and postoperative care is given. (Nursing assessments when a patient has any immobilizing device are listed in Chapter 50.)

Splints

A temporary splint is used immediately after an injury to immobilize a part before treatment is begun or until swelling subsides. Splints are used for therapeutic purposes also; these are discussed in Chapter 89. Emergency first aid splinting is discussed in Chapter 31.

A common splint is the half-cast, in which a full cast

is applied, then sawed in half (bivalved). The bottom half of the cast may be used alone, or both halves may remain in place. Half-casts are held in place with an elastic roller bandage, which may also be used alone after healing begins, to give support. The half-cast may be taken off at intervals and reapplied or it may remain in place for the full period of immobilization.

Another type of splint is the *inflatable splint.* Although most often used in emergency first aid, it may also be used in the hospital. It consists of a plastic bag inside a second plastic bag, with a zipper on one side. Sizes are available to fit parts of the body such as the leg, ankle, and arm. If it is to remain in place for some time, a light stockinette is loosely applied to the extremity, after which the splint is applied, zipped up, and inflated just enough to immobilize the part. It is comfortable for patients because it is light, and convenient for physicians and technicians because it is transparent and does not need to be removed when x-rays are taken. Care must be taken not to puncture the bag.

Other splints include the Thomas or ring splint (which may be used in combination with traction), molded aluminum splints, and other metal splints. Nursing care of a patient in a splint is similar to that of a patient in a cast.

Casts

The cast is applied and remains on the person until bones have joined together, called fusion. You may be asked to assist with cast application. Specific in-service training is usually required regarding local protocol. General principles in preparation for casting are:

- ♦ Gather all materials beforehand, including stockinette and padding materials. You will also need a source of water.
- ♦ Follow manufacturer's instructions regarding preparation of cast or splint material.
- ♦ Wear gloves if blood is involved in the fracture or to protect your hands from the casting materials.
- ♦ Prepare the injured area. In many cases the area is washed (without soap), carefully dried, and shaved. An astringent or alcohol is often applied.
- ♦ Lubricate the area, as ordered.
- ♦ Have sterile dressings available for an open compound fracture.
- ♦ Position the patient as directed.
- ♦ Assist or restrain the patient as needed.
- ♦ Reassure the patient during the procedure.

The patient will often have a follow-up x-ray taken after the cast is applied. When the patient is returned to the unit, be sure the patient is comfortable and has a call light within reach. Clean up immediately after the procedure, before the cast or splint material hardens. A special sink with a plaster trap is usually available. *Do not* put plaster or cast material in a regular sink.

Nursing care of the patient in a cast is discussed under Nursing Process in the next section.

The Plaster Cast. A cast must be cared for properly so it immobilizes the injured part without causing further damage or injury. A plaster cast remains wet for 24 to 48 hours. Because it must dry in the same shape as when it was applied, it should be supported with pillows to preserve its original contour. It is kept uncovered, and the patient is turned so that all sides of the cast will dry. (Turning also helps prevent other complications.)

The wet cast is handled with the *palms* only, not with the fingertips. *(Rationale: Finger pressure can dent the cast and create a pressure point.)* It is best to move the extremity by grasping on either side of the casted area. Do not grasp the cast unless absolutely necessary.

In some instances a cast dryer may be used. However, care must be taken not to apply intense heat because this could burn the patient, crack the cast, or dry the outside of the cast while the inside stays wet and becomes moldy.

The patient may complain of being cold while the cast is drying. Cover the rest of the patient's body with a blanket and prevent drafts. If the weather is hot, the patient may complain of being too warm. Cool liquids, a cool cloth applied to the forehead, and a somewhat lower room temperature may help. Ice packs may be used around the cast to offset heat given off by drying plaster.

If the edges of the cast are rough, they can be covered with tape, a procedure called *petaling* (Fig. 70-1). If a stockinette is in place inside the cast, you can cover the rough edges by pulling the edge of the stockinette out, folding it over the edge of the cast, and taping it in place. This helps prevent irritation caused by plaster crumbs and rough cast edges.

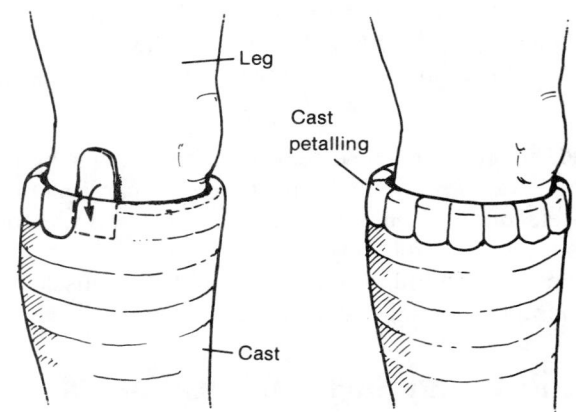

Figure 70-1. Cast petaling protects the patient's leg from rough cast edges. (Skale N. Manual of Pediatric Nursing Procedures. Philadelphia, J.B. Lippincott, 1992)

A cast near the genital area must be protected from moisture. Even after a plaster cast is dried, it must not become wet or the plaster will dissolve.

Key Concept

If a cast or splint becomes dented, softened, or broken, it will not serve its purpose: immobilization of a body part.

Synthetic Casting Materials. Light synthetic casting materials are colorful and are often more convenient than plaster casts. They are sometimes more durable; they take less time to dry. The most commonly used material is fiberglass. The synthetic cast is lighter and stronger than plaster and can be exposed to some water. X-rays can be taken through this material.

Cast Removal. The cast is removed with a cast saw. The saw oscillates back and forth although it appears to be rotating. The blade moves only a fraction of an inch and will not cut the patient. Because this can be a frightening experience, it will help if the nurse explains the procedure beforehand. Patients who realize there is no danger from removal of the cast will be able to tolerate the noise and dust. The nurse wears gloves and, sometimes, protective eyewear for this procedure.

After a cast is removed, the patient may be instructed to wear a brace for an additional week or two. This helps give additional stability to the injured area.

Traction

Another means of immobilization is traction. Traction may be used with other means of immobilization, such as internal fixation.

Traction exerts a pulling force to keep bone fragments in good position so they will heal properly. The strength of pull on the bones by means of weights must be enough to counteract the overall pull of the muscles. The physician will determine how much weight should be applied. The direction of pull holds the bones in alignment and is controlled by the type of traction.

The amount of traction is controlled by application of principles of physics. The direction and degree of pull are controlled by weights, location and number of pulleys, and counterbalance measures. An overhead frame attached to the bed holds the traction pulleys and equipment. A trapeze should also be attached so the patient can pull his or her head and shoulders off the bed.

The two types of traction, skin and skeletal, are outlined in the accompanying box and discussed briefly here. Nursing care for the patient in traction is discussed in the Nursing Process section.

Skin Traction

In skin traction, the pull is applied to the skin. An example of skin traction is illustrated in Figure 70-2. A belt, head halter, foam rubber wrapped with an elastic bandage, or a foam boot is applied to the skin before being attached to traction. Traction on the skin transmits the pull to musculoskeletal structures.

Skeletal Traction

In skeletal traction, the traction is applied directly to the bones. The pin sites in skeletal traction are cared for like any other incision, to prevent infection. If signs of infection develop, they must be reported immediately. Infection in the incision site can spread to the bone, causing the serious complication of *osteomyelitis*.

Skull Tongs. When skull tongs are used, an incision is made in the scalp and holes are drilled on either side of the skull bone. The tongs are inserted into these holes as shown in Figure 70-3. The patient is then kept in bed and must remain immobile until the injury heals, surgery is performed, or a halo vest is applied. The following points outline the steps used to apply skull tongs and special precautions needed:

◆ Patient teaching and support are essential. *(Rationale: If the patient has sustained a sudden injury, he or she will be frightened and may be newly paralyzed. Thus, it is important to remain with the patient during the entire procedure.)*
◆ The physician will either shave the area around tong insertion sites or instruct the nurse on the specific area to be shaved. Wear gloves. Under local anesthesia, shallow holes are drilled into the sides of the skull. There may be some pain during the drilling although most patients feel pressure rather than severe pain. The noise of the drilling will be uncomfortable because sound is conducted by bone.
◆ Once the tongs have been inserted, nursing care includes giving attention to the insertion sites. Any signs of infection must be reported at once. This is vital with skull tongs because the tongs are in close proximity to the brain. Headache can be a serious danger sign because it could indicate encephalitis or osteomyelitis.
◆ The patient is usually in an antidecubitus bed (see Chapter 44).
◆ The patient's level of consciousness and PERRLA (eye signs) are routinely checked (see Chapters 50 and 71).

The Halo Apparatus. The halo apparatus is a form of skeletal traction that allows the patient to move about (see Fig. 70-3). The pins holding the halo in place pen-

Types of Traction

Skin Traction

BUCK'S TRACTION (BUCK'S EXTENSION)

The leg is wrapped with an elastic roller bandage or tape and traction is applied through a weight attached to a spreader bar below the foot. A foam boot may also be used. The traction pull is toward the pulley at the bottom of the bed.

CERVICAL HEAD HALTER TRACTION

For neck pain, neck strain, and whiplash, traction can be applied to the cervical spine by means of a head halter. The pull of cervical skin traction should be felt as an upward pull on the back of the neck. A slight change in the level of the head of the bed is often the key to correct application of this type of traction. Because this is a form of skin traction, it cannot be used for prolonged periods. This type of traction is often used by the patient at home.

RUSSELL'S TRACTION (BALANCED TRACTION)

Downward pull, as in Buck's traction, may be applied to the leg, but an additional overhead pulley system is incorporated into the traction apparatus with the leg supported by a sling. The pull is up (toward the ceiling) and toward the foot of the bed.

PELVIC TRACTION

Used in pelvic fractures to support separated bones. This traction may be applied by either a belt or a sling. The pelvic belt causes downward pull on the pelvis, while the pelvic sling supports the pelvis off the bed. With a pelvic belt, the upper rim of the belt should rest at the top of the iliac crest and not around the abdomen. This type of traction is used in treating a herniated intervertebral disk or muscle spasm of the back. It is usually applied intermittently, on 2 hours, off 2 hours, while the patient is awake. Weights on the traction are increased gradually.

The weights on *any* traction device should never be removed or changed without a physician's order.

Skeletal Traction

SKULL TRACTION OR HEAD TRACTION

This form of skeletal traction is accomplished by inserting the points of a skull tong device (such as Vincke or Crutchfield tongs) into the skull bone. It is used to reduce a fracture of the cervical vertebrae. This type of traction is often used only temporarily until a halo device can be placed.

THE HALO DEVICE

This form of skeletal traction allows the patient to move about. The combination of the halo, which is attached to the skull, and the vest, which is worn on the body, provides the traction. It is used in vertebral fractures.

THE STEINMANN PIN OR KIRSCHNER WIRE

Either of these devices is drilled through the shaft of a bone (commonly in a leg fracture) and attached to the traction apparatus.

In any type of skeletal traction, good skin care at the site of insertion is vital, as is maintaining the patient in the correct position.

etrate the skull only a fraction of an inch. The four pins enter the scalp in four different areas. Nursing care during application of the halo and after application is summarized in the Nursing Process section.

Common Surgical Techniques

Attached External Fixation

Casts and splints were the traditional treatments for fractures until the advent of the *external fixator.* This device consists of pins held together outside the body and placed into the bone and held in the proper place by metal components (Fig. 70-4). These components are adjusted to maintain traction on the fracture to hold the fracture in proper alignment. The alignment must be maintained until bone healing occurs. External fixators are often used when there is a wound in the fracture area. *(Rationale: The wound is easier to treat because it is not covered by casting material.)*

Nursing care is consistent with care of the patient with a fracture and also includes care of the pin site. The physician will order the type of pin care required. Generally, pin sites are cleaned three times daily with hydrogen peroxide (or Betadine). If dressings are in place, they are changed, using sterile technique. The nurse wears gloves when caring for any wound. General care of any patient in an immobilization device is covered later in this chapter.

Rejection, an adverse reaction to the nails, screws, or plates used, can occur even though they are made of a special metal alloy that, in most cases, is nonirritating.

Internal Fixation

Another method of immobilizing a fracture is internal fixation, whereby a device is put into or onto the bone to keep it reduced or immobilized, or both. Internal fixation is done as a surgical procedure, by open reduction, so the surgeons can see the bones and determine exactly how to put them back together. This procedure is called open reduction, internal fixation (ORIF). It is the treatment of choice in certain fractures such as those of the hip, where casting is generally impossible. Internal fixation also eliminates the need for traction and usually for a cast. The patient is able to be up and about sooner as well.

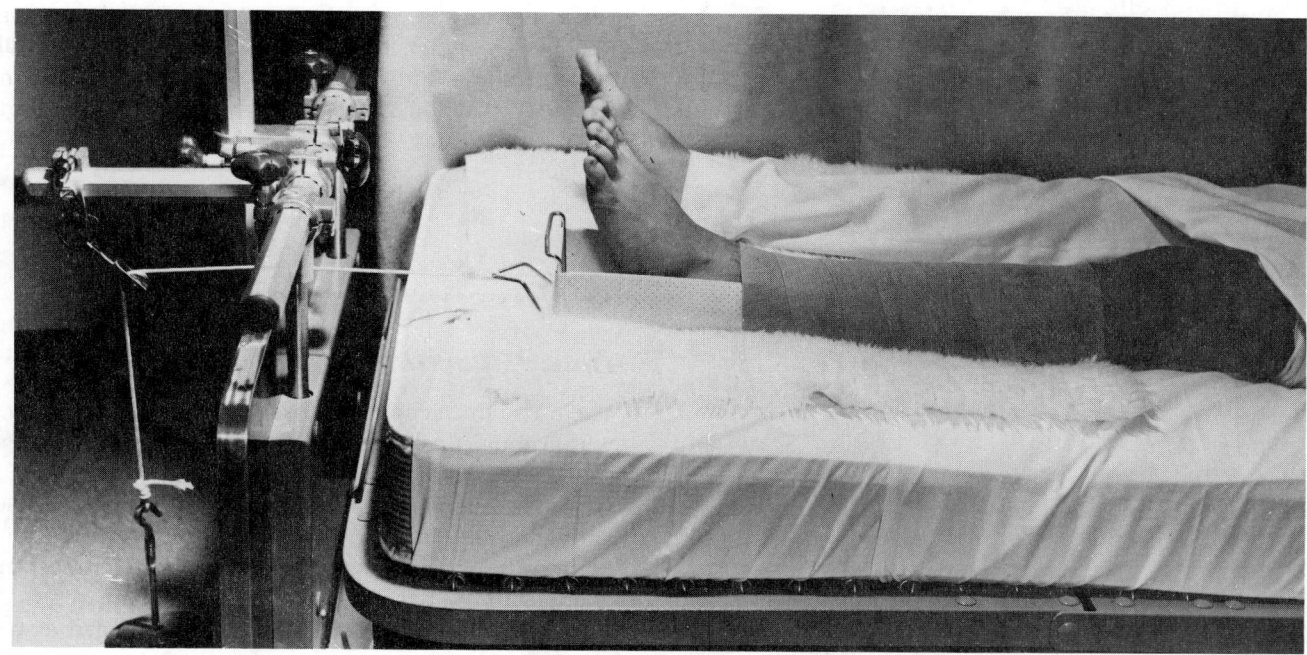

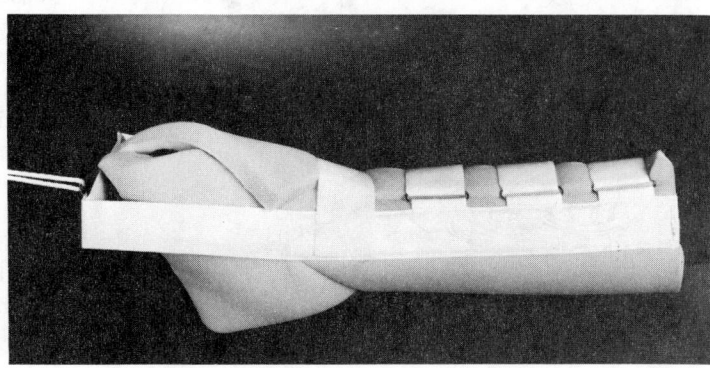

Figure 70-2. In Buck's extension, traction is placed on the lower extremity. The pull is toward the pulley at the bottom of the bed. A prepadded boot may be used in Buck's extension. (Photo of boot courtesy of All Orthopedic Appliances.)

Internal fixation is accomplished with a variety of devices. A nail or long spike may be driven the length of the bone. This method is used more frequently in the long bones of the leg, in which case the spike is called an *intermedullary nail.* Usually internal fixation is done if there is more than one transverse fracture or if the patient's history indicates that fractures do not align or heal easily with casting.

A metal plate may be applied with screws to the outside of a bone; it is often intended to remain in place permanently. This is often done if the bone is fractured in several places. Screws are sometimes inserted to hold the bone fragments in place without the use of a plate. Wires may be used to wire fragments of bone together.

The patient with internal fixation may have no visible form of immobilization; the nurse must keep in mind that there is a fracture and the patient must be handled carefully. However, internal fixation is sometimes combined with another form of immobilization, such as traction, splinting, or partial casting.

Arthroscopy

Arthroscopy is a surgical procedure that is usually performed on an outpatient basis. Arthroscopy allows the surgeon to view and operate on the interior of a joint using only a very tiny incision (a "stab wound"). This is performed through a scope, which is called an *arthroscope.* The procedure is known as a "closed" procedure because the joint does not need to be laid open.

Examples of procedures that are performed by arthroscopy include removal of foreign or loose objects, such as a piece of cartilage or a bone spur. It is also possible to perform a shaving procedure to make a rough and worn joint smooth and more comfortable. A torn meniscus or torn ligament can be diagnosed and sometimes can be repaired through arthroscopy. In some cases, a miniature television camera is passed through the scope and is used to improve the surgeon's view of the joint.

Arthroscopic surgery is much safer and more comfortable for the patient than is open surgery. Therefore, it is used whenever possible.

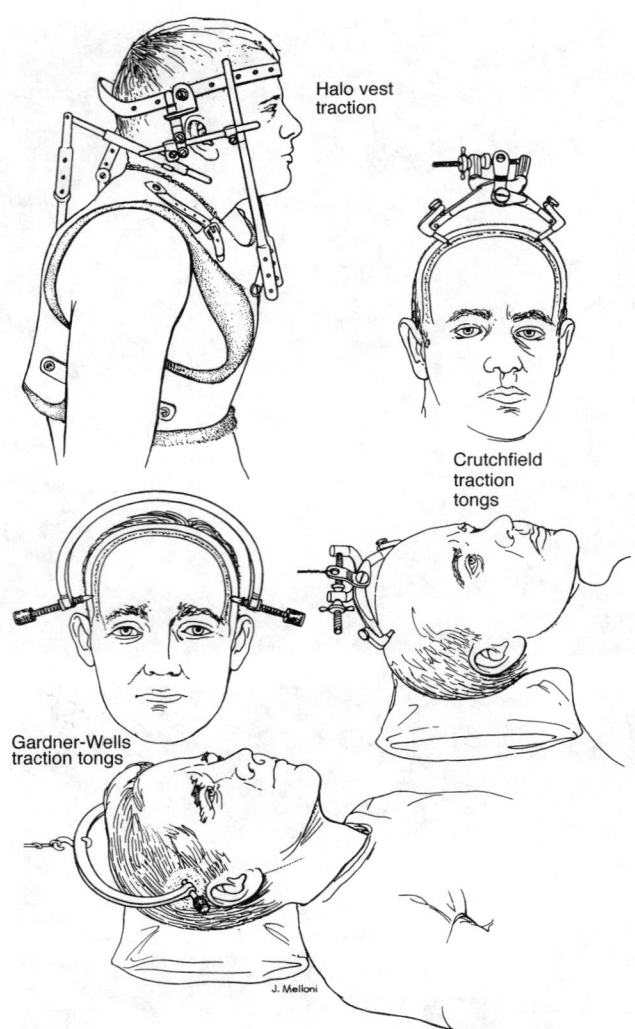

Halo vest
traction

Crutchfield
traction
tongs

Gardner-Wells
traction tongs

J. Melloni

Figure 70-3. Methods of cervical traction. (From Suddarth DS. The Lippincott Manual of Nursing Practice, Ed 5. Philadelphia, J.B. Lippincott, 1991.)

Total Joint Replacement or Arthroplasty

Repair or replacement of a joint is called **arthroplasty**. Several joints can be replaced totally. In some cases of fractured hip, the femoral head is replaced. In other cases, the hip socket is also replaced with a studded cup, which may be cemented into a deepened hip socket. This is known as a *total hip replacement* or total hip arthroplasty (THA). Other joints that can be totally or partially replaced are the ankle, the knee, the shoulder, the elbow, and the wrist. Total joint replacements are used in some severe injuries and in severe degenerative arthritic disorders, when joints become injured, fused, or too malformed to be functional. Postoperative care is similar to that described for open reduction of the hip or other joint.

Shoulder joint replacement has not been as successful as hip joint replacement because the shoulder joint is not as well supported and not as stable, due to minimal bony contact. The shoulder joint is also more subject to trauma and disease. In a patient with minimal shoulder damage, a *hemiarthroplasty* may be done; in this procedure, only the head of the humerus is replaced.

❖ *Nursing Process*

Data Collection

The nurse must carefully observe and assess the patient with a musculoskeletal disorder. Chapter 50 describes physical examination and nursing assessment. This assessment establishes a baseline for future comparison and determines the presence of suspected muscle, joint, or bone complications. The nurse should report any changes in the baseline level.

When doing a musculoskeletal assessment, the nurse assesses the range of motion in all joints. The patient may be referred to a specialist if limited mobility is suspected. Gait and balance are observed, as well as the ability to safely use mobility aids such as the wheelchair, walker, cane, or crutches. The use of these devices is described in Chapter 43.

The nurse also observes the patient's emotional response to the disorder or disease. Does the patient need assistance to meet daily needs? Does the disorder affect social activities or self-esteem? Is the patient anxious or fearful of the outcome?

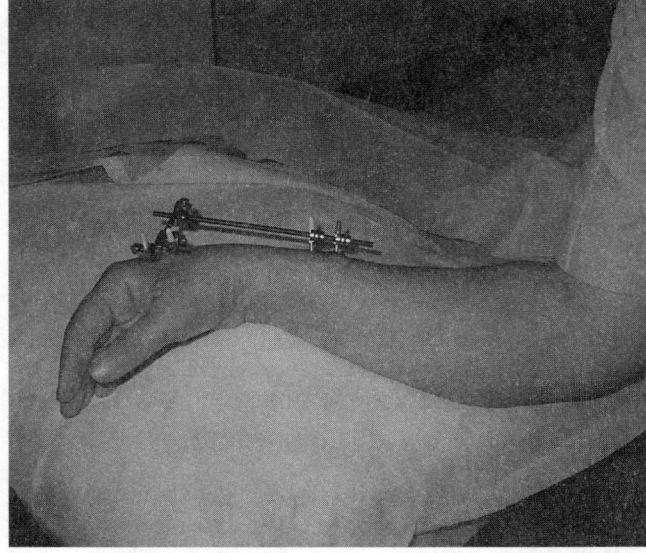

Figure 70-4. An external fixator in place to immobilize several fractures in the lower arm and wrist. (Photo courtesy of R. Heeter, MD, and Ronald L. Christensen.)

ASSESSMENT WITH IMMOBILIZATION DEVICE IN PLACE. Many orthopedic patients have some sort of immobilization device in place. It is particularly important for the nurse to assess these patients, so that any complications can be prevented or treated immediately. Assessment factors are categorized in the accompanying box. Complications are discussed later in the chapter after the Nursing Process.

The nurse's major concern while observing the patient in an immobilization device is to watch for signs of pressure (Fig. 70-5). Undue pressure of any kind can cause serious *neurovascular compromise.* This term means damage to nerves or blood vessels. Pressure, and its accompanying lack of blood or nerve supply, can cause tissue necrosis (death) and other complications discussed in this chapter.

The extremity is evaluated for *color, motion,* and *sensitivity* (CMS). These factors are sometimes referred to as *circulation, movement, and sensation.* Color relates to the part of the limb distal to the injury; motion is the ability to move fingers or toes; sensitivity is feeling in fingers or toes. The pulses in the extremity, distal to the cast, are checked frequently. The patient is asked to wiggle the fingers and toes; and the nurse touches them to make sure the patient can feel the touch and to make sure they are warm.

Sometimes, drainage from an infection can be seen through the window in the cast or may soak through the cast. It is also important to check the lowest part of the cast for drainage because it will flow in the direction of gravity. If a stain appears on a cast, notify the team leader or charge nurse. Then, draw a line around the edges of the stain. Be sure to use a *waterproof* pen. This line is used as a guide for later observation and comparisons.

Nursing Alert

Wear gloves when performing assessments or other care for patients with a compound fracture, wound infection, or possibility of infection or hemorrhage.

Keys to Nursing Assessment
Neurovascular Assessment in Musculoskeletal Conditions*

Complications of Pressure

- Edema. Swelling at the edges of the device and in parts beyond.
- Blanched or cyanotic skin color. Fingers and toes are inspected frequently and separately for signs of circulatory impairment.
- Movement or sensory disorders. The patient should be able to wiggle the fingers or toes and identify specifically which digit is being touched. Symptoms include numbness, tingling, and inability to move. Patient should be able to flex foot (dorsiflexion and plantar flexion).
- Temperature of digits. If there is pressure, fingers and toes will be colder on the affected side.
- Severe pain. If severe pain is unrelieved by medication; swelling is probably present.
- Lack of distal pulse. A lack of distal pulse indicates blood is not flowing properly.

Wound Infection

- Elevated vital signs
- Odor of decaying tissue
- Elevated white blood cell count
- Drainage of blood or serous fluid from the fracture area (may be seen in cast window or may soak through cast)
- Redness and swelling in surrounding tissues
- Pain
- Swelling

Infection of the Bone (Osteomyelitis)

- Fever
- Pain
- Redness and heat
- Elevation in lymphocytes (white blood cells)
- Nausea, with or without vomiting
- Headache
- Swelling and pressure

Pulmonary Embolism

- Petechiae on the chest, particularly just under the collar bone on the affected side (in the intraclavicular fossa), in the axilla, and on the soft palate
- Petechiae may also be seen on the abdomen and on the sides of the body (the flanks)
- Rapid respirations; dyspnea
- Confusion, restlessness, anxiety (due to hypoxia)
- Fever
- Tachycardia
- Death can occur very quickly.

Hemorrhage

- Fast pulse
- Lowered blood pressure
- Rapid respirations
- Symptoms of shock
- Panic

Carefully document observations and patient's statements.

* Especially in traction, splinting, and casts

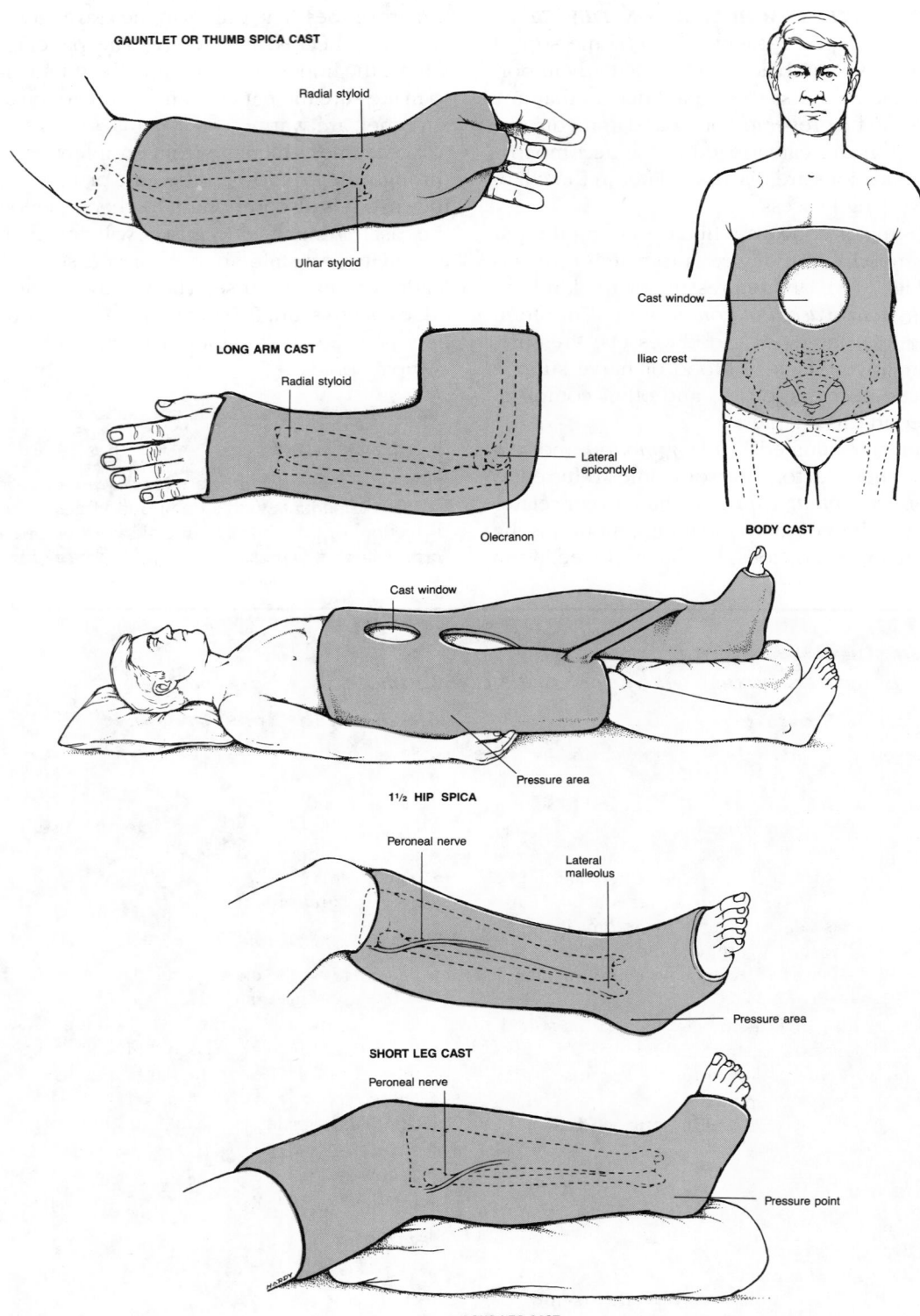

Figure 70-5. Pressure areas in different types of casts.

Nursing Diagnosis

Based on data collection, the following nursing diagnoses may be established for the patient with a musculoskeletal disorder. Some diagnoses may have several causal factors.

- ◆ Altered Nutrition: Less Than Body Requirements related to the need for high levels of protein and calcium
- ◆ High Risk for Infection related to invasive immobilization devices or compound fracture
- ◆ High Risk for Trauma related to immobilization device, poor calcification of bones, previous fracture, improper gait, or inability to use crutches, walker, wheelchair properly
- ◆ High Risk for Disuse Syndrome related to immobility, pain, spica cast
- ◆ Impaired Skin Integrity related to fracture, cast
- ◆ Altered Sexuality Patterns related to immobilization device, spica cast
- ◆ Impaired Physical Mobility related to pain, immobilization device, inability to use adaptive equipment
- ◆ Impaired Home Maintenance Management related to immobility, pain
- ◆ Body Image Disturbance related to amputation, long-term disability resulting from trauma

Planning and Implementation

The patient and nurse plan together for effective care to meet patient needs. The nurse provides preoperative and postoperative care for the patient undergoing orthopedic surgery, including lumbar decompression, joint replacement, insertion of a fixation device, or placement of a prosthesis. The patient with a musculoskeletal disorder may also require assistance in mobility, pain control, cast care, meeting nutritional needs, dealing with emotional problems, and understanding more about the disorder, its prognosis, and its treatment. A nursing care plan is developed to meet these needs.

Caring for Patients in Casts

The patient with a new cast may feel helpless. The nurse reassures the patient that someone is there to care for him or her. At the same time the nurse helps the person learn to provide as much self-care as possible. The accompanying box lists some aspects of nursing care for the person in a synthetic cast or spica cast.

The patient may be discharged shortly after receiving the cast. Patient and family teaching is important so the person can learn to adjust to living with a cast for several weeks. Some of the things to be taught the person in a cast are given in the accompanying patient teaching box.

The extremity and the cast should be supported at all times. A sling will support an arm cast. A person with a leg cast can use a wheelchair with an adjustable leg support.

If the break is such that a walking cast can be applied, the patient may be able to get around with the help of a cane at first. Otherwise, the patient may use crutches or a walker following a leg fracture. The physician decides how much movement and weight bearing are allowed. A *cast boot* is usually worn over the cast (Fig. 70-6).

Special Considerations in the Aging
Casts

Sometimes the older patient does not move sufficiently to counteract the dangers of hypostatic pneumonia. The nurse encourages deep breathing exercises with an incentive spirometer as a good preventive measure. The older person may have difficulty in learning crutch walking or to use other mobility aids safely.

Caring for Patients in Traction

The patient in traction will require careful nursing interventions. Self-care will be at a minimum, and the patient's needs must be met. The accompanying box gives guidelines for providing care.

THE PATIENT IN A HALO VEST. The nurse may be asked to assist the physician in application of the halo appliance. Explain to the patient what will be done and provide the physician with the halo, the vest, a special wrench and positioning plate, a regular wrench, and Xylocaine. Sterile technique is used and gloves are worn.

The patient is often in a special bed before the halo device is applied. Give care to the patient, being extremely careful not to change the alignment of the head or neck. Support the patient's head and neck while the patient is moved and during application of the halo and vest. After the halo and vest are applied, help the patient to sit up slowly. *(Rationale: The patient may become dizzy or faint.)* Support the patient in a sitting position while the physician adjusts the vertical bars of the halo.

Nursing care includes care of the patient following the application of the halo device. Good skin care around the vest and pin sites must be given. The pins are cleansed several times daily with an antiseptic, usually hydrogen peroxide. Even though the insertion sites are small, infection is possible and must be watched for. Gloves are worn when giving care.

The patient may have some mild discomfort, which is usually relieved by Tylenol. If it is not easily relieved, this should be reported at once.

Nursing Skill Guidelines
Caring for Patients in Casts

Synthetic Cast

- Check for rough edges. Petal as necessary, as shown in Figure 70-1. A sock or nylon stocking can be pulled over the cast to prevent it from snagging on clothing.
- Total immersion of these casts is not recommended, but it is not necessary to prevent all contact with water. (*Rationale: Although the cast is not likely to dissolve, the padding will become wet and may become rotten. Also, the underlying skin can itch or necrose.*)
- The fiberglass cast is solid. It does not give at all, as does a plaster cast. The fiberglass cast, as a result, may be too tight for patient comfort.
- Good skin care around the cast is essential.
- The person must be cautioned against being too active. (*Rationale: The cast can break and the extremity injured further.*)

Spica (Body) Cast

- Turn the patient frequently. (*Rationale: It is important to prevent pressure points, venostatis, and circulatory complications.*)
- Reassure the patient as you turn him or her. (*Rationale: Turning may cause apprehension and fear of falling.*)
- Be sure no crumbs or other foreign substances get inside the cast. (*Rationale: This would cause itching and skin breakdown.*)
- Provide air conditioning if possible. In hot weather it is particularly difficult to make the patient comfortable.
- Give special attention to elimination and the area near the buttocks.

- Use a fracture bedpan for elimination. These bedpans need to be removed slowly. (*Rationale: They overflow easily.*)
- Powder or lotion may be applied to the bedpan before placing it under the patient. (*Rationale: This helps to slip the pan into place.*) Protect the bed with a waterproof pad.
- Report symptoms such as abdominal pain and a bloated feeling. The area of the cast over the stomach should be cut out. (*Rationale: This helps to prevent superior mesenteric syndrome, also known as "body cast syndrome."*) If the stomach area is not cut out, the stomach has no place for expansion after eating or if the person has gas. This could lead to partial or complete strangulation of the bowel.
- Encourage the patient to exercise as much as possible. *Isometric exercises* should be done inside the cast. (*Rationale: This encourages circulation and helps prevent complications.*)
- Move the patient out of the room on a litter or a standing wheelchair.
- Encourage diversional activities.
- Use several people or a hydraulic lift or chair to move the patient. (*Rationale: This helps prevent injury to staff and the patient.*)
- Encourage the patient to do self-care as much as possible. (*Rationale: This helps improve self-image and provides meaningful exercise.*)

> **Nursing Alert**
> Severe headache is a specific danger sign with the halo.

The patient may complain of difficulty in swallowing, inability to open the mouth all the way, or persistent neck pain; this should be reported at once because these symptoms are signs that the vertical connecting bar is too long.

The patient may complain that he or she cannot see straight ahead. This is a sign that the apparatus is not on straight. If any complications occur, the apparatus should be readjusted by the physician.

Nursing care should be directed at patient teaching and emotional support. Always encourage patients to be as independent as possible.

The halo device will probably be worn for 10 to 12 weeks, during which time the patient or family will be responsible for care. Patients will require teaching related to care while the appliance is used. Subjects to be taught are listed in the accompanying box. Carefully document all teaching.

Preventing Disorders of Immobility

Prolonged bed rest is dangerous, and many complications may occur. Prevention of complications and patient teaching are aspects of nursing care. The orthopedic nurse works closely with the physical therapist in helping the patient regain mobility.

Providing Comfortable Positioning and Proper Alignment

Some orthopedic patients must remain in bed. Maintaining proper body alignment is essential. (It helps if you think of the patient in bed as standing; position the person with that in mind.) The patient is turned frequently to prevent skin breakdown. A footboard helps prevent footdrop; and pillows, sandbags, splints, and trochanter rolls help prevent contractures and maintain the patient's position. Passive and active range-of-motion exercises promote and maintain joint mobility and muscle strength. Encourage the patient to move independently as much as possible.

Providing Skin Care

The skin must be kept in good condition and protected from irritation. When bathing the patient, use as little soap as possible around the casted area. Use lotion for cleansing and for soothing dry skin. For pressure areas, use lamb's wool padding. In general, sheets should be very smooth and cleared of crumbs after a meal. Special beds, air mattresses, foam pads, and flotation pads may be used, but these should not be substituted for frequent skin care.

If the patient has an incision or pins in place, give special care to these breaks in the skin. Use the protocol prescribed by your hospital. Wear gloves. The neurovascular assessment and skin care can be performed during routine patient repositioning.

Providing Adequate Nutrition

The patient's diet should be high in protein to promote healing. It should contain bulk and liberal amounts of fluids to aid in elimination. Intake and output records are kept, and the patient observed for signs of urinary infection or constipation. The patient may be receiving intravenous fluids. These patients often receive nutritional supplements, such as Resource or Ensure.

Providing Activity and Exercise

The nurse must know just how much activity the patient is allowed. Overexercise can be harmful also. Patients confined to bed should have a trapeze on the bed frame so they can help lift their bodies for nursing care. The patient can also use the trapeze for exercise. Encourage the patient to exercise other parts of the body as much as possible.

Passive and active range of motion are provided, as described in Chapter 43. Remind the patient in a cast or splint to move frequently. Fingers and toes can be wiggled. The patient should also be taught to do *isometric* (muscle-setting) exercises of the immobilized part. Isometrics should be done as frequently as possible. A continuous passive motion (CPM) machine is sometimes used to exercise extremities. The patient is assisted to be out of bed as much as possible. Usually, a casted extremity will be more comfortable if it is elevated as much of the time as possible. The patient may need assistance to use crutches, a walker, or other assistive devices (Chapter 43).

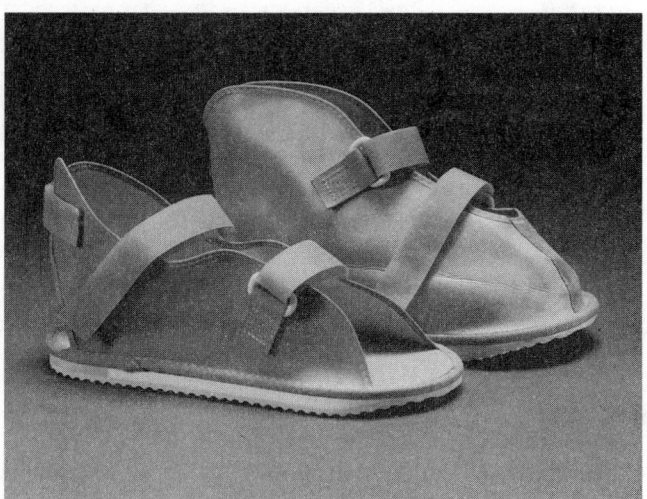

Figure 70-6. Usually, a cast is reinforced on the bottom to make it a "walking cast." Then, a cast walking shoe/cast boot (shown) is worn over the cast. The cast boot comes in several sizes and is adjustable by use of the Velcro closures. It is available in open-toe or closed-toe models. (Product photo courtesy of 3M Health Care.)

Nursing Skill Guidelines
Caring for Patients in Traction

◆ Follow the physician's order for the exact amount of weight to be used.
◆ Be sure weights are hanging free; they must never rest on the bed or the floor. *(Rationale: Releasing the pull defeats the purpose of traction.)*
◆ When adding weights or attaching traction, release the weights gradually onto the rope. *(Rationale: Suddenly adding weights causes an uncomfortable jerk and may disrupt alignment of the fracture.)*
◆ Never remove weights without an order. *(Rationale: Traction usually is ordered to be continuous.)*
◆ If the footpiece is touching the pulleys at the bottom of the bed, report it at once. The patient should be moved up in bed when this happens. *(Rationale: This would negate the effects of traction.)*
◆ Inspect pulleys and ropes regularly. *(Rationale: The ropes can slip out of their grooves or become untied.)*
◆ Be certain you fully understand the physician's orders, regarding the patient's body positioning, that is, the degree to which the head of the bed may be elevated and to which side the patient with a fracture may turn. *(Rationale: This will prevent complications and maximize effects of the treatment.)*
◆ Do not use a pillow under an extremity in traction unless specifically ordered by the physician. *(Rationale: Placement of the pillow might counteract the effects of the traction.)*
◆ Encourage the patient to exercise the feet periodically. *(Rationale: Every effort should be made to prevent footdrop, a deformity caused by nerve damage, because the foot has been allowed to remain in an abnormal position.)*

◆ Reposition frequently as needed. *(Rationale: The weight of the traction may tend to pull the patient out of alignment.)*
◆ Maintain the patient's body alignment. Be sure to obtain specific guidelines from the physician before allowing the patient to change positions.
◆ Guide the weights if the patient is allowed to use a trapeze to slide up in bed. *(Rationale: This ensures that the weights hang freely and are not impeded when the patient moves.)*
◆ Follow the physician's orders for ROM exercises. If ROM is not ordered for the patient, find out what kind of exercise or positioning is needed.
◆ Provide diversional activities for the patient.
◆ Use the fracture bedpan. *(Rationale: It can be slipped under the patient's hips more easily than the large conventional pan.)*
◆ Maintain skin integrity. It is important to be sure that the rubber strips, roller elastic bandage or tape does not irritate the patient's skin.
◆ Apply lotion to the patient's elbows. Good skin care is required. *(Rationale: These measures prevent skin breakdown.)* If the elbows become irritated, you may want to apply elbow protectors.
◆ If the patient has skeletal traction, pin site care is given, as ordered. Wear gloves when caring for the patient with skeletal traction.

Evaluation

Periodically, the nurse, the patient, the family, and other members of the healthcare team evaluate the outcomes of care. Have short-term goals been met? Are long-term goals still realistic? Planning for further nursing care considers the patient's prognosis, as well as any complications and the patient's response to care given.

Orthopedic Complications

Orthopedic complications were briefly discussed under Nursing Assessment earlier in the chapter. More details are given here.

Neurovascular Pressure

If assessment factors indicate there is pressure from a cast or splint (see Fig. 70-5), measures must be taken to relieve the pressure *immediately*. It may be necessary for the physician to remove all or part of a cast or splint. In some cases, the cast is cut in half lengthwise (bivalved) and held together by an elastic roller bandage. This relieves pressure while maintaining the immobilization. Other causes of pressure may be a dent, swelling, or crutches that are too long.

Wound Infection

In any compound fracture or open reduction, there is a break in the skin. Infection is a possibility. Always use gloves when caring for the patient with any wound. The nurse must observe carefully for signs of infection, as indicated in the earlier Nursing Assessment.

Acute Osteomyelitis

Osteomyelitis is a serious infection of bone. Acute osteomyelitis may be due to a compound fracture exposing the bone to infection or to organisms such as staphylococcus or streptococcus that are carried by the bloodstream from infection elsewhere. Pus forms in the shaft of the bone and under the covering (periosteum), separating the periosteum from the bone. Fragments of dead bone loosen (**sequestration**) and must be removed (sequestrectomy). Early detection of osteomyelitis is imperative to prevent bone necrosis. When osteomyelitis is suspected, vigorous antibiotic therapy is begun at once. When the offending organism is isolated, specific antibiotics are given intravenously or directly into the wound. A catheter may be placed in the wound for irrigation and drainage. Careful attention to rest, nutrition, fluid intake, elimination, and skin care is vital. The patient should move about to prevent problems associated with prolonged bed rest; however, absolute rest of the affected part is necessary. Surgical drainage is sometimes performed to remove the exudate. If healing becomes impaired, remaining dead bone tissue (sequestrum) must be removed surgically.

Nursing Considerations. Osteomyelitis is so painful that the affected part is sensitive to the slightest touch or motion. It should not be moved any more than absolutely necessary, and when it must be moved, it should be supported and splinted with a pillow, and lifted and moved with the rest of the body. Sandbags, a cast, or a brace help immobilize the limb. Again, extreme care should be taken to avoid jarring the bed.

The prescribed diet is high in proteins, calcium, carbohydrates, and fats to improve resistance and is high in fluids as well. Modern antibiotics have greatly improved chances for recovery.

Swelling, redness, or pain in another part of the body may be a sign that infection is spreading and should be reported. Pathologic fractures are possible although they may not be recognized because the pain is eclipsed by the greater pain of the osteomyelitis. Growth of new bone may lengthen the infected bone, or bone destruction may shorten it. A break in aseptic technique when dressings are changed could introduce outside organisms into the wound. Every attempt is made in orthopedic practice to prevent osteomyelitis.

Chronic Osteomyelitis

If the antibiotics given are not effective in killing the offending organism, an abscess may form or the organism may build up resistance to the antibiotic. In these cases, chronic osteomyelitis occurs. These are reasons for doing a culture and sensitivity test *before* beginning a course of antibiotic therapy. Acute osteomyelitis may also become chronic in the immunosuppressed patient (such as one on chemotherapy or with acquired immunodeficiency syndrome).

Another type of chronic osteomyelitis is caused by the tubercle bacillus, which settles in the bone (*tuberculosis osteomyelitis*). If the spine is affected, this is known as *Pott's disease.*

Hypostatic Pneumonia and Atelectasis

Another complication that must be prevented is hypostatic pneumonia or *atelectasis* (collapse of all or part of a lung). Encourage the patient to move about as much as possible and to cough and take deep breaths; respiratory therapy is usually prescribed.

Pulmonary Embolism

An *embolism* is the sudden blockage of an artery by a piece of foreign material. The foreign material (*embolus*) can be a blood clot, a clump of bacteria, an air bubble, a piece of tissue, or a piece of an intravenous catheter. The most common embolism in fractures is a bolus of fat. The *fatty embolism* is most common in young people with multiple injuries, particularly fractures of the long bones (such as the femur and humerus). This embolism travels through the circulation and causes an obstruction in the brain, the heart, or most commonly, the lungs. This is an emergency and requires immediate corrective action. Specific symptoms of embolism are consistent with the blockage of blood supply to the affected area.

Treatment is symptomatic. The physician is notified immediately; oxygen is given. Blood gas determinations are made. Give the patient emotional support and calmly explain what is being done. Emergency surgery may or may not be life-saving.

Deep Vein Thrombosis (DVT)

Venostasis (standstill of blood flow) occurs when a patient is immobile for a long period of time. This predisposes to clot formation, called *thrombosis.* Venous thrombosis occurs most often in the legs and pelvis. This situation can be fatal if the clot moves and obstructs a vital blood vessel. This is one of the primary complications of bed rest and is the reason for doing passive exercises and for encouraging the patient to move as soon and as much as possible.

Hemorrhage

In many fractures, bone fragments damage blood vessels. The nurse should be alert to signs of hemorrhage.

Compartment Syndrome and Related Complications

In Chapter 17, the muscle compartments of the extremities are discussed. These compartments can be severely damaged by pressure, resulting in any of the following complications: **compartment syndrome**; *Volkmann's contracture* (also called *Volkmann's paralysis*), *Volkmann's syndrome*, and *ischemic muscular atrophy* (affecting the fingers and sometimes the wrist); as well as *pressure palsy* or *pressure paralysis*. The pressure may result from a tight cast or may result from swelling between the tight bands of fascia between the muscle compartments. Excision of the fascia (*fasciotomy*) may be needed to relieve internal pressure.

If left uncorrected, permanent damage results in approximately 6 hours and complete muscle death in 24 to 48 hours. The cause of this damage is the occlusion of circulation in a major artery (*ischemia*), which in turn affects the nerves in the limb, often without affecting other muscle compartments.

Nursing Considerations. In caring for any patient with a cast, a severe sprain, or any other condition that causes swelling in an extremity, the nurse must be alert to symptoms of nerve compression. If the patient is in a cast, removal of the cast will probably alleviate the symptoms. However, if the swelling is internal and cannot be relieved, emergency measures must be instituted at once.

Nursing Alert

Never ignore a complaint of pain or pressure from a person in a cast or splint. Check the CMS, elevate the extremity, and report the situation immediately.

Other Complications

Confusion is not uncommon, especially in the elderly. Most often it occurs at night, when patients are more confused and restless. Nerve or blood vessel compression or compartmental syndrome can lead to paralysis.

Constipation can occur because of age, inactivity, poor eating habits, and insufficient fluids. Kidney stones may form because of poor nutrition, as a result of changes in mineral composition that may occur during the healing process, or because of inactivity or overmedication with salicylates. Skin breakdown may result from poor circulation, immobility, infrequent turning, or poor skin care.

Sometimes bones do not fuse and the break does not heal. This is a common complication of fractures. It may be due to poor physical condition, including malnutrition, poor circulation, or age. Contractures, footdrop, and external rotation may be caused by poor positioning or lack of exercise.

Musculoskeletal Disorders

Amputation

Amputation is the absence of or removal of a limb or part of a limb. An amputation may be congenital, the result of injury, or surgically performed. Reasons for surgical amputation include progressive malignancy or neurovascular compromise as a result of diabetes or cardiovascular disease.

An amputation becomes the treatment of choice only when the disease process cannot be controlled or arrested by other means. In these cases, the amputation is often a lifesaving measure. In malignant disease, such surgery may offer comfort, increased function, and potential longevity not otherwise possible. Amputation is not always curative in malignancies.

Level of Amputation

Terminology used for levels of amputation is relatively descriptive. Amputations are classified according to the affected limb and the level of the amputation. The level of amputation is determined by the specific process of deformity for which the procedure is deemed necessary. An amputation of the hand is called a below-the-elbow amputation (BEA); an above-the-elbow amputation is abbreviated AEA. Below-the-knee amputation is abbreviated BKA and above-the-knee amputation, AKA (Fig. 70-7). Sometimes, only a finger or toe is amputated. An example of this description is "amputation of first finger, right hand, below second knuckle."

Phantom Limb

The sensation that the amputated limb is still there and is painful or itches is a frequent aftermath of amputation. Patients may be too embarrassed to mention it. Encourage a patient who seems to be disturbed and uneasy for no apparent reason to talk. If phantom pain or discomfort is causing distress, explain that it is not uncommon, that it is due to damage to the nerves in the stump, and that it will disappear in time. It is often helpful to tell the patient to "move the missing limb." By activating the damaged nerves leading to the amputated limb, the patient usually feels great relief. If this is not helpful, the patient should receive medication for the pain. Persistent pain can interfere with prosthesis fitting.

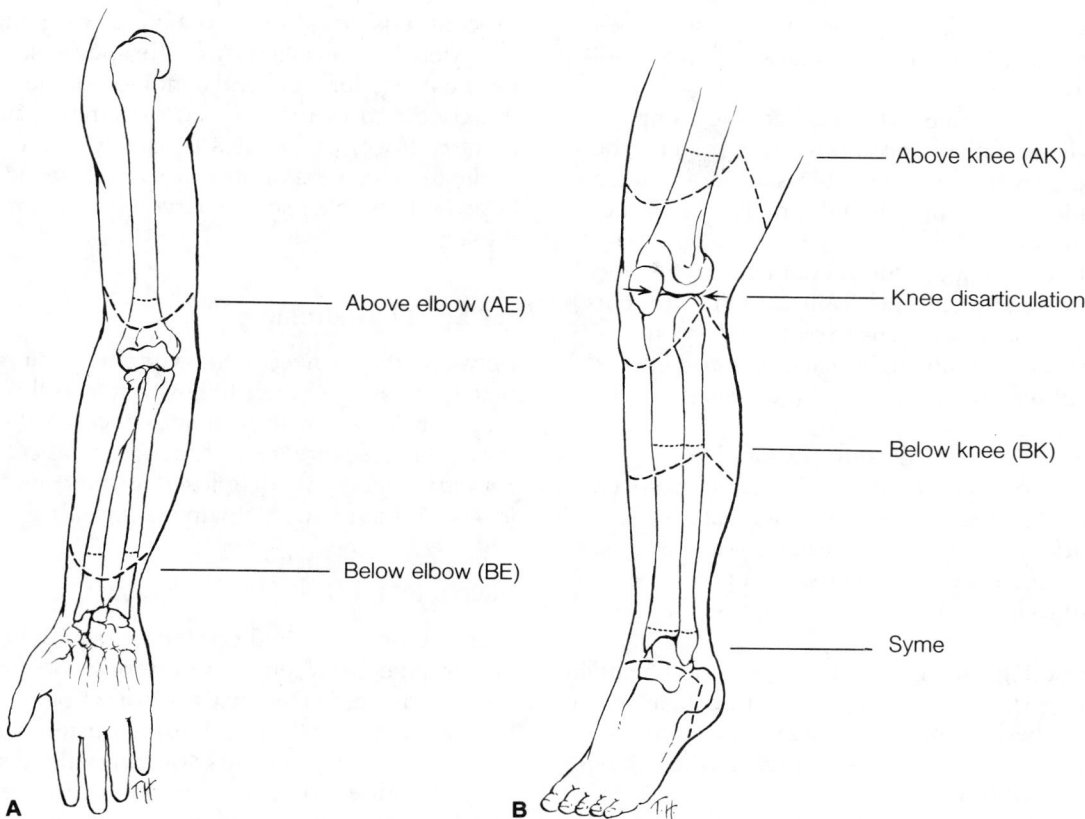

Figure 70-7. Levels of amputation are determined by circulatory adequacy, type of prosthesis, function of the part, and muscle balance. **(A)** Levels of amputation of upper extremity. **(B)** Levels of amputation of lower extremity.

The Prosthesis

The patient is fitted with a prosthesis as soon as possible after surgery; sometimes a temporary prosthesis is attached while the patient is still anesthetized. Leg prostheses have proven successful. Skirts or trousers conceal a leg prosthesis, which can be equipped with a shoe that matches the one on the opposite foot.

An arm prosthesis is more conspicuous because the hand end is difficult to cover and still be useful. It is difficult to make an artificial hand look real. A practical prosthetic hand is fashioned with a mechanical hook consisting of metal prongs placed opposite each other to replace the fingers and thumb. The opposition placement is essential to allow the amputee to hold articles in a normal manner. These devices are activated by movements within a shoulder harness.

Nursing Considerations

As soon as the incision is healed, and sometimes, immediately after surgery, elastic bandages are applied to the stump to shrink it. It shrinks rapidly at first, but some shrinkage usually continues for a year or more. Two sets of roller bandages are needed because the bandage is changed at least twice a day, and more often if the patient perspires freely. The patient and a member of the family are taught how to apply the bandage. Correctly wrapping the stump is important to the later use of a prosthesis and to reduce edema. The stump is wrapped so it forms a cone shape. You will need instruction in the recommended wrapping in each individual case.

Prevention of Complications. Four potential complications following an amputation are hemorrhage, infection, failure of the stump incisions to heal, and (after leg amputation) hip contractures. The following nursing skills are used in preventing complications.

- ◆ Keep a tourniquet within reach at all times.
- ◆ Observe the dressing for bleeding.
- ◆ Use aseptic technique when changing dressings.
- ◆ If drains have been inserted by the surgeon, drainage must be assessed for amount and color and the container emptied as ordered.
- ◆ Take care not to dislodge drains when turning patient.
- ◆ When changing dressings, check the incision closely for signs of healing. Notify the physician of any blackened or opened areas along the incision

line, any unusual drainage, or if the incision does not show signs of healing. (A black area may indicate gangrene.)

◆ Encourage the patient who has had a leg amputated to lie in a prone position, rather than on the back. To prevent hip contractures, do not place pillows under the stump when the patient is on the back. The foot of the bed may be elevated after amputation to reduce stump edema.

◆ If ordered, skin traction is applied to the stump as soon as the patient returns from the operating room. A cast of lightweight material is sometimes applied to the stump to maintain the shape of the stump.

◆ If no cast is in place, the stump should be cleansed, thoroughly dried, and carefully inspected each day. Any redness or irritation must be reported at once because any irritation or skin breakdown will interfere with the use of a prosthesis and may lead to infection.

Patient Teaching. Prosthesis self-care should be taught and encouraged as soon as possible. The arm amputee manipulates the prosthesis by means of a harness extending around the opposite shoulder; a wire arrangement connects the harness to the prosthesis. The amputee thrusts the shoulder forward to open the prongs and relaxes to close them. Although these movements are barely noticeable, a patient can learn how to use them effectively. Because of new materials and new computer programs, prostheses are becoming much more functional.

Emotional Support. The patient who has an amputation has a natural grief reaction and may exhibit irritability, anger, depression, or other emotions. Allow the patient time to ventilate these feelings. Listen to the patient's concerns and offer support.

Exercise. In the foot or leg amputation, preparations for walking are begun almost as soon as the patient recovers from the anesthetic. Exercises to increase arm strength for crutch walking may have been started preoperatively. The physical therapist may instruct in exercising by showing the patient how to maintain muscle tone and directing the nurse in efforts to help the patient prevent contractures. Usually, by the first or second postoperative day, the patient is helped to sit up at the edge of the bed and soon progresses to a wheelchair. Periodic bed rest is advisable because prolonged sitting may cause contractures.

Reattachment of Severed Limbs

With the advent of microvascular surgery, some patients who have suffered traumatic amputations have successfully had the limb reattached. However, this procedure is not always possible. Factors that must be considered are availability of the specialist, equipment for the procedure, general condition of the patient, and the condition of the severed extremity. The reattachment of lower extremities is usually not as successful as the reattachment of upper extremities because of the large and complex sciatic nerve system that innervates the legs.

Facet Joint Syndrome

Between the bones of the vertebral column are flat places where the bones lightly touch each other, called facet joints. When these joints become dislocated or misaligned, severe pain can occur. *Facet joint syndrome* is commonly diagnosed as the cause of chronic low back pain (chronic pain syndrome).

Intervertebral Disk (IVD) Disease

Pressure on the spinal cord, occurring when the disk of cartilage between two vertebrae becomes weakened and presses against the spinal nerves, is called herniated disk or "slipped disk." Currently, back pain is seen more often because of competitive sports, job-related injuries, degenerative joint disease, and progressive bone disorders, such as osteoporosis in elderly patients.

Diagnostic Tests. The diagnosis of a herniated disk can be made with a CT scan or MRI. This is performed in conjunction with the presentation of a positive patient history and physical examination. Sometimes, water-soluble myelography is also done to outline nerve root filling. This is particularly useful in patients who have had prior surgery. The CT scan also helps to define cervical stenosis (narrowing) of either the central or the lateral foramina. This type of stenosis may produce nerve compression and symptoms of low back or radiating pain similar to those of a herniated disk.

Medical and Surgical Treatment. The patient is rarely immobilized. Instead, patients are encouraged to proceed with exercises as outlined by a physical therapist. The therapist sets up a regular walking program and aquatic (water) exercises. Lumbosacral corsets or braces, if used, are only worn for a short time, because reliance on these devices weakens the supporting abdominal musculature (muscles). Antispasmodic medications may be helpful.

Another approach to treatment of the patient with a herniated IVD is injection of a drug, specifically chymopapain (Chymodiactin), directly into the disk. This drug is contraindicated if the patient is obese, elderly, or allergic to the drug. This treatment also cannot be used if the patient has more than two herniated discs or if the patient has lateral foraminal narrowing. (The foramina [openings] on the sides are narrower than normal.) When a drug is injected into the disk, the disk collapses. If the openings are narrowed, the nerves could then be compressed by the bones. Therefore, drug injection is a treatment for only a select few patients.

Spinal cord injuries or disorders are treated surgically by removing the cause of the pressure, if possible. The surgeon removes a portion of the vertebra to expose the spinal cord and takes out the bone fragment, the herniated disk, the tumor, or the clot pressing on the cord. This operation is called *lumbar decompression.* The term lumbar decompression applies to any of the necessary procedures used to relieve pressure on the nerves.

Sometimes the weakened vertebra is strengthened by attaching a steel rod or by grafting a piece of bone (from the tibia or iliac crest, or donated bone) onto several vertebrae or between a vertebra and the sacrum. This is called spinal fusion; when the graft heals, the spine will be stiff in that area.

Another surgical procedure is the interbody fusion. In this procedure, bone grafts or substitutes are placed between the vertebrae, after the disk space is cleaned out. The specific type of fusion to be done is determined after careful testing to determine the cause of spinal instability.

Nursing Considerations: Postoperative Care. Attention is given to routine postoperative care, along with management of accompanying pain. Meticulous wound care must be given so that the wound will not become contaminated; infection could lead to meningitis. Watch closely for signs of bleeding and other drainage, leakage of cerebrospinal fluid, or shock caused by trauma. Neurologic evaluation is done at frequent intervals. (See Chapter 71.) When a lumbar decompression has been performed, it is important to observe sensation and mobility in the legs, to detect further complications; one complication is nerve damage during surgery. Any complaints of tingling, numbness, or difficulty in moving the legs should be reported immediately. Another complication is edema, which may cause pressure on the spinal cord or which may cause fluid to collect in the legs. The accompanying box lists assessments to be made in postlumbar decompression. If a cervical laminectomy or decompression has been performed, the assessments mentioned above remain important; in addition, the patient's upper extremities can show signs of nerve damage and respiratory function can be impaired.

Adequate rest to the back is required; however, movement is recommended for the patient to prevent respiratory complications. *Logroll* turns are done. The

---

Keys to Nursing Assessment
Postlumbar Decompression

◆ Nerve damage: Change in sensation or mobility of legs; tingling, numbness of legs
◆ Edema: Collection of fluid in legs; severe pain, which could indicate edema within spinal column
◆ Change in level of consciousness: could indicate encephalitis or meningitis.
◆ Muscle spasms: Leg pain; can be prevented by exercises
◆ Thrombophlebitis: Leg pain; can be prevented by surgical stockings, exercises, and ambulation
◆ Additional injury: Prevented by avoiding heavy lifting for a period of time.

Following *cervical* decompression, in addition to the preceding, *also* observe for:

◆ Nerve damage: Difficulty or change in sensation of arms; difficulty in moving arms; difficulty in breathing

Other observations include those made for any postsurgical patient.

---

patient can be taught to help the nurse carry out the proper turning procedures by holding the body straight and keeping the arms crossed over the chest; the nurse rolls the patient over as a single entity. Two nurses may work together to logroll the patient. A turning sheet may be used. Analgesics are given for pain and should be offered before the patient is moved or turned.

When a bedpan is offered, the patient should never be lifted, but rather should be rolled onto the pan. A fracture bedpan should always be used. (*Rationale: It is smaller and the patient does not arch the back when using it.*) The patient should be taught never to reach or stretch for articles.

During the first few postoperative days, muscle spasms may develop, especially in the legs. The physician may order exercises to relieve these spasms. The patient may also be taught isometric (muscle-setting) exercises for the quadriceps because these exercises can be performed without moving in bed.

The patient may wear antiembolism stockings or have the legs wrapped in Ace bandages because immobility could lead to thrombus formation.

Patients are allowed out of bed in gradual progression from sitting upright, to dangling, and eventually to ambulating. This procedure usually begins on the first postoperative day following a lumbar or cervical decompression. Occasionally, the patient wears a brace or a corset to give support to the back; when a brace is applied, a thin cotton shirt is put on first to protect the skin. The most common is called the "clam-shell" brace.

It is also called the TLSO brace (thoracolumbar sacro-orthosis). Be sure to smooth all wrinkles so the skin is kept intact. Then, with the patient on the side, place the middle of the brace over the spine; roll the patient onto it. After the brace is fastened, help the patient to the edge of the bed, so the legs will fall over the side when he or she sits up; then assist him or her to sit up slowly. The patient needs the support of the brace to maintain the effect of the surgery.

After a lumbar decompression, the patient will gradually be allowed to do light work but must always avoid heavy lifting. Caution should be used when doing any lifting for a least a year after the operation. Emphasize to the patient that if he or she disregards this precaution even once during convalescence, injury may result.

If a spinal fusion has been done, the patient may have more limitations. It is usually necessary for the patient to wear a brace or corset whenever he or she gets out of bed. Sometimes, the physician applies a body cast. Occasionally, the physician orders the brace to be worn even when the patient is in bed. Prolonged sitting should be avoided because it puts extra strain on the back. Never attempt to move a patient unless you have been given permission and have been taught how to do it. The patient who is paralyzed also needs care appropriate to the degree of paralysis (see Chapter 71).

Temporomandibular Joint Disorders

Temporomandibular joint disorders (TMJ), which involve the joint of the lower jaw, are treated with braces or surgery (see Chapter 81).

Systemic Disorders With Musculoskeletal Manifestations

Gout (Hyperuricemia)

Substances called *purines* are produced during protein metabolism. If the body is unable to metabolize these substances, uric acid accumulates in the bloodstream and forms crystal deposits in the joints. This condition, called gout, is more common in men. It usually affects the big toe, the instep, the ankle, or the knee, but it may appear in any joint.

Signs and Symptoms. Gout attacks periodically, causing swelling and pain; eventually motion in the affected joint becomes limited. Renal damage and vascular damage (especially atherosclerosis) can follow.

An attack of gout begins with severe pain, swelling, and redness. It lasts from 3 to 14 days, after which it disappears suddenly. It may return any time; other-wise the joint is normal. The slightest touch or weight is unbearable during an attack. As time goes on, repeated attacks damage the joint permanently. The list of triggering agents includes alcohol, allergy, surgery, injury, infection, nitrogenous or fatty foods, a fasting diet, emotional stress, or a change in the patient's environment.

Medical Treatment. Gout cannot be cured, but the attacks can be controlled and prevented. Patients must follow the routine prescribed and see their physicians regularly. Diet is the most important treatment. High-purine foods (such as liver) must be avoided.

Colchicine (Colsalide) is usually effective in relieving gout symptoms. If given early enough, it relieves the pain and other symptoms in 12 to 24 hours. Side effects include gastrointestinal disturbances, (nausea, vomiting, abdominal pain, and diarrhea). *Probenecid* (Benemid) is used in long-term management because it prevents the reabsorption of uric acid into the kidney. *Allopurinol* (Zyloprim) inhibits uric acid formation. The patient taking any of these medications must ingest 3 liters of fluids each day to promote a large urine volume. When taking these medications, aspirin or any other salicylate should *not be taken* because they counteract the other gout-relieving drugs.

Nursing Considerations. A bed cradle protects the affected joint. Preventing the affected part or the bed from being bumped or jarred is so important that a warning sign may be hung in a prominent place. Gentle application of warm or cold compresses is sometimes ordered, and elevating the affected joint may make the patient more comfortable. To prevent the joint from stiffening, exercise should be started as soon as the pain and the redness have cleared.

Systemic Lupus Erythematosus

Systemic lupus erythematosus (lupus, SLE) is a systemic disorder that shows symptoms in many systems of the body. There are two types of lupus erythematosus: discoid and systemic. *Discoid lupus erythematosus* is a chronic disease with skin manifestations of disklike patches with raised, reddish edges and depressed centers. SLE is an acute or subacute febrile disease found primarily in women. It causes widespread damage to the collagen system and can affect any organ system, such as kidneys, heart, or lungs. It is marked by remissions and exacerbations; it can be chronic and mild or rampant and fatal. A characteristic skin rash occurs in a butterfly formation around the eyes; a rash also occurs over other parts of the body.

Lupus also shows arthritic symptoms, including joint pains and aching muscles. Other symptoms include anorexia, nausea, vomiting, swollen glands, and general malaise. In severe cases, the inflammatory process may involve the lining of the lungs and heart and can damage the kidneys, nervous system, or brain. SLE has no known cure, but early intervention can often prevent serious joint damage.

Medical Treatment. There is no specific cure. Treatment is based on manifestations of symptoms. Salicylates on a regular basis, systemic corticosteroids, and sometimes immunosuppressive drugs are methods of treatment. Generally, patients are advised to avoid sunlight because it can intensify skin manifestations. A sunscreen lotion (of at least SPF 22) should be used if exposure to the sun cannot be avoided. It is important for the patient to get adequate rest and not become overtired. Treatment of the musculoskeletal symptoms is like that of other types of arthritis (drugs, exercise, physical therapy).

Scleroderma (Progressive Systemic Sclerosis)

The term **scleroderma** means hard skin; it is considered a collagen disorder. It involves chronic hardening and shrinking of all the connective tissues in the body, including blood vessels, muscles, and the digestive tract. The disorder begins on the face and hands, where the skin becomes hard and unwrinkled and cannot be pinched up from the underlying structures. The condition slowly spreads.

The patient often has joint pains and difficulty in movement. A common early symptom is Raynaud's phenomenon, which is described in Chapter 74 (the fingers are very sensitive to cold). Scleroderma may be generalized (*systemic, diffuse*), limited to distal parts of extremities and face (*acrosclerosis*), to fingers and toes (*sclerodactyly*), or localized into small areas (*morphea*). This condition most often affects women and usually begins in middle age. However, the most severe forms commonly affect men, African Americans, and older people. It may have an autoimmune component.

Symptomatic treatment is offered; joint manifestations are treated the same as other arthritic conditions. The nurse must take into consideration the hardened skin when giving injections. Smoking is contraindicated because of lung involvement.

Rickets

Rickets is a nutritional disease caused by a lack of vitamin D in the diet during childhood. This vitamin deficiency causes faulty absorption of calcium or phosphorus, both of which are needed for normal bone hardening. In rickets, the bones remain soft and become distorted; when they finally do harden, they remain in this deformed state. Bow legs is a good example of the effect of rickets on the bones. Children with rickets are slow to walk and cut teeth; they are pale, irritable, and inactive. Rickets is both prevented and treated at an early age by exposure to sunshine and vitamin D. Milk with vitamin D also helps prevent rickets. The adult form of vitamin D deficiency, which results in softening of the bones, is called *osteomalacia*.

Degenerative Disorders

Muscular Dystrophies

The cause of muscular dystrophies, which are degenerative and hereditary diseases of skeletal muscles, is unknown; some researchers believe they are related to a disruption in enzyme production. Treatment centers on support of the patient, who should be encouraged to continue all activities as normally as possible. Exercise programs and splints may be used to prevent deformities. Often, special braces can be used to permit ambulation. The patient should be informed of the need to prevent upper respiratory infections, to maintain ideal weight, and to strive for general good health. Chapter 67 covers the muscular dystrophies in more detail because they often affect children.

Osteoporosis

Osteoporosis is a condition in which bone mass is decreased, most commonly in postmenopausal women. It can cause pathologic bone fractures, difficulty in weight bearing, loss of height, and a curvature of the spine most commonly known as *kyphosis*. Many women take oral calcium in an effort to prevent osteoporosis. Taking the hormones estrogen and progesterone is advised by some physicians. This condition will be discussed in detail in Chapter 85, in connection with care of older people.

Inflammatory Disorders

Arthritis

Arthritis means inflammation of a joint. More than 100 arthritic disorders are known. The most common types of arthritis are:

◆ *Rheumatoid arthritis* (RA)
◆ *Osteoarthritis:* degenerative joint disease (DJD), osteoarthrosis, hypertrophic arthritis
◆ *Ankylosing spondylitis:* rheumatoid spondylitis, rheumatoid arthritis of the spine
◆ *Gout*
◆ *Systemic lupus erythematosus:* SLE, lupus
◆ *Scleroderma:* progressive systemic sclerosis

Arthritis affects more than 18 million people in the United States. *Monoarticular* arthritis affects one joint;

polyarticular arthritis affects many joints. Most types of arthritis (except ankylosing spondylitis and gout) are more common in women.

Arthritis may be due to several factors:

◆ *Infectious arthritis:* infection of a joint by a virus or microorganism
◆ *Traumatic arthritis:* direct injury to a joint
◆ *Degenerative arthritis:* degeneration or deterioration of a joint
◆ *Metabolic arthritis:* metabolic disorder such as gout

Many researchers believe that arthritis has an autoimmune component. In many cases it is not known what causes arthritis or how to cure it. However, it is usually possible to control it and prevent or correct the crippling effects of the disorder. Both *acute* and *chronic* forms of arthritis occur. Acute exacerbations may also occur with chronic forms of the disease.

The incidence of arthritis is divided as follows:

◆ *Monocyclic* (35% of cases): has sudden onset; may never return; and usually responds well to medications
◆ *Polycyclic* (50% of cases): is marked by exacerbations and remissions
◆ *Progressive* (15% of cases): keeps getting worse; does not stop with treatment

Signs and Symptoms. The following are warning signs of arthritis:

◆ Persistent pain and stiffness on arising for 6 weeks or more; stiffness aggravated by damp weather or strenuous activity
◆ Pain or tenderness in the joints, often symmetrical
◆ Swelling in the joints
◆ Recurrence of symptoms, particularly when more than one joint involved
◆ Obvious redness and warmth in a joint
◆ Unexplained weight loss, fever, or weakness combined with joint pain
◆ In degenerative joint disease—Bouchard's nodes (enlargement of proximal interphalangeal joints) or Heberden's nodes (growths on the terminal phalangeal joints)

The accompanying box describes goals and pain management in arthritis.

Rheumatoid Arthritis

Signs and Symptoms. Rheumatoid arthritis (RA) is probably the most painful and the most crippling form of arthritis. It occurs worldwide and is three times more common in women than men. Theories suggest that a triggering mechanism in the body (possibly a virus) causes the immune system to be overactive. Although RA is not genetic, there seems to be a genetic pre-

Management of Arthritis

Goals

◆ Relieve inflammation (medication)
◆ Relieve pain (medications, local treatments)
◆ Maintain optimal functioning (exercise, adaptive devices)
◆ Educate the patient (prevention, treatment)

Pain Management

◆ Splinting/casting/night splinting/traction
◆ Positioning
◆ Heat (paraffin baths, diathermy)
◆ Cold (ice packs)
◆ Physical therapy
◆ Massage (if joint not acutely inflamed)
◆ Medications (most commonly salicylates)
◆ Low-impact exercise; isometric exercises (improves muscle strength without overexerting joints)
◆ Rest (physical and emotional)
◆ Avoid fatigue and overexertion (10 or more hours rest daily)
◆ Sleep on firm bed
◆ Have bed and chair at same level, to facilitate transfer
◆ May need chair that helps patient to stand up
◆ Have chair 3 to 4 inches higher than regular chair, to avoid bending too much at hips. (Do not use pillow in the chair; this promotes slouching, which is tiring.)
◆ Emotional support

disposition to the disorder; several members of one family may be affected. Table 70-1 compares RA and osteoarthritis.

In RA, extra synovial fluid is secreted within the joints. The capsule swells, the synovial membrane becomes inflamed, and the cartilage is eaten away. An overgrowth of synovial lining occurs. When the cartilage and bone erode, the joint becomes painful because bone rubs against bone. If the joint becomes calcified, movement is impossible. The condition of an immovable joint is called **ankylosis**. This does not occur in all RA patients, however. Deformities of RA include joints hyperextended because of contracted tendons, swollen joints, hammer toes (cock-up toes), knock knees, gait problems, and bone spurs on the soles of the feet. If the opening in the spinal column becomes calcified, its diameter gets smaller, a condition called *spinal stenosis.* This can cause pressure on the spinal cord.

Medical Treatment. Treatment includes drug therapy (Table 70-2), exercise, and physical therapy. The goal of treatment is to reduce inflammation before the joint is permanently damaged. Exercise helps prevent con-

Table 70-1. Comparisons Between Rheumatoid Arthritis and Osteoarthritis*

Rheumatoid Arthritis	*Osteoarthritis (DJD)*
Systemic (fatigue, weight loss, anemia)	Not systemic (results from wear and tear)
Fever	No fever
Systemic inflammation	Local inflammation (joint only)
Probably autoimmune origin	Most common arthritis
3:1 in women	2:1 in women
Affects young adults (ages 20–30)	Affects older and elderly adults (over age 45)
	Common in women after menopause
	More common in obese people
Affects small and large joints (symmetrical); most common in fingers, knees, elbows, ankles	Affects primarily large weight-bearing joints and knuckles (knees, hips, knuckles, spine)
May remain the same for life	May be progressive
Causes inflammatory process in other parts of body (lungs, kidneys, eyes)	Sets up local inflammation
	Can be hereditary
Surgery does not help (condition returns)	May surgically replace or fuse joints (last choice for treatment)
May have lumps (nodules) on joints, which are painful	Often have lumps, but do not restrict activity and are not painful
Fingers may swell; joints feel cold and moist; bluish color; muscles may become weakened	Joints usually don't swell; muscles remain firm
Joints distorted and dislocated	Not as likely to be disabling; may remain localized in body
Joints may ankylose (fuse)	Joints usually don't ankylose
Abnormal laboratory values (rheumatoid factor, sedimentation rate high; hemoglobin low)	

* Source: Arthritis Foundation.

tractures and strengthens muscles to provide joint stability. Patient teaching is outlined in the accompanying box. In some cases, excess synovial fluid may be aspirated. Measures to increase body resistance, such as rest and a well-balanced diet, are helpful.

Osteoarthritis or Degenerative Joint Disease (DJD)

Osteoarthritis is believed to have a genetic cause or predisposition. It causes faulty connective tissue formation in the joints. The cartilage degenerates first. Next, bony hypertrophy (overgrowth) occurs, with the creation of bone spurs. Particles of cartilage break off and float in the joint, making movement painful. The bones wear down and may actually be less painful when they become smooth. **Synovectomy**, which is excision of the synovial membrane, helps to prevent further inflammation in some cases. Total joint replacement (*arthroplasty*) is the last resort, but in many cases, is effective. In other cases, the joint must be fused to prevent pain. (See Table 70-1 for comparison of osteoarthritis with RA.)

Nursing Alert

Many of the drugs used to treat arthritis have serious side effects. Be sure to check your reference sources *before* administering any drugs. You must be alert to possible side effects and report any difficulties immediately.

Ankylosing Spondylitis

Ankylosing spondylitis is sometimes called *rheumatoid arthritis of the spine* because it primarily affects the facet joints and the stabilizing ligaments of the spinal column. It is also called Marie-Strümpell disease. It mainly affects young men and almost always appears before the age of 50. The most common early symptoms are hip and low back pain and stiffness. In some cases, the neck and hips become fused and breathing may be impaired because chest expansion is impeded. In severe cases, stiffening of the spine also occurs, with resultant humpback and curvature of the chest. Neck stiffness may make it impossible for patients to turn their heads.

Table 70-2. Medications Used in Arthritis*

Medications	Examples	Descriptions	Side Effects
Salicylates	Aspirin, acetylsalicylic acid	Should be taken with food Patients often take 12 or more daily. Should be taken even if symptoms have subsided. May be enteric-coated, buffered, or delayed-release to meet patient needs. Patient should increase fluid intake.	Minor GI upsets Formation of kidney stones Some anticoagulant action
Nonsteroidal anti-inflammatory drugs (NSAIDs)	Ibuprofen (Motrin, Advil, Nuprin) Indomethacin (Indocin) Piroxicam (Feldene) Sulindac (Clinoril)	Should be taken with food. Patient often takes four daily. Regular blood counts needed.	Stomach irritation May cause visual disturbance, headache, dizziness Edema if patient has cardiac disorder Contraindicated if taking hepatotoxic drugs, such as lithium
Gold salts	Aurothioglucose (Solganal) Gold sodium thiomalate (Myochrysine)	May be combined with aspirins or NSAIDs. Should not be combined with penicillamine or antimalarials. May be given IM monthly (more effective, but more side effects). Used in RA Blood and urine must be monitored.	Pruritus, GI upsets, purpura, anemia, hepatitis
Antimalarials	Hydroxychloroquine sulfate (Plaquenil sulfate) Chloroquine (Aralen)	Used in RA and SLE	Eye damage
Penicillamine	Cupramine, Depen Titratabs	Not frequently used, but sometimes effective in RA	
Coricosteroids	Cortisone, hydrocortisone, prednisone	Taken orally May be injected directly into joint (reduces side effects) in severe flare-up. Effective in counteracting symptoms, but do not arrest disease process.	Many undesirable side effects: cataracts, diabetes mellitus, osteoporosis (see Chapter 56)
Immunosuppressives	Methotrexate (Amethopterin) Asathioprine (Imuran) Cyclophosphamide (Cytoxan)	Dangerous drugs Used as a last resort, most often in severe RA. Monthly examination of blood (hemoglobin, hematocrit, WBC, platelets), and liver function monitored	Many undesirable side effects: bone marrow depression with resulting infection, hemorrhaging in the bladder, fever, anemia, predisposition to cancer

* Listed in order of preference. The first listed are the most commonly used, have the least desirable side effects, and are tried first.
GI, gastrointestinal; RA, rheumatoid arthritis; SLE, systemic lupus erythematosus; WBC, white blood cell count.

The treatment is basically the same as for other types of arthritis. Phenylbutazone (Butazolidin) is sometimes given. The patient should refrain from lying on the side to prevent excess sideways curvature of the spine.

Other Inflammatory Disorders

Bursitis

A *bursa*, a sac filled with synovial fluid, pads bony prominences in the joints. **Bursitis** is inflammation of a bursa; there is an increase in fluid, and this causes dis-

tention. Eventually the wall of the bursa hardens and becomes calcified. One type of bursitis is the result of long-continued irritation or friction in a joint; this type is comparatively painless and not disabling. With chronic inflammation, calcification may result; there is pain and tenderness in the joint, and movement is limited.

The usual treatment for bursitis includes heat and rest of the affected part. Anti-inflammatory medications may be indicated. Injection of the bursal sac with corticosteroid medications may give relief in severe cases.

If these treatments are not effective, the bursa must be excised surgically.

Tenosynovitis

Tenosynovitis is inflammation of a tendon sheath. It may be due to an infection that particularly affects the wrist or the ankle. The infected tendons swell and are painful and disabling. *Noninfectious tenosynovitis* is caused by strains or blows or by the prolonged use of a particular set of tendons, as in piano playing or keyboarding over long periods. The symptoms are pain and tenderness, especially with movement. (Incidentally, this is not the same thing as "writer's cramp.") Treatment includes the following:

♦ Resting the affected body part
♦ Application of ice to decrease swelling
♦ Occasional physical therapy
♦ Nonsteroidal anti-inflammatory drugs (NSAIDs), when indicated
♦ Surgery (may be needed)
♦ Antibiotics (may be helpful)

It is important to eliminate activities that exacerbate symptoms during the inflammatory phase.

Musculoskeletal Trauma

Types of Injuries

Sprain and Strain

A **sprain** is an injury to the ligaments around a joint, causing the ligaments to stretch and tear. Sprains are painful but seldom serious. They cause swelling and interfere with movement. Rupture of the nearby blood vessels makes the skin black and blue. The usual treatment is to elevate the injured art and to provide a firm support for it, such as an elastic bandage. The pain and swelling can be relieved by applying ice for 48 to 72 hours. Warm moist packs may be used after the first 48 to 72 hours.

A **strain** involves damage to the muscle body or the tendon attachment. A sprain is a more severe injury than a strain. The sprain is often associated with joint disability, whereas the strain is not.

Dislocation

When a ligament gives way so completely that a bone is displaced from its socket, the joint is said to have a **dislocation**. Dislocations cause severe pain, an abnormal position of the bone, and inability to manipulate the joint. Following an x-ray examination, the physician is able to put the bone back into position. This is sometimes done under anesthesia by stretching the ligaments and manipulating the joint. Occasionally, the physician cannot reduce the dislocation, and the

area must be surgically opened and realigned. A splint, a brace, or an elastic bandage is then applied to immobilize the parts until they heal. Ice is applied to reduce swelling. It may take several weeks for the joint capsule and surrounding ligaments to return to their normal position.

Fracture

Any break or crack in a bone is called a **fracture**. It occurs when stress placed on a bone is greater than the bone can withstand. Bones may beak spontaneously in such diseases as osteomalacia and osteomyelitis. But most fractures are caused by trauma. Usually underlying structures such as muscles, blood vessels, and so forth are damaged in a fracture.

Accidents are the chief causes of broken bones. A fracture can occur when a hard surface is struck accidentally, or by a hard fall, as can happen in sports activities, automobile accidents, and accidents with machinery. Up to the age of 45, more men than women have fractures; after this time, more women are affected because hormonal changes of menopause may cause decalcification of bones (osteoporosis). Slippery floors and bathtubs, loose rugs, and dark stairways or corners are hazardous, especially to older persons.

Types and Patterns of Fractures. The following are basic types of fractures:

Keys to Patient/Family Teaching
Use of Exercise in Arthritis

Patient teaching for the person with arthritis includes:

♦ Body should be kept in best possible physical condition. Control weight, rest, and exercise.
♦ Exercise daily even if there is pain. Do specific exercises and not just daily work.
♦ Heat should be applied before exercise to lessen pain. Don't overdo the exercising because of lessened pain.
♦ Prepare for exercise with gentle stretching. Stretching and exercise better done actively (self-movement) rather than passively (by nurse or therapist).
♦ When possible do active exercise. If not possible do isometrics or have someone do passive exercise. May use continuous passive motion (CPM) machine.
♦ Do low-impact exercises, such as swimming, slow walking, or bicycling.
♦ Stop exercising if pain becomes too severe.
♦ Adaptive devices or a corrective corset or brace may be used.
♦ Prevent contractures: turn doorknobs to radial (thumb) side when possible. Flatten hand as much as possible.

◆ *Complete:* entire cross section of bone is involved; bone usually displaced
◆ *Incomplete:* portion of the cross section of bone is involved, or can be a longitudinal fracture
◆ *Closed:* skin is not broken in the fracture; sometimes called *simple fracture*
◆ *Open:* skin is broken directly to the fracture; sometimes called *compound fracture;* various grades of tissue involvement

Some fractures are defined by the pattern of the break. For instance, there are transverse, oblique, and spiral fractures. A fracture may be depressed, in which bone splinters are driven into underlying tissue. In a compression fracture, the bone collapses in on itself. In a greenstick fracture, one side of the bone breaks while the other side bends. These types and patterns are illustrated in Figure 70-8.

Signs and Symptoms. The most pronounced symptom of a broken bone is *pain* that becomes more severe with movement of the part, with pressure over the fracture. Pain may be accompanied by loss of function and *deformity* (an unnatural position of the part). Other symptoms include swelling over the part and discoloration caused by bleeding within the tissues. First aid for fractures is described in Chapter 31.

Medical and Surgical Treatment. An x-ray is taken of the injured area to determine the extent of the fracture and the positions of the bone fragments. A portable high-quality video machine is now available to make the first determination of fractures. Such a machine is helpful in sports injuries because it can be carried onto the field before the person is moved.

The bone is restored to correct alignment so it can heal properly. The method chosen will depend on the place and extent of the break and the condition and age of the patient. The object is to bring the fragments back into place (*reduction*) and to hold them in that position (*immobilization*) until the break is healed. The two types of reduction are *closed* and *open.* In *closed reduction,* bone ends are realigned through external manipulation; in *open reduction,* the realignment is accomplished through surgery.

The different types of immobilization devices include casts, internal and external fixation, splints, and traction. These treatments and related nursing care are discussed earlier in this chapter. The use of computers helps determine the exact type of prosthesis or reconstruction needed in some cases.

If a patient has a compound fracture, surgery usually will be performed. The wound is *debrided* (dead and damaged tissue removed) and *irrigated* (with antibiotics, peroxide, normal saline, or other solutions). The bones are then *immobilized* with various internal fixa-tion devices. Often, if a cast is applied, a "window" is cut out over the incisional area, so the condition of the wound can be routinely assessed.

Hip Fracture

Hip fractures include fractures of the head and neck of the femur or of the trochanter. These fractures often heal poorly because nutrition is disrupted by the healing process in such large bones. In addition, hip fractures are common in older people, whose bones heal more slowly and who are more likely to have the bone degeneration of osteoporosis (particularly older women.) The sample Nursing Care Plan illustrates the use of nursing process in the care of a patient with a fractured hip.

Signs and Symptoms. Whenever an older person falls or complains of pain in the hip, groin, or knee, an assessment for hip fracture should be done. The location of the fracture causes the symptoms to vary somewhat. However, many hip fractures involve shortening of the leg on the affected side and external rotation of the foot.

In most cases, if the fracture is in the neck of the femur, the patient will complain of severe pain, made worse by movement. If the head of the femur is compacted onto the neck, the patient may not have much pain and may even be able to bear weight. For this reason, a physician should examine any older person who falls. If the fracture is in the trochanter, the patient will usually have muscle spasms, obvious shortening of the leg, external rotation of the foot, complaints of severe pain, and a large bruise on the hip. Specific diagnosis is made by x-ray. The hemoglobin level may be decreased because of bleeding; blood glucose and enzyme levels may be elevated because of trauma.

Medical and Surgical Treatment. The fracture will first be immobilized by traction. If the patient cannot undergo surgery, this traction continues for about 6 weeks. However, if at all possible, surgery with open reduction of the fracture and internal fixation is done as soon as possible. This allows the patient to become mobile soon after the injury, thus preventing severe complications of immobility, which particularly affect the older person.

Open reduction of the fracture is done in the operating room. An incision is made and the bone ends lined up. The bones are fixated together (*internal fixation*) by use of pins, nails, screws, or metal plates (sometimes called *hip pinning*), or by the use of an *intermedullary nail.* If these devices cannot provide stabilization, the head of the femur is removed and replaced with a *prosthesis.* Some surgeons implant a prosthesis on all fractured hips. The hip prosthesis provides stabilization and also prevents complications, such as nonunion of bones and death of the joint, which can

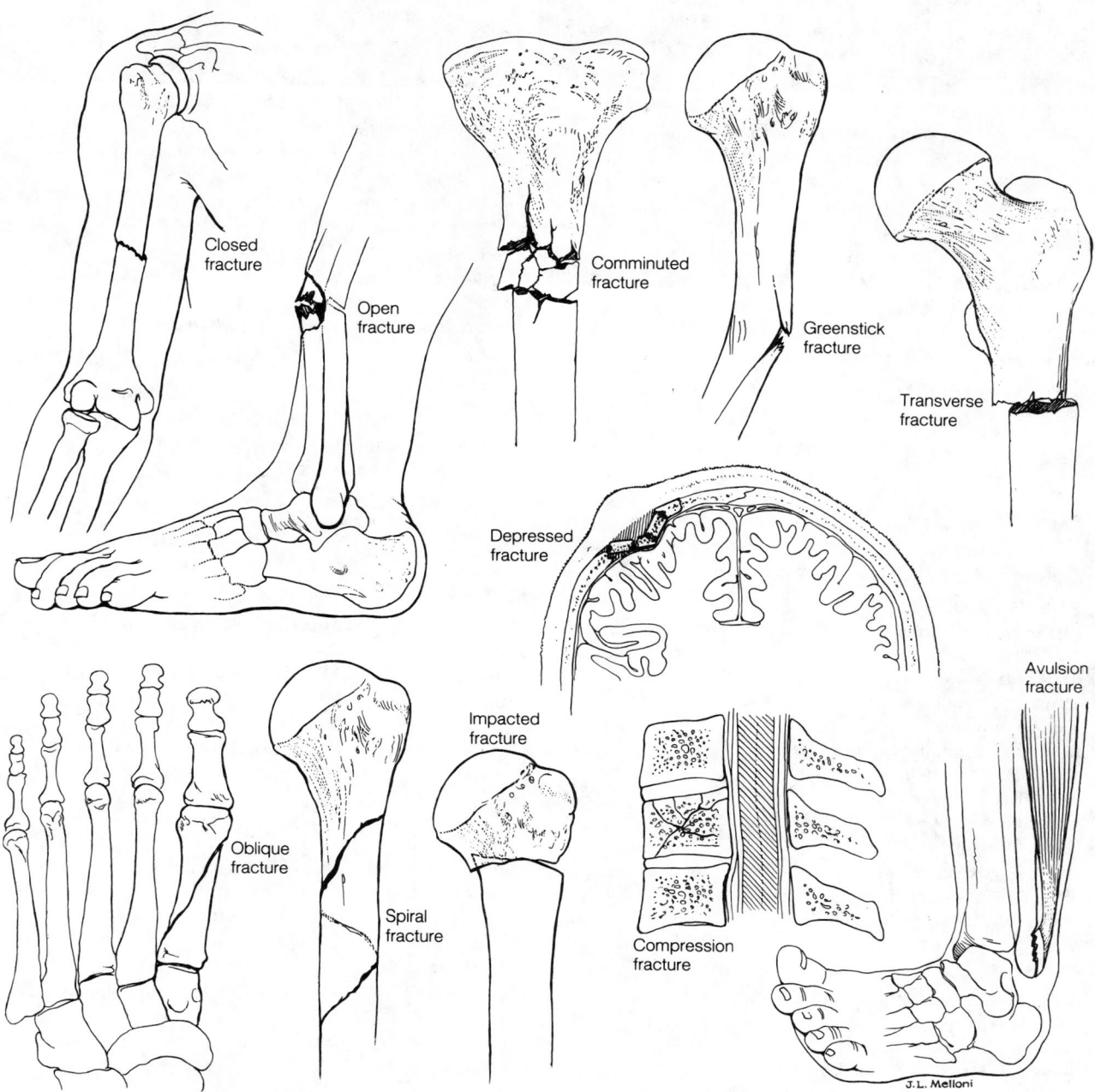

Figure 70-8. Types and patterns of fractures. (From Suddarth DS. The Lippincott Manual of Nursing Practice, Ed 5. Philadelphia, J.B. Lippincott, 1991.)

occur as a result of poor blood supply to the joint or bone. (In many cases today, total hip arthroplasty or replacement is done, which provides even more comfort and quicker mobility.)

Nursing Considerations: Preoperative and Postoperative. Routine preoperative care is carried out, with special attention to nutrition and hydration. The patient is carefully instructed in routine postoperative procedures, as well as special precautions (such as flexion limitations

or restrictions concerning how much weight can be supported on the affected side). Nursing skills in caring for the patient with a hip replacement are given in the accompanying box.

Frequent turning in bed is important. A special pillow called an *abduction pillow* should be placed between the patient's legs when turning the patient (Fig. 70-9). *(Rationale: This pillow prevents adduction, which could result in dislocation of the prosthesis.)*

Ida McBride is a 65-year-old widowed female with a history of osteoporosis who was hospitalized after falling at home and fracturing her left femur. At the time of the fall she was living independently in her own home, frequently baby-sitting for her daughter's children. She is 5 days postsurgery: an open reduction with internal fixation. She has begun physical therapy with the goal of progressive ambulation and return to her prefracture level of independence in everyday activities. One of the nursing diagnoses from her plan of care is featured below.

Nursing Diagnosis: *Physical Mobility, related to musculoskeletal impairment following fractured hip repair*

Goal 1: Patient verbalizes the physician's instructions about position and activity

Goal 2: Whenever observed the patient's position is compatible with restrictions

Goal 3: Patient correctly demonstrates quadriceps settings, gluteal settings, breathing exercises, exercises for the upper extremities, and exercises for the unoperated extremities

Goal 4: Patient progresses from simple standing to walking with a walker (11/3) to walking with one person (11/7)

Nursing Actions (assess/do/teach)	Rationale	Evaluative Statement
1. Carefully check the physician's instructions about position and activity. Before moving the patient explain what you are going to do and how the patient can help. General guidelines: Keep the leg abducted, avoid acute flexion, prevent external rotation of the leg on the operated side.	These instructions usually depend on the operative approach.	11/2; Goal 1 met; patient able to describe position and activity restrictions and explains their rationale. 11/4; Goal 2 partially met; patient still crosses her ankles and forgets to keep her legs abducted.
2. Teach exercises the patient can do in bed prior to beginning ambulation.	Exercises prepare the muscles for walking and facilitate good venous return.	11/2; Goal 3 met; patient correctly demonstrates the exercises and is frequently observed exercising in bed; strong motivation to regain independence.
3. Reinforce the ambulation skills the patient is learning in physical therapy and use them when assisting the patient out of bed to the bath room or for walks. Ensure that proper safety precautions are taken with each interaction. Praise the progress the patient is making and celebrate the achievement of milestones: independent balance, use of walker, one-person assist, etc.	Ambulation will increase muscle mass, tone and strength and facilitate mastery. Patient's history of osteoporosis places her at high risk for reinjury. These activities promote self-esteem and confidence in ability to continue.	11/3; Goal 4 met; patient began walking with walker today but is terrified she will fall and moves reluctantly. Continue to assist and encourage.
4. Refer the patient to social service for discharge planning if help will be needed once the patient returns home.		

◆ Routine postoperative care is provided. This includes deep breathing, high-protein diet, and oral fluids in addition to intravenous fluids.

◆ Neurovascular assessments usually are done every 15 minutes for 1 hour, every hour for 24 hours, every 4 hours for 24 hours, and every 8 hours thereafter.

◆ Anticoagulant therapy may be initiated, and antiembolism stockings are worn.

◆ Frequent turning in bed (from unaffected side to back) is important.

◆ Care is provided to prevent the most common complications: infection and dislocation of the prosthesis or pins.

◆ The incision and drainage are evaluated frequently. If a drainage device is in place, it is emptied frequently and the drainage measured.

◆ Dressings are changed as needed, using sterile technique.

◆ Good skin care is essential; the skin must be kept dry. Pressure areas must be relieved to prevent skin breakdown.

◆ Frequent back care is given every 2 hours while the patient is in bed.

◆ Following insertion of a hip prosthesis and sometimes following open reduction, the leg usually is maintained in an abducted position and in neutral or slight external rotation. The surgeon's orders for positioning and movement must be followed precisely.

◆ Active and passive range of motion (ROM) exercises are given as ordered.

◆ A trapeze should be placed on the overhead frame. This will help in using the bedpan and in moving.

◆ Early mobility is vital, particularly in the older person. Complications of immobility cause more deaths than the surgery itself.

◆ The patient should be assisted into a chair two or three times a day. Check with the physician for any flexion restrictions before getting the patient into a chair.

◆ Progressive ambulation usually begins on the day after surgery. The physician will determine how much weight the patient is allowed to bear on the operative side. Do not ambulate the patient before checking on this information. A walker is often used.

◆ The patient is instructed in routine postoperative procedures and precautions.

◆ Turn the patient to the *unaffected side* with a pillow between the knees to provide good alignment.

◆ Position the patient comfortably and support with pillows or sandbags and trochanter rolls so the body is in correct alignment and contractures will not develop. The patient may usually be allowed to remain in this position for 2 hours.

◆ Turn onto the back again. The patient usually remains in this position for an hour.

◆ Elevate the head of the bed at least 30° when the patient is on his or her back. *(Rationale: This prevents aspiration.)*

◆ The patient is again turned to the *unaffected* side. (*Note:* The patient with a hip fracture is usually *not* placed on the affected side, although some surgeons allow this.)

◆ A special fluidized or airflow bed may be used (see Chapter 44.)

Neoplasms

Bone Tumors

Bone tumors are of two types: primary and metastatic. *Primary* bone tumors are those that originate in the bone. They may be benign or malignant. *Benign* bone tumors are usually well circumscribed, slow growing, and seldom spread. Benign bone tumors include osteomas, chondromas, giant cell tumors, cysts, and osteoid osteomas. Primary *malignant* bone tumors are rare. They include osteogenic sarcoma and multiple myelomas. These are extremely malignant and metastasize early, often to the lungs.

Metastatic bone tumors are those that travel to the bone *from some other part of the body*. This type of bone tumor is relatively common. Metastatic bone tumors come from primary lesions in the lung, breast, prostate, kidney, ovary, or thyroid. Carcinomas tend to metastasize to bone more commonly than do sarcomas. The prognosis with metastatic bone disease is poor.

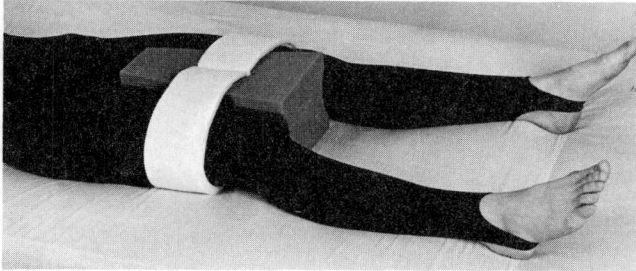

Figure 70-9. An abduction pillow may be used after a total hip replacement to prevent dislocation of the prosthesis.

Nursing skills for turning the patient with a hip replacement are:

◆ Any turning for the patient who has had a hip fracture surgically stabilized should be specifically ordered by the surgeon.

The symptoms of a bone tumor include pain, swelling, restricted motion, and aching. One of the most significant signs of a malignant bone tumor is *pathologic fracture*. The bone fractures because it is weakened, even though there has been no external trauma.

Diagnosis of bone tumors is made by x-ray, biopsy, frozen section, and laboratory evaluations. Whenever malignant tumors are suspected, chest films are routinely taken to look for pulmonary metastases (spread to the lungs). A skeletal radiologic survey (bone scan, scintiscan), MRI, or CT scan is done to locate additional bone lesions.

Treatment may consist of surgical removal of a primary tumor, chemotherapy, or radiation therapy. Metastatic bone lesions are usually treated with palliative measures (as opposed to curative). Nursing care is centered on patient comfort, pain control, and prevention of pathologic fractures.

Keys for Review

Key Questions for Critical Thinking

1. You work on the orthopedic floor. An 80-year-old man has a closed fracture of the leg. Formulate a teaching plan for him. Contrast your teaching of the 80-year-old man with an 8-year-old boy with the same type of fracture. Describe your teaching of the boy's parents.
2. List orthopedic complications and their prevention. Identify medical treatment given for each complication. Outline nursing care with rationale.
3. Your patient has arthritis in the hands. Describe how you would explain her condition to her. Identify adjustments she will have to make to the condition and explain to her how best she can live with the arthritis and adjustments.
4. Compare a hip fracture in a 30-year-old person and an 80-year-old person. Contrast medical and surgical treatment of each. Identify differences in nursing care between the two patients. Discuss the possible prognosis for each.

Key Readings

Beaver BM (Guest Editor). Trauma Symposium in Nursing Clinics of North America, March, 1990

Berkow R (Ed). The Merck Manual of Diagnosis and Therapy, Ed 16. Rahway, NJ, Merck & Co, 1992

NANDA Nursing Diagnoses: Definitions and Classifications 1992. Philadelphia, North American Nursing Diagnosis Association, 1992

O'Toole M (Ed). Miller-Keane Encyclopedia and Dictionary of Medicine, Nursing, and Allied Health, Ed 5. Philadelphia, W.B. Saunders, 1992

Rodts MF (Guest Editor). Orthopedic Nursing Symposium in Nursing Clinics of North America, March, 1991

Rodts MF (Guest Editor). Sports Nursing Symposium in Nursing Clinics of North America, March, 1991

Key Readings (continued)

Smeltzer SC, Bare BG. Brunner and Suddarth's Textbook of Medical-Surgical Nursing, Ed 7. Philadelphia, J.B. Lippincott, 1992

Suddarth DS. The Lippincott Manual of Nursing Practice, Ed 5. Philadelphia, J.B. Lippincott, 1991

Taylor C, Lillis C, LeMone P. Fundamentals of Nursing: The Art and Science of Nursing Care, Ed 2. Philadelphia, J.B. Lippincott, 1993

Thomas CL (Ed). Taber's Cyclopedic Medical Dictionary, Ed 17. Philadelphia, F.A. Davis, 1993

Keys to Learning More

Chapter 71: nervous system disorders
Chapter 76: cancer
Chapter 81: digestive disorders, TMJ, tooth disorders
Chapter 85: geriatric disorders
Chapter 89: rehabilitation

Key Resources

Arthritis Foundation
1314 Spring Street, NW
Atlanta, GA 30309
404/872-7100

March of Dimes Birth Defects Foundation
1275 Mamaroneck Avenue
White Plains, NY 10605
914/428-7100

Muscular Dystrophy Association
3561 Sunrise Avenue
Tucson, AZ 85718
602/529-2000

Key Resources (continued)

National Institute of Arthritis and Musculoskeletal and
Skin Diseases
  National Institutes of Health
  Bethesda, MD 20892
  301/496-4000
National Multiple Sclerosis Society
  205 East 42nd Street
  New York, NY 10017
  212/532-3060

Key Resources (continued)

National Scoliosis Foundation
  93 Concord Avenue
  PO Box 547
  Belmont, MA 02178
Osteoporosis Foundation
  612 North Michigan Avenue, Suite 510
  Chicago, IL 60611
Scoliosis Association
  PO Box 51353
  Raleigh, NC 27609
  919/846-2639

71 Nervous System Disorders

Keys for Learning

Learning Objectives

♦ Briefly review neuroanatomy, using related terminology and acronyms.
♦ Describe neurologic diagnostic tests.
♦ Describe and demonstrate care of the patient who has a craniotomy.
♦ Discuss the significance of increased intracranial pressure, its signs and symptoms, and the role of the nurse in observing for it.
♦ Identify the major classifications of seizures, seizure precautions, and nursing care during a seizure.
♦ Describe the most common chronic and acute disorders of the brain and nervous system.
♦ Describe nursing considerations related to care of the person with a head injury.
♦ Describe general principles of nursing care for patients with any type of paralysis.
♦ Apply the nursing process to the person with disorders of the nervous system.

Key Terms

ataxia	intracranial pressure
aura	laceration
autonomic dysreflexia	meningitis
cephalalgia	neuralgia
concussion	opisthotonos
contusion	paraplegia
craniotomy	quadriplegia
epilepsy	seizure
hematoma	vertigo

Keys to Understanding This Chapter

Chapter 18: nervous system anatomy and physiology
Chapter 28: special diets
Chapter 32: sudden death and CPR

Keys to Understanding This Chapter
(continued)

Chapter 43: body mechanics and positioning, including assistive devices
Chapter 44: special beds
Chapter 46: bladder and bowel retraining
Chapter 50: head-to-toe nursing assessment
Chapter 52: patient comfort and pain management
Unit Ten: surgical intervention
Unit Eleven: pharmacology and medication administration
Unit Thirteen: neurologic considerations in pediatrics

Key Points

♦ Because the brain and nervous system control the body's movements, disorders may cause unwanted movement or immobility.
♦ Increased intracranial pressure may have many causes. It is a significant sign of brain and spinal cord disorders. One of the first and most important signs of increased intracranial pressure (or other disorders of the brain) is a change in the level of consciousness.
♦ Seizure disorders may have different manifestations, ranging from generalized tonic–clonic movements to an uncontrolled movement without loss of consciousness.
♦ Degenerative disorders of the nervous system may cause difficulties in movement, sensory deficits, or varying degrees of alteration in mental status.
♦ Infectious disorders of the nervous system can quickly become life-threatening.
♦ Brain and spinal cord injuries can result in a range of physical and mental deficits, including paralysis.
♦ Most brain tumors are nonmalignant. Benign tumors, however, cause pressure on the brain and can be fatal.

Rosdahl CB: Textbook of Basic Nursing, 6th ed. © 1995 J.B. Lippincott Company

Key Learning Activities

◆ Interview a person who is paralyzed. Report to the class about the patient's rehabilitation and feelings.
◆ Make a poster for your facility emphasizing prevention of head injuries. Examples include automobile air bags, seat belts, child restraint seats, and motorcycle/ bicycle helmets.
◆ Following interviews of several nurses, make a list of "tips for feeding patients who have difficulty chewing and swallowing."

The medical specialty related to the nervous system is neurology (neuro). The physician trained in this specialty is a *neurologist*; surgeons are called *neurosurgeons*. The nurse specializing in care of people with a disorder of the nervous system is called a *neurologic nurse*.

Anatomy and Physiology Review

The nervous system is divided into two major parts: central nervous system (CNS), consisting of brain and spinal cord, and the peripheral nervous system, consisting of cranial and spinal nerves. These major systems control voluntary and involuntary movements. The autonomic nervous system consists of a specialized group of peripheral fibers that regulate involuntary actions, such as heart actions.

Nervous tissue is made up of cells called neurons. No two neurons are alike. Electric and chemical reactions occur within the body's three types of neurons (sensory, motor, and interneurons), thus carrying messages to and from all parts of the body and the brain.

Diagnostic Tests

Many x-rays and other diagnostic tests are used to determine the integrity or functioning of the brain, spinal cord, and nerves.

X-ray Evaluation

Computerized Tomography

Computerized tomography (*CT scan*), also called *computed tomography*, is a technique that incorporates x-rays and computer technology to produce an image of a transverse plane of the body. (It was formerly called CAT scan, computerized axial tomography.) The x-ray beam passes through the desired plane and is picked up by a scintillator, which feeds the computer the information. The computer can display the black and white images on a TV screen or can produce a permanent printout or photograph. Because it is non-invasive and therefore safer for the patient than a lumbar puncture, tomography is becoming more widely used for detecting neurologic abnormalities. An injec-

Key Abbreviations and Acronyms: Neurologic Nursing

ADL	Activities of daily living
ALS	Amyotrophic lateral sclerosis
ANS	Autonomic nervous system
C-2, C-3, etc.	Refers to level of injury in the cervical section of the spinal cord
CNS	Central nervous system
CSF	Cerebrospinal fluid
CT	Computed tomography, (CAT-computed axial tomography)
EEG	Electroencephalogram, electroencephalograph
HD	Huntington's disease
ICP	Intracranial pressure (↑ ICP = increased intracranial pressure)
IPPB	intermittent positive pressure breathing
IVD	Intervertebral disk
L-1, L-2, etc.	Refers to level of injury in the lumbar area of the spinal cord
LOC	Level of consciousness
LP	Lumbar puncture
MRI	Magnetic resonance imaging
MG	Myasthenia gravis
MS	Multiple sclerosis
PCA	personal care attendant
PERRLA	Pupils equal, round, react to light, accommodation OK (+C-eyes coordinated)
PET scan	Position emission tomography
PNS	Peripheral nervous system
PROM	Passive range of motion
T-1, T-2, etc.	Refers to level of injury in the thoracic area of the spinal cord

tion of radiopaque dye can be used to visualize the brain or spinal cord. (Radiopaque dyes *cannot be used* if the patient is allergic to shellfish or iodine. See Chapter 50 for added precautions.)

This test is not appropriate for the patient who:

◆ Is claustrophobic or very large (the machine is small)
◆ Cannot cooperate (unless sedated)
◆ Has a head tumor
◆ Cannot lie still for 20 to 30 minutes

Positron Emission Tomography

Positron emission tomography (*PET scan*) is a type of tomography used to study changes within the brain, in which glucose containing a radioisotope is injected.

The patient is kept flat in bed for a few hours after this test and is observed for signs of irritation, such as a stiff neck or pain when bending the head forward. The patient is also observed for signs of anaphylaxis (severe allergic response).

Magnetic Resonance Imaging

Magnetic resonance imaging (*MRI*) is the most current development in imaging. Many radiologists feel that MRI will replace CT scanning in certain cases. MRI does not use ionizing radiation; thus, it is not believed to be biologically hazardous. It is particularly sensitive in identifying multiple sclerosis plaques and the other abnormal changes in demyelinating diseases. MRI can distinguish normal from abnormal tissue and can predict such occurrences as stroke, heart attack, and cancerous lesions before they appear with clinical symptoms.

Because MRI uses a strong magnetic field, it is contraindicated in any patient who:

◆ Has any metallic implant (such as hip prosthesis, metal plates) or internal surgical clips
◆ Has gold fillings in the teeth
◆ Has a pacemaker or heart valve prosthesis
◆ Has a metal intravenous intracatheter
◆ Is a metal worker (may have tiny metal fragments in the body)
◆ Is extremely claustrophobic
◆ Cannot lie on his or her back for 45 to 60 minutes
◆ Has a severe head tremor
◆ Is not able to cooperate (unless sedated)

The following are considerations:

◆ Do not carry metal scissors, flashlight, or similar objects if you are accompanying the patient to the test.
◆ Have the patient remove all jewelry.
◆ Explain to the patient that he or she will be totally enclosed in the machine for about an hour.
◆ Explain that a clicking noise will be heard throughout the procedure.
◆ Explain that the inside of the machine is very shiny and bright. It will be more comfortable if the eyes are kept closed.
◆ Make sure the patient understands that a technician will be monitoring the entire test and will not leave him or her alone.

Special Considerations in Children
MRI And CT Scan

◆ The child may be permitted to take a favorite toy or blanket along for the test. (For MRI, make sure there is no metal in the toy.)
◆ Sedation is often required.
◆ Maintain safety.

Cerebral Angiography and Arteriography

In rare instances, angiography or arteriography may be done. An *angiogram* is an x-ray of any blood vessel, and an *arteriogram* is an x-ray of an artery. The nurse should obtain a baseline neurologic assessment before beginning this procedure because one risk of this invasive procedure is the possibility of dislodging a thrombus, which could cause a stroke (cerebrovascular accident). The procedure involves injecting a radiopaque substance into the carotid or femoral artery; x-rays are then taken of the blood vessels in the brain to detect tumors or abnormal conditions in the blood vessels. The nurse should be alert for any signs of allergy to the drug injected for the test. *Severe* anaphylaxis usually occurs immediately, if it is going to occur.

The nurse observes for symptoms of muscular weakness or twitching in the face or extremities or respiratory difficulty. If any of these occur, the physician must be notified immediately.

After the x-ray, ice or a sandbag is applied to the insertion site to reduce edema and to prevent hematoma formation. The area is checked for bleeding every 30 minutes for several hours. The color, temperature, and pedal pulse of the leg are observed if the femoral artery was used as the injection site. Because of the radiopaque dye used, fluids should be encouraged, unless contraindicated.

Myelography

In some cases, it is necessary to visualize the spinal cord further by taking a *myelogram*. A lumbar puncture is done and a radiopaque substance is injected into the spinal canal. The patient, in the prone position, is tilted so the dye will flow around the spinal cord; then x-rays can be taken to detect tumors or a ruptured intervertebral disk. The radiopaque substance used today is *water soluble*.

Brain Scan

Although largely replaced by the CT scan, the radioactive brain scan (scintiscan) is still done occasionally. A radioactive substance is injected, after which a scintillator is used. The rationale for this procedure is that a site of pathology will accumulate the radioisotope to a greater degree than normal brain tissue.

Other Diagnostic Tests

Lumbar Puncture

The lumbar puncture (LP, spinal tap) is usually done to obtain a specimen or measure pressure of cerebrospinal fluid (CSF). Other reasons are included in the list below. The LP is performed using a hollow needle with a *stylet* (guide) inside. This apparatus is inserted into the subarachnoid space in the lumbar region of the spinal canal, using strict aseptic technique (Fig. 71-1).

Reasons for lumbar puncture include:

◆ To measure pressure of CSF
◆ To obtain a sample of CSF for culture and sensitivity, blood, pus, or other substance levels (eg, protein, glucose)
◆ To inject an anesthetic or other drug
◆ To inject air for special tests

Lumbar puncture is performed by the physician under strict sterile conditions. The nurse assists during the procedure, as outlined in the following skill.

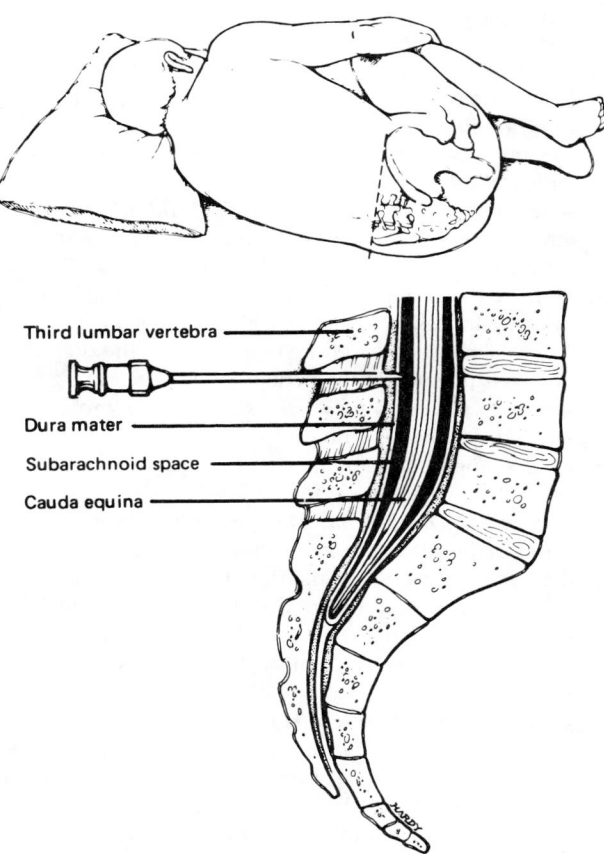

Third lumbar vertebra

Dura mater

Subarachnoid space

Cauda equina

Figure 71-1. Technique of lumbar puncture. The interspaces between the spines of L-3 and L-4 are just below the line joining the anterosuperior iliac spines.

Nursing Skill
Assisting During a Lumbar Puncture

Supplies and Equipment

Sterile gloves; unsterile gloves
Dressing materials
Local anesthetic solution (sterile), usually lidocaine (Xylocaine)
Bath blanket
Prepacked sterile, disposable lumbar puncture kit
Antiseptic solution
Specimen labels
External light source (may be needed)

Procedure

See Chapter 54 for a review of sterile technique.

1. Make sure a signed permit has been obtained from the patient. Nursing students do not witness these.
2. Be sure the procedure has been thoroughly explained to the patient. The patient needs to know that a small amount of CSF will be withdrawn for testing and that the site will be anesthetized. *(Rationale: No invasive procedure can be done without informed consent.)*
3. Wash your hands. Wear gloves. *(Rationale: To prevent the spread of microorganisms.)* The physician will wear sterile gloves and will often use goggles or a face shield, per universal precautions.
4. Bring all equipment to the bedside. Have the patient empty the bladder. *(Rationale: To avoid the discomfort of a full bladder.)*
5. Identify the patient. *(Rationale: Make sure you have the right patient.)*
6. Assess the patient's vital signs before the procedure begins. *(Rationale: To provide a baseline assessment for later comparison.)*
7. Remove the patient's clothing. Put on a hospital gown, opening in the back. Drape with a bath blanket or sheet. When the procedure begins, move the drape to uncover the back of the patient. *(Rationale: The gown gives easy access to the proper site. Draping provides privacy and warmth, if needed.)*
8. Place equipment within reach of the physician. Open packs and make sure extra sterile gloves are available. *(Rationale: This will make the procedure more efficient.)*
9. Position the patient on the side with the lower part of the back at the edge of the bed. Help the patient to draw the knees up toward the chin and bend the head forward as shown in Figure 71-1. Explain to the patient that this will enhance comfort. Tell the person to lie very still. You may need to hold the person in place. *(Rationale: This position increases the space between the lower vertebrae and makes needle insertion easier. Any sudden movement is dangerous and could cause spinal cord damage.)*
10. Explain the procedure; offer reassurance. *(Rationale: This procedure can be frightening. The patient needs to be relaxed.)*
11. Assist as requested. You may be asked to remove caps of bottles, to label specimens, or to assist in bandaging the insertion site. *(Rationale: This speeds up the procedure and ensures accurate specimen identification.)*
12. Note the beginning CSF pressure, as measured by the physician. Assess the color and clarity of the CSF; it should be a pale color and clear. *(Rationale: This information is important in diagnosing the patient's disorder.)*
13. Assess the patient for any difficulty. *(Rationale: Untoward side effects are rare, but they can occur.)*
14. After the procedure, return the patient to a comfortable position in bed. Keep the patient's head flat (supine) for at least 6 hours, or as otherwise ordered. *(Rationale: This lessens the possibility of CSF leakage and postpuncture headache.)*
15. Remove and dispose of equipment. (Wear gloves.) Finish labeling specimens and completing request forms: send to the laboratory immediately in an approved biohazard bag. Properly dispose of your gloves. Wash your hands. Document the procedure carefully. *(Rationale: It is important to the healthcare team that this procedure was done.)*
16. Assess the patient's vital signs and neurologic signs. Compare to baseline data. Assess for level of consciousness (LOC). Report any unusual findings to the physician. *(Rationale: To assess for side effects from the procedure.)*
17. Encourage fluids, unless contraindicated. Intake and output is often ordered for 24 hours. The patient is often encouraged to lie flat. *(Rationale: It is important to rehydrate the patient; fluids and not elevating the head help minimize headache.)*
18. Monitor the insertion site for leakage of CSF, hematoma formation, or edema. *(Rationale: These are possible unwanted results of LP.)*
19. Assess severity of headache. Report severe headache, which is unrelieved by mild analgesics, as ordered. Report any headache that lasts more than 24 hours. *(Rationale: These may be symptoms of potential complications.)*

> **Special Considerations in Children**
> ### Lumbar Puncture
>
> ◆ The nurse will have to hold the child. Sometimes the parents are willing to help hold the child; this is less frightening to the child.
> ◆ Because the needles are smaller, insertion may be easier in children.

Potential complications after LP are:

◆ Severe pounding headache, unrelieved by mild analgesics
◆ Malaise
◆ Nausea, with or without vomiting
◆ Irritation/hematoma at injection site
◆ Leg or buttock pain (temporary)

◆ CNS infection
◆ Brain herniation (most severe complication)

Electroencephalography

Electroencephalography (EEG) records the electrical impulses generated by the brain. It is used frequently in the diagnosis of seizure disorders, brain tumors, blood clots, infections, and sleep disorders. Another important use of the EEG is to provide confirmation of brain death (electrocerebral silence).

The electroencephalograph is the machine that makes the graph (*encephalogram*) of these impulses. It is connected to electrodes placed on the patient's forehead and scalp by means of a special glue called *collodion*. In some cases, a cap containing the electrodes is placed on the head; in a few clinics, tiny needles are used. The procedure is painless, has no after effects, and requires 1 to 2 hours. (If needles are used, there is a slight possibility of infection. A shampoo may be needed to remove collodion.) The preparation of the patient may involve sedation or the patient may be requested not to sleep for a period of time. These measures will allow a sleeping or resting EEG to be done.

Explain to the patient that no electric shock will be felt and the EEG procedure cannot determine thoughts or mental ability. Tell the person that he or she will be asked to open and close the eyes and sometimes, to perform other movements on command.

In some cases, lights will be flashed, the patient will be asked to watch a repeating pattern on a TV monitor, or a small electrical stimulus will be given. The brain's responses to these stimuli are recorded. These responses are called *evoked responses*.

Videotelemetry Monitoring

Hospitals specializing in neurology and seizure disorders use a diagnostic tool called videotelemetry monitoring. Videotelemetry monitoring involves video, au-

dio, and EEG monitoring of a person 24 hours a day or all night. When the patient experiences a seizure, it can be seen and heard on videotape as well as electrically by EEG.

When the seizure begins, be sure to provide the usual safety for the patient. In addition, make sure the patient is within camera range, so the event will be filmed. It is also important to uncover the patient, if possible, so the entire body can be visualized.

Medical and Surgical Treatment

Common Medical Treatment

Neurologic procedures are described with specific disorders.

Common Surgical Treatment

Surgery may be performed on the brain by entering the skull, may be performed on the spinal cord itself, or may be performed on other nerves. (The treatment of disorders in the bones of the spinal column is discussed in Chapter 70.)

Craniotomy

Surgical entry into the skull (cranium) is called a **craniotomy**. This invasive procedure is performed for many reasons. One of the most common is brain tumor. (Any tumor must be removed because it places pressure on the brain.) A *craniectomy* is a procedure that removes a portion of skull bone.

The patient is reassured that there is little pain involved in brain surgery because the skin is locally anesthetized. The procedure is noisy because the surgeon will drill out a part of the skull bone; but there will be no pain from the skull or brain because the brain has no sensory nerves. The patient is almost certain to be apprehensive. The nurse's concerned, competent preoperative care helps reassure the patient. The family also needs reassurance.

❖ Nursing Process

Data Collection

Chapter 50 describes a head-to-toe assessment, including that of the nervous system. This assessment establishes a baseline for future comparison. The nurse should report any changes in the baseline level.

The nurse assesses the general appearance and mobility level of the patient, LOC, muscle tone and strength, balance, coordination, protective reflexes, eye signs, and an overview of the function of some of the cranial nerves. The box on page 1019 lists some of the components of a neurologic nursing assessment.

Additionally the nurse observes the patient's emotional response to the situation. Does the disorder affect social activities, self-care, and self-esteem? Does the patient seem anxious or fearful of outcomes?

Nursing Diagnosis

Most nursing diagnoses found in neurology patients are a result of a specific neurologic dysfunction. Some diagnoses may be the same but have different causal factors. The following are examples of nursing diagnoses that may appear on nursing care plans of neurologic patients:

◆ Self-care Deficit related to sensory-motor deficits
◆ Social Isolation related to unpredictability of seizures
◆ Altered Oral Mucous Membrane related to effects of medication, trauma during a seizure
◆ Altered Health Maintenance related to insufficient knowledge of condition and treatment
◆ Chronic Low Self-esteem related to change in body image
◆ High Risk for Disuse Syndrome related to effects of immobility
◆ Fear related to changes in role responsibilities
◆ Anxiety related to threat to self-concept
◆ Altered Nutrition: Less Than Body Requirement related to (1) difficulty in obtaining and preparing food, (2) chewing and swallowing difficulties
◆ High Risk for Urinary Infection related to invasive procedures, immobility
◆ High Risk for Constipation related to immobility
◆ Hopelessness related to deteriorating physiologic condition
◆ High Risk for Injury related to unsteady gait, uncontrolled movements
◆ Activity Intolerance related to generalized weakness

Planning and Implementation

The patient and nurse plan together for effective care to meet needs based on the nursing diagnosis. The nurse provides preoperative and postoperative care for the patient undergoing a craniotomy. The patient with a neurologic disorder may need help also in doing activities of daily living (ADL), performing exercises, finding comfortable body alignment and positions, controlling elimination needs, meeting nutritional needs, dealing with sensory and emotional problems, and understanding more about the disorder, its prognosis, and its treatment. A nursing care plan is developed to meet these needs. Two sample nursing care plans for a pa-

tient with a neurologic disorder are given later in the chapter.

Providing Preoperative Care

Before a craniotomy, routine preoperative preparation is followed. In addition, the patient's head or a portion of it is shaved; the patient must be informed before it is done. (Often the hair is not shaved until the patient is in the operating room area.) A special permit must be signed by the patient or a legal guardian before hair can be removed or surgery done. (The hair is shaved and put into a paper bag and labeled. It can be used for a wig or hairpiece if the patient desires.)

If the patient is to remain awake during a craniotomy, he or she should be informed of this before the surgery. Medications may be given that sedate the patient yet allow him or her to be aroused, so that when the surgeon stimulates various parts of the brain during the surgery, the patient can respond. The patient should be advised beforehand whether the surgeon will ask questions or ask for specific movements during surgery.

Surgery may take from 2 to 6 hours. Anything the nurse can do to make the waiting period more bearable for the family will be helpful. Taking time to say a few words to them at intervals will let them know that they are not forgotten.

Providing Postoperative Care

During the immediate postoperative period, the patient requires expert observation and nursing care, usually provided by intensive care nurses. Comparisons are made continually between the patient's present condition and the findings of the initial neurologic examination (the baseline assessment). It is important to note any changes, such as signs of increasing ICP.

The patient's vital signs and respiratory status are monitored regularly. The head of the bed is elevated and nasogastric suction usually is in place to help prevent aspiration. The patient should be positioned according to the physician's orders and the dressings should be checked for bleeding and CSF, especially in the back and on the side. Frequent craniotomy checks are vital. These include noting the patient's neurologic signs, LOC, orientation to time and place, and ability to speak clearly. It is important to check the patient's ability to grasp equally in both hands and to check the ability to move each foot in any position on command. If the patient is allowed out of bed, the patient's ability to stand with the eyes closed (Romberg test) is checked. The patient should be able to stand on each foot without holding on to anything. Any deviation from normal must be reported immediately. If in doubt, consult your team leader; the patient's neurologic status can change very rapidly.

During convalescence, the patient needs encouragement and understanding. For example, the patient may find that it takes time to regain control of bodily movements, or that he or she may spill food and drop things and may become dizzy when walking. The patient is reassured. To ensure the patient's safety, assistance is given as needed.

Providing Exercise

It is important to provide the patient with as much active and passive exercise as possible to prevent contractures, muscle atrophy, and other *disuse deformities.* Many devices are used to assist patients who are paralyzed or otherwise physically challenged. These include the patient lift, wheelchair, braces, and splints (see Chapters 43 and 89).

Assisting with ADL

The patient may need assistance with ADL. These include skin care, special eye care, mouth care, and care of the nails and hair (see Chapter 45). The may also need assistance to manage bowel or bladder elimination (see Chapter 46). It is important to maintain adequate nutritional status to rebuild strength and to prevent further breakdown (see Chapter 28).

Providing Comfort With Special Devices

Several special beds may be used for immobilized patients. These include the Clinitron, the Restcue, the Kin-Air, and others. The most important goals of such beds are to prevent skin breakdown and alleviate pain.

For example, one of the beds, the Kin-Air, operates on the principle of varying levels of air inflation. It has many configurations for optimum patient comfort and safety (such a bed is pictured in Chapter 44). It is important to follow the manufacturer's specifications when using any of these special beds.

Special Considerations in Aging
Skin Care

Often the skin of the older person is very fragile, and skin care is even more important. Special antidecubitus beds or mattresses may be ordered as a routine in the fragile elderly neurologic patient.

Special "neuro" chairs also aid in transferring patients in and out of bed and serve as a comfortable place for the patient to rest when out of bed. These chairs are adjustable to various positions and can be placed in high Fowler's or Trendelenburg positions if necessary. Various commercial reclining chairs are also used.

The following method is used when *assisting the patient to move, using the "neuro chair"*:

◆ To get the patient out of bed, put the chair in the flat position and raise it to the same level as the bed. (*Rationale: It will be easier to transfer an immobile patient if the bed is in high position and flat, to match the bed.*)
◆ Lock the wheels of the chair and the bed.
◆ Make sure you have enough help so the patient will not fall. Use a "bridge" if the patient is immobile.
◆ Move the patient from bed to the flattened chair, using proper body mechanics. Adjust the chair to a sitting position.
◆ Apply a patient safety device, if needed, to provide patient safety. (*Rationale: The patient may have spastic movements or seizures.*)
◆ Place the call light within reach.
◆ To return the patient to bed, reverse the process.

Implementing Seizure Precautions

A **seizure** is a spontaneous alteration in function resulting form an abnormal discharge of neurons in the brain. (Seizure disorders are discussed under Craniocerebral Disorders in the next section). When a patient is admitted to the healthcare facility with a history of seizures or when taking certain medications, he or she is placed on "seizure precautions." This means that special steps are taken to ensure that an injury will not occur as a result of a seizure. Seizure precautions must be tailored to the type of seizure experienced. Equipment, as listed in the accompanying box, is kept at the bedside.

Assessing Intracranial Pressure

Intracranial pressure (ICP) is the pressure exerted inside the cerebrospinal cavity by the brain, blood, and CSF. An increase in pressure occurs when one of these

---

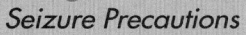

Nursing Skill Guidelines
Seizure Precautions

Bedside Equipment

◆ Oral airway. (*Rationale: To assist in maintaining a patent airway.*) *Note:* Do not insert if seizure activity has begun.
◆ Four side rails up and padded. (*Rationale: To prevent falls and promote safety.*)
◆ Suction set-up. (*Rationale: In case the patient has difficulty in handling secretions.*)
◆ Set-up of piggy-back port on an open IV. (*Rationale: In case the patient needs emergency drugs.*)
◆ Rectal or tympanic temperature probe. Oral temperatures are not as safe.

is altered in size or shape. This alteration causes reciprocal changes of the other contents because the skull is rigid and there is no extra space. The ICP may also be raised by normal body functions, such as straining at stool (the Valsalva maneuver); it may temporarily reach well over 100 mm Hg at this time.

The concern here is *abnormally* increased ICP (IICP, ↑ICP). Normal ICP is 4 to 13 mm Hg. (Sustained ICP over 15–20 mm Hg is considered "abnormally high".) Examples of conditions that may abnormally increase ICP include head injury, brain tumor, CNS infection, brain surgery, stroke, and hydrocephalus.

When one of the contents of the cerebrospinal cavity enlarges, the first consequence is venous compression. Then, displacement of the brain/spinal cord occurs. If the rise in ICP is not arrested, blood flow decreases, causing decreased oxygen to sensitive brain tissue (*cerebral hypoxia, cellular hypoxia*).

Increased ICP can occur suddenly and can progress rapidly. Usually, ↑ICP begins on one side of the brain, although both sides are quickly involved. IICP is a potential complication of many neurologic disorders; it can be fatal. It is important to detect and treat ↑ICP early, before complications occur. The earliest and most important sign of ↑ICP is *any change in LOC*. Other signs are presented in the accompanying box.

Keys to Nursing Assessment
Signs of Increased Intracranial Pressure

- Any change in *level of consciousness* (loss of consciousness, lethargy, confusion, seizures)
- Any change in *sensory/motor function* (slowed reflexes, slowed response time, restlessness, ataxia, aphasia, slowed speech)
- *Headache,* which becomes progressively worse or is aggravated by movement
- Change in *eye signs* or vision (change in pupil size, unequal pupils, slowed or no response to light, inability to follow examiner's finger, difficulty seeing)
- Change in *vital signs* (pulse below 60 or above 100; increased blood pressure; widening of pulse pressure; increased or lowered body temperature)
- Change in *respiration/respiratory distress* (occurs late—caused by pressure on brain stem)
- *Elevated intracranial pressure* (ICP), recorded on a monitoring device

Other signs/symptoms include:
- Nausea and vomiting (especially projectile vomiting)
- Urinary incontinence
- Bulging fontanels (in infant); elevation of bone segments
- Sudden changes in condition
- Leakage of CSF (clear yellow or pinkish) from nose or ear

ICP MONITORING. In special circumstances, the ICP is monitored by surgically inserted devices. These include the *intraventricular catheter* (most common), *subarachnoid* (*subdural*) *bolt* (or screw) and *epidural sensor* (least invasive). These devices are placed using strict sterile technique and sense ICP; a computer calculates it and prints it out. This information is used by the neurologist to determine the plan of care.

The catheter and screw may also be used to drain off CSF, which can be sent for laboratory analysis, or may be drained to relieve pressure.

Nursing Alert

Any break in an ICP monitoring system must be reported to the physician *immediately.* The system *must* remain sterile. Never move the patient's head up or down without specific physician's orders.

Evaluation

Periodically the nurse, patient, and family evaluate outcomes of care. Have short-term goals been met? Are long-term goals still realistic? Planning for further nursing care considers prognosis, complications, and patient response.

Craniocerebral Disorders

Herniation of the Brain

When ↑ICP exerts enough pressure to displace a portion of the brain, herniation can occur. *Herniation,* in this case, is a downward or sideways (lateral) pushing of a portion of the brain through an opening. This opening can be a natural intracranial opening, such as the foramen magnum. In this case, the brain would herniate through the large foramen (opening) in the occipital bone, which lies between the cranial cavity and the spinal cavity. Herniation can also occur through a previous craniotomy site or through an opening caused by trauma. Herniation is a dangerous and potentially fatal complication.

If the ICP is elevated enough, herniation of the brain can be precipitated by the withdrawal of even a small amount of CSF by LP. Therefore, a safer method of determining ICP in the person with suspected ↑ICP is ICP monitoring, discussed previously.

Headache

Headaches can be a minor discomfort or extremely painful. Some people suffer from chronic headaches. Although there are many types of headaches, only the more common types will be discussed here.

Headache as a Symptom

Headache (**cephalalgia**) is one of the most common symptoms of a neurologic disorder. It is also associated with many other diseases and disorders. Headache is not a disease in itself, but it is a *symptom* of an underlying disorder.

Headache often appears with such conditions as eye strain, sinusitis, muscle strain, ligament strain, cervical degenerative changes, or emotional tension and stress. It is also associated with brain tumors, hypertension (high blood pressure), and ↑ICP. Persistent or recurring headaches are frequently associated with true neurologic diseases or disorders such as brain tumors and aneurysms. Occasional headaches that disappear after an analgesic is taken should not be confused with a persistent headache.

Migraine Headache

Although migraine headache has been identified for years, its specific cause is still not known. It seems to be a result of a vascular disturbance, in which the blood vessels in the brain dilate abnormally.

The person may have a warning or premonition (aura) that a headache will occur. These warnings may include mood changes, anorexia, or numbness of a part of the body. In some cases, if treated immediately, the headache can be prevented. Medications used in migraine headaches are listed in the accompanying box.

Often migraine headaches are common in other family members; migraine occurs more frequently in people who have asthma, hay fever, and food allergies. It may be brought on by stress and is more common in the rigid, compulsive individual. Migraine may be aggravated by caffeine (or its sudden withdrawal), chocolate (which contains caffeine), nicotine, cheese, alcohol, or certain food preservatives such as monosodium glutamate. Fasting and missing meals may serve as a trigger, as does premenstrual fluid retention. Certain drugs, including hormonal contraceptives and reserpine (Serpasil), an antihypertensive agent, also may bring on migraines. Migraine headaches often occur on only one side of the head and are described as "throbbing"; many times, they are accompanied by nausea and vomiting.

Sometimes, an ice pack applied to the back of the neck, at the base of the skull, helps with the pain. A promising treatment is that of *biofeedback*. In this case, the patient needs special instructions in the technique. Acupuncture has been helpful to many people.

Cluster Headache

The cluster (histamine) headache is sometimes known as a cluster migraine because it tends to occur in groups or clusters, often at night. Like the migraine, it seems to be a result of a vascular disturbance. This

Key Medications

for Migraine Headache

- General analgesics: codeine, A.S.A. (aspirin), ibuprofen (Advil, Motrin), and acetaminophen (Tylenol)
- Combination drugs: acetaminophen and other drugs (such as Darvon compound)
- Vasoconstrictors or drugs that prevent vasodilation: ergot alkaloids
- Oxygen
- Sumatriptan (Imitrex), can be self-administered sub Q by patient at home
- Propranolol HCl (Inderal)
- Mild diuretics (to control fluid retention associated with menses)

Nursing Considerations

- Many of these drugs can be habit forming.
- Some of these drugs, particularly vasoconstrictors, have unpleasant side effects.
- All of these drugs are most effective if given immediately at the first sign of a headache.

can be a severely disabling headache. Cluster headaches are more common in men.

The onset of the headache is sudden and severe. It is often on one side only and involves the eye, neck, and face on that side. The eye may appear to bulge out and other symptoms of vasodilation are seen, such as edema, lacrimation (tear formation), rhinorrhea (runny nose), diaphoresis (sweating), and flushing of the affected side of the face. The pupil constricts, and the face and head are sensitive to external touch. The condition may disappear as suddenly as it occurs, although it may also continue for several days. Some drugs have been effective in selected cases, although no specific cure is known. These drugs include vasoconstrictor drugs, corticosteroids, and indomethacin (Indocin).

Seizure Disorders

An abnormal discharge of neurons in the brain will initiate a seizure. Seizures are also described as an "electrical storm" in the brain. The term **epilepsy** refers to a chronic seizure disorder. It is estimated that more than two million Americans have epilepsy.

As knowledge and techniques develop, classification systems for seizures have arisen over the years. The most practical classification used currently is the revised International Classification of Epileptic Seizures. The revision was made by Gastaut in 1969.[1] A classification

[1] Gastaut H. "Clinical and electroencephalographical classification of epileptic seizures." Epilepsia 11:102, 1970.

adapted from Gastaut's classification is given in the accompanying box. The classification is based on the clinical nature of the seizure's onset.

Under this system, there are two major classifications of seizure disorders:

♦ Partial—involve only part of the brain
♦ Generalized—involve the entire brain

It is believed that seizures may not be simply of one type. Some seizures begin with one type and progress to another.

Partial seizures involve part of the brain and may be classified as either simple partial seizures or complex partial seizures. There is one main difference between these two types. In a *simple partial seizure*, there is no alteration in consciousness. In a *complex partial seizure*, consciousness is impaired and symptoms are complex.

Generalized seizures involve the entire body and brain. They are the same on both sides of the body.

Nursing Alert

The role of the nurse during a seizure is to *protect* and *observe*.

Signs and Symptoms. During a *simple partial seizure*, a rhythmic jerking begins in one part of the body. The individual is aware that the seizure is occurring and is unable to stop or control the movement. The seizure is usually brief, lasting less than a minute. Types include Jacksonian (clonic movements starting in one muscle group and spreading), adversive (the person may become combative), or sensory (the person has unpleasant hallucinations, talks unintelligibly, or experiences vertigo).

Complex partial seizures are characterized by a motionlessness or repetitive movements such as lip smacking or chewing or swallowing movements or behaviors such as picking at clothes or rubbing the nose. After a complex partial seizure, the individual usually experiences a period of confusion and does not remember the incident.

Generalized seizures can take several forms, as described in the box. The individual experiencing a *tonic–clonic* seizure may cry out at the onset of the seizure; an aura may be experienced. An **aura** is a premonition or forewarning of an impending seizure. Recent information indicates that an aura may actually be a simple partial seizure occurring before a tonic–clonic episode. The onset is followed by a fall and rigid contraction of body muscles (tonic phase); then followed by rhythmic jerky movements. The episode of a seizure is called the ictal phase. Following the seizure (postictal phase), the person may fall into a deep sleep lasting minutes or hours.

The *absence seizure* is characterized by an altered LOC lasting no longer than 10 seconds. There is a sudden cessation of all activity, accompanied by a blank stare. The individual is not aware that the seizure has occurred and continues with whatever activity he or she was performing. Absence seizures are difficult to spot because the individual appears to be daydreaming. A person can experience as many as 100 absence seizures in one day.

Myoclonic seizures are characterized by quick, often repetitive muscle jerks, involving the extremities and facial muscles. In *atonic seizures*, the muscles become momentarily flaccid and the individual drops to the floor. *Infantile spasms* are characterized in infants by clusters of rapid spasmlike movements of the extremities, with neck flexion and extension of the arms. Any of these generalized seizures may occur individually or in clusters.

Nursing Alert

Every patient during a seizure must be observed for *respiratory depression*.

Diagnostic Tests. Diagnosis of seizure disorders is made on the basis of patient history, physical examination, laboratory tests, and EEG findings. An accurate description of the seizure itself is essential to identifying the type of seizure and appropriate treatment.

The EEG is a useful tool in diagnosing seizures because different seizure types produce specific electrical wave patterns. Just because the EEG looks normal does not necessarily mean that the person is not experiencing seizures.

Videotelemetry monitoring is helpful to the physician in diagnosing the specific seizure type.

Other diagnostic procedures include:

♦ CT scan and MRI to identify a tumor or brain lesion
♦ Angiogram to differentiate between a brain tumor and a blood vessel malformation
♦ Blood work to indicate electrolyte imbalance, drug toxicity, or underlying disorders

---

Key Concept

The EEG of person with a seizure disorder may look normal, especially if there is no seizure occurring at the time the EEG is done.

Medical and Surgical Treatment. The primary treatment of seizures is the use of a group of medicines referred

Classification of Seizures

I. Partial seizures (seizures with a local origin)
   AY. Simple (elemental symptoms; usually no loss of consciousness)
      1. Focal motor (without Jacksonian march)
      2. Jacksonian
      3. Adversive
      4. Focal sensory (somatic sensory, visual, auditory, gustatory, and vertiginous)
      5. *Epilepsia partialis continua*
   BY. Complex (symptoms usually include impairment of consciousness)—temporal lobe seizures (psychomotor seizures)
   C. With secondary generalized seizure
II. General seizures (generalized bilateral without focal onset)
   AY. Tonic–clonic seizures
   B. Absence seizures
   C. Myoclonic seizures
   D. Infantile spasms
   E. Tonic seizures
   F. Atonic seizures
   G. Akinetic seizures
III. Unclassified epileptic seizures (including all seizures that cannot be classified due to inadequate or incomplete data)

Adapted from Gastaut's adaptation of the International Classification of Seizures. Adapted by Hickey JV. The Clinical Practice of Neurological and Neurosurgical Nursing, Ed 3. Philadelphia, J.B. Lippincott, 1992. From Gastaut H. "Clinical and electroencephalographical classification of epileptic seizures." Epilepsia 11:102, 1970.

to as antiepileptic drugs (see accompanying box). These drugs work by raising the seizure threshold in an individual. The choice of drugs is based on the type of seizure experienced. Sometimes several drugs are used in combination to control the seizures. Routine blood levels of the drug are monitored to ensure a therapeutic dose.

Surgery may be performed in certain circumstances in which the seizure focal point can be clearly identified in the brain. Electrodes are placed directly on the brain to obtain more specific information as to where the seizure is originating. The surgery involves actual removal of the brain tissue that is thought to be initiating the seizure. Great care must be taken to ensure that healthy brain tissue is not damaged during the surgery. A procedure called *brain mapping* is done before surgery to identify the important brain structures to be avoided.

Nursing Considerations. Care of the patient during a seizure should focus on prevention of injury and accurate observation. Precaution procedures are discussed in the Nursing Process section earlier in the chapter. The accompanying box describes nursing actions to maintain patient safety.

Careful documentation of the seizure is important, so the physician can best develop a treatment plan. Some hospitals have an "event form," on which all seizures are documented. Documentation must include: what the patient was doing at the onset of the seizure, where the seizure began, how the person fell, time of day, triggering events, seizure progression and symmetry, eye response, patient responsiveness, results of commands and memory test, duration, direction of eye gaze and eye movements, confusion, incontinence, drooling, and diaphoresis. Document what the patient says about the seizure and how he or she behaves; check eye signs and LOC. Describe clusters of seizures.

Teaching in seizure disorders is essential for the patient and family. Suggestions for information to be taught are included in the accompanying box. The patient should learn to adapt life-styles to the disorder, living as normally as possible. Most people with seizure disorders are well controlled. It is important for them to understand the importance of regular medication administration in the maintenance of a seizure-free life.

Status Epilepticus

Status epilepticus is defined as a seizure or series of seizures, lasting 30 minutes or longer, in which the person does not regain consciousness. Any type of seizure can develop into status epilepticus; however, tonic–clonic status epilepticus is perhaps the most life-threatening.

Nursing Alert

Status epilepticus is a *medical emergency.*

Treatment of status epilepticus includes expert nursing and medical care, including intravenous medications. Key medications are listed in the accompanying box.

Nerve Disorders

Neuralgia

The term **neuralgia** literally means "pain in a nerve." It is often applied to fleeting pains in the shoulder and upper arm that are caused by angina, spinal tumor, or herniated intervertebral disk, as well as by other conditions. If application of external heat and administration of analgesics, such as aspirin, do not relieve the pain, medical evaluation is needed.

Carpal Tunnel Syndrome

Repeated movements of the wrists or continuously holding the wrist in an abnormal position cause edema of tissue in and around the carpal tunnel, which is located in the wrist. (The carpal tunnel is the passageway for the median nerve and the flexor tendons that attach to the carpal [finger] bones.) Most commonly affected are physicians, secretaries, and computer operators. The edema causes pressure on the nerve, resulting in pain, muscle weakness, and abnormal sensations in the hand. The area aches at night. The muscles of the hand may begin to atrophy. A common symptom is the frequent sensation of numbness in the hand.

The initial treatment involves immobilization of the wrist and hand, to rest the wrist joint and allow the edema to be absorbed. Antiinflammatory medications are given. If this is not effective, surgery may be done. Most patients recover quickly and have normal use of the hand after surgery.

Trigeminal Neuralgia (Tic Douloureux)

Sometimes, generally in older people, the route of the trigeminal nerve (the fifth cranial nerve) becomes painful. Nobody knows why this happens, but the pain is excruciating and comes in spasms that last for 2 to 15 seconds. The pain may be triggered by the slightest touch to various parts of the face or even by a breeze, a change in temperature, or a mouthful of food, depending on where the trigger zone is. Some drugs may help temporarily, but surgery is the most satisfactory treatment. Partial removal of the nerve roots eliminates the pain permanently, although it may leave burning, tickling sensations for several weeks or months. Following surgery, various symptoms may occur, depending on which branches of the nerve were sectioned. The patient may have some eye irritation or may have difficulty eating, in addition to adjusting to a certain amount of numbness. The patient is taught to avoid situations that previously triggered pain.

Bell's Palsy

Bell's palsy is emotionally upsetting for the patient because it produces a paralysis of part of the face (affecting the facial nerve; the seventh cranial nerve). Usually affecting one side of the face, it gives the patient a lopsided look. The eye on the affected side will not close, so special eye care may need to be given. The mouth on the affected side cannot be controlled or turned up when the patient smiles. This lack of control often causes the patient to drool. A Bell's palsy-type syndrome may occur as the result of a brain lesion, although most often the cause of Bell's palsy is unknown. This condition is treated with heat and massage. It may

Key Medications
Antiepileptic Drugs and Seizure Type

- carbamazepine (Tegretol): tonic–clonic, complex partial, mixed
- clonazepam (Klonopin): absence, akinetic, myoclonic
- mephobarbital (Mebaral): tonic–clonic, absence
- phenobarbital (Barbita, Luminal): all adult types, febrile seizures in children
- phenytoin (Dilantin): generalized tonic–clonic, status epilepticus, Reye's syndrome, and non epileptic seizures
- primidone (Mysoline): tonic–clonic, complex-partial
- trimethadione (Tridione): absence seizures not responsive to other drugs
- valproate (Depakene, Depakote): simple and complex absence and mixed seizure types

Nursing Considerations

- Blood disorders may occur.
- Respiratory depression may occur; the patient must be observed carefully.
- The patient is cautioned not to drink alcohol.
- Patient must consult an obstetrician during pregnancy and lactation because many of these drugs can be dangerous, especially to the fetus or infant.
- Orthostatic blood pressures are checked, at least daily.
- Careful oral hygiene is necessary.
- Many of these drugs are taken by a patient for life, to prevent seizures

also be treated, in the early stages, with prednisone (Meticorten, Orasone). Usually, the symptoms subside gradually, but they may take months to do so.

Shingles (Herpes Zoster)

Shingles is an acute viral disease caused by the varicella zoster virus, the same virus that causes chickenpox. The disease results from reactivation of latent virus cells residing in dorsal root or cranial nerve ganglion cells. Shingles is sometimes associated with other diseases, such as pneumonia or a lymphoma. Sometimes an injury or an injection of a drug may trigger the inflammation. Shingles appears as a vesicular eruption that follows the distribution of sensory nerves and causes excruciating pain. The eruption is usually confined to one side of the body, although it may encircle the trunk.

The appearance of shingles is frequently preceded by mild to moderate pruritus (itching), tenderness, or pain. Some patients also experience gastrointestinal upset and general malaise. The interval between pain and eruption of vesicles averages 3 to 5 days. Lesions erupt

Nursing Skill Guidelines
Maintaining Patient Safety During a Seizure

◆ Protect from nearby hazards. Move the overbed tray table and other dangerous items away from the patient. *(Rationale: The patient will not be able to control muscle movements or reactions during the seizure.)*

◆ Loosen restrictive clothing, such as ties or shirt collars. *(Rationale: It is important to maintain an unobstructed airway.)*

◆ Do not place anything in the person's mouth after a seizure has begun. *(Rationale: The tongue cannot be swallowed, and the teeth may be broken and aspirated by forcing an object into the mouth.)*

◆ Do not attempt to restrain the patient. *(Rationale: Injury may occur as a result of forcibly restraining, against the contraction of the muscles.)*

◆ Place a small soft padding beneath the head, such as a folded jacket. *(Rationale: To protect the head from injury.)*

◆ Turn the patient's head to the side. *(Rationale: To maintain a clear airway and to prevent aspiration.)*

◆ Monitor the seizure activity and location carefully. Note the exact time the seizure begins and ends. Test the extremity strength and tone. *(Rationale: This can give the physician a better idea of the exact type of seizure.)*

◆ Call the patient's name. Give a simple command, such as asking the patient to grab your hand and to let go. *(Rationale: The patient's responses to these evaluative techniques assist the physician to evaluate the type and severity of the seizure.)*

◆ Give the patient a "memory test" by asking him or her to remember two unrelated words. *(Rationale: Whether or not the patient is able to remember the words helps the physician to determine the type of seizure.)*

◆ After the seizure, ask the patient if there was an aura (warning). *(Rationale: The patient may be taught to take protective measures before a seizure occurs.)*

◆ Check the tongue and oral cavity for any bite injuries. *(Rationale: To determine the severity of the seizure and if any treatment is necessary.)*

◆ Observe and document carefully. *(Rationale: This will assist the physician to treat the patient.)*

◆ Offer reassurance and emotional support. Seizures can be frightening to the patient and family or visitors. The patient is often embarrassed. *(Rationale: The person may be incontinent or confused. Many people are frightened by witnessing a seizure.)*

Keys to Patient/Family Teaching
Seizure Disorders

Patient/family teaching for the patient with seizures includes:

◆ Explanation of seizure disorder
◆ Specific information about the particular seizure type experienced by the patient
◆ Safety and prevention of injury during a seizure
◆ Care of the patient during and after a seizure
◆ Importance of taking medications as prescribed
◆ Medication side effects
◆ Importance of family observation of seizure, so it can be fully described to the neurologist.
◆ Importance of adequate sleep, balanced diet, and suitable physical activities
◆ Avoidance of situations that can precipitate a seizure
◆ Importance of wearing a Medic-Alert tag
◆ Importance of regular follow-up with physician
◆ Importance of having blood drawn to determine blood levels of antiepileptic medications

the nerves *after* a herpes infection) may cause pain and discomfort for 8 or more weeks. This is most common in patients older than 60 years of age.

In rare cases, the infection may invade the eyes and cause conjunctivitis. If this cannot be checked, blindness may result in the affected eye (*ophthalmic zoster*). In patients with serious underlying conditions that suppress the immune system, a much more severe disease may develop (see Chapters 77 and 78).

Treatment is aimed at giving symptomatic relief from the pain and pruritus. Analgesics should be used to relieve

Key Medications (IV)
Status Epilepticus

◆ diazepam (Valium)
◆ lorazepam (Ativan)
◆ phenobarbital (Luminal)
◆ phenytoin (Dilantin)
◆ thiopental sodium (Pentothal)

Nursing Considerations

◆ When these drugs are given intravenously for status epilepticus, there is danger of overdose.
◆ Be alert for CNS signs such as drowsiness and lethargy, for respiratory depression, and for cardiovascular signs, which may range from hypotension to cardiovascular collapse.
◆ Some of these drugs may also cause kidney damage.

for several days and are usually gone within 3 to 4 weeks. Shingles is a self-limiting, localized disease that causes discomfort for several days but usually heals without complications. However, some scarring may occur. In addition, *postherpetic neuralgia* (pain along

the pain. Occasionally, narcotics may be necessary. Wet dressings with Burow's solution may be useful in the vesicular stage of the infection. Calamine lotion and antihistamines may be useful in treating pruritus. Intravenous acyclovir (Zovirax) has improved the rate of healing of skin lesions and shortened the period of pain. Oral corticosteroids have been used in patients aged 50 to 60 years and older to decrease postherpetic neuralgia.

Spinal Cord Disorders

The nurse must understand several basic concepts when caring for the person with a spinal cord injury:

◆ The spinal cord connects the brain to the rest of the body. (Without the spinal cord, communication between the brain and the rest of the body is literally cut off.)
◆ The spinal cord lies in an enclosed and confined space—the vertebral column. (Any invasion into this space can cause devastating effects.)
◆ The spinal cord is responsible for the *reflex arc* (see Chapter 18). The reflex arc is a built-in protective mechanism. (It allows, for example, a person to quickly jerk the hand away from a hot stove, thus bypassing the brain and preventing further injury.)

Application of these concepts will help the nurse better understand the care required for spinal cord injuries.

Categories of Spinal Cord Disorders

Spinal cord problems can be divided into three main categories: congenital defects, tumors, and trauma.

Congenital Defects. *Congenital defects* of the spinal cord are malformations that occur in the developing fetus. These most often have an impact on the CNS by disrupting the flow of CSF and are discussed further in Chapter 65.

Tumors. A spinal cord *tumor* is located within the vertebral column, taking up space and causing compression of the cord. This interferes with the blood supply and the circulation of CSF. Tumors may be surgically removed. The resulting neurologic deficit will vary, depending on the type of tumor and length of time compression has occurred. If a tumor involves the cord itself, the damage is usually more severe and is often permanent.

Trauma. *Trauma* to the spinal cord is usually caused by a penetrating object, including a displaced vertebrae or other foreign object, such as a bullet. Transection (severing) of the cord can be incomplete (partial) or complete. If the transection is *complete*, there is loss of all sensation

and voluntary movement below the site of injury. A *partial* or *incomplete* transection has a better prognosis. In the latter case, the resulting deficits will depend on whether *ascending* (sensory) or *descending* (motor) nerve tracts have been severed. The spinal cord also may be *bruised,* in which case function may be regained.

Level of Injury

The level of the spinal cord at which injury occurs determines which body functions are affected (Fig. 71-2). **Paraplegia** is a paralysis of the legs and lower body and is usually the result of injury to the cord below the first thoracic vertebrae. **Quadriplegia** is a paralysis of all four extremities and is usually the result of an injury above the first thoracic vertebrae.

The extent of all spinal cord injuries depends on the location and severity of the injury. Injuries occurring at the second and third cervical vertebrae are usually fatal. Any damage at the level of C-4 and above requires respiratory assistance because nerve innervation to the respiratory muscles is affected.

Effects of Injury

A number of things may occur with damage to the spinal cord. Deficits in sensation range from complete loss of sensation to numbness and tingling of the extremities. Movement disabilities can also range from muscle weakness to partial or complete paralysis. Loss of mental function varies from mild confusion to coma, sometimes involving loss of speech, sight, or hearing. Complications of spinal cord injury may include impaired circulation, bowel and bladder incontinence, bone demineralization, skin breakdown, anemia, muscle spasms, contractures, increased body temperature, gastric distention, and respiratory complications. Blood clots may develop in the legs. The lower the cord transection, the fewer the complications.

Any damage to the spinal cord is frightening to the patient and family. There is always a possibility of temporary or permanent paralysis. Sometimes the final outcome of a spinal cord injury is uncertain for a long period of time; this is particularly stressful.

Once the diagnosis of paralysis is made, the emotional shock to the person and family is devastating. Adjustments ranging from minor modifications to a total change in life-style must be made. Changes needed may include adaptations in the physical setup of the home, installation of elevators and ramps, change of employment, adaptations so the person can drive a car, assistance with ADL, and adaptations so the person can move about.

Medical and Surgical Treatment. To prevent further damage, extreme care is taken when moving the patient immediately after the injury. The patient must be handled and moved by trained rescue personnel; the nurse *never* moves such a patient unless no other professional

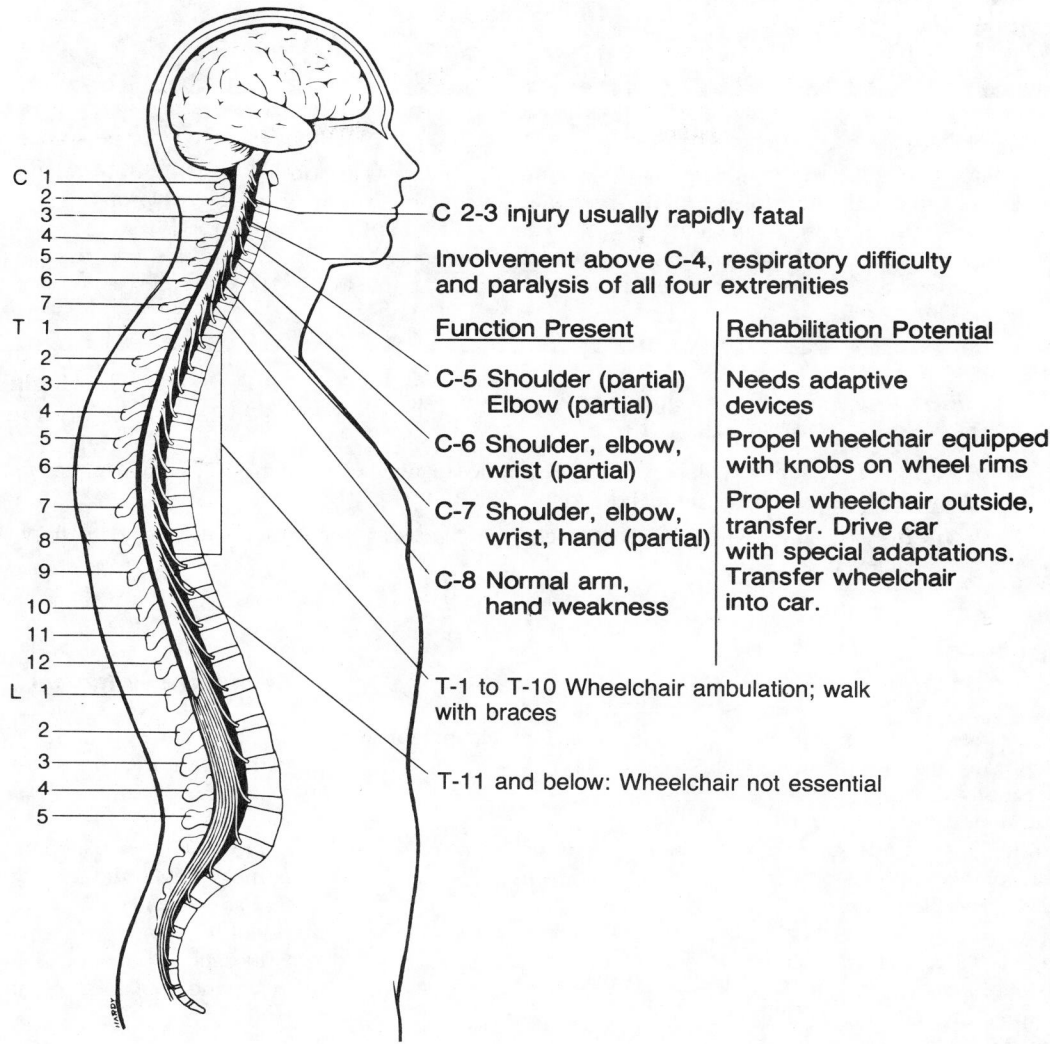

Figure 71-2. Results of spinal cord injury at various levels.

assistance is available. The patient should be kept flat on a firm surface, with the head, neck, and spinal cord stabilized before being moved. *Never lift the patient with a spinal cord injury by the head, shoulder, or feet.* Most likely the patient will need treatment for shock and hemorrhage.

Diagnostic Tests. X-ray examination to determine the extent of injury is done first. If the cause of paralysis is trauma, skeletal traction may be applied to immobilize the damaged cervical vertebrae. This is done with several different devices, described and illustrated in Chapter 70.

Pain may be caused by nerve damage or it may be aggravated by injections, kidney stones, or fecal impactions. Pain may be felt in a paralyzed area of the body or it may occur in a ringlike fashion at the level of injury. Temporary relief may be gained by injection of a local anesthetic such as lidocaine hydrochloride (Xylocaine).

Surgery may be necessary to remove a portion of vertebral bone that is pressing on the spinal cord, or it may be done to determine if the cord is severed (cut all the way through—a *complete cord transection*). If the spinal column is not stable, spinal fusion is done to prevent further damage to the spinal cord and to enable the patient to have more mobility later.

Rehabilitation must begin *immediately* on hospitalization. Cardiac and pulmonary reserves must be maintained. The patient must be rehabilitated in all spheres—body, mind, and spirit. It is best for the patient with a spinal cord injury to be admitted to a rehabilitation center as soon as possible; usually the general hospital is not equipped to handle all the problems that may arise.

Nursing Considerations. The nurse is a vital link in the continuing assessment of a patient with spinal cord

Mr. Charles Riggins is a 27-year-old white man who sustained a spinal cord injury from a gunshot wound at level T-8, resulting in paraplegia. After Mr. Riggins was stabilized he was transferred to the Regional Spinal Cord Center. Mr. Riggins was a construction worker and very proud of his physical abilities before this injury; now he is paralyzed from the waist down. He has outbursts of anger during which he becomes abusive, loud, and vulgar. Just as abruptly as these periods occur they end, and he becomes very apathetic. Two of the nursing diagnoses developed for Mr. Riggins follow.

Nursing Diagnosis: *High Risk for Impaired Skin Integrity Related to Impaired Mobility and Spasticity as Evidenced by Altered Sensations*

Goal 1: By 8/7 patient will identify those techniques that will enable him to actively participate in reducing and preventing skin breakdown.

Goal 2: By 8/14 patient will demonstrate techniques necessary for maintaining his skin integrity at its optimal level.

Nursing Actions (assess/do/teach)	Rationale	Evaluative Statement
1. Emphasize to Mr. Riggins that he is responsible for his own health and that complications such as pressure sores are continuous threats.	To make the patient accountable for his own well-being	8/7 Goal 1 met; patient collaborated with healthcare team to establish a plan to help maintain his skin integrity.
2. Assist Mr. Riggins to understand the importance of continuous observation and effective skin care.	To help prevent problems	8/14 Goal 2 met; patient is actively participating in reducing those risks that are potential threats to the integrity of his skin.
3. Encourage Mr. Riggins to plan and participate in a regularly scheduled program of pressure-relieving lift-offs and weight shifting techniques. To promote participation	To promote participation	8/14 Catalog of adaptive equipment given and explained to patient.
4. Teach safety measures to help avoid shearing forces, friction, or dermal injury.	To identify methods that enable the patient to control his own well-being.	8/20 Personal care attendant (PCA) obtained to assist Mr. Riggins with ADLs.
5. Encourage Mr. Riggins to obtain and use appropriate protective devices to maintain adequate circulation, eliminate pressure, and avoid injury.	To help maintain his well-being	

(continued)

injury. The nurse observes the patient daily as nursing care is given. It is possible for the nurse to observe minute changes in the patient's condition not yet evident to the patient or others. A sample nursing care plan for a patient with paraplegia provides some considerations.

Rehabilitation focuses on preventing disabilities from increasing and on strengthening and making the most of whatever powers remain. It *begins immediately* with preventing disorders such as skin breakdown and disuse disorders such as footdrop. Passive and active exercises are begun immediately to develop muscle strength and movement. The degree of success depends on the nature and the extent of nerve damage as well as the patient's own perseverance. Despite paralysis, many patients are able to move about and do ADL. With today's new equipment and techniques, many paralyzed people are able to live independently.

Nursing Diagnosis: *Powerlessness Related to Losses Resulting From the Accident and Increased, Unwanted Dependency as Evidenced by Alternating Periods of Apathy, Anger, and Resistive Behavior.*

Goal 1: By 8/7 patient will identify factors that he can control.

Goal 2: By 8/10 patient will participate in decisions related to his plan of care.

Nursing Actions (assess/do/teach)	Rationale	Evaluative Statement
1. Assess the degree of powerlessness exhibited by Mr. Riggins and his family. Recognize nonproductive behavior. Identify methods of communication or lack of.	To establish an individual plan of care	8/7 Goals 1 and 2 are met; patient recognizes that he can control areas of his own care collaborating with the healthcare team to establish a plan.
2. Allow Mr. Riggins time to work through and express his feelings. Provide a nonjudgmental atmosphere—one of mutual respect and trust. Provide emotional support.	A nonjudgmental atmosphere facilitates verbalization of patient's feelings.	8/10 Patient was visited by a member of a local support group.
3. Assist Mr. Riggins to identify those factors which he can control; give him a degree of power for his present and future well-being.	To help the patient identify his capabilities, not just his limitations. This empowers and motivates the patient.	
4. Determine Mr. Riggin's resources, interests, values, goals, coping patterns, and support system. Assist patient to achieve his optimal level of functioning. Refer to appropriate community resources as indicated.	To provide focus points and goals for the patient. This helps identify what he will need to achieve his goals.	
5. Assess family support system and help them adapt to the changes imposed by the present situation. Refer to support groups and/or counseling as necessary.	Care will be ongoing and at times exhausting. Emotions and relationships can become strained. They will need care and support, if they are to remain effective and healthy.	

The patient should be encouraged to make every effort to maximize abilities and apply self-care. Improvement can be expected, but strong willpower and perseverance may be required to accomplish even the simplest task. Often the patient will be discouraged. The nurse helps most by letting the patient express frustration and discouragement and by acknowledging these feelings.

Many patients with spinal injury now survive who previously would have died from their injuries. These patients require careful nursing care. Guidelines for such are given in the accompanying box. (Patients who are paralyzed due to other causes need much the same care.)

Autonomic Dysreflexia

Autonomic dysreflexia (sudden, dangerous hypertension) can occur at any time resulting in a seizure, a stroke, or hemorrhage. Autonomic dysreflexia can be triggered by such common occurrences as a distended bladder or fecal impaction. Signs and symptoms of autonomic dysreflexia are:

- Elevated blood pressure (a particularly significant sign)
- Sudden, throbbing headache
- Chills
- Pallor
- Goose flesh ("goose bumps")
- Nausea, with a metallic taste

If the patient displays these signs and symptoms, the nurse notifies the physician immediately, because this can be an emergency situation. The nurse immediately elevates the patient's head and may also lower the feet. This lowers the patient's blood pressure. The patient and family are taught preventive measures.

Nursing Skill Guidelines
Caring for the Paralyzed Patient

- Use measures to prevent footdrop. Splints are commonly used.
- Change the patient's position frequently and provide passive and active range of motion. (*Rationale: To prevent disorders caused by immobility–disuse disorders*).
- Give respiratory care as needed. (*Rationale: To prevent respiratory complications. Pneumonia is a particularly dangerous complication.*)
- Encourage the patient to sit up as much as possible, with adequate support. A standing wheelchair, tilt table, or "neuro" chair is used as soon as possible. (*Rationale: This will prevent respiratory complications and will help the patient to maintain self-esteem.*)
- Use special devices (beds, chairs, and other mechanical devices in the early phases of treatment. Trochanter rolls and sandbags may also be used. (*Rationale: To maintain proper body alignment and positioning to prevent orthopedic deformities.*)
- Give special skin care. Make sure the sheets are smooth and the bed is clean. (*Rationale: To prevent pressure areas or skin breakdown.*)
- If cervical traction, tongs, or a halo device is in place, assess the pin site. Site care is given if ordered by the physician. Incisional care is given postoperatively. (*Rationale: To prevent infection. Infection can be particularly dangerous to paralyzed person whose physical condition is already compromised.*)
- Teach the patient the warning signs of genitourinary infection. (*Rationale: This is a common complication of immobility.*)
- Encourage fluid intake. (*Rationale: To prevent kidney stones and bladder infections.*)
- Institute bladder retraining and rehabilitation early, if possible. (*Rationale: This helps restore the patient to independence and self-esteem.*)
- If urinary retention is present, use a urinary appliance, retention cathether, or self-catheterization. (*Rationale: The patient may not be able to tell when the bladder is filled. Retention of urine can lead to autonomic dysreflexia, infection, or hydronephrosis.*)
- If a catheter is used, make sure it is draining properly and is handled in as clean a manner as possible. (*Rationale: To avoid bladder infections.*)
- Teach the patient/family to care for the indwelling catheter or urinary appliance as early as possible, if bladder retraining is not an option. (*Rationale: This will reinforce self-care.*)
- If disposable pads or incontinence products are used, special attention must be given to keep the skin clean and dry. (*Rationale: This will help to prevent skin irritation, pressure areas and infection.*)
- Teach the patient to do manual disimpaction for a fecal impaction. (*Rationale: Damage to the bowel can trigger autonomic dysreflexia.*) Some patients do a manual disimpaction daily, as their bowel maintenance program.

- Give injections above the level of injury, if possible. (*Rationale: Circulation is impaired below the level of injury and the action of the drug is delayed. The skin is more subject to breakdown below the level of injury.*)
- Avoid applying external heat to areas of decreased sensation, particularly to the penis or testes. Take care to avoid decubiti, ingrown toenails, or sharp objects touching the patient. Monitor temperature of bath water. (*Rationale: Burns occur easily because of lack of circulation and sensation: the patient would not feel the injury; and skin stimulation can cause autonomic dysreflexia.*)
- Maintain nutritional status. (*Rationale: To maintain health and to promote healing.*)
- Establish some sort of communication system if the patient cannot speak. This can involve blinking the eyes, moving a finger, or using a computer. (*Rationale: The person's mind is usually active; there must be some way for the person to make needs, wants and thoughts known to others.*)

Special Considerations in Female Patients

- Menses usually resume within 3 months following the injury. (*Rationale: It takes a period of time for the body to adjust.*)
- The use of tampons for menstrual flow is dangerous. (*Rationale: The woman may forget that a tampon is in place because she has no sensation.*)
- The use of birth control pills is not recommended. (*Rationale: They can lead to thrombus formation, particularly because this woman is not exercising. Effectiveness often decreases because of interactions with other medications.*)
- The use of intrauterine devices is not recommended. (*Rationale: They can promote thrombus formation or infections. This woman would not be able to tell if the device had fallen out. She also would not be able to feel the pain associated with a perforated uterus.*)
- Labor and childbirth may be dangerous. (*Rationale: The woman may not be aware of beginning labor. The likelihood of a cesarean birth is increased because the woman may not be able to assist with the delivery and the uterus may not have adequate muscle tone. Labor and delivery may serve as a trigger for autonomic dysreflexia.*)

Special Consideration in Sexuality

- Many persons with varying degrees of paralysis have active sex lives. Adaptations and understanding on the part of the partner may be necessary. It is possible for a paralyzed man to father a child and for a paralyzed woman to bear a child.

Autonomic disturbances may be treated with atropine-like drugs, which block the unwanted effects of the vagus nerve.

Degenerative Disorders

In addition to all the physical problems displayed by the person with a degenerative disorder, the patient will often show major emotional and psychological problems. The patient may exhibit profound mood swings and may behave with outbursts of frustration or anger. Inappropriate sexual behavior may be exhibited. The patient may also show signs of regression, even infantile behavior. The nurse can help by allowing the patient and family to express their feelings and anxieties.

There are support groups for most degenerative disorders. These groups are made up of other patients and families. The addresses of local and national groups are easy to obtain. The nurse assists the patient and family to find an appropriate support group. The nurse encourages the patient and family members to talk with other persons who have faced a similar situation. Talking with others can offer reassurance and give helpful suggestions for management of the patient.

Multiple Sclerosis

Multiple sclerosis (MS) is one of the most common nerve disorders in the United States. It is most common in young adults and in people living in the northern temperate climate. In MS the myelin sheath covering the nerves is destroyed. Because the white matter of the brain and the spinal cord is destroyed, normal transmission of impulses is disrupted. The cause of MS is unknown, although cold weather seems to aggravate it; thus, it may be an environmental disease. Others believe it is viral in origin; a current theory proposes that it is an autoimmune disease.

Signs and Symptoms. Several parts of the body may be affected. MS usually causes a slow paralysis and a slowly developing disturbance of speech and vision. Symptoms are few at first; then they increase in both number and seriousness.

It is difficult to diagnose MS until certain symptoms appear together and create widespread disturbance of the nervous system. Some common symptoms are poor balance and difficulty in walking, weakness and clumsy movements, tremor, blurred or double vision or blindness, slurred speech, paraplegia, and bowel and bladder incontinence or retention. The patient may have sudden emotional upsets, becoming either depressed or exuberant and euphoric. The patient may be dizzy or nauseous and may vomit; or the patient may have spastic paraplegia and muscle tremor.

The symptoms may disappear in the early stages, and the patient may appear normal and well for years. Each time symptoms reappear, they are more severe and of longer duration. Thus, the disease is marked by *remissions* and *exacerbations*. A patient may live 20 years or more after the disease is diagnosed, but disabilities develop with time.

Diagnostic Tests. MRI is the diagnostic study that best detects changes in the myelin sheath. MRI shows the plaque changes, and these correlate well with the patient symptoms, if the person has MS.

Medical Treatment. Although MS cannot be cured, much research is being conducted in an attempt to isolate the cause and to find a cure. Authorities agree that it is important to build up the patient's general health by providing plenty of rest and a balanced diet and by avoiding excitement and exposure to infection. Physical therapy helps prevent physical deformities and maintain muscle strength.

During significant exacerbations, patients may be treated with intravenous ACTH. This may be done on an outpatient or inpatient basis. ACTH is given for 6 to 7 days and then decreased, with weekly injections for another month.

Recently, it has been discovered that the drug, interferon, is effective in treating MS. It treats the disease itself rather than just the symptoms.

Nursing Considerations. Skin care is important. The body becomes wasted, causing susceptibility to complications from immobility such as skin breakdown or pneumonia. Body position of the patient must be changed frequently and deep breathing must be practiced to prevent pneumonia. Attention should be given to maintain proper body alignment; paralysis and weakness can lead to body deformities. Elimination problems usually occur; therefore, diet and fluid intake must be monitored. The patient may be incontinent of urine or may have urinary retention. Care of the patient with an indwelling catheter must focus on avoidance of infection. Because constipation often occurs, a bowel training program can be initiated as discussed in Chapter 46.

Unless it is physically necessary, the patient does not need to stay in bed; instead, the person should be encouraged to lead as normal a life as possible. The MS patient can live at home as long as physical care can be carried out independently or can be provided for the patient. Sometimes work can be found for the patient to do at home until the advancing disease makes this impossible.

The MS patient and family need support. Persons who live with the MS patient on a daily basis need to alter aspects of their life-styles and to readjust goals in accordance with the patient's condition.

Parkinson's Disease

Parkinson's disease, also called parkinsonism, is the second most common neurologic disease of the elderly. It is a progressive brain disease, characterized by slowness of movement (bradykinesia) and a fine, rhythmic tremor.

The disease affects automatic movements, such as blinking, eating, talking, walking, and maintaining posture. Features are tremors, rigidity, slowing of voluntary movement, shuffling and unsteady gait, unstable posture, and masklike facial appearance (Fig. 71-3).

Mental changes often accompany this disease, but they vary in intensity. Common changes are emotional lability (fluctuations) and a slowed thinking process. Parkinson's disease is considered a progressive disease, and it may lead to a state of immobility. Many of these patients are clinically depressed.

Parkinsonism affects slightly more men than women, usually appearing in people in their 60s. The cause is unknown in most persons. The idiopathic form seems to be caused by a disruption in a specific neurotransmitter called *dopamine* (a substance that sends impulses from one neuron to another).

Signs and Symptoms. Symptoms appear gradually; it may be years before the patient becomes alarmed and consults a physician.

Tremors are regular but so mild they are scarcely noticeable. They may affect only one side, then spread to the other side; this may happen immediately or after as long a period as 15 years. Tremors may start in the fingers, then extend to the arm and finally spread to the entire body. Severe tremor is constant—two to five shakes in a second with the thumb beating against the fingers in a sort of "pill-rolling" movement. The tremors become worse if the patient gets excited, but the shaking may cease if he or she moves voluntarily. The tremors disappear when the patient is asleep, except in the final stages of the disease. All the muscles become rigid. The limbs are flexed slightly, and all movements are slowed. Because the disease affects the spine and neck, the patient sits or stands in a stooped position. The arms no longer swing when he or she walks, and the person is unable to shift position quickly to keep balance; he or she shuffles along when walking to keep from falling. If pushed a little, the person loses balance and goes faster in the direction of the push. Movement of the small muscles that control changes in facial expression is affected. The patient cannot blink the eyes or smile, and the face is masklike. The person with parkinsonism often drools.

Medical and Surgical Treatment. The most effective antiparkinsonism drug found to date is levodopa (L-dopa). The accompanying box lists precautions and consid-

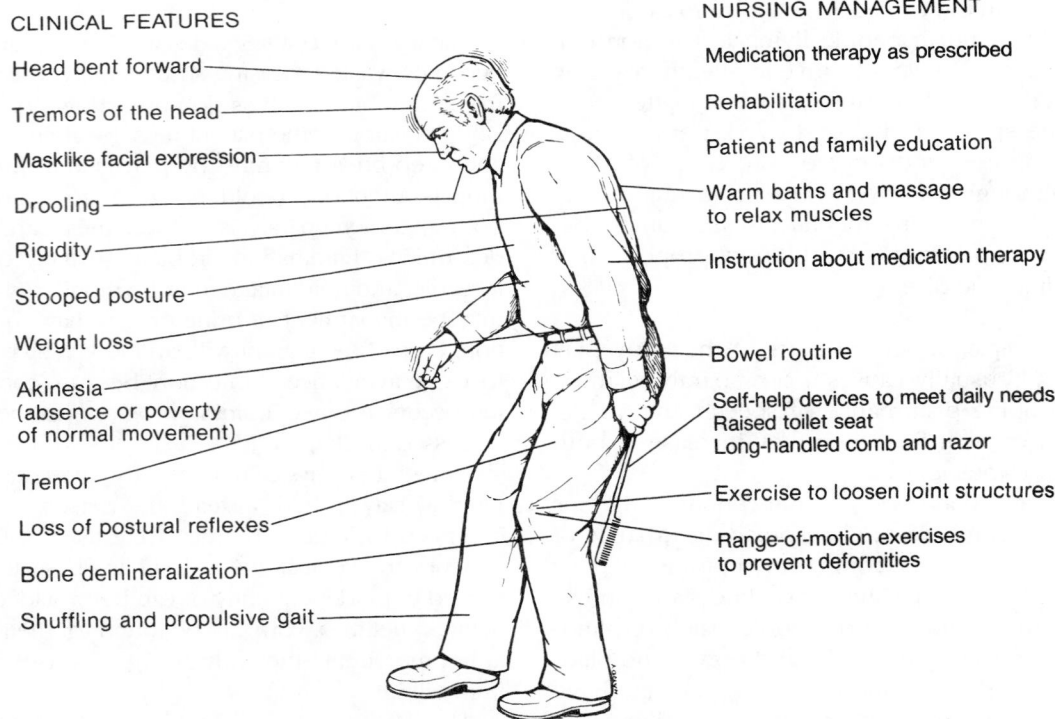

CLINICAL FEATURES

Head bent forward
Tremors of the head
Masklike facial expression
Drooling
Rigidity
Stooped posture
Weight loss
Akinesia (absence or poverty of normal movement)
Tremor
Loss of postural reflexes
Bone demineralization
Shuffling and propulsive gait

NURSING MANAGEMENT

Medication therapy as prescribed
Rehabilitation
Patient and family education
Warm baths and massage to relax muscles
Instruction about medication therapy
Bowel routine
Self-help devices to meet daily needs: Raised toilet seat Long-handled comb and razor
Exercise to loosen joint structures
Range-of-motion exercises to prevent deformities

Figure 71-3. Clinical manifestations and nursing management of the patient with parkinsonism. (Smeltzer SC and Bare BG. Brunner and Suddarth's Textbook of Medical-Surgical Nursing, Ed 7. Philadelphia, J.B. Lippincott, 1992)

Key Medications
for Parkinson's Disease

♦ levodopa (Dopar, Larodopa, L-dopa): replenishes missing dopamine, a neurotransmitter found in the brain

Nursing Considerations

♦ L-Dopa may cause hemolytic anemia.
♦ L-Dopa must be used carefully in patients with glaucoma. If L-dopa is given, the intraocular pressure must be carefully monitored. *(Rationale: One of the side effects of L-dopa is increased intraocular pressure.)*
♦ L-Dopa is contraindicated in undiagnosed skin lesions. *(Rationale: The drug may aggravate these conditions.)*
♦ The patient taking L-dopa must avoid certain foods. These include high-protein foods (which retard absorption of the drug) and foods high in vitamin B_6, (which quickly counteracts positive effects of L-dopa). This patient must not take multivitamins.
♦ The patient cannot use drugs classified as monoamine oxidase (MAO) inhibitors. MAO inhibitors often potentiate or counteract L-dopa effects. The patient can become hyperactive and hyperexcitable with increased parkinsonian symptoms and hypertension.

erations needed when the patient is receiving this drug. For example, vitamin B_6 in foods or multivitamins renders L-dopa ineffective. Monoamine oxidase (MAO) inhibitors, which are usually given to counteract depression, should be discontinued several weeks *before* L-dopa is administered.

Physical therapy helps keep the patient active and enables him or her to feed and dress himself or herself and get in and out of bed or a chair. The patient can be taught how to exercise legs and fingers, how to maintain balance, and how to keep neck muscles from contracting. Exercises do not eliminate the tremor, but they do help prevent rigidity.

Because handling food, chewing, and swallowing are difficult, the patient may not eat enough nutritious food. Specific vitamins (except vitamin B_6) and a high-calorie, high-protein diet are prescribed.

Surgery may be performed in carefully selected cases. Surgery involves the deliberate production of a lesion in the thalamus. The procedure is used less frequently than in the past because of the effectiveness and greater safety of L-dopa.

Nursing Considerations. The nurse provides teaching for the patient and family (see accompanying box). While the patient is in the healthcare facility, the nurse can check the consistency of food and teach the patient and family about food preparation. Food should be prepared so that it is easy to chew and swallow. Meat should be ground and potatoes mashed; a straw should be provided for liquids. Be careful to prevent burns. The patient will be embarrassed by the difficulties of eating, so he or she must be encouraged to eat. The patient is helped to make menu selections that are agreeable and safe. A sample nursing care plan outlines some care factors.

Constipation may develop because of the lack of saliva, the lack of physical activity, the lack of roughage in the diet, or because of various medications taken by the patient. Usually a stool softener is given. Fluid intake is encouraged (at least four to six glasses of water and juice each day).

The nurse helps the patient learn how to use adaptive techniques and devices (see Chapter 89). The family can be helped in making adaptations to the home and in homemaking.

Home Care Adaptations
Parkinson's Disease

♦ Dangerous items, such as throw rugs and highly waxed floors, should be removed from the home. *(Rationale: This patient has poor balance and can easily fall.)*
♦ It may be necessary to arrange for bathroom facilities and a bedroom on the first floor. *(Rationale: To avoid stair climbing, which can be dangerous and may be impossible.)*
♦ Install handrails as needed in bathroom, stairs, and hallways. Use a nightlight. *(Rationale: The patient can be more self-sufficient.)*

Keys to Patient/Family Teaching
Parkinson's Disease

Patient/family teaching in parkinsonism includes:

♦ Encouragement of the patient to be as independent as possible
♦ Suggestions to protect the patient from unnecessary stress and fatigue
♦ Use of adaptive techniques and devices
♦ Importance of protecting the patient from injury
♦ Importance of taking medication on time
♦ Foods to be avoided when taking medication
♦ Importance of adequate nutrition and fluids
♦ Ways to prevent constipation
♦ Importance of regular eye examinations; intraocular pressure to be checked
♦ Pertinent exercises and how to maintain balance
♦ Use of adaptive feeding utensils, when indicated

Ms. Eileen O'Brien is a 76 year old, white, widowed woman. She was admitted to a long-term care facility because the clinical manifestations of her Parkinson's disease had progressed to a point that greatly incapacitated her. Ms. O'Brien had fallen 15 times within the past 3 months. Although she did not sustain any serious physical injuries, she becomes very frightened of falling whenever she tries to walk. She cries frequently and prefers others to assume all responsibility for any activity that requires walking. In addition, her drooling has increased. This, combined with her muscle weakness and tremors, makes it difficult for her to maintain adequate nutrition, which is evident by her increasing weight loss. The following nursing diagnoses focus on two of her disabling symptoms.

Nursing Diagnosis: *High Risk for Injury (falls), Related to Increasing Rigidity, Decreasing Postural Reflexes, Deteriorating Sense of Balance and Sluggish Reactions as Evidenced by her Increasing Episodes of Recent Falls.*

Goal: By 12/1 the patient will demonstrate behaviors to reduce injury from falls.

Nursing Actions (assess/do/teach)	Rationale	Evaluative Statement
1. Have physical therapy and Ms. O'Brien outline a program to maximize her muscle strength, enhance her coordination, help her compensate for deficient automatic movements, and enhance her joint mobility.	To involve patient in her program	12/1 Goal met; patient is using learned techniques to avoid falling. 12/7 OT made home visit.
2. Encourage Ms. O'Brien to learn and use postural and gait training techniques.	To help patient compensate for her shuffling gait and leaning forward while walking	
3. Obtain and teach Ms. O'Brien to use the safety aids prescribed by occupational therapy (grabrails on tub, reciprocal walking frame, etc).		
4. Decrease the potential for orthostatic hypotension and advise the patient to take frequent rest periods.	To help prevent fatigue, weakness, and dizziness	
5. Keep room hazard free.		
6. Assess the home environment for safety.		

(continued)

Myasthenia Gravis

Myasthenia gravis (MG) is a chronic disorder that affects younger women more commonly or men when they are older. It is not a common disease. It affects the response of voluntary muscles. In some cases, medication can restore some or all of the lost muscle function. Although the cause is not known, research tends to favor an autoimmune or genetic origin. Certain medications may also be involved.

Myasthenia gravis may persist for years, or it may be rapidly fatal. With the mild form, the patient can remain active as long as he or she avoids activities that are very tiring. With the severe form, the patient may need total assistance.

Signs and Symptoms. The disease usually evolves gradually; the patient notices that certain muscles seem to be weak immediately after they have been

Nursing Diagnosis: *Altered Nutrition: Less Than Body Requirements, Related to Muscle Weakness and Tremors as Evidenced by Difficulty in Chewing and Swallowing, Drooling, Frequent Choking Episodes, and Weight Loss.*

Goal 1: By the end of first week (12/1) patient will increase oral nutrition as evidenced by cessation of weight loss.

Goal 2: By the end of second week (12/8) patient will regain 1 lb of lost weight.

Nursing Actions (assess/do/teach)	Rationale	Evaluative Statement
1. Modify consistency of food as necessary, serve small frequent feedings, provide dietary supplements, ensure a pleasant relaxed atmosphere, and allow for frequent rest periods during prolonged eating periods.	To minimize unpleasant aspects of eating and promote nutritional intake	12/1 Goal 1 met; patient's intake has increased and she is maintaining her present weight.
2. Use assistive devices that will minimize any obstacles for adequate nutritional intake (stabilized plate, non-spill cup, flexible plastic straw, and electrical warming tray).		12/8 Goal 2 met; patient has regained 1 ½ lbs of her lost weight.
3. Encourage Ms. O'Brien to consciously think through the swallowing process. Assist Ms. O'Brien to use methods to control the buildup of saliva. Maintain patient in sitting position for 30 minutes after eating/feeding.	To prevent choking and/or aspiration	
5. Monitor patient's weight on a weekly basis.		
6. Continue to monitor patient's capabilities.		Changes that·increase patient's limitations can be noted and can be responded to in a timely manner.

exercised, but muscle strength returns with rest. The eye muscles are often the first affected. The patient looks sleepy, the face is expressionless, the eyelids droop, and the person has double vision. The muscles of the face may be affected, especially those used in chewing, swallowing, coughing, and speaking. If the muscles of respiration are affected, it is difficult for the person to breathe. If the person is unable to expectorate secretions, pneumonia may develop.

A *myasthenic crisis* occurs rapidly and is considered an emergency. *Dysphagia* (difficulty in swallowing), *dysarthria* (difficulty in speaking), *ptosis* (drooping eyelids), *diplopia* (double vision), and *respiratory distress* are the accompanying symptoms. Maintaining an open (patent) airway can be lifesaving.

Medical Treatment. Drugs are given to increase strength by intensifying muscular response to nerve impulses (see the accompanying box). The nurse and patient must be aware of the danger of overmedication or of temporary resistance to the drug. Intermittent positive pressure breathing treatments (IPPB) are often indicated. In the case of severe respiratory involvement, a tracheostomy may be performed.

Nursing Alert

An important precaution in myasthenia gravis is to avoid sedatives, tranquilizing drugs, and morphine; these drugs may cause respiratory or cardiac depression.

Key Medications
for Myasthenia Gravis

- neostigmine methylsulfate (Prostigmin)
- pyridostigmine bromide (Mestinon, Regonol)
- ambenonium chloride (Mytelase): used only if patient cannot take either of the others

Nursing Considerations

Because these medications play a vital role in the patient's ability to swallow and to handle respiratory secretions:

- Medications *must* be given on time.
- Medications are vital—they play a role in the patient's ability to swallow and to handle respiratory secretions.
- Give medications with food (to minimize side effects).
- Report any side effects immediately.

Home Care Adaptations
Huntington's Disease[2]

- Lamps with a "touch" base or the "Clapper" can be used.
- If handrails are being installed, ensure they can support full body weight. Also be sure handrails are at the proper height.
- An electric razor and electric toothbrush can be used. To steady the hands and arms, the patient may sit down and rest the elbows on a table when shaving or brushing the teeth.
- If the person can swallow thin liquids, two straws can be used. Straws are cut to just above the rim of the glass.
- Cut a spot out of a styrofoam cup for the person's nose. This makes drinking easier and safer. (*Rationale: The person does not have to tip the head back to drink, thus preventing choking.*)

Nursing Considerations. The patient may need to be fed by tube or TPN. Suction may be necessary to remove secretions. An oral suction machine should be kept at the bedside of the patient; it may be lifesaving in the case of choking or threatened aspiration.

The patient should be forewarned of the signs of myasthenic crisis and instructed to take precautions regarding medical assistance before the crisis develops. A Medic-Alert tag should be worn and a self-dialing telephone should be within easy reach. (A voice-activated phone is necessary if the patient cannot dial or hold the receiver.) The patient should also be aware that emotional upsets and infections can intensify the disease and precipitate a crisis. Patient teaching is an important aspect of care, as outlined in the accompanying teaching box.

Huntington's Disease

Huntington's disease (HD), also known as *Huntington's chorea*, is hereditary and involves a combination of physical and mental symptoms that usually start with fidgeting, jerking, and spasms. The personality changes include irritability, loss of judgment, and carelessness. These symptoms progress to greater weakness, severe personality disorders, psychosis, and death. Death usually occurs from pneumonia or from another disorder related to lack of mobility.

Symptoms generally do not appear until the patient is past age 30. About 50% of children of an affected parent contract the disease; other children may be carriers. Couples at risk are wise to have genetic counseling before deciding whether to have children. No cure is known, although some tranquilizing and psychotropic drugs provide symptomatic relief. Home care adaptations can be made for a better quality of life.

Keys to Patient/Family Teaching
Myasthenia Gravis

Patient/family teaching for the patient with myasthenia gravis includes:

- Importance of wearing a Medic-Alert tag.
- Use of a self-dialing phone or cellular phone. (*Rationale: To enable the patient to call for help in an emergency.*)
- Importance of taking medications on time. Use an alarm clock. (*Rationale: A constant blood level must be maintained for the medications to be effective.*)
- Importance of maintaining a regular exercise schedule: conserve energy for essential activities.
- Avoidance of exposure to extremes in temperature. (*Rationale: This may trigger myasthenic crisis.*)
- Importance of a well balanced diet to maintain optimum health and strength.
- Importance of avoiding infections.
- Signs of myasthenic crisis (respiratory distress, muscular weakness, dysphagia, fever, and general malaise).
- Interventions to avoid a myasthenic crisis (can be triggered by infection, stress, surgery or inaccurate dose of medication); keep suction available for emergency.
- Treatment of myasthenic crisis—*first,* maintain the airway.

[2] Adapted from "HSDA Hotline." Huntington's Disease Society of America/Minnesota Chapter, PO Box 23632, Minneapolis, MN 55423, April 1993.

In March 1993 scientists announced they had discovered the HD gene. This discovery does not mean that there is a cure; more research is needed to determine the exact mechanisms of brain cell death.

Amyotrophic Lateral Sclerosis

Amyotrophic lateral sclerosis (ALS) is a rapidly progressive neurologic disorder resulting in destruction of cortical, brain stem, and spinal cord motor neurons. ALS, also known as Lou Gehrig's disease, usually occurs between 50 and 70 years of age and affects more men than women.

Early in the disease process, the individual experiences weakness, fatigue, and spasticity of the upper extremities. As the disease advances, muscles atrophy and flaccid quadriplegia and eventual involvement of the respiratory muscles occur. The course of the disease is consistent with no remission. ALS is always fatal, usually because of respiratory dysfunction.

Key Concept

The individual with ALS retains intellectual and sensory function throughout the course of the disease.

Ataxia

Ataxia refers to defective muscular coordination. The term refers to a lack of coordination, difficulty in walking, or a progressive condition characterized by a marked spasticity. It can occur in a variety of related disorders.

Both *Friedreich's ataxia* and *Marie's ataxia* are progressive neuromuscular disorders of genetic origin. Onset is usually before age 20 in Friedreich's and before age 40 in Marie's ataxia. These conditions are characterized by sclerosis of the spinal cord, which causes progressive difficulty in walking, with a peculiar swaying gait; slurred speech; scoliosis; myoclonic muscle contractions; and progressive muscular weakness, ending in paralysis.

Symptoms appear in the lower extremities first, forcing the patient to be in a wheelchair for the last few years of life. The affected person usually dies at an early age from complications such as pneumonia or infection.

The patient with ataxia needs extensive nursing care. The patient and family need emotional support. Genetic counseling is highly recommended for family members.

Inflammatory Disorders

Brain Abscess

A brain abscess is a collection of pus that may develop as a result of an infection of the ears, mastoid, sinus, or skull. It can also occur as a direct result of injury to the brain or from brain surgery. If left untreated, this encapsulated "pus pocket" eventually ruptures and spreads, causing further abscesses and meningitis.

The symptoms of a brain abscess mimic those of a brain tumor. The patient may also experience a fever if the primary infection site is still infected. The patient with a brain abscess is at risk for ↑ICP and seizures, as well as a spread of the infection. Surgical treatment is necessary to drain the abscess. Massive doses of IV antibiotics are given preoperatively and postoperatively. The patient may be left with some brain damage or may be completely cured.

Meningitis

Meningitis is an inflammation of the meninges (membranes that cover the brain and the spinal cord). Infection can travel to the meninges from nearby structures, such as the sinuses or the middle ear, or it may be carried by the bloodstream. The infection is caused by viruses, fungi, or bacteria. The causative organism of meningitis is age related. People of different ages tend to be infected by different organisms. It is a serious disease to which children are particularly susceptible.

Three organisms (meningococci, pneumococci, and *Haemophilus influenzae*) cause about 70% of *bacterial* meningitis. *Viral* meningitis is commonly caused by the mumps virus. A condition known as *aseptic meningitis complex* or *benign viral meningitis* (summer grippe) occurs in young children, usually in the summer; it is often accompanied by a rash. In this case, meningeal irritation exists, but no pyogenic organism can be found in the CSF.

Signs and Symptoms. Meningitis usually appears abruptly. Most symptoms are due to ↑ICP. The patient's LOC and eye signs may be altered, and the person may have seizures.

Signs and symptoms of meningitis include fever, chills, severe headache, nausea and vomiting, *nuchal rigidity* (stiff neck), and irritability. Two neurologic signs are present: positive Kernig's sign and positive Brudzinski's sign. Photophobia (intolerance to light) and pain when the eyes are moved from side to side occur. The patient may have seizures. A petechial-purpuric rash is also possible. **Opisthotonos** (an acute spasm in which the body is bowed forward, with the head and heels bent backward) is often present. Additionally, children have tense or bulging fontanels and a high-pitched cry.

Diagnostic Tests. The physician diagnoses meningitis based on a general neurologic examination and two special neurologic signs: Kernig's and Brudzinski's signs.

Kernig's sign: The patient lies on the back and one of the legs is brought up so the hip and knee are both flexed to 90°. The knee is then straightened (the sole of the foot toward the ceiling). If the patient experiences pain or resistance, this indicates meningeal and spinal root inflammation and Kernig's sign is considered *positive.*

Brudzinski's sign: The patient lies on the back and the head is brought forward toward the chest. If the patient experiences pain or resistance, this indicates meningeal irritation, arthritis, or a neck injury. If the patient responds by flexing the hips and knees, meningeal inflammation is indicated and Brudzinski's sign is considered *positive.*

Once a diagnosis of meningitis is made, LP is done to determine the causative organism.

Medical Treatment. After the causative organism has been determined, the physician prescribes large doses of appropriate antibiotics. Antibiotics are highly effective in treating meningitis in adults. If the infection is exceedingly virulent, the drugs may prove useless and the patient may die. Sometimes the nerves of sight and of hearing are damaged as a result of a meningitis attack. Appropriate treatment is instituted.

Nursing Considerations. Nursing care is provided with the awareness that the patient is critically ill. A hypothermia blanket and antipyretic medications may be ordered for high fever, and intravenous fluids and nourishing liquids are given. Tube feedings or total parenteral nutrition may be necessary. Side rails should be in place and padded for the patient's protection. The patient is on seizure precautions. The head of the bed is elevated to at least 30°, unless otherwise ordered. The patient's respiratory status is carefully monitored; tracheostomy is a possibility. The patient should be kept quiet to reduce irritability and to help in relaxation. Traffic in and out of the patient's room should be kept to a minimum. It is important to monitor the disoriented patient. Otherwise the patient should be instructed not to flex the neck because this can obstruct venous flow and increase the ICP. The patient should also avoid acute hip flexion because this can cause increased intraabdominal and intrathoracic pressure. These increased pressures interfere with cerebral blood vessel drainage and cause increased ICP.

Because meningitis is a communicable disease, isolation precautions should be carried out. Meningococcal meningitis is particularly contagious because the causative organisms are present in the throat as well as in the CSF. The incubation period is 2 to 10 days.

Encephalitis

Encephalitis, sometimes called sleeping sickness, is an inflammation of the brain and the meninges caused by viruses, bacteria, or chemical poisoning (such as lead poisoning). It is characterized by destruction of nerve cells. It may follow vaccination or a viral infection such as measles. Encephalitis seems to be more prevalent after influenza epidemics. It may be transmitted by mosquitoes and ticks.

Some types of viral encephalitis are more lethal than others; the death rate has varied from 5% to 70%, depending on the cause of the infection. Many patients who recover from encephalitis are left with mental changes, with seizure disorders, or with parkinsonian symptoms, all of which become increasingly disabling.

Signs and Symptoms. Viral encephalitis attacks suddenly, causing violent headache, fever, nausea, vomiting, and drowsiness. The patient may show muscular weakness and may have tremors or visual disturbances.

Medical Treatment. No drug specific for treating encephalitis has been found. Treatment consists of reducing the fever and maintaining a quiet environment. Tube feedings or total parenteral nutrition are necessary for the nonresponsive patient. If acute respiratory distress occurs, a tracheostomy and mechanical ventilation are required. Warm, moist packs may be ordered to relieve muscle spasms. Side rails should be in place. The patient and family needs instructions for patient safety to prevent falls. The patient is also subject to seizures and may exhibit mental changes.

Guillain-Barrè Syndrome

The cause of Guillain-Barrè syndrome, also called *polyneuritis,* is unknown. It is characterized by inflammation of the nerve roots and the spinal cord, with varying degrees of motor weakness and absent reflexes. Disability ranges from muscle weakness to total paralysis. The onset is often sudden. It usually begins in the lower extremities, ascends, and may progress to total paralysis.

Excellent nursing care is necessary to maintain adequate ventilation, elimination, and nutrition and to prevent deformities. Recovery is usually slow, depending on the severity of the symptoms. Emotional support is essential. This condition is frightening for the patient. If the patient is correctly managed during the acute phase of the disease, however, recovery is often complete.

Poliomyelitis

Poliomyelitis, commonly called *polio*, is caused by a virus that attacks neurons affecting the motor nerves between the brain or the spinal cord and the muscles. The virus usually enters the body through the mouth or the nose and travels along the nerve fibers to the nerve cells connected with a group of muscles. Cells may be damaged temporarily or may be destroyed. If enough nerve cells are destroyed, the muscle becomes paralyzed.

A vaccine is available: Sabin oral vaccine (OPV). It prevents polio in most cases. Because of complacency, however, the number of cases in the world is increasing.

Postpolio Syndrome

A number of people who had polio in the 1940s and 1950s are now experiencing mild to severe muscle weakness as a delayed complication of the first infection. The muscles affected may be the same as those affected earlier, or they may be different. No treatment is yet known, although the disorder is sometimes treated with the same medications as used for an autoimmune disorder.

Acute Transverse Myelitis

Acute transverse myelitis is an inflammatory condition affecting the spinal cord. It occurs as a result of inflammation or destruction of the myelin of the spinal cord neurons. Impairment of bowel and bladder function, generalized weakness of the extremities, and loss of sensation is experienced.

Acute transverse myelitis has several causes. If the disease is diagnosed as *postinfectious*, it usually begins 5 to 20 days after a viral infection. The cause may also be related to collagen vascular disease, syphilis, or acquired immunodeficiency syndrome (AIDS). The prognosis for these patients varies. Some individuals will recover fully, and others will not.

Nursing care for the patient with acute transverse myelitis is aimed at supportive and preventive care. The nurse must be alert for urinary retention, constipation, skin breakdown, thrombus formation, and other complications of immobility.

Trauma

The brain is protected from injury by the thick bones of the skull, as well as by the tough outer membrane of the meninges, the *dura*. In addition, the CSF acts as a shock absorber. A violent blow to the head, however, can cause several kinds of injury to the brain and skull.

> **Nursing Alert**
>
> Serious symptoms can appear up to several days after a head injury. The patient must be observed carefully.

Hematoma

Hemorrhage and edema may occur with laceration or contusion. As a result, there may be a dangerous elevation in ICP. When blood vessels are ruptured within the skull a **hematoma** can result. This swelling or mass of blood compresses the brain tissue and creates further damage.

There are several classifications of hematomas. An *epidural hematoma* is an accumulation of blood, usually from an artery, between the dura and the skull (Fig. 71-4**A**). The pressure of an epidural hematoma can cause seizures and paralysis; one or both of the pa-

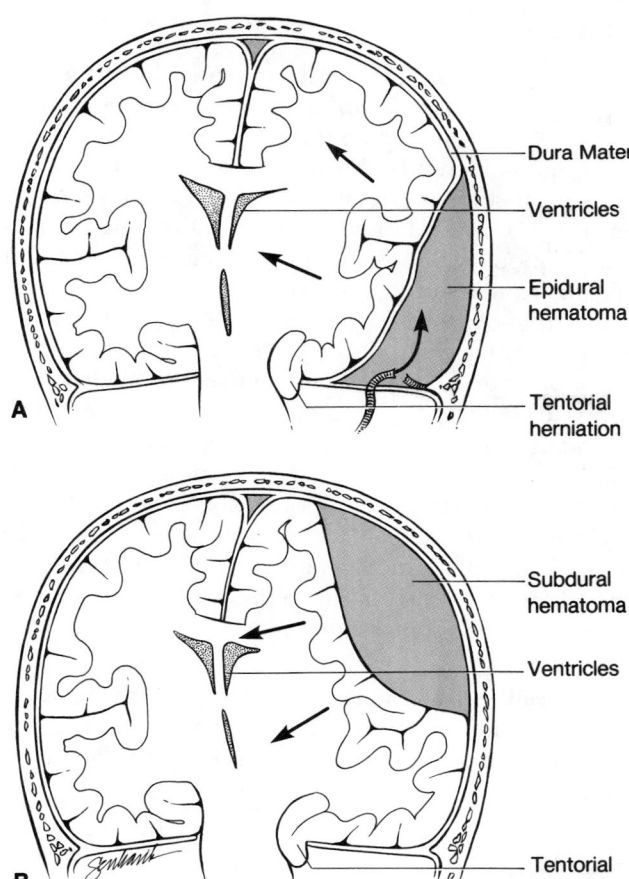

Figure 71-4. Epidural and subdural hematomas. **(A)** Epidural hematoma. Note the broken blood vessel and the shift in the midline structures of the brain. **(B)** Subdural hematoma. (Jackson DB and Saunders RB. Child Health Nursing: A Comprehensive Approach to the Care of Children and Their Families. Philadelphia, J.B. Lippincott, 1993)

tient's pupils may be dilated. Usually, the patient is unconscious immediately after the injury, then lucid for a brief period, then unconscious again as blood accumulates in the epidural space and causes pressure. Epidural hematomas are more common in children.

A *subdural* (below the dura) *hematoma* is typically slow forming. It is caused by an accumulation of blood, usually from a torn vein on the brain's surface (see Fig. 71-4**B**). Symptoms vary with the size and location of a subdural hematoma. The patient may feel drowsy or lose consciousness; there may be seizures, paralysis, and muscle weakness. Speech may be affected. The patient may be confused. Symptoms may not appear for days or even weeks, after the accident.

The nurse must observe carefully for any signs of elevated ICP. Specific signs and symptoms are determined by the area of the brain affected and the extent of any neurologic damage.

Acceleration, Deceleration, and Coup-Contrecoup Injuries

Two types of injury may occur in closed head trauma. The first is the *acceleration–deceleration* injury (Fig. 71-5**A**). This occurs when the head is thrown forward and then suddenly backward, as in an auto accident when a car stops suddenly and the head is thrown forward and backward or strikes something. The brain is moved about within the skull, striking the bones and causing a variety of injuries to the brain.

In *coup-contrecoup* injuries, the site of impact (coup) is not the site of the greatest cerebral damage. In coup-contrecoup, there are injuries both below and opposite the site of the impact (Fig. 71-5**B**). Because the brain is partially anchored at the brain stem and floats freely in CSF, the brain may be hit on one side (*coup*) and then bounce (rebound) off the other side of the skull (*contrecoup*). Blood vessels, nerve tracts, brain tissue, and other structures are bruised and torn. Serious injuries may also occur to the brain stem because of the rebound (contrecoup) action.

Penetrating Head Injuries. In a penetrating head injury, the amount of damage is dependent on the size and location of the penetrating object, such as a bullet.

Skull Fracture

A fracture may be *open* or *closed*, depending on whether the scalp is intact. Many skull fractures are minor, being no more than cracks in the bone. Usually these heal without difficulty. A severe blow to the head, however, may break the bone and force the broken edges to press against the brain (*depressed skull*

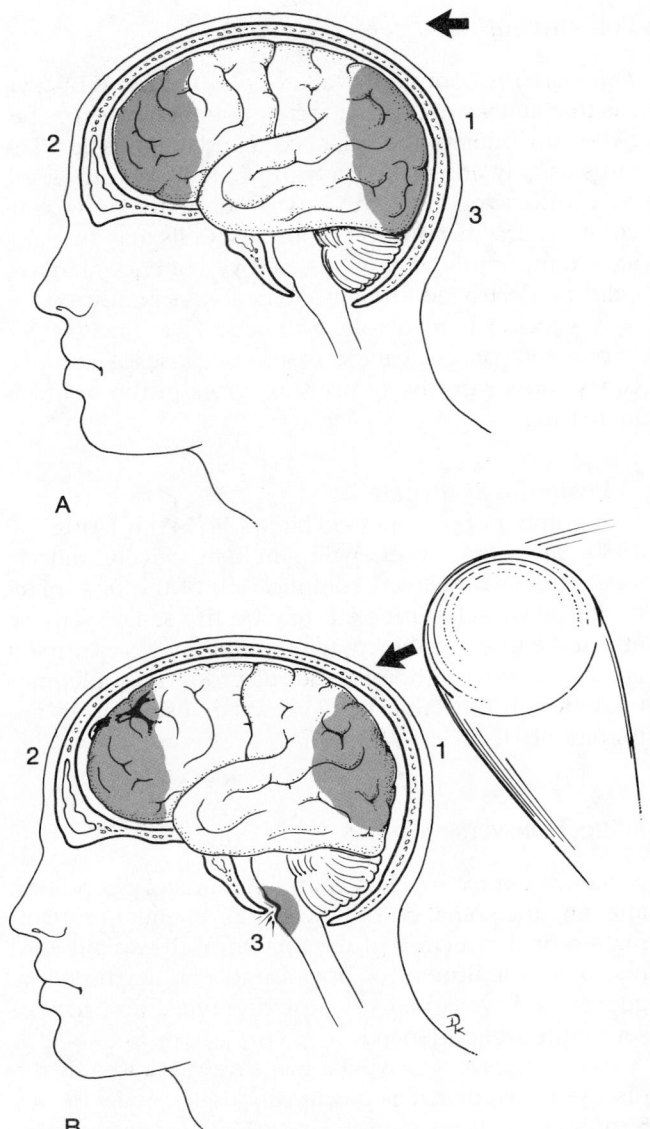

Figure 71-5. Head injuries. **(A)** Acceleration and deceleration injury. The head is hurled forward (and stops suddenly when hitting an immobile object, such as a car dashboard). The brain is hit by the accelerated skull (*1*). The brain then is hurled forward and smashes against the halted skull (*2*). The brain then rebounds (*3*). The brain is bruised and may change shape in response to the impact. Bleeding may also result. **(B)** Coup and contrecoup injury. The brain is injured at the original site of injury (coup injury) (*1*). As the brain shifts from impact and rebounds to the other side, the contrecoup injury occurs. Blood vessels supporting the brain may rupture (*2*) and nerve tracts, brain tissue, and other structures may be bruised and torn. The most serious effects frequently are in the area of the brain stem (*3*).

fracture). Effects will vary with the severity and location of the brain injury. If, for example, the bone fragment is pressing on the brain's speech center, the patient's speech may be impaired until the pressure is relieved.

Any fracture at the base of the skull may injure the nerves entering the spinal cord or interfere with the circulation of the CSF. Or it may damage the cerebellum, which is an especially dangerous situation. Blood, air, and pus are damaging to brain tissue. Brain cells exposed to these substances are destroyed. Infection usually results.

Concussion

A **concussion** is the result of any blow to the head. The concussion may not cause any damage to the structures of the brain, but temporary unconsciousness may result. How long the person remains unconscious varies. Some patients recover from concussions with no apparent ill effects; others may have blurred vision or a severe headache. A patient who has had other than a very minor concussion should see a physician immediately for a thorough neurologic examination.

A *postconcussion syndrome* may persist for several weeks to months after the original injury. The symptoms include headache, anxiety, fatigue, or **vertigo** (a sensation of rotation of oneself or one's surroundings; not true dizziness).

Laceration and Contusion

A **laceration** is a tearing of the brain tissue caused by direct impact or penetrating injury. Lacerations are commonly associated with depressed skull fractures. In **contusion**, the brain tissue is bruised.

Medical and Surgical Treatment in Head Injury. When the patient with an epidural hematoma enters a cycle of consciousness and unconsciousness, immediate neurosurgery usually is necessary to prevent death. Usually surgery is required in the patient with a subdural hematoma. Surgery involves tying off the bleeding vessel and removing the blood clot. Burr holes may be made in the skull or an intraventricular catheter inserted, to relieve excess ICP, by draining off CSF or blood.

Nursing Considerations. Loss of consciousness does not always follow a severe head injury. Every patient who has suffered a blow to the head, as minor as it may appear, needs to be carefully observed until it is certain that the injury has not damaged the brain, because the symptoms of damage do not always appear immediately.

The patient who is conscious should be kept absolutely quiet, should have complete bed rest, and should be observed for the following signs of ↑ICP: headache, dizziness, visual impairment, hearing loss, nausea, or clear or bloody drainage from the ears, nose, or mouth. The patient should also be observed for changes in blood pressure, changes in pupillary signs, and other indications of increasing ICP. The hospitalized patient should be checked frequently for LOC, eye signs, or personality changes, as well as for nausea or dizziness.

A patient released after receiving first-aid treatment following a head injury should be advised to see a physician immediately if he or she has any of the recurring symptoms mentioned earlier. The family should be taught these symptoms also, because the patient may not be able to detect deterioration of functioning (see the accompanying box).

Neoplasms of the Brain

Brain tumors occur in all age groups. Only a small percentage of brain tumors are malignant, and they may be the result of metastasis from another part of the body. Even a benign brain tumor can be fatal, however, because of its pressure on the brain. Benign tumors may

---

Keys to Patient/Family Teaching
Head Injuries

Patient/family teaching for the patient with head injury includes:

◆ Important factors: (1) the patient may not be coherent enough to recognize dangerous symptoms, (2) symptoms may not appear until several days, weeks, or even months following a head injury.

◆ The patient should relax for 24 hours so the brain has a chance to recover. A member of the family should determine the patient's orientation to time and place every 2 hours for the first 24 hours following any blow to the head.

Symptoms to be reported to the physician:

◆ Unusual or increased drowsiness
◆ Weakness of arms or legs; muscle twitching
◆ Nausea and vomiting (especially forceful or projectile vomiting)
◆ Headaches—localized or generalized, unrelieved by mild analgesic
◆ Dizziness
◆ Visual or hearing disturbances, abnormal eye movements
◆ Difficulty arousing from sleep, particularly during the first 24 hours
◆ Personality changes such as forgetfulness, irritability, speech difficulties
◆ Bleeding or clear drainage from the mouth, nose, or ears
◆ Seizures
◆ Blood pressure changes
◆ Any other signs of ↑ ICP

also later become cancerous. Regular follow-up care is essential following treatment for any brain tumor.

Signs and Symptoms. The symptoms of brain tumors are headache, sudden projectile (with great force) vomiting, and visual abnormalities, all caused by ↑ICP. Additional symptoms may develop, depending on which area of the brain is affected. For example, if the motor area is affected, numbness or twitching in the arm may occur; a tumor on the brain's frontal lobe causes personality changes and affects memory or the ability to reason. Often a seizure is the first symptom of a brain tumor. If elevated ICP near the brain stem is not relieved, severe respiratory difficulties and possible death from respiratory failure may occur. As brain tumors grow, the symptoms become progressively worse.

Diagnostic Tests. Neurologic assessment is important. Especially important to diagnosis is the neurologic history. By questioning the patient and family, the physician can determine the progress of any neurologic deficits. Diagnostic tests, such as the CT scan and EEG, are performed, to determine the location, size, and neurologic effects of the tumor.

Medical and Surgical Treatment. Treatment options include surgery, chemotherapy and radiation therapy, or a combination of these. The specific treatment is determined according to the type and location of the tumor.

Surgery (craniotomy) is discussed at the beginning of this chapter. Success of surgery for a brain tumor depends on the location of the tumor and whether it can be removed without causing brain damage. Some tumors are inoperable, that is, impossible to remove without causing severe brain damage or death. Even "successful" brain surgery can result in neurologic deficits.

Nursing Considerations. Preoperative and postoperative care in craniotomy is discussed at the beginning of this chapter in the Nursing Process section.

Keys for Review

Key Questions for Critical Thinking

1. Differentiate among CT scan, PET scan, and MRI. Describe nursing care for each with rationale.
2. Discuss normal and abnormal ICP. Describe the earliest and most important sign of abnormal ICP. Identify other signs and symptoms of IICP and explain why they are significant.
3. Outline the responsibilities of the nurse when a person has a seizure.
4. You are caring for a patient who is paralyzed. Describe nursing care for the patient paralyzed from the waist down. Compare with care for the patient paralyzed from the neck down.
5. Explain why a brain tumor is life threatening, whether it is malignant or benign.

Key Readings

Berkow R (Ed). The Merck Manual of Diagnosis and Therapy, Ed 16. Rahway, NJ, Merck & Co, 1992

Engel J. Seizures and Epilepsy. Philadelphia, F.A. Davis, 1989

Key Readings

Hickey JV. Neurological and Neurosurgical Nursing, Ed 3. Philadelphia, J.B. Lippincott, 1992

NANDA Nursing Diagnoses: Definitions and Classifications 1992. Philadelphia, North American Nursing Diagnosis Association, 1992

Nursing '93 Drug Handbook. Springhouse, PA, Springhouse, 1993

O'Toole M (Ed). Miller-Keane Encyclopedia and Dictionary of Medicine, Nursing, and Allied Health, Ed. 5. Philadelphia, W.B. Saunders, 1992

Snyder M. A Guide to Neurological and Neurosurgical Nursing, Ed 2. Albany, NY, Delmar Publishers, 1991

Taylor C, Lillis C, LeMone P. Fundamentals of Nursing: The Art and Science of Nursing Care, Ed 2. Philadelphia, J.B. Lippincott, 1993

Smeltzer SC, Bare BG. Brunner and Suddarth's Textbook of Medical-Surgical Nursing, Ed 7. Philadelphia, J.B. Lippincott, 1992

Keys to Learning More

Chapter 74: cardiovascular disorders, including CVA

Chapter 76: cancer

Chapter 86: dementias in the aging

Chapter 87: psychiatric nursing

Chapter 88: substance abuse, which can permanently alter neurologic function

Chapter 89: rehabilitation

Chapter 90: death and dying

Key Resources

American Parkinson's Disease Association Inc.
116 John Street
New York, NY 10038
212/732-9550

American Spinal Injury Association
2020 Peachtree Road, NW
Atlanta, GA 30309

Epilepsy Foundation of America
815 15th Street, NW, Suite 528
Washington, DC 20005
202/638-5229

Guillain-Barrè Foundation
129 North Carolina Avenue, SE
Washington, DC 20003
202/387-2216

Huntington's Disease Society of America
140 W. 22nd Street
New York, NY 10011-2420
1-800/345-HDSA

Key Resources (continued)

National Association to Control Epilepsy
22 East 67th Street
New York, NY 10012

National Head Injury Foundation
333 Turnpike Road
Southborough, MA 01722
508/485-9950

National Hydrocephalus Foundation
22427 South River Road
Joliet, IL 60436

National Parkinson's Foundation
1501 NW 9th Avenue
Miami, FL 33136
305/547-6666

National Spinal Cord Injury Association
600 West Cumming Park, #3200
Woburn, MA 01801
1-800/962-9629

Parkinson's Disease Foundation
Medical Center
William Black Medical Research Bldg.
640 West 168th Street
New York, NY 10032
212/923-4700

Spina Bifida Association of America
1700 Rockville Pike, Suite 250
Rockville, MD 20852

72 Endocrine Disorders

Keys for Learning

Learning Objectives

- Describe tests that evaluate endocrine function and nursing care related to these tests.
- Discuss symptoms and treatment of overproduction and underproduction of hormones and nursing care required for each disorder.
- Define the major classifications of diabetes mellitus, symptoms and treatment related to each type, and required nursing care.
- Discuss and demonstrate administration of insulin.
- Describe precautions related to insulin and oral hypoglycemic agents.
- Explain the interactions of diet, exercise, and diabetes medications in the treatment of diabetes mellitus.

Key Terms

cretinism	hyperglycemia	ketoacidosis
diabetes insipidus	hyperparathyroidism	myxedema
diabetes mellitus	hyperthyroidism	polydipsia
endocrinologist	hypoglycemia	polyphagia
exophthalmos	hypoparathyroidism	polyuria
goiter	insulin	thyroidectomy
Graves' disease		

Keys to Understanding This Chapter

Chapter 15: anatomy and physiology of integumentary system

Chapter 16: fluid and electrolyte balance

Chapter 19: anatomy and physiology of endocrine system

Chapter 23: anatomy and physiology of digestive system

Chapter 26: food and its functions

Chapter 28: diet therapy and special diets

Chapter 31: first aid

Chapter 38: signs and symptoms of illness or injury

Chapter 45: personal hygiene and skin care

Keys to Understanding This Chapter
(continued)

Chapter 46: elimination

Chapter 47: specimen collection

Chapter 50: head-to-toe nursing assessment

Chapter 57: administration of medications

Chapter 61: complicated pregnancy, including the diabetic mother

Unit Thirteen: childhood disorders, including endocrine disorders

Chapter 69: disorders in fluid or electrolyte balance

Key Points

- Endocrine glands secrete hormones that influence metabolism, growth, and development.
- Many tests may be used to diagnose an endocrine disorder.
- Physical appearance may also play a part in diagnosis, due to a defect in growth or development.
- The pituitary gland is referred to as the "master gland" because its secretions affect the functioning of every other gland.
- The thyroid is the largest endocrine gland; it secretes hormones that stimulate catabolism (cell breakdown).
- The parathyroid glands regulate bone formation.
- The adrenal glands secrete epinephrine (part of the "flight-or-fight" response to danger). They also secrete various steroid hormones, which control many vital functions related to fluid and electrolyte balance and regulation in development of sex characteristics.
- Diabetes mellitus occurs when the pancreas does not make enough insulin or the body becomes resistant to insulin.
- Endocrine disorders result from overproduction or underproduction of hormones. Symptoms relate to the above functions.

Key Learning Activities

◆ Interview patients with various endocrine disorders. Report on their initial symptoms, diagnosis, and response to treatment.
◆ Seek a patient with diabetes who is new to using insulin. Observe a staff nurse teaching the patient (insulin administration, self-monitoring of blood glucose). Observe teaching by the dietitian.

The endocrine system is intricately involved in regulating nearly all body processes. The physician trained in this specialty is called an **endocrinologist**, although other specialists also treat endocrine disorders.

Anatomy and Physiology Review

The endocrine glands (ductless glands) are groups of cells that produce chemical substances called hormones (see Chapter 19). They secrete the hormones directly into the bloodstream where they play a part in metabolism and influence growth and activity of cells and body systems. Normally, they produce, store, and release hormones as needed. It is known that many endocrine glands are sensitive to stimulation from each other.

The major endocrine glands are the pituitary (anterior and posterior), thyroid, parathyroid, adrenal, gonads, and specialized cells within the pancreas. Examples of hormones are ACTH, ISH, oxytocin, and insulin.

Diagnostic Tests

Many blood and urine tests are done to diagnose an endocrine disorder because the components of blood and urine are important indicators of endocrine function. Direct observation also plays a part in diagnosis

of endocrine problems. Some endocrine disorders lead to defects in growth or appearance and can be identified by the physical appearance of the patient.

> **Key Concept**
>
> Endocrine disorders are usually caused by overproduction or underproduction of hormones.

Tests of Thyroid Function

Laboratory Tests
Blood Tests. In assessing thyroid function, usually a combination of blood tests is done because there are various hormones secreted and no single test can give a complete picture. Thyroid function tests (TFTs) include:

◆ FTI—free thyroxine index
◆ LATS—long-acting thyroid stimulation
◆ T_4—serum thyroxine
◆ T_3—serum triiodothyronine
◆ RT_3U—T_3 resin uptake
◆ TSH—thyroid-stimulating hormone

Protein-Bound Iodine (PBI). The quantity of PBI (a constituent of thyroid hormone) in the blood is measured by this test. This test is not reliable and is not done often.

Key Abbreviations and Acronyms for Endocrine System

ACTH	Adrenocorticotropic hormone
ADA	American Diabetes Association
ADH	Antidiuretic hormone (vasopressin)
FBS	Fasting blood sugar (fasting blood glucose)
FSH	Follicle-stimulating hormone
GDM	Gestational diabetes mellitus
GH	Growth hormone
GTT	Glucose tolerance test
IDDM	Insulin-dependent diabetes mellitus
IGT	Impaired glucose tolerance
LH	Luteinizing hormone
MSH	Melanocyte-stimulating hormone
NIDDM	Non–insulin-dependent diabetes mellitus
PBI	Protein-bound iodine
PPG	Postprandial glucose
PTH	Parathyroid hormone (parathormone)
RAI	Radioactive iodine uptake (test)
SIADH	Syndrome of inappropriate antidiuretic hormone
STH	Somatotropic hormone (somatotropin)
TFT	Thyroid function test
TSH	Thyroid-stimulating hormone
U-100	100 units of insulin per mL (U.S. insulin strength)

X-ray Evaluations

Thyroid Scan (Radioscan or Scintiscan). For a thyroid scan, the patient ingests radioactive iodine or sodium pertechnetate. (See Chapter 50 for precautions when dye is used.) After the dye is taken, a "scanogram" (x-ray) is taken to indicate the amount of radioactivity in the entire body. If a great deal of the radioactive iodine is taken up by the thyroid, this indicates that the thyroid is hyperactive. If a deceased amount of iodine is in the thyroid, a malignancy might be present. This test may also indicate locations of thyroid malignancy metastases to other parts of the body.

Radioactive Iodine Uptake (RAI). This test measures thyroid gland activity. The patient drinks a small amount of a radioactive iodine dissolved in distilled water or swallows a capsule of the radioactive substance. At various intervals, up to 24 hours, a scan of the thyroid gland is taken to measure the amount of radioactive material removed from the bloodstream and taken up by the thyroid. A normally active thyroid will remove from 15% to 45% within that period; in hyperthyroidism it may remove as much as 90%. Factors that can influ-

ence accuracy of a radioactive iodine test are use of oral contraceptives, anticoagulants, salicylates, and propylthiouracil (PTU) derivatives. Make certain the patient is not allergic to iodine or shellfish. This test should not be done on pregnant women.

Other *contraindications* include:

◆ Recent x-ray studies using contrast dye
◆ Person taking thyroid or antithyroid medications
◆ Person taking iodine
◆ Person who recently has had other radioactive study

It is important to know how much iodine the patient usually consumes (ocean shellfish, iodized salt, SSKI—saturated solution of potassium iodide, Lugol's solution), if the patient uses iodine-containing antiseptics, or if the person has had a recent x-ray using iodine-based contrast media. Ask patients if they are taking the contraindicated medications as above, or if they take thyroid-stimulating hormone (TSH), estrogen, or barbiturates. These substances should not be used for a week before the test.

Pretest preparation may include fasting or a light breakfast. Patients must know exactly when to return to the laboratory. Teach the patient that the dose of radiation is not dangerous.

Other Tests

Thyroid Ultrasound (Thyroid Echogram). This test determines the size, shape, and position of the thyroid gland. Abnormal findings may indicate a cyst or a solid nodule, which is often cancerous. The test may also be done periodically during treatment to determine the effectiveness of therapy. The test may also be done to evaluate the thyroid during pregnancy because RAI examination is dangerous for the fetus.

The ultrasound examination will not hurt; there will be no disturbance of breathing or swallowing. The test takes approximately 15 minutes. The patient will be lying on the table; a liberal amount of gel will be applied to the neck to ensure transmission of sound waves. Photos and computer printouts will be evaluated by the physician.

After the test, the patient may need assistance to remove the gel from the skin.

Tests of Parathyroid Function

Blood Tests

Blood tests are done to evaluate parathyroid function. These include serum parathormone, parathyroid hormone (PTH) levels and serum phosphate, and calcium levels.

Other Diagnostic Tests

Ultrasound, magnetic resonance imaging (MRI), thallium scan, and fine-needle biopsy can be used to evaluate the function of the parathyroids and to localize parathyroid cysts, tumors, and hyperplasia (abnormal increase in size). Chapter 71 describes some of these tests.

Tests of Adrenal Function

Laboratory Tests

Blood Tests. Blood tests are done to determine adrenal function. These include the ACTH stimulation test, serum ACTH test, and plasma cortisol test.

Urine Tests. Urine tests are also done to evaluate adrenal function. Measurement of metabolites of catecholamines in the urine is useful in diagnosis. Urinary metanephrine is the most diagnostic urine test of adrenal medulla function. A 24-hour specimen of urine may be collected for determining vanillylmandelic acid (VMA), a metabolite of catecholamines. Additionally, a 24-hour specimen of urine may be collected for determining other metabolites, such as 17-hydroxycorticosteroids, 17-ketosteroids, and 17-ketogenic steroids, all of which are diagnostic of adrenal cortical function.

X-ray Evaluations

Radiographic evaluations of adrenal function include the adrenal angiogram and venogram, computed tomography (CT) scan of the adrenals, as well as x-ray study of the sella turcica. These examinations detect benign and malignant tumors of the adrenal glands, as well as hyperplasia.

Adrenal Angiogram/Venogram. These tests involve insertion of a catheter and injection of dye so that x-ray contrast studies can be done. Allergy to dye should be determined before the test and other precautions, as listed in Chapter 50, observed. The patient is usually NPO before the test. The major complication is an allergic reaction to the dye. To prevent this complication, propranolol (Inderal), diphenhydramine (Benadryl), or other medications may be administered for several days before and after the test. The test may also cause hemorrhage or dislodging of an atherosclerotic plaque from the wall of the blood vessel used for dye injection. This may cause an infarction. If hemorrhage occurs within the adrenal glands, Addison's disease may result. If surgery is needed later, it is more difficult when any of these events have occurred.

Contraindications are:

◆ Pregnancy
◆ Allergy to dye
◆ Unstable patient
◆ Hemophilia, bleeding disorder
◆ Measurable atherosclerosis
◆ Uncooperative patient

Tests of General Pancreatic Function

Laboratory Tests

Serum Amylase. The serum amylase is a blood test that reveals the amount of amylase enzyme that is present. Amylase is secreted in the pancreas and is necessary for digestion. Urine may also be tested for the presence of amylase. The amylase level in urine remains elevated for a longer time than that of serum. These tests are indicated when pancreatitis is suspected.

Serum Lipase. Lipase is another enzyme secreted by the pancreas. The lipase level may also be determined; elevations of serum lipase suggest pancreatitis. Related disorders are discussed in Chapter 81.

Specific Tests for Diabetes Mellitus

Laboratory Tests

Blood Tests. A number of blood tests indicate the functioning of the endocrine portion of the pancreas. Most of these are specifically related to detection and evaluation of diabetes mellitus. They include:

◆ Fasting blood glucose level (FBS)
◆ GTT—glucose tolerance test
◆ HgbA$_{1c}$—glycosylated hemoglobin (glycohemoglobin)
◆ Plasma insulin assay
◆ Serum glucose test
◆ 2-Hour PPG—2-hour postprandial (after a meal) blood glucose

Urine Tests. Urine tests for glucose and acetone are sometimes done.

Tests for Glucose Levels

Fasting Blood Glucose Level. The fasting blood glucose level is used as a screening procedure. This test was formerly called *fasting blood sugar* and is often abbreviated FBS. In most cases, an elevated fasting (without eating) or nonfasting blood glucose level is an indication of diabetes mellitus. The FBS level is defined as the amount of glucose (sugar) present in the blood when the patient has been fasting for the prescribed length of time (6–8 hours). The normal range for fasting blood glucose is 65 to 115 mg/dL. The abbreviation dL means *deciliter*—1/10 of a liter, which equals 100 milliliters. Normal blood glucose values for adults are given in Table 72-1.

Two-Hour Postprandial Blood Glucose Level. Two-hour postprandial (after a meal) blood glucose level deter-

Table 72-1. Normal Blood Glucose Values for Adults*

Fasting blood glucose	<115 mg/dL
Blood glucose level after 75-g oral glucose intake	After 30 min, 1 h, and 1½ h— <200 mg/dL
	After 2 h, <140 mg/dL

* The values may differ for pregnant women.

mination is also a common test to determine how well sugar is handled by the body. This test is usually done at home by a person with known diabetes, who can use his or her own glucose meter. It is not a commonly used tool for initial detection of diabetes.

The role of the nurse is often to teach this procedure to the patient.

◆ The patient has nothing to eat or drink after midnight. First, a fasting blood specimen is drawn.
◆ A high-carbohydrate breakfast (a measured amount of carbohydrate) is given. It is important that the patient eat the whole meal quickly. The dietitian can make a list of foods to be eaten.
◆ One blood test is done 2 hours after this meal to determine the glucose level in the blood. In nondiabetic people, the blood glucose level is not elevated 2 hours after a meal, but the level of a person with diabetes remains elevated. This test is not to be confused with routinely testing blood glucose immediately before a meal.
◆ The results are reported to the physician.

Glucose Tolerance Test. The glucose tolerance test (GTT) is a timed test used when the fasting blood glucose level falls above normal, but below the diagnostic level for diabetes. It is also used in gestational diabetes screening in both the 1-hour and 3-hour formats. Functional hypoglycemia is diagnosed through the GTT.

◆ The patient should ingest at least 150 g carbohydrate daily for 3 days before the test (most individuals following a good general diet will easily meet this criterion).
◆ Tests of both blood and urine are taken during the fasting state.
◆ The patient drinks 75 to 100 g glucose. It is important that the patient consume this glucose completely and as quickly as possible because this is a timed test and the starting point must be as precise as possible.
◆ Blood and urine specimens are again taken at prescribed intervals: ½ hour, 1 hour, 2 hours, and 3 hours. The collection of specimens is timed from the point of ingestion of glucose.
◆ The test begins with an empty bladder, although the pretest urine specimen is also saved as one of the fasting specimens to be examined.

◆ The laboratory technician takes the blood and urine specimens, labels them, and indicates the time when each was collected.
◆ The patient may have water to drink while the test is going on; this makes the patient more comfortable and makes it easier to void frequently.
◆ No juice or other fluids or food is permitted.
◆ The patient is not allowed to smoke. Smoking can affect digestion of food and glucose metabolism.
◆ The patient cannot chew gum. It contains sugar and stimulates digestion.
◆ Some factors may affect the test (because they elevate glucose levels). These include thiazide diuretics, oral contraceptives, lithium, caffeine, and nicotinic acid.
◆ Normal plasma glucose levels peak at 160 to 180 mL within 30 minutes to 1 hour after administration of an oral glucose test dose and return to fasting levels or lower within 2 to 3 hours. Urine glucose tests should remain negative throughout.

Glycosylated Hemoglobin. Glycosylated hemoglobin reflects the mean average blood glucose level over the previous 6 to 10 weeks. It is measured by determining the amount of glucose attached to a certain portion of hemoglobin in red blood cells. It is invaluable in monitoring of blood glucose control and allows the patient and healthcare team to set a measurable goal. Although normal ranges vary depending on the laboratory, most physicians will try to have their patients in the range of 5% to 8%, depending on which exact subfactors are measured.

Urine Tests. Normal urine is free from sugar (glucose), acetone, and protein, but any of these may be present in the urine of the diabetic patient. Excess glucose in the blood spills over into the urine; acetone appears as a by-product of faulty metabolism. With the availability of a variety of sophisticated, but easy-to-use, blood glucose monitors, urine testing is done infrequently, both in the healthcare facility and at home. The most common need for urine testing is the test for ketones if the blood glucose level is consistently high.

Keto-Diastix. This convenient test measures glucose and acetone at the same time. (Acetone is a ketone body that is present when the body cells are starving because of faulty metabolism. Buildup of acetone leads to ketosis, which in turn leads to acidosis. Vomiting or excessive perspiration can alter electrolyte balance.)

The procedure for using Keto-Diastix is as follows:

◆ Wear gloves.
◆ Dip the test strip quickly into the urine. Take the reading for glucose and acetone, using the color chart on the bottle. *Note:* It is important to keep the bottle tightly closed because moisture in the air can render the strips ineffective.

♦ A *double-voiding* technique must be used for diabetic urine tests to obtain a true determination of the amount of glucose and ketones spilled in the urine at any particular time. The patient should void and discard that specimen. The procedure begins with an *empty* bladder.

♦ Then, ½ hour later, another freshly voided specimen should be collected and used for testing. *Note:* The specimen from a catheter must be obtained from the tubing and not from the bag. (These are *current* samples.) The bag contains older urine.

Nursing Alert

The test for acetone is especially important if the patient is vomiting, has a fever, or has a high concentration of glucose in the blood (above 240 mg/dL).

Medical and Surgical Treatments

Common Medical Treatments

Because there are such a variety of disorders with an endocrine basis, the medical treatments are discussed with each condition. (Table 56-4 lists many hormones and other drugs which affect the endocrine system.)

Common Surgical Treatments

Thyroidectomy

Thyroidectomy is the surgical removal of the thyroid gland. Generally, about five sixths of the gland is removed (*subtotal thyroidectomy*) so that some thyroid hormone production can continue postoperatively.

Lugol's solution (iodine and potassium iodide in water) is given for a limited time (10 days to 2 weeks) before surgical removal of the thyroid. The patient must be observed for "iodism" (iodine toxicity) evidenced by rash, excessive salivation, and swelling of the buccal mucosa. Lugol's solution should be given through a straw because it stains the teeth; it should be mixed with milk or fruit juice to mask the taste. The purpose of giving Lugol's solution is to make the gland smaller, firmer, and less vascular before surgery and to prevent further release of thyroid hormones into the circulatory system. This also helps prevent a thyroid crisis postoperatively. The accompanying box gives guidelines for nursing care in thyroidectomy.

A subtotal thyroidectomy usually prevents recurrence of hyperthyroidism because only enough of the gland is left to maintain normal function. If a total thyroidectomy is done (because of injury or malignancy), thyroid extract must be given to the patient for life.

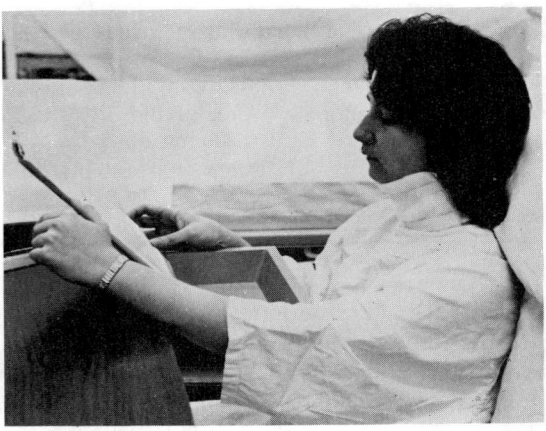

Figure 72-1. In making the thyroidectomy patient comfortable in a chair, the nurse sees that the head and neck are well supported with pillows. The overbed table enables the patient to reach frequently needed articles without turning her head. It also is convenient to use this table when respiratory therapy treatments are given.

The patient should be encouraged to rest and avoid excessive physical activity. The patient must be taught the importance of continued medication therapy. It is also important to teach and document the teaching of signs and symptoms of hypofunction and hyperfunction of the thyroid gland and the necessity for close follow-up after surgery. Thyroid function tests must be given at periodic intervals.

Postoperative Complications. *Tetany* is generalized continuous muscle spasm of the entire body. It is most often caused by accidental removal of the parathyroid glands during thyroidectomy and is a dangerous development. PTH is administered, along with calcium gluconate, to treat the condition. If the parathyroid glands have been totally removed, administration of PTH must continue for life.

Thyroid crisis (thyrotoxicosis or thyroid storm) is possible, either in the hospital or, occasionally, after discharge. It is caused by a sudden increase in thyroxine. It is dangerous and the nurse must be alert for symptoms, both preoperatively and postoperatively. Symptoms of thyroid crisis include tachycardia, anxiety, and an abrupt increase in temperature, respiration, pulse, and blood pressure. This extreme form of thyrotoxicosis can cause death from heart failure. Sedatives, tranquilizers, and cardiotonics are prescribed to treat it. The goal of management is to maintain oxygen and glucose levels in body cells, while reducing fever.

Thyroid storm is not so prevalent postoperatively with antithyroid drugs or iodine preparations, such as Lugol's solution. In some cases, corticosteroids are given.

Nursing Skill Guidelines
Providing Care After Thyroidectomy

Preoperative Care

♦ A high-calorie, high-protein, high-vitamin diet is given. The patient is weighed daily. *(Rationale: to check for edema.)*

♦ Radiation—generally in the form of radioactive iodine that will localize in the thyroid—may be given. *(Rationale: to attempt to destroy part of the thyroid.)*

♦ The pulse is checked frequently. *(Rationale: The patient's heart rate may be affected.)*

♦ Adrenergic-blocking agents (such as propranolol hydrochloride—Inderal) may be given in the severely hyperthyroid patient. *(Rationale: to regulate heart rate.)*

♦ In every possible way, the nurse should maintain a quiet environment, control visitors, and move unhurriedly when giving care. *(Rationale: This helps relax the patient and prevents excitement. The patient is in a "hyper" state because of the disease.)*

♦ The patient should be informed that there will be some discomfort when swallowing after surgery. The person should anticipate having to turn, breathe deeply, and use the incentive spirometer after surgery. *(Rationale: Preoperative preparation and practice help the patient to be more cooperative postoperatively.)*

♦ Patients may be concerned about a scar. Actually, the scar is a thin line and a scarf or necklace can camouflage it.

Postoperative Care

♦ Postoperatively, the patient is placed in semi-Fowler's position with the head elevated and supported by pillows. *(Rationale: this alleviates strain on the suture line.)* *(Fig. 72-1.)*

♦ Narcotics are prescribed for pain. Temperature, pulse, and blood pressure are checked frequently for example, every 15 minutes until stable. The patient is monitored closely for signs and symptoms of hemorrhage and thyroid storm. *(Rationale: These are the two most common complications following thyroidectomy.)*

♦ The patient can have ice chips or sips of water as soon as nausea ceases.

♦ Occasionally, a patient is given oxygen to make breathing easier. Noisy breathing or cyanosis must be reported immediately—a tracheostomy might be necessary. A tracheostomy set should be kept at the bedside. *(Rationale: It is vital to maintain a patent airway.)*

♦ The nurse should observe for signs of hoarseness. The quality of a patient's voice should be assessed every 30 to 60 minutes during the immediate postoperative period. The nurse should report any voice changes at once. *(Rationale: Voice change could be the first sign of edema or injury to the laryngeal nerve.)*

♦ Suction might be needed, especially after an aerosolized respiratory therapy treatment (such as IPPB). *(Rationale: This helps relieve excessive secretion of mucus and prevents choking.)*

♦ Cold fluids are usually tolerated well. (Do *not* give milk; it will form a film in the throat.) A soft diet may be given as soon as the patient can swallow. A well balanced, high-calorie diet is given to help the patient regain lost weight.

♦ Usually, the patient is allowed out of bed the day after surgery. When the patient sits in a chair, make sure the head and neck are supported. An overbed table makes it convenient to reach for needed articles without turning the head. *(Rationale: Turning the head is uncomfortable and might dislodge the suture line; see Fig. 72-1).* The patient is usually discharged from the hospital on the third or fourth postoperative day.

Nursing Alert

Internal hemorrhage, following thyroidectomy, is a threat. Dressings are inspected for excessive bleeding. The nurse should check for edema in the neck or bleeding at the back of the neck. An endotracheal tube should be kept available in the patient's room, both preoperatively and postoperatively, because swelling may obstruct the airway, causing respiratory distress. In this event, the endotracheal tube is inserted and the patient is taken to the operating room for a tracheostomy.

❖ Nursing Process

Data Collection

The nurse observes and assesses patients for possible endocrine disorders. Chapter 38 describes signs and signs and symptoms of illness and Chapter 50 describes physical examination and nursing assessment. This assessment establishes a baseline for future comparison and determines the presence of suspected endocrine-related complications. The nurse should report any changes in baseline levels.

Many assessments of endocrine function are based on laboratory examination of blood. Other testing, such as x-ray or ultrasound, is also done. It is the role of the nurse to check reports of these evaluations and call the physician's attention to abnormal reports. The nurse often does blood testing for glucose and occasionally may do urine glucose or acetone testing.

The nurse may observe signs and symptoms of endocrine disorders while caring for patients. Any signs or symptoms should be brought to the attention of the physician. In addition, the nurse observes the patient's emotional response to the disorder or disease. Does the patient need assistance to meet daily needs? Is the patient anxious or fearful of the outcome? Does disorder-related teaching need to be done? Is the person having difficulty accepting the long-term nature of a disorder?

Nursing Diagnosis

Based on data collection, the following sample nursing diagnoses may be seen on nursing care plans for patients with endocrine disorders. Nursing diagnoses may have more than one causal factor.

- ◆ Altered Nutrition: Less Than Body Requirements related to endocrine dysfunction
- ◆ Altered Nutrition: More Than Body Requirements related to metabolic dysfunction
- ◆ Impaired Skin Integrity related to diabetic ulceration, poor tissue healing following surgery or trauma, impaired circulation
- ◆ Ineffective Individual Coping related to chronic disorder, lifelong administration of insulin or other hormone
- ◆ Ineffective Management of Therapeutic Regimen as evidenced by failure to follow prescribed regimen of diet, exercise, and insulin
- ◆ Impaired Physical Mobility related to foot ulcers, impaired circulation, amputation
- ◆ Impaired Home Maintenance Management related to low activity tolerance, impaired mobility, pain
- ◆ Knowledge Deficit related to management of hormonal disorder, diet, exercise, medication administration
- ◆ Body Image Disturbance related to amputation of limbs, loss of mobility, chronic disorder

Planning and Implementation

The patient, family, and nurse plan together for effective care to meet patient needs, based on the nursing diagnosis. The nurse provides preoperative and postoperative care for the patient undergoing thyroidectomy or other surgery. It is also important to correctly prepare patients for diagnostic tests.

Because disorders of the endocrine system can affect most functions of the body, it is difficult to list all the nursing implications. An endocrine disorder can be a simple imbalance that is successfully treated by administration of hormones or other medications. However, in some cases, such as end-stage renal disease caused by diabetes mellitus, the patient may need total nursing care and assistance to meet all needs, including those related to death and dying.

The patient also may have difficulty accepting the fact that an endocrine disorder is chronic and that treatment, such as insulin injections, must continue for life. Most patients need to be taught about their disorder, its prognosis, and its treatment. A nursing care plan is developed to meet individual patient needs. A sample nursing care plan for a patient with an endocrine disorder is provided later in the chapter with the discussion of Graves' disease.

Testing for Blood Glucose Level

Many nurses in various healthcare facilities do the blood glucose monitoring. The Nursing Procedure outlines the skills used in performing the test. These steps can also be used in teaching the patient how to self-monitor blood glucose levels.

Evaluation

Periodically, the nurse, patient, family, and other members of the healthcare team evaluate the outcomes of care. Have short-term goals been met? Are long-term goals still realistic? Planning for further nursing care considers the patient's prognosis, any complications, and the patient's response to care given. Patient and caregiver teaching is an important component of nursing care. Do they understand the treatment required and the underlying reasons? Has adequate patient/family teaching been done and documented?

Pituitary (Hypophysis) Disorders

The pituitary gland is tiny, but it has tremendous influence in the body and affects the operations of every other gland. For this reason, it is sometimes called the "master gland." It lies in the sphenoid bone at the base of the brain and has three parts, the anterior, the middle, and the posterior lobes.

Anatomy and Physiology of the Anterior Pituitary

The anterior lobe alone produces or releases the following hormones: growth hormone (GH), adrenocorticotropic hormone (ACTH), thyroid-stimulating hormone (TSH), prolactin, follicle-stimulating hormone (FSH), and luteinizing hormone (LH). These hormones are of vital importance in growth, maturation, and reproduction of human beings.

(Text continues on page 1057)

Testing for Blood Glucose Level

Supplies and Equipment

Blood glucose testing strips
Glucose testing meter
Sterile lancet
Lancet activating device (optional)
Cotton balls
Alcohol swab
Gloves

Suggested Procedure and Rationale

1. Wash hands.
   (Rationale: Handwashing prevents the spread of organisms.)

2. Gather supplies.
   (Rationale: Organization facilitates performance of the skill.)

3. Explain procedure to patient.
   (Rationale: Providing information fosters patient cooperation.)

4. Have patient wash hands with warm water.
   (Rationale: Handwashing cleanses the puncture site and warm water promotes vasodilation.)

5. Assist patient to a comfortable position.
   (Rationale: Puncture site should be easily accessible.)

6. Remove test strip from container. Turn glucose-testing meter on. Check that code number on strip matches code number that initially appears on monitor screen. (or follow manufacturer's instructions).
   (Rationale: Matching code numbers on strip and meter ensure that machine is calibrated correctly.)

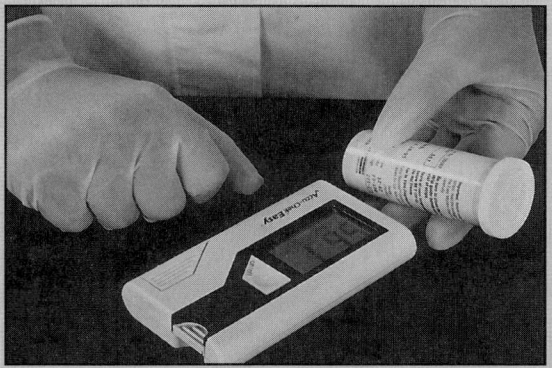

Step 6 Comparing the test strip code number to the number on the monitor

7. Prepare lancet by twisting cap off. Arm automatic device by pushing back the plunger until it clicks. Attach lancet. Remove cap. Keep tip sterile.
   (Rationale: This reduces transmission of organisms to puncture site.)

8. Put on gloves.
   (Rationale: Gloves act as a barrier.)

9. Select site on finger for puncture. Gently massage finger toward the intended puncture site, keeping finger in dependent position.
   (Rationale: Massage and dependent position encourage blood flow to the area.)

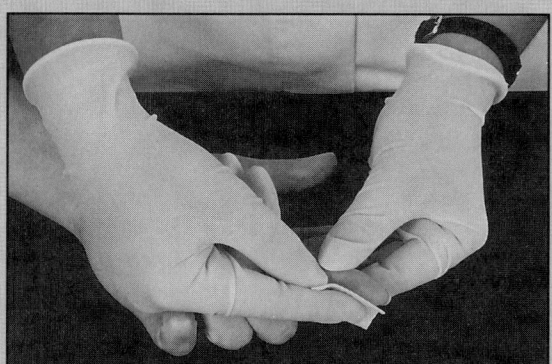

Step 9 Preparing the puncture site

10. Clean site with alcohol prep and allow to dry thoroughly. (Patients are sometimes taught to omit this step at home.)
    (Rationale: Alcohol can affect the blood sample and cause destruction of some red blood cells.)

(continued)

11. Prick side of finger with lancet and squeeze gently. Use cotton ball to wipe away first drop of blood if recommended for particular meter that is used. *(Rationale: Directions for some meters indicate that first drop of blood should not be used because it may be diluted by serum and give a false reading.)*

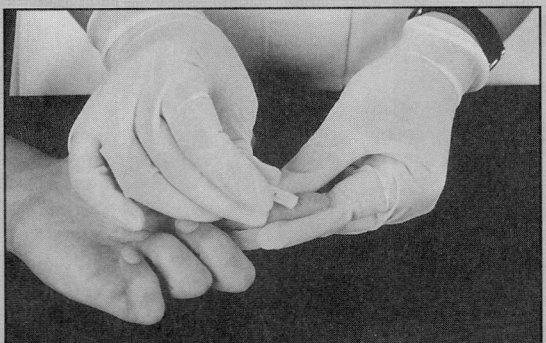

Step 11 Using a lancet to prick the finger

12. Gently touch drop of blood to target area of strip or use pipette, as instructed. *(Rationale: Blood must color entire target area but should not be smeared on strip or test results will be inaccurate.)* Have patient hold clean cotton ball on the puncture site for a few seconds. *(Rationale: The person with diabetes often has slowed clotting.)*

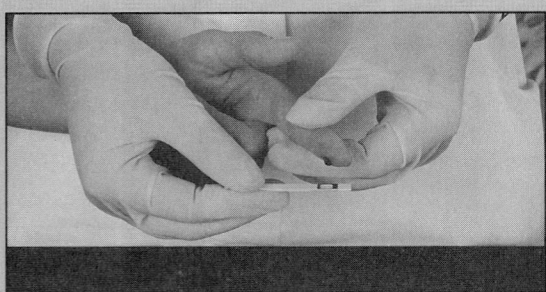

Step 12 Placing a blood drop on the target area of the strip

13. Insert strip as far as it will go into meter with target area facing red dot on meter (or follow manufacturer's directions for specific meter). *(Rationale: Strip must be inserted correctly for machine to determine blood glucose level.*

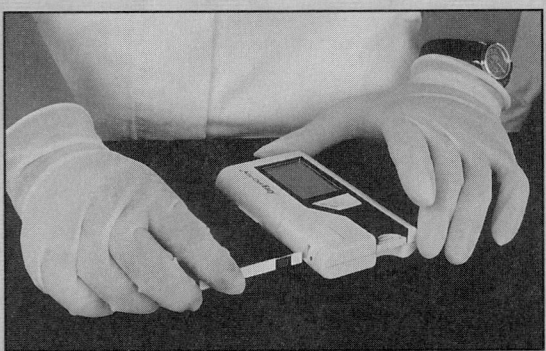

Step 13 Placing the strip in the meter

14. Read test results in 15 to 60 seconds on meter face. Remove strip and turn meter off. *(Rationale: Individual meters read test results within varying time frames.)*

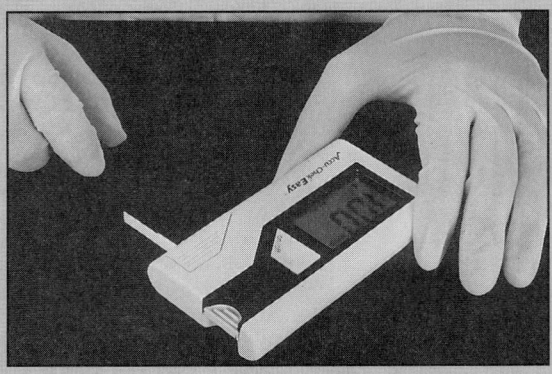

Step 14 Reading the results (Photos © B. Proud.)

15. Dispose of equipment properly. Remove gloves and wash hands. *(Rationale: Proper disposal of equipment and handwashing prevent the transmission of organisms.)*
16. Record blood glucose reading on proper forms. Check to see if the patient is on insulin coverage. *(Rationale: Documentation provides coordination of care. Blood glucose reading may necessitate insulin coverage.)*
17. Meters used in hospitals require a daily quality control check.

Overproduction of Anterior Pituitary Hormones: Giantism and Acromegaly

Disturbances of the anterior lobe of the pituitary gland may cause overproduction of the growth hormone, somatotropin (STH). If overproduction occurs in childhood, it causes excessive growth of bones, or *giantism*. In an adult, an excess of STH causes overgrowth of tissues, called *acromegaly*. The victim's features coarsen; the person develops a massive lower jaw, thick lips, a bulbous nose, a bulging forehead, and hands and feet that seem to be enormous. In women, facial hair also appears (hirsutism) and the voice deepens. Headaches are common and partial loss of vision may develop. The spleen, heart, and liver enlarge; muscles weaken, and joint pain and stiffness appear. There may be impotence or amenorrhea.

Acromegaly is treated by irradiation of the pituitary gland or surgical intervention. Recently, certain drugs have shown promise in lowering the levels of growth hormone. Treatment can stop the progress of the disease, but therapy cannot alter abnormal growth that has already occurred.

Absence of Anterior Pituitary Hormones: Simmonds' Disease

Simmonds' disease is rare; it is also called *panhypopituitarism*. It occurs when hormones normally released by the anterior pituitary gland are absent. Simmonds' disease can be caused when the pituitary gland is destroyed by a tumor, by surgery, or by postpartum emboli. The genitalia become atrophied, and the patient ages prematurely and becomes wasted. Treatment depends on the cause. Hormones must be given to the patient, once the pituitary gland is removed or destroyed; the combination of hormones, however, is individualized and difficult to determine.

The Middle Lobe

The middle lobe of the pituitary gland produces the melanocyte-stimulating hormone (MSH), which functions in skin coloration. Disorders are related to pigmentation of the skin.

Anatomy and Physiology of the Posterior Pituitary

The posterior lobe of the pituitary gland secretes and releases hormones that affect blood pressure and control water balance in the kidney tubules. The hormones it releases are antidiuretic hormone (ADH or vasopressin) and those that stimulate uterine contractions and release of milk by the breasts when the baby nurses (oxytocin).

Underproduction of ADH: Diabetes Insipidus

Diabetes insipidus is a disease caused by underproduction of the hormone ADH, which regulates the passage of water through the kidneys.

Primary nephrogenic insipidus is a rare disease caused by kidney dysfunction, due to a deficiency in ADH or to a lesion in the midbrain. *Secondary central diabetes insipidus* results from a tumor in the gland itself or pressure in the pituitary area from head trauma or other tumors. It may also occur following pituitary surgery.

In diabetes insipidus, urine is copious; the patient may void as much as 15 to 20 liters in 24 hours. The patient is constantly thirsty; restricting fluids has no effect. The urine is dilute, with a specific gravity less than 1.006, and contains no sugar or acetone. The nurse must keep accurate intake and output records to make sure the volume of output is being replaced; electrolyte levels must be closely monitored. Despite an abnormally large appetite, the patient is weak and the nurse might need to assist the patient with self-care. Treatment consists of giving ADH, vasopressin (Pitressin) subcutaneously or intramuscularly to control the output of urine.

> **Nursing Alert**
>
> Pitressin administration must be monitored closely because it can cause coronary artery constriction.

Syndrome of Inappropriate Antidiuretic Hormone (SIADH)

This disorder involves the excessive secretion of ADH from the pituitary gland. Patients with SIADH cannot excrete a dilute urine. Fluid retention and sodium deficiency occur. SIADH can result from central nervous system disorders, chemotherapy, ADH production by some cancers, and overuse of vasopressin therapy.

Urine output is decreased. The patient may complain of a headache or experience confusion, lethargy, seizures, and possibly coma if the sodium deficiency is severe. Weight gain also occurs.

Close monitoring of fluid intake and output, daily weights, and mental status is necessary. The nurse should institute safety measures to reduce the risk of possible injury.

Neoplasms of the Pituitary

Neoplasms of the pituitary gland can affect various aspects of body function. An *overgrowth of eosinophilic cells* in the pituitary can result in giantism. A *basophilic* tumor in the pituitary can upset production of the hormone that regulates the adrenals, leading to hyperadrenalism and Cushing's syndrome (described later). A *chromophobic* tumor can destroy the pituitary and result in hypopituitarism. A patient with this disorder has fine, scanty hair, lowered basal metabolism rate, lowered body temperature, and a tendency to be obese and move very slowly.

The pituitary may be removed for a variety of reasons. It may be malignant; it may be removed to decrease diabetic retinopathy. Occasionally it is removed to control pain associated with metastatic carcinoma of the breast or prostate. Surgical removal of the pituitary is called *hypophysectomy.* Routine preoperative and postoperative care is given. Usually, the patient is admitted to the intensive care unit postoperatively.

Anatomy and Physiology of the Thyroid Gland

The thyroid gland is located just below the larynx in the anterior middle part of the neck. It lies on either side of and anterior to the trachea. It consists of two lobes connected by a strip called the isthmus. The thyroid is the largest of the endocrine glands and secretes the hormones thyroxine (T_4) and triiodothyronine (T_3), which regulate metabolism by stimulating catabolism (the breakdown of cells and foods, with release of energy). Too much of these hormones makes the tissues burn oxygen rapidly; too little causes the reverse. The thyroid gland requires iodine to produce these hormones. A pituitary hormone also contributes to their production. The thyroid gland also produces calcitonin, which helps to maintain calcium balance in the plasma.

Overproduction of Thyroid Hormone: Hyperthyroidism

Hyperthyroidism is also called **Graves' disease** or *exophthalmic or toxic diffuse goiter.* It is a condition in which the metabolic rate is increased by overproduction of T_4. The exact cause of this overactivity is not known, but it may develop as a result of physical or emotional strain, infection, or changes related to adolescence or pregnancy. Current theories point to an autoimmune origin in which the person forms antibodies against thyroid cells, specifically the TSH receptor cells. It occurs most frequently in women.

Signs and Symptoms. The patient is highly excitable and overactive and may have tremors that make it impossible to eat without help. The pulse is rapid; the person may have heart palpitations and increased incidence of arrhythmias. These will cause damage if not treated. The systolic blood pressure is elevated. The person feels hot, eats voraciously, yet loses weight because calories are burned so rapidly. The skin takes on a characteristic salmon color. In women, menstruation may cease.

Another common system is bulging eyes (**exophthalmos**). Figure 72-2 illustrates a woman with Graves' disease. The cause of this symptom is not fully understood. It can lead to blindness caused by stretching of the optic nerve or corneal ulceration. The neck is swollen, and the pressure from the gland may cause difficulty in swallowing or hoarseness.

If untreated, this disorder may cause intense nervousness, delirium, and finally death as a result of persistent cardiac overload.

Medical and Surgical Treatment. The treatment for hyperthyroidism may be medical or surgical. Medical treatment consists of prescribing antithyroid drugs to block secretion of the thyroid hormone. Propylthiouracil or methimazole (Tapazole) may be given either as part of a medical treatment or as preparation for sur-

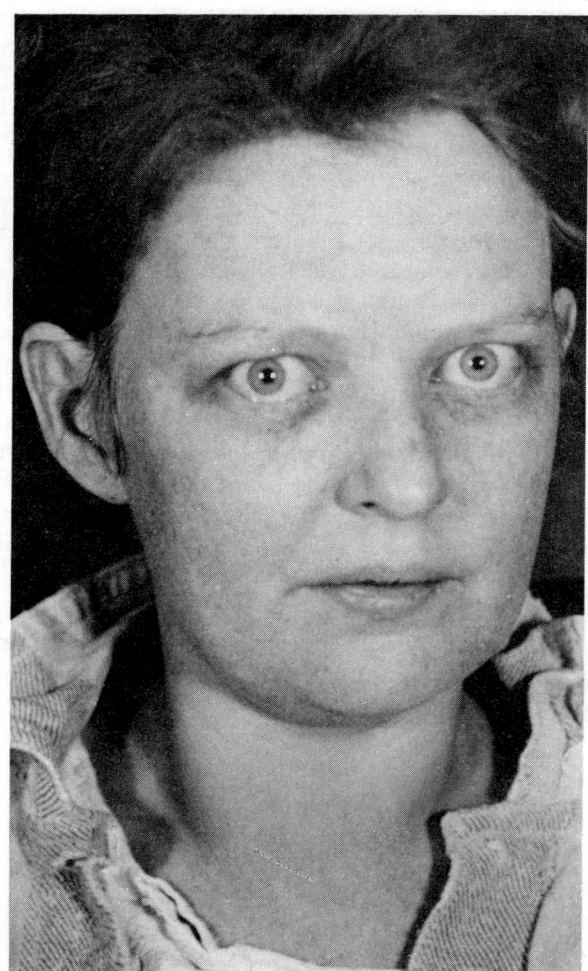

Figure 72-2. A woman with Graves' disease. Note the exophthalmos and enlarged thyroid gland. (Chaffee E.E. and Lytle I.M. Basic Physiology and Anatomy, Ed 4. Philadelphia, J.B. Lippincott.)

gery. If prescribed as medical therapy, these drugs are given daily, generally over a long time. They may have toxic effects—fever, skin rash, and enlarged lymph nodes, with an increase in white blood cells.

Therapeutic doses of radioactive iodine may also be prescribed. These are administered as an oral solution that is absorbed by the gastrointestinal tract. The radioactive iodine is transported to the thyroid gland, where it destroys the gland's ability to make T_4 and T_3. Surgical removal of the thyroid is no longer the treatment of choice and is done only after antithyroid drugs and radioactive iodine have proven unsuccessful, or when the goiter is so large it constricts structures in the neck region.

Nursing Considerations. The nursing care for the patient with hyperthyroidism focuses on minimizing overactivity, improving nutritional status, maintaining a normal body temperature, and improving self-esteem.

The nurse should assist in providing a calm environment and minimizing the patient's expenditure of energy by helping with activities and encouraging alternating periods of rest and activity. Increased calories and nutritional support are provided to help improve nutritional status. If exophthalmos is present, eye protection, such as patches, drops, or artificial tears, can be used. If body temperature is elevated, acetaminophen and cooling blankets may be used to reduce body temperature. Because the patient is experiencing changes in appearance, appetite, and weight along with the overactivity, it is important to convey to the patient an understanding of concern and willingness to help. The Nursing Care Plan gives care for several nursing diagnoses for a woman with Graves' disease.

Underproduction of Thyroid Hormone: Hypothyroidism

Hypothyroidism occurs when a deficiency of T_4 slows down metabolic processes. It may be due to removal of the thyroid gland or to a decrease in its activity. It is more likely to affect women than men. The congenital form of this deficiency causes a condition called **cretinism.** Advanced hypothyroidism in the adult is called **myxedema.**

Signs and Symptoms. *Cretinism.* Untreated cretinism results in arrested physical and mental development and dystrophy of bones and soft tissues. The person is dwarfed and has a large head, short arms and legs, puffy eyes, and protruding tongue. The person also has dry skin and movements are uncoordinated; sterility occurs in almost all cases. Mental retardation/intellectual impairment ranges from moderate to severe. If discovered early, this condition can often be successfully treated with administration of thyroid extract, which must be continued for life.

Myxedema. Symptoms of hypothyroidism in adults include slowing of physical and mental activity, accompanied by forgetfulness and chronic headache. The patient's expression becomes masklike, the skin is dry, hair coarsens and tends to fall out, the voice is hoarse and low, and the patient gains weight. The patient may become chronically constipated and anemic, and heart rate may be affected. The radioactive iodine uptake rate will almost always be normal; menorrhagia (excessive menstrual flow) may occur.

Treatment. Oral thyroid extract or synthetic thyroid hormones may be given to supply the hormone deficiency; synthetic preparations are being used increasingly. The results are dramatic. The patient becomes more alert and the appearance becomes normal. This replacement therapy must be done gradually because a rapid change can be dangerous; for example, the heart rate may increase too rapidly and show signs of strain from increased activity.

Nursing Considerations. Anyone with a thyroid deficiency is more susceptible to respiratory depression from sedatives or hypnotics. Some people have to take thyroid replacement preparations all their lives, but with well regulated treatment, they stay normally well and healthy. Such a patient must see the physician for periodic examinations.

Long-term untreated hypothyroidism can result in *myxedema coma,* a medical emergency necessitating immediate but careful administration of thyroid hormone. This must be followed by treatment of any depressed respiratory function that occurs and by close monitoring of cardiac function.

The nursing care of a patient with hypothyroidism focuses on improving activity tolerance and independence, resuming normal bowel function, improving mental activity, and adhering to medical regime.

Nursing Alert

◆ Sedatives, narcotics, and hypnotic drugs should not be given to the person with hypothyroidism, or should be given in very small doses. *(Rationale: The respiratory and heart rates are slowed and additional heart depressants could cause respiratory or cardiac arrest.)*

◆ Be alert for signs of myocardial infarction. *(Rationale: This is due to the long period of slowed circulation to heart muscle.)*

◆ Anginal pain often occurs when thyroid hormone therapy is begun; it is a dangerous development and must be reported at once. The patient must also be taught the signs and symptoms of angina. *(Rationale: This pain can be the first sign of a myocardial infarction. A clot might be blocking a portion of the coronary circulation.)*

Mari Hassan is a 35-year-old, married East Indian woman who was diagnosed with Graves' disease (hyperthyroidism) 6 months ago. The diagnosis was based on her physical appearance (enlarged neck, protruding eyes, agitated expression); symptoms of agitation, restlessness, and weight loss; and laboratory findings (elevated serum thyroid hormone, 24-hour radioiodine uptake, and T_3 resin). She was placed on antithyroid medication. She was admitted to the hospital because of a worsening of her symptoms: profuse diaphoresis, tachycardia, cyclic mood swings, amenorrhea, and extreme fatigue. During the nursing history the nurse discovers that Mrs. Hassan has not been taking the antithyroid medication regularly because for the first time in her life she has been losing weight effortlessly—as a result of her quickened metabolism. "I've always had a weight problem and I didn't want to do anything now that would cause me to gain back the weight I've lost over the past year. I want to look more like my American friends." The patient's understanding of the gravity of her illness is limited. A major nursing priority is patient education to prevent the complications of Graves' disease: exophthalmos, heart disease, and thyroid storm. Two nursing diagnoses from her plan of care are highlighted below.

Nursing Diagnosis: *Noncompliance with Medical Regimen Related to Deficient Understanding of the Gravity of the Illness and a Desire to Continue to Lose Weight as Evidenced by Progression of her Symptoms and Self-Report.*

Goal 1: Prior to discharge patient will describe the relationship between taking her antithyroid medication and the prevention of exophthalmos, heart disease, and thyroid storm.

Goal 2: Prior to discharge patient will verbalize her willingness to follow the proposed medical regimen.

Long-term goal: The patient's laboratory values and clinical picture will demonstrate compliance with medical regimen and adequate management of hyperthyroidism.

Nursing Actions (assess/do/teach)	Rationale	Evaluative Statement
1. Carefully assess the patient's knowledge of Grave's disease and the seriousness of the complications that accompany lack of treatment; explore the multiple reasons that underlie her past choice to not take the prescribed antithyroid medication; refrain from being judgmental.	Teaching and counseling to be effective must be based on an accurate grasp of the patient's knowledge base and values.	3/6 Goal 1 met; patient accurately describes the progression of symptoms in untreated Grave's disease. 3/6 Goal 2 met; patient verbalizes a willingness to take antithyroid medication, reports she had no idea so much was at stake.
2. Explain the many ways in which an excess secretion of thyroid hormone can influence her physical and mental well-being; project into the future and describe the typical progression of the untreated disease; be sensitive to her ability to understand and process the information given and where possible, link teaching to her values.	Only with accurate knowledge can persons make informed treatment decisions.	
3. Respect her right to make autonomous decisions about her treatment; where possible, support the decisions she makes; affirm "healthy" choices.	Persons are entitled to make autonomous decisions about their care.	

(continued)

Nursing Diagnosis: *Chronic Low Self-Esteem Related to Physical Appearance (Obesity) and Unsatisfactory Interpersonal Relationships as Evidenced by Noncompliance for Weight Loss Reasons and Numerous Self-Deprecatory Statements.*

Goal 1: Prior to discharge, patient makes more positive statements about herself.

Goal 2: Prior to discharge, patient describes a plan for developing her personal strengths.

Nursing Actions (assess/do/teach)	Rationale	Evaluative Statement
1. Establish a trusting, caring relationship with the patient and communicate that she is valued for herself.	Unconditional acceptance is often lacking for persons with low self-esteem.	3/7 Goal 1 partially met; negative statements are decreased but there are few positive verbalizations.
2. Help the patient to explore and maximize her strengths. Develop a positive plan of action to develop these strengths and to convert weaknesses to strengths (*e.g.,* weight reduction program that incorporates exercise and that can also meet social needs). Communicate the belief that the patient has within herself all the resources she needs to enhance her self-esteem.	These are empowerment strategies; simply having someone else believe that "I have the personal resources to turn my life around" can be a powerful stimulant.	3/7 Goal 2 partially met; patient is beginning to show a willingness to develop plans to promote self-esteem.
3. Discuss the "self-fulfilling prophecy" syndrome with the patient and explore the potential effects of longstanding negative self-evaluation and feelings about self and capabilities.	We instruct others how to perceive us by our posture, confidence, verbalizations. Cultural considerations may interfere with progress for this patient (ie, role of women in East Indian society and increased acceptance of female obesity in contrast to some other cultures).	

An Autoimmune Thyroid Disorder: Hashimoto's Thyroiditis

Hashimoto's thyroiditis is a condition of the thyroid believed to be autoimmune in origin. It is of the type of autoimmune disorders known as *organ specific* because the body builds up antibodies against thyroid tissue only (see Chapter 78).

Nontoxic Thyroid Enlargement: Simple Goiter

Sometimes the thyroid gland, even though enlarged, does not cause toxic symptoms, in which case it is called a *colloid goiter* or a simple **goiter**. The thyroid gland is enlarged and the distended spaces are filled with colloid, a gelatinous material. No symptoms of T_4 deficiency are noted. If symptoms of too much T_4 occur (hyperthyroidism), the goiter is referred to as a *toxic goiter.*

Colloid goiter affects women more commonly than men and may appear during pregnancy or adolescence or with an infection. Except for its appearance, a colloid goiter usually does not have a harmful effect on health, unless it becomes so large that it interferes with swallowing or breathing.

Usually, a simple (colloid) goiter is caused by a deficiency of iodine in the diet. The thyroid gland must have iodine to produce thyroid hormones. If a sufficient supply is not available, the gland enlarges in an effort to produce the hormone. Sea (salt) water contains iodine, as does some soil and inland drinking water. Noncoastal areas, such as mountainous areas, the Pacific Northwest, and the Great Lakes region, are deficient in iodine.

Treatment. Goiter is treated by giving iodine for a period of 2 to 3 weeks and repeating the treatment three or four times during the year, if the diet is deficient in iodine. The administration of iodine does not cure the simple goiter; it will *prevent* simple goiter or stop its progress.

It is not difficult to reinforce the body's supply of iodine because it needs such a very small amount. The most economical, suitable, and reliable goiter prevention program is the use of iodized table salt. Surgery may be necessary if a goiter causes excessive pressure.

Neoplasms of the Thyroid

Benign Neoplasms. A liquid or semisolid cyst sometimes forms in the thyroid. This can be located by ultrasound. A simple cyst can be aspirated. A semisolid cyst is most often malignant and must be surgically removed.

Malignant Neoplasms. A malignant tumor can occur any time from childhood to late adulthood. If a thyroid tumor is cancerous, it must be removed surgically or treated by irradiation with radioactive isotopes. A biopsy will tell whether such a growth is malignant. Most common thyroid cancers are slow growing, although a fast-growing adenocarcinoma may metastasize and be unresponsive to radiation therapy.

Anatomy and Physiology of the Parathyroid Glands

The parathyroids are tiny bean-shaped glands (four, six, or eight in number) located on either side of the underparts of the thyroid gland. They secrete the parathyroid hormone, parathormone (PTH), which, aided by vitamin D, regulates the amount of calcium and phosphorus in the blood, and thus regulates bone formation.

Overproduction of Parathormone: Hyperparathyroidism

Hyperparathyroidism is an excess of parathormone, the parathyroid hormone, causing elevated calcium levels in the blood; this results in depletion of calcium in the bone (osteomalacia). Bone tissue becomes softened and weakened, leading to skeletal tenderness. The bones tend to break easily, even in the absence of pressure or injury (pathologic fractures) and the skull may enlarge. Muscles are weak, and the patient is tired, nauseated, and constipated. Kidney stones, urinary tract infections, and uremia may develop. The person may become disoriented and paranoid and may lose consciousness. This condition may be secondary to chronic nephritis.

Hyperparathyroidism is detected by a consistently high level of blood calcium and by x-ray indications of skeletal changes or pathologic fractures.

A diuretic agent such as furosemide (Lasix) and large amounts of fluids are often given to prevent renal disorders. Phosphates may be carefully given to reduce serum calcium. A lobectomy, to remove part of the gland, may be done. Preoperatively, the patient should be encouraged to exercise to help prevent some calcium from being released from the bones. The diet is limited in calcium in some cases. If, after the operation, muscle spasm (tetany) appears, the patient is given calcium gluconate to restore the calcium–phosphorus balance in the blood.

A tracheostomy tray and intravenous calcium are kept at the bedside for use in an emergency. The postoperative diet is high in calcium, fat, and carbohydrate. The patient needs special care to avoid injury (bumps or pressure) until bones have become recalcified.

Underproduction of Parathormone: Hypoparathyroidism

Hypoparathyroidism is a deficiency of PTH. It is caused by a lowered production of the hormone, with a consequent reduction of the amount of calcium available to the body and an accumulation of phosphorus in the blood. Hypoparathyroidism may be caused by accidental removal of the parathyroid glands during a thyroidectomy.

The lack of calcium causes tremors and muscle spasms (tetany), which is the characteristic sign of hypoparathyroidism. Cardiac output is decreased. Latent tetany is suggested by a positive Trousseau's sign (carpopedal spasm caused by blocking the blood flow to the arm for 3 minutes using a blood pressure cuff) or a positive Chvostek's sign (twitching of the mouth, nose and eye after tapping the area over the facial nerve just in front of the parotid gland and anterior to the ear). This extreme muscular irritability may be so pronounced as to cause laryngospasm or seizures. Other symptoms include loss of hair, coarsening of skin, brittle nails, arrhythmias, and possible heart failure.

The treatment is to increase the serum calcium level. Calcium salts (calcium gluconate) must be given, usually intravenously. (Calcium preparations are *never* given intramuscularly because they would injure tissues.) Large doses of vitamin D are also given because of the regulatory effect vitamin D has on calcium levels in the body. It may also be necessary to administer sedatives or anticonvulsants in the acute phase of hypoparathyroidism (to prevent seizures). Patient teaching about medications and need for follow-up is important.

Anatomy and Physiology of the Adrenal Glands

The adrenals (suprarenals) are small three-cornered glands, one atop each kidney. Each has two parts. The medulla secretes the hormones epinephrine (adrenaline) and norepinephrine and is stimulated by the sympathetic nervous system. When quick action is needed, epinephrine is secreted instantly to increase the flow of the blood to the brain, heart, muscles, and other vital organs. The cortex (outer covering) secretes various types of steroid hormones. They control many vital functions: regulating metabolism to supply quick energy, helping maintain fluid and electrolyte balance, and regulating the development of secondary sex characteristics.

Disorders of the Adrenal Cortex

Hyperfunction of the Adrenal Cortex

Cushing's syndrome is not common. It is caused by overproduction of hormones secreted by the adrenal cortex. It may be precipitated by steroid therapy, by a tumor of the adrenal glands, or by a tumor of the pituitary.

Fat distribution is abnormal: the face is rounded ("moon face") and the abdomen is heavy and hangs down, but the arms and legs are thin. As the disease progresses, the patient becomes weaker, the bones soften, and the patient might have a backache. Edema develops and urinary output is reduced. High sodium and low potassium blood levels and hyperglycemia follow. The patient is hypertensive. Wounds do not heal and the patient bruises easily. Mood swings are common; the patient may be irritable or euphoric.

If hyperadrenalism occurs in childhood, male puberty comes early. A girl develops masculine traits because of increased secretion of male sex hormones by the adrenal glands.

Treatment depends on the cause. Surgical removal of the adrenal gland may be indicated. Adrenocortical hormones will be given as indicated. After surgery, the patient is treated as for Addison's disease (see next section). If the cause is pituitary in origin, there are various methods of treatment, not without controversy. Nursing care is usually aimed at treatment of symptoms.

Measures to protect the patient from injury and infection, such as assessing skin integrity, promoting good hygiene, and removing or minimizing environmental hazards, are instituted. The patient's weight is monitored daily and vital signs are assessed frequently. Electrolyte and glucose levels are checked for changes.

Primary Aldosteronism

Primary aldosteronism is a rare condition of the adrenal cortex, characterized by excessive secretion of aldosterone. Symptoms include hypertension and muscle weakness because of low potassium levels. If tumors or excessive growth of the adrenal glands exist, surgery is the treatment of choice.

> **Nursing Alert**
>
> Many young people, especially athletes, use large doses of steroids to enhance muscle development. This is a dangerous practice that often leads to long-term disability and can cause death. In addition to sexual dysfunction, heart arrhythmias, and many problems in later life, the person is at risk for severe behavior problems. In some cases, the person becomes aggressive, loses touch with reality, or shows manic symptoms.

Hypofunction or Destruction of the Adrenal Cortex

Destruction or degeneration of the adrenal cortex causes a condition called *Addison's disease*. It is comparatively rare. Tuberculosis, cancer, or a massive infection can be the underlying cause, but in most cases, the gland atrophies (wastes away) due to unknown causes. It may be a secondary response to pituitary malfunction. In this case, ACTH is not produced in sufficient amounts by the pituitary gland; thus, adrenal function is diminished.

Signs and Symptoms. Addison's disease decreases the production of adrenal hormones, with the result that fluid and electrolyte balance in the body is upset and the blood sugar level is lowered (hypoglycemia). In addition, thyroid function is abnormally low and the blood is low in sodium and high in potassium.

The first symptom is usually a darkening of skin and oral mucous membranes, so that the skin looks bronzed. The patient becomes dehydrated and anemic and loses weight. Blood pressure drops. The hair becomes thin. Strain or stress of any kind may cause adrenal shock, with abnormally low blood pressure, nausea and vomiting, diarrhea, headache, and restlessness. Tremors and disorientation may arise, progressing to loss of consciousness and seizures.

Treatment. Treatment consists of supplying needed hormones in an effort to restore normal fluid and electrolyte balance. Patient teaching is vital. The patient must cooperate by seeing the physician regularly and by avoiding strain or excitement of any kind, such as overwork, infection, or exposure to cold. By protecting his or her health, the patient with Addison's disease can do very well.

> **Key Concept**
>
> The patient should wear an identification tag with instructions for hormone dosage in case the prescribing physician cannot be contacted.

Nursing Considerations. The diet is usually high in protein and salt and low in fluid. *(Rationale: When salt (sodium) is lost, water is also lost from the body.)* Because this patient is dehydrated, retention of fluid is the goal. Because sodium has been lost as a result of previous hormone imbalance, it is replaced in the diet. Water intake is restricted. *(Rationale: Water overloads the system.)*

Five or six small meals may be prescribed, or the patient may be given between-meal snacks of milk and crackers. *(Rationale: The person may be too weak to eat a large meal at one time. The diet is planned to combat dehydration.)*

The person should be watched for dizziness or lowered blood pressure and should be protected from falling. An accurate record of food and fluid intake is vital, with the type and amount of all fluids and food being recorded, as well as the volume and specific gravity of each voiding. *(Rationale: All of these measurements help to determine the fluid and electrolyte balance of the body. Therapy is continued until these values are normal.)*

Addisonian Crisis (Adrenal Crisis)

Addisonian crisis occurs when adrenal function falls to a critically low point; it is marked by nausea, vomiting, weight loss, and extreme hypotension. A stressful situation is usually the underlying cause. Time is crucial in treating the patient because of the possibility of fatal vascular shock. Hydrocortisone (Cortef, Hydrocortone), given intravenously, is the immediate treatment. Vasopressors, such as dopamine hydrochloride (Dopastat, Intropin), are sometimes given to raise blood pressure. Salts (sodium and potassium ions) that have been lost by vomiting are replaced in an intravenous solution of saline with electrolytes added. The exact solution to be given is prescribed several times daily by the physician; the ratio of electrolytes is based on laboratory tests.

Disorders of the Adrenal Medulla

Neoplasms

Pheochromocytoma is a tumor, usually benign, that originates in the adrenal medulla. A tumor of the adrenal medulla increases secretion of the hormones epinephrine and norepinephrine. This, in turn, causes hypertension, tremor, headache, nausea and vomiting,

dizziness, and increased urination. The treatment for this condition is surgical removal of the tumor—a dangerous operation because it may cause sudden and extreme changes in blood pressure. If the patient has a bilateral adrenalectomy, he or she must be treated for Addison's disease postoperatively; adrenal hormones must be supplied artificially for life.

An Endocrine Disorder of the Pancreas: Diabetes Mellitus

Diabetes mellitus is a chronic disease characterized by abnormal metabolism of carbohydrate, protein, and fat. It often leads to a variety of complications affecting the circulatory and nervous systems.

Anatomy and Physiology Review

Insulin is a hormone produced by the *beta* cells in the islets of Langerhans located within the pancreas. Insulin is used by the body to regulate metabolism. Without this hormone, glucose cannot enter the fat cells, blood glucose levels rise, and the individual may begin to experience symptoms of hyperglycemia. The *alpha* cells in the pancreas secrete glucagon, which raises blood glucose levels. The *delta* cells secrete somatostatin, which regulates the release of insulin and glucagon from alpha and beta cells.

At least 12 million people in the United States are believed to have diabetes, half of whom have not yet sought medical attention. The numbers have increased in recent years because so many Americans are overweight as a result of their sedentary life-styles. Also, the accuracy of testing has improved, thus confirming more cases. The number of people with diabetes is expected to double as more people live to middle and old age, when most cases are discovered.

Signs and Symptoms of Diabetes. Diabetes can present a wide variety of symptoms. Classic symptoms include the "three polys":

- **Polyuria** (excessive urination)
- **Polydipsia** (excessive thirst)
- **Polyphagia** (excessive hunger)

Classic symptoms are more likely in type I diabetes and come on rapidly. Other signs and symptoms include:

- Fatigue
- Blurred vision
- Mood changes

- Numbness and tingling in extremities
- Dry skin
- Infections (urinary tract, vaginal yeast infections)
- Weight loss (most often in type I)

Classification of Diabetes Mellitus

Diabetes mellitus is classified in the following ways:

- *Type I:* Insulin-dependent diabetes mellitus (IDDM)
- *Type II:* Non—insulin-dependent diabetes mellitus (NIDDM)
- *Impaired glucose tolerance* (IGT): Elevated fasting blood sugar
- *Gestational diabetes mellitus* (GDM): Occurs during pregnancy and disappears on delivery

Both young people and older people can develop any of the types. The current classification replaces the previously used term "juvenile diabetes."

Key Concept

- In type I diabetes, insulin injections are required to maintain life; no insulin is produced.
- In type II diabetes, insulin may or may not be required.
- In impaired glucose tolerance (IGT), the blood glucose level is above normal but does not meet diagnostic criteria for diabetes.
- Women with gestational diabetes mellitus (GDM) have a 25% to 60% chance of developing type II diabetes later in life.

Type I Diabetes Mellitus

Type I diabetes (IDDM) may occur at any age, although it is most often diagnosed when the patient is under 30 years of age. Because these patients have deficiency of insulin, it is essential to initiate insulin therapy to prevent rapid and severe dehydration, ketoacidosis, and death.

Type I diabetes accounts for approximately 10% of diabetes cases in the United States. Recent research has determined there is an inherited tendency to develop the disease and that other environmental factors are often needed to trigger the disease process. These specific factors and how they work are as yet unknown, but a variety of drugs and viruses are suspect.

There also appears to be an autoimmune influence because antibodies to insulin and islet cells are present at the time of diagnosis. In addition, there is a greater-than-chance association of type I diabetes with some other autoimmune diseases.

Signs and Symptoms. These patients are usually lean and experience the "classic" symptoms of diabetes:

- Significant weight loss
- Thirst
- Frequent urination
- Fatigue

Treatment. The goal of treatment in type I diabetes at diagnosis is to achieve metabolic stabilization, restore body weight, and relieve symptoms of hyperglycemia. Ongoing goals are to achieve and maintain normal metabolic functions and to minimize the negative impact of diabetes on the person's life.

Type II Diabetes Mellitus

Type II diabetes (NIDDM) may occur at any age but is most likely after age 30. More than 80% of patients are overweight and they usually do not have classic symptoms. The pancreas is often still functional at diagnosis and insulin levels may be normal, low, or elevated. Insulin resistance, a decreased tissue sensitivity to insulin, is usually present. Patients with type II diabetes do not depend on insulin injections to sustain life, but they may require insulin for adequate glucose control.

Approximately 90% of diabetes cases in the United States are type II. It is more prevalent in the African American, Native American, and Hispanic populations.

Risk factors for type II diabetes include heredity, obesity, age, and stress. As with type I diabetes, there seems to be an inherited tendency to develop type II diabetes, which is usually triggered by an environmental factor. (Type II diabetes carries about twice the heredity risk of type I.) The etiology of type II is still unknown.

Treatment. The major goals for treatment of type II diabetes are to achieve metabolic control and prevent vascular complications. Recommended treatment includes meal planning, a planned exercise program, and diabetes medication, if needed. Weight management is of primary concern because losing even 5 to 10 lb may lead to a significant improvement in blood glucose control. Table 72-2 outlines differences between type I and type II diabetes mellitus.

Impaired Glucose Tolerance

Impaired glucose tolerance (IGT) is a condition in which glucose levels are above normal but not high enough to be considered diagnostic for diabetes mellitus. About 25% of patients with IGT will develop diabetes mellitus later.

Gestational Diabetes Mellitus

Gestational diabetes mellitus (GDM) occurs in 2% to 5% of pregnant women, usually in the second or third trimester. Related to pregnancy hormones that stimulate insulin resistance, every pregnant patient between

Table 72-2. Comparison of Type I and Type II Diabetes Mellitus

	Type I	Type II
Age of onset	Under age 30	Over age 30
Classic symptoms	Nearly always present	Usually not present
Hereditary factors	Occasionally present	Usually present
Weight	Normal or underweight	Usually overweight
Prone to ketoacidosis	Yes	No
Usual treatment	Insulin, meal plan, exercise	Meal plan, exercise, may need oral hypoglycemics or insulin

24 and 28 weeks' gestation should be screened for GDM. It usually disappears after delivery, but these women carry a 25% to 60% risk of developing type II diabetes later in life.

Diagnostic Tests

Diagnostic tests for diabetes mellitus were included at the beginning of this chapter. They include blood and urine tests and tests for glucose levels. Diagnostic criteria for diabetes mellitus are given in the accompanying box.

Medical Treatment of Diabetes Mellitus

The insulin-requiring person with diabetes must maintain a carefully planned regimen of diet, exercise, and insulin therapy. The patient's understanding and compliance with the treatment plan greatly improves its effectiveness.

Goals of diabetes management are:

Diagnostic Criteria for Diabetes Mellitus

In *nonpregnant adults,* one of the following must be present:

◆ Random blood glucose level of at least 200 mg/dL *and* classic signs and symptoms
◆ Fasting blood glucose level of at least 140 mg/dL on two different test days
◆ Fasting blood glucose below 140 mg/dL *and* elevated blood glucose levels during two or more oral glucose tolerance tests

In *pregnant women,* diagnosis of gestational diabetes is made if two or more blood glucose levels meet or exceed the following during a 100-g oral glucose tolerance test:

Fasting	105 mg/dL
1 h	190 mg/dL
2 h	165 mg/dL
3 h	145 mg/dL

◆ Relieve symptoms
◆ Maintain normal weight
◆ Achieve normal activity
◆ Maintain blood glucose levels between 80 and 130 mg/dL
◆ Achieve normal glycosylated hemoglobin
◆ Prevent long-term and short-term complications
◆ Prevent hypoglycemic and hyperglycemic reactions

Diet

Diet is one of the most important factors in control of diabetes. More carbohydrates than the body can use or store will cause development of ketosis or acidosis. With too little food, the person will be undernourished, and if taking insulin, the person will be threatened with hypoglycemia. Therefore, the person with diabetes must have the right type and amount of food to prevent these complications.

The clinical dietitian calculates the diet for the individual diabetic patient in relation to age, sex, activity, health, cultural background, and usual dietary habits. Essential amounts of vitamins, minerals, and calories for the individual are included. It is helpful if food intake and exercise are approximately the same each day. If the patient will be doing strenuous exercise, extra food is eaten.

The American Diabetic Association and the American Dietetic Association have compiled quantitative diets that use exchange lists. This diet is often called the ADA diet. A booklet, *Exchange Lists for Meal Planning,* helps plan the diet. It provides six lists of food: milk, vegetables, fruits, starch/breads, meat and substitutes, and fats. The list is given in Appendix D. Each list shows equivalents that can be exchanged, which allows the patient a greater variety of food and freedom of choice.

An essential component of the ADA diet is a *reduction in the level of saturated fat.* (Generally, American diets contain too much fat.) Diabetic patients are more at risk for atherosclerosis than the general public. Atherosclerosis contributes to heart disease. Salt should also be reduced to avoid fluid retention.

The dietary allowance is usually divided among three meals plus snacks. It is best if these are eaten at the same time each day. The patient must regulate intake. If deviations occur, the balance between diet and insulin dosage will be upset. The dietitian may want to distribute carbohydrates in different proportions throughout the meals if the person is extremely hungry.

It is important that diabetic patients participate in their own planning. They must have a clear understanding of food choices so they can continue with meal management at home. The hospital dietitian instructs the patient before discharge or on an outpatient basis.

Sugarless products are on the market in increasing numbers, but some physicians feel that a patient with diabetes should learn to adjust the diet while using regular foods. Many of the special products are more expensive and have no nutritional advantages. Patients are usually allowed to use a sugar substitute in tea or coffee or to add to foods. If sugar substitutes are added to foods during cooking, the food may taste bitter. Recent controversy surrounds the use of some sugar substitutes. Sugar-free beverages are available, as are cookies and candies made with artificial sweeteners.

Saccharin is high in sodium and should be limited. New laws have been passed in an attempt at more accurate and consistent labeling; sugar, fat, and protein content are usually identified on the label. The word *dietetic* on the label is not enough.

Exercise

Because diabetes is a disorder of metabolism, a proper balance of diet, exercise, and insulin is needed every day. The insulin-dependent patient should be taught how and when to exercise and the relationship of exercise to food intake and insulin use.

Without this balance, serious problems will occur because the patient's body cannot compensate for changes. Moderate aerobic exercise (20–30 minutes daily) enables the well controlled individual with diabetes to make more efficient use of available insulin and glucose. Exercise also increases circulation, helps control weight, helps decrease blood pressure, and reduces stress. Some persons must be careful of exercise because of increased risks of eye damage and vascular problems. The hospitalized patient will not have the usual amount of exercise; thus, the disease may quickly get out of control. The nurse should be alert for symptoms of hypoglycemia or hyperglycemia.

Insulin Therapy

Years ago, a person with IDDM could not expect to live. Now the outlook for management with insulin is very good. Insulin is available in several forms to meet individual needs. All forms are given subcutaneously because the digestive enzymes destroy its effectiveness if taken by mouth. When insulin is present in the blood, it enables glucose to pass through the capillary membrane and thus be used by cells for energy. Insulin also helps the liver convert glucose to glycogen and increases the use of oxygen by the cells.

Types of Insulin. Table 72-3 lists the classifications of insulin and their actions (see also Table 56-4). Regular insulin and semilente insulin are quick acting and are given 15 to 30 minutes before a meal so they will reach the bloodstream at about the same time as the glucose from the meal. Quick-acting insulins, if used alone, usually have to be repeated during the day because their effects do not last as long as those of other forms of insulin.

Intermediate-acting insulins are usually given 30 minutes before breakfast, supper, and at bedtime. Their action will handle the glucose from meals during the day. Regular insulin is often combined with intermediate and long-acting insulin for the best glucose management. One strength, U-100, is widely available to the public in the United States. U-100 means that 1 mL contains 100 units of insulin.

Syringes for giving insulin are marked in units for measuring the dose of insulin. A U-100 syringe is used. Different types of syringes are available.

◆ 1-mL, $\frac{1}{2}$-mL, and the 3/10-mL disposable syringe, with a needle. The latter syringes should be used for very small dosages because they are more accurate.
◆ Dial-a-dose prefilled syringes with short-acting (regular) insulin
◆ Dial-a-dose prefilled syringes with long and short-acting insulin mixed in a ratio of 70% to 30% (70% NPH and 30% regular insulin). One type, called Novolin 70/30, comes in prefilled syringes and multiple-dose vials. It contains 70 units of NPH and 30 units of regular insulin per milliliter.

Other types of injectors are available:

◆ Novo-pen or Novolin-pen is a cartridge that looks like a pen. The patient dials the desired dose of insulin.
◆ Jet injector does not use a needle. This method is not painless; the depth of injection must be set carefully, and a fair amount of maintenance is involved.

Care of Insulin. Insulin deteriorates if it is exposed to excessive heat, light, or agitation. Constant refrigeration is not needed, but the patient should be instructed to refrigerate extra bottles until needed. Insulin should not be frozen. Insulin in current use should be kept at room temperature.

Insulin preparations may be mixed to meet the needs of individual patients. A patient using NPH insulin alone at breakfast may have an elevated glucose level by

Table 72-3. Insulin Actions

Action	Type of Insulin	Onset (h)*	Peak (h)	Duration (h)	Time When Hypoglycemia Most Likely to Occur	Characteristics
Rapid-acting†	Regular, clear	½–1	2–5	5–8	Before lunch	Always clear or colorless. Can be combined with all other insulins.
	Semilente	½–1	2–4	12–16	Before lunch	Almost colorless; slightly cloudy. Cannot be mixed with NPH. Not used in emergency.
Intermediate-acting‡	NPH (isophane)	1–3	6–15	18–28	Late afternoon During night	Milky white. Can be mixed with regular, but not lente or semilente.
	Lente	2	6–12 (peaks about 2–4 h later than NPH)	24–28	Late afternoon During night	Can be mixed with regular or semilente. Cloudy.
	Globin (globin zinc)	2	6–8	18	Late afternoon	Yellowish
Long-acting	Protamine zinc (PZI)	6–7	14–24	36+	Night and early morning	Milky; white or cloudy
	Ultralente (very slow)	4–7	12–24	24–36	Night and early morning	Cloudy
Mixed	70% intermediate 30% regular	½–1	2–12	18–24		Cloudy
Buffered Regular	BR	Continuous administration			Less likely in stable diabetics	Used *only* in insulin pumps.

* Administration is subcutaneous. Times are given in hours.

† Rapid-acting: These insulins may be mixed with longer lasting insulin to give all-day coverage. Regular and semilente insulin are often used in combination to treat diabetic ketoacidosis.

‡ Intermediate: Patients must have a noon meal and a midafternoon snack to prevent insulin reaction.

** Long acting: These insulins must be mixed thoroughly before the syringe is drawn up. The patient will often need a bedtime snack to avoid insulin reaction.

noon. To correct this condition, a small amount of regular insulin may be given with the NPH. These mixtures can be given in the same syringe. The syringes may be prepared up to 3 weeks in advance and refrigerated. If 70/30 is the right proportion, Novolin 70/30 or Humulin 70/30 can be used.

Key Concept

If types of insulin are to be mixed, the *regular* insulin is drawn up first, after injecting air into both vials. *Remember:* "Clear to partly cloudy."

It is important to roll and invert prefilled syringes before administration to mix the solution well. Insulin vials are also rolled between the hands and inverted. *Do not shake a vial.* Shaking causes air bubbles to form, which would alter the dosage given.

Vials or prefilled syringes that are not crystal clear (regular insulin) or milky white or that do not easily resuspend when the vial is rolled should be discarded. Other signs of unusable insulin include "frosting" (coating on the bottle), especially with NPH, and any setting or clumping. The expiration date printed on the side of the vial should be noted and contents not used after that date. It is important to make sure insulin is not decomposed. *If in doubt, throw it out!* The accompanying box gives precautions for nurses giving insulin in the hospital; however, the guidelines can also be used for patient teaching.

Nursing Alert

Many hospitals require insulin to be double-checked by another nurse before it is administered. Even if your facility does not have such a policy, it is a good idea. Even a tiny error in insulin dosage can cause serious adverse reactions.

The development of two types of human insulin, Humulin and Novolin, has decreased autoimmune (aller-

Nursing Skill Guidelines
Giving Insulin

◆ Test the patient's blood glucose each time before giving any insulin. Insulin is usually given before meals. *(Rationale: To make sure the patient is not getting too much or too little insulin.)*

◆ Give the insulin on time. *(Rationale: The dosage depends on the schedule. Alteration in the time is dangerous to the patient.)*

◆ Give the correct type of insulin. Wear gloves. *(Rationale: The wrong type of insulin could be fatal.)*

◆ Prepare the correct unit dosage. U-100 is used in the United States.

◆ Use a U-100 insulin syringe. Never use a regular hypodermic syringe for giving insulin. *(Rationale: The dosage is too delicate and cannot be measured accurately in another type of syringe.)*

◆ Mix insulin properly and be sure that regular or globin insulin is not cloudy. *(Rationale: Cloudiness indicates that the insulin is breaking down.)*

◆ Gently roll and gently invert the bottle to mix insulin; do not shake it. *(Rationale: Shaking may cause foam or bubbles to develop that would change the potency or alter the dosage.)*

◆ If you are mixing types of insulin, remember that regular insulin can be mixed with all other types of insulin; semilente cannot be mixed with NPH. If using a combination of insulins, the regular should be drawn into the syringe first.

◆ Be sure there are no air bubbles in the syringe. *(Rationale: They would displace insulin.)*

◆ Check syringe and medication administration record before giving the injection. All insulin should be double-checked by another nurse. *(Rationale: To double-check time and dosage and to make sure no one else has given the insulin.)*

◆ Check whether the patient is NPO. *(Rationale: Administration of insulin might lower the blood sugar too much, or the dosage may need to be altered.)*

◆ Cleanse the skin with alcohol or another antiseptic and allow the alcohol to dry slightly before injecting the needle. *(Rationale: Drying helps prevent pitting of the skin caused by alcohol and insulin.)*

◆ Give the injection subcutaneously, rotating injection sites. Most hospitals have a body diagram on the chart, so that each nurse can indicate the injection site. Current recommendations suggest rotating sites within the abdomen only. The abdomen is highly recommended because it has a large area and the absorption is even. *(Rationale: If the injection is given in the same site each time, tissue might necrose. Scarring can develop, and malabsorption occurs [lipodystrophy].)*

◆ Insert the needle at a 90° angle, using a 28- 29-gauge short needle, approximately 1.27 cm or 1/2 inch. If the patient is a child or is very thin, the angle is 45° to 60°. *(Rationale: The administration is intended to be subcutaneous; a longer needle would probably lead to intramuscular administration. You might hit bone.)*

◆ Withdraw the needle at the angle at which it was inserted. *(Rationale: To prevent intradermal injury and tissue trauma.)*

◆ Chart the insulin dose on the diabetic management sheet in the chart. Record the blood sugar level.

◆ Assess for symptoms of hypoglycemia or hyperglycemia. *(Rationale: These reactions can occur at any time. They are more likely to occur in the hospitalized patient because another disease process is often present. The diet is different than at home, and the patient often is not exercising.)*

---

gic) reactions in diabetes. Antibody levels with human insulin are lower than with beef or pork (animal) insulin. Therefore, diabetic patients may require lower dosages of human insulin because it is used better by the body. The breakdown of fat tissue with scarring and malabsorption (*lipodystrophy*) and allergic reactions are rare with human insulin.

All newly diagnosed patients are given human insulin, and many previously diagnosed patients have been switched to human insulin.

Insulin Coverage. Many diabetics experience difficulty with their insulin regulation when they become ill, particularly in the case of infection. For this reason, the hospitalized diabetic patient, no matter what the con-

ditions for hospitalization, will almost always have routine blood testing for glucose and will often have "insulin coverage" to control elevated blood glucose levels. The physician determines a sliding scale of regular insulin, based on the glucose levels in the blood. The patient receives this coverage three to six times per day, in addition to the usual intermediate-acting dose. Many patients who are usually well controlled on oral hypoglycemic agents must be controlled on insulin alone during the course of an operation, a pregnancy, or a systemic disease. Insulin requirements increase during events of disease and stress.

The Insulin Pump. These are mechanical devices that inject insulin automatically. These pumps attempt to

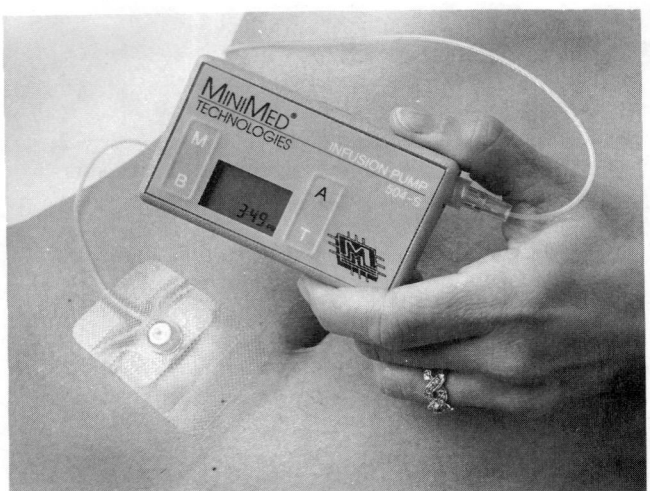

Figure 72-3. MiniMed insulin pump. (Courtesy of MiniMed Technologies, Sylmar, CA.)

mimic pancreatic function and distribute the insulin to maintain an acceptable blood glucose level (Fig. 72-3). They release insulin continuously; the patient also may inject a bolus before eating. Development continues with small implantable devices that automatically monitor blood glucose levels and deliver the appropriate insulin directly into the bloodstream. An insulin called buffered regular (BR) is often used in the pump. This insulin is not used in any other way.

Pancreas Transplantation

Experimentation with pancreas transplantation on patients with diabetes has been underway for many years. Success has been limited because of the high rate of rejection, but with new antirejection medications, transplant results are improving. Research has also shown some success in implanting only the beta cells from the islets of Langerhans.

Oral Hypoglycemic Agents (Sulfonylureas)

Insulin itself is not effective when given by mouth, but several products that can be given orally lower the blood glucose levels of some patients with diabetes. It is not fully understood how these agents work, but they are thought to stimulate the pancreas to produce more insulin, to improve the use of insulin at receptor sites on the cell, or to increase the effectiveness of existing insulin. These agents are not an oral form of insulin and are not to be regarded as a substitute for insulin (see Table 72-4).

Oral hypoglycemic agents are used only in the treatment of stable, uncomplicated, type II NIDDM. Oral agents act within 2 to 6 hours after being given, with the effects lasting between 8 to 60 hours. Some oral hypoglycemics are given two or three times per day. Table 72-4 briefly describes some of the sulfonylureas.

Nursing Alert

The patient receiving first-generation oral hypoglycemics should be advised not to drink alcohol. The reaction between the drug and alcohol may cause the face to flush and may cause nausea and vomiting.

Complications of Diabetes Mellitus

Hypoglycemic Reaction

The dose of insulin is calculated to control an individual's blood glucose level. Too much insulin in relation to the amount of glucose will reduce this level to below normal and will cause a reaction called **hypoglycemia**. This was formerly called insulin shock.

Signs and Symptoms. In hypoglycemia, the patient feels the symptoms of *excess adrenalin*, which is released in response to low blood sugar. The person is weak, cold, and suddenly exhausted; the patient is hungry and nervous and trembles and perspires. The patient may also experience headache, drowsiness, nausea, and vomiting. Without treatment, other symptoms develop, such as dizziness, confusion, and loss of speech. The patient is unable to control body movements, has double or blurred vision, and if still untreated, may have seizures

---

Table 72-4. Sulfonylurea Agents for Control of Type II Diabetes Mellitus

Name	Dose	Duration of Action	When Given
acetohexamide (Dymelor)*	250–1500 mg	12–18 h	q.d. or b.i.d.
chlorpropamide (Diabinese)*	100–500 mg	up to 60 h	q.d.
tolazamide (Tolinase)*	100–1000 mg	12–24 h	q.d. or b.i.d.
tolbutamide (Orinase)*	500–3000 mg	6–12 h	b.i.d. or t.i.d.
glyburide (Diabeta, Micronase)†	2.5–20 mg	16–24 h	q.d. or b.i.d.
glipizide (Glucatrol)†	5–40 mg	12–24 h	q.d. or b.i.d.

* First generation drugs
† Second generation drugs (have fewer side effects)

and lose consciousness. The blood pressure is elevated, and pulse is rapid. If the patient remains untreated, there may be permanent damage to the brain, most likely causing death.

Key Concept

All persons with diabetes should wear a Medic-Alert tag at all times.

Nursing Considerations. Hypoglycemia can develop so rapidly that the patient may be having seizures or may become unconscious before anyone knows what is wrong. The nurse should be quick to recognize the early symptoms of hypoglycemia as given in Table 72-5.

Carbohydrates must be given to counteract insulin reaction. If the patient is conscious, sugar in some form (4 oz orange juice, 4 oz regular soft drink, 6 to 8 Lifesavers, honey, or Karo syrup) is given. Individually packaged glucose tablets are available at the pharmacy. It is easier and safest to give sugar in liquid form. The unconscious patient is given glucose intravenously. This is available as Glucagon for Injection (USP), both in intravenous and intramuscular preparations. If there is no response within 5 to 10 minutes after the injection, 50 mL of 50% glucose is administered intravenously. In some areas, the use of 50% glucose is the initial treatment of choice.

Nursing Alert

Chocolate bars should be avoided as treatment for hypoglycemic reaction because of their high fat content.

An insulin reaction requires emergency treatment, followed by adjustment of the patient's carbohydrate intake and insulin dosage to regulate the disturbed metabolism. This is not easy in the first 24 hours following the reaction, and the patient must be under close observation for recurrence of symptoms. Blood glucose levels should be checked frequently.

If medical care is not available, a substance called Instant Glucose may be used. It is packaged in a tube containing 25 g pure glucose. The glucose is squeezed into the patient's mouth. In an unconscious patient, the glucose is placed between the lower lip and the front teeth and will be absorbed through the oral mucous membranes. (*Rationale: This prevents aspiration.*) The absorption in this manner is much slower than if the glucose were given intravenously.

The Somogyi phenomenon occurs when hypoglycemia is followed by compensatory period of rebound hyperglycemia as the body attempts to correct the problem by increasing glucose production. This phenome-

non most commonly occurs late at night or early in the morning when the patient is asleep. During this time insulin continues to be absorbed from the injection site, although not enough glucose is available for the insulin to act on it. As a result, the body secretes glucagon, norepinephrine, and corticosteroids to correct the hypoglycemia but exceeds the necessary amounts, resulting in hyperglycemia. Treatment involves reducing insulin dosages until the optimum level is reached.

Hyperglycemia (Diabetic Ketoacidosis)

Diabetic ketoacidosis results from a lack of effective insulin, causing hyperglycemia. Glucose no longer enters the muscle cells. To make up for the loss of sugar as a source of energy, the body uses more fats and proteins, which are broken down into ketones and sent to the muscles to provide energy. If too much of these ketones accumulate (ketosis), the body fluids will not be in balance, and a condition called **ketoacidosis** will follow. In the process, a volatile substance called acetone is produced; it has a characteristic sweetish odor (like nail polish remover) that can be detected on the patient's breath in later stages of ketosis. Any condition that interferes with storage of glycogen in the liver and increases the body's need to burn fat and energy, such as lack of insulin, vomiting, surgery, or anesthesia, may increase production of ketone bodies.

Signs and Symptoms. Hyperglycemia comes on over a period of time. The patient with **hyperglycemia** experiences weakness, drowsiness, vomiting, thirst, abdominal pain, and dehydration and has flushed cheeks and dry skin and mouth. The breath may have the sweetish odor mentioned earlier; breathing may become rapid and deep; pulse may be rapid and weak; and blood pressure low. Unconsciousness may follow. Sometimes the unresponsive patient who is admitted to the hospital has not been aware of having diabetes. Or a person may have a diabetic condition that is hard to control and gets out of hand, even when the patient follows the regimen faithfully. For a comparison of hypoglycemia and hyperglycemia, see Table 72-4.

Treatment and Nursing Considerations. Intervention must include intravenous fluids such as 0.9% sodium chloride (normal saline) with electrolytes as well as insulin replacement. While laboratory examination of blood and urine specimens is being completed, blankets are applied to the unresponsive patient to support warmth and combat shock. The blood pressure, temperature, pulse, and respiration are checked frequently.

Continuous intravenous infusion of low-dose regular insulin, with a controlled-flow mechanism, is used. By lowering the production of ketones, insulin makes more carbohydrate available to tissues and builds up

Table 72-5. Hypoglycemia Versus Hyperglycemia

	Hypoglycemic Reaction* (Insulin Reaction)	Hyperglycemia (Acidosis, Diabetic Ketoacidosis, "Diabetic Coma")
Reason	Too much insulin (blood sugar too low). Also caused by too little food or too much exercise.	Too little insulin (a frequent occurrence during a systemic infection); Ketosis results from upset in acid–base balance.
Onset	Sudden (may occur with patient on insulin or on oral hypoglycemics.)	Slow—several hours to days (more rapid in active child)
Causes	Omitted meal, overdose of insulin, overexertion, vomiting, excessive dieting	Omitted dose of insulin, spoiled insulin, error in dosage, improperly mixed insulin, increased need for insulin due to stress of illness, exposure, surgery, or improper diet. Also, undiagnosed diabetic. Not following diet plan (especially active child or adolescent)
Symptoms†		
Skin	Pale, moist, cool and clammy, sweating	Flushed, dry, hot, no sweating
Behavior	Shaky, nervous, irritable, trembling, confused, disoriented, strange actions, difficulty in problem-solving. Later, unconsciousness (rarely, seizures). May first be evidenced by a personality change or drowsiness	Drowsy, lethargic, dizzy, weak; later, delirium and loss of consciousness. Anorexia
Breath	Normal odor	Fruity odor (acetone)
Respiration	Normal, rapid, and shallow	Air hunger (Kussmaul breathing), labored, slow
BP	Increased	Decreased
Pulse	Increased	Increased
Hunger	Great hunger, often sudden in onset	Anorexia, nausea—may have time of excessive hunger
Thirst	None	Great thirst
Vomiting	Absent	Present, with abdominal pain
Sugar in urine	Absent in second voiding (in unusual circumstances, sugar may be spilled, depending on type and time of insulin administration and kidney function)	Present in high concentrations
Acetone in urine	Absent	Usually present
Urination	Small amount	Frequent, copious, diluted
Blood sugar level	Low, below 60	High, over 140
Chemistry	Electrolytes usually within normal limits	Blood electrolytes and BUN elevated
Other	Blurred or double vision, dizziness, headache, sleepiness	Ringing in ears
Response to treatment	Rapid	Slow
Treatment	Glucose, stop exercising. Take simple sugar (regular soft drinks upset the stomach less than does orange juice). Glucagon for injection available; 50% glucose; glucose tablets	Force fluids (usually IV), give antiemetics, keep patient warm. Intravenous regular insulin in low dosage
Nursing considerations	Prepare to assist with blood samples, urine collection, IV administration of glucose. Remain with patient until he or she is fully conscious and watch for symptoms of recurrence. Patient is often nauseated after a reaction; nursing measures should prevent complications of emesis. Institute seizure precautions.	Prepare to insert catheter, assist with IV, gastric lavage, ECG. Prepare to deal with circulatory or respiratory complications and later, with nausea. Remain with patient and observe

* Note: *The symptoms of the hypoglycemic reaction are those of adrenalin overdose, because the body secretes adrenalin when the blood sugar gets too low, in an attempt to raise blood sugar.*

† *A slow drop in blood sugar is most likely to result in confusion, sleepiness, and headache. A rapid drop in blood sugar (such as caused by exercise) is more likely to result in shakiness, pallor, rapid heart rate, and sweating.*

the glycogen supply in the liver. Regular insulin acts quickly.

Following the initial emergency, blood specimens are tested for sugar hourly and a record is kept of fluid intake and output. Blood levels of potassium, chlorides, and bicarbonates are also monitored hourly. Sodium levels are checked every 8 hours. Urine or blood ketones are checked every 4 to 8 hours. All of these tests are necessary to evaluate the patient's progress and so the physician knows how much insulin to give and which electrolytes to replace. When the patient's metabolism is in balance again, the physician prescribes a regimen specifically designed for the individual patient.

Nursing Alert

If you are outside the hospital and do not know whether a person is having a hypoglycemic or hyperglycemic reaction, *give sugar. (Rationale: If you give sugar, and it is incorrect, an already high blood sugar would only go up a small amount. However, if you give insulin and the blood sugar is already too low, the reaction is faster, more severe, and more long-lasting. Death is much more likely if insulin is incorrectly given.)*

Nonketotic Hyperosmolar State

The patient in nonketotic hyperosmolar state has a blood glucose level in the vicinity of 1,000 mg/dL, without typical symptoms of ketosis. It occurs more frequently in older adults without a history of diabetes or with a history of mild type II diabetes. The mortality rate is 65%. Only 50% of these patients are unconscious. The underlying causes of nonketotic hyperosmolar state are advanced age, severe stress, diuretics, undiagnosed diabetes, or response to hypnotic sedative or anticonvulsant drugs.

The patient experiences hyperglycemia, hyperosmolarity, severe dehydration, and coma. There is some, but not enough insulin. The hyperglycemia results in severe loss of water and electrolytes, which in turn causes water to shift from the intracellular to the extracellular fluid, resulting in intracellular dehydration.

The treatment is a continuous low-dose infusion of insulin and aggressive fluid and electrolyte replacement.

Nursing Considerations. The goal of nursing care is to restore the fluid volume and correct the hyperosmolar state. Intravenous fluids and electrolyte replacements are administered. Fluid and electrolyte balance, intake and output, and daily weights are monitored. Blood and urine glucose levels are evaluated frequently.

Infections

Infections aggravate diabetes. When blood vessels are damaged due to increased glucose concentration, the patient is more susceptible to infections. Patients with diabetes are particularly susceptible to yeast and fungal infections, carbuncles, and furuncles, as well as the common cold and influenza. Because of sugar in the blood and reduced circulation, it is difficult for them to fight infection. Good diabetes management minimizes blood vessel damage and reduces infections. It is important to prevent injury as well because the person with diabetes heals slowly.

Surgical Complications

The person with diabetes is considered a greater surgical risk because of circulatory problems associated with diabetes and difficulty in regulating insulin balance after surgery. The person with diabetes is also more prone to infections from any wound, including the surgical incision, and does not heal as readily because of impaired circulation.

Postoperative nursing care includes frequent glucose monitoring, watching for possible complications, encouraging fluids, and following measures to prevent respiratory, circulatory, and wound complications. This person is more prone to skin breakdowns. Practice meticulous skin care. Persons with type II diabetes who do not usually take insulin may require insulin during the perioperative period to control the blood glucose elevations.

Neuropathy

Many diabetic patients experience peripheral neuropathy (changes in the nervous system) that result from microvascular changes (thickening of the capillary basement membrane). The symptoms, most often in the feet and leg, are bilateral (on both sides) and symmetrical (same on each side). Patients often complain of pains that awaken them during the night, but they do not have pain during the day. Pain is relieved by walking.

Nephropathy

Kidney disease may develop in the person with diabetes as a result of microvascular changes. This is a serious situation and can lead to death from kidney failure. The first signs often are kidney infections or albumin or blood in the urine. These must be followed up immediately.

Retinopathy

Many physicians recommend yearly eye examinations for the person with diabetes because of microvascular changes that can occur. Circulatory problems may appear first in the retinal arteries (in the retina of the eye) in the form of hemorrhage or inflammation. The disorders in the blood vessels of the retina can usually be seen with the ophthalmoscope. The condition of retinal blood vessels is considered to reflect the general status of the entire circulatory system.

Laser beams are used to curtail pathologic changes in the eye. Damage already done cannot be reversed, but further damage can often be prevented. Cataracts often appear and can be removed surgically if retinal damage is not too great.

Arteriosclerosis and Atherosclerosis

High blood glucose levels may cause an increase in arteriosclerosis. These conditions affect the peripheral blood vessels, especially in the lower extremities, and the vessels of the kidney and heart. The poor circulation causes the tissues to be deprived of oxygen. In turn, this causes complications such as hypertension, coronary artery disease, peripheral vascular disease, myocardial infarction, and stroke. The person with diabetes is two to six times more likely to have a stroke and twice as likely to have a myocardial infarction as the general population. Skin breakdown and a greatly slowed healing process are also due to poor circulation and lack of oxygen. It is also believed that elevated glycosylated hemoglobin is stickier than normal hemoglobin, so it is more likely to clump or clot and occlude small blood vessels in the brain, heart, and kidneys.

Nursing Alert

Uncontrolled diabetes mellitus makes the person much more prone to long-term complications such as hypertension, stroke, heart, kidney disorders, blindness, and amputation secondary to gangrene. Control of the blood glucose level greatly reduces the possibility of these complications.

Patient Teaching

Because the patient will ultimately be responsible for self-care, the most important aspect in long-term management is educating the person and family to understand the disease and its management. Much of this teaching is the responsibility of the nursing staff or the diabetes educator. The accompanying box gives guidelines for general patient teaching in diabetes mellitus.

It is easiest for the patient to understand the disease if it is explained in terms such as: "The body needs sugar for energy; insulin is needed to convert sugar into energy. In diabetes, the body does not have enough insulin, so it gets weaker from lack of sugar. The result is that you are hungry, but your body is unable to use food eaten. As you eat more, sugar accumulates in the blood and urine, causing you to become thirsty because

---

Keys to Patient/Family Teaching
Teaching the Patient and Family About Diabetes Mellitus

◆ Assess the patient and family knowledge about diabetes.
◆ Start with the basics. Build on what the person already knows.
◆ Explain everything in terms the patient can understand.
◆ Give ample opportunity for the patient to ask questions and be willing to repeat information given.
◆ Ask for return demonstrations. Make sure the person is not "agreeing" just to be cooperative.
◆ Use booklets and pictures and give the patient materials to keep.
◆ Include the patient's family if possible.
◆ Recognize each patient as an individual with individual needs.
◆ Structure information to meet individual needs. People learn in different ways and at different rates of speed.
◆ Promote independence. It increases self-esteem and is safer for the patient.
◆ Stress that seemingly trivial problems can be serious and the physician should be notified immediately.
◆ Survival skills that each person with diabetes must be taught are: basic meal planning, self-monitoring of blood glucose, recognition of hypoglycemia, and insulin preparation and administration (if appropriate).

---

your body craves water to dissolve the sugar. Some of the sugar is spilled over into the urine."

The patient should understand that diabetes is never cured, but it is considered *controlled* or *managed* when the following conditions exist:

◆ The person feels well.
◆ The person maintains normal weight on a balanced diet.
◆ The blood glucose level is maintained within 80 to 130 mg/dL (normal).

The patient needs to understand that long-term complications may be reduced if blood glucose levels are controlled. The person should prevent injuries. Special care and regular examinations are necessary for the feet, hands, teeth, and eyes. Illness can cause diabetes to go quickly out of control.

The patient will be responsible for managing food selection, blood testing, and insulin administration. It is important for the nurse to observe the patient's performance of these procedures. The nurse will then be able to assess the patient's understanding and ability to perform the task. It is important for the nurse to give reinforcement in procedures that are being done correctly and to assist in areas in which the patient is not proficient.

Physician Contact. The physician will help the patient determine the most appropriate schedules of insulin dosage, as well as diet and exercise management. Patients should not attempt to adjust insulin dosage on their own. Symptoms such as loss of appetite, hunger, or any gastrointestinal upset severe enough to keep the patient from eating or to cause diarrhea or vomiting should be reported to the physician if it persists for more than 24 hours.

Glucose Monitoring. Patients will be taught to use one of the glucose monitoring devices. They may be taught to test urine for ketones. They should notify the physician if the blood sugar is consistently above 240 mg/dL for 3 days. The nurse should teach the patient to do these tests and document the results. These records should be taken to physician appointments.

Self-monitoring of blood glucose (SMBG) is an important tool in the daily routine for the individual with diabetes. It allows the patient to evaluate the diabetes management, aids in problem-solving and insulin adjustments, and provides invaluable information to the physician.

Numerous blood glucose meters are available. With recent advances in technology, these meters have become easier to use and some models are made specifically for the visually impaired. Although quick and highly accurate results are obtained, it is an expensive monitoring program.

Every meter is different and teaching a patient how to use a meter should only be done by a healthcare provider highly skilled in the use of the particular meter chosen by the patient. Two basic methods of blood glucose testing are commonly used today:

◆ *Visual* (compare test strips to color chart)
◆ *Meter* (test strip is inserted into an electronic device)

Visual testing is commonly used for non—insulin-requiring patients and they often test relatively infrequently (eg, 2–4 days a week). Meter testing is strongly recommended for all patients requiring insulin because of the need for precise, accurate results. Guidelines for blood glucose monitoring are in the accompanying box.

Step-by-step directions for blood glucose testing were given in the Nursing Process section of this chapter (see Nursing Procedure 72-1). Although these are steps identified for the nurse, the nurse can teach these steps to the person who is doing self-monitoring.

The Meal Plan. The meal plan should be explained to the patient and family in terms that can be easily un-

Common Guidelines for Blood Glucose Monitoring

◆ The calibration number (code or lot number) on the strip bottle must match the meter. The meter calibration can easily be changed if they do not match.
◆ Make sure the test strips are not outdated.
◆ Do not expose the meter or strips to extremes of temperature, light, or air more than necessary.
◆ Check the meter with the procedure and control solution, as indicated by the manufacturer.
◆ Hands should be washed with soap and water and dried well.
◆ If alcohol is used, be sure to let it dry. Repeated use of alcohol will toughen the fingertips and make lancing more difficult.
◆ Use the *lateral* aspect of any fingertip for testing. *(Rationale: The lateral aspects of the fingers have more blood vessels, so blood will be easy to obtain. The lateral aspects of the fingers also have fewer nerve endings, thus making the procedure more comfortable.)*
◆ Rotate the sites. *(Rationale: If sites are not rotated, one site will become irritated and may become infected; the area may also become so hardened that it is impossible to use.)*
◆ Always recap the strip container immediately after removing the strip.
◆ If the testing procedure calls for removal of blood from the strip, be sure to use the correct material and method (eg, wiping with a cotton ball versus blotting with a tissue).
◆ Dispose of test strips, lancets, and other materials according to universal precautions. Wear gloves.
◆ Test as often as prescribed by the physician.
◆ Certain meters require a high degree of maintenance. Check the operator's manual for procedure and frequency of cleaning.

derstood and followed. Many children are allowed to eat foods that formerly were forbidden and are able to control their disease by taking insulin. Cultural background also should be considered (see Chapter 27). The patient should understand the relationship between diet, insulin, and exercise. Alcohol may be allowed, in moderation, unless the patient is taking first generation oral hypoglycemics.

Social Factors. Patients may have many questions about the effect of diabetes on their life-styles. Patients should be assured that they can participate in activities, as long as they make allowances for changes in exercise levels and control their blood sugar level. They should avoid fatigue. Genetic counseling may be advisable before deciding whether to have children.

Keys to Patient/Family Teaching
Foot Care and Diabetes Mellitus

Patient/family teaching for foot care in diabetes mellitus includes:

◆ Inspect feet daily. If necessary, use a mirror to check the undersides of the feet or areas that are difficult to see. (*Rationale: Daily inspection allows for prompt intervention should a problem arise.*)

◆ Wash feet daily. *Do not soak.* (*Rationale: Soaking softens the skin too much. It becomes more easily damaged.*)

◆ Dry thoroughly yet gently, especially between the toes. (*Rationale: to prevent cracking and infections.*)

◆ Massage gently with a good quality lotion. Do *not* use lotion between toes. (*Rationale: To keep the skin soft.*)

◆ Do not attempt to treat an ingrown toenail. See a podiatrist.

◆ Cut nails only with the physician's permission. Cut nails straight across with a blunt-tipped scissors. See a podiatrist for treatment of corns and calluses. Self-treatment in any form is dangerous and absolutely forbidden. (*Rationale: To prevent complications.*)

◆ Never pick at sores or rough spots on the skin.

◆ Do not walk barefooted. (*Rationale: To prevent cuts.*)

◆ Put lamb's wool between overlapping toes. (*Rationale: To prevent rubbing and irritation.*)

◆ Exercise daily. (*Rationale: To improve circulation.*) Walking is the best exercise. If the person is unable to walk, sit on the edge of the bed, point toes upward, then downward. Do this 10 times. Make a circle with each foot 10 times.

◆ Make sure that shoes fit well, are of high quality, and give good support. Inspect the inside of shoes for any rough areas. (*Rationale: To prevent any ulcerations or breaks in the skin of the feet. The circulation of the feet may be poor and any ulceration is often difficult to heal.*)

◆ Wear new shoes only for a short period each day for a few days. (*Rationale: To avoid irritation.*)

◆ Never wear constrictive stockings or socks. Avoid sitting with knees crossed. (*Rationale: These items restrict circulation.*)

◆ Do not use adhesive tape on the skin. (*Rationale: To prevent abrasion when it is removed.*)

◆ For cold toes, use warm socks and extra blankets at night. Select stockings that allow toe motion. Heating pads and hot water bags are dangerous. (*Rationale: Because circulation is poor and neuropathy may be present, the person can be burned more easily.*)

◆ See a physician for a cut or burn, no matter how small it is (Fig. 72-4). If first aid treatment is necessary, cleanse the area gently with soap and water. Do not use harsh antiseptics. Apply a dry, sterile dressing. It is essential to see a physician as soon as possible. (*Rationale: Vigorous therapy is necessary to prevent complications. Because of impaired circulation, gangrene is a possibility. This would necessitate amputation.*)

◆ Instruct patients to get the answers to questions from the physician or nurse.

Smoking. Smoking is definitely contraindicated because the vasoconstrictor effect of nicotine increases the likelihood of circulatory disorders. The person with diabetes should be strongly urged and assisted to stop smoking.

Insulin Injection. The diabetic patient must be taught about the type of insulin and syringe, along with dosages and how to self-administer insulin. It might be helpful for the nurse to draw up the insulin the first time and immediately let the patient inject it to get over the initial fear of injection. The nurse should use the type of syringe that will be used at home.

Nearly all patients are able to learn to give their own insulin. Children over the age of 7 or 8 are usually able to give their own insulin (see Figure 66-3.)

The patient must learn that injection sites must be rotated. Injections should never be given within an inch of the same spot twice in the same month. The abdomen is recommended for most people.

Hypoglycemia and Hyperglycemia. The patient must understand the symptoms of hypoglycemia and hypergly-

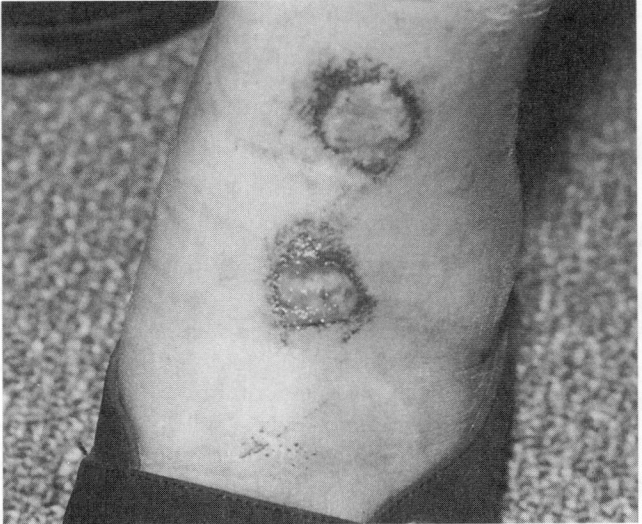

Figure 72-4. Ulcerations, particularly on the legs or feet, are serious for the diabetic patient. In many cases, an ulceration heals very slowly or may not heal. Gangrene is a serious threat and usually necessitates amputation. (Photo by Kimberly Malcolm, Courtesy of Fairview Northland Regional Home Care, Princeton, Minnesota)

cemia (see Table 72-5) and be aware of the treatment if they should occur. The patient should carry sugar in case he or she experiences frequent reactions. These reactions can be dangerous and the patient must know how to manage them. A glucagon/glucose emergency kit is recommended for patients on insulin.

Sexuality. Many diabetic men experience impotence. Approximately 50% of diabetic men are unable to achieve a satisfactory erection; the cause is believed to be neurogenic. The difficulty in many men is retrograde ejaculation (semen is not propelled to the outside). Chapter 83 describes means of treating impotence. Hormones and other therapy are not effective in alleviating impotence. Many diabetic men need some sort of penile implant or prosthesis. There is very little literature related to sexual dysfunction in diabetic women, although it occurs.

Exposure to Cold. The patient should also be aware that exposure to extreme cold slows circulation of blood, especially in the extremities, due to vasoconstriction. Frostbite or hypothermia is a danger, especially because this person does not heal well.

Vision Impairment. The patient with diabetes must appreciate the importance of a regular eye examination to avoid impairment of vision. Many assistive devices are available for use by the vision-impaired diabetic patient (see Chapter 73). Furniture can also be placed where it is less likely to be bumped—a bump can cause a break in the skin.

Dental Examination. It is important for the diabetic person to have regular dental examinations. Dental caries can lead to infection and rough edges can irritate the mouth, exposing the mouth to infections.

Foot Care. The person with diabetes should be warned against injury. The accompanying box describes diabetic foot care. An injury to the foot may lead to the necessity for amputation. It is essential to teach the patient about preventive foot care (see Fig. 72-4).

Traveling. The person with diabetes who plans to travel a great distance, perhaps across several time zones, should consult the physician before the trip. Often, the daily insulin dose is adjusted during travel days, until the person is on the regular morning schedule again. Diet and exercise must be considered in this plan. People taking insulin and testing blood glucose levels should keep medications and equipment with them in carry-on luggage and give a spare supply to a companion, in case checked luggage gets lost. They should also carry a fast-acting sugar and some food with them when traveling. They will probably be asked for a prescription if they try to buy syringes, even though this is not required by law.

Identification. Every person with diabetes should wear a tag, such as a Medic-Alert tag, which gives immediate and positive identification of the problem. Many times, the card in the billfold is not easily found. The tag worn on the body gives immediate information to healthcare personnel.

Key Concept

The person with diabetes is able to have a relatively normal life and to live longer than in the past. A sensible life-style will help prevent complications. It is important to balance diet, exercise, and insulin.

Keys for Review

Key Questions for Critical Thinking

1. You are with a patient who is suspected of having diabetes mellitus. Outline the tests he or she probably will receive. Identify the care you will be expected to provide.
2. Your patient was diagnosed with diabetes mellitus. He has had instruction from a diabetic instructor. He is not clear on how to do the self-monitoring of blood glucose. Outline what you will tell him.

Key Questions for Critical Thinking
(continued)

3. Your patient is a child with diabetes mellitus. The parents ask you to explain the differences in the various kinds of diabetes mellitus. Describe what you will tell them.

Key Readings

American Diabetes Association. Physician's Guide to Insulin-Dependent (Type I) Diabetes: Diagnosis and Treatment. 1988

American Diabetes Association. Physician's Guide to Non—insulin-Dependent (Type II) Diabetes; Diagnosis and Treatment, Ed 2. 1988

Berkow R (Ed). The Merck Manual of Diagnosis and Therapy, Ed 16. Rahway, NJ, Merck & Co, 1992

Fain JA (Guest Editor). Diabetes Symposium in Nursing Clinics of North America 28(1), March, 1993

Jackson DB, Saunders RB. Child Health Nursing: A Comprehensive Approach to the Care of Children and Their Families. Philadelphia, J.B. Lippincott, 1993

NANDA Nursing Diagnoses: Definitions and Classifications 1992. Philadelphia, North American Nursing Diagnosis Association, 1992

Nursing '94 Drug Handbook. Springhouse, PA, Springhouse, 1994

O'Toole M (Ed). Miller-Keane Encyclopedia and Dictionary of Medicine, Nursing, and Allied Health, Ed 5. Philadelphia, W.B. Saunders, 1992

Porth CM. Pathophysiology: Concepts of Altered Health States, Ed 4. Philadelphia, J.B. Lippincott, 1994

Smeltzer SC, Bare BG. Brunner and Suddarth's Textbook of Medical Surgical Nursing, Ed 7. Philadelphia, J.B. Lippincott, 1992

Enrichment Keys

Garg SK, Chase P, Marshall G, and Hoops SL. Oral contraceptives and renal and retinal complications in young women with insulin-dependent diabetes mellitus. JAMA April 13, 1994. Vol. 271 #14, 1099–1102

Keys to Learning More

Chapter 73: sensory disorders, including diabetic retinopathy and glaucoma

Chapter 74: cardiovascular disorders

Chapter 81: digestive disorders

Chapter 85: geriatric disorders

Chapter 89: rehabilitation, needed for the person who has an amputation

Key Resources

American Diabetes Association
    National Center
    1660 Duke Street
    Alexandria, VA 22314
    1-800/232-3472

Eli Lilly and Co.
    Educational Resource Program
    PO Box 10 B
    Indianapolis, IN 46206

Juvenile Diabetes Foundation International
    432 Park Avenue South
    New York, NY 10016

73 Sensory Disorders

Keys for Learning

Learning Objectives

- Describe the diagnostic procedures used for sensory disorders, particularly of the eye and ear.
- Describe nursing procedures related to patients with sensory disorders.
- Outline patient and family teaching related to these procedures.
- Describe and demonstrate special preoperative and postoperative procedures for eye and ear surgery.
- Describe common disorders of the eye, including symptoms, treatment, and nursing care.
- Describe types of contact lenses.
- Describe common disorders of the ear, including symptoms, treatment, and nursing care.
- State the definition and significance of vertigo.

Key Terms

blepharitis	entropion	otology
cataract	enucleation	otosclerosis
chalazion	glaucoma	presbycusis
conjunctivitis	hyphema	ptosis
diplopia	keratoplasty	refraction
ectropion	Meniere's disease	

Keys to Understanding This Chapter

Chapter 5: basic human needs

Chapter 15: sensory receptors in the skin

Chapter 18: nervous system anatomy and physiology

Chapter 20: sensory system anatomy and physiology

Chapter 21: circulatory system anatomy and physiology

Chapter 31: first aid

Chapter 38: signs and symptoms of illness or injury

Chapter 49: hot and cold applications, including those to the eye

Chapter 50: nursing assessment and physical examination

Keys to Understanding This Chapter
(continued)

Chapter 57: administration of medications, including eye and ear medications

Unit Thirteen: pediatric nursing

Chapter 71: nervous system disorders

Key Points

- The sensory system is important in enabling the patient to receive information from the surrounding environment.
- Most eye and ear surgeries are done on an outpatient basis. Careful teaching enables the patient to rapidly resume daily activities. The family must be included in teaching.
- The visually impaired and hearing-impaired person may have difficulties carrying out activities of daily living including personal hygiene. Self-esteem problems and body image disturbance may develop.
- Early recognition and treatment of glaucoma are essential to prevent visual changes and blindness.
- Hearing deficits may occur at any age and are caused by diseases and congenital and environmental factors. Determination of the cause of a hearing deficit is important because it may point to a serious problem.

Key Topics Outline

Anatomy and Physiology Review

Diagnostic Tests for Auditory and Eighth Cranial Nerve Disorders

Medical and Surgical Treatments of the Eyes
　Common Medical Treatments
　Common Surgical Treatments

Medical and Surgical Treatments of the Ears
　Common Medical Treatments
　Common Surgical Treatments

Key Learning Activities

◆ Place soft earplugs in your ears and carry on a conversation or watch television with the earplugs in place. How well were you able to understand what was being said or what was going on?
◆ Blindfold a partner and place a plate of food in front of him or her. Describe the location of items on the plate and on the table. Observe your partner's ability to eat. What assistance was needed?

The sensory system involves those organs and structures that give a person information about the surrounding world through the senses of touch, smell, taste, sight, and hearing. The receptors for these senses are located in the peripheral parts of the body. The impulses are then transmitted to the brain where they are interpreted.

Any defect in the sensory organ, the transmission of nerve impulses to the brain, or the brain itself can cause an apparent malfunction in the sensory system. Specific disorders of the nervous system and brain are discussed in separate chapters. This chapter discusses disorders related to the senses of sight and hearing, as well as a brief overview of other special senses.

Anatomy and Physiology Review

The Eye and Vision

In Chapter 20, you learned that the eye is the organ of vision or sight. The eye is well protected by the bony orbit, eyelids, eyelashes, lacrimal glands, and conjunctiva. The layers of the eyeball are the sclera and cornea, the choroid, and the retina. The sclera (white of the eye) and the cornea (transparent section in the front of the eye) protect the eye. The cornea and lens refract light rays so they can focus on the retina. The choroid layer brings oxygen and nutrients to the eye and carries wastes away from the eye. It also contains muscles that adjust the lens and it secretes aqueous humor (which maintains intraocular—within the eye—pressure). The pupil regulates the amount of light entering the eye. The retina contains the specialized neurons or receptor

cells, the rods and cones, as well as the optic nerve, which transmits the visual impulses to the brain for interpretation.

The Ear and Hearing

In Chapter 20, you learned that the ear provides the sense of hearing. The external ear (pinna) gathers and guides sound waves into the auditory canal. The sound vibrations are picked up by the eardrum (tympanic membrane) and transmitted via the ossicles (hammer, anvil, stirrup) in the middle ear to the inner ear. The inner ear contains the cochlea (true organ of hearing), as well as the vestibule and semicircular canals (involved in balance). Sound is transmitted to the brain for interpretation by the cochlear division of the auditory (acoustic, vestibulocochlear) nerve. Information about balance and body position is transmitted by the vestibular division of the auditory (vestibulocochlear) nerve. The eustachian tube con-

Key Abbreviations and Acronyms Related to the Senses

db	Decibel
ERG	Electroretinogram
IOL implant	Intraocular lens implant
OD	Right eye (oculus dexter)
OS	Left eye (oculus sinister)
OU	Both eyes (oculi unitas)
PE tubes	Polyethylene tubes
RGP lens	Rigid gas permeable lens

nects the middle ear with the nasopharynx; its function is to equalize pressure, but it may become infected.

Diagnostic Tests for Auditory and Eighth Cranial Nerve Disorders

There are many tests of hearing and visual acuity. Some of the basic screening procedures such as audiometry, the use of the Snellen chart, and screening for color vision are described in Chapter 50 because they are part of a physical examination.

Caloric Test or Caloric Study

This test is designed to determine if there is an alteration in the vestibular origin of the acoustic nerve. If the test is found to be abnormal, it suggests a diseased labyrinth or a tumor of the acoustic nerve. It can differentiate these disorders from disorders of the brain stem.

Procedure. The patient is either seated or supine and water is irrigated into the external ear canal. Sometimes, warm and cold water are alternated. The affected side is tested first because less reaction might be expected to occur here.

The normal response to this test is nystagmus (rapid, rhythmic eye movements), nausea, vomiting, vertigo (a feeling of spinning), and a feeling of falling. A decreased or absence of response within 3 minutes indicates an abnormality.

Contraindications. Water cannot be used for this test if the patient's eardrum is punctured. Cold air may be substituted. The patient who is having an attack of Meniere's disease should not be tested until the symptoms improve.

Nursing Considerations. Anticipate nausea and vomiting. Keep the patient NPO or on clear liquids before the test and provide an emesis basin. The patient is usually returned to the room by wheelchair or allowed to lie down until the nausea subsides (usually no more than an hour).

Electronystagmography

Electronystagmography (ENG) places electrodes near the patient's eyes to assess for alterations of the vestibular system. In ENG, the caloric test is performed while the eye movements are recorded on a graph. The other components of the test are the same as for the caloric test.

Other Tests

Magnetic resonance imaging (MRI) is used to detect tumors of the eighth cranial nerve. Chapter 71 contains the procedure and contraindications for MRI. An elec-

troencephalogram (EEG) with evoked responses can be used to detect abnormalities of the nerve pathways between the eighth cranial nerve and the brain stem. This procedure is also discussed in Chapter 71. Another test of the function of the vestibular system and the semicircular canals involves placing the patient into a chair that revolves in several planes and then evaluating the functioning of the proprioception sense and the vestibular system.

Medical and Surgical Treatments of the Eyes

Common Medical Treatments

Eye Patching

In some cases the physician will order one or both eyes to be patched. Several types of patches are available. A simple patch may be used to keep the eye covered for rest or protection. A pressure patch may be used to keep the eye closed; this is securely taped in place. A metal shield is also commonly used to protect the eye.

> **Key Concept**
>
> If both eyes are patched, the patient must be cared for in the same way as a nonsighted person. This patient may be apprehensive. An older person may also become confused if both eyes are patched.

Common Surgical Treatments

Since the advent of effective suture materials and more advanced surgical methods, most surgical procedures on the eye are performed on an outpatient basis. In many cases, the patient has local anesthesia and is awake during the procedure. These procedures are very exacting; they are done with the aid of an operating microscope. Patient cooperation is essential. Therefore patient and family teaching is important. Teaching and preoperative and postoperative nursing care are discussed in the Nursing Process section of this chapter.

Medical and Surgical Treatments of the Ears

Common Medical Treatments

A dry wipe may be ordered to clean drainage out of the external auditory canal and the auricle. An ear irrigation may be performed to rinse drainage or medication from the ears and to remove wax or other foreign body. It is done only on a physician's order and it is not done if a patient's eardrum is punctured. Nursing skills in performing both of these procedures are given in the Nursing Process section of this chapter.

Common Surgical Treatments

Because a great deal of surgery on the ear is done on an outpatient basis, nursing care centers around patient and family teaching. If the patient is in the hospital, the same principles apply. Nursing care is included in the Nursing Process section.

Cochlear Implant

The cochlear implant is a surgically implanted device that emits an auditory signal, bypassing the damaged cochlear system and stimulating the remaining auditory nerve tissue. This procedure is for the profoundly deaf and allows the perception of sound. There are several classifications of implants: from the location and transmission of the signals, to the types of electrodes and stimulation. Patient selection includes an otherwise healthy individual with no evidence of mental retardation or psychological disorder. The patient must not be able to recognize words spoken away from the line of vision and be realistic and optimistic about the results.

Patients are encouraged to talk with others who have had the surgery to learn both the positive and negative aspects. Postoperatively the patient is treated similarly to other patients with middle ear surgery. Within a few weeks after the surgery, the controls on the implant are adjusted and the rehabilitation process begins. The patient must learn to discriminate sounds and voices, learning to listen.

❖ Nursing Process

Data Collection

The nurse must carefully observe and assess the patient with a sensory disorder. This may involve a disruption in vision, hearing, or one of the other special senses. Chapter 50 describes assessment, including some aspects of vision and hearing. This assessment establishes a baseline for future comparison and determines the presence of suspected complications. The nurse should report any changes in the baseline level. The accompanying box lists some components of nursing assessment.

In addition, the nurse observes the patient's emotional response to the disorder or disease. Is the patient nonsighted? Is the patient able to hear? If vision or hearing has been lost, is the patient able to communicate?

Keys to Nursing Assessment
Sensory System
General: Vision and Hearing

- Nursing history, including information from family
- Presence of recent infections
- Medication use and recreational drug use
- General appearance of eyes/ears; examination with ophthalmoscope or otoscope
- Presence of foreign objects
- History of trauma to eyes/ears
- Assessment of cranial nerve function
- Neurologic status
- Signs of cardiovascular disorder (such as stroke)

Hearing and Ear Assessment

- Prolonged noise exposure
- Presence of chronic respiratory infections
- Screening with audiometer or similar instrument
- Symptoms and history of hearing loss

Visual and Eye Assessment

- Vision assessment with Snellen chart or similar tool (gross determination of visual acuity if person has poor vision)
- Screening for color blindness
- Screening for visual field deficits
- Screening for extraocular muscle disorder
- Symptoms and history of vision loss
- Direct observation of disorders such as ptosis

Is the patient able to work? Can the person move from place to place? Does the patient need assistance to meet daily needs? Does the disorder affect social activities or self-esteem? Is the disorder correctable?

Nursing Diagnosis

This section lists nursing diagnoses that may appear on nursing care plans related to visual, hearing, and other deficits. The same diagnoses may have several causal factors. The following are examples of nursing diagnoses for the person with a visual disorder.

- High Risk for Altered Nutrition: Less Than Body Requirements as evidenced by difficulty in buying, preparing, and eating food related to loss of vision
- Social Isolation related to blindness, visual disorder, inability to drive
- Diversional Activity Deficit related to loss of vision, inability to read or sew, inability to drive
- Anxiety/Fear related to plans for future, self-care abilities, rehabilitation, loss of employment, inability to drive

Based on data collection, the following nursing diagnoses may be established for the person with a hearing disorder.

♦ High Risk for Infection related to ruptured eardrum, chronic respiratory infections
♦ High Risk for Injury related to lack of hearing, hearing deficit, Meniere's disease (risk of falling)
♦ Impaired Verbal Communication related to congenital deafness, hearing disorder
♦ Chronic Low Self-esteem related to loss of hearing
♦ Pain related to trauma, otitis and other infections, punctured eardrum

Based on data collection, the following nursing diagnoses may be established for the patient with a disorder of one of the special senses of taste, touch, or smell.

♦ High Risk for Altered Nutrition: Less Than Body Requirements related to lack of olfactory sense and lessened appeal of food
♦ High Risk for Trauma related to lack of sensory perception and impaired nerve transmission from sensory receptors as manifested by inability to feel or recognize pain, pressure, heat, cold
♦ Knowledge Deficit related to specific disorder and its treatment

Planning and Implementation

The patient, nurse, and healthcare team plan together for effective care to meet patient needs, based on the nursing diagnosis. The nurse provides preoperative and postoperative care for the patient undergoing eye or ear surgery. Because the suture line is delicate in many of these operations, it is important to assist the patient to protect it. Most of these operations are done on an outpatient basis and teaching of the patient and family is essential. These nursing interventions follow.

The patient with a disorder in hearing may require assistance in communication, maintaining balance, and in meeting social and recreational needs. The nonsighted person may need assistance in moving about or in learning to read Braille or meet daily needs. Persons with a disruption in vision often need rehabilitation to resume self-care. They may need assistance in transportation and employment.

Patients with hearing or vision loss may need assistance in dealing with the emotional aspects of the disorder. All patients are helped to understand more about the disorder, its prognosis, and its treatment. Rehabilitation is designed to promote self-care. A sample nursing care plan for a patient with a sensory disorder is provided later in the chapter.

Providing Preoperative Care in Eye Surgery[1]

Because many patients for eye surgery are older and may be confused, both family and patient teaching is needed.

♦ Make sure all teaching is done and documented. Patient and family teaching is included in the accompanying box. The following are other nursing skills used in preparing the person for eye surgery.
♦ Make sure all items on the preoperative checklist are checked off. The patient must sign an *informed* consent *before* any preoperative medications are given.
♦ The patient may have been asked to take a laxative or enema the night before surgery. Make sure the person was NPO after midnight for an early procedure.
♦ Assist the patient if he or she is confused or if a sedative has been given.
♦ Wash the patient's face with surgical soap as ordered. The male patient is often asked to shave immediately before surgery. Instill eye drops if ordered.
♦ If eyelashes are to be clipped, use a blunt scissors coated with petrolatum. (*Rationale: The petrolatum catches the eyelashes and prevents them from falling into the eye.*)
♦ Be sure to report any signs of a respiratory infection. (*Rationale: Infection may necessitate cancelling the surgery.*)
♦ The physician may order that the patient's eyes be patched. Be sure to find out what type of patch is to be used.
♦ Explain the reasons for the patching to the patient. (*Rationale: Explanations reduce apprehension and confusion.*)
♦ Have the patient bring a hearing aid if one is worn. This may be worn during the surgery. (*Rationale: The patient must be able to hear the surgeon's instructions.*) Be sure to document this on the preoperative checklist.
♦ Make sure preoperative teaching is done and documented. Answer any questions the patient or family may have.

Providing Postoperative Care in Eye Surgery

Because the patient usually goes home soon after surgery, postoperative care centers around patient and family instruction. Postoperative care is designed to prevent complications, including hemorrhage, in-

---

[1] Preoperative and postoperative care instructions adapted from information submitted by Frederick S. Brightbill, MD, Madison, Wisconsin.

Keys to Patient/Family Teaching
Preparation for Eye Surgery

Patient/family teaching for the person who will undergo eye surgery includes:

Instructions for Preoperative Care

◆ Activities permitted before surgery and restrictions following the procedure
◆ Eye drops or other medication prescribed to dilate the eye or treat an infection. The patient and family must be taught how to administer these medications and possible side effects.
◆ Other procedures such as eye patching
◆ Steps in the procedure: what will be done and what is expected of the patient
◆ If the patient will be awake during the procedure, he or she must be aware of this preoperatively.
◆ Review of postoperative care before surgery
◆ Assistance is needed to drive patient home after surgery and probably to help him or her for at least a day or two postoperatively.

Instructions for Postoperative Care

◆ Eye dressings are left in place.
◆ Eye medications are not used until the patient sees the surgeon (usually on the first postoperative day). The patient should bring eye medications to that appointment.
◆ A metal shield is often worn while sleeping or napping, for up to 4 weeks to protect the eye from being accidentally bumped or touched.
◆ If both eyes are patched, the family must know how to assist the person who is temporarily nonsighted.

◆ The person does not sleep on the operative side for one week. This avoids accumulation of fluids and pressure on the suture line.
◆ After the first postoperative day, the patient is often instructed to clean the eye gently to remove mucus. Cotton balls or tissue are used and are moistened with tap water.
◆ The patient should be careful to avoid disrupting the suture line. Instructions often include to avoid any sudden movements; not to press on or rub the operative eye; and to avoid bending over with the head below the waist for about 2 weeks; avoid straining at stool; avoid activities such as coughing, sneezing, nose blowing; avoid vomiting; do not lift more than 20 lbs for about a week; try not to bump or shake the head vigorously; and to shampoo as in a "beauty shop" (with head back) for at least a week.
◆ Falls and jolts are to be avoided. The patient must be careful walking on ice or up and down stairs. (Depth perception may be altered postoperatively.)
◆ Water or soap should be avoided in the operative eye. Bathing and showering is permitted.
◆ The person may read, watch TV, and may ride in or drive a car, as vision permits.
◆ Stitches may be removed or may be absorbable. Follow the surgeon's instructions.
◆ Glasses will probably be fitted in about 6 weeks. They may need to be changed during the first year, as the eyes adjust.
◆ Any excess drainage, sudden pain, or bleeding must be reported to the surgeon immediately.

---

creased intraocular pressure, stress on the suture line, and infection. Common components of postoperative nursing instructions were listed in the patient and family teaching box.

Providing Preoperative Care in Ear Surgery

Patient and family instructions for ear surgery are similar to those for eye surgery. The patient and family should be prepared for what will be done and what to expect before and after the surgery. The patient often is awake for surgery and must be able to follow instructions. The patient should be aware of this preoperatively. Ear drops may be instilled and the ear may be packed with cotton.

Providing Postoperative Care in Ear Surgery

If the patient is to go home immediately after surgery, the patient and family must be taught how to perform care. Usually the patient is allowed out of bed as soon as he or she leaves the recovery area. Someone must be available to drive the patient home. Other items in patient and family teaching are included in the accompanying box on patient teaching for ear surgery.

If dressings are to be changed or medications instilled by the nurse, strict aseptic technique must be followed. *(Rationale: You want to prevent infection. Meningitis or encephalitis is possible because of the close proximity to the brain.)* The patient usually is instructed not to remove dressings.

Nursing Alert

Report any paralysis of the face, paralysis on the operative side, or ptosis (drooping eyelid) immediately. *(Rationale: These may indicate damage to the facial nerve or the presence of edema.)*

Procedure

1. Make sure you have adequate light. *(Rationale: The ear is a delicate organ and you must be able to see the canal to give careful care.)*
2. Wash your hands and don gloves. *(Rationale: Drainage may be infectious.)*
3. Explain the procedure to the patient. *(Rationale: A patient who understands a procedure usually is more cooperative.)*
4. Straighten the ear canal, as directed in Chapter 57 and as shown in Figure 73-1.
5. Insert the sterile cotton-tipped applicator only as far as you can see. *(Rationale: You could puncture the eardrum if you go further than you can see.)*
6. Use each applicator only once, drawing it out and rotating it. *(Rationale: Applicators are not reused because they can spread infection.)*
7. Dispose of the soiled applicators and gloves according to body substance isolation precautions. *(Rationale: You do not want to spread infection.)*
8. Wash your hands.
9. Document the procedure. Indicate any observations regarding amount, color, odor, and consistency of drainage.

Irrigating the Ear

The nurse may follow the physician's order to irrigate the patient's ear. Irrigation is not used if the patient's eardrum is punctured. There is a difference in straightening the ear canal of an adult and a child, as illustrated in Figure 73-1. Gloves may or may not be worn, depending on the facility's protocol and whether universal precautions or body substance isolation is used.

Keys to Patient/Family Teaching
Postoperative Care in Ear Surgery

Patient/family teaching for the patient undergoing ear surgery includes:

◆ Dressings and packs must remain in place for several days to avoid disruption of the delicate suture line and to prevent infection.
◆ Watch for signs of dizziness or prolonged nausea; these are symptoms of inner ear disturbance.
◆ Vomiting is to be avoided. Antiemetics are taken as ordered. (Vomiting is a violent action and can disrupt the delicate suture line.)
◆ Abrupt changes in position are avoided. Do not sit up quickly. This may overstimulate or upset the semicircular canals of the inner ear.
◆ Avoid sudden movement, straining, lifting or acts such as sneezing or coughing. These may disrupt the suture line.
◆ The patient should not blow his or her nose. In addition to the danger of disrupting the suture line, this can lead to infection, spread via the eustachian tubes.
◆ Observe for bleeding, complaints of pressure or pain, and indications of lowered blood pressure. Hemorrhage is a possible complication.
◆ The patient should follow the surgeon's orders regarding positioning. Lying on the operative side facilitates drainage. Lying on the nonoperative side prevents fluid/blood accumulation and stretching of the suture line when grafts have been done.
◆ Monitor for fever, headache, vertigo or ear pain. Any of these may indicate infection, hemorrhage, edema, labyrinthitis or irritation of the auditory nerve.
◆ The patient may bathe but should not allow water to enter the operative ear.
◆ All normal activities usually can be resumed about 2 weeks after being checked by the surgeon.

Using a Dry Wipe

The physician may order a dry wipe to clean drainage out of the external auditory canal and auricle.

Nursing Skill
Using a Dry Wipe

Supplies and Equipment

Gloves
Cotton-tipped applicators

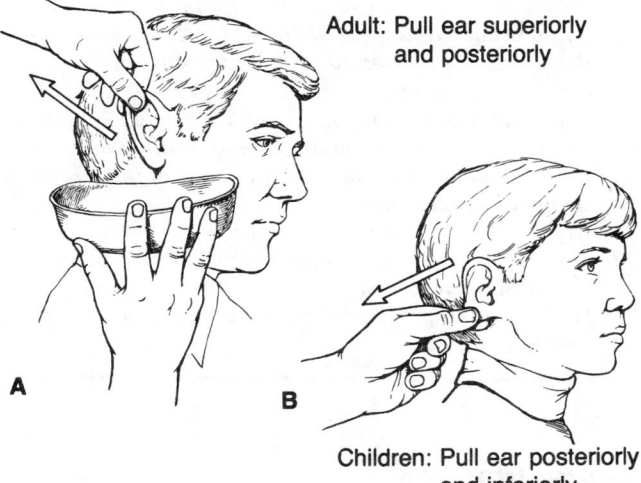

Figure 73-1. Technique for irrigation of the external auditory canal. Note the difference in direction of pull on the pinna between the adult (**A**) and the child (**B**).

Nursing Skill
Irrigating the Ear

Supplies and Equipment

Gloves (optional)
Plastic cover
Towel
Large emesis basin
Solution
Sterile rubber-bulb syringe in sterile large volume medication syringe

Procedure

1. Warm the solution to body temperature. *(Rationale: Hot or cold solutions can stimulate the inner ear and cause nausea or dizziness.)*
2. Wash your hands and don gloves if required.
3. Tell the patient what you are going to do. *(Rationale: An informed patient usually is more cooperative.)*
4. Help the patient sit up and provide adequate back support. Have the patient turn toward the affected side so fluid can drain out.
5. Drape the patient with a plastic cover and with a towel. Have patient hold a large emesis basin under the ear to be irrigated. *(Rationale: This will keep the patient's clothing from being soiled.)*
6. Straighten the ear canal, as shown in Figure 73-1. *(Rationale: This position provides better access to the ear canal.)*
7. Expel air from the sterile syringe. Draw up the irrigating solution. *(Rationale: A sterile syringe is used because it is important not to introduce new organisms into the ear.)*
8. Insert the syringe as far as you can see into the meatus. Do not plug the canal with the syringe. *(Rationale: The solution must be allowed to flow out freely. You do not want to build up too much pressure.)*
9. Irrigate gently with the prescribed solution. Note the patient's reaction. Stop the procedure if the patient finds it very uncomfortable. *(Rationale: This procedure can cause sudden and great discomfort. A person can become dizzy or nauseated.)* If this happens, let the patient rest before you continue.
10. Allow the patient to lie on the affected side. *(Rationale: It is important to prevent any great pressure on the eardrum; it might be ruptured. Lying on the affected side allows the fluid to drain.)*
11. Dry the canal and ear.
12. Discard waste and gloves per your facility's protocol and wash your hands.
13. Document the procedure, including any patient reaction.

Evaluation

The nurse, patient, family and other members of the healthcare team evaluate outcomes of care. Have short-term goals been met? Are long-term goals still realistic?

Is the patient able to perform self-care? Are family members available to assist? What type of rehabilitation, education, or assistive aids are needed? Planning for further nursing care considers the patient's prognosis, as well as any complications and the patient's response to care given.

The Eye and Vision Disorders

Several specialists are involved in the treatment of the eye.

- An *ophthalmologist* has received a Doctor of Medicine (MD) degree and has completed at least 3 years of postgraduate training in diseases and surgery of the eye. This physician is licensed to diagnose and treat eye disorders, prescribe medication, perform surgery, and fit glasses or contact lenses.
- An *optometrist* has received a Doctor of Optometry (OD) degree following undergraduate and graduate studies and is licensed to examine eyes, prescribe eyeglasses or contact lenses, and in many states, treat some eye diseases with medication.
- An *optician* is responsible for grinding lenses and fitting spectacles as specified by either the ophthalmologist or optometrist.
- *Ophthalmic technicians* are certified by the Joint Commission on Allied Health Personnel to assist the ophthalmologist in performing tests on patients.

Refractive Errors

To see objects clearly, light rays entering the eye must come to a focus point on the retina. Table 73-1 summarizes the causes and types of improperly focused light rays—refractive errors.

Holding objects at a distance, squinting, and headaches are some of the signs that indicate refractive errors and the need for corrective lenses. To diagnose and treat refractive errors, the examiner must perform an examination called a **refraction**.

Refractive Examination

The pupils may or may not be dilated for examination. Drops such as cyclopentolate HCl (Cyclogyl), phenylephrine HCl (Mydfrin, Neo-Synephrine), scopolamine hydrobromide (Isopto Hyoscine), or tropicamide (Mydriacyl) are used to dilate the pupils. This provides a better view of posterior structures and paralyzes accommodation in younger patients. This allows more accurate testing for spectacles (*refraction*). The *phoropter* simulates different corrective lenses and is placed in front of the patient's eyes. Light from the examiner's retinoscope is streaked across the eye, while the lenses from the phoropter are adjusted until the

Table 73-1. Refractive Errors of the Eye

Type	Cause	Result
Myopia (nearsightedness)	Elongation of the eyeball	Light rays focused at a point in front of the retina; blurred distant vision.
Hyperopia (farsightedness)	Shorter than normal eyeball	Light rays focused at a point behind the retina; blurred close vision
Astigmatism	Unequal curvature in shape of lens or cornea	Light rays focused on two different points on the retina; distorted vision
Presbyopia	Loss of elasticity of lens (poor *accommodation*)	Light rays focused at a point behind the retina; decreased close vision

light streak is neutralized. The final corrective lenses are selected by alternating similar lenses and having the patient indicate which lens provides the clearest vision.

The Ophthalmoscopic Examination. The *ophthalmoscope* is an instrument used for viewing the retina and other interior structures of the eye (Fig. 73-2). The examination reveals information about the blood vessels of the inner eye, especially those of the retina, as well as information as to the presence of tumors and condition of the optic nerve. The blood vessels of the eyes indicate the general condition of blood vessels throughout the rest of the body. Atherosclerotic and hypertensive changes in the blood vessels are usually a sign that the same conditions exist elsewhere. (Complications of diabetes mellitus can often first be seen in the eyes).

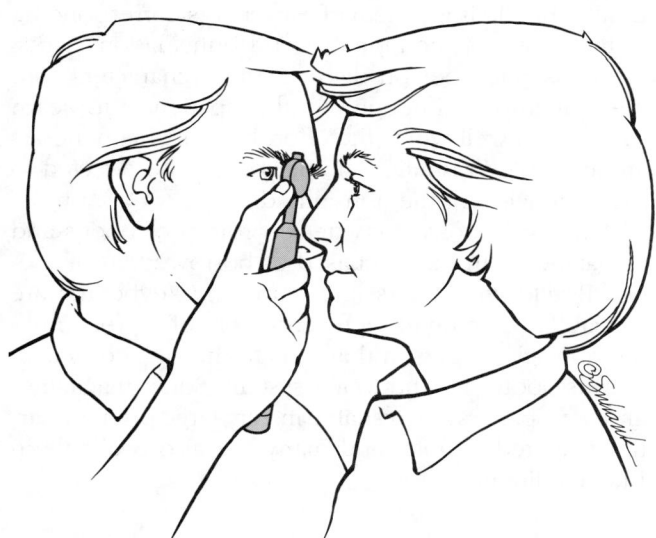

Figure 73-2. Technique for the proper use of the ophthalmoscope. The right eye of the examiner looks into the patient's right eye. The index finger is used to adjust the lens for proper focus. (Smeltzer SC and Bare BG. Brunner and Suddarth's Textbook of Medical-Surgical Nursing, Ed 7. Philadelphia, J.B. Lippincott, 1992)

Slit Lamp Examination. The slit lamp is a special type of microscope that directs a beam of light onto or through the cornea to view the anterior structures of the eye. Abnormalities of the conjunctiva, cornea, anterior chamber, iris, lens, and anterior vitreous can be identified. The slit lamp may also be used in association with a type of magnifying lens to view the posterior structures of the eye.

Tonometry. Intraocular pressure, the pressure within the eye, is measured indirectly by an instrument called a tonometer. Two devices, the *Schiotz tonometer* and the more accurate *applanation tonometer*, are used to detect glaucoma. Glaucoma is a disease of insidious onset, usually occurring after age 40 and having familial tendencies.

Other Tests. Other tests may be done to evaluate the function of the eyes and vision in specialized situations. The *retinal angiogram* is a visual depiction of the blood vessels in the retina, following the injection of radiopaque dye. Ultrasound may also be used (*ocular ultrasound*).

The *electroretinogram* (ERG) records the minute electrical impulses given off by the retina when it is struck by light (in much the same way as an electroencephalogram is recorded). The ERG determines whether the retina is functioning. Before the test, tell the patient that a contact lens containing the measuring device (electrode) will be placed on the eye, after local anesthesia. The patient's head will be under a "cone" and much of the test will be done while the room is dark. The ERG can confirm a diagnosis of retinitis pigmentosa (see Chapter 66) before the condition can be determined by other means.

Assistance for the Visually Impaired

Among your patients you will at times have a visually impaired patient. The following skills will help you give professional nursing care to the visually impaired.

◆ Encourage patients to gradually assume responsibility for their own care.

- Identify yourself when you enter the room.
- Speak before touching patients to prevent frightening them.
- Speak in a normal tone to the person, not about him or her.
- Keep the call light within reach and place the bed in the lowest position.
- Place food on the plate in the same "clock positions" for every meal. Tell the person what is being served and where it is located on the plate.
- When ambulating, walk slowly and allow the person to take your arm. (Do not push.)
- Orient the patient to the location of objects in the room such as furniture, the door, grooming articles, and the water pitcher; keep these objects in the same place.
- Let the patient know when you are leaving the room.
- Never pet or play with a guide dog. This may create a dangerous situation for the visually impaired person if the dog is distracted.

Eyeglasses. Eyeglasses (spectacles) may be prescribed to correct myopia, hyperopia, astigmatism, and presbyopia and for some low-vision (legally blind) individuals. Bifocals, two lenses in one, may be prescribed to correct the problem of presbyopia because each lens is ground separately; one corrects the defect in the near vision, the other in the far vision. Trifocals are also available and provide arm-length viewing in addition. *Presbyopia*, vision loss resulting from loss of lens elasticity, is a condition which occurs with aging. It is discussed further in Chapter 85.

Contact Lenses. Contact lenses are designed to fit directly on the cornea where they float on a layer of tears. Contact lenses may provide better vision than eyeglasses by eliminating minification (myopia) or magnification (hyperopia) of objects. Newer *hard contact lenses* are made of rigid gas-permeable plastic (RGP) and are paper thin. They are kept in place by capillary attraction and by the upper eyelid. They are usually worn for daily wear only and require special cleaning, rinsing, and storage solutions for care.

Soft contact lenses are made of hydrophilic plastic of a larger diameter and greater flexibility than rigid gas-permeable lenses. Soft contacts are apt to cause corneal ulceration more frequently than hard lenses because they are more difficult to care for and are far more likely to be damaged than are RGP lenses.

Extended-wear soft contact lenses allow oxygen and carbon dioxide to pass freely through the lens and may be worn for up to 2 weeks before removal. Recent studies, however, reveal a 10 to 15 times greater risk of infection than in daily wear use. Some soft lenses are disposable and are discarded after a period of time for a new set of lenses.

Many people take contact lenses for granted. It is important for contact lens wearers to realize infections and injuries can be caused by prolonged wear or improper care of contacts and contact lens containers. In some cases, blindness may result from *infectious keratitis* (inflammation of the cornea). Patients should be cautioned not to put contacts into the mouth to wet or clean them. This can transfer unwanted pathogenic organisms to the eye.

The greatest danger with the use of any type of contact lens is the possibility of injury to or infection of the cornea, which can permanently affect vision. In the case of accident or unconsciousness, the wearer could become blind if hard contact lenses are not removed. When the eyes are closed, tears cannot circulate freely and corneal ulcers can quickly develop. For this reason, contact lenses should not be worn when sleeping unless they are designed to be worn continuously. If the person wearing contact lenses is hit in the eye area, injury to the cornea may result. It is almost impossible for the lenses to break while they are in place because the eyeball will "give" with the blow and because the eye is protected by the surrounding bony structure. However, in the event of injury, severe swelling, or infection of the eye, it may be necessary for the physician to remove the lenses.

Reading Aids. One of the hardest things for a recently blinded person to become accustomed to is the inability to read. This can be remedied by learning to read Braille. Braille is a system of raised dots corresponding to the letters of the alphabet and punctuation marks; the nonsighted person discerns these characters with the fingertips. Although it takes patience to learn Braille, it is well worth the effort because many books are available in Braille. The person can be directed to local agencies for the nonsighted.

"Talking" books (cassette recordings of books and magazines) can be purchased or borrowed; also, special Braille typewriters and computer keyboards are available. Learning to type is no more of a problem to the nonsighted person than it is to the sighted person because both use the touch system. Some magazines and newspapers are available in very large print for partially sighted people, and many are also available in Braille editions.

The Guide Dog. Many nonsighted people use a *seeing eye dog* also called a *leader dog* or *guide dog*. The guide dog is taught to recognize danger spots such as curbs, obstacles, or holes. The dog is taught to be careful of traffic. The dog wears a harness fitted with a U-shaped handle that the nonsighted person grasps; dog and master can then communicate through the movements of the harness. These trained dogs are recognized everywhere and are accorded certain privileges. The dog is allowed to enter restaurants, subways, hotels, and other public places that might be off-limits to pets. If the master is not moving, the dog will lie quietly nearby. Airlines often reserve space for the dog.

A nonsighted person who wishes to use a guide dog must live at a training center for a period of time to learn how to use and take care of the dog.

The White Cane. A white cane is a signal that the person carrying it is nonsighted. Only a nonsighted person is allowed to use a white cane, and the person has the right-of-way over all traffic. Some nonsighted persons, however, are reluctant to use a white cane unless absolutely necessary.

One type of collapsible cane that can be carried in a purse or pocket is longer than a normal walking cane and has a metal or plastic tip that transmits sound and thus provides some guidance about the person's surroundings. As a part of the rehabilitation process, nonsighted people are taught to use these canes to locate curbs and other obstructions.

Nursing Alert

Lions International has vision and hearing improvement as a major goal. If you come into contact with someone who needs eyeglasses, a guide dog, a hearing aid, or surgery but cannot afford it, put the person in contact with their local Lions Club.

Inflammation and Eye Infections

Conjunctivitis

Conjunctivitis, also called pink eye, is inflammation of the conjunctiva, the membrane lining the eyelids and covering the sclera. It causes pain, redness, swelling, itching, and sometimes purulent discharge (pus). The discharge may be so profound the eyelids are stuck together. Conjunctivitis may be caused by a bacterial, viral, or rickettsial infection, as well as an allergy. Following appropriate cultures, antibiotic eye drops or ointments are prescribed for bacterial infections and antiviral medications for viral infections. The treatment of conjunctivitis caused by allergy includes avoiding the offending allergen, taking antihistamines and undergoing desensitization. Boric acid or saline solution irrigations or warm soaks may be given to remove discharge, reduce swelling, and decrease pain and itching (see Chapter 49). Conjunctivitis is contagious. Proper handwashing, use of gloves, and disinfection of the patient's linen are essential to prevent the spread of infection.

Blepharitis

Blepharitis is an inflammation of the eyelid caused by excessive dryness of the eyes, excessive oiliness of the skin, or infection. This condition is usually manifested by red lid margins and purulent drainage. The treatment of blepharitis consists of applying warm packs to the eye to help loosen crusted drainage. The eyelid is cleansed gently with a mild soap and water once or twice a day. An antibiotic ophthalmic ointment may be applied to resolve infection and prevent recurrence.

Stye

A *stye*, called hardeolum, is an acute inflammation of an oil or sweat gland of the eyelid. Styes are red, raised, swollen, and painful. They contain pus, and once drained, the pain is relieved and healing begins. The treatment of a stye includes hot, wet compresses applied to the area to help localize the infection and application of a topical antibiotic ointment. In severe cases, the abscess is incised and drained. The patient must be taught not to squeeze a stye, which could spread infection.

Chalazion (Meibomian Cyst)

A **chalazion** is an accumulation of lipid (fatty) material from a chronically obstructed meibomian gland. If the lesion is small and does not affect vision, no treatment is necessary. However, if it becomes infected or interferes with vision or closure of the eyelid, it may be necessary to incise and drain the area.

Trachoma

Trachoma is another form of conjunctivitis found in hot, dry climates. It is caused by the organism *Chlamydia trachomatis*, which may also cause the oculogenital infection *inclusion conjunctivitis*. Trachoma is highly communicable and is one of the leading causes of preventable blindness in the world. The treatment of trachoma includes topical and systemic antibiotics, which are very effective. Trachoma is rarely seen in the United States today.

Keratitis

Keratitis is an inflammation of the cornea caused by bacterial, viral, or fungal infections, often after trauma to the cornea. Keratitis is manifested by pain, sensitivity to light (photophobia), blurred vision, purulent drainage, and redness of the sclera. Corneal ulceration is a common sequela. The treatment consists of appropriate cultures and eye drops to dilate the pupil. Medications include fortified antibiotic drops given hourly for bacterial disease and antiviral or antifungal therapy as necessary. *Herpes simplex keratitis* is the most common cause of unilateral visual loss from infectious keratitis in the United States.

Structural Eye Disorders

Structural eye conditions may occur as a result of the aging process, injury, or nervous disorder. These include ectropion, entropion, and ptosis (Table 73-2). **Ectropion** refers to a turning of the eyelid outward due to the aging process. The eye is no longer able to drain effectively and tearing occurs. Surgical intervention is necessary. **Entropion** is also more common in the elderly and is an inward turning of the lid margin. The lower lashes are turned inward and are often not visible, but they irritate the conjunctiva and cornea. Corrective surgery may also be necessary. **Ptosis** of the eyelid is the drooping of the upper eyelid. Ptosis may be due to muscular weakness, damage to the oculomotor nerve, or interference with the sympathetic nerves, which maintain the smooth muscle tone of the lid. Depending on the cause, corrective surgery and correction of the neurologic disorder may be necessary.

Progressive Structural Disorders of the Eye

Glaucoma

Glaucoma is a condition of increased pressure of the fluid within the eye (aqueous humor) and is one of the leading causes of blindness in the United States. It is caused by a disturbance in the normal balance between production and drainage of eye fluid. This results in increased intraocular pressure, which permanently damages the retina and the optic nerve and, if left untreated, can result in visual changes and blindness (Fig. 73-3**B**). Early diagnosis and treatment are of the utmost importance to prevent loss of vision.

Chronic Open-Angle Glaucoma. Chronic open-angle glaucoma is the most common type of glaucoma. In this condition, there is inadequate drainage of the aqueous humor through the *trabecular* (supporting) meshwork, located in the angle of the anterior chamber of the eye. This results in a buildup of aqueous fluid, which causes an increase in intraocular pressure.

The onset of chronic open-angle glaucoma is slow and often symptoms are absent, mild, or intermittent. Therefore, a serious loss of vision may occur before the condition is discovered. When symptoms occur, they include discomfort of the eyes, temporary blurring of vision, reduced peripheral vision, and the appearance of halos around lights. Glaucoma is often diagnosed at a routine eye examination when increased intraocular pressure is discovered.

The medical treatment of open-angle glaucoma may include eye drops to increase aqueous outflow or oral medication, such as acetazolamide (Ak-Zol, Dazamide, Diamox) to decrease production of aqueous humor. Laser treatment is often used to facilitate the drainage of aqueous humor. In some cases, filtration surgery is required.

Narrow (Closed)-Angle Glaucoma. Narrow-angle glaucoma is an emergency requiring immediate recognition and treatment to prevent irreversible visual changes and blindness. In narrow-angle glaucoma, the aqueous humor is blocked by a bulging of the iris at the anterior chamber before it filters through the trabecular meshwork. This results in an accumulation of aqueous humor, with resultant increased intraocular pressure. In some cases, dilating the pupils with medications induces a closed-angle glaucoma. Symptoms usually occur suddenly, but they may occur gradually and be intermittent. These consist of blurred vision, halos around lights, severe eye pain, headaches, and occasionally nausea and vomiting.

The treatment of narrow-angle glaucoma consists of miotic eye drops (which constrict the pupil). They are given immediately to allow drainage of the aqueous humor and decrease intraocular pressure. Analgesics are given to relieve pain and the patient is kept on bed rest. Early surgical intervention is indicated and consists of an *iridectomy.* This procedure involves making a hole in the iris so the aqueous humor can flow uninhibited from the posterior to anterior chamber. Iridectomy is performed with a laser or by traditional surgery.

Secondary Glaucoma. Secondary glaucoma is usually the result of swelling, infection, hemorrhage, or trauma of the eye. It usually develops gradually and is painless.

Table 73-2. Structural Eye Disorders

Disorder	Result	Possible cause	Treatment
Ectropion	Eyelid turned outward	Aging process	Corrective surgery
Entropion	Eyelid turned inward	Spasm	Corrective surgery
Ptosis	Drooping of upper eyelid	Injury; neurologic disorder	Corrective surgery
			Correction of neurologic disorder (may be permanent damage; may require surgery)

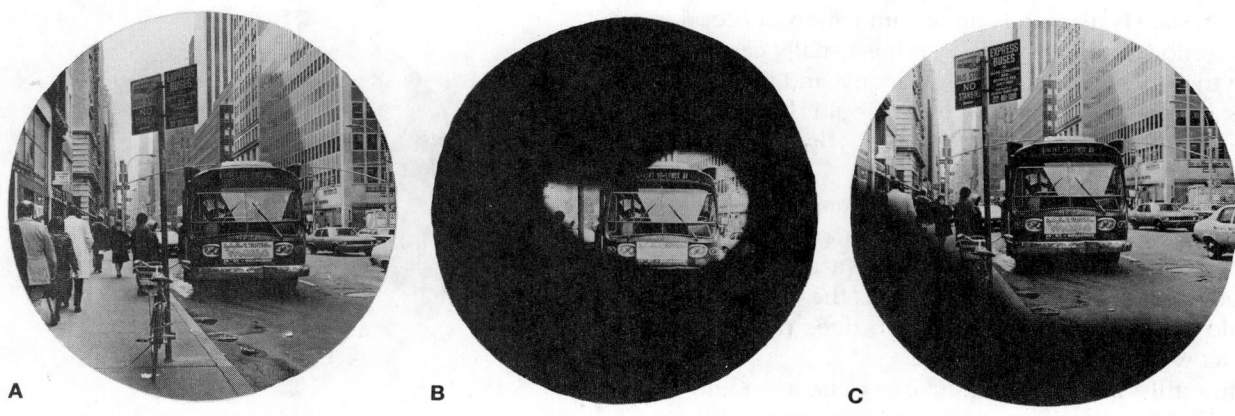

Figure 73-3. Vision and effects of eye diseases with the camera representing the right eye. **(A)** A street scene viewed by a person with normal 20/20 vision. **(B)** The same scene viewed by a person with advanced glaucoma. Glaucoma involves loss of peripheral vision but the individual still retains most of the central vision. **(C)** The street scene viewed by a person with a cataract. Cataract is diminished acuity from an opacity of the lens. The field of vision is unaffected, but the person has an overall haziness of the view, particularly in glaring light conditions. (Photos courtesy of The Lighthouse, The New York Association for the Blind.)

The treatment for secondary glaucoma is the same as for open-angle glaucoma. Patient education is important because the prescribed eye medications should be instilled as ordered. The patient may be instructed to avoid excessive fluid intake and all medications containing atropine. Frequent follow-up examinations by the ophthalmologist are imperative.

Cataracts

A **cataract** is an opacity or cloudiness of the lens of the eye. Because light entering the eye must pass through the lens to reach the retina, vision is impaired when the lens loses its transparency (see Fig. 73-3**C**). Cataracts may be congenital, may be caused by injury to the eye, or may occur as part of the aging process. When a cataract occurs due to trauma it usually develops quickly. A majority of cataracts, however, are associated with changes in the eye related to aging and develop slowly. Cataracts have been associated with excessive exposure to ultraviolet rays and radiation, certain drugs such as steroids, and systemic diseases including diabetes mellitus. One of the earliest symptoms of cataract is seeing halos around lights. The patient may also notice decreased visual acuity and double vision (**diplopia**).

Treatment. The only remedy for cataracts is surgery to remove the lens. This is one of the most frequently performed surgical procedures in the United States. Visual acuity in the person with cataracts, which cannot be corrected better than 20/60 with eyeglasses, is an indication for a cataract extraction. However, the main indication for surgery is when the patient complains that the loss of vision interferes with the activities of daily living.

Several types of surgical procedures are used to remove the lens. An *extracapsular cataract extraction* may be performed. This involves removal of the anterior capsule of the lens, followed by intact removal of the lens nucleus through a larger incision. Another alternative is *ultrasonic fragmentation* (*phacoemulsification*) of the nucleus through a smaller incision. An *intraocular lens implant* (IOL) is used with each procedure. Cataract surgery is usually done as an outpatient procedure using a local anesthetic.

Eye Trauma

Contusion and Hematoma. A blunt injury to the eye may cause swelling and bleeding into the soft tissues surrounding the orbit, resulting in a contusion or hematoma, also known as a "black eye." Cold packs are applied for the first 12 to 24 hours to decrease bleeding and edema. Warm packs may be used after 24 hours to hasten the absorption of the blood from the tissues.

Foreign Bodies. Foreign bodies may be external (on the corneal or conjunctival surface) or internal (penetrating through the cornea or sclera and entering the inside of the eye). The latter are most often the result of pounding metal on metal. *Never* attempt to remove a penetrating object from the eye. This could damage internal ocular structures. A topical anesthetic may be ordered for severe ocular pain until the object can be removed. Ultrasound may be used to locate an embedded foreign body and an electromagnet or surgery may be necessary for removal. The emergency removal of foreign bodies is discussed in Chapter 3l.

Hyphema. Hyphema is an accumulation of blood in the anterior chamber of the eye. It is usually caused by blunt trauma and can lead to glaucoma and vision loss. Signs of bleeding in the eye should be reported immediately.

Chemical Burns of the Eye. If an irritating acid or alkali chemical comes in contact with a person's eye, irrigation with water should be done for a minimum of 5 minutes. During irrigation of the eye, the flow of water should be directed so the solution does not come in contact with the other eye.

After this initial irrigation, the patient should be brought immediately to a hospital emergency department or an ophthalmologist's office for further treatment. The eye is then lavaged (flushed out) for an extended period of time. This prolonged irrigation is important because acids and alkalis can continue to "melt" the eye, even after it seems that thorough irrigation has been performed. After irrigation is complete, a topical antibiotic ointment is instilled and ophthalmologic consultation continued.

Corneal Abrasions. Corneal abrasions involve the outer (epithelial) layer of the cornea and are often caused by tree branches, fingernails, paper, and contact lens injuries. Symptoms include severe pain, redness, and tearing (lacrimation). Corneal abrasions are easily diagnosed by their green appearance following fluorescein dye instillation, while viewing with a cobalt blue light.

Treatment of corneal injuries includes instillation of antibiotic drops or ointment and pressure patching. These measures should result in healing within 24 to 48 hours. If healing does not occur, prompt follow-up is required to prevent complications. A serious complication is corneal destruction, which often requires corneal transplantation.

Keratoplasty. If severe visual impairment results from irreversible changes in the cornea, vision might be restored by corneal transplantation (**keratoplasty**). Keratoplasty involves the replacement of damaged corneal tissue with human donor tissue that is obtained within 6 hours after death.

Detached Retina. A detached retina is a separation of the retina from the choroid, thus depriving the image-receiving layer of its blood supply. Separation of these layers usually follows a hole or tear in the retina, the result of a blow or injury, myopia, degenerative changes, surgery, tumor, diabetic retinopathy, or extreme hypertension. Because the sensory layer can no longer receive visual stimuli, vision in the affected area is lost (Fig. 73-4).

Symptoms may occur suddenly or gradually. If a large part of the central retina is affected, the loss of

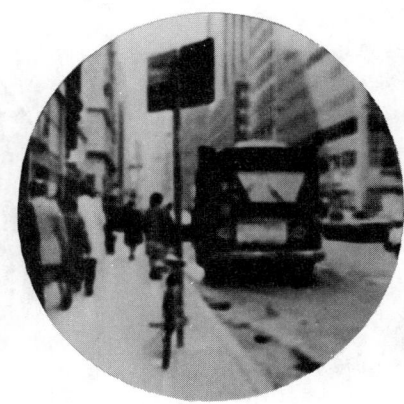

Figure 73-4. Retinal detachment causes a field of vision defect. Detachments are most often superior so the shadow or defect is perceived as inferior. Compare with normal vision in Figure 73-3. (Photo courtesy of The Lighthouse, The New York Association for the Blind.)

vision is greater than if the outer edges are destroyed. The patient may see flashes of light (*flashers*) or moving spots (*floaters*); vision may be blurred or it may seem as though a shade has been pulled over part of the vision. There is usually no pain with a detached retina.

One possible treatment for detached retina is a surgical procedure called *scleral buckling*. This operation shortens the sclera, thus allowing contact between the retina and the choroid. Procedures involving use of a laser beam (*photocoagulation*) and the application of extreme cold (*cryosurgery*) are also used to create an inflammatory reaction and promote healing.

Enucleation

Enucleation is removal of the eyeball. This procedure may be done when the eye has been destroyed by disease or injury or if a malignant tumor develops. After the eye is removed, a metal or plastic implant is buried in the empty eye capsule. It is moved by the eye muscles attached to the capsule. After healing is complete, a glass or plastic prosthesis shaped like a shell is fitted over the buried implant, for cosmetic purposes. This shell is painted to match the other eye.

Care of the Prosthetic Eye

The patient must learn how to insert and remove the eye and how to care for it. Some types of prostheses are removed at night and placed in a solution. When practicing insertion and removal of the eye, the person leans over a soft or padded surface to prevent possible breakage of the eye. The more current versions of prostheses are made of plastic and are not easily broken.

To insert a prosthetic eye:

◆ Wear gloves.
◆ Wet the prosthesis. *(Rationale: This action allows it to slip in easily.)*
◆ Lift the upper eyelid. Slip the eye up under the top lid.
◆ Hold the prosthesis while pulling down gently on the lower lid. Slip the lower lid over the edge of the prosthesis. Have the patient blink. This should slip the lids over the prosthesis and seat it in place.

To remove the prosthesis:

◆ Pull down on the lower lid.
◆ Press inward on the bottom of the prosthesis. This should allow the prosthesis to slip out.
◆ Be sure to work over a soft surface to avoid breaking the prosthesis.

In care of the eye socket, the physician's instructions are followed. Rinsing with tap water or a mild solution available for this purpose is usually recommended.

The Ear and Hearing Disorders

The branch of medicine concerned with diseases and disorders of the ear is called **otology**; the physician in this specialty is known as an *otologist*. The otologist tests hearing, examines the ear for signs of disease, and determines the treatment. The *audiologist* tests hearing by various means. The *otorhinolaryngologist* or *otolaryngologist* treats disorders of the ear, nose, and throat.

Hearing Loss

Types of Hearing Loss

Impaired hearing may occur at any age. Many children have been branded as slow learners, when the real problem was an undetected hearing defect. Injuries can affect hearing and cause deafness. Hearing may also be impaired by disease, by exposure to excessive noise, or by congenital factors. Hearing loss may vary from slight to moderate or may be complete.

Conductive Hearing Loss. A conductive hearing loss is sometimes referred to as a *transmission* hearing loss. This is an interference with the conduction of sound waves to the organs of hearing. It may be caused by a disorder in the auditory canal, the eardrum, or the ossicles (tiny bones of the middle ear). Fluid in the middle ear is the most common cause of conductive hearing loss. Types and causes of conductive losses are listed in the accompanying box. Conductive hearing losses are further classified:

◆ *Air conduction loss* is due to a defect in the external auditory canal.

Types and Common Causes of Hearing Loss

Conductive Losses

◆ Otitis media; middle ear disease
◆ Perforated eardrum
◆ Otosclerosis
◆ Defects of external auditory canal
◆ Obstructions of external auditory canal (ie, foreign body or cerumen)

Sensorineural Losses

◆ Excessive noise
◆ Presbycusis (related to aging)
◆ Ototoxic drugs
◆ Tumors (eg, acoustic neuroma)
◆ Meniere's disease
◆ Congential factors
◆ Trauma, skull fractures, brain damage (eg, cerebrovascular accident)
◆ Viral infections (eg, meningitis)

◆ *Bone conduction loss* is due to a defect in the bones of the middle ear.

Sensorineural or Perceptive Hearing Loss. Perceptive or sensorineural hearing loss involves a disturbance of the organs of the inner ear or of the transmitting nerve. A sensorineural hearing loss involves the organ of Corti (cochlea) or the auditory nerve (eighth cranial nerve). Types and causes of sensorineural losses are listed in the box. Sensorineural hearing loss is further tested to differentiate whether it is the following:

◆ *Sensory* (cochlea). Cochlear loss can be caused by factors such as trauma, viral infections, toxic drugs, or Meniere's disease. The sensory conditions are usually not fatal.
◆ *Neural* (eighth cranial nerve defect). A sensorineural hearing disorder can be caused by a tumor of the cranial nerve known as an *acoustic neuroma*. These tumors are potentially fatal.

Other causes of sensorineural hearing loss include excessive noise and congenital predisposition.

A person who is losing hearing because the organs of hearing are impaired has little chance of escaping deafness, unless the cause of the difficulty is discovered before damage occurs. This process is generally not reversible.

Central Hearing Loss. Central hearing loss refers to the brain's inability to interpret sounds once they have been transmitted. This sometimes occurs in atherosclerosis or after a cerebrovascular accident.

Functional Hearing Loss. In functional deafness, no organic cause can be found and there is no visible damage to the auditory nerve. It is believed to stem from some underlying psychological problem. Professional counseling sometimes helps.

Prevention of Hearing Loss

People should be made aware of the dangers of infections and noise to their hearing. Nurses can do preventive teaching in their work with patients, as outlined in the accompanying teaching box.

Prompt treatment of infectious diseases, such as upper respiratory infections that can spread to the ear, helps to prevent deafness. The use of antibiotics early in the course of an ear infection also helps to arrest the disease and to prevent later complications.

Noise pollution is of great concern, particularly in young people and in industry. Many hearing disorders can be prevented by the wearing of protective ear devices. The Occupational Safety and Health Act (OSHA) has established standards for industries in general. The loud volume generated from radios and stereo equipment is often harmful to young people's hearing.

Assistance for the Hearing Impaired

Total deafness usually cannot be corrected. (In some cases, a cochlear implant has proven helpful.) Deafness is often congenital and associated with inability to speak or with speech that is very difficult to understand. A person with a marked hearing loss cannot hear sounds that warn of danger. This person loses the thread of a conversation and may ask questions or make comments that have no relation to the discussion. This can become embarrassing, and often, the person with a hearing loss lapses into a silence that makes him or her seem uninterested or inattentive. People who are unable to hear their own voices may talk very loudly or in a monotone. Most people are generally less tolerant of hearing loss than they are of vision loss and become impatient when they are asked to repeat their words. Some people with impaired hearing stubbornly refuse to admit that they do not hear well, and they deny themselves the help of a hearing aid because of embarrassment. Hearing loss that is due to advancing age (**presbycusis**) cannot be restored, but there are ways of compensating.

Occasionally you will have patients who are hearing impaired. The following skills will help you give professional care to hearing-impaired persons. The Nursing Care Plan is an example of care of a person with suspected hearing loss.

- Get the patient's attention before you begin to speak.
- Face the patient on the same level.
- Place yourself in good light so your mouth can be seen clearly.
- Do not chew, smoke, put objects in your mouth, or cover your mouth while talking.

Keys to Patient/Family Teaching
Prevention of Hearing Problems

Patient/family teaching regarding prevention of hearing problems includes:

- Excessive noise (eg, "boom" boxes, TV, stereos, work environment) is to be avoided. Keep volume down and wear protective gear if working in a noisy area.
- Ears should be protected on cold and windy days. Be aware of dangers of riding with car windows open, motor boats, motorcycles, and so forth.
- Ear plugs should be worn for swimming if the person has ear problems.
- Ears to be dried thoroughly after bathing or swimming.
- Foreign objects should not be placed in ears.
- Ears should not be cleaned excessively. The person should not pick or pull ears excessively.
- Infection should be prevented and treated immediately. Ear infection not to be treated personally; see a professional.
- Ear piercing should be done by a physician or trained technician; follow instructions for follow-up care.
- At symptoms of hearing loss, a physician should be seen immediately.

- Decrease background noises, such as television and radio.
- Speak slowly and clearly; repeat entire phrases rather than specific words.
- Restate the conversation in different words.
- Use contextual clues such as objects, persons, and hand motions to facilitate the conversation.
- Verify that the person understood the conversation.

Lip Reading and Sign Language. The person with a hearing loss can learn lip reading; it includes watching facial expressions as well as lips. To understand lip reading, the hearing-impaired person must be directly facing the speaking person.

Another means of communication is sign language (signing). Letters of the alphabet and words are formed by certain movements of the fingers and hands. People who use sign language constantly are able to speak rapidly with their fingers.

Hearing Aids. The physician will determine whether a hearing aid will help and which type will be the most beneficial. Unfortunately, a hearing aid usually is not as effective in improving hearing as glasses are in improving vision. It takes time and patience to get used to wearing a hearing aid and to learn to adjust it.

Sample Nursing Care Plan
The Hearing Impaired Person

Stella Snow is an 85-year-old widowed Native American resident in a long-term care facility. Her medical diagnoses include hypertension, coronary artery disease, glaucoma, and degenerative joint disease. You have recently noted that she does not always respond when spoken to, and on assessment you suspect a hearing deficit that is more severe on the left. Mrs. Snow is scheduled for a hearing examination. In the meantime, you add the diagnosis below to her plan of care.

Nursing Diagnosis: *Sensory/Perceptual Alteration: Auditory, Related to Effects of aging (?— Etiology Yet to be Established) as Evidenced by Change in Usual Response to Auditory Stimuli and Inappropriate Responses*

Goal: By 5/9 patient's hearing acuity is diagnosed and treatment initiated as needed.

Long-term Goal: Patient's responses to auditory stimuli demonstrate adequate ability to perceive and respond to auditory stimuli.

Nursing Actions (assess/do/teach)	Rationale	Evaluative Statement
1. The first priority after detection of a hearing problem is its accurate diagnosis. Report your observations to a physician who can order a hearing examination and follow through on the recommended treatment. Evaluate Mrs. Snow's response to the proposed treatment; if a hearing aid is necessary, ensure that Mrs. Snow understands how it works and what she needs to do to keep it functioning properly.	Careful assessment provides a basis for treatment	5/9 Goal met; Mrs. Snow has a sensorineural hearing loss (presbycusis) and use of a hearing aid is being evaluated.
2. Before speaking to Mrs. Snow, orient her to your presence by standing in front of her and gently touching her. Talk directly to the patient while facing her so that she can see your lips; decrease background noises if necessary; remember not to chew gum, cover your mouth, or turn your face away from the patient while speaking to her.	These actions prevent startling the patient. These interventions facilitate comprehension.	

Hearing aids operate on either the principle of bone conduction or air conduction, depending on the type of hearing loss. The device amplifies sounds and a tiny receiver is inserted in the ear. An earpiece is molded to the wearer's ear. Many hearing aids today are so tiny they are barely noticeable. The wearer can regulate the volume and the intensity of sounds. One difficulty encountered with hearing aids is that distracting sounds are amplified along with the significant sounds. However, difficulties can be overcome if the patient perseveres and wears the aid at all times, not just occasionally. The earpiece should be washed every day with mild soap and water and dried well; a pipe cleaner will help in cleaning the cannula.

Disorders of the External Ear

Most external ear disorders are more annoying than serious. If proper treatment is given, the condition tends to be healed without difficulty. Unfortunately, many people attempt to treat these disorders by themselves, and consequently complications could develop.

Impacted Earwax. Impacted earwax (*cerumen*) in the auditory canal is one example of a condition requiring medical attention. The wax will be removed by irrigating the outer ear with a solution warmed to body temperature (37°C or 98.6°F). This procedure is outlined earlier in this chapter.

The patient should be instructed not to attempt to remove wax or other objects from the ear. Pushing on a foreign object may damage the eardrum. If the patient has a perforated eardrum, irrigation might force the wax and the solution into the middle ear and cause infection. Poking at the wax with a finger, a hairpin, or an applicator may injure the canal and cause infection, or it may push the wax further in.

Furuncles. Furuncles (boils) are infections in the auditory canal, often the result of picking at the ear to remove wax. They are intensely painful. Heat may be applied, and antibiotics are given.

Foreign Objects. Objects are often put into the ear canal by children or persons with an intellectual impairment. They must be removed by a physician because pushing on the object may push it in further or rupture the eardrum. If the foreign object is a food substance such as a pea, bean, or corn, moisture will cause it to swell and cause extreme pain and will often damage the eardrum.

Sometimes insects enter the auditory canal. If they remain, they cause extreme distress by their fluttering and buzzing. If a flashlight is held to the ear, the light may draw the insect out; sometimes a few drops of mineral oil, alcohol, or anesthetic jelly will anesthetize or kill the insect and it will float out if the patient's head is turned to the affected side. If none of these expedients works, the patient should see a physician at once. It is dangerous to try to remove an insect with forceps; removing an insect from the ear is a delicate process that requires great skill.

External Otitis. External otitis, sometimes called swimmer's ear, is characterized most commonly by chronic external ear inflammation. It is caused by prolonged exposure to water. The patient is usually given antibiotics and advised to avoid swimming until the infection clears. Ear plugs should be worn when swimming. Prevention can be accomplished with application of ear drops, composed of substances such as acetic acid (Domeboro Otic, VoSol Otic), boric acid (Aurocaine 2, Ear-Dry, Swim-Ear), or chloramphenicol (Chlormycetin Otic).

Fungus Infections. These infections in the auditory canal tend to occur in warm, damp climates, especially when the auditory canal has not been completely dried. Most are opportunistic and feed on cerumen or dead skin cells. Fungus infections can be treated with ear drops containing antifungal medications, alcohol, and glycerin. Such infections are resistive to treatment; often it is necessary to continue treatment for a number of weeks.

Punctured Eardrum. A punctured or perforated eardrum is a serious threat to hearing later in life, as well as a possible source of middle ear infection. While the perforation will often heal spontaneously, surgery is sometimes necessary. Occasionally, *myringotomy* (surgical incision into the eardrum) is done for therapeutic reasons.

Piercing the Earlobes. This procedure, performed for cosmetic purposes, should be done by a physician or a trained technician using the correct sterile equipment and following sterile technique. Patient teaching is important. After the ears are pierced, the patient is advised to keep the original earrings in place for at least 2 weeks, to turn them frequently, and to cleanse the earlobes often with an antiseptic solution, such as alcohol. The practice of piercing the external ears above the lobes is often more painful, but not as likely to cause infection, because the earlobes are thicker and not as quick to heal.

Disorders of the Middle Ear

Otitis Media

The ear is especially susceptible to upper respiratory infections, which can travel through the auditory tube (eustachian tube) from the nose and throat. Children are especially vulnerable to these infections because their auditory tubes are straighter and shorter. *Otitis media* is an inflammation of the middle ear.

Serous Otitis Media. Fluid collects in the middle ear as a result of obstruction of the auditory tube—a condition that may be caused by infection, allergy, tumors, or sudden changes in altitude. The symptoms are crackling sensations and fullness in the ear, with some hearing loss. If this condition is not treated promptly, the pressure of the fluid may rupture the eardrum. The treatment of choice remains controversial. It consists of antibiotic use or of surgical incision into the tympanic membrane and drainage (*myringotomy*). This is followed by analysis and treatment of the original cause of the difficulty, such as removal of a tumor in the nasopharynx.

Acute Purulent Otitis Media. Acute *purulent* otitis media is caused by an upper respiratory infection spreading through the auditory tube. Pus forms and collects in the middle ear to create pressure on the eardrum. Symptoms are fever, earache, and impaired hearing. The eardrum is inflamed and bulging and may rupture. This is often treated initially with antibiotics. *Myringotomy* may also be indicated to prevent rupture of the eardrum. In this procedure, an incision is made into the tympanic membrane to relieve pressure and drain pus. If spontaneous rupture of the eardrum occurs, scarring, which disrupts normal ossicle vibrations, can result. Often this permanently impairs hearing.

If acute purulent otitis media is not treated promptly, it can lead to chronic otitis media. In the past, mastoiditis was also a complication; however, it is rarely seen today, thanks to the discovery of antibiotics. Meningitis is also a possibility if the infection spreads to the meninges of the brain. Other problems include nausea and vomiting, dizziness, injury to the facial nerve causing facial paralysis, or a brain abscess—all of which may start with a simple earache. Fortunately these serious complications are less frequent with improved treatment for acute infections.

Chronic Purulent Otitis Media. Chronic purulent otitis media is usually associated with a punctured eardrum or may be a complication of acute otitis media, mastoiditis, or a severe upper respiratory infection. Symptoms include ringing in the ears, hearing loss, pain, and purulent drainage. Antibiotics are prescribed, and a mastoidectomy may be necessary in some instances. Steroids may be given to reduce inflammation.

Treatment for Middle Ear Infections

Myringotomy. Puncture of the eardrum (*myringotomy*) is the common procedure used to treat otitis media. It releases the pressure and relieves the pain, and healing proceeds rapidly. Discharge from the ear is bloody at first, then purulent. The ear should not be plugged tightly with cotton; this would interfere with drainage. A small piece of cotton can be placed in the outer ear to absorb the drainage. It should be changed frequently. Appropriate antibiotics are given, and rest, adequate diet, and prevention against chilling are recommended.

Polyethylene Tubes. Sometimes, a polyethylene (PE) tube is inserted through the eardrum into the middle ear. This procedure is most commonly done in children with recurrent ear infections. The tubes allow continuous drainage from the middle ear. In this case, the patient must use care to prevent water from entering the ear. Swimming and showering are *contraindicated.*

Tympanoplasty. A more recent procedure than radical mastoidectomy involves reconstruction of the middle ear (*tympanoplasty*) to preserve vital parts, with less impairment of hearing. Tympanoplasty is the plastic reconstruction of the bones of the middle ear; it is done when infection or tumor has destroyed the tiny bones

of the middle ear. The bones are so reconstructed as to again extend from the oval window to the eardrum. It is a delicate procedure performed with the aid of the operating microscope.

Otosclerosis

Otosclerosis is a bony fixation of the stapes, one of the three bones in the middle ear that transmits sound to the inner ear. This condition interferes with the vibration of the stapes and impairs or destroys hearing. It is usually slow to develop. Otosclerosis seems to have some hereditary basis because there is a familial tendency to its development. It is the most common cause of conductive deafness.

Signs and Symptoms. One of the first symptoms is *tinnitus* (ringing in the ears), which is accentuated in quiet surroundings. It may go on for some time before the patient notices a hearing loss. The patient may not notice that he or she is losing the ability to hear until it gets to the point where ordinary conversation becomes difficult to hear, especially when others speak in low tones. The patient with this condition may be aided by surgery or by use of a hearing aid.

Treatment. Surgery to restore vibration of the stapes (*stapes mobilization*) may or may not be effective; therefore, it is usually left to the patient to decide whether or not to have surgery. The operation is done under local anesthesia with an operating microscope. It frees the stapes so that it can vibrate. A more common procedure today is the removal of the stapes (*stapedectomy*) and replacement by a prosthesis.

Many patients are able to hear immediately after the prosthesis is placed, but the return of hearing is not necessarily permanent; deafness may suddenly occur. Such deafness is due to an infection or to formation of scar tissue. If stapedectomy is not successful, *fenestration* (creation of a new oval window in the ear) may be done.

Disorders of the Inner Ear

Almost every disorder of the inner ear is difficult to treat. Neither surgery nor hearing aids help inner ear deafness (*perceptive deafness*). Drugs used by a person to treat conditions of the body unrelated to the ear can be harmful to the inner ear (ototoxic) and may be a cause of inner ear disorder. Streptomycin, for instance, may injure the auditory nerve. Some diseases or the aging process may also cause inner ear damage. Treatment often consists of preventing further injury and training in speech reading.

Meniere's Disease

Meniere's disease is a disturbance of the semicircular canals in the inner ear, a body mechanism that is important in maintaining body balance. Although not fatal, it is not curable. There is no known cause, but the fluid distention in the labyrinth leads to destruction of the cochlear hair cells.

Signs and Symptoms. The symptoms are devastating and alarming. The patient has sudden attacks of severe and true *vertigo*, which is a sensation of spinning or rotating, either of oneself or of one's surroundings. (Vertigo is not the same as simple dizziness, although sometimes the terms are interchanged.) Meniere's disease also is characterized by nausea, vomiting, and tinnitus. The person may not be able to walk and definitely should not drive. If the condition is untreated, hearing eventually deteriorates. Bed rest during an acute attack is sometimes necessary. The sudden attacks of Meniere's syndrome are violent; they may last only a few minutes or several weeks, during which time the quantity of fluid in the space between the semicircular canals increases.

Treatment. Medical treatment of Meniere's syndrome is aimed at relieving the symptoms. To decrease edema and pressure on the inner ear, the patient may be put on a low-sodium diet, although how beneficial this diet is remains controversial. The person may be given sedatives or tranquilizers to subdue apprehension and accompanying anxiety. Drugs may be given to relieve vertigo and nausea. The patient is advised to omit alcohol, coffee, tea, cola drinks, chocolate, and tobacco. Sometimes, when only one ear is affected, an operation to cut the auditory nerve is performed, which results in complete deafness in the affected ear.

Nursing Considerations. When caring for these patients, it is important to avoid jarring the bed, making sudden movements, turning on bright lights, or making loud noises. *(Rationale: These actions may precipitate an attack.)* Everything must be done slowly and explained to the patient before it is done. Protect the patient from falls. *(Rationale: If the vertigo is severe, the patient is in danger of falling.)* Side rails should be up and the bed kept in low position at all times to protect the patient from dangerous falls.

Give fluids and foods in small amounts. *(Rationale: The nauseated patient is better able to tolerate small amounts.)* Remember, the attacks are so devastating that the patient is understandably apprehensive. It is important to reassure the patient that relief is possible if he or she keeps quiet and follows the physician's instructions.

> **Key Concept**
>
> The person with Meniere's disease is often frightened. Vertigo can occur at any time and can occur without warning.

Disorders of Other Special Senses

In addition to hearing and vision, the special senses include the senses of touch, taste, and smell.

Sense of Touch

The sense of touch (*tactile sense*) includes the sensations of softness, pressure, pain, heat, and cold. This sense also identifies the position and movements of the body in space and assists the inner ear to maintain balance. The muscles and tendons of the body give information to the labyrinth, which is involved in maintenance of balance. This information about the position of the body in space is called *proprioception.*

A disorder in the tactile sense is often the result of a neurologic disorder. The person with a spinal cord injury, nerve transmission deficit, or disorder in the sensory area of the brain may not be able to feel or interpret pain. Thus, this patient may be endangered because he or she cannot react appropriately to an injury or an internal disorder. This person may be easily burned, for example, and not be aware of the danger. In some cases of chronic pain, nerve transmission may be intentionally interrupted. In other cases, the person is not able to maintain balance and may easily fall or may be dizzy much of the time.

Sense of Taste

The sense of taste is called the *gustatory* sense or gustation. It involves the sensations of sweet, salty, sour, and bitter, as well as others. Disorders in this sense are usually not life-threatening. An absence or alteration in the sense of taste may reduce the person's interest in eating.

Sense of Smell

The sense of smell (*olfactory* sense or olfaction) greatly affects the sense of taste. Disorders in olfaction are usually not life-threatening, but they may reduce pleasurable sensations in eating or in smelling flowers or perfumes. In certain cases, such as in gas leaks, the lack of olfactory sense may be dangerous to the person.

Keys for Review

Key Questions for Critical Thinking

1. You have patient who is undergoing eye surgery. Describe your preparation of the person, including preoperative and postoperative care and teaching.
2. Formulate a lesson plan for teaching high school seniors how to prevent hearing and vision loss. Include what you will teach and how you will teach it.
3. Among the patients on the floor on which you work are a hearing-impaired person and a vision-impaired person. Identify ways in which your care would be the same for these two patients. Determine ways in which care would be different. Explain how the care would be different if the person were both hearing and visually impaired.

Key Readings

Bartley GB, Liesegang TJ (Eds). Essentials of Ophthalmology. Philadelphia, J.B. Lippincott, 1992

Beare PG, Myers JL. Principles and Practice of Adult Health Nursing. St. Louis, C.V. Mosby, 1990

Berkow R (Ed). The Merck Manual of Diagnosis and Therapy, Ed 16. Rahway, NJ, Merck & Co, 1992

Craven RF, Hirnle CJ. Fundamentals of Nursing: Human Health and Function. Philadelphia, J.B. Lippincott, 1992

Earnest VV. Clinical Skills in Nursing Practice, Ed 2. Philadelphia, J.B. Lippincott, 1993

Fischbach F. A Manual of Laboratory and Diagnostic Tests, Ed 3. Philadelphia, J.B. Lippincott, 1992

NANDA Nursing Diagnoses: Definitions and Classifications 1992. Philadelphia, North American Nursing Diagnosis Association, 1992

O'Toole M (Ed). Miller-Keane Encyclopedia and Dictionary of Medicine, Nursing, and Allied Health, Ed 5. Philadelphia, W.B. Saunders, 1992

Scherer JC. Introductory Medical-Surgical Nursing, Ed 6. Philadelphia, J.B. Lippincott, 1995

Smeltzer SC, Bare BG. Brunner and Suddarth's Textbook of Medical-Surgical Nursing, Ed 7. Philadelphia, J.B. Lippincott, 1992

Suddarth DS. The Lippincott Manual of Nursing Practice, Ed 5. Philadelphia, J.B. Lippincott, 1991

Key Readings (continued)

Taylor C, Lillis C, LeMone P. Fundamentals of Nursing: Art and Science of Nursing Care, Ed 2. Philadelphia, J.B. Lippincott, 1993

Keys to Learning More

Chapter 85: disorders of aging and prevention of accidents

Chapter 89: rehabilitation

Key Resources

American Foundation for the Blind
15 West 16th Street
New York, NY 10016
212-620-2000

American Speech-Language-Hearing Association
10801 Rockville Pike
Dept AP
Rockville, MD 20852
301-897-5700

American Tinnitus Association
PO Box 5
Portland, OR 97207
503-248-9985

Lions International
300 22nd Street
Oak Brook, IL 60521-8842
708-571-5466

National Society to Prevent Blindness
500 East Remington Road
Schaumburg, IL 60173
312-843-2020

Retinitis Pigmentosa Foundation Fighting Blindness
1401 Mt. Royal Avenue
4th Floor
Baltimore, MD 21217-4245
410-225-9400

Self Help for Hard of Hearing People
4848 Battery Lane, Dept. E
Bethesda, MD 20814
301-657-2248

74 Cardiovascular Disorders

Keys for Learning

Learning Objectives

♦ List at least five predisposing factors to coronary artery disease and describe the relationship between each factor and cardiovascular disorders.
♦ Explain the purpose of diagnostic tests in cardiovascular disorders.
♦ Discuss the role of the nurse in diagnostic tests.
♦ Discuss the role of the nurse in surgical interventions used in cardiovascular disorders.
♦ Describe at least five common disorders of the heart and discuss related nursing care.
♦ Describe at least four disorders of the blood vessels and discuss related nursing care.
♦ Describe the four types or stages of cerebrovascular accident. Identify nursing considerations for the acute phase in this disorder.

Key Terms

aneurysm	echocardiography	necrosis
angina pectoris	embolus	pancarditis
angiogram	endocarditis	pericarditis
aphasia	hemiplegia	phlebitis
arrhythmia	hypertension	stenosis
arteriosclerosis	ischemia	stent
atherosclerosis	myocarditis	thrombophlebitis

Keys to Understanding This Chapter

Chapter 5: basic human needs
Chapter 21: anatomy and physiology of cardiovascular system
Chapter 22: anatomy and physiology of respiratory system
Chapter 28: diet therapy and special diets
Chapter 31: emergency care
Chapter 32: sudden death and cardiopulmonary resuscitation
Chapter 38: signs and symptoms of illness or injury

Keys to Understanding This Chapter
(continued)

Chapter 42: vital signs
Chapter 50: physical examination and nursing assessment
Chapter 52: pain management
Chapter 53: pre- and postoperative care
Chapter 54: sterile technique, used in many areas of cardiovascular nursing
Unit Eleven: pharmacology and medication administration
Chapter 61: complications of pregnancy, including the mother with cardiovascular problems
Chapter 65: heart problems in children

Key Points

♦ Hypertension can lead to such serious problems as myocardial infarction, kidney damage, congestive heart failure, and cerebrovascular accident.
♦ Some types of heart disease can be cured, whereas others can be controlled by treatment.
♦ Coronary artery disease develops over many years and therefore prevention of controllable risk factors should begin early in life.
♦ Angina or angina pectoris is a *temporary* loss of oxygen to the heart muscle. If this loss of oxygen supply continues, the result is *ischemia* (or prolonged deficiency of oxygenated blood), whereas death of heart tissue is called *myocardial necrosis.*
♦ Patients should be medicated promptly as ordered by the physician when complaining of chest pains, to prevent further extension of damage to heart muscle due to anoxia (lack of oxygen).
♦ Congestive heart failure means the heart is failing, has lost its pumping ability, and is unable to do its work. It is a syndrome (group of symptoms) that affects individuals in different ways and to different degrees.

Rosdahl CB: Textbook of Basic Nursing, 6th ed. © 1995 J.B. Lippincott Company

Cardiovascular disorders include those conditions that interfere with the heart's ability to pump, those that disrupt blood flow within the coronary or cerebral vessels, and those peripheral vascular diseases that disrupt blood flow to a localized area such as an extremity. Together, they are the leading cause of death in the United States among persons over age 25 and the second leading cause of disability among younger persons. The specialty is called *cardiology;* the physician is called a *cardiologist.*

Anatomy and Physiology Review

The cardiovascular system, described in Chapter 21, consists of the heart, blood and lymph vessels, and the fluid blood and lymph.

The heart has four chambers, two atria and two ventricles, which are separated by specialized valves and by the septum. The atria are the uppermost chambers and *receive* blood. The lower chambers, the ventricles, pump blood *out of the heart* into arteries. The right ventricle pumps unoxygenated blood into the pulmonary arteries and on into the lungs (pulmonary circulation). The left ventricle pumps oxygenated blood into the aorta, the largest artery in the body, and on into the body (systemic circulation). The heart muscle itself is supplied by the coronary arteries. A complex electrical system sends impulses to heart muscle, causing contractions (heartbeats). Blood pressure and pulse are vital signs that help evaluate heart action.

The blood vessels are called arteries, arterioles, capillaries, venules, and veins. The systemic arteries carry blood, nutrients, and oxygen to body cells; veins carry wastes and carbon dioxide away from cells.

Diagnostic Tests

Laboratory Tests

Blood Tests

An important blood screening in heart disorders includes the measurement of levels of serum enzymes. These include *creatinine phosphokinase* (CPK), *lactic dehydrogenase* (LDH), and *aspartate aminotransferase* (AST), formerly called serum glutamic oxaloacetic transaminase (SGOT). These enzymes are released into the bloodstream when muscle damage occurs, as in myocardial infarction (MI). Levels of these enzymes rise and fall in the serum at specific times and therefore must be correlated with the patient's medical history, as well as with other diagnostic tests.

Blood lipid studies may be ordered to determine *hyperlipidemia* (excess fat in the blood). Cholesterol is a blood lipid (fat) often associated with coronary artery disease.

Other important tests are the *serum electrolytes,* such as potassium, sodium, and magnesium. A decrease in the level of these electrolytes can cause heart arrhythmia.

Key Abbreviations and Acronyms Used in CV Care

AST	Aspartate aminotransferase
CAD	Coronary artery disease
CCU	Coronary care unit
CHF	Congestive heart failure
CICU	Coronary intensive care unit
CS	Completed stroke
CVA	Cerebrovascular accident
CVP	Central venous pressure
ECG, EKG	Electrocardiogram
EPS	Electrophysiology studies
HR	Heart rate
MI	Myocardial infarction
PTCA	Percutaneous transluminal coronary angioplasty
RIND	Reversible ischemic neurologic deficit
SBE	Subacute bacterial endocarditis
SIE	Stroke in evolution
TIA	Transient ischemic attack
t-PA	Tissue plasminogen activator

Nursing Alert

Ask if the patient is allergic to shellfish or iodine before any test using radiopaque dye is done. This dye could cause a severe anaphylactic reaction (see Chapter 50).

X-ray Evaluations

Angiocardiogram and Arteriogram

An **angiogram** (angiocardiogram) is an x-ray of the heart and major vessels after a radiopaque dye has been injected into a vessel. It shows the course of the dye from the heart to the lungs, back to the heart, then out through the aorta. This procedure can provide information about structural abnormalities and calcifications within the vascular system. An *arteriogram* is an x-ray of any artery. Because it is uncomfortable and carries some risk, the patient must sign a permission form before either procedure can be done. Nursing care in these procedures is discussed in the Nursing Process section of this chapter.

Other Diagnostic Tests

Electrocardiogram

An *electrocardiogram* (ECG) is a graphic record or tracing that represents the heart's electrical action (Fig. 74-1). It provides essential information about the state of the heart, heart rate, heart rhythm, and the presence of certain disorders.

The ECG may be done at the patient's bedside or in a room set aside for this purpose. Patients should be told that the test is painless and that they must lie very still. Leads, or electrodes, are placed on the patient's skin (the chest, wrists, and ankles) and connected to a machine called an electrocardiograph. The graph or tracing (ECG) is placed on the patient's chart after the cardiologist has interpreted it and written a statement and summary of the findings. The patient does not usually require any special treatment either before or after the procedure. The person interpreting the ECG must be informed of any cardiac medications the patient is receiving. It is also valuable to have data regarding the patient's age, sex, blood pressure, height, weight, and symptoms available for the cardiologist.

Stress Test

The purpose of the *stress test* is to assess the severity of symptomatic and asymptomatic (without symptoms) cardiac disease. The patient pedals a stationary bicycle or walks on a treadmill while ECG and blood pressure measurements are taken. Various chemicals or medications (thallium, dipyridamole [Persantine], dobutamine HCl [Dobutrex]) may also be injected before or during the test, or used instead of the exercise. The response of the heart to physical activity or the medi-

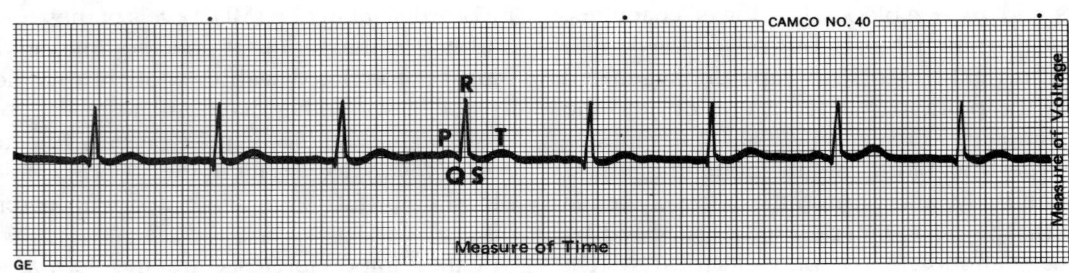

Figure 74-1. An electrocardiogram provides valuable information about the heart's ability to conduct impulses. (Craven RF and Hirnle CJ. Fundamentals of Nursing: Human Health and Function. Philadelphia, J.B. Lippincott, 1992)

cation is determined and an appropriate exercise program or method of treatment is prescribed for the individual.

Trendelenburg Test

The *Trendelenburg test* assesses the efficiency of the valves in the superficial veins. It is diagnostic for varicose veins. The patient lies down with the legs elevated. A tourniquet is applied to the upper thigh, and the patient is asked to stand. The pattern of blood flow while the tourniquet is in place and after its removal indicates the degree of valvular competence in the legs. The physician can then decide what treatment is to be given.

Echocardiogram

Echocardiography uses sound waves to produce a three-dimensional view of the heart and its blood flow. There is no radiation exposure. The test can assess heart size, detect the presence of excess fluid in the pericardial sac, assess valvular function, and even show the size of individual heart chambers. It is especially useful in the diagnosis and differentiation of heart murmurs. In many cases, this noninvasive test has replaced invasive tests.

Nuclear Scan

The nuclear scan will determine the pumping ability of the heart. A weak radioactive chemical (thallium or technetium) is given intravenously during the scan to provide a better view of the heart's chambers or myocardium.

Electrophysiology Study

The electrophysiology study (EPS) provides valuable information in locating the source of an **arrhythmia** (irregular heartbeat) and determining the most effective medication to control it. The EPS is done in the cardiovascular laboratory and takes approximately 2 to 3 hours. The cardiologist will attempt to recreate the patient's abnormal heart rhythm by using a temporary pacemaker. The leads for the pacemaker are inserted through a catheter that is threaded into the major vessels of the heart. Once the arrhythmia occurs, various medications are administered to see which will best prevent it. Nursing care is discussed under Nursing Process in this chapter.

Cardiac Catheterization

The purpose of cardiac catheterization is usually to obtain information about congenital or acquired defects of the heart, to measure oxygen concentration, to determine cardiac output, or to assess the status of the heart's structures and chambers. Some special procedures can also be done via cardiac catheter.

In this procedure, a long, flexible catheter is passed into the heart through a large blood vessel. The pressure is measured as the catheter passes through each location and blood specimens are taken in each area. A dye may also be injected. The procedure is performed by a team of physicians, nurses, and technicians and takes from 1 to 3 hours. Nursing care for cardiac catheterization is discussed under Nursing Process in this chapter.

Medical and Surgical Treatments

The coronary care unit (CCU) or coronary intensive care unit (CICU) is a special hospital unit designed for the care of patients with heart disorders. The staff is specially trained in coronary care and emergency measures.

Training in coronary care includes normal anatomy and physiology of the heart, normal and abnormal ECG readings, laboratory tests and their significance, emergency drugs and resuscitation measures, use of special equipment (such as cardiac monitors and defibrillation equipment), and the special emotional aspects of coronary care nursing. A detailed discussion of patient care in a CICU is beyond the scope of this text.

Common Medical Treatments

Thrombolytic Therapy

Pharmacologic agents such as streptokinase (streptase), urokinase (Abbokinase, Win-kinase), as well as alteplase, also known as tissue plasminogen activator, t-PA (Activase) have been shown to dissolve clots in the coronary arteries. These clots cause occlusion (blockage) of the blood flow in situations such as acute MI (myocardial infarction). The specific drugs are usually given through a peripheral vein by nurses in the emergency room or ICU. Patients for thrombolytic therapy are selected by the following criteria:

- History of chest pain within the past 6 hours. *(Rationale: Studies have shown that the sooner the pharmacologic agent is administered, the less heart muscle damage results.)*
- ECG changes indicating **ischemia** (lack of blood supply) to the heart that persists even after the administration of sublingual nitroglycerin
- No recent history of surgery, organ biopsy, cardiopulmonary resuscitation, cerebrovascular accident (CVA), or bleeding abnormalities

The patient generally feels relief of chest pain if the procedure is successful. The patient is assessed for complications including arrhythmias, bleeding, allergic reactions, and fever. The patient will be in the CCU for 1 to 2 days to facilitate close observation.

Common Surgical Treatments

Percutaneous Transluminal Coronary Angioplasty

In percutaneous transluminal coronary angioplasty (PTCA), a balloon-tipped catheter is inserted into a narrowed coronary artery. The steps in the procedure are illustrated in Figure 74-2. A radiopaque dye is injected to allow clear viewing of the coronary arteries by x-ray so the surgeon can see the procedure.

Sometimes this procedure is simply called angioplasty. Angioplasty widens the opening (lumen) of the artery and improves blood flow to the muscles of the heart. Another type of angioplasty involves use of a cutting device.

In some cases angioplasty does not maintain arterial patency; the artery closes. Some surgeons are finding long-term success by doing an angioplasty and placing a **stent**. A stent is a wire coil that looks like that in a ball point pen. This coil is left in the artery when the balloon catheter is removed and keeps the artery open. Researchers state that the use of stents reduces closing of the artery by a third.

Cardiac Surgery

Some patients with heart disease may be helped by heart surgery. *Closed-heart surgery* refers to surgical procedures that may be done without stopping the heart. *Open-heart surgery* involves opening or operating on the heart in such a way that the heart must be stopped and the circulated blood oxygenated by a device, such as the pump oxygenator (heart–lung pump). This is known as *extracorporeal* (outside the body) *circulation*. As blood circulates through the machine, carbon dioxide is removed and oxygen is added through osmosis, filming, or bubbling. The machine also keeps the blood warmed to body temperature. A trained cardiopulmonary technician maintains the machine and determines if the blood is being properly oxygenated. A patient can be maintained for several hours on the heart–lung pump. Various types of heart and blood vessel surgery may be done with the use of the pump oxygenator, or it may be used as a support device in other types of surgery. In some cases, heart surgery is done after the patient's body temperature is lowered (surgical hypothermia) or under higher-than-normal atmospheric pressure with hyperoxygenation (in the *hyperbaric chamber*). Nursing care in cardiac surgery is discussed in the Nursing Process section of this chapter.

Heart Valve Replacement

Heart valves can become damaged by disease or a congenital situation. In some cases, artificial or mechanical valves are transplanted to replace damaged valves. In other cases, human heart valves are used. Human heart valves have several advantages: 1) they do not need to be replaced as soon (about 10 years for artificial valves); 2) they better control pressures within the heart; 3) they are quiet (some artificial valves click);

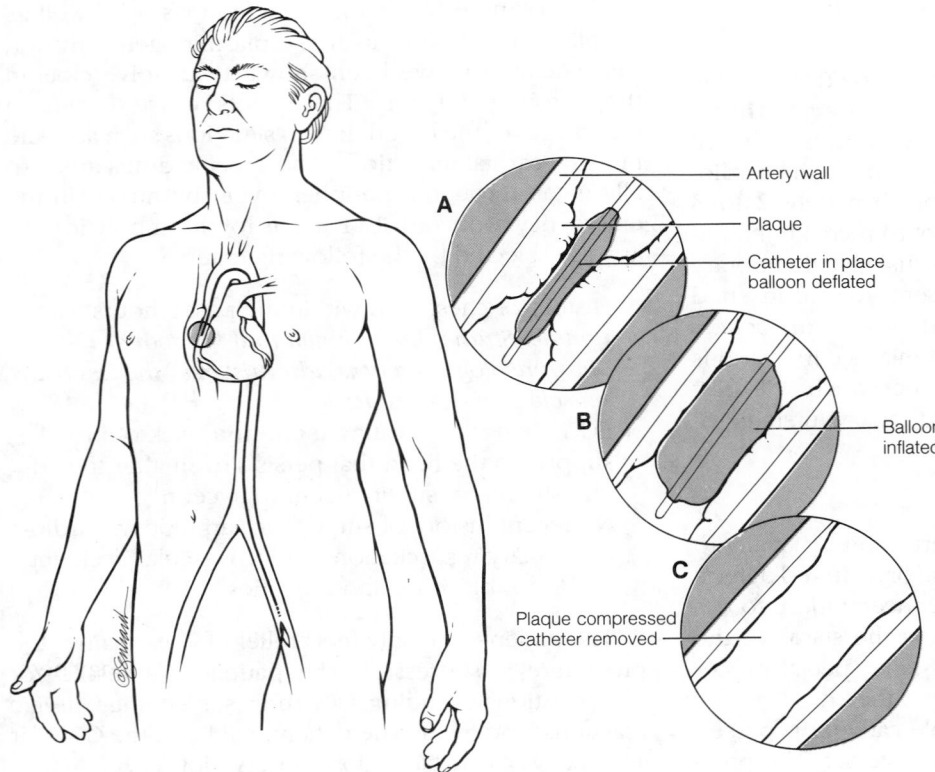

Figure 74-2. Percutaneous transluminal coronary angioplasty is a less invasive procedure than coronary artery bypass surgery in selected patients. **(A)** A balloon-tipped catheter is passed into the affected coronary artery and placed within the atherosclerotic lesion. **(B)** The balloon is then rapidly inflated and deflated with controlled pressure. **(C)** After the plaque is compressed, the catheter is removed, allowing improved blood flow in the vessel.

Labels in figure:
A — Artery wall, Plaque, Catheter in place balloon deflated
B — Balloon inflated
C — Plaque compressed catheter removed

and 4) they can be preserved until needed. In addition, human heart valves grow with a child recipient. However, because human valves are foreign tissue, more antirejection drugs may be needed by the recipient.

Heart Transplantation

Many problems are associated with heart transplantation, the greatest of which is *rejection* by the body of any foreign object or protein substance. This normal defense mechanism fights infection, but in the case of transplantation, it works against the well-being of the patient, so the normal antibody response must be offset by drugs or the new heart will be rejected. Antirejection or immunosuppressive drugs (drugs that suppress the immune response), such as cyclosporine (Sandimmune) and FK 506, are given. The success rate in heart transplantation continually improves. Medical and nursing care in heart transplantation is specialized and beyond the scope of this book.

❖ *Nursing Process*

Data Collection

The nurse must carefully observe and assess the patient with a cardiac or blood vessel disorder. Chapter 50 describes physical examination and nursing assessment, including that of the cardiovascular system. This assessment establishes a baseline for future comparison and determines the presence of suspected cardiovascular complications. The nurse should report any changes in baseline assessments.

A complete cardiovascular assessment begins on admission of the patient. The nursing assessment includes a complete nursing history, as well as observations made by the nurse. When taking the health history, it is important to ask about any potential risk factors (smoking, exercise, rest, nutrition). The nursing assessment also includes determination of issues that might interfere with the patient's ability to perform activities of daily living.

When doing a cardiovascular assessment, the nurse assesses the apparent function of the heart and blood vessels. Components of the nursing assessment include heart sounds, blood pressure, and pulse. Certain signs and symptoms such as shortness of breath may be observed while taking the patient's vital signs. Difficulty breathing, orthopnea, edema, cyanosis, pain, and fatigue are other possible indications of heart disorders. The nurse also observes the patient's emotional response to the disorder or disease and the person's understanding of ongoing treatment needed. See the accompanying box for signs and symptoms of cardiovascular disorders.

Keys to Nursing Assessment

Signs and Symptoms of Cardiovascular Disorders

- ◆ Changes in the rate, quality, and rhythm of the pulse
- ◆ Rise or fall in blood pressure or central venous pressure
- ◆ Edema, especially in the feet and the ankles (faulty heart action causes the collection of fluids in the tissues)
- ◆ A gain in weight from excess fluid in the tissues
- ◆ Difficulty in breathing and the presence of a cough, often due to pulmonary edema
- ◆ Cyanosis, due to lack of oxygen in the blood or to a circulatory disorder
- ◆ Clubbing of the fingers; needing to squat to breathe
- ◆ Pain (a significant symptom)
- ◆ Fatigue, for no apparent reason
- ◆ Intermittent claudication, which denotes a decrease in blood supply to the legs and feet (a person with arterial blockage will feel pain within 1 minute after beginning to walk)

Nursing Diagnosis

Based on data collection, the following are examples of nursing diagnoses that may appear on nursing care plans of patients with cardiovascular disorders:

- ◆ Fluid Volume Excess related to excess sodium retention or intake, as evidenced by edema
- ◆ Impaired Social Interaction related to limited physical ability, pain
- ◆ Fatigue related to inadequate circulation, discomfort
- ◆ Sleep Pattern Disturbance related to orthopnea
- ◆ High Risk for Peripheral Neurovascular Dysfunction related to circulatory disorders, coronary insufficiency

Planning and Implementation

The patient, nurse, and family plan together for effective care to meet patient needs based on the nursing diagnosis. The nurse provides preoperative and postoperative care for the patient undergoing diagnostic tests such as cardiac catheterization and for procedures such as angioplasty. The patient with a heart or blood vessel disorder may also require assistance in meeting daily needs. The person who has had a stroke may need total assistance and nursing care temporarily or on a long-term basis. The person with a chronic disability such as hemiplegia or a damaged heart may need assistance in dealing with emotional problems. Many patients need to understand more about the disorder, its prognosis, and its treatment. A nursing care plan is developed for each patient to meet individual needs. A sample nursing care plan for a patient with a cardiovascular disorder is provided later in the chapter.

Providing Care During Diagnostic Tests

Nurses assist persons in preparing for diagnostic tests and give instructions to the patient and family about the tests.

ANGIOCARDIOGRAM AND ARTERIOGRAM.
Usually the patient's breakfast is omitted before the procedure. A sedative may be given an hour before the test is scheduled. The groin area is often used for catheter insertion; it is prepped and may be shaved. Other routine preoperative procedures are carried out. The patient voids just before the test.

The patient may have an allergic reaction to the dye after the procedure. The patient must be watched for signs of a delayed reaction after returning to the room. Signs to watch for include rapid pulse, diaphoresis, shakiness, skin rash, or a drop in blood pressure. The patient may complain of a swollen throat or having difficulty swallowing. The dye is irritating if it comes in contact with the skin, and sometimes the injection site becomes swollen and painful. Ice packs may be prescribed to relieve discomfort. (See Chapter 50 for special precautions when dye is used.)

The patient is kept on bed rest until fully awake and is instructed not to bend the leg or flex the hip for approximately 8 hours. This injection site (where the catheter was inserted) must be closely observed for bleeding. Vital signs are carefully monitored to check for internal hemorrhage. Peripheral pulses distal to the injection site are checked. It is possible for the patient to develop a clot or other blockage in the blood vessel. If pulses are absent, emergency measures must be taken. Color and warmth of the affected extremity are also checked.

ELECTROPHYSIOLOGY STUDY.
Before the procedure, a consent form must be signed by the patient. The patient will be NPO after midnight. A sedative is sometimes ordered to relax the patient before and during the procedure.

After the procedure, a sandbag is placed on the arterial site. The patient will be on bed rest for 1 to 2 hours after the procedure. Vital signs are checked every 15 minutes initially and less frequently after they are stable.

Cardiac Catheterization.
The patient may be apprehensive about the procedure. It will help to explain that the procedure is really not painful, although the patient may be a little uncomfortable. A local anesthetic is given during the procedure. The patient is warned there may be a sensation of warmth and a "fluttering" feeling of the heart, as the catheter is passed through the blood vessels during the procedure.

A signed permit is required and the patient is NPO for at least 6 hours before the procedure. Exceptions to the NPO order are specific medications ordered by the physician.

Cardiac catheterization usually has no complications, but it is not entirely without danger. Assess the catheter insertion site for bleeding or hematoma. Sandbags are often placed on the arterial site. The patient's peripheral pulses are checked every 15 minutes for an hour after the test and frequently after that for several hours. Some physicians keep the patient in bed for the rest of the day.

> **Nursing Alert**
>
> After any study in which the femoral site is used, the patient should lie flat for about 8 hours. This helps to avoid swelling, bruising, and bleeding at the puncture sites.

> **Nursing Alert**
>
> A rapid or irregular pulse after cardiac catheterization must be reported immediately. This may indicate heart or valve damage, clot formation, or hemorrhage. Any complaint of chest or insertion site pain must be reported at once also.

Providing Care During Cardiac Surgery

Usually, patients come into the hospital who have been under intensive medical treatment for several weeks before surgery. This allows time to prepare them physically and emotionally for the experience. Many patients welcome heart surgery as a new chance at life because often no other treatment can help them. New methods of treatment and new surgical techniques are giving a chance to live a normal life to many people who would not have survived in previous years.

Preoperatively, the important considerations are good nutrition; extra oxygen for the body, which has been deprived of an adequate oxygen supply; vitamin therapy; antibiotic therapy; and routine procedures, such as laboratory and x-ray examinations, heart catheterization, ECGs, and practice in deep breathing. The reason for all these procedures is to build the patient up to the best possible physical condition before surgery.

Registered nurses are usually responsible for the immediate postoperative nursing care following open-heart surgery; the LPN or nursing student assists. The first 2 days after surgery are the most critical to survival. Goals of postoperative nursing care are:

◆ Provide adequate tissue oxygenation
◆ Assess cardiac function
◆ Maintain fluid and electrolyte balance
◆ Control chest drainage with suction
◆ Monitor body temperature
◆ Relieve pain

Communicating With the Aphasic Patient

Some disorders, such as cerebrovascular accident (CVA), cause aphasia (usually refers to inability to speak). It is essential that a communication system be established with all patients. The two major nursing goals in aphasia are to assist the patient to communicate nonverbally and, if possible, retrain the person to speak. The following nursing skills will help you and the patient communicate:

◆ If the patient can write, supply a tablet and pencil or provide a board on which he or she can write.
◆ If the patient cannot write, provide a board or chart on which is printed or on which you have written key words and phrases. The patient can point to these words and phrases to make needs known.
◆ The patient may be able to move a finger or in some way let you know that he or she understands what is being said.
◆ If the patient cannot move at all, a common system of communication is that of blinking. The patient can blink once for "yes" and twice for "no."
◆ Talk to the patient even if the person cannot answer. Chat while you perform daily nursing care.
◆ Do not talk down to the patient.
◆ Never talk about the patient to another person, including healthcare personnel, in the patient's presence. The patient may be able to hear and understand everything although unable to speak.
◆ Some patients unable to speak are able to use a computer. Assistive devices are available for those who cannot use a conventional keyboard.

Speech therapy should begin as soon as possible. Once the speech therapist has decided what procedures to use, the nursing staff should reinforce what the speech therapist has taught.

Teaching Regarding Prevention

To aid the patient in preventing cardiovascular disorders, the nurse teaches about predisposing factors (eg, fat buildup in the arteries and hypertension). Prevention involves a healthy diet to keep weight and the cholesterol level down, exercise for the strengthening the heart, and cessation of smoking.

The aims of prevention of and care in hypertension and many other cardiovascular disorders are to reduce weight if necessary; eliminate or sharply reduce dietary salt intake; encourage a healthy pattern of sleep, rest, and relaxation; and avoid emotional upsets. If the patient is taking antihypertensive drugs, teaching involves the necessity of taking the prescribed medications despite the fact that the patient feels well. Antihypertensives help relieve emotional stress, relax the blood vessels, and reduce tissue fluid and blood volume. Possible side effects of the medications should be included in the teaching (see Chapter 56).

The nurse may suggest a nutritionist for consultation or a support group for helping the patient lose weight or maintain an ideal weight. Counseling about fat in the diet may be helpful.

Aerobic exercise (if not too stressful) is good for cardiovascular conditioning. Walking, especially at a good pace, is effective and inexpensive. The greatest risk in exercising is avoiding it. The nurse can teach how to warm up and cool down before and after exercising. Smoking cessation programs may be necessary for those who wish to stop smoking.

Often patients are taught to measure blood pressure at home. Many authorities believe that with the patient involved more directly in self-care, there is greater compliance with the medication and required routine. A person can alter the life-style to make it more healthy. The accompanying box describes teaching factors and actions the individual can take to reduce the risk of cardiovascular disease.

ABNORMAL CONDITIONS THAT CAN LEAD TO SERIOUS CARDIOVASCULAR CONDITIONS. Some types of heart disease can be cured, whereas others can be controlled by treatment. A patient's attitude toward heart disease has a tremendous effect on recovery. Some patients are so frightened that they are afraid to move. Other patients deny the seriousness of their diease and disregard orders about diet, rest, and smoking. Several types of heart conditions are are discussed here that, if not treated, can lead to more serious cardiovascular conditions. Individuals should understand the seriousness of these conditions and the value of diet, exercise, and medication. Patient teaching is of utmost importance.

Arteriosclerosis and Atherosclerosis. **Arteriosclerosis** applies to several pathologic conditions in which there is thickening, hardening, and loss of elasticity in the walls of arteries. Often it is referred to as "hardening of the arteries." **Atherosclerosis** is the most common type of arteriosclerosis. It is characterized by fatty deterioration of the arterial smooth muscle

Prevention of Cardiovascular Disorders

Patient/family teaching regarding prevention of cardiovascular disorders includes:

◆ Harmful effects of smoking. *(Rationale: Nicotine is a vasoconstrictor. It also increases heart rate and blood pressure.)*

◆ Reduction of sodium (salt). *(Rationale: Salt restriction minimizes fluid retention.)*

◆ Maintenance of weight within standardized guidelines. *(Rationale: Obesity places a strain on the circulatory system.)*

◆ Harmful effects of cholesterol. Avoid foods high in animal fats. *(Rationale: Excess cholesterol can form plaque in blood vessels.)* Choose foods according to the Food Guide Pyramid (see Chapter 26).

◆ Harmful effects of foods containing caffeine. Avoid coffee, cola drinks, and chocolate. *(Rationale: Caffeine is a vasoconstrictor.)*

◆ Value of "plenty of fluids." *(Rationale: Fluids help the body eliminate wastes.)*

◆ Exercise regularly and moderately. Walking is a healthful exercise. *(Rationale: Exercise stimulates circulation and builds cardiac strength and endurance.)*

◆ Short periods of exercise are alternated with periods of lying down or standing. Avoid crossing legs at the knees when sitting. *(Rationale: Crossing legs at the knees hampers circulation.)*

◆ Both feet should comfortably touch the floor when a person is sitting. *(Rationale: This position avoids constriction of blood vessels in the groin area.)*

◆ For a few minutes in the morning and evening the feet should be elevated. It is best to be lying down with the entire body lower than the feet. *(Rationale: This position encourages venous return.)*

◆ Constrictive garments, especially around the legs, arms, and waist, are to be avoided. Women should not wear garters or girdles that fit tightly. *(Rationale: These items restrict circulation.)*

◆ Proper-fitting shoes are important. *(Rationale: Irritation and skin breakdown are prevented with proper fitting shoes. An ulcer on the foot or leg is difficult to cure if peripheral circulation is impaired.)*

◆ Environmental stress and anxiety-producing factors should be avoided or minimized. *(Rationale: Stress causes release of substances called catecholamines, which constrict blood vessels and, thus, elevate blood pressure.)*

◆ Importance of following regimen for prescribed medications.

◆ Plenty of rest is necessary. Learn how to relax.

walls. Gradually, over a period of years, as walls absorb increasing amounts of circulating fats or lipids and the lumen of the arteries narrows (**stenosis**). This buildup of fat and mineral deposits is called *plaque*. The lumen may close completely. The artery with a narrowed lumen compared to the normal coronary artery is illustrated in Figure 74-3. Often the terms arteriosclerosis and atherosclerosis are used interchangeably. These diseases may affect the heart valves and may lead to hypertension or coronary artery disease.

A diet high in saturated fat is usually associated with an increased cholesterol level in the blood. It has been found that unsaturated fats, such as corn oil and cottonseed oil, do not raise the blood cholesterol level as much as do the saturated fats found in butter, eggs, and meats. Some people seem to metabolize cholesterol differently than others. In treating cardiovascular disorders, the physician periodically measures blood cholesterol levels and may attempt to control the amount of cholesterol by diet, medications, and exercise. It is now believed that the *balance* between high-density lipoprotein (HDL or "good cholesterol") and low-density lipoprotein (LDL or "bad cholesterol") is more important than is the actual total cholesterol value. However, as the total level rises above 150, the risk of coronary artery disease increases.

Hypertension. **Hypertension** is high blood pressure. It is estimated that 50% of all Americans over the age of 65 have hypertension. Under the age of 50, it is more common in men. It has been found that African Americans are likely to get hypertension earlier in life, at higher levels, and twice as often as white people.

Hypertension can lead to MI, kidney damage, congestive heart failure, and CVA, commonly known as stroke. A consistently high blood pressure leads to heart damage. With advancing age, blood pressure tends to rise, although the reasons for this are not completely clear. One thing is certain: the condition of the heart and blood vessels has the greatest effect on blood pressure. Although hypertension cannot be cured, with treatment blood pressure usually can be brought within the normal range.

Hypertensive heart disease (high blood pressure) is predominantly a spasm of small arterioles. These spasms increase the blood pressure and thus contribute to arteriosclerosis, a vicious circle. Because the heart must pump harder to force blood through the arteries, the result is *hypertrophy* (enlargement) of the heart muscle. Hypertension may exist from a known cause—such as kidney failure, malformations of blood vessels, certain tumors, and some specific endocrine disorders—or the cause may be unknown.

In most cases, the cause of high blood pressure is unknown; this is classified as *essential hypertension.* Symptoms other than elevated blood pressure may not

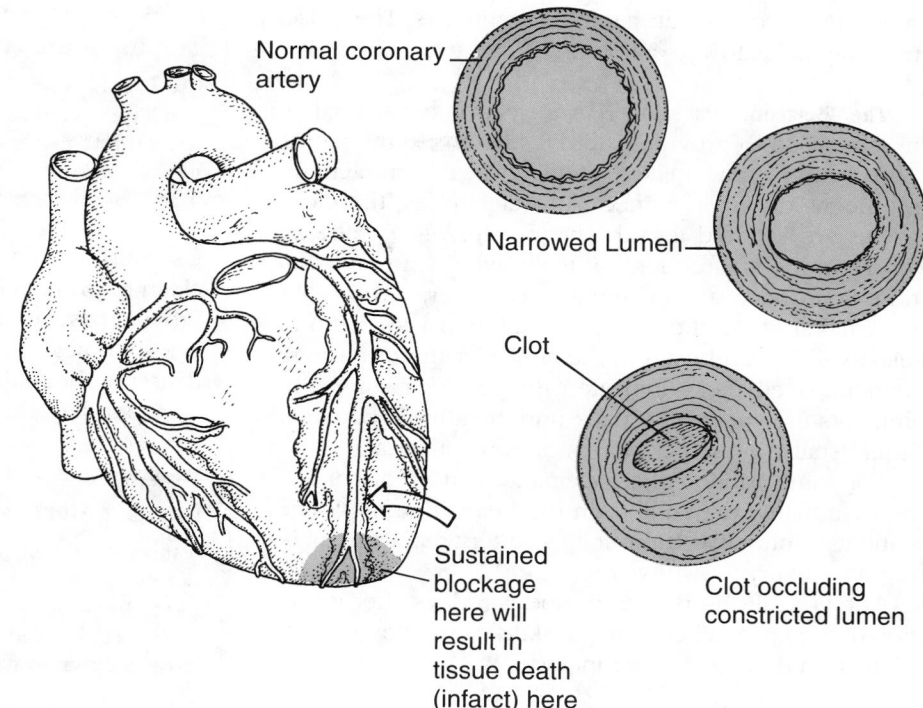

Normal coronary artery

Narrowed Lumen

Clot

Sustained blockage here will result in tissue death (infarct) here

Clot occluding constricted lumen

Figure 74-3. Atherosclerotic plaque: a buildup of fat, cholesterol, fibrin, cellular waste products, and calcium on the endothelial lining of an artery. (Craven RF and Hirnle CJ. Fundamentals of Nursing: Human Health and Function. Philadelphia, J.B. Lippincott, 1992)

occur for years, and no restrictions are imposed until other symptoms develop. Patients are encouraged to exercise in moderation, observe moderation in eating, and avoid tension and anxiety. They are advised not to smoke, not to drink alcoholic beverages, and to avoid caffeine and sodium. Symptoms of hypertension may become severe, with headache, fatigue, dyspnea, edema, and nocturia.

Malignant hypertension, which is not a cancer, is most often seen in younger people. The incidence is highest in African Americans, especially men under age 40. The onset is sudden, and the disease progresses rapidly. In many cases it is difficult to determine the cause. Malignant hypertension is known to cause rapid necrosis (death) in vital organs, such as the heart, brain, and kidney. Most patients with malignant hypertension survive less than 2 years.

Evaluation

The nurse, the patient, and the family evaluate the outcomes of care. Have short-term goals been met? Is the patient stabilized following the initial emergency? Are long-term goals still realistic? Will this patient need long-term nursing care or short-term rehabilitation placement? Does the patient need home health aide/homemaker services or regular in-home medication administration? Has the patient been referred to a "stop smoking" program? Is a support group needed for patient or family members? Planning for further nursing care must consider the patient's prognosis, as well as any complications and the patient's response to care given.

Heart Disorders

Cardiac Arrhythmias

An **arrhythmia** is an irregularity in the rhythm of the heartbeat. It is a complication of MI, as well as of other heart and circulatory disorders. It may also be caused by severe trauma or electric shock. Common arrhythmias are:

◆ *Sinus tachycardia:* Heartbeat is 100 or more. (This rate is normal in children.) It can be present in instances of high fever, extreme emotion, overactive thyroid, strenuous exercise, and shock.
◆ *Sinus bradycardia:* Heartbeat is 60 or less. (This may occur in athletes as a *normal* phenomenon.) If it occurs with digitalization, it is a symptom of heart block (an abnormal situation).

Atrial and ventricular fibrillation are discussed later in this section.

Atrioventricular Heart Block

Heart block is not a disease in itself but is associated with many types of heart disease, especially disease of the coronary arteries and rheumatic heart disease. In atrioventricular (AV) heart block, the contractions of the heart are weakened and do not have enough force to send blood from the atria into the ventricles. The pulse rate may be as low as 30 bpm.

The Electronic Pacemaker. An electronic pacemaker may be used to provide external stimulus to the heart. The electronic pacemaker stimulates heart contractions by means of wires connected to electrodes; the electrodes are inserted into the heart (Fig. 74-4). Patients who experience frequent difficulty with heart contractions may have a permanent pacemaker. A portable pacemaker about the size of a small transistor radio is also available and used in the clinical setting. If a permanent pacemaker is indicated, the physician surgically implants the pacemaker pack underneath the patient's skin, usually in the pectoral or abdominal area.

For some patients the pacemaker can be discontinued gradually, depending on the heart rhythm. Other patients cannot live without it. A battery replacement is required every 5 to 10 years.

The critical observation period is 3 days after insertion of the pacemaker. Nursing skills care following implantation of a pacemaker include:

◆ Carry out routine postoperative care.
◆ Check all electrical equipment in the room for grounding.
◆ Carefully assess the pulse, including cardiac rhythm and rate. The heart rate should correspond to the setting on the pacemaker. Any deviation must be reported at once.
◆ Assess for neck vein distention or muffled heart sounds (cardiac tamponade), serious signs that should be reported at once.

Nursing Alert

Use of rubber (latex) gloves is recommended when handling pacemaker terminals or generators. *(Rationale: Care is necessary to prevent an electrical shock, which could upset the heart rate or stop the pacer.)*

◆ Use sterile technique and keep the incision site clean to prevent infection.
◆ Provide passive or active range-of-motion and incentive spirometer treatments, to prevent complications.
◆ Reassure the patient. Many find it difficult to adjust to dependence on a machine.

Nursing Alert

If the patient with a pacemaker notices any symptoms of dizziness or lightheadedness, he or she should be instructed to move at least 6 feet away from the source of any electrical interference.

A patient with a pacemaker should wear a Medic-Alert tag. The patient should be taught how to count the pulse, and any deviation should be reported at once.

Telecommunications or *teletransmission* of the ECG is now possible for the patient with a pacemaker. At a prescribed time and frequency, the person with a pacemaker can use a special modem to transmit the heart rate, rhythm, and battery life to a central location, usually the hospital, which then transforms the patient's heart rate and rhythm onto ECG paper for interpretation and follow-up.

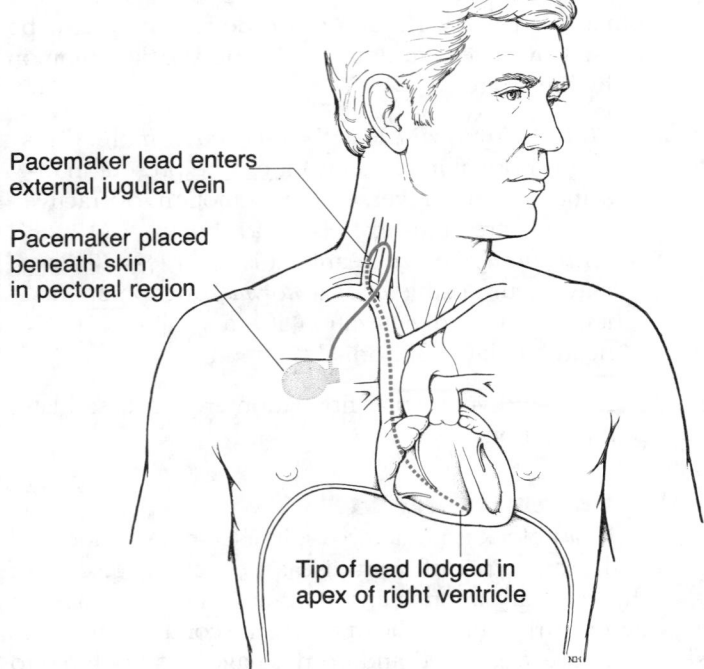

Pacemaker lead enters external jugular vein

Pacemaker placed beneath skin in pectoral region

Tip of lead lodged in apex of right ventricle

Figure 74-4. Pacemaker therapy. The pacemaker delivers an electrical impulse to the heart at specified intervals, causing the heart to beat.

Fibrillation

A disorganized twitching of atrial muscles is known as *atrial fibrillation*. It is sometimes seen in patients with atherosclerosis and rheumatic heart disease. The pulse is irregular because the coordination between the atrium and ventricle is interrupted. The treatment depends on the cause, but unless it is life-threatening, the physician usually prescribes digitalis preparations.

Ventricular fibrillation is a twitching of the heart in which the rhythm is totally disorganized and blood does not circulate. This is the most dangerous type of fibrillation. Ventricular fibrillation is an emergency situation and is fatal if not treated because it leads to cardiac arrest. The treatment is electrical *defibrillation*, which is done by a physician or a trained CCU nurse. In defibrillation, a high-voltage electric current is passed through the patient's body in an attempt to shock the heart back into a regular beat (Fig. 74-5).

Nursing Alert

The nurse and everyone else present must be very careful not to touch the patient or the bed while electrical defibrillation is being done or they too will receive the shock and may be injured.

External cardiac compression and cardiopulmonary resuscitation may be needed until the code team arrives to perform electrical defibrillation (see Chapter 32).

Conditions Affecting the Heart's Pumping Function

Congestive Heart Failure

Congestive heart failure, also known as *cardiac decompensation, cardiac insufficiency*, and *cardiac incompetence*, means that the heart is failing and unable to do its work; it has lost its pumping efficiency. Congestive heart failure is a syndrome (a group of symptoms) that affects individuals in different ways and to different degrees. The heart will try to keep up with demands made on it; treatment will help the heart make a satisfactory adjustment. Abnormal conditions in the heart may make continued treatment necessary or signs of heart failure will appear again.

When the heart is failing we say it is *decompensated*. After treatment, when it is able to carry its normal load, we say that the heart is *compensated*.

Congestive heart failure is the result of strain on the heart, which may be caused by heart disease, blood vessel disease, hypertension, renal insufficiency, congenital defects, or other diseases, such as hyperthyroidism, which speeds up heart action, or rheumatic fever, which damages heart valves. Older people are subject to heart failure because of arteriosclerosis.

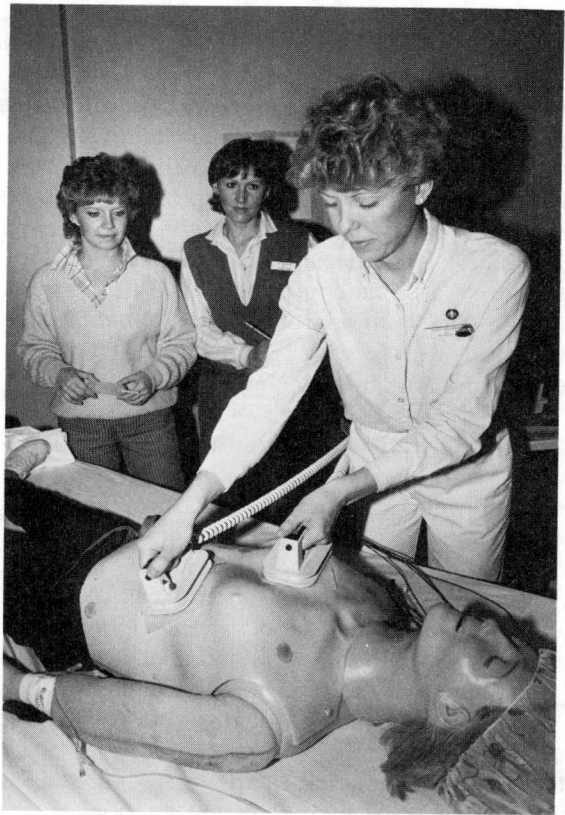

Figure 74-5. Nursing students observe as their instructor demonstrates the paddle placement for *electrical defibrillation*. An electrical current is passed through the heart in an attempt to reestablish an effective heartbeat. It is important that all personnel stand clear of the bed, to avoid receiving a shock themselves. (Photo © Bistram Photography; courtesy of Unity Medical Center, Fridley, Minn.)

Signs and Symptoms. Failure of the right ventricle to pump results in congestion in the systemic circulation. The main cause of right heart failure is left heart failure. The first signs of a failing heart that the patient may notice are excessive fatigue and dyspnea; the person may have to rest after walking halfway up the stairs or may need two pillows at night to breathe comfortably. Many people develop a persistent cough, which indicates the start of *pulmonary edema*. The ankles may swell during the day, and although this swelling disappears overnight, it recurs as soon as the person is on the feet again (*dependent edema*). Sudden weight gain may be caused by an accumulation of fluid in the tissues. Some parts of the body, especially feet and ankles, may become swollen; pressing on a swollen part leaves an indentation that lasts for a time (pitting edema). Other symptoms include numbness or tingling in the fingers, albuminuria, cyanosis, engorgement and visible pulsation of neck veins, and engorgement of the liver, with or without jaundice. (The heart attempts to compensate by *dilation, hypertrophy, and tachycar-*

dia.) If a patient has failure of one side of the heart, he or she will eventually have failure on the other side, unless successfully treated.

Pulmonary edema is the most serious symptom and occurs as a result of left-sided heart failure. When the left heart does not effectively pump, the pulmonary circuit becomes congested. The symptoms of pulmonary edema include cough, moist rales (gurgling or crackling lung sounds), dyspnea, and heart palpitations. The patient sounds asthmatic and may have blood-streaked sputum. Acute pulmonary edema is a *medical emergency* and is treated with IV morphine, oxygen under pressure, and a high-Fowler's position.

Diagnostic Tests. The usual tests for detecting heart disease are performed, such as *electrocardiography*, x-ray examination, echocardiography, and, in some cases, cardiac catheterization. Circulation time and arterial and venous blood pressure are measured also. Urine output is diminished (oliguria), the specific gravity is elevated, and albumin (albuminuria), blood (hemoglobinuria), and casts are found in the urine. Blood chemistry shows nitrogen retention by elevated blood urea nitrogen (BUN), uric acid, and creatinine concentrations.

Hemodynamic Monitoring. Heart pressures are increased and will need to be hemodynamically monitored. The use of the Swan-Ganz catheter to measure internal pressures is called *hemodynamic monitoring*. Placement of the catheter is an invasive procedure and is not without risk. It is able to measure the movement and pressures of blood in the heart and its blood vessels.

Medical Treatment. Treatment and nursing care are aimed at easing the load on the heart. Rest and sedation, if needed, are important. Cardiotonic glycosides (such as digoxin) are often used to slow the heart rate, increase the force of systole, and decrease heart size. *Digitalis* is a cardiotonic glycoside that is given to slow the heart rate, strengthen the heartbeat, and regulate heart rate. If these goals are accomplished, systemic circulation will be improved, and this will increase urine output and reduce dyspnea and edema. Diuretics help the body rid itself of excess fluid and salts. Salt (sodium) in the diet is restricted, and fluids may be restricted to about 1,800 mL/d.

Nursing Considerations. The nurse measures intake and output and the patient's weight daily to determine the extent of edema. Oxygen is given if the blood is not getting enough from the lungs. High Fowler's position usually aids breathing.

Use massage and a foam rubber pad or sheepskin for the buttocks because the patient will be sitting up much of the time. This person is susceptible to skin breakdown because of lack of movement and poor circulation. A footboard may be used to prevent footdrop.

A CPM machine to provide leg movement and promote circulation may be used.

Nursing skill guidelines for using digitalis are:

◆ The amount of digitalis or its derivatives (eg, digoxin) administered is larger at first (*loading dose*) than it will be later.

◆ The dosage is gradually decreased, until the amount needed to stabilize the heartbeat (*maintenance dose*) is found. If the amount is too large, the patient will have undesirable side effects. When the heart rate is slowed sufficiently, the patient is said to be *digitalized*.

◆ Before administering digitalis preparations, the nurse should take the apical pulse for 1 full minute. Do not give the medication if the pulse is below 60 (70 for a child), and report this immediately. (*Rationale: The low pulse may indicate overdigitalization.*)

◆ Nursing care includes accurate measurement and documentation of intake and output; close observation of the patient's color, noting the presence of dyspnea or edema; and accurate daily weighings. (*Rationale: Any change in these signs might indicate overdigitalization or a worsening of the underlying disorder.*)

◆ Side effects and adverse reactions of digitalization include gastrointestinal symptoms, such as nausea and vomiting; headache; and blurred vision, with a yellow appearance to everything. Bradycardia also occurs when the digitalis slows the heart too much. This is the reason the apical pulse is counted before each dose of any cardiotonic drug. In some facilities, all digitalis preparations are checked by two nurses before the drug is given to the patient.

◆ If the patient is discharged from the hospital and prescribed a digitalis preparation, patient teaching for discharge should include how to count pulse rate, symptoms of digitalis toxicity, and the significance of notifying the physician of any changes or symptoms. Document patient teaching.

Nursing Alert

◆ When giving digitalis preparations, the nurse must be aware of the different names. Be careful not to confuse *digitalis, digitoxin,* and *digoxin. Digoxin* is fast acting and more rapidly eliminated than digitoxin. The dosages of these different preparations vary considerably.

◆ When setting up a digitalis derivative, pour it into a separate medicine cup and keep it in its sealed package. It is then identified as the digitalis preparation. (*Rationale: By setting it up in this manner, if you need to withhold it, you will know for certain which medication is the digitalis.*)

Infectious and Inflammatory Heart Disorders

Chronic Rheumatic Heart Disease

Although young adults may contract rheumatic fever, it usually is seen in children between the ages of 5 and 15 years. (Acute rheumatic fever is discussed in Chapter 65.) Fewer than 10% of persons with rheumatic fever develop rheumatic heart disease.

The aftermath of childhood rheumatic fever may be malfunctioning of heart valves. This chronic condition usually does not show up until about age 40. Symptoms include **myocarditis** (inflammation of the muscular walls of the heart), **endocarditis** (inflammation of the inner lining of the heart, usually involving the valves), or **pancarditis** (inflammation of the entire heart).

The first signs to be noticed are difficulty in breathing, a cough, and sometimes cyanosis and expectoration of blood. If the condition grows worse, the patient's feet and ankles swell, the liver enlarges, and the abdominal cavity fills with fluid—signs of heart failure. The systolic blood pressure may fall.

The most common problem in chronic rheumatic heart disease is a narrowing of the mitral valve. This is called *mitral stenosis.* Blood collects in the chambers of the heart and enlarges them, causing congestion in the lungs (pulmonary edema). The left side of the heart is the first to be affected. The condition progresses to the right side and leads to heart failure.

The surgical insertion of a valve may be indicated. The physician determines the particular valve design that best fits the patient's clinical need.

Prevention of Recurrence of Rheumatic Fever. The best protective measures for a person who has had rheumatic fever are to avoid exposure, colds, and streptococcal infections; keep up resistance; get adequate sleep; and eat a balanced diet. Complications may result from a tooth extraction, oral surgery, or major surgery. Some persons take a daily maintenance dose of penicillin G as a prophylactic measure. It is important to prevent strep infections or recurrence of rheumatic fever because each time the person has rheumatic fever, cardiac complications become more likely.

Bacterial Endocarditis

The membrane that lines the chambers and valves of the heart is called the endocardium. Infection of this membrane causes a condition known as *endocarditis.* *Subacute bacterial endocarditis* (SBE) is a serious disease that was once nearly always fatal. Although antibiotics have changed this gloomy picture, bacterial endocarditis is still a health problem. However, modern treatment helps control it and keep it from disabling the patient.

People with damaged heart valves, especially those who have had rheumatic fever or who have congenital heart defects, are more susceptible to infection. The extraction of an infected tooth, childbirth, an upper respiratory infection, or "mainlining" street drugs may release disease organisms into the bloodstream that then attack damaged heart valves. A streptococcal organism is a frequent offender.

One of the first signs of bacterial endocarditis is a low-grade fever, which gradually increases. The patient has chills and perspires, loses appetite, and loses weight. The person's face has a brownish tinge, and tiny reddish purple spots (*petechiae*) appear on the skin and mucous membranes. Usually, the patient is anemic. As the disease progresses, signs of congestive heart failure appear.

The course of bacterial endocarditis is rapid, and the disease can be fatal if untreated. However, 90% of patients treated can be cured without ill effects. Blood cultures (culture and sensitivity, C&S) can usually identify the specific causative organism. Then large doses of antibiotics to which the causative organism is sensitive are given.

Nursing Considerations. The nurse makes the person as comfortable as possible and conserves the person's energy. The rate and quality of pulse should be noted frequently. *(Rationale: A change could indicate complications.)* Observe closely for fluctuation in body temperature and for any symptoms of complications. *(Rationale: Hematuria, pain, or impaired circulation in an extremity might be the result of a blood clot originating in the diseased valve.)*

Pericarditis

Pericarditis is an inflammation of the sac surrounding the heart. Its causes may be nonspecific, infectious, allergic, malignant, or traumatic in origin. It is characterized by pain in the precordial area (over the heart and lower thorax), which is aggravated by breathing and twisting movements. A *friction rub* is a sign associated with pericarditis and is audible on auscultation. Pericardial infections are treated with antibiotics in most cases.

Coronary Artery Disease

People over age 50 are the most common victims of coronary artery disease (ischemic heart disease), although younger people are not immune. During the early middle years, more men than women are affected; after menopause, women are affected as often as men. There seems to be a familial tendency toward the disease. However, it is believed that coronary artery disease develops over many years, so precautions should begin early in life. More attention is given now to discovering the disease early, before an attack has occurred and before atherosclerosis has severely damaged the heart.

Angina Pectoris

Angina pectoris, usually referred to as angina, literally translated means "pain in the chest." Angina occurs suddenly when extra exertion calls for an increase in blood supply to the heart that the narrowed arteries are unable to provide. Consequently, the heart muscle suffers.

In angina there is a temporary loss of oxygen to the heart (*anoxia*). If this loss of oxygen supply continues, the result is **ischemia** (prolonged deficiency of oxygenated blood) and **necrosis** (death of heart tissue), or MI (myocardial infarction).

There are several types of angina pain. *Intractable angina* does not respond to therapy and often is so persistent that the patient cannot work. *Unstable angina* is that type of pain that increases and decreases in frequency, duration, and intensity. *Nocturnal* angina occurs at night; *decubitus* angina is felt when lying down and relieved by sitting up.

When the underlying disease is coronary atherosclerosis, the prognosis may be more encouraging than when other factors are involved. The earlier the age of onset, the poorer the prognosis.

Signs and Symptoms. The pain is more severe over the heart, although it may spread to the shoulders and arms, neck, or jaw. The patient often describes the

---

Keys to Patient/Family Teaching
Prevention of Angina Pectoris

Patient/family teaching regarding prevention of angina pectoris includes:

♦ Proper use of medications:
   Take medication at same time every day.
   Do not stop or change dosage without physician's approval.
   Nitroglycerin deteriorates when exposed to sunlight or moisture.
   Nitroglycerin should be kept in the original container.
   A fresh supply of nitroglycerin should be purchased every 3 months.
   Check with physician before taking nonprescription medications. They may cause harmful side effects with the cardiac medication.
♦ Adjustments to life-style may need to be made: what can or cannot be done. Try to determine what brings on the attacks, so those activities can be curtailed.
♦ Smoking must be stopped.

Post-MI Rehabilitation Plan

♦ In hospital, gradual increase in activity as ordered by physician
♦ Exercise tolerance test and exercise progression
♦ Graded exercise program—monitor tolerance by checking blood prssure, pulse
♦ Emotional support and counseling
   ♦ Stress management
   ♦ Sexual counseling
   ♦ Life-style changes, if any
♦ Risk factor management
   ♦ Dietary: low-fat diet for hyperlipidemia, weight control
   ♦ Smoking cessation
   ♦ Hypertension control
♦ Medication as ordered

---

sensation as tightening, viselike, or choking. Indigestion is often the first complaint. The pain is more likely to be felt in the left arm because this is the direction of aortic branching, but it may be felt in either arm. The patient may be pale, may feel faint, or may be dyspneic. The pain often stops in less than 5 minutes, but it is intense while it lasts. It is a warning that the heart is not getting enough blood and oxygen. People who ignore this warning are risking serious illness or sudden death if they do not immediately seek a physician's care. The patient may have recurrent attacks of angina, but treatment lessens the danger of a fatal attack.

Diagnostic Tests. Diagnosis is made on the basis of ECG, specific blood tests (especially enzymes), x-ray examinations, the patient's medical history, and specific symptoms. If nitroglycerin relieves the attack, it is considered angina. Angina is often precipitated by exercise or exertion, eating, emotions, or exposure. In a diabetic person, the pain may not be felt because of peripheral neuropathy.

Nursing Alert

If the pain of angina lasts for more than 15 minutes, it is considered to be an MI until proved otherwise. Repeated attacks of angina can be a sign of or can contribute to MI.

Medical and Surgical Treatment. The patient who is under a physician's care knows what to do for angina. The patient usually carries nitroglycerin tablets and has been instructed to dissolve a tablet under the tongue as soon as an attack begins. It brings quick relief by dilating the coronary arteries; patients can use this drug safely for many years with no ill effects. Topical nitroglycerin ointment or nitroglycerin-impregnated pads (*transdermal*) are widely used to protect against anginal pain and promote its relief. Amyl nitrite is also effective in relieving angina. It comes in ampules that are broken in a handkerchief and inhaled. Medication used in angina pectoris and MI are listed in Table 74-1.

If the patient's anginal attacks cannot be controlled by medication or PTCA, coronary artery bypass surgery may be considered as a lifesaving measure.

Nursing Considerations. The nurse can help the patient by teaching about angina pectoris and how to prevent further attacks. Patients who know that certain things bring on an attack can learn to be more careful. If anginal pain becomes more frequent and or more severe, the patient may have to curtail certain activities. The best approach for the patient is to follow rules for treatment, learn what can and cannot be done, and live accordingly.

It is important for the patient to quit smoking because nicotine constricts coronary arteries, increases blood pressure, and increases pulse rates. Some teaching points are listed in the accompanying box.

Myocardial Infarction

An MI, also known as *heart attack, coronary thrombosis,* or coronary occlusion, is the sudden blocking of one or more coronary arteries. If it involves an extensive area, the person will die. If it is less extensive, there will still be necrosis of heart tissue and subsequent scarring, but other vessels can take over for the injured area (*collateral circulation*).

The prognosis after any MI is guarded for 3 to 4 weeks, although the first 2 weeks are the most life-threatening time.

The major complications of MI are life-threatening arrhythmias and cardiac standstill. Abnormal heart rates and rhythms in the patient with a recent MI often mean the left ventricle is not pumping adequately. As a result, congestive heart failure may occur.

Signs and Symptoms. The attack begins suddenly, with sharp, severe pain in the chest, sometimes radiating to the left arm and shoulder. It is like angina but sometimes lasts longer and is more severe; exertion may have nothing to do with the onset. Unlike angina, it is not relieved with rest, and nitroglycerin or amyl nitrite does not help. Because it may imitate indigestion or a gallbladder attack with abdominal pain, definite diagnosis often is difficult.

Common symptoms of MI include restlessness; confusion; a sense of impending death; skin that is ashen, cold, and clammy; dyspnea; cyanosis; rapid, thready, and irregular pulse; drop in blood pressure; and drop in body temperature. Nausea and vomiting may be present, and the person is often in shock. A silent coronary (one that shows no symptoms) is common, especially among diabetic patients, and may result in damage to heart muscle. *Denial* occurs in almost all cases; the patient cannot believe that he or she is having an MI.

Diagnostic Tests. Tests help determine the nature of the attack. An ECG will be done and several diagnostic blood tests will be made to assess the duration and severity of the infarction. The sedimentation rate of the red blood cells almost always is higher after MI, as is the AST level. Cardiac isoenzyme levels will also be elevated after MI. These include fractional CPK (creatine phosphokinase) enzymes, especially CPK-MB; and LDH (lactic dehydrogenase) or HBD (hydroxybutyric dehydrogenase). Serum myoglobin is tested to estimate

---

Table 74-1. Common Drug Therapy: Ischemic Heart Disorders

Type	*Reason for Use*
Anticoagulant: warfarin sodium (Coumadin)	Prevents clot formation and the extension of further clots
Narcotic: morphine sulfate	Prevents pain. If pain is controlled, patient is able to relax, thus aiding the treatment process.
Nitrates and Nitrites: nitroglycerine preparation; sublingual, topical, or IV (Follow protocol of health agency when administering nitroglycerin, which may include blood pressure measurement at specific times.)	Vasodilator to control angina (can cause hypotension and shock)
Antiarrhythmics: lidocaine (Xylocaine)	Control irregular rhythm, ie, premature ventricular contractions
Diuretics: furosemide (Lasix)	Control fluid retention

the amount of heart muscle damage and must be done within a very specific time frame after the MI in order to be accurate.

Medical Treatment. Patients should be medicated promptly when complaining of chest pains to prevent further extension of damage to heart muscle. Pain indicates *anoxia*—lack of oxygen. Drugs dilate blood vessels to allow more oxygen to reach heart muscle. Pain medication is often given at regular times at first rather than PRN. Medications used for MI and angina are summarized in Table 74-1.

Oxygen by cannula or mask may be administered to relieve pain and assist the patient to breathe. A low-cholesterol and restricted-sodium diet is usually ordered. Caffeine-containing beverages usually are not allowed. The patient is informed of the hazards of smoking and is encouraged to quit as soon as possible.

Nursing Considerations. *Immediately Post-MI.* Continuous nursing care in the CCU is vital until the patient's condition stabilizes. The patient is usually on a cardiac monitor, which continuously records ECG, blood pressure, pulse, and pulse pressure. Hemodynamic monitoring is used. Alarms are set to alert the staff if one reading deviates from preset limits. Nursing care includes:

- Frequent vital signs
- Electronic cardiac monitoring
- Intake and output *(Rationale: Lowered urine output may be a sign of fluid retention or kidney disorders secondary to MI.)*
- Careful observation for restlessness, dyspnea, or chest pain *(Rationale: These are signs that tissue damage is worsening.)*
- Assessment for signs of congestive heart failure (dyspnea, frequent cough, chest rales, edema)
- Assessment of skin color *(Rationale: Pallor or cyanosis may indicate anoxia because of impaired circulation.)*
- Medications to promote pain relief and improve functioning of the heart. Medications may be given on a scheduled basis, rather than PRN to *prevent* pain.
- Emotional support and stress reduction
- Monitoring diet, intravenous fluids, or total parenteral nutrition.
- Planned daily exercise program according to the cardiac rehabilitation program, as shown in the accompanying box
- If the patient is taking antihypertensive drugs, teaching should emphasize the necessity of taking prescribed medications despite the fact that the patient feels well. Be sure to discuss potential side effects when teaching.

During Recovery from MI. Rest comes first (up to approximately 72 hours after an MI). The injured heart must have time to repair. The damaged spot in the heart takes from 3 to 6 weeks to heal. Tough scar tissue forms after about 8 weeks. The Nursing Care Plan shows the development of two nursing diagnoses and interventions in an MI patient. Nursing care includes:

- Patients are allowed to use a commode at the bedside for a bowel movement. The commode is preferable to a bedpan. *(Rationale: The patient is more likely to strain on the bedpan.)* Stool softeners are usually prescribed. *(Rationale: Stool softeners prevent straining with a bowel movement.)*
- Aid the patient in doing isometric (muscle-setting) exercises. *(Rationale: They provide muscle exercise without overtiring the patient.)*
- Use thromboembolic (antiembolism) stockings, as prescribed by physician. *(Rationale: Proper use of stockings prevents thrombophlebitis.)*
- Place all items convenient to the patient's reach. Be sure the call light is available. *(Rationale: The patient must not stretch or strain for necessary items.)*
- Perform physical care (ie, baths and backrubs). *(Rationale: You want the patient to rest and be comfortable.)*
- After giving the bath and before making the bed, allow the patient to rest for a while. Positioning the patient in semi-Fowler's position is often preferred. *(Rationale: This helps assist in breathing and relieve pain.)*

Patients who are admitted with a diagnosis of "Rule out MI" will be placed on complete bed rest until it is determined whether they have had a heart attack. Patients who do not have pain may feed themselves, even in the acute phase. Activities are planned to promote maximum relaxation and to reduce stress.

The patient who has had an MI can live a normal life and can often go back to previous employment. The goal is not to change the patient's life-style but to make modifications. The patient and the family should be instructed before discharge how to follow a pattern of healthy living and how to recognize emotional and physical stress. The patient and family are taught signs and symptoms that require immediate medical help (see accompanying box). This teaching must be carefully and completely documented.

Blood Vessel Disorders

Inflammatory Disorders and Complications

Thrombophlebitis

Thrombophlebitis is the inflammation of the wall of a vein, in which one or more clots form. *Venous thrombosis* defines the condition wherein a blood clot

Michael Fleck is a 37-year-old single white male accountant who presented in the emergency department with crushing chest pain that was promptly diagnosed as myocardial infarction (anterior wall of the left ventricle). He was admitted to the coronary care unit, where care was directed to resolution of the acute attack and prompt relief of pain, prevention of complications and further attacks, and rehabilitation and education. Two of the nursing diagnoses developed for Mr. Fleck follow.

Nursing Diagnosis: *Alteration in Tissue Perfusion: Cardiopulmonary Changes Related to Heart Tissue Damage and Decreased Cardiac Output as Evidenced by Unstable BP; Frequent PVCs (Abnormal Heart Rhythm—more than 5/min); and Cool, Pale Skin*

Goal: By 7/5 patient will demonstrate stable hemodynamics: (1) BP within the range of 110–130/64–74; (2) rare to absent premature ventricular contractions (PVCs); (3) hourly urine output greater than 30 mL/h.

Nursing Actions (assess/do/teach)	Rationale	Evaluative Statement
1. Monitor BP and P (at least every 1–2 h until stable), VS, I & O daily weights, (for signs of fluid overload), lab values; record and interpret rhythm strips q4h (done by RN); monitor postural BP and HR (heart rate) once patient is out of bed (OOB)	To provide a basis for treatment	7/5 Goal met; patient's BP within his range of normal; less than 1 PVC/min; urine output, 50–60 mL/h
2. Administer prescribed medications, documenting patient response	Need for medication can change literally from minute to minute	
3. Increase activity as ordered, using respiratory assessments as guides	To increase demands on heart gradually	
4. Plan interactions so patient has undisturbed periods of rest (1–2 h intervals); keep environmental stress to a minimum	To facilitate healing	7/9 Social Service referral to evaluate and help plan financial support for future

(continued)

(*thrombus*) has formed inside a blood vessel. The blood clot forms in response to the initial inflammation (see Fig. 74-3). **Phlebitis** is the inflammation of a blood vessel without clot formation.

Thrombophlebitis and thrombosis may be caused by excessive coagulability of the blood in some situations (eg, following trauma, childbirth, MI, or cancer surgery). Obesity is also a predisposing factor. Women who use birth control pills are believed to have a higher than average chance of developing blood clots.

Venous thrombosis may be caused by pressure or by prolonged inactivity, such as might occur after surgery or in any illness in which the patient remains in one position for long periods of time. The legs are most likely to be affected. The venous blood does not move fast enough to prevent clotting; this is known as *venous stasis* or venous standstill. This is a major reason for early ambulation in illness. Any condition that requires prolonged immobilization is now commonly being treated by physicians with low-dose prophylactic anticoagulation. (Some physicians recommend that adults take 1 or 2 aspirins daily, as a preventive measure.)

Most thrombi form in veins because venous blood moves more slowly than arterial blood. However, a thrombus may form in an artery (*arterial thrombosis*); this is usually related to arteriosclerosis, but may be due to infection or injury, or may be a consequence of diabetes mellitus.

Nursing Diagnosis: *Anxiety Concerning the Future Related to Lack of Knowledge as Evidenced by Statements Such as "I Suppose this Means I'll Never be Able to do all the Things I Really Enjoy any More," or "I Pulled Through This One but the Next One Just Might get me."*

Goal 1: Prior to discharge patient accurately describes (1) the nature of coronary artery disease (CAD) and (2) a rehabilitation program designed to prevent complications or recurrence

Goal 2: Before discharge patient reports feeling less anxious about the future and more in control of his life

Nursing Actions (assess/do/teach)	Rationale	Evaluative Statement
1. Assess what the patient knows about coronary artery disease and correct any misconceptions; be especially sensitive to unfounded fears.	Allows you to tailor your teaching to the unique needs of *this* patient	7/9 Goal 1 met; patient able to verbalize the process of CAD and has identified life-style factors he can improve (diet, exercise, stress management) to prevent recurrence
2. Select an optimal teaching moment (involve significant others if possible) and instruct the patient about the nature of CAD and specific life-style changes that will decrease the likelihood of complications and recurrence of an MI; use questioning to ensure that the patient understands the basic reasons for life-style changes and the benefits to be obtained; provide written materials if available	Knowledge is a powerful antidote to anxiety and enables the patient to participate maximally in the plan of care and regain a sense of control.	7/9 Goal 2 met—but patient says life will never be the same for him since he's had this "brush with death"; states he is determined to use this to motivate more healthy living

Special Considerations in Aging

Elderly patients or those with heart disease or varicose veins are most susceptible to thrombophlebitis. Prolonged sitting may also be a contributing factor. Older people should be informed that it is important to change position frequently. A rocking chair gives some exercise for people who find walking difficult.

Keys to Patient/Family Teaching:
When to Seek Medical Help Post-MI

Patient/family teaching regarding medical help after an MI includes:

- Chest pain unrelieved with sublingual nitroglycerin
- Severe shortness of breath
- Faintness or dizziness
- Unusual fatigue or weakness
- Irregular or rapid heartbeat

Signs and Symptoms. The symptoms of thrombophlebitis include pain in the affected leg, redness and swelling, fever, and the symptoms that usually go with fever, such as fatigue and loss of appetite. *Homans' sign* is a specific test for thrombophlebitis. In this test, calf pain is greatly increased when the foot is dorsiflexed.

Medical Treatment. Opinions differ about the treatment of thrombophlebitis. In superficial thrombosis, most physicians want the leg elevated, with heat applied, and complete rest. Occasionally, nonstrenuous

The Relationship Between Smoking and Vascular Disease

Smoking is contraindicated in all vascular disease because nicotine causes spasm of arteries. The connection between arteriospasm and smoking is so definite that many physicians tell patients that treatment will not be helpful unless smoking is stopped.

exercises are recommended to promote circulation. Anticoagulant drugs are usually given.

Nursing Considerations. All patients in bed should be provided with an exercise plan as early as possible. The simplest exercise that the patient can do is to periodically contract and relax the leg muscles and move the toes and feet. (Muscle-setting and isometric exercises are sometimes prescribed.) The bedcovers must be loose enough to permit free movement. The patient can also push the feet against the footboard (isometric). Most patients who must maintain bed rest wear antiembolitic stockings and may have the foot of the bed elevated to help prevent venous stasis. Passive range-of-motion exercises (PROM) or the continuous passive motion (CPM) machine should be used if the patient is unable to exercise actively.

◆ If exercise is ordered, wriggling the toes, bending the knees, and turning the ankle back and forth are easily done by the patient.
◆ In deep thrombophlebitis, the affected part should be immobilized.
◆ Prevent the patient from coughing vigorously or breathing deeply (because of the danger of embolism; see next section). Try to keep the patient from straining when defecating; stool softeners are given for this purpose.
◆ Warm, moist packs (low temperature) may be used. *(Rationale: Gently stimulate circulation and dissolution of the clot, but avoid overdilation of blood vessels.)*
◆ Enforce bed rest. *(Rationale: Moving could cause embolism.)* Elevate the affected leg on soft pillows. *(Rationale: This promotes comfort and enhances venous return from the leg.)*

Nursing Alert

Never massage or rub a patient's leg. *(Rationale: Rubbing could dislodge a clot and cause embolism.)*

If the patient is on anticoagulant therapy, follow the general nursing precautions and procedures. The patient is usually given intravenous heparin during the acute phase and warfarin (Coumadin) as a prophylactic measure later. Routine prothrombin times (or other clotting time tests) are done. If the patient is to wear an antiembolitic stocking or an elastic bandage, it should be applied with even pressure from the toes up to the thigh. *(Rationale: Uneven pressure could cause another clot to form.)* Elastic stockings or bandages are removed at least once per shift for a short time. The extremity is gently cleansed, and lotion may be applied. The ex-

tremity should be carefully inspected at that time for any skin changes. (See Chapter 48.)

The patient may have to stay in bed for several weeks. If so, help him or her to progress *gradually* from complete bed rest to ambulation, according to physician's orders. Constantly observe the patient for any signs of embolism.

Embolism

Embolism is a severe complication of thrombophlebitis. An **embolus** is a blood clot that may be carried in the circulation to some vital organ and can lodge in a blood vessel.

Pulmonary Embolism. If the obstruction occurs in a large pulmonary blood vessel (the most common site for embolism from the legs), it may cause sudden death. The obstruction of a small vessel may not be so damaging. The patient who has a pulmonary embolism is likely to complain of a sudden, sharp chest pain, breathing difficulty, violent cough, and bloody sputum. The patient will become cyanotic, and symptoms of shock develop rapidly. The immediate treatment is to administer oxygen and to provide for complete bed rest in a high semi-Fowler's position. Continuous intravenous anticoagulation therapy with heparin is now a widely used treatment. Pain relief with the use of intravenous morphine sulfate is also indicated.

Coronary Embolism. If the embolus lodges in a blood vessel within the heart, the heart tissue distal to the blockage will die (necrose). Depending on how large the vessel is, the necrosed area may cause instant death. Symptoms of a lesser blockage are sudden severe chest pains and other characteristic symptoms of MI. This situation is covered earlier in this chapter.

Cerebral Embolism. In cerebral embolism, the clot blocks one of the blood vessels in the brain. The amount of damage done depends on the size and location of the vessel. This situation is commonly known as a CVA, or stroke, and is covered later in this chapter.

Peripheral Embolism and Thrombosis in a Limb. The embolism can lodge in a blood vessel leading to an extremity. In this case, the first symptom is severe pain at the site of the blockage. The extremity becomes pale and cold to the touch; pulses distal to the blockage are lost. The limb becomes white and cold. Other symptoms of shock are seen if the blood vessel is large. Amputation below the level of the blockage may be necessary if a clot in a large vessel cannot be dissolved quickly or removed surgically because without circulation, gangrene will occur.

Surgical Treatment. Certain surgical procedures may be carried out to combat the danger of embolism. Emboli can be removed from pulmonary arteries, although this is a rare procedure. If the thrombus is located in the femoral vein, the blood vessel is ligated (tied off) at that point in a procedure called a femoral ligation. Sometimes, the vena cava is made smaller (vena cava ligation) or a filter inserted in the vein to prevent clots from moving to the heart.

Peripheral Vascular Disorders

Most peripheral vascular disorders are evidenced at one time or another by the following symptoms:

◆ *Intermittent claudication:* There is no pain when the person is at rest, but exercise, particularly walking, causes excruciating pain, which disappears when the limb is again at rest. Smoking, vascular spasm, and atherosclerosis aggravate this condition. Intermittent claudication caused by venous stasis is called *venous claudication.*

◆ *Tingling and numbness:* The extremity or part of the extremity becomes numb, or the person feels a persistent tingling sensation. It is caused by poor circulation.

◆ *Coldness and difference in size:* The extremities may feel cold to the touch or the patient may sense that the hands and feet are cold. One leg may be markedly different in size, color, and temperature from the other.

◆ *Lack of new tissue growth:* The skin may become paper thin, shiny, and easily subject to breakdown. Blood vessels can be seen.

Nursing Considerations. Peripheral vascular diseases may be prevented or arrested by simple changes in everyday life. The nurse can help by teaching the patient. See Patient Teaching: Prevention of Cardiovascular Disorders in the Nursing Process section of the chapter. General nursing care in peripheral vascular disease is outlined in the accompanying box.

Buerger's Disease

Buerger's disease (*thromboangiitis obliterans*) is the result of inflammation that causes obstruction of the veins and the arteries of the extremities, especially the legs. It is more common among men than women, and heavy smokers especially are affected. It is aggravated by chilling. It is much less common today than in the past two decades.

Usually the first sign the patient notices is cramps in the calf muscles, which are brought on by exercise and disappear when the patient rests. Other symptoms include tingling, burning, numbness, and edema, which may develop into pitting or brawny edema. There are hardened, painful areas along the course of blood vessels. When the feet and legs hang down, they take on

---

Nursing Skill Guidelines
Caring for Patients With Peripheral Vascular Disease

◆ Protect the patient's feet and legs from undue pressure of linens. (*Rationale: This prevents discomfort and skin breakdown.*)

◆ Take great care in trimming the toenails. (*Rationale: Cuts or abrasions on the feet are difficult to heal.*)

◆ Be sure to dry carefully between the toes after washing them. (*Rationale: An infection heals much more slowly when circulation is poor.*)

◆ Be very careful about application of heat. Use extra clothing rather than external heat to warm the extremities. (*Rationale: This person is easily burned.*)

◆ Report skin breakdown immediately. (*Rationale: Ambitious therapy will be needed.*)

◆ A warm bath may help increase the circulation; be sure the water is not hot. (*Rationale: Heat helps dilate blood vessels. This patient is very susceptible to burns.*) Use a bath thermometer; the maximum temperature is 100°F or 37.8°C.

◆ Do not attempt to treat corns or calluses. (*Rationale: You may accidentally cut the patient.*)

---

a mottled purplish red hue; when raised, they become abnormally pale. Ulcers then may develop that could result in gangrene. As the disease progresses, the pain continues even when the patient is resting.

Medical and Surgical Treatment. The patient must be careful to avoid anything that makes this condition worse, especially chilling of hands and feet. Tobacco in any form is dangerous because nicotine constricts blood vessels. The patient should be advised to stop smoking or using smokeless tobacco immediately.

The patient may exercise mildly if this is not painful. For this purpose, the Buerger-Allen exercises are prescribed. They consist of alternately raising, lowering, and resting the legs. Sometimes cramps occur with exercise, a condition called *intermittent claudication*. An electrically operated rocking bed (oscillating bed) may be used if the patient cannot exercise actively. Antibiotics and analgesics may be necessary for infection and pain. External heat is not used. Extra clothing may be worn instead. Fluid intake should be encouraged; usually up to 20 glasses of fluids per day are needed to stimulate circulation and kidney activity. Tight clothing should be avoided.

Sometimes a *sympathectomy* is performed, whereby the sympathetic nerves, which innervate the smooth muscles, are cut. This relieves vasospasms and increases blood flow to the lower extremities. If ulcers become infected, gangrene may develop and make an amputation necessary.

Raynaud's Phenomenon

Raynaud's phenomenon has an unknown cause but is characterized by spasmodic constriction of arteries supplying the extremities. It especially affects fingers and toes. Often only the fingers are involved. It affects women more frequently than men, especially young adults. Cold and emotional stress are the usual precipitating factors.

The symptoms of Raynaud's phenomenon are distressing. The patient's hands are blanched and cold, and they perspire and feel numb and prickly. Later they become blue—especially the fingernails—and are painful. As heat restores blood flow, the hands become red and warm. In the early stages, these symptoms disappear after an episode, and the hands seem normal again. But as the disease progresses, the cyanosis persists between attacks, and ulcers, which are slow to heal, may develop on the fingertips. The skin looks tight and shiny, and the nails become deformed. There may be gangrene of the fingertips.

The most important aspect of treatment is to avoid chilling at all times. The person must always wear warm clothing out of doors in the winter, such as wool gloves, socks, and insulated boots. A goosedown or other comforter at night provides steady warmth. Electric blankets may be dangerous because they may be too hot. Emotional upsets and tension of any kind should be avoided. Smoking is definitely contraindicated. Drugs to relieve spasm of arteries and dilate blood vessels provide considerable relief. A sympathectomy may be necessary.

Varicose Veins of the Legs

Varicose veins result from a weakening of the valves of the veins so blood pools in the legs or another dependent area. Normal veins fill from below because of valvular action. Varicose veins fill abnormally because they are not able to drain out the blood. (Hemorrhoids and esophageal varices are also varicose veins.) Predisposing factors are heredity and weakening of the vein walls resulting from prolonged standing, poor posture, repeated pregnancies, round garters, obesity, tumors, high blood pressure, and chronic diseases such as those of the liver or kidneys. Varicose veins may also occur as an aftermath of thrombophlebitis. Women are more commonly affected with varicosities of the legs than are men, especially if they have had several pregnancies.

Signs and Symptoms. The main symptom of varicose veins in the legs is the appearance of dark, tortuous superficial veins that become more prominent when the person is standing and appear as dark protrusions in the legs. These superficial veins can sometimes rupture, causing a *varicose ulcer.* Internal or deep varicose veins cause symptoms such as pain, fatigue, a feeling of heaviness, and muscle cramps. Symptoms are much more severe in hot weather and at high altitudes. A diagnostic test involves putting the patient into the Trendelenburg position to test blood drainage. If, on standing, the leg veins do not fill normally, this is a sign of varicose veins.

Medical and Surgical Treatment. Treatment includes elevating the legs for a few minutes at 2- to 3-hour intervals throughout the day. It also includes avoiding constriction, standing for long periods, or restrictive clothing. The patient should wear support stockings. These measures are all aimed at promoting venous drainage from the legs.

Most commonly in more severe cases, surgical ligation and stripping of varicose veins is done. The larger veins are surgically ligated, or tied off, and smaller ones are stripped out.

Sclerosing solutions are occasionally used in the physician's office or day surgery clinic for small varicosities. The solution is injected into the vessel; this causes an irritation and eventually a fibrosis.

Nursing Considerations. Patient teaching is vital. The patient must be taught measures that promote venous drainage. In this way, surgery might be prevented.

If surgery is done, antiembolitic stockings are applied to the leg postoperatively, and the foot of the bed is elevated to encourage return of venous blood. Analgesics may be ordered. Aspirin is often the drug of choice because of its anticoagulant action.

Early ambulation is important after this operation. Often the nurse is instructed to get the patient out of bed to walk as soon as the patient recovers from anesthesia. The patient may be alarmed at the idea of walking so soon after the operation, while the legs are stiff and sore, and will most likely need reassurance and an explanation of the need for moving about. The order is often written for the patient to walk 5 to 10 minutes out of each hour during the day and several times at night. The patient must be assisted and encouraged to keep up this regimen.

Discharge teaching for the patient after venous stripping appears in the accompanying box. The patient is instructed on how to apply antiembolitic stockings correctly. Knee-high stockings and socks with elastic tops are to be avoided. If weight reduction is suggested, the clinical dietitian probably will give instructions.

Telangiectasia (Spider Veins)

Telangiectasia is described as a group of small dilated blood vessels. It is treated by scleropathy, the injection of a weak sodium chloride solution into nonfunctioning veins. Pressure is applied at specific points and the veins stick together and are gradually absorbed. The lines almost disappear. The treatment is relatively painless.

Aneurysms

An **aneurysm** is an outpouching of a blood vessel. Although it may occur in any vessel, the most common site is the aorta. An aneurysm here or in a cerebral vessel represents an *extreme emergency*. If it ruptures, surgical intervention may be done if the aneurysm is in an operable site. However, if it is not done immediately, the person will hemorrhage and may die. If the aneurysm is discovered before it ruptures, it is treated by surgical repair or removal. Usually, a synthetic graft is substituted for the portion of the vessel affected.

Aneurysms may be congenital, may occur after trauma such as an automobile accident, or may develop as a result of the increased pressure of arteriosclerosis. Unknown cerebral aneurysm rupture is often the cause of sudden death in healthy athletes.

Cerebrovascular Accident and Transient Ischemic Attack

A sudden or gradual interruption of blood supply to a vital center in the brain is a CVA, also known as a *stroke* or a *central vascular accident.* A CVA may cause complete or partial paralysis or death. In the United States, thousands of people die every year following a CVA. Although there is much controversy over this issue, it is believed that use of birth control pills over an extended period could be a precipitating factor of CVAs in women. Postmenopausal women are more likely to have CVAs than are younger women. Both of these situations seem to be related to hormones.

Direct causes of CVAs include:

- Cerebral thrombosis: the most frequent cause of CVA, in which a blood clot blocks an artery that supplies a vital center in the brain, usually as a result of arteriosclerosis.
- Cerebral hemorrhage or aneurysm: an artery in the

brain bursts because of a severe rise in blood pressure or arteriosclerosis.
- Cerebral embolism: a blood clot breaks off from a thrombus elsewhere in the body and is carried to the brain, where it lodges in a blood vessel and shuts off blood supply to part of the brain.

There are four specific types or stages of CVA:

- Transient ischemic attack (TIA) is a sudden, short-lived attack. The person recovers within 24 hours. The TIA is often a warning that another, more serious stroke will occur later. The risk of completed stroke for this person is 25% to 35% greater than normal.
- Reversible ischemic neurologic deficit (RIND) is similar to TIA, except that the symptoms last for as long as a week. Recovery is complete or nearly so. This is also a warning that a more serious stroke is more likely in this person.
- Stroke in evolution (SIE) is a gradual worsening of symptoms of brain ischemia.
- Completed stroke (CS) occurs when symptoms of stroke are present and stabilize over a period of time. At this point, active rehabilitation can begin.

Signs and Symptoms. The symptoms of a CVA depend on the cause. In some cases of *thrombosis*, the patient has had dizzy spells or sudden loss of memory for some time before the actual CVA. No pain accompanies these symptoms, so they are often ignored. A *cerebral hemorrhage* may give warning. It causes dizziness and ringing in the ears (tinnitus), as well as a violent headache, often with nausea and vomiting. A hemorrhage may follow unusual exertion, such as shoveling snow, heavy eating, or vigorous exercise. *Embolism* usually occurs without warning, although the patient often has a history of heart or blood vessel disease.

The sudden CVA is usually more severe. The victim becomes unconscious; the face is red; breathing is noisy and becomes difficult. The pulse is slow, but full and bounding. Blood pressure is elevated, and the patient may be in a deep coma. The coma may deepen progressively until the person dies, or the person may gradually regain consciousness and eventually recover. Patients who are unresponsive for a long period of time are less likely to recover. The first few days after onset are critical. The patient who is responsive may show signs of memory loss or inconsistent behavior; he or she may be easily fatigued, may lose bowel and bladder control, or may have poor balance.

Results of Cerebrovascular Accidents

Hemiplegia. The most common result of a CVA is **hemiplegia**, which is paralysis of one side of the body. Other functions may be affected by hemiplegia such as hearing, general sensation, and circulation;

Laurine Miller is a 55-year-old African American married woman with a history of hypertension admitted to the hospital with the diagnosis of left cerebrovascular accident (CVA) secondary to thombosis. This is her sixth hospital day and her physician believes that the acute phase of the stroke is resolved and that she is now ready for more aggressive rehabilitative therapy. She has right hemiplegia and expressive (motor) aphasia. Obvious nursing priorities include her impaired mobility, potential for injury, self-care deficits, nutrition and elimination alterations, impaired adjustment, and sense of powerlessness. The following diagnoses focus on her altered thought processes, speech problem, and sensoriperceptual alterations.

Nursing Diagnosis: *Altered Thought Processes Related to Interrupted Circulation to the Brain as Evidenced by Inaccurate Interpretation of Environment and Non-Reality-Based Thinking*

Goal: At the end of the first week of rehabilitative therapy the patient is consistently oriented to person, place, and time and accurately interprets environment.

Nursing Actions (assess/do/teach)	Rationale	Evaluative Statement
1. Continually reorient the patient; offer simple explanations of where she is, why, and what is currently happening; gently correct the patient's misperception of objects, persons, events; use clocks, calendars, and familiar objects to reorient the patient; educate family members so that they can assist with reorientation instead of reinforcing the confusion.	Mental stimulation helps prevent intellectual regression and disorientation	11/2 Goal partially met; patient is oriented ×3 but continues to misinterpret reality (eg, she believes she is in the hospital to deliver a baby)

(continued)

the degree of impairment depends on the part of the brain affected.

Generally, hemiplegia progresses through three stages: 1) the flaccid stage, in which there is limpness and weakness on the affected side; 2) the spastic stage, in which muscles are contracted and tense, and movement is difficult; and 3) the recovery stage, when therapy and rehabilitation methods are most successful.

Aphasia and Dysphagia. Many patients with CVA are aphasic. **Aphasia,** a result of damage to the speech center in the brain, is a condition in which people are unable to speak. This can be frustrating and frightening because mental functioning usually is unimpaired. Nursing skills in communicating with aphasic patients are given in the Nursing Process section earlier in this chapter.

A more complicated disorder is *dysphagia*, an inability to say what one wishes to say. Many patients regain some power of speech, but others never do.

Brain Damage. The extent of brain damage resulting from a CVA determines a patient's chances for recovery; if the damage is slight, recovery will be more rapid and complete. Also, the chances of recovery are better for a younger person who suffers a CVA.

Hemianopsia (Hemianopia). *Hemianopsia* is defined as visual blindness in half of the visual field of one eye or both eyes. It is a common occurrence in CVAs. This condition must be considered in all aspects of care. For instance, the patient is approached from the unaffected side. The patient is taught to scan (move the head from side to side) to see things.

Pain. Usually there is very little pain associated with CVA. Existing pain may be aggravated by other prob-

Nursing Diagnosis: *Impaired Verbal Communication Related to Decreased Circulation to the Brain (Thrombosis) as Evidenced by Difficulty Expressing Thought Verbally and Inappropriate Verbalization*

Goal: At the end of the first week of rehabilitative therapy, the patient displays 10% accuracy with yes and no responses.

Nursing Actions (assess/do/teach)	Rationale	Evaluative Statement
1. Realize that the patient can understand what is spoken to her (do not shout) but that she has difficulty finding the correct words to respond; name familiar objects for her and request her to repeat the name after you (eg, *watch, hand*)	It is important to use every encounter to encourage and support communication; practice facilitates retention.	11/4 Goal met; patient displays 20% accuracy with yes and no responses
2. Be sensitive to the patient's frustration level and respect her fatigue; be calm, gentle, and patient; assist family members in their attempts to communicate and role-model effective strategies.	The attention span may be limited; frustration may lead to abandoning the project.	
3. Praise the patient's successes in using words correctly and communicate confidence that she can resolve her speech problem	Praise promotes self-esteem and empowers her with the confidence she needs to be successful.	

(continued)

lems such as infection, bladder calculi, fecal impaction, or emotional disturbances. Temporary relief may be obtained by the injection of a local anesthetic.

Autonomic Disturbances. The patient with a CVA may also have autonomic disturbances, such as perspiration or "goose flesh" above the level of the paralysis. The patient may have dilated pupils, high or low blood pressure, or headache. Disturbances of this kind may be treated with atropine-like drugs.

Personality Changes. Personality changes may be functional or organic. The functional type occurs as a result of frustration, such as not being able to speak or walk, or as a result of other people's attitudes. In either case the patient may feel useless or helpless.

Organic changes may result from blockage of blood supply to part of the brain. This often occurs in CVA patients. In this instance the person may cry or be excited easily. These conditions cannot be consciously controlled.

Nursing Considerations

The CVA patient often is admitted in an unresponsive state. This is known as a *stroke in evolution* (SIE). The quality of nursing care given during the acute phase often has considerable bearing on how much rehabilitation is possible and how fast it can be accomplished. Nursing care skills in this stage include:

♦ Note any changes in the patient's level of consciousness (LOC) and any other changes from neurologic findings indicated in the initial neurologic examination.
♦ Document every sign of improvement or lack of it.
♦ Position the unresponsive patient to keep the airway open and prevent aspiration, on the unaffected side. (*Rationale: Proper positioning prevents contractures and undue pressure on any part.*)
♦ Provide adequate support for the affected limbs. Extremity splints are now routine for this patient. (*Rationale: Positioning, support, and splints will help prevent contractures.*)

Nursing Diagnosis: *Sensory/Perceptual Alteration: Kinesthetic, Related to Physiologic Changes Associated with CVA*

Goal: By the end of the first week of rehabilitative therapy the patient demonstrates awareness of the right side of her body

Nursing Actions (assess/do/teach)	Rationale	Evaluative Statement
1. Use position changes, transfers, and assisted ambulation to assess for hemianesthesia (loss of sensation), paresthesia (feelings of heaviness, numbness, tingling), and loss of muscle-joint sense; carefully assess potential for injury and use appropriate safeguards.	Such alterations on the affected side of her body place her at high risk of injury.	11/2; Goal met; patient is visually scanning her affected side and demonstrating awareness
2. Use interactions with patient to reinforce adaptive strategies patient is learning in physical therapy.	Reinforcement facilitates mastery of new skills.	
3. Teach the patient to scan her right side visually and to check for correct positioning.	During the period of adjustment, vision may need to compensate for her impaired kinesthetic awareness.	

- Avoid placing the unresponsive patient on the back. *(Rationale: The tongue may fall back and occlude the airway and secretions may accumulate in the back of the throat if the patient is on his or her back.)*
- Turn the patient often, at least once every 2 hours, keeping the body in proper alignment.
- Provide suctioning as necessary. A mechanical airway or tracheostomy may be required. Probably oxygen will be administered.
- Monitor vital signs carefully. *(Rationale: An elevated temperature and lowered pulse and respiration rates are signs of increased intracranial pressure, which must be reported.)*
- Carefully observe eye signs and LOC (see Chapter 71).
- Keep the patient's eyes lubricated with soothing eye drops as ordered.
- Talk to the patient and explain everything you are doing as if the patient were responsive. *(Rationale: Although the patient is not responding, he or she hears. Hearing is the last sense to be lost.)*

At the end of the emergency phase the person is said to have a *completed stroke* (CS). Nursing skills in caring for the patient in a CS who has regained consciousness are:

- Continue to turn the patient often, now from the unaffected side to a back position.
- Encourage coughing and deep breathing.
- Encourage the patient to move if possible. *(Rationale: Movement prevents hypostatic pneumonia, formation of kidney stones, fecal impaction, urinary retention, and other complications.)*
- Provide PROM exercises as ordered.
- Encourage the patient to cooperate with the physical therapist.
- Administer ordered drugs (usually heparin, dicumarol, or coumadin) with care. Watch for side effects. *(Rationale: These drugs usually are given to prolong clotting time and to prevent further clots from being formed. However, there is danger of hemorrhage with their use.)* The patient usually does not need pain medication.
- Begin bowel and bladder retraining as the patient is ready for it.

The nurse must be aware of the various results of CVAs mentioned previously. The nurse deals with them in a kind and understanding manner. The patient needs, most of all, support and reassurance, and needs to feel accepted as he or she is right now.

The Rehabilitation Phase

Immediately on admission of the patient, the hospital staff should begin planning for rehabilitation. The quality of nursing care given during the acute phase will often have considerable bearing on how much rehabilitation is possible and how fast it can be accomplished. If contractures were prevented, the patient can learn to walk again that much faster. If the skin was kept intact, the patient will not have to contend with ulcerations and infections. If bowel and bladder training were begun, the patient will be well on the way to independence. The goal of all rehabilitation is to return the patient to as much self-care as possible in activities of daily living (ADL). As soon as possible, the patient is taught ADL, such as transferring from bed to chair or to toilet, and dressing and feeding. Speech therapy also begins as soon as possible. The accompanying Nursing Care Plan illustrates the rehabilitative care of a patient who has had a stroke. Chapter 89 describes some specific rehabilitation techniques and assistive devices.

Members of the family play a vital role. They need to know what the patient can do and how to encourage the person after discharge from the hospital. They should also understand that, because of brain damage, the person may behave differently after a stroke. Whatever the patient's disability, members of the family should recognize their own and the patient's emotional needs. They also need to be taught how to do various procedures that are helpful to the patient, while allowing the person to do as much as possible. The family needs a great deal of emotional support to deal with the patient's limitations.

Many resources are available to assist in rehabilitation, including local social service agencies, the American Heart Association, and the state Division of Vocational and Occupational Services. The local public health nursing service can often be of great assistance in helping the family to prepare for the patient's homecoming, as well as in assisting the patient to perform self-care at home.

Keys for Review

Key Questions for Critical Thinking

1. Discuss predisposing factors to coronary artery disease. Formulate a plan you could use to teach a patient to prevent these factors.
2. Define congestive heart failure and outline signs and symptoms. Describe nursing care for CHF. Differentiate between a compensated and decompensated heart.
3. Describe nursing care of patients undergoing CVAs during the phases of stroke in evolution and completed stroke. Give rationales for interventions.
4. Differentiate between angina pectoris and MI. Determine how medical treatment and nursing care is different in each. Explain why immediate relief of chest pain is important when caring for patients with MI.

Key Readings

Baas LS. Essentials of Cardiovascular Nursing. Gaithersburg, MD, Aspen, 1991

Berkow R (Ed). The Merck Manual of Diagnosis and Therapy, Ed 16. Rahway, NJ, Merck & Co, 1992

Key Readings (continued)

Craven RF, Hirnle CJ. Fundamentals of Nursing: Human Health and Function. Philadelphia, J.B. Lippincott, 1992

Fuller J, Schaller-Ayers J. Health Assessment: A Nursing Approach, Ed 2. Philadelphia, J.B. Lippincott, 1994

Nursing '94 Drug Handbook. Springhouse, PA, Springhouse, 1994

O'Toole M (Ed). Miller-Keane Encyclopedia and Dictionary of Medicine, Nursing, and Allied Health, Ed 5. Philadelphia, W.B. Saunders, 1992

Smeltzer SC, Bare BG. Brunner and Suddarth's Textbook of Medical-Surgical Nursing, Ed 7. Philadelphia, J.B. Lippincott, 1992

Taylor C, Lillis C, LeMone P. Fundamentals of Nursing: The Art and Science of Nursing Care, Ed 2. Philadelphia, J.B. Lippincott, 1993

Underhill SL, Woods SL, Froelicher ESS, et al. Cardiovascular Medications for Cardiac Nursing. Philadelphia, J.B. Lippincott, 1990

Enrichment Keys

Levin RF. "Caring for the cardiac spouse." American Journal of Nursing 93(11):51–53, 1993

Wingate S. Cardiac Nursing: A Clinical Management and Patient Care Resource. Gaithersburg, MD, Aspen, 1991

Keys to Learning More

Chapter 75: blood and lymph disorders
Chapter 77: allergic and immune disorders
Chapter 79: respiratory disorders

Keys to Learning More (continued)

Chapter 80: oxygen therapy and respiratory care
Chapter 85: geriatric nursing
Chapter 89: rehabilitation and home care

Key Resources

American Heart Association
National Center
7320 Greenville Avenue
Dallas, TX 75231
214-748-7212

75 Blood and Lymph Disorders

Keys for Learning

Learning Objectives

- Describe common blood disorders, their causes, treatment, and related nursing care.
- Differentiate between acute and chronic leukemia, including the treatment and prognosis for each.
- List the various blood components and products used in blood transfusions.
- Describe symptoms of a transfusion reaction and associated nursing care.

Key Terms

agranulocytosis
allogeneic
anemia
autologous
crossmatched
cytapheresis
hematology

hematopoietic
leukemia
lymphoma
oncologist
purpura
splenectomy

Keys to Understanding This Chapter

Chapter 16: fluid and electrolyte balance
Chapter 19: endocrine system
Chapter 21: cardiovascular system, including blood information
Chapter 22: respiratory system
Chapter 30: medical asepsis and universal precautions
Chapter 38: signs and symptoms of illness or injury
Chapter 42: vital signs
Chapter 47: specimen collection
Chapter 50: physical examination and nursing assessment
Chapter 52: pain management
Chapter 54: surgical asepsis
Unit Eleven: pharmacology and medication administration

Keys to Understanding This Chapter
(continued)

Chapter 65: care of the child with blood or lymph disorders
Chapter 69: fluid and electrolyte disorders
Chapter 72: endocrine disorders
Chapter 74: cardiovascular disorders

Key Points

- Blood transfusion is common treatment for blood disorders. It can cause serious reactions requiring careful observation of the patient.
- Anemias deprive a person of energy and oxygen to carry out the activities of daily living.
- White blood cell disorders can affect a person's ability to fight infections.
- Blood disorders affecting clotting factors can cause serious and life-threatening bleeding problems.

Key Topics Outline

Anatomy and Physiology Review
Diagnostic Tests
    Laboratory Tests
    Other Diagnostic Tests
Medical and Surgical Treatments
    Common Medical Treatments
    Common Surgical Treatments
Nursing Process
    Data Collection
    Nursing Diagnosis
    Planning and Implementation
    Evaluation
Disorders of Red Blood Cells: Anemias
Disorders Involving White Blood Cells and Lymph
    Agranulocytosis
    The Leukemias
    Lymphomas
Bleeding Disorders
    Purpura

Rosdahl CB: Textbook of Basic Nursing, 6th ed. © 1995 J.B. Lippincott Company

Chapter 21 describes the circulatory system, in which blood and lymph play a major role. The medical specialty related to blood and lymph is **hematology**. The physician trained in this specialty is the hematologist.

Blood and lymph are closely related to many other systems and disorders of the body. For example, cancer can occur in the blood or can be spread or localized in lymphatic tissue. Thus, blood and lymph disorders are often treated by a cancer specialist, the **oncologist**.

Some blood and lymph disorders have systemic consequences and symptoms. In addition, the general condition of many body systems and many disorders can be revealed by laboratory examination of blood. The *medical technologist* and other laboratory personnel perform these determinations.

Anatomy and Physiology Review

The **hematopoietic** system is composed of blood-forming organs, such as bone marrow, lymph nodes, and the spleen. The elements of blood and lymph (red blood cells, white blood cells, platelets, plasma, and clotting factors) are responsible for carrying oxygen and nutrients to all body cells and carrying wastes away from the cells. The blood also carries substances such as electrolytes, hormones, and enzymes to selected areas of the body. The lymphatic system collects fluids and proteins from interstitial fluid and returns these to the general circulation. (Lymph only carries fluids away from tissues.)

In addition, specialized components of the blood protect the body from infection and hemorrhage. The heart pumps blood through the blood vessels.

The ABO system has four blood groups. The letters correspond to antigens found in erythrocytes. These groups are A, B, AB, and O. Additional antigens may be present. One such antigen is Rh factor. If the Rh antigen is present, the person is type Rh+. If it is absent, the person is type Rh−. Approximately 85% of us are Rh+.

Diagnostic Tests

Laboratory Tests

Many laboratory tests can be done to determine the numbers and types of cells and their condition. The presence of abnormal cells or any other abnormality such as clotting problems can also be detected.

The Complete Blood Count

The complete blood count (CBC) is a common analysis of blood. The CBC often gives valuable diagnostic information. A CBC usually includes a numerical esti-

Key Abbreviations and Acronyms in Blood-Related Disorders

ACT	Activated clotting time
ALL	Acute lymphocytic leukemia
AML	Acute myelogenous leukemia
APTT	Activated partial thromboplastin time
CBC	Complete blood cell count
CLL	Chronic lymphocytic leukemia
CML	Chronic myelogenous leukemia
Cryo	Cryoprecipitate
DIC	Disseminated intravascular coagulation
ESR, Sed Rate	Erythrocyte sedimentation rate
FFP	Fresh frozen plasma
Hct	Hematocrit
Hgb	Hemoglobin
HTLV-I	Human T-cell leukemia (lymphotropic) virus, type I
IG	Immune globulin
IVIG	Intravenous immune globulin
PPF	Plasma protein fraction
PT, Pro-time	Prothrombin time test
RBC	Red blood cell
WBC	White blood cell

mate of numbers of red blood cells (RBCs), white blood cells (WBCs), and platelets. These numbers reflect the functioning of bone marrow, ability to carry oxygen to cells, and the patient's infection-fighting status and clotting abilities. Deficiencies or excesses of these cells indicate specific problems. The physician will then evaluate the laboratory studies compared to the patient's symptoms.

The test for hemoglobin (Hgb) identifies the amount of hemoglobin in an RBC; this determines the patient's ability to carry oxygen to cells. The hematocrit (Hct) identifies the percentage of RBCs in the blood. A study of the color and size of blood cells may also be done as a routine part of the CBC. Specific types of anemia can be diagnosed, using the CBC.

White Blood Cell Count and Differential

Because in some diseases, WBCs increase in number (*leukocytosis*) or decrease in number (*leukopenia*), a WBC count is a valuable aid to diagnosis. A laboratory technician views a drop of blood under the microscope and estimates the number of WBCs. The normal count of 5,000 to 10,000/mm³ increases to 25,000/mm³ or higher when infection is present. In some diseases, the relative proportion of the kinds of WBCs varies, and therefore a differential count (diff) is made, in which the number of granular leukocytes is compared with the number of nongranular leukocytes. This count gives further diagnostic clues to the physician. The WBC and differential counts (WBC and diff) are often done at the same time.

Normal response to injury or an invading pathogen is *leukocytosis*. Abnormal leukocytosis may be further identified in relationship to the particular type of WBC involved (eg, *mononucleosis* is an increase in monocytes.) A well-known disorder is called *leukemia*, a disorder of leukocytes.

Prothrombin Time (PT Test, Pro-time)

The prothrombin level indicates the activity of certain factors found in the plasma. These factors are important in blood clotting (factors V, VII, X, prothrombin, and fibrinogen). Initially, the normal prothrombin level is approximately 12 seconds depending on the standards of the individual laboratory. After anticoagulant therapy with drugs such as coumarin derivatives (Coumadin), the patient's prothrombin time is maintained at $1\frac{1}{2}$ to 2 times the normal level.

It is important to measure the prothrombin level daily when the patient begins drug therapy. Once the blood level of anticoagulant is stabilized, the prothrombin level can be determined less often (approximately every 2 weeks).

Nursing Considerations. Nursing care is important to the patient receiving anticoagulants. Following are essential nursing skills:

- ◆ Assess for signs of:
  - ◆ Bleeding, no matter how slight
  - ◆ Headache
  - ◆ Unexplained abdominal pain
  - ◆ Changes in the neurologic signs or level of consciousness
- ◆ Avoid intramuscular injections and needle sticks, if possible.
- ◆ Do not take temperatures rectally.
- ◆ Do not give daily dose of anticoagulant until after blood specimen for the prothrombin time is drawn.
- ◆ Report results of test to physician (in case dosage needs to be adjusted).

Activated Partial Thromboplastin Time (APTT)

This test detects coagulation deficiencies related to several clotting factors. This test is frequently used to monitor the activity of heparin. As with coumarin, when heparin therapy is initiated, APTT levels are monitored every day. The results are reported to the physician, who decides the doses needed to regulate the APTT levels. The nurse should watch for any signs of bleeding.

Bleeding Time

This test gives a global index of coagulation capacity. When standard technique is used, the normal bleeding time is usually less than 9 minutes. An abnormally high bleeding time may indicate a platelet disorder or vascular disease.

Sedimentation Rate

Erythrocyte sedimentation rate (ESR or "sed rate") measures the speed (in mm/h) that RBCs (erythrocytes) settle to the bottom of a tube of unclotted blood in exactly an hour. The normal rate varies with age, sex, and the method of testing. Inflammation alters the blood proteins, resulting in heavier-than-normal RBC. The speed with which they fall to the bottom of the tube corresponds to the degree of inflammation. Although the ESR is a nonspecific test, it is useful in diagnosing many occult (not seen) diseases.

When performed in conjunction with a WBC count, the ESR can indicate infection. It is also used to monitor the course of inflammatory activity. The ESR is useful in diseases such as rheumatic fever, rheumatoid arthritis, and acute myocardial infarction.

Bleeding/Clotting Time

Other tests that may be ordered include *activated clotting time* (ACT), *thrombin time, reptilase time,* and *platelet count.*

Blood Culture

A blood culture is done to discover whether any organisms are present in the patient's blood or to determine which antibiotics would be most effective against a specific organism. The nurse must follow the parameters established by the physician for the proper timing of obtaining a blood culture. The blood is usually obtained while the patient is experiencing the most severe symptoms that have brought him or her to the hospital. If the patient is in the hospital for a fever of unexplained origin (FUO), the culture should be taken when the patient has a fever. It is the nurse's responsibility to notify the laboratory technician when an elevated temperature occurs.

The culture should be obtained before any antibiotic therapy is started to avoid interference with test results. Because this test requires special collection procedures, the blood is usually drawn by the laboratory staff.

Other Diagnostic Tests

Bone Marrow Aspiration or Biopsy

In bone marrow aspiration or biopsy, a large needle is inserted into the iliac crest (the flaring portion of the hip bone) to draw a sample of bone marrow. The iliac crest contains more marrow than the sternum (breast bone), which is less frequently used. If the patient has had previous radiation to the pelvis, the sternum is used.

These tests are done to determine whether or not the bone marrow is manufacturing blood cells normally. They are done most often in blood disorders such as leukemia and anemia. The nurse assists the physician in bone marrow studies. Nursing skills include:

◆ Be sure to wear gloves and follow universal precautions.
◆ Have all necessary equipment ready before the procedure is begun.
◆ Explain what is being done and provide support to the patient.
◆ Forewarn that a slight "give" may be felt as the needle enters bone and a sharp pain (like a burning sensation) as marrow is aspirated.
◆ Inform the patient that procedure takes only a few minutes.
◆ Help the patient to lie still during procedure.
◆ Observe the patient after test. (Few complications occur, but there might be some bleeding at the puncture site).
◆ Have the patient rest for at least 30 minutes after the procedure.

Medical and Surgical Treatments

Common Medical Treatments

Blood Transfusion

Intravenous (IV) therapy was introduced in Chapter 57. The administration of blood and blood components intravenously is called a *blood transfusion*. The prin-

ciples of intravenous therapy apply, with several added precautions. These precautions, as part of nursing skills, are listed in the accompanying box.

Blood and Blood Component Solutions. *Whole blood* is rarely used today except to treat massive acute hem-

---

Nursing Skill Guidelines
Precautions During
Blood Transfusions*

◆ Follow all procedures for intravenous therapy PLUS . . .
◆ Take and record baseline vital signs before transfusion is started, after first 15 minutes, hourly, at end of transfusion, and 1 hour later (or as required by hospital policy).
◆ Assess patient's understanding of procedure and obtain informed consent according to hospital policy.
◆ Instruct patient to report unusual symptoms immediately.
◆ Remain with patient and observe for reactions during first 15 minutes and monitor patient for reactions throughout entire transfusion.
◆ Provide emotional support to patient throughout transfusion.
◆ Do not store component in nursing unit or other unmonitored refrigerator; do not keep blood out of a monitored refrigerator for more than 30 minutes before transfusion is started.
◆ Do not warm blood in an unmonitored water bath or sink or microwave oven.
◆ Do not allow any solution other than 0.9% normal saline to come in contact with the blood component or administration set.
◆ Never add medications, including those intended for intravenous use, to blood or components or infuse through the same administration set as the blood component.
◆ Document thoroughly, including the *absence* of signs and symptoms.
◆ Return empty blood containers to the transfusion service, if this is facility policy. Many hospitals discard blood containers according to a specific protocol.
◆ Never administer a blood component without a blood filter.
◆ Do not use the same blood filter for more than 4 hours.
◆ Do not transfuse a single unit of blood for more than 4 hours.

* Adapted from: Transfusion Therapy Guidelines for Nurses, National Blood Resource Education Program; Office of Prevention, Education, and Control; National Heart, Lung, and Blood Institute; National Institutes of Health, Public Health Service; U.S. Department of HHS, 1990

Drug Reference for Blood

> The Food and Drug Administration (FDA)-approved drug reference that *must* be used by anyone administering blood or caring for a transfused patient is the Circular of Information for the Use of Human Blood and Blood Components.* Copies are obtained from the hospital blood bank or transfusion service.
>
> * *See "Transfusion Therapy Guidelines for Nurses" (p. 1131) and Enrichment Keys (p. 1140).*

orrhage. The normal circulating blood volume in an adult is approximately 6 liters (8–10 pints). Whole blood can be stored refrigerated for up to 35 days.

Packed RBCs are the most common component transfused; they are produced by removing the plasma from whole blood. Packed cells can be stored refrigerated for up to 42 days, with the addition of a special preservative. They are given to the patient with anemia who does not need increased circulating volume. One unit provides 250 to 300 mL.

With the use of special equipment, some blood banks are able to treat RBCs to freeze them for up to 10 years. However, when frozen RBCs have been used, they lose approximately 20% of their effectiveness. Units of rare blood types are often handled this way.

Platelet concentrate and *cryoprecipitate* (factor VIII: antihemophilic factor) are used to treat clotting deficiencies. They are produced by separating them from a unit of plasma. Platelets are given in leukemia and other illnesses that affect the ability to clot. Cryoprecipitate is transfused to patients with hemophilia A.

Plasma can be fresh frozen (FFP) to preserve labile (easily broken down) clotting factors. Many deteriorate within a day if just refrigerated. Plasma is thawed just before transfusion. FFP is given to correct clotting deficiencies. Because of the slight risk of transmitting infectious disease, FFP should not be used as a blood volume expander.

Blood Derivative Solutions. FFP is also used to produce various derivatives. These products are safer than blood and blood components because they are treated to inactivate blood-borne microorganisms such as the human immunodeficiency (HIV) and hepatitis viruses.

Serum albumin (Albumisol) and *plasma protein fraction* (PPF) are used in hypovolemic shock (low blood volume) or to replace albumin lost because of burns or kidney and liver diseases. A synthetic (not from blood) plasma expander, *Dextran*, is also available.

Factor VIII and other clotting factors are used to treat hemophilia and other clotting disorders.

Immune globulins (IG) are given to a person who has been recently exposed to an infectious disease. An example is the nurse who is exposed to a patient's blood and receives immune globulin containing antibodies against hepatitis B. Vaccines (Recombivax) are also available to protect healthcare workers from hepatitis B. Anti-Rh (D) immune globulin (RhoGam) is administered to Rh(D)-negative women, to prevent fetal blood incompatibility problems. Most immune globulins are given intramuscularly, but one form, intravenous immune globulin (IVIG) must be given intravenously.

Special Blood Products. Autologous blood is self-donated; it is the safest blood for the patient. It can be collected when surgery is planned far enough in advance. *Directed* or *designated* blood donations are from donors selected by the patient, such as a family member. However, studies have shown that directed donations are no safer than blood from the community blood supply.

> ### Key Concept
>
> New tests and procedures for screening blood and selecting blood donors have improved the safety of blood transfusions. However, blood-borne diseases such as HIV virus, which causes acquired immunodeficiency syndrome (AIDS) and hepatitis can still be transmitted, even though more rarely than in the past. The nurse handling tested blood still must always use universal precautions.

Type and Crossmatch. Blood of different types is often incompatible when mixed. The wrong type of blood could easily kill the patient. Blood is *typed* to determine the ABO group and to determine the presence or absence of Rh factors (see Chapter 21). The blood for transfusion is then **crossmatched**, that is, a small amount of the patient's blood is mixed with a small amount of the blood from the particular unit of blood for transfusion to determine compatibility. Even with these safeguards, the nurse must observe the patient very carefully while blood is being given because dangerous reactions can still occur. The precautions for administration of blood are presented earlier in this chapter.

> ### Nursing Alert
>
> The patient receiving a blood transfusion and the unit of blood itself *must* be positively identified by two licensed personnel. A patient identification bracelet should be put on *before* the laboratory staff draws the blood sample for type and crossmatch testing, with *no exceptions*. Misidentification of the patient with the wrong test sample or blood unit can be fatal. Most fatal transfusion reactions are caused by *human error*, not from a problem with the blood itself.

Blood Administration. Blood transfusions are usually administered by registered nurses. Because any transfusion can be potentially fatal, the patient receiving a transfusion needs special care.

Transfusion Reaction. Several types of transfusion reactions can occur during or after the transfusion. Symptoms of severe reaction usually appear during the first 50 mL or less of blood infused.

Nursing Alert

Reactions from both mild and life-threatening causes can exhibit *similar* symptoms. Therefore, every symptom should be considered potentially serious. The transfusion should be discontinued until the cause of the symptom can be determined.

The accompanying box lists signs and symptoms to look for in a patient receiving a transfusion. If any of these symptoms occur, guidelines should be followed in conjunction with hospital policy.

Common Surgical Treatments

Bone Marrow Transplantation

One method of treatment having great success in certain circumstances is that of bone marrow transplantation. It is effective in many cases. Two approaches are used to obtain bone marrow.

The **autologous** approach involves taking the patient's own bone marrow and storing it in a frozen state, while intensive chemotherapy and radiation therapy are administered to the patient. Subsequently the patient's own bone marrow is reinfused. This allows for recovery from the intensive therapy treatments and prevents allergic or rejection reactions.

The other approach, called **allogenic** transplantation, involves obtaining bone marrow from a normal

---

Blood Transfusion Reactions*

Possible signs and symptoms (changes from pretransfusion data)

General

- Fever (rise of 1°C or 2°F)
- Chills
- Muscle aches, pain
- Back pain, chest pain
- Headache
- Heat at site of infusion or along vein

Nervous System

- Apprehension, impending sense of doom
- Tingling, numbness

Respiratory system

- Respiratory rate (slower or faster)
- Dyspnea (painful breathing)
- Cough, wheezing, rales

Gastrointestinal System

- Nausea, vomiting
- Pain, abdominal cramping
- Diarrhea (may be bloody)

Cardiovascular System

- Heart rate (slower or faster)
- Blood pressure (lower, raised, shock)
- Peripheral circulation (cyanosis, facial flushing, cool/clammy, hot/flushed/dry, edema)
- Bleeding (generalized, oozing at surgical or transfusion site)

Renal System

- Changes in urine volume (less, none)
- Changes in urine color (dark, concentrated, shades of red/brown/amber)

Integumentary System

- Rashes, urticaria (hives), swelling, itching
- Diaphoresis (sweating)

Signs of Reaction in an Unconscious Patient

- Weak pulse, faster or slower
- Fever
- Drop in blood pressure
- Dark red/brown urine
- Decreased or no urine output
- Oozing at surgical site

Managing a Transfusion Reaction

If a transfusion reaction occurs:

1. STOP THE TRANSFUSION IMMEDIATELY.
2. Keep the IV open with 0.9% normal saline.
3. Report the reaction to both the transfusion service and attending physician immediately.
4. Do clerical check at bedside of patient identification band, blood bag, and accompanying materials.
5. Treat symptoms per physician's order and monitor vital signs.
6. Send blood bag with attached administration set and labels to the transfusion service.
7. Collect blood and urine samples and send to laboratory.
8. Document thoroughly on transfusion reaction form and in patient chart.

* *Transfusion Therapy Guidelines for Nurses,* ibid.

compatible donor, usually a blood relative. The donor bone marrow is crossmatched in a manner similar, but much more complex, to that used for blood transfusion. The donor marrow is then transplanted into the patient, following chemotherapy and radiation.

Because chemotherapy and radiation destroy the patient's own marrow, this patient is susceptible to infections. Also, large numbers of blood transfusions are required as part of treatment.

Key Concept

Because it is so difficult to match bone marrow donors and potential recipients, bone marrow donors are always in demand. Contact your local blood bank or donor organization if you wish to donate.

Splenectomy

The spleen is involved in blood formation, in the destruction of old RBCs, in the storage of RBCs, and in influencing bone marrow and antibody formation in infection. **Splenectomy** or removal of the spleen is sometimes done as a therapeutic measure. Spleen removal may sometimes slow down related disease processes; this is especially true if the spleen has been hyperactive. In some types of disease, such as hemolytic disease, removal of a hyperactive spleen may slow down the progression of the disease. In other conditions, when a hyperactive spleen is the actual cause of the disease, its removal will be curative. In Hodgkin's disease, the spleen may be removed as part of the staging procedure, which determines the stage of progression of the disease. (In this case, splenectomy is *not* a treatment for the disease itself.)

❖ *Nursing Process*

Data Collection

The nurse must carefully observe and assess the patient with a disorder of the blood or lymph. Chapter 50 describes physical examinations and nursing assessment. Normal blood values appear in Appendix C. Assess the patient's skin for petechiae, bruises, or evidence of other abnormal bleeding. Measure the blood pressure and pulse. Obtain a thorough nursing history including nutritional status, dyspnea, elimination difficulties, difficulty in walking or moving, and pain. Does the person get frequent infections? Are injuries common? Signs and symptoms in these areas may indicate a blood or lymph disorder.

The nursing assessment establishes a baseline for future comparison and determines the presence of suspected blood, lymph, or other disorders. The nurse

should document and report any changes in this baseline level.

In addition, the nurse observes the patient's emotional response to the disorder or the disease. Some blood or lymph disorders are chronic; some are life-threatening. What types of assistance does the patient require? Is counseling needed? Will the person need assistance to meet daily needs; will home care be needed after hospital discharge? Is the patient anxious or fearful about the outcome? Does the person understand the medication and treatment regime?

Nursing Diagnosis

Based on data collection, nursing diagnoses are established for the patient with a disorder in the blood or lymph. Some diagnoses may have more than one causal factor. The following are examples of nursing diagnoses that may appear on nursing care plans of patients with a blood or lymph disorder:

♦ High Risk for Infection related to impaired immune system
♦ Fluid Volume Deficit related to hemorrhage
♦ Diarrhea related to medication side effects
♦ Impaired Physical Mobility related to injuries, bruising, bleeding into the tissues, fatigue
♦ Activity Intolerance related to leukemia, anemia, general weakness
♦ Body Image Disturbance related to purpura, other visible bleeding disorders
♦ Chronic Pain related to sickled cells, bone marrow aspiration, transfusion reaction
♦ Anticipatory Grieving related to chronic or fatal condition, genetic nature of disorder

Planning and Implementation

The patient, nurse, and family plan together for effective care to meet patient needs, based on the nursing diagnosis. The nurse provides pretest, preoperative, post-test, and postoperative care for the patient undergoing procedures such as bone marrow aspiration or bone marrow transplant. The patient with a blood or lymphatic disorder may also require nursing care ranging from assisting with some daily activities to total nursing care.

In the case of a chronic, genetic, or fatal disorder, the patient and family are assisted to deal with the diagnosis and prognosis and emotional problems. Patients and family members are taught about the disorder, the prescribed medications, precautions, and treatments to be carried out in the hospital and at home. A nursing care plan is developed to meet these needs. A sample nursing care plan for a patient with a blood or lymph disorder is provided later in the chapter.

Evaluation

The nurse, patient, and other members of the health-care team evaluate the outcomes of care. Have short-term goals been met? Are long-term goals still realistic? Is the prognosis the same or has it changed? Is the patient in remission at this time or is a long-term cure anticipated? Will home care, social services, respite care, or rehabilitation services be necessary? Planning for further nursing care and community services considers the patient's prognosis, as well as complications and the patient's response to care given.

Disorders of Red Blood Cells: Anemias

Anemia can refer to any of the following RBC conditions:

◆ Reduction in total number of cells
◆ Deficiency of hemoglobin
◆ Malfunctioning of cells

Anemia can be caused by:

◆ Loss of RBCs in hemorrhage
◆ Destruction of RBCs due to causes such as RBC defects (eg, sickle cell anemia) or hemolysis (eg, in malaria)
◆ Interference with the production of RBCs due to deficiencies of iron or certain vitamins, or injury to bone marrow, such as damage from drugs or chemicals (eg, benzene)
◆ Other diseases such as cancer, rheumatoid arthritis

Although anemia is actually a symptom of other diseases, it sometimes is regarded as a disease in itself.

The seriousness of the disease depends on such factors as the speed of onset, whether it is chronic, and the patient's overall general health and nutritional status. The more rapidly anemia develops, the more serious it is likely to be.

Signs and Symptoms. There are several types of anemia, but the symptoms are essentially the same. Signs and symptoms can include any or most of the following:

◆ Pallor
◆ Fatigue, weakness
◆ Faintness
◆ Loss of appetite
◆ Symptoms of congestive heart failure
◆ Gastrointestinal complaints
◆ Jaundice
◆ Rapid pulse (heart tries to compensate for lack of oxygen to cells)

◆ Chills (reduced oxygen, low blood volume)
◆ Decreased hemoglobin, hematocrit
◆ Hypotension

Diagnostic Tests. The simplest method of diagnosing anemia is by determining the hemoglobin content of the blood. If the hemoglobin is below 14 g (to 16 g) per 100 mL in a man or 12 g (to 14 g) per 100 mL in a woman, the person is considered anemic.

Anemia From Blood Loss

Hemorrhage or continued slow bleeding will cause anemia. If the loss of blood is chronic, as from an ulcer, the cause of the bleeding must first be determined and treated. The usual treatment is to administer iron supplements. If the patient does not respond, transfusions of packed RBCs may be considered for treatment. The patient who is hemorrhaging as a result of trauma is more likely to show symptoms than is the person who is bleeding slowly. The patient with a massive hemorrhage will also show symptoms of shock.

Iron Deficiency Anemia

Young people are likely to develop this most common type of anemia. It may result from faulty eating habits, such as poor diet or hurrying meals. With the anemia comes a poor appetite. A deficiency caused by faulty eating habits can be remedied easily by taking extra iron and by eating foods high in iron. Under certain conditions, the body needs more iron, such as during adolescence or pregnancy. Women also need more iron than men because they lose blood in menstruation. The accompanying box lists nursing skills for administering iron supplements.

Pernicious Anemia

The patient with pernicious anemia lacks a substance in the gastric fluids called *intrinsic factor*, which is produced in the stomach. The intrinsic factor is re-

---

Nursing Skill Guidelines
Administering Iron Supplements

◆ Give oral iron preparations with meals. *(Rationale: Iron is irritating to the gastrointestinal tract; it can have an unpleasant metallic taste and is easier to take if given with food.)*
◆ Give citrus juices with the iron preparation. *(Rationale: Vitamin C enhances absorption of iron.)*
◆ Give liquid iron through a straw. *(Rationale: Use of a straw avoids discoloring teeth and minimizes unpleasant taste.)*
◆ Explain to patient that iron will make stools black and might cause constipation. Stool softeners may be prescribed.

quired for vitamin B$_{12}$ to be absorbed from food in the small intestine. Vitamin B$_{12}$ is needed for proper absorption and utilization of iron in the body as well as protection of nerve fibers. Most cases of pernicious anemia begin during late middle age. It is most often seen in people of northern European descent. The disease is diagnosed through the Shilling test.

Signs and symptoms are:

◆ Digestive disturbances
◆ Sore mouth
◆ Diarrhea

Signs of nerve damage include:

◆ Numbness and tingling in extremities
◆ Irritability
◆ Depression
◆ Confusion
◆ Loss of balance

Diet alone is not an effective treatment. The patient must take vitamin B$_{12}$ (cyanocobalamin) for life. Vitamin B$_{12}$ cannot be given orally to patients with pernicious anemia because they lack the intrinsic factor necessary to absorb the B$_{12}$. Thus, it is given intramuscularly. Once replaced, an injection every 4 weeks is usually sufficient to maintain adequate levels of B$_{12}$ in these patients.

Sickle Cell Anemia

Sickle cell anemia is an inherited disorder in which the RBCs become sickle shaped (sickled) when hypoxic (lacking oxygen). This is due to the presence of abnormal hemoglobin called hemoglobin-S (Fig. 75-1). Because sickled cells are shaped differently than normal RBCs, they become caught in the capillaries, causing an obstruction to blood flow. The sickled cells are also destroyed more rapidly than normal cells. Sickled cells are able to carry oxygen, but the transport of oxygen to the tissues is impaired because of the obstruction in the capillaries.

In the United States, sickle cell anemia is found predominantly in African Americans. The gene for sickling in hemoglobin is found in 1 of 9 African Americans. However, because the disease is a recessive trait, a person must have the gene from both parents to develop the actual disease. Therefore, the sickled hemoglobin *trait* is carried by about 11% of African Americans, but most of them do not have the disease. The actual disease of sickle cell anemia is present in *many fewer people.*

Symptoms in the person who actually has sickle cell anemia (*sicklemia*) can include episodes, from early childhood, of fever, with pain in the arms, legs, and abdomen. The patient may be jaundiced and is more susceptible than normal to infections. During a crisis period, the patient's abdomen is tender and rigid. Headache, paralysis, and seizures may result from cerebral thrombosis.

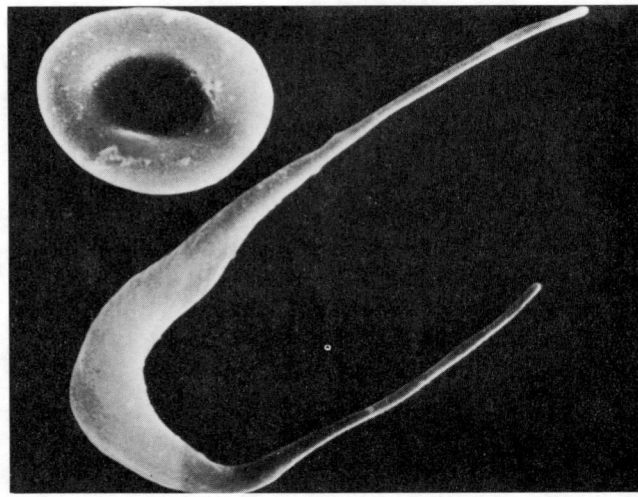

Figure 75-1. A sickled and a normal red blood cell. (Courtesy of Comprehensive Sickle Cell Center, University of Miami.)

A regime of frequent blood transfusions can contribute to a more normal growth rate and better general health in the affected child. Associated risks include the possibility of iron overload and disease transmission through transfusions. The patient is treated with iron chelating agents to remove excess iron from the blood and counteract iron overload. These patients are encouraged not to fly, especially in non-pressurized planes, because they might become hypoxic.

Aplastic Anemia

Aplastic anemia results from disease of the bone marrow where most blood cells are produced. Aplastic anemia is characterized by *pancytopenia* (decreased RBCs, WBCs, and platelets). Some possible causes include excessive radiation, various drugs, tumors, insecticides, chemicals, and environmental toxins. Sometimes it appears without any apparent cause. Some researchers believe that some cases of aplastic anemia are autoimmune in origin. The patient with aplastic anemia is extremely ill and becomes weak, tired, and short of breath, with even the least exertion.

Bone marrow transplantation is the most successful therapy. Aplastic anemia has a poor prognosis, with a high mortality rate from complications, without bone marrow transplantation. However, the prognosis is improved dramatically if bone marrow transplantation can be done.

Nursing Considerations. The patient with aplastic anemia is extremely susceptible to infection and bleeding. Nursing care should include:

◆ Administration of antibiotics per doctor's order
◆ Aseptic technique in all invasive procedures

♦ Careful handling of patient
♦ Cautioning patient to avoid bruises and cuts (strong bleeding tendency)
♦ Temperatures not taken rectally
♦ Use of reverse isolation during exacerbations of the disease

Disorders Involving White Blood Cells and Lymph

Agranulocytosis

In **agranulocytosis**, the production of WBCs is decreased, causing severe neutropenia (lack of neutrophils in the blood). One cause of this condition is the toxic effects of certain drugs, especially barbiturates, tranquilizers, chloramphenicol, and sulfonamides.

Signs of this disease are chills and fever, headache, and ulcers on the mucous membrane of the mouth, nose, throat, rectum, or vagina. Treatment begins by removing the drug causing the trouble. Because WBCs are depleted, the person is more susceptible to infection, and extreme care is taken to protect this person from exposure. If the cause is not a neoplastic disorder, bone marrow function may resume in 2 to 3 weeks.

The Leukemias

Leukemia is a neoplastic disorder in which WBCs (leukocytes) increase in abnormal abundance. Usually an increase in WBCs is a sign that the body is fighting disease, but this is not true in leukemia. The increase is so abnormally high that it reduces the number of other cells in the blood, including blood platelets and erythrocytes, which are essential to prevention of bleeding and anemia.

Leukemia is identified as *lymphocytic* or *myelogenous*, according to the type of WBC involved.

Leukemia affects both children and adults. Most authorities define leukemia as a cancer of the blood or blood-forming organs (the bone marrow, lymph nodes, and spleen). It is the most common form of childhood cancer (see Chapter 65). Scientists have identified a retrovirus, human T cell leukemia virus, type I (HTLV-I), as the cause of one form of human leukemia.

The increase in the number of cases of leukemia is attributed to several factors. It may be that because people now live longer, there is a greater chance for the disease to develop. Also, it has been discovered that people whose work exposes them to considerable radiation run a greater risk of developing leukemia.

Acute Leukemia

Two types of acute leukemia are known: *acute lymphocytic leukemia* (ALL), which is most common in people under 20 years of age, and *acute myelogenous*

leukemia (AML), which is most common in adults. ALL usually has a more favorable prognosis. These disorders, as they affect children, are discussed in detail in Chapter 65.

Signs and Symptoms. The symptoms of acute leukemia appear suddenly, often with an acute respiratory infection. Blood tests reveal that many WBCs are not fully developed. In about 60% of cases, the patient's blood shows an unusual increase in WBCs. However, in about 40% of cases, the WBC count in the peripheral blood may be decreased at the time of diagnosis of acute leukemia. Sometimes symptoms disappear temporarily, perhaps for several months, but most often in acute leukemia they grow steadily worse, unless treated.

Medical and Surgical Treatment. Treatment with chemotherapy has greatly improved survival. Children commonly are surviving 5 years and many are cured. Adults with some types of leukemia still hold a guarded prognosis for survival beyond a year; however, some forms of leukemia respond well to treatment.

Chemotherapeutic drugs are given to slow the rapid production of leukocytes. (Note: These drugs can interfere with production of normal blood cells and often have toxic side effects. The use of these drugs is described in Chapter 76.) However, in the treatment of acute leukemia, it seems necessary to give chemotherapy to the extent that essentially all cells in the bone marrow are temporarily "wiped out." Because the WBC count is very low, and therefore, body defenses are low, antibiotics are given to prevent secondary infections.

> **Nursing Alert**
> Drug therapy in leukemia must be balanced so that it does the most damage to abnormal cells without harming the patient.

In some cases of acute leukemia, therapeutic **cytapheresis** may be performed. This procedure removes the excess cells and is followed by treatment of the bone marrow.

Nursing Considerations. Nursing care in acute leukemia is aimed at supportive treatment and prevention of complications. Because of the diversity of the illness and its response to treatment, no single plan can be established. Blood transfusions are given to provide more RBCs, hemoglobin, and platelets. Rectal temperatures are not taken because patients have very few platelets and may hemorrhage. Patients also have difficulty fighting infections because the WBCs are ineffective.

Chronic Leukemia

The two forms of chronic leukemia are *chronic lymphocytic leukemia* (CLL) and *chronic myelogenous leukemia* (CML).

Signs and Symptoms. Often the first signs of chronic leukemia are swollen lymph nodes in the neck, axilla, or groin, or a swelling in the upper left side of the abdomen, which makes the patient's abdomen feel heavy. This abdominal swelling is caused by enlargement of the spleen. The patient has all the symptoms of anemia, along with difficulty in breathing, if the spleen is enlarged. Eventually, the person becomes very weak, bleeds easily, has fever, and is susceptible to secondary infections, such as pneumonia.

Medical Treatment. Treatment includes transfusions, antibiotics, and chemotherapeutic drugs to slow production of leukocytes. Radiation is sometimes used. The general purpose in prescribing drugs is to retard processes that cause the disease and aid its development. Improvement after treatment is often dramatic.

Nursing Considerations. Leukemia is frightening and may carry a guarded prognosis. Referral to counseling or a support group may be beneficial. The patient should be encouraged to return to a normal life insofar as possible. Activity is not harmful, nor will complete rest halt the progress of the disease. Guidelines for nursing care in leukemia and lymphoma are presented in the accompanying box.

Lymphomas

Lymphomas are neoplastic diseases of the lymphoid system. They are currently classified as Hodgkin's disease and non-Hodgkin's lymphomas. Of the lymphomas, Hodgkin's disease is the most common. The onset of Hodgkin's disease is usually 20 to 40 years of age; in non-Hodgkin's lymphomas, age of onset is 50 to 60 years. Lymphomas affect more men than women.

Hodgkin's Disease

The cause of Hodgkin's disease is not known. Hodgkin's lymphomas may be categorized as *lymphocytic* or *histiocytic.*

Signs and Symptoms. Hodgkin's disease begins with a painless enlargement of the lymph nodes in the neck (cervical) and less commonly in the groin (inguinal). As the nodes get larger, they press on surrounding tissues and cause pain. The patient loses weight, has a poor appetite, and feels weak and tired. Often the patient

---

Nursing Skill Guidelines
Caring for the Leukemia or Lymphoma Patient

♦ The nurse should plan nursing care so as to conserve the patient's strength and provide rest periods. (*Rationale: The patient is generally exhausted.*)

♦ The patient should eat a high-protein diet. (*Rationale: Protein provides energy.*)

♦ During a bleeding episode, the patient should rest and have gentle pressure applied to the bleeding site. Cold compresses should be applied where indicated. When injections are given, very small gauge needles should be used and injection sites must be rotated carefully. Wear gloves. (*Rationale: This patient is prone to bleeding.*)

♦ Do not serve irritating foods or beverages; use a soft toothbrush; and keep the patient's lips moist with oil or another preparation, as ordered. Give frequent mouth care, especially before and after meals. (*Rationale: The mucous membranes are very fragile.*)

♦ The patient should have a bed cradle to hold covers off the legs and feet. (*Rationale: Pain in bones and joints is very common.*)

♦ Analgesics and other drugs may be given, although the nurse should attempt to relieve pain with nursing measures first. The patient should be kept as comfortable as possible and should not suffer needlessly.

♦ Antipyretic drugs and frequent bed baths with cool sponges are given; the patient's room is kept cool. (*Rationale: Leukemia and lymphoma are inflammatory processes; often there is fever.*)

♦ Keep the patient's fingernails short; use soap sparingly; and use lotion liberally. (*Rationale: This person's skin is very friable.*)

♦ Good skin and back care is vital. (*Rationale: The skin is particularly friable; this patient is often relatively immobile.*)

♦ The nurse must use good handwashing technique and medical asepsis. (*Rationale: This patient is particularly susceptible to infection, because of the disorder of white blood cells or lymph.*)

---

complains of chills, night sweats, and itching. The patient may have a fever and develop anemia and a tendency to bleed.

Diagnostic Tests. Hodgkin's disease is diagnosed by microscopic examination of tissue from an affected lymph node and from results of a bone marrow biopsy. The specific diagnosis is made when a malformed cell, called the Reed-Sternberg cell, is present.

Medical Treatment. Treatment is based on the staging of the disease, according to symptoms present; the four stages are listed in the accompanying box. Radiation therapy in early-stage Hodgkin's disease is curative in 80% to 90% of cases. The lymphatic system can usually tolerate larger doses of radiation than the rest of the body. However, radiation can lead to permanent sterility.

Chemotherapy is usually used for late stages, with a long-term remission rate of 50% to 80%

Nursing Considerations. Nursing care for Hodgkin's disease is similar to that for leukemia.

Non-Hodgkin's Lymphomas

In non-Hodgkin's lymphomas, prognosis and treatment approaches vary considerably, depending on how it is classified. Just as with Hodgkin's disease, correct staging is essential in determining the treatment regimen.

Localized lymphomas may not require any therapy initially, and the patient may survive for several years without significant difficulty. The intermediate- and late-stage lymphomas generally require combination chemotherapy. Although they require more aggressive therapy, they are potentially curable with combination chemotherapy.

Bleeding Disorders

Purpura

Purpura is the term used to describe small hemorrhages in the skin, mucous membranes, or tissues under the skin. Purpura has many causes. *Idiopathic thrombocytopenic purpura* is one type of thrombocytopenia, a decrease in the number of platelets in circulating blood.

Purpura sometimes appears as tiny red spots (*petechiae*), or the spots may extend over larger areas. These hemorrhages are caused by decreased numbers of

Ann Arbor Staging Classification of Hodgkin's Disease

STAGE I	The disease is limited to a single node and surrounding structures. (Radiation treatment has been most effective at this stage.)
STAGE II	The disease involves more than a single node, but is confined to one side of the diaphragm (above or below).
STAGE III	The disease is present both above and below the diaphragm, but does not extend beyond lymph node chains, spleen, or the mouth, nose, and throat areas.
STAGE IV	The disease has extended to the bone marrow, lung, skin, and other areas of the body.

Keys to Patient/Family Teaching
Hemophilia

Patient/family teaching for the patient with hemophilia includes:

◆ Maintenance of safety
◆ Injury prevention
◆ Life-style changes to meet patient's limitations
◆ Medication teaching: medications must be taken as prescribed
◆ Signs and symptoms of difficulties
◆ Methods of administering factor VIII concentrate at home, if appropriate

platelets in the blood or by defective platelet functioning. They are signs that the patient has a tendency to bleed; the person may bleed from the nose, the mouth, or intestinal tract. Treatment may include transfusions of platelets or removal of the spleen. Some patients recover without treatment.

Nursing Alert

◆ Because the blood does not clot correctly in a patient with a bleeding disorder, even a slight injury can result in a serious hemorrhage.
◆ Watch for signs of internal bleeding such as unusual pallor, rapid pulse, restlessness, and drop in blood pressure.
◆ Protect the patient from falls or bumping into objects.

Hemophilia

Hemophilia is an X-linked genetic condition in which the blood is slow to coagulate, due to lack of factor VIII (hemophilia A) or factor IX (hemophilia B) in blood plasma. These factors are substances essential for clotting of blood. Almost all affected individuals are males. A mother may inherit the trait and pass it on to a son. The trait is not passed on by a father to his sons.

Unchecked bleeding may be severe; in hemophiliacs, even a pinprick may cause prolonged oozing of blood. The most minor surgical procedure is risky and is usually preceded by a transfusion of the appropriate blood factor.

Medical Treatment. Factor VIII and IX concentrates are now available for transfusion. Cryoprecipitated antihemophilic factor (obtained from FFP) is another source of factor VIII for treatment of hemophilia A. Some individuals are taught to administer their own concentrate at home. This can quickly control bleeding episodes.

Until recently it was not uncommon for a child to die from hemophilia, but with proper management of symptoms and use of replacement therapy of the missing blood factor, many hemophiliacs now live well into adulthood. Some patients with hemophilia who received treatment with factor concentrates before they began to be heat treated in 1984 have become infected with the HIV virus. If this develops into AIDS, life expectancy is shortened.

Nursing Considerations. In addition to providing prescribed treatments, emotional support is important. It is particularly vital that the patient and family be taught measures to prevent bleeding episodes. The accompanying box lists major teaching subjects.

Disseminated Intravascular Coagulation

Disseminated intravascular coagulation (DIC) is a potentially fatal condition marked first by widespread clotting in small blood vessels and secondarily by hemorrhage. It is a response to some underlying disease or condition, such as a hemolytic transfusion reaction. An essential first step in treatment is to remove the cause. DIC is most often treated in the intensive care unit. It can be rapidly fatal.

Keys for Review

Key Questions for Critical Thinking

1. Identify the blood components and derivatives used in blood transfusions. Explain when blood transfusions are used.
2. Describe the signs and symptoms of a transfusion reaction, including nursing action for each. Identify the most common cause of a fatal transfusion reaction.
3. Compare acute and chronic leukemia, including signs and symptoms, medical and surgical treatment, nursing care, and prognosis.
4. Explain why clotting disorders are dangerous for patients.
5. Compare the anemias. Include the differences in treatment and nursing care for each.

Key Readings

Berkow R (Ed). The Merck Manual of Diagnosis and Therapy, Ed 16. Rahway, NJ, Merck & Co, 1992

Fischbach F. A Manual of Laboratory and Diagnostic Tests, Ed 3. Philadelphia, J.B. Lippincott, 1992

NANDA Nursing Diagnoses: Definitions and Classifications 1992. Philadelphia, North American Nursing Diagnosis Association, 1992

Nursing '94 Drug Handbook. Springhouse, PA, Springhouse, 1994

O'Toole M (Ed). Miller-Keane Encyclopedia and Dictionary of Medicine, Nursing, and Allied Health, Ed 5. Philadelphia, W.B. Saunders, 1992

Smeltzer SC, Bare BG. Brunner and Suddarth's Textbook of Medical-Surgical Nursing, Ed 7. Philadelphia, J.B. Lippincott, 1992

Smith-Temple AJ, Johnson JY. Nurses' Guide to Clinical Procedures, Ed 2. Philadelphia, J.B. Lippincott, 1994

Taylor C, Lillis C, LeMone P. Fundamentals of Nursing: Art and Science of Nursing Care, Ed 2. Philadelphia, J.B. Lippincott, 1993

Thomas CL (Ed). Taber's Cyclopedic Medical Dictionary, Ed 17. Philadelphia, F.A. Davis, 1993

Enrichment Keys

American Association of Blood Banks (AABB), American Red Cross (ARC), and Council of Community Blood Centers (CCBC). Circular of Information for the Use of Human Blood and Blood Components, 1992

National Blood Resource Education Program Nursing Education Group. "Transfusion nursing: trends and practices for the '90s." American Journal of Nursing 91(6) June, 1991

Keys to Learning More

Chapter 76: cancer
Chapter 77: allergic and immune disorders
Chapter 78: HIV, AIDS, and autoimmune disorders
Chapter 79: respiratory disorders
Chapter 85: geriatric disorders
Chapter 90: death and dying

Key Resources

American Heart Association National Center
    7320 Greenville Avenue
    Dallas, TX 75231
    214-748-7212

National Association for Sickle Cell Disease
    4221 Wilshire Boulevard, Suite 360
    Los Angeles, CA 90010
    213-936-7205

National Hemophilia Foundation
    110 Greene Street, Suite 406
    New York, NY 10012
    212-219-8180

76 Cancer

Learning Objectives

- Differentiate between carcinoma, sarcoma, leukemia, and lymphoma. State at least five factors believed to contribute to cancer.
- State the seven danger signals of cancer (CAUTION).
- Describe means used to diagnose cancer and discuss nursing actions in each.
- Identify the four major treatments for cancer and describe related nursing care in each modality.
- Discuss emotional aspects of cancer and nursing actions pertaining to these.

Key Terms

antineoplastic	carcinoma	oncogene
benign	cytology	oncology
biotherapy	leukemia	palliative
biopsy	lymphoma	Pap test
cancer	metastasis	sarcoma
carcinogens	neoplasm	therapeutic

Keys to Understanding This Chapter

Chapter 21: normal blood and lymph structure and function

Chapter 27: assisting the patient to meet nutritional needs

Chapter 28: diet therapy and special diets

Chapter 30: medical asepsis

Chapter 36: therapeutic communication

Chapter 43: body mechanics and positioning

Chapter 45: personal hygiene and skin care

Chapter 46: assisting with elimination

Chapter 50: physical examination and nursing assessment

Chapter 51: infection control techniques

Chapter 52: patient comfort and pain management

Chapter 53: the person who has surgery

Chapter 54: surgical asepsis

Keys to Understanding This Chapter
(continued)

Unit Eleven: pharmacology and medication administration

Chapter 65: leukemia in children

Chapter 75: blood and lymph disorders

Key Points

- Cancer is an abnormal acceleration of cell growth (uncontrolled, progressive replication).
- Cancer can affect any system of the body.
- Cancer can spread to nearby tissues or can metastasize throughout the body.
- The four major types of cancer are carcinoma, sarcoma, leukemia, and lymphoma.
- Many cancers can be cured, if detected early.
- Cancer is treated by chemicals/drugs (chemotherapy), biotherapy (immunotherapy), irradiation, radiation therapy (external or internal), and surgery.
- The leading cause of cancer death is lung cancer, which is often caused by smoking.
- All persons should be taught the seven warning signs of cancer.

Key Topics Outline

General Cancer Information
Diagnostic Tests
    Laboratory Tests and Blood Studies
    X-ray Evaluations
    Other Diagnostic Tests
    Invasive Diagnostic Techniques
Medical and Surgical Treatments
    Common Medical Treatments
    Common Surgical Treatments
Nursing Process
    Data Collection
    Nursing Diagnosis
    Planning and Implementation
    Evaluation

Millions of dollars are spent each year by frantic patients and their families in an effort to cure cancer. Many of these people could have been treated effectively if they had gone to a reputable physician early in the course of the disease.

The medical specialty concerned with cancer and its treatment is **oncology**. The specialist is called an *oncologist* and the nurse is an *oncology nurse*. Because the spread of cancer is often via the blood and lymphatic system, and because the treatment of many blood and lymphatic disorders uses the same modalities as treatment for cancer, the specialist treating the cancer may also be called a *hematologist*. Closely associated with these specialties is the *radiologist*, who administers radiation therapy.

General Cancer Information

Cancer, also known as **carcinoma**, is a group of more than 150 diseases characterized by abnormal alteration in cell growth. The one thing that distinguishes all cancer cells from normal cells is *uncontrolled, progressive replication* (reproduction). Cancer is a disorderly growth of body cells that undermines and spreads through normal tissues. For this reason, it is also referred to as **neoplasm**, which means "new growth."

Not all growths or tumors are cancers. Noncancerous tumors are identified as **benign** or *nonmalignant.* They are often self-contained and usually do not spread a great deal. Neoplasms, when malignant, usually are not confined within a capsule and can spread to nearby tissues. They also spread to other parts of the body through the blood and the lymph systems. This is called **metastasis**.

The four major groups of cancer are identified in the accompanying box.

Some types of cancer grow more rapidly than others.

Cancer Progression

The place where the cancer starts is called the *primary site*; the metastatic sites are known as *secondary sites* or secondary lesions. Cancer may spread through the body by:

◆ Extending directly into nearby tissue or a body cavity, such as the abdomen or chest (the most frequently affected sites)
◆ Traveling through blood vessels to other parts of the body, especially the lungs, bones, and liver (Fig. 76-1).

Prognosis

Generally, if cancer is detected early, while in the primary site, prognosis for a cure is favorable. In certain malignancies, even in advanced states, cure is also possible. Examples include acute leukemias, some forms of advanced lymphomas, and advanced carcinomas, such as testicular carcinoma. In these situations, cure is currently possible for a significant percentage of patients. The treatment in these cases is usually combination therapy—several different modalities used together.

The definition of *cure* when referring to cancer is variable, based on the cancer type. Currently over 8 million Americans are alive who have had cancer. According to the American Cancer Society (ACS) definition, 5 years without symptoms following treatment is usually considered as "cured." It is appropriate, however, to view cancer as a chronic illness because for many types of cancer a 5-year time line is not significant.

Incidence of Cancer

One in three Americans now living will have cancer during their lifetime. Cancer is second only to heart disease as a cause of adult deaths in the United States. Many of these deaths might have been saved with early detection and treatment. Cancer incidence and mortal-

Four Major Groups of Cancer

◆ **Carcinomas,** such as lung or colon cancer, arise from *epithelial* tissues.
◆ **Sarcomas,** including those of bone and muscle, arise in *connective* tissue.
◆ **Leukemias** arise from *blood-forming organs* (bone marrow, spleen).
◆ **Lymphomas** originate in the *lymphoreticular* system (lymphatic tissue).

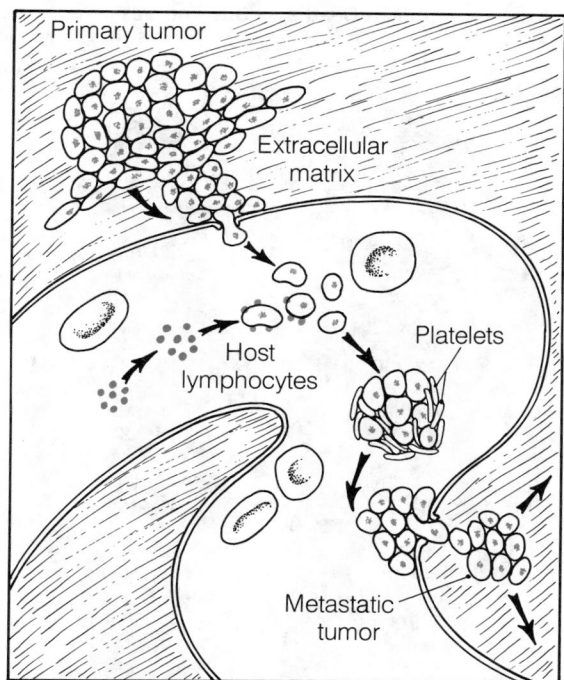

Figure 76-1. Mechanism of hematogenic metastasis. Adapted from Kumar V., et al. Basic Pathology, 6th ed. Philadelphia, W.B. Saunders, 1992.

ity rates are generally higher for African Americans than for white Americans. This trend is thought to occur because cancers in African American population are often diagnosed at a later stage.

Figure 76-2 illustrates cancer incidence and deaths by site and gender.

Lung cancer has now overtaken breast cancer as the leading cause of cancer deaths in women, even though breast cancer currently has the highest incidence. The increase of lung cancer is attributed primarily to cigarette smoking. The second leading cause of cancer deaths in women is breast cancer, with cancer of the colon and rectum being the next most frequent.

Cancer deaths in men occur, in order of descending frequency, as follows: lungs, prostate gland, and colon and rectum. It should also be noted that prostate cancer is the leading site of incidence. This emphasizes the need for early detection and treatment.

Causes of Cancer

Authorities believe that cancer develops from a combination of causes, rather than from any one factor. **Carcinogens** are substances known to cause or promote cancer. Some carcinogens are created by human beings (eg, cigarette smoke, smog). Other carcinogens are found naturally in our environment (eg, viruses, ultraviolet radiation). Carcinogens can work in either of two ways.

♦ Cause changes that turn a normal cell into a cancer cell
♦ Create conditions that influence other factors to cause the cancer

> **Key Concept**
>
> The leading cause of cancer deaths in both men and women is *lung cancer,* which is directly related to cigarette smoking.

Asbestos, cigarette smoke, benzene, and mustard gas are just a few substances that have been shown to have a direct causal relationship between exposure and the development of cancer. Although not an actual agent, chronic irritation can predispose to the development of cancer. Examples of chronic irritation include pipe smoke, sunlight, friction on a mole, and cervical irritation.

Cancer Research

Many cancers develop slowly, often 5 to 40 years after exposure to a carcinogen. In contrast, some people exposed to carcinogens never develop cancer. Researchers continue to conduct studies to help us better understand the role of carcinogens in cancer development.

Human clinical trials are the basis for research. They are systematic evaluations of new cancer treatments, begun only after the treatment has been shown to be beneficial in animal or laboratory testing. Researchers use clinical trials to determine the effect of the therapy on a tumor, to compare different combinations of treatments, or to determine the most effective dose of a drug.

Research into cancer prevention has provided new hope for persons facing higher risks for developing cancer. *Quality of life studies* are also conducted as part of the clinical trials. The following are examples of current research.

Oncogenes are bits of genetic material transmitted on chromosomes, which control the development of inherited characteristics. Researchers believe oncogenes are present in every body cell and remain harmless until triggered. Once triggered, however, oncogenes transform normal cells into cancerous cells.

Research using *genetic engineering* allows correction of impaired immune systems or transplantation of normal copies of genes into cells that have mutated genes.

Research into cancer prevention has provided new hope for persons facing higher risks for developing cancer. *Hormonal manipulation,* commonly referred to as "the tamoxifen study," is currently being studied in women who have a high risk for developing breast cancer.

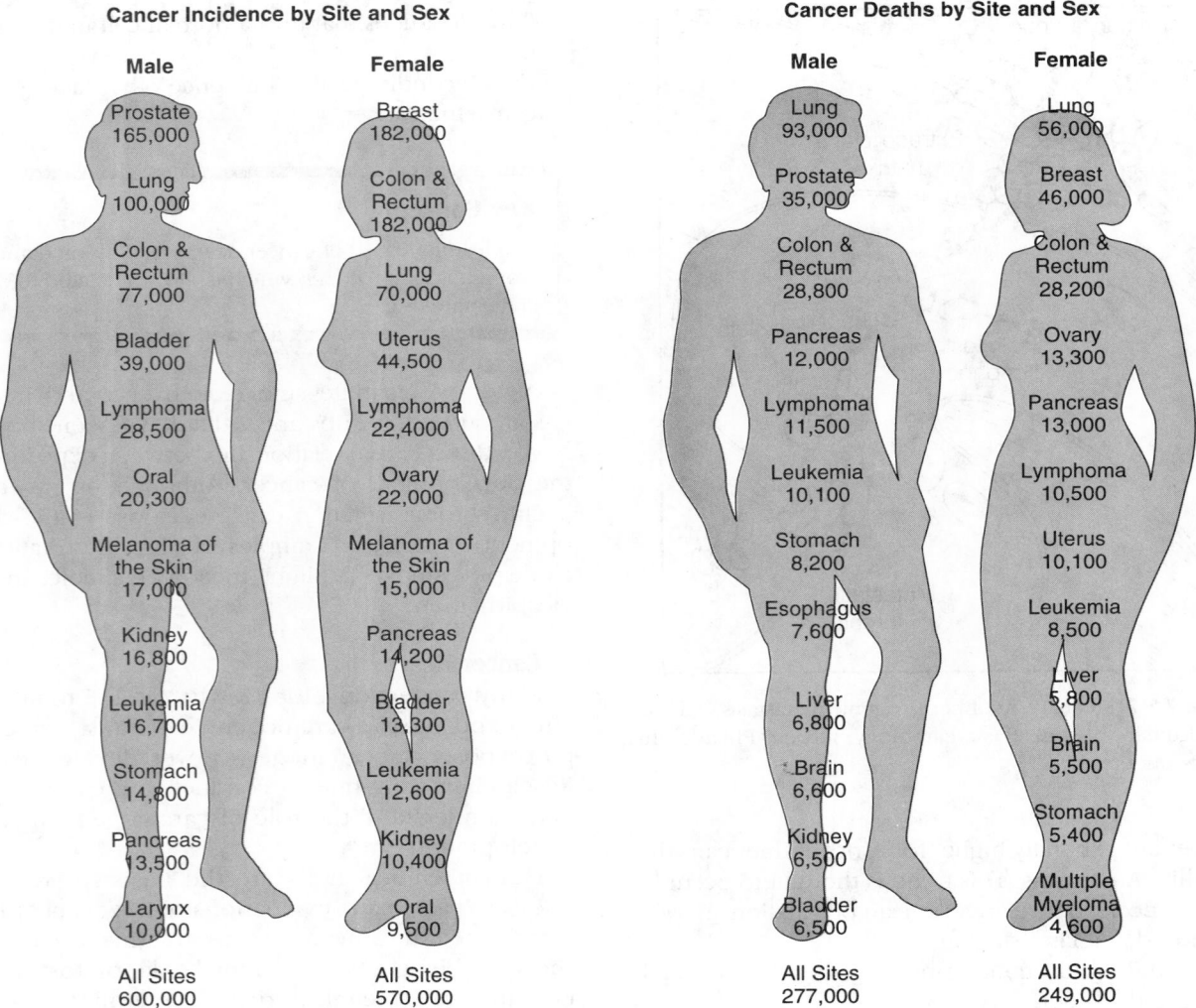

Figure 76-2. Leading sites of cancer incidence and death in males and females. Data from American Cancer Society: Cancer Facts and Figures, 1993.

Nurses, too, are performing cancer research. Research is ongoing and covers the spectrum from understanding attitudes regarding cancer prevention through measuring the effects of cancer treatment on long-term survival.

> ### Key Concept
>
> Early detection promises the highest rate of survival for patients with cancer. Periodic physical examinations and self-examinations are important components of early detection.

Cancer Prevention

In addition to eliminating known carcinogens from the environment, the National Cancer Institute and the ACS have proposed dietary guidelines. Following these

guidelines is believed to lower the incidence of cancer. The major points of these guidelines are:

- Avoid obesity
- Reduce fat intake
- Increase fiber intake
- Include vegetables and fruits in the diet
- If you drink, limit consumption of alcohol
- Limit consumption of salted, pickled, smoked, and nitrite-cured foods

Diagnostic Tests

Diagnostic evaluations can evoke fear and anxiety in patients and their families. The nurse can play a major role in providing information and support. The first step in providing this support is to accurately assess both the patient's and the family's desire to know, as well as

Key Abbreviations and Acronyms in Cancer

ACS	American Cancer Sociey
BRM	Biological response modifiers
BSE	Breast self-examination
CA	Cancer
CAF	Cytoxan, Adriamycin, fluorouracil
CEA	Carcinoembryonic antigen
CMF	Cytoxan, methotrexate, fluorouracil
CSF	Colony-stimulating factors
5-FU	5-Fluorouracil
IFN	Interferon
Pap test	Papanicolaou test (smear)
PCA pump	Patient-controlled analgesia pump
PIC line	Peripheral indwelling catheter
PICC	Peripherally inserted central catheter
PSA	Prostate specific antigen
TSE	Testicular self-examination

their ability to understand, the reason for the procedure. Specific nursing considerations for each diagnostic test are contained in the chapter in which the procedure is presented.

Laboratory Tests and Blood Studies

Laboratory tests and blood studies help to diagnose cancer. Some malignancies can alter the chemical composition of the blood or alter the hematologic status of the patient. There may be distinct changes. For example, in cancer of the prostate, a specific antigen is present in the blood, the PSA, prostate-specific antigen. The PSA provides a valuable screening test.

Cytology. The study of cells (**cytology**) can contribute to diagnosis. A cytologic examination is done on sputum, bronchial washings, vaginal and cervical secretions, prostatic secretions, pleural secretions, or gastric washings. This method is less accurate than biopsy, but has proven value, particularly in cancer of the cervix and uterus. The test most frequently used to detect cancer of the cervix and uterus is the **Pap test**, named after Dr. Papanicolaou, who developed a method for examining body secretions for malignant cells. The Pap test should constitute an important part of the physical examination of every woman who is over age 20 or who is sexually active.

Tumor Markers. Tumor markers are specific proteins, antigens, genes, hormones, and enzymes released by tumors. These substances can be found in the blood

and can be helpful in monitoring the response of a tumor to treatment, assessing the extent of tumor involvement, or detecting recurrent cancer. These tumor markers can lack specificity. Therefore, they are often a poor screening tool to detect the initial presence of cancer.

One commonly used tumor marker is CEA (carcinoembryonic antigen), which is present in the fetus, but not normally after birth. It is often produced in cancer. However, it may also be initiated by liver disorders, benign tumors, and chronic heavy smoking. Therefore, it is useful in monitoring response to cancer treatment, but not in initial diagnosis.

X-ray Evaluations

Radiologic studies allow for visualization of the internal structures of the body. These radiographs may view the function of an entire organ system such as a gastrointestinal series of the digestive system. They may also be site specific, such as a chest x-ray or a mammogram.

Tomography. Computed tomography (CT) scanning can provide sectional views of the various structures of the body. It is one of the most useful tools in the staging of malignancies. Many malignancies are "staged," that is, the extent of tumor invasion or involvement is categorized, according to predefined criteria. An example of staging is the Ann Arbor Staging Classification of Hodgkin's Disease, as shown in Chapter 75. By staging a malignancy, the physician can better determine the treatment of choice. CT scanning is most useful for tumors in the chest, abdominal cavity, and brain.

Other Diagnostic Tests

Ultrasonography. This noninvasive technique uses sound waves that can be directed into specific tissues. This is most applicable in detecting tumors within the pelvis, retroperitoneum, and peritoneum. Ultrasound has many clinical diagnostic applications and is discussed in relationship to pregnancy, as well as in diagnosing disorders of all body systems.

Magnetic Resonance Imaging. Magnetic resonance imaging (MRI) can also provide sectional images of the body but without the use of ionizing radiation. With the use of magnetic fields it can aid in detecting, localizing, and staging malignant disease in the central nervous system, musculoskeletal system, spine, head, and neck.

Invasive Diagnostic Techniques

Endoscopy. Periodic physical examination is important. Many Americans follow the ACS recommended guidelines. Sometimes, physicians find an abnormality and need to evaluate findings more closely. Instruments such as the sigmoidoscope, vaginal speculum, colonoscope, gastroscope, bronchoscope, and laryngoscope may be used for visual observation of internal organs. Examinations with these scopes are discussed in the chapters of this unit related to specific body systems.

Exploratory Surgery and Biopsy. In some cases, surgery must be done to visualize, examine, and take a sample **biopsy** of internal lesions or lymph nodes. *Biopsy is the most important means of diagnosing cancer.* The pathologist studies a small sample of tissue removed from the organ in question. In almost all cases, it can be determined whether the lesion is benign or malignant.

Frozen Section. When a biopsy has been done of a nodule or a total specimen has been excised, the tissue is quickly frozen and sliced very thin; the pathologist studies the specimen under the microscope. This method can be done while the patient remains anesthetized. The pathologist reports the findings to the surgeon who then decides the type of surgery needed.

Medical and Surgical Treatments

Common Medical Treatments

Chemotherapy

The term *chemotherapy* means the use of chemical agents to destroy cancer cells. There are several therapeutic indications for chemotherapy:

◆ Chemotherapy can be used to treat widespread or metastatic disease because it is a systemic rather than a local treatment.
◆ Chemotherapy can provide a *cure* for patients with certain types of cancer, even in advanced stages. Examples include acute leukemias, some types of lymphomas, and testicular cancer.
◆ Chemotherapy is used for temporary control and palliation of tumor-related difficulties.
◆ Chemotherapy may be used after surgery to treat metastases or in an attempt to prevent metastases from occurring (*adjuvant therapy*).

Nursing skills in caring for patients receiving chemotherapy are discussed in the Nursing Process section of this chapter.

Chemotherapeutic Agents. There are two basic classifications of **antineoplastic** (against cancer) chemotherapeutic agents. These are:

◆ *Cell-cycle specific:* actions are most effective during cell proliferation
◆ *Cell-cycle nonspecific:* actions are independent of cellular cycles

Examples of both of these are given in the accompanying box.

To understand how chemotherapeutic agents break the cycle of cell division and replication, it is necessary to understand the cell cycle (Fig. 76-3). Cancer cells have a proportionally higher number of cells dividing at any one time than do normal cells because their replication and growth are uncontrolled and progressive. Chemotherapeutic agents are generally most effective when cells are dividing. Therefore, malignant cells are

---

Key Medications
for Cancer Chemotherapy

Examples of Cell-Cycle Specific Agents

◆ *antimetabolites:*
—fluorouracil, 5-fluorouracil, 5-FU (Adrucil, Efudex)
—mercaptopurine, 6-mercaptopurine, 6-MP (Purinethol)
—methotrexate, methotrexate sodium (Folex, Mexate)
◆ *vinca alkaloids:*
—vinblastine sulfate, VLB (velban, Velsar)
—vincristine sulfate (Oncovin)

Examples of Cell-Cycle Nonspecific Agents

◆ *alkylating agents:*
—chlorambucil (Leukeran)
—cisplatin, cis-platinum (Platinol)
—cyclophosphamide (Cytoxan, Neosar)
—mechlorethamine HCl, nitrogen mustard (Mustargen)
—thiotepa (Thiotepa)
◆ *nitrosureas:*
—lomustine, CCNU (CeeNu)
—streptozocin (Zanosar)
◆ *hormones* (ACTH, cortisone, prednisone, sex hormones)
◆ antineoplastics that *alter hormone balance:*
—aminoglutethimide (Cytadren)
—flutamide (Eutexin)
—tamoxifen citrate (Nolvadex, Tamofen)
◆ *antitumor antibiotics:*
—dactinomycin (Cosmegen)
—doxorubicin HCL (Adriamycin, Rubex)
—mitomycin-C (Mutamycin)
—plicamycin, mithramycin (Mithracin)

Examples of Frequently Used Combinations

—CMF: cytoxan, methotrexate, fluorouracil
—CAF: cytoxan, Adriamycin, fluorouracil
(Both are often combined with an antiemetic and a corticosteroid)

Nursing considerations relating to administration of chemotherapeutic drugs are discussed in the text. *Note:* Most patients receive *combinations*.

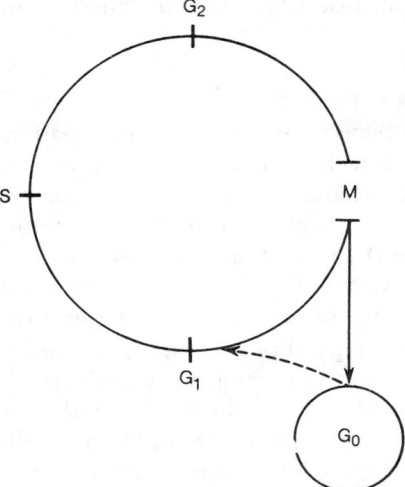

Figure 76-3. Phases of the cell cycle. The cycle represents the interval from the midpoint of mitosis to the subsequent end point in mitosis in a daughter cell. G_0 is the resting or dormant phase of the cell cycle. G_1 is the postmitotic phase during which RNA and protein synthesis is increased and cell growth occurs. The S phase represents synthesis of nucleic acids with chromosome replication in preparation for cell mitosis. During G_2, RNA and protein synthesis occurs as in G_1. Cell division occurs in M (mitosis). (Porth C.M. Pathophysiology: Concepts of Altered Health State, Ed 4. Philadelphia, J.B. Lippincott, 1994.)

more susceptible to chemotherapeutic agents than are normal cells.

Cell-cycle specific agents are most effective against rapidly growing tumors. Examples are given in the accompanying box. The action of *cell-cycle nonspecific agents* is not confined to a specific phase of cell division. Therefore, they may be effective on large tumors that have fewer actively dividing cells. They may also be combined with other agents for broader coverage (see accompanying box.)

Another chemotherapeutic approach to treating cancer involves the use of *hormone* and *steroid* compounds. Hormone therapy can produce temporary regression of metastatic cancers, especially those that originate in reproductive organs (breast or prostate carcinomas). Alteration of the endocrine environment of the body seems to reduce some malignancies or prevent them from proliferating.

Recent research has shown that the most effective treatment for many cancers is a *combination* of several chemotherapeutic drugs. The drugs may be rotated in accordance with the reactions of the cells or the action of the drug. One way of measuring the cellular reactions is by studying tumor markers.

Administration Routes and Devices. Chemotherapeutic agents can be administered by a variety of routes. These include the oral, intramuscular, intracavitary, intraperitoneal, topical, intra-arterial, intrapleural, and intravenous routes.

Vascular Access Devices. If chemotherapy is to be given intravenously or intra-arterially, a vascular access device is often used. Because chemotherapeutic agents can damage tissue and many patients have poor veins, these devices are ideal. They are more convenient, more comfortable for the patient, and also eliminate the danger inherent in repeated venipunctures. Selection of a vascular access device considers frequency of use, length of treatment, integrity of veins, and patient preference. Vascular access devices include:

♦ Peripheral access device, peripheral indwelling catheter (PIC) line, PICC line (peripherally inserted central catheter)
♦ Central venous access (subcutaneous port)
♦ External catheters (Hickman, Broviac)

Chemotherapy Infusion Pump. In some cases chemotherapeutic agents are administered on a constant basis by means of a chemotherapy infusion pump. A small pump (about the size of a hockey puck) is surgically implanted under the patient's skin in the abdomen. This technique can administer the drug directly into the cancerous organ. The pump can also be external and can be managed with relative ease by the patient or home care nurse.

When the patient has an implantable chemotherapy pump, the nurse must be alert constantly for side effects. Possible side effects include chemical hepatitis and gastritis. With this method of administration, the patient may show undesirable side effects more quickly and the symptoms are much more difficult to alleviate. When the implanted pump is empty, it is filled with normal saline through the Silastic port on the pump or is removed, if therapy is completed.

Key Concept

The person undergoing chemotherapy for cancer has both physical and emotional needs. Follow the protocol for treatment, as established by your healthcare facility. Be supportive. A referral to professional counseling or chaplaincy services may be beneficial to the patient and/or family.

Biologic Therapy (Immunotherapy)

Nurses must be knowledgeable about the use of biologic therapies to properly administer the drugs and evaluate side effects. Patients must be taught relevant self-care strategies.

Evidence indicates that host immunity is an important factor in resistance to cancer. The immune response is a process of surveillance, recognition, and attacking foreign cells. The manipulation of the immune response is called **biotherapy** or *immunotherapy* and is the newest modality for cancer treatment. The substances used are called *biological response modifiers* (BRM).

Biotherapy can be *active* (intradermal injection of irradiated tumor cells), *passive* (injection of antibodies) or *nonspecific* (improving the entire immune system). Substances can be used to boost or direct the immune system or to restore the body's normal defenses. Research into this field continues and it is thought that with time, biologics will demonstrate the most efficacy when used in combination with other modalities of cancer treatment.

Monoclonal Antibodies. These are biologics produced by genetically fusing cancer cells with normal cells. The "new" cells seek out specific targets on cancer cells. Their use in cancer diagnosis and treatment is being studied. Use of these cells carries risk of serious allergic reactions. Other side effects include headaches, wheezing, fever, chills, rash, nausea, vomiting, and tachycardia.

Interferons (IFN). Interferons yield an antiviral effect by interfering in RNA synthesis. They convert inactive immune cells into active cells that attack tumor cells directly. Interferon may also directly inhibit (slow) the proliferation (growth) of malignant cells. The most common side effects are flulike symptoms including headaches, fever, chills, muscle aches, weakness, and tachycardia. This type of reaction typically decreases in severity with continued treatment. In larger doses, IFN can cause lowered blood counts, gastrointestinal symptoms, central nervous system disturbances, and hair loss.

Interleukin-2. This biologic is essential for the growth of infection-fighting T cells. It has demonstrated some value in treatment of renal cancer, melanomas, and non-Hodgkin's lymphoma. Toxicities are more severe, causing treatments to be given primarily in the acute care setting. Increased capillary permeability can occur, which causes hypotension, ascites, and edema (including pulmonary edema). Interleukin-2 can also cause flulike symptoms.

Colony-Stimulating Factors (CSFs). These encourage growth and maturation of blood cell components including granulocytes, macrophages, lymphocytes, monocytes, erythrocytes, and platelets. Accelerated recovery of these cells following the damage caused by cancer treatment has decreased the resulting *neutropenia* (decreased neutrophils). It also allows patients to tolerate higher doses, with less *myelosuppression* (reduction in bone marrow function.) Side effects of CSFs

generally include bone pain or flulike symptoms and rash.

Radiation Therapy

In addition to its use in diagnosis, radiation is used for therapy in cancer. Radiation therapy is indicated in many cases of cancer and may be used as either a **therapeutic** (curative) treatment or a **palliative** treatment (relief without cure). In radiation therapy, the organ is exposed to radioactive agents that destroy malignant cells.

Three types of rays are involved in radiation diagnosis and therapy: alpha, beta, and gamma rays. *Alpha* and *beta* rays can penetrate only the upper layer of the skin. *Gamma* rays, on the other hand, can penetrate deeply into body tissues. In addition to natural radioactive isotopes of certain elements such as radium, radioactive isotopes of elements such as iodine and gold are produced artificially.

There are two types of radiation therapy, external beam radiation and internal (implanted) radiation.

External Beam Radiation. In therapy, both deep and surface x-rays are used, as well as cobalt, radium, and radioactive isotopes of other elements. Extreme precautions are taken to protect both patients and staff and healthy cells from the hazards involved in administering radiation therapy. Linear accelerators have made it possible to deliver high doses of irradiation to deep-seated malignancies, without damaging critical body organs and without causing severe surface skin reactions.

Nursing care is directed toward ensuring the patient's safety and carrying out measures that provide relief of side effects, which often occur. Undesirable side effects include decreased appetite, abdominal cramping, and diarrhea. Some of the special nursing care is described in the Nursing Process section of this chapter.

Internal Radiation—Implanted/Injected Radioactive Isotopes. Radioactive substances can be targeted internally to a specific cancerous site to destroy it from within. Implanted isotopes can be placed close to cancer cells. Such implants may be in the form of "seeds" containing a radioactive source. One example is that of strontium 89, which is used for metastatic bone cancer. Because the radioactive isotope is bone seeking, it seeks out the cancerous lesions. Implantable radioactive isotopes are also implanted directly into the cervix to treat cancer there.

Internal radiation has several advantages over external radiation therapy:

- ◆ It exposes and damages fewer normal cells.
- ◆ A higher dose can be given to the tumor.
- ◆ Other tissues are less likely to be exposed to radiation.
- ◆ Radiation can be given over a shorter period of time.

Nursing considerations are given in the Nursing Process section of this chapter.

The keys to safety with radiation are *time*, *distance*, and *shielding*. Limit the *time* spent near the source of radiation. Increase the *distance* you stand from the source and use available *shielding* to block radiation.

Common Surgical Treatments

The nurse's role is cancer surgery includes preoperative care and patient teaching as described in Chapter 53 and elsewhere. The importance of patient teaching cannot be overemphasized. If postoperative exercises are recommended, such as those following mastectomy, the patient can be taught the exercises preoperatively to be able to do them more effectively after surgery.

It is necessary to allow patients to participate in their own treatment plan as much as possible. Patient adaptation depends on the person's own security and self-image. Kindness, understanding, and active listening on the part of the nurse can provide an atmosphere in which patients are free to express themselves.

Removal of Cancerous Tissues. Complete removal of all malignant tissue before it metastasizes is the ideal treatment. Surgery usually involves removal not only of the tumor, but also of an area of surrounding tissue. This is done to determine if the cancer has spread, as well as to remove any malignant cells that may have spread to the surrounding area.

Prophylactic Surgery. Surgery may also be used as a preventive measure in cancerous lesions, such as hairy moles. This is called *prophylactic* or *preventive surgery.* In addition, some of the endocrine glands known to influence the development of specific cancers can be removed, such as in testicular cancer. In some cases, if cancer is discovered in one breast, both breasts are removed, as a prophylactic measure.

Palliative Surgery. Palliative measures are performed to relieve the complications of malignancies that cannot be totally excised. The goal of this type of surgery is not to cure, but to promote comfort for the patient.

Bone Marrow Transplant and Other Specialized Procedures. In some cases of leukemia, bone marrow transplant is effective. This procedure is discussed in Chapter 75.

Other specialized procedures are described in the discussion of disorders of specific body systems throughout this unit.

❖ Nursing Process

Data Collection

Chapter 50 describes some basic nursing assessment techniques. This assessment establishes a baseline for future comparison and determines the presence of suspected disorders, such as cancer. The nurse should report any changes in baseline level. The accompanying box lists some components of the nursing assessment for symptoms of cancer.

A patient may report unexplained loss of weight, a general feeling of discomfort, or a change in elimination habits or other normal function. Everyone should be taught to *report immediately* any of the warning signs identified by the ACS, as presented in the accompanying box. People do not always pay attention to slightly uncomfortable sensations that serve as warnings. These are not normal; if they last for any length of time, they should be investigated.

Usually, pain does not appear until the later stages of cancer, when the tumor enlarges enough to cause pressure on surrounding tissues.

Self-examination techniques are important skills for nurses to teach their patients. Pamphlets, which reinforce patient teaching techniques, are readily available from the ACS. Cancer screening guidelines are also available; these encourage the public to participate in decisions regarding screening tests applicable for them based on age, sex, and risk factors.

In addition, the nurse observes the patient's emotional response to the disorder or disease. Does the patient need assistance to meet daily needs? Does the disorder affect social activities or self-esteem? Is the disorder life-threatening? Is the patient anxious or fearful of the outcome? Is ongoing counseling, rehabilitation, or home care needed? Is a support group available? What are the reactions of family members? Will the patient be a candidate for hospice care?

Nursing Diagnosis

Based on data collection, nursing diagnoses are formulated for the person with cancer. These nursing diagnoses can relate to any body system, depending on the location of the cancer. Some diagnoses have several causal factors. Examples of nursing diagnoses that may be seen on a patient's nursing care plan are:

- Pain related to progression of disease, diagnostic procedures
- Chronic Pain related to bone metastasis, disdain for pharmacologic remedies, need to self-control pain
- Altered Nutrition: Less Than Body Requirements related to anorexia, vomiting, nausea
- Impaired Skin Integrity related to radiation therapy, incontinence
- High Risk for Infection related to inadequate secondary defenses, malnutrition, chronic disease process
- Spiritual Distress related to challenged belief system
- Anticipatory Grieving related to anticipated loss of life, family, friends, possessions
- Altered Thought Processes related to adjustment to morphine, brain metastases

Planning and Implementation

The patient and nurse plan together for effective care to meet patient needs, based on the specific nursing diagnosis. The nurse provides preoperative and postoperative care for the patient undergoing various surgical procedures. The nurse also provides supportive care during testing and treatment modalities.

The patient with cancer may require assistance in meeting many needs, ranging from activities of daily living to total nursing care. Because the diagnosis of cancer is threatening to most patients, the person may need assistance or professional counseling to deal with emotional problems. Teaching is important so the patient and family understand more about the disorder, its prognosis, and treatment. A nursing care plan is developed to meet these needs. A sample Nursing Care Plan for a patient with cancer is presented.

Providing Care During Chemotherapy

Chemotherapy should be administered by specially trained nurses. Care must be taken during administration because antineoplastic drugs kill normal cells in addition to cancer cells. Nursing skills to provide nursing safety during parenteral administration of chemotherapeutic drugs are:

- Wear gloves, gowns, and protective eyewear when preparing and administering these medications. *(Rationale: This protects nurse from personal injury.)*
- Do not allow these drugs to come in contact with your eyes or mucous membranes. If this should occur, rinse the part thoroughly with clear water for at least 5 minutes. Obtain first aid immediately.
- Be knowledgeable about medications being administered. *(Rationale: This provides quality patient care.)* No chemotherapeutic agent should be administered without careful review of administration guidelines and side effects.
- Chemotherapeutic agents can be administered orally. No special handling precautions are needed in this case.

Nursing skills related to care of the patient receiving chemotherapy are summarized in the accompanying box.

Providing Care During Radiation Therapy

Special care is necessary for the patient receiving radiation. Again the nurse protects herself or himself from radiation rays. The accompanying box lists nursing care of patients receiving external beam therapy and radioactive implant.

Helga Borne is a 78-year-old woman with a history of cancer of the left breast, which was diagnosed and treated through modified radical mastectomy 4 years ago. Her admitting diagnosis is fracture of T-12 and L-1 secondary to bone metastasis. She is receiving radiation therapy and physical therapy to facilitate ambulation with a brace. Bone scans reveal extensive metastasis and her prognosis is limited. She reports constant pain. She and her husband live in a small apartment and are visited at least weekly by a daughter who lives about 30 miles away. Fiercely independent and stoic in regard to pain, she is only beginning to ask questions about what the future holds for her and voicing doubts about her ability to manage. Two nursing diagnoses are developed here.

Nursing Diagnosis: *Knowledge Deficit Regarding Radiation Therapy Related to Lack of Previous Experience*

Goal: By 10/6 patient correctly describes: a) what to expect during radiation therapy, b) the goal of therapy, c) common side effects and what can be done to minimize their occurrence or severity, and d) what she can do to facilitate healing during this time.

Nursing Actions (assess/do/teach)	Rationale	Evaluative Statement
1. Assess both the patient and family's knowledge level regarding radiation therapy; carefully elicit any misconceptions and anxieties.	Teaching is most successful when specifically directed to the individual's learning needs.	10/5; Goal met; patient accurately described radiation therapy, noting her role and common side effects.
2. Teach the patient and family what radiation therapy is, its goal, what will be expected of the patient during treatment, common side effects to be alert for and what can be done to minimize their occurrence or severity; offer pertinent reading materials.	Accurate knowledge is an antidote for anxiety and prepares the patient to participate maximally in her treatment	
	Anxiety during a teaching session can compromise learning; reading materials will reinforce what was taught and provide a ready reference.	

(continued)

Adequate explanation of therapy to the patient is necessary. The patient should understand that the treatment will not hurt, it will only take a few minutes, and the area being treated will not feel hot. The patient has a right to understand the goal of therapy and the possible side effects of radiation.

Although it may be frightening to the patient to be alone during the radiation therapy, much of this anxiety can be minimized by explaining before therapy is begun the need to avoid radiation exposure to healthcare personnel.

When caring for a patient who has a radioactive implant (and in some cases after intravenous administration of a radioactive isotope), you should first become familiar with the policies and procedures of the institution. Take precautions to protect yourself and the patient's visitors from excessive radiation, by following general safety principles.

Assisting the Patient to Receive Nourishment

Cancer can deplete the body of proteins and affect total nutrition. The diet must be high in proteins, carbohydrates, and vitamins. The importance of good nutrition and maintenance of fluid/electrolyte balance cannot be stressed enough, particularly for patients on intensive radiation or chemotherapy. Chapters 27 and 28 give hints for assisting with nutrition. Eating several small

Nursing Diagnosis: *Impaired Adjustment Related to Grave Prognosis and Limited Time to complete "Unfinished Business"*

Goal 1: By 10/6 the patient will feel free to express her concerns about the future.

Goal 2: By 10/8 the patient will begin to explore possible options for care as her ability to manage independently decreases.

Nursing Actions (assess/do/teach)	Rationale	Evaluative Statement
1. Share with the patient that it is "normal" to have many concerns about the future at a time like this; use statements like, "it must be hard for you to think ahead to the future . . . ?" to elicit her concerns; evaluate her knowledge of care options during the terminal phase of her illness (home health care, hospice, hospitalization) and counsel appropriately.	Normalizing anxieties and fears makes them easier to discuss. Open-ended statements communicate your care and willingness to share her struggle.	10/6; Goal 1 met; patient has expressed how fearful she is of losing control and needing to be dependent on others. 10/7; Goal 2 partially met; patient knew very little about hospice care but has been talking about this option and reading literature
2. Communicate to the patient that there is no need for her to face this life challenge alone and that there are many supports she can draw on; educate about community resources.	Diffuses the overwhelming stress of what might happen in the future and that it might possibly be beyond the patient's control.	

meals is easier than eating large meals. Nutritional supplements may also be ordered.

It is important for patients undergoing chemotherapy or radiation to be placed on an intensive vitamin regimen. This regimen usually includes β-carotene (beta-carotene), vitamins E and C, and a daily multivitamin. B vitamins are often not given because they become toxic when combined with chemotherapy.

Minerals are also important. The patient is advised to eat liver and other red meats, good sources of iron to rebuild red blood cells. If the patient is not able to eat liver, gelcaps containing liver amino aids (but not fat) are available. The patient may be advised to take other mineral supplements, such as selenium or potassium, and is encouraged to eat yogurt. A dietary supplement, MXM, contains garlic and nutrients found in cruciferous vegetables (broccoli, cauliflower); it may be taken as a protective measure if the patient is not eating.

One problem in the patient receiving chemotherapy or radiation is destruction of platelets, which are necessary for blood clotting. Blood counts are done regularly. Therapy may need to be canceled if the patient's platelet count becomes too low.

Key Concepts

- ◆ Dietary preferences may change during therapy. If a mineral or vitamin is missing from the diet, it should be replaced with supplements.
- ◆ Patients on chemotherapy are often excessively thirsty. They should be taught to vary fluids taken and not to drink only plain water. *(Rationale: Excessive plain water can cause electrolyte imbalances.)*
- ◆ Eating fresh parsley is one of the few known means of building up the platelet count. Encourage the patient to eat as much as 1/2 cup of fresh parsley daily. You can assist the patient to find palatable ways to prepare it. If all else fails, gelcaps containing parsley are available, although fresh parsley works better.

Managing Nausea and Vomiting

Many patients on chemotherapy or radiation therapy are nauseated. Some have great difficulty in eating or in keeping food down. Sometimes therapies such as guided imagery help with this. The patient can be distracted or may have visitors during meals. In addition, many patients are placed on antiemetics, either as a precautionary measure of if nausea actually occurs. Table 76-1 lists commonly prescribed antiemetics.

Providing Special Skin Care

Because some cancer patients cannot eat, they lose weight and become emaciated. In addition, therapies such as radiation and chemotherapy may make the skin more friable. Many aspects of skin care are presented in Chapter 45. Skin care in external radiation therapy is presented earlier in the current chapter in a box.

Teach the patient to keep the skin clean and dry. A good moisturizing lotion should be used. After radiation treatments for cancer of the pelvis or abdomen, the skin over the sacrum needs special attention.

If the patient is incontinent, help the person to manage the problem through the use of absorbent pads and frequent toileting. Aim to keep the skin as clean and dry as possible.

Assisting With Special Mouth Care

The patient on radiation or chemotherapy is subject to mouth sores, including mucositis, canker sores, and esophageal ulcers. The patient would be more comfortable using a mouthwash of salt or soda water because commercial products may contain alcohol or other substances that may cause irritation. Eating acidic foods may also aggravate the problem. Regular administration of L-lysine may help prevent mouth ulcerations.

If ulcerations and irritation persist, a "swish and swallow" medication may be prescribed. These liquid medications are often a mixture of diphenhydramine (Benadryl), viscous Xylocaine, and sometimes an antacid such as Mylanta.

Preventing Secondary Infections

Radiation or chemotherapy frequently renders the patient more susceptible to infections, because the white blood cell count is depressed. In addition, cancerous cells deprived of food and oxygen die. As this dead tissue sloughs, it may leave a raw open area or an ulcer, which may bleed if the cancerous growth involves blood vessels. This open surface provides an excellent entrance for bacteria.

Regular blood counts are done to determine the effectiveness and safety of continuing therapy. Means of building the platelet count are discussed in the dietary

Nursing Skill Guidelines
Caring for Patients During Radiation Therapy

Care of Patients Receiving External Beam Radiation Therapy

♦ Provide frequent rest periods. *(Rationale: The treatment and the disease often cause fatigue.)*

♦ Encourage nutrient intake. *(Rationale: A diet high in calories, protein and vitamins is recommended to increase strength and help offset nausea and diarrhea. Proteins are needed to build new tissue.)* Individuals vary in their tolerance to food during radiation therapy. (Guidelines for management of nausea and vomiting are presented elsewhere in this chapter, as well as in Chapters 46, 90, and 91.)

♦ Provide good oral hygiene. *(Rationale: This helps prevent breakdown of oral mucosa.)*

♦ Provide special skin care. Steps in skin care are outlined in the next section. (See also Chapter 45.)

♦ Keep the radiation site dry and free from irritation. The patient's clothing should fit loosely. *(Rationale: Friction may cause irritation.)*

♦ Avoid invasive procedures. Procedures such as rectal temperatures and injections should be avoided if possible. These measures must be particularly avoided in the radiation field.

♦ Follow supportive routine nursing measures for side effects, such as gastrointestinal symptoms. If these symptoms are severe, radiation treatment may need to be discontinued or postponed.

*Skin Care During External Radiation Therapy**

♦ Use only plain tepid water on the skin.

♦ Use a soft washcloth. Do not scrub.

♦ Assess skin in the treatment area for erythema, pain, and dry or moist peeling.

♦ If a moisturizing lotion is prescribed, be sure the physician determines the type of lotion to be used.

♦ Do not remove marks placed on the skin by the radiologist. *(Rationale: These marks are used as the guide for locating the treatment site.)*

♦ Do not use deodorant, powder, soap, perfume, cosmetics, scented lotion, or other skin preparations on the treatment area.

♦ Do not wear tight clothing over the treatment area.

♦ Wear cotton clothing next to the skin. *(Rationale: Wool or synthetics may irritate.)*

♦ Do not use any heating or cooling devices on the treatment area. Caution the person to prevent burning, such as in the shower.

♦ Protect the skin from sun (use at least an SPF-15 sunscreen).

♦ Protect also from wind and cold. *(Rationale: This person can be burned or frostbitten easily. The skin in the treatment area may be permanently hypersensitive.)*

Self-Care and Care of Patients With Implanted Radioactive Isotopes

♦ Ask to be reassigned if there is any possibility that you are pregnant.

♦ When giving nursing care, do not stay with the patient longer than necessary.

♦ Plan ahead so that as few trips as possible are made into the patient's room.

♦ Keep a record of time spent with the patient or wear a "radioactive sensor" badge. Usually, a chart is placed on the door to the room and nurses and physicians sign in and out.

♦ Do not stand close to the patient longer than necessary. Lead aprons or shields are used to minimize radiation exposure to staff.

♦ In addition to universal precautions, handle drainage and dressings with extra care. *(Rationale: There may be residual radioactivity.)*

♦ Check whether the implant is in place after necessary nursing measures have been completed. All equipment such as bedpans, emesis basins, and linens must be routinely checked before being removed from the patient's room. *(Rationale: The implant might become dislodged, in which case it could be lost. If not handled properly, it is dangerous to others. In addition, the patient would not be receiving the needed treatment.)*

♦ If an implant does fall out, do not touch it unless absolutely necessary. Notify radiology department staff at once. If you must move an implant, touch it only with a long forceps. A lead container is kept at the bedside for storage, in the event of an emergency.)

♦ Provide as much diversionary activity for the patient as possible. Encourage friends and family to telephone, if the patient's physical condition allows this. Provide a television. Encourage friends to write. *(Rationale: This will lessen the patient's sense of isolation.)*

♦ Teach family members the procedures to follow. Visiting time is limited. *(Rationale: Their safety must be ensured.)*

♦ The radiology department will check the room and must declare it safe before another patient can be admitted. In some hospitals, the room is not cleaned by housekeeping until declared safe by the radiology personnel.

---

* *Adapted from A Cancer Source Book for Nurses, American Cancer Society, 1991.*

Table 76-1. Commonly Prescribed Antiemetics Used With Chemotherapy

Antiemetic Drug	Dosage Range	Route of Administration
prochlorperazine (Compazine)	5–10 mg q4–6h	IV/IM/PO
	10–15 mg (extended-release) b.i.d.	PO
	25 mg q12h	PR (per rectum)
dexamethasone (Decadron)	10–20 mg q4–8h	IV/PO
metoclopramide (Reglan)	10–20 mg q4–6h	IV/PO
	1–2 mg/kg 30 min before chemo, then q2h × 2, then q3h × 3	IV
trimethobenzamide (Tigan)	250 mg q4h	PO
	200 mg Q4–6H	PR/IM
dronabinol (Marinol)	5 mg/meter squared before chemo, 2–4 h after chemo, then 4–6 doses qd	PO
ondansetron HCl (Zofran)	0.15 mg/kg before chemo, then 4 & 8 h after chemo	IV
	32 mg—1 dose before chemo	IV
	8–30 mg before chemo, then 4 & 8 h after, then b.i.d. × 1–2 d	PO
lorazepam (Ativan)	2–6 mg daily in divided doses (max: 10 mg/d) smaller doses IV	PO, IM, IV

section. A drug called filgrastim, or granulocyte colony-stimulating factor (G-CSF) (Neupogen), helps build the white blood cell count (specifically the neutrophils).

The nurse must be sure to wear gloves when handling any dressing or drainage and follow universal precautions or body substance isolation closely. As infection decreases, the patient's general condition may also improve.

Managing Odor

An offensive odor may be given off by infected lesions. The most effective way to control odor is to remove the source. Therefore, it is important to provide good skin, perineal, and mouth care. Other helpful measures include changing dressings or pads as often as possible, irrigating the wound as ordered, and removing used dressings and bed protective pads immediately from the room. Commercial deodorants may be used, in addition to good nursing care.

Assisting Patients to Manage Stress

The diagnosis of cancer, in combination with the various treatments, can be stressful. The nurse can assist in dealing with stress. Many people with cancer have experienced relief by using a technique called guided relaxation or imagery.

THERAPEUTIC VISUALIZATION. In addition to stress relief, some patients with cancer have experienced pain relief using therapeutic visualization or guided imagery. Audio or videotapes are used to guide patients toward teaching their bodies to respond to cues and become more proficient at lessening stress, relieving pain, or even combatting cancer cells.

The growing belief in a link between the immune system and cancer has given credibility to these techniques. Allowing the patient control over this aspect of treatment is believed to be an added bonus. Diversional activities are important.

The patient may also enjoy occupational therapy, music therapy, exercise, or pet therapy as stress relievers.

Assisting With Pain Control

Many patients with advanced cancer have pain, yet studies show that nearly all cancer-related pain can be managed. Follow the physician's orders about giving morphine or other pain-relieving drugs when the patient needs them. It is often advised to give pain medications at the first hint of pain; prolonged pain is unnecessary. Sedatives are sufficient to keep some patients comfortable; everything you do to make the patient comfortable will help to make any medication more effective. Chapter 52 describes general management of pain and Chapter 91 discusses pain management in the hospice setting.

Many patients in acute pain manage their own pain control with a patient-controlled analgesia pump (PCA pump). The stigmas surrounding the use of narcotics for cancer pain are gradually being corrected and nurses play an important part in the patient's understanding of the significance of taking pain medications on a regular schedule. The type and dose of pain medication prescribed by the physician are influenced by the origin of pain, as well as its severity.

Special Considerations in Aging
Pain

Misconceptions of reported pain may affect elderly people. They may underreport pain or the pain may be misconceived as deriving from normal aging. A disease process such as stroke may interfere with pain perception or with the ability of the person to express the discomfort.

Assisting With Other Concerns

HOT FLASHES. Many patients, both men and women, experience "hot flashes" while on chemotherapy and sometimes while on radiation. One reason for this is the use of hormonal agents for therapy or radiation to the gonads. Hot flashes can be uncomfortable, unexpected, and frightening, especially to men.

TEMPERATURE DYSREGULATION. Patients often complain of "going hot to cold" and back. Suggest dressing in layers, so clothes can be removed or put back on.

INSOMNIA. Many patients have great difficulty sleeping while on therapy. Because of thirst, they have to get a drink or go to the bathroom frequently. Hot flashes or pain may wake them. They may be anxious about the condition; people are more likely to worry or be confused at night.

EXHAUSTION. The patient often complains of being exhausted during therapy. Much of this is due to the physical stress of having cancer and receiving foreign substances (radiation, chemicals). In addition, red and white blood cell counts are lowered by the treatments. If the red blood cell count is low, the amount of oxygen received by body cells is decreased.

HAIR LOSS. Patients receiving radiation or chemotherapy often lose their hair. This includes eyelashes and hair on other parts of the body. Encourage the person to purchase an attractive wig or hat. The woman may wish to wear false eyelashes as well.

BONE SCANS AND FOLLOW-UP. Follow-up x-rays and bone scans are usually done regularly to determine if treatment has been successful. This may be anxiety-producing for the patient.

Providing Patient/Family Education

The key to nursing care of the patient with cancer is to involve the patient and the family in education and management of treatments, procedures, and all decisions, to the extent they are able and willing to be involved. Begin by asking patients what information they are missing. Follow through by ensuring they receive information in a manner they can understand. It would be beneficial to supply educational pamphlets as a reference for the patient and family. Also provide information about support and educational services available.

Evaluation

The nurse, patient, and family evaluate outcomes of care. Have short-term goals been met? Are long-term goals still realistic? What types of therapy or rehabilitation will be needed? Planning for further nursing care considers the patient's prognosis, as well as any complications and the patient's response to care given.

Cancers in specific systems of the body are discussed throughout this book, in conjunction with the chapters on each body system. Cancers in children are described in Unit Thirteen. Hospice nursing is discussed in Chapter 91.

> ### Key Concept
>
> The mere diagnosis of "cancer" provokes fear for most people. It is important to offer reassurance and support. It is also vital to emphasize that most cancers are curable, especially if treatment is begun early. Care of the person with cancer will give you an opportunity to use all of your nursing skills, as well as your interpersonal skills.

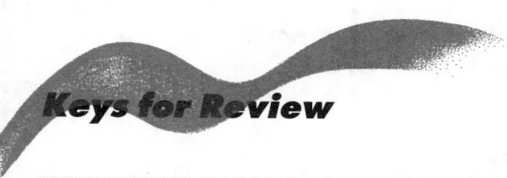

Keys for Review

Key Questions for Critical Thinking

1. Your patient has colon cancer. He says his cousin had a lymphoma and treatment was different. Determine how you would explain the difference between the two types of cancer. Include treatments in your explanation.
2. Describe five or more factors believed to contribute to cancer development. Determine how you would explain these factors to a patient.
3. State the seven danger signals of cancer. Explain the significance of each.
4. Explain the significance of time, distance, and shielding in caring for patients undergoing radiation treatment.
5. You are caring for a patient who has implanted radioactive isotopes. She is crying because she is lonely in her room. She states, "No one—not even the nurse—comes to talk to me." Discuss what you should say to her and other care you could provide.

Key Readings

Altman R, Sarg M. The Cancer Dictionary. New York, Facts on File, 1992

American Cancer Society. A Cancer Source Book for Nurses, Ed 6. Atlanta, GA, American Cancer Society, 1991

American Cancer Society. Cancer Facts and Figures—1993. Atlanta, GA, American Cancer Society, 1993

Belcher AE. Cancer Nursing. St. Louis, Mosby-Yearbook, 1992

Berkow R (Ed). The Merck Manual of Diagnosis and Therapy, Ed 16. Rahway, NJ, Merck & Co, 1992

Dollinger M, Rosenbaum E, Cable G. Everyone's Guide to Cancer Therapy. Kansas City, Andrews & McMeel, 1991

Fischbach F. A Manual of Laboratory and Diagnostic Tests, Ed 3. Philadelphia, J.B. Lippincott, 1992

Johnson J, Klein L. I Can Cope: Staying Healthy with Cancer, Revised. Minneapolis, Chronimed, 1994

NANDA Nursing Diagnoses: Definitions and Classifications 1992. Philadelphia, North American Nursing Diagnosis Association, 1992

Nursing '94 Drug Handbook. Springhouse, PA, Springhouse, 1994

Porth CM. Pathophysiology: Concepts of Altered Heath States, Ed 4. Philadelphia, J.B. Lippincott, 1994

Ryder B (Ed). The Alpha Book on Cancer and Living. Alameda, CA, Alpha Institute, 1993

Key Readings (continued)

Scherer JC. Introductory Medical-Surgical Nursing, Ed 5. Philadelphia, J.B. Lippincott, 1991

Smeltzer SC, Bare BG. Brunner and Suddarth's Textbook of Medical- Surgical Nursing, Ed 7. Philadelphia, J.B. Lippincott, 1992

Taylor C, Lillis C, LeMone P. Fundamentals of Nursing: The Art and Science of Nursing Care, Ed 2. Philadelphia, J.B. Lippincott, 1993

Keys to Learning More

Chapter 77: allergic and immune disorders

Chapter 78: HIV, AIDS and autoimmune disorders

Chapter 80: oxygen therapy

Chapter 83: male reproductive disorders

Chapter 84: female reproductive disorders

Chapter 89: rehabilitation, ambulatory and home care nursing

Chapter 90: death and dying

Chapter 91: hospice nursing

Key Resources

American Cancer Society
1599 Clifton Road NE
Atlanta, GA 30329
404/320-3333

Candlelighters Foundation
7910 Woodmont Avenue
Suite 460
Bethesda, MD 20814

Leukemia Society of America
600 Third Avenue
New York, NY 10016
617/482-2256

National Alliance of Breast Cancer Associations
1180 Avenue of the Americas, 2nd floor
New York, NY 10036

National Cancer Institute
Office of Cancer Communications
Building 31, Room 10A24
National Institutes of Health
Bethesda, MD 20892
1-800/4-CANCER

Skin Cancer Foundation
245 Fifth Avenue, Suite 2402
New York, NY 10016

77 Allergic and Immune Disorders

Keys for Learning

Learning Objectives

- ◆ Discuss ways in which allergens enter the body.
- ◆ Define immunity, immune response, and autoimmunity.
- ◆ List six types of disorders of the normal immune response and define and give examples of each type.
- ◆ State the purpose of skin tests for allergies.
- ◆ State the symptoms of anaphylaxis and describe first aid.
- ◆ List at least four types of allergies.
- ◆ Identify three allergic reactions with a systemic response.
- ◆ State the symptoms of bronchial (allergic) asthma and briefly describe nursing care.
- ◆ Name four possible symptoms indicative of a drug allergy.

Key Terms

allergens	eczema
allergy	histamine
anaphylaxis	hives
angioedema	immunity
antibodies	immunogens
antigen	immunosuppression
autoimmunity	urticaria

Keys to Understanding This Chapter

Chapter 21: cardiovascular system
Chapter 22: respiratory system
Unit Five: nutrition and diet therapy
Chapter 31: first aid
Chapter 32: cardiopulmonary resuscitation
Chapter 38: signs and symptoms of illness and injury
Chapter 50: nursing assessment
Unit Eleven: pharmacology and medication administration

Keys to Understanding This Chapter
(continued)

Chapter 65: allergies in children
Chapter 68: skin disorders
Chapter 69: fluid and electrolyte disorders
Chapter 70: musculoskeletal disorders
Chapter 72: endocrine disorders
Chapter 75: blood and lymph disorders
Chapter 76: cancer

Key Points

- ◆ The immune system leads the "battle" against invading microbes and malignant cells that contact or enter the body.
- ◆ The major defenders include lymphocytes and B cells, which react to antigens by secreting antibodies.
- ◆ Antigens are foreign protein substances that enter the body and stimulate the production of antibodies.
- ◆ Individuals can be allergic to almost anything.
- ◆ Common manifestations of allergic reactions vary; they may range from mild to life-threatening (anaphylaxis).
- ◆ Treatment of allergies is directed toward removal of the allergen and counteracting the antibody response.

Key Topics Outline

Anatomy and Physiology Review
Immunity and Autoimmunity
    Immunity
    Autoimmunity
Diagnosis of Allergies
Treatment of Allergies
    Common Medical Treatments
    Emergency Treatment of Anaphylaxis
Nursing Considerations in Immune Disorders

Rosdahl CB: Textbook of Basic Nursing, 6th ed. © 1995 J.B. Lippincott Company

Key Learning Activities

♦ Select a common allergen to study. Go to the local grocery store and make a list of products you find containing those ingredients.
♦ Find the emergency equipment at your affiliating clinical agency. List the medications and equipment available for treating a patient experiencing a severe allergic reaction.
♦ If you (or a family member) has an allergy, list everything you know about it: cause, prevention, treatment. Did you have allergy tests? Were you able to identify causative factors yourself? Is there more you would like to know about it?

The immune system is complex and protects an individual from "foreign invaders." This is called the *immune response*. Sometimes this system acts against the person's best interests, and an allergy or disorder of immunity results.

Allergy is defined as *hypersensitivity* to one or more substances; it is common. The allergy is acquired as a result of exposure to these offending substances and involves the action of the *immune system*. The physician who treats these disorders is called an *allergist*, although internal medicine and family practice specialists treat these patients as well. Pediatricians also see many children with allergies.

Anatomy and Physiology Review

The immune system consists of the spleen, lymph nodes, thymus, bone marrow, appendix, tonsils, and adenoids, along with B cells and T cells (lymphocytes) and macrophages. Chapter 21 briefly introduces the concept of immunity. The immune system is closely related to blood in that both share their origin in bone marrow. In addition, the bloodstream carries the components of the immune system throughout the body.

When an **antigen** (a foreign protein substance) touches or enters the body, the body reacts by producing **antibodies** for protection against that antigen. Subsequent contact with this antigen amy result in an allergic reaction and a wide variety of symptoms. This *antigen–antibody reaction* results in the release of chemical mediators, the most frequently mentioned being **histamine**. These mediators initiate a series of physiologic events in the organs of the body, resulting in the allergic reaction. Because antibodies form after contact with a substance, the allergic reaction cannot occur at the first exposure.

Antigens that cause an immune response in the body are known as **immunogens**. However, at times, a tissue reaction may occur, in which case the antigens are known as **allergens**. We say that the person is sensitive or allergic to the allergen.

Allergens can enter the body in various ways. The following lists ways and gives examples of each:

♦ Inhalation: pollen, dust, mold, and animal dander
♦ Ingestion: drugs (aspirin, penicillin), foods (chocolates, eggs, seafood, strawberries), preservatives
♦ Injection: drugs, insect stings or bites, immunizations, or blood transfusions
♦ Direct contact: poison ivy, cosmetics, dyes, metals, latex rubber, nylon, wool

The tendency toward an allergic response is thought to be inherited, but this does not mean a specific allergy is inherited. The manifestation of allergy is tied to many factors, including hormonal responses, type and concentration of allergen, body part involved, exposure to the antigen, and concurrent illness. The symptoms of allergy can occur at any age and vary in response from mild to life-threatening (as in *anaphylaxis*).

Immunity and Autoimmunity

Immunity

Immunity is a normal adaptive state of the body designed to protect the body from a disease.

Development of Immunity

Immunity can be natural or acquired. *Natural immunity* is present at birth, is more or less permanent, and appears to be species specific. For this reason, people do not contact animal diseases, such as canine parvovirus. It is the result of natural factors and involves heredity, race, and sex.

Acquired immunity develops after birth. It results from exposure to an antigen, thus activating an immune response. Acquired immunity can be active or passive, depending on whether the immune response occurs in the host or a donor. *Active immunity* is an immunity developed by the body. It is acquired from actually having the disease or from being inoculated with a vaccine containing antigens of the disease. *Passive immunity* is immunity of a temporary nature borrowed from another source. The fetus receives immunity (antibodies) from the mother in utero and the infant through the mother's breast milk. Passive immunity is also acquired through injection of antiserum or through the use of pooled gamma globulin.

Disorders of Immunity

Usually the body's immune system is working well on the body's behalf. The point at which a person becomes ill is when, for some reason, the immune system fails or does not operate as it should. Some immune disorders are:

◆ Infectious disease: the invading organism group is stronger (more virulent) or more numerous than the immune system antibodies.
◆ **Immunosuppression:** depression of the immune system, caused by disease, injury, shock, radiation, or drugs. It may also be congenital (agammaglobulinemia).
◆ Overproduction of gamma globulins: may be indicative of malignant blood diseases or chronic infection.
◆ Severe immune response to an invading antigen (**anaphylaxis**).
◆ *Rejection response* to a beneficial foreign substance placed in the body, such as graft versus host disease after organ or tissue transplant.
◆ Autoimmune response: allergic response to one's own cells (AIDS, SLE, some arthritis).

Many of these disorders of immunity are also discussed elsewhere in this book in connection with the study of various body systems.

Autoimmunity

Sometimes the body does not recognize or tolerate self as "self." The body begins to make antibodies against its own healthy cells or inhibits normal cell function. This is called **autoimmunity**. The result is damage to the body tissues by the immune system. The resulting diseases can affect almost any cell or tissue of the body. Although the mechanisms behind autoimmunity are not totally recognized, the following factors have been suggested:

◆ Genetic predisposition and influence of certain antigens in rejection of a person's own tissue
◆ Interaction with physical, chemical, and biologic agents that trigger an abnormal immune response
◆ Abnormalities in immune cells that lead to an inappropriate immune response

Examples of autoimmune diseases are diabetes mellitus, rheumatoid arthritis, multiple sclerosis, hemolytic anemia, myasthenia gravis, and systemic lupus erythematosus.

Diagnosis of Allergies

It is often difficult to find out what is causing an allergy. The antigen–antibody response may vary with fatigue, seasons, or hormones. A detailed medical history, physical examination, laboratory studies, and skin testing are means used to establish a diagnosis.

Medical History

The history includes data regarding the onset, duration, nature, and progression of allergy symptoms; factors that aggravate and alleviate symptoms; data on environmental exposure on the job, and by smoking, hobbies, household activities, and animals; history of family allergies; and medication usage.

Physical Examination

The physical examination includes assessing the skin for color, including erythema, cyanosis, and pallor; temperature; rashes; pruritus; and hives. The respiratory system is examined for nasal edema and congestion, sneezing, rhinorrhea, conjunctivitis, edema of the oropharynx, hoarseness, stridor, cough, dyspnea, wheezing, hypoxia, tympanic membrane bulging or retraction, and fluid levels. The gastrointestinal tract is assessed for nausea, vomiting, altered peristalsis, cramping, or diarrhea. Evaluation of cardiovascular status may reveal tachycardia, hypotension, syncope, signs of shock; and of the nervous system, signs of anxiety, confusion, seizures, or temperature elevation. An allergy can also affect the kidney or bladder; ask about sudden weight gain or retention of water (edema). Behavior can also change.

Laboratory and Skin Tests

Laboratory Tests. Laboratory tests include a complete blood count with white blood cell differential and eosinophil count, an eosinophil smear of secretions, and measurement of blood levels of immune response factors such as IgE (immunoglobulin E).

Skin Tests. Skin tests are done to confirm suspected allergies or to determine the causes of allergic reactions (Fig. 77-1). Several antigens are tested at one time, with each antigen injected *intradermally* (see Chap. 57) or applied to a small *scratch* on the skin (*epicutaneous* method). These are then labeled or otherwise identified. After 20 minutes, the allergist reads the skin tests in much the same way that a tuberculin test is read. Erythema (redness) and most commonly an induration (a lump, wheal, or edema) indicate a positive skin test. The degree of edema, measured in millimeters, indicates the severity of the reaction. In this way, the allergist can identify which substances are causing the patient's allergic reaction and to what extent the patient reacts to each allergen. However, despite a positive skin test, an allergen may not always cause an allergic reaction. Antihistamines may be ordered by the physician for the patient's comfort when tests are done. Assessment of skin tests is contained in Chapter 50.

The patient is observed closely during a skin test because occasionally a test will cause a severe reaction. Such a reaction is unusual because the amount of allergen used is very small; however, it can happen if the patient is highly sensitive to the allergen. The symptoms of a severe allergic response (anaphylaxis) are reviewed later in this chapter. Symptoms and treatment of anaphylaxis are described in Chapter 31.

Treatment of Allergies

Once the offending antigen is identified, treatment can be started. Treatment depends on numerous factors, but generally includes the following common medical treatments.

Common Medical Treatments

Avoidance of the Substance

It is not always easy to avoid an allergen. For instance, although it is no problem to stop eating shrimp, it is more difficult to eliminate white flour from the diet or dust from the environment. However, other types of allergens can be avoided. Foam rubber or polyester fiber can be substituted for feather pillows, and antiallergenic or hypoallergenic cosmetics are available. Encourage the person with allergies not to rake leaves. Some people are able to relocate to a pollen-free area during the pollen season. Other people may have to give up their pet. Many nurses are allergic to *latex* and must avoid rubber gloves, catheters, and other latex-based materials. Nevertheless, some allergens cannot be avoided, and it is also known that severe emotional reactions can precipitate or aggravate an allergic reaction.

Desensitization

Desensitization or hyposensitization *immunotherapy* consists of giving minute doses of allergens subcutaneously. The doses are gradually increased to enable the patient to slowly develop a tolerance to the allergen. Sometimes this treatment eliminates the allergy, with the injections being given weekly or more often. If desensitization is being done to treat a seasonal allergy, it must be started at least 3 months before the specific allergy season. If the allergy is not seasonal, injections are continued throughout the year. This treatment is fairly expensive, but it is particularly helpful to those with pollen or dust allergies. Treatment may last from 1 to 2 years or longer; some may last for 5 years.

Nursing Alert

Patients should remain in the physician's clinic for 20 minutes following an injection for desensitization because of the possibility of severe reactions.

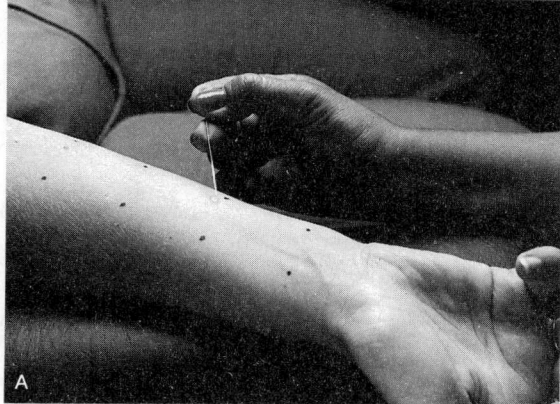 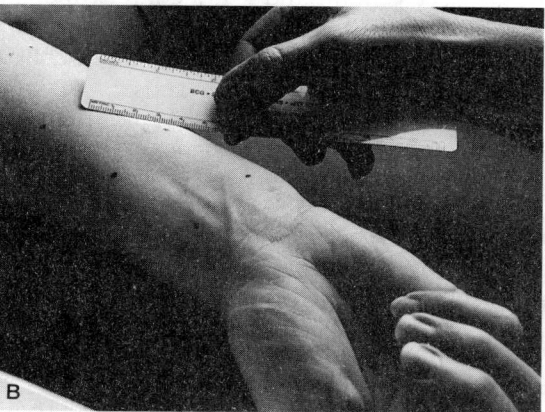

Figure 77-1. Skin testing by prick method. **(A)** The volar surface of the forearm is marked and drops of antigen are applied 3 to 4 cm apart. The skin is penetrated through the antigen with a pricking device. **(B)** The wheal-and-flare reaction is measured with a millimeter ruler. (From Suddarth DS. The Lippincott Manual of Nursing Practice, Ed 5. Philadelphia, J.B. Lippincott, 1991, p. 877.)

Drug Therapy

Drugs may be given to specifically counteract the allergy or to treat allergy symptoms.

Antihistamines. Antihistamines are effective because they inhibit the action of histamine within the body. However, they give only temporary relief and must be used frequently if the patient is to remain free of symptoms. They should not be used for allergies that are not seasonal because prolonged use of antihistamines also has undesirable effects. These drugs may cause drowsiness, and in asthma, they may dry up the secretions so much that the patient cannot swallow or expectorate.

Drugs Used to Treat Symptoms. The type of drug used will depend on the symptoms. *Epinephrine* may be given in an emergency to neutralize adverse effects of histamine. It is used to relieve or reduce bronchospasms and to reduce congestion of bronchial mucosa by dilating the bronchi. It constricts small blood vessels in the skin and it counteracts symptoms of shock. Epinephrine is also used in severe anaphylaxis to treat vasodilation and bronchial constriction. Lung symptoms may be relieved by bronchodilators and expectorants.

Cortisone preparations and other anti-inflammatory agents may be given to reduce itching and inflammation in skin lesions. External medications may be applied to the skin for their cooling and antiseptic effects and to reduce itching and other symptoms.

Emergency Treatment of Anaphylaxis

Anaphylaxis refers to a hypersensitivity reaction to an antigen. Severe reactions may lead to vascular collapse, laryngoedema, shock, and death. It can be caused by anything to which the person is allergic. Common causes include antibiotics, aspirin and other drugs, vaccines, foods, insect venom, and x-ray contrast media containing iodine. The accompanying box lists symptoms of anaphylaxis. See Chapter 31 for more details regarding first aid treatment for anaphylaxis.

Nursing Alert

During skin testing and allergy shots, there is a risk of systemic reaction to the allergen. Epinephrine in 1:1,000 concentration, syringe, tourniquet, and emergency equipment should be kept available.

Treatment. Treatment must be started immediately because more severe reactions begin very quickly. If the cause is an injection or insect bite, a tourniquet is applied above the site to slow the rate of absorption of the antigen into the system. An ice pack to the site will

---

Symptoms of Anaphylaxis

Anaphylaxis is an emergency situation. Notify the physician *immediately* if you observe these symptoms in your patient:

◆ Sneezing (continuous)
◆ Edema, itching at site of injection or sting
◆ Rash (hives)
◆ Apprehension, choking sensation, airway obstruction
◆ Hypotension
◆ Weak, rapid, and thready pulse
◆ Diaphoresis (profuse sweating)
◆ Pallor or cyanosis
◆ Pupillary dilation (eyes)
◆ Loss of consciousness
◆ Seizures
◆ Dyspnea

---

also slow absorption. The immediate problems are *airway obstruction* from laryngeal edema and *vasodilation*, resulting in hypotension and hypoperfusion of organs. The cardiac output falls and the heart cannot pump enough blood and oxygen to the tissues. This results in anaerobic metabolism and lactic acidosis. The brain is particularly sensitive to alterations in perfusion and oxygen content. Severe bronchospasms may also occur.

The treatment of anaphylactic shock involves removal of the causative agent and administration of antihistamines to block the effects of histamine on the blood vessels, bronchioles, and gastrointestinal tract. In severe cases, epinephrine may be used to counteract the vasodilation that occurs. Epinephrine also relaxes the smooth muscle of the airways and inhibits further mediator release.

Nursing Considerations. The nurse follows the emergency protocol when dealing with anaphylaxis:

◆ *Open the airway*—an endotracheal tube, oxygen, or suction may be needed.
◆ *Support the circulation*—an IV, Trendelenburg position, or CPR may be needed.
◆ *Administer medications.* These include epinephrine, aminophylline, antihistamines, and corticosteroids.

❖ *Nursing Process*

It is important that the nurse report any allergies the patient describes or exhibits. For the patient's protection, drug allergies must be noted in large letters on the front of the chart and on the medication record when the patient is admitted. The patient wears a special identification band. A person can have an allergic reaction to any drug. A reaction will be manifested faster and more dramatically if the drug is administered parenterally. No drug should be given without first making sure that the patient is not allergic to it. If there is any doubt, or if the patient has a history of allergies or asthma, the physician may do a skin test (intradermal) first. Even then, the nurse must be prepared to deal with possible anaphylaxis.

Nursing can play a large role in the care of the patient with allergies, from identification of suspected allergens, to treatment of allergic responses, to the prevention of future reactions through patient education.

Data Collection

The nurse must carefully observe and assess the patient with an allergic or immune disorder. Chapter 50 describes head-to-toe nursing assessment, including a brief outline for assessment of the immune system. This assessment establishes a baseline for future comparison and determines the presence of suspected allergies or immune disorders. The nurse should document and report any changes in this baseline level.

The patient with an *immune disorder* will generally present with vague symptoms such as fatigue or dyspnea, frequent or recurrent infections, slow wound healing, joint pain, skin rashes, or visual disturbances. Ask the patient about any family history of cancer or immune disorders. The physician and other staff can further evaluate any reported abnormalities.

Assessment of the immune system also includes the administration and evaluation of skin tests. These may be administered intradermally (described in Chapter 57) or by a scratch test (see Fig. 77-1). The patient's medical history is particularly important in assessing allergic and immune disorders. In addition, the nurse observes the patient's emotional response to the disorder. Does the disorder interfere with the person's daily life? What assistance is needed?

Nursing Diagnosis

Disorders of the immune system are believed to contribute to or cause many systemic symptoms and disorders. Allergies are responsible for symptoms ranging from rhinorrhea and skin rash to asthma or a total anaphylactic response. The most well known autoimmune disorder is the human immunodeficiency virus (HIV) infection and full-blown acquired immunodeficiency syndrome (AIDS; discussed in Chapter 78). Therefore, nearly any nursing diagnosis is possible, depending on the specific immune disorder. The following are samples of nursing diagnoses that may appear on a nursing care plan for a patient with an allergy. Some diagnoses represent more than one causal factor.

♦ Diarrhea related to food allergy
♦ Impaired Skin Integrity related to pruritus
♦ High Risk for Caregiver Role Strain related to a chronic disorder
♦ Sleep Pattern Disturbances related to pruritus, dyspnea
♦ Fatigue related to asthma
♦ Altered Growth and Development related to childhood asthma
♦ Self-esteem Disturbance related to rash, itching, difficult breathing

Examples of nursing diagnoses for anaphylaxis include:

♦ Anxiety/Fear related to inability to breathe
♦ High Risk for Suffocation related to airway nonpatency
♦ Altered Thought Processes related to loss of consciousness

Planning and Implementation

The patient, nurse, and family plan together for effective care to meet patient needs based on the nursing diagnosis. The nurse provides supportive care and continuously monitors the patient's status. The patient with an allergy or asthma may require assistance in activities of daily living and in dealing with the emotional aspects of having a chronic disorder. The nurse teaches the patient and family about the disorder, its prognosis, and treatment. Some teaching factors are listed in the accompanying box. A nursing care plan is developed to meet these needs. A sample Nursing Care Plan for a patient with a disorder of immunity is presented also.

Keys to Patient/Family Teaching
Allergic Conditions

Patient/family teaching for the patient with allergic conditions includes:

♦ Name of allergen and how and where it occurs.
♦ Relationship between symptoms and exposure to causative allergens.
♦ Medication and food labels are to be read carefully.
♦ Proper administration of medications, including inhalers and self-injections.
♦ Observations for delayed responses to immunotherapy (allergy shots).
♦ Compliance and self-responsibility are important focuses.
♦ It may take weeks to months to obtain optimal results.

John Miller is a 33-year-old single man who, while hospitalized with a herniated disc, complained of localized itching, edema, and sneezing. He reported that there is a strong history of various allergies in his family and that he himself has hay fever that he treats with OTC (over-the-counter) drugs. A consult to a dermatologist was placed immediately. The nursing diagnosis below was added to his plan of care.

Nursing Diagnosis: *Knowledge Deficit: Allergy Management Related to Previous Lack of Interest in Learning, as Evidenced by Self-Report*

Goal: Prior to discharge patient verbalizes steps he can take to prevent future problems with allergic reactions.

Nursing Actions (assess/do/teach)	Rationale	Evaluative Statement
1. Conduct a careful allergy history to determine possible allergies including known drug, insect, food, or pollen sensitivities; explain the process of skin testing if this is recommended.	The hallmark of allergy is the recurrent development of manifestations associated with distinct factors in the environment.	11/4 Goal met; patient verbalizes feeling more "in charge" of his allergies and is confident of his ability to manage future recurrences of problems.
2. Stress the importance of promoting optimal health as a defense against future allergic reactions (good nutrition, balance between exercise and rest, positive thinking, good stress management skills). If allergens are known, develop strategies to avoid them (environmental control). Explain the purpose of immunotherapy, if this is recommended, and answer questions the patient may have.	Enhances natural defenses	
3. Always record known allergies clearly on the patient's chart, nursing Kardex, and plan, or as dictated by agency policy.	Anaphylaxis is life-threatening and prevention is the key; high-risk patients must be identified.	

Evaluation

The nurse, patient, and family evaluate the outcomes of care. Have short-term goals been met? Are long-term goals still realistic? Planning for further nursing care considers the patient's prognosis, as well as any complications and the patient's response to care given. The seriousness of the immune disorder influences the future planning for care and rehabilitation.

Types of Allergies

Allergic reactions may affect the skin and mucous membranes, the respiratory passages, and the gastrointestinal tract. They can result in a rash, edema, itching, dys-

pnea, contractions of the smooth muscles, and in severe cases total shock and death (anaphylaxis).

Edema is a symptom that may be related to allergy or to emotional factors. It may occur in one part of the body, such as the lips and eyelids, or it may be generalized. If the swelling presses on a vital organ, such as the larynx, it can severely impair the person's ability to function, in this case, respiration.

Allergies With a Respiratory Response

Allergic Asthma

Spasms of smooth muscles of the bronchi, in addition to edema, create difficulty in breathing, which causes a cough, an accumulation of mucus, and wheezing. In a severe attack, the patient may become cyanotic. Chapter 79 describes asthma in more detail.

Bronchial Asthma

Bronchial asthma is a common condition, characterized by recurring paroxysms of dyspnea of the wheezing type, caused by a narrowing of the lumen of the smaller bronchi and bronchioles. It is associated with an allergic reaction in the bronchioles.

Bronchial asthma has several classifications, including *extrinsic asthma* (a reaction to inhaled allergens), *intrinsic asthma* (in which there is no eliciting allergen, but it may be related to infections or environmental stimuli, such as air pollution), and *mixed asthma*. There is also asthma induced by such factors as exercise, aspirin, or occupational factors including fumes, dust, and gases.

Symptoms of bronchial asthma include periods of dyspnea, a sense of tightness in the chest, wheezing, cough, tenacious sputum, cyanosis, profuse perspiration, and increased pulse rate and respirations. It can be a frightening disorder; the person can have a sensation of suffocation. Death can occur in extreme situations.

Treatment of asthma includes the use of bronchodilators, corticosteroids, antihistamines, and anticholinergics. Inhalation therapy with beta-adrenergic agonists, cromolyn sodium (Intal, Nalcrom, Opticrom), and steroids is convenient and easy to use. Narcotics are contraindicated; they cause respiratory depression. Additional treatments include control of the environment (such as dust, fumes, and animal dander). Learning to control precipitating factors is essential. Dietary control may be necessary for sensitive persons. Exercise is encouraged rather than discouraged. Patients should be instructed to use their inhaler before exercise (to avoid bronchospasm). Patients may be cautioned to wear a face mask in extremely cold weather.

Allergic Rhinitis

Hay fever is an inflammation of the nasal passages caused by an allergen. Additional responses include sneezing, watery rhinorrhea; edema, burning, itching and watering of the eyes; fullness and itching of the ears; as well as itching of the throat and palate. Potential allergens include all inhalants, pollen, molds, dust, dust mites, perfumes, and animal dander. The symptoms may be seasonal or perennial.

Allergies With a Skin Response

Urticaria (Hives)

Reddened areas (erythema), itching (pruritus), and burning around swollen patches on the skin may appear. The swellings are called **hives** or **urticaria**. They appear suddenly and they disappear after a few hours or may last for a period of days or weeks. Hives may result from a variety of causes including foods, additives, medications, infections (viral, bacterial, or parasitic), or from stress factors (heat, sun, cold, emotional stress). Management includes identification of the causative factor and medications such as antihistamines, epinephrine, or steroids.

Eczema

In **eczema**, the skin is covered with tiny blisters that itch and ooze, usually in the folds of the neck, the elbow, and the knees. In chronic eczema, the skin becomes scaly and thickened (see Chapter 68).

Contact Dermatitis

A common allergen is poison ivy. In contact with the skin, the oils of the plant cause itching, swelling, redness, and blisters. Other allergens include soaps, detergents, perfumes, cosmetics, metals in jewelry, leathers, wool, and latex products.

Gastrointestinal Allergy

In this type of allergy, also called a *food sensitivity*, the immune system reacts to an otherwise harmless substance. Common food allergens include dairy products, eggs, wheat, soybeans, fish, shellfish, chocolate, nuts, seeds, corn, beer, citrus fruits, and many food additives and preservatives. Common manifestations of food allergies are nausea and vomiting, diarrhea, abdominal pain and tenderness, swelling of the lips and throat, itching of the palate, rhinoconjunctivitis, sneezing, wheezing, urticaria, and migraine headaches. In many cases, a food that causes burping often also causes allergy. It is also believed that a woman craves foods to which she is allergic in PMS, thus aggravating the situation. **Angioedema** is a condition characterized by development of urticaria and edema in areas of skin and mucous membranes.

Drug Allergy

Adverse Drug Reactions. A true drug allergy results from the antigen–antibody response, but an adverse drug reaction is a noxious or unintended effect of a medication. Drug reactions are linked to about 3% of hospitalizations and 15% to 30% of hospitalized patients have adverse drug reactions. Symptoms vary depending on the drug. The nurse should pay close attention if a patient claims to be allergic to a substance or drug. A careful history of the previous reaction should be obtained and documented in the medical record. Persons who are allergic to certain medications or have had severe reactions should be encouraged to wear Medic-Alert tags.

Serum Sickness or Serum Reaction. A serum reaction may be caused by administration of certain drugs. The antiserum used for rabies treatment may cause a severe serum reaction. Symptoms occur 7 to 14 days after receiving a drug against which the patient has no immune bodies. These symptoms include itching and inflammation at the point of injection, skin rash, enlarged lymph nodes, and sometimes, swollen joints, as well as a feeling of general weakness and an elevated temperature. Treatment usually includes antihistamines, with corticosteroids being given in more severe cases.

Keys for Review

Key Questions for Critical Thinking

1. Explain the difference between an antibody and an antigen. Describe the immune response.
2. Identify ways allergens can enter the body. Discuss how each method can be prevented.
3. Describe autoimmunity in relationship to immunity and the immune response.
4. List four types of allergies and give an example of each.

Key Readings

Berkow R (Ed). The Merck Manual of Diagnosis and Therapy, Ed 16. Rahway, NJ, Merck & Co, 1992

Hafen BQ, Karren KJ. Prehospital Emergency Care and Crisis Intervention, Ed 2. Englewood Cliffs, NJ, Prentice Hall, 1992

Jackson DB, Saunders RB. Child Health Nursing: A Comprehensive Approach to the Care of Children and Their Families. Philadelphia, J.B. Lippincott, 1993

NANDA Nursing Diagnoses: Definitions and Classifications 1992. Philadelphia, North American Nursing Diagnosis Association, 1992

Nursing '94 Drug Handbook. Springhouse, PA, Springhouse, 1994

O'Toole M (Ed). Miller-Keane Encyclopedia and Dictionary of Medicine, Nursing, and Allied Health, Ed 5. Philadelphia, W.B. Saunders, 1992

Porth CM. Pathophysiology: Concepts of Altered Health States, Ed 4. Philadelphia, J.B. Lippincott, 1994

Smeltzer SC, Bare BG. Brunner and Suddarth's Textbook of Medical-Surgical Nursing, Ed 7. Philadelphia, J.B. Lippincott, 1992

Key Readings (continued)

Smith AJ, Johnson JY. Nurses' Guide to Clinical Procedures, Philadelphia, J.B. Lippincott, 1990

Taylor C, Lillis C, Lemone P. Fundamentals of Nursing: Art and Science of Nursing Care, Ed 2. Philadelphia, J.B. Lippincott, 1993

Thomas CL (Ed). Taber's Cyclopedic Medical Dictionary, Ed 17. Philadelphia, F.A. Davis, 1993

Keys to Learning More

Chapter 78: HIV, AIDS and autoimmune disorders
Chapter 79: respiratory disorders

Key Resources

American Academy of Allergy and Immunology
611 Wells Street
Milwaukee, WI 53202
414/272-6071

Asthma and Allergy Foundation of America
1717 Massachusetts Avenue, NW, No. 305
Washington, DC 20036
1-800/7-ASTHMA

National Institute of Allergy and Infectious Diseases
Building 10, National Institutes of Health
Bethesda, MD 20892
301/496-4000

National Jewish Center for Immunology and Respiratory Medicine
1400 Jackson Street
Denver, CO 80206
1-800/222-LUNG

78 HIV, AIDS, and Autoimmune Disorders

Keys for Learning

Learning Objectives

- Define autoimmunity and autoimmune disease.
- Define HIV and describe the method of categorizing HIV infections according to the Centers for Disease Control and Prevention.
- Describe AIDS and its treatment. State the most common opportunistic infections and cancer of AIDS.
- Describe nursing precautions to protect against AIDS.
- Describe nursing care and special needs of patients with AIDS.

Key Terms

acquired immunodeficiency syndrome (AIDS)

B cells

human immunodeficiency virus (HIV)

Kaposi's sarcoma

lymphocyte

non–organ-specific

opportunistic infections

organ-specific

pandemic

Pneumocystis carinii pneumonia

retrovirus

systemic

T cells

Keys to Understanding This Chapter

Chapter 21: immunity and the blood

Chapter 30: medical asepsis

Chapter 36: therapeutic communication

Chapter 38: signs and symptoms of illness or injury

Chapter 50: nursing assessment

Chapter 51: infection control techniques

Chapter 52: pain management

Chapter 54: surgical asepsis

Unit Eleven: pharmacology and medication administration

Chapter 62: disorders of the neonate

Chapter 63: sexually transmitted diseases

Chapter 68: skin disorders

Chapter 75: blood and lymph disorders

Chapter 76: cancer

Chapter 77: allergic and immune disorders

Key Points

- Autoimmune disorders occur when the body fails to recognize its own cells as "self" and begins to destroy those cells.
- It is important for the body to seek a balance between suppressing the immune response that is causing an illness and maintaining enough immunity to fight the invasion of threatening foreign substances.
- The terms HIV and AIDS are not synonymous. HIV causes AIDS, but the person who is HIV positive does not automatically have AIDS.
- The Centers for Disease Control and Prevention has updated the definition of AIDS to include diagnosis based on a count of 200 T cells per cubic millimeter of blood.
- Universal precautions are used to protect healthcare workers and minimize the risk of contracting HIV and other infections.

Key Topics Outline

Anatomy and Physiology Review
Diagnostic Tests
Nursing Process
    Data Collection
    Nursing Diagnosis
    Planning and Implementation
    Evaluation
Disorders in Autoimmunity
Human Immunodeficiency Virus
    HIV and Acquired Immunodeficiency Syndrome

Key Learning Activities

- In your clinical facility, review the policy on universal precautions. Memorize and apply them.
- Attend seminars in your community featuring keynote speakers on the topic of AIDS.
- Attend an AIDS support group. What is the purpose of the group? What support is given?

As you learned in Chapter 77, the immune system protects the body from adverse effects of invasion by microorganisms. It also regulates the removal of damaged cells and disposes of abnormal cells that arise within the body. One specific disorder of immunity is an autoimmune disorder.

This chapter lists several common autoimmune disorders and gives a brief overview of the human immunodeficiency virus (HIV), as it relates to acquired immunodeficiency syndrome (AIDS).

Anatomy and Physiology Review

As described in Chapters 21 and 77, the immune system normally functions to protect the body. Normally the body is able to distinguish "self" from "not self" and to take steps to eliminate substances in the "not self" category that enter the body. The difficulty in an *autoimmune disorder* is that the body fails to recognize its own cells as "self" and begins to destroy its own cells. The reader *should* review the first part of Chapter 77 before studying this chapter.

The condition called AIDS is related to the autoimmune disorders because the HIV virus weakens the immunity-producing cells of the body. The body then cannot fight off infections and the person becomes susceptible to "opportunistic" infections.

Diagnostic Tests

Blood tests are available to detect the HIV virus. These include the *ELISA* (enzyme-linked immunosorbent assay), which detects antibodies to the HIV proteins. If the ELISA is positive, a test called a *Western blot* will be performed. The Western blot is accurate and specific for detection of HIV. The ELISA is less specific for HIV and can react positively to other viruses. A procedure is available that can differentiate between the presence of the HIV antigen and the antibody, the PCR (polymerase chain reaction). For example, many infants of HIV-positive mothers are born with HIV antibodies only. It is believed that they will not develop AIDS. This could be the beginning of the search for a vaccine.

❖ Nursing Process

Data Collection

The nurse must carefully observe and assess the patient with a diagnosed or potential autoimmune disorder. It is difficult to list specific signs and symptoms because an autoimmune disorder can affect most systems of the body. Chapter 50 describes physical examination and nursing assessment, which establish a baseline for future comparison and determine the presence of suspected complications. The nurse should document and report any changes in this baseline level.

Autoimmune disorders are often chronic and can be fatal. Therefore, the nurse also evaluates the patient's emotional response to the disorder or disease. Does the patient need assistance to meet daily needs? Does the disorder affect social activities or self-esteem? Is the disorder life-threatening? Are medications being taken as prescribed? Is the patient anxious or fearful of the outcome? What support services are needed for the patient or the family? Is professional counseling or a support group recommended? Are rehabilitation or home care services needed?

Nursing Diagnosis

Based on data collection, the following nursing diagnoses are samples that may be seen on nursing care plans for patients with many autoimmune disorders:

◆ Chronic Pain related to development of disease
◆ Altered Nutrition: Less Than Body Requirements related to inability to digest nutrients, anorexia
◆ Impaired Skin Integrity related to diarrhea, reaction to sun, medications
◆ Impaired Physical Mobility related to decreased strength and endurance

Because of the destruction of tissue all over the body in HIV and AIDS, almost all nursing diagnoses will be used at one time or another. The following are samples, showing multiple causal factors:

◆ Altered Nutrition: Less Than Body Requirements related to opportunistic infections, anorexia, persistent diarrhea, and general body tissue wasting
◆ Ineffective breathing pattern related to PCP (*Pneumocystis carinii*) pneumonia.
◆ High Risk for Infection related to distressed immune system
◆ High Risk for Disuse Syndrome related to immobility, fatigue, decreased level of endurance
◆ Hopelessness related to deteriorating condition, feeling of abandonment, long-term stress
◆ Impaired Tissue Integrity related to medications, thrush, shingles, athlete's foot, other fungal infections, altered nutritional status, suicide attempts
◆ Impaired Social Interactions related to fear, fatigue, pain debilitation
◆ Ineffective Individual Coping related to lack of adequate support system, reaction to terminal illness
◆ Altered Thought Processes related to AIDS dementia, suicidal ideation, depression

Planning and Implementation

The patient, nurse, and support persons plan together for effective care to meet patient needs, based on the nursing diagnosis. Most autoimmune disorders are chronic; many are progressive. Thus, this patient may require assistance in meeting all basic and healthcare needs, as well as in dealing with the chronic and terminal nature of the disorder. The nurse teaches the patient and family about the disorder and the prescribed medications and treatment. Counseling, social services, home care, and other community agencies are often involved. A nursing care plan is developed to meet identified needs. A sample Nursing Care Plan is provided here.

Evaluation

The nurse, patient, and support person evaluate outcomes of care. Have short-term goals been met? Are long-term goals still realistic? What community services are required? Does the patient need financial assistance? Planning for further nursing and healthcare considers the patient's prognosis and the patient's responses to care.

Disorders in Autoimimmunity

Normal immunity is based on the ability of the body to recognize foreign proteins and to marshal its defenses to destroy that foreign matter. However, immune mechanisms are not always positive or beneficial to the host. Under certain conditions, they may produce tissue injury and clinical disease. The difficulty in an autoimmune disorder is that the body fails to recognize its own cells as "self" and begins to destroy those cells.

Types

Autoimmune disorders range from those that are **organ-specific** (affecting one organ), **systemic** (affecting the entire body), to those that are **non–organ-specific** with lesions affecting one or more organ.

Organ-specific autoimmune disease is characterized by chronic inflammatory changes in a specific organ.

Examples include thyrotoxicosis or Graves' disease (thyroid), insulin-dependent diabetes mellitus (pancreas), and autoimmune thyroiditis.

Systemic autoimmune disorders are characterized by widespread pathologic changes in many organs and tissues. Examples include systemic lupus erythematosus (SLE), rheumatoid arthritis (RA), and myasthenia gravis (MG).

Non–organ-specific autoimmune disorders combine the features of systemic and organ-specific diseases. Examples include primary biliary cirrhosis and chronic active hepatitis (Table 78-1.)

Persons at Risk

Research has indicated that autoimmune diseases other than AIDS show a highly significant familial tendency. Relatives of a patient with a diagnosed autoimmune disease, such as SLE or RA, are known to be at high risk for developing the same disease. Also, multiple autoimmune disorders are known to occur in the same patient. Women are more likely to develop autoimmunity than men, often reaching a 10:1 (female:male) ratio or greater in certain diseases. Scientists believe that thymic hormones, sex hormones, and corticosteroids play a significant role in this ratio.

Examples of Autoimmune Disorders

These disorders may be considered allergies with a systemic response.

Rejection of a Transplanted Organ. To discuss in detail the procedure of organ transplantation is beyond the scope of this book. However, it is important to understand that a transplanted organ is a foreign substance in relation to the recipient's body, and the recipient's bodily defenses will reject this foreign substance unless specific measures are taken to prevent that rejection. Tissue typing before transplant is done in much the same manner as blood typing to obtain the most genetically compatible match between donor and recipient. Another measure taken to suppress the rejection is giving immunosuppressive drugs. Signs of rejection can be similar to other antigen–antibody responses and in-

---

Table 78-1. Autoimmune Disorders

Organ Specific	*Non-organ Specific*	*Systemic*
Thyrotoxicosis	Primary biliary cirrhosis	Systemic lupus erythematosus
Scleroderma	Chronic active hepatitis	
Inflammatory bowel disease		Multiple sclerosis
Insulin dependent diabetes mellitus		Pernicious anemia
Autoimmune thyroiditis		Rheumatoid arthritis
Organ transplant rejection syndrome		Myasthenia gravis

Ms. Carla Hurbison, a 39-year-old white woman, was admitted to Medical Center Hospital complaining of anorexia and weight loss due to herpes virus lesions of mouth, esophagus, and lower extremities and diarrhea secondary to acquired immunodeficiency syndrome (AIDS). Ms. Hurbison repeatedly talked about the fact that she was getting more ill more frequently and that her weight loss, fatigue, and pain were also increasing in severity. She cried about the fact that her family seemed to be becoming exhausted as time goes on. The following nursing diagnoses were developed for Ms. Hurbison's plan of care.

Nursing Diagnosis: *Altered Nutrition: Less Than Body Requirements Related to Oral/Esophageal Lesions, Anorexia, and Diarrhea*

Goal: 10/2 patient will verbalize understanding of factors that decrease nutritional intake and institute necessary interventions to eliminate those factors.

Nursing Actions (assess/do/teach)	Rationale	Evaluative Statement
1. Assess nutritional status by weighing patient, monitoring intake, calorie count, and appropriate laboratory levels. Have patient consult with dietitian to develop a plan to facilitate adequate nutritional intake. Encourage patient input into dietary regime.	Good nutrition is necessary for healing. If patient has input into and participates in planning her own dietary regime, she is more likely to adhere to it.	Goal met; 10/2 is implementing techniques to improve her nutritional intake and decrease her diarrhea.
2. Teach patient techniques to lessen pain associated with oral/esophagal lesions such as: avoiding acid-type and highly seasoned foods; taking blenderized foods, liquid supplements, and small frequent feedings.	These techniques will lessen the pain associated with eating and will help increase food intake. They may also maximize limited absorptive capacity.	
3. Use mouth rinses as directed. Use ice or anesthetic gel before eating.	These have a numbing affect, which will decrease pain associated with eating.	
4. Advise patient to take frequent rest periods and to eat during times when she is feeling better.	These actions will maximize intake.	
5. Encourage patient to monitor stools in relation to what she eats and to avoid those foods that cause diarrhea due to increased motility, bulk, irritation, or sensitivity.	In addition to foods that increase motility, add bulk, and cause irritation, each individual has certain foods that cause sensitivity in their digestive system, which can cause diarrhea.	10/4 Diarrhea has lessened with altered diet and medication.
6. Drink water at room temperature.		

(continued)

clude fever, chills, diaphoresis, hypertension, hypotension, edema, and signs of organ involvement.

Systemic Lupus Erythematosus. Systemic lupus erythematosus (SLE) is a chronic systemic disorder. It is believed to be caused by development of antibodies that fight the body's own tissues and cells. The result is widespread damage to connective tissues; the hematologic system; and the skin, kidneys, heart, and brain. Evaluation of SLE includes laboratory tests to document the antibodies and extent of end-organ involvement. Treatment involves education in rest and stress management, and the use of anti-inflammatory agents and steroids.

Nursing Diagnosis: *Ineffective Family Coping Related to Prolonged Disease Progression with Overwhelming Responsibilities that are Exhausting Their Ability to be Effective Care Givers.*

Goal: 10/2 family will identify the need for outside assistance and seek help.

Nursing Actions (assess/do/teach)	Rationale	Evaluative Statement
1. Identify role of patient in family and how illness has changed the family roles, noting how they feel about these changes.	Emotional needs are as important as physical needs.	Goal partially met; 10/2 patient and family met with Social Services and identified several areas that would be beneficial for them to seek help.
2. Note factors, other than illness, that may be affecting family's ability to provide effective care.	Past relationships, time schedules, available space, and finances are some factors that may affect the family's effectiveness.	Goal met; 10/6 family contacted Home Health Agency and counselor in an effort to lighten their responsibilities and resolve some of their emotional conflicts.
3. Assess information available to and understood by the family regarding outside help.	This basic information will enable the nurse to provide appropriate referral and to encourage the family to seek the help they need.	
4. Request Social Services consult regarding available resources and services and services both for patient and family needs (caregivers, housekeeping, support groups/counseling, financial, spiritual).	Social Services has a wide knowledge base.	

Rheumatoid Arthritis. This disorder, characterized by an inflammation of the joints, may also have systemic manifestations. Its origin is generally believed to the autoimmune. It is primarily a disorder of the musculoskeletal system.

Key Concept

Autoimmunity is related to many disorders. It is now thought that autoimmunity plays a role in many other previously unexplained disorders.

Treatment

General treatment of autoimmune diseases is, for the most part, symptomatic (ie, the specific symptoms are treated as they occur). General treatment includes the use of *mild analgesics* to provide relief from pain and to reduce inflammation, *corticosteroids* to treat inflammation (many conditions respond specifically to these drugs), and *radiation* to suppress the abnormal antigen–antibody responses to the body. Systemic autoimmune disorders are difficult to treat successfully because a balance must be sought between suppressing the immune response that is causing the illness and maintaining enough immunity to fight off invasions of actual threatening foreign substances.

Human Immunodeficiency Virus

Human immunodeficiency virus (HIV) was recognized in the United States in 1983 and has reached **pandemic** proportions. This means it is affecting a particularly wide geographical area.

Prevention of HIV Transmission in Healthcare Workers

The risk of HIV infection and AIDS among healthcare workers is small, but a definite risk. However, you are only at risk if you are *directly* exposed to blood or other body fluids of HIV-infected persons. *Universal Precautions* established by the Centers for Disease Control (CDC) in Atlanta must be consistently applied to *every and all patients*. It is necessary to practice these precautions with each patient, because medical history and examination alone will not reveal all persons infected with the HIV virus.

Action of the HIV Virus

This virus is defined as an infectious human retrovirus. A **retrovirus** overtakes the biosynthesis of living cells to duplicate itself. Two types of cells commonly associated with this retrovirus are **T cells** (**lymphocytes** that mature in the thymus) and **B cells** (lymphocytes originating in the bone marrow). T cells and B cells produce antibodies for specific immune responses. The HIV retrovirus specifically invades and depletes the T_4 lymphocytes, thereby rendering the body's immune system inoperable. The person is then vulnerable to many **opportunistic infections**, which are invasions of microorganisms that proliferate wildly because the immune system is defective. Such infections, which rarely cause disease in people with healthy immune systems, account for 90% of the mortality of AIDS.

Key Concept*

◆ AIDS is the leading cause of death in men (and the fourth leading cause of death in women) between the ages of 25 and 44 in the United States.

◆ AIDS is the leading cause of death among African American women between the ages of 25 and 44 in the United States.

◆ Women and children are the fastest growing groups to become infected with the HIV virus.

◆ Between 1991 and 1992, the incidence in the United States rose by 13%.

Information as of July 1994 (CDC)

Signs and Symptoms

The HIV can remain dormant for 3 to 11 years (the average is 8 to 11 years for an adult male) before causing the characteristic signs and symptoms:

◆ Persistent lymphadenopathy
◆ Fever
◆ Night sweats
◆ Diarrhea
◆ General malaise
◆ Anorexia
◆ Weight loss

Once the virus becomes active, the patient will usually progress through the several stages of the disease.

Nursing Alert

The HIV infection can remain dormant for a long time, or presenting symptoms may not readily identify the patient as having HIV or AIDS. Therefore, it is important to learn and rely on universal precautions to protect yourself from unknown risk.

CDC Classification System

The Centers for Disease Control and Prevention (CDC) in Atlanta, Georgia has developed a system of classifying HIV infections. The 1994 clinical categories are presented in the accompanying box.

These measures are used to guide clinical treatment of HIV-infected persons. Antiretroviral drugs have been shown to be most effective within certain levels of immune dysfunction. These and other drugs used in treatment of HIV infections are presented later in this chapter.

HIV and Acquired Immunodeficiency Syndrome

Over the past decade **acquired immunodeficiency syndrome** (AIDS) has become one of the most pressing public health problems in the world. More than one million Americans are infected with HIV. The number of people infected worldwide is several times that number.

The term AIDS is defined by the CDC as: "the presence of a reliably diagnosed disease at least moderately indicative of underlying immunodeficiency, where there is no known cause other than HIV."

Currently, scientists believe that virtually all persons with the HIV antigen will eventually develop AIDS, most within 5 years. The virus has a lengthy incubation period and it is believed that infected persons remain able to transmit the disease for the rest of their lives. It may take as long as 6 to 12 months after infection before

---

CDC Classification of HIV Infections

Clinical Categories

Category A: Positive HIV test, persistent generalized lymphadenopathy, history of acute HIV infection.

Category B: symptomatic conditions: oral thrush, cervical dysplasia or invasive carcinoma, constitutional symptoms such as fever or diarrhea lasting longer than one month, herpes zoster (shingles) involving at least two distinct episodes, peripheral neuropathy.

Category C: secondary infectious diseases and cancers; encephalopathy (HIV-related), Kaposi's sarcoma, lymphoma, recurrent pneumonia.

Classification Using T_4 Lymphocyte Count*

Category 1: T_4 count $\geq$ 500/mm³ cubic millimeter of blood

Category 2: T_4 count 200–499/mm³ blood

Category 3: T_4 count < 200/mm³ of blood. A T-cell count below 200 is considered *full-blown AIDS*.

* mm³ = cubic millimeter

oral thrush, shingles, and severe athlete's foot are common. As immunity diminishes, serious infections are likely to develop. *Opportunistic infections* include:

- **Pneumocystis carinii** pneumonia (PCP pneumonia): a protozoan infection of the lungs
- Cryptococcal meningitis: caused by a fungus
- Toxoplasmosis: a parasitic brain infection
- Tuberculosis (TB): rapidly increasing in the HIV+ population
- **Kaposi's sarcoma:** an opportunistic cancer prevalent in homosexual men with AIDS
- A variety of fungal, viral, and bacterial infections may also surface, causing constitutional disease

---

Key Concept

In an immunosuppressed person, a very small reaction to the PPD test for TB may be considered positive. This person is considered *anergic;* (the test *appears to be negative* because the person's body cannot appropriately respond to the antigen). This does not mean the person has not been exposed to TB; the PPD may *mistakenly be read as negative.*

In the anergic person, a *two-step* skin test may be done. Two tests are done, a week apart. This boosts the person's immune system so they can accurately respond to the antigen.

Controls are also used. Candida and mumps are injected at the same time as PPD. This evaluates the body's ability to respond to *any antigen.* A person with a healthy immune system should respond to candida and/or mumps. The immunosuppressed person does not respond to any of the tests.

---

antibodies or antigens can be detected by a blood test (up to 18 months for infants).

Persons at Risk

Who is at risk for HIV infection? Male homosexuals or bisexuals and their sexual contacts and intravenous drug users who share needles remain at greatest risk. The infection is becoming much more widespread among the heterosexual population, however. (As mentioned above, infants of HIV-infected mothers often have HIV antibodies, but only about 1 of 4 go on to develop the symptoms of AIDS. The results of HIV testing in these infants cannot be reliably done until they are 9 to 18 months of age.) The risk of contracting HIV infection from processed blood and blood products is now greatly reduced, with widespread screening for HIV antibodies in blood donors.

The HIV in the heterosexual population is transmitted primarily sexually. The use of condoms in all sexual contacts is recommended to help prevent the spread of the disease. Women and children are currently the fastest growing group of patients. This is often related to intravenous drug abuse in the mother or her sexual partners.

Nursing Alert

Condoms do not guarantee "safe sex." They provide *safer* sex.

Opportunistic Infections in AIDS

When the T cell count falls to 200 to 400/mm³, the first opportunistic infections usually appear. Initial infections of the skin and mucous membranes such as

---

Key Medications

HIV Infections

CDC recommendations for administration of antiviral drugs (ZDU or DDC):

T-cell count > 500; no medications

T-cell count 200–500 without symptoms; medications may be discussed with physician; not recommended

T-cell count 200–500 with symptoms; ZDU recommended

T-cell count < 200; ZDU and DDI or DDC on a rotating basis

- acyclovir (Zovirax): chronic herpes simplex infections
- amphotericin B (Fungizone): antifungal [acute cryptococcal meningitis]
- bleomycin (Blenoxane), doxorubicin HCl (Adriamycin), vincristine (Oncovin): systemic chemotherapies to control Kaposi's sarcoma, in some cases
- didanosine (DDI, Videx): used for patients who are intolerant to ZDU, action is similar to ZDU
- dideoxycytidine (DDC): potent antiviral action
- INH, isoniazid (Nydrazid, Laniazid): to treat tuberculosis (TB) in persons with HIV infections
- ketoconazole (Nizoral): for oral thrush
- loperamide HCl (Immodium): to treat diarrhea associated with HIV enteropathy
- prednisone (Meticorten, Orasone, Deltasone): for severe inflammation or immunosuppression
- rifampin (Rifadin, Rimactane): bacterial tubercular infection
- stavudine, D₄T: newly approved by FDA, blocks virus replication. Used in patients who have failed on other drugs or to rotate with other drugs.
- trimethoprim and sulfamethoxazole (Septra, Bactrim): to treat *Pneumocystis carinii* pneumonia
- zidovidine (ZDU [formerly called AZT], Retrovir): slows progression of HIV-related disease (not curative)

NOTE: many of these drugs cause serious adverse side effects. CDC recommends that ZDU and DDI or DDC be rotated to prevent resistance to the drugs.

(weight loss, diarrhea, fever) and neurologic disorders (dementia, muscle and nerve weakness)

Treatment. Antiviral drugs such as zidovudine, ZDU (Retrovir), do not eradicate HIV completely, but they do slow the rate of T_4 lymphocyte depletion, to assist the immune system to fight opportunistic infections.

Mortality Rate. The mortality rate for persons with AIDS continues to be extremely high. No single treatment or drug therapy is available to cure this disease or restore lost immune function. Researchers are working to develop a vaccine to help combat the virus.

Key Concept

The treatment of AIDS cannot be defined specifically. The patient is treated *symptomatically*, that is, each of the symptoms is treated, because each patient shows different symptoms and groups of symptoms.

Medications in HIV Infections and AIDS. Medical researchers agree that the ideal approach to the management of AIDS symptoms involves the prevention of and early treatment of potentially fatal opportunistic infections. Drugs are often given in combination form and many produce serious side effects. Many drugs are tolerated only for a short period of time because of potential toxicity. Medications and related information are listed in the box on p. 1173.

Nursing Considerations. The social, economic, and medical impact of HIV and AIDS will be prominent feature of American medicine for the next generation.

Key Concept

An economist for the U.S. Department of Health and Human Services has estimated the cost of treating an HIV-positive person at $5,150 per year. This compares with treatment costs of $32,000 annually for a person with AIDS. Average lifetime cost is $85,300, higher than previously estimated due to prophylactic treatment and early positive HIV diagnosis (which help to prolong patients' lives).[1]

Patients with AIDS are burdened with a host of problems that require special nursing considerations. Because of their weakened condition, many require total nursing care. AIDS dementia is becoming an increasing problem (see Chapter 86). AIDS is a terminal disease, so it is important to focus on patient comfort. Emotional support, combined with technical skills, will help to provide patients with the ability to cope with their illness while hospitalized.

Until the AIDS virus is defeated, hope for improving the quality of a patient's life rests on the ability of healthcare workers to treat them with respect and dignity. The accompanying box summarizes subjects to teach the AIDS patient and their support persons.

---

[1] Hollinger FJ. "Costs in dollars and lives continue to rise." Journal of the American Medical Association, August 29, 1991.

Keys for Review

Key Questions for Critical Thinking

1. Compare immune disorders and autoimmune disorders. Describe medical and nursing care in each.
2. Identify the difference between HIV and AIDS. Describe how treatment would differ in each. Identify both physical care and psychological care the nurse should provide, especially in AIDS.
3. Identify opportunistic infections associated with AIDS. Discuss how they start and how they can be prevented. Include kinds of care that can be given.
4. State the cost of AIDS from various sociologic standpoints.
5. State information about universal precautions: purpose, when used, who uses it, how applied. Discuss how you can show concern for a patient when you are wearing a mask and gloves. Suggest how this applies to children and to the aging.

Key Readings

Berkow R (Ed). The Merck Manual of Diagnosis and Therapy, Ed 16. Rahway, NJ, Merck & Co, 1992

Centers for Disease Control and Prevention. "Revised classification for HIV." Morbidity and Mortality Weekly Report 41, 1993

DeVita VT, Hellman S, Rosenberg S, et al. AIDS: Etiology, Diagnosis, Treatment and Prevention, Ed 3. Philadelphia, J.B. Lippincott, 1992

Fischbach F. A Manual of Laboratory and Diagnostic Tests, Ed 3. Philadelphia, J.B. Lippincott, 1992

NANDA Nursing Diagnoses: Definitions and Classifications 1992. Philadelphia, North American Nursing Diagnosis Association, 1992

Nursing '94 Drug Handbook. Springhouse, PA, Springhouse, 1994

O'Toole M. (Ed). Miller-Keane Encyclopedia and Dictionary of Medicine, Nursing, and Allied Health, Ed. 5. Philadelphia, W.B. Saunders, 1992

Porth CM. Pathophysiology: Concepts of Altered Health States, Ed 4. Philadelphia, J.B. Lippincott, 1994

Smeltzer SC, Bare BG. Brunner and Suddarth's Textbook of Medical-Surgical Nursing, Ed. 7. Philadelphia, J.B. Lippincott, 1992

Key Readings (continued)

Taylor C, Lillis C, LeMone P. Fundamentals of Nursing: Art and Science of Nursing Care, Ed. 2. Philadelphia, J.B. Lippincott, 1993

Enrichment Keys

Collins P, Newland A. "Treatment modalities of autoimmune disorders." Seminars in Hematology 29:(1), 1992

Kampf LP. Who could have known? RN vol. 6, #3, June/July 1994, 29

Keys to Learning More

Chapter 79: respiratory disorders
Chapter 86: dementia-type disorders
Chapter 87: mental health/psychiatric nursing
Chapter 89: rehabilitation and home care
Chapter 90: death and dying
Chapter 91: hospice nursing

Key Resources

Centers for Disease Control and Prevention
  Department of Health and Human Services
  US Public Service
  Atlanta, GA 30333
  404/639-3534

Hearing-Impaired AIDS Hotline
  1-800/243-7889

National HIV and AIDS Hotline (CDC)
  1-800/342-AIDS

National AIDS Information Clearing House
  1-800/458-5231

Spanish AIDS Hotline
  1-800/344-7432

US Public Health Service
  202/245-6867

79 Respiratory Disorders

Keys for Learning

Learning Objectives

- Describe possible abnormal findings of a respiratory assessment.
- Discuss the purpose of diagnostic tests related to the respiratory system and the related nursing care.
- Describe and demonstrate care of the patient recovering from chest surgery.
- Identify the most common acute, chronic, and infectious respiratory disorders, their related signs and symptoms, and nursing and medical management.
- Describe the specific types of tuberculosis, their associated symptoms, and treatment.
- Discuss the principles of prevention and the nursing implications of tuberculosis.
- Identify the signs and symptoms of cancers of the lung and larynx and describe their medical treatment and related nursing care.
- Discuss the impact of trauma on the respiratory system.

Key Terms

anergic	paracentesis
asphyxiation	pleurisy
asthma	pneumothorax
bronchiectasis	pulmonary emphysema
bronchitis	rhinitis
empyema	rhinoplasty
hyperventilation	strangulation
hypoxia	suffocation
laryngectomy	thoracentesis
laryngectomee	

Keys to Understanding This Chapter

Chapter 5: basic human needs, of which breathing is prominent

Chapter 21: cardiovascular system

Chapter 22: anatomy and physiology of respiratory system

Keys to Understanding This Chapter
(continued)

Chapter 30: medical asepsis

Chapter 32: cardiopulmonary resuscitation

Unit Seven: nursing process

Unit Eight: communication and documentation

Chapter 38: signs and symptoms of illness or injury

Chapter 42: vital signs

Chapter 47: specimen collection

Chapter 50: physical examination and nursing assessment

Chapter 51: isolation techniques

Chapter 52: patient comfort and pain management

Chapter 53: the person who has surgery

Chapter 54: surgical asepsis

Unit Eleven: pharmacology and medication administration

Chapter 62: respiratory distress and resuscitation of newborn

Chapter 68: respiratory disorders in children

Chapter 74: cardiovascular disorders

Chapter 77: allergic and immune disorders

Key Points

- The respiratory and cardiovascular systems are vital to the functioning of the entire body because of their roles in providing and transporting oxygen to the cells and wastes away from cells.
- The nursing assessment of a patient with a respiratory disorder is critical in determining the severity of respiratory distress, the immediacy of the situation, and the necessary nursing care.
- Disorders of the respiratory system may be caused by infections (bacteria, virus, fungi), irritants (smoking, allergens, environmental chemicals), masses (cancerous tumors), or trauma.

Rosdahl CB: Textbook of Basic Nursing, 6th ed. © 1995 J.B. Lippincott Company

Key Points (continued)

- ◆ Respiratory disorders may be characterized by multiple clinical manifestations such as cough, changes in respiratory pattern, and abnormal breath sounds.
- ◆ When hypoxia (lack of oxygen) occurs, subsequent changes in the neurologic and cardiovascular systems may develop.
- ◆ Key elements in the treatment of respiratory disorders include medications specific to the disease; oxygen administration; postural drainage; positioning; turning, coughing, and deep breathing (TCDB); and breathing exercises.
- ◆ The goals of nursing management for patients with respiratory disorders are a patent (open) airway, an effective breathing pattern, and improved gas exchange.

Key Topics Outline

Anatomy and Physiology Review
Diagnostic Tests
    Laboratory Tests
    X-ray and Fluoroscopy Examinations
    Other Diagnostic Tests
Medical and Surgical Treatments
    Common Medical Treatments
    Common Surgical Treatments
Nursing Process
    Data Collection
    Nursing Diagnosis
    Planning and Implementation
    Evaluation

Key Topics Outline (continued)

Infectious Respiratory Disorders
    Pneumonia
    Pleurisy
    Histoplasmosis
    Tuberculosis
    Empyema
Chronic Respiratory Disorders
    Chronic Obstructive Pulmonary Disease
Trauma
Neoplasms
    Benign Neoplasms
    Lung Cancer
Disorders of the Nose
    Inflammatory Disorders
    Structural Disorders
    Nasal Trauma
Disorders of the Throat
    Trauma
    Neoplasms

Key Learning Activities

- ◆ Search for articles in healthcare journals that discuss respiratory disorders. Learn to identify each disorder.
- ◆ Interview a person with asthma. Describe the emotional and physical aspects, the medications used, and the warning signs of an impending asthma attack.
- ◆ Interview a patient with a total laryngectomy who uses esophageal speech. Describe the emotional and physical aspects. What is the person's current status?

Healthcare professionals may specialize in the field of respiratory care. A physician specializing in the area of respiratory disorders is called a *pulmonologist.* A related field is *respiratory care,* with technicians and therapists.

Anatomy and Physiology Review

In Chapter 22, you learned that the respiratory system consists of the upper respiratory tract (nose, sinuses, pharynx, and trachea) and the lower respiratory tract (bronchi and lungs). This system provides oxygen to the cells throughout the body and eliminates carbon dioxide (a waste product) from the body. This exchange of inhaled oxygen for carbon dioxide wastes from the cells occurs at the alveolar level in the lungs.

Because the blood carries oxygen and carbon dioxide, both the cardiovascular and the respiratory systems must be functioning for life to continue. A person can survive for only a few minutes without oxygen; it is the most vital basic need of people and animals.

Diagnostic Tests

Laboratory Tests

Sputum Specimen. Sputum specimen tests determine if any organisms or blood are present in the sputum. The nurse should collect the specimen early in the morning because at that time it most likely will contain sputum, rather than just saliva. The procedure for collecting a sputum specimen is presented in Chapter 47.

> **Nursing Alert**
>
> Precautions should be taken in care and disposal of sputum. Gloves should be worn when collecting specimens and hands washed after contact with sputum. A mask and eye shield should be worn if splashing is likely. All used facial tissues are discarded as contaminated material.

Lavage Specimens. If the patient is unable to cough up sputum, a specimen may be obtained by *bronchoalveo-*

Key Abbreviations and Acronyms Used in Respiratory Conditions

ABGs	Arterial blood gases
ARDS	Adult respiratory distress syndrome
CPT	Chest physiotherapy
CHF	Congestive heart failure
COPD	Chronic obstructive pulmonary disease
CPAP	Continuous positive airway pressure
CPR	Cardiopulmonary resuscitation
CXR	Chest x-ray
pH	Hydrogen ion concentration
PPD	Purified protein derivative
SOB	Short (shortness) of breath
TB	Tuberculosis
TCDB	Turn, cough, deep breathe
TCH	Turn, cough, hyperventilate

lar lavage. In this procedure, sterile saline is pumped into a bronchus. Then, cells and fluid from the bronchioles and alveoli are removed by bronchoscope, along with the saline. The cells are analyzed in the laboratory, most often to diagnose pulmonary tuberculosis (TB).

Throat Culture. A sample of both the mucus and the secretions from the back of the throat is obtained on a cotton-tipped applicator and applied to a slide or culture medium, which is then incubated in the laboratory to determine if organisms are present. Drug sensitivity determinations may also be done to determine which drug is most effective against a particular organism. This is known as a culture and sensitivity (C&S) test or *throat culture.* The procedure for collecting a throat culture is also explained in Chapter 47.

A full culture will determine all organisms present in the specimen. This test takes several days because the organisms must have time to grow.

A culture may be done within a matter of hours to rule out the presence of the streptococcus organism. This test does not rule out any other organisms. This "quick strep" test is done in cases of suspected strep infection so that appropriate antibiotic therapy can be initiated quickly.

Blood Gas Determinations. The best indicator of oxygen deficiency is the level of arterial blood gases. The partial pressure of oxygen (Pao_2) value is generally considered normal when it is between 90 and 100 mm Hg (millimeters of mercury). Severe oxygen deficiency exists when the Pao_2 is less than 40 mm Hg. The laboratory can analyze an arterial blood sample and determine the relative amounts and partial pressure of oxygen (Pao_2)

and carbon dioxide ($Paco_2$) in the blood, as well as the hydrogen ion concentration (pH) of the blood. The physician, nurse, and respiratory therapist then evaluate the blood gas results and plan the most effective treatment for the patient.

Key Concept

Blood Gas Determinations

Arterial blood gas (ABG) values measure partial pressure of oxygen (Pao_2) and partial pressure of carbon dioxide ($Paco_2$). These are reported as *mm Hg* (millimeters of mercury).

Values for Pao_2:
 Normal Pao_2
  80–100 mm Hg
Mild oxygen deficiency
  60–80 mm Hg
Moderate oxygen deficiency
  40–60 mm Hg
Severe oxygen deficiency
  < 40 mm Hg

X-ray and Fluoroscopy Examinations

Chest X-ray. The chest x-ray is no longer done routinely on all patients who are admitted to the hospital. It is, however, ordered to determine abnormalities in the lungs or heart. Abnormalities that can be observed on x-ray include lung tumors or other growths, lung abscess, TB, foreign objects in the lungs, pneumonia, or an enlarged heart.

CT Scan. The computed tomography (CT) scan is a series of x-rays taken to provide a cross-sectional view of the chest or other part of the body. The procedure is described in more detail in Chapter 71. CT scanning is valuable in diagnosis of TB, lung abscesses, or lung tumors.

Lung Scan. After a radioactive drug is introduced into the system by injection or inhalation, a lung scan (scintiscan) is done. This test yields a two-dimensional map representing various organs or tissues. Disorders are often revealed as a difference in density from normal tissue. Sometimes, when the gas is inhaled, this is called a *ventilation scan.*

Lung Perfusion Scan. Albumin tagged with a radioactive material is injected intravenously. These particles pass through the venous system and the heart, but when they reach the lungs they lodge in the capillaries. Different views are illustrated by the scan. Lesions, pneumonia, and other disorders can then be located.

Pulmonary Angiography. This test involves injection of radiopaque dye into the pulmonary blood vessels to determine pathology. Chapter 50 describes nursing precautions in the use of radiopaque dye.

Other Diagnostic Tests

Magnetic Resonance Imaging (MRI). As with many other body systems, MRI can be used to diagnose disorders in the lungs and bronchi. This test is a noninvasive nuclear procedure and can produce images of tissues with high fat and water content, which often cannot be seen by conventional x-ray. Thus, it is useful in diagnosis of lung disorders. The MRI allows the physician to distinguish between cancerous, trauma-induced, and normal tissues because it gives information about their chemical composition. The nursing precautions involved in MRI are presented in Chapter 71.

Pulmonary Function Test. The pulmonary function test measures the amount of air inhaled (*inspiration*) and exhaled (*expiration*) in one breath and assesses the patient's general respiratory status. Many large hospitals have pulmonary function laboratories for this purpose. Besides measuring *tidal volume* (volume of air in an average breath), inspiratory volume, and expiratory volume, the pulmonary function test measures total lung capacity, *vital capacity* (amount of air that is forcibly exhaled after a maximum breath), and *residual volume* (amount of air remaining in the lung after forced exhalation). The ratios between specific measurements can be determined. The machine used for these tests is the *spirometer*.

Key Concept

Do not confuse the spirometer and the incentive spirometer. The spirometer measures pulmonary function. The incentive spirometer also measures pulmonary function, in a sense, but is used by the patient. The incentive spirometer helps the postoperative patient to perform respiratory exercises to maintain lung function.

The pulmonary function test is used to diagnose disorders and to assess therapy. The test helps the physician and respiratory therapist assess pulmonary pathology at an early stage and indicates whether the patient has a cardiac or a respiratory disease. The test can evaluate the effectiveness of respiratory therapies and bronchodilator drugs and can indicate the surgical risk involved in many cases.

The nurse may act as a "cheerleader" when this test is administered, encouraging the patient to breathe as deeply as possible or to follow other instructions.

Bronchoscopy. Bronchoscopy is an invasive procedure in which a scope is passed through the mouth and pharynx into the trachea and bronchi (*bronchoscope*). The purposes of this test are to observe lung tissue, to obtain a biopsy or bronchial washings, to remove mucous plugs or foreign objects, and to determine the location and extent of a mass (tumor). Two types of bronchoscopes are used, the rigid and the fiberoptic. The fiberoptic scope is smaller and more flexible, which is more comfortable for the patient and which allows the physician to better visualize the lung within the smaller airways (Fig. 79-1).

Before the test, the patient's throat is anesthetized and medications (such as Versed) are administered intravenously to help the patient relax. These medications may cause the patient to have a temporary memory lapse. The patient may not remember having the test, for example. It is important to alert the patient to this possibility before the test.

Food and fluids are withheld for 6 to 8 hours before a bronchoscopy and mouth care is given immediately before the procedure. The procedure must be explained to the patient, who will most likely remain awake. Dentures should be removed and any loose natural teeth noted because a tooth may become loosened or dislodged by the bronchoscopy, and this could lead to aspiration. A mild sedative is usually given intravenously, just before the procedure.

The patient remains NPO until the gag reflex returns and is positioned on the side. (*Rationale: It is important to keep the airway open and to prevent choking and aspiration.*) The anesthetic numbs the throat, so the patient's reflexes do not react and allow the person to cough out secretions. The side-lying position helps to facilitate drainage. Edema of the throat, bleeding, and dyspnea should be noted because if the airway becomes obstructed, an emergency tracheostomy may be needed. In most cases, a sterile endotracheal tube is kept at the bedside until the patient is fully awake. In a respiratory emergency, the endotracheal tube can be placed to assist in keeping the airway open temporarily. The patient should be at rest and should eat soft foods for 24 hours following this procedure. Clear liquids may be given as soon as the gag reflex returns.

Because most bronchoscopy procedures are performed on an outpatient basis, the patient and family must be taught careful observational skills. They should particularly observe for:

◆ Any swelling of the throat
◆ Difficulty in swallowing
◆ Any breathing difficulty
◆ Any bleeding

Be sure all teaching is completely documented.

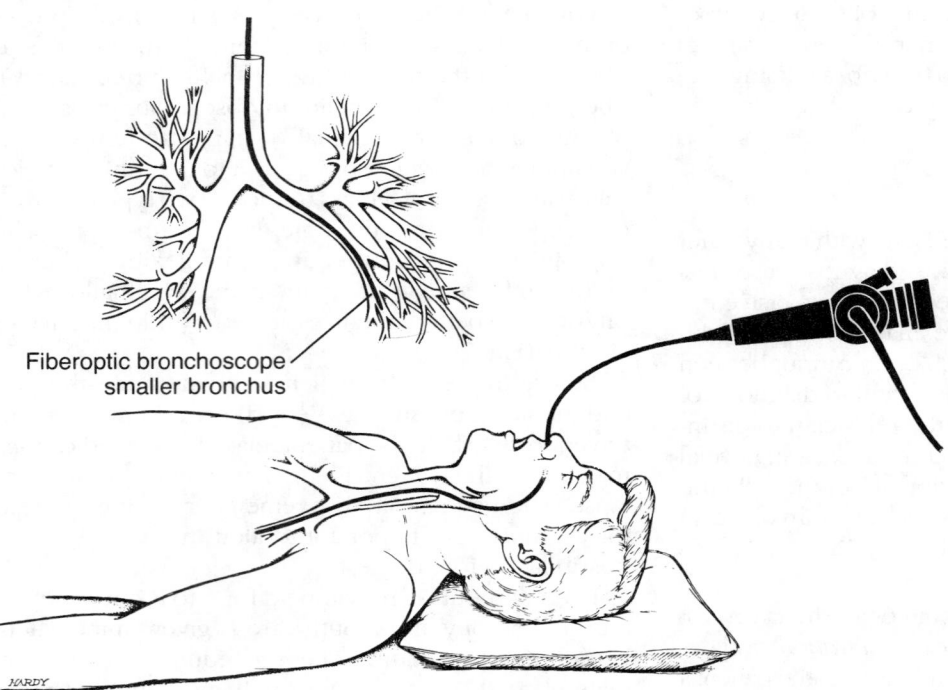

Figure 79-1. Fiberoptic bronchoscopy.

Fiberoptic bronchoscope
smaller bronchus

Skin Tests

Skin tests are commonly used to determine if a person has been exposed to TB or other disorders, such as histoplasmosis. The procedure is the same as for administering tests to determine allergies to medications or other allergens. (Intradermal injection is described and illustrated in Chapter 57; assessment of skin tests is described in Chapter 50.)

PPD Tuberculin Test. The tuberculin test indicates whether a person has ever been exposed to the tubercle bacillus. Approximately 0.1 mL tuberculin serum (PPD—purified protein derivative) is injected intradermally, with a syringe and needle. The injection site is examined for edema (induration) and redness (erythema) 2 and 3 days (48 and 72 hours) after the injection. Erythema alone does not indicate a positive reaction; the degrees of positive readings are based on the area of induration, sometimes combined with erythema (see Chapter 50).

A positive tuberculin test does not necessarily mean that a person has active TB; it simply means that the person has been exposed to the bacillus at some time. A person who is a positive reactor usually remains so for life. Thus, the PPD test is usually not repeated. In addition, some individuals may develop a severe allergic reaction to the test. If a person has a positive reaction to the PPD, a chest x-ray should be done to determine if the lungs are affected.

The Use of Controls. Candida and mumps antigen sera may be injected at the same time as the PPD to deter-

mine a person's ability to respond to *any foreign agent* (antigen). Persons with healthy immune systems should respond to candida and/or mumps. If this does not occur, the person is considered **anergic**. In this case, the PPD may have been mistakenly read as negative. In other words, in the anergic person, the PPD *appears to be negative* because the person's body cannot appropriately respond to any antigen. This does not mean that the person has not been exposed to TB.

If the person is judged to be anergic, a *two-step PPD test* may be necessary. The two-step PPD test involves doing two PPD tests, 1 or 2 weeks apart. This method attempts to boost the person's immune system to appropriately respond to the antigen. Many public health departments now do the two-step test routinely.

Special Considerations in Aging
PPD Tests

A negative result on the PPD test in an elderly person does not necessarily indicate that the person has never been exposed to TB or does not have active TB. Persons over age 65 may be anergic because of immune system failure (*not* an immunodeficiency disease). If an elderly person tests PPD negative, other tests may be necessary to confirm a diagnosis of TB (sputum culture, chest x-ray, or two-step PPD test).

Tine Test. Another method of tuberculin testing is the tine test, which is simply a different method of injecting the tuberculin. It is often used in mass screening. A sterile stainless steel disk with four tines is impregnated with PPD; the tines are pressed into the patient's skin. The disks are packaged individually and are disposable; thus, they offer a practical advantage when testing a large group of people.

Histoplasmosis Test. A similar skin test may also be done to detect the presence of the histoplasmosis fungus.

Medical and Surgical Treatments

Common Medical Treatments

Postural Drainage

Postural drainage uses gravity to help the patient cough up secretions and mucus from the lungs. The patient adopts a head-downward position (Fig. 79-2),

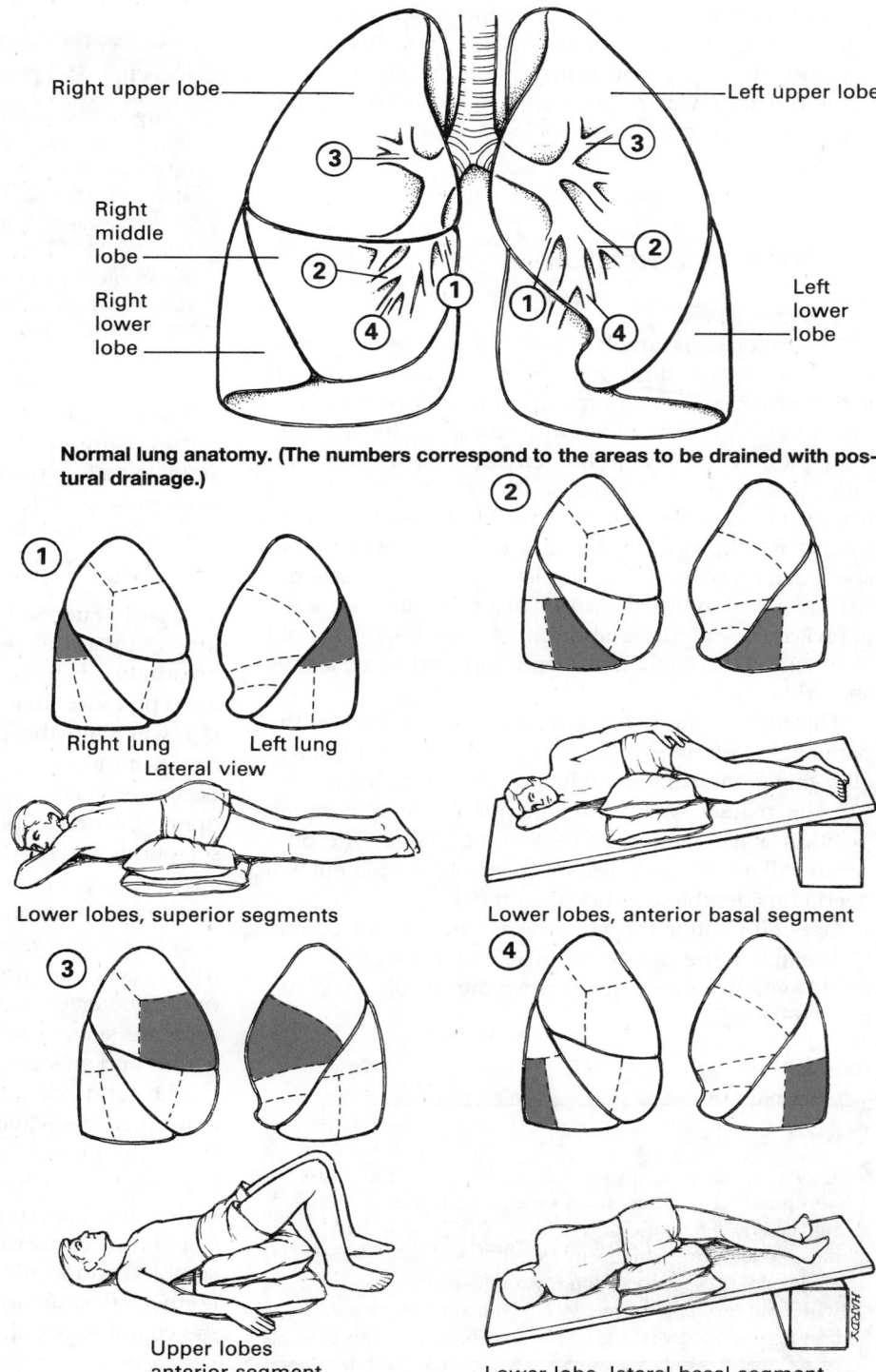

Normal lung anatomy. (The numbers correspond to the areas to be drained with postural drainage.)

① Right lung   Left lung
Lateral view
Lower lobes, superior segments

② Lower lobes, anterior basal segment

③ Upper lobes anterior segment

④ Lower lobe, lateral basal segment

Figure 79-2. Postural drainage. Usually the bronchi of the lower and middle lobe empty most effectively when the patient's head is down. The force of gravity helps drain secretions from the smaller bronchial airways to the main bronchi and the trachea. The patient then is able to cough up the secretions. This procedure is most effective if done in early morning.

which allows the secretions to run far enough into the trachea from the bronchi so that they can be coughed out. The patient's exact position will depend on the portion of the lung to be drained. Treatments generally last about 15 to 20 minutes. This is called chest physiotherapy (CPT). The nurse should receive specific instructions from the respiratory therapist, physical therapist, or pulmonary physician before performing these procedures.

Often postural bronchial drainage is done in combination with other respiratory treatments such as inhalations to loosen and bring up secretions from the lungs and to prevent respiratory complications. Nursing considerations appear in the Nursing Process section of this chapter.

Common Surgical Treatments

Thoracentesis

Thoracentesis involves puncturing the chest wall to remove excess fluid or air from the pleural cavity. It is done for diagnostic purposes or to relieve breathing difficulties in patients with tuberculosis, cancer of the lung, pleural effusion, pulmonary edema, and chest injuries. Using sterile technique, the physician inserts a trocar (large needle with obturator) into the pleural cavity and withdraws fluid. As the needle is withdrawn, the specimen is collected in a sterile container. The amount of fluid withdrawn is measured in a graduate. The specimen is then sent to the laboratory for analysis. The fluid is considered contaminated and appropriate measures should be taken.

Throughout the procedure, the nurse will assist the patient and offer support. The procedure is similar to abdominal paracentesis, which is described in Chapter 81. The patient will be most comfortable in a sitting position while leaning on the overbed table. The physician will need very little assistance, but the patient will need considerable emotional support.

Generally, after the procedure, the patient is able to breathe more easily because the pressure of the fluid, which often causes respiratory distress, has been relieved.

Nursing Alert

Thoracentesis is an invasive procedure. A permit must be signed. The patient must be watched carefully for signs of fluid leakage or infection. The patient may have some pain, which can usually be relieved by an analgesic. Be sure to watch for respiratory depression when any drugs are used. A rare but serious complication is pneumothorax (collapse of a lung).

Paracentesis

Paracentesis is defined as the puncturing of a body cavity for aspiration of fluid; however, this process most commonly refers to puncture of the abdominal cavity. Removing fluid from the abdomen can relieve breathing difficulties. Abdominal distention from excess fluid immobilizes the diaphragm and interferes with breathing.

Nursing Alert

A large amount of fluid withdrawal (over 1,000 mL) during paracentesis or thoracentesis can result in vasodilation and *hypovolemia* (decreased circulating fluid volume). This can cause *syncope* (temporary loss of consciousness, fainting) and shock. The nurse should take the blood pressure and pulse immediately after paracentesis or thoracentesis and every 15 minutes until readings are stable and at an adequate level.

Thoracotomy

Lung surgery is often called *thoracotomy*, which is an incision into the thorax or chest cavity. Nursing care in chest surgery is outlined in the Nursing Process section of this chapter.

Closed Water-Seal Drainage. After chest surgery, the lungs must be reinflated and kept inflated. The breathing mechanism operates on the principle of negative pressure, that is, the pressure in the chest cavity is lower than the pressure of the outside air, which causes air to rush into the lungs. Thus, a vacuum must occur artificially within the chest, after it has been opened, to reestablish negative pressure. In addition, secretions and blood that may have accumulated in the chest cavity must be removed. The most common method of reestablishing negative pressure is by *closed water-seal drainage*. In this procedure, one or more catheters are inserted into the chest cavity. If more than one catheter is inserted, each may be connected to a separate suction setup, or they may all be joined together and attached to one suction setup.

The term "closed" means that no air is allowed to enter the chest cavity; otherwise, the lungs would collapse. By putting the drainage tubes under water, air is prevented from backing up into the chest. The most widely used apparatus is the disposable system, often called the Pleur-Evac (Fig. 79-3). This system comes assembled and sterile, with instructions for use. It can be connected to suction, and provides a water seal. When the chamber is full, it is discarded and replaced with a new one.

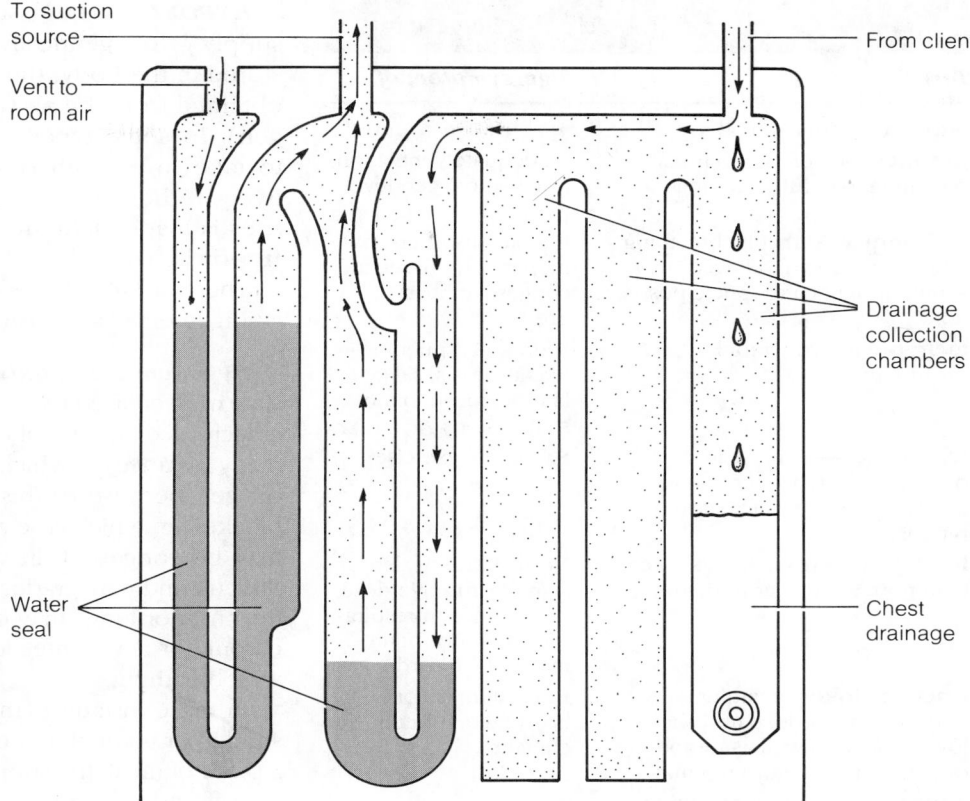

Figure 79-3. The Pleur-Evac system of underwater drainage. This system operates using the same principles as the three-bottle system, but the Pleur-Evac is much safer and more convenient. It is prepackaged and sterile and is thrown away after use. The arrows indicate the flow of air when the lung is inflated properly. The drainage is measured in the device before it is emptied.

Labels in figure:
To suction source
Vent to room air
Water seal
From client
Drainage collection chambers
Chest drainage

❖ *Nursing Process*

Data Collection

The nurse must carefully observe and assess the patient with a respiratory disorder. Because adequate oxygenation is vital to life, a disorder in the respiratory system can be quickly life-threatening. Chapter 50 describes physical examination and assessment, including that of the respiratory system. This assessment establishes a baseline for future comparison and determines the presence of suspected complications. The nurse should report any changes in the baseline level.

When doing a nursing assessment of the respiratory system, the nurse assesses the breathing and oxygenation level of the patient. The accompanying box lists some of the components of the respiratory nursing assessment.

In addition, the nurse observes the patient's emotional response to the disorder or disease. Is enough oxygenation occurring to support life? Is emergency resuscitation required? Does the patient need assistance to meet daily needs? Does the disorder affect social activities or self-esteem? Is the patient anxious or fearful about the outcome?

Alterations in Respiratory Status

Various events can alter the respiratory st... patient. These may be caused by illness... are discussed here; others are liste...

ASPIRATION. Patholo... ment of fluid, mucu... lungs. This can c...

HYP... pati...

Keys to Nursing Assessment
Respiratory System

- ◆ Nursing history
- ◆ Respiratory rate, depth, and character
- ◆ Respiratory status
- ◆ Respiratory distress/signs or dyspnea or poor oxygenation
- ◆ Signs/symptoms of hypoxia (lack of oxygen)
- ◆ Symptoms such as cough, hemoptysis
- ◆ Lung sounds/breath sounds
- ◆ Assessment of skin tests related to tuberculosis or other lung conditions
- ◆ Observation of mouth and throat by visualization and palpation

Table 79-1. Key Terminology Related to Respirations

Term	Sign/symptom of:
eupnea—normal breathing	
dyspnea—labored or difficult breathing, painful breathing	Inadequate ventilation, lowered oxygen level in blood
orthopnea—difficulty breathing while lying down, relieved by sitting upright (orthopneic position)	Cardiac disorders, pulmonary emphysema, congestive heart failure
tachypnea—very rapid breathing	High fever, pneumonia, alkalosis, salicylate overdose, brain stem lesions
hyperpnea—increase in depth of breaths, maybe increase in rate (no feeling of increased respiratory effort)	Strenuous exercise
bradypnea—respiration slower than normal, regular in rhythm	Normal during sleep; sign of drug overdose, disturbance in respiratory center of brain, metabolic disorder
Cheyne-Stokes breathing—combination of deep and shallow breaths, as well as periods of apnea (may be up to 3 min)	Brain stem lesion, heart failure, brain damage
apnea—cessation of breathing	
—*central apnea:* no brain drive to breathe	Undeveloped respiratory center in preterm infants, adult brain stem lesion, high spinal cord injury
—*obstructive apnea:* no air flow due to upper airway obstruction	Foreign object in airway, excessive secretions, absent cough reflex
—*mixed apnea:* centr[...] immediately follo[...] struction	
—*adul[...]* and[...]	[...]ctive (tongue or [...]ructures re-[...]sity [...]ain damage, [...] [...]losis, re-

HYPERVENTILATION. In **hyperventilation,** the [...]ent breathes abnormally fast or deeply, resulting in [...]cause lung disorders or death. [...]gic or another substance is the move[...] [...]s or injury. Some [...]d in Table 79-1.

HYPOXIA. The tissue cells must have a constant supply of oxygen to live, but because oxygen is not stored in the body, the supply of oxygen is normally obtained from the air (air is approximately 21% oxygen). In some types of illness, the body is unable to take in enough oxygen or cannot use it effectively. When the level of oxygen in the body tissues is inadequate, the patient is said to suffer from **hypoxia**.

There are four types of hypoxia: hypoxemic, circulation, anemic, and histotoxic.

Hypoxemic Hypoxia. Hypoxemic hypoxia is a state of decreased oxygen level in the blood, leading to a decreased amount of oxygen in the tissues. There are many instances in which the body does not get enough oxygen because of this disorder: the airway may be blocked, in which case respiration will cease; the lungs may be congested, in which case respiration will be difficult and may gradually become worse; an injury to the chest or lungs may cause difficulty in breathing; or chronic or acute infections in the lungs may interfere with breathing.

In these instances, the decrease in oxygen may be sudden or gradual. For example, if a person chokes on a piece of meat, the supply of air or oxygen is suddenly cut off and the person will die if the airway is not restored within a matter of minutes. In many infectious or chronic conditions of the lungs, breathing is impaired but not stopped completely. In these instances, most of which are not emergencies, the nurse can help to maintain life by assisting the patient to breathe or to obtain oxygen.

Circulation Hypoxia. *Circulation hypoxia* is due to inadequate blood circulation. If blood cannot get to tissues, the oxygen supply is cut off. The two chief circulatory disorders that account for a decrease in oxygen supply are failure of the heart to pump and blockage or rupture of a blood vessel.

Failure of the heart to pump may be caused by a lack of blood to the heart itself, by a weakening of the heart muscle, by stoppage, or by wild, uncontrolled beating of the heart (fibrillation). If the blood cannot get through a blood vessel because of a clot or stricture or because of developing atherosclerosis, the blood supply is reduced or stopped completely. This happens in a *cerebrovascular accident* (stroke) and in a *thrombosis*. In a ruptured *aneurysm*, the vessel explodes and the channel for blood is absent.

Anemic Hypoxia. *Anemic hypoxia* is due to re-[...]uction in the oxygen-carrying capacity of the blood. [...]ygen is carried to the tissues by hemoglobin, a [...]tituent of red blood cells. A lack of hemoglobin [...]ed *anemia*. Anemia can occur through de-[...] blood volume, because of decreased hemoglobin within the red blood cells, or because of inability of the hemoglobin to take on oxygen. In sickle cell anemia, the malformed red blood cells cannot pass through the capillaries. Carbon monoxide poisoning is a form of anemic hypoxia because the carbon monoxide combines with hemoglobin, leaving no room for oxygen.

Histotoxic Hypoxia. *Histotoxic hypoxia* is due to inability of the tissues to use oxygen. Under the influence of certain chemicals, the cells are unable to use oxygen; this is known as histotoxic hypoxia. The most common example is cyanide poisoning. Persons who have suffered smoke inhalation often have inhaled cyanide gas and may have histotoxic hypoxia.

Signs and Symptoms of Hypoxia. One of the most obvious signs of oxygen deficiency is shortness of breath (SOB). When expressed by the patient, SOB is known as *dyspnea*. SOB can also be assessed by the nurse through clinical observation: restlessness, apprehension, an anxious facial expression, panic, fatigue, or impaired coordination. As the need for more oxygen continues, the patient's rate and depth of respiration may increase.

Severe oxygen deficiency can be observed by the patient's use of accessory breathing muscles of the neck and upper chest. Gasping, wheezing, or retractions of the breastbone or intercostal spaces are also late signs of hypoxia.

Mental changes, confusion, stupor, and unconsciousness are all signs of oxygen deprivation. Check the level of consciousness on all patients who show signs of hypoxia.

Cardiac symptoms may develop due to hypoxia. The basic problem is inability of the heart to provide blood, thus oxygen, to the tissues. The heart often overworks. In addition, the heart itself does not get enough oxygen. Symptoms include rapid pulse, arrhythmias, fibrillation, and cardiac standstill (cardiac arrest). The body's first response to hypoxia is to increase the pulse in an effort to get more oxygen. Heart *arrhythmias* are a common early sign of hypoxia.

Changes in skin color are another indication of difficulty. *Cyanosis* is the bluish or dusky discoloration of the skin, nail beds, and mucous membranes that results from either a marked lack of oxygen or a severe loss of blood. It is often seen in shock. *Pallor*, very pale skin, also indicates oxygen lack or severe loss of blood. Assessment for these signs is described in Chapter 50.

Nursing Diagnosis

Based on data collection, the following sample nursing diagnoses may be seen on a nursing care plan for the patient with a respiratory disorder. Multiple causal factors are listed.

- Fluid Volume Excess related to compromised respiratory mechanism
- Impaired Gas Exchange related to lung disorders, obstruction, trauma, altered oxygen supply
- Ineffective Airway Clearance related to obstruction, trauma, painful/ineffective cough, excess secretions, cerebrovascular accident, infection, or spinal cord injury
- Ineffective Breathing Pattern related to neurologic disorder, obstruction, trauma, pain
- Altered Oral Mucous Membrane related to mouth breathing
- Impaired Verbal Communication related to tracheostomy, laryngectomy, obstruction, trauma, physical barriers, brain damage
- Activity Intolerance related to imbalance between oxygen supply and demand, pain, lung disorders, emphysema, asthma
- Anxiety related to inability to breathe

Planning and Implementation

The patient, nurse, and family plan together for effective care to meet patient needs, based on the nursing diagnosis. The nurse provides preoperative and postoperative care for the patient undergoing various types of lung and chest surgery. It is especially important to manage chest suction in the patient who has had open-chest surgery. The patient with a respiratory disorder may be anxious. This person may also require assistance in management of portable oxygen. The person may need assistance to meet some or all basic needs, in dealing with emotional problems, and understanding more about the disorder, its prognosis, and its treatment. A nursing care plan is developed to meet these needs. A sample nursing care plan for a patient with a respiratory disorder is provided later in the chapter.

Caring for the Patient With Chest Surgery

Before chest surgery, it is important that the patient be taught deep-breathing techniques, as well as range-of-motion (ROM) exercises, because the extent of the patient's participation in postoperative care will directly reflect the quality of preoperative care given. Postoperative exercises are vital to recovery.

The patient is given routine preoperative and postoperative care. Other skills in postoperative care are summarized in the accompanying box.

The *immediate postoperative* concern for the patient who has had lung surgery is to maintain an adequate airway, whether it is ordered that the patient be in the intensive care unit (ICU) to receive mechanical ventilatory assistance or is on a regular nursing station and is to receive supplemental oxygen. In

Nursing Skill Guidelines
Caring for the Person Who Has Had Chest Surgery

◆ Always wear gloves.
◆ Turn the patient often. *(Rationale: This will help facilitate drainage and prevent hypostatic pneumonia and other complications. The wound will drain the most when the patient is lying on the affected side; however, because this can be uncomfortable for the patient, coordinate turning to this side with the time when the pain medication effectiveness is optimum.)*
◆ Be sure the patient turns and coughs and uses the incentive spirometer, as ordered.
◆ Encourage patient to breathe deeply.
◆ Assess for dyspnea, rate of respiration, cyanosis, increased heart rate, chest pain, restlessness, orthopnea, or hemoptysis. *(Rationale: These symptoms could indicate that the chest suction is manfunctioning.)*
◆ Help the patient sit comfortably in the chair while the chest suction is operating.
◆ If the patient is up walking with tubes and drainage bags or bottles, the hemostatic clamps must go along. *Rationale: The patient must always be within reach of the clamps in case of accidental dislodgement of tubes.)*
◆ Make sure the patient is passing flatus rather than having gas pains or distention difficulties. *(Rationale: Abdominal distention can cause difficulty in breathing and extreme discomfort.)*
◆ Encourage ambulation and exercises *(Rationale: This will help the patient recover more quickly and will decrease any risks of complications.)* It is important to maintain a level of comfort acceptable to the patient, so that deep breathing and coughing can and will be done.

Nursing Assessment: Danger Signs

Be alert for the following:

◆ Leakage of air into the drainage system, whether in a simple water-seal type or a mechanical suction type, is indicated by constant *bubbling* in the *water-seal* system or bottle, once the patient's lungs have been initially expanded. There will be bubbling in the *control* bottle—the one connected to suction. If bubbling in the control bottle stops, the suction pressure is too low.
◆ There may be an air leak at the insertion site of the chest tube, in connections, in the bottles, or in the stoppers in three bottle suction; there may also be a leak in the closed drainage system itself.
◆ To check the location of an air leak, pinch the tubing for a few seconds at intervals between the chest tube and drainage connection. If the bubbling stops, the air leak is due to the system (check all connections). If the bubbling continues, pinch off tubing at intervals between the patient and the system. when the pinching is between the source of the air leak and the water chamber, the bubbling will stop.
◆ Keep all tubes, bags and other devices *below* the level of tube insertion. *(Rationale: This position prevents reflux—back flow.)*
◆ If the patient shows signs of cyanosis or dyspnea, or complains of chest pain, investigate the situation immediately. This is an emergency!

---

any event, care is directed at preventing respiratory complications.

Vital signs are recorded frequently; the patient is turned often to prevent complications of immobility. The patient must be encouraged to breathe deeply and to cough (TCDB) at least every 2 to 4 hours. The patient usually uses the incentive spirometer. It is easier to cough if the patient is in an upright position and if the incision is splinted with a pillow or is held tightly with both hands. (See Chapter 53.)

The patient must exercise soon after surgery because many muscles have been incised during chest surgery and function must be restored; exercise also prevents complications related to immobility. The nurse carries out passive ROM exercises for the patient, and within a few days the patient actively participates in ROM. Full ROM exercises, including isometric (muscle-setting) exercises, must be provided

for the operative shoulder and arm; these exercises may be initiated *immediately* following surgery. It is important that movement be discontinued at the point of pain or great resistance. The muscles should not be overextended or overtired.

Nursing Alert

If a patient with any disorder of the respiratory system is receiving a narcotic, the nurse must be particularly watchful for respiratory depression. Depressed respirations can be an undesirable side effect in any patient, but the situation is most dangerous for the patient whose respiratory function is already compromised.

CHEST SUCTION. Patients have chest suction following lung surgery. Care must be taken to preserve the negative pressure within the chest cavity. *(Rationale: If the negative pressure is lost, the lungs will collapse.)* The nurse must assess the signs of shock, dyspnea, pain in the chest, or a rapid increase in chest tube drainage and must report these symptoms immediately. *(Rationale: The most serious postoperative complications are hemorrhage into the lung cavity [hemothorax] or collection of air in the pleural cavity, causing collapse of all or part of a lung [pneumothorax.])* In a hemothorax the fluid (blood) collects in the lower part of the pleural cavity. In pneumothorax, the air rises to the top (see Fig. 79-5**C**). See the accompanying box for guidelines.

Pneumothorax. A serious complication in any patient who is undergoing chest drainage with tubes is **pneumothorax**, which is the presence of air in the pleural cavity or between the pleura and the chest wall, usually causing the collapse of a lung. This is an *emergency situation*; the tubing should be double-clamped immediately and a physician notified. Signs of pneumothorax are:

◆ Shortness of breath or dyspnea
◆ Chest not symmetrical
◆ Mediastinal shift toward the affected side
◆ Sudden, sharp chest pain
◆ Drop in blood pressure
◆ Weak, rapid pulse
◆ Cessation of breathing movement on affected side
◆ Cyanosis
◆ Change in level of consciousness

If any of these signs occur, clamp the chest tubes and *get help immediately.*

Nursing Alert

The integrity of the suction apparatus must be maintained at all times. The water seal must be maintained. *Refill* the chamber if the fluid level gets low. The nurse must report *at once* if the patient has any complaints of severe pain or dyspnea. A clamp is kept with the patient to clamp off the chest tubes in case of emergency. (DO NOT clamp chest tubes unless there is a specific physician's order.)

If a bottle breaks, the closed system will be disrupted. This is an emergency situation! Clamp the chest tubes immediately and summon help.

Caring for the Patient With Nasal Surgery

Most surgery on the nose is performed on an outpatient basis. Therefore, patient and family teaching is essential. Be sure to carefully and completely document all teaching.

The nose is vascular; hemorrhage is always a possibility. The family and patient must know what to watch for. The procedure can also be painful. In addition, the patient may be anxious because nasal procedures can interfere with respiration. The accompanying box identifies guidelines for nursing care in nasal surgery.

Relieving Respiratory Distress

ORTHOPNEIC POSITION. Many patients will not be able to breathe unless they are in a sitting or semisitting position (orthopneic position). The nurse should position this patient with pillows so the back is supported. Sometimes, it helps if the patient leans on a padded overbed table while in this position or sleeps in a lounge chair, because it may be required that the patient remain in the sitting position while sleeping (see Figure 72-1).

TURNING, COUGHING, DEEP BREATHING (TCDB). The importance of TCDB was explained in Chapter 53. TCDB is vital for any patient who is in bed for a long time. Lung complications can occur when a patient is immobile and will develop more quickly when a respiratory problem is present. To prevent such complications, you must be sure that the patient continually ventilates and expands the lungs as much as possible.

Administering Respiratory Treatments

POSTURAL DRAINAGE. Because postural drainage uses gravity, the patient is placed in a head-downward position, as shown in Figure 79-2. Request training from the respiratory therapist specific to the individual. *(Rationale: Positions vary from patient to patient because of the specific disorder and the area of the lung being drained.)* The accompanying box details nursing skills in postural bronchial drainage.

BREATHING EXERCISES AND INCENTIVE SPIROMETER. The physician will probably order breathing exercises to help the patient build up respiratory capacity. This is usually done with the aid of the incentive spirometer. Instructions to the patient depend on the particular type of device used. This procedure is described more fully in Chapter 53 and is illustrated in Figure 53-5. One of the main reasons for doing postoperative incentive spirometry is to prevent *atelectasis* (see Fig. 79-5**B**). Atelectasis is an airless or potentially collapsed state of the lung due to obstruction by mucus or a foreign object.

The patient may be instructed to do other exercises to increase respiratory capacity and function and may be taught the technique of abdominal breathing—pushing the abdominal wall out during inspiration and pulling it in during exhalation.

INTERMITTENT POSITIVE PRESSURE BREATHING (IPPB) TREATMENT. This treatment is not often used today, unless aerosolized medications are to be given. The most common use of IPPB is in cystic fibrosis. IPPB is briefly described in Chapter 80.

Nursing Skill Guidelines
Caring for the Patient Having Chest Suction

♦ Always wear gloves.
♦ Never attempt to set up any chest suction without assistance. *(Rationale: In most hospitals, at least two people must check a suction setup before it can be connected to the patient. This is a safety precaution.)*
♦ Never disconnect or change chest suction without being absolutely certain about what to do. *(Rationale: A patient's life depends on the ability to maintain the integrity of the pleural space.)*
♦ Wear gloves when working with chest suction.

Preventing Air Leakage

♦ Never disconnect chest tubes! *(Rationale: These provide the suction that keeps the lungs inflated. If they are disconnected the lungs will collapse.)*
♦ Clamps or hemostats should be kept with the patient, either clipped to the bedding or to the patient's gown (when using the three-bottle system). With the disposable system, a clamp is attached with the tubing. Thus, additional clamps are not necessary. If the patient gets out of bed, the clamps go along. *(Rationale: The tubes are clamped as an emergency measure in case the tubes become accidentally disconnected.)*
♦ If the tubes become disconnected, double-clamp all tubes close to the chest wall and summon assistance immediately. *(Rationale: This is an emergency situation!)*
♦ If air enters the chest cavity, the patient's lungs will collapse. You must obtain help immediately.
♦ Clamping chest tubes may cause a tension pneumothorax. *If any untoward symptoms occur, call for help immediately.*
♦ Never empty drainage in a closed system. The amount is noted as ordered. The entire system is discarded when full.
♦ Never use pins to fasten the tubes to the bed. *(Rationale: A pin might puncture the tube.)*
♦ Never change a chest dressing. *(Rationale: The dressing may be helping to maintain the integrity of the chest wall.)*
♦ Never take the plugs out of the bottles without assistance and never pull on chest tubes. *(Rationale: These actions may result in air entering the chest cavity.)*
♦ Tape all connections to make sure they are airtight.

Keeping the Tubes Open (Patent)

♦ Chest tubes do not need to be stripped unless there are clots or very thick drainage. In this case, stripping the tubes may be necessary to maintain patency.
♦ Hold the tube in place while you are stripping or milking it. *(Rationale: Holding the tube between your hands and the patient's chest keeps you from pulling on the tubes and possibly displacing them.)*

♦ Chest tubes should not be stripped more than 7 to 9 inches at a time. *(Rationale: This will prevent possible tearing of the pleura.)*
♦ Use short strokes rather than one long stroke.
♦ If a chest tube becomes kinked, report it immediately.
♦ To set up the drainage after it is inserted, wrap a piece of cloth tape around the tube and then attach the tape to the edge of the bed, so the tube hangs straight down into the bottle. *(Rationale: Straight drainage provides the best drainage flow.)*
♦ The remainder of the tubing is in the bed with the patient. *(Rationale: The excess tubing allows the patient to turn in bed and move about.)*
♦ Be sure the patient does not lie on the tubing. *(Rationale: This might obstruct the flow of the drainage.)*

Caring for the Bottles or Containers

♦ Drainage containers must remain lower than the level of the patient at all times. *(Rationale: To facilitate drainage and to prevent backflow.)*
♦ If bottles are used, a stand is provided for safety with the three-bottle system. Sometimes they hang in a rack provided for this purpose and are attached to the bed. (This system is rarely used.)
♦ The disposable closed system is safer than the bottle system. *(Rationale: The plastic container is much less likely to break and the tubes are more secure in the drainage container.)*

Nursing Assessment and Documentation

♦ It is your responsibility for accurate observation and reporting. The amount, color, and consistency of the drainage is vital information; inform the physician or team leader if there is a marked change.
♦ Observe for excessive bleeding or for abrupt absence of drainage. *(Rationale: Hemorrhage is a dangerous complication, and abrupt absence of drainage often means that the system is not operating properly.)*
♦ Document any changes in respiratory status, or respiratory distress.
♦ Document milking of the tubes.
♦ Put a piece of tape on the drainage bottle to indicate the fluid level, and record the level of the drainage as ordered.
♦ Discard all drainage tubes and other equipment as required by universal precautions.

Nursing Skill Guidelines
Caring for the Patient Who Has Had Nasal Surgery

◆ Wear gloves.
◆ Precautions must be taught to the patient or family and teaching carefully documented. (*Rationale: Most nasal surgery is done on an outpatient basis. The patient will be going home immediately after surgery.*)

Promoting Respiration

◆ The patient is often very uncomfortable. (*Rationale: The initial postoperative period can be very painful. The person will probably have to breathe through the mouth.*)
◆ Give frequent oral hygiene. (*Rationale: Breathing through the mouth is very drying to the mucous membranes.*)
◆ Elevate the head of the bed. (*Rationale: This facilitates breathing.*)
◆ Observe carefully for choking. Suctioning may be needed. (*Rationale: Considerable mucous drainage is usual, because the nasal mucosa has been irritated.*)
◆ Observe for signs of respiratory distress. (*Rationale: Swelling or bleeding may cause respiratory difficulties. Aspiration into the lungs is always a threat.*)

Assessment for Hemorrhage

◆ Observe for nausea, coffee-ground emesis, dark-colored emesis, frequent spitting of blood, blood on the dressing and any signs of shock. (*Rationale: The nose is very vascular and may bleed profusely. In surgery of the nose or nosebleed [epistaxis], blood may run down the back of the throat and be swallowed.*)
◆ At regular intervals, examine the back of the throat for draining of blood by using a flashlight and tongue depressor.
◆ The nostrils are usually packed with gauze, which is removed 24 to 48 hours following surgery. Observe carefully for hemorrhage after removal of a pack.
◆ The mustache dressing, a gauze pad impregnated with petrolatum and held in place with strips of adhesive, is applied beneath the nostrils. (*Rationale: This is applied to absorb drainage.*)

AEROSOL TREATMENT. A mask or mouthpiece apparatus is attached to oxygen or compressed air and aerosolized medication is administered. This treatment is further discussed in Chapter 80.

OXYGEN. Many patients with respiratory and other problems receive supplemental oxygen by cannula or mask. This assists them to breathe more easily and provides a higher concentration of oxygen than does room air. It is important for the nurse to provide emotional support because this is a frightening experience for pa-tients and families. The administration of oxygen is illustrated and described in detail in Chapter 80.

Administering Nasal Treatments

NASAL MEDICATIONS. Nasal sprays and nose drops are often used for patients with respiratory disorders. Procedures for administering nasal medications are described and pictured in Chapter 57.

NASAL IRRIGATION. A purulent discharge may form crusts in the patient's nose; these can be removed by nasal irrigation. The irrigation solution flows into one nostril and out through the other. The important point to observe in giving a nasal irrigation is to use the correct amount of pressure—too much pressure may force the fluid into the sinuses and the eustachian tube, thus spreading the infection. This is not a common procedure. If you are asked to do it, request specific instructions.

Suctioning to Remove Oral–Nasal Secretions

Many patients with respiratory problems must be suctioned to remove excess secretions and mucus from the airway (Fig. 79-4). Suctioning may also be indicated in unconscious patients or in patients with an ineffective

Nursing Skill Guidelines
Assisting With Postural Drainage

◆ Always wear gloves.
◆ Explain to the patient why the head-downward position is necessary for much of the treatment (*Rationale: This position may be uncomfortable, but if the patient understands the reason, he or she will be more likely to cooperate.*)
◆ Improve drainage by striking the patient between the shoulder blades with cupped hands (*pummeling*) or by "*vibrating*" the patient. (*Rationale: This helps loosen the secretions.*)
◆ Have tissues available. (*Rationale: The patient will probably cough up secretions.*)
◆ Wear gloves and handle all soiled tissues as contaminated material. (*Rationale: This patient may be infectious. Body substance precautions are observed.*)
◆ Have pillows and pads available. (*Rationale: The various positions are easier to assume if a movable bed and pillows are available.*)
◆ Perform this procedure before the patient eats. (*Rationale: The patient may gag, choke, or vomit. This will help to prevent vomiting and aspiration.*)
◆ Give the patient oral hygiene following the procedure. (*Rationale: The stagnant or infected mucus may have a foul taste and odor.*)
◆ Dispose of all materials properly. Wash your hands. Document the procedure and the patient's reactions.

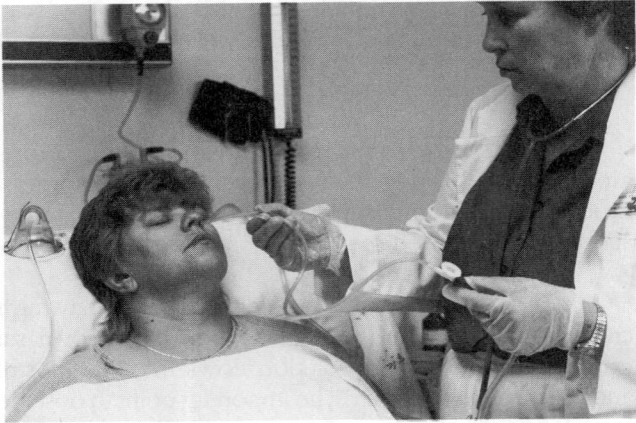

Figure 79-4. Nasotracheal suctioning. The nurse gently inserts the tube, *without* suction. To begin the suctioning, the thumb of the left hand is placed over the white port on the tube. This stops the intake of air and creates a vacuum. The tube is withdrawn fairly rapidly, while rotating and applying suction. (Craven RF and Hirnle CJ. Fundamentals of Nursing: Human Health and Function. Philadelphia: J.B. Lippincott, 1992)

cough. A new sterile suction kit is used each time the patient is suctioned so that organisms are not introduced into the lungs. The following nursing skill outlines oral–nasal suctioning. The patient who cannot swallow may require only oral suctioning. In this case, a "tonsil suction" is used and clean technique is followed. The procedure for suctioning a tracheostomy is similar and is presented in Chapter 80.

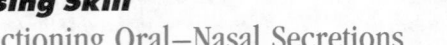

Nursing Skill
Suctioning Oral–Nasal Secretions

Supplies and Equipment

Sterile, disposable suction tube
Gloves
Sterile suction machine in the room

Procedure

1. Assemble equipment and explain procedure to patient.
2. Place conscious patient in semi-Fowler's position to prevent aspiration.
3. Wash hands and set up equipment, opening sterile suction package.
4. Put on sterile or clean gloves, as ordered. Wear eye protection, if indicated. *(Rationale: This prevents introducing organisms into the respiratory tract.)*
5. Pick up sterile catheter and connect to suction tubing that is held with the nondominant hand. This hand is now unsterile (sterile to clean-contaminated).
6. Moisten the catheter with sterile saline to increase patient comfort. Check functioning of suction machine.
7. Gently insert the catheter through the nostril with the suction off as illustrated in Figure 79-4. *(Rationale: Both*

the catheter and the suctioning can be irritating to mucous membranes.)
8. Once the catheter is inserted down to the end of the trachea (stimulating the cough reflex), begin suctioning, which lasts about 10 to 15 seconds. The entire process of entering, suctioning, and withdrawal should not exceed a total of 20 seconds. *(Rationale: Suctioning stops oxygen inhalation and hypoxia may result. It is also very uncomfortable.)*
9. Withdraw the catheter fairly rapidly in a rotating motion while suctioning continues. *(Rationale: Rotation helps clean all surfaces of the respiratory passageways.)*
10. Repeat suctioning until the mucus disappears, with the patient given time to rest and breathe normally between suctionings. The patient may be given oxygen before and after passage of the catheter to relieve panic.
11. Flush the catheter with sterile normal saline between suctionings. *(Rationale: Flushing cleans and clears catheter and lubricates it for next suctioning.)* Suctioning pressures of 80 to 100 mm Hg are used for the adult patient. *(Rationale: A vacuum pressure in excess of 120 mm Hg causes trauma to the delicate respiratory mucosa; bleeding can occur.)*
12. Properly dispose of all materials and make sure the patient is comfortable. Wash your hands.
13. Document the procedure and the patient's reactions. *(Rationale: This can be a frightening and uncomfortable procedure.)*

Nursing Alert

Suctioning can cause *dysrhythmia* (irregular heartbeat) and *desaturation* (loss of oxygenation). The nurse must continuously assess the patient being suctioned.

Evaluation

The nurse, patient, and family evaluate outcomes of care. Have short-term goals been met? Are long-term goals still realistic? Planning for further nursing care considers the patient's prognosis, as well as any complications and the patient's response to care given.

Infectious Respiratory Disorders

The Common Cold (Acute Rhinitis)

The common cold is also known as acute **rhinitis**. Colds are caused by one or more filterable viruses; as many as 100 cold viruses have been identified. Colds are easily spread by talking, coughing, or sneezing. Individuals are contagious 48 hours before the appearance of the first symptoms. If a person's resistance is lowered by fatigue, chilling, or substances that continually irritate the nasal membranes (such as smog), susceptibility to the virus is increased.

The usual symptoms of a cold are sneezing, nasal discharge or congestion, headache, sore throat, general malaise, cough, and sometimes a slight fever. The senses of smell and taste are blunted. This unpleasant condition usually lasts from 5 days to 2 weeks.

Treatment. The most important treatment for a cold is rest. This also aids in keeping the person from infecting others. Rest during a cold is especially important for infants, the elderly, and debilitated people because they are more susceptible to serious complications.

Drinking plenty of a variety of fluids is essential to help reduce fever, to replace lost fluids, and to thin secretions. Strict attention is given to washing the hands and using disposable tissues to prevent spreading the infection to others. The nose should be blown gently. *(Rationale: To prevent the infection from spreading into the sinuses, the ears, or the eustachian tubes.)* Aspirin, acetaminophen, or ibuprofen help to relieve discomfort and reduce fever. Some authorities believe that vitamin C is helpful in preventing and treating colds. Nose drops should be used with discretion. Antibiotics are ineffective against the cold virus.

Special Considerations in Children
Use of Salicylates

Infants and children should not be given aspirin or other salicylates to control fever because of the danger of Reye's syndrome. Acetaminophen (Tylenol) is used.

The person should consult a physician if the fever continues for more than 2 days; if severe headache is unrelieved by a mild analgesic; and if severe coughing, earache, or chest pain occurs. A physician should be immediately consulted if dark or bloody sputum is coughed up. In some cases, a throat culture is done. Sometimes this indicates a strep throat, but a negative culture for streptococci does not necessarily mean that a strep infection is not present. The patient with a chronic respiratory condition, such as asthma, should consult a physician at the first sign of a cold.

If the infection enters the lower respiratory tract, complications such as laryngitis, bronchitis, and pneumonia can result.

Nursing Alert

Usually a nurse who has a cold may continue working if he or she feels well. However, it is essential to follow all the principles of good personal hygiene, especially handwashing. Some facilities require this nurse to wear a mask and not be assigned to high-risk patients.

Streptococcal Sore Throat

"Strep throat" was mentioned in Chapter 65. Physical symptoms are more widespread than in the ordinary sore throat, with general physical weakness and malaise, high fever, pus on the tonsils, and a headache. Many adults who have recurrent streptococcal throat infections have permanently plugged eustachian tubes, so any change in atmospheric pressure is uncomfortable for them. Penicillin is the specific antibiotic prescribed for strep throat unless the person has an allergy or a penicillin-resistant streptococcal infection. The most dangerous complications of strep throat are rheumatic fever and glomerulonephritis, which are discussed in Chapters 65 and 82.

Influenza

Influenza, commonly called flu, is an active contagious respiratory disease caused by one of several strains of filterable viruses, types A, B, C, D and others. Flu strains may also be described using the name of the place of origin, such as the Hong Kong or Asian flu. Influenza occurs in periodic epidemics, usually due to virus types A and B. Most patients recover, but some die from complications such as heart disease, pneumonia, or encephalitis. Patients may develop parkinsonism many years after having had flu.

The most dangerous complication of influenza is pneumonia. The patient is particularly susceptible to any lung disorder after the flu because of general debility. Other complications are chronic disorders such as bronchitis, sinusitis, and ear infections.

Special Considerations in Children and Aging
Complications in Influenza

Infants and elderly people are at a much higher risk for developing complications from influenza than are other people.

Signs and Symptoms. The patient becomes suddenly very ill, with muscle pains, fever, headache, sensitivity to light and burning eyes, and chills. The person may sneeze, cough, have a nasal discharge, complain of sore throat, feel nauseous, and vomit often. Fever is high (100°–103°F; 37.8°–39.4°C) and lasts for 2 to 3 days, but the other symptoms, especially the cough, persist longer. A cough may persist for several weeks after the person has had the flu.

Treatment and Nursing Considerations. The patient is given large quantities of fluids, including fruit juices and plenty of water. Fluids help the body to flush out wastes created by the virus. (Milk is not given because it tends to form a film in the throat.) The patient may be given a regular diet although he or she is often anorexic (without appetite). Bedrest is prescribed, as well a mild analgesic, to relieve headache, fever, and muscular pains. Cough syrup may be given to relieve the dry cough; the narcotic contained in some cough preparations may also assist the patient to sleep. The patient should be kept warm and should avoid exposure to other diseases. The nurse must watch for signs of secondary infection, such as chest pains, purulent or rose-colored sputum, a rise in temperature, and an increase in pulse rate.

Prevention. Individuals at high risk for acquiring influenza are encouraged to be vaccinated yearly in the fall to provide protection from this infection. The elderly, persons with chronic disease, immunosuppressed persons, and healthcare workers are encouraged to have the inoculation. The vaccine is synthetic, alleviating side effects seen in the past.

During an outbreak, people are urged to stay away from crowds, and public gatherings are sometimes suspended. Visiting patients at healthcare facilities should be avoided during this time.

Laryngitis

The larynx (voice box) lies below the pharynx and contains the vocal cords. Laryngitis is an inflammation of the larynx. It often accompanies respiratory infections or may result from overuse of the voice or excessive smoking. The patient coughs, is hoarse, and may lose the voice. Talking and smoking should be avoided, and high-humidity inhalations are given to soothe the mucous membranes of the throat. If laryngitis is a complication of another infection, antibiotics may be given.

Chronic laryngitis may be a complication of chronic sinusitis or chronic bronchitis or may follow repeated attacks of acute laryngitis. Continued irritation of the throat by public speaking, smoking, or irritating gases may contribute to the problem. Patients with chronic laryngitis must be carefully examined for signs of cancer, particularly if they smoke cigarettes.

Acute Bronchitis

Bronchitis is an inflammation of the bronchial tubes (bronchi). Acute bronchitis often follows a respiratory infection, especially during the winter months. A dry cough is an early symptom; later, the cough produces mucus and pus. Other symptoms are fever and malaise.

Treatment includes bed rest, a nutritious diet, and plenty of fluids. Humidifiers help by moistening the air, whereas dry air aggravates the cough. Antibiotics are given to treat the infection, and precautions are taken to prevent the infection from spreading. Salicylates are sometimes given.

As in any respiratory disease, the patient is instructed to cover the mouth when coughing, and the sputum is disposed of in the manner prescribed by universal precautions. Acute bronchitis, if untreated, will often develop into chronic bronchitis.

Lung Abscess

A lung abscess is a localized area of infection in the lung that breaks down and forms pus. It can be caused by a foreign body in the lung or by aspiration of oral fluids or respiratory secretions; it may follow pneumonia. Symptoms are chills and fever, with a loss in weight and a cough productive of purulent sputum that has a foul odor. It is treated by establishing drainage, for which surgery may be required. If the cause of the abscess is an aspirated object, the object usually can be removed by bronchoscopy. Antibiotics usually are effective in treating the disease, after the offending cause is eliminated.

Pneumonia

Pneumonia is an inflammation of the lung with consolidation or solidification (see Fig. 79-5**A**). The lung becomes firm as the air sacs are filled with exudate. In past years, one of four persons who had pneumonia died, but modern treatment has greatly reduced the death rate.

Special Considerations in Aging
Pneumonia

Pneumonia accounts for 10% of all hospital admissions in the United States and is often a cause of death in the elderly.

Pneumonia is now classified according to the causative organism. It may be bacterial, viral, fungal, or chemical in origin. It may also be caused by aspiration of fluid or a foreign object into the lungs. Goals in treatment of pneumonia are:

- ◆ Appropriate antibiotic therapy
- ◆ Respiratory assessment to measure effectiveness of therapy
- ◆ Administration of oxygen
- ◆ Adequate fluid intake
- ◆ Small, frequent meals
- ◆ Positioning to aid breathing
- ◆ Turning, coughing, and deep breathing (TCDB)
- ◆ Intake and output records
- ◆ Frequent mouth care for comfort

Signs and Symptoms. The onset is characterized by a severe, sharp pain in the chest (pleurisy), and a chill, followed by fever that may be as high as 105°F or 106°F (40.6°C or 41.1°C). There is a painful cough, with tenacious sputum and pain on breathing. The patient's pulse is rapid. Respiration is rapid and expiration difficult. The patient feels very ill and may be cyanotic. The white blood cell count is high. Mental changes, such as delirium or anxiety, may be apparent.

Blood cultures and sputum cultures are taken, and the sputum is analyzed to determine the causative organism. Sensitivity tests are done to determine which antibiotic is most effective against that organism. A chest film will show what part of the lung is affected and to what degree.

Treatment. Antibiotics have revolutionized the treatment of pneumonia. They are usually administered intravenously for rapid action and to maintain a blood level that is effective in eradicating the causative organism. In 24 to 48 hours, the fever usually disappears and the other symptoms improve dramatically. Antibiotics are discussed in Chapter 56.

Nursing Considerations. Nursing skill guidelines are outlined in the accompanying box. Gradually, the patient is allowed more activity and convalesces slowly while resistance is built up. An x-ray is taken to make sure that the infection in the lungs has cleared completely.

Bacterial Pneumonia

Persons who are not in good general physical health or who are physically inactive, as well as older people or those with chronic lung disorders, seem to be susceptible to infectious bacterial pneumonia. Substance abusers, such as alcoholics and persons who "snort" cocaine, are particularly susceptible.

Viral Pneumonia

Viral pneumonia is caused by a variety of the influenza virus. Antibiotics are not effective against viral pneumonia. However, antibiotics are often used to treat or prevent the secondary infections sometimes seen in viral pneumonia. The patient is treated symptomatically. Viral pneumonia is rarely fatal, but it may leave the patient in a weakened condition.

Pneumocystis carinii Pneumonia

Pneumocystis carinii pneumonia (PCP) is caused by organisms that are not totally known. Some authorities believe that the causative organism is a protozoa; others blame yeastlike fungi. PCP pneumonia is most commonly seen as one of the opportunistic diseases in the patient with an advanced human immunodeficiency (HIV) infection or acquired immunodeficiency syndrome (AIDS).

Nursing Skill Guidelines

Caring for the Patient With Pneumonia

- ◆ Always wear gloves.
- ◆ Be alert for increasingly labored respirations. *(Rationale: If the patient has difficulty breathing, he or she is given oxygen, usually by mask or cannula.)*
- ◆ Adjust the patient's position. An orthopneic position may be necessary. *(Rationale: This helps the person to be more comfortable and to breathe more easily.)*
- ◆ Place a pillow lengthwise under the back. *(Rationale: This helps the person to expand the chest more fully.)*
- ◆ Place a blanket around the shoulders if the person has chills. Keep the patient's bed dry. Assess the patient's vital signs at least every 4 hours. Attempt to control fever and discomfort with acetaminophen or ibuprofen, if ordered. Tepid sponges may also be ordered. *(Rationale: Fever is often very high; this can be dangerous.)*
- ◆ Maintain the intravenous site or heparin lock. *(Rationale: This patient is probably receiving IV antibiotics.)*
- ◆ Put side rails up if there is any sign of confusion, especially in the older person. *(Rationale: The high fever, the medications, and the disease process may contribute to confusion and lead to injury.)*
- ◆ Encourage the patient to cough and to expectorate secretions while splinting the chest. *(Rationale: It is vital to keep the lungs as free of secretions as possible. Splinting the chest helps to relieve the discomfort of coughing.)*
- ◆ Encourage the patient to breathe deeply. Aerosolized treatments or incentive spirometry may be prescribed. *(Rationale: The lungs must be expanded as much as possible.)*
- ◆ Measure intake and output and daily weights, if ordered. *(Rationale: Some patients may have edema. Some patients will need total parenteral nutrition to maintain hydration and nutrition.)*
- ◆ Give small amounts of fluids frequently. *(Rationale: To encourage intake.)*
- ◆ Give mouth care frequently; put water-soluble lubricant (not oily) on the patient's lips. *(Rationale: A fever causes the mucous membranes to be very dry; this patient also has probably been breathing through the mouth. Oil might be aspirated and is not used with oxygen.)*
- ◆ Keep the patient's surroundings quiet. *(Rationale: Rest promotes healing.)*

Chemical Pneumonia

Chemical pneumonia is largely associated with aspiration of a chemical substance. The nurse should be aware that a patient may aspirate into the lungs without any obvious evidence of vomiting. Some persons are at an extremely high risk for this. They include the elderly, the alcoholic, the debilitated, the postanesthesia patient, and those with swallowing impairments.

Aspiration Pneumonia

If the person vomits or inhales a foreign object, or substances such as water or large amounts of mucus, the material may be drawn into the lungs. This aspiration not only causes the infectious process, but it can cause additional edema and complications because of the acidity of the gastric contents.

Complications of Pneumonia

Complications from pneumonia seldom occur today, except in the elderly, debilitated, or immunocompromised patient. If the infection does spread, it also may cause inflammation of the pleura, the middle ear (otitis media), sinusitis, or bronchitis.

Pleurisy

Pleurisy, an inflammation of the pleura (the double membrane covering the lungs), can be a complication of pneumonia, caused by a spread of the infection from the lungs. The pleura becomes thickened, and the two membrane surfaces rub together.

There is a sharp pain with every breath. Later, as fluid forms, the pain diminishes, and a dry cough takes its place, accompanied by shortness of breath and exhaustion after the slightest effort. (Pleuritic pain may occur with other diseases such as rheumatic fever, lupus erythematosus, and polyarteritis.)

The treatment of pleurisy is much like that for pneumonia: bed rest and restriction of activity. The patient is encouraged to cough, but because this is painful, applying hot or cold packs over the area or having the patient lie on the affected side may help to make him or her more comfortable.

When the collection of fluid in the pleural space increases, the patient is said to have a *pleural effusion* (Fig. 79-5**D**). The patient may exhibit the same symptoms as pleurisy, but often becomes dyspneic and has a rapid pulse. Pleural effusion can be a result of congestive heart failure; of pulmonary infections, including TB; and of malignancies. The treatment is directly related to the underlying cause and may be geared to treating specific symptoms.

Histoplasmosis

Because histoplasmosis mimics "summer flu," it is often misdiagnosed. The causative fungus is inhaled in dust from soil rich in the fungus (eg, chicken houses, barns, caves). In the United States, it is most common in the midwestern states.

Signs and Symptoms. The lungs become inflamed from invasion by foreign material, and this damages the lymph glands and lungs. As a result, scar tissue and calcium deposits may form.

Special Considerations in Children and Aging
Histoplasmosis

Very young children and older men are most likely to contract histoplasmosis, and they are especially susceptible to the form that spreads from the lungs to other parts of the body.

Symptoms are much like those of the flu. Many people are infected with the disease without knowing it because the symptoms are so mild. Most people recover after a few weeks. In more severe cases, weight loss and weakness occur, and a very long convalescence is required. In the chronic form, the disease spreads throughout the body, causing weight loss, bleeding, and other severe problems. It is occasionally fatal.

The fungus may be identified by isolation in culture, and in some cases, both sputum and urine must be cultured. A skin test, administered intradermally, can indicate the presence of the fungus in the body.

Treatment. In the mild form of the disease, treatment is similar to that for the flu. Usually, the symptoms clear by themselves. In more severe cases, amphotericin B (Fungizone) or another antifungal drug, is given. The drug must be given intravenously for several weeks.

Tuberculosis

Cases of TB are increasing. The following factors increase the risk for TB infection:

◆ HIV positive
◆ Chronic renal failure
◆ Advanced age
◆ Immunosuppression from steroids or cancers
◆ Unclean living conditions
◆ Homelessness
◆ Poor diet

Immigrants from certain parts of the world seem to be more vulnerable. Men are affected more than women.

Key Concept

The number of cases of TB has increased dramatically over the last several years because of the large number of persons with HIV infection who are susceptible and infected with TB.

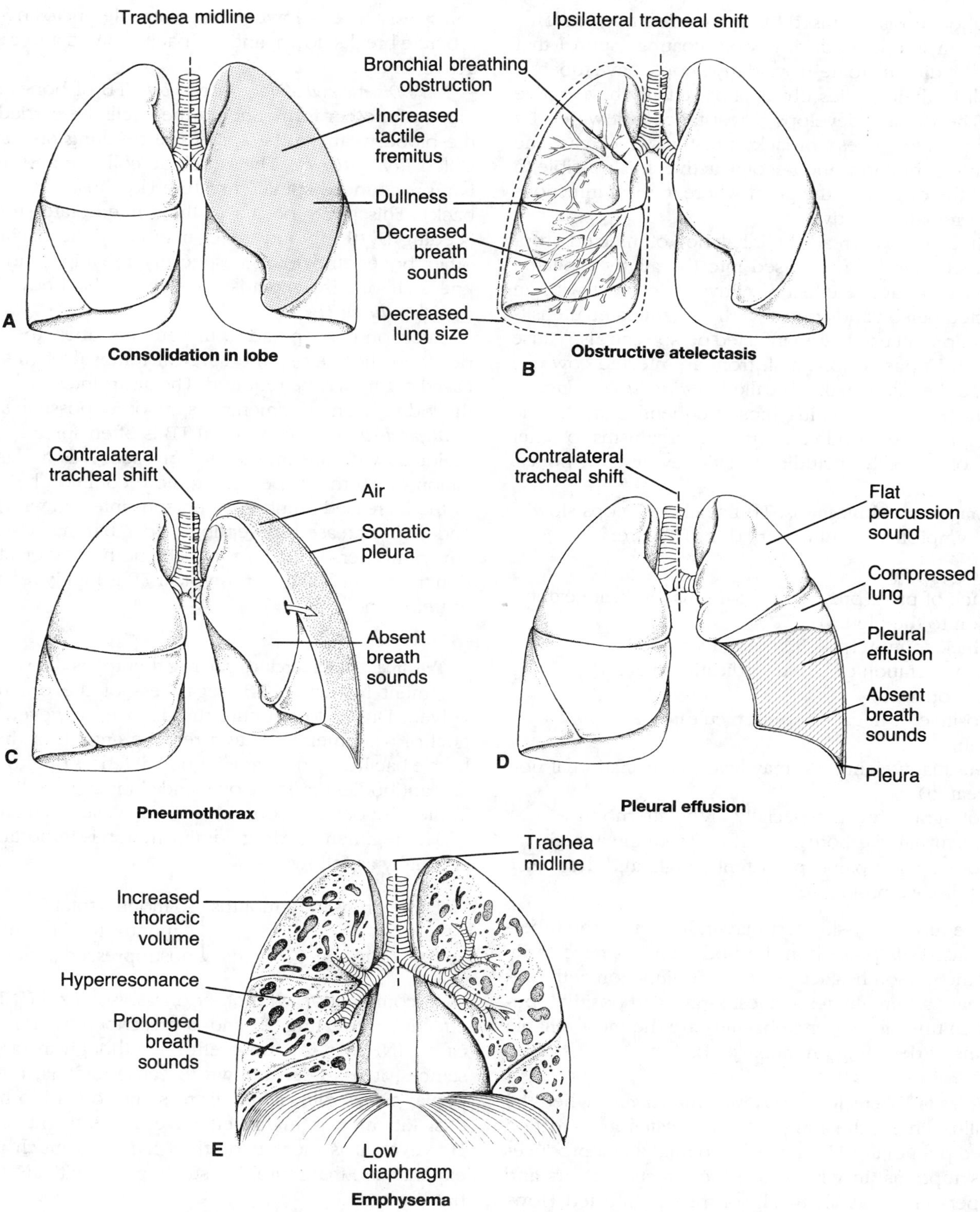

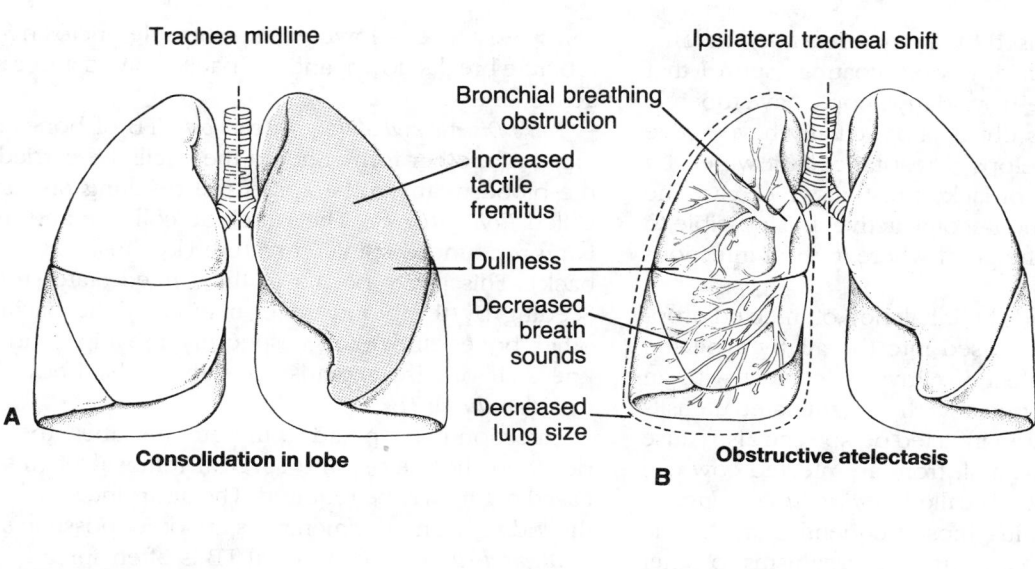

Trachea midline

Ipsilateral tracheal shift

Bronchial breathing obstruction

Increased tactile fremitus

Dullness

Decreased breath sounds

Decreased lung size

A

Consolidation in lobe

B

Obstructive atelectasis

Contralateral tracheal shift

Air

Somatic pleura

Absent breath sounds

C

Pneumothorax

Contralateral tracheal shift

Flat percussion sound

Compressed lung

Pleural effusion

Absent breath sounds

Pleura

D

Pleural effusion

Trachea midline

Increased thoracic volume

Hyperresonance

Prolonged breath sounds

Low diaphragm

E

Emphysema

Figure 79-5. Respiratory system disorders and their comparative effects on the lungs. **(A)** Consolidation within a lobe: trachea in center, dull sound in affected lobe. **(B)** Obstructive atelectasis: trachea shifts to affected (ipsilateral) side; decreased lung size, decreased breath sounds. **(C)** Pneumothorax: trachea shifts to other (contralateral) side; breath sounds absent on affected side. **(D)** Pleural effusion or hemothorax (fluid or blood pooling in pleural cavity): trachea shifts to other side; absent breath sounds in affected lobe; lung compressed. **(E)** Emphysema: enlarged (barrel) chest, prolonged breath sounds, hyperresonance (echo), trachea in center.

Tuberculosis is caused by the *tubercle bacillus*. This organism is enclosed in a waxy coating (spore) that makes it difficult to destroy. Many people have tubercle bacilli in their bodies but do not actually have active TB. The disease develops if resistance is lowered by poor nutrition, stress, or lack of rest, in which case the organisms multiply and become active. It is possible to arrest the disease to the point where it is not infectious and it remains inactive.

Tuberculosis spreads by inhalation of infected droplets that have been released into the air by a person who has an active infection. Physical contact with an infected person and contact with contaminated utensils or equipment used by an infected person can also cause spread. Unpasteurized milk from an infected cow can spread the disease; this is called *bovine tuberculosis*.

The tubercle bacillus most frequently attacks the lungs, but the blood can carry the organisms to other parts of the body, including the kidneys and the bones.

Symptoms and Diagnosis. TB usually develops slowly. The symptoms of pulmonary (lung) TB are:

◆ Cough
◆ Lack of pain (presence of pain may indicate extension to the pleura)
◆ Thick sputum (possibly blood streaked)
◆ Expectoration of blood (indicating pleural hemorrhage)
◆ Positive or negative sputum culture
◆ Fatigue
◆ Gradual weight loss (may lead to emaciation, if not treated)
◆ Low-grade fever, especially in the afternoon
◆ Nocturnal diaphoresis (profuse sweating at night)
◆ Severe chest pains, persistent cough, and dyspnea as disease progresses

The tuberculin skin test may indicate that the tubercle bacillus is present in the body but not necessarily that the person has active TB. In conjunction with preliminary tuberculin tests, chest x-rays and positive sputum cultures for tubercle bacillus are the most reliable means of detecting pulmonary TB.

Types of Tuberculosis. *Pulmonary Tuberculosis.* When the bacillus enters the lungs, it precipitates an infection called pulmonary TB. It may be so mild that it produces no symptoms, in which case the infection clears and the person is unaware that he or she was infected. However, the tuberculin test will be positive and a chest film will reveal a small scar, a sign that at some time the bacillus was active. The scar is the end result of efforts of the white blood cells to surround and destroy the bacilli. The bacilli are then encased in lump called a *tubercle*. The tubercle (known as the primary lesion or primary TB), may remain inactive for life, but if the person's resistance is lowered, the capsule enclosing the tubercle breaks down, and the bacilli spread and cause active illness.

Pott's Disease and Miliary Tuberculosis. TB of bones and joints is another form. Should the bacilli be carried by the bloodstream to the spine, the resulting disease is called *Pott's disease*. The vertebrae collapse and there is a pronounced spinal curvature (kyphosis or humpback). This rarely occurs in the United States today. Seeding by the bloodstream may carry the bacilli to other bones and joints, especially the hips and the knees. If disease spreads throughout the body, it is called *miliary TB*.

Infection may spread to the uterine tubes, the ovaries, and the uterus, and surgical removal of the diseased organ may be required. The gastrointestinal tract, the kidneys, and the meninges are other possible sites.

Atypical Tuberculosis. Atypical TB is often spread to individuals who are immunosuppressed. It is a classification of TB that is becoming more common because of the increased numbers of persons infected with HIV and their increased susceptibility to TB. It may also occur in the person undergoing chemotherapy or radiation treatment for cancer. Atypical TB is highly resistant to treatment.

Treatment of Tuberculosis. Drug therapy is the specific treatment for active TB, regardless of the organ involved. Drugs do not cure the disease, however. The goal of drug therapy is to arrest the growth of the tubercle bacillus so the natural body defenses (leukocytes and antibodies) can take over and eliminate the disease. Table 79-2 outlines some of the drugs used to treat TB.

The regimen for drug administration is important. It is usually as follows:

◆ Three drugs for 2 months ⎱ (6 months total–
◆ Two drugs for 4 months ⎰ 9 months total for immunosuppressed patients)

In combination with other drugs, isoniazid (INH) is effective in treating TB and is prescribed in almost all cases. INH has few toxic effects, although in rare instances, it has been known to cause anemia, neutropenia, or gastrointestinal distress and to lead to hepatitis. Rifampin is highly effective in treatment of TB. However, it is more toxic than INH and much more expensive. Ethambutol is usually given with INH and has low toxicity.

Because effective drugs are now available, surgery is rarely necessary. Surgical procedures include total pneumonectomy (removal of an entire lung), partial pneumonectomy (removal of the affected part of a lung), lobectomy (removal of a lobe of a lung), and wedge resection or segmental resection (removal of one or more bronchopulmonary segments).

Table 79-2. Key Medications: Tuberculosis

Drugs of Choice	Nursing Considerations
isoniazid/INH (Nydrazid, Lani-azid)	Inexpensive, few side effects, used in most cases
ethambutol (Myambutol)	Usually given with INH, low toxicity
pyrazinamide/PZA (PMS Pyrazinamide, Tebrazid, Zinamide)	Used in retreatment of TB, more toxic effects
rifampin (Rimactane, Rifadin)	Higer potential for adverse effects, as well as more undesirable interactions with other drugs
streptomycin sulfate	Usually used only if other drugs are ineffective; can only be given to patients with normal renal (kidney) function; must encourage fluids; often given in combination with other drugs. Given IM (never give IV). Use cautiously in elderly patients. Can cause hearing damage. When used for primary treatment of TB, it is discontinued when sputum becomes negative.

Nursing Considerations. TB is a long-term illness. Nursing care consists of several elements:

◆ Careful administration of medications. Following a time schedule is important to build up a blood level of the drugs. Give at the same time each day, if a QD dose, or spread doses throughout the day. (If b.i.d., instruct the patient to take every 12 h; if t.i.d., take every 8 h; if q.i.d., take every 6 h, rather than 8-12-4-8, for example.) Teach the patient the importance of continuing medications, even if the symptoms seem to have subsided.
◆ A well-balanced diet, high in protein and vitamins A and C
◆ Prevention of spread of the disease, with careful handwashing, and use of personal protective equipment (ie, gloves, mask; use of this equipment is described in Chapter 30.)
◆ Respiratory isolation measures, if disease is active (see Chapter 51).
◆ Plenty of rest
◆ A smoke-free environment
◆ Diversionary activities

Prevention. Nurses can take an active part in community health by seeking ways to prevent TB. The following are some suggestions:

◆ Educate the public in good, general health practices.
◆ Burn all used tissues. (The TB bacillus can survive for months in dried sputum.)
◆ Trace active cases and start early treatment of contacts to stop further spread of the disease.
◆ Follow-up on all persons who have had active TB. Regular examination is necessary for life to determine if there is a recurrence and to treat it immediately.
◆ Screen members of high-risk groups such as immigrants from Southeast Asia.
◆ Give nursing home residents the PPD tuberculin test on admission and at intervals thereafter.
◆ Screen healthcare workers yearly.

The American Society of Thoracic Physicians believes that prophylactic medication treatment (long-term administration of antituberculosis medications) should be recommended for the following people:

◆ Household members and other close contacts of the person with recently diagnosed TB
◆ Persons with positive tuberculin tests who have chest x-ray findings indicative of TB
◆ Newly infected persons
◆ Persons with positive TB tests who have been on steroids, have received immunosuppressant drugs, and have hematologic diseases, silicosis, or diabetes mellitus
◆ Others who have positive reactions, such as infants, teens, and elderly people
◆ Persons who are immunosuppressed as a result of HIV or AIDS

Empyema

Empyema, sometimes called pyothorax, is a collection of purulent exudate in the pleural cavity.

Acute Empyema

Acute empyema is a secondary infection that may follow TB, lung abscess, or pneumonia. It may also result from an infection of the chest wall or other surrounding tissue or may be introduced directly by a wound of the chest or by surgery. Because it is almost always a secondary infection, empyema is difficult to diagnose; symptoms are usually masked by the primary problem.

The symptoms of empyema are chest pain (usually on one side), cough, fever, dyspnea, and general malaise. If empyema is suspected, more decisive information can be obtained by a chest x-ray and by thoracentesis. The offending organism can also be determined by a culture and sensitivity test on fluid aspirated by thoracentesis.

Antibiotics to combat the infection and measures to drain the empyema cavity are started. The latter may be done by closed drainage or by thoracentesis, in which case an antibiotic may be injected into the pleural cavity. Bedrest and sedative cough preparations are also given. If this is not successful, open drainage is done.

Chronic Empyema

Chronic empyema may be a complication of acute empyema or may be caused by bronchopleural fistula, osteomyelitis of the rib cage, or an aspirated foreign body. It may also be a complication of TB or a fungus infection of the lungs.

Soft rubber drainage tubes are inserted in the wound, and large, absorbent dressings and pads are applied. Usually the drainage is profuse at first, so the dressings have to be changed frequently. In open drainage, usually a rib is removed, and this can cause some pain.

Chronic Respiratory Disorders

Snoring

Snoring or *stertorous breathing* is a respiratory disorder that is common in some people when they sleep. It is usually not a serious problem but is considered a pathologic condition if the person is not relieved of the snoring, no matter what sleeping position is used; if the snoring can be heard two or three rooms away; and if the partner has to move to be able to sleep. In extreme cases of snoring, surgery may be done. A procedure called the palatopharyngoplasty, which removes extra material from the upper throat, has been successful in some cases. Other remedies include elevating the head of the bed, using a special pillow, sewing an object such as a ball on the back of the pajamas (so the person does not sleep on the back), not eating a heavy meal in the evening, not smoking, not taking sleeping pills or drinking alcohol, losing weight and using decongestants.

Sleep Apnea Syndrome

Sleep apnea syndrome causes the person to wake up many times during the night. It is most common in middle-aged, overweight men. The formal definition of sleep apnea is "more than five cessations of airflow for at least 10 seconds each per hour of sleep."[1] It is believed to occur because soft tissues at the back of the throat fall back and occlude the air-

way. This airway occlusion can last as long as 90 seconds. The person suddenly awakens because of lack of oxygen. This can occur hundreds of times during a single night.

Diagnosis is based on symptoms and history, including:

◆ Extreme tiredness
◆ Difficulty in concentration
◆ Loss of memory
◆ Inability to perform one's job
◆ Falling asleep during the day
◆ Episodes witnessed by sleeping partner

Almost all people with sleep apnea snore, although the reverse is not necessarily true. The person has problems including:

◆ Danger of auto accidents or industrial accidents
◆ Increased risk of high blood pressure with related disorders
◆ Social and employment problems

Treatment. Recommended treatment includes the following measures:

◆ Lose weight
◆ Stop smoking
◆ No alcohol, especially before bedtime
◆ Elevate the head of the bed
◆ Continuous positive airway pressure (CPAP) oxygenation
◆ Possible surgery (this treatment is controversial)

Respiratory stimulant medications have not proven helpful. In severe cases, tracheostomy (which is plugged during the day) may be required to bypass upper airway obstruction.

CPAP Oxygenation. The CPAP apparatus is commonly used to assist persons with sleep apnea. This machine looks like an oxygen-delivery system and is usually used at night, so the person can sleep. It delivers gas to the patient at a positive pressure, so the alveoli are held open. (They usually close at the end of expiration.) This positive pressure prevents respiratory obstruction, increases oxygenation, and reduces breathing effort.

Allergic Rhinitis (Hay Fever)

Rhinitis is an inflammation of the nasal mucous passages. Hay fever and allergic rhinitis are conditions occurring when the inflammation is an allergic reaction caused by a protein substance. It may be due to pollen from weeds, flowers, or grasses at certain seasons, or it may be a reaction to dust, feathers, or scales from animal skin. People with a family history of allergy are more susceptible to hay fever, as are those who have asthma or eczema. The number of people with a hereditary ten-

---

[1] O'Toole M (Ed). Miller-Keane Encyclopedia and Dictionary of Medicine, Nursing and Allied Health, Ed 5. Philadelphia, W.B. Saunders, 1992:1379.

dency comprises about 10% of the U.S. population. Persons of all ages are affected; it may appear suddenly at any age and may just as suddenly disappear.

Signs and Symptoms. Allergic rhinitis is a disagreeable and inconvenient disease. Symptoms are edema, an itchy nose, excessive sneezing, and profuse, watery discharge from the nose and eyes. It is aggravated on windy days and is worse in the morning and the evening. It takes a great deal of testing to determine the cause, and detailed questioning and many skin tests may be needed to identify the offending substance. Sometimes several substances are the offenders. Chapter 77 discusses allergies and describes and illustrates allergy tests in more detail.

Treatment. The first step in treatment is to avoid the offending substance. This may mean eliminating a food from the diet, avoiding contact with animals, or avoiding dusty places. Air conditioning and filtering or purifying air also helps. Antihistamines relieve the symptoms, and desensitization injections may eliminate them entirely. Cortisone and ACTH may be given for severe attacks. An untreated allergy of this kind may lead to asthma, sinusitis, or nasal polyps.

Dust Diseases (Pneumoconioses)

Pneumoconioses are caused by habitual inhalation and retention in the lungs of certain heavy, harmful dusts. The most common among these diseases is silicosis, common in miners, which is caused by breathing silica, or quartz dust. Asbestosis is another common form. As dangerous dusts are inhaled, they eventually slow down or stop the ciliary action in the nose and lungs, and the dusts accumulate in the lungs. The dusts can cause irritation, allergic reaction, or chemical reaction.

Usually the first symptom of dust diseases is dyspnea. Later, the patient develops a chronic cough; the offending particles will be expectorated in the thick mucus. Chest pains are often a later result. Serious complications include TB, pneumonia, chronic bronchitis, and emphysema. Vast evidence now indicates that asbestos is directly related to a specific lung cancer (mesothelioma).

Treatment focuses on prevention because these diseases are difficult to treat once extensive areas of the lungs are involved. The only treatment at present is to reduce exposure to the dust. Damage previously done cannot be reversed.

Chronic Obstructive Pulmonary Disease

Chronic obstructive pulmonary disease (COPD) is also called chronic obstructive lung disease (COLD). It is a broad classification of disorders that includes bronchial asthma, bronchiectasis, chronic bronchitis, and pulmonary emphysema. Each of these is discussed in the following pages. COPD is irreversible and is associated with persistent dyspnea on exertion and reduced airflow of less than one half normal. It affects 25% of the adult population and is the fifth most common cause of death in the United States. The accompanying Nursing Care Plan illustrates the use of nursing process with two nursing diagnoses in providing care for a person with a respiratory disease.

Care of the patient with COPD involves physical, psychological, and environmental measures. The goals of treatment are to improve ventilation and to overcome hypoxic states through the following measures:

- ◆ Avoidance of irritants: smoking, allergens, industrial chemicals
- ◆ Use of medications: bronchodilators, expectorants, liquefying agents
- ◆ Postural drainage
- ◆ Fluid intake (2–3 qt/d)
- ◆ Cautious use of oxygen
- ◆ Breathing exercises
- ◆ Activity as tolerated
- ◆ Avoidance of extremes of heat and cold
- ◆ Positioning to facilitate breathing (Fowler's or orthopneic)
- ◆ Small, frequent meals

Fluid intake is important. The patient is encouraged to drink 2 to 3 quarts daily to thin mucus and make it easier to expectorate.

Nursing Alert

It may not be possible for the patient with acute or chronic congestive heart failure to increase fluid intake to this extent.

Oxygen is administered with caution. Persons with COPD have adapted to higher carbon dioxide levels instead of oxygen levels. When administering oxygen to a patient with COPD, the amount should not exceed 3 L/min.

Breathing exercises, combined with other respiratory treatments, increase the volume of air that the patient is able to exhale. Inhaling and holding the breath also improve breathing. Practicing pursed-lip breathing, especially during periods of dyspnea, is effective. (*Rationale: This technique forces air into the lungs.*) The patient must be faithful in consistently carrying out breathing exercises.

Bed rest should be discouraged. The patient is advised to keep active. (*Rationale: The patient must be given support and direction to enable him or her to accept the fact that therapy is a lifelong commitment.*) It is important to remember that activities should be

Mr. Aaron Greenberg is a 70-year-old widowed man with a history of chronic obstructive pulmonary disease (COPD) recently exacerbated by bronchitis. He presented at the hospital after experiencing increasing shortness of breath and rib pain for 2 days. He has a productive cough (green sputum). Crackles and rhonchi are present bilaterally. His orders on admission are for bed rest with bathroom privileges (BRP), oxygen at 2 liters per minute (O_2 at 2L) sputum for culture and sensitivity, chest x-ray, blood cultures, and Alupent 0.3 cc in nebulized normal saline every 4 hours. Two nursing diagnoses from his plan of care follow.

Nursing Diagnosis: *Ineffective Airway Clearance Related to Tracheobronchial Infection, Increased Secretions, and Fatigue as Evidenced by Crackles, Rhonchi, and Fear of Coughing (Pain)*

Goal: By 9/15 patient maintains clear, open airway (abnormal breath sounds absent)

Nursing Actions (assess/do/teach)	Rationale	Evaluative Statement
1. Assess VS q4h (note elevated temperature or heart rate)—listen for abnormal breath sounds.	This establishes a baseline for treatment and helps in monitoring effectiveness of treatment.	9/15 Goal met; crackles and rhonchi notably decreased bilaterally
2. Instruct about the importance of effective coughing; keep a sputum cup and tissues at the bedside; suction PRN if patient is unable to move secretions; observe the color, quality, and quantity of sputum; send the sputum specimen to the lab and monitor results.	These actions facilitate expectoration.	
3. Provide emotional support and use comfort measures liberally.	Pain interferes with deep coughing and facilitates the pooling of secretions.	
4. Explain the importance of frequent position changes to the patient on bed rest and encourage ambulation when permitted.	Position changes prevent the pooling of secretions and other complications related to inactivity.	
5. Monitor the patient's fluid intake and guard against dehydration; encourage the patient to drink at least 3000 mL water/day. Do not give milk.	Dehydration contributes to thick, tenacious secretions that are difficult to expectorate. Water is the best expectorant; milk increases mucus production.	
6. Schedule and maintain respiratory therapy.	Respiratory therapy helps promote effective airway clearance.	
7. Administer the prescribed medication to fight infection.		

(continued)

limited to whatever the heart and breathing capacities can tolerate. The patient has the potential to lead a fairly active life if he or she chooses.

Persons with COPD have special needs because of the chronic nature of the disease. Nurses can assist these persons to live optimally by:

♦ Assisting to develop energy-conserving measures in their day-to-day living
♦ Teaching relaxation techniques to use in situations of respiratory distress
♦ Teaching management of acute exacerbations of disease and when to call for help

Nursing Diagnosis: *High Risk for Impaired Gas Exchange Related to Poor Ventilation and Lung Aeration*

Goal: Patient's blood gases remain within the range of normal

Nursing Actions (assess/do/teach)	Rationale	Evaluative Statement
1. Observe the respiratory rate, pattern, characteristics, and use of accessory muscles; monitor VS, breath sounds, arterial blood gases (ABGs); assess for signs of hypoxia (skin color, capillary refill), dyspnea, exertion at rest; observe for subjective indications of hypoxemia and hypercapnea; notify the physician if the chest x-ray report uses the words *infiltrate* or *atelectasis*.	Early detection of impaired gas exchange facilitates treatment. These words are indicative of pneumonia.	9/17 Goal met; ABGs remain WNL (within normal limits)
2. Encourage turning, deep breathing, and other mobilization maneuvers.	These actions prevent the pooling of secretions.	

♦ Helping the patient to identify situations or other factors that "trigger" symptoms and assist them to find ways to modify or remove these triggers

Bronchial Asthma

Asthma is an intermittent bronchial spasm accompanied by swelling of the membrane lining the bronchi and by a thick mucous secretion. The spasm traps the air in the alveoli and shuts out fresh air. An asthma attack is a frightening experience for the patient struggling to get air into the lungs. (Chapter 65 briefly describes asthma in children.)

Signs and Symptoms. The onset of an asthma attack is sudden. There is a feeling of chest tightness and choking. The patient is dyspneic, especially on expiration, and pale. In a severe attack the person may become cyanotic and may perspire and wheeze. As the attack subsides, the person coughs up thick, white mucus.

Asthma attacks may be occasional or frequent, but the patient is usually symptom free between episodes. Frequent attacks may lead to emphysema. Those who have hay fever or bronchitis are especially susceptible, and asthma can occur at any age and at any time. Asthmatic children usually have fewer symptoms as they grow older, but the symptoms of asthmatic adults grow worse with age. A sudden change in temperature, extreme physical exertion, contact with animal dander,

overeating, emotional stress, and exposure to antigens may trigger attacks.

An attack that persists for more than 24 hours and that does not respond to treatment is called status asthmaticus, which is a medical emergency and can lead to death.

Treatment. The main objective of treatment is to relieve breathing difficulties. Several classifications of medications may be used in treatment of asthma. These are listed in the accompanying box. Many people with asthma have the condition well controlled.

Nursing Considerations. Asthma is a frustrating and frightening disorder. The person may worry or become anxious about having an asthma attack, and this stress alone can precipitate the attack. Professional counseling may be needed to deal with the emotional aspects of this disease. The nurse must be calm and supportive and promptly administer the prescribed medications. Chapter 57 gives guidelines for the use of inhalers. Patient teaching subjects are suggested in the accompanying box.

Bronchiectasis

Bronchiectasis is a chronic dilation of the bronchi in which the walls of the bronchi become permanently distended. The main cause is infection following TB,

Key Medications
for Asthma

◆ Beta (β) agonists: these medications dilate bronchial airways: epinephrine (Adrenalin, Sus-Phrine); albuterol (Proventil, Ventolin)
◆ methylxanthines: bronchodilators: aminophylline/theophylline ethylenediamine (Cardophyllin, Phyllocontin); theophylline (Theo-Dur, Slo-Phyllin, Aerolate); cromalyn sodium (Intal)
◆ anticholinergics: atropine methylnitrate
◆ corticosteroids: prednisone (Meticorten, Orasone, Deltasone), beclomethasone (Vanceril, Beclovent, Beconase)

Nursing Considerations

◆ Many of these drugs can cause tremor, dizziness, restlessness, insomnia, or headache. More serious reactions may lead to seizures.
◆ These drugs should not be used with other CNS stimulants.
◆ They are used cautiously in patients with cardiac disorders; they may cause cardiac arrhythmias and other difficulties.
◆ They can react negatively with propranolol (Inderol) and other β blockers.
◆ Elderly patients often require a reduced dosage.
◆ Smokers often require a higher dosage.
◆ Patients with congestive heart failure or liver disorders usually require a lower dosage.

Keys to Patient/Family Teaching
Asthma

Patient/family teaching related to the use of inhalers for asthma include:

◆ Inhalers are used before meals so breathing is easier during eating.
◆ Rinsing the mouth with water after using a steroid inhaler helps prevent fungal infections of the mouth.
◆ Inhaler mouthpiece is rinsed daily for same reason.
◆ Proper technique for using inhalers. Inhalers are not helpful if used incorrectly. Proper techniques are summarized in Chapter 57.
◆ Importance of taking medications and taking them on time. Using medications regularly helps to prevent difficulties and complications.

influenza, pneumonia, chronic sinusitis, an upper respiratory infection, measles, or aspiration of a foreign body from the upper respiratory system. Often it begins in young adulthood and progresses slowly over a long period of time. In a child, it may be a complication of cystic fibrosis and immunodeficiency diseases. It is rarely fatal but may have serious complications. It is usually chronic; the patient must adopt a different lifestyle.

Symptoms. The characteristic symptom of bronchiectasis is a chronic cough, most often occurring when the patient arises in the morning; it produces greenish yellow sputum with a foul odor. As the disease progresses, the amount of sputum increases, and sometimes blood is coughed up. In fact, bronchiectasis is the most common cause of hemoptysis (bloody sputum). The patient loses weight because of poor appetite and may experience chronic fatigue.

Treatment. Drainage of the purulent material is part of the treatment. This is accomplished by postural drainage, in which the head is lower than the chest (see Figure 79-2). The patient is encouraged to cough and breathe deeply. Humidification of air is recommended

to help thin secretions and make expectoration easier. Antibiotics are given to control the infection. Expectorant cough medicines may be prescribed. Good nutrition, fresh air, and rest are also important. The person should not smoke. Special mouth care is needed to overcome the offensive taste and breath odor and to make food more palatable. Prompt attention to such conditions as bronchial asthma and bronchitis helps to prevent bronchiectasis. Surgical intervention may be necessary for individuals who continue to have bouts of pneumonia after treatment. Because bronchiectasis can be prevented, it is seen less frequently than in the past. Patient teaching is summarized in the accompanying box.

Chronic Bronchitis
Chronic bronchitis is more serious than acute bronchitis. It often develops so gradually that the patient disregards its most significant symptom, a chronic cough. Consequently, the disease is firmly established

Keys to Patient/Family Teaching
Prevention of Bronchiectasis

Patient/family teaching related to prevention of bronchiectasis includes:

◆ Children should be vaccinated against whooping cough (pertussis) and measles.
◆ Adults should be vaccinated against influenza.
◆ Give good care in pulmonary disorders to prevent complications.
◆ Maintain general health at optimum level.
◆ Prompt reaction if a foreign object is aspirated into lungs.

before the patient decides that treatment is needed. Chronic bronchitis is a form of COPD. It usually leads to pulmonary emphysema, which is described later. (Repeated attacks of acute bronchitis may lead to a chronic condition, or it may develop after an acute respiratory infection such as influenza or pneumonia.)

Cigarette smoking is one of the most common causes of bronchial irritation; air pollution may also be responsible. People exposed to irritating dusts or chemicals seem to be more likely to develop bronchitis. It affects all ages but is most common in persons over age 40 (the tendency to postpone treatment could be one reason for this).

Signs and Symptoms. Chronic bronchitis begins with a dry cough, also known as smoker's cough, which is most severe when the patient gets up in the morning. As time goes on, the person coughs up mucus and pus, sometimes with streaks of blood. SOB becomes apparent with exertion; as the disease progresses, it persists even when the patient is quiet. The patient's history of a cough as well as living habits helps the physician in making a diagnosis. The diagnosis is also aided by x-rays of the chest, fluoroscopic examinations, and sputum tests.

Treatment. Treatment is a slow and continuous process; no drugs will work a miracle. However, treatment will reduce the symptoms and help to prevent complications. Untreated, the disease may progress until the bronchioles of the lungs are permanently damaged, or it may lead to asthma, emphysema, or heart failure. Aerosolized treatments, postural drainage, and chest percussion are done. These treatments help to facilitate removal of secretions. It is important to build up the patient's general health and to use precautions to avoid exposure to respiratory infections. The patient should have plenty of rest and be free from emotional stress. If the work environment exposes the person to excessive dust or other factors that aggravate the bronchitis, it may be necessary to change jobs. Cigarette smoking must also be avoided. Antibiotics will help to clear coexisting respiratory infections that complicate the condition.

Pulmonary Emphysema

Pulmonary emphysema is an overdistention of the alveoli that causes loss of elasticity and destroys alveolar tissue (see Figure 79-5**E**). It is a form of COPD. It is in the alveoli that the exchange of carbon dioxide and oxygen occurs. In emphysema, air becomes trapped in the alveoli by excessive, thick mucus. The patient is unable to exhale, the lungs become distended, and the muscles suffer from lack of oxygen and become less elastic. The condition becomes worse as more and more air is trapped in the alveoli and cannot

be exhaled. As a result, the heart must work harder to pump blood through the body and get oxygen to the muscles and other body tissues. The end result of emphysema is often congestive heart failure or right heart failure.

Authorities believe that chronic bronchitis is the direct cause of chronic pulmonary emphysema, although it may also follow chronic bronchial asthma, TB, and bronchiectasis. The number of cases of emphysema is directly related to cigarette smoking. Recent evidence also indicates that some families carry a deficiency of a substance that protects the lung tissue during respiratory tract infections and that these families are prone to development of emphysema.

Special Considerations in Aging
Emphysema

Some cases of emphysema occur in older people simply because the lungs have lost their elasticity due to the aging process.

Some of the less common types of emphysema include *hypoplastic emphysema* (a developmental defect in which there are fewer alveoli, but they are abnormally large), *interlobular emphysema* (accumulation of air between the lobules of the lungs), and *interstitial emphysema* (escape of air from the alveoli, caused by chest trauma or bronchiolar obstruction).

Congenital or *infantile lobar emphysema* causes respiratory distress in infants and is characterized by lung overinflation. Another type of emphysema that occurs in young adulthood is caused by the *congenital deficiency of* α_1 *(alpha-one) antitrypsin*, a plasma protein.

Signs and Symptoms. The first symptom of emphysema is difficulty in breathing after exertion. As the condition progresses, the person has persistent difficulty in breathing. Other symptoms are wheezing and a chronic cough. The patient is pale and drawn and is afraid of choking. Many patients use abdominal muscles as well as other accessory muscles to aid in breathing. The patient is afraid to lie down, so sits up, leaning forward and contracting the muscles of the neck with every breath. The patient also raises the shoulder girdle and shows retraction above the clavicles when breathing. The chest becomes barrel shaped, and the patient looks anxious. In the advanced stages, as carbon dioxide accumulates in the blood, the person becomes listless and drowsy. The disease runs its course over a period of many years.

Prevention. Preventive treatment is most important to correct the conditions that cause emphysema because changes in lung tissue or the blood vessels of the lungs are *irreversible*. This means, for one thing, alerting the public to the danger signs, such as morning cough or smoker's cough.

Adult Respiratory Distress Syndrome

Adult respiratory distress syndrome (ARDS) is also called *noncardiogenic pulmonary edema*. ARDS is a state of progressive lack of oxygenation following a serious illness or injury. Causes include aspiration, drug overdose, cardiac surgery (especially bypass), pancreatitis, ESRD, embolism, major surgery, and trauma. The person is in acute respiratory failure and usually must be maintained on mechanical ventilation and the blood pressure maintained with medications. If the cause can be determined, it can be treated. However, the mortality rate is greater than 50%.

Key Concept

Cigarette smoking causes or predisposes to many of the diseases of the respiratory system and of other parts of the body. It is the single most important factor in causation of disease in the United States today.

Trauma

An accident may cause respiratory problems or death. If there is no air exchange in the lungs, the person will die within a matter of minutes.

Absence of Air Exchange

Asphyxiation is the condition in which there is a lack of oxygen in the blood and an excess of carbon dioxide in the blood and tissues. It can be caused by any form of suffocation.

Suffocation is stoppage of breathing and the asphyxia that results when breathing stops. Suffocation may be caused by externally applied pressure to the throat (strangulation), by drowning (aspiration), by electric shock, or by gases that enter the lungs and prevent the exchange of oxygen and carbon dioxide. Choking on a foreign object that plugs the airway or covering the nose and mouth with an object, such as a pillow or plastic bag, also causes suffocation. Sudden infant death syndrome (SIDS) or crib death is also believed to be a form of suffocation, which results when the infant stops breathing and does not restart spontaneously.

Strangulation refers to the arrest of respiration because of an obstruction of the air passage. Most commonly, this term is applied to trauma to the person by another person, by hanging, or by an accident.

Chest Trauma

Asphyxiation can result from a sudden blow to the chest. This may result in a collapsed lung or blockage of the airway. Accumulation of blood in the lungs can cause asphyxiation by drowning.

A puncture wound to the chest caused by a foreign object such as a knife or a bullet is an emergency and must be treated immediately. If a foreign object is in place, do not remove it. Get emergency assistance immediately. *(Rationale: The object may plug the hole and maintain the negative pressure within the lungs until help arrives.)*

If an object, such as a bullet, has caused an open hole in the chest wall, plug the hole immediately. *(Rationale: If you leave the hole open, the lungs will collapse because the negative pressure will have been lost.)* You can keep the hole plugged until emergency assistance arrives.

Nursing Alert

Cardiopulmonary resuscitation (CPR) is not effective if the airway is blocked or if there is an open wound of the chest. The nurse must clear the airway or apply pressure to occlude an open chest wound *before* initiating CPR.

Respiratory Complications in Drug Poisoning

In many cases of drug overdose, the respirations are depressed. In some cases, death is caused by the depression of the respiratory system to the point of apnea. This is called *respiratory arrest*. The drugs most likely to cause these symptoms are the narcotics (such as codeine, morphine, and heroin) and the depressants (such as barbiturates).

In the case of an overdose of *stimulants* (such as cocaine or amphetamines), the respirations may be increased. In this type of overdose, the overstimulation may lead to seizures, hypertension, stroke, and death.

Drowning

One type of drowning occurs when water or another liquid enters the respiratory passages. The medical term for fluid in the lungs is *aspiration*. Death is caused by suffocation because the fluid is heavier than air and settles in the alveoli. The presence of the fluid prevents air exchange in the lungs. A very small amount of fluid can cause death. Aspiration can also lead to aspiration pneumonia, a serious complication.

Another type of drowning, called dry drowning, occurs when the person is under the water, but neither air nor water can get into the lungs because of bronchospasm. In this case, the person dies because of the lack of oxygen and inability to breathe but no water is in the lungs.

Neoplasms

Benign Neoplasms

A benign lung tumor, os characterized on the x-ray film by smooth edg harply defined margins. If the tumor is periphe are usually no symptoms. If the tumor is in nchi, there may be obstruction, causing infe atelectasis distal to the obstruction (see Fig. 79 nchoscopy and biopsy are usually done to de he reason for an abnormal shadow in the lu nent is symptomatic.

Lung Cancer

Lung cancer affects m en than women. However, the American ety reports that lung cancer is now the lea f cancer death in both men and women (see!). Lung cancer is most common between th and 70.

The Surgeon Ge sory Committee reported that in the m cancer deaths, persons were cigarette n available research, curtailing smoking is entive measure. Another cause of these eved to be air pollution. That there are m ple in the population today may partly ac gh incidence of lung cancer because it is primarily of young people.

It is hard to dete the early stage because the symptom until the disease is well advanced. A ry will often reveal the cancer. Lung c ses in the bronchi and produces no s enlarges.

The first indicati erally occurs when the patient begins ucus and blood-streaked sputum. T perience dyspnea, chills, and fever. E nt may think he or she is merely smok may resolve to cut down. Later, fati weight loss, and chest pains occur. ician is consulted,

the disease is likely to be in an advanced stage. Bronchoscopy, chest x-ray, sputum examination, and lung scan confirm the diagnosis.

Treatment. If the tumor is localized, immediate surgery, with removal of part or all of the lung, may be successful. If the tumor is extensive and involves lymph nodes, radiation or chemotherapy (or both) may be used. These treatments will not usually cure the disease, but they often improve the quality of life for the patient.

If the patient has widespread lung cancer, with metastasis to other organs, a combination of chemotherapeutic drugs may be instituted. Responses to this treatment vary. At this time, no chemotherapeutic agent can cure lung cancer, but it is useful in controlling pain and in reducing the pleural effusions caused by the cancer.

Disorders of the Nose

Inflammatory Disorders

Sinusitis

Sinusitis is inflammation of one or more of the sinuses located in the head. The maxillary sinus (antrum) is the one most frequently affected by infection spreading from the nasal passages. If the patient's resistance is low, the person is more susceptible to sinus infection. A sinus infection is uncomfortable. Allergy, frequent colds, and nasal obstruction of any kind increase susceptibility to repeated attacks of sinusitis. If neglected, sinusitis becomes chronic and damages the mucous membranes; treatment is then less effective. Of all the possible complications of sinusitis, infections of the middle ear or the brain are the most serious. Sinusitis may also lead to bronchiectasis or osteomyelitis in the adjacent bone. Early treatment is important to prevent these complications.

Acute Sinusitis. Acute sinusitis begins with pain and pressure. Pain is felt in the cheek or the upper teeth if the maxillary sinuses are affected. Frontal sinus pain occurs over the eyes. The patient may have a low-grade fever, fatigue, and a poor appetite. A purulent nasal discharge is accompanied by a postnasal drip, which is irritating to the throat. Sinus congestion shows on x-ray. Treatment includes forced fluids, antibiotics to control infection, analgesics to relieve pain, and, in severe cases, bed rest. Nose drops containing phenylephrine (Neo-Synephrine) and ephedrine are often used to shrink the swollen turbinates and to encourage drainage; antihistamines are also used. Steam inhalation or hot moist packs to the forehead can be effective.

If drainage is obstructed in an acute sinus infection, the sinus may be irrigated with warm saline solution, a comparatively painless procedure. However, it may be necessary to puncture the bony wall between the nose and the sinus cavity (Caldwell-Luc procedure) or to enter the frontal sinus through the inner aspect of the eyebrow. These surgical procedures are painful for the patient, who may become frightened and feel dizzy or faint.

Chronic Sinusitis. Many people mistakenly think that nothing can be done for sinusitis, and unfortunately, they allow it to become chronic. Chronic sinusitis is characterized by repeated flare-ups of the infection, despite treatment. Symptoms of chronic sinusitis include:

◆ Cough, due to postnasal drip
◆ Chronic headaches in the affected area
◆ Facial pain
◆ Nasal stuffiness
◆ Fatigue

Sometimes a relatively simple operation to create a new sinus opening may be ordered. Because many cases of chronic sinusitis are allergic in nature, allergy tests may be done and desensitization injections given (see Chapter 77).

Structural Disorders

Deviated Septum

The nasal septum is a partition made of bone and cartilage that divides the nose into right and left cavities. The septum is rarely absolutely straight, but unless the deviation is marked, it usually causes no trouble. An unusually crooked septum can interfere with drainage in one nostril or with the insertion of a nasogastric tube. An injury that causes a deformity in the septum should have the attention of a physician; if it is not corrected, it can cause sinusitis. The operation to correct such a deformity is called a *submucous resection or septoplasty*. Nursing care in nasal surgery is discussed in the Nursing Process section of this chapter.

Nasal Polyps

Polyps are tumors that look like small bunches of tiny grapes. Nasal polyps obstruct breathing and sinus drainage. They are easily removed by surgery under local anesthesia, but tend to return, in which case the operation has to be repeated. A biopsy of the tissue should be done to determine if the growth is malignant.

Plastic Surgery

Plastic surgery of the nose (**rhinoplasty**) may be done for cosmetic reasons or to correct deformities resulting from injury. Nasal surgery is described earlier in this chapter.

Nasal Trauma

Fractures

A fractured nose is a relatively common occurrence. It should be set (moved back into place) promptly, to avoid later deformity. Usually, no other treatment is needed.

Nosebleed (Epistaxis)

Irritation or injury to a small mass of capillaries on the nasal septum may cause bleeding. Hypertension can give rise to bleeding, in which case the bleeding is more likely to be severe and easily controlled. Certain blood disorders, cancer, and rheumatic fever are other possible causes. Nosebleed is a fairly common occurrence, but when severe can be serious.

First aid for nosebleed is a nursing skill in Chapter 3. If initial treatment is not effective, the nasal cavity may be packed with gauze to create pressure on the bleeding area. Nasal packing is usually accomplished by passing string through the nose and bringing it out the mouth. Then, the pack is tied on the string and the string is pulled back through the nose until the pack is in the back of the nasal cavity. The other end of the string extends out through the nostril.

Bleeding points may also be treated with silver nitrate or other solutions that stop bleeding, or they may be cauterized to coagulation.

Disorders of the Throat

The throat (pharynx) is the tube communicating with the nasal cavity (nasopharynx), the oral cavity (oropharynx), and the larynx cavity (laryngopharynx). Two throat disorders common in children but occurring occasionally are tonsillitis and streptococcal sore throat (strep).

Trauma

Aspiration of Foreign Body

A foreign body lodged in such a fashion that the patient cannot breathe is an emergency situation. In most cases, a sharp blow between the shoulder blades while the person is lowered, or the abdominal thrust (Heimlich) (Chapter 32), will dislodge the object. If these fail and the patient cannot breathe, an esophagostomy or intubation with an airway if persons are available who can perform it. Artificial ventilation will probably be needed if the airway is opened. Tracheostomy is covered in Chapter 80.

A small object may be aspirated without causing asphyxiation; this condition and atelectasis of all or part of the lung (see Fig. 79-5**B**). It must be removed. For this, bronchoscopy usually is effective. Open-lung surgery may be performed if the object has lodged deep in a bronchus.

> **Nursing Alert**
>
> If a person is not breathing, CPR must be given. This is done with an airway and a manual breathing bag if available. (*Rationale: This is often more effective; it is less strenuous for the rescuer; and it prevents the spread of infection from the patient to the healthcare worker.*) If an airway and manual breathing bag are not available, mouth-to-mouth breathing is required.

Neoplasms

Cancer of the Larynx

Cancer of the larynx most often afflicts men over the age of 45, although it is increasing in women who smoke. Those who have chronic laryngitis, strain their voices, or are heavy drinkers or smokers are the most likely to develop cancer of the larynx. It is also believed that hereditary tendencies play a part.

The symptoms are chronic hoarseness of the voice, and, in some instances, inability to speak above a whisper.

Treatment. If the condition is detected early, radiation may be an effective method of treatment. Surgery is often successful in inducing a complete cure. The operation consists of removing either the tumorous part or the entire larynx. The surgery is called **laryngectomy**. A person who has a total laryngectomy is referred to as a **laryngectomee**. If the cancer has spread beyond the vocal cords, a simple or radical neck dissection is done.

After the larynx is removed, air enters and leaves through the trachea. Provision for this is made by inserting a tube into the trachea through an opening in the lower part of the neck. This procedure is called a tracheostomy; it is permanent, even after the airway tube is removed.

Nursing Considerations. Patient teaching and support are of great importance. The patient faces not only the knowledge that he or she must permanently breathe through a hole in the neck, but also the possibility that the tumor may be malignant. Fears about never speaking again may be reduced by assuring the patient that, although the natural voice will be lost, voice training (esophageal and pharyngeal speech) will make it possible to carry on a conversation. If the patient has had only a partial laryngectomy, reassure him or her that speech will most often return quickly. It may be helpful

for the patient to be visited by another person who has made a good recovery after a laryngectomy. Because reconstruction of the esophagus is likely, the patient should be told that, for a time, feeding may be done through a nasal or gastrostomy tube (until the esophagus heals) and that the tracheostomy opening will be permanent. Good oral hygiene is needed; it helps the patient to be more comfortable and helps to keep the surgical site as clean as possible.

When respiratory passages become irritated, mucous secretion increases; this must be removed frequently by suction through the tracheostomy tube. A suction machine is kept at the patient's bedside, and it is important the patient never be left alone without a call light. A member of the family may stay with the patient for the first few postoperative days. The procedure for suctioning and care of the "trach" tube is presented in Chapter 80.

Because the patient cannot cry out for help, he or she is fearful of choking and of not being able to breathe. If oxygen is to be administered, it is applied by mask over the tracheostomy tube. There is also the danger of hemorrhage, as evidenced by hemoptysis (coughing or spitting up of blood) or by symptoms of shock.

The drainage from the wound following a neck dissection or other procedure in this area is usually handled by a portable wound suction device. This device stays with the patient at all times. The nurse empties and measures the drainage. Management of the portable wound suction device (such as Hem-O-Vac) is described and pictured in Chapter 54 (see Figure 54-2).

The patient probably will be allowed out of bed the first postoperative day, and soon will be taught how to suction the tube and take care of it. Everybody involved in the patient's care should know how to perform this procedure. When the airway becomes obstructed, the patient becomes cyanotic quickly and could die within a few minutes if the obstruction is not removed. In this emergency, call for help and suction the tracheostomy opening. Unless the physician has previously instructed the charge nurse as to what emergency procedures to use, the physician should be consulted to see if the tracheostomy tube can be removed as an emergency measure.

The patient usually loses the sense of smell temporarily after surgery, but this will begin to return as he or she learns to breathe through the tracheostomy tube. However, the sense of smell will be best recovered in the patient who learns esophageal speech.

Subjects to be included in patient teaching are listed in the accompanying box.

Communication. Before the surgery, the method of postoperative communication should be discussed with the patient. If the patient knows that some type of communication after surgery is guaranteed, much of the fear

---

Keys to Patient/Family Teaching
Laryngectomy

Patient/family teaching for the person recovering after a total laryngectomy includes:

- Care of the tube (cleaning, suctioning, if necessary, and how to handle emergencies)
- Communication techniques
- Support groups available for persons/families after laryngectomies and/or a diagnosis of cancer
- Assistance with smoking cessation, if applicable
- The permanent laryngectomy opening may be covered by a necktie, a crew or turtle neck shirt, a scarf, or jewelry.
- Methods of ensuring free entry of air.
- Prevention of aspiration of fluids or foreign objects into the laryngectomy tube. Showering must be done with care and swimming is often prohibited.
- In extremely cold weather, the person should wear a scarf over the opening. The person may still have difficulty because the normal warming and humidifying action of the nose is absent.
- Thin, filmy scarves should not be worn, because they may be sucked into the tracheostomy and obstruct breathing.

---

will be allayed. Immediately postoperatively, a workable communication system must be set up. Provide the patient with writing materials. If the patient is trying to tell you something, make every attempt to find out what it is.

Key Concept

Sometimes, the patient must write notes to communicate. In this case, make sure the person's dominant hand is not encumbered with an intravenous apparatus. A child's "Magic Slate" often works well on a temporary basis. Alphabet cards and picture cards are also available.

Make sure this person's signal light is answered immediately because he or she will not be able to tell you what is wrong on the intercom. (The person may be given a tap bell to use for emergencies.)

Speech Therapy and Training. Speech therapy should begin as soon as possible. The technique of esophageal speech consists of swallowing air and using the swallowed air to make speech sounds while regurgitating the air. It takes patience and constant practice to learn how to do this; some patients learn the technique in 2 or 3 weeks. Esophageal speech is not smooth although it is the easiest to learn.

Most patients progress to pharyngeal speech. The air used in this case is that which enters the nose and mouth; it is blocked by quick tongue action. The pharynx becomes the sounding board. Pharyngeal speech takes much more practice, but it is smoother and has a more natural sound than esophageal speech.

The third speech technique is devised for the patient who is unable to learn esophageal or pharyngeal speech. It is the artificial larynx, an electronic device that the patient holds against the throat. Currently, many physicians during surgery are implanting an electronic device that aids in making speech sound more normal.

Tracheoesophageal puncture is another alternative to speech after a total laryngectomy. Voice is produced by movement of air from the lungs through a puncture in the posterior wall of the trachea, into the esophagus, and out of the mouth. A prosthesis is placed over the puncture site once it has healed. In some patients, speech is possible by placing a finger over the tracheostomy opening, after taking a breath.

Identification. It is absolutely vital that the laryngectomee wear an identifying tag, such as the Medic-Alert tag, so others will know that he or she breathes through an opening in the neck. This is especially important if speech training has not yet begun. Remember, if the opening is plugged, the laryngectomee will die of asphyxiation.

Resources. Some communities have clubs and organizations available to laryngectomees. The clubs are sponsored by the International Association of Laryngectomees. In this way, members are able to give each other encouragement and emotional support. They are often willing to visit laryngectomy patients in the hospital, which gives the patients encouragement to begin rehabilitation.

Water Dangers. Anyone who has a tracheostomy or a permanent laryngectomy tube must always be careful to prevent water from getting into the opening; this person must use great caution in showering. A snorkel device is available to fit over the stoma of the laryngectomee to allow patients to swim, in which case extreme caution must be used. Strenuous water sports are contraindicated.

Keys to Review

Key Questions for Critical Thinking

1. Describe how chest tubes function. Identify warning signs that something is wrong when chest tubes are used.
2. Describe abnormal sounds heard on auscultation. Determine what each indicates and give medical and nursing interventions for each.
3. Compare the four types of hypoxia, giving the signs and symptoms for each. Determine what nursing assessments and interventions should be made in hypoxia.
4. Describe COPD and four disorders associated with it. Determine how the disorders differ. Identify medications used in treatment. Outline patient teaching involved.
5. Suggest nursing measures to be taken to prevent the spread of TB to others. Identify important teaching factors.

Key Readings

Belcher AE. Cancer Nursing. St. Louis, Mosby-Yearbook, 1992

Berkow R (Ed). The Merck Manual of Diagnosis and Therapy, Ed 16. Rahway, NJ, Merck & Co, 1992

NANDA Nursing Diagnoses: Definitions and Classifications 1992. Philadelphia, North American Nursing Diagnosis Association, 1992

Nurse Review. Respiratory Problems. Springhouse, PA, Springhouse, updated 1993

Nursing '94 Drug Handbook. Springhouse, PA, Springhouse, 1994

O'Toole M (Ed). Miller-Keane Encyclopedia and Dictionary of Medicine, Nursing and Allied Health, Ed 5. Philadelphia, W.B. Saunders, 1992

Scherer JC. Introductory Medical-Surgical Nursing, Ed 5. Philadelphia, J.B. Lippincott, 1991

Sexton D. Nursing Care of the Respiratory Patient. Norwalk, CT, Appleton-Lange, 1990

Smeltzer SC, Bare BG: Brunner and Suddarth's Textbook of Medical-Surgical Nursing, Ed 7. Philadelphia, J.B. Lippincott, 1992

Suddarth DS. The Lippincott Manual of Nursing Practice, Ed 5. Philadelphia, J.B. Lippincott, 1991

Enrichment Keys (continued)

Taylor C, Lillis C, LeMone P. Fundamentals of Nursing: Art and Science of Nursing Care, Ed 2. Philadelphia, J.B. Lippincott, 1993

Enrichment Keys

Allen MA, Ownby K. "Tuberculosis: the other epidemic." Journal of Association of Nurses in AIDS Care 2(4): 1991

Della Bella LA. "Steroidophobia and the pulmonary patient. American Journal of Nursing, 92(2):26–29, 1992

Reinke L, Hoffman L. "Breathing space: how to teach asthma co-management." American Journal of Nursing, 92(10):40–51, 1992

Bloch AB, Cauthen GM, Onorato I, et al. "Nationwide survey of drug-resistant tuberculosis in the United States." Journal of the American Medical Association 271(9):665–671, 1994

Keys to Learning More

Chapter 80: oxygen therapy

Unit Fifteen: geriatric nursing

Chapter 89: rehabilitation, ambulatory and home care nursing

Unit Seventeen: death and dying

Key Resources

American Lung Association
1740 Broadway
New York, NY 10019
212/315-8700

Cystic Fibrosis Foundation
6931 Arlington Road
Bethesda, MD 20814
1-800/FIGHT-CF

National Jewish Center for Immunology and Respiratory Medicine
1400 Jackson Street
Denver, CO 80206
1-800/222-LUNG

80 Oxygen Therapy and Respiratory Care

Keys for Learning

Learning Objectives

- State major goals of oxygen therapy.
- Discuss safety factors in oxygen administration.
- List key points in nursing assessment of the patient who is receiving oxygen.
- Describe the use of the pulse oximeter.
- Discuss nursing care of the patient receiving oxygen, on mechanical ventilation, or with an artificial airway.
- Be able to set up basic oxygen equipment.

Key Terms

ambu bag	pulse oximeter
artificial airway	respirator
nasal cannula	ventilator
non-rebreathing mask	

Keys to Understanding This Chapter

Chapter 5: basic human needs
Chapter 6: optimum health
Chapter 21: cardiovascular system
Chapter 22: respiratory system
Chapter 29: safety
Chapter 30: medical asepsis
Chapter 32: sudden death and CPR
Chapter 42: vital signs
Chapter 54: surgical asepsis
Unit Eleven: pharmacology and medication administration
Chapter 64: fundamentals of pediatrics (oxygen administration)
Chapter 74: cardiovascular disorders
Chapter 79: respiratory disorders

Key Points

- The most urgent or vital basic need is that of oxygen. Without oxygen, a person will die in a matter of minutes.

Key Points (continued)

- Therapeutic oxygen is considered a drug. It must be prescribed by a physician and has associated dangers.
- Oxygen administration can be used to assist a person to breathe or to totally support life.
- Oxygen is administered in several ways: nasal cannula, simple mask, partial-rebreathing mask, non-rebreathing mask, Venturi mask, intermittent positive pressure breathing, and aerosol mist.
- Oxygen supports combustion; great care must be taken when using oxygen—a fire can be explosive.
- The nurse works with the respiratory care department in oxygen administration.

Key Topics Outline

Oxygen Provision
    Sources of Oxygen
The Patient Who Is Having Difficulty Breathing Adequately
    Types of Oxygen Delivery Devices
Administering Oxygen to the Patient Who Is Unable to Breathe Without Assistance
    The Manual Breathing Bag
    Ventilatory Support
    Assisting the Patient on a Mechanical Ventilator
    Assisting the Patient Who Has a Tracheostomy

Key Learning Activities

- Design a chart showing types of oxygen delivery devices, when each is used, dangers/precautions, and special nursing considerations.
- Review administration of oxygen to children (see Chapter 64).
- Interview a patient who has received oxygen. How did the person feel? What were the patient's concerns? What was the most difficult thing about the treatment?

Rosdahl CB: Textbook of Basic Nursing, 6th ed. © 1995 J.B. Lippincott Company

Oxygen is a gas vital to life. It is the most urgent basic need. If a person is deprived of oxygen, death will occur in a matter of minutes. Normally, we all extract sufficient oxygen from the air we breathe. Therapeutic (supplemental) oxygen is necessary only when insufficient oxygen is available for the body's needs, due to a breathing or blood deficiency. Excess oxygen is not helpful; in fact, it can be harmful. Therefore, oxygen is prescribed like a drug and administered to the patient under controlled conditions. Furthermore, the more oxygen in the air, the greater the danger of fire. Oxygen is necessary for anything to burn and increasing oxygen will make common flammable materials able to burn faster and hotter. Therefore, safety is of the utmost importance. This chapter discusses the patient who is receiving supplemental oxygen, as well as the person whose breathing is supported by a mechanical ventilator or who has an artificial airway.

Oxygen Provision

Oxygen is administered to patients who have an oxygen deficiency. By increasing the concentration of oxygen the patient inhales, more oxygen can be made available for the body's consumption. Oxygen is used in such conditions as pneumonia, carbon monoxide poisoning, severe asthma, heart failure, heart attack, or after surgery of the chest or abdomen. It makes the patient more comfortable; the patient breathes more easily.

Goals of Oxygen Therapy

Three goals can be accomplished by increasing the concentration (or percentage) of oxygen the patient inhales:

◆ To reverse hypoxemia (low oxygen concentration in the blood).
◆ To decrease the work of the respiratory system. If supplemental oxygen is given, the respiratory muscles need not work as hard to pump air in and out of the lungs to maintain sufficient oxygen supply in the blood.
◆ To decrease the work of the heart in pumping blood. The heart tries to compensate for hypoxemia by increasing output. Giving oxygen can ease the load on the heart.

Hazards of Oxygen Therapy

Like other medications, certain hazards are associated with oxygen (O_2) administration. Oxygen given in high concentration over a period of days can result in oxygen toxicity, which manifests itself with changes in lung tissue. (You have already learned that excess oxygen in neonates can cause vision difficulties.) In some patients, increased oxygen concentrations may also affect the ventilatory

Key Abbreviations and Acronyms for Oxygen Administration

ABG	Arterial blood gases
ARDS	Adult respiratory distress syndrome
CO_2	Carbon dioxide
CPAP	Continuous positive airway pressure
ET	Endotracheal tube
HBO	Hyperbaric oxygenation
IPPB	Intermittent positive pressure breathing
LPM	Liters per minute
NRM	Non-rebreathing mask
O_2	Oxygen
PRM	Partial rebreathing mask
PSI	Pounds per square inch
PSV	Pressure support ventilation
SIMV	Synchronized intermittent mandatory ventilation
trach	Tracheostomy

drive control mechanisms, actually weakening the stimulus to breathe. Therefore, oxygen should be considered a drug, to be administered with the same care that is used in administering other drugs. A physician should evaluate the patient's need for oxygen and write specific orders for oxygen therapy with the appropriate dosage. The administration of oxygen by mask or cannula is expressed in liters per minute (LPM); some devices can control the specific concentration of oxygen to be administered. With mechanical ventilators, oxygen concentration can be more accurately controlled.

Everyone, including the patient, visitors, and other patients in the unit, must know and follow the necessary precautions when oxygen is being used. If oxygen comes in contact with any combustible material, even a small spark can ignite an explosive fire. See the list of precautionary measures in the accompanying guidelines box.

Assessment of Respiratory Status

Whenever a patient is receiving oxygen, respiratory status must be constantly monitored to make sure the treatment is having the desired effect. The accompanying box lists skills in nursing assessment of respiratory status. (See also Chapter 50 for adults and Chapter 62 for infants.) If any signs of respiratory distress occur, the physician should be notified immediately.

Use of the Pulse Oximeter. The **pulse oximeter** is a convenient monitor used to measure the degree of oxygen saturation in the blood. Using a finger clip or an ear probe, it shines a light beam through soft tissue. This measurement is noninvasive (unlike drawing blood for arterial blood gas analysis) and can be

Nursing Skill Guidelines
Providing Oxygen

Precautionary Measures

◆ Explain to the patient the dangers of lighting matches or smoking cigarettes or pipes. Be sure the patient has no matches, cigarettes, or smoking materials in the bedside table.

◆ Make sure that warning signs (OXYGEN-NO SMOK-ING) are posted on the patient's door and above the patient's bed (even if the entire facility is nonsmoking.)

◆ Use caution with all electrical devices, such as heating pads, electric blankets, or the ordinary signal light. Hospitals usually provide a signal light with a grounding device or give the patient a tap bell.

◆ Do not use oil on oxygen equipment. *(Rationale: Oil can ignite if exposed to oxygen.)* Be sure there are no traces of oil on your hands before adjusting oxygen apparatus.

◆ Be aware of all potential sources of sparks, especially when administering oxygen by means of a containment device (such as a tent or isolette). NOTE: Items that appear innocuous (such as friction toys, electric razors) have proven to cause an explosive fire.

General Care

◆ Reassure and gain cooperation of the patient. The patient should be informed of the therapeutic uses of oxygen before the equipment is brought into the room. Reassure the patient and family. *(Rationale: They may be afraid because people often believe that the use of oxygen is a sign of deteriorating condition. Oxygen need will be reduced if the patient is relaxed.)*

◆ Instruct the patient not to change the position of the mask, cannula or any of the equipment, once it is in place. *(Rationale: This could change the amount of oxygen being delivered.)*

◆ Maintain a constant concentration of oxygen for the patient to breathe; monitor the equipment at regular intervals.

◆ Give pain medications as needed, prevent chilling and try to ensure that the patient gets needed rest. Be alert to cues about hunger and elimination. *(Rationale: The patient's physical comfort is important.)*

◆ Watch for respiratory depression/distress.

◆ Encourage or assist the patient to move about in bed. *(Rationale: This prevents hypostatic pneumonia or circulatory difficulties.)* Many patients are reluctant to move, because they are afraid of the oxygen apparatus.

◆ Make sure the tubing is patent at all times and the equipment is working properly.

◆ Assess, document and report the patient's condition regularly.

◆ Provide frequent mouth care. Make sure the oxygen contains proper humidification. *(Rationale: Oxygen can be drying to mucous membranes.)*

◆ Keep in mind that oxygen does not control every breathing difficulty. However, where it is indicated, it can dramatically improve the patient's condition. The person breathes more easily, the pulse rate drops, and an anxious attitude may change to a relaxed one.

◆ Discontinue oxygen only after the patient has been evaluated by a physician. Generally, oxygen given in medium to high concentrations (above 30%) should not be abruptly discontinued. It should be gradually decreased in stages, and the patient's arterial blood gases or oxygen saturation level monitored. *(Rationale: These steps determine whether continued support is needed.)*

◆ Wear gloves any time you might come in contact with the patient's respiratory secretions. *(Rationale: Spread of infection is prevented.)*

---

used continuously or intermittently. The oximeter is read as percent oxygen saturation (O_2 sat). The pulse oximeter has limited accuracy and its reading must be interpreted with knowledge of the patient's blood components and other variables. Still, it is a useful adjunct to other evaluations of the patient's respiratory status. The use of the pulse oximeter is described and illustrated in Chapter 53.

Sources of Oxygen

The oxygen source most frequently used in hospitals is the large bulk storage tank, with its convenient in-room piping system. However, small oxygen tanks (cylin-

ders) or oxygen "strollers" are still necessary to provide a portable supply or an emergency backup. In some smaller hospitals, in nursing homes, and in parts of the hospital where oxygen is used infrequently, cylinders are used.

Wall Outlet. With bulk storage and piping systems, a wall outlet is installed next to each patient's bed. The nurse should be familiar with the wall outlet system used by the hospital. Wall outlets and adapters vary, not only by type of gas supplied, but from manufacturer to manufacturer. Shapes, colors, and connection methods may change. Therefore, the nurse should practice inserting the adapter into the outlet so that it can be

Respiratory Status of a Patient Who is Receiving Oxygen

◆ Observe patient's respirations. Assess rate, depth, and character of respirations.

◆ Document difficulty in breathing. (Abnormal movements, retraction, irregular breathing patterns, abnormal breathing sounds.)

◆ Assess lung sounds. (Document abnormal lung sounds.) See Chapter 50.

◆ Assess level of patient comfort. (If the patient is anxious, very restless, may not be getting enough oxygen.)

◆ Measure pulse rate often. (In respiratory distress, pulse rate often rises.)

◆ Monitor results of arterial blood gases (ABG), which are often drawn and analyzed regularly. This involves an arterial stick (as opposed to a venipuncture) and drawing of blood from an artery.

◆ Check pulse oximeter readings, often used to determine the patient's oxygen saturation. This is a noninvasive procedure.

◆ If indicated, monitor the patient electronically (pulse, respiration, blood pressure, oxygen saturation).

◆ Assess for presence of cyanosis. (blueness, duskiness of skin and mucous membranes.)

◆ Monitor bag and mask for proper fit, proper usage, and no leakage.

◆ Observe the patient whose oxygen has been discontinued closely. If the patient becomes short of breath, if pulse rate increases markedly, or if patient shows signs of cyanosis, the physician should be called at once and oxygen resumed.

done quickly and easily during an emergency. The suggested procedure follows:

◆ Obtain a flowmeter and firmly push the adapter into the outlet.

◆ Give a gentle pull outward. (*Rationale: This ensures that the adapter is locked in place.*)

◆ Once the adapter is inserted, check to see that no oxygen is leaking around the edges. If oxygen is escaping, remove and reinsert the adapter.

◆ To remove adapter, push in slightly, then firmly pull out. Do not be startled by the loud popping sound made by the release of pressure of the contained oxygen behind the wall source.

Oxygen Cylinders. Although oxygen cylinders are available in many sizes, they can be grouped into two categories: large and small. Large cylinders can be identified not only by their relative size, but also by the presence of a metal cap screwed onto the top of the cylinder, to protect the valve from damage. Also, the valve itself has an attached handle and threaded connection site. Large cylinders are generally used when high flow rates are to be used or when oxygen is needed for an extended period of time.

Small cylinders can be identified by the rectangular valve, with no handle and three holes on one side. Small cylinders are used for transporting a patient or for emergency use of short duration. Many patients have small cylinders to use at home.

Care in the handling and use of cylinders makes them safe. Because the gas contained within a cylinder is under extremely high pressure, the pressure must be reduced to a safe level before the cylinder is connected to a patient; this is done by means of the regulator. Attached to most regulators are a flowmeter and a pressure gauge. The flowmeter is either round or similar to the flowmeter used with wall outlets; it indicates oxygen flow to the patient in LPM. The pressure gauge is round, but usually smaller than the (round) flowmeter and indicates the pressure in the cylinder in pounds per square inch of pressure (PSI units).

Safety in using oxygen cylinders is vital. They are under high pressure. If you must move a cylinder, it *must* be secured on a cylinder cart; if the top breaks off, it becomes "jet-propelled." Be sure to turn the valve "OFF" when not in use. Be sure to keep cylinders *away* from heat. If you are asked to administer oxygen or another gas using a cylinder, request instruction in the application and management of the regulators.

Oxygen Strollers. Portable oxygen can also be provided by a liquid oxygen "stroller." They have also been nicknamed "walkers" or "companions" by their manufacturers. The liquid oxygen portable unit consists of a Thermos vessel in a shoulder bag or small carrying case. Liquid oxygen is much more dense than is the gas, so a liquid portable stroller can carry more oxygen and yet be lighter and more compact than a steel gas cylinder. The liquid oxygen is allowed to evaporate within a warming coil into its gaseous state; it is then metered to the patient through a tubing to an oxygen cannula or other device. Liquid oxygen strollers are generally quite safe.

Guidelines for operating a liquid portable oxygen stroller are:

◆ Keep the tank upright at all times. (*Rationale: If tipped, the tank will vent the oxygen contents quickly.*)

◆ Strollers can be refilled from a larger stationary reservoir unit.

◆ Whether a stroller is full or empty is determined by its relative weight.

◆ Strollers will gradually empty by themselves; as the liquid oxygen warms, it evaporates. For this reason, strollers cannot totally replace cylinders as sources of emergency portable oxygen.

The Oxygen Concentrator. The oxygen concentrator is widely used in home care and extended care settings. It compresses room air and extracts oxygen. It can provide concentrated oxygen at flows in the range of 1 to 5 LPM and is much safer and more convenient than an oxygen tank. It also does not need to be refilled, but it does require periodic maintenance by a technician. It needs electricity to operate and is not portable.

The Hyperbaric Chamber. Some large hospitals have a hyperbaric chamber, which simulates deep-sea diving, by increasing atmospheric pressure. This is called *hyperbaric oxygenation* (HBO) or *high-pressure oxygenation*. In the chamber, oxygen can be taken into the body in concentrations higher than possible at normal atmospheric pressure. With the increased pressure, hemoglobin as well as blood components other than hemoglobin can carry oxygen. HBO is used in carbon monoxide poisoning, to treat anaerobic infections (such as gas gangrene), to administer some types of radiation therapy for cancer, and to perform some surgery (especially heart surgery).

The Patient Who Is Having Difficulty Breathing Adequately

When administering oxygen to a patient who is having difficulty breathing adequately, the type of device used is of critical importance. The primary concern is the concentration (percentage) of oxygen desired. Blood gases are monitored. Other considerations are patient comfort, patient compliance, and safety.

Types of Oxygen Delivery Devices

Oxygen delivery devices can be classified into two types: low-flow devices and high-flow devices. *Low-flow oxygen devices* do not provide an exact oxygen concentration. The patient's breathing pattern has a major influence on the concentration of oxygen a particular patient obtains from the device. Low-flow oxygen devices include the nasal cannula, simple mask, partial-rebreathing mask, and non-rebreathing mask. In *high-flow oxygen devices*, the oxygen percentage is constant (provided it is set up properly). One high-flow device is the Venturi mask.

With all oxygen devices, except the Venturi mask and sometimes the partial rebreathing mask, humidification should be provided. The rationale in humidification is that oxygen from a tank or bulk system is absolutely dry and somewhat irritating to the respiratory mucosa. The humidifier sends oxygen through small holes into water, to create bubbles that add molecules of water to the gas. The humidifier is connected to the threaded outlet at the bottom of the flowmeter or regulator. A small universal connector extends from the front or top of the humidifier for connection to the oxygen device.

Humidifiers need not be used with a Venturi mask. The amount of room air contained provides enough humidity. A wing nut and tailpiece are used to connect the Venturi mask to the flowmeter or regulator.

Nasal Cannula

The **nasal cannula** (nasal prongs) is the device that most patients prefer for small to moderate increases in oxygen concentration. The cannula has two short tubes, one fitting into each naris (nostril). The cannula is a low-flow device that can deliver 24% to 44% oxygen at flow rates of 1 to 6 LPM. Patients prefer cannulas over masks because they are less confining and do not interfere with eating or talking.

Cannulas should be used with caution on patients with irregular breathing patterns because the percentage of oxygen reaching the lungs varies with the rate and depth of respirations. Nursing actions regarding the use of nasal cannulas are described in the accompanying Nursing Procedure.

Simple Mask

The simple mask is a transparent green mask with a simple nipple adapter (Fig. 80-1). It is fitted over the nose, mouth, and chin. It is a low-flow oxygen delivery device providing an oxygen concentration in the 40% to 60% range, at liter flows of 6 to 10 LPM. Nursing skills in supplying oxygen with a simple mask are:

Nursing Skill
Supplying Oxygen With a Simple Mask

Supplies and Equipment

Oxygen mask
Source of oxygen
Gloves

Procedure

1. Wash your hands and wear gloves. (*Rationale: These actions prevent transmission of microorganisms.*)
2. Explain the procedure and the need for oxygen to the patient. (*Rationale: Patient has a right to know what is happening and why; this also helps to decrease anxiety.*)
3. Attach the humidifier to the threaded outlet of the flowmeter or regulator.
4. Connect the tubing from the simple mask to the nipple outlet on the humidifier.
5. Set the oxygen at the prescribed flow rate. (*Rationale: The oxygen must be flowing before applying the mask to the patient.*)

Supplying Oxygen With the Nasal Cannula

Supplies and Equipment

Flowmeter
Oxygen source
Nasal cannula and tubing
Humidifier and sterile water (optional)
Oxygen in use sign ("No Smoking")
Gloves

Suggested Procedure and Rationale

1. Gather supplies.
   (*Rationale: Organization facilitates performance of the skill.*)
2. Wash hands. Wear gloves.
   (*Rationale: Handwashing prevents the spread of organisms.*)
3. Explain procedure to patient.
   (*Rationale: Providing information fosters patient cooperation.*)
4. Prepare the oxygen equipment:
   a. Plug the flowmeter into the wall outlet or oxygen tank.
   b. Attach the humidifier to the flowmeter.

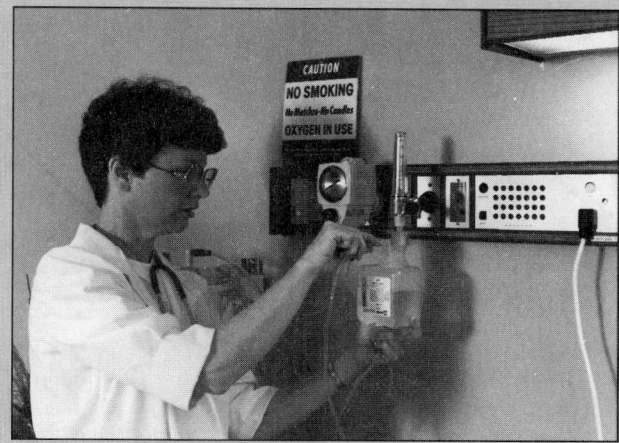

Step 4d   Attaching the connecting tubing to the humidifier nozzle

5. Adjust flowmeter setting to the ordered flow rate. Check that oxygen is flowing out of prongs. Rate via cannula should not exceed 6 L/min (LPM).
   (*Rationale: Higher rates may cause excess drying of nasal mucosa.*)
6. Insert prongs into patient's nostrils. Adjust tubing behind ears and slide plastic adapter under chin until comfortable.
   (*Rationale: Proper position allows unobstructed oxygen flow and eases the patient's respirations.*)

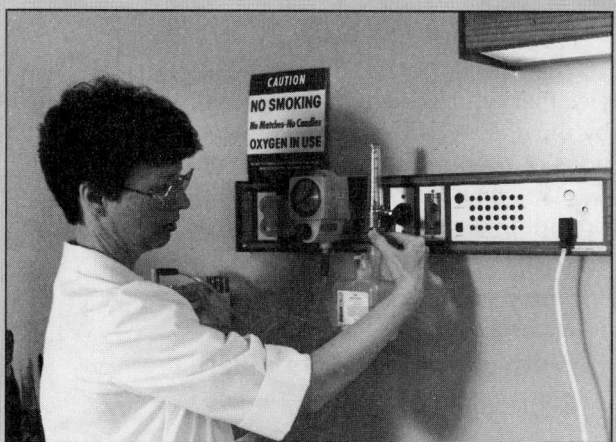

Step 4b   Attaching the humidifier to the flowmeter

   c. Fill the humidifier with sterile water.
   d. Attach cannula with connecting tubing to adapter on humidifier.
   (*Rationale: Humidification prevents drying of nasal mucosa. Agency policy dictates whether low flow oxygen (3 liters or less) requires humidification.*)

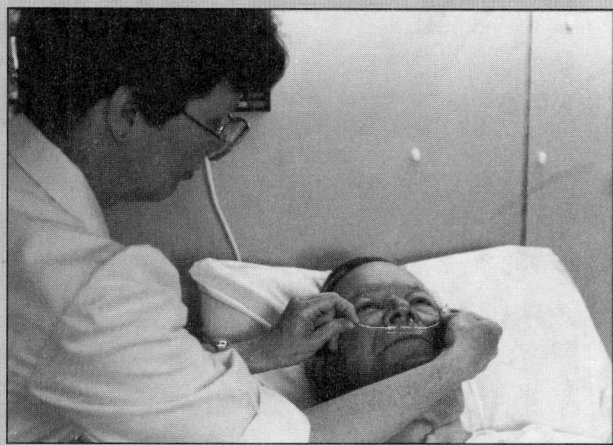

Step 6   Inserting prongs into the nostrils

7. Encourage patient to breathe through nose rather than mouth.
   (*Rationale: More oxygen is inhaled into trachea and less likely to be exhaled through the mouth.*)

(continued)

8. Assess patient's comfort level. Leave call signal within reach.
(Rationale: Anxiety increases the demand for oxygen.)
9. Wash hands.
(Rationale: Handwashing prevents the spread of organisms.)
10. Place "No Smoking" sign at entry into room.
(Rationale: Sign warns patient and visitors that smoking is prohibited because oxygen is combustible.)

11. Dispose of gloves and wash your hands. Document the procedure and record the patient's reaction.
(Rationale: Documentation provides for coordination of care.)
12. Check oxygen setup including water level in humidifier. Clean cannula and assess nares at least every 8 hours.
(Rationale: Sterile water needs to be added when level falls below line on humidification container. Nares may become dry and irritated and require use of a water-soluble lubricant.)

---

6. To apply the mask, guide the elastic strap over the top of the patient's head, bring the strap down to just below the patient's ears. (Rationale: This position of the elastic will hold the mask most firmly.)
7. Gently, but firmly, pull the strap extensions to center the mask on the patient's face with a tight seal. (Rationale: The seal prevents leaks, as much as possible.)
8. Make sure that the patient is comfortable. (Rationale: Comfort helps relieve apprehension.)
9. Put the call signal within the patient's reach before leaving the room. (Rationale: The patient may not be able to call for help with the mask in place.)
10. Remove and properly dispose of gloves; wash your hands. (Rationale: Respiratory secretions are considered contaminated.)
11. Document the procedure and record the patient's reactions.
12. Check the patient periodically for depressed respirations or increased pulse.

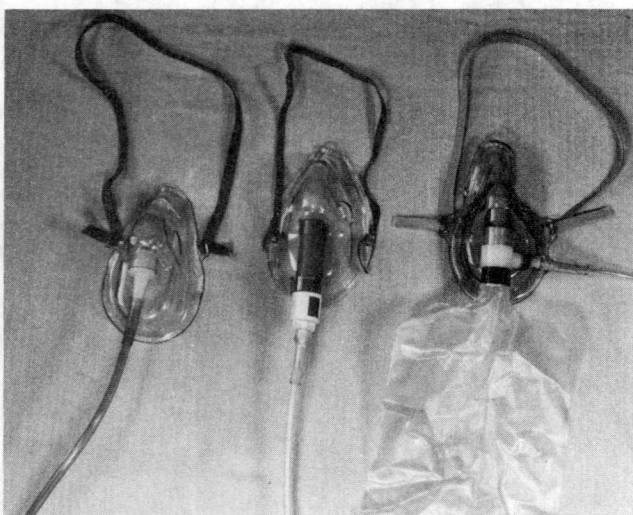

Figure 80-1. The three most common face masks used to administer oxygen. (*Left*) Simple mask. (*Center*) Venturi type mask. (*Right*) Partial rebreathing or reservoir mask. All are disposable. (Photo by Paul Montague.)

13. Check for reddened pressure areas under the straps.
(Rationale: The straps, when snug, put pressure on the underlying skin areas.)

Nursing Alert

The simple mask requires a minimum oxygen flow rate of 6 LPM to prevent carbon dioxide buildup.

Partial-Rebreathing Mask

The partial-rebreathing mask (PRM) is a low-flow device that can be identified by the presence of a bag and by the absence of valves (see Figure 80-1). Concentrations of 60% to 90% oxygen can be achieved with this device. The following nursing skill summarizes steps in providing oxygen with the PRM.

Nursing Skill
Providing Oxygen With a Partial-Rebreathing Mask

Supplies and Equipment

Mask
Oxygen source
Gloves

Procedure

1. Wash your hands and wear gloves.
2. Explain the procedure and need for oxygen to the patient. (Rationale: The patient has a right to know what is happening and why; this also helps to decrease anxiety.)
3. A humidifier is not necessary and often is not recommended. (Rationale: The humidifier can restrict enough airflow so the device cannot keep up with the patient's demand.) Attach to oxygen source.
4. Set the oxygen flow rate at 12 to 15 LPM.

5. Place your finger inside the mask over the hole that leads out of the bag. *(Rationale: This will cause the bag to inflate with oxygen.)*

6. Place the mask over the bridge of the nose and bring the mask down over the chin. Guide the elastic strap over the head and secure as with the simple mask.

7. Ask the patient to take a few breaths, and observe to make sure that the bag deflates with each inspiration, but *not to less than one third full. (Rationale: If the bag does not inflate and deflate, it is either malfunctioning or not correctly sealed.)*

8. Reduce or raise the flow rate to the minimum possible level at which proper deflation occurs (but *not less than 6 LPM). (Rationale: Regulation of the flow rate is based on the breathing of the patient, as related to the bag's deflation and inflation.)*

9. Make sure that the patient is comfortable. Put the call signal within the patient's reach before leaving the room.

10. Remove and dispose of gloves; wash your hands. *(Rationale: These actions prevent the transmission of microorganisms.)*

11. Document the procedure, recording the patient's reactions.

12. Check the patient periodically.

Key Concept

◆ The PRM is never run at a specific oxygen flow rate; rather, it is run at whatever flow rate the patient requires to keep the bag at least one-third inflated. *(Rationale: This prevents the patient from rebreathing his or her own carbon dioxide.)*

◆ A minimum flow rate of 6 LPM is required with this mask, however.

Non-rebreathing Mask

The **non-rebreathing mask** (NRM) can be distinguished from the PRM by the presence of valves on the outside of the mask, as well as valves between the mask and bag. The NRM can provide oxygen in the 90% to 100% range. Like the PRM, the NRM is never run at a specified liter flow. The bag of the NRM must also remain at least one third inflated.

To use the NRM, follow the same procedures as for the PRM. Continuous observation of the patient's respirations and proper bag deflation are essential. Cardiac monitoring, with alarms, is strongly suggested.

Nursing Alert

The NRM is used only in intensive care units or in a one-to-one patient care situation. *(Rationale: insufficient oxygen flow or accidental interruption in oxygen flow will seal the mask against the patient's face and potentially suffocate the patient.)*

Because of the extremely high oxygen concentrations produced by the NRM, oxygen toxicity may occur in as little as 72 hours. **NEVER** LEAVE THIS PATIENT ALONE.

Venturi Mask

The high-flow Venturi mask provides the most reliable and consistent oxygen enrichment of all the facial devices (see Fig. 80-1). The Venturi mask can be identified by the presence of a hard plastic adapter, with large "windows" on the sides of the adapter.

Venturi masks offer specific oxygen concentrations in the 24% to 50% range. The exact concentration offered varies with the manufacturer. By drawing room air in through the windows, the Venturi mask mixes a low flow of gas (oxygen) with a high flow of room air. This produces a high flow of gas to the patient, with a specific oxygen concentration. Oxygen concentrations are changed by changing adapters, by changing the window opening, or by combining these changes. Because of the number of possibilities, the nurse should refer to the directions accompanying the mask. The directions also specify the oxygen flowmeter setting to use for each desired oxygen percentage. The respiratory care personnel should be consulted as well. Nursing skills in use of the Venturi mask are presented.

Nursing Skill
Providing Oxygen With the Venturi Mask

Supplies and Equipment

Mask
Oxygen source
Gloves

Procedure

1. Wash your hands and wear gloves.

2. Explain the procedure and need for oxygen to the patient. *(Rationale: The patient has a right to know what is happening and why; this also helps to decrease anxiety.)*

3. Attach the wing nut and tailpiece to the threaded outlet of the flowmeter.

4. Connect the tubing from the Venturi mask to the tailpiece. Attach to oxygen source.

5. Attach the appropriate adapter or set the window openings, in accordance with the manufacturer's directions for the prescribed percentage of oxygen.

6. Set the flowmeter to the manufacturer's recommended flow rate for the prescribed oxygen percentage.

7. Place the mask over the bridge of the patient's nose and then down onto the chin. Guide the elastic strap over the patient's head and secure as for the simple mask.

8. Make sure the patient is comfortable. Put the call signal within the patient's reach.

9. Place the bed linen so as not to cover the Venturi adapter. (*Rationale: The linens could plug the windows and disrupt the concentration of oxygen desired.*)

10. Remove and dispose of gloves; wash your hands. (*Rationale: These actions help to prevent transmission of microorganisms.*)

11. Document the procedure, recording the patient's reaction.

12. Check the patient periodically for depressed respirations and increased pulse.

13. Check for reddened pressure areas under the straps. (*Rationale: The straps, when snug, put pressure on the underlying skin areas.*)

Nursing Alert

◆ Humidifiers should NOT be used with Venturi masks. (*Rationale: Significant back-pressure may cause activation of the safety pressure valve on the humidifier and may cause some humidifiers to burst. In addition, the large amount of room air used by these devices humidifies the gas adequately.*)

◆ The windows must remain exposed to room air. The oxygen flow can be occluded if the windows or the end of the adapter are covered by sheets or blankets. (*Rationale: This would alter the oxygen concentration.*)

The IPPB Treatment

Intermittent positive pressure breathing (IPPB) may be ordered for children or adults with chronic lung conditions. It is most often used for patients with cystic fibrosis. These treatments are often administered by the nurse, after instruction by respiratory care personnel.

The goal of IPPB is to assist the patient to breathe more easily, because mucus is liquefied. This mechanical device forces room air or oxygen-rich air, combined with medications, deep into the airway. Thus, the patient's lungs are expanded more completely, secretions are able to be removed, and respiratory disorders can be treated or complications prevented. Nursing guidelines for IPPB are listed in the accompanying box.

Aerosol Mist Treatment

Aerosol mist treatment refers to a suspension of microscopic liquid particles in the air. It is used to add humidity to certain oxygen delivery devices, hydrate thick sputum, administer bronchodilator medications to relax bronchioles narrowed by bronchospasm, administer anti-inflammatory or asthma prevention medications, or deliver antibiotics to the lungs to fight infection.

The mini-nebulizer is a hand-held apparatus commonly used for aerosol therapy. Mini-nebulizers are

Nursing Skill Guidelines
Using Intermittent Positive Pressure Breathing

◆ Obtain specific instructions for operation of the machine being used.

◆ Use IPPB *only with* aerosolized medications.

◆ The pressure may be ordered by the physician (usually 10–20 cm H_2O). If pressure is not ordered, use your discretion.

◆ Instruct the patient to take slow, deep breaths 7 to 10 times per minute. (*Rationale: Diaphragmatic breathing causes more air to enter the lungs.*)

◆ Each inspiration and expiration should last 2 to 4 seconds. Forceful exhalation is not necessary and may be harmful. (*Rationale: Forcing exhalation may cause lung damage. You do not want the patient to hyperventilate.*)

◆ Encourage the patient to cough up mucus. Suctioning may be necessary, to ensure that mucus is removed. (*Rationale: Mucus could be aspirated or cause further obstruction; it also provides a culture medium for pathogens.*)

◆ Combine IPPB with postural drainage when instructed, for additional removal of secretions (see Chapter 79).

◆ Continue IPPB treatment for 10 to 20 minutes. The treatment is finished when the prescribed amount of medication is used up, or if the patient cannot tolerate further therapy.

◆ Assess the patient carefully for signs of difficulty. (*Rationale: Bronchodilators, as well as the treatment itself, can cause tachycardia, and dysrrhythmias and may lead to dizziness, headache, nausea or palpitation.*)

commonly used for patients with chronic obstructive pulmonary disease (COPD) and asthma to deliver inhaled medications. A mask or mouthpiece apparatus is attached to a chamber containing the prescribed solution. The chamber is attached via tubing to oxygen or a compressed air source. When used, a visible mist appears. The patient inhales the medication in the form of the mist.

Administering Oxygen to the Patient Who Is Unable to Breathe Without Assistance

The Manual Breathing Bag

The manual breathing bag or manual resuscitator (sometimes called the **ambu bag** after a popular brand) affords high oxygen concentrations and more effective and sanitary resuscitation than the mouth-to-mouth method. The face mask of the manual breathing bag is placed over the patient's nose first, and then over the mouth. Room air may be used; for more oxygenation, the bag can be connected to an oxygen source. The most important thing is to make sure that patient's airway is patent (open) and to start treatment immediately.

Sudden death may occur in acute respiratory failure. Resuscitation must be initiated at once or brain death will usually occur within 4 to 6 minutes. When the nurse first notices that a patient is not breathing, he or she must *immediately* initiate respiration and circulation, if necessary. Call a "code," so you get assistance.

Ventilatory Support

A patient in a state of ventilatory failure (not able to breathe adequately alone) will need the support of a mechanical ventilator. A **ventilator** (sometimes called a **respirator**) is a machine that forces air into the lungs.

The Negative Pressure Ventilator

The negative pressure ventilator encloses all or part of the body. By lowering the pressure around the chest, it causes the chest to expand and air to flow into the lungs. Because negative pressure ventilators (such as the iron lung) are cumbersome and restrict access to the patient, they are seldom used today. A small device of this type may be used in the patient's home, however.

The Positive Pressure Ventilator

The positive pressure ventilator pushes air into the lungs through a circuit joining the machine to the patient. Positive pressure ventilators are classified into two types, volume and pressure. They are further classified as to whether they assist in breathing or control breathing.

The Volume Ventilator. This type of positive pressure ventilator delivers a consistent, preset volume of air with each breath, so adequate breathing is ensured.

The Pressure Ventilator. This ventilator pushes air into the lungs until a preset pressure is reached. The pressure ventilator is not always as effective as the volume ventilator.

The Assisted-Breath Ventilator. This type of ventilator helps support patients who are breathing on their own, but who are too weak to breathe adequately. This support may be necessary to avoid ventilatory failure or hypoxia.

The Controlled-Breath Ventilator. This ventilator breathes for the patient. It forces a breath at set time intervals. (Controlled-breath ventilators lock the patient out of any control over his or her own breathing.)

Key Concept

An **artificial airway** is the general term for an endotracheal tube (ET), nasotracheal tube, or tracheostomy tube. The tube keeps the patient's natural airway from being blocked or closed off and allows the flow of air for breathing.

Assisting the Patient on a Mechanical Ventilator

Patients may be placed on mechanical ventilators to support breathing in conditions where they are unable to move enough air in and out of the lungs on their own. This may be caused by an acute situation (surgery, trauma, drug overdose, or other causes). Some patients may also need chronic mechanical ventilation due to neuromuscular disease (such as a spinal cord injury) or lung disease (such as emphysema). Most patients need ventilatory support for a short time and are withdrawn from it, as their condition improves. The respiratory care department usually provides technical and patient care support to a patient on a mechanical ventilator. The nurse should consult with respiratory care staff if there are any questions about the patient's care or about operation of the ventilator.

Ventilator patients should be assisted to turn from side to side at least every 2 hours to improve lung function and to prevent disorders of immobility, such as pressure areas or thrombophlebitis. Many of these patients are on special airflow beds. These patients also require suctioning of lung secretions, which they are unable to mobilize because of the artificial airway.

Key Concept

- ◆ The patient on a ventilator is usually sedated, which will decrease the patient's responsiveness and ability to communicate. Sedation may also depress the respiratory effort, however.
- ◆ The patient will also have an artificial airway placed, which prevents the patient from speaking.
- ◆ The nurse must be sensitive to the patient's needs. For patients on long-term ventilation, various communication aids (chalk board, letter-pointing board, "Magic Slate") are used. It is essential that the nurse continue to talk to the patient and still explain everything that is being done.

Weaning From the Ventilator

As the patient begins to improve and breathe without assistance, the number of positive pressure breaths is gradually reduced. The patient who has been on a ventilator for some time may need to be removed gradually (weaned) from ventilatory support. This can be done in several ways, depending on the situation. Some patients have a difficult time breathing after having been on a ventilator. This may be a result of true physical inability to breathe, but often has an emotional basis (ventilator dependency and fear). Emotional support and encouragement are needed. If the patient has required a high degree of ventilatory and oxygen support, he or she may show signs of adult respiratory distress syndrome (ARDS), which may make weaning more difficult. (This condition is briefly described in Chapter 79; it is frequently fatal.)

Methods of Weaning From the Ventilator. One strategy to facilitate weaning from the ventilator uses *synchronized intermittent mandatory ventilation* (SIMV). SIMV gives the patient a preset number of mechanical breaths at a certain volume. In addition, the patient can take as many breaths at his or her own volume as desired. As the patient progresses, machine-controlled breaths are decreased in volume or rate. Thus, the patient takes on more of the work of breathing gradually and progresses to being able to breathe without mechanical assistance. Another ventilatory mode used is called *pressure support ventilation* (PSV). In PSV, constant pressure is applied as the patient inspires. This lessens the inspiratory effort or work needed by the patient. *Continuous positive airway pressure* (CPAP) allows inspiratory and expiratory airway pressures to be maintained above atmospheric pressure. This helps keep the patient's lungs inflated and tends to improve lung function, even though the patient breathes spontaneously.

Assisting the Patient Who Has a Tracheostomy

Insertion of the Tracheostomy Tube

A tracheostomy tube may be inserted directly into the trachea as an emergency lifesaving measure when there is sudden blockage of the mouth or throat, or it may be a permanent breathing orifice (opening) for the person who has had throat surgery. The nurse in the intensive care unit or emergency room may be asked to assist the physician with the tracheostomy ("trach") procedure. Most often, an endotracheal airway is placed first and the patient is transported to the operating room for this sterile procedure.

The tracheostomy ("trach") tube has three parts: an outer tube (outer cannula) with a cuff (an inflatable attachment designed to occlude the space between the trachea walls and the tube for mechanical ventilation), an inner tube (inner cannula), and a solid rounded-end obturator. The obturator is inserted into the outer cannula *only during insertion*. The outer cannula and obturator are then inserted, as one unit, into the tracheal opening. When the outer cannula is in place, the ob-

turator is withdrawn. The obturator is then replaced by the inner cannula (tube), which is locked in position. Cloth tape is attached to each side of the outer tube and tied behind the neck, to hold it firmly in position. The following nursing skills outline nursing measures when assisting at a tracheostomy procedure.

Nursing Skill

Assisting at a Tracheostomy Procedure

Supplies and Equipment

Sterile, disposable tracheostomy tray
Local anesthetic, such as procaine hydrochloride (Novocain) or lidocaine (Xylocaine)
Syringes and small-gauge needles
Sterile and clean gloves for physician and nurse
Strong light
Emergency breathing apparatus (such as manual-breathing bag)
Source of suction
Source of oxygen

Procedure

1. Set up the equipment, which usually comes as a disposable "trach tray." (*Rationale: The nurse must know what is supposed to be on the tray and anticipate other needs for the procedure.*)
2. Explain the procedure to the patient. (*Rationale: The patient who understands can better cooperate and relax.*)
3. Put on clean gloves. The physician will gown and don sterile gloves. (*Rationale: Gloving helps prevent transmission of microorganisms and cross contamination.*)
4. Hold the patient's head during the procedure, if requested by physician. A folded towel may be placed behind the neck to hyperextend it and expose the surgical site. (*Rationale: The site must be immobilized during the procedure.*)

> **Nursing Alert**
>
> Spinal cord injury patients should not have their necks hyperextended. (*Rationale: Further injury may be done.*)

---

5. Provide strong emotional support. (*Rationale: The patient must lie very still throughout this frightening procedure. Lack of oxygen causes the patient to be extremely apprehensive.*)
6. Provide oxygen through an endotracheal tube while the tracheostomy is being done, if needed. This is most often done with a manual-breathing bag.
7. Dispose of equipment according to universal precautions. Dispose of gloves. Wash your hands.
8. Record pertinent information about what was done and by whom.

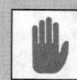
Suctioning and Providing Tracheostomy Care

Supplies and Equipment

Tracheostomy suctioning kit containing the following sterile supplies:

Gloves
Suction catheter
Basins or containers
Sterile normal saline
Portable or wall suction apparatus
Sterile tracheostomy dressing
Twill tape or Velcor trach ties
Hydrogen peroxide
Sterile gauze pads
Cotton-tipped swabs
Disposable inner cannula (optional)
Goggles and gown (optional)
Clean towel or plastic drape (optional)

Suggested Procedure and Rationale

1. Gather supplies.
   (Rationale: Organization facilitates performance of the skill.)
2. Explain procedure to patient.
   (Rationale: Providing information fosters patient cooperation.)
3. Wash hands.
   (Rationale: Handwashing prevents the spread of organisms.)
4. Adjust bed to a comfortable working height.
   (Rationale: Bed at proper height prevents back strain.)
5. Assist patient to semi or high-Fowler's position if conscious. Place on side facing you if unconscious.
   (Rationale: Upright positions promote drainage and prevent airway obstruction.)
6. Place towel or drape across patient's chest. Put on gown or goggles (optional). Turn suction on to appropriate level. Put on gloves if you will be positioning the patient.
   (Rationale: Gown, goggles, and gloves act as a barrier and protect nurse from patient's secretions.)
7. Prepare suction equipment:
   a. Open sterile tracheostomy suctioning kit and cleaning supplies on bedside tray or table.
   b. Pick up sterile container, open it, and pour sterile saline into it.
   c. Put on sterile gloves.
   d. Pick up sterile suction catheter with dominant hand.

   e. Use nondominant hand to connect wall or portable suction catheter tubing to sterile suction catheter.
   (Rationale: Surgical asepsis decreases the potential for introducing organisms into the respiratory tract. Nondominant hand becomes unclean once it touches nonsterile suction tubing.)

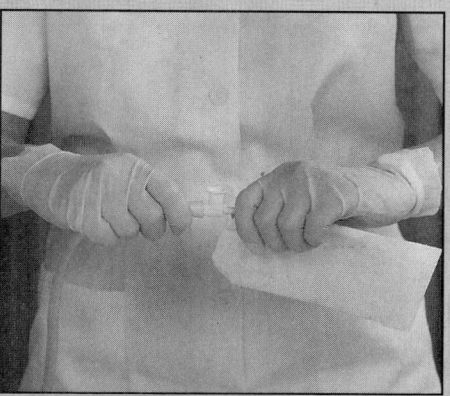

Step 7e   Connecting the sterile catheter to the suction tubing

8. Dip suction catheter into basin with sterile saline. Use nondominant hand to occlude suction port.
   (Rationale: Occluding port applies suction and ensures that equipment is functioning.)

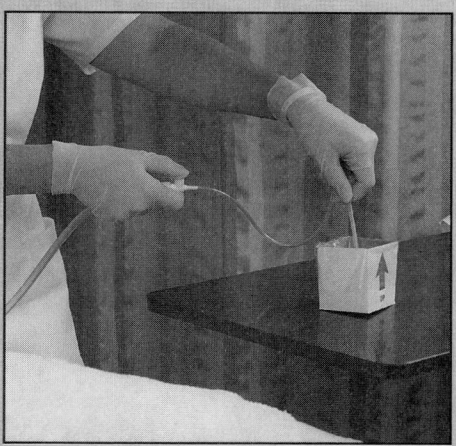

Step 8   Dipping the catheter into the sterile saline and occluding the suction port with the nondominant hand

(continued)

9. Remove oxygen delivery system with nondominant hand.
   (Rationale: This facilitates tracheostomy tube suctioning.)
10. Use dominant hand to insert catheter into trachea for 4 to 5 inches or until patient coughs. Do not apply suction while inserting the catheter.
    (Rationale: Applying suction while inserting catheter may damage mucosa in trachea and promote hypoxia.)

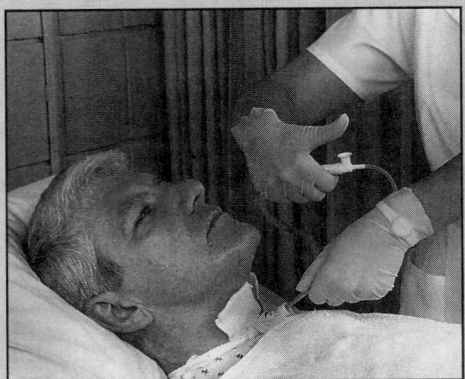

Step 10 Inserting the catheter with the suction off

11. Occlude suction port with nondominant hand while rotating and removing catheter. Suctioning should not continue for longer than 10-second intervals.
    (Rationale: Rotating the catheter provides for effective removal of secretions from the trachea. Limiting suctioning to 10-second intervals reduces development of hypoxia.)
12. Dip catheter into saline solution while applying suction. Repeat suctioning procedure if necessary. Allow 1 minute between suctioning and reapply oxygen delivery system while waiting to continue procedure.
    (Rationale: Saline clears the catheter. Interval between suctioning reduces development of hypoxia. Reapplying oxygen system maintains oxygen supply.)
13. Before removing gloves, cleanse cannula. If inner cannula is disposable, remove and replace with clean cannula. For replaceable cannula:
    a. Unlock cannula and carefully remove it.
    b. Hold over sterile basin
    c. Rinse with sterile saline.
    d. Gently replace inner cannula and lock in place.
    (Rationale: Rinsing with saline prevents accumulation of tracheal secretions.)

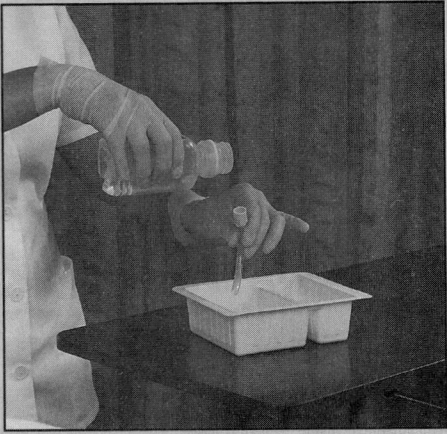

Step 13 Rinsing the inner cannula with saline

14. Cleanse around tracheostomy stoma and under tracheostomy tube faceplate with sterile cotton-tipped swabs dipped in hydrogen peroxide.
    (Rationale: Hydrogen peroxide aids in the removal of accumulated and encrusted secretions.)

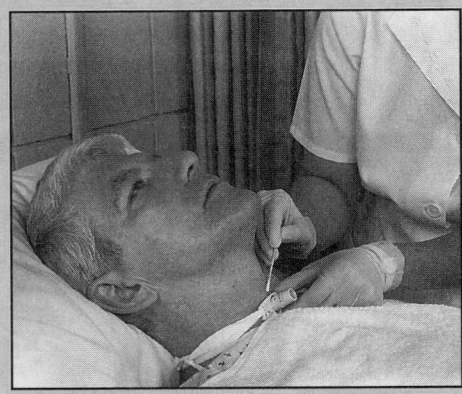

Step 14 Cleansing underneath the faceplate

15. Rinse area using cotton-tipped swabs moistened in normal saline.
    (Rationale: Normal saline removes hydrogen peroxide and additional secretions.)
16. Dry area with sterile gauze pad.
    (Rationale: Moisture provides a medium for growth of bacteria.)

(continued)

17. Change tracheostomy tube tape if necessary:
    a. Have assistant hold trach tube in place with sterile hand or, if unassisted, leave soiled tapes in place until new ones are inserted and secured.
    b. Pass ends of tape through opening on faceplate and bring behind patient's neck to other opening on opposite side of faceplate.
    c. Insert through opening, pull securely, and tie or Velcro in place.

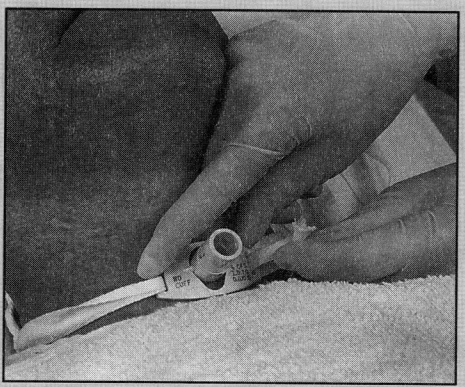

Step 17c Inserting the tracheostomy tape through the opening and pulling through (Photos © B. Proud.)

d. If necessary, remove soiled tape.
    (Rationale: Keeping tracheostomy tube secure while changing the tape prevents the patient from accidentally coughing up the tube.)

18. Place sterile tracheostomy dressing under faceplate. Tegaderm may be applied under gauze.
    (Rationale: Sterile dressing absorbs drainage.)
19. Reattach oxygen delivery system over tracheostomy tube.
    Rationale: This provides for adequate oxygenation.)
20. Remove gloves, goggles, and gown, (if worn). Reposition patient. Lower the bed.
    (Rationale: These measures ensure patient's comfort and security.)
21. Wash hands.
    (Rationale: Handwashing prevents the spread of organisms.)
22. Dispose of equipment according to agency policy.
    (Rationale: Proper disposal prevents transmission of organisms.)
23. Document suctioning procedure, nature and amount of secretions, and patient's response. Record respiratory assessments following suctioning procedure.
    (Rationale: Documentation provides for coordination of care.)

Nursing Alert

Observe for a leaking cuff. Listen for a wheezing or a "squeaking" sound. Observe for signs of respiratory distress and report these immediately.

---

9. After the procedure, assess for swelling, difficulty swallowing, or bleeding. *(Rationale: Any of these situations could impede respiration.)*
10. Make sure the patient is now able to breathe freely. *(Rationale: A patent airway is the purpose of the tracheostomy.)*

Care of the Tracheostomy Tube

If the cannula is accidentally coughed out, which rarely happens, it must be replaced immediately by a physician or nurse trained in the procedure and the physician notified. An extra tracheostomy set should be kept in the patient's room at all times, in case of emergency.

All equipment for cleaning and caring for the tube should be kept at the bedside. Each hospital has specific routines for trach care. For the person with a temporary tracheostomy tube, the air to be breathed must be warmed and moistened artificially by a humidifier. *(Rationale: In normal breathing, air is warmed and cleansed by the action of the nose and throat. Humid-*

ification helps to prevent secretions from becoming dry and tenacious.) If a person has a permanent trach, the body becomes adjusted to room air.

Suctioning is a sterile procedure. A new catheter is used each time the patient is suctioned. A sterile container for the solution is contained in the suctioning kit, as are sterile gloves.

The patient will need continued reassurance. *(Rationale: Until becoming accustomed to breathing through the tube, the patient may be very apprehensive, easily upset by coughing, and concerned about not being able to communicate verbally.)*

A signal cord must be kept within the patient's reach at all times. *(Rationale: This patient cannot talk or call out for help.)* Provide the patient with some means of communicating (a "Magic Slate" talking board or pad and pencil. Sometimes, the patient can whisper into a stethoscope and you can hear.)

Assess for signs of respiratory difficulty, and take immediate action should respiratory distress occur. Suctioning may be needed.

According to the healthcare facility protocol, the nurse suctions the tube and provides other tracheostomy care. These measures are explained in the accompanying Nursing Procedure.

Keys for Review

Key Questions for Critical Thinking

1. One of your patients needs assistance in breathing. Explain oxygen as a basic need. The patient is receiving oxygen by nasal cannula. State teaching that should be done with this patient. Identify teaching needed for the visitors.
2. Describe four types of oxygen masks. Describe the difference in their use and identify when each is used.
3. You have a patient under your care who needs a tracheostomy. Describe what a tracheostomy is. State your responsibilities during the procedure.

Key Readings

Craven RF, Hirnle CJ. Fundamentals of Nursing: Human Health and Function. Philadelphia, J.B. Lippincott, 1992

Earnest VV. Clinical Skills in Nursing Practice, Ed 2. Philadelphia, J.B. Lippincott, 1993

Key Readings (continued)

Kacmarek R. Essentials of Respiratory Care, Ed 3. St. Louis, Mosby-Yearbook, 1990

Smeltzer SC, Bare BG. Brunner and Suddarth's Textbook of Medical-Surgical Nursing, Ed 7. Philadelphia, J.B. Lippincott, 1992

Smith AJ, Johnson JY. Nurses' Guide to Clinical Procedures, Ed 2. Philadelphia, J.B. Lippincott, 1994

Taylor C, Lillis C, LeMone P. Fundamentals of Nursing: The Art and Science of Nursing Care, Ed 2. Philadelphia, J.B. Lippincott, 1993

Keys to Learning More

Unit Fifteen: geriatric nursing

Chapter 89: rehabilitation and home care nursing

Unit Seventeen: death and dying

81 Digestive Disorders

Keys for Learning

Learning Objectives

- Describe procedures used to diagnose gastrointestinal disorders, and describe the related preoperative and postoperative nursing care.
- Describe the nursing actions in nasogastric suction, gastrostomy tube care, total parenteral nutrition, colostomy, and ileostomy care.
- Outline patient and family teaching related to the diagnostic procedures; discuss emotional aspects.
- Describe common disorders of this system (including ulcers, irritable bowel syndrome, inflammatory bowel disease, diverticulosis, hernia, appendicitis, bowel obstruction, cancer of the intestinal tract, cirrhosis, hepatitis, gallbladder disease, and pancreatitis).
- Describe and demonstrate related nursing care, including preoperative and postoperative care, for the above disorders.
- Differentiate between Crohn's and ulcerative colitis, and describe their possible complications. Identify appropriate medication therapy, and outline the related patient and family teaching plan for Crohn's disease and ulcerative colitis.
- Define the five known types of viral hepatitis, and describe their mode of transmission and long-term consequences.
- Describe the eating disorders of obesity, bulimia, and anorexia nervosa; describe symptoms, treatment, and related nursing care.

Key Terms

achalasia	hiatal hernia
cholecystitis	ileus
cholelithiasis	lavage
diverticulosis	leukoplakia buccalis
diverticulitis	obese
endoscopy	peritonitis
fistula	pilonidal cyst
gastrectomy	pyorrhea
gastritis	stoma
hemorrhoids	ulcer

Keys to Understanding This Chapter

Chapter 5: basic human needs
Chapter 16: fluid and electrolyte balance
Chapter 23: digestive system
Chapter 26: food and its functions
Chapter 28: diet therapy and special diets
Chapter 30: medical asepsis and universal precautions
Chapter 32: CPR, including obstructed airway
Chapter 38: signs and symptoms of illness or injury
Chapter 45: personal hygiene and skin care
Chapter 46: elimination
Chapter 47: specimen collection
Chapter 50: physical examination and nursing assessment
Chapter 51: isolation techniques
Chapter 52: patient comfort and pain management
Chapter 53: the person having surgery
Chapter 54: surgical asepsis
Unit Eleven: pharmacology and medication administration
Chapter 65: digestive disorders of children
Chapter 69: disorders in fluid and electrolyte balance
Chapter 76: cancer

Key Points

- The normal gastrointestinal (GI) tract is responsible for the digestion of food, absorption of nutrients, and elimination of metabolic waste material.
- The intact GI tract helps defend the body against pathogens as is demonstrated by the low pH of gastric acid (which destroys most bacteria in its presence).
- Peristalsis, the regular wavelike contractions within the normal GI tract, provides the necessary propulsion for the contents to move through and interact with each area and to carry out each specific and necessary GI function.

Diseases and disorders of the digestive tract may affect the mouth, throat, stomach, intestines, or rectum and also the accessory organs, such as the gallbladder or liver. The specialist in this area is called a *gastroenterologist,* although specialists in internal medicine also treat these patients. The *enterostomal therapist* (ET) is a nurse who assists people who have an ileostomy, colostomy, ureterostomy, or gastrostomy. The ET nurse also is a consultant in specialized skin care for other patients. The department or clinic dealing with disorders of the digestive system is usually called digestive care or GI care.

Anatomy and Physiology Review

In Chapter 23, the digestive system was described. The major organs of digestion include those of the digestive tract, which opens to the outside on both ends. The mouth (buccal, oral cavity) includes the teeth, tongue, taste buds, and salivary glands. Here, much of the *mechanical* digestion is carried out (chewing), and *chemical* digestion begins with the action of the amylase-ptyalin. The food (bolus) then passes through the pharynx and esophagus to the stomach by the action of peristalsis. In the stomach, gastric juices mix with the food to form chyme. Mechanical digestion continues, and chemical digestion is carried out with the addition of pepsin, hydrochloric acid, and other secretions. In the small intestine (duodenum, jejunum, ilium), the major digestion and absorption of nutrients is carried out. The last portion of the GI tract is the large intestine (cecum, colon, rectum, anus), which is approximately 6 ft long. Here, water, vitamins, and minerals are reabsorbed, and solid wastes are prepared for excretion.

The accessory organs of digestion include the liver, gallbladder, and pancreas. The liver has many functions, including production of amino acids, production of glycogen and bile, and storage of nutrients and several vitamins. The gallbladder stores bile until needed by the body, and the pancreas secretes three enzymes needed in digestion (amylase, trypsin, and lipase) and insulin, which is important in carbohydrate metabolism.

Diagnostic Tests

Laboratory Tests

The special tests commonly used in diagnosing GI difficulties include laboratory examination of blood, urine, vomitus, stomach contents, and feces. Stomach contents may be examined to detect bacteria, blood, organic acids, and acid salts. The nurse's part in these procedures is to collect specimens, assist the physician with examinations, and prepare and reassure the patient during procedures that are often tedious and uncomfortable.

Blood Tests for Liver Disorders.

◆ Serum *liver profile or liver function tests* (LFTs), which commonly include total bilirubin, albumin, total protein, alkaline phosphatase, serum gamma-glutamyl transpeptase (GGT), serum aminotransferase (AST; formerly SGOT), serum alanine aminotransferase (ALT; formerly SGPT), lactate dehydrogenase, cholesterol, and trigyceride levels, are valuable as indicators and trending of abnormal liver processes. When the physician orders "LFTs," check your facility's lab manual to determine exactly which tests are included.

◆ *Hepatitis profile* identifies the presence of antibody and antigen for the hepatitis A, B, or C virus. Recent exposure, past contact, and the clearing of virus from the body can be determined by this test.

◆ *Iron saturation studies* help differentiate such diagnoses as hemochromatosis (a hereditary condition with excessive tissue iron storage) or Wilson's disease (a hereditary condition with defective secre-

Key Abbreviations and Acronyms

BE	Barium enema x-ray
CS	Cardiac sphincter
CT	Computed tomography
CUC	Chronic ulcerative colitis
DTAD	Drain tube attachment device
EGD	Esophagogastroduodenoscopy
ERCP	Endoscopic cholangiopancreatography
ET	Enterostomal therapist
GI	Gastrointestinal
HAV	Hepatitis A virus
HBV	Hepatitis B virus
HCV	Hepatitis C virus
HDV	Hepatitis D virus
HEV	Hepatitis E virus
IBD	Inflammatory bowel disease
IBS	Irritable bowel syndrome
LES	Lower esophageal sphincter
LFTs	Liver function tests
NG	Nasogastric
NPO	Nothing by mouth
PEG tube	Percutaneous endoscopic gastrostomy tube
SBFT	Small bowel follow-through x-ray
TAC	Time, amount, character
TMJ	Temporomandibular joint
TPA	Total parenteral alimentation
TPN	Total parenteral nutrition

tion of copper into bile and its storage in the liver, which can eventually cause liver damage).

◆ *Blood urea nitrogen* (BUN) and *creatinine levels* determine kidney function and damage.

◆ *Prothrombin time* will assess the blood's ability to clot. (If the coagulation time is dangerously slow, vitamin K can be given—an important step to lessen the danger of hemorrhage if an operation is necessary.)

◆ *Serum globulins and immunoglobulin levels* are blood proteins associated with antibodies and immunity of the body.

Urine Test for Liver Disorders. The urine test for *bilirubin,* which is the by-product of red blood cell breakdown, can assess liver function. (Care should be taken to submit fresh voided specimens to the laboratory for the most accurate results.) *Liver biopsy* is the only true diagnostic tool to identify and differentiate liver disease.

Stool Specimens. Laboratory examination of stool specimens detects disease organisms, parasites, eggs (ova), blood, and fat. The procedure for collecting a stool specimen is discussed in Chapter 47.

Tests for Occult Blood. *Occult blood* is blood that is not visible on observation. (*Frank blood* is blood that is visible to the eye.) The *guaiac* test of feces or other excreta may be done to ascertain the presence of blood. The guaiac is simple to perform and is often done at the nursing station or in the laboratory. Gloves must be worn while performing this procedure. Some physicians do not feel that the guaiac test is accurate enough for general use.

Hemoquant stool testing not only determines the presence of blood, but also quantifies the amount of blood (fecal hemoglobin). The hemoquant is more accurate than the guaiac. The hemoquant can be done only in the laboratory, however. Thus, it is not as quick or convenient as the guaiac. Each method of testing has its own manufacturer's instructions that must be followed to obtain accurate results.

X-ray and Fluoroscopic Examinations

X-ray (roentgenography) and fluoroscopy make it possible to photograph and view the gross anatomy of any area of the GI tract.

The stomach and intestine are soft tissues. To view their contour, the patient must be given a radiopaque substance, such as barium sulfate, which x-ray films will not penetrate. It is administered orally or rectally, depending on the area to be investigated. The progress of this substance through the GI tract is noted on films at suitable intervals and on the fluoroscopic screen. The physician observes how long it takes the barium to pass through the tract and notes any abnormalities in the contour of organs or passages that might indicate ulcers or tumors.

Barium Swallow. For examination of the stomach and duodenum, an upper GI series (*upper GI* or *barium swallow*) is undertaken. The patient drinks a preparation of barium; it is thick and chalky, and some people find the consistency unpleasant. After 1 or 2 hours, x-rays are taken of the small bowel. The rate at which the barium travels through the small intestine is significant in some digestive tract diseases.

In an upper GI series, the area to be examined also may be positioned under the fluoroscope as the patient drinks the fluid, and the outline of the stomach, its outlet, and the intestinal tract may be observed as the fluid progresses through the GI tract. X-ray films also are taken at definite intervals as a permanent record of the outline of the stomach and intestine.

Barium Enema. The barium preparation is given rectally if the colon is to be examined and is known as a *barium enema* or *lower GI* series. If a barium enema is to be given, the solution will be administered by enema. The patient may worry about being able to retain the solution. Tell the patient that there will be a chance to go to the bathroom immediately following the procedure. One more x-ray will be taken after the solution is expelled.

Key Concept

♦ An *informed* consent is required for any invasive procedure.

Following any barium procedure, observe the patient's stools:

♦ Note if barium is passed (white, chalky).
♦ Observe for constipation.
♦ Watch for signs of bowel obstruction.

Give laxatives or stool softeners as ordered.

Bowel Preparation for Diagnostic Procedures. The entire alimentary tract is prepared for a barium enema or colonoscopy examination by emptying it as thoroughly as possible. This is done using cathartics and sometimes enemas.

Because these procedures are usually performed on an outpatient basis, patient teaching is important. The patient must understand the dietary and bowel preparation and should know what the procedure entails.

A substance commonly used to cleanse the bowel is called GoLYTELY. It contains electrolytes, which cause complete evacuation of the bowel. The patient is required to drink several quarts of this mixture in divided doses the evening before the procedure. This is commonly called the "bowel prep." Tell the patient to mix the solution beforehand, carefully following the package instructions. It is usually easier to drink if it is chilled first. Caution the patient to have a bathroom readily available during the preparation process.

With GoLYTELY, the patient is instructed to eat a light supper (some physicians require clear liquids) in the evening and then to have nothing by mouth (NPO), except for the bowel prep, after supper. The patient may brush the teeth but is requested not to drink any water.

Another alternative if the patient is not able to drink the large amount of fluid is Fleet Phospho Soda. This involves drinking about two thirds of a glass of fluid in the evening and again in the morning. This preparation is more violent and is contraindicated in the patient with abdominal pain, heart disorders, impaired renal function, rectal or anal lesions, or who is pregnant. (The patient must drink clear liquids along with this preparation because it removes electrolytes and can cause dehydration.)

Before colonoscopy, the patient is instructed not to take aspirin or ibuprofen for 1 week prior to the test because of the possibility of bleeding. The patient will need encouragement to follow the instructions for any bowel preparation.

Nursing Considerations. The following are nursing considerations when assisting with a barium enema:

◆ Wear gloves.
◆ Be sure that the area around the rectum is clean before the patient goes for the examination.
◆ The patient should have a clean gown.
◆ If you are asked to take the patient to the x-ray department, use a litter or wheelchair, depending on the patient's condition.
◆ Remain with the patient until someone in the x-ray department takes over. Offer encouragement.
◆ If you are required to stay during the examination, you will assist the patient when moving out of and into the wheelchair or to and from the x-ray table and the litter.
◆ *Be sure* to protect yourself during the procedure by wearing a lead apron. If there is any possibility that you are pregnant, particularly in the first trimester, *do not assist with x-rays.*
◆ Check with the x-ray department to make sure that the series has been completed before giving the patient anything to eat or drink.

Gallbladder X-rays. An x-ray study (*cholecystogram* or *gallbladder series*) or an ultrasound will show the outline of the gallbladder and stones if they are present. (Ultrasound is discussed later in this chapter.)

Nursing Considerations. Because this test is usually done on an outpatient basis, patient teaching and documentation of teaching is important.

The following are nursing considerations when assisting with gallbladder x-rays:

◆ The patient is instructed to eat a fat-free supper the night before the x-ray is taken.
◆ The patient usually takes a dye by mouth. (See Chap. 50). The physician will specify the time it is to be taken. (*Rationale: The liver excretes this dye into the bile, which then goes to the gallbladder.*)
◆ The patient has nothing to eat for the next 12 hours. (*Rationale: This gives time for the dye to concentrate in the gallbladder.*)
◆ The patient is NPO, except for water, until bedtime, after which nothing is allowed.
◆ Smoking and chewing gum are discouraged. (*Rationale: They cause premature emptying of the dye from the gallbladder.*)
◆ A small enema may be given in the morning.
◆ If the patient vomits, the test may be postponed.

(*Rationale: Some of the dye may have been lost, and the test would be inaccurate.*)
◆ Sometimes after the initial x-ray series, the patient is given a fatty meal, and another x-ray is taken. (*Rationale: This shows how well the gallbladder is contracting.*)

Endoscopy

Endoscopy is the direct visualization of the interior of the body through the intestinal tract using specialized instruments. These instruments are called *endoscopes* and consist of a soft flexible tube containing specially designed fiberoptic strands that are connected to a light source. The fiberoptic scope (fiberscope) transmits light rays so that a clear image of the internal tissue is directed back up the scope to the lens and eyepiece, which the physician (endoscopist) manipulates. This technology is known as *fiber illumination.* The introduction of video imaging now allows viewing of internal tissue on a monitor or television-like screen. The physician, nurse, assistant, and even the patient can now see inside the intestinal tract. Excellent colored photography can document a patient's condition and healing process. Rapid advancement of endoscopic technology and its related equipment makes endoscopy a safe and effective diagnostic tool and provides many and various therapeutic applications.

Various procedures may be performed by endoscopy. Polyps or tumors may be biopsied or excised (cut out). Strictured areas may be stretched (dilated). Active hemorrhaging or bleeding may be localized and stopped. Biliary stones may be removed or crushed. Palliative measures, such as stent and tube placement, can ease the symptoms caused by tumor obstruction in the biliary tract. Feeding tube placement into the GI tract can allow nutritional support to a debilitated patient. The most common types of endoscopy include *esophagoscopy* (esophagus), *gastroscopy* (stomach), *colonoscopy* (colon), and *sigmoidoscopy* (sigmoid colon).

Because these procedures are done on an outpatient basis, the patient must be informed that he or she will need someone to drive him or her home after the test. (*Rationale: The sedation may make driving unsafe. There also may be some discomfort from the gas used to inflate the bowel and from the procedure itself.*)

General Preparation for Endoscopy. The nurse carries out any prescribed preparations for the patient, but the examination is usually performed in a separate endoscopy department by a trained endoscopist. This may be a gastroenterologist, surgeon, or internist. The patient should be well-informed and instructed by the physician on the particular endoscopy procedure because a consent must be obtained. No incisions are made for routine endoscopy procedures. The adult patient is

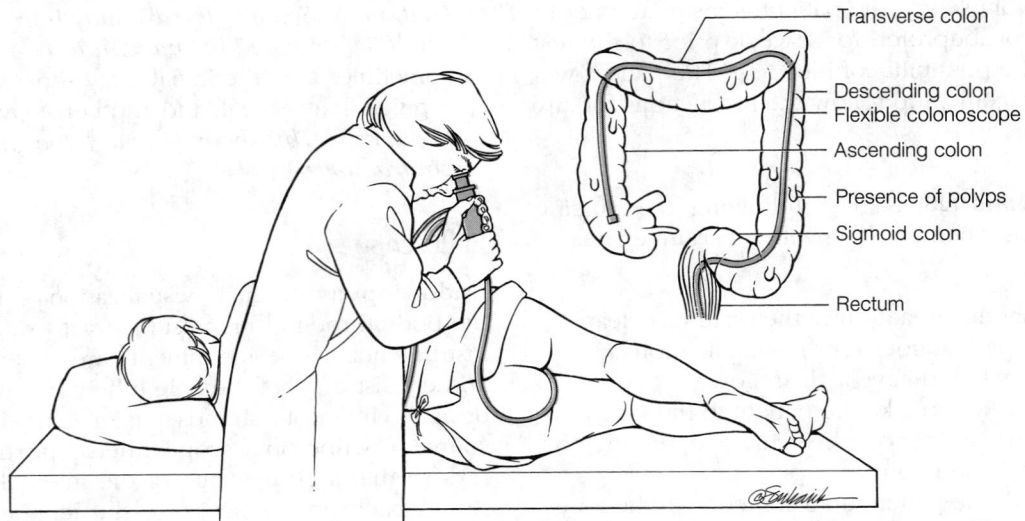

Figure 81-1. In colonoscopy, a flexible scope is passed through the rectum and sigmoid colon into the descending, transverse, and ascending colon. Smeltzer SC, Bare BG. Brunner and Suddarth's Textbook of Medical-Surgical Nursing, Ed 7. Philadelphia, J.B. Lippincott, 1992.

usually sedated with a short-acting intravenous analgesic (such as fentanyl [Sublimaze]) or a sedative such as midazolam (Versed). This use of drugs is called *conscious sedation* and allows introduction and manipulation of the endoscopes, yet provides a relaxed patient who is able to respond and maintain vital functions.

Oral Endoscopy

Esophagoscopy visualizes the esophagus, and *gastroscopy* visualizes the stomach and duodenum. These procedures allow identification of growths, strictures, ulcers, or inflammatory disease. This type of procedure is called *oral endoscopy* because the scope is passed through the patient's mouth.

Nursing Considerations

♦ In preparation for the procedure, the nurse instructs the patient to remain NPO after midnight; the procedure is fully explained.

♦ The nurse must wear gloves during the procedure.

♦ The throat will be sprayed with a topical anesthetic in the procedure room.

♦ A mouthpiece protects the patient's mouth and the endoscope tube.

♦ The nurse stresses to the patient that normal breathing is not hindered by the endoscope tube.

♦ The procedure takes 15 minutes to 1 hour.

♦ The patient will feel fullness and pressure because air is instilled into the stomach. *(Rationale: It is important to expand the stomach fully, so the entire interior surface can be visualized by the physician or endoscopist.)*

♦ After oral endoscopy, the patient in observed

closely for dyspnea (difficult breathing). *(Rationale: The passage of the tube may irritate the throat or cause swelling.)*

♦ If the patient has undergone a dilatation (stretching) procedure, the nurse should observe for bleeding, pain, dysphagia (difficulty in swallowing), dyspnea, or a change in vital signs.

♦ *The nurse must not give any food or fluids* until the gag reflex returns and the patient is fully aware.

Colonoscopy

Colonoscopy allows visualization of the entire colon to the level of the terminal ileum. This scope is passed into the patient's body through the rectum (Fig. 81-1). Colonoscopy can help identify growths and inflammatory disease. Small polyps and lesions may be excised (cut out) or cauterized (sealed off by heat or electric current). Growths also may be biopsied. The colonoscopy can be used to follow up on abnormal x-rays; foreign bodies can be removed. Various specialized tools are available for use with endoscopes. They are built so they can be passed down the channel of the scope.

Nursing Considerations

♦ This is usually an outpatient procedure, so careful teaching is necessary (see p. 624). The colon should be clear of any waste material. This can be accomplished by the bowel preparation described previously.

♦ The nurse prepares the patient according to agency protocol.

♦ The nurse must be sure to wear gloves.

◆ Colonoscopy is performed with the patient lying on the back or left side. The procedure takes 30 minutes to 1 hour.

◆ Most patients feel the air being instilled into the bowel (insufflation) and the endoscope tube being passed. This is usually described as a mild cramping sensation or pressure. *(Rationale: This sensation is mainly caused by the passage of the tube through the anal sphincter and the colon.)*

◆ The colonoscopy procedure is the most uncomfortable when the scope "goes around the turns" in the colon. The nurse can assist by encouraging the patient to take a few deep breaths and to relax each time the scope is passed around one of these corners in the large bowel.

◆ After the procedure, vital signs should be taken and recorded. The patient is usually free to leave when vital signs are stable.

◆ Teach the patient that lying on the right side with the knees bent and relaxed will promote the passage of residual air in the colon. Walking and a warm bath also help. *(Rationale: This will help to make the patient more comfortable.)* It is important for the nurse to be sensitive to the patient's privacy at this time.

◆ Instruct the patient that the first meal should be light. *(Rationale: Acccumulated air may cause cramps.)*

◆ Stools should be observed for gross bleeding for 2 to 3 days after the procedure, particularly if polyps were removed or biopsies taken.

A rare complication is perforation of the colon. The patient is instructed to contact the physician if experiencing fever, chills, rectal bleeding, or severe abdominal pain.

Key Concept

Screening tests, such as the rectal examination, proctoscopy (sigmoidoscopy), and colonoscopy, can discover cancer early. They are often recommended for patients older than age 40 who are at risk. Risk factors include the following:

◆ Family history of cancer, especially of the rectum, bowel, or female reproductive organs
◆ Family history of ulcerative colitis
◆ Presence of precancerous or bleeding polyps
◆ Change in bowel habits
◆ Rectal bleeding or blood in the stool

Sigmoidoscopy

Sigmoidoscopy can visualize approximately 18 inches (27–30 cm) up the left side of the colon and permits the biopsy and removal of premalignant pol-yps. Besides its use in diagnosing lower colon symptoms and problems, this examination is recommended as a routine colon cancer screening test for people older than 50 years (American Cancer Society).

Nursing Considerations

◆ Sigmoidoscopy is commonly performed in clinics and outpatient settings.
◆ The nurse must wear gloves during the procedure. At least one enema is given prior to the examination.
◆ It is not necessary to withhold food, because its presence in the upper GI tract will not interfere with the examination.
◆ The patient will be relieved to know that he or she will be lying on the back or left side during the exam. Only the near-obsolete rigid proctoscope requires the knee-chest position on a "procto" table, as in years past.
◆ Sigmoidoscopy takes less than 20 minutes. The patient is usually comfortable without sedation.
◆ Usually no special care is required after this procedure. Stools should be observed for gross bleeding.

Key Concept

Patient teaching before any endoscopy is important. Patients need to know what to expect before, during, and after the procedure and what complications are possible. Be sure to document all teaching.

Colon Biopsy

The endoscopy procedures of the lower bowel allow biopsies to be taken. The removed tissue is examined for the presence of cancer cells and other abnormalities.

Polypectomy

Endoscopy of the lower bowel, including colonoscopy, allows polyps to be removed and examined. This is called polypectomy. In many cases, polyps are considered to be precancerous.

Endoscopic Retrograde Cholangiopancreatography (Pancreas and Ducts)

Endoscopic retrograde cholangiopancreatography (ERCP) is an upper endoscopy procedure that allows the radiographic (x-ray) visualization of the ducts and related structures of the liver and pancreas. This test specifically diagnoses disorders of the pancreas. The patient undergoes gastroscopy, and a small-caliber catheter is introduced into Oddi's sphincter. (This sphincter is located just past the duodenum and allows bile and pancreatic enzymes into the intestine.) Dye is carefully injected; the resulting films diagnose structural defects, retained stones, or tumors. (See Chapter 50 for precautions when dye is used.)

The patient needs support during this procedure, as it may be uncomfortable, particularly if a structural defect exists. Patients must be observed following the ERCP for hemorrhage, infection, and particularly for pancreatitis. (Pancreatitis is characterized by fever, pain, nausea, vomiting, and elevated amylase levels in the blood.)

Other Invasive Tests

Abdominal Paracentesis

In abdominal paracentesis (abdominal tap), the abdominal cavity is punctured to obtain a specimen or drain off excess fluid. The procedure may be *diagnostic* (fluid is withdrawn for microscopic study or cultures) or *therapeutic* (fluid is withdrawn to relieve pressure in the abdominal cavity).

The diagnostic puncture is performed when bleeding or infection is suspected. It is not done if the bowel is obstructed or distended or if the patient has a blood-clotting defect. Therapeutic abdominal tap is done when the patient is distended with fluid (*ascites*). Because the patient also may have difficulty breathing, removal of this fluid will frequently relieve the condition. The patient is usually sitting up for the procedure, with the feet on a foot stool. Leaning on an overbed table may increase comfort. The fluid is obtained from the lower portion of the abdomen. Sometimes a catheter is inserted into the abdominal cavity for continuous drainage.

Nursing Considerations

◆ The abdomen is scrubbed in preparation.
◆ The patient is asked to void immediately before the procedure. (*Rationale: This helps to avoid rupture of the urinary bladder by the needle.*) Be sure to wear gloves.
◆ Monitor vital signs during and after the procedure. Watch for fainting or dizziness.
◆ Measure the amount of fluid obtained.
◆ Send the appropriate specimens to the laboratory.
◆ After the procedure, observe the patient for bleeding or any signs of shock.
◆ Check the dressing to make sure it is tightly applied and dry. (*Rationale: It is important to prevent and check for bleeding.*)
◆ Keep the patient in Fowler's position, unless ordered otherwise. (*Rationale: This facilitates drainage and assists breathing.*)
◆ Observe urine output. Check the scrotum of the male for edema. (*Rationale: This helps evaluate the effectiveness of the procedure and determine if complications exist.*)

◆ Tell the outpatient to observe for any signs of infection.
◆ Document the procedure and all teaching carefully.

Liver Biopsy

A liver biopsy is most often done to verify suspected cancer of the liver or to detect other liver disorders. However, a biopsy is not done if the patient has a bleeding tendency. (*Rationale: The liver is a highly vascular organ.*)

A small sample of liver tissue is obtained using a long needle with an inner cutting cannula. The needle is inserted with the aid of a stylet inside the needle. The stylet is then withdrawn, and the inner cannula is inserted beyond the end of the needle and rotated to obtain a specimen. The specimen is then withdrawn. A sample also may be obtained by suction. The sample is examined microscopically. Locating a specific liver site or suspected tumor can require radiologic (x-ray) or ultrasound assistance to aid the physician to perform the liver biopsy.

Nursing Considerations

◆ Explain the procedure, and assist the patient to maintain the proper position while the procedure is in progress. Wear gloves.
◆ The skin is anesthetized before the large needle is inserted. Instruct the patient not to breathe during insertion of the needle. (*Rationale: This facilitates insertion and prevents puncturing other structures.*)
◆ Stay with the patient, and offer encouragement and support during the procedure. (*Rationale: This procedure is often uncomfortable.*)
◆ Following liver biopsy, position the patient on the right side. Apply pressure to the biopsied site (usually the right side) for 4 to 6 hours, using a sandbag or folded bath blanket. (*Rationale: This helps prevent bleeding.*)
◆ Vital signs are usually taken every 15 minutes for 1 hour and then every 30 minutes for 4 hours. They are then taken hourly for 8 hours. The patient is observed closely for signs of bleeding. Hemorrhage may be into the abdomen (watch for signs of shock) or from the puncture site.

Gastric Analysis

The stomach contents are analyzed to determine how much free hydrochloric acid is present. Too much hydrochloric acid may indicate a peptic ulcer; too little could be a sign of cancer or pernicious anemia. Gastric analysis can be performed by examining a specimen of vomitus or a portion of the stomach contents that has been aspirated by a syringe attached to a previously inserted nasogastric tube. The patient is NPO from 8 PM, and the test is done before breakfast.

Tomography

Tomography (computed tomography) is a technique that allows three-dimensional visualization of the density of tissues by which abnormalities can be precisely located. This procedure is discussed in Chapter 71.

Abdominal Ultrasonography

Ultrasonography (ultrasound) uses high-frequency sound waves that are directed back toward a transducer placed over the abdomen. The sound waves are interpreted as electrical impulses that display on a special monitor. Gallstones within the gallbladder and tumors of the abdomen can be identified by abdominal ultrasound. This test is becoming the preferred diagnostic tool, especially to rule out gallstones. No preparation, other than NPO after midnight, is required for ultrasound.

Medical and Surgical Treatments

Common Medical Treatments

Gastric Suction

Suction is used for periodic or continuous drainage in the following GI conditions:

◆ To obtain a specimen of stomach or intestinal contents for examination
◆ To treat intestinal obstruction
◆ To prevent and treat distention after surgery by removing gas and toxic fluid materials from the stomach or the intestines
◆ To empty the stomach prior to emergency surgery or after swallowing poisons
◆ To protect the suture line following GI surgery

GI tubes are inserted through the nostril and may terminate in the stomach or intestine. This is called a *nasogastric* tube (Fig. 81-2). The outer end might have a clamp attached, or a plastic connection might link it to a longer tubing attached to an electric suction machine. Suction may be continuous or intermittent, depending on the type of tube. Table 81-1 describes several tubes commonly used for nasogastric suction. Nursing skills related to gastric suction appear in the "Nursing Process" section of this chapter.

Gastric Lavage

If a patient has ingested a caustic poison, it may be necessary to place a large single- or double-lumen tube into the stomach to dilute or neutralize (charcoal) the poison, remove the stomach contents, and wash out the stomach. This is called **lavage.** The procedure is basically the same as that for inserting the nasogastric tube,

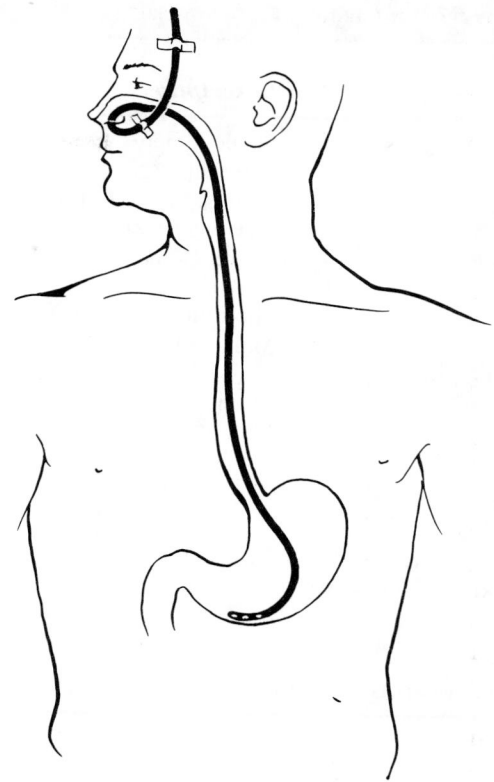

Figure 81-2. One type of nasogastric tube: Levin. It remains in place in the stomach. The tube is taped to the face and attached to suction. It is used to keep the stomach emptied or to obtain a specimen of stomach contents.

except that the lavage tube is large and is inserted through the mouth, rather than through the nose. The stomach is then irrigated or "washed" of its contents.

For acute bleeding stomach ulcers and, less commonly, bleeding esophageal varices, the stomach is lavaged with saline or tap water to clear blood and stomach contents prior to performing endoscopic procedures to arrest and treat GI bleeding. (Iced lavage is not often used today. This is believed to inhibit platelet function, thus prolonging bleeding.)

Tube Feedings (Enteral Nutrition)

It is sometimes necessary to assist in nutritional intake when a patient is unable to take adequate calories or appropriate nutrients, solid foods, or liquids by mouth. Many of these patients' nutritional status can be greatly improved, with shorter healing and recovery times, if they receive nutritional support. In some cases, enteral nutrition is life-sustaining or life-saving. If the stomach is functioning normally, it is safer and more appropriate to access it directly than to give fluids and nutrients into the circulatory system (parenteral nutrition).

The specific procedures for administering a tube feeding and related nursing care of the patient are given

Table 81-1. Common Gastrointestinal Suction Tubes*

Tube Type	Description	Purpose	Nursing Considerations
Levin or Wangensteen	Single lumen Short tube (20–24 in) Multiple holes at distal tip (see Fig. 81-2)	Provides intermittent suction of gastric contents	Irrigate frequently with small amounts of saline or air to keep patent.
Salem Sump	Double lumen (two ports) Short tube (20–24 in) Multiple holes at distal tip	One port provides air flow. Second port allows suction of gastric contents with continuous suction	Clear the air port with air to keep open and prevent distal tip from sucking against the wall of the stomach and causing irritation.
Sengstaken-Blakemore	Triple lumens consisting of one channel and two balloons	One channel provides irrigation and intermittent suction of gastric contents. One balloon provides pressure on the cardiac sphincter area when inflated just inside the stomach. Second balloon provides pressure along the wall of the esophagus to stop bleeding varices.	Nastrotracheal suction is often needed, because swallowing is impossible.

* Mercury-weighted tubes are no longer used for any internal body placement (because of the risk of mercury poisoning). Tungsten-weighted tubes may be used.

in Chapter 28. It is important to give site care to maintain the skin surrounding a through-the-skin feeding tube. Special skin care is addressed later in this chapter with the discussion of ostomies; a daily skin care is discussed in Chapter 45.

Total Parenteral Nutrition

Total parenteral nutrition (TPN) is sometimes called *total parenteral alimentation* (Fig. 81-3). (This is sometimes called *hyperalimentation,* which is incorrect terminology—the amounts given are not excessive.) TPN is a method by which large quantities of fluids and nutrients are administered to a patient directly into the circulation. This method is referred to as *parenteral nutrition* because it does not access the digestive system. TPN may provide total nutritional support, or it may be supplemental. By this means, the desired carbohydrate, protein, fat, water, electrolytes, vitamins, and minerals can be provided. Nursing care for TPN is discussed in the "Nursing Process" section of this chapter.

The Peripheral Line. A long catheter is inserted into a blood vessel (usually the subclavian vein). The catheter can be made of several substances, including plastic and teflon. The catheter is inserted by a physician under strict sterile techniques. The catheter is advanced into the superior vena cava.

The Central Line. A central line also may be surgically placed. This involves a small catheter that is placed directly into a large blood vessel—often the superior vena cava—and sutured in place. This is called a central line; it allows long-term accessibility and unrestricted movement of the patient when the line is not being used.

The Hickman catheter is one such device. It leaves a small-caliber tube exiting 10 to 14 inches from the upper chest. The Port-a-Cath system is accessible by a special needle and is just under the surface of the skin, again on the upper chest. Both systems require periodic heparinization (injection of a dilute solution of intravenous heparin) to keep the blood from coagulating. Similar lines are used for cancer chemotherapy and when long-term administration of intravenous antibiotics is necessary.

Common Surgical Treatments

Colostomy and Ileostomy

Many disorders of the intestinal tract require surgery and an artificial opening into the bowel. An incision is made in the abdomen, and a loop of intestine is brought through the incision and opened to allow for drainage of feces. The opening is called a **stoma** or *ostomy.* A *colostomy* is an opening into the colon, whereas an *ileostomy* is an opening into the ileum. A person also may have a urinary diversion, such as a *ureterostomy.* The person with an ostomy of any type is referred to as an *ostomate.* A stoma may be an *end* (one stoma), *double-barreled* (two stomas—both cut ends of the intestine are brought to the outside), or *loop* (the bowel is not completely severed, so the one stoma has two openings). A colostomy or an ileostomy may be temporary if treat-

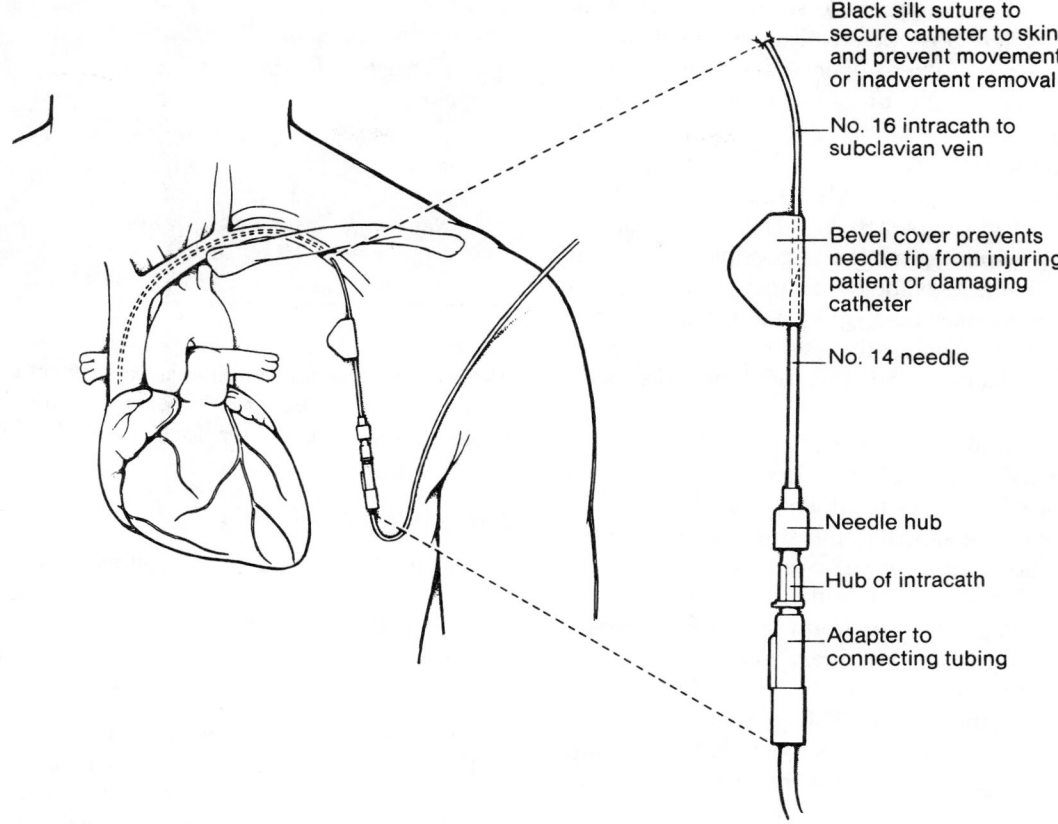

Black silk suture to secure catheter to skin and prevent movement or inadvertent removal

No. 16 intracath to subclavian vein

Bevel cover prevents needle tip from injuring patient or damaging catheter

No. 14 needle

Needle hub

Hub of intracath

Adapter to connecting tubing

Figure 81-3. Technique of total parenteral nutrition (TPN). A large catheter is inserted into the circulatory system, usually entering the subclavian vein and then being passed into the superior vena cava. By this means, all nutrients can be infused directly into the patient's bloodstream in carefully measured amounts.

ment to eliminate or relieve the underlying condition is successful. In this case, an operation to close the intestinal and abdominal openings is performed later; the feces are then excreted through the normal rectal outlet. The second operation is called a *takedown*. If treatment necessitates removal of the colon or the rectum, the colostomy or ileostomy will be permanent.

Description of Stoma and Appliance. Placement of the stoma depends on how much of the bowel was removed. A colostomy in the transverse colon is usually a temporary measure and is located on the right, left, or midline of the abdomen. A permanent colostomy is usually made at the level of the descending or sigmoid colon and is usually located on the left side of the abdomen. An ileostomy (after total removal of the colon) has a stoma that is usually located on the lower right side of the abdomen.

The new stoma, which is mucous membrane, should be moist and ranges from dark red to rich pink. It looks like pursed lips, and immediately after surgery, it is swollen and may bleed occasionally.

As the stoma decreases in size, holes of correct size are cut in the disposable pouches that are applied. After approximately 6 weeks, the stoma can be measured for a permanent appliance. (The appliance must fit properly or it will leak.) Leaking of fecal material onto the skin causes *periostomal* (around the stoma) skin irritation and can result in skin breakdown. Nearly all ostomy supplies used today are completely disposable. After a prescribed number of days, the entire pouch is removed and discarded.

Emotional Adjustment and Teaching. The patient who is to have a colostomy or ileostomy may need assistance to adjust. Naturally, the patient wonders how heavily life will be disrupted and may be particularly concerned about the effect on sexual relationships, the care of the colostomy or ileostomy, and the acceptance of family and friends. Most hospitals have *certified ET nurses* who are specially trained to teach patients with ostomies and to provide supportive counsel. The staff nurse should contact the ET nurse before the patient's surgery. This ET nurse assists the patient and family, aids in patient teaching, answers questions, and discusses with the surgeon optimum placement for the stoma. The ET nurse also visits the patient postoperatively to assist in teaching and patient support. Other nursing care is discussed in the "Nursing Process" section of this chapter.

The Continent Ostomy

A continent ostomy is possible.* This concept also is discussed briefly in Chapter 82 in relation to urinary diversion. If a continent diversion is possible, the patient can manage drainage without the use of the external pouch. The patient must be cooperative and must be psychologically able to manage the ostomy. This procedure is discussed in relation to inflammatory bowel disease.

Gastrectomy and Other Surgery for Ulcers

Gastrectomy is a surgical procedure to remove a stomach ulcer when other treatments fail. Two-thirds to three-quarters of the stomach, the pylorus, and the first part of the duodenum are removed (subtotal gastrectomy), and the remaining part of the duodenum is joined to the stomach. A *gastrojejunostomy* joins the stomach to the jejunum. A *vagotomy* is surgery to divide the vagus nerve; this reduces the stimulus to create hydrochloric acid, reducing gastric acidity. (This procedure is usually done at the same time as gastric surgery because it limits the stomach's ability to produce secretions.)

❖ *Nursing Process*

Data Collection

The nurse must carefully observe and assess the patient with a GI or digestive disorder. Chapter 50 describes physical examination and nursing assessment, including that of the digestive system and accessory organs. This assessment establishes a baseline for future comparison and determines the presence of suspected complications. The nurse should report any changes in the baseline level.

When assessing the GI system, the nurse assesses the patient's height compared with weight and subjective information about eating habits and recent weight gain or loss. The nurse determines whether the person is able to chew and swallow and whether food preparation is a problem. The accompanying box lists some of the components of the GI nursing assessment.

In addition, the nurse observes the patient's emotional response to the disorder or disease by asking the following questions: Does the patient need assistance to meet daily needs? Does the disorder affect social activities or self-esteem? (For example, does the patient have a colostomy?) Is the disorder life-threatening? Is the patient anx-

---

> ### *Keys to Nursing Assessment*
> ## Digestive Disorders
>
> ◆ Nutritional history
> ◆ Recent weight gain or loss
> ◆ Ability to purchase, prepare, and store food
> ◆ Ability to chew and swallow
> ◆ Any symptoms of digestive disorders
> ◆ Pattern of bowel elimination

ious or fearful of the outcome? Is a support group, home health nursing, Meals on Wheels, or other community program appropriate after discharge from the hospital?

Nursing Diagnosis

Based on data collection, the following sample nursing diagnoses may be seen on the nursing care plan established for the patient with a digestive disorder. Some diagnoses may have more than one causal factor.

◆ Activity Intolerance related to abdominal surgery, diarrhea, generalized weakness
◆ Bowel Incontinence related to inability to digest food
◆ Altered Nutrition: Less than Body Requirements related to inability to digest food, inability to absorb nutrients
◆ Body Image Disturbance related to weight loss or gain, colostomy
◆ Knowledge Deficit related to diagnostic tests, tube feeding, ostomy
◆ Pain related to abdominal surgery
◆ High Risk for Fluid Volume Deficit related to diarrhea, intestinal obstruction, indwelling tubes, medications
◆ High Risk for Impaired Skin Integrity related to ileostomy or colostomy, TPN feeding, physical immobilization, cancer treatment

Planning and Implementation

The patient, nurse, and family plan for effective care to meet patient needs based on the nursing diagnosis. The nurse provides preoperative and postoperative care for the patient undergoing endoscopy, liver biopsy, or surgery on the stomach or related organs. The patient with a digestive disorder also may require assistance in meeting nutritional or self-care needs. Many digestive disorders have a strong emotional component, either aggravating the disorder or related to the course of the disease. This can include the emotional components of disorders, such as IBD, ulcer, or bulimia, or acceptance of a permanent colostomy or ileostomy. Patients often need assistance to understand more about the disorder,

---

* Adapted from Erwin-Toth P and Florute CV. Nursing Management of Continent Ostomy Diversions. Progressions, vol. 5, no. 3, 1993.

its prognosis, and its treatment. Special procedures may be required at home; thus, patient teaching is vital. A nursing care plan is developed to meet each patient's needs. A sample nursing care plan for a patient with a digestive disorder is provided later in this chapter.

Aiding in Elimination of Feces

ENEMAS. The patient with a disorder of the digestive system may need an enema to prepare for a diagnostic test or surgery, alleviate symptoms of constipation or distention, or administer specific medications and fluids (see Chapter 46).

DIGITAL REMOVAL OF FECAL IMPACTION. Digital removal of a fecal impaction is done for severely constipated patients. The procedure is done only after attempts have been made to remove the mass by means of stool softeners or enemas. Fecal impaction can develop after a barium enema or barium swallow and should be considered a possible complication from these procedures. Chapter 46 explains the symptoms of a fecal impaction and the procedure for its removal.

Caring for the Patient With a Nasogastric Tube

The nurse should never insert a nasogastric tube without having been carefully instructed in the procedure. The nursing student generally is not asked to insert the nasogastric tube but might be asked to assist. Be sure to explain the procedure to the patient before beginning.

The nasogastric tube will be connected to a mechanical intermittent suction machine, such as the Gomco suction. The nurse must be alert and report any failure of the mechanical apparatus. Nasogastric suction is usually intermittent and low pressure unless specifically ordered otherwise by the physician. Place the stopper in the bottle firmly to prevent spilling and to ensure a good vacuum. Secure suction bottles in the clips of the stand.

IRRIGATING THE NASOGASTRIC TUBE. A physician's order is needed for irrigating the nasogastric tube. This order should include the type and amount of solution to be used and the frequency of irrigation (sometimes it is "as needed—PRN"). Patient condition and different surgical procedures dictate the specific methods to be used. Although this procedure is not always done, the nursing skill is presented here.

Nursing Skill
Irrigating the Nasogastric Tube

Supplies and Equipment

Irrigation set
Normal saline solution
Stethoscope
Disposable pad or bath towel
Clamp
Disposable gloves

Procedure

1. Wash your hands, following clean technique. (When supplies are set up for the first time, they are sterile.) In many facilities a new setup is used each time. Precautions are needed to prevent the spread of infection from person to person, but sterile technique is not necessary. (*Rationale: The digestive tract is not sterile.*)
2. Assemble the appropriate equipment and solutions at the bedside, and explain to the patient what you are going to do.
3. Wear gloves during this procedure.
4. Pour the ordered solution into the irrigation bottle. The most commonly used solution is normal saline at room temperature. Measure the amount of solution used. (*Rationale: It is important to subtract the amount of any solution not aspirated from the total amount of drainage for the day so that the intake and output record will be accurate.*)
5. Disconnect the nasogastric tube from suction, and check to make sure it is in the stomach. (If in the lungs, death can result.) This procedure is described in the next section.
6. Slowly introduce the solution using the specified irrigating syringe. Do not use excessive force to avoid damage to the suture line.
7. Reconnect the tube to gentle suction. The tube should be kept open without putting undue stress on the suture line. The gastric contents should return freely when the tube is reconnected to suction.
8. Note the amount, color, and consistency of any drainage. If the fluids do not return freely, this may be a sign of a plugged nasogastric tube and should be reported immediately. (Distention can burst sutures.)
9. Dispose of gloves, wash your hands, and properly dispose of equipment.
10. Document the procedure, noting the time, description of the drainage, and relevant patient reactions. Note the amount of fluid instilled or aspirated on the intake and output sheet.

Nursing Alert

The danger of aspiration cannot be overemphasized; it can be a *fatal* complication. Other complications from nasogastric tubes include otitis media, pneumonia, infection of the stomach or small intestine, inflammation of the nose or mouth, and ulceration of the nose or larynx.

If the patient has aspirated fluids into the lungs, you would withdraw fluid with a syringe through a nasogastric tube as well. If there is any question about placement of a nasogastric tube, have it checked by an experienced professional nurse or physician. An x-ray may be required to determine tube placement.

NURSING ASSESSMENTS. The patient and drainage must be assessed. Verify placement of the tube in the stomach by aspiration of a small amount of stomach contents or by auscultation. Inject a small amount of air (15–20 mL) while you are listening with a stethoscope approximately 3 inches (8 cm) below the sternum. If the tube is in the stomach, you will be able to hear the air enter (a "whooshing" sound).

Nursing Alert

If the tube is coiled in the esophagus, it will be difficult or impossible to inject the air. In addition, injection of air often causes the patient to belch immediately.

If the tube is in the larynx, the patient usually is not able to speak.

If either of these situations occur, notify the physician immediately.

Other nursing assessments are listed in the accompanying box.

Vomiting must be reported at once; it often indicates a malfunction of the suction apparatus. If the suction apparatus appears not to be functioning properly, report it at once, and note the situation on the patient's chart.

The nurse should give soothing mouth rinses and apply a lubricant to the patient's lips and nostril and K-Y jelly to the catheter where it touches the nostril (because the patient's nose and throat may become irritated and dry). A humidifier should *not* be used because of bacteria in the air. If possible, the patient should brush his or her own teeth and should be instructed to rinse the mouth well with mouthwash but not to swallow.

Be sure to reposition the tape and give good skin care to prevent skin breakdown on the nose or cheek.

REMOVING THE NASOGASTRIC TUBE. The tube is temporarily clamped before being removed to make sure that the patient can tolerate its absence. Usually, the physician removes a long tube. The nurse may be instructed to remove shorter tubes. The tube is removed by deflating any balloons and simply pulling out, slowly at first, then rapidly when the patient begins to cough. Resistance is seldom encountered. The tube should not be removed if there is any resistance. Generally, if difficulty is encountered, another attempt in an hour or so will be successful.

Keys to Nursing Assessment
Checking Drainage in Gastric Suction

- Check the hookup of bottle and its level of fluid
- Check the drainage for the following characteristics:
- Color
    - Normal—greenish yellow
    - More yellow after injury or surgery and becoming darker and brownish as bile secretion returns
    - Maroon or red (with smell like blood) if blood is present
- Odor
    - Normal—acidic or sour
    - Foul—indicates presence of infection
    - Bloodlike—indicates gastric bleeding.
- Consistency: thin, thick, tenacious, presence of chunks, particles, strands of mucus
- Amount (if tube is irrigated or patient has oral fluids, these amounts must be deducted from output)
- Presence of vomitus (amount and character)—add to output
- Check fluid intake and output, including drainage.
- Check for symptoms of electrolyte imbalance. Monitor daily blood level results.
- Check daily weights, if ordered.
- Assess time, amount, and characteristics of stools, if any.
- Assess for any other symptoms (including pain, cramping, nausea, edema, or jaundice).

Conceal the tube after you have removed it. The nurse should be sure to remove any tape marks from the patient's face; acetone may be necessary. The nurse should provide mouth care and be alert for complaints of discomfort, distention, or nausea after the tube has been removed. Liquids and food are not given without a physician's order.

Caring for the Patient Receiving Total Parenteral Nutrition

The nurse must observe certain precautions when caring for the patient receiving TPN (Fig. 81-3). Strict sterile techniques *must* be followed during changes of bottles, tubing, filters, and dressings. Because the catheter is placed directly into a large blood vessel, any contamination would be quickly disseminated throughout the body. Dressings at the insertion site *must* be sterile. Nursing assessments include observation as follows. The catheter must be taped securely at the insertion site to prevent dislodgement. All connections must be secure. The patient's hands may need to be restrained if pulling on the tube is a problem. Assess and document the integrity of the skin and tube at least each shift.

The rate of flow is carefully controlled using a volumetric infusion pump because the rate of infusion for TPN must be constant to prevent episodes of circulatory overload, hypoglycemia, or hyperglycemia. Any unused nutrient solution is discarded after 24 hours to reduce the chance of infection.

Be sure to check the procedure manual at your agency regarding TPN. Most health facilities have a specific protocol for administration of nutrients by TPN. Nursing assessment factors are listed in the accompanying box.

Patients may go home on TPN and manage these lines at home. Discharge planning is directed toward teaching the patient or the family how to manage and become confident in the care of the lines. Document all teaching.

Assisting With Management of a Colostomy or Ileostomy

When the patient returns from the operating room, the stoma is covered by a plastic disposable pouch, which opens at the bottom. This pouch is held in place by a skin barrier that adheres to the abdominal skin. The bottom of the pouch is clamped with either a special ostomy closure clamp or binder clip. When the pouch is $\frac{1}{3}$ to $\frac{1}{2}$ full with stool or flatus, it is emptied. To do this, the patient sits on the toilet, removes the closure clamp, and empties the pouch contents between the legs into the toilet.

OSTOMY MANAGEMENT. General nursing care skills are outlined in the accompanying box. A second box lists factors in assessing the stoma.

Stoma Condition in the New Colostomy or Ileostomy

Abnormal and Danger Signs

- Abnormal sounds
- Excessive bleeding (more likely to occur in ileostomy)
- Darkening in color (indicating stenosis around the stoma, which cuts off the blood supply)
- Blanching or extreme lightening in color (indicating lack of circulation to the stoma)
- Drying of the stoma
- Edema of the stoma
- Prolapse (stoma pulls back into abdomen)
- Skin irritation around stoma (see guidelines for skin care)
- Signs of infection
- Herniation around stoma

Routine Assessments

- Size of the appliance. (It must be large enough so that it does not cut off circulation but small enough so that it does not leak.)
- Intake and output records
- Daily weights
- Electrolyte balance or imbalance; results of blood work
- Amount, character of stool
- Vital signs

tains nerves and to prevent irritation, it is important not to apply a leather belt over it. Men who have their stoma site at the beltline may be required to use suspenders. (This is one of the important reasons for the ET nurse to discuss the placement of the stoma preoperatively.) Patients can wear the ostomy pouch tucked into their underwear, or they can wear bikini underwear beneath the pouch.

Immediately after surgery, many patients choose to wear loose-fitting clothing. However, patients will discover that even when wearing tight-fitting clothing or jeans, the presence of the pouch underneath is not noticeable.

Bathing. All pouching systems are waterproof, so a patient can take a bath or shower or go swimming with the pouch on. Patients may choose to remove the soiled pouch and shower without it. However, this is not advisable for the person with an ileostomy. *(Rationale: Bowel function in ileostomy is fairly frequent and unpredictable.)*

Activity. Heavy lifting is prohibited for 6 to 8 weeks following any abdominal surgery. Nothing heavier than 5 lb is suggested during this important period of tissue healing. This is particularly important in the ostomate to avoid hernias, which can develop in the incision or around the stoma. After this initial

The Pouch. Skin barriers on pouching systems eventually will deteriorate. Depending on the brand of pouch used, the pouch should be changed one to two times per week. *(Rationale: Following the recommended wear time guidelines will prevent deterioration of the pouch adhesive and prevent skin breakdown around the stoma.)*

There are many different styles and sizes of ostomy pouches (Fig. 81-4). The ET nurse will assist the staff nurse and patient in choosing the appropriate pouch, depending on abdominal contours and amount and type of drainage. The patient will be fit into a *cut-to-fit* pouch while in the hospital (so the size of the stoma opening can be adjusted as stoma edema decreases). After approximately 1 month to 6 weeks, the ET nurse can fit the patient into a *precut* pouch (to eliminate the need for cutting out each pouch prior to changing it). Ostomy equipment is stocked at medical suppliers, although some pharmacies also carry it. Most insurance companies cover at least part of the cost.

Clothing. Most patients will return to wearing the same clothes as before surgery. Because the stoma con-

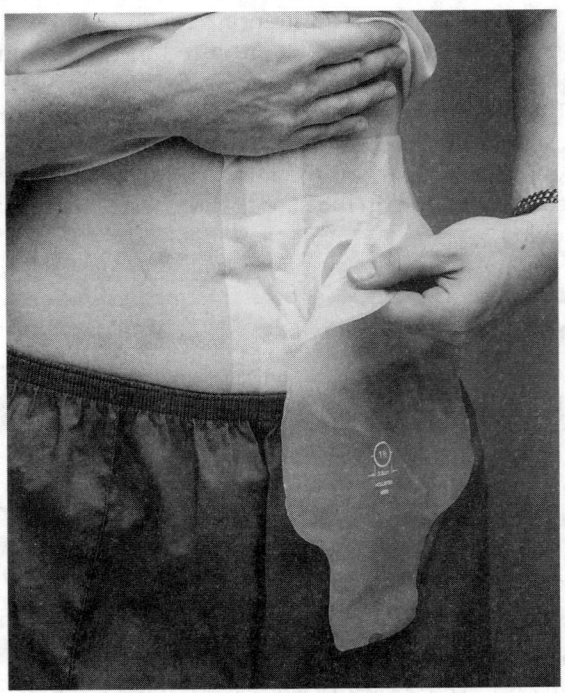

Figure 81-4. One type of disposable ostomy pouch. This pouch is flat and is easily concealed under clothing. (Product photo courtesy of 3M Health Care.)

postoperative period, there are no activity limitations for the ostomate.

Diet. Following any bowel surgery, it is recommended that the patient be on a low-fiber diet for approximately 1 month. *(Rationale: The bowel becomes edematous with surgery, and high-fiber foods may have difficulty passing through this edematous bowel.)* After 1 month, the person with a colostomy can return to a regular diet.

The person with an *ileostomy* needs to monitor the diet more closely than the person with a colostomy. The most common complication following an ileostomy is food blockage. (Foods that tend to cause blockage include dried fruits, popcorn, many vegetables, nuts, and meats in casings, such as frankfurters.) Undigested food obstructs the bowel just prior to the stoma, and this prevents passage of stool. It is particularly important for a person with an ileostomy to chew his or her food very well. This person may also have difficulty with odor from flatus; eliminating common gas-forming foods usually helps.

It is important for the person with an ileostomy to drink plenty of fluids. This person has a less-formed stool and therefore loses more fluids during the digestion process. In addition to losing increased water, this person tends to lose sodium and potassium in the stool. Therefore, it is important not to drink just plain water, but to drink fluids that contain electrolytes, such as Gatorade, soda pop, and broth.

CHANGING THE OSTOMY APPLIANCE. The nurse will assist and teach the patient as needed (Fig. 81-5). The goal is to promote self-care.

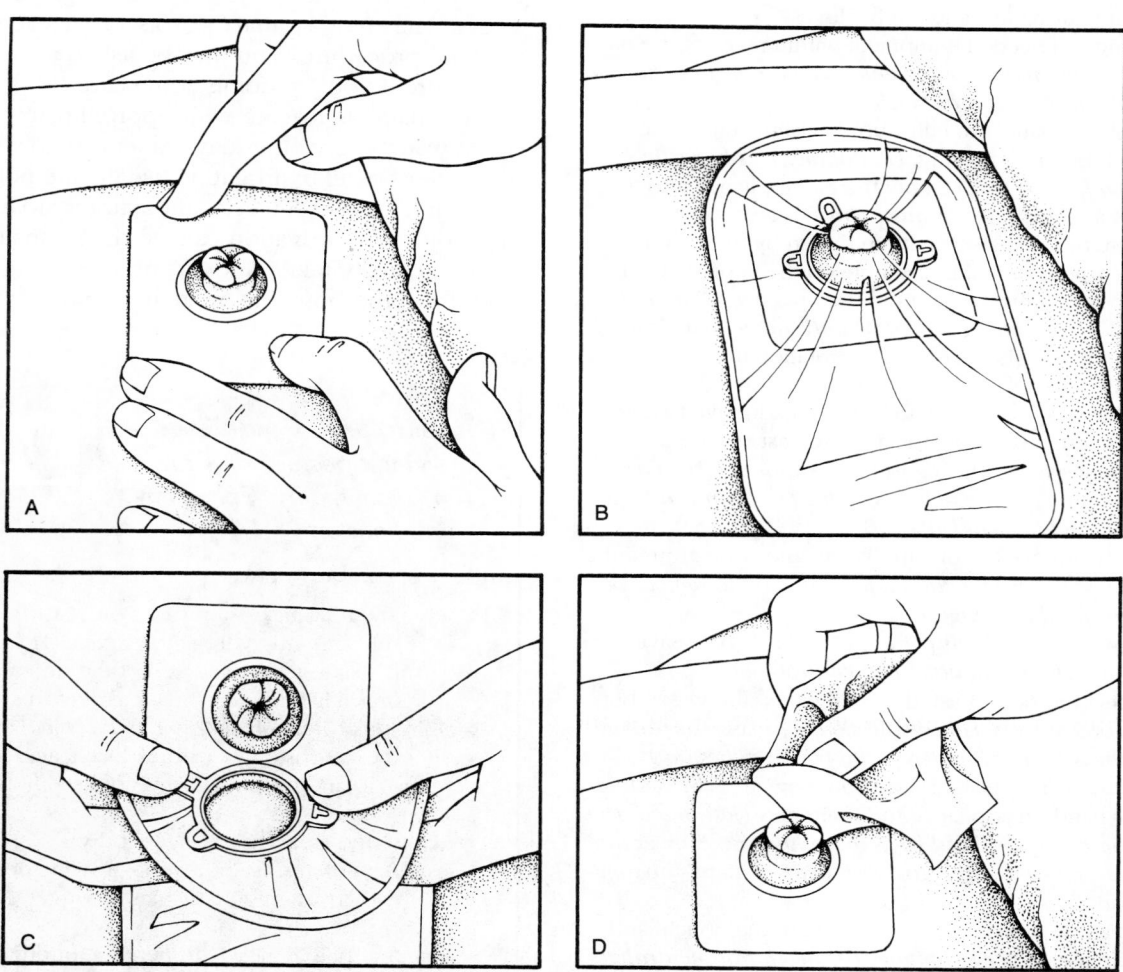

Figure 81-5. Ostomy care. **(A)** A Stomahesive wafer with flange ($1\frac{1}{2}$, $1\frac{3}{4}$, $2\frac{1}{4}$, $2\frac{3}{4}$) can be applied directly to the periostomal area after it has been thoroughly cleaned and dried. **(B)** An opaque or transparent drainable pouch is positioned at the desired angle over stoma. **(C)** Pouch may be removed without removing wafer. **(D)** Stoma may be assessed without removing wafer. (Adapted by permission from ConvaTec, a Division of ER Squibb & Sons, Inc.)

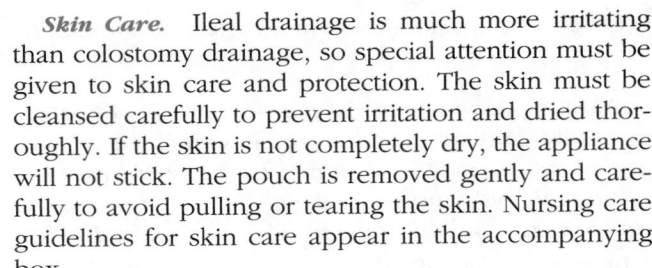

Nursing Skill
Changing the Ostomy Appliance

Supplies and Equipment

Pouch or pattern
Pouch adhesive wafer
Closure clip
Stomahesive paste (optional)
Cotton balls or gauze
Scissors
Pen or pencil
Tissues
Water
Soft towel
Liquid deodorant
Plastic waste bag
Gloves

Procedure

1. Wash your hands, and apply gloves.
2. Arrange all needed equipment within reach of the patient. (*Rationale: The patient must become accustomed to self-care as soon as possible.*)
3. Teach the patient to cuff (turn back) the tail of the pouch before emptying. (*Rationale: This keeps the pouch free of stool.*) Empty the old appliance into the toilet and flush. (*Rationale: This removes odor.*)
4. Locate the stoma size pattern drawn by the ET nurse. With a pen, trace this size hole on the paper backing of the pouch adhesive. Cut out the opening. (*Rationale: The pouch opening should be only ¹⁄₁₆ inch larger than stoma size. This prevents skin irritation from chronic exposure to stool.*)
5. Remove paper backing from pouch adhesive (wafer). Apply a thin bead of Stomahesive paste to the edge of the adhesive you have just cut. (*Rationale: The paste is a kind of caulking to help seal the pouch around the stoma and prevent leakage.*)
6. Gently remove the old appliance, and wipe around the stoma with tissue. (*Rationale: You want to remove mucus or fecal drainage.*)
7. Dispose of the old appliance in a plastic bag. Save the closure clip. (*Rationale: This controls odor.*)
8. Inspect the skin. Wash the area with warm water, but do not use soap. (*Rationale: Soap can leave a residue on the skin that interferes with pouch adhesion.*)
9. Carefully dry the skin. Apply the new appliance. Hold your hand on appliance for 2 minutes. (*Rationale: The warmth of your hand helps warm the skin barrier and paste so the adhesives seal well to the patient's abdominal wall.*)
10. Add a few drops of the deodorant to the pouch, and clamp it closed. (*Rationale: The deodorant neutralizes odors.*)
11. Properly dispose of waste material and gloves.
12. Wash your hands, and document the procedure, noting patient reactions.

Skin Care. Ileal drainage is much more irritating than colostomy drainage, so special attention must be given to skin care and protection. The skin must be cleansed carefully to prevent irritation and dried thoroughly. If the skin is not completely dry, the appliance will not stick. The pouch is removed gently and carefully to avoid pulling or tearing the skin. Nursing care guidelines for skin care appear in the accompanying box.

COLOSTOMY IRRIGATION. Colostomy irrigation is another type of bowel management. This enables the person to regulate the colostomy so he or she does not need to wear a pouch. Prior to the widespread use of disposable, odor-proof ostomy equipment, nearly all patients with colostomies used irrigation for bowel management.

Colostomy irrigation is similar to an enema (see Chapter 46). It is usually done with a cone tip and bag; the fluid drains into the toilet through an irrigating sleeve. The enterostomal therapist often teaches the patient the procedure. You may be asked to perform this procedure if you are doing home care.

Most patients irrigate with approximately 1,000 mL of tap water every other day. Patients who wish to regulate their bowel by irrigating usually are not taught to do so until at least 6 weeks after surgery to allow healing. Colostomy irrigation can be time consuming, because it usually takes 1 to 1½ hours to irrigate all the stool from the bowel. Now that ostomy equipment is

---

Nursing Skill Guidelines
Giving Special Skin Care in Gastrostomy, Colostomy, and Ileostomy

Protocol may vary between facilities.

♦ Wipe the new gastrostomy or stoma, as ordered, with half-strength hydrogen peroxide (H_2O_2).
♦ Carefully assess the condition of the stoma and surrounding skin daily (see box earlier in this section).
♦ Do not use alcohol. (*Rationale: It is too drying.*)
♦ After the gastrostomy or stoma has healed, clean it with soap and water. (Soap is not used if it irritates the patient's skin.)
♦ Expose the area to air to keep it dry.
♦ If redness or a yeast-appearing growth appears, treat with an antibiotic, such as nystatin (Mycostatin) powder.
♦ A wafer of Stomahesive to peritube (around the tube) skin will protect it from drainage. Stomahesive paste may be used in addition.
♦ A drain tube attachment device (DTAD) can help to secure the tube.

odor proof, most patients elect the easier and less time-consuming option of wearing a pouch.

Evaluation

The nurse, patient, family, and other members of the healthcare team evaluate outcomes of care by answering the following questions: Have short-term goals been met? Are additional teaching or rehabilitative measures needed? Is additional treatment or surgery necessary? Are long-term goals still realistic? Are community services required? Planning for further nursing care takes into consideration the patient's prognosis, complications, and responses to care given.

Cancer of the Gastrointestinal Tract

Cancer within the GI tract can arise anywhere, although it is rarely seen in the small intestine. The general symptoms are similar to those found with cancer in any other part of the body: fatigue, weight loss, weakness, and anemia. Unfortunately, pain often does not occur in the early stages. Cancers of the mouth, esophagus, and stomach affect more men than women. However, men and women have an approximately equal chance of contracting cancer of the colon.

Disorders of the Mouth

Mouth disorders may not seem to be dangerous, but they are uncomfortable, often painful, and at times disfiguring or cosmetically unattractive. They also interfere with nutritional intake or lead to other undesirable or more serious conditions.

Miscellaneous Oral Disorders

Dental Caries
Dental caries (tooth decay) are the result of an erosive process that breaks down tooth enamel and later invades the pulp of the tooth, causing discomfort and sometimes necessitating removal of the tooth. The major cause of dental decay is bacteria nourished by food particles left on the teeth as a result of faulty brushing. The following factors play a part in the decay process: the acids in the mouth and their effectiveness in destroying bacteria, presence of plaque on the teeth and sugar in the mouth promoting bacterial growth, susceptibility of the teeth to decay, and the length of time between brushings.

Good brushing is essential for the development of a healthy mouth and the prevention of tooth decay. Many dentists recommend using fluoridated water or having fluoride applied by the dentist. Flossing helps prevent gum disease. Professional dental care also is important. Adults should have their teeth checked twice a year.

Dentures
Many people put off having infected teeth removed because they dread replacing them with dentures. Meanwhile, they are exposing themselves to generalized infection. In some cases, dentures are the best solution to dental problems. At other times, reconstructive partial inserts can be used. Dentures may be slightly uncomfortable when they are first fitted, but the dentist can remove sources of irritation. The only way to become accustomed to dentures is to wear them all the time, especially when awake. This also helps preserve the normal shape of the face. The term for "without teeth" is *edentulous*.

Infectious Disorders

Herpesvirus Simplex Infections
Cold sores or fever blisters are painful vesicles occurring on the face, lips, perioral (around the mouth) area, cheeks, and nose and are usually caused by the herpes simplex virus type I. (Herpes simplex virus type II is the agent usually responsible for genital herpes infections.) Cold sores usually disappear after a few days, and treatment is not usually required.

Medication may be prescribed for comfort but is not curative. Zovirax ointment (5% acyclovir ointment) may be applied to the lesions. The lesions are infectious, so gloves should be worn. Although this may not speed healing, it may decrease the shedding of the virus. Drying agents, such as ether or alum, also may be applied to the lesions to speed healing. Cold sores often may become secondarily infected by bacteria. Topical antibiotic ointments may be prescribed to treat bacterial infections.

Canker Sores (Aphthous Stomatitis)
Canker sores are recurrent, small, white, painful ulcers that appear on the inner cheeks, lips, gums, tongue, palate, and pharynx. No one knows exactly what causes them; however, many local and systemic factors, such as food and drug allergies and physical and emotional stress, have been suggested.

Dental trauma is the most common factor in inducing recurrent canker sores. Premenstrual flare-ups and remissions during the third trimester of pregnancy are common. Canker sores may be associated with chronic ulcerative colitis, Crohn's disease, and malabsorption syndromes. Herpes simplex virus is usually not cultured from canker sores, although it is believed that the cause is viral.

No effective treatment has been found. The sores usually heal on their own in a few days. The use of topical anesthetics (eg, benzocaine or lidocaine) may help to relieve the pain. Silver nitrate stick application destroys nerve endings and may provide relief of pain. Application of a solution of tetracycline may improve healing in some patients. Oral lysine also is believed to be helpful.

Periodontal Diseases

Periodontal disease affects the bones and the tissue around the teeth. It can be the result of poor oral hygiene, inadequate dental care, or poor nutrition.

Gingivitis

Gingivitis is inflammation of the gums. General symptoms include bleeding gums, swelling, tenderness, and difficulty chewing. It has many causes, among them accumulation of food particles in the teeth, vitamin deficiencies, anemia, and leukemia. It can lead to more serious disorders, such as inflammation of the tissues directly surrounding a tooth. Proper care of teeth and gums, including daily flossing, and an adequate diet are the best preventive measures.

Pyorrhea Alveolaris

Pyorrhea is an inflammation of the gums and teeth, sometimes with a purulent discharge. It usually begins with *periodontitis* (inflammation of the tissues around and supporting the teeth). This is caused by the collection of food, bacteria, and tartar deposits between the gumline and the tooth root. Untreated, periodontitis spreads to the underlying bony structure. The teeth loosen because their support structure breaks down, making chewing impossible.

Treatment includes impeccable tooth, gum, and mouth care, including regular flossing; surgical scraping and drainage of the infected area; antibiotics; or extraction of the affected teeth. Surgical scraping is very painful, so other measures are tried first. Left untreated, pyorrhea can result in an abscess or a systemic infection.

Oral Trauma

Various types of injuries, such as fracture of the jaw, laceration of the lips, and traumatic loss of teeth, can cause injury to the mouth. First aid for traumatic loss of teeth *(avulsion)* is described in Chapter 31.

Lacerations of the lips heal without complications with simple suturing because of a good blood supply. However, if the entire lip is severed, there might be problems with lip movement.

For a jaw fracture, usually the upper and lower jaws are wired or fastened together so that they will heal without displacement. This is called *intermaxillary fixation.* This patient cannot open his or her mouth. Consequently the nurse must be ready to assist as neces-

sary. The patient needs help at meals because foods are sipped through a straw or from a spoon. Intravenous or nasogastric tube feedings and TPN may be necessary.

A wire cutter must be kept with the patient at all times for emergency use. If the patient is choking or vomiting, the wires must be cut, or the patient could die. The patient's head should be slightly elevated, and oral suctioning equipment should be available. Antiemetic drugs are usually administered for the first few days after injury. A tracheostomy or an airway might be required as an emergency measure.

If an *extraoral* (outside the mouth) device is in place, special attention is given to the position of the patient's head for maximum comfort. The device often goes around the patient's head. The patient is instructed not to roll onto the device to avoid bending or dislodging the wires.

Temporomandibular Joint Disorders

The joint where the lower jaw (mandible) and the temporal bone of the skull join is called the *temporomandibular joint* (TMJ). Disorders of this joint are caused by structural defects, malignant lesions, trauma, and infection. Myofascial pain, sometimes referred to as *TMJ syndrome,* is becoming more common as the stress of daily living increases. The TMJ disorder is more common in women than in men. It is a result of clenching the jaw or grinding the teeth *(bruxism),* usually as a result of stress. Symptoms include a clicking or grinding of the jaw when it is moved and pain around the ears. It may be impossible or painful to open the mouth.

A soft, nonchewy diet is prescribed, along with warm, moist packs or diathermy. The patient is advised not to move the jaw, and a dental retainer or bite-plate may be fitted so that the patient is not able to clench the jaw or grind the teeth. Braces may be helpful. Muscle relaxants and analgesics might be prescribed. Surgery may be needed in extreme cases.

Neoplasms

Precancerous Lesions

The most common precancerous lesion is **leukoplakia buccalis** (smoker's patch), a creamy white patch on the mucous membranes of the mouth or tongue, often seen in middle-aged people who smoke or have dental caries. It often disappears if the patient stops smoking.

Cancer of the Mouth

Cancer of the mouth can be successfully treated if discovered early. However, many people tend to ignore sores or irritations in the mouth because they think such symptoms are not significant. Cancer of the mouth may be treated with surgery, radium implants, or deep x-ray therapy.

If possible, the malignancy is removed with as wide an excision as necessary to remove all infected structures and lymph nodes. The most extreme surgical procedure is called a *radical neck dissection*. If extensive surgery is necessary, edema might interfere with breathing, and a tracheostomy might be done. Nasogastric or gastrostomy feedings might be indicated. The operation is often followed by reconstructive surgery to correct facial defects.

Nursing Considerations. Postoperatively, secretions are suctioned, and the head of the bed is elevated to make breathing easier. As the nurse supports the patient's head by placing hands on either side, the patient is instructed to breathe deeply and use the incentive spirometer. Coughing is not encouraged unless congestion is present. These measures are needed to prevent hypostatic pneumonia. An emergency airway should be available at the bedside.

Mouth care is carefully given to improve patient comfort and prevent odor. Great care must be taken to prevent disruption of the suture line. Liquids are given through a nasogastric tube until the patient is able to swallow. Self-care is the goal.

Disorders of the Esophagus

Structural Disorders

Esophageal Varices
Esophageal varices are outpouchings of the blood vessels of the esophagus, most often associated with cirrhosis of the liver. Treatment is imperative—untreated varices can hemorrhage profusely, and the patient may die. Varices are further discussed later in this chapter.

Sclerotherapy is an endoscopy procedure whereby caustic agents are injected into the tissue near the varices. This procedure, done in a series of treatments, causes scar tissue to form and stops hemorrhaging. The patient must be assessed for hemorrhage after each treatment and before and after surgery.

Band ligation is another endoscopy procedure in which small rubber bands are placed on and around bleeding varices on the wall of the esophagus. These bands stop the bleeding, and when the tissue is healed they slough off, leaving scar tissue less likely to rebleed.

Esophageal Diverticulum
Esophageal diverticulum or *Zinker's diverticulum,* is an outpouching of the esophagus, usually where the esophagus passes through the neck area. The patient first complains of bad breath, which is caused by bits

of food that have built up in the diverticulum. The nature and location of the outpouchings are determined by x-rays.

The patient's dietary status is evaluated; blenderized meals are usually given with supplemental vitamins. The patient is treated medically with a bland diet, antacids, antiemetics, and other measures to prevent reflux (return flow) of food and fluid. Surgery may be necessary if symptoms do not diminish with conscientious medical management.

Nursing measures include placing the patient in a semi-Fowler's position, serving small meals, and fitting the patient with loose clothing. The patient is encouraged to maintain appropriate weight to keep an enlarged stomach or excess fatty tissue from pushing up on the esophagus.

Heartburn
Heartburn is a common GI symptom. Also known as *acid indigestion*, it is an uncomfortable burning sensation in the lower chest, so named because of its proximity to the heart. It has no relationship to the heart, however. Other symptoms of heartburn include nausea, belching, a bloated feeling, or a sore throat from acid reflux. Heartburn occurs when the lower esophageal sphincter (LES) leading into the stomach is weak or relaxes inappropriately, allowing the acidic stomach contents to move back up into the esophagus.

Some drugs and food aggravate this condition, including aspirin, chocolate, peppermint, spicy foods, coffee, tomato products, citrus fruits, and fried foods. Cigarette smoking greatly decreases the lower esophageal sphincter pressure and aggravates heartburn. Drinking alcohol and overeating also aggravate the condition. Antacids, such as Mylanta, Rolaids, or Tums, can temporarily relieve heartburn. The patient also should be instructed not to lie down after a large meal and not to wear tight belts or waistbands.

> **Nursing Alert**
>
> It may be difficult to differentiate between heartburn and the pain of a heart attack. *If there is any question, the patient must seek medical care immediately.*
>
> Significant symptoms of heart attack that are *different* from heartburn are intense chest pain, often radiating to the neck, jaw, back, or arms; difficulty breathing or breathlessness; fainting; numbness in a limb; sudden nausea and vomiting; and cold, clammy skin accompanied by sweating.

Hiatal Hernia
Hiatal hernia is a condition in which part of the stomach protrudes through the esophageal hiatus (gap or cleft) of the diaphragm (Fig. 81-6). The most com-

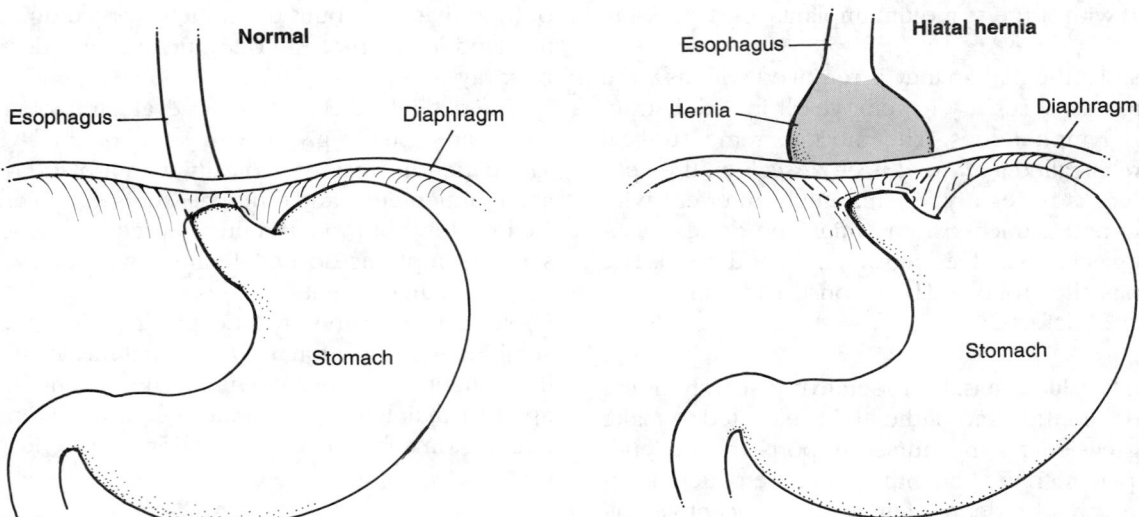

Figure 81-6. Diagram of the normal esophagus and diaphragm meeting the stomach, compared to an esophagus, diaphragm, and stomach with a hiatal hernia.

mon cause is increased pressure in the abdominal cavity caused by coughing, straining at stool, sudden physical exertion, or lifting heavy objects. Many people older than age 50 have hiatal hernias without symptoms. A large hiatal hernia is likely to cause symptoms, however.

Signs and Symptoms. Signs and symptoms of hiatal hernia include a feeling of fullness, abnormal stomach sounds, ulceration, bleeding, and pain. (*Note:* Hiatal hernia does *not* cause heartburn, although a person with a hiatal hernia may have heartburn from another cause.)

Treatment. Management is directed at keeping the acid contents of the stomach from maintaining long contact with the lining of the esophagus. If a hernia is small and does not cause distress, no treatment is necessary. Surgical treatment is needed only in large hiatal hernias. Postoperative care is routine, except that edema of the stomach and esophagus may make eating problematic for the first few days.

Nursing Considerations. After surgery, the patient is fed intravenously or with TPN for several days. The nurse should assess nasogastric tube drainage carefully, looking particularly for blood. A small amount of blood may be evident immediately after the operation, but after this disappears, the drainage should have the yellowish-green color of normal gastric secretions. Frank bleeding signals a hemorrhage. If the patient has had chest surgery, special attention should be given to chest tube management and deep breathing; the incentive spirometer is used. Oxygen is administered, and

care is given to the chest drainage site. Other postoperative care is routine.

Observe carefully for vomiting or aspiration, particularly when the patient begins to take solid or semisolid foods. (*Rationale: Regurgitated food may irritate the suture line, and aspiration can cause postoperative pneumonia.*) Special patient teaching is presented in the accompanying box.

Chronic Disorders

Achalasia

Achalasia is a motility disorder of the lower two-thirds of the esophagus in which the food cannot pass into the stomach. Causes include absence of effective or coordinated peristalsis of the body of the esophagus or failure of the cardiac sphincter to relax.

The most prominent symptom of achalasia is difficulty in swallowing. Achalasia is chronic and progressive. Patients often use large volumes of fluids or bulk in an attempt to force the cardiac sphincter to open and allow food to move into the stomach. Thus, malnutrition and vitamin deficiencies may develop. These patients also are susceptible to respiratory problems caused by aspiration of the regurgitated esophageal contents.

A special test called *esophageal manometry* is used to measure and record the motility patterns of the esophagus. A barium swallow with esophagoscopy may be done to assist the diagnosis. These procedures also can be used to monitor the progression of the disorder.

Treatment. Surgical treatment often involves dilation of the cardiac sphincter, which is dilated to the point of weakening or disrupting its ability to close. This is done by endoscopy with a variety of balloons and dilators. Medical treatment is directed toward educating the patient.

Nursing Considerations. Teaching involves improving dietary and eating habits. The patient must be taught to eat slowly and in a peaceful setting. Chewing food thoroughly and drinking plenty of liquids during the meal help food move into the stomach. See the "patient teaching" box related to esophagitis, hiatal hernia, and achalasia for added suggestions.

Inflammatory Disorders

Esophagitis

Esophagitis is the acute or chronic inflammation and irritation of the lining of the esophagus. Symptoms may include pain, heartburn, indigestion, nausea, or regurgitation because the esophagus often responds to physical irritation, such as exposure to alcohol, caffeine, spices, hot or cold liquids, or smoking. Bacterial or yeast infections also may be a cause.

Most commonly, however, esophagitis is caused by the reflux (backwash) of hydrochloric acid and gastric contents into the esophagus from the stomach. Cardiac sphincter (CS) incompetence (weakness) is a frequent cause. This means that the sphincter that leads into the stomach is unable to close completely or to stay closed. Thus, stomach contents can be regurgitated up into the esophagus. Another condition that allows esophagitis to occur is hiatal hernia.

Barrett's esophagus is the condition of extreme and chronic irritation of the lower esophagus. This results in a change in esophageal lining cell formation from the normal squamous cell type to the columnar cell type, which is found in the wall of the stomach. This is thought to be a precancerous condition that requires annual endoscopic surveillance and careful medical management to heal and minimize esophagitis.

Treatment of esophagitis is directed at alleviating or minimizing the causes. Nursing measures include elevation of the head of the bed, avoidance of gastric irritants, small meals, loose clothing, and encouragement of proper weight maintenance. If the patient's diet is aggravating the condition, nutritional counseling is in order. The patient should *not* smoke.

Neoplasms

Cancer of the Esophagus

Cancer of the esophagus is most common in men and in people who smoke. It is distressing because any attempt at swallowing causes food to be regurgitated, creating a disagreeable taste and odor in the patient's mouth and discomfort. Often the patient needs parenteral fluids, including TPN. Surgery is the only effective method of treating the cancer and allowing the patient to eat normally.

Often the malignancy is not curable because it may be in an inoperable area or may have been discovered after the cancer metastasized. Metastasis is fairly common because the esophagus is close to other vital structures.

Persistent difficulty in swallowing should be brought to the attention of a physician, because this is often the first sign of esophageal cancer. Diagnosis is made on the basis of an *esophagogram* (x-ray of the esophagus), upper GI series, and laboratory cytology. Esophagoscopy or bronchoscopy may be done to visualize the tumor and take a biopsy.

Innovative developments in chest surgery have resulted in rapid advances in treatment in recent years. All the malignant tissue that can be isolated is removed. This may be curative in an early stage. Radiation therapy is usually included before or after surgery or at both times. Even if it is impossible to remove all of the cancerous tissue because the disease has spread, surgery may help the patient eat normally. One palliative procedure is to create a bypass for food and fluids.

Disorders of the Stomach

Inflammatory Disorders

Gastritis

Gastritis, which is inflammation of the stomach, is often called indigestion. It occurs in acute, chronic, and toxic forms. *Acute gastritis* is caused by overeating, ingestion of irritating drugs (such as aspirin or steroids), food poisoning, overuse of alcohol, or a microbe. The major symptom is abdominal pain, often with anorexia and nausea. Enteritis (inflammation of the intestine) is often present as well. Offending foods or drugs are removed, and a bland diet of liquids or soft foods is given, along with antacids.

Chronic gastritis continues over time. Pain may occur after eating, but often there is no pain. Causes include excessive alcohol use, vitamin deficiencies, hiatal hernia, ulcers, and abnormalities in gastric secretions. Treatment is similar to that of peptic ulcer.

Toxic gastritis follows ingestion of poison or a corrosive. It is evidenced by burning stomach pain, cramps, nausea, vomiting, and diarrhea. The emesis or diarrhea may be bloody. This is an emergency situation; the patient is treated by poison-control specialists in the emergency room. The poison is either flushed out by gavage or neutralized, if possible with a substance such as activated charcoal.

Ulcers

An **ulcer** is an open sore occurring in the skin or mucous membrane and accompanied by sloughing of inflamed and necrotic tissue. A *peptic ulcer* is a break in the integrity of the mucosa of the esophagus, stomach, or duodenum. *Duodenal ulcers* (ulcers in the duodenum) are characterized by high gastric secretion of hydrochloric acid. *Gastric ulcers* (ulcers in the stomach) are thought to be the result of a break in the mucous barrier mechanisms that normally protect the lining of the stomach (Fig. 81-7). The overgrowth and presence of the microorganism *Helicobacter pylori* in the mucosa of the stomach and duodenum have been strongly associated with antral gastritis, duodenal ulcers, and to a lesser degree, gastric ulcers. The antral area is the proximal, expanded part of the pylorus. Treatment regimens using bismuth compounds (such as Pepto-Bismol) and antibiotics to eradicate the microbe are proving effective in healing and preventing recurrence of ulcers and gastritis.

A simple and quick test called *Clotest* can diagnose the presence of *H. pylori* from a gastric mucosal biopsy taken at the time of upper endoscopy. Also, a serum

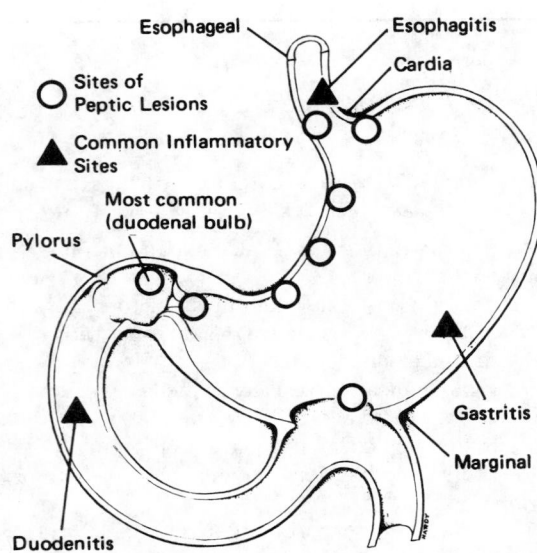

Figure 81-7. "Peptic" lesions may occur in the esophagus (esophagitis), stomach (gastritis), or duodenum (duodenitis). Note peptic ulcer sites and common inflammatory sites.

blood test (serum *H. Pylori* Immunoglobulin G) is specific for the bacterium. It identifies the presence of antibodies (which validates the bacterium's existence in the GI tract). Differentiatiation between gastric and duodenal ulcers is shown in the accompanying box.

Signs and Symptoms. Symptoms of peptic ulcer are given in Table 81-2.

Melana (black stool) is a significant finding. Blood from a stomach ulcer will make the stools black and tarry because partial digestion has taken place before excretion. Occult blood is demonstrated by a guaiac, Hemoquant, or other specific diagnostic test. Gastroscopy and x-rays help to diagnose peptic ulcer and differentiate it from a cancerous lesion.

> ### Key Concept
> Cigarette smokers are twice as likely to have ulcers as nonsmokers. Alcohol use also predisposes to ulcer formation.

Treatment and Nursing Considerations. The goals in ulcer treatment are to eliminate irritation of the lesion, reduce acidic secretions, reduce activity of the stomach and intestine, and reduce emotional stress. Patient teaching is an important part of management (see the box).

Diet. Recent research has shown that the frequency of meals is as important as their content. A bland diet may be given while pain is present but usually is not continued thereafter. For the first few weeks, the diet

Characteristics of Peptic Ulcers

Gastric Ulcer

- ◆ Most common in people over age 65
- ◆ Most common in elderly women
- ◆ Lifestyle risk factors: stress, alcohol abuse, smoking
- ◆ Nonsteroidal anti-inflammatory drugs and aspirin use (commonly prescribed for arthritis), which contributes to gastric ulcer formation
- ◆ High epigastrium pain 1 to 2 hours after meals; eating may not relieve
- ◆ Weight loss
- ◆ High mortality rate; higher incidence of malignancy than duodenal ulcer

Duodenal Ulcer

- ◆ Most common in people under age 65
- ◆ Three times more common in men than women
- ◆ Lifestyle risk factors: stress, alcohol abuse, smoking
- ◆ Risk factor conditions: pulmonary disease, cirrhosis of the liver, chronic pancreatitis, chronic renal failure
- ◆ Midepigastrium pain 2 to 4 hours after meals and during night; often relieved by eating
- ◆ Weight gain
- ◆ More likely to perforate than gastric ulcer
- ◆ Four times more common than gastric ulcers

Keys to Patient/Family Teaching
Management of Ulcers

Patient and family teaching for the patient with ulcers includes the following:

- ◆ Three meals with a bedtime snack should be routine.
- ◆ Meal size and portions should be a comfortable and tolerated level. Avoid overdistension.
- ◆ Foods that aggravate symptoms should be determined and eliminated.
- ◆ Foods should be eaten slowly and chewed well.
- ◆ The physician should be contacted if diarrhea or increased discomfort occur or if the person is not improving.
- ◆ Methods of relaxation should be used.
- ◆ Concerns should be verbalized.
- ◆ A personal balance should be established between exercise and physical and emotional rest, especially during stressful periods.

eliminates gas-forming foods, highly seasoned foods, and those high in roughage, such as fresh fruits, popcorn, and nuts. Because coffee, tea, cola beverages, chocolate, and alcohol stimulate secretion of hydrochloric acid, they also are omitted.

Milk and cream may be included, although not in large quantities. Many adults cannot digest the lactose in milk or cream and require a different type of diet.

The trend today is toward prescribing three normal meals and a bedtime snack rather than six small feedings used previously.

Medications. Antacid preparations buffer (neutralize) gastric hyperacidity. Antacids containing aluminum hydroxide (such as Amphogel) may cause constipation, and those containing magnesium hydroxide (such as Mylanta) may cause diarrhea. Maalox and Gelusil are a combination of magnesium and aluminum salts and are less likely to cause electrolyte depletion. Because antacids can disrupt the electrolyte balance, they are often rotated to maintain acid–base balance. The nurse should inform the patient that bicarbonate of soda (baking soda) should not be used on a regular basis, be-

Table 81-2. Differences in Symptoms of Ulcers and Stomach Cancer

Symptoms of Ulcer	Symptoms of Stomach Cancer
◆ Frequent dyspepsia	◆ Sudden dyspepsia
◆ Burning sensation in stomach (may be seasonal)	◆ Absence of pain until cancer is advanced ("silent neoplasm")
◆ Pain that always begins in same place	
◆ Pain relieved by eating	◆ Pain unrelieved by eating
◆ Pain that may be relieved by vomiting	◆ Pain unrelieved by vomiting
◆ Black, tarry stools (melana)	◆ Coffee-ground emesis
◆ Free hydrochloric acid in stomach	◆ Absence of free hydrochloric acid in stomach
◆ Tenseness, irritability	◆ Weakness, lethargy
◆ Difficulty in sleeping	◆ Tiredness much of the time
◆ Weight often maintained	◆ Unexplained weight loss
	◆ Cancer cells possibly visible in slides of gastric contents

cause it upsets the acid–base balance more than commercial antacids. Chewable antacids must be chewed slowly before being swallowed to obtain maximum benefit.

Histamine (H_2) receptor antagonists inhibit acid secretion in response to all stimuli. Therefore, they cause reduced gastric acid secretions. See the accompanying box for examples. These drugs also are called H_2 blockers. The H_2 blockers have largely replaced the anticholinergic drugs that were formerly used because the H_2 blockers are safer and have fewer undesirable side effects. The H_2 blockers are well absorbed from the GI tract and begin working within 30 to 60 minutes. Intravenous administration is possible for a faster effect. The H_2 blockers usually provide healing for acute gastric and duodenal ulcers in 6 to 8 weeks. They also have been proven safe and effective in long-term management of chronic gastric ulcers and related conditions, such as esophagitis and gastritis.

Omeprazole (Prilosec) is a new acid secretory inhibitor that binds to the proton pump of the parietal cell of the stomach to inhibit the secretion of acid. It has been classified as a "proton pump inhibitor." Omeprazole is a more potent drug used when other ulcer drug therapies have not been effective or lasting. Like the H_2 blockers, omeprazole is safe and has few side effects. Gynecomastia (development of breast tissue in men) and sexual dysfunction have been infrequently reported. Capsules should be swallowed whole and not opened or crushed.

Misoprostal (Cytotec) is a synthetic prostaglandin (hormone-like drug) that is prescribed in conjunction with necessary nonsteroidal anti-inflammatory drug (NSAID) therapy for arthritis conditions. It enhances gastric mucosal defenses and inhibits gastric secretion to prevent gastric ulcers. Arthritis patients are at greater risk of gastric ulcers, especially if they are female and older than 65 years. Diarrhea and loose stools are the most common reported side effects of misoprostal.

Sucralfate (Carafate) provides an additional protective mucous coating to the lining of the stomach and duodenum. This allows healing of ulcers or gastritis. The most common side effect of sucralfate is constipation.

Rest. Most ulcers can be controlled without surgery. Rest is important, although it does not necessarily imply rest in bed. Relaxation is even more important; many patients are hospitalized at the outset of treatment to force relaxation. Tranquilizers also may be prescribed. Once the course of treatment is established, the patient maintains the routine at home.

Management of Stress. The nurse helps the patient to rest and relax. The patient should be encouraged to verbalize concerns, rather than internalize them. Physical activity also helps to alleviate frustrations. Stress management workshops and support groups are often helpful.

Complications of Peptic Ulcers

Nursing Considerations. In the event of complications, the patient will have a nasogastric tube inserted, to which suction is attached. Nothing is given by mouth for at least 24 hours, and fluids are administered intravenously.

Massive doses of antibiotics will be given to counteract abdominal infection. Continued distention without the passage of flatus or feces is a sign of serious interference with peristalsis, causing intestinal paralysis (*paralytic ileus*).

Hemorrhage. Hemorrhage is one of the most serious and frequent complications of ulcers. It occurs when an ulcer penetrates a blood vessel. If the blood vessel is small, the bleeding may be so slight that it is not noticed. Vomiting blood or passing tarry stools is evidence of more extensive hemorrhage. If bleeding is massive, the signs of shock appear: pallor, weak and rapid pulse, low blood pressure, faintness, and collapse. A significant sign is *coffee-ground emesis* (an emesis of partially digested blood). If the blood loss is large and sudden, the patient is most likely to vomit; if it is small and grad-

---

Key Medications
for Ulcers

- *Antacids:* Amphogel, Mylanta, Maalox, Gelusil, Di-Gel, Riopan
- *Histamine (H_2) receptor antagonists* (H_2 blockers): cimetidine HCl (Tagamet), ranitidine HCl (Zantac), famotidine HCl (Pepsid), nizatidine (Axid)
- *Acid secretion inhibitor* (proton pump inhibitor): omeprazole (Prilosec)
- *Mucus enhancer* or gastric secretion inhibitor (protects against drug-induced ulcer formation): misoprostal (Cytotec)
- *Added mucous* coating to stomach lining: sucralfate (Carafate)
- *Antibiotics:* Drug chosen is based on specific pathogen present (most common pathogen causing ulcers is *Helicobacter pylori*).

Nursing Considerations

- Remind the patient to allow at least 1 hour between eating or taking doses of antacid and the H_2 blocker medication. (*Rationale: Actacids and food delay absorption of the H_2 blockers, although the therapeutic effect will eventually be the same.*)
- Some of these drugs, such as Zantac and Tagamet, can cause leukopenia. Other side effects include constipation, diarrhea, headache, and dizziness.
- Other considerations are presented in the accompanying text.

ual, the blood will more likely be passed in a stool (*tarry stools*).

> **Special Considerations in Aging**
> **Bleeding With Ulcers**
> The risk of bleeding is greater in older people, especially if they are taking NSAIDs, such as ibuprofen.

Endoscopic procedures can be performed to seal off bleeding vessels with a small heat probe or bipolar cautery probe passed down an inner channel of an endoscope. Injection of epinephrine by schlerotherapy technique also will stop acute bleeding. Treatment of a bleeding ulcer also includes rest, enforced by sedatives. Blood transfusion and intravenous fluids are often necessary. Surgery will probably be necessary if bleeding continues. Above all, the patient must be kept quiet and reassured.

Aspiration. Aspiration of stomach acid may cause asthma, pneumonia, and chronic lung disease. The use of omeprazole may lessen this risk.

Perforation. Perforation occurs when an ulcer penetrates the wall of the stomach or intestine, allowing the contents to escape into the abdomen and cause *peritonitis*. **Peritonitis** is inflammation of the serous membrane lining the walls of the pelvis and abdomen. Peritonitis is discussed later in this chapter in the section on appendicitis. The symptoms of perforation are startling, beginning with a sudden, viciously sharp pain in the abdomen. Physical signs include pallor and diaphoresis. The abdomen becomes hard and is tender and painful. The patient breathes rapidly with the knees drawn up in an attempt to relieve the pain. The face later becomes flushed and feverish. This condition can be fatal. It demands immediate surgery to close the perforation. A perforation can occur without warning and may not be preceded by marked signs of digestive disturbance.

Obstruction. Obstruction may occur when scar tissue builds to the point where it obstructs the passage of food through the pyloric sphincter. The symptoms include vomiting of undigested food and stomach pain. This pain is relieved only by vomiting. Peritonitis is a major threat.

Caring for the Patient Having a Gastrectomy. Preoperative nursing care for the patient undergoing gastrectomy includes the following:

◆ Administer antibiotics or sulfonamides as ordered.

(Rationale: This eliminates bacteria from the bowel and lessens the likelihood of postoperative infection.)
◆ Provide preoperative teaching. *(Rationale: The patient will need to follow a dietary regimen after surgery.)*
◆ Encourage the patient to verbalize feelings and relax as much as possible. The social worker or chaplain might help the patient solve personal, financial, and family problems and help to relieve worry.
◆ Encourage the patient to eat what is offered and to practice good oral hygiene. Vitamin and mineral supplements might be given. *(Rationale: These will build the patient up for surgery.)*
◆ A nasogastric tube may be inserted, perhaps for several days. Enemas may be given. TPN may be given. *(Rationale: The stomach and colon must be empty when the patient arrives in the operating room. The NG tube and TPN help to rest the stomach.)*

Postoperative nursing care includes the following:

◆ Use nasogastric suctioning for 2 to 3 days as ordered. *(Rationale: This keeps the operative area clean and eliminates pressure from accumulated fluids.)*
◆ Keep the nasogastric tube patent at all times. Drainage is assessed carefully. It may be tinged with bright red blood at first. If the amount of red blood increases or remains bright red, this should be reported. *(Rationale: This is a sign of hemorrhage.) The nasogastric fluid should progress toward normal color (greenish-yellow).*
◆ Irrigate the nasogastric tube as ordered. It is usually irrigated with approximately 20 mL of normal saline. Keep the patient in semi-Fowler's position. *(Rationale: If the nasogastric tube is irrigated incorrectly, the suture line could be disrupted. This position facilitates drainage.)*
◆ Provide routine postoperative care, including attention to early ambulation (usually the operative or first postoperative day), deep breathing, and incentive spirometer. Encourage the patient to cough gently if congestion in the lungs develops. The patient may be reluctant to deep breathe or cough because of incisional pain. Support the incision and give pain medications as prescribed. *(Rationale: Early exercise prevents complications; medications facilitate exercise.)*
◆ Assess dressings for excess drainage. Reinforce as needed. Usually the initial dressing change is not done by the nurse. *(Rationale: Excess drainage indicates infection or a rupture of the suture line. The surgeon observes the incision and does the first dressing change.)*

◆ Keep the patient NPO (usually) the first day. When bowel sounds return to normal, the nasogastric tube is often removed. (Sometimes it is clamped and left in place.) Clear liquids begin when bowel sounds are present. The diet progresses as tolerated. Feedings are decreased if the patient complains of nausea or abdominal distention. *(Rationale: These are signs of complications. The nasogastric tube may need to be reinserted.)*

Postoperative Complications. The suture line is delicate and may rupture and hemorrhage. Signs of shock will appear with massive hemorrhage. The nurse must assess the gastric drainage carefully for signs of bright red or partially digested blood. It is vital that the nasogastric tube be operating properly to avoid distention.

Too much food or eating foods that are not recommended will usually cause the patient immediate discomfort. This syndrome is called *dumping*. Symptoms of dumping include palpitation, sweating, faintness, excessive weakness, and diarrhea or vomiting. Symptoms of shock also can occur. Small, frequent, dry meals (without liquids) usually lessen this problem. Antispasmodic drugs also help. Foods most likely to cause dumping are those high in carbohydrates and electrolytes, especially salt. Chinese food containing monosodium glutamate is often particularly irritating.

Evisceration (protrusion of abdominal contents out of the body through the suture line) is a possible, although rare, complication following any abdominal surgery. Should it occur, the physician must be consulted. Immediate first aid consists of applying a large sterile compress soaked in saline. Sterile technique must be observed. The nurse should *never* attempt to push the abdominal contents back into the abdomen.

Some patients, especially those who have had a vagotomy, are susceptible to diarrhea, which may become chronic. Treatment is symptomatic.

Other complications specific to a gastrectomy include a leaking anastamosis (the place where the two ends of the digestive system are joined together), indicated by an increase in body temperature and *edema*. *Regurgitation* also may be caused by an obstruction.

Neoplasms

Cancer of the Stomach

The treatment of cancer of the stomach (the "silent neoplasm") usually involves surgery to completely remove the stomach and join the esophagus to the jejunum (total gastrectomy). If the tumor is small, only part of the stomach may be removed.

The most important symptom is sudden dyspepsia (indigestion) not relieved by eating. In addition, there is unexplained weight loss and general weakness. "Coffee-ground" emesis and absence of free hydrochloric acid in the stomach are other significant signs (see Table 81-2). Microscopic examination of gastric contents may show cancer cells, while other routine laboratory and x-ray studies confirm the presence of a neoplasm and its exact location.

Gastrectomy for Stomach Cancer. Removal of the entire stomach is called *total gastrectomy;* removal of part of it is called *subtotal gastrectomy*. Because metastasis to the spleen is a common occurrence, it is usually removed as well. The prognosis is often not good because metastasis has usually occurred before the cancer is discovered.

Nursing Considerations. Nursing care for subtotal gastrectomy is essentially the same as that for peptic ulcer. However, total gastrectomy requires the following differences:

◆ Because the chest cavity must be opened, procedures similar to those following any chest surgery must be carried out (see Chapter 79). This includes management of chest tubes and chest suction.
◆ Drainage from the nasogastric tube is small. *(Rationale: This drainage normally comes from stomach secretions.)*
◆ Malnutrition may cause anemia or other deficiency disorders. Vitamins and minerals are usually supplemented; vitamin B_{12} must be given for life. *(Rationale: The stomach is no longer present to secrete the "intrinsic factor" necessary to metabolize vitamin B_{12} from foods.)*
◆ The patient is instructed to increase gradually the amount of food eaten at one time until three meals a day are tolerable.
◆ The patient should plan regular rest periods. *(Rationale: To prevent overexertion.)*
◆ Regular medical follow-up is essential.

Disorders of the Small or Large Bowel

Structural Disorders

Diverticulosis and Diverticulitis

Diverticulosis refers to outpouching (diverticula) along the intestine. It is asymptomatic (without symptoms). **Diverticulitis** means inflammation of these outpouchings, usually due to impaction of fecal materials. Symptoms of diverticulitis are nagging pain, usually in the left lower quadrant, and temperature elevation. A barium enema can confirm the presence of diverticula.

Stool softeners, enemas, and bulk-forming agents, such as psylliun (Metamucil), help to provide a soft, nonirritating, and unforced bowel movement. When fever and abdominal pain are present, indicating infection along with inflammation, antibiotics are prescribed. A low-residue diet, including avoidance of milk products, is recommended.

When active diverticulitis has been resolved, the patient should begin adding high-fiber foods to the diet and continue using the bulking agents. Adequate water intake of six to eight glasses each day is considered important. Regular bowel habits, including regular exercise and plenty of fruit, vegetables, and fiber, are key to preventing future problems for people with diverticulosis.

Abdominal Hernia

An *abdominal hernia* is a protrusion of the intestine through the abdominal wall; the layman's name for this condition is *rupture* (Fig. 81-8). The abdominal wall is weak in spots, and it is at these points that a hernia can develop. Often it is possible to push the intestine back by lying down and pressing on the abdomen, thus *reducing* the hernia.

Types of Hernia. Congenital defects are responsible for a large number of hernias; thus, a hernia may be seen in an infant. An acquired hernia may be the result of heavy lifting, pregnancy, coughing, or sneezing. Later in life, obesity and muscle weakness may be the cause. The most common types of hernia are *incisional* (in the incisional area following surgery), *inguinal* (through the inguinal area in the groin, especially in males), *femoral* (into the femoral canal that carries blood vessels and nerves into the thigh), and *umbilical* (through the umbilicus).

Signs and Symptoms. The symptoms of hernia vary, depending on the location. Some hernias are asymptomatic, although if untreated, they often become larger and cause pain. If the condition is allowed to progress, the intestine often becomes constricted, and the blood supply is cut off. This is a *strangulated hernia,* a possibly fatal condition that requires emergency surgery.

Treatment. A hernia can usually be repaired by surgery (*herniorrhaphy*). Hernia repair is likely to be neglected because a hernia is often not a painful condition, and the person puts up with the discomfort. If it has gone untreated for many years, the traditional repair may not hold, because the tissues are weakened and will not heal easily. In this case, a *hernioplasty* may be done. This reconstructive repair includes reinforcement with mesh. Herniorrhaphy can now be done using the laporoscope after inflation (insufflation) of the abdomen with carbon dioxide. The patient will only have two or three small "stab wounds" instead of an abdominal incision.

Nursing Considerations. Usually nursing care in herniorrhaphy is not complicated; the patient is allowed out of bed the day of the operation and can have food and fluids. In some cases, this procedure is done on an outpatient basis. In a male, the scrotum may become swollen and painful after inguinal hernia repair, and an ice pack and a suspensory support may be ordered for relief. The patient is taught that some discomfort is the result of the CO_2 insufflation and will dissipate quickly. A warm shower or pack to the abdomen may help.

Every precaution is taken to avoid sneezing or coughing postoperatively, and the patient is instructed to press a hand firmly over the area of the incision or the hernia when sneezing or coughing. This is to prevent the sudden movement and pressure from causing recurrence of the hernia. The patient is encouraged to move around but to avoid straining and lifting for several months. The bed should be adjusted to its lowest position to avoid strain when the patient gets out of bed. Recovery after laparoscopic surgery, especially if mesh reinforcement was used, is faster.

When the patient returns to work depends on the nature and extent of the hernia, age and weight, and the type of work the patient does. If the work is heavy or strenuous, vocational counseling and retraining might be needed. (If a repair with mesh has been done, the person will most likely *not* have any long-term lifting restrictions.) A referral to the local public health nursing service and the state Division of Vocational Services may be helpful.

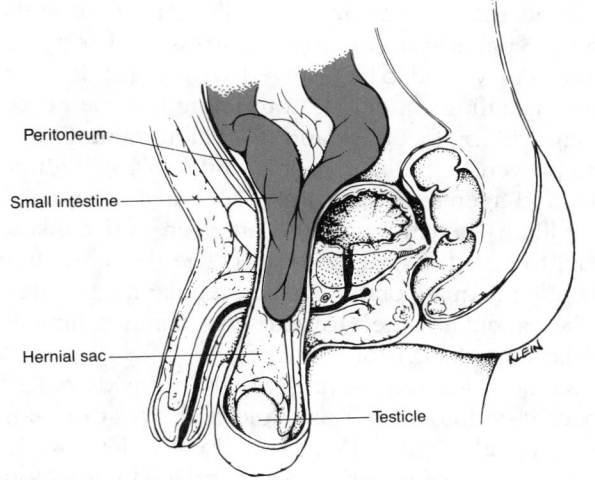

Peritoneum

Small intestine

Hernial sac

Testicle

Figure 81-8. Inguinal hernia. Note that the sac of the hernia is a continuation of the peritoneum of the abdomen and that the hernial contents are intestine, omentum, or other abdominal contents that pass through the hernial opening into the hernial sac. Smelter SC, Bare BG. Brunner and Suddarth's Textbook of Medical-Surgical Nursing. Ed 7. Philadelphia, J.B. Lippincott, 1992.

Intestinal Obstruction

Ileus is obstruction of the intestine. The obstruction may be due to a mechanical or chemical difficulty and occurs when gas or fluid cannot move through the bowel normally. A mechanical obstruction can be caused by *adhesions* (scars from previous surgery), *volvulus* (twisting of the bowel), a foreign body in the bowel (such as a fruit pit), *intussusception* (telescoping of the bowel), muscle spasm (spastic ileus), edema, a strangulated hernia, fecal impaction, or a tumor. A vascular obstruction, such as atherosclerosis, also can cause gradual cessation of peristalsis because of decreased blood supply.

A tumor in the intestine becomes larger, finally blocking the passage. If the obstruction is high in the GI tract, the patient will vomit. This is nature's way of emptying the stomach of accumulated digestive fluids. As these materials continue to accumulate, the vomitus becomes thick, dark, and foul smelling because the number of bacteria normally present in the digestive tract increases. If the obstruction is further down, vomiting may be absent; the patient becomes dehydrated and is unable to take fluids by mouth.

Paralytic obstruction (paralytic ileus) is caused by a decrease or interruption of the nerve stimulus to the intestine and may result from postanesthesia paralysis, trauma to the autonomic nervous system, complications from peritonitis, inactivity, large doses of narcotics, or other nerve damage.

The accompanying Nursing Care Plan uses the nursing process in caring for a patient with small bowel obstruction.

Signs and Symptoms. Symptoms of intestinal obstruction include severe cramping pain, nausea and vomiting (the emesis may contain fecal material), listlessness and general weakness, thirst, distention and a feeling of fullness, constipation, severe halitosis, and a foul taste in the mouth. Repeated vomiting of food eaten the day before is a strong indication of an obstruction. If not treated, the patient will become very ill, with symptoms of dehydration and shock. The symptoms of *small* bowel obstruction develop and progress rapidly; those of *large* bowel obstruction progress more slowly.

Treatment. Blockage may be partial or complete. Complete obstruction in the small intestine usually necessitates surgery; obstruction in the lower part of the large intestine may be treated medically. Treatment of the obstruction will depend on what is causing the obstruction. Medical treatment includes *intestinal decompression,* involving intubation (with a nasogastric tube) and constant suction to keep the intestine empty and allow the bowel to rest.

Nursing Considerations. The nurse assists with replacement of fluids, electrolytes, intravenous glucose, and con-

stant monitoring. If the condition deteriorates, emergency surgery becomes necessary. Postoperative nursing care follows the protocol for abdominal surgery.

Nursing Alert

An intestinal obstruction can be an emergency and must be treated *immediately*.

Chronic Disorders

Irritable Bowel Syndrome

Spastic colon, spastic colitis, mucous colitis, and *irritable colon* are terms patients have been given for what is medically known as *irritable bowel syndrome* (IBS). This condition is the most common GI complaint seen by the family physician. IBS is a functional, not pathologic, disorder of the small or large intestine. The disorder affects the structure of the intestine, but the specific cause is not known. IBS does *not* lead to or cause ulcerative colitis or cancer.

Signs and Symptoms. This disorder in motility of the intestine causes alternately tense and flaccid segments of bowel. The resulting symptoms are abdominal pain, cramps, flatulence (gas), constipation, or diarrhea. The symptoms will vary in intensity and pattern for each patient. Tests such as the upper GI series, barium enema, and sigmoidoscopy help to diagnose IBS. These tests also eliminate other pathology with similar symptoms.

Treatment. Patients must be willing to explore their lifestyle patterns and emotional stressors. Lifestyle situations may need to be changed to manage this chronic and frustrating condition. Counseling may be needed, along with biofeedback and relaxation training, which has proven helpful for people with IBD. A high-fiber diet and agents that add bulk (such as Metamucil, Effersyllium) help to promote an even and consistent stool to pass through the bowel. The diet also should include adequate oral fluids and regular meal patterns. If the patient is subject to lactose intolerance, limitation of dairy products is often helpful.

Medications may be prescribed to provide relief for specific symptoms. For example, sedatives or tranquilizers (eg, alprazolam [Xanax]) help to quiet bowel activity and relax the patient. Dicyclomine hydrochloride (Bentyl) is an antispasmodic drug that can relieve pain and cramping symptoms if used routinely during periods of increased bowel irritability. Common side effects are dry mouth, blurred vision, and dizziness. Some patients do require occasional antidiarrheal agents, such as loperamide (Imodium), to help them maintain normal activity. Some stressful or even happy events can

Mr. Antanapolis is a 71-year-old white married man admitted to the hospital with the diagnosis "R/O (rule out) small bowel obstruction." For several days prior to being hospitalized he experienced nausea and vomiting, abdominal distention, and abdominal pain. On physical examination, a massive prominent gastric bubble was noted, suggestive of partial small bowel obstruction. His admission orders included the following: NPO, Salem sump to low Gomco suction, CT scan in A.M., colonoscopy, and orders for IV fluids. Surgery will be done if his condition does not stabilize quickly. This is the first hospital admission for Mr. Antanapolis. Two of the nursing diagnoses developed for his plan of care follow.

Nursing Diagnosis: *Fluid Volume Deficit Related to Nausea and Vomiting (Decreased Fluid Intake) as Evidenced by Increased Serum Sodium Levels, Dry Mouth, and Dry Skin*

Goal 1: Patient's IV fluid intake is 2,400 mL daily.

Goal 2: By the third hospital day, the patient's fluid output approximately equals the fluid intake.

Goal 3: By the third hospital day, the signs of dehydration are decreased or absent: serum sodium levels return to normal limits; mouth and skin regain moisture.

Goal 4: Patient will be stabilized if surgery is required.

Nursing Actions (assess/do/teach)	Rationale	Evaluative Statement
1. Monitor VS every hour until stable and fluid intake and output every shift; assess for signs of fluid and electrolyte imbalance. Daily weight.	This helps detect quickly a worsening of fluid volume deficit.	7/5, All goals are met; fluid output averages 2,200 mL daily; decreased signs of fluid deficit.
2. Administer IV fluids as ordered: $D_5 \frac{1}{2}$ NS $\bar{c}$ 30 mEq KCl @ 100 mL/h.	This rehydrates and compensates for deficient oral intake.	Electrolyte levels WNL (within normal limits).
3. Offer frequent mouth care.	These are comfort measures.	
4. Offer frequent skin care.		

Nursing Diagnosis: *Knowledge Deficit Regarding Diagnostic Tests Related to no Prior Experience With Hospitalization and Testing*

Goal 1: When questioned, the patient can explain the nature and purpose of the scheduled diagnostic test; what he can expect by way of preparation, experience during the test, and aftercare; and ultimately what has been learned from the test.

Goal 2: The client verbalizes any questions or fears he has about the diagnostic procedure.

(continued)

trigger unwanted symptoms that would keep patients homebound without medication.

Nursing Considerations. Remind the patient to be consistent and willing to follow his or her prescribed treatment plan closely. Too often, these patients get so discouraged by seemingly slow improvement or small setbacks that they never allow the bowel to establish a more normal pattern. Keeping a log or diary can be helpful in tracking progress or identifying needed treatment plan changes.

Nursing Alert

Rectal bleeding and fever are not associated symptoms of IBS. Such presenting symptoms should be reported to a physician for evaluation.

Nursing Actions (assess/do/teach)	Rationale	Evaluative Statement
1. Determine what the patient knows about a diagnostic procedure before initiating teaching; clarify any misperceptions, and respond to specific fears and concerns (see p. 624).	Teaching can then be individualized; patient senses that he is valued as an individual.	7/4, Goal 1 partially met; patient still confused about some tests (eg, CT scan) and sees no need for so many "machines"; basically understands what is happening, however.
2. When the patient demonstrates "readiness" for learning (not overly anxious, in pain, sleepy, etc.), explain the nature and purpose of the proposed study and what he can expect by way of preparation, actual experience, and aftercare; be sure to allow time to respond to his questions. Give written information.	Knowledge empowers the patient to participate better in the plan of care.	7/6, Goal met; patient openly questions staff about his care and voices fears (and anger!).
3. Make the time to explain the results of diagnostic procedures in language he understands, and relate these results to the treatment he is receiving.	This gives the patient a sense of control over the experience.	

Chronic or Acute Constipation

Constipation is a condition in which the patient has infrequent, hard bowel movements accompanied by mucus. The patient may have a fecal impaction with diarrhea around it. This condition may be caused by cancer, chemical dependency, or mechanical obstruction. It also may be a psychosomatic disorder.

The patient should be encouraged to drink a great deal of fluids, take prune juice or eat bran, increase the amount of bulk in the diet, exercise, and follow a regular schedule for defecation. Everyone should be educated to evacuate the bowel when they feel the urge. Postponing the act desensitizes the bowel to the presence of feces.

Because prolonged constipation can be a sign of serious difficulty, such as intestinal obstruction or paralytic ileus, immediate action is needed to determine the cause. The patient should be warned not to strain while having a stool. The patient also should be encouraged to avoid worrying about constipation because undue concern can lead to further inability to defecate.

Diarrhea

Signs and Symptoms. Many patients complain of diarrhea, in which stools are liquid or semiliquid, very light colored, foul-smelling, and accompanied by severe stomach cramps and much flatus. Stools may contain undigested food and mucus. The person often experiences severe anal cramps or spasms (*tenesmus*). If chronic and not self-limiting, diarrhea symptoms must be evaluated for possible causes (particularly before the patient self-medicates). A bacterial infection and IBD should be ruled out. Often, the cause points to IBS, which was discussed previously in this chapter.

The nurse assesses the patient's intake and output and weight. Electrolyte levels should be monitored because diarrhea can severely disrupt electrolyte balance. Record the exact time, amount, and character (TAC) of each stool. The patient's diet may be restricted to clear liquids and then advanced slowly to observe for improvement or worsening. (*Note:* When diarrhea continually awakens a patient from normal sleep, this often indicates intestinal pathology.) Medications are listed in the accompanying box.

Special Considerations in Children
Giardiasis

Giardiasis, caused by the protozoan *Giardia lamblia*, is commonly associated with contaminated water or food. Day-care centers have had outbreaks associated with poor handwashing between diaper changes and children sharing toys that have been in their mouths. Symptoms may be mild or severe with nonbloody diarrhea, abdominal pain, and distention most often present. Metronidazole (Flagyl) for adults and furazolidine (Furoxone) for children are the usual antibiotic treatments. The entire family or day care may need stool testing to completely irradicate *Giardia* infection.

Inflammatory Disorders

Inflammatory Bowel Disease

IBD is a general term for the diseases sometimes known as ulcerative colitis and Crohn's disease. *Ulcerative colitis* is the inflammation and ulceration of the lining of the colon. (When localized to the rectum, it is called *ulcerative proctitis*.) Chronic ulcerative colitis (CUC) implies long-standing disease. The risk of colon cancer increases if CUC lasts longer than 8 to 10 years. *Crohn's disease* can occur in any part of the intestinal tract. Unlike colitis, it involves inflammatory processes of the entire thickness of the bowel wall. It is usually patchy and often skips over segments of healthy bowel. The risk of cancer in Crohn's is the same as that of the general population.

Signs and Symptoms. Typical symptoms of ulcerative colitis and Crohn's disease are diarrhea, blood and mucus in the stool, abdominal pain, cramps, bowel incontinence, loss of appetite, weight loss, fever, nausea, and vomiting. Electrolyte imbalance may result from loss of body fluids. Symptoms may develop gradually or suddenly. Patterns of exacerbation (attacks) and remission can be expected for most patients.

Research suggests that environmental, immunologic, hereditary, age, and cultural factors may influence this disease. However, the cause and cure of IBD are unknown.

Complications. In ulcerative colitis and Crohn's, bowel obstruction and perforation are threats. They may be caused by scar tissue or a **fistula** (abnormal channeling between loops of bowel) and are the most serious outcome of these diseases. Perforation is an emergency. Results include hemorrhage and peritonitis; removal of the colon and permanent ileostomy are often required. Symptoms of perforation include rapid, thready pulse; extreme anxiety; severe abdominal pain; fever; abdominal rigidity (boardlike); and cold, clammy skin. Symptoms of peritonitis are discussed later in this chapter in relation to appendicitis.

Treatment. The patient who presents with severe symptoms is weak, miserable, and often frightened by the seriousness of the illness. Nursing care and medical management are aimed at optimal bowel rest. The patient is NPO or limited to clear liquids. TPN is often used, and oral supplements may be given. Advances in medical treatment allow most patients to manage and cope with their disease.

Medications. Steroids (such as cortisone), which reduce inflammation and generate healing, are given intravenously, orally (tablets), or rectally (foam, suppositories, or enema). Sulfasalazine (Azulfidine) is the most commonly used drug to treat IBD, especially ulcerative colitis. It is composed of sulfa and aspirin-like salicylate. The problematic common side effect of sulfa intolerance (headache, rash, and depressed white blood cell count) has been helped by the introduction of 5-amino salicylic acid (5-ASA) drugs, such as Asacol, olsalazine Na (Dipentum), and Pentasa. The sulfa has been removed and replaced by other carrier agents to deliver the active ingredient, 5-ASA, to the colon where it is absorbed and activated. *Mercaptopurine* (Purinethol) is a potent immunosuppressent drug that is useful in treating fistulas. Close monitoring of blood count and clinical condition is necessary with this drug. Intravenous antibiotics may be indicated during severe flare-up. Antidiarrheal medication can be helpful to allow the patient to maintain normal work and daily activity patterns.

Nursing Alert

Patients are weaned off steroid medications slowly and systematically and must be told not to stop them suddenly. Steroids suppress normal secretions of the adrenal gland, and abrupt discontinuation can trigger life-threatening adrenal insufficiency problems. Milder withdrawal symptoms of yawning, goose flesh, and muscle aches and pains are often reported by patients during weaning. See Chapter 56 for side effects of steroids.

Surgery. Approximately two-thirds of Crohn's patients require surgery, and 40% of these require a second surgery. This is due to the typical recurrence of Crohn's disease. Ulcerative colitis, on the other hand, is eliminated by removal of the entire colon, which is the treatment of choice when surgery is needed. The standard ileostomy allows fecal waste to be collected in an appliance attached to the abdomen. Care of the ileostomy is discussed earlier in this chapter.

For some IBD patients and patients with noninvasive cancer of the colon, a procedure called the *ileoanal reservoir* has been effective. This has not been effective in Crohn's. The ileoanal reservoir is the surgical creation of a pouch fashioned from the small intestine that collects ileal drainage. One type is called the Parks S pouch (shaped like an S) or the Parks J pouch (shaped like a J). The Parks procedures are usually done in two stages; if the patient is quite ill, three stages may be done. In stage 1, the entire colon and lining of the rectum are removed, and the reservoir is fashioned. The anal sphincter is retained, and the reservoir (pouch) is sewn to it. A temporary ileostomy is done. The patient then eliminates stool through the ileostomy stoma for 6 weeks to 3 months, and the bowel is rested. The stage 2 surgery is the take-down of the ileostomy. The Parks pouch acts as the sigmoid colon, and the patient usually achieves sphincter control. The ileoanal reservoir procedure requires a longer recuperation time than the standard ileostomy but greatly improves the quality of life for patients in whom it can be used. The person will pass stool four to eight times in 24 hours and does not have a permanent stoma.

Another procedure, called the *Kock pouch* or the *continent ileostomy,* is often more acceptable than the standard ileostomy. In the Kock procedure, the colon, rectum, and anus are removed. A permanent ileostomy is done, and an internal abdominal reservoir is fashioned from about 45 cm of the small intestine. This reservoir is attached to the ileostomy and collects the stool. A one-way nipple valve is created with the ileal tissue and a flush (flat) stoma is present on the abdominal wall. Postoperatively, the pouch is catheterized and irrigated with 20 to 50 mL of normal saline every 2 hours. The returns flow out by gravity. The skin around the stoma and the tube are checked several times daily and dressings changed. The catheter must be securely anchored. This procedure is usually not possible if the patient is obese, high-risk, or has Crohn's disease, toxic megacolon, diabetes mellitus, or active colitis. The patient is usually able to achieve the same continence as with a colostomy by periodic catheterization and wearing a small absorbent patch.

Complications of either internal pouch procedure include stool seepage and *pouchitis* (inflammation of the pouch).

In another procedure, *total colectomy with ileorectal anastamosis*, the colon is removed, and the ileum is sewn to the rectum. The patient eliminates stool through the anus. There is, however, a risk of cancer in the retained rectum. Stools usually number three to eight daily. In other cases, the ileum is sewn directly to the anus. In this case, continence may not be as good, but still there is no stoma.

Surgery for unperforated Crohn's disease is often necessary, but removal of diseased bowel is not usually a cure. This is because Crohn's disease often recurs in another segment of bowel. The risk of cancer follows the incidence figures of the normal population, however.

Nursing Considerations. The prescribed diet for the person with IBD will probably be low-residue and lactose-restricted to help prevent recurrence. Some patients do well on a regular diet. Recent studies have shown that IBD patients do not show significantly more emotional illness than normal, thus dispelling a common misconception. However, emotional stress can aggravate and stimulate the physical symptoms. The nurse must be sensitive and supportive to help the patient cope with the disease-related stressors: symptoms, diagnostic tests, bowel preparation, dietary restrictions, activity limitations, and medication side effects.

Appendicitis

The appendix is a slender blind tube, approximately 10 cm (4 inches) long, which opens off the tip of the cecum. Nobody knows why it is there. It may become obstructed by a hard mass of feces with subsequent inflammation, infection, gangrene, and possible perforation. A ruptured appendix is serious because intestinal contents can escape into the abdomen and cause peritonitis or an abscess.

Signs and Symptoms. An acute attack of appendicitis usually begins with progressively severe generalized pain in the abdomen, which later localizes as pain and tenderness in the lower right quadrant midway between the umbilicus and the crest of the ilium (Mc-Burney's point). *Rebound tenderness* usually is present; that is, when the abdomen is palpated, the pain is greater when the pressure is released quickly than when the examiner pushes down. The quality of the tenderness is related to the exact location of the appendix. Usually the pain is accompanied by fever, nausea, vomiting, and an increase in white blood cells—a sign of resistance to infection. Ultrasound can often diagnose an enlarged appendix. An attack of appendicitis may subside and recur.

Treatment. Prompt surgical treatment is necessary to remove the appendix before it ruptures. A newer trend toward minimally invasive surgery techniques, such as *laparoscopic appendectomy,* have given the patient the advantage of decreased chance of wound infection, smaller incisions, and shorter recovery periods. In most instances, the patient recovers rapidly and is permitted fluids and food and allowed out of bed soon after the operation. The patient may go back to work in 10 to 15 days with cautions to avoid heavy lifting.

If the appendix has ruptured, treatment for peritonitis is necessary. This includes an incisional drainage tube and large doses of intravenous antibiotics. This is a serious and possibly fatal complication. However, modern treatment with suction devices, irrigation of the peritoneum, intravenous fluids, and antibiotics has greatly reduced the danger.

Nursing Considerations. Many people mistake abdominal pain, nausea, and vomiting as a temporary intestinal upset. Everyone should be taught what to do and especially what *not* to do for severe abdominal pain (see accompanying box).

Peritonitis

Peritonitis is inflammation of the peritoneum, the membrane that lines the abdominal cavity and covers the abdominal organs. In the upper abdomen, peritonitis is usually the result of a perforation of the intestine or appendix, by which intestinal contents escape into the abdomen. Because the intestinal tract is normally filled with bacteria, the resulting perforation may cause inflammation and infection of the peritoneum.

The most common causes of perforation are appendicitis, ulcer, IBD, abscessed diverticula, and cancer. Pelvic peritonitis may be due to an infected uterine tube, a ruptured tubal pregnancy, or a ruptured uterus.

Keys to Patient/Family Teaching
Actions To Take in Severe Abdominal Pain

Patient and family teaching should include the following:

◆ Do not take an enema or a cathartic. *(Rationale: They increase peristalsis, and the result may be a perforated appendix and peritonitis.)* If an enema is ordered as a preoperative measure, it must be given low and very slowly.
◆ Do not take anything by mouth, not even water.
◆ Call a physician for any attack of severe pain or for pain that persists.
◆ Do not apply heat to the abdomen. *(Rationale: Heat could spread infection.)*
◆ Do not take Aspirin or any other analgesic. *(Rationale: They tend to mask symptoms. Aspirin and ibuprofen are anticoagulants.)*

Peritonitis may be generalized, extending throughout the peritoneum, or it may be localized as an abscess.

Signs and Symptoms. Peritonitis often develops suddenly, with severe abdominal pain; nausea and vomiting; a gradual rise in temperature; a weak, rapid pulse; and low blood pressure. The patient's respirations are shallow because breathing hurts the abdomen; the patient tries to avoid moving the abdomen, drawing the knees up to prevent pressure from the bedclothes and to relieve the pain. The abdomen is tense and boardlike and becomes very distended. Flatus and intestinal contents are stationary in the intestinal tract, and paralytic ileus may develop. If the infection does not respond to treatment, the patient grows weaker. The pulse is thready, breathing becomes more shallow, temperature falls, and death follows.

Treatment. Surgery is sometimes necessary to close the perforation and promote drainage, although the perforation may close by itself. During surgery, the peritoneum is irrigated, usually with a saline and antibiotic solution.

Nursing Considerations. Postoperative treatment centers on the following:

◆ Replacing fluids and electrolytes and fighting infection by administering massive doses of antibiotics
◆ Analgesics to relieve pain and provide rest
◆ Elevating the head of the bed (Fowler's position). *(Rationale: To promote drainage.)*
◆ Monitoring a drain (wick) or abdominal drainage tube, which is connected to a portable wound suction or an electric suction machine

◆ Closely observing pulse and temperature. *(Rationale: To assess for infection.)*
◆ Documenting incisional drainage (amount, type), vomiting, drainage through the GI tube, intake and output of fluids, and gas and feces passing through the rectum
◆ Preventing abdominal distention using a rectal or a nasogastric tube *(Rationale: Excess distention is uncomfortable and can disrupt the suture line or cause other difficulties from pressure.)*
◆ Giving special attention to mouth care because the patient has no fluids by mouth *(Rationale: Fever and the GI tube make the mouth dry and parched.)*
◆ Using siderails. *(Rationale: To prevent falls.)*
◆ Proceeding carefully with all care *(Rationale: The least movement, touching, or jarring of the bed intensifies pain.)*

Peritonitis is less common today, and recovery is more likely, largely due to improvements in surgery and the use of antibiotics.

Neoplasms

Cancer of the Small Intestine

Cancer can occur anywhere in the intestinal tract, although it rarely occurs in the small intestine. If a cancer does occur in the small intestine, the prognosis is usually poor because the disease is difficult to discover in the early stage. There are usually no symptoms in the early stages. As the cancer advances, pain may be present. The patient may have diarrhea (with or without blood), anorexia, nausea, and vomiting. Perforation or obstruction may occur.

The portion of the bowel containing the tumor may be removed and the ends of the bowel joined. Such rejoining, or *reanastamosis,* is not possible if the malignancy is extensive. Suction relieves distention, intravenous fluids are given, and antibiotics may be prescribed. Postoperative nursing care is routine.

Cancer of the Colon

Colon cancer is believed to arise from a single polypoid lesion. Early detection requires surveillance for polyps. The American Cancer Society recommends screening procedures in an effort to locate polyps and thus prevent colon cancer. These are presented in the accompanying box.

TNM Staging for Colon Cancer.[1] Staging of the tumor (stage of the disease) is necessary for the physician to

[1] Some material in this section is adapted from "Cancer of the Colon and Rectum: Research Report," U.S. Dept of Health and Human Service, NIH Publication #92-95, 1991.

American Cancer Society Recommendations for Colorectal Cancer Screening

◆ Digital examination after the age of 40
◆ Fecal occult blood test annually for anyone over the age of 50
◆ Flexible sigmoidoscopy every 3 to 5 years for people over the age of 50
◆ For people with a family history of colorectal cancer, an examination of the entire colon by colonoscopy or an x-ray technique of double contrast barium enema every 5 years starting at age 35 or 40
◆ Anyone with previous malignant or adenomatous polyps removed from their colon, colonoscopy every 3 to 5 years

plan treatment. Because there are several different staging systems, the actual number may vary slightly, but the theory is the same (as the numbers increase, the cancer has become more invasive and life-threatening). One example is TNM staging:

T: Tumor size
N: (lymph) Node involvement
M: (presence of) Metastasis

Stages of colon cancer and common treatment measures are presented in Table 81-3. Treatment depends on staging of the cancer and on the age and general health of the patient.

Patients also are encouraged to participate in clinical trials of newer therapies. Treatment consists of surgery, chemotherapy, radiation, biologic therapy, or combinations of these (see Chapter 76).

Surgery. Types of surgery include *local excision* (removal of a small polyp or cancerous area using endoscopy), removal of a cancerous segment and reanastamosis (sewing the ends back together), *wedge resection* (removing only a small amount of bowel), and *bowel resection* (removing a larger portion of the bowel). A temporary or permanent *colostomy* also may be required.

Chemotherapy and Other Therapies. Chemotherapy is systemic treatment given orally or parenterally, including injection directly into the tumor.

Three chemotherapeutic agents, 5-fluorouracil (5-FU), leucovorin (folinic acid), and interferon, are becoming accepted protocol for colon cancers, especially those of stage I and II. 5-FU or related compound, such as floxuridine (5-FU deoxyribonucleoside), is often used in combination with other drugs to increase its effectiveness. Leucovorin, a form of folic acid, enhances the ability of 5-FU to kill cancer cells and reduces unwanted side effects of 5-FU. In some cases, the drug is

Table 81-3. Staging of Colon Cancer

Stage	Description	Common Treatment
Stage 0, carcinoma in situ (Dukes' A colon cancer)	• Very early, superficial, only in innermost lining of colon (mucosa); not spread to submucosa (where blood and lymph vessels are located)	• Local excision • Wedge resection • Polypectomy
Stage I (Dukes' B_1 colon cancer)	• Spread to second or third layers of colon, involves inside wall of colon; has not spread through outer wall of colon or outside colon; *or* • Penetrates all layers of bowel wall, with or without invasion of adjacent tissues; has not spread into lymph nodes	• Bowel resection, may be combined with chemotherapy
Stage II (Dukes' B_2 colon cancer)	• Spread outside colon to nearby tissue but *not* to lymph nodes	• Bowel resection with chemotherapy or radiation or with chemotherapy and biologicals
Stage III (Dukes' C colon cancer)	• Spread to nearby (regional) lymph nodes but not to other parts of body; *or* • Extends to nearby tissues without spread to lymph nodes	• Bowel resection with chemotherapy • Clinical trials evaluate other protocols, including radiation combined with interhepatic injection of chemotherapeutic agents
Stage IV (Dukes' D colon cancer)	• Cancer has spread to other organs of body (distant sites); most commonly liver and lungs	• Bowel resection (may be palliative to relieve pain or allow passage of stool) • Surgery to remove metastases • Radiation, chemotherapy, clinical trials

given for 7 days, then stopped for 21 days, and the cycle repeated. In other cases, the regimen seems to be more effective if it is continuous.

Other chemotherapeutic agents used include the following:

♦ Interleukin-2 (IL-2), used to stimulate growth of lymphocytes. The lymphocytes are removed from the patient's body or from the tumor itself and are treated with IL-2. They are then reinjected into the patient, along with more IL-2.
♦ Biologic response modifiers. These biologics improve the body's normal responses to foreign invaders, including cancers. One is *levamisole,* which stimulates the immune system.

Other therapies include radiation, internal or external. Adjuvent therapy is often given; medications are used to kill cancer cells that were undetectable.

Follow-up Tests to Determine Effectiveness of Chemotherapy for Colon Cancer. There are two major tests for tumor markers specific for colon cancer. These tests are not diagnostic for undiagnosed cancer but can help to evaluate the response of colon cancer to treatment. Usually, the tumor markers are high before treatment and then fall after treatment. If a repeat assay shows a rise later, this may indicate a recurrence of the cancer. These tumor markers may be high also in people without cancer, especially in smokers and those with noncancerous growths or imflammation of the digestive tract. Tumor markers used to evaluate therapy for colon cancer follow:

♦ *Carcinoembryonic antigen assay* (CEA assay)— should be found only in minute amounts in the healthy adult
♦ *Carbohydrate antigen 19-9* (CA 19-9)

Disorders of the Sigmoid Colon and Rectum

Structural Disorders

Hemorrhoids

Hemorrhoids are swollen (varicose) veins of the anus or rectum. External hemorrhoids protrude as lumps around the anus (Fig. 81-9). They are painful, especially if the patient is constipated and is in the habit of straining to have a bowel movement. They may alternately appear and disappear. Usually, external hemorrhoids do not bleed, but they may become large, painful, and itchy. The pressure of the uterus on the rectum during pregnancy, intra-abdominal tumors, constipation and diarrhea, obesity, congestive heart failure, and portal hypertension are the major causes of hemorrhoids.

Signs and Symptoms. Internal hemorrhoids develop inside the anal sphincter; they may bleed but are less likely to be painful if they do not protrude. Signs of bleeding may be no more than a drop of blood on the toilet paper, or bleeding may be so extensive and continuous that it causes anemia. Internal hemorrhoids almost always protrude with defecation, but at first they can be pushed back with the finger. As they grow larger, this is no longer possible, and they discharge blood and mucus. Bleeding is one of the signs of cancer, and this symptom should never be ignored. The analscope makes it possible to inspect the inside of the rectum; in this way, the hemorrhoids can be visualized and a biopsy taken.

Treatment. Sometimes hemorrhoids disappear without treatment. Often they can be relieved by warm sitz baths, anesthetic ointments, or witch hazel compresses (Tucks). It is important to keep the stools soft by proper diet and stool softeners. Correcting constipation may prevent and eliminate hemorrhoids.

If surgery is necessary, the veins are tied off and excised (*hemorrhoidectomy*) or are cauterized. Sometimes a solution is injected to shrink (sclerose) the tissues. Occasionally, hemorrhoidectomy must be done as an emergency procedure if the hemorrhoid is thrombosed, causing vascular obstruction. This is not a life-threatening situation; surgery is done to relieve pain.

Nursing Considerations. The patient takes a cleansing enema at home the night before surgery, and enemas are given "until clear" the morning of the operation. The rectal area is cleansed and may be shaved, in addition to other prescribed routines.

When the patient returns from the operating room, positioning on the side or abdomen will help relieve pressure on the operative area. Analgesics are given for pain. A liquid diet is permitted for the first meal after the operation; thereafter, a full diet is allowed.

The patient is allowed to sit up. This is painful, and a rubber ring or flotation pad under the buttocks helps relieve pressure on the operative area. It is necessary for the patient to move as soon as possible to prevent complications postoperatively. On the operative day or the next day, the physician will want the patient to ambulate.

Several daily sitz baths may be ordered. The patient must have assistance when getting in and out of the tub. The heat of the bath may make the person feel faint. The patient stays in the bath for 20 minutes, with the temperature of the water at 110°F (43.3°C). It is best if the water is circulating (see specific procedure in Chapter 49).

Because removal of hemorrhoids involves excision of portions of blood vessels, bleeding may occur. The nurse must assess for signs of bleeding, either on the dressings or as indicated by symptoms of faintness, weakness, lowered blood pressure, or other signs of shock.

Special care is needed to assist with the first bowel movement following any rectal surgery. The patient is naturally apprehensive. The nurse should explain that stool softeners are given to make the bowel movement easier. There will be some pain but probably much less than imagined. Encourage the patient to heed the urge to defecate; otherwise, constipation may develop. Toi-

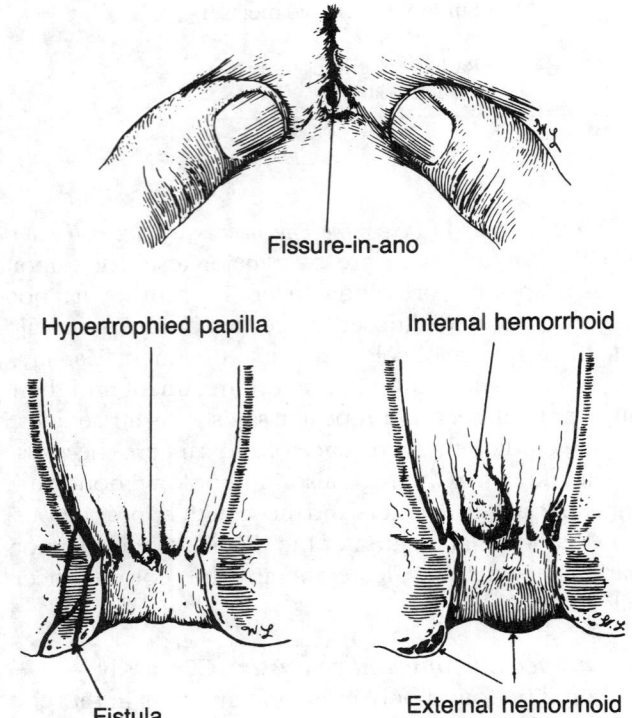

Fissure-in-ano

Hypertrophied papilla

Internal hemorrhoid

Fistula

External hemorrhoid

Figure 81-9. Various types of anal lesions.

let paper should not be used because it may damage the suture line. "Tucks" (pads impregnated with witch hazel) are often used to cleanse and soothe the anal area and to relieve itching. Petrolatum applied around the rectal area when moist compresses are being used helps maintain elasticity and integrity of the skin. If the patient is unable to defecate by the second postoperative day, this should be reported to the physician. If defecation has not occurred by the third day, an enema will probably be ordered.

Because the surgery was performed in close proximity to the urinary structures, anesthesia or manipulation may make it difficult to void. If the patient does not void, distention could cause complications and discomfort, and catheterization will be needed.

> ### Key Concept
>
> If the patient goes home early, these procedures must be part of patient or family teaching.

Anal Abscess and Anal Fistula

Infection of the tissues around the rectal area causes anal abscess. This condition is painful and may be accompanied by fever and chills. The abscess is usually incised and drained, or it may rupture spontaneously. An anal abscess may form an *anal* **fistula**, a small tunnel in the tissues that discharges pus and feces through one or more openings onto the skin (see Fig. 81-9). Surgery is necessary to open the fistulous tract; it is then packed with gauze to keep the edges of the wound apart. This allows the tissues to heal by granulation and thus eliminates the fistula. The fistula must heal from the *inside out,* or another abscess will form.

In general, the nursing care for an anal fistula is similar to that for any patient after rectal surgery, with the following differences. The fistula wound is packed with petroleum gauze, which is changed every day. The drainage from the abscess is profuse, purulent and foul smelling. The gauze dressing on the wound and cellucotton pads need to be changed frequently. Dressings must be disposed of properly and gloves worn to prevent the spread of disease. The fistula must be kept draining; if it stops draining before the entire area is filled in with granulation tissue, another abscess has formed.

Anal Fissure

An *anal fissure* is an ulcer in the skin of the anal wall (see Fig. 81-9). It causes severe pain on defecation and sometimes slight bleeding. The patient may dread the pain so much that defecation is delayed, and the person becomes constipated. Sitz baths and local anesthetic ointments are commonly used to treat anal fissure; a stool softener also helps. The only cure for this condition is surgical removal of the ulcer.

Pilonidal Cyst (Pilonidal Sinus Tract)

A **pilonidal cyst** is common in males and often exists for many years without causing any trouble. It is a closed fistula, usually containing hair follicles. It is located in the lower sacral or perineal area. If it becomes infected and opens and drains, it is surgically excised. There are often several sinus tracts, all of which must be excised. In many cases, the area of incision is large and must heal by granulation (from the inside out). Postoperative management is aimed at the prevention of pain by proper and careful positioning, sitz baths, and analgesic medications. Early ambulation is encouraged to prevent complications. Because pilonidal cysts may recur, the operation may need to be repeated.

Neoplasms

Cancer of the Rectum

If the cancerous growth is in the upper part of the rectum, it can be removed without removing the rectal sphincter, so ultimately the bowel will continue to function normally. If the tumor involves the rectal opening, a dual operation is necessary through the abdomen from above (including a colostomy) and through the perineum from below. This second type of surgery is called an *abdominal-perineal resection.*

With surgical staplers and other newer instruments, some surgeons have had success retaining the rectal sphincter and doing a low resection and anastamosis to eliminate the need for a permanent colostomy.

Nursing care for this patient is extensive. Vital signs must be carefully assessed. Dressings must be checked for bleeding at regular intervals. The danger of shock following this surgery is great. Care often includes caring for a colostomy, administering parenteral fluids (including blood transfusion), nasogastric suctioning, caring for bladder drainage (a Foley catheter is usually inserted in the bladder), and irrigating and caring for drainage from the perineal wound. The patient must be turned frequently to prevent respiratory complications and thrombophlebitis, and it is difficult to find a comfortable position. If the condition permits, the patient should be encouraged to ambulate as soon as possible postoperatively, usually within 2 days. The recovery is much faster if the patient ambulates soon. Assistance will be needed to accomplish this.

Disorders of the Liver

The liver is the largest, most vascular, and busiest organ in the body. It is responsible for the metabolism of carbohydrates, proteins, fats, and steroids. It stores many important vitamins, such as vitamins A, the B complexes, and E. Prothrombin and fibrinogen are produced in the liver and are needed to clot blood. Detoxification of foreign and toxic substances is a unique function of the liver.

Signs and Symptoms. *Jaundice* results from an excessive concentration of bile salts in the bloodstream, which causes a yellow discoloration of the tissues. Anything that interferes with the work of the liver or obstructs the flow of bile into the intestines causes bilirubin to accumulate, and jaundice is a sign of the increased bilirubin in the blood (bilirubinemia). This yellow discoloration of the tissue is particularly noticeable in the whites of the eyes. Jaundiced skin is easily observed in the white or African American patient, but it is difficult to detect in Asian Americans. A deficit of bile in the intestines interferes with fat digestion, causing the stools to float and to appear pale and fatty and have a disagreeable odor. The bile salts that have escaped into the tissues make the skin itch; the urine is dark. Treatment depends on the cause of jaundice.

Liver failure (hepatic coma), characterized by tremors and mental changes, including stupor or coma, is serious. It may occur after massive GI hemorrhage, as a complication of some surgical procedures, after massive infections, and following an overdose of certain drugs. It also occurs in the patient with cirrhosis. Treatment of liver failure is symptomatic, including control of bleeding, a low-protein diet, and careful management of the fluid and electrolyte balance. Antibiotics may be given, and in some cases, adrenocortical (steroid) drugs. The prognosis is guarded, and the possibility of successful treatment decreases with each episode.

Nursing Considerations. Because jaundice and liver failure are signs of a liver disorder, general nursing care addresses these situations. The accompanying box gives general nursing skills when caring for any patient with a liver disorder.

Chronic Disorders

Cirrhosis

In cirrhosis, the normal architecture of the liver is destroyed until ultimately the liver can no longer do its work. In an effort to repair itself, the liver may become so enlarged (*hepatomegaly*) that the blood vessels serving it become obstructed. This leads to indigestion, vomiting of blood, blood in the stool, constipation, fluid in the abdomen (*ascites*), and an enlarged spleen. Esophageal varices may develop—an extremely dangerous condition.

Alcoholism is blamed in more than half the cases of cirrhosis in the United States. Drinking leads to poor eating habits, and good nutrition is essential for keep-

> ### Nursing Skill Guidelines
> #### Caring for the Person With a Liver Disorder
>
> ◆ Use starch baths, calamine lotion, and tepid sponging for relief from itching.
> ◆ Place calamine lotion and cotton at the bedside, so the patient can apply lotion to spots that itch. (*Rationale: Pruritus is a common symptom in liver disorders.*)
> ◆ Assess for signs of blood in the stools and urine or on the toothbrush when the patient brushes the teeth. Look for black-and-blue marks. (*Rationale: These are signs of a bleeding disorder, a common complication of liver disease.*)
> ◆ Exert pressure on the puncture site for a longer time than is usual after the needle is withdrawn after an intravenous procedure. (*Rationale: This prevents a hematoma that would ooze blood and make it impossible to use the vein again. This is important, because people with liver conditions need frequent blood tests.*) A central line or heparin lock is often in place. (Pressure is applied to the site of an intramuscular injection as well.)
> ◆ Provide support and explanation concerning jaundice. (*Rationale: The sense of self-worth can be impaired because of the patient's yellow appearance.*)

ing the liver working properly. However, doctors are puzzled to find that alcoholics who are adequately nourished also have cirrhosis; the exact cause of cirrhosis is not known. Cirrhosis is more prevalent among men than women and occurs most often in people 45 to 65 years of age. Cirrhosis can be caused by drugs or toxins and by certain general anesthetics. Viral hepatitis also can lead to cirrhosis. Whatever the cause, liver disease is increasing in frequency. It may be that the increased use of certain antibiotic drugs is partly responsible. These drugs must be excreted by the liver, and the added burden may be more than it can carry.

Diagnosis. Diagnosis of cirrhosis is made on the basis of symptoms; damage is evaluated in terms of circulatory disturbances, disturbances in bile drainage, and actual damage to the functioning liver cells as measured by laboratory tests.

Signs and Symptoms. Cirrhosis may develop so gradually that the patient may not realize that anything is wrong or may not have any signs of the disease. The patient may not be aware of a low-grade fever or notice a loss of weight because the weight loss is offset by an increase in abdominal girth (circumference). This is caused by *ascites,* an abnormal accumulation of fluid in the peritoneal cavity. As the disease advances, the fever increases, the patient has abdominal pain, the pulse becomes rapid, and breathing becomes difficult because of the enlarged abdomen. The patient tends to bleed easily. Blood appears in vomitus or as a nosebleed, and veins are dilated because of portal hypertension. The patient is jaundiced, and the skin is dry. The patient feels weak, mentally dull, and confused. Hemorrhaging and infection may develop.

Esophageal varices often rupture, causing massive *hematemesis* (bloody emesis). The body's defenses are reduced, and the patient is more susceptible to infection. Uncontrolled cirrhosis may result in hepatic coma.

Treatment. Treatment for cirrhosis of the liver is aimed at helping the liver repair itself.

Treatment extends over a long period. In the patient with liver failure, at least 2 months are needed before improvements can be noted. With careful attention to diet and the omission of alcohol or other toxic substances, the cirrhosis patient may live for many years.

Nursing Considerations. Frequent mouth and skin care must be given. Emollient baths may be ordered to reduce pruritus (itching) and to soothe the skin. Blood transfusions are given to combat anemia. A transfusion of concentrated human serum albumin is often administered.

The diet is high in vitamins, moderate in carbohydrates and fats, and low in sodium; the amount of protein depends on the functional level of the liver. If these essential nutrients are not supplied, the body burns up its store of protein, thus increasing the accumulation of ammonia (a waste product) in the blood. Alcohol, tobacco, and fatty foods (pork, bacon, gravies, pastries) are omitted. Small liquid or semisolid meals are given frequently. This is more appealing to a person with a poor appetite. The diet is often supplemented with multivitamins and vitamin B_{12}. Vitamin K (usually intramuscularly) is given to reduce the risk of hemorrhage. Watch for bleeding following an injection.

Diuretics and reduced sodium intake are ordered. Daily weights and accurate intake and output indicate if the liver is functioning. Daily abdominal girth measurements are often ordered. The patient should be positioned in semi-Fowler's position to aid breathing. Good skin care and other nursing measures to reduce itching are vital (see Chapters 64 and 68).

Great care should be taken to prevent complications associated with bed rest, such as pneumonia and thrombophlebitis. Paracentesis (aspiration of fluid from the abdomen with a large syringe and needle) may be necessary to relieve ascites.

Fulminent Hepatic Failure

Fulminent hepatic failure involves progressive multisystem failure resulting from massive liver cell death. Patients are confused, somnolent, or comatose and usu-

ally have ascites, edema, coagopathy (clotting disorder), and a shrinking liver. The mortality rate is high, and care is supportive.

Hepatic Encephalopathy

Hepatic encephalopathy (hepatic coma) is a complication of chronic liver disease caused by the accumulation of ammonia in the brain tissue. There are several progressive stages, starting with mild confusion, aberrant behavior, motor dysfunction, and finally a complete lack of response to stimuli. The goal of treatment is to stop or delay the progression of symptoms.

These patients need much attention and monitoring. Restricting dietary protein and maintaining electrolyte balance will help lower ammonia levels. *Lactulose* (Cephulac) will promote ammonia retention and excretion through the GI tract. Providing a safe and controlled environment will prolong and stabilize their condition. Alcohol avoidance is a must.

Inflammatory Disorders

Hepatitis

Hepatitis is an acute or chronic condition of liver inflammation that also may be accompanied by liver tissue damage. Viruses are the most prevalent cause of hepatitis, affecting several hundreds of millions of people throughout the world. In the last decade, the knowledge of hepatitis has expanded, as has the ability to identify serologically (with blood tests) the distinct and unrelated human viruses causing most hepatitis. Alcohol, some drugs, and some autoimmune conditions cause some forms of hepatitis. There are at least five main types of viral hepatitis: hepatitis A (HAV, formerly called "infectious hepatitis"), hepatitis B (HBV formerly called "serum hepatitis"), hepatitis C (HCV, formerly called "parenterally non-A, non-B hepatitis"), hepatitis D (HDV), and hepatitis E (HEV). Some of the less frequent viruses that case hepatitis-like symptoms are Epstein-Barr virus, cytomegalovirus, rubella, rubeola, herpes simplex viruses, varicella zoster virus, and mumps virus.

The symptoms of hepatitis are varied and are often subtle; this makes diagnosis and prevention difficult. Common presenting signs and symptoms are listed in the accompanying box.

Hepatitis A

HAV is the most common form of viral hepatitis. It is spread by the fecal–oral route and transmitted by contaminated food, water, or infected food handlers. Oral–anal sexual practices also can transmit the virus. It primarily affects children and young adults. This disease is attributed to poor sanitation, crowded conditions, and difficulty in recognizing carriers of the disease.

Common Presenting Signs and Symptoms of Hepatitis

- ◆ Fatigue and lethargy
- ◆ Nausea (sometimes vomiting and diarrhea)
- ◆ Loss of appetite
- ◆ Abdominal pain
- ◆ Joint and muscle aches
- ◆ Mild fever (more common in hepatitis A)
- ◆ Malaise (generalized feeling and complaint of illness)
- ◆ Jaundice
- ◆ Liver enlargement (hepatomegaly)
- ◆ Dark urine

In HAV, the greatest excretion of the virus occurs before jaundice is apparent. As the disease runs its course and jaundice appears, the person becomes less infectious. Thus, the patient may have unknowingly spread the disease to other people. A person who has been exposed may be given immune serum globulin as a prophylactic measure; this is effective against HAV.

Generally the patient is noninfectious approximately 1 month after having become ill. A person may harbor the virus without actually having the clinical disease. No adequate protection against carriers is known. Patients generally recover fully in 4 to 6 weeks with rest and supportive care. They acquire a life-long immunity to HAV infection and do not develop chronic hepatitis.

Hepatitis B

HBV is transmitted by three mechanisms: percutaneous transmission by way of infected blood, blood products, or instruments; sexual transmission in semen or saliva; or perinatal transmission from infected mother to her child at birth. Individuals at risk of exposure to HBV include intravenous drug users who share needles, sexually active homosexuals, patients receiving hemodialysis, patients of mental institutions, and infants of women who are HBV carriers. Healthcare workers are at significant risk. Universal Precautions must be followed religiously and rigorously by healthcare workers to protect themselves against viral hepatitis. The Centers for Disease Control and Prevention (CDC) has recommended preexposure HBV vaccination for people working in medical, dental, laboratory, and associated groups that have increased risk of exposure to blood and blood products. The synthetic vaccinations, *Recombivax-B or Engerix-B*, are given in three intramuscular injections at 0, 1, and 6 months. A blood test confirms the presence of antibodies. If the vaccine recipient does not produce antibodies, one booster may be given. If antibodies are still not formed,

the person is classified as a "non-reactor." A significant percentage of healthy people are non-reactors; the reason is unknown. Many institutions are providing these vaccinations for their "at-risk" healthcare workers free of charge.

Becase the incubation period of HBV is from 60 to 110 days, it is often difficult to trace the exact source of the disease. The acute symptoms of HBV are more clinically severe and longer lasting than HAV, although they may include any of those listed in the previous section. Recovery and resolution of HBV infection occurs in all but approximately 17% of infected people. Overwhelming acute HBV infection and liver tissue damage can progress to fulminent hepatic failure and death within weeks of clinical onset. Also, a small percentage (5%–10%) of people do not clear the virus from their blood within 6 months and become chronic carriers of HBV. Persistent HBV infection also increases one's risk of liver cancer.

Hepatitis C

The primary cause of parenterally transmitted non-A, non-B hepatitis has been seriologically distinguished as HCV. Patients, such as hemophiliacs who require blood and blood products and intravenous drug users are at greatest risk of HCV infection. After the incubation of the virus for 35 to 70 days, the clinical manifestations of HCV are again typical of the other viral hepatitis infections.

Often the symptoms are mild enough to be overlooked by the patient, and medical intervention is not immediately sought. However, 50% of these patients later present with chronic disease, and of those, 20% will develop cirrhosis of the liver. Half of all people newly infected with HCV will become lifetime carriers of the virus.

Hepatocellular carcinoma also is associated with HCV. *Interferon alfa-2b* (Intron), an antiviral medication, and steroid drugs are used to ease symptoms and slow the progression of chronic hepatitis. These patients are often good candidates for liver transplants.

Hepatitis D

Only individuals infected with HBV can contract HDV as a coinfection or a suprainfection (at the same time). The severity seems to be related to the severity and virulence of the HBV infection. Interferon is helping those who have developed the chronic form of HDV. Transmission, expected recovery outcomes, and prevention are the same as for HBV.

Drug-Induced or Toxic Hepatitis

Liver injury can result from ingestion or exposure to certain known or unknown drugs, chemicals, or fumes. The liver tissue is damaged, or the chemical collects in the body and the liver cannot excrete it. These events may cause no symptoms other than elevated liver function tests or the patients may demonstrate fully developing fulminent hepatic failure. The liver has great regenerating ability, and treatment is focused on clearing the offending agent. Supportive rest and care while monitoring liver function and electrolyte balance are necessary.

> **Special Considerations in Children**
> ### Overdose on Acetaminophen
> Patients who overdose on *acetaminophen* (Tylenol) are at risk for fulminent hepatic failure. Small children who accidentally ingest even a few tablets could have significant problems. Appropriate therapy should be activated within 24 hours of ingestion.

Hepatitis E
Althrough HEV has not been identified in the United States, it is epidemic and sporadic in places such as India, Pakistan, Mexico, and Peru, all of which have poor water and sanitation systems. World travel must be undertaken with a clear understanding of the prevailing conditions and the necessary precautions for safe and healthy travel. The physician should be alerted if a patient with symptoms reports international travel in suspect countries. The mode of transmission is fecal–oral and HEV resembles HAV in symptom presentation and clinical course. Recovery is usually complete, and lifetime immunity to HEV occurs. There is a high mortality in infected pregnant women, however.

Nursing Considerations. Treatment and nursing care are similar for all forms of viral and nonviral hepatitis. Supportive care emphasizes bed rest and avoidance of any strenuous physical activity during the acute phase of infection and presenting symptoms, especially when jaundice, abdominal discomfort, and abnormal liver tests are present.

The elderly or those who develop ascites or encephalopathy may require in-hospital management. This treatment includes a nutritionally balanced diet, intravenous hydration, and electrolyte management. Injections of vitamin K and fresh frozen plasma may be beneficial. Medications are used sparingly, and alcohol is avoided completely.

Overexertion must be avoided when the patient begins to feel better. Too much activity too soon is likely to bring on a recurrence of symptoms. This may be a boring time, especially if the person was active before the illness. Helping the patient to gain knowledge of liver disease and understanding of their particular virus infection will help them to consider possible consequences and lifestyle changes. This can be a frightening

or enlightening time for these patients. Supportive listening is an effective tool to help patients recover from hepatitis.

Care must be taken when handling rectal thermometers, bedpans, or the feces of a person with viral hepatitis. Gloves should always be worn. Universal Precautions must be closely observed when caring for these patients.

The patient should be warned never to donate blood if they have ever had an HBV infection. *(Rationale: The virus can be present in the blood and body fluids for an entire lifetime.)*

Liver Abscess
Liver abscesses are caused by the spread of infection from some part of the intestinal tract, perhaps from the appendix or gallbladder, or by obstruction of the bile tracts. The symptoms of liver abscess are chills, a temperature that fluctuates (intermittent fever), extreme loss of weight, nausea and vomiting, abdominal distention, and right-sided pain in the abdomen and shoulder. Jaundice is frequent. Pain over the liver is a later symptom. If the abscess bursts, it scatters infection through the abdominal or chest cavity. Antibiotics are given, and the outcome depends on how successful the person is at combatting the infection. Sometimes an attempt is made to establish drainage by surgery. Universal Body Substance Precautions help to prevent the spread of infections.

Trauma

Frequently, the liver is injured in an accident. Extensive damage is likely to be fatal, and the patient may die from hemorrhage before reaching the hospital. Sometimes surgery is necessary to control bleeding or to remove a portion of the damaged liver. One great danger accompanying liver surgery is shock, because the liver is such a vascular organ. Nursing care includes careful monitoring of vital signs and assisting in treating shock. Careful sterile technique is used to prevent infection. The nurse should observe the color of the wound drainage for indications of bile or blood; either could indicate a rupture of the suture line. Many patients with a ruptured liver die.

Neoplasms

Cancer of the Liver
The liver is rarely the site of a primary cancer; more often cancer of the liver is *metastatic*. A cancer that does begin in the liver can be removed surgically by removing the affected part of the liver. If cancer is due to metastasis, surgery is not indicated; the patient usually is treated palliatively with radiation or chemother-

apy (antineoplastic drugs may be infused directly into the liver—intrahepatic).

Liver Transplantation

Life-threatening liver diseases have been treated with liver transplants. The success of this technique is related closely to the body's acceptance of a foreign organ, technical difficulties, the hazards of immunosuppression, and the availability of a well-functioning liver for transplantation. Further discussion of liver transplantation is beyond the scope of this book.

Gallbladder Disorders

The gallbladder lies on the undersurface of the liver. It is the storage reservoir for bile, which the liver manufactures. Fat digestion cannot take place without bile.

Inflammatory Disorders

Cholecystitis and Cholelithiasis

Two common forms of gallbladder disease are inflammation of the gallbladder (**cholecystitis**) and gallstones (**cholelithiasis**). Cholecystitis and cholelithiasis often occur together, and each aggravates the other. The stones may block the duct that leads from the gallbladder. The stones may injure the wall, leading to infection. Bacterial contamination of bile often develops and is the cause of serious complications. The most likely victims of gallbladder disease are obese women older than age 45. Frequent pregnancies also seem to make women more susceptible. Asian Americans seldom have cholecystitis or cholelithiasis.

The cause of gallstones (calculi) is unknown. Formation of most gallstones is believed to be due to abnormally thick bile, which is high in cholesterol and low in bile acids. The gallbladder absorbs water, causing the bile to change into *crystals,* then *sludge,* and then *gallstones.* Some gallstones also have a calcium base; they are harder than cholesterol-based stones.

Sometimes the infected gallbladder fills with pus (*empyema of the gallbladder*) and may rupture, causing peritonitis. Chronic gallbladder disease also may permanently damage the liver.

Signs and Symptoms. The symptoms of cholecystitis or cholelithiasis include the following:

◆ Indigestion, due to lack of bile. The patient complains of feeling "full" after eating. Fatty foods make this condition worse.
◆ Light-colored stools, due to lack of bile pigment. The stools float in the toilet because they contain fat (which is normally broken down by bile) and

are foul smelling. Stools are accompanied by excessive flatus.
◆ Fever and malaise
◆ Jaundice (yellowing of the sclera), caused by stones obstructing the bile passages or by a spasm of the common bile duct. Bile backs up in the gallbladder; the liver stops manufacturing bile, and the bilirubin it would normally use in this process goes into the bloodstream. Very dark urine coexists with jaundice for this reason.
◆ Gallstone colic, a sharp pain over the gallbladder, which sometimes extends to the back or to the right shoulder. The pain usually comes on suddenly a few hours after a heavy meal when the gallbladder is trying to contract to send bile into the intestine to help digest the food. If this effort forces a stone into the cystic duct, the pain is excruciating. Usually, the patient vomits, which causes further distress instead of relief. If gallstones (*calculi*) are small, a person may be only slightly uncomfortable, or he or she may never feel any pain.

> ### Key Concept
> Some patients describe the pain of gallstone colic as the feeling of a "huge bubble" in the upper abdomen or chest area. It is important to differentiate between gallstone colic and the chest pain related to heart attack.

Medical Treatment. The diet is restricted to nonfatty foods. Such foods as cheese, cream, greasy fried foods, fatty meats, and gas-forming vegetables are not given. The patient may have lean meat (never fried), plain mashed or baked potato, or rice. Alcoholic beverages are contraindicated.

Immediately after an attack, the patient is given liquids only. If the attack is severe, meperidine (Demerol) may be given. Morphine should not be used, because it is believed to increase the spasms.

In some cases, drugs may be effective in dissolving cholesterol-based gallstones. Chenodiol (Chenix) has been used for several years. A new drug, ursodiol (Actigall), is a naturally occurring bile acid that is taken orally and dissolves noncalcium stones by diluting the thick bile that is present.

> ### Nursing Alert
> Strenuous dieting and rapid weight loss can precipitate a gallbladder attack or the formation of stones. The lack of fat in the diet causes the bile to pool in the gallbladder because it is not needed for fat digestion.

Surgical Treatment. Cholecystectomy is often done through a laparoscope. The gallbladder is excised by laser and removed through the scope. Recovery is usually fast following this procedure.

Surgical procedures include *cholecystostomy* (opening and draining the gallbladder), *cholecystectomy* (removal of the gallbladder), *choledochostomy* (incision into the common bile duct), and *choledocholithotomy* (incision into the duct and removal of calculi).

Nursing Considerations. The nurse assists with various diagnostic and x-ray tests. The patient may receive vitamin K, either orally or deep intramuscularly, or blood transfusions to promote blood clotting and maintain the blood and hemoglobin levels. If the patient is unable to eat, intravenous fluids or total parenteral nutrition will be used. It is necessary to get the patient into as good physical condition as possible. Other preoperative preparations are as for other abdominal procedures. It is especially important to tell the patient about the tubes and drains that will often be in place postoperatively.

Postoperative nursing care in cholecystectomy depends on what surgical approach is used. If abdominal laparotomy is done, nursing care is essentially the same as for any major surgical procedure, except that care for bile drainage from the wound is necessary. The patient is expected to turn, deep breathe, and use the incentive spirometer to prevent pneumonia. If the patient is congested, the nurse helps with gentle coughing by placing the hands firmly on either side of the incision, making a "splint."

A nasogastric tube is often in place to empty the stomach immediately postoperatively. Many surgeons place a tube into the wound for drainage following surgery. Others allow the ducts to readjust and take over bile drainage spontaneously. If the patient has a drainage tube (most often a T-tube), the physician may order the drainage bag to be kept at floor level for a short time to allow for the release of excess bile. Later, the bag is raised. The level of the container is noted on the Kardex or nursing care plan, and the patient is gradually "weaned" from the drainage tube. The amount and character of the bile should be measured and recorded every 24 hours. If the amount does not diminish in a few days, it may be an indication that the bile is not beginning to enter the intestine properly. (*Note:* The patient may go home with the T-tube in place. The nurse must teach the patient clamping procedures and what to watch for before discharge. Document all teaching.)

Teach the patient to maintain low Fowler's position to facilitate drainage. Monitor the tube closely to prevent blockage or dislodgement of the T-tube. After the T-tube has drained for 24 hours, it may be clamped for 1 to 2 days before it is removed. The patient must watch for signs of jaundice or discomfort when the tube is clamped or removed. The skin surrounding the tube should be protected with zinc oxide or petrolatum. The stools and urine of the postoperative patient should be observed for the presence or absence of bile. The bile should disappear, and the stools and urine should become normal in color and consistency as function returns. Accurate fluid intake and output also are documented.

Most physicians order a regular diet, as tolerated, after surgery. Most patients have no trouble digesting a small amount of fat. Generally, the patient who has had gallbladder surgery should avoid foods that caused preoperative discomfort. Gas-forming foods and alcohol are avoided. The patient may be referred to a dietician for counseling.

Common Bile Duct Obstruction

A patient may retain or develop biliary stones that block bile flow within the common bile duct. This may even occur following a cholecystectomy (removal of the gallbladder). The patient with a common bile duct obstruction is very ill. The person complains of severe abdominal pain, nausea, and vomiting. On examination, other symptoms include fever, jaundice, elevated white blood count, or elevated liver and pancreatic enzymes.

The endoscopy procedure ERCP is commonly done to diagnose the condition. (This procedure is described earlier in this chapter.) If the stone is small, the sphincter (the opening to the intestine from the gallbladder, liver, and pancreas) is cut to enlarge the opening (*sphincterotomy*). This will facilitate the passage of the stone. Surgical intervention is indicated if this cannot be accomplished by ERCP with sphincterotomy.

The patient's condition must be assessed carefully after an ERCP with sphincterotomy. Routine vital signs, intravenous hydration, intravenous antibiotics, and follow-up laboratory work are important for the next 12 to 24 hours. Pain intensity and effective response to analgesics must be monitored closely. Pancreatitis and hemorrhage are the most common complications.

Neoplasms

Cancer of the Gallbladder

Early cancer of the gallbladder is not easily detected. Symptoms are similar to those in cholecystitis. Surgery might be tried, but because the liver is often invaded as well, prognosis is usually poor. More women than men develop cancer of the gallbladder.

Disorders of the Pancreas

Inflammatory Disorders

Pancreatitis

The pancreas, a gland immediately behind the stomach, secretes pancreatic juice, which aids digestion. The pancreas also contains the islets of Langerhans, groups of cells that secrete the hormone insulin. (Disorders of this portion of the pancreas are discussed in Chapter 72.) Normally, bile does not enter the pancreas; if it does, pancreatitis may develop. This process destroys pancreatic tissue and leads to hemorrhages, edema, and severe pain. Pancreatitis is also caused by pancreatic enzymes being secreted directly into the pancreas, rather than into the duodenum. It also may be caused by a gallstone that travels backward in the duct. Analgesics are ordered to relieve pain and spasm. The prescribed diet is low in fat and high in protein and carbohydrates. If the islets of Langerhans are affected, treatment for diabetes mellitus is also necessary. If stomach distress is severe, a nasogastric tube may be inserted, and the patient may be given intravenous fluids or TPN. Rest and freedom from emotional strain and upsets are important. Because the pain is so intense, narcotics may be given.

Neoplasms

Cancer of the Pancreas

Tumors of the pancreas are usually malignant. Cancer of the body or the tail of the pancreas is usually not detected until metastasis has occurred. The prognosis is poor. In addition to other symptoms of biliary obstruction, jaundice is sometimes the first symptom of cancer of the pancreas. The only hope of cure is to remove the cancerous growth. ERCP can diagnose the presence and specific location of a tumor in the head or tail of the pancreas. This is helpful preoperative information for the surgeon.

Before the operation, attention is concentrated on building up the patient's resistance. The patient might need to gain weight, but the appetite is usually poor. Total parenteral nutrition is now frequently used to restore nutritional deficits.

After surgery (*pancreatectomy*), the patient must be maintained with insulin and digestive enzymes.

Conditions of Overnutrition and Undernutrition

Obesity

Charts of "desirable weight" are available, usually from insurance companies. They list desirable weights in relation to height, bone structure, sex, and age. The ideal percentage of body fat in an adult male is 20%; in an adult female, the percentage is 25%. A person exceeding this amount is *overfat*. Some people, such as athletes, may be *overweight* (exceeding the figures on the chart), but the weight may be from muscle tissue and not excess fat. Therefore, they are not overfat. The percentage of fat is estimated by using calipers to measure skin fold thickness or is measured directly by weighing the person underwater on a special scale.

Obesity is the condition of being overfat. If a person is 20% over the ideal weight, he or she is said to be **obese.** *Morbid* or *massive* obesity exists when a person is many pounds overweight (frequently identified as 100 lb [55 kg]) or twice normal weight.

Complications

Obesity contributes to many physical disorders. The person runs a greater than normal risk of having circulatory disorders, such as arteriosclerosis, atherosclerosis, hypertension, heart attack, or stroke; diabetes mellitus (four times the rate than for people of normal weight); and general respiratory difficulties, ranging from shortness of breath and dyspnea to actual lung pathology. The obese person often suffers from musculoskeletal disorders and is more susceptible to contagious diseases. Hyperlipidemia (excess fat in the blood) develops, and fat is deposited in the liver, causing liver damage. Dermatitis in moist skin folds, chafing, excessive perspiration, and heat intolerance are associated problems.

Causes

Obesity occurs when the number of calories taken into the body exceeds the number of calories expended on physical activity by the body. Eating the wrong types of foods, especially fats, and emotional stress factors contribute to this unbalance. Obesity usually occurs with time, and successful weight loss also takes time.

Treatment

If a physical cause for the obesity is found, it is treated. A nutritionally sound diet and exercise program are planned. The patient must be seen at regular intervals to be sure that the weight loss and new eating patterns are being maintained and that no other physical problems develop. Any person wishing to lose a large amount of weight should do so under a physician's supervision.

Nursing Alert

Weight loss programs requiring ingestion of large amounts of water may be dangerous to the person with glaucoma (it may increase intraocular pressure) or certain kidney or liver disorders. The nursing mother should not be on a drastic weight loss program because toxins and pollutants, which are stored in fat tissue, can pass to the baby.

Weight Loss Programs

Various diets and group counseling systems (such as Weight Watchers or a weight loss center) are available. One of these may be all a person needs to reach and maintain a sensible body weight. If this is not successful, the patient may seek medical assistance. Many physicians prescribe a diet, but the morbidly obese person needs much emotional support as well. Guidelines for nursing care of obese patients in the hospital are presented in the accompanying box.

Key Concept

Most diet recommendations include *reduction of fat* in the diet. It is believed that controlling fat gram intake is more important and leads to more permanent weight loss than "counting calories." Many obese people try "crash diets," but the problem with these is that the person does not change long-term eating habits. After the diet is stopped, the weight is usually regained. This "yo-yo" effect of fast weight loss and immediate weight gain can be almost as dangerous as the original obesity. Patient reeducation is vital in the long-term maintenance of weight lost.

The Bariatric Clinic

Bariatric clinics, under the direction of a physician, have been established to help people lose weight or maintain weight. The nurse has a role in this type of clinic. Various medical and nursing procedures are performed when the patient first seeks assistance. A complete physical examination is done, which includes an electrocardiogram at rest and after exercise, a phonocardiogram (a graphic record of heart sounds), weight, height, blood pressure, photographs from side and front, a complete metabolic function test, a complete laboratory workup, liver function test, a complete visual test, and pulmonary function tests. Certain body measurements are taken, such as body girth and skin fold thickness. These form a baseline for treatment. The patient and spouse often benefit from counseling if a large amount of weight is to be lost.

Surgical Treatment

Surgery may be performed in cases of extreme obesity that are resistant to all other forms of treatment. The most common procedure is gastric partitioning or stapling, in which the stomach volume is reduced by 90%. In-depth teaching and pre- and postoperative counseling is required for this patient. The person must understand the added surgical risk and must alter eating patterns, or the weight will be regained.

Life-Threatening Eating Disorders

Obesity is an eating disorder that results in excess weight. Two other eating disorders usually result in severe underweight and often cause functional malnutrition. Anorexia nervosa and bulimia often begin during

---

Nursing Skill Guidelines
Caring for the Hospitalized Obese Patient

- Two gowns may be needed, one forward and one backward. Help the patient tie the gown.
- One hospital bed may not be large enough; securely tie two beds together and place the mattresses crosswise. Keep the beds in low position and the siderails up at the "foot" of the bed.
- An overbed trapeze helps the patient to move in bed. The person may need to sit up to breathe. Blocks may be placed under the head of the bed, because the gatch mechanism is not appropriate. If the person is in one bed, he or she may be too heavy to lift if a crank-style bed is used or the electric gatch may not work.
- When assisting the patient to get up, get help if needed. (*Rationale: You will not be able to support the patient alone.*) *Always* use a transfer belt; you can join two together if needed.
- Put the bed in a position so the feet just touch the floor. (*Rationale: If it is too high, the patient may fall; if it is too low, the patient may not be able to stand up.*)
- Have the patient wear rubber-soled shoes (not slippers); assist the person to tie the shoes.
- Use a heavy-duty walker, wheelchair, or litter. A commode or wheelchair with removable arms may be needed. (*Rationale: This will allow the patient to fit.*)
- A mirror may be needed so the person can see the feet when walking.
- Assist the person with personal care; dressing alone may be impossible. The patient may not be able to comb the hair. (*Rationale: Because of the weight of the arm.*)
- Skin care is particularly important in skin folds and perineum. (*Rationale: The patient often cannot reach to do self-care, and chafing is common.*)
- A shower is usually safer than a bath in the tub; help the patient to sit in the shower.
- Use a large enough blood pressure cuff, and keep the cuff at the bedside to ensure consistency.
- Use longer needles for intramuscular injections.
- Use a bedpan rather than a specimen bottle for urine specimens. (*Rationale: The person will not be able to place the bottle.*)
- If the apical pulse is difficult to hear, use the cone side of the stethoscope, and mark the chest at the optimum location.
- Consider the self-esteem needs of the person. Accentuate the person's achievements and skills.

---

the adolescent years and are most common in women. They are briefly discussed in Chapter 66.

Anorexia Nervosa. Anorexia nervosa is characterized by a self-imposed starvation. No physiologic cause has been found. The person (95% are young females) believes that she is fat, when actually she is very thin, often to the point of emaciation. The major physical problem becomes one of malnutrition, along with electrolyte imbalances. However, other conditions, such as dental caries, muscle wasting, slow pulse and hypotension, blotchy skin, loss of hair (alopecia) or abnormal hair growth (hirsutism), and susceptibility to infections also are common. Anorectic women almost always experience amenorrhea (absence of menses). The person may be hyperactive, even though she is undernourished. The mortality rate is from 5% to 15%, usually caused by circulatory collapse or cardiac failure secondary to the electrolyte imbalances.

Bulimia. It is estimated that approximately one-third of all anorectic patients become bulimic. Bulimia is known as the "binge" syndrome. The bulimic person may either binge (gorge with food) or binge–purge. In the binge–purge form of the disorder, the bulimic eats thousands of calories at one sitting and then in an effort to avoid weight gain, purges her body of the food, either by self-induced vomiting or by excessive doses of laxatives. The nonpurging bulimic is obese. The person who binges and purges is extremely thin, often to the point of starvation. As in anorexia nervosa, a high percentage of these people are young women.

Signs and Symptoms

Symptoms and conditions common to anorexia nervosa and bulimia follow:

- Higher incidence of depression, obesity, and chemical dependency in the family than in the general population
- Overprotective parents with rigid rules and high expectations
- Usually very good students and school leaders
- Feeling of helplessness or being out of control, yet manipulative behavior
- Intense fear of becoming "fat"
- Inaccurate self-image
- Low self-esteem, but unrealistically high goals

- Often great weight loss in a short time with no physical disorder
- Electrolyte imbalances (see Chapter 69)
- Hiding or hoarding of food
- Preoccupation with food or gourmet cooking
- "Playing" with food; moving it around on the plate without eating it
- Shyness about eating with others
- Secretive behavior
- Going to the bathroom immediately after each meal
- Spending of a great deal of time locked in the bathroom
- Going to various physicians, requesting prescriptions for vague physical complaints
- Hiding medications

Nursing Considerations

During a crisis, treatment is symptomatic, with enforced feeding, tube feeding or TPN IV or oral, replacement of missing electrolytes, and oxygen given to assist with respiration. Daily nursing assessments include regular vital signs, daily weights, and accurately documenting calorie intake and output (food and fluids). Be sure to explain all procedures and the reasons for them to gain the patient's cooperation. Explain the abnormal laboratory findings and their relationship to diet and to physical well-being. The person needs to understand the functions of electrolytes in the body and the consequences of starvation. Offer small amounts of high-protein food or fluids often. High-protein, high-calorie liquids may be more tolerable than solids. Monitor fluid intake, so the person takes a variety of fluids, including fruit juices; make sure the person does not drink excessive amounts of plain water. *(Rationale: To avoid electrolyte imbalance.)* After the crisis, extensive psychotherapy and family counseling are needed. Group therapy is often helpful.

Key Concept

Anorexia nervosa, bulimia, and obesity can be life-threatening.

Keys for Review

Key Questions for Critical Thinking

1. State the role endoscopy has in diagnosing GI disorders. Contrast its use to that of x-rays.
2. List factors that are known to aggravate digestive conditions. Explain how you can use these factors in instructing a patient to prevent problems with hiatal hernia.
3. Contrast therapy for a patient with diverticulosis and a patient with diverticulitis. Explain why therapy is different.

Key Readings

Baillie J. Gastrointestinal Endoscopy: Basic Principles and Practice. Oxford, Butterworth-Heinemann, 1992

Beck M, Evans N (Ed). Gastroenterology Nursing: A Core Curriculum. St Louis, Mosby-Yearbook, 1993

Berkow R (Ed). The Merck Manual of Diagnosis and Therapy, Ed 16. Rahway, NJ, Merck & Co, 1992

Fischbach F. A Manual of Laboratory and Diagnostic Tests, Ed 3. Philadelphia, J.B. Lippincott, 1992

Gilbert G, Chao C, Eapen T. "Peptic Ulcer Disease: How to Treat it Now" Postgraduate Medicine 89(4), 1991

North American Nursing Diagnosis Association. Nursing Diagnoses: Definitions and Classifications 1992. Philadelphia, North American Nursing Diagnosis Association, 1992

Nursing '94 Drug Handbook. Springhouse, PA, Springhouse, 1994

O'Toole M (Ed. Miller-Keane Encyclopedia and Dictionary of Medicine, Nursing, and Allied Health, Ed 5. Philadelphia, W.B. Saunders, 1992

Philadelphia College of Pharmacy and Science. Hepatitis, the Elusive Disease. Kenilworth, NJ, Schering Corp, 1991

Porth CM. Pathophysiology: Concepts of Altered Health States, Ed 4. Philadelphia, J.B. Lippincott, 1994

Selby J. "How Should We Screen for Colorectal Cancer?" Journal of the American Medical Association 3:1294-1295, 1993

Smeltzer SC, Bare BG. Brunner and Suddarth's Textbook of Medical-Surgical Nursing, Ed 7. Philadelphia, J.B. Lippincott, 1992

Key Readings (continued)

Taylor C, Lillis C, LeMone P. Fundamentals of Nursing: The Art and Science of Nursing Care, Ed 2. Philadelphia, J.B. Lippincott, 1993

Thomas CL (Ed). Taber's Cyclopedic Medical Dictionary, Ed 17. Philadelphia, F.A. Davis, 1993

Enrichment Keys

Bosworth T. "Study Suggests Eradication of H. Pylori— Healing of Many Duodenal Ulcers" Gastroenterology and Endoscopy News 1, 1993

McConnell EA. "Loosening the grip of intestinal obstructions." Nursing '94 24(3):34-42, March 1994

Keys to Learning More

Unit Fifteen: geriatric nursing
Unit Seventeen: death and dying

Key Resources

American Anorexia/Bulimia Association Inc.
133 Cedar Lane
Teaneck, NJ 07666
201/836-1800

American Liver Foundation
1425 Pomptom Ave
Cedar Grove, NJ 07009
1-800/223-0179

Digestive Diseases Clearinghouse
1555 Wilson Blvd., Suite 600
Rosslyn, VA 22209-2461
(Includes PDQ search and information service:
1-800/4-CANCER)

Journal Available to Nurses
Progressions, ConvaTec
c/o Mosby-Yearbook
St. Louis, MO 53146

National Foundation for Ileitis and Colitis
444 Park Ave South
New York, NY 10016
212/685-3440

United Ostomy Association
36 Executive Park, Suite 120
Irvine, CA 92714

82 Urinary Disorders

Keys for Learning

Learning Objectives

- List main categories of information to be attained in a urologic history.
- Describe the major diagnostic tests used to evaluate the function of the urinary system.
- Discuss the rationale behind nursing care of the patient with urologic disorders.
- Identify the categories of incontinence and goal of treatment for each type.
- Review the care of patients with suprapubic catheters, indwelling catheters, and intermittent catheters.
- Describe the difference between cystitis, pyelonephritis, and glomerulonephritis.
- Describe the implications of obstructive disorders on renal function.
- Describe the care of a patient with an ileal conduit.
- Describe the phases of acute renal failure, and describe nursing care.
- Differentiate between acute renal failure and chronic renal failure.
- List the advantages and disadvantages of peritoneal dialysis, hemodialysis, and kidney transplantation.

Key Terms

anuria
calculi
crystalluria
cylindruria
cystitis
cystogram
dialysis
glomerulonephritis
hemodialysis

ileal diversion
incontinence
lithiasis
lithotripsy
nephrectomy
nephrologist
pyuria
renal failure
residual urine volume

Keys To Understanding This Chapter

Chapter 5: basic human needs
Chapter 16: fluid and electrolyte balance

Keys To Understanding This Chapter
(continued)

Chapter 24: anatomy and physiology of urinary system
Chapter 25: anatomy and physiology of male reproductive system
Unit Five: nutrition and diet therapy
Chapter 30: medical asepsis
Chapter 38: signs and symptoms of illness or injury
Chapter 45: personal hygiene and skin care
Chapter 46: elimination
Chapter 47: specimen collection
Chapter 50: physical examination and nursing assessment
Chapter 52: pain management
Chapter 53: the person who has surgery
Chapter 54: surgical asepsis
Unit Eleven: pharmacology and medication administration
Unit Thirteen: pediatric nursing
Chapter 69: fluid and electrolyte disorders
Chapter 71: neurologic disorders
Chapter 72: endocrine disorders
Chapter 76: cancer

Key Points

- The kidneys are sensitive to disruption of blood flow.
- All body systems affect urinary function, and disorders of the kidneys will affect all body systems.
- Incontinence is treatable.
- Nursing care of the patient with urinary disorders focuses on maintaining and preserving renal function, decreasing discomfort, preventing infection, promoting skin integrity, and maintaining fluid balance.
- Early symptoms of renal disease are subtle, and the nurse's ability to detect small changes in the patient is crucial to early treatment.

Rosdahl CB: Textbook of Basic Nursing, 6th ed. © 1995 J.B. Lippincott Company

Key Learning Activities

◆ Interview a person having hemodialysis. What were his or her symptoms before dialysis? How does he or she cope with the disease, his or her fears, and the limitations of lifestyle? If the person has end-stage renal disease, how has this changed his or her life and future plans?

Diseases and disorders of the urinary system are treated by a urologist, a specialist in urinary tract disorders. The urologist also may treat disorders of the male reproductive system because the two systems are closely related. Disorders of the urinary system also may be treated by a **nephrologist**, a specialist in the medical aspects of kidney disease. Combining forms in urology are explained in the accompanying box.

The effective functioning of the upper urinary system is driven by blood flow to the kidneys. Therefore, any systemic condition affecting blood flow to the kidneys will affect the ability of the kidneys to function. These systemic conditions include hypertension, congestive heart failure, trauma, and changes

Anatomy and Physiology Review

When considering the urinary tract, it is helpful to divide the urinary system into the *upper* urinary tract (kidneys and ureters) and the *lower* urinary tract (bladder and urethra).

The upper urinary tract acts as a filtering system for the by-products of metabolism and adjusts the fluid and electrolyte balance of the body. It also delivers urine to the lower tract. The lower urinary tract acts as a storage area until micturition (voiding, urination) occurs. Structures of the upper tract include the paired kidneys, within which the nephrons are the functional units. The urine then flows through the ureters into the urinary bladder (lower urinary tract) and out of the body through the urethra.

Combining Forms in Urology

Because many terms in urology are similar, they are confusing. The following are several of the more common combining forms that appear in this chapter:

Prefixes:

nephr(o)-	pertaining to the kidney
lith(o)-	stone
urethr(o)-	pertaining to the urethra (from bladder to outside the body)
ureter(o)-	pertaining to the ureter (tubes from kidneys to bladder)
cyst(o)-	pertaining to any bladder
vesic(o)-	pertaining to a bladder, usually the urinary bladder
pyel(o)-	pertaining to the renal pelvis

Suffix:

-tripsy	crushing

Table 82-1. Conditions Indicated by Abnormalities in the Urine

Abnormality or Abnormal Substance in Urine	Possible Conditions
Abnormal pH	Gout, calculi (stones), infections
Abnormal specific gravity	Kidney disease, electrolyte imbalances, liver disorders, burns
Proteinuria or albuminuria (protein)	Nephritis, kidney stones, renal circulatory difficulties, infection, trauma, preeclampsia (of pregnancy)
Glycosuria (sugar)	Diabetes mellitus, shock, head injury
Ketonuria (ketones)	Diabetes, starvation, bulimia, other digestive disturbances (such as faulty fat metabolism)
Bilirubin	Liver dysfunction, biliary obstruction, hepatitis
Hemoglobinuria or hematuria (blood)	Infection, calculi, cancer, trauma, overdose of an anticoagulant, bleeding disorder

in the small blood vessels related to diabetes mellitus. On the other hand, damage to the lower system usually occurs due to obstruction or sphincter incompetence. Although damage to the upper system is life-threatening, damage to the lower system is rarely so. However, damage to the lower system can greatly affect the patient's quality of life.

Key Concept

Many kidney disorders are actually circulatory disorders that cause renal vascular insufficiency.

Diagnostic Tests

Laboratory Tests

Urine Tests

Routine Urinalysis. Urinalysis gives much information about the condition of the kidneys and how well they are working. It tells whether disease is interfering with the function of different parts of the kidneys (renal tubules, nephrons, and glomeruli). It shows whether pathogenic organisms are at work in the kidney or bladder, and it shows whether food materials that should go to body cells are escaping into the urine. Routine urinalysis includes tests for pH, specific gravity, glucose (sugar), acetone, albumin (protein), blood, and bilirubin.

The urine is collected by nursing personnel and promptly sent to the laboratory for urinalysis. The urine collected may consist of a single random specimen, a fractional specimen, or a 24-hour collection (see Chapter 47). The specimen may be collected as a clean, voided specimen; as a midstream specimen; or by catheterization.

Urine normally has a specific gravity of 1.010 to 1.025

Key Concept

Gloves are worn when obtaining urine specimens.

and a pH ranging from 4.6 to 8. There is no glucose, ketones, blood, albumin, or bilirubin in normal urine. When examined microscopically, there should be no red blood cells, crystals, white blood cells (WBCs), or casts (epithelial, fatty, or waxy material abnormally forced out of the renal tubules). An abnormal reading in any of the aforementioned tests indicates a dysfunction. Table 82-1 discusses conditions that are indicated by abnormalities found in urine.

Urine Culture. A urine culture is done by placing some urine on a special substance (culture medium) and allowing it to incubate (grow). Any organisms present in the urine will thereby be revealed. The nurse must be careful not to contaminate the specimen with any outside organisms so that a true culture of only the patient's urine will be obtained. Generally, the urine is collected by a midstream specimen voided into a sterile container. (The physician may order a catheterization to obtain a sterile urine specimen for culture, although this carries the risk of introducing new organisms into the bladder.) Once the urine is collected for culture, it must be sent to the laboratory immediately. See Chapter 47 for the specific procedure. *(Rationale: If the urine is allowed to stand, microorganisms can grow in it, thereby defeating the accuracy of the test.)*

If a culture reveals that an organism is present in the urine, the organism is tested with various drugs to see which one (usually an antibiotic) is most effective in eradicating the organism (sensitivity test). That drug is then given to the patient. Culture and sensitivity (C & S) tests on urine are usually ordered together.

Creatinine Clearance. The creatinine clearance test shows how efficiently the nephrons are filtering urea from the blood. Urea is the chief nitrogenous constituent of urine metabolism. The amount of urea excreted matches the amount of protein in the diet. Creatinine clearance is one of the most valuable tests identifying early kidney disease and is useful in following renal function of patients with known kidney disease. A 24-hour urine collection is made, noting the exact time the collection is started and completed. *(Rationale: Exactness is vital to obtain the full 24-hour specimen.)* A venous blood sample is also drawn during this period. Chapter 47 describes 24-hour collection procedures.

Other Urine Tests. The laboratory also will test the urine casts (**cylindruria**) for crystals (**crystalluria**), and for pus (**pyuria**) or WBCs, which would indicate infection. Urine calcium may be measured to help detect bone disease; high amounts of calcium indicate degeneration of bone tissue. The urine also may be tested for the presence of other minerals, various drugs, and other abnormal components. The nurse may strain all urine for the presence of **calculi** (stones).

Residual Urine Volume. After a patient voids, it is important to determine if the bladder was emptied or not (the emptying ability of the bladder).

Before beginning the test, the patient voids as much as possible. Some hospital protocols require a voiding, followed by a second voiding 5 minutes later. This is referred to as *double voiding technique.* The patient is then immediately catheterized with a straight catheter (one that is inserted to obtain a specimen and then removed) to collect whatever urine remains in the bladder that cannot be excreted by the patient. This is called the **residual urine volume**.

If the residual volume is greater than 150 to 200 mL, a disorder of the bladder is probably causing urine retention. The physician may order a catheter to be left in place if the residual is over a certain amount. In this case, a retention catheter, such as a Foley, is used for the initial procedure.

Blood Tests

Blood Chemistry. A blood chemistry test may indicate the amounts of other electrolytes in the blood, such as potassium, calcium, and sodium, which reflect the overall fluid and electrolyte balance and help measure renal and liver status. Determining how much of these substances is in the blood will help to determine how well the kidney is filtering.

Blood Urea Nitrogen. The blood urea nitrogen (BUN) test is an analysis of a specimen of blood, which determines how efficiently the glomeruli are removing the nitrogen portion of urea. The most common cause of an elevated BUN is kidney disease, although it also may be elevated in diabetes, some malignancies, and cases of improper protein metabolism.

Serum Creatinine. Creatinine is a product of energy metabolism and is related to muscle mass. Normally, it is excreted by the kidneys. The glomerular filtration rate must be reduced by at least 50% for significant elevation of the serum creatinine to occur. Therefore, monitoring serum creatinine is a much more accurate measurement of renal function than monitoring the serum BUN. If the serum creatinine is elevated, this usually indicates a serious kidney disorder, such as impaired kidney function or an obstruction.

Key Concept

Diagnostic tests without a thorough history are merely tests. An accurate medical and nursing history will give clues to diagnosis and may eliminate the need for costly tests.

X-Ray Evaluations

Kidney-Ureter-Bladder X-Ray. The kidney-ureter-bladder x-ray, commonly referred to as a KUB plate, provides an overall view of the urinary system.

Intravenous Pyelogram. An intravenous pyelogram (IVP) is composed of a series of x-rays taken after a

Key Abbreviations and Acronyms

ATN	Acute tubular necrosis
BPH	Benign prostatic hyperplasia
BUN	Blood urea nitrogen
CAPD	Continuous ambulatory peritoneal dialysis
CMG	Cystometrogram
C & S	Culture and sensitivity
CT	Computerized tomography
EMG	Electromyogram
ESRD	End-stage renal disease
ESWL	Extracoporeal shock wave lithotripsy
IVP	Intravenous pyelogram
KUB	Kidney-ureters-bladder X-ray
ROM	Range of motion
TURPT	Transurethral resection of a prostate tumor
UA	Urinalysis
UPP	Urethral pressure profile
UTI	Urinary tract infection

radiopaque dye has been intravenously injected. The x-rays reveal the outline of the kidneys, ureters, and bladder. Before the IVP is done, the radiologist must determine whether the patient is allergic to iodine or shellfish, because the dye is iodine-based (see Chapter 50 for precautions when dye is used).

The patient is allowed nothing by mouth (NPO) for 8 to 10 hours before the tests. A laxative is usually given the night before to rid the bowel of any gas, because this could obstruct the view of urinary structures. The patient may brush the teeth in the morning but should be instructed not to swallow any water.

In the x-ray department, one x-ray is taken and developed. A radiopaque dye is then intravenously injected, and several more x-rays are taken at intervals to visualize the concentration of dye in the kidneys.

Nursing assessment includes observing for untoward reactions to the dye. Fluids should be forced for 24 hours to help remove the dye and relieve any dehydration that may have resulted from the patient not having had anything by mouth prior to the test.

Nephrotomogram. The tomogram, commonly used today, allows x-rays to be taken of a section (plane) of the body with a rotating x-ray tube after intravenous injection of a contrast medium. The *nephrotomogram* is a study of the kidney. Preparation and care of the patient are the same as for IVP.

Cystogram. A **cystogram** is an x-ray of the bladder and urethra, made possible by the instillation of a dye directly in the bladder through a catheter. It will show the outline of the bladder and any backflow of urine into the ureters. A crystogram may be done to show the outline of the urethra while the patient is voiding (*voiding cystogram*). A *cystourethrogram* is an x-ray showing both the urethra and the bladder.

Renal Arteriogram. Contrast dye is injected through a catheter into the aorta at the level of the renal blood vessels. The kidneys are thereby visualized to determine the presence of a pathologic condition such as a tumor. The care of the patient after this examination is the same as for patients having any arteriogram (see Chapters 50 and 74).

Computed Tomography. Computed tomography (CT scan) is a noninvasive technique that allows cross-section views of kidney anatomy to locate abnormalities, such as cysts, tumors, or calculi. The x-ray beams pass through the body at many different angles, and a computer collects and displays the data. (Tomography is discussed in further detail in Chapter 71.)

Retrograde Pyelogram. After the bladder is outlined by instillation of a dye by catheter, smaller catheters are introduced into the ureters and then passed into the kidney pelvis, where dye is injected into them. X-rays are then taken that show the kidneys and ureters. This procedure is combined with cystoscopy (described later in this chapter). Preparation includes giving a low-residue diet the day before and a laxative or enema in the evening and immediately before the test. Observation following the test is the same as that required for any other test using dye (see Chapter 50).

Radioactive Renogram (Renal Scan). Sometimes the kidneys are tested by means of radioactive substances. If a lesion is present, it will "pick up" more of the radioactive isotope than normal tissue; therefore, it will be visible on the scan.

Bone Scan. In a bone scan (scintiscan), a radioisotope is injected in an intravenous bolus. The patient is instructed to drink 1 L of fluid to assist the bones to take up the isotope. X-ray images are obtained 2 hours after the injection. A bone scan is indicated when bony metastases are suspected in cases of renal, bladder, or prostatic cancer. If bony metastases exist, they will demonstrate increased uptake of the radioisotope.

Nursing Alert

Because many diagnostic and minor urologic surgical procedures are performed on an outpatient basis, aggressive patient and family teaching is needed. They must be taught how to perform the preoperative preparation and untoward signs after the procedure. This teaching must be carefully documented.

Urodynamic Tests

Urodynamic testing involves tests that determine the function of the *detrusor* muscles of the bladder (which push the urine out), the external sphincter muscle, and the pubococcygeal muscles. Urodynamic tests also evaluate the ability of these muscles to work in sequence.

Uroflowmetry. *Uroflowmetry* is a noninvasive assessment of the status of micturition (voiding). The patient is asked to void into a funneled commode that is connected to an electronic device. This device calculates the rate at which the urine flows, time taken to void, and volume voided. This information is recorded on a graph.

Before the test, the patient should be instructed to void in the same fashion as usual. Leave the patient alone, if possible. This will help to eliminate "bashful bladder syndrome." Further testing will be needed to differentiate between bladder outlet obstruction and hypotonic bladder (poor muscle tone).

Cystometrogram. A *cystometrogram* (CMG) is a measurement of bladder pressure during bladder filling and emptying (voiding). For the test, a urethral catheter is inserted, and the bladder is filled either with a liquid, such as normal saline, or with x-ray contrast media. The patient is instructed to notify the physician or nurse when he or she begins to feel a sense of fullness and again when the bladder actually feels full. The patient is then asked to begin to urinate and is asked to stop at a certain point. Normally, bladder pressure remains the same during bladder filling, until the volume is approximately 500 mL. When the patient is asked to void, the pressure should increase abruptly because of bladder contraction. The pressure should then fall to the previoiding level when the patient is told to stop voiding. The bladder is now relaxing.

Perineal Electromyogram. The perineal electromyogram (EMG) is a test of urinary muscle function. Several methods are used to record perineal EMG. Patch electrodes are much more common today than the needle electrodes previously used. (Patch electrodes are more comfortable for the patient.) The perineal EMG is usually combined with the CMG because the major function of the EMG is to evaluate the relationship of perineal muscle activity and detrusor contraction. (A detrusor is a muscle that pushes down.)

Urethral Pressure Profile. A urethral pressure profile (UPP) assists in evaluating smooth muscle activity along the urethra. This procedure is often done following a CMG. For the UPP, the bladder is filled either with a fluid, such as normal saline or water, or with contrast media using a catheter. A puller mechanism provides a slow, even rate of catheter withdrawal, while resistance exerted by the urethral wall is registered as a pressure rise on a graph.

Key Concept

Urodynamic tests are safer than x-ray procedures, which require intravenous dye. These non–x-ray procedures are becoming the test of choice in many cases.

Endoscopy

Cystoscopy

A cystoscopy examination allows the physician to view the inside of the bladder through a tubular instrument, the cystoscope, which has a mirror and an elec-

tric lamp or fiberoptic lens on the end of it. The cystoscope is passed into the bladder through the urethra. This examination will detect bladder inflammation or a tumor in the bladder that may or may not be causing blood to appear in the urine. The openings of the ureters into the bladder are also visible; fine opaque wax catheters can be threaded into these openings for collection of separate specimens of urine from each kidney to determine which kidney is diseased. Dye also may be instilled through these catheters.

The cystoscope may be used just to view the ureters while inserting ureteral catheters. The cystoscopy also may be done to remove a polyp or a tumor, do a biopsy, or remove kidney stones. Electrosurgery (*fulguration*) also may be performed through a cystoscope to remove small tumors or to coagulate (cauterize) small, bleeding blood vessels.

Because a cystoscopy is usually done in a special operating room, the patient requires routine preoperative preparation (Chapter 53). A cystoscopy may be performed with general anesthesia. Local anesthesia involves administering a tranquilizer or sedative before the examination to relax the patient and instilling xylocaine jelly into the urethra.

Urine specimens obtained are examined in the laboratory. A mild analgesic may be prescribed after the procedure because voiding may be uncomfortable for 1 to 2 days. Also, sitz baths may be ordered to assist in voiding and to soothe the affected area.

The urine has a reddish tinge immediately after cystoscopy. If this lasts more than 24 hours or the urine becomes darker, it should be reported. The patient is encouraged to drink fluids to prevent urinary stasis and flush any remaining dye out of the system.

Nursing Alert

Chills and fever should be reported. *(Rationale: These are signs of an infection.)* Other symptoms of complications include sharp abdominal pain, hematuria (blood in the urine, as opposed to red dye), **anuria** (absence of urine formation), dysuria (painful urination), or urine retention.

Needle Biopsy

For a specific diagnosis following x-ray studies, a needle biopsy of the kidney may be done. The kidney is located by x-ray or ultrasound and the patient's back marked so that the needle can be inserted into the correct place.

The patient is given a sedative and placed in a prone position; a sandbag is placed under the abdomen. *(Rationale: This helps bring the kidney into a more accessible position.)* A local anesthetic is injected into the skin, and the biopsy needle is inserted.

After the procedure, pressure should be applied to the biopsy site to minimize bleeding. The patient should be kept lying flat for 24 hours and watched *very carefully* for any signs of hemorrhage. *(Rationale: Hemorrhage is a complication of a needle biopsy. The kidney is very vascular.)* Blood pressure, pulse, and respirations should be taken and documented at frequent intervals.

> ### Nursing Alert
> Assess the patient carefully for hemorrhage following a biopsy or other renal procedure. The kidney is a vascular organ. Signs of hemorrhage include decreased blood pressure, increased pulse rate, and other symptoms related to shock.

Observe for hematuria. *(Rationale: Bleeding would first occur in the kidney and then would be excreted in the urine.)*

Medical and Surgical Treatments

A Common Medical Treatment: Dialysis

Dialysis is a process that takes on the work of the kidney temporarily when a damaged kidney is not functioning. It can work on a long-term basis when the kidneys cease to function as a result of disorders, such as acute kidney disease, shock, diabetes mellitus, or chronic hypertension. Patients with severe drug overdose or poisoning also are treated with dialysis in many cases.

The purpose of dialysis is as follows:

♦ Removes waste products of protein metabolism from the blood
♦ Removes poisons or toxins from the blood
♦ Removes excess water
♦ Establishes or maintains proper levels of electrolytes
♦ Maintains acid–base balance
♦ Instills drugs (such as antibiotics), electrolytes, or other substances

Some people are maintained for many years on intermittent dialysis. People who are awaiting a kidney transplant are maintained on dialysis until a suitable kidney is available.

The two types of dialysis are *peritoneal dialysis and hemodialysis,* both of which remove body wastes through a semipermeable membrane by osmosis, diffusion, and ultrafiltration.

Nursing care during dialysis is found in the nursing process section of this chapter.

Peritoneal Dialysis

In peritoneal dialysis, the intestinal wall (peritoneum) serves as the semipermeable membrane. Peritoneal dialysis is not used if the patient has a known peritonitis or has had recent abdominal surgery. It is most often used on a short-term basis (eg, in the case of poisoning).

Procedure. A catheter is inserted into the visceral cavity through which the dialysis solution (*dialysate*) is instilled into the abdominal cavity. The solution is allowed to remain in the peritoneum for the time specified by the physician. It is then allowed to flow freely out of the catheter into the container, which is lowered to facilitate gravity flow. This process may be continuous or repeated intermittently.

Possible complications of peritoneal dialysis follow:

♦ Bacterial or chemical peritonitis—cloudy, odoriferous outflow
♦ Pain—abdomen, back, or shoulder (referred)
♦ Shortness of breath
♦ Protein loss
♦ Fluid overload or loss
♦ Electrolyte imbalance
♦ Constipation
♦ Infection
♦ Bleeding—bloody returns

A permanent access device to the peritoneum has been developed; this may expand the concept of peritoneal dialysis for the patient with end-stage renal disease (ESRD), discussed at the end of this chapter.

Outpatient Peritoneal Dialysis. Continuous ambulatory peritoneal dialysis (CAPD) is used for home dialysis. The dialysate remains intraperitoneally and is exchanged by the patient four to five times per day. This procedure offers the advantage of being free from the constriction of machines. Other advantages are that steady blood chemistry levels can be obtained easily, it is a shorter and more inexpensive process, and the training is less complicated than that for home hemodialysis (dialysis by way of blood circulation).

Hemodialysis

In **hemodialysis**, an artificial semipermeable membrane is contained within the dialysis machine.

Procedure. Hemodialysis is performed by circulating blood from the patient through a machine outside the body. This procedure is also known as *extracorporeal hemodialysis.* The prefix "hemo" refers to blood; thus, this type of dialysis removes wastes directly from the blood.

Shunt Placement. A shunt or fistula usually is inserted internally to facilitate repeated hemodialysis. The *shunt* consists of a U-shaped tube, which is usually between the radial artery and the cephalic vein in the arm. The patient's nondominant arm is used for this process. This shunt allows the circulation to bypass the capillary network in that area and provides access to the arterial system. At the time of dialysis, two venipunctures are made into the shunt, one for the arterial blood source and the other for the venous return. Hemodialysis is conducted within the machine by means of blood flow from the patient. This shunt remains in place because the patient needs dialysis treatment two or three times per week to maintain life.

The Cannula. Other access sites for hemodialysis can include a cannula or a subclavian catheter. A *cannula* is an *external* device composed of two small plastic tubes. One tube is placed in an artery and the other into a vein. This cannula is located in the patient's arm or leg. Each tube comes through the skin at an exit site and rests outside the body. When the patient is not on dialysis, the two parts of the cannula are connected together with a plastic connector and usually covered with an occlusive dressing. The blood can then flow from the artery to the vein through this shunt. A *subclavian catheter,* an intravenous device, is fairly large and is placed into subclavian blood vessels in the neck region. It has two ports, one for the arterial blood source and one for the venous return.

Complications. Possible complications include the following:

◆ Septicemia
◆ Air emboli
◆ Hemolytic anemia
◆ Disequilibrium syndrome
◆ Hepatitis
◆ Hypotension
◆ Pain, cramps
◆ Nausea and vomiting
◆ Exsanguination (severe, immediately life-threatening hemorrhage)

General complications of dialysis are described in more detail in the accompanying box.

Key Concept

◆ Dialysis: Waste products are removed from the body in cases of serious renal dysfunction.
◆ Peritoneal dialysis: The dialyzing solution is introduced into the peritoneal cavity. The semipermeable membrane is the person's own peritoneum.
◆ Hemodialysis (extracorporeal hemodialysis): The dialyzing solution is circulated through a machine outside the body, as is the patient's blood. The semipermeable membrane in this case is made of synthetic material and is within the machine.

Complications of Continued Dialysis

◆ The cannula can fall out—the patient might bleed to death. Less severe bleeding also can occur because the cannula is heparinized.
◆ The membrane within the dialysis machine can rupture, causing hemorrhage.
◆ If the chemical agents used are the wrong ones or if the chemistry workup is incorrect, the patient's electrolyte balance will be disrupted even further.
◆ Because most patients on dialysis have high blood pressure (caused by renal damage), they may go into shock when connected to the machine.
◆ The blood in the machine must be warm, or the patient can suffer cardiac arrest from the shock of cold blood.
◆ Infection or septicemia is always a possibility. Because this patient has especially low resistance, infection can be dangerous.
◆ Blood can clot in the cannula and cause phlebitis.
◆ Male patients often become impotent, although this may correct itself as the condition is stabilized.
◆ Excesses in alcohol or food intake will not be excreted between dialysis runs.

Common Surgical Treatments

Extracorporeal Shock Wave Lithotripsy

Extracorporeal (outside the body) *shock wave lithotripsy* (ESWL) is becoming the treatment of choice in cases of stones in the kidney or upper ureter. It may be used for stones in other parts of the body as well (such as gallstones).

In this treatment, the stones are "blasted" by shock waves that are so intense that the stones are broken into small, gravel-like fragments. If the stone is in the lower ureter, it can be pushed up into the upper ureter or kidney and treated with ESWL. (ESWL is not used in the lower ureter or bladder because it can be traumatic, and these tissues are more delicate.) ESWL is a specialized and potentially hazardous procedure that must be performed by carefully trained physicians and technicians. Nursing considerations in ESWL appear in the nursing process section of this chapter.

Kidney Transplant

Surgeons can take a kidney from a well human being or a recent cadaver and transplant it to the body of another person to replace a diseased organ.

The kidney is "typed" before transplant to get as good a match between donor and recipient as possible. This process is similar to that used in blood typing for a transfusion. Tissue typing of this sort allows the most suitable match for the patient. Often, living relatives have compatible tissue matches and may be considered as kidney donors. The donor must have two well-functioning kidneys and must have no underlying disease.

Medical authorities have agreed that a kidney transplant should be attempted only when it has a reasonable chance to succeed and when all other options have been attempted. Transplant surgeons have special training. The surgery is less complex than that in other types of transplants.

More kidney transplantation is done than any other type of organ transplantation, and a high percentage of these transplants are successful. A major advantage of kidney transplantation is that a live donor is able to sacrifice one kidney and continue to live without difficulty. Also, cadaver donors can supply two kidneys for two potential patients. Moreover, the patient can be carefully prepared for a long time because they can be maintained by renal dialysis.

Rejections of Transplanted Organs. The chief difficulty with transplants is dealing with the body's natural reaction to reject foreign substances (see Chapters 77 and 78). Certain factors cause rejection. For example, if the person has been exposed to foreign proteins in the process of previous transplant attempts or multiple blood transfusions, rejection is more likely. However, many drugs are available today to suppress rejection, and transplanted organs have much greater promise. The rejection syndrome in kidney transplantation is usually easier to manage than in other organ transplants.

Complications of Antirejection Medications. There are side effects to drugs that suppress tissue rejection because they also suppress immune response. Assessment includes observation for the following:

Keys to Nursing Assessment
Urologic Conditions

- Urinary history
- General health history
- Family health history
- Exposure to toxins
- Presence of related disorders (insulin-dependent diabetes mellitus, heart or blood vessel disorders, infections, cancer)
- Character of urine
- Intake and output amounts
- Urinary residual
- Difficulty or pain in voiding
- Any incontinence and type
- Sudden weight gain or loss
- Diet
- Presence of symptoms, such as edema, poor skin turgor

- Development of malignancies
- Susceptibility to viruses
- Susceptibility to infections of all types
- Gastric ulcers
- Gastrointestinal bleeding
- Psychiatric disorders
- Bone disorders

If the patient rejects the first kidney transplant, a second transplant may be performed.

Key Concept

A concern in all transplants today is that of transmission of diseases, such as acquired immunodeficiency syndrome, to the recipient. Specific tests are becoming more accurate in detecting the human immunodeficiency and hepatitis B viruses and thus preventing the transplantation of an infected organ.

❖ Nursing Process

Data Collection

The nurse must carefully observe and assess the patient with a urinary disorder. Chapter 50 describes physical examination and nursing assessment, including that of the urinary system. This assessment establishes a baseline for future comparison and determines the presence of suspected complications. The nurse should report any changes in the baseline level; it is important to recognize and treat kidney malfunctions early. The accompanying box lists some components of the urologic nursing assessment.

In addition, the nurse observes the patient's emotional response to the disorder or disease by asking the following questions. Would a support group be helpful? Does the patient need assistance to meet daily needs? Do family caregivers understand medications and treatments needed? Is home care or public health nursing necessary after discharge? Does the disorder affect social activities or self-esteem? Is the condition chronic or life-threatening? Is it reversible or treatable? Does the patient need periodic dialysis or other regular treatment? Is the patient anxious or fearful of the outcome?

Special Considerations in Children
Complete History

It is important to get an accurate history when admitting pediatric patients. Voiding patterns and behaviors may be the only clue to detecting anomalies. Encourage the child to describe his or her toileting habits for you. (*Rationale: Frequently children do not recognize something is abnormal, so they don't know to tell their parents about their symptoms.*)

Keys to Patient/Family Teaching
Intermittent Self-Catheterization (Clean Procedure)

Patient teaching for intermittent self-catheterization includes the following step-by-step method:

◆ Gather equipment: water-based lubricant, catheter, container for urine, bag for catheter, and soap and water.
◆ Wash hands. (The patient will colonize the bladder with his or her own bacteria.)
◆ Lubricate catheter.
◆ Insert the catheter slowly until the urine flows. *Males:* Hold penis up while inserting the catheter 1 to 2 inches more once the urine begins to flow. *Females:* Use a hand mirror to help locate urinary meatus.
◆ When urine flow stops, squeeze catheter closed and remove.
◆ Measure urine if instructed to do so, and empty and rinse basin.
◆ Wash catheter in warm soapy water, rinse thoroughly, and dry outside well with a clean towel. Store catheter in clean zip-lock bag.
◆ Wash hands.
◆ Replace worn, cracked, or encrusted catheters as necessary.
◆ Monitor for signs of urinary tract infection: pain, burning, frequency and urgency, and cloudy or strong smelling urine.

Note: It is easier for many people if the catheter is attached to a bag before insertion. This helps to prevent spilling of urine.

Nursing Diagnosis

Based on data collection, the following nursing diagnoses may be established for the patient with a urologic disorder:

◆ High Risk for Infection related to dehydration, excess of wastes in the body, tissue breakdown and damage
◆ High Risk for Fluid Volume Deficit or Excess related to inability of kidney to effectively concentrate urine, fluid restrictions, electrolyte imbalance
◆ Stress Incontinence/Reflex Incontinence/Functional Incontinence related to sphincter incompetence, neurologic disorders, impaired mental status, medications, fistula, cancer, surgery, trauma, obstruction
◆ Urinary Retention related to obstruction, sphincter incompetence, cancer, trauma
◆ Impaired Tissue Integrity related to dehydration, mucous membrane friability and breakdown, general malaise
◆ Social Isolation related to incontinence, presence of appliance

◆ Altered Sexuality Patterns related to indwelling catheter, dialysis
◆ Pain related to surgery, invasive diagnostic tests, urinary tract infections, pyelonephritis, calculi

Planning and Implementation

The patient, nurse, and family plan together for effective care to meet patient needs based on the nursing diagnosis. The nurse provides preoperative and postoperative care for the patient undergoing lithotripsy, renal surgery, dialysis, or invasive diagnostic tests. The patient with a urinary disorder also may require total assistance in meeting daily needs, dealing with emotional problems, and understanding more about the disorder, its prognosis, and treatment. A urinary disorder may be chronic. Renal disease may require regular dialysis or a kidney transplant, or it may be life-threatening with minimal treatment available. A nursing care plan is developed to meet individual patient needs. A sample nursing care plan for a patient with a urinary disorder is provided later in the chapter. Damage to the kidneys can be life-threatening if not recognized and treated promptly. The goal of nursing care is to prevent further damage or worsening of function.

Caring for the Patient With a Urologic Problem

General nursing procedures in caring for patients with urologic problems include the following;

◆ Administration of prescribed diuretics, mineral supplements, and antibiotics
◆ Attention to skin and mouth care (because of dehydration, edema, and general tissue friability)
◆ Management of pruritus (see Chapter 68)
◆ Assessment of skin condition, tissue turgor, presence of edema or dehydration
◆ Measurement and recording of intake and output, recording color and clarity
◆ Urine-specific gravity
◆ Daily weights to assess for edema, urinary retention
◆ Monitoring of fluid intake, fluid restrictions (to help control edema and electrolyte imbalances)
◆ Encouragement of fluid intake, if not contraindicated, to dilute urine and lessen dysuria
◆ Assistance in voiding
◆ Management of dysuria
◆ Urinary catheterization
◆ Management and care of indwelling catheter, suprapubic cystocath
◆ Management of incontinence, frequency, urgency, and other urinary symptoms
◆ Management of continuous irrigation systems

◆ Sitz baths, warm moist packs to offset pain and encourage voiding
◆ Movement and activity to prevent disorders of immobility, such as deep vein thrombosis, pneumonia, and urinary tract infections
◆ Obtaining frequent vital signs, especially blood pressure
◆ Management of related symptoms, such as diarrhea, nausea, vomiting, headache

Straining Urine for Calculi

If kidney or other urinary tract stones are suspected, the physician will order all urine to be strained (see Chapter 46). In Chapter 46, nursing care of the patient with urinary incontinence is also discussed, along with bladder rehabilitation techniques. In the current chapter, causes of incontinence will be explored.

The nurse is also responsible for assisting the person to manage a urethral or suprapubic catheter (see Chapter 46). The sterile insertion, removal, and irrigation of urethral catheters are described in Chapter 54; the physician places suprapubic and other types of catheters. In some cases, the patient is taught to perform regular self-catheterization.

Assisting the Dialysis Patient

The nurse in any unit of the hospital may be asked to prepare a patient for dialysis or care for the patient following a dialysis run. Some of the nursing care follows.

Some patients have dialysis machines at home and do their dialysis during the day or at night. In this case, a family member must be trained to assist and to recognize complications. In some cases, specially trained dialysis nurses assist in the home. Many smaller hospitals are served by regional dialysis centers, which send trained personnel to assist in the smaller hospitals on a rotating basis. In this way, patients can be treated in their own towns.

Nursing Considerations. Before the dialysis run, be sure the patient is wearing a name band. Measure and record vital signs and weight. The patient is often NPO after midnight for a morning run. Blood may be drawn on call to dialysis.

During the peritoneal dialysis run, keep the puncture site and the dialysate (dialysis fluid) sterile. The nurse is responsible for documenting the dialysis process, including patient intake and output through normal body orifices and a complete record of the dialysate. Carefully record the amount and type of solution used and received back, the drugs or electrolytes added, and the times the solution was instilled and drained. (The hemodialysis run will be monitored by specially trained personnel.)

In all types of dialysis, monitor and document vital signs, including temperature, apical pulse, respiration rate, blood pressure, daily weight, and level of consciousness. Although not common, complications can occur, either as a result of the dialysis itself or as a result of the underlying disease. During the procedure, the patient often must remain in bed for an extended time (Fig. 82-1).

Following the run, vital signs are taken frequently. The nursing care plan includes frequent turning, deep breathing, good skin care, and careful oral hygiene.

Nursing Alert

Nursing assessment in peritoneal dialysis includes observation for signs of drug reactions, abdominal distention or pain, bleeding or shock, respiratory problems, infection, and leakage around the catheter leading into the peritoneum.

When a patient is on dialysis, strict dietary restrictions must be enforced. For example, alcohol cannot be excreted and therefore should not be consumed by the patient.

Meticulous sterile technique is used when caring for the hemodialysis shunt. *(Rationale: Because the shunt is inserted within the circulatory system, any infection would quickly spread throughout the body.)* The shunt must be kept clean and dry and must be observed frequently for clotting and signs of infection. Other nursing guidelines are given in the accompanying box.

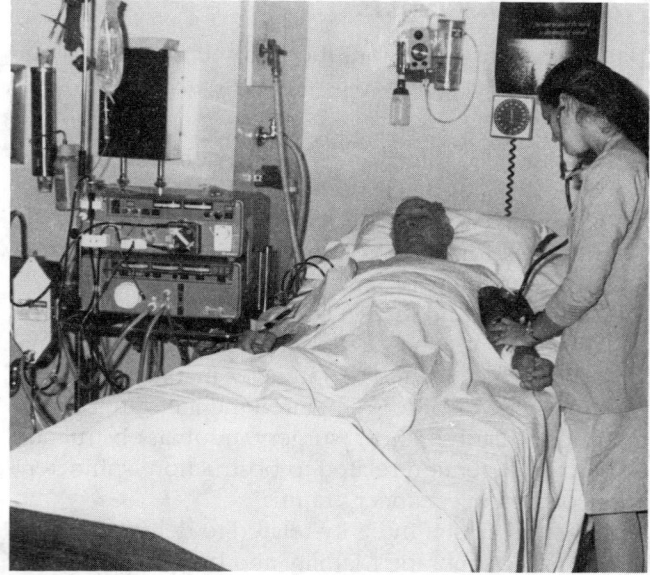

Figure 82-1. Nurse monitoring the patient undergoing hemodialysis in the hospital. (Georgetown University Medical Center)

Nursing Care Guidelines
Caring for the Patient Receiving Dialysis

◆ Always wear gloves. You will be exposed directly to the patient's blood.

◆ Check the shunt every 2 to 4 hours for vibration (*thrill*), which can be felt. Listen with a stethoscope for the whooshing sound of blood moving through the shunt (*bruit*). This is recorded as follows: "RAG (right arm Gortex) ++." (The ++ indicates that you can feel and hear the blood movement.)

◆ Notify the physician immediately if there is a change in the intensity of these sounds or sensations or if they are absent.

◆ Two clamps should be kept on the dressing over the external cannula at all times. (*Rationale: In case of cannula separation.*)

◆ Do not draw blood on the arm with a cannula or fistula to avoid disturbing the shunt.

◆ Do not take blood pressures on the arm with a cannula or fistula to prevent cannula separation.

◆ Blood pressure may need to be taken with an electronic device. (*Rationale: You may not be able to hear it with a stethoscope.*)

◆ If an A-V fistula bleeds, pressure must be applied until bleeding stops. (*Rationale: This can be a life-threatening emergency.*)

◆ The port usually is not flushed.

◆ Many of these patients also are diabetic and require insulin.

◆ These patients usually will not void. (*Rationale: They are not making urine because of lack of kidney functioning.*)

◆ Do not give orange juice; give apple juice or grape juice. (*Rationale: Orange juice is high in potassium.* Elevated potassium is common in these patients and is very dangerous. *Hyperkalemia* [elevated potassium] can cause fluid overload, shortness of breath, and irregular heartbeat, which can lead to cardiac arrest.)

◆ Blood for potassium and other electrolyte levels are usually drawn daily.

◆ Follow medication times exactly to maintain therapeutic blood level and avoid overload.

◆ Measure daily weights to evaluate fluid retention.

◆ Blood pressure is often elevated; monitor carefully.

◆ "Guaiac all stools" is often ordered.

◆ Teach the patient and family about care of the fistula or cannula and other aspects of care. They must understand that disconnection of the fistula is an emergency and the emergency action that must be taken.

◆ Carefully and completely document all teaching.

Nursing Alert

A serious complication of dialysis treatment is separation of the cannula or displacement of the arterial cannula, although this occurs rarely. This is a medical emergency because the patient can *exsanguinate* quickly.

Caring for the Patient Undergoing Lithotripsy

The patient must be taught about ESWL prior to the procedure. Tell the patient that he or she may be immersed in water in a large tub, similar to the Hubbard tank (a large butterfly-shaped whirlpool). Water helps to localize, transmit, and buffer the shock waves. If the submersion tank is used, small water wings are placed on the patient's arms to keep them afloat and out of the way. (Newer methods use a fluid-filled bag and submersion is not required.) A mild sedative is usually given prior to the procedure. The procedure is not totally without discomfort. Patients describe the sensation as like being struck by a blow to the body. Document all teaching.

Nursing assessment includes observation of urine. Following ESWL, the patient will have slightly bloody urine for 24 to 48 hours. The color is most often described as rosé. This is due to ureteral trauma that is caused as the gravel-like stone fragments are being passed in the urine. Urine is strained, and fluids are encouraged. The patient may be bruised or "black and blue" in the area of the lateral pelvic bones.

Certain precautions are followed after discharge from the hospital. The patient is urged to force fluids and strain all urine (see Chapter 46). After ESWL, intake of certain foods is limited, depending on the analysis of the stones. The patient is taught to report any untoward symptoms to the physician. The patient who has had one kidney stone has an increased chance of forming another one.

Caring for the Postoperative Patient

Whether surgery is done for stone removal, cancer, or kidney transplantation, deep breathing and turning can be painful postoperatively (*Rationale: A flank incision is usually used for a ureterolithhotony or a nephrotomy incision.*) Care of the patient who has undergone urologic surgery follows normal nursing postoperative care (Chapter 53). Additional care includes the following:

◆ Patients need the prescribed pain medication prior to turning and deep breathing. Encourage the use of the incentive spirometer.

◆ The patient may have multiple tubes for urinary drainage postoperatively. The nurse must be aware of the location, size, and kind of tubes and the ex pected drainage from each. Each tube and its drainage are assessed regularly.

◆ Assessment also includes careful observation for any indication of excessive bleeding. Hemorrhage can easily occur after surgery for renal calculi because the kidneys are so vascular.

◆ There may be large amounts of urinary drainage on dressings after urologic surgery, but *drainage should not be bright red;* bright red drainage indicates frank bleeding. The color most often used to describe normal bloody discharge following nephrolithotomy is "rosé."

◆ The patient will often have a urinary catheter or suprapubic cystocath postoperatively. See Chapter 46 for a description of nursing care involved with these devices.

Evaluation

The nurse, patient, and family evaluate outcomes of care. Have short-term goals been met? Are long-term goals still realistic? Will the patient be able to be cared for at home? Are home nursing services required? Is a support group indicated? Do the patient and caregivers understand and plan to follow the treatment plan? Does the patient have a way to get to dialysis, or will it be done at home? Planning for further nursing care considers the patient's prognosis, any complications, and the patient's and family's responses to care given.

Urinary Incontinence

Urinary incontinence refers to involuntary voiding or loss of urine. In men, two well-defined sphincter muscles control the voiding of urine. The *internal* sphincter muscles control the opening of the bladder into the urethra, and the external sphincter controls the opening of the outer end of the urethra. In women, only the *internal* sphincter muscle functions well. Normally when sufficient urine collects in the bladder, the involved nerve endings are stimulated, and the person feels a desire to urinate (void). When control of this function is lost, incontinence occurs. For the patient's physical and emotional well-being, it is important to achieve *continence,* if possible.

Many classifications of incontinence exist. However, to make it easier to understand treatment and etiologies, the following classes of incontinence are discussed:

◆ Transient incontinence
◆ True (total) incontinence
◆ Stress incontinence
◆ Reflex or urgency incontinence
◆ Overflow (paradoxical) incontinence

Transient Incontinence

Transient incontinence is caused by temporary and usually reversible factors, such as changes in mental status, infections, medications, fluid intake, mobility problem, or stool impaction. Once the precipitating cause is discovered and modified, the incontinence usually resolves without further intervention.

True (Total) Incontinence

True, or total, incontinence is defined as urinary leakage that is nearly continuous. Causes of true incontinence include the following:

◆ Injury to the external (voluntary) urethral sphincter in the male
◆ Injury to the perineal musculature (muscles) of the female
◆ Congenital or acquired neurogenic disease, such as spina bifida or spinal cord injury
◆ Congenital anomaly in which the urinary bladder is exposed on the lower abdomen (*exstrophy*)
◆ Abnormally placed ureteral orifices in the female (opening distal to the neck of the bladder or into the vagina)
◆ Vesicovaginal fistula, secondary to situations such as obstetric (related to childbirth) injuries and surgical injuries (which may include injury during surgery or defects that are caused by an infection following surgery)
◆ Invasive cancer of the cervix or prostate
◆ Radiation injury following treatment of cervical cancer
◆ Surgical removal of the prostate in the male
◆ Abdominal perineal resection for rectal cancer in the male or female

The most common cause of true incontinence in the male is surgical removal of the prostate (prostatectomy). This procedure is described in Chapter 83.

Treatment. *Electrocautery.* If incontinence is caused by a small fistula, a urologist can treat it with electrocautery. In this procedure, the defective tissue is cauterized (destroyed) by an electrode that emits either alternating or direct electrical current. (The term electrocautery refers to the procedure and also to the instrument that is used.)

Kegel Exercises. Various incontinence patterns can be managed with Kegel exercises (see the patient teaching box in Chapter 84). These exercises are designed to increase sphincter tone. The patient will need to wear a disposable pad during the training period to catch the urine. If after 1 year this conservative mode of treatment is not effected in retraining the bladder, the patient may opt for surgery.

Surgical Treatment. If a fistula is large or if it is caused by radiation therapy or invasive cancer (and in certain other situations), the patient may require *ileal diversion* (urinary diversion) to correct the incontinence (described later in this chapter). Abnormally placed ureteral orifices can be corrected by surgical *ureteral reimplantation.* In this procedure, the urologist attaches the ureters to the urinary bladder.

Kegel exercises can be used in postsurgical and other types of true incontinence. If the Kegel exercises are not effective in controlling urine flow, *sphincter implantation* is possible. An artificial sphincter is inserted surgically. This device consists of a cuff, which is placed around the neck of the bladder. It contains two bulbs—one to inflate the device to maintain continence and one to deflate the device when the patient wants to empty the bladder. These are placed in the scrotum in the male and in the vulva in the female. This device was originally designed for the patient with a neurogenic bladder disorder.

Stress Incontinence

Stress incontinence leads to leakage of urine following a sudden increase in intra-abdominal pressure (such as coughing, sneezing, or other physical strain). Stress incontinence primarily affects women with pelvic relaxation caused by childbirth trauma, loss of tissue tone, or aging. Hemodynamic tests are often used to confirm or rule out stress incontinence.

Medical Treatment. Conservative (medical) treatment is usually of no value in severe cases, although it has been effective in less serious cases, especially in younger people. These measures are primarily used for patients who are poor surgical risks or do not wish to undergo surgery. Conservative treatment includes Kegel exercises, vaginal cones, and drug therapy (such as phenylpropanolamine and tricyclic antidepressants). Other treatment choices include the use of alphaadrenergic agents and estrogen therapy for women with vaginal atrophy. If these conservative measures fail, surgical repair will be necessary, unless the patient chooses to continue to wear a peripad or incontinent briefs for urinary containment.

Surgical Treatment. Many operative procedures are used to correct stress incontinence. The underlying principles of these procedures are the same; by elevating the neck of the bladder and suturing it into place, the normal curvature of the bladder is restored. With the curative of the bladder neck restored, continence is usually regained.

Reflex and Urge Incontinence

Urge (urgency) incontinence is the involuntary loss of urine that follows a sudden, strong desire to urinate. Patients with this condition usually cannot stop their urinary stream once it starts and often cannot get to their bathroom in time.

Reflex incontinence and urge incontinence are similar in that both types of patients experience urgency before voiding. This is caused by bladder spasm. However, urge incontinence is due to irritation of the bladder wall or irritation from urine components. Reflex incontinence is due to bladder instability secondary to upper motor lesions or neuropathies.

Often the patient with urge incontinence will reduce his or her fluid intake to decrease incontinent episodes. This concentrates the urine further and causes increased spasms. Patients with urge incontinence also will use the toilet frequently and in small amounts to prevent incontinent episodes. This ultimately decreases the functional capacity of the bladder. If this practice continues for a long time, the muscles become weakened. Distention of the bladder then causes it to spasm at lower volumes. Therefore, this becomes a vicious cycle.

Treatment and Nursing Considerations. Nursing measures for urge and reflex incontinence include encouraging fluids. This dilutes urine and flushes irritating substances out of the bladder. Bladder retraining is used to increase the time between voidings and thus to increase

---

Keys to Patient/Family Teaching
Bladder Retraining

- The patient must be able to follow one-step commands.
- Use a voiding diary (to determine frequency and continence status).
- Establish a baseline pattern of voiding with the voiding diary.
- Set the interval goal slightly shorter than the average interval between incontinent or voiding episodes, as shown in the voiding diary.
- Once the patient consistently empties his or her bladder when toileting, begin to increase the interval between toileting times.
- Encourage the patient to resist the urge to toilet for 5 to 10 minutes (by using distraction or relaxation techniques).
- Gradually increase the length of time the patient is to resist the urge to toilet until a target goal is reached (usually 20 minutes).
- Gradually increase the length of time between voidings to the target goal of 3 to 4 hours.

functional bladder capacity. Nursing skills in bladder training are given in the accompanying box. More detailed discussion is in Chapter 46. The following medications may be prescribed to inhibit bladder spasms:

◆ Propantheline bromide (such as Norpanth, Pro-Banthine)
◆ Oxybutynin chloride (Ditropan)
◆ Calcium channel-blockers (nifedipine [Procardia])
◆ Imipramine (Tofranil)

Biofeedback and Kegel exercises are often used as an adjunct to bladder retraining, so the patient learns to contract the pubococcygeal muscles until near toileting facilities. If these measures do not work, surgery for bladder augmentation (*augmentation cystoplasty*) may be considered to increase the functional size of the bladder.

Overflow (Paradoxical) Incontinence

The name paradoxical describes the condition; the bladder operates opposite to normal. It collects urine but does not empty when full. This type of incontinence also is called overflow incontinence, because the patient typically has a large, distended bladder but dribbles urine.

This dribbling incontinence results when the bladder muscles have decompensated, which can be caused by an obstruction or an injury. Examples of obstruction that can cause this muscle decompensation include benign prostatic hyperplasia (BPH), cancer of the prostate that presses on the urethra, and postoperative urinary retention. This is the reason that observation of voiding is so vital following surgery. A flaccid neurogenic bladder also can cause paradoxical incontinence. Causes of neurogenic bladder disorder include spinal cord injury or lesions, usually below the T_{12} level.

Treatment. The only treatment for paradoxical incontinence caused by an obstruction is relief of the obstruction. Surgery is usually needed. If the incontinence is a result of a neurogenic bladder, the problem may be treated with medications and a bladder retraining program. This may include double voiding, prompted voiding, and controlled fluid intake.

Nursing Considerations. The patients typically have a large residual urine volume, and the bladder is distended. If the cause of the distention is postoperative urine retention, one or two catheterizations will usually resolve the problem. Other noninvasive methods of assisting the patient to void are discussed in Chapter 46. Patient teaching is outlined in the box.

Credé's Maneuver. In Credé's maneuver (pronounced "krā-dáz,") the nurse applies firm, gentle pressure to the bladder, with hands held flat, starting at the umbilicus and moving down to the symphysis pubis. This procedure is repeated several times, with the final pres-

---

Keys to Patient/Family Teaching
Incontinence

Patient and family teaching in incontinence includes

◆ Teach Principles of bladder retraining, including the Credé maneuver, if necessary.
◆ Self-catheterization may be required for long-term management.
◆ The patient may wear an appliance, condom catheter, or incontinent briefs or pads.
◆ Appliances should be washed regularly.
◆ Skin care is important to maintain good skin integrity.
◆ Teach female patients to wipe from front to back to help prevent urinary infections.
◆ Wash hands after toileting.
◆ An incontinent pad is used on the bed and wheelchair to prevent soiling.
◆ Incontinence is often correctable and usually can be reduced.

---

sure being applied directly over the bladder. Bladder incontinence is more difficult to control than bowel incontinence, but with perseverance, control can be established for many patients.

Infectious Disorders

Cystitis

Cystitis, in this context, means inflammation of the urinary bladder. Normally the inside of the bladder is sterile, but bacteria can enter it from infected kidneys and lymphatics or from the urethra. Women are more susceptible than men to cystitis because of the shorter urethra. As indicated previously, one reason for using sterile technique during catheterization is to prevent introduction of bacteria into the bladder. Cystitis is usually the result of infection elsewhere in the urinary tract or in the reproductive system. Systemic disease may make a person more susceptible to bladder infection.

Signs and Symptoms. The patient with cystitis has a desire to urinate frequently, although the bladder does not need emptying. Very small amounts are voided each time. Urination is accompanied by a painful, burning sensation; sometimes there is blood in the urine, and the patient complains of a "heavy feeling" in the abdomen or perineum. The cardinal signs of urinary tract infection are frequency, dysuria, hematuria (or other abnormal components of urine, such as WBC or pus), and a positive urine culture.

Nursing Considerations. A urine for culture and sensitivity is obtained by the nurse. Antibiotics or sulfonamides are given. The specific drug is selected on the basis of the culture and sensitivity results. Some medications given for urinary tract infections cause a discoloration of the urine. For example, phenazopyridine hydrochloride (Pyridium) causes the urine to be orange–red and may stain fabric and toilet fixtures. Patients should be informed of this before administration of these medications.

Fluid intake 3 to 4 L/d is recommended, unless contraindicated, *(Rationale: The additional fluid intake helps dilute the urine, thus lessening burning with urination. It also encourages elimination, thus preventing stasis of urine in which bacteria can multiply. The flushing out of the system prevents formation of crystals, which may develop a result of sulfonamide therapy.)* Cranberry juice is given to increase the amount of acid in the urine. Warm sitz baths are ordered. The nurse should remind female patients always to wipe from front to back to help prevent urethral contamination from stool.

Special Considerations in Aging
Urinary Tract Infections

◆ The only presenting symptom of a urinary tract infection in the elderly often is a *change in mental status*. Suspect this type of infection in all elderly patients who present with sudden, acute changes in mental status.

◆ The elderly do not metabolize medications as quickly or as well as younger patients. The nurse should account for this change when choosing doses and times for medications given PRN (as needed).

◆ The elderly often have several chronic disorders. Always be aware of how these disorders influence kidney function. Be alert to subtle changes in behavior or personality or daily functioning, and report these changes to the physician. Document your assessments carefully.

Pyelonephritis

Acute Pyelonephritis

Acute pyelonephritis or simple inflammation of kidney and renal pelvis, is the most common form of kidney disease. It is usually the result of infection by organisms that have migrated from another part of the body. They may reach the kidney through the bloodstream, causing inflammation, edema, and sometimes many small abscesses. Pyelonephritis also may result as an ascending infection from the lower urinary tract.

The patient with this condition is very ill, with accompanying pain, pyuria (pus in the urine), chills, fever, nausea, vomiting, headache, and flank pain. If the bladder is also infected, he or she will have a desire to urinate frequently, and burning will accompany voiding. A urine test reveals bacteria in the urine (bacteriuria) as well as WBCs (leukocytes) and casts (epithelial, fatty, or waxy material extruded in the urine).

Nursing Considerations. Bedrest, plenty of fluids, attention to mouth and skin care, proper nourishment, and change of position are important. All these measures are directed toward patient comfort and prevention of deformities or infection. If the patient has nausea or vomiting, an intravenous line will be started to prevent dehydration. Antibiotics, sulfonamides, or urinary antiseptics are given to combat specific organisms. Every effort is made to prevent this condition from becoming chronic by eliminating the infection and by comprehensive patient teaching.

Chronic Pyelonephritis

Chronic pyelonephritis may develop if the infection recurs or an obstruction interferes with the passage of urine. The kidney becomes permanently damaged, and kidney tissue is not replaced. The treatment of chronic pyelonephritis consists of continued efforts to prevent more damage. If it is severe, chronic pyelonephritis can lead to death.

Key Concept

Damage to the kidney can be life-threatening if not treated promptly.

Glomerulonephritis

Glomerulonephritis is a group of diseases in which the kidneys are damaged and partly destroyed by inflammation of the glomeruli. When medical personnel speak of nephritis, they are most often speaking of glomerulonephritis. It is believed that some, if not all, forms of glomerulonephritis are autoimmune in origin. In this case the person forms antibodies against his or her own glomerular basement membrane (see Chapter 78).

Acute Glomerulonephritis

Often the signs of acute glomerulonephritis appear approximately 2 or 3 weeks after an upper respiratory infection or after scarlet fever. The organism is usually the same *Streptococcus* that causes "strep" throat. This form of glomerulonephritis is most common in children.

Signs and Symptoms. The patient may not notice the symptoms of glomerulonephritis at first. Members of the family may be the first to sense that something is wrong when they become aware of the patient's pale, puffy face and swollen tissue (edema). The patient gets up many times at night to void. The urine will be diluted because of lack of proper filtering in the glomeruli. Hematuria or smoky urine may be present. The patient experiences headaches and irritability. Erythrocytes, albumin, and casts are present in the urine. The blood pressure often rises, and the patient may have seizures. In the absence of treatment, serious complications, and possibly death, may follow.

Treatment and Nursing Considerations. The goal in treatment of acute glomerulonephritis is to restore kidney function to the best extent possible. The patient must stay in bed, sometimes for several weeks, to rest the body and put as little strain on the urinary system as possible. Dietary management correlates with laboratory test results. Accurate intake and output and daily weighing must be documented. Fluids are given to balance output. The patient receives antibiotics, such as penicillin, to counteract any existing infection. Skin care and oral hygiene are needed to prevent skin breakdown and infection; this patient's skin is friable (fragile). Passive or active exercises help prevent respiratory and circulatory complications.

With treatment, almost all patients recover from acute glomerulonephritis; they are not considered well until the urine has been continuously free of albumin and red blood cells (erythrocytes) for several months.

Chronic Glomerulonephritis

Chronic glomerulonephritis may develop immediately after an episode of acute nephritis or after the patient has been free of symptoms for an extended time. It also is possible for a person to contract chronic nephritis without having been aware that he or she had acute nephritis.

Signs and Symptoms. Chronic glomerulonephritis is much more serious than acute glomerulonephritis, because it causes permanent damage to the kidney by destroying nephrons and thereby disrupting kidney function. The symptoms are similar to those in glomerulonephritis. In the beginning stage, there are few physical symptoms, other than mild general malaise; albumin in the urine; pale, dilute urine; slight anemia; hypertension; and marked edema throughout. The disease flares up at intervals, but the patient usually feels well between attacks. During the course of the disease, which may be 10 to 30 years (with symptoms under control), signs of renal insufficiency develop. If ESRD, end-stage renal disease, also known as chronic renal failure, develops, the patient may die quickly.

Treatment. Treatment includes attention to edema through salt and water restrictions and antihypertensive medications. If ESRD occurs, as evidenced by the previous symptoms and elevated BUN and serum creati-

nine, the patient is given the same treatment as that for chronic renal failure. Renal failure is discussed later in this chapter.

> **Nursing Alert**
>
> The person with chronic glomerulonephritis is very ill and needs excellent nursing care. The person may be placed in protective isolation.

In the advanced stages of the disease, complications are blurred vision, followed by blindness. Nosebleed (epistaxis) and gastrointestinal bleeding are not unusual in the terminally ill patient.

Nursing Considerations. When signs of a flare-up of chronic glomulonephritis appear, the patient is placed on bedrest. Salt intake is lowered, and protein and fluid are limited in the diet. Exposure to infection of any kind must be avoided. Transfusions may be given for anemia. The patient is placed in the orthopneic position to facilitate breathing. With this treatment, the symptoms usually subside in approximately 3 weeks, and the patient gradually returns to a normal routine.

In the absence of dialysis or a kidney transplant, the prognosis in the chronic form of the disease is poor.

> **Nursing Alert**
>
> Chronic glomerulonephritis can have serious complications. These may include pulmonary edema, increased blood pressure, anemia, cerebral hemorrhage, congestive heart failure, and renal failure.

Obstructive Disorders

Obstructions in the urinary system may be caused by a stone (calculi), a growth, a spasm of the ureter, a kink in the ureter or infectious scarring (Fig. 82-2). In males, an enlarged prostate gland also can interfere with the passage of urine. Causes of urinary obstruction may be any of the following: meatal stenosis, calculus, blood clot, tumor, BPH, fibrosis, urethral stricture, neurogenic bladder, precipitates (materials precipitated out of urine), adhesions, or scar tissue.

Hydronephrosis

When urinary obstructions eventually block the outflow of the kidneys, a condition called **hydronephrosis** develops. In this condition, urine is formed but urinary flow out of the kidney is obstructed. Depending on where the obstruction occurs, waste products can

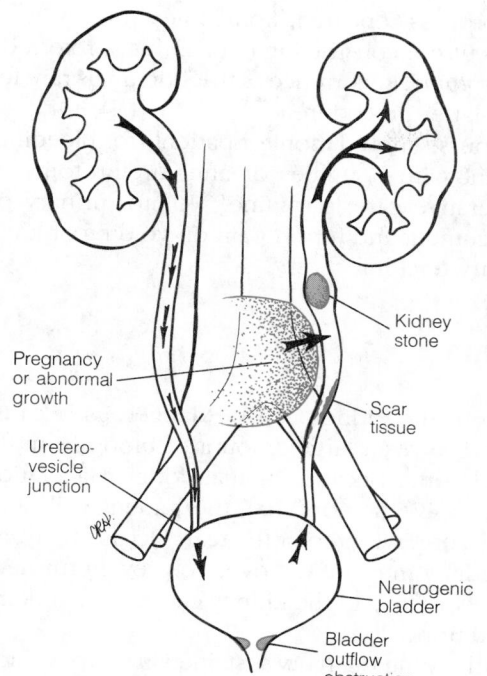

Figure 82-2. Locations and causes of urinary tract obstruction. Porth CM. Pathophysiology: Concepts of Altered Health States. Ed 4. Philadelphia: J.B. Lippincott, 1994.

accumulate in the kidney and back up into the blood; this leads to ESRD.

Hydronephrosis is a complication of an obstructive process. If the obstruction is in the ureter, only one kidney will be involved; if it is in the urethra, urine is abnormally retained in the bladder. Usually in urethral obstruction, both kidneys are affected. A bladder infection also is likely because the urine is allowed to stagnate.

Hydronephrosis may be gradual, partial, or intermittent. Generally, acute hydronephrosis is reversible, but the cause of the obstruction must be removed as soon as possible to prevent the development of chronic hydronephrosis.

Stones (Calculi) in the Urinary Tract

Urine contains various salts, including uric acid, calcium, and oxaline, which, if they do not dissolve, form stones. This condition is called **lithiasis**. Stones (calculi) form primarily in the kidneys and descend through the urinary passages. No one knows exactly why stones form, although it is believed that infection, dehydration, and urinary stasis (standstill) are contributing factors. People susceptible to calcium stones are usually allowed only a limited amount of milk because the high content of calcium contributes to the stone formation. Often the stones are analyzed for mineral content so

that certain minerals can be restricted in the diet. Patients with a long-term illness who are immobilized for extended periods also are vulnerable. Adequate hydration will help prevent the formation of kidney stones.

Signs and Symptoms. Pain in the region of the obstruction is the primary symptom of renal calculi. Often this pain is called *colic,* an excruciating pain that comes in waves as the ureter tries to force the obstructing stone onward. This pain is violent and unbearable. Only a strong analgesic will relieve it; antispasmodics also may be ordered. If the stone is very small, the spasm may move it along, allowing the patient to pass it. Hematuria also may be present.

Nursing Considerations. Urine containing gravel or small stones should be saved for laboratory examination. If colicky attacks recur, surgery is usually necessary to remove the obstruction. In some cases, stones have been dissolved with medications. (This procedure is not widely used at this time.) Gross hematuria may occur if the stone has traumatized the ureter. Signs of urinary tract infection may be present.

The nursing care plan involves monitoring for signs of infection, observing for hematuria, giving medications, applying warm packs for pain, and encouraging fluids. When a patient is admitted with a possible diagnosis of calculi, all urine should be strained. The nurse or the patient can do this by pouring the urine through gauze, cheesecloth, or a strainer. The calculi must be saved. Usually, the urine is measured and discarded, and the material strained out is saved for examination by the physician or the laboratory.

Surgical Treatment of Ureteral Calculi

Usually once a stone passes through the ureter into the bladder, the patient has no difficulty passing it out of the body in the urine. If the stone does not pass through the ureteral channel spontaneously, it must be surgically removed.

Urethroscopic Calculi Removal. In some cases, it is possible to remove a stone without crushing it. This can be accomplished using a *urethroscopy* procedure. The stone is grabbed and pulled out of ureter, using a special tonglike instrument called a stone basket. Some bleeding is not unusual following this procedure because of the trauma caused by the passing of the scope or stone.

Lithotripsy. The term **lithotripsy** refers to the crushing of stones (calculi). This can be done in the bladder or the urethra by the older method of passing a crushing instrument into the urethra or urinary bladder through the urethroscope. The newer shock wave techniques allow lithotripsy to be accomplished in the ureters or the kidneys as well. (This procedure is discussed previously in this chapter.) The purpose of crushing the stone is to make the fragments small enough to be passed in the urine.

Surgical Removal of Calculi. In rare cases, a stone blocking a ureter requires an incision to remove it. The incision into the ureter with removal of a stone is called *ureterolithotomy*. Preoperative and postoperative care are basically the same as for other abdominal procedures, with careful observation and straining of the urine and care of drainage tubes postoperatively.

Treatment of Calculi in the Kidney

The treatment of **nephrolithiasis** (calculi in the kidney) can be treated in three ways.

Extracorporeal Shock Wave Lithotripsy. The most common treatment today is ESWL. This procedure is discussed previously in this chapter.

Percutaneous Nephrolithotomy. Another means of removing kidney stones is called *percutaneous nephrolithotomy*. In this procedure, a small stab wound is made in the flank, and a catheter is inserted. An ultrasonic probe is inserted through the catheter. Then ultrasound waves are directed at the stone. These waves break the stone into pieces that are small enough to be withdrawn through the catheter. After the procedure, the catheter is left in place for 1 or 2 days, until edema subsides. At this time, normal passage of urine into the ureter and bladder can resume.

Surgical Nephrolithotomy. The method of kidney stone removal least likely to be used today is *surgical nephrolithotomy*. This involves major surgery that includes an incision into the kidney and removal of the stone. However, most calculi can be removed using ESWL or ultrasound, both of which are much safer and less invasive.

Urethral Strictures

Fibrous bands can form anywhere along the urethra to narrow it and interfere with the passage of urine. These conditions are most common in men because their urethra is longer.

Urethral strictures cause difficulty voiding. This patient wants to void frequently, but voiding is accompanied by an intense burning sensation. A urethral stricture can be stretched by inserting metal instruments (sounds, boughies) of graduated sizes into the urethra, beginning with the size that will go past the strictures and gradually increasing to larger ones. Because strictures have a tendency to reform, the patient will need to return to the hospital periodically to have this dila-

tation process repeated. Sometimes surgery is necessary to cut the constricting bands; this is referred to as a *urethrotomy*. Recurrence of the stricture is rare following this latter procedure.

The nurse should monitor patients for bleeding after treatment with boughies or after urethrotomy. Other postoperative care is routine. Monitor urinary output and document and report pain on voiding or any signs of urinary tract infection.

Trauma

Trauma to the kidney can be dangerous because the kidney receives a large amount of blood from the abdominal aorta. Because a small kidney laceration can cause massive hemorrhage, the patient will need immediate surgery to repair the tear. Occasionally, a damaged kidney must be removed to prevent further hemorrhage. Bruising of the kidney can result in edema and blocked urine flow.

A fairly common injury sustained in motor vehicle and other accidents is bladder rupture. This results in shock, sepsis, and hemorrhage. The patient must have emergency surgery, after which a urinary drainage system and other drains will be in place. Postoperative care is routine, with special attention to urinary drainage. Complications later may include impotence or incontinence.

General health teaching includes attention to frequent voiding, to keep the bladder empty when traveling or participating in sports or other dangerous activities.

Neoplasms

Bladder Tumors

The bladder is the most common site of urinary system cancers. Bladder cancer occurs most often in men between the ages of 50 or 70 years. Tumors may be embedded in the bladder wall or may appear as small warts on the inside surface, Most tumors of the bladder are malignant.

Occupational exposure to chemicals increases the risk of this cancer. Cigarette smoking and lung cancer also are associated with increased incidence of bladder cancer. There also seems to be a correlation between coffee drinking or other caffeine intake, taking analgesics containing phenacetin, and the use of certain artificial sweeteners and the occurrence of bladder cancer.

Most often, the presenting sign of bladder cancer is painless hematuria (bloody urine). Bladder cancer is diagnosed by CT scan, x-ray, or cystoscopy.

Treatment. The treatment for bladder cancer varies, depending on the extent of the tumor. Superficial tumors are removed by endoscopic resection (cutting out) or fulguration (cauterization, destruction by electricity). A special cystoscope called a *resectoscope* may be used. It is inserted into the bladder through the urethra. This is known as *transurethral resection of a bladder tumor* (TURBT). Laser therapy also may be used. Patients with this type of tumor return at 6-month intervals for cystoscopic examination to determine if there is tumor recurrence or further tumor development. Radiation therapy or chemotherapy may be given as a preventive measure.

Larger or more extensive tumors are removed through an incision made into the bladder (*cystotomy*). If the tumor is large and invasive, the entire bladder may be removed (cystectomy).

Bladder tumors often metastasize to the lymph nodes, then to the bones of the pelvis, ribs, and vertebrae, and sometimes to the kidneys, liver, or lungs. Radiation therapy and chemotherapy are usually combined with surgery to prevent or minimize metastases.

Urinary Diversion. If the bladder is removed, some sort of urinary diversion is required (Fig. 82-3). An ileal conduit is the most commonly used method for excretion of urine. This requires that the patient wear an appliance over the stoma to contain urine. There is often no voluntary control of urinary flow.

Types of Urinary Diversion. Types of urinary diversion are presented in the accompanying box. Many factors influence the choice of the type of urinary diversion to be used. In the ileal conduit (see Fig. 82-3**A**), a loop of ileum is connected to the ureters and brought out through the skin. In another procedure, called a *ureterosigmoidostomy,* the ureters are connected to a loop of bowel, the sigmoid colon, so urine can drain out through the rectum (see Fig. 82-3**B**). In another procedure, a tube may be placed into the kidney and brought out through the skin (*cutaneous nephrostomy*) or if the bladder is not totally removed, placed in the bladder and brought out through the skin (*cutaneous cystostomy* or *suprapubic cysto-*

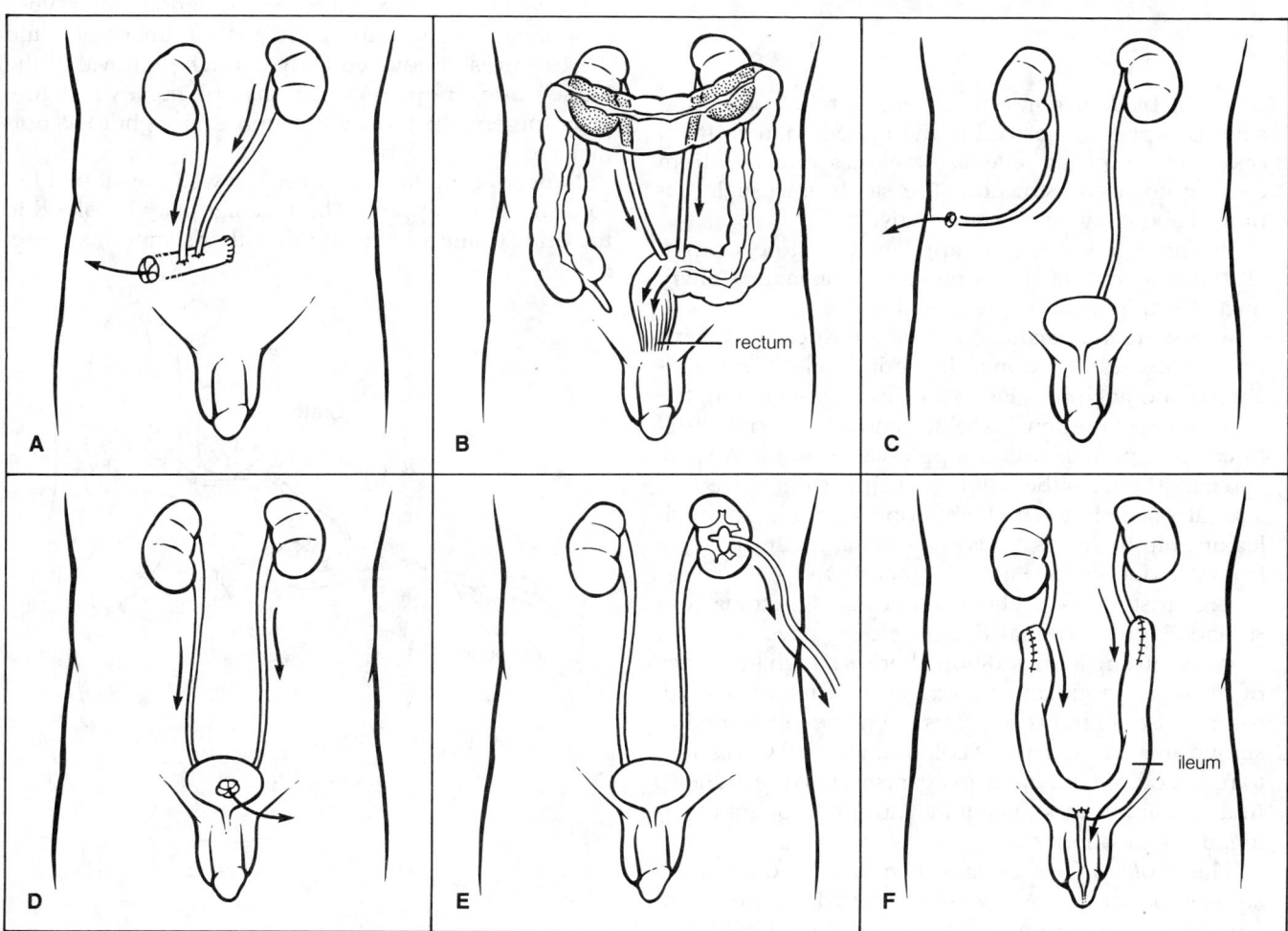

Figure 82-3. Methods of urinary diversion. (**A**) Ileal conduit. (**B**) Ureterosigmoidostomy. (**C**) Cutaneous ureterostomy. (**D**) Vesicostomy. (**E**) Nephrostomy. (**F**) Camey Procedure. Smeltzer SC, Bare BG. Brunner and Suddarth's Textbook of Medical-Surgical Nursing. Ed 7. Philadelphia, J.B. Lippincott, 1992.

Types of Urinary Diversion

Ileal Conduit: Segment of ileum close to the ileocecal valve resected; ureters reanastamosed to it.
    Proximal end of ileal segment closed; distal end brought to abdominal wall as stoma
Ureterostomy: Ureters brought to abdominal wall as stoma
Ureterosigmoidostomy: Transplantation of ureters into intact sigmoid colon; urine and stool elimination controlled by anal sphincter
Continent diversion (Kock Pouch): Two ileal limbs present; each is intussuscepted to create nipple valve.
    Efferent limb brought to skin as stoma.
    Ureters stitched to afferent limb, which prevents reflux
Continent diversion (Indiana pouch): Segment of cecum and ileum resected from the bowel.
    Ureters tunnelled into colon to prevent reflux.
    Continence maintained by ileocecal valve.
    Ileum brought to skin as stoma (pleated to be smaller)
Neobladder: Internal urinary reservoir that empties through urethra

cath). In bladder removal, a stent (a tube- or spring-shaped support) is placed in the ureters to keep them open. This prevents edema or excess drainage from causing urinary obstruction. The stents are usually removed about 2 weeks postoperatively.

In urinary diversion, an appliance must be worn at all times to collect the continuous drainage. Urinary tract infection must be prevented.

A *continent diversion* (such as the Kock or Indiana pouch) also can be done, depending on patient preference and anatomy (Fig. 82-4). In this operation, the midportion of the ileum is folded and opened onto itself to create a pouch, with a nipple-valve stoma. A small gauze pad covers the stoma, which is catheterized on a regular schedule. The high reoperation rate to repair leaking nipple valves tends to discourage many patients from this option. (See also Chapter 81.)

Ureterostomy is rarely done because the stoma constructed is often so small that the elderly have a difficult time visualizing it. In addition, there is a high incidence of stricture, necessitating reoperation. Ureterosigmoidostomy also is rarely done. Postoperative follow-up has shown an increased risk of colon cancer and sepsis, due to reflux of *Escherichia coli* organisms into the kidneys. In addition, the stool is liquid, causing frequent toileting, if not incontinence.

The *neobladder* is a relatively new procedure. It is a surgical option for only a select few who have no involvement of the tumor in the base of the bladder so that the urethra can be salvaged (rather than removed).

Nursing Considerations. Urinary diversion may strongly affect the person's body image. Bladder removal for men is often associated with permanent sexual dys-

function. Adapting to cancer, loss of the bladder, and loss of body image can be devastating. The nurse must be supportive. Patient teaching is an important aspect of nursing care (see box).

Benign Renal (Kidney) Cysts

Cysts of the kidney may be multiple (polycystic disease) or single (monocystic). They are usually benign. Polycystic disease has been found to be a familial problem. It may progress to ESRD or chronic renal failure.

Cancer of the Kidney

Tumors of the kidney are almost always malignant. They occur more frequently in men and rarely before age 30. Renal cancer is aggressive, and patients often have distant metastases and local invasion of nearby organs. Renal cancer accounts for about 2% of all cancers.

A cancer of the kidney is referred to as a *nephroma*. A primary cancer of the kidney is called a *hypernephroma*. Other prefixes are used to denote other types of kidney tumors. If the kidney is a primary site, and the cancer is discovered early enough, removal of the kidney using **nephrectomy** may be curative. Before such surgery, the kidney function is brought to as normal a level as possible.

Cancer of the kidney is usually well developed before signs of it appear. The first sign may be blood in the urine (painless hematuria). Other symptoms are fe-

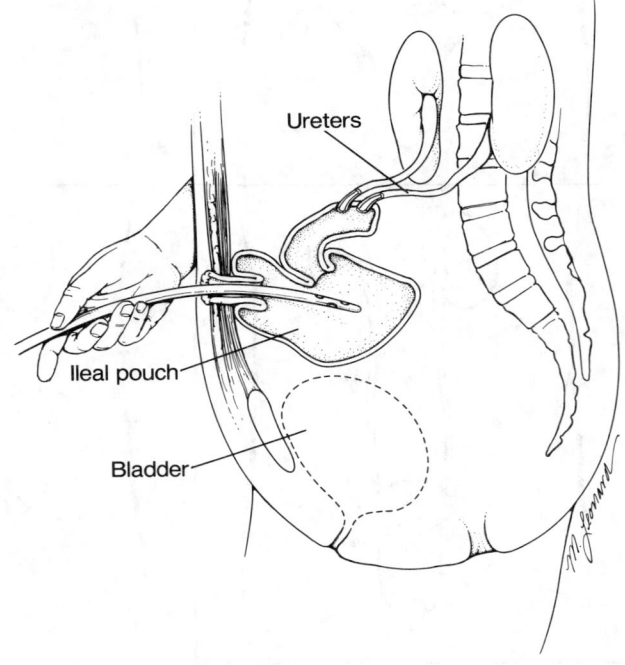

Figure 82-4. Continent ileal urinary reservoir (Kock pouch). Insertion of a catheter through the valve to drain stored urine. Smeltzer SC, Bare BG. Brunner and Suddarth's Textbook of Medical-Surgical Nursing. Ed 7. Philadelphia, J.B. Lippincott, 1992.

Care of the Ileal Conduit

Patient and family teaching about the ileal conduit includes the following:

- Change appliance every 5 to 7 days.
- Use solvent to loosen appliance; do not "tear" the appliance off.
- Clean the skin with water and mild soap.
- To remove encrustations, use gauze soaked with a 1-to-3 part solution of vinegar and water.
- Examine the stoma; healthy stoma tissue is deep pink to dark red and shiny. If the stoma is macerated, dusky, or wet looking, notify the physician.
- Dry the skin area gently, but thoroughly, before applying the appliance.
- If the tissue is excoriated, apply medication as ordered by the enterostomal therapist.
- Use a synthetic barrier cream that contains little or no karaya (urine destroys karaya).
- Instruct the patient that there may be strands of mucus in their urine (from the mucus-producing cells of the ileum).
- Patients should increase their fluid intake to 3 L/day (to flush out sediment and mucus and to prevent clogging of the stoma).

ver, loss of weight, and malaise; a palpable flank mass and pain may appear later.

After x-rays, CT scan, renal arteriography, or ultrasound have confirmed the diagnosis, the kidney may be surgically removed, provided that the other kidney is healthy. Radiation and/or chemotherapy is used when the cancer has spread to the lymph nodes.

Renal Failure

Changes in renal (kidney) function may be considered on a continuum that ranges from impairment to insufficiency to failure.

Renal Impairment, Insufficiency, and Failure

Renal impairment is identified by specific urine concentration and dilution tests. *Renal insufficiency* becomes apparent when the kidneys cannot meet the demands of dietary or metabolic stress. **Renal failure** exists when normal everyday demands cannot be met. As renal function diminishes, the kidney loses its ability to adapt to varying intakes of foods and fluids.

Early in renal failure, the creatinine clearance test provides a convenient means of evaluating the effectiveness of therapy. Later, in chronic renal failure, the serum creatinine level reflects the level of renal func-

tion. As the disease progresses, the serum creatinine level increases.

Causes of Renal Failure. Renal failure is the inability of the kidneys to remove waste products from the blood and body cells and excrete them in the urine. It is a toxic condition associated with renal insufficiency and retention of nitrogenous substances in the blood. This may be the result of kidney disease or urinary tract disturbances. It also may follow acute glomerulonephritis; drug overdose or poisoning; excessive inhalation of a highly toxic substance, such as sulfur or carbon tetrachloride; severe transfusion reactions; and other severe shocks to the system. It also may result from an injury that decreases blood supply to the kidneys. Insulin-dependent diabetes mellitus often leads to chronic renal failure.

A relatively common cause of acute renal failure is acute drug overdose or poisoning. Renal failure also may occur more slowly as a result of *nephrotoxic* drugs given for unrelated disorders. Common nephrotoxic drugs are listed in the accompanying box.

Substances and Common Drugs That Can Become Nephrotoxic

Common Drugs and Possible Renal Damage

- Penicillins: allergic reactions
- Sulfonamides: allergic reactions
- Cephalosporins (eg, cefaclor, cefazolin Na [Ancef], cefoxitin Na [Mefoxin], cephalothin Na [Keflin], cephradine [Velosef]): damaged kidney cells
- Allopurinol (Zyloprim, Lopurin): allergies, also altered liver function
- Aminoglycosides (eg, gentamicin, neomycin, streptomycin): damaged kidney cells
- Amphotericin-B (Fungizone): used to treat fungal infections: can cause permanent renal damage
- Lithium (psychiatric drug): renal toxicity
- Cimetidine (Tagamet): used to treat peptic ulcer; can cause creatinine elevation
- Phenytoin (Dilantin): used to control seizures; can cause toxic hepatitis
- Nonsteroidal anti-inflammatory, analgesic drugs (eg, ibuprofen, indomethacin [Indocin], ketoprofen [Orudis]): used to control pain; can cause acute renal failure or nephrotic syndrome
- Antineoplastics: used to treat cancers; can damage renal cells

Other Substances Toxic to the Kidneys

- Heavy metals
- Aniline dyes
- Iodine-based contrast media
- Carbon tetrachloride
- Ethylene glycol
- Benzene

> **Key Concept**
>
> The nephrotoxicity of any drug must be determined before giving it to a patient. Whenever administering medications, watch for signs of kidney dysfunction, and report this to the physician at once.

Acute Renal Failure

Acute renal failure is sudden in onset. It may be caused by factors outside the kidney (*prerenal failure*), as when the cardiovascular system fails to perfuse the kidneys adequately with blood. (Perfusion is the pouring through of blood in the renal circulation.) Acute renal failure also may be caused by obstructions in the flow of urine (*postrenal failure*) or by damage to the kidney tissue (*intrinsic failure*). Tubular damage, referred to as *acute tubular necrosis*, is the most common form of intrinsic renal dysfunction.

Acute renal failure is characterized by three phases: oliguria, diuresis, and recovery. The *oliguric phase* occurs when the urinary output is less than 400 mL per 24 hours. In this case, laboratory values for serum sodium are decreased, and the serum creatinine and BUN are elevated. This phase may last from 8 to 14 days. In the *diuretic phase*, production of urine is increased. Although urine volume increases, the nurse must be aware that the quality of this urine is inadequate, and the body still is retaining waste products. This is evidenced in the remaining elevation of the BUN and the serum creatinine levels. The *recovery phase* begins when the BUN stabilizes or is in the normal range. In this case, urine volume is normal, and the patient returns to normal activity. This may take several months. However, some patients do not improve and develop chronic renal failure.

During acute renal failure, laboratory studies are performed frequently to monitor BUN, creatinine, and sodium and potassium levels. Early dialysis is often effective for the patient with this disorder.

Dietary measures should be instituted to help control the complications of the condition. Sodium, potassium, protein, and fluids may need to be controlled.

Chronic Renal Failure or End-Stage Renal Disease

Chronic renal failure is known as ESRD. ESRD is an irreversible kidney disease. By definition, this condition includes chronic abnormalities in the internal environment of the kidneys. Chronic renal failure requires maintenance with dialysis or kidney transplantation if the patient is to survive. See the nursing assessment box for symptoms of ESRD. If the underlying condition cannot be corrected, it is possible that the patient will die. Ideally, once a patient is known to have ESRD, he or she should be referred to a dialysis center where the

> **Keys to Nursing Assessment**
> ### Symptoms of ESRD
>
> End-stage renal disease includes any or all of the following symptoms:
>
> ◆ Anemia
> ◆ Itching (pruritus)
> ◆ Uremic frost (waste products crystallizing on the skin)
> ◆ Loss of appetite (anorexia)
> ◆ Hiccups (singultus)
> ◆ Nausea
> ◆ Vomiting
> ◆ Fatigue
> ◆ Fluid accumulation (edema)
> ◆ Generalized body edema (anasarca)
> ◆ Potassium retention
> ◆ Sodium retention
> ◆ Hypertension (high blood pressure)
> ◆ Gastrointestinal bleeding
> ◆ Bleeding disorders
> ◆ Bone disease
> ◆ Nerve conduction defects
> ◆ Congestive heart failure
> ◆ Inflammation of the pericardial sac
> ◆ Decreased immune response
> ◆ Decreased platelet function
> ◆ Retardation of growth in children
> ◆ Dementia
> ◆ Sexual dysfunction
> ◆ Malnutrition
> ◆ Decreased vitamin metabolism
> ◆ Metabolic acidosis

patient and family will be helped to decide whether the patient will receive no treatment, peritoneal dialysis or hemodialysis for life, or kidney transplantation.

The nursing and medical care plans are designed to treat the primary cause of ESRD and to treat the symptoms as they occur. The patient is kept in as normal a state as possible, and attempts are made to prevent further kidney damage.

Nursing Considerations. Nursing considerations in ESRD are the following:

◆ Sedatives are given for restlessness, transfusions for anemia, and digitalis for tachycardia or dysrhythmias.
◆ Fluids are restricted because the kidneys are not excreting urine. Fluids must be varied. Urge the patient to spread the fluid allowance throughout the day.
◆ Alkaline solutions are given for acidosis, and the patient is put on a diet high in fat and carbohydrates and low in protein, sodium, and potassium.
◆ Fluid and electrolyte balance should be maintained

Shirley Downes is a 74-year-old African-American woman admitted to the hospital with the diagnosis of chronic renal failure. She has a history of hypertension, dementia, chronic renal insufficiency, right CVA with left hemiparesis, glaucoma, anemia, and hypothyroidism. Prior to this admission she has been living with her daughter and three grandchildren. There is every reason to believe that the family relationship is loving and that the patient's daughter has consistently acted in her mother's best interests. Until now the patient's renal insufficiency has been treated conservatively with fluid and dietary adjustments. The medical team has approached the daughter for her consent to begin dialysis treatments for her mother. The medical resident has explained to the daughter that dialysis should correct the patient's electrolyte and metabolic imbalances but that, given her multiple medical problems, there is no guarantee that her quality of life will be significantly improved. Conservative management will be less effective and may lead to a more rapid death. The daughter appears to be overwhelmed by the implications of this decision. Prior to this hospitalization she had begun seeking nursing home placement for her mother, believing that she could no longer minister to her mother's needs at home. The following nursing diagnosis addresses the daughter's decision-making dilemma.

Nursing Diagnosis: *Decisional conflict (initiation of dialysis) related to uncertainty about what is in the patient's best interests and fear of making the wrong decision (guilt) as evidenced by statements reflecting ambivalence, fear, distress*

Goal: By 10/3 the patient's daughter will express a decision regarding dialysis treatments for her mother that she believes are in the mother's best interests

Nursing Actions (assess/do/teach)	Rationale	Evaluative Statement
1. Attempt to elicit what the daughter believes the best course of action for her mother will be; explore each option, discussing possible consequences for both the patient and her family; clarify any misunderstandings the patient and daughter have (*eg*, should withholding dialysis result in an earlier death, it would not be the daughter's decision that "killed" the mother, but rather the disease process)	The qualities of the nurse–patient–family relationship make the nurse a key player in these types of decisions	10/2 Goal met; the daughter informed the medical staff that she believes that her mother would not wish dialysis but that conservative management should continue to be employed; "My mother has lived a full and a good life but she was never one for doctoring—she often used to say that she was in the Lord's hands and ready for Him whenever he'd call. I don't think she'd go for all these treatments."
2. Help the daughter to understand (a) the difference between a treatment that is *efficacious* (will alter the course or progression of the disease) and one that is *beneficial* (truly in the patient's broadest best interests); and (b) that no one is obligated to consent to a treatment of questionable efficacy and benefit	Lacking medical information and possibly confused about the patient's best interests versus overall family interests, the daughter may need assistance drawing helpful distinctions	
3. Once the daughter has made her decision (refer her to the hospital ethics committee, a spiritual counselor, or other counselor if indicated), support her decision and be an advocate if necessary	Caretaker fatigue is frequently observed in the adult children of dependent older persons; support may be necessary to bolster their confidence and self-esteem	

if at all possible. Frequent blood chemistry studies will be done, and the physician needs the reports as soon as possible. Adjustments can be made by intraveneously administering electrolytes.

◆ Accurate documentation of intake and output is vital because it is important to determine exactly how much urine the kidneys are secreting. This helps to determine the extent of the disease.

◆ Daily weights are taken to detect the presence of fluid retention or edema.

◆ Good skin care and special mouth care are impor-

tant. To relieve the itching and crusting brought on by pruritus and uremic frost, the patient should bathe with tepid water, use no soap, and place a small amount of vinegar or baking soda in the bath water.

◆ Chilling and exposure to infections should be prevented because the patient has few natural defenses to fight off infection. Also, many antibodies are excreted through the kidneys. It is important to be alert for respiratory or cardiac complications. These are serious signs.

Keys for Review

Key Questions for Critical Thinking

1. Describe the difference between a continent diversion and an ileal conduit. State how nursing differs in the two.
2. Explain why inflammations of the urinary tract are treated so aggressively. Identify teaching you would use in prevention of urinary tract infections.
3. Compare the classes of incontinence. Describe the goals of care for each class and the primary treatment for each.
4. Develop a plan of care for teaching bladder retraining to a 70-year-old woman.

Key Readings

Belcher AE. Cancer Nursing. St. Louis, Mosby-Yearbook, 1992

Berkow R (Ed). The Merck Manual of Diagnosis and Therapy, Ed 16. Rahway, NJ, Merck & Co, 1992

Doughty DB. Urinary and Fecal Incontinence: Nursing Management. St. Louis, Mosby-Yearbook, 1991

Fischbach F. A Manual of Laboratory and Diagnostic Tests, Ed 3. Philadelphia, J.B. Lippincott, 1992

Gray M. Genitourinary Disorders. St. Louis, Mosby-Yearbook, 1992

Jeter K, Faller N, Norton C. Nursing for Continence. Philadelphia, W.B. Saunders, 1990

NANDA Nursing Diagnoses: Definitions and Classifications 1992. Philadelphia, W.B. Saunders, 1990

Nursing '94 Drug Handbook. Springhouse, PA, Springhouse, 1994

O'Toole M (Ed). Miller-Keane Encyclopedia and Dicttionary of Medicine, Nursing, and Allied Health, Ed 5. Philadelphia, W.B. Saunders, 1992

Smeltzer SC, Bare BG. Brunner and Suddarth's Texbook of Medical-Surgical Nursing, Ed 7. Philadelphia, J.B. Lippincott, 1992

Key Readings (continued)

Taylor C, Lillis C, LeMone P. Fundamentals of Nursing: Art and Science of Nursing Care, Ed 2. Philadelphia, J.B. Lippincott, 1993

Thomas CL (Ed). Taber's Cyclopedic Medical Dictionary, Ed 17. Philadelphia, F.A. Davis, 1993

Enrichment Keys

Urinary Continence Guideline Panel. Urinary Continence in Adults: Clinical Practice Guidelines. AHCPR Publication #920038.

Agency for Health Care Policy and Research, Public Health Service, US Department of Health and Human Services, Rockville MD, March, 1992

Keys To Learning More

Chapter 83: male reproductive disorders

Chapter 84: female reproductive disorders

Unit Fifteen: geriatric nursing

Chapter 89: rehabilitation, ambulatory and home care nursing

Unit Seventeen: death and dying

Key Resources

National Association of Patients on Hemodialysis and Transplantation
    211 E. 43rd Street
    New York, NY 10017
    212/867-4486

National Kidney Foundation
    30 East 33rd Street, Suite 1100
    New York, NY 10016
    212/889-2210

United Network for Organ Sharing (UNOS)
    3001 Hungary Spring Road
    Richmond, VA 23228
    804/289-5380

83 Male Reproductive Disorders

Keys for Learning

Learning Objectives

♦ Discuss the results of prostate surgery on the function of the genitourinary system.
♦ Describe the postoperative care of the patient who has had a radical prostatectomy.
♦ Define impotence and its treatment.
♦ Describe the implications of impotence on human sexuality.
♦ Explain why not correcting cryptorchidism will result in sterility.

Key Terms

cryptorchidism
epididymitis
epispadias
hesitancy
hydrocele
hypospadias
impotence
orchiectomy

orchitis
phimosis
plication
priapism
prostatectomy
seminoma
urologist
varicocele

Keys to Understanding This Chapter

Chapter 19: endocrine system
Chapter 24: urinary system
Chapter 25: male reproductive system
Chapter 30: medical asepsis
Chapter 38: signs and symptoms of illness or injury
Chapter 45: personal hygiene and skin care
Chapter 46: elimination
Chapter 47: specimen collection
Chapter 50: physical examination, including the male reproductive system
Chapter 53: the person who has surgery
Chapter 54: surgical asepsis
Chapter 63: sexuality and sexually transmitted diseases
Chapter 72: endocrine disorders

Keys to Understanding This Chapter
(continued)

Chapter 76: cancer
Chapter 78: HIV, AIDS, and autoimmune disorders
Chapter 82: urinary disorders

Key Points

♦ Impotence is generally psychogenic in nature, but it can have organic components.
♦ Chronic prostatitis is resistant to antibiotic therapy.
♦ Unrelieved torsion of the spermatic cord results in necrosis of the affected testicle.
♦ Recurrent or chronic infection will destroy sperm production.
♦ Most testicular cancer occurs between ages 18 and 35. Testicular self-examination should be performed by all men from early adolescence.
♦ Patients with benign prostatic hyperplasia should avoid decongestants, antihistamines, and diet pills because these medications increase the tendency to develop acute urinary retention.
♦ Patients contemplating surgical treatment of benign prostatic hyperplasia should be told that they may experience some incontinence and/or impotence after the operation.
♦ A sudden increase of bleeding after surgery is a medical emergency.

Key Topics Outline

Anatomy and Physiology Review
Diagnostic Tests
    Laboratory Tests
    Tests to Diagnose Penile Disorders
    Other Diagnostic Tests
Medical and Surgical Treatments
    Common Medical Treatments
    Common Surgical Treatments

Rosdahl CB: Textbook of Basic Nursing, 6th ed. © 1995 J.B. Lippincott Company

Key Learning Activities

- Observe a patient with a transurethral resection of the prostate (TURP).
- Interview a patient who has had a TURP (at least 6 months ago). Has he had any complications? What are his major concerns? How has he adjusted? What suggestions would he make to other patients?
- Make a chart listing sexually transmitted diseases and indicating their effects on the male reproductive system.

The male reproductive system is closely intertwined with the urinary system. For this reason, disorders of the male reproductive system are often treated by the **urologist.**

Anatomy and Physiology Review

Chapter 25 discusses the male reproductive system and how it functions. The male reproductive system includes the testes (which produce sperm—the male gamete) and the epididymides (which transport the sperm to the vasa deferentia where the sperm is stored). The two paired vas deferens also produce the components of semen. The prostate produces nutrients for the sperm, and the seminal vesicles propel the sperm and semen through the penis during ejaculation.

In this chapter, the prostate is considered separately from the rest of the reproductive system, because it is also considered a part of the urinary system.

Diagnostic Tests

Laboratory Tests

The Prostate-Specific Antigen Level

The prostate-specific antigen (PSA) test is specific for prostate cancer. The PSA is usually elevated before cancer can be detected by external examination. In other words, the PSA is elevated *prior to* the onset of clinical symptoms. Thus, prostatic cancer can be discovered and treated early for a much improved prognosis. This test should be included in all physical examinations of men older than 40 years.

Other Laboratory Tests

Other tests, such as the sperm count or DNA determination may be done.

Tests to Diagnose Penile Disorders

Several diagnostic tests are used to evaluate the function of the corpus cavernosum of the penis. These tests are most often part of a testing battery for impotence.

Cavernosography

This is an x-ray examination of the corpus cavernosum. *Dynamic infusion cavernosography* involves injection of the radiopaque contrast medium or saline solution directly into the corpus cavernosum. It allows evaluation of the corpus and associated blood vessels and can detect venous leaks.

Key Abbreviations and Acronyms for Male Reproductive Disorders

ARRP	Anatomic retropubic radical prostatectomy
BPH	Benign prostatic hyperplasia
PSA	Prostate-specific antigen
PUS	Prostate ultrasound
TURP	Transurethral resection of the prostate
UTI	Urinary tract infection

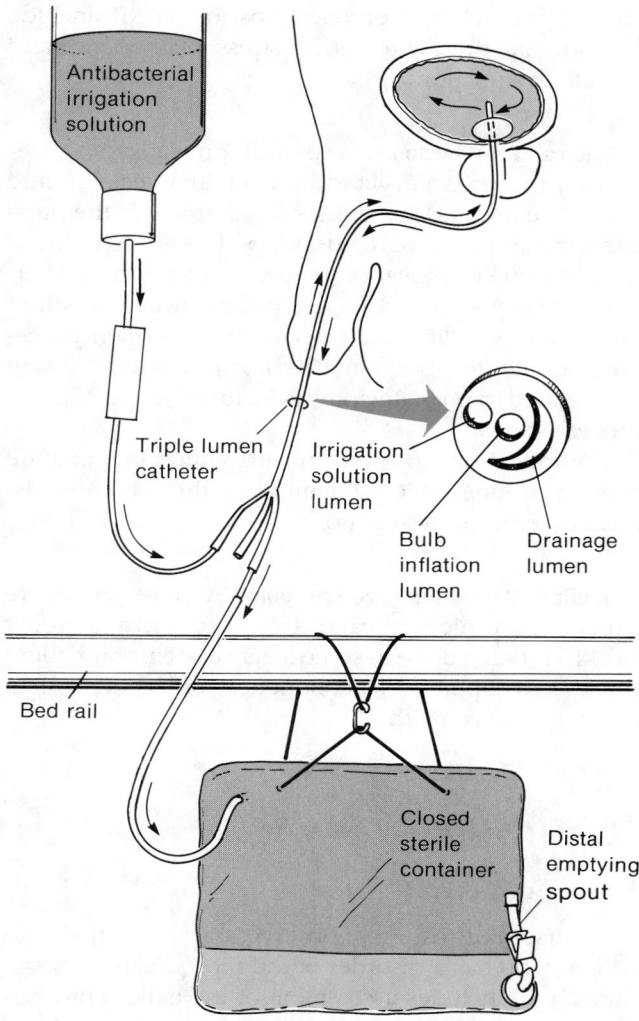

Figure 83-1. The closed sterile drainage system, used in transurethral resection of the prostate (TURP).

Labels in figure: Antibacterial irrigation solution; Triple lumen catheter; Irrigation solution lumen; Bulb inflation lumen; Drainage lumen; Bed rail; Closed sterile container; Distal emptying spout

Cavernosometry

This test measures the pressures in blood vessels of the corpus. *Dynamic infusion cavernosometry* allows the physician to study a graphic representation of the pressures within the corpus as a function of infused volume.

Nursing Considerations. The usual precautions relating to radiopaque dyes are taken, if these are to be used (see Chapter 50 for precautions when dye is used). There may be some discomfort when the dye or saline is injected. The man should be told that these procedures will usually induce an erection.

Other Diagnostic Tests

Prostatic Biopsy

To diagnose prostatic cancer following a suspicious rectal examination, a *transrectal biopsy* may be done. This is an ultrasound technique. The ultrasound probe

used for this test is combined with a special bioptic needle that is activated by a rapid-firing spring. The biopsy needle obtains a tissue sample in a fraction of a second. Because this procedure is so fast, the patient does not feel pain. The probe, inserted through the rectum, gives a clear picture of the prostate on a television screen. This allows the urologist to guide the biopsy needle to the location of the suspected cancer.

> **Key Concept**
>
> The male patient may be embarrassed and concerned about any disorder related to the reproductive system. He may see the disorder as a threat to his manhood. The female nurse must be especially conscious of these concerns and be sensitive to the patient's feelings when caring for him.

Medical and Surgical Treatments

Common Medical Treatments

Continuous Bladder Irrigation

Following removal of the prostate, the patient will, almost without exception, return from the operating room with a special TURP irrigation setup in place (Fig. 83-1). This device may also be used following some other genitourinary procedures.

In the operating room a special catheter with three lumina (separate tubes or openings) is inserted. One lumen is used to inflate the balloon that holds the catheter in place. Another lumen allows fluids to run into the bladder for irrigation; and the third carries drainage from the bladder to the drainage bag. The irrigation may be continuous after surgery or it may be intermittent.

The purpose of postoperative TURP bladder irrigation is to keep the catheter patent. Continuous irrigation washes out blood before it can form clots; intermittent irrigation washes out clots that plug the catheter. If clots plug the catheter and are not irrigated out, overdistention of the bladder results. In many cases, the flow is controlled by a computerized pump or controller. Nursing care related to TURP follows in the Nursing Process section.

Radiation Therapy

Following a prostatectomy, the patient may receive radiation therapy or chemotherapy particularly if there was local invasion of nearby organs or lymph nodes by the cancer. Key medications are listed in the box. Chapter 76 contains a more detailed discussion of chemotherapy.

y Medications

for Chemotherapy

♦ diethylstilbestrol (Stilbestrol)
♦ ketoconazole (Nizoral)
♦ spironolactone (Aldactone)

Nursing Considerations

♦ Side effects of these agents include edema, impotence, and gynecomastia (abnormal development of breasts).

Common Surgical Treatments

Prostatectomy

The usual treatment for benign prostatic hyperplasia and prostatic cancer is surgical removal of the excess or abnormal prostate tissue (prostatectomy).

The prostate can be dissected through an incision over the bladder (a suprapubic prostatectomy or suprapubic resection), by perineal incision (perineal prostatectomy or perineal resection), or by transurethral resection of the prostate (TURP). It also can be done through cystoscope (resectoscope) through the urethra.

Suprapubic Prostatectomy. The suprapubic procedure is usually performed if the gland is greatly enlarged (more than 100 g), and it may be done in two stages. First, a cystostomy (incision into the bladder) is done to relieve retention of urine; second, the prostate tissue is removed. After the two-stage suprapubic operation, the patient returns with two indwelling catheters in place, one in the urethra and the other in the suprapubic wound (a suprapubic cystocath). These catheters are attached to separate drainage containers, allowing for more accurate measurement. The wound catheter is attached to an irrigation apparatus and the urethral catheter is attached to a closed drainage system. (The physician may prefer that any bladder irrigation be done through the urethral catheter.)

Perineal Prostatectomy. If the gland tissue is removed by perineal prostatectomy, catheter drainage is through the perineal incision only. In this case, the man will find it difficult to sit up.

Transurethral Resection of the Prostate. The most common procedure, particularly for older men or those who are poor surgical risks, is TURP. The prostate tissue is removed through the urethra by means of a resectoscope, which has a cutting edge or electric wire that slices the prostate away bit by bit. Because the operation is done through the urethra, no incision is made. The recovery period after TURP is shorter than that with

other approaches. Complications of TURP include hemorrhage, urinary retention, stress incontinence and erectile dysfunction.

Radical Prostatectomy. A radical prostatectomy (removing the prostate gland, the seminal vesicles, and part of the urethra) sometimes cures cancer of the prostate if metastases have not developed. Often an orchiectomy is done (removal of the testes) or hormone therapy (estrogens) may be given to slow down growth of the tumor. A radical prostatectomy is an open procedure because an abdominal incision is needed. Nursing care related to prostatectomy is included in the Nursing Process section.

Complications of radical prostatectomy include stress incontinence, epididymitis, urethral stricture, fistula and erectile dysfunction.

Radical Retropubic Prostatectomy. A new procedure called anatomic radical retropubic prostatectomy (ARRP) is being done in some locations. This procedure causes less impotence, incontinence, and bleeding than more traditional methods.

❖ *Nursing Process*

Data Collection

The nurse must carefully observe and assess the male patient who has a disorder of the reproductive system. Chapter 50 includes assessment of the male reproductive system. This assessment establishes a baseline for future comparison and determines the presence of suspected complications. The nurse should report any changes in the baseline level. The accompanying box lists some components of nursing assessment of the male reproductive system. Because of the close relationship between the male urinary and reproductive systems, many of the same questions are asked. It is

Keys to Nursing Assessment

Male Reproductive System

♦ Urinary and reproductive history
♦ General health history
♦ History of sexually transmitted diseases or exposure
♦ Sexual dysfunction
♦ Urinary dysfunction
♦ Inspection of external reproductive structures
♦ Prostate examination
♦ Testicular examination

also important to realize that some patients are embarrassed in discussing reproductive health.

The nurse observes the patient's emotional response to the disorder or disease. A sexual dysfunction has major emotional components. Does the man need assistance to meet daily needs? Is the disorder correctable? Does it affect social activities or self-esteem? Is it life-threatening? Is the man anxious or fearful of the outcome? What additional services are needed?

Nursing Diagnosis

Based on data collection, nursing diagnoses are established. Some diagnoses may have different causal factors. The following are examples of nursing diagnoses that may appear on nursing care plans for male patients with reproductive disorders:

◆ Altered Urinary Elimination related to prostate enlargement
◆ Urinary Retention related to prostate enlargement, surgical trauma
◆ Impaired Tissue Integrity related to prostatic disorders, radiation therapy
◆ Sexual Dysfunction related to impotence, medications, altered body image
◆ Altered Sexuality patterns related to impotence, structural defects, infections, surgical trauma
◆ Situational Low Self Esteem related to impotence
◆ Fear related to poor prognosis

Planning and Implementation

The patient, nurse and healthcare team plan together for effective care to meet patient needs based on the nursing diagnosis. The nurse provides preoperative and postoperative care for the patient. The male patient with a reproductive disorder may also require assistance in meeting daily needs, dealing with emotional problems, and understanding more about the disorder, its prognosis and treatment. A nursing care plan is developed to meet these needs. A sample nursing care plan for a male patient with a reproductive disorder is provided later in the chapter.

Preoperative Preparation for Prostatectomy

As part of the preoperative preparation for a radical prostatectomy, the nurse should prepare the patient and his sexual partner for the strong possibility of sexual dysfunction postoperatively. About 90% of men are impotent after surgery except those who have the ARRP procedure. (Depending on age, the impotence rate with ARRP is only about 30%, with younger men less likely to become impotent.) Because 80% of prostate cancers are androgen dependent, one of the treatment goals will be to decrease circulating androgens and this

will further impact the ability of the male erection.

The patient who wishes to have childre couraged to consider sperm banking. Revie of penile implants available and how they

Discussion should include the possibilit patient will have a suprapubic cystoscopy (suprapubic cystocath) and some sort of c bladder irrigation for 2–3 days following surge

Before the prostatectomy, the patient ma a catheter inserted for continuous drainage of to prevent accumulation of stagnant urine in the der. He is given plenty of fluids, with proper die rest to build up his resistance, and often antib prophylactically.

Providing Postoperative Care

The patient will require routine postoperative care suc as antiembolytic stockings, early ambulation, and in centive spirometry. Fluids are encouraged. The patient will have continuous bladder irrigations for several days. Stool softeners will be given, as well as antispasmodics for bladder spasms.

Sitz baths are usually ordered following a perineal prostatectomy. After a bowel movement, care must be taken to avoid contaminating the wound. Perineal cleansing should be done by the nurse, using meticulous aseptic technique.

Patients who have had a radical prostatectomy have a urethral catheter in place for approximately 2 weeks. This helps splint the vesicoureteral (bladder and ureter) incision. Accidental removal of the catheter may require that the patient return to surgery for its reinsertion.

After removal of the catheter, these patients usually have difficulty with incontinence until they are able to retrain their external urethral sphincters to do the work of both the internal and external sphincters. The nurse can assist in this sphincter retraining by instructing the patient in Kegel exercises.

Some urine will dribble onto the dressings after the wound catheter is removed, so attention must be given to keeping the skin clean and dry. It may take a month or more for the wound to heal.

Postoperative care of the patient who has a radical prostatectomy includes pain management (aspirin is not used because of its anticoagulant effects), maintaining traction on the irrigation balloon (to maintain hemostasis and prevent hemorrhage), managing bladder spasm with medication, monitoring intake and output, monitoring the color of the irrigation returns, and preventing urinary obstruction or retention. The postoperative patient will have bloody drainage, but the amount of the blood in the drainage should steadily decrease. Because hemorrhage is a major postoperative complication, any sudden increase of blood in the drainage should be reported and documented.

13

e will be taught pelvic floor
taining continence. An ex-
se (see box in Chapter 84).
nt and his partner deal with
A sample Nursing Care Plan
ndergone a radical prostatec-

nt With Side Effects From

common problem with radiation
ectomy. It is treated by increasing
spasmodics and analgesics.
experience *proctitis* with preoper-
ctitis is an inflammation of the rec-
e of the low-residue diet and anti-
ions may help alleviate symptoms.
y experience *urethral stricture*, due to
mportant to teach the patient the signs of
ion and to monitor urine output closely.
dition must be monitored during radiation
Patients are prone to excoriation and yeast in-
. Other considerations in assisting the patient
g radiation are presented in Chapter 76.

Managing Continuous Bladder Irrigation

TURP irrigation, which is usually used following
prostatectomy, is illustrated in Figure 83-1. Nursing
skills related to TURP irrigation are listed in the accompanying box. The patient is often discharged early.
Teach the patient and family about postoperative
observations.

Nursing Alert

When caring for a patient with a continuous TURP
bladder irrigation, *shut off the irrigation* if:

♦ The patient complains of bladder fullness.
♦ The patient complains of urinary urgency.
♦ The patient complains of bladder or flank pain.
♦ The drainage from the TURP tube stops.

Check to see if there is an order for a manual irrigation.

Teaching Testicular Self-Examination

Every man should be taught to do a testicle self-examination. The examination is performed when the man
is relaxed. The shower is a good place to perform the
exam. The testes can be palpated for lumps or nodules.
If any abnormalities are found, a physician should be
considered at once. The accompanying box concerns
patient teaching for testicular self-examination.

Evaluation

Periodically the nurse, patient, family and other members of the healthcare team evaluate outcomes of care.
Have short-term goals been met? Are long-term goals
still realistic? Planning for further nursing care takes into
consideration the patient's prognosis, as well as any
complications and the patient's response to care given.
Emotional aspects of reproductive disorders are dealt
with; the person may be referred to a support group or
other community service for follow-up.

Erectile Disorders

Impotence

Impotence is the inability of the male to achieve or
maintain an erection sufficient to complete sexual intercourse. Men with *primary impotence* have never
achieved an erection; men with *secondary impotence*
have previously had erections. Episodes of transient impotence increase with age. Half of all adult males have
experienced impotence at some point in their lives.
Psychogenic causes underlie 80% of all impotence. It is
important to reassure your patient that this is a common
problem and is unlikely to be permanent.

Transient Impotence
There are three types of transient impotence:

♦ *partial*—unable to have a full erection
♦ *intermittent*—sometimes potent with the same
partner
♦ *selective*—potent only with certain sexual partners

Causes or factors related to impotence are listed in
the accompanying box. Men with diabetes mellitus are
likely to sustain permanent impotence due both to neuropathy and microvascular changes, as the diabetes
progresses. In this man, impotence has a slow, insidious onset and is usually irreversible. On the other hand,
impotence due to vascular problems only may respond
to revascularization surgery or vasodilating agents.

Medical and Surgical Treatment. Erection is caused by
spinal reflex arcs activated by tactile stimuli and psychogenic factors (auditory, visual, and psychological
stimulation). If the patient is able to achieve an erection
during his sleep or when masturbating, it is likely the
dysfunction is psychogenic in nature. Frequently, counseling will help these patients. If the patient can't
achieve erection by these means, a complete workup
is done. This includes endocrine studies, as well as biopsies, infusion cavernosometry and cavernography
and ultrasound studies. Drug therapy may be helpful
in some cases. Key medications are listed in the box
on p. 1307.

Mr. Francis Orio, a 63-year-old white, married male presented with the following symptoms: hesitancy and straining on urination, decrease in size and force of stream, frequency, and nocturia. Further diagnostic studies revealed prostatic cancer. The course of treatment pursued was a radical prostatectomy, which rendered Mr. Orio impotent. The patient often expressed concerns regarding his sexual inability in relation to his marriage and fears of the cancer recurring. A nursing diagnosis developed for Mr. Orio follows.

Nursing Diagnosis: *Situational Low Self-Esteem related to effects of surgery*

Goal: 7/7, patient will verbalize coping strategies regarding sexual disfunction and incorporate change into self-concept in a positive manner to enhance his self-esteem.

Nursing Actions (assess/do/teach)	Rationale	Evaluative Statement
1. Encourage patient to verbalize his concerns and sexual needs—listen to his comments about the situation and what it means for him. Have him describe himself, noting how he sees and how he believes others see options. Be aware of patient's self-concept in relation to cultural or social values.	These actions allow the patient to vent his feelings and help the nurse understand how the patient perceives himself and his problems.	7/7, Goal partially met; patient and wife are requesting information regarding their various options. 7/10, Goal met; patient is confident and comfortable with himself. He and wife are openly discussing their options.
2. Allow patient to go through the grieving process; be open and receptive to behavior changes during this time. Expect some expression of negative feelings.	Each patient goes through it in their own way and in their own time.	
3. Recognize behavior of overconcern with body and its processes. Set limits on maladaptive behavior. Help patient learn how to deal with his feelings and release his emotions in a positive manner.	Limits provide structure and direction.	
4. Assess interaction of patient and wife. Encourage open communication of their feelings with each other.	Good communication is the basis of all good relationships.	
5. Assess patient and wife's knowledge regarding options related to impotency. Help patient and wife to obtain information regarding coping strategies. Provide information at patient and wife's level of acceptance.	They will be able to make informed decisions regarding what alternatives are best for them.	7/10 Patient received booklet about penile implants.

A vacuum device, although cumbersome, is noninvasive, while penile implants are permanent and may subject the patient to potential complications of surgery such as infection, pain, swelling, and erosion of tissue around the device.

Penile Implants. There are many different implants; the semirigid rod, mechanical devices, the self-contained prosthesis, and finally, the inflatable prosthesis. Each type of device has its own advantages and disadvantages. The semirigid rod is the easiest device to implant, yet the least natural. The inflatable prosthesis mimics a natural erection best, yet it is the most expensive. The patient who has a penile implant must be counseled to avoid sexual activity for six weeks. *(Rationale: The site*

Nursing Skill Guidelines
Managing Continuous TURP or Bladder Irrigation

♦ Record the amount of irrigating solution instilled into the bladder and the total output. *(Rationale: In this way, an accurate record of the patient's actual urinary output can be determined. The amount of irrigation solution is subtracted from the total output to determine urine volume.)*

♦ The nurse must carefully monitor the TURP setup to make sure all the tubes are open and that they are not twisted or kinked.

♦ Because many men who have TURPs are older and may become confused, the nurse must make sure patients do not pull on the catheters or change rates of flow of the solutions—a physician's specific order for protective devices (restraints) may be needed. Catheters must remain taped in place.

♦ Often the physician orders that traction be placed on the penis, which is kept taped securely in place on the hip or abdomen and is not allowed to hang down. This facilitates drainage and prevents clotting, but may be uncomfortable.

♦ It may be necessary to irrigate the catheter manually. Be sure the physician has written an order. There is often a standing order to irrigate the catheter PRN.

♦ The nurse must take special note if the patient complains of a feeling of fullness, urgency, or bladder or flank pain, or if the drainage stops flowing from the tube. In any of these situations, the continuous irrigation must be shut off and the team leader or physician notified immediately.

needs time to heal completely.) If injection therapy is to be used, the patient should be told that, priapism, which is prolonged, uncomfortable erection, may result.

Penile Revascularization. The other surgical procedure is the penile revascularization. Only recently has this type of surgery not been considered experimental. Only about 5% of all impotent men are candidates for penile vascular surgery. Such surgery involves the reconstruction of arterial blood supply or the removal of veins that drain blood from the penis too rapidly.

Priapism

Priapism refers to an abnormal and persistent erection of the penis without sexual desire. Prompt treatment is vital.

Priapism may have many causes, including penile or spinal cord injury or tumor and cerebrospinal syphilis. Pelvic vascular thrombosis is most often identified as the cause. However, priapism may also result from pro-

Keys to Patient/Teaching
Testicular Self-Examination

Patient teaching for testicular self-examination includes the following:

♦ This examination should be performed monthly.
♦ The glans of the penis are examined and palpated for lumps, lesions, blisters, or discharge.
♦ The penile shaft is examined and palpated in the same manner. Pay particular attention to the base and underside of the shaft.
♦ Examine the skin of the scrotum for lesions, discolorations, or varicosities.
♦ Palpate each testicle for lumps, swelling, tenderness, or irregularity.

longed sexual activity, leukemia, sickle cell anemia, or other blood dyscrasias. It is very possible in infections such as prostatitis, urethritis or cystitis, particularly if complicated by the presence of calculi. It may be a side effect of drugs including trazodone (Desyrel), chlorpromazine (Thorazine), prazosin (Minipress) and tolbutamide (Orinase), as well as certain antihypertensives, anticoagulants, and corticosteroids. This condition may also be an undesirable result of therapy for impotence.

Signs and Symptoms. The patient has pain and tenderness, as well as emotional discomfort. The corpora cavernosa contain thick, dark venous blood; the corpus spongiosum and glans penis are not involved.

Medical and Surgical Treatment. Priapism is difficult to treat and treatment may be unsuccessful. It may be relieved by caudal or spinal anesthesia. Certain medications, such as anticoagulants, may be effective if used immediately. Estrogens are not effective. *Cavernostomy* with a large needle (to allow drainage) and irrigation

Factors Related to Male Impotence

Drug use: hormones, immunosuppressive agents, diuretics, anti-Parkinson's agents, antihypertensives, antidepressants, psychotropics, tobacco, alcohol, amphetamines, barbiturates, marijuana, cocaine

Chronic diseases: renal failure, heart failure, atherosclerosis, multiple sclerosis

Endocrine disorders: diabetes mellitus, thyroid disorders, adrenal disorders, pituitary disorders

Trauma: spinal cord injury

Cardiovascular disorders: stroke, heart disorders, inadequate vascularization

Surgery: prostatectomy, ileostomy, colostomy

may be used, or surgery may be required. Surgical approaches include creation of a fistula between the glans and corpus and semipermanent diversion with a saphenous vein shunt.

Structural Disorders

Undescended Testicle (Cryptorchidism)

A small percentage of male babies are born with testicles that have not descended to their normal position in the scotum (**cryptorchidism**). Sometimes the testicles descend without treatment; but if this does not happen, they should be correctly positioned to allow for successful sperm production. The internal body temperature is too warm for sufficient sperm production.

If both testes have remained in the abdomen past puberty, they may be malformed and the secondary sex characteristics of the male may not develop, because the appropriate hormones have not been secreted. Hormones must then be given throughout the patient's lifetime. If the testes lodge in the inguinal canal, they may secrete adequate hormones, but most likely will not produce spermatozoa; however, it is unusual for both testes to be undescended. If one testis is descended normally, the man will most likely not be sterile.

This condition can often be treated medically by hormonal therapy. If this is not effective, corrective surgery *(orchiopexy)* is usually done between the ages of 5 and 7. (After puberty, an operation for two undescended testicles will not be effective in preventing sterility.) Orchiopexy involves suturing of the testes to the scrotal sac to fixate them.

Abnormal Placement of the Urethra

If the urethral meatus is located on the underside of the penis, this condition is known as **hypospadias;** if

the meatus is located on the upper surface, the condition is known as **epispadias.** These are congenital conditions and are usually repaired surgically at a young age if they are severe.

Phimosis

Many men who have not been circumcised at birth develop a condition known as phimosis in which the foreskin becomes so tight that it will not retract over the glans penis. **Phimosis** may also be caused by an injury. The condition is relieved by circumcision. Circumcision may also be done for aseptic reasons or if the sexual partner has a stubborn vaginal infection.

Torsion of the Spermatic Cord

Torsion of the spermatic cord is the twisting of the spermatic cord, resulting in interruption of testicular blood supply. This condition can result in necrosis of the testicle if left untreated for more than a few hours. Torsion is fairly uncommon and occurs most often in adolescent boys and young men. It may be caused by bilateral and congenital absence of the lateral attachments of the testes and epididymis to the scrotum. Torsion often follows an activity that puts a sudden pull on the cremasteric muscle, the muscle that elevates the testis. This may be caused by extreme cold, such as jumping into very cold water. Occasionally, torsion may be spontaneous or it may occur during sleep.

The symptoms of torsion are nausea, vomiting, abdominal pain, and a sudden severe scrotal pain, which is unrelieved by rest or support. Torsions cause the left testes to rotate clockwise and the right one counterclockwise.

This condition can be treated with a surgical detorsion and bilateral orchiopexy (surgical fixation of the testes). This will fixate each testis and prevent recurrence of another torsion. If the torsion has caused a testicle to be necrotic, it must be removed (orchiectomy). An orchiopexy is then performed on the unaffected side to prevent torsion of that testis.

Varicocele

A **varicocele** is caused by the dilatation of the veins in the scrotum (pampiniform plexus). A varicocele may be unilateral or bilateral, yet is more commonly seen on the left side. This probably occurs because the left spermatic vein is longer than the right, resulting in fewer competent valves. If there is an associated infertility problem, the varicocele may be blamed, because of increased intrascrotal heat. A varicocele that appears suddenly, later in life, is suggestive of a renal tumor that has invaded the renal vein. This interferes with venous drainage from the testicle. Dilatation of the veins can be increased by the Valsalva maneuver (such as is performed when straining at stool). The veins will empty when the patient is lying flat. The symptoms of a varicocele are swelling and a nagging pain in the scrotum. It is treated by surgical ligation or removal of the cause of the observation.

Hydrocele

A **hydrocele** is an accumulation of fluid in the space between the membrane covering the testicle and the testicle itself. It may be due to infection **(orchitis)** or to an injury. The scrotum enlarges but does not cause pain unless the hydrocele is a sudden development, in which case there may be pain and swelling. It may be treated by aspirating the fluid, although this is rarely satisfactory in the adult. Sometimes the sac is removed surgically. **Plication,** the stitching of folds or tucks in the hydrocele wall to reduce its size will usually prevent redevelopment of the hydrocele.

Symptomatic treatment includes applying cold packs, providing emotional reassurance, providing support for the scrotum, and keeping the dressings changed to prevent skin irritation. A drain will often be used if a plication is not performed.

Hernias

A hernia is a protrusion of the abdominal contents through a defect in the abdominal wall. *Inguinal hernias* are the most common type of hernia in males, as the inguinal canal is a natural area of weakness (see Chapter 25). On examination, the nurse will note an area of bulging in the groin area when the patient coughs or bears down, if an inguinal hernia is present. If the hernia does not move into position, it is called an *irreducible hernia*. This is a medical emergency, as the compromised blood supply can cause necrosis of the bowel tissue. Most hernia repairs are done in day surgery, on an outpatient basis. Hernias are discussed in Chapter 81.

Inflammatory Disorders

Epididymitis

Epididymitis is an inflammation of the tube that carries sperm cells away from the testes. It is usually due to gonorrheal, staphylococcic, streptococcic, or colon bacillus infections, and often follows an infection of the urinary tract or prostate gland. Chlamydia is now becoming the most common cause; it can lead to sterility.

The symptoms are redness, pain, and swelling in the scrotum, sometimes accompanied by chills, fever, nausea, and vomiting. Antibiotics are administered, and support and cold packs are applied to the scrotum. If an abscess forms, it usually is incised and drained sur-

gically. Repeated or chronic infection or application of heat will destroy sperm production.

Orchitis

Orchitis, inflammation of the testes, may be the result of an infection or an injury, Mumps after puberty may cause orchitis, which causes sterility. The symptoms of orchitis are pain and swelling in the scrotum and, sometimes, urethral irritation. A scrotal support is used to support the testes, and an ice bag is applied to the scrotum. Heat is not used.

Prostatitis

Prostatitis is inflammation of the prostate gland, due to the ascent of bacteria up the urethra. Acute prostatitis may also be caused by massage of the prostate in a patient with chronic prostatitis.

Acute Prostatitis

The patient with acute prostatitis presents with an exquisitely tender, enlarged and asymmetrical prostate, as determined on digital rectal examination. The patient may also complain of chills, fever, myalgia (muscle pain), general malaise, low back pain, perineal pain and post-ejaculatory pain. Urinary symptoms include urgency on urination or obstructive symptoms including nocturia, hesitancy or dribbling after urination. Acute prostatitis is treated with antibiotics for 4–6 weeks. If inadequately treated, chronic prostatitis may develop.

Chronic Prostatitis

Diagnosis of chronic prostatitis is made with divided urinalysis, urine culture and prostate ultrasound. The white blood count will be elevated. The patient with chronic prostatitis is usually asymptomatic, but may complain of back or perineal pain. These patients are treated with a long course of antibiotics, usually 3–6 months.

Nursing Considerations. Nursing measures include pain control and warm compresses or sitz baths for discomfort. Once the acute period is over, the patient is instructed to increase numbers of ejaculations, to decrease pressure. The patient is instructed to increase fluid intake, to flush bacteria out of the bladder, and takes stool softeners to prevent constipation.

Neoplasms

Benign Prostatic Hyperplasia (BPH)

Cancer of the prostate is the most commonly occurring cancer in men. However, not all enlargements of the prostate gland are malignant. Many men experience normal enlargement of the prostate with aging. In fact, most men by the age of 50 have some prostatic enlargement. This enlargement is correctly known as *benign prostatic hyperplasia* (BPH). Benign prostatic hyperplasia often impinges on the urinary stream.

Signs and Symptoms. The first symptoms may be difficulty in urinating. The patient does not empty his bladder completely when he voids and finds that he must void during the night. He may also find it increasingly difficult to start to void and may notice traces of blood in his urine. This may lead to cystitis. BPH is associated with age and testicular function.

The physician can assess the effects of prostatic enlargement on the urinary system by examining a catheterized specimen of urine and by cystoscopy. A blood chemistry test will also indicate how well the kidneys are functioning.

Diagnostic Tests. BPH is diagnosed by digital rectal exam, urodynamic testing, endoscopy and prostate ultrasound. Severe cases will show changes in the UA/UC (urinalysis, urine culture) and in the serum creatinine and BUN. Complications of untreated BPH include obstruction, with acute urinary retention, pain and increased frequency of UTI (urinary tract infections).

Nursing Alert

If the patient experiences an episode of acute urinary retention at home, he can try a warm shower or bath to relax the sphincter muscles. Advise him to allow the urine to flow in the shower or tub if this works. If a shower or bath does not work, he should go to the emergency room for immediate treatment.

Medical and Surgical Treatment. Treatment of BPH includes watchful waiting until the patient is symptomatic and drug therapy (with estrogen, luteinizing hormone or alpha-adrenergic agents). Surgical procedures which do not remove the prostate include balloon dilatation of the prostatic urethra or implantation of a prosthetic stent (a device to hold the urethra open).

Prostatectomy (removal of the prostate) procedures include retropubic, suprapubic, perineal, or transurethral prostatectomy (TURP).

Malignant Neoplasms

Cancer of the Prostate

Cancer of the prostate is the most common cancer in men. All men over 40 should have a yearly examination.

Signs and Symptoms. The first signs of prostatic cancer involve difficulty in voiding. This occurs because the prostate gland surrounds the urethra and the tumor growth presses on the urethra and impedes the urinary stream. Signs of difficulty in voiding include the following;

◆ Urgency
◆ Frequency
◆ Nocturia
◆ **Hesitancy** (difficulty in starting the stream)
◆ Dysuria (painful voiding) in some cases

In addition, hematuria (blood in the urine) is a frequent sign.

The patient may have other symptoms before, but when he notes blood in the urine, he finally consults the physician. A biopsy determines the diagnosis. If the patient does not seek medical advice for these symptoms, complete urinary retention may result. This can be an emergency situation. Another problem that may be caused by an enlarged prostate is severe intractable constipation (*obstipation*).

Diagnostic Tests. The prostate gland is palpated for nodular growths. The examiner can palpate these growths through the wall of the rectum. On examination, a cancerous prostate feels irregular and may have hard nodules. The yearly examination is particularly important if the person has a family history of prostatic cancer. Cancer of the prostate is distinguished from prostatitis with a prostate biopsy. The PSA level will also be elevated in prostate cancer.

Medical and Surgical Treatment. Treatment of prostate cancer includes radical prostatectomy and radiation therapy. These were discussed at the beginning of the chapter, and nursing actions were discussed in the Nursing Process section.

Radiation can be used for cancer of the prostate. It may be used to reduce tumor size or actually to cure some stages of cancer of the prostate. It may also be considered as a palliative measure for the patient with bony metastases, thus alleviating some of the pain.

Pain Management in Advanced Disease

If the patient has distant metastases, the goal of management usually focuses on providing comfort and providing support for family members. Analgesics should be given on a routine schedule (not PRN). Narcotics are often prescribed. Oral administration is preferable because it allows the patient more control in his pain management. In later stages of the disease, continuous morphine may be intravenously given for pain control.

Chapters 90 and 91 describe care of the patient who is terminally ill.

Cancer of the Testes

Although not common, cancer can occur in the testes. Testicular cancer most frequently occurs in men between 18 and 25 years of age. The incidence of testicular cancer is higher in men with undescended testicles. There are two difficult categories of testicular tumors, each treated differently. The first type of testicular tumor is the **seminoma.** After a unilateral **orchiectomy** (removal of the testis on one side), any residual tumor will be irradiated. The second type of testicular tumor is the **non-seminoma.** After a unilateral orchiectomy is performed, the patient will undergo a retroperitoneal (behind the peritoneum) lymph node dissection. This involves removal of the lymph nodes along the aorta, the iliac vessels, and the inguinal area on the affected side. Further treatment for possible residual tumor involves the administration of chemotherapy or radiation therapy.

Cancer of the Penis

Cancer of the penis is relatively rare, especially in men who have been circumcised. It is treated locally, as a skin cancer, but occasionally, amputation of the penis is necessary as a lifesaving measure.

Special Considerations in Aging

Sexual Problems

- ◆ Sexual activity tends to decrease with age, the more sexually active a male was in his youth, the more likely that he will continue sexual activity into old age.
- ◆ The incidence of erectile dysfunction increases with age. This is mainly caused by medication side effects, neuropathy, or vascular problems.
- ◆ Although sperm viability decreases with age, sperm production continues at the same level throughout life.
- ◆ Erection takes longer to achieve and ejaculation is less intense, with aging.

Keys for Review

Key Questions for Critical Thinking

1. Differentiate among the different kinds of prostatectomies. Explain how it is determined which one will be used. Describe preoperative and postoperative teaching for each.
2. Your 75-year-old patient has a TURP irrigation system in place. Identify the most common complication of a TURP and of this type of drainage. Describe when continuous irrigation should be stopped. Develop a teaching plan for the patient and his family.

Key Readings

Andreoli TE, Carpenter CJ, et al. Cecil's Essentials of Medicine, Ed 2. Philadelphia, Saunders, 1990

Belcher AE. Cancer Nursing. St Louis, Mosby-Yearbook, 1992

Berkow R (Editor). The Merck Manual of Diagnosis and Therapy, Ed 16. Rahway NJ, Meck & Co, 1992

Doughty DB. Urinary and Fecal Incontinence: Nursing Management, St Louis, Mosby-Yearbook, 1991

Fischbach F. A Manual of Laboratory and Diagnostic Tests, Ed 3. Philadelphia, Lippincott, 1992

Gray M. Genitourinary Disorders. St Louis, Mosby-Yearbook, 1992

NANDA Nursing Diagnoses: Definitions and Classifications 1992. Philadelphia, NANDA, 1992

Key Readings (continued)

Nursing 93 Drug Handbook. Springhouse PA, Springhouse, 1993

O'Toole M (Editor). Miller-Keane Ency. & Dic. of Medicine, Nursing, and Allied Health, Ed 5. Philadelphia, Saunders, 1992

Smeltzer, S.C., and Bare, B.G.: Brunner and Suddarth's Testbook of Medical-Surgical Nursing, ed.7 Philadelphia: J.B. Lippincott, 1992.

Morales A. "Nonsurgical Management Options in Impotence" in Hospital Practice, Vol 30, No 3,1993

Morgantaler A. "Current Diagnosis and Management of Impotence" in Comprehensive Therapy, Vol 17, No 7, 1991

Morley JE, "Management of Importance" in Postgraduate Medicine, Vol 93, No 3, 1993

Keys To Learning More

Chapter 84: female reproductive disorders

Unit Fifteen: geriatric nursing

Chapter 89: rehabilitation, ambulatory and home care nursing

Unit Seventeen: death and dying

84 Female Reproductive Disorders

Keys for Learning

Learning Objectives

- Describe diagnostic tests and common surgical procedures related to gynecologic disorders.
- Describe nursing care related to surgical procedures.
- Demonstrate the ability to teach patients regarding gynecologic disorders and their prevention.
- Name common diseases or disorders of the female reproductive system, and identify treatment.
- Describe and demonstrate nursing procedures related to female reproductive disorders.
- Describe the most common types of cancer in the female reproductive tract, and describe detection and treatment.
- Describe nursing care related to cancers of the female reproductive tract.

Key Terms

amenorrhea	mammography
cervicitis	mammoplasty
culdoscopy	mastalgia
cystocele	mastectomy
dilation and curettage	menorrhagia
dysmenorrhea	metrorrhagia
endometriosis	rectocele
gynecology	vaginitis
hysterectomy	vulvitis
laparoscopy	

Keys to Understanding This Chapter

Chapter 5: basic human needs
Chapter 25: female reproductive system
Chapter 30: medical asepsis and Universal Precautions
Chapter 45: personal hygiene and skin care
Chapter 47: specimen collection
Chapter 49: heat and cold application
Chapter 50: assisting with a physical examination and nursing assessment

Keys to Understanding This Chapter
(continued)

Chapter 51: isolation techniques
Chapter 52: comfort and pain management
Chapter 53: surgery
Chapter 54: surgical asepsis
Unit Eleven: pharmacology and medication administration
Unit Twelve: maternal and newborn nursing
Chapter 63: sexually transmitted diseases and fertility control
Chapter 76: cancer

Key Points

- Healthy sexual function and reproduction is a fundamental need in women and an important loss if dysfunctional.
- A sexual history is important in defining areas of concern.
- Breast self-examination and observation of one's own menstrual cycle are helpful to the physician in early diagnosis of female reproductive disorders.
- Diagnostic studies are a necessary, although sometimes uncomfortable, process. The nurse is invaluable in preparing the patient and relieving her concerns.
- Nursing skills performed to assist the female patient include perineal care, vaginal irrigation, and insertion of vaginal suppositories.
- The nurse is an important link in assisting the woman to prevent problems through clear and understandable patient teaching.
- Explanation and follow-up with a patient who must undergo surgical treatment is important. The patient may not have heard or understood all that was explained to her.
- High cure rates exist in certain cancers if discovered early (especially breast and cervix).

Key Learning Activities

- Discuss with an experienced nurse how he or she obtains a sexual history from a female patient.
- Practice breast self-examination as illustrated in this chapter or taught in class.
- Teach breast self-examination to a friend or classmate.

Gynecology is the branch of medicine that is concerned with genital and breast conditions in women. The physician who is a specialist in this field is the *gynecologist*. Disorders of the reproductive system usually occur during adult life; however, menstrual difficulties may occur during early adolescence. A major consideration in the treatment of gynecologic conditions during the childbearing years is to maintain fertility without endangering the patient.

> **Key Concept**
>
> Unless the nurse is specially trained in sexual counseling, the nurse's interventions center around teaching regarding anatomy, self-care related to hygiene, and breast self-examinations.

Anatomy and Physiology Review

The female reproductive system is a complex and specialized set of organs, as described in Chapter 25. At conception, the genitals of both sexes are similar. Because of the influence of hormones, the male and female reproductive systems develop their unique characteristics. The female reproductive system becomes fully functional and able to reproduce at *puberty*, which includes *menarche*, the onset of menstruation.

The organs of the female reproductive system are the two ovaries, which produce the eggs (ova) and secrete female sex hormones. During the monthly cycle, ovulation occurs, at which time the egg is released and travels down the oviduct (uterine tube) to the uterus. If fertilization occurs, the ovum implants in the uterus and develops into a fetus. If fertilization does not take place, menstruation occurs. The vagina is the opening to the outside.

The breast also is part of the reproductive system. It is affected by the hormones produced by the reproductive organs. The breast is a glandular organ filled with blood and lymph vessels. After pregnancy, it manufactures milk from certain substances in the blood, which is called *lactation*. Progesterone, an ovarian hormone, and prolactin, a pituitary hormone, stimulate lactation. Estrogen, another ovarian hormone, suppresses lactation.

Diagnosis of Female Reproductive Disorders

The Pelvic Examination

Every woman past puberty should have a complete pelvic examination, including a Pap test, at least every 1 to 3 years or more often if any pathology is present or if there is a family history of pathology (Fig. 84-1). The pelvic examination offers the physician the opportunity to visualize the cervix, vagina, and perineum.

The physician also can do a biopsy of the cervix during a pelvic examination, or a portion of the cervix can be cauterized, removed, or coagulated with electricity or laser.

In preparation for the gynecologic or pelvic examination, the patient is asked to empty her bladder. Discomfort can be minimized if she breathes deeply and relaxes during the examination. You will need to provide a vaginal speculum and gloves. The patient is placed in the lithotomy position, and the external genitalia are examined. The physician *palpates* the uterus and ovaries by inserting a gloved finger into the vagina and placing the other hand on the abdomen. The examination also may include *rectovaginal* examination, in which one finger is placed in the vagina and another finger is inserted into the rectum. This palpation can evaluate abnormalities of the rectal area and problems or the posterior genital organs.

Laboratory Tests

Pap Test

A malignant growth in the uterus or cervix sometimes sheds cells into the uterine and vaginal secretions. By microscopically examining a smear from these secretions, it is possible to detect these cells before symptoms of cancer appear. This examination is known as the Pap (Papanicolaou's) test or Pap smear. It is believed to be more than 90% accurate in detecting cervical cancer. It is less accurate in detecting cancer of the endometrium of the uterus.

Cancer of the cervix is one of the most common forms of cancer in women. If the Pap test is positive or the cervix looks suspicious, further testing is necessary. With early detection, successful treatment of cervical cancer is common.

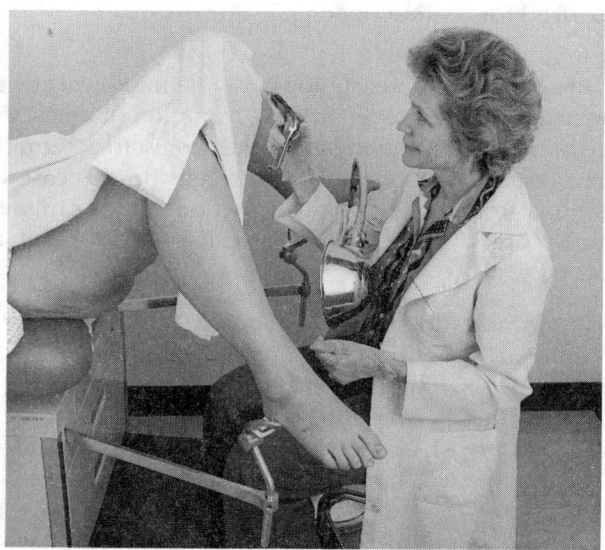

Figure 84-1. Lithotomy position for patient used in pelvic examination. Examiner's position. Fuller J, Schaller-Ayers J. Health Assessment: A Nursing Approach. Ed 2. Philadelphia, J.B. Lippincott, 1994.

The National Institutes of Health now recommend that the Pap smear be done every 1 to 3 years if the two previous test results were negative. They state that regular testing should begin at puberty, especially if the person is sexually active, and should continue to at least age 65. The American Cancer Society and the American College of Obstetricians and Gynecologists continue to recommend yearly Pap tests.

The nurse often will be asked to assist the physician in performing the Pap test. The procedure for positioning the patient is the same as for any routine pelvic examination. The equipment needed includes—in addition to the equipment for the pelvic examination—glass slides and the applicator or Y-shaped wooden stick that is inserted through the speculum to obtain a smear of cervical mucosa. This material is smeared onto the glass slide; a special spray fixative or hair spray is sprayed over the slide to "fix" the specimen to the glass.

> **Nursing Alert**
>
> Pap tests should be done between menstrual periods, because they become less accurate when a woman is menstruating. Some women have a higher than normal chance of contracting cervical cancer. These women should be screened regularly, sometimes more often than once a year.

If a patient has an abnormal Pap test, this does not necessarily mean she has cancer. However, abnormal findings indicate that further testing and evaluation are necessary.

> **Key Concept**
>
> It is important for all women to understand the importance of regular Pap tests, because early treatment of cervical cancers is effective in a high percentage of cases. The patient also should be taught that an abnormal Pap test does not necessarily mean she has cancer.

Tests for Endometrial Cancer

A Pap test may indicate endometrial cancer. However, in 30% to 40% of cases, the Pap test shows a false negative for this type of cancer. Aspiration of the endocervix (the internal portion of the cervix) is more accurate (approximately 70%) for endometrial cancer. A biopsy of the endometrium itself has proven more than 90% accurate.

Blood Tests Used in Female Reproductive Cancers

Several blood tests are used in conjunction with biopsy (cervix and breast) to determine the type of cancer present. These include the *estrogen* and *progesterone-*

Key Abbreviations and Acronyms Used in Gynecologic Disorders

AP	Anterior-posterior (repair)
BSE	breast self-examination
D&C	Dilation and currettage
DES	Diethylstilbestrol
GYN	Gynecology
HPV	Human papillomavirus
NIH	National Institutes of Health
Pap	Papanicolaou
PID	Pelvic inflammatory disease
PMS	Premenstrual syndrome
TSS	Toxic shock syndrome

receptor analysis. Blood tests also are used to determine effectiveness of cancer treatment. They are not used for initial screening to determine whether a patient has cancer.

Breast Examination

A woman should have a breast examination by her caregiver at least once a year or more often if she has a cystic disorder. However, if any unusual symptoms appear, the woman should have her breast examined immediately. The physician will do essentially the same palpation examination as the woman has done in her self-examination and also may do other procedures. Breast self-examination is discussed later in this chapter.

Mammography

Mammography is an x-ray examination of the breasts that is capable of detecting some breast cancers 1 to 2 years before they reach palpable size. Up to 40% of all early breast cancers are discovered in this manner.

A baseline mammogram is recommended for women between the ages of 35 and 40 years. The recommendation for women 40 to 50 years old is a mammogram every 1 to 2 years. Women older than 50 years are encouraged to have a mammogram every year. Routine mammography is strongly recommended for women who have any of the following characteristics:

◆ Previous cancer
◆ Cystic breast disorders
◆ No children
◆ First child after age 30
◆ Family history of breast cancer
◆ Strong family history of any type of cancer
◆ Female hormone (estrogen) therapy

◆ Extreme fear of cancer (need mammography for reassurance)

Procedure. The procedure is simple and does not require the injection of dye. However, a specially trained radiologist must interpret the mammary x-rays.

Some laboratories request that the patient refrain from using deodorant or powder prior to the test because they may contain zinc or other metals that interfere with the x-ray. The patient wears a gown that opens in the front and is asked to remove neck jewelry and clothing above the waist. The nurse can be helpful by explaining to the patient that she will be asked to assume several positions that will allow her to place her breasts flat on the x-ray plate. A compressor is pressed from above or the side to flatten each breast as much as possible. The procedure may be uncomfortable but should not be painful.

Interpretation. Tumor tissue will show up on mammography as denser-than-normal breast tissue. However, only tumors in which calcium deposits or abnormal breast duct patterns exist will show up on mammography (these comprise approximately 70% of breast tumors that can be diagnosed). The radiologist can often speculate whether a tumor is malignant or benign by its shape, location, and size. If a lesion is present, a biopsy is usually done.

Breast Ultrasound

The ultrasound examination can distinguish a breast cyst from a solid mass, which usually requires a biopsy to determine if it is malignant. The breast ultrasound is not used for routine screening.

Breast Biopsy. A breast biopsy is a definitive means of determining if cancer is present. A portion of breast tissue or fluid is examined by the pathologist to determine the presence and type of cancer cells. In the case of tissue, a frozen section is usually done and examined microscopically. Breast biopsy can be performed in several ways:[1]

◆ *Aspiration* (fine-needle aspiration)—Cells from a lump are drawn into a syringe. (In the case of some cysts, fluid is aspirated, collapsing the cyst. Often, this cyst requires no further treatment.)
◆ *Needle biopsy*—A needle with a cutting edge is inserted into a lump and rotated to remove a core sample.
◆ *Excisional biopsy*—An entire lump is removed and

---

[1] Adapted from "Breast Biopsy: What you should know." National Instututes of Health, 1990.

analyzed. If cancer is localized in this lump, no further treatment may be required.

♦ *Incisional biopsy*—Part of a lump is removed as a sample.

Abdominal Ultrasound and X-Ray Evaluations

Ultrasonography

Ultrasonography uses high-frequency sound waves directed back at a transducer placed over the abdominal or pelvic region. The sound waves are converted to electrical impulses, which can be viewed on a special monitor. By scanning the abdomen and viewing the results on the screen, the physician can evaluate reproductive conditions, such as tumors, cysts, and other pelvic diseases. A secondary approach for ultrasound can be made with a special probe through the vagina (vaginal ultrasound) to allow another view of the pelvic organs that could not be seen any other way.

X-Ray Examinations

Several x-ray procedures determine patency of the uterine tubes or the presence of abnormalities in the uterus and tubes. The most common of these is the *hysterosalpingogram*, in which the uterus and tubes can be visualized following an injection of contrast dye (see Chapter 50). The ovaries also may be visualized. These procedures are most often necessary to locate the cause of infertility or to determine if a tumor is present.

Laparoscopy

Laparoscopy provides direct visualization of the uterus and accessory organs of the uterus, including the ovaries and the uterine tubes (Fig. 84-2).

Procedure. For this procedure, a small incision is made in the area of the umbilicus, and the abdomen is then distended (insufflated) with approximately 2 L of carbon dioxide or oxygen. The gas is used because it allows for a better view of the organs; it separates the intestines from the pelvic organs. The laparoscope is inserted into the peritoneal cavity, and the physician can view the internal organs. Laparoscopy is usually performed using general or spinal anesthesia. There may be two or three small incisions. An absorbable suture is placed in the incisions.

The patient usually ambulates on the operative day. Patient and family teaching must be documented, particularly if the patient is to be discharged from the day-surgery center to home. Several things to be taught are listed in the box.

Culdoscopy

Culdoscopy furnishes direct visualization of the uterus, uterine tubes, broad ligaments, colon, and small intestine. It is performed by passing an instrument (the endocope) through the vaginal wall behind the cervix, after a small incision is made in the posterior vaginal cul-de-sac. The procedure is usually done in the operating room with the patient in a knee-chest position. The patient may have local, regional, or general anesthesia. Usually, no sutures are involved, and routine postoperative care is given.

During the culdoscopy, photographs may be taken of the cervix and the vaginal vault; cold conization of the cervix also may be done. This procedure also is used to diagnose pelvic pain, tubal pregnancy, and pelvic masses.

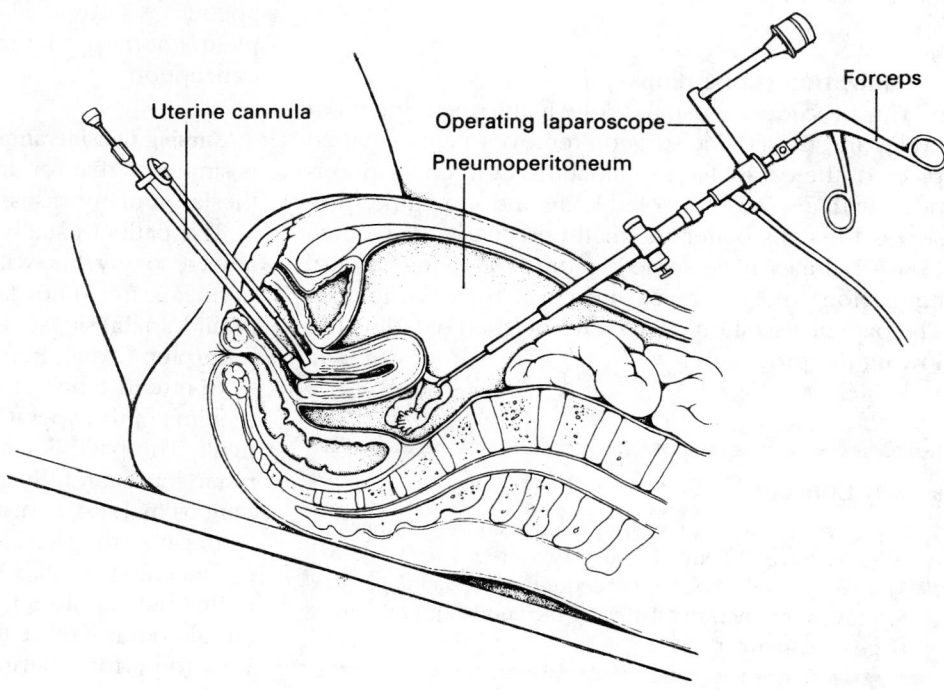

Figure 84-2. Laparoscopy. In this case, a tubal ligation is being done. The only incision will be a tiny one near the umbilicus.

Colposcopy

High-risk women often are screened routinely with colposcopy, which allows better visualization of the vagina and cervix than the regular speculum. Many physicians feel that the results are more reliable than those from the Pap test. The culposcope is a lighted, magnifying speculum that is inserted into the vaginal vault. Accurate diagnosis often requires biopsy, however.

Cervical Biopsy

A cervical biopsy is the microscopic examination of a small piece of tissue from the cervix. It is performed when the physician observes irregularities in the cervix or when a suspicious Pap smear is obtained. One means of obtaining the tissue is through a "punch" procedure (punching out a button of tissue for examination).

Conization (Cone Biopsy)

This procedure is usually done in the operating room under anesthesia. The surgeon removes a cone-shaped piece of the cervix for examination. Cold conization is done with a specially cooled knife and sometimes preserves the cells better. A small percentage of women (3%–12%) may have some bleeding following cervical conization, and the nurse must watch for symptoms. The patient also should watch for delayed bleeding following the procedure.

Key Concept

Some women who have cervical conizations or other biopsies have difficulty in carrying a pregnancy later. They may need a special procedure, called *cerclage*, to prevent premature dilation of the cervix and miscarriage (see Chapter 61).

Medical and Surgical Treatments

Common Surgical Treatments

Some of the diagnostic surgical procedures mentioned previously also may be used for treatment. These include laparoscopy, culdoscopy, colposcopy, and biopsies of the cervix, uterine lining, or breast.

Dilation and Curettage

Dilation and curettage (D&C) is the most frequently performed gynecologic surgery. It can be used to diagnose disorders and for treatment of some disorders. In D&C, the cervix is *dilated* (widened) using calibrated rods. A spoon-shaped instrument (curette) is then passed into the uterus, and the endometrial lining is scraped out *(curettage)*. D&C takes approximately 15 minutes; it is often done in the day-surgery department.

Purposes. D&C is used as a diagnostic procedure in cases such as abnormal vaginal bleeding or to obtain tissue for examination following a positive Pap test. The uterine scrapings are examined for evidence of malignant or nonmalignant growths or other abnormalities. Sometimes a D&C is done just before the menstrual period in an effort to find the cause of female infertility. The D&C is frequently used to evaluate *endometrial hypoplasia* (incomplete development of the uterine lining), **menorrhagia** (excessive menstrual flow), and **metrorrhagia** (bleeding between menses). In some cases, the D&C is all that is needed to eliminate the problem.

D&C is used as treatment in other instances. It may be used after an abortion, whether spontaneous or therapeutic. A D&C is always performed after an incomplete abortion to remove the retained products of conception.

Nursing Considerations. The preoperative preparation is similar to that for any patient about to receive anesthesia. In many cases, general anesthesia is used.

The patient usually makes an uneventful postoperative recovery. She will wear a perineal pad and require perineal care. Minor discomforts are usually relieved by a mild analgesic, such as acetaminophen (Tylenol) or ibuprofen (Advil, Rufen).

In rare instances, the vagina is packed with gauze at the time of the operation, which may make voiding difficult. The pack is usually removed the next day. The nurse must carefully assess the patient or teach the patient to make sure distention does not occur.

Because the D&C is often done on an outpatient basis, teaching is vital. Vaginal discharge will be bloody at first but should quickly become serosanguinous and should not last more than a few days. Teach the patient how to perform perineal care. Teach signs of abdominal distention. The patient is instructed to call the physician if any problems occur. All teaching must be carefully documented.

Hysterectomy

A **hysterectomy** is the surgical removal of the uterus. It may be performed for a variety of reasons: cancer of the cervix, ovaries, or uterus or to treat uterine fibroids, severe endometriosis, or prolapsed ("fallen") uterus. In some cases, such as a ruptured uterus during labor, an emergency hysterectomy must be performed. The uterus may be removed by means of a *vaginal* hysterectomy (through the vagina) or an *abdominal* hysterectomy (through an abdominal incision). Nursing care for hysterectomy patients is discussed in the nursing process section of this chapter.

Types of Hysterectomy. If the entire uterus, including the cervix, is removed, it is called a *total hysterectomy (panhysterectomy)*. Rarely today is the cervix left in place; if this is done and the body and fundus of the uterus are removed, it is called a *subtotal hysterectomy*. If the surgeon also removes the attached ovarian tubes, this is a *salpingectomy*, the total procedure is called a *panhysterosalpingectomy*. If the removal of both ovaries is combined with total removal of the uterus and both tubes, this is known as a *panhysterosalpingo-oophorectomy*. If one ovary is removed, the operation is a *unilateral* oophorectomy; if both are removed, it is *bilateral*.

If cancer has metastasized to the entire abdomen, radiation therapy, with or without chemotherapy, may be used palliatively, and surgery may not be necessary. In some cases, however, radical surgery is done.

Cosmetic Breast Surgery

Corrective surgery may be performed on normal breasts. A plastic surgery revision of the breast is referred to as a **mammoplasty.** If the breast is to be made larger, the term *augmentation* mammoplasty is used; if the breast is to be made smaller, the appropriate term is *reduction* mammoplasty. Following breast surgery, *reconstructive* mammoplasty is often done. Usually, these operations are not serious and do not cause any adverse effects. Occasionally, however, the materials implanted in the augmentation mammomplasty are rejected by the body and must be removed. For example, silicone implants are not recommended for use at this time.

❖ Nursing Process

Data Collection

The nurse must carefully observe and assess the woman with a reproductive disorder. Chapter 50 describes physical examination and assessment, including that of the male and female reproductive systems. This assessment establishes a baseline for future comparison and determines the presence of suspected disorders and complications. The nurse should report any changes in the baseline level.

When performing a nursing assessment of the female, the nurse obtains a reproductive and sexual history, which assists the physician in making a diagnosis. The accompanying box lists some of the components of the nursing assessment.

Many patients are reluctant to discuss sexual or reproductive concerns. One objective of the nurse is to express concern and to put the patient at ease when discussing sexuality or sexually related concerns. In addition, the nurse observes the patient's emotional response to the disorder or disease. Does the patient need assistance to meet daily needs? Is the disorder life-threatening? Does the disorder affect social activities, sexual identity, or self-esteem? Is the patient anxious or fearful of the outcome?

Nursing Diagnosis

Based on data collection, the following sample nursing diagnoses may be seen on nursing care plans for the female patient with a reproductive disorder. Some diagnoses may have more than one causative factor.

- ♦ High Risk for Altered Body Temperature related to infection
- ♦ Altered Urinary Elimination related to female structural abnormalities, pregnancy, multiple pregnancies, pelvic inflammatory disease (PID), surgical trauma, abdominopelvic malignancy
- ♦ Impaired Tissue Integrity related to PID, injury, radiation therapy
- ♦ Altered Tissue Perfusion: Peripheral (right or left arm) related to mastectomy
- ♦ Altered Sexuality Patterns, Sexual Dysfunction related to genital infection, genital deformities, injury, altered self-esteem, sexually transmitted disease

---

Keys to Nursing Assessment
Female Reproductive System

- ♦ Sexual history
- ♦ Reproductive history
- ♦ Method of birth control used
- ♦ Menstrual history; date of last menstrual period
- ♦ History of sexually transmitted diseases or high-risk lifestyle
- ♦ Visual observation of external genitalia
- ♦ Breast examination; teaching of breast self-examination

- Body Image Disturbance, Self-Esteem Disturbance related to mastectomy, sexual dysfunction, inability to conceive, sexually transmitted disease
- Diarrhea, Bowel Incontinence, Constipation related to structural abnormalities, infection, multiple child-birth injuries

Planning and Implementation

The patient, nurse, and healthcare team plan together for effective care to meet patient needs based on the nursing diagnosis. The nurse provides preoperative and postoperative care for the patient undergoing procedures such as hysterectomy and mastectomy. The patient with a reproductive disorder also may require teaching about preventive measures, such as breast self-examination. The patient may need assistance in meeting needs, dealing with emotional problems, and understanding more about the disorder, its prognosis, and its treatment. A nursing care plan is developed to meet these needs. A sample nursing care plan for a female patient with a reproductive disorder is provided later in this chapter.

Teaching Feminine Hygiene

The nurse, particularly the female nurse, is in an excellent position in the examining room or the hospital to teach the patient personal hygiene. Many women do not realize that after urinating or defecating they should *wipe from front to back* to prevent urinary tract and vaginal infections. The nurse also can stress the importance of thorough handwashing. The nurse can teach the patient the procedure for breast self-examination and reaffirm the necessity of a yearly Pap test, breast examinations, and serology tests for sexually transmitted diseases. The woman who is susceptible to infections should be cautioned against using bubble baths or bath oils and nylon panties or panty hose. Menstrual discharge also is an excellent culture medium for microorganisms. It is also important to stress adequate vitamin D and calcium intake, as well as fruits and vegetables. The patient should be taught the dangers of smoking. These and other important points are presented in the accompanying box.

Teaching Breast Self-Examination

The American Cancer Society recommends that each woman examine her breasts monthly, approximately 1 week following the menses, to determine if there are any lumps or nodules or any thickening (Fig. 84-3 and p. 1319). If the woman is postmenopausal, she should examine her breasts on the same date each month. The key is to note any *change from the previous month*. Self-examination of the breasts is done in several steps. The flat of the hand, rather than the fingertips, is used to

---

Keys to Patient Teaching
Prevention of Vaginal Infections

All women should be taught the following preventive measures:

- Wipe from front to back after going to the bathroom.
- Wash hands thoroughly after using the bathroom or changing perineal pads.
- Change tampons or sanitary pads frequently. Dispose of them safely. They should be placed in sealed plastic bags in the trash or burned, if possible.
- Pull panties, with perineal pad attached, straight down to avoid spreading infection during menses.
- Remove tampon immediately, and call physician if any signs of toxic shock syndrome appear (fever, nausea, vomiting, diarrhea, weakness).
- Douche only when absolutely necessary. Use the cleanest technique possible. Dispose of all equipment each time in a safe way.
- Clean the bathtub carefully before use, or take showers.
- Do not use bubble bath or bath oil, especially if prone to infection.
- Wear only cotton panties; avoid nylon panties.
- Wear only ventilated pantyhose or hose with garters.
- Avoid tight pants or jeans.
- Avoid nonventilated clothes or tight exercise clothing.
- Change out of a wet bathing suit immediately after swimming. Stay out of swimming pools or hot tubs if you are prone to infection. (The chlorine in the pool may predispose to infection. An infected person also can spread the infection to others.)
- Cut down on sugar.
- Do not use vaginal deodorant sprays or scented powders.
- Have the male partner wear a condom when having sexual relations. A water-soluble lubricant, such as K-Y jelly, may be needed to increase comfort and prevent irritation.
- Check with physician at earliest sign of infection. (Sexual partner should be checked also.)
- Consult physician regarding use of oral contraceptives or other hormones.
- Do not use colored or scented toilet tissue.
- Do not use deodorant tampons.

---

perform breast palpation. The woman should check the nipples for lumps, tenderness, discharge, or any changes. The entire procedure is described and illustrated in a booklet entitled "*How to Examine Your Breast,*" which is published by the American Cancer Society. The accompanying box describes the steps as you might describe them to a patient.

Keys to Patient Teaching
Breast Self-Examination

Step 1. In the Shower

♦ Examine breasts during bath or shower. *(Rationale: Hands glide more easily over wet skin.)*

♦ Keeping fingers flat, move gently over every part of each breast. Use right hand to examine left breast, left hand for right breast. Check for any lump, hard knot, or thickening.

♦ Check the axillae for any unusual signs (rash, lesions, absence of hair, unusual pigmentation).

Step 2. Before a Mirror

♦ Inspect breasts with arms at sides. One breast (usually the left) may be slightly larger.

♦ Raise arms high overhead. Breast movement should be equal and free on both sides.

♦ Look for any changes in contour of each breast (a swelling, dimpling of skin, one-sided flattening, or changes in the nipple).

♦ Rest palms on hips and press down firmly to flex chest muscles. Left and right breast will not exactly match. Few women's breasts do. Regular inspection shows what is normal and will give confidence in the examination.

♦ If the breasts are large or pendulous, stand or lean forward. Both breasts should move freely.

Step 3. Lying Down

♦ To examine left breast, put a pillow or folded towel under left shoulder.

♦ Place left hand behind head. *(Rationale: This distributes breast tissue more evenly on the chest.)*

♦ With right hand, fingers flat, press gently in small circular motions around an imaginary clock face. Begin at outermost top of left breast for 12 o'clock, then move to 1 o'clock, and so on around the circle, back to 12. (A ridge of firm tissue in the lower curve of each breast is normal.)

♦ Move in an inch toward the nipple, and keep circling to examine *every part of breast,* including the nipple. This requires at least three more circles.

♦ Repeat procedure on right breast. Notice how the breast structure feels.

♦ If any abnormalities are noted, measure the distance and direction from the nipple and report to the physician.

Step 4. Nipple Check

♦ Squeeze the nipple of each breast gently between thumb and index finger. Any discharge, clear or bloody, should be reported to the physician immediately.

Adapted from "How to Examine your Breasts," published by the American Cancer Society, 1992, and "Assessing Patients: Examining the Breasts." Nurses' PhotoLibrary, Springhouse, 1993.

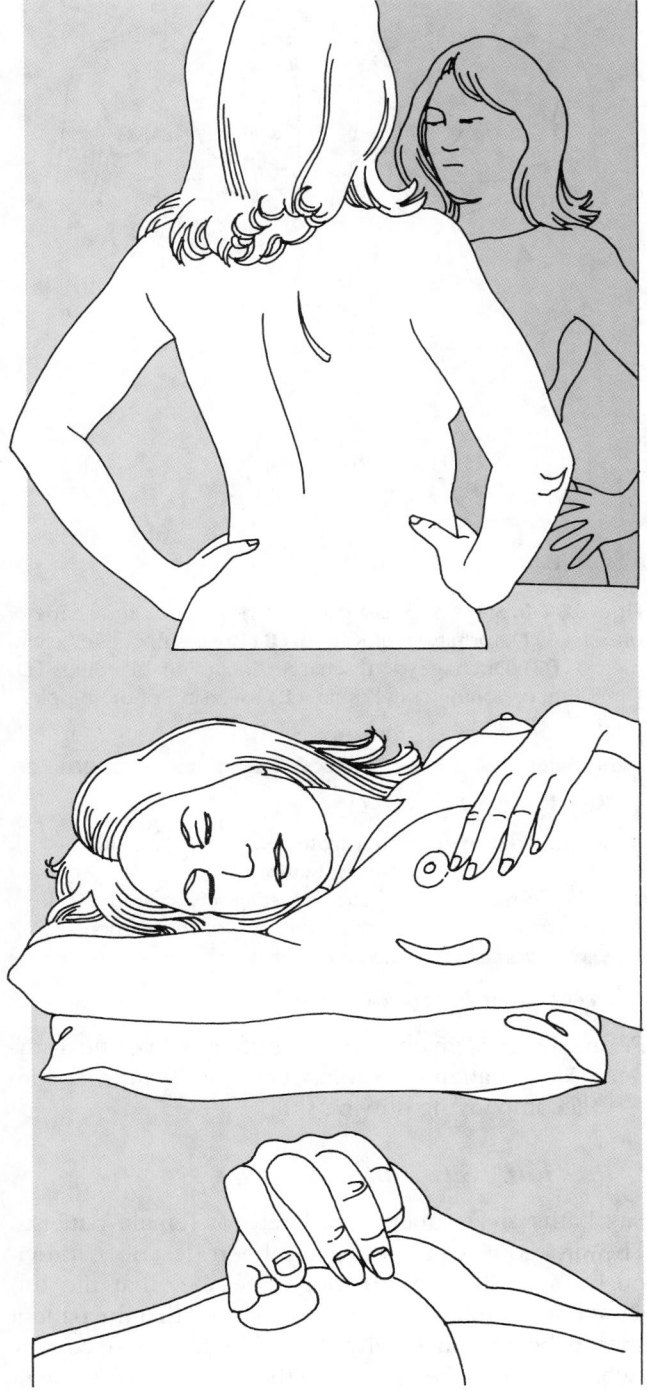

Breast self-examination, performed once a month, before a mirror (step 2). Attention is given to contours. Pressing down on hips serves to tense pectoralis major muscles to inspect for retraction of skin. Step 3 is performed in supine position with elevation by a pillow or blanket. Step 4 involves a nipple check to detect abnormal discharge. Art from Taylor C, Lillis C, LeMone P. Fundamentals of Nursing: The Art and Science of Nursing Care. Ed 2. Philadelphia, J.B. Lippincott, 1993.

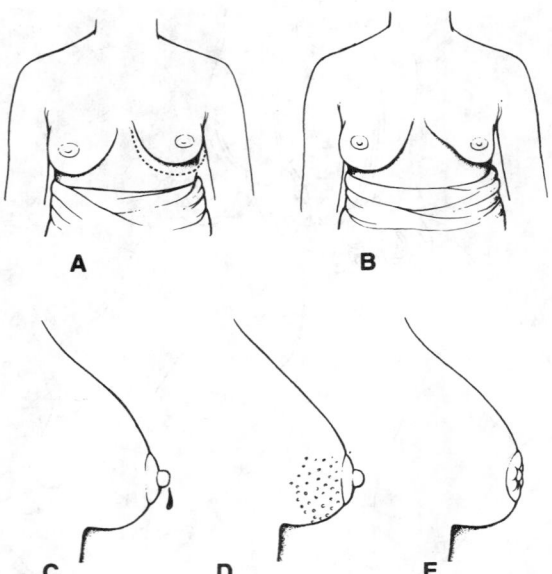

Figure 84-3. Signs of breast cancer. Uneven size and shape of breast: **(A)** Deformity or elevation. **(B)** Breasts not alike (asymmetry). **(C)** Drainage or discharge, including bleeding. **(D)** Dimpling, or "orange peel" skin. **(E)** Inversion of the nipple.

Key Concepts

Women discover approximately 90% to 95% of all breast cancers by self-examination.

A woman who has had a mastectomy should check the scar area. This is a common site for recurrence.

Providing Perineal Care

Perineal care is given to patients after any perineal surgery. Many patients need instruction in this procedure (see accompanying nursing skill).

Providing Sitz Baths

Sitz baths are frequently ordered for female patients. The procedures involved have been described previously (see Chapter 49), but remember that the tub should be disinfected after each use and that the patient should be informed why the procedure is necessary (whether it is done to cleanse the area, to aid the healing process, or to make the patient more comfortable).

Performing a Douche or Vaginal Irrigation

The douche or vaginal irrigation is not as frequently prescribed as in the past. It is believed that frequent douching irritates the vaginal mucosa and predisposes the patient to infection. (The secretions from the mucous membrane protect the area from infection. Therefore, it is not desirable to wash away these secretions unless necessary.)

Nursing Skill Guidelines
Providing Perineal Care

◆ Teach the patient to always cleanse from front to back with toilet tissue or sponges. *(Rationale: This method avoids fecal contamination in the vaginal or urethral area.)*
◆ With the patient seated on the toilet or bedpan, a perineal bottle ("peri bottle") is filled with warm tap water, sterile water, or saline, and the perineal area is thoroughly sprayed or squirted. Spray from front to back. *(Rationale: This keeps the area free of infection.)*
◆ Sometimes cotton balls or Zephiran sponges are used. Zephiran sponges are used only by physician's order. The patient should use each cotton ball or sponge only once. *(Rationale: This helps prevent spreading infection by contaminated materials.)*
◆ Teach the patient to wipe the lateral areas first, saving the last sponges for the urethral area. *(Rationale:The urethral area is the cleanest area.)*
◆ This procedure should be repeated each time the perineal pad is changed, each time the patient uses the toilet or bedpan, or more often as ordered or needed for comfort.

PURPOSE AND PROCEDURE. If the physician orders a vaginal irrigation, the procedure and purpose should be explained to the patient. The vaginal irrigation cleanses the vaginal canal of excess discharge, supplies heat or medication, and relieves pain and inflammation.

The physician orders the solution to be used. Frequently used are povidone-iodine (Betadine), saline solution, sterile water, or a solution of acetic acid (vinegar). Disposable douches also are available. The accompanying nursing skill outlines the procedure.

Nursing Skill
Giving a Douche or Vaginal Irrigation

Supplies and Equipment
Gloves
Irrigating bag, tubing, and clamp or disposable douche
Disposable douche tip
Bedpan
Solution, as prescribed
Standard (short intravenous stand)
Bath thermometer
Protective pad for the bed (such as Chux)
Perineal pad (sanitary napkin), if needed
Tissues

Bath blanket
Mineral oil, if needed

Procedure

1. Wash your hands, and put on gloves. Goggles may be used. (*Rationale: These actions prevent the spread of infection.*)
2. Have the patient void. (*Rationale: A full bladder will interfere with the insertion of the douche nozzle and may cause discomfort. The douche may stimulate voiding if the bladder is full.*)
3. Protect the bed. Have the bedpan ready before preparing the solution. (*Rationale: The fluid will cool; it is important to administer it at the correct temperature. Some fluid might be spilled; you can avoid having to change the linens by protecting the bed.*)
4. Prepare approximately 1,500 mL of the prescribed solution at the required temperature, 100°F to 110°F (37.8°C to 43.3°C), according to the purpose of the treatment. (*Rationale: Heat relieves inflammation, but a solution that is too warm will burn the mucous membranes and the skin around the meatus when flowing back.*)
5. If the solution is ordered at a temperature above 105°F (40.6°C), mineral oil or petrolatum should be applied to the vulva and perineum. Maximum temperature is 115°F (46.8°C). (*Rationale: The vulva and perineum are more sensitive than the vagina.*)
6. Carefully inspect the douche tip to make sure it is not cracked or rough. (*Rationale: delicate vaginal tissue might be injured.*)
7. Have the patient lie back with a rolled bath blanket under her head, and place her on the bedpan. (*Rationale: In this position, gravity will help direct the solution over the entire vagina.*) A douche also may be given while the patient is sitting on the toilet.
8. Place the irrigating bag slightly above the level of the patient's hips, never more than 18 inches (48 cm). (*Rationale: This ensures a continuous, but gentle, flow of the solution. If the bag is higher, it can drive infection into the uterus.*)
9. Release the clamp to let the air out to the tubing before you insert the nozzle. (*Rationale: Air might distend the uterus or vagina.*)
10. Separate the labia, and gently insert the nozzle, directing it downward and backward. (*Rationale: This is the direction that the vaginal canal slants.*) A small amount of water-soluble lubricant, such as K-Y jelly, may be used to aid insertion.
11. Gently release the clamp, and allow the fluid to flow slowly. Rotate the nozzle gently during the treatment. (*Rationale: A natural pocket is formed between the cervix and the rear wall of the vagina. Rotating the douche tip rinses material out of this pocket and directs fluid over all parts of the vagina.*)
12. Clamp the tubing, and gently withdraw the tip from the vagina.
13. Discard the entire douche system in the prescribed manner. (*Rationale: This helps prevent the spread of infection.*)
14. If the patient is able, have her sit up on the bedpan for a few minutes. (*Rationale: This will help to drain the fluid from the vagina.*)
15. Place a sanitary napkin over the vulva. (*Rationale: This helps to protect bed and patient from additional drainage.*)
16. Properly dispose of gloves. Wash your hands, and document the treatment on the patient's chart.

Inserting a Vaginal Suppository

Medication is applied to the vaginal canal by means of vaginal suppositories. Most suppositories must be kept refrigerated until ready for use.

◆ Unwrap the suppository just prior to insertion. Be sure to wear gloves. (*Rationale: The medicine is usually incorporated in a cocoa butter base, which melts at body temperature and dispenses the medication. Room temperature allows the suppository to soften and lose its shape, making insertion difficult or impossible.*)
◆ With the patient lying on her back or side, insert the suppository full length, rounded end first, into the vagina. This will be at least 2 inches (4.5 cm). (*Rationale: It is necessary to clear the external vaginal muscles or the suppository will be expelled.*)
◆ Dispose of materials properly. Wash your hands, and document the procedure, indicating the patient's reactions.

Caring for the Patient Undergoing a Hysterectomy

PREOPERATIVE CONSIDERATIONS. In addition to the usual preparation for abdominal or perineal surgery, the patient may have a vaginal irrigation or douche. She will most likely have an enema to cleanse the colon of feces.

This patient will probably come into the hospital on the morning of surgery. The clinic nurse must give instructions in the administration of the enema and other procedures to be done the evening before surgery. It also is the clinic nurse who will be available to answer the patient (and her partner's) questions before surgery.

A Foley catheter is often inserted in the surgical preparation room to lessen the danger of bladder perforation during removal of the uterus. The Foley catheter is usually removed on the first postoperative day and is not replaced unless the patient cannot void. If the bladder also is repaired, the surgeon may place a suprapubic cystocath during surgery to drain urine and rest the bladder. Thromboembolic disease (TED) stockings are often placed on the legs to prevent thrombophlebitis and are left in place for several days.

All of the patient's questions should be answered fully. The husband or significant other should be included in all patient teaching. The hospital chaplain or the patient's spiritual leader can be a source of needed

Janine White Bear, a 32-year-old Native American woman was admitted with severe vaginal bleeding due to uterine fibroid. Her hemoglobin and hematocrit were 8.7 and 36.6, respectively. She had a history of deep vein thrombosis (DVT) after the delivery of her second child. A hysterectomy was performed. She returned from surgery with a Foley catheter in place, intravenous infusion running, and antiembolitic hosiery on. The catheter was removed in 48 hours. Two nursing diagnosis incorporated in her plan of care follow.

Nursing Diagnosis: *Altered Urinary Elimination Related to Decrease of Bladder Sensation*

Goal: 2/6, Patient will urinate quantities sufficient each 8 hours with 100 mL residual at any one voiding.

Nursing Actions (assess/do/teach)	Rationale	Evaluative Statement
1. Maintain patency of Foley catheter while in place. Prevent pulling on urethra, avoid improper drainage due to dependent loops of catheter tubing.	Prevent distention of bladder or bladder infection.	Goal met: 2/6, Patient voided 700 mL urine in 8 hours with a residual of not more than 50 mL for any one voiding.
2. Monitor intake and output carefully. Encourage fluid intake when able to take orally. Infuse intravenous fluids as ordered.	This keeps patient hydrated and decreases risk of infection.	
3. Assess for bladder distention, especially if catheter drainage decreases and when catheter is removed.		
4. Catheterize Ms. White Bear as necessary for discomfort with pelvic distention or if she has not urinated within 8 hours.	Catheterization will prevent stress on suture line.	
5. Catheterize for residual urine immediately after voiding until residual remains 100 mL or less.	Eliminating residual urine prevents stagnation of urine in bladder, thus decreasing chances of developing a bladder infection.	
6. Encourage patient to empty bladder periodically, not just when the urge is present.	Emptying bladder helps regain bladder sensation and tone.	
7. Monitor for any signs of bladder infection.		

(continued)

support and reassurance. Be sure to document all teaching.

POSTOPERATIVE NURSING CONSIDERATIONS. Nursing care is planned according to the type of hysterectomy. The patient who has had an abdominal hysterectomy is treated like any patient who has had an abdominal incision. The patient recovers more quickly from a vaginal procedure than from the abdominal procedure.

Routine postoperative care is given to prevent complications. Early ambulation is important. The patient often has a urethral or suprapubic catheter. Make sure the patient is able to void after the catheter is removed.

The patient wears perineal pads, with tapes that stick to the panties. Be sure to teach her to pull the panties

Nursing Diagnosis: *Altered Tissue Perfusion (Renal) Related to Increased Risk Factors as Noted by Past Medical History*

Goal: 1/2, Patient will demonstrate methods that improve peripheral circulation to prevent any postoperative circulatory complications.

Nursing Actions (assess/do/teach)	Rationale	Evaluative Statement
1. Assess for positive Homan's sign, and perform neurovascular assessments. Document and report any suspicious findings.	Early identification of problems allows for initiation of early treatment.	1/3, Goal met; patient wearing antiembolitic stocking, doing leg exercises while in bed, and up and ambulating in hallway. Shows no signs of any postoperative circulatory problems.
2. Have patient apply antiembolitic stockings and change position while in bed at least every 2 hours. Teach and encourage patient to do leg exercises while in bed, and assist patient to ambulate as soon as permitted.	These activities help maintain venous return from lower extremities.	
3. Teach patient to avoid placing any pressure under knees and not to rub the calves of her legs.	This decreases the risks of thrombus and embolism.	

and pad straight down to avoid fecal contamination of the operative area. Assess the amount, color, and odor of vaginal drainage. Frequent perineal care is given, and the use of the peri bottle will keep the perineum clean and the patient more comfortable. The patient is taught how to perform the procedure. Frequent sitz baths also are given to increase patient comfort.

A vaginal pack is often in place following surgery. This is usually removed on approximately the first or second postoperative day. The patient may complain of severe back pain while the pack is in place. The nurse can reassure her that the pain will be much relieved by the removal of the packing.

Before discharge from the hospital, the patient should be informed of complications that might occur and when to notify the physician. All teaching must be carefully documented.

Evaluation

The nurse, patient, and family evaluate outcomes of care. Have short-term goals been met? Are long-term goals still realistic? Does the patient need follow-up care or education? Is long-term therapy required? Planning for further nursing care takes into consideration the pa-

tient's prognosis and any complications and the patient's response to care given.

Breast Neoplasms

Most breast lesions are benign. Malignant lesions are more likely than benign lesions to be irregularly shaped and hard and often show secondary signs, such as enlarged lymph nodes in the axillary area, asymmetry of the breast, retraction of the nipple, discharge or bleeding, dimpling, or elevation of one breast (see Fig. 84-3). Benign lesions are more likely to be round or oval with a smooth border and usually show no secondary signs. Furthermore, benign lesions are likely to be movable, while malignant lesions are often attached to the surrounding skin, the underlying structures, or breast tissue.

Benign Neoplasms

Chronic Cystic Mastitis

Cystic disease is the most common breast disorder in women between the ages of 30 and 50. It is believed to be the result of a hormonal imbalance and is related to the activity of the ovaries. It is rare after menopause.

Breast tissue cells collect together and form a mass. This cell mass shuts off the ducts and forms cysts. These masses may form fibrous tumors (*fibromas*) or lumps in the breast. A biopsy is performed to rule out cancer. Most lumps removed from the breast are benign. A cyst may be excised or drained without removal of any of the surrounding tissue. If there are numerous cysts, the physician may do a simple **mastectomy**, in which only the breast is removed as a preventive measure, because cysts are sometimes precancerous. Caffeine aggravates cyst formation. Women with a cystic condition are therefore advised to avoid coffee, tea, chocolate, and cola drinks. It is often suggested that these women have a yearly mammogram.

Breast Cancer

Cancer of the breast is the most common type of cancer and the second most common cause of cancer death in women. (Lung cancer is the most common cause of cancer death, due to cigarette smoking.) Approximately one in nine women will develop breast cancer at some time in their life.[2] More than 142,000 American women develop breast cancer every year. More than half are cured, but the number would be higher if more cases were discovered and treated earlier. Research shows that if breast cancer is treated within 3 months of its discovery, the 5-year survival rates are much higher. Breast cancer also may occur in men, but this is rare. Factors predisposing to breast cancer are presented in the accompanying box.

Key Concept

Approximately 95% of all women with a palpable breast lump discover it by breast self-examination.

Signs and Symptoms. Signs of breast cancer are usually evident before pain appears (see Fig. 84-3). Women are urged to consult a physician if they notice a lump or any other change in the breast. Other signs and symptoms include nipple discharge, history of pain or tingling without a palpable mass, breast enlargement or thickening during adulthood, nipple retraction, or puckering in any area of the breast.

Prompt action may mean the difference between life and death. The American Cancer society states that more than two-thirds of women who consult a physician immediately after finding a lump in the breast are

Predisposing Factors in Breast Cancer

The following categories of women have an increased risk of developing breast cancer:

◆ Onset of menstruation (menarche) prior to age 12
◆ Late menopause (over age 50)
◆ Long or irregular menstrual cycles
◆ Women over age 40 (approximately 25% are between ages 40 and 49; approximately 70% are over age 50)
◆ Family history of breast cancer, especially mother, maternal grandmother, maternal aunt, sister, or daughter
◆ History of fibrocystic breast disease
◆ History of cancer of the other breast
◆ History of endometrial or ovarian cancer
◆ Women who have never had a baby
◆ Women who had their first baby after age 30
◆ Women who have not nursed babies
◆ Women on antihypertensive therapy
◆ Radiation exposure before age 30
◆ Diet high in fat
◆ Obesity
◆ Alcohol and tobacco use
◆ Previous breast surgery (biopsies, implants, cosmetic mammoplasty)

alive 5 years later; less than one-third of those who delayed more than 3 months live that long.

Diagnostic Tests. A mammogram will often show a lump or mass and may help to indicate the type of lesion. Breast ultrasonography also may be helpful to differentiate between malignant and nonmalignant lesions. Breast biopsy is diagnostic for breast cancer. In addition, estrogen-receptor and progesterone-receptor analyses are done to determine the type of tumor present. Approximately two-thirds of patients with breast cancer test estrogen-receptor positive.[3]

Key Concept

According to research done in Minnesota, some breast cancers may exist for as long as 6 years before being detected by palpation. Thus, regular mammography, in conjunction with breast self-examination, is recommended by many physicians.

Surgery. Prior to surgery for a malignant lesion, the surgeon discusses available treatment with the patient

---

[2] Meyer WC, Jensen PA. Breast Cancer Detection, Quarterly Check-Up. Minneapolis, Paul larson OB-GYN Clinic, 1992.

[3] Berkow R (Ed). Merck Manual of Diagnosis and Therapy, Ed 16. Rahway, NJ, Merck & Co., Inc., 1992.

and her spouse or significant other. The treatment mode depends on the type of tumor, extent of the disease at the time of diagnosis, age of the client, medical condition of the client, and client's feelings related to body image and self-esteem. It is imperative that a malignant lesion be treated *as soon as possible* to prevent its spread.

The extent of the surgery varies, and much controversy exists about how much is necessary. If the malignancy in confined to one lump, a *simple lumpectomy* will usually be performed. If the cancer involves more tissue, a *partial mastectomy* may be done, or the entire breast may be removed in a *simple mastectomy.* If the cancer has spread beyond the breast, a *radical mastectomy* may be necessary, although this is rarely done today. In the *total radical mastectomy,* the total breast is removed, along with the overlying skin, the axillary channels, the lymph nodes that drain the area, and the pectoral muscles. A *modified radical mastectomy,* which leaves pectoral muscles intact, is more common today. In some cases, if one breast is affected, the other breast also is removed in a *prophylactic mastectomy.* In other cases, a breast insert (*prosthesis*) is placed during surgery; however, there is great controversy concerning the safety of these prostheses. In most cases, reconstructive surgery is done, either as part of the initial procedure or later.

Key Concept

If breast cancer is localized to the breast at the time of detection, the 5-year survival rate is more than 90%.

Prognosis. If the lymph nodes contain cancer cells, the finding is referred to as "node positive," and the pathologist identifies the number of nodes involved. If the lymph nodes are not involved, then the patient's prognosis is good. However, if all the nodes are involved, the prognosis is guarded. The fewer the nodes involved, the better the prognosis. Current research also indicates that if breast surgery is performed during or just before ovulation, a cure may be more likely.

Radiation and Chemotherapy. Radiation or chemotherapy may be given to prevent further spread of the cancer. In some cases, radiation therapy is used instead of mastectomy to destroy cancer cells. When chemotherapy or biologicals are used after surgery as a preventive measure, this is called *adjuvant systemic therapy.*

Postmastectomy hormone therapy has been used extensively in recent years. This is especially important if lymph nodes are affected. Hormone therapy involves altering the woman's hormonal environment. For example, if the patient is not past menopause and has had

a mastectomy, a second operation may be performed to remove the ovaries to eliminate the source of estrogen, which is thought to stimulate tumor growth.

Various other chemotherapy regimens also are used. These are usually combinations of drugs, such as the "CMF regimen," which is listed in the accompanying box. These agents also may be combined with biologic agents (biologic response modifiers). The initial round of chemotherapy may be from 6 months to 2 years.

Adjuvant tamoxifen therapy is often used, especially in women older than 50 years or potmenopausal women. This therapy is believed to prolong survival and help prevent cancer on the contralateral (opposite) side. It also may help reduce cardiovascular disease and osteoporosis but may increase the incidence of uterine cancer. Tamoxifen has been shown to delay recurrence in premenopausal women but does not seem to prolong the overall survival rates.

If axillary lymph nodes are all negative, the oncologist may not treat with adjuvant therapy, because mastectomy or lumpectomy may be considered curative.

In the premenopausal patient with positive lymph nodes, some form of chemotherapy (such as the CMF regime) and radiotherapy are given for approximately 6 months. In postmenopausal women with positive nodes (especially those with estrogen-receptor positive tumors), adjuvant tamoxifen therapy is often given for 2 to 5 years.

Any therapy must be thoroughly discussed with the oncologist. Decisions are made on the basis of the type and extent of the tumor and the patient's wishes. Chapter 76 describes cancer treatments and their side effects in more detail.

Skin Grafting, Plastic Revision, and Reconstructive Surgery. Because radical mastectomy involves removal of a large area of skin, it may be necessary to take a skin graft from the thigh to close the wound. The patient's arm may be bandaged against her body to avoid pull on the graft, with her elbow bent at a right angle and the arm supported by a pillow or sling. If there is no skin graft,

---

Key Medications
for Breast Cancer Chemotherapy

◆ CMF regimen (combination chemotherapy): cyclophosphamide (Cytoxan), methotrexate (Mexate), 5-fluorouracil (5-FU)

◆ Changes in hormonal balance following removal of ovaries: male hormones, corticosteroids

◆ Prevention of spread and recurrence: tamoxifen (Nolvadex, Tamofen)

Nursing considerations are contained in the accompanying test and in Chapter 76.

the arm is free. Sometimes, the patient has the mastectomy first and comes in at a later date for a plastic revision of the wound. Plastic surgery or skin grafting improves the appearance or skin coverage of the wound. Skin grafting and plastic revision performed later are often the treatment of choice, because the plastic surgery is more likely to be successful and easier after the initial wound has healed and the edema has abated. Radiation also is damaging to new grafts.

In reconstructive breast surgery, the surgeon implants a suitable prosthesis and reconstructs the nipple area with a graft. Reconstructive surgery also may be done at the same time as the original surgery. Reconstructive surgery is easier to do following less widespread surgery, such as lumpectomy.

Newer therapy involves instillation of saline over a period of weeks to gradually stretch the skin of the chest. When optimal size is reached, a permanent prosthesis is implanted. The nipple is constructed and the areola area can be tattooed for a more natural appearance.

Prosthesis. A prosthesis can be fitted to duplicate the remaining breast, so there will be no change in the patient's appearance. Until the physician decides the patient is ready for the prosthesis, the patient can purchase a padded bra or she can pad her bra. A surgical supply house and corsetiere where prostheses are sold usually have an experienced fitter on their staff. The physician often recommends a particular store or medical supply house where the prosthesis can be fitted. One adaptable type of prosthetic breast is made of foam rubber and is light and washable. Another is filled with a heavy liquid, and it looks and feels much like a normal breast. The latter is the more realistic looking prosthesis, because it does not tend to ride up as does the lightweight foam rubber one. However, it is heavy and hot in the summer. Care must be given not to puncture the bag or the fluid will be lost.

Nursing Considerations. *Preoperative Care.* Preparation of the patient in the physician's office begins as soon as she is told that she will need surgery. She needs to understand her alternatives and the surgery the physician is recommending. She also must understand the procedure for a biopsy and for a frozen section; she needs to understand that most breast lesions are benign. However, she also needs to understand that if the frozen section is positive, the surgeon may do more extensive surgery immediately.

Physical preoperative preparations are done. The entire area of breast tissue is shaved and prepared, and all preparations for major surgery are made. The most common procedure is to keep the patient in the operating room while biopsy is done; if cancer is present, surgery can be done immediately.

Preoperative teaching includes information about turning, deep breathing, and early ambulation, as with any other preoperative patient. The nurse should teach postmastectomy exercises and allow the patient to practice. The patient also should be informed that lifelike breast prostheses are available. The patient's partner and other family members are included in discussions if possible.

Addressing Patient Concerns. The patient who is going to have a breast operation is understandably apprehensive. Will it be cancer? Will the breast be removed? The understanding nurse listens and supports the patient and family. Extreme emotional reactions are possible; talking with another person who has had breast cancer may be helpful for the patient. This disease affects the entire family, and each family member may need reassurance.

Postoperative Care. Routine postoperative care is given. Treatments are designed to prevent complications and to rehabilitate the patient as soon as possible. The patient should be encouraged to walk and move around. She also needs to be encouraged to do her postmastectomy exercises.

If drains are placed in the surgical wound to drain excess fluid and prevent edema, the nurse should be aware of this so that a large amount of drainage can be anticipated. The dressings must be checked frequently. Another method of drainage is to connect the suction tube to a suction machine or other device that exerts gentle suction on the wound catheter as it expands (Hem-O-Vac).

The affected arm should be kept elevated for several days to minimize the development of edema. Some edema is expected if the surgery involves the lymphatic system. Occasionally a snug elastic sleeve will be used to decrease or prevent swelling. A low-sodium diet and diuretics also may be ordered.

The postmastectomy patient will need much emotional support. It is normal for her to experience grief due to loss of a body part, and she may direct her anger at the nursing staff or family members.

> **Nursing Alert**
>
> The blood pressure of the postoperative mastectomy patient should never be taken on the operative side. Also, the patient should not receive an injection or have blood drawn from the affected side. Infection of the wound is possible. Although some edema in the arm is normal after a radical mastectomy, it may be a sign of infection if it persists. (Edema does not disappear as rapidly in obese patients.) Signs of infection in the arm or the hand should be reported immediately.

Postoperative Exercises. If radical surgery is performed, postmastectomy exercises are needed to prevent shortening of muscles, contracture of joints, and loss of muscle tone. By improving lymphatic circulation, exercise causes the edema of the arm on the affected side to be reduced. If a skin graft has been done, exercises to restore normal use of the arm are started as soon as the arm is freed. In other cases, exercises should begin on the operative day or the first postoperative day. Encourage the patient to keep her shoulders level and relaxed and not to hunch toward the affected side. It may be difficult to get the patient to move her affected arm away from her body, but it is important to keep the muscles from becoming permanently contracted.

Meanwhile, the patient should be encouraged to use the arm on the affected side. She should use that hand to wash her face, brush her hair, and eat. She may need assistance to cut her meat or butter her bread.

Key Concept

Steady, persistent exercise every day is necessary to stretch the muscles gradually. The exercises should be done for a short time, three or four times a day to avoid fatigue and unnecessary pain.

The American Cancer Society publishes a booklet, "Reach to Recovery—Exercises after Mastectomy," that describes postmastectomy exercises that can be done at home. Some exercises can be combined with ordinary daily activities, such as sliding a towel back and forth to wipe the back, brushing the hair, and reaching with the arms when making a bed. The patient should have a good start in learning how to exercise the muscles before she goes home. Some hospitals offer postmastectomy classes so that patients can exercise together. Exercises may include wall hand-climbing, rope-turning, rod or broom exercises, and pulley exercises.

Key Concept

It is helpful to have a representative from the American Cancer Society's "Reach for Recovery" program visit the patient while she is still in the hospital. This person can recommend places that sell prostheses. They often try to bring a padded bra for the patient to wear home from the hospital. They also can offer much-needed emotional support and answer questions.

Disorders Related to the Menstrual Cycle

Disturbances of Menstruation

The most common menstrual disorders are amenorrhea, menorrhagia, metorrhagia, dysmenorrhea, extreme irregularity, and premenstrual syndrome (PMS).

Amenorrhea

Ammenorrhea is the absence of or abnormal stoppage of menses (menstruation). If the menses have not been established by the 15th year, the patient should be examined. The difficulty may be hormonal or emotional, and it should have the attention of a specialist. Amenorrhea also may be due to nutritional or emotional causes or to malformations of the female organs. (The menses are normally absent in pregnancy and after menopause.) After evaluating the cause of the patient's amenorrhea, the physician prescribes appropriate treatment.

Nursing Alert

Women in a "starvation" situation often experience amenorrhea, a serious symptom. This may also be a sign of anorexia or bulimia. Women in intensive athletic training also are amenorrheal in many cases. They should be under the supervision of an experienced sports medicine specialist.

Menorrhagia

Menorrhagia is excessive bleeding in amount or duration during menstruation. The excessive loss of blood results in anemia. If this irregularity occurs in a young girl, it may adjust itself, but it should be watched. If it occurs during menopause, it may indicate pathology. Menorrhagia also may occur in the patient with an intrauterine device (IUD) for birth control. In excessive bleeding unexplained by organic causes, hormone therapy may be helpful. A D&C also may be performed as therapeutic treatment.

Metrorrhagia

Metorrhagia is bleeding between menstrual periods. It is abnormal and should be brought to the attention of a physician, because it may indicate cancer or retained placental tissue in the postpartum patient or in the patient who has had a spontaneous or induced abortion. Metorrhagia may indicate fibroid tumors and is frequently associated with the use of oral contraceptives; in this instance, it is referred to as *breakthrough bleeding.*

Dysmenorrhea

Dysmenorrhea is painful menstruation. Normal menstruation should not be painful. Functional causes of menstrual pain may stem from constipation, insufficient exercise, poor posture, fatigue, or improper placement of a tampon. These conditions can be remedied easily. If pain is very severe, it may be due to an increase in prostaglandin secretion, which intensifies uterine contractions. Medications such as ibuprofen (Motrin) or mefenamic acid (Ponstel) effectively block prostaglandin production. These drugs are taken at the beginning of menstruation and regularly for 48 hours thereafter. Dymenorrhea often fades by itself after childbearing but occasionally can be a symptom of displaced uterus, tumors, endocrine disturbances, or endometriosis.

Extreme Irregularity

Extreme irregularity of menses should be evaluated, because it may indicate a hormonal deficiency that could result in later *sterility.*

Premenstrual Syndrome

PMS, also called *premenstrual tension,* is associated with symptoms that are common to as many as 40% to 50% of women, with more severe symptoms occurring in women older than 35 years. In some cases, the PMS symptoms increase with age.

Signs and Symptoms. The signs and symptoms of PMS are cyclic in nature, generally developing 7 to 14 days prior to the onset of menses and disappearing with its onset. More than 100 symptoms of PMS have been identified; these fall into the general categories of mood alterations, symptoms related to fluid retention, and neurologic, vascular, gastrointestinal, and respiratory symptoms. Common symptoms include abdominal distention, backache, headache, generalized edema, abnormal sleep patterns, acne, visual disturbances, food cravings, occasional vomiting, irritability, and moodiness. **Mastalgia** (breast pain) is a common symptom. A diminished chemical in the brain, serotonin, has been linked to many PMS symptoms. PMS also seems to be an allergic reaction in some cases.

In many women, PMS is replaced by dysmenorrhea at the onset of menses. Menstrual headache in some instances is severe and may need to be treated with medications.

Treatment and Nursing Considerations. There is often some relief with the use of a low-salt diet for 1 to 2 weeks during the premenstrual cycle and with medications that increase the excretion of sodium ions. (The accompanying box lists key medications.) Increasing protein and decreasing sugar also are helpful in many cases. If allergens can be identified, their elimination can greatly reduce symptoms. Positive stress management is helpful, especially when combined with an active exercise program and omission of caffeine. If the condition becomes severe, tranquilizers may be prescribed. A support group may be helpful in extreme cases.

Toxic Shock Syndrome

The use of tampons, particularly those with plastic inserters, has been associated with a serious syndrome of symptoms known as toxic shock syndrome (TSS).

> ## Key Medications
> *for PMS*
>
> ♦ Diuretic medications: hydrochlorothiazide (HydroDIURIL, Esidrix)
> ♦ Hormones: oral contraceptives, progesterone
> ♦ Tranquilizers: alprazolam (Xanax), diazepam (Valium)
> ♦ Supplements: vitamin B supplements especially pyridoxine; magnesium supplements

---

TSS is believed to be caused by a bacterial toxin *(Staphylococcus aureus).* Toxic shock syndrome is characterized by fever of 102°F (38.8°C) or greater, with vomiting or diarrhea. There may be a sudden drop in blood pressure and accompanying weakness and dizziness. A red rash may occur, which later may result in peeling of the skin. The blood count may drop. Urine output is diminished. (Wound infections also may be caused by the same "staph" organism that causes TSS.)

If any of these symptoms occur, the patient is instructed to remove the tampon and to call her physician *immediately.* This can be a life-threatening disease.

The chance of developing TSS is negligible if tampons are not used. If the patient does use tampons, instruct her about changing them frequently and using them intermittently during menstruation. Tampons need to be inserted carefully to avoid abrasions of the vaginal tract.

The instances of TSS have dropped dramatically since 1980 when efforts were made to decrease the absorbency of tampons and to make them from materials less likely to support the growth of bacteria. However, the risk is still present.

> ## Nursing Alert
>
> A serious infection or TSS may develop if a tampon is forgotten or moves so high it cannot be removed by the woman. If the string breaks or a tampon cannot be removed for another reason, the woman should see her physician immediately.

Discomforts of Menopause

Menopause (climacteric) is the cessation of menstruation and occurs usually between the ages of 45 and 50, although it may occur earlier or later. Menopause signifies that the production of estrogen and progesterone has stopped and that ovulation has ceased. Menopause is a normal body change and should not cause difficulties. However, some women experience difficulties as a result of hormonal changes, namely a decrease in estrogen and progesterone. Generally, one of the first signs of menopause is a change in the menses. The amount of flow becomes less, and the cycle becomes irregular. Finally, the menses stop altogether. In a few women, bleeding becomes heavier for a time. Because the ovaries are producing less estrogen, the levels may be inadequate. This may cause symptoms.

The most common symptom is the "hot flash," with accompanying perspiration, palpitation, and fatigue. While hot flashes are not serious, they are annoying and embarrassing to the patient. Another possible symptom of menopause is vaginal dryness and atrophy. The vagina losses its normal lubrication and elasticity. Some women experience weight gain, skin dryness, sagging breasts, and signs of calcium deficiency (osteoporosis).

Sometimes women experience psychological symptoms during menopause. These include insomnia, anxiety, crying spells, fatigue, mood swings, and depression. Menopause can be difficult in a society that emphasizes youthfulness.

Treatment. Occasionally, mild sedatives or tranquilizers may be necessary. Hormone therapy may be prescribed to treat severe symptoms and discomforts. This therapy delays symptoms of menopause and can help the woman's body adjust more gradually. Some research has theorized that using hormones increases the woman's tendency toward uterine cancer. Other research asserts that conjugated estrogens (Premarin), in combination with medroxyprogesterone acetate (Provera), help reduce the risk of later developing breast or cervical cancer.

Nursing Considerations. A woman often needs emotional support during menopause. She should be educated to realize that menopause is a normal physiologic function. Teach the woman helpful health measures: a well-balanced diet, stress-relieving exercise, adequate rest, leisure activities, and relaxation techniques.

Induced Menopause. After hysterectomy (removal of the uterus) and bilateral oophorectomy (removal of both ovaries) or radiation therapy for cancer, artificial or surgical menopause occurs. If only the uterus has been removed, there will be no menstrual flow; however, normal hormonal cycles will continue. A young woman who has had both ovaries and the uterus removed will often be maintained on estrogen therapy.

Key Concept

The premenopausal woman who experiences surgical menopause may have more difficulties than the older woman who undergoes a normal menopause. The younger the woman is, the more likely she is to have difficulties with surgical menopause without estrogen-replacement therapy.

Structural Disorders in Pelvic Organs

Vaginal Fistula

A fistula is an opening between two organs that normally do not open into each other. It is the result of an ulcerating process, such as cancer or irritation or a childbirth injury. A fistula may develop between the ureter and the vagina *(ureterovaginal)*, between the bladder and the vagina *(vesicovaginal)*, or between the vagina and the rectum *(rectovaginal)*.

Any fistula is a most troublesome condition. If it is between the ureter or the bladder and the vagina, urine will leak into the vagina. If it is between the rectum and the vagina, it causes fecal incontinence. A long-standing fistula is difficult to repair successfully because the tissues are eroded. Infection can become an additional problem.

In many cases, particularly in young women, an attempt is made to surgically repair the fistula. A successful repair is difficult because of the associated problems. The incision must granulate from the *inside out* to prevent an abscess. The closeness of the urinary tract to the bowel makes infection a common postoperative complication. Repaired fistulas tend to recur because of continued irritation.

Efforts are made to assist the healing process by building up the patient's resistance and by keeping the patient as clean as possible, without perineal irritations. The patient with an unrepairable fistula is distressed by the odor and constant drainage. Sitz baths and deodorizing douches help maintain cleanliness.

Cystocele

Cystocele is the downward displacement of the bladder toward the vaginal orifice. It is most often seen in women who have experienced frequent deliveries or deliveries close together. Sometimes it is the result of injuries during childbirth.

Cystocele can cause nagging discomforts: pelvic pain, backache, fatigue, and a sagging weight in the pelvis. The patient may experience *stress incontinence*, the dribbling of urine if she coughs, strains, sneezes, or laughs. She also may have urgency, frequency, and residual urine.

If the condition is not advanced, perineal exercises (Kegel) may be prescribed to strengthen the muscles (see box). Surgery may be necessary whereby the anterior vaginal wall is repaired *(anterior colporrhaphy* or *anterior repair)* and the bladder returned to its normal position.

Rectocele

Rectocele is the upward displacement of the rectum toward the vaginal orifice. Rectocele may be caused from injuries during childbirth. The patient with recto-

---

Keys to Patient Teaching
Kegel Exercises

- Locate the muscles surrounding the vagina by sitting on the toilet and starting and stopping the flow of urine.
- Test the baseline strength of the muscles by inserting a finger in the opening of the vagina and contracting the muscles.
- Exercise A—Squeeze the muscles together and hold the squeeze for 3 seconds. Relax the muscles. Repeat.
- Exercise B—Contract and relax the muscles as rapidly as possible 10 to 25 times. Repeat.
- Exercise C—Imagine sitting in a pan of water and sucking water into the vagina. Hold for 3 seconds.
- Exercise D—Push out as during a bowel movement, only with the vagina. Hold for 3 seconds.
- Repeat exercises A, C, and D 10 times each and exercise B once. Repeat the entire series three times a day.

Regular practice of the Kegel exercises can restore muscle tone. Benefits are control of stress incontinence, increased vaginal lubrication during sexual arousal, relief of constipation, increased flexibility of episiotomy scars, and stronger gripping of the base of the penis during intercourse.

---

cele will experience backache, fatigue, heaviness in the pelvic region, and bowel difficulties. There will be incontinence of flatus and a fluctuation between constipation and diarrhea. Surgical repair of the posterior vaginal wall with a return of the rectum to its normal position is known as *posterior colporrhaphy* or *posterior repair*. The woman who has repair of a cystocele *and* a rectocele is said to have had an anterior-posterior (AP) repair.

Another procedure that is sometimes necessary is called the Marshall-Marchetti. In this operation, the urethra is supported by sutures through the anterior wall of the vagina on either side of the urethra. The sutures are then passed through the outer covering layer (periosteum) of the pubic bone and secured.

Preoperative Nursing Considerations in GYN Surgery. Prior to an AP repair or other gynecologic procedure, the patient is given an enema, and a catheter is inserted, unless a suprapubic cystocath will be used. For the anterior colporrhapy, the catheter is left in place for several days, and a residual urine volume or culture may be ordered once the catheter is removed. Showers and sitz baths promote comfort and healing. The patient will be instructed to avoid lifting, sexual intercourse, and prolonged sitting and standing until full healing has occurred (usually 6–8 weeks).

Prolapsed Uterus

A prolapsed uterus is one that sags or herniates into the vagina or in severe cases, even outside the vagina. The most common cause is damage during childbirth; the menopausal woman or one nearing menopause is the most likely candidate. The woman is examined while standing or bearing down. The prolapse is classified as first degree (cervix, without straining or traction, can be seen when labia are spread), second degree (cervix protrudes out to the level of the perineum), or third degree or procidentia (entire uterus or most of it protrudes out of the vagina onto the perineum).

The patient with a prolapse complains of nagging backache, constipation, and stress incontinence. There may be pain with intercourse *(dyspareunia)*. The cervix may be irritated by rubbing on the underwear. A hysterectomy may be performed to eliminate a severe prolapse. Some physicians prefer to resuspend the uterus back into its normal position, particularly in a younger woman.

If surgery is contraindicated because the woman is elderly or in poor physical condition, a *pessary* may be indicated. The pessary is a ring-shaped device, which may be one of several types. It is inserted snugly against the cervix and prevents the uterus form moving downward. It is inserted much as is a diaphragm. However, there is some discomfort when the pessary passes through the vaginal muscles because of its larger size and firmer consistency. The patient should be taught to insert and remove the pessary. It should be removed and cleaned with warm, soapy water at least once a week. Most pessaries also must be removed to have comfortable sexual intercourse and sometimes to have a bowel movement.

Abnormal Flexion of the Uterus

A displaced uterus is usually congenital, but it may be the result of childbearing. Backward displacement is called *retroversion* or *retroflexion*. Forward displacement is called *anteversion* or *anteflexion*. A displaced uterus may cause backache, dysmenorrhea, or sterility. Uterine displacement can be corrected by surgery in which the uterus is sutured in its proper position.

Inflammatory Disorders

Infections of the Female Reproductive Tract

Vulvitis

Vulvitis, inflammation of the vulva, may be the result of trauma due to scratching, improper cleansing, birth control pills, or an irritating vaginal discharge. Most often, it is caused by some type of infection. Severe itching and burning; pain during urination, defecation, or intercourse; and swelling and redness are usually associated with vulvitis. The goal of treatment is to determine the causes and eliminate them.

Vaginitis

Vaginitis is an inflammation of the vagina. Normally the secretions of the vagina protect it from infection. However, two organisms often do cause vaginal infection: *Trichomonas vaginalis* and *Candida albicans* (formerly known as monilia and commonly known as "yeast infection"). Trichomoniasis is likely to be transmitted sexually, whereas candidiasis can more easily be spread in other ways. However, both are considered sexually transmitted infections.

The most prominent symptom of vaginitis is a whitish vaginal discharge called *leukorrhea*. The discharge is odorous and profuse (more so in trichomoniasis) and makes the perineum, vagina, and urethra burn and itch. The discharge may be frothy or thick and whitish.

In trichomoniasis and candidiasis, the sexual partner must be treated at the same time so that the infection will not be spread back and forth ("ping-pong" infection; see the key medications box). Circumcision of the male may be necessary to help control a recurring infection (see Chapter 83).

Trichomonas Vaginalis (Trichomoniasis).

This infection is caused by a one-celled parasite. The prominent feature of the *Trichomonas* infection is the very foul-smelling discharge that is foamy white or greenish yellow in the female; the male usually has no symptoms. The condition may be persistent and difficult to cure. Trichomoniasis is considered a sexually transmitted disease, but the organism can survive for several hours on moist objects, such as toilet seats and towels.

Trichomoniasis is most often treated with oral tablets of metronidazole (Flagyl), taken by both sexual partners simultaneously. The patients should abstain from alcohol during treatment, because severe gastrointestinal distress almost always results. Sometimes, if the infection is stubborn, metronidazole or antibiotics are inserted vaginally.

> ### Nursing Alert
>
> If a pregnant woman contracts trichomoniasis, treatment is necessary, although it is usually postponed until the second or third trimester because of the unknown effects of the drug on the developing fetus. Untreated trichomoniasis can lead to a fragile cervix that will not be able to withstand delivery.

Candidiasis.

Candidiasis is a stubborn and difficult-to-cure fungus infection. It is often referred to as a "vaginal yeast infection." It is common; three-fourths of all

> ### Key Medications
> *for Vaginal Infections*
>
> ◆ Treats trichomonas and bacterial vaginosis: metronidazole (Flagyl)
> ◆ Treats candidiasis: nystatin (Mycostatin, Nilstat); miconazole nitrate (Monistat, Micatin)

women will have at least one such infection. Candidiasis may be transmitted sexually or in other ways.

The causative organism (*Candida albicans*) is often present in the vagina under normal circumstances, but certain factors or changes can activate the infection. The two major factors that lead to infection are the presence of glucose or glycogen in the urine and a change in vaginal pH. The factors that influence development of a vaginal yeast infection include the following:

◆ Change in vaginal pH
◆ Hormonal changes during menstrual cycle
◆ Hormonal changes during pregnancy
◆ Hormonal changes for any other reason (such as taking exogenous hormones, estrogens, steroids)
◆ Long-term use of birth control pills
◆ Use of systemic antibiotics
◆ Diabetes mellitus
◆ Spilling of sugar in the urine, whether diabetic or not
◆ Compromised immunity

Signs and Symptoms. Women with candidiasis complain of vaginal itching, which ranges from mild to intense. The itching is inside the vagina and on the outer structures in approximately 80% of cases. The woman often complains of soreness, irritation, and burning, especially during sexual intercourse. Vaginal discharge may be profuse; it is often clumpy and white and may resemble cottage cheese. There may be redness or a rash around the vagina.

The male partner often has no symptoms. However, he may have a red, blotchy rash on the penis, which may or may not itch. An abnormal discharge also may be present. He should be sure to tell the physician his partner has a yeast infection.

Treatment Considerations. Women in the following situations should consult their primary caregiver at the first sign of a vaginal infection:

◆ First vaginal infection
◆ Not sure it is a yeast infection
◆ At risk for human immunodeficiency virus or acquired immunodeficiency syndrome
◆ Diabetic
◆ Fever over 100°F (oral)
◆ Girls younger than age 12

◆ Pregnancy
◆ New pain, including lower abdomen, back, or either shoulder
◆ Malodorous vaginal discharge

Nursing Considerations. Frequent bathing provides temporary relief from irritation and itching. Over-the-counter medications, such as nystatin (Mycostatin, Nilstat) and miconazole nitrate (Monistat, Micatin), are available. Various systems of medication delivery are available. These include creams with several different types of applicators, tablets that dissolve inside the body, and suppositories. A combination pack containing suppositories and cream is available to treat internal and external symptoms. The nurse is a key person in teaching women how to use the medication.

Patient teaching is particularly important, because many patients will treat their own infection at home and may not see the physician. Instructions are basically the same in all treatment systems. These instructions are listed in the patient teaching box.

Women who are treating a vaginal infection should consult their caregiver in the following cases:

◆ No signs of improvement after 3 days of treatment
◆ Worsening of symptoms within 3 days
◆ Complete relief from all symptoms not occurring in 7 days of treatment
◆ Return of symptoms within 2 months

The latter cases indicate the presence of an infection or condition other than candidiasis.

Bacterial Vaginosis

Bacterial vaginosis (formerly called nonspecific vaginitis) is a relatively common vaginal disorder that is believed to be caused by a combination of organisms. It is a complex condition that is not completely understood. The patient complains of increased white, gray, or yellowish vaginal discharge with or without irritation. An unpleasant "fishy" odor occurs, which increases after intercourse or washing with soap. Redness and edema are not usually significant.

The usual treatment consists of a 7-day course of an oral antibiotic, most commonly metronidazole. This infection may be sexually transmitted; therefore, simultaneous treatment of the sexual partner is recommended.

Atrophic (Senile) Vaginitis

This condition often occurs in postmenopausal women. It is caused by atrophy of the vaginal mucous membranes and decreased mucus and other vaginal secretions, which results from lowered estrogen production. This disorder is highly irritating and is discussed further in Chapter 85.

Keys to Patient Teaching
Self-Care in Vaginitis

In all treatment systems the following instructions are given to the patient:

◆ Read and follow the instructions on the package carefully.
◆ Insert the full dosage of medication at bedtime.
◆ Cream is used during the day to control external itching.
◆ Use the treatment for 7 *consecutive* days.
◆ Do not skip treatment during menses.
◆ Refrain from sexual intercourse during treatment and for at least 3 days after treatment is completed.
◆ A condom or diaphragm used during treatment will not be effective (because latex is weakened by the medication).
◆ Use only unscented sanitary napkins during treatment.
◆ Do not use tampons during treatment (because they absorb some medication, reducing the dosage; tampons are irritating).

Atrophic vaginitis is treated by using a water-soluble lubricant (such a K-Y jelly) during intercourse. An estrogen-based cream also may be helpful.

Vaginitis is difficult to cure. It can be extremely irritating and persists for a long time. Recurrence is fairly common. Early and persistent treatment is the only way to prevent this disorder from becoming chronic. The patient may find it necessary to wear sanitary napkins to absorb the profuse drainage. Frequent napkin replacement, perineal care, and sitz baths will help to prevent odor and irritation. Sometimes, mild tranquilizers or mild analgesics are given to lessen the effects of pruritus. Patient teaching measures presented earlier in this chapter are particularly important for this patient.

Cervicitis

Inflammation of the cervix, **cervicitis**, is caused by several organisms, notably *Staphylococcus*, *Streptococcus*, or *Gonococcus*. It occurs quite often during childbirth because of trauma and sometimes tearing of the cervix. It also can be related to frequent douching, sexually transmitted disease, or a forgotten tampon. Cervicitis also may result from continued use of contraceptive foam or jelly. The main symptoms are leukorrhea and bleeding. Pain on sexual intercourse also may be a symptom.

Unless cervicitis is treated promptly, it may be difficult to cure. Periodic vaginal examinations help in diagnosis. The major treatment is the administration of antibiotics. Sometimes the cervix must be cauterized. After cauterization, a watery discharge appears, which may become foul smelling. It takes about 6 to 8 weeks for the area to heal after cauterization. Some of the precautions taken to prevent vaginal infection also help to prevent cervical infections.

Endometriosis

Normally endometrial tissue is confined to the inside of the uterus. In **endometriosis**, tissue resembling endometrial tissue appears in various places in the pelvic cavity: on the ovaries, ovarian tubes, bladder, intestine, rectum, or pelvic wall.

The patient has pelvic pain, abnormal uterine or rectal bleeding, symptoms of pressure in the pelvis, and dymenorrhea. She also may be sterile and may have pain on sexual intercourse (dyspareunia). The cause of endometriosis is unknown, but it usually affects women between the ages of 25 and 45. There is an especially high incidence in women who have never experienced childbirth.

Treatment is directed toward relief of symptoms. Physicians often recommend pregnancy for two reasons. First, endometriosis eventually may result in sterility and inability to get pregnant; second, because endometriosis is influenced by hormonal changes, the symptoms often improve after pregnancy.

If pregnancy is not desirable, medications may be used to shrink the endometrial tissue, thereby decreasing the symptoms. (The accompanying box outlines some of these medications.) Sometimes, the endometriosis recurs when the medication is stopped. Extensive and chronic endometriosis may require drastic surgical treatment, such as hysterectomy, salpingectomy, and oophorectomy. A woman experiencing this condition will require a great deal of emotional support.

Pelvic Inflammatory Disease

PID, an infection of the ovaries (*oophoritis*), ovarian tubes (*salpingitis*), uterus, or pelvic cavity, enters the body through the vagina, peritoneum, lymphatic system, or bloodstream. *Gonococcus* is often the cause of pelvic infection, although PID also may be caused by *Streptococcus*, chlamydial infections (approximately half of all PIDs), and other disease processes. The microorganisms most often pass up through the vagina and uterus and are more common in women who have had an abortion or those with an IUD in place.

A foul-smelling vaginal discharge is a common symptom of PID. The patient also complains of backache, pelvic pain, fever, chills, malaise, nausea, and vomiting.

Treatment. Antibiotics are usually effective in destroying the causative bacteria, unless the PID is caused by herpesvirus II, which is not affected by antibiotics. The antibiotics used to treat PID are often administered intravenously. The sexual partner is also examined, because

---

Key Medications
for Endometriosis

- ◆ Hormones:
- ◆ Combination (estrogen-progestin) oral contraceptives
- ◆ Progestins
- ◆ Synthetic estrogen, danazol (Danocrine, Cyclomen)
- ◆ Gonadotropin-releasing hormone agonists (cause lowered estrogen levels):
- ◆ Leuprolide (Lupron)
- ◆ Nafarelin acetate (Synarel)
- ◆ Medications used to treat endometriosis can cause any or all of the following side effects: abdominal swelling, breast tenderness, breakthrough bleeding, atrophic vaginitis, weight gain, edema, hot flashes, emotional lability

---

he too may be infected and need treatment. Sexual intercourse is discouraged as long as the woman has any trace of infection. If PID is not treated, it may become chronic and cause sterility in the woman, due to the formation of scar tissue that blocks the ovarian tubes.

Nursing Alert

A woman who has had PID is more likely to have an ectopic pregnancy than a woman with normal health.

Nursing Considerations. The patient with PID in the hospital is usually placed in Fowler's position. (*Rationale: This helps encourage pelvic drainage.*) Sitz baths may be ordered. (*Rationale: This helps relieve the pain.*)

Precautions must be taken to dispose of soiled pads and dressings as contaminated material. Always wear gloves when caring for this patient, and follow the other procedures in Universal Precautions. The patient should have perineal care after removing the pad and after using the bedpan. Sometimes an abscess forms, and the surgeon institutes drainage through an incision in the abdomen.

During the active disease process, douches and sexual intercourse should be avoided. Patient teaching and the cooperation of the sexual partner are vital in the treatment of PID.

Vulvodynia[4]

Although not actually an infection, vulvodynia can cause great discomfort. Only recently has treatment been known for this disorder.

---

[4] Solomons CC, Melmed MH, Heitler SM. Calcium Citrate for Vulvar Vestibulitis (Vulvodynia): A Case Report. Journal of Reproductive Medicine 36(12):879–882, 1991.

Vulvodynia causes extreme and disabling pain in the vulvar area. Most women with vulvodynia are between ages 20 and 40, and most are white. This disorder has not been seen in African American women.

The pain is believed to be caused by excess calcium oxylate crystals in the urine. Calcium citrate is given orally to block formation of oxylate. Calcium citrate also prevents formation of calcium oxalate kidney stones. In addition, some patients are helped by following a low-oxylate diet, which eliminates spinach, green beans, celery, sweet potatoes, tomato sauce, peanuts, chocolate, tea, and coffee. The patient's treatment must be managed by a physician.

Sexually Transmitted Diseases

Many sexually transmitted diseases cause inflammation or other disorders of the female reproductive tract. These are discussed in Chapter 63.

Trauma

Many women are victims of trauma, including battering by others, automobile accidents, and falls. Many times, this trauma involves the reproductive organs.

Most rapes occur in women and may cause physical disorders, including vaginal, cervical, or anal bruising or tearing; tampon impaction, or sexually transmitted disease. Rape is discussed briefly in Chapter 63. Childhood sexual abuse is discussed in Chapter 65. Psychiatric sequelae are discussed in Chapter 87.

Other trauma can cause various types of injury to the reproductive organs. These are diagnosed and treated symptomatically, depending on the nature of the injury.

Neoplasms of the Lower Reproductive Tract

Tumors of the Ovary

Benign Ovarian Tumors

Also known as *cysts*, these benign growths may form from fluid retained in the ovary or from other causes. Although they usually do not cause any trouble, cysts may enlarge and press on other abdominal organs and cause pain if they rupture or twist.

Cancer of the Ovary

Women who have a personal or family history of cancer have a higher than average chance of developing ovarian cancer. Cancers that seem the most predictive of ovarian cancer are breast, uterus, colon, and ovary. If a woman has had a tubal ligation, this seems to decrease the incidence of ovarian cancer (to one-third the risk of other women). Some researchers believe this is because carcinogens travel up the uterine tubes to the ovaries.

Diagnosis can be made by vaginal ultrasound and the Ca 125 blood test. Cancer of the ovary often displays no early symptoms and usually is detected only after metastasis of the cancer has occurred. This is a fairly frequent cause of death in young women because it is often not discovered in time to provide a long-term cure.

Cancer of the ovary is treated surgically. The procedure will involve a total abdominal hysterectomy and removal of both tubes and both ovaries. Hormones are not given, because they seem to nourish this particular type of cancer cell. Radiation therapy or chemotherapy is usually prescribed after the surgery.

Tumors of the Uterus

Benign Uterine Tumors

The *fibroid tumor* is the most common tumor of the uterus. These tumors are of all sizes; they usually grow slowly and arise from muscle cells. They are believed to develop as a result of hormonal influences. The first symptom to appear is abnormal vaginal bleeding, associated with a feeling of heaviness and pressure in the pelvic region. The fibroid tumor, or *myoma*, may become so large that it presses on the urethra or bowel, causing retention of urine or constipation.

Treatment. Treatment for fibroids depends somewhat on the patient's age. Often it is possible to remove a nonmalignant tumor from the uterus without removing the uterus itself. This is important for a woman during childbearing years, especially if she plans to have children. Other treatments include medroxyprogesterone (Depo-Provera) injections or oral contraceptives to suppress the uterine lining, thus shrinking the tumors. Leuprolide (Lupron) injection therapy is showing promise in shrinking fibroids as well.

Key Concept

Most nonmalignant tumors shrink after menopause; hence, postmenopausal bleeding is seldom caused by a myoma.

Cancer of the Endometrium

The fundus, the body of uterus, is not attacked as frequently by cancer as the cervix; however, malignant growths do occur in the endometrium and fundus. Cancer of the fundus and the endometrium are most likely to occur in women older than 50 years or after meno-

Factors Placing Women at Risk for Developing Cervical Cancer

♦ Presence of human papillomavirus infection (HPV)
♦ Sexual activity at a young age
♦ Frequent sexual activity
♦ Multiple sexual partners
♦ Presence of genital warts (condyloma)
♦ Presence of genital herpesvirus II
♦ Maternal history of cancer, especially cervical cancer
♦ Mother took diethylstilbestrol (DES) during pregnancy with this daughter (particularly if mother had toxicity to DES)

pause. There also is an increased risk in women who have previously taken estrogens. Therefore, hormone therapy is prescribed with caution.

Vaginal bleeding is the first symptom of uterine cancer; this may begin as a watery, blood-tinged discharge. If it occurs before menopause, it may be mistaken for menstrual irregularity. A diagnostic curettage to obtain scrapings from the uterus is performed if the Pap test suggests cancer. If the test results of the scrapings are positive, a hysterectomy is performed, followed by radium implantation, x-ray therapy, or both to the pelvic cavity. This patient also may have postoperative chemotherapy but usually not with hormones.

Cancers of the Cervix

Cancer of the cervix is a common cause of cancer in women. (Only breast cancer is more common among reproductive cancers in women.) Cervical cancer occurs most commonly between ages 40 and 55. The accompanying box lists factors that place women at a higher risk of developing cervical cancer.

In the past, it was believed that there was a connection between cervical cancer and uncircumcised sexual partners, but this has not been proven. In addition, some researchers believe that there is a causative relationship between long-term use of female hormones, including many oral contraceptives, and development of cervical cancer. This also is unproven. Women at risk should be followed carefully by a gynecologist and should have frequent Pap tests.

Signs and Symptoms. Bleeding is the first sign of cervical cancer, but it does not occur in the early stages when a positive Pap test would indicate the presence of cancer cells. The bleeding usually appears first as spotting between periods or following intercourse. The condition also can occur after menopause.

Staging of Cervical Cancer. Cervical cancer has been staged similar to many other types of cancer to stan-

dardize treatment. The accompanying box describes some of the stages.

Treatment. Early cervical cancer (in situ and some types of stage I) is susceptible to radiation therapy (usually radon implantation). In addition, early cervical cancer is more easily localized and therefore more easily excised. In these early states, conization by "cold knife" (cryosurgery) or laser conization is frequently used. If conization is used, Pap tests should be done every 3 months for the first year and every 6 months after that. These are outpatient procedures in selected cases. Hysterectomy also may be done for early cervical cancer if the woman does not wish to remain able to reproduce.

In the early and middle stages, conization or hysterectomy may be done. In the middle stages, hyster-

Staging of Cervical Carcinoma (Overview)

♦ *Stage 0.* Carcinoma in situ (in place). The cancer is limited to the epithelial layer and shows no signs of invasion of deeper tissue or of surrounding areas. This may be treated by biopsy or conization alone. (A biopsy may remove all of the cancer tissue.) Laser treatment also is used. Ninety-five percent of these patients survive for more than 5 years.
♦ *Stage I.* The cancer is confined to the cervix and is usually treated by conization or hysterectomy. These may be combined with radiation or chemotherapy.
♦ *Stage II.* Carcinoma extends beyond the cervix but not into the pelvic wall, or it involves the vagina but not the lower one-third. (Stage IIA carcinoma shows no obvious parametrial involvement; stage IIB shows obvious parametrial involvement.) These cancers are usually treated with hysterectomy, combined with radiation or chemotherapy.
♦ *Stage III.* Carcinoma extends to the pelvic wall, involves the lower one-third of the vagina; Stage III also includes all cases with hydronephrosis and nonfunctioning kidney. (Stage IIIA shows extension onto the pelvic wall; stage IIIB shows extension onto the pelvic wall and hydronephrosis or nonfunctioning kidney or both.) These cancers are often treated with total hysterectomy, salpingectomy, oophorectomy (panhysterosalpingo-oophorectomy), and other abdominal surgery as needed. The surgery would be combined with radiation or chemotherapy.
♦ *Stage IV.* The cancer is widely spread throughout the pelvic region or throughout the body. This stage is generally inoperable, except for palliation. It is generally treated with radiation.

International Federation of Gynecology and Obstetrics, 1987.

ectomy is the treatment of choice. Many of these surgical procedures are combined with radiation or chemotherapy, particularly in stages other than cancer in situ.

Cervical Cancer in the Pregnant Woman. If a woman is pregnant and cervical cancer in situ is discovered, treatment is delayed until after delivery, which may be allowed to occur vaginally. If invasive cancer is discovered early in the pregnancy, the pregnancy is terminated, and the cancer is treated as in the nonpregnant woman. If invasive cancer is discovered late in pregnancy (third trimester), treatment is delayed until the fetus is viable, and cesarean delivery is done.

> **Nursing Alert**
>
> One cannot emphasize too strongly the importance of the Pap test for women past puberty, particularly if they are sexually active. Cancer of the cervix is almost 100% curable if it is discovered early and treated before it spreads.

Pelvic Exenteration

In some cases of advanced malignancy, especially if the patient is young, the entire contents of the pelvis are removed. This is a complex procedure with a high mortality rate. The patient will have urine and feces draining through openings on the abdominal wall postoperatively.

Keys for Review

Key Questions for Critical Thinking

1. Suggest how you would approach and reassure an adolescent who is having her first gynecologic examination. Discuss, in addition to your approach, specific actions you would take.
2. Formulate teaching plans for feminine hygiene to a clinic patient who is having a routine gynecologic examination and to a woman for whom you are providing perineal care following birth. Discuss how your approaches would differ and why.
3. While teaching a woman to do breast self-examination, you also want to emphasize the importance of doing these examinations regularly. Determine important points the woman should know. State how the teaching would differ between a 28-year-old woman and a 60-year-old woman.
4. Your patient has frequent vaginal infections. State important points to be used in teaching prevention.

Key Readings

Berkow R. (Ed). The Mercke Manual of Diagnosis and Therapy, Ed 16. Rathway, NJ, Mercke & Co., 1992

Earnest VV. Clinical Skills in Nursing Practice, Ed 2. Philadelphia, J.B. Lippincott, 1992

Everson L. "An Update on Breast Imaging." Colleagues. Minneapolis, University of Minnesota Hospital Medical Bulletin, #5, 1992

North American Nursing Diagnosis Association. Nursing Diagnoses: Definitions and Classifications 1992. Philadelphia, North American Nursing Diagnosis Association, 1992

Key Readings (continued)

Nursing '94 Drug Handbook. Springhouse, PA, Springhouse, 1994

O'Toole M (Ed). Miller-Keane Encyclopedia and Dictionary of Medicine, Nursing, and Allied Health, Ed 5. Philadelphia, W.B. Saunders, 1992

Reeder SJ, Martin LL, Koniak D. Maternity Nursing: Family, Newborn, and Women's Health, Ed 17. Philadelphia, J.B. Lippincott, 1992

Taylor C, Lillis C, LeMone P. Fundamentals of Nursing: The Art and Science of Nursing Care, Ed 2. Philadelphia, J.B. Lippincott, 1993

Enrichment Keys

Dumas L. "Women's health." Symposium in The Nursing Clinics of North America 27(4):821–969, December 1992

American Cancer Society. "How to examine your breasts." September 1992

Reingold AL. "Toxic shock syndrome: An update." American Journal of Obstetrics and Gynecology 165(4), Part 2:1236–1239, October 1991.

Wolenski, Marianne and Pelosi, Marco A. "Laparoscopic Hysterectomy." Today's OR Nurse, November 1991. 23-29.

Keys to Learning More

Chapter 85: geriatric nursing
Unit Seventeen: death and dying

Unit *15* Assisting the Older Person

85 Geriatrics: The Aging Adult

Keys for Learning

Learning Objectives

- Review and recall from Chapter 13 the changes involved in aging.
- Review and recall from Unit Four the anatomic and physiologic changes occurring in the person as he or she ages.
- State at least five care settings for the older adult. State at least two advantages and disadvantages of each.
- Describe the characteristics of a good nursing home.
- Describe nursing measures to assist an older person to meet nutritional needs, meet the need for elimination, and maintain personal hygiene.
- State nursing measures to assist an older person to compensate for impaired proprioception.
- State nursing measures to assist an older person to meet communication needs.
- Discuss the importance of relationships and stimulation.
- Describe the special aspects of depression and chemical dependency as they affect the older person.
- Discuss elder abuse and the vulnerable adult.

Key Terms

aphasia

edentulous

elder abuse

friable

geriatrics

gerontology

halitosis

kyphosis

osteoporosis

presbycusis

presbyopia

proprioception

respite

Sjögren's syndrome

vulnerable adult

Keys to Understanding This Chapter

Chapter 3: services available to the older adult through healthcare delivery services

Chapter 4: legal aspects and patient rights; the vulnerable adult

Chapter 5: basic human needs of all people

Keys to Understanding This Chapter
(continued)

Chapter 6: health habits that apply to all people

Chapter 7: community health and its services

Chapter 13: lifestyle changes and developmental tasks specific to aging

Unit Four: anatomy and physiology of systems, including physical changes occurring in normal aging

Unit Five: diet therapy

Unit Six: importance of safety to the aging

Unit Nine: basic patient care skills

Unit Eleven: administration of medications

Unit Fourteen: disorders of the adult

Key Points

- Normal aging does not cause specific illness. However, lifestyle adjustments are needed to compensate for physical changes.
- Most seniors live at home. A small minority live in special adapted living situations.
- Approximately one-third to one-half of all health problems in the elderly relate directly or indirectly to nutrition. Water is a substance that frequently must be encouraged and supplemented.
- Adjustments to basic personal hygiene measures may be needed for the senior. Skin care, nail and foot care, and adapted clothing are concerns.
- Appropriate care for constipation includes adequate fiber and fluids; laxative use should be avoided.
- Anatomic changes may lead to problems with voiding or bowel and bladder incontinence.
- Communication may be hindered due to presbyopia, presbycusis, or aphasia.
- Safety is a concern, due to loss of the sense of proprioception.
- The elderly must remain physically and mentally active to prevent anxiety, depression, and disorders due to immobility.

Rosdahl CB: Textbook of Basic Nursing, 6th ed. © 1995 J.B. Lippincott Company

Key Learning Activities

♦ Visit a long-term care facility for adults. What is the age range? What activities are available? What type of staff work there? What is the cost?

♦ Interview three people older than 75 who live in their own homes. What do they do for recreation? What community resources do they use? What work or volunteering do they do?

♦ Obtain an Elderhostel brochure. What courses are available? Where are they located? What is the cost?

♦ Volunteer as a driver or accompany a driver for "Meals on Wheels." Why does a person do this task? What did you learn?

Previous chapters describe many normal emotional and physical changes of aging. These changes occur to some extent in every person as they age. This chapter discusses needs of the aging adult as a result of *normal aging*. The next chapter discusses assistance of the person with the additional challenge of confusion or dementia. These are *abnormal* disorders that develop in some aging people.

Gerontology is the study of the effects of normal aging and age-related diseases on the human. **Geriatrics** is the branch of medicine concerned with problems and illnesses of aging and their treatment. Care of the older person is called *geriatric nursing*.

Normal aging does not cause specific illnesses. The majority of elderly are active, healthy adults. While chronic illnesses are more common in seniors, acute illnesses are less common. It is important to be aware of the differences between normal aging and its effects on the individual and the pathologies associated with disease. Normal aging changes are given in tables at the end of every Chapter from 15 through 25. Many problems commonly associated with aging are disease processes resulting from combinations of heart disease, poor dietary habits, and lack of exercise.

Changes related to normal aging processes are as follows:

♦ Decreased functioning of organs
♦ Change in visual and auditory acuity
♦ Decreased reaction time
♦ Unsteady gait, decreased sense of balance
♦ Decreased tactile sensations
♦ Stiff joints
♦ Increased emotional and physical losses
♦ Decreased capacity for recovery from injury or illness

The nurse who is aware of processes of normal aging is better able to assist seniors to meet basic needs resulting from these changes. Normally, seniors retain the ability to learn, adapt, and change.

Care Settings for Older Adults

When developing a plan of care, it is important to observe and assess the person's current lifestyle. Remember that a very high percentage of seniors live in their own homes. However, some need assistance or special care. Care settings for seniors are highly variable; each has advantages and disadvantages. Cultural differences and finances often dictate choices available to the individual person. The person's ability for self-care and potential for rehabilitation also are issues that require assessment. Some of the care settings for the elderly are home care, adult day care centers, retirement communities, board-and-care facilities, acute hospitals, long-term facilities, and hospice care.

Factors determining the choice of residence for an aging adult include any of the following:

♦ Ability to provide for physical, financial, and emotional self-care needs
♦ Physical, financial, and emotional support from family and friends
♦ Access to healthcare and rehabilitation services, including availability and transportation
♦ Need for safety and legal assistance

Home Care

The majority of seniors live in their own homes and independently care for their own needs. The current trend in healthcare is to provide needed care for these people in their homes. To some degree, such things as financial aid, Medicaid, food stamps, and rental and fuel assistance help the aging stay in their homes longer.

Home health agencies have a substantial variety of services available 24-hours a day. Complicated physical needs may be provided in the home. Other services, such as home health aide or homemaker or occupational, physical, speech, or respiratory therapy also are available (Fig. 85-1). Homebound meals and transportation are also available.

Circumstances may require the older adult to move into the home of one of their children. In this situation, roles are reversed. The child is now the caregiver, and the parent is the care receiver.

Senior Day Care

Senior day-care centers provide social and self-care activities for seniors, while providing relief (**respite**) for adult children.

Retirement Complexes

Many independent living complexes have been designed and built exclusively for elderly people. These are not nursing homes; generally, they do not provide

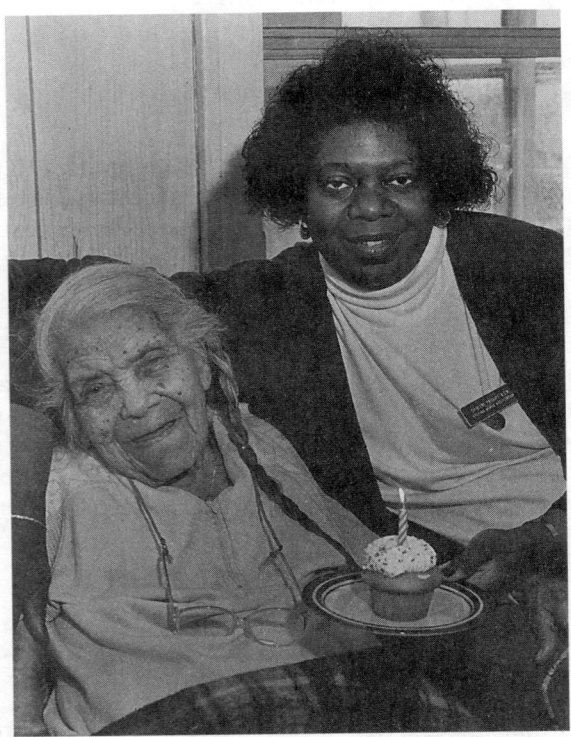

Figure 85-1. This home care nurse helps the elderly woman celebrate her birthday. Everyone needs to feel that someone cares. Photo courtesy of MCOSS Inc., Red Bank, NJ.

nursing services. Meals may be available in a common dining room, although a small kitchen is available in the senior's living quarters as well. Laundry services are often available. Generally, the rent is lower than in board-and-care or extended-care facilities. Some have "sliding scale" rent. The older person has the advantage of living in close proximity to other people of his or her age group, while having access to assistance when needed.

Long-Term Facilities

Long-term care facilities have developed into specialized areas for care of elderly and chronically ill younger people. Choice of facility depends on availability of services, finances, and client needs. The facility should provide the best possible nursing care, in as homelike an atmosphere as possible (see accompanying box). Long-term facilities offer three general levels of care:

◆ *Board-and-care facility*—room and board, laundry, and some personal nursing services. Standards and regulations vary.
◆ *Rehabilitative care facility*—often a unit within another facility. A client may go here from an acute-care facility and receive physical, occupational, or speech therapy. Twenty-four-hour care is provided for a few weeks or months, but the client plans to return home after recovery from a disabling (eg, cerebrovascular accident) or traumatic (eg, hip fracture) experience.
◆ *Extended-care facility* (ECF) or *skilled nursing facility* (SNF)—often referred to as a "nursing home". This type of facility offers care from nurses and other healthcare workers under the direction of a physician. In recent years, extensive regulations have been instituted; care given in these facilities has improved greatly. The bedside nurse is extensively used in these facilities. Special knowledge of aging is essential to provide adequate patient care.
◆ *Intermediate care facilities* (ICF) provide less care than the skilled nursing facility.

Helping The Older Person Meet Basic Needs

The older person may need assistance from nurses or other healthcare workers to meet basic needs because of limitations due to changes of aging. Each client requires the nurse to be aware of specific variations in needs and of the surroundings in which care is given. For example, 24-hour care available in a skilled facility has resources and limitations that differ from those when caring for seniors in their own homes.

Characteristics of a Good Skilled Care Nursing Home

♦ Is licensed by state or local government and regularly inspected
♦ Meets Medicare or Medicaid requirements
♦ Has a physician who makes regular visits
♦ Has a staff of licensed nurses available 24 hours a day, 7 days a week
♦ Provides other healthcare and therapeutic care
♦ Provides special services for residents, such as a beautician or barber
♦ Provides rehabilitation services by trained personnel and encourages all residents to work toward rehabilitation
♦ Has an inservice program for all staff members
♦ Conducts routine staff member evaluations
♦ Maintains high standards of safety for residents
♦ Provides nutritionally adequate food and special diets if needed

♦ Provides for social needs of the residents in a home-like atmosphere
♦ Has a well-planned and purposeful activities program
♦ Provides a recreational program
♦ Maintains a medical record, Kardex, and nursing care plan for each resident
♦ Makes provisions for obtaining necessary diagnostic laboratory and radiology services for the residents
♦ Encourages family and friends to visit often
♦ Encourages visits by young children (and many times by pets)
♦ Recognizes and provides for spiritual needs of residents
♦ (Many of these characteristics apply to less skilled levels of geriatric facilities as well.)

Nutritional Needs

Satisfactory nutritional status must be maintained to prevent body systems from premature deterioration. It is estimated that one-third to one-half of all health problems of seniors are directly or indirectly related to nutrition and inadequate fluid intake. Basic nutritional needs of all people are discussed in Chapter 26. The nurse considers nutritional adaptations of each person when planning care. Good nutrition results in increased energy and a healthy mental outlook. In addition, medical or surgical conditions heal faster with fewer complications when nutrient needs are met.

Proper nutrients must be available to build the thousands of compounds needed to maintain the body. Nutrients consumed also must be absorbed, stored, reorganized, or otherwise converted into useful substances. This requires a healthy gastrointestinal system, pancreas, and liver. It also presumes that a malabsorption disorder does not exist.

Geriatric Considerations

Special factors are involved in nutrition in the aging. Nutrients are absorbed more slowly; caloric needs are reduced. Fewer calories should be consumed, while retaining specific nutrient requirements.

Nutrient requirements in healthy seniors vary only slightly from younger people. *Protein* requirements are unchanged. A minimum of 1 g protein for each kilogram of body weight is necessary for maintenance. However, building and repairing tissues after injury (eg, pressure ulcers) or illness (eg, cancer) greatly increase daily protein requirements. *Fat* intake should be no more than approximately 35% of total caloric intake.

Fats with essential fatty acids are more nutrient-dense than empty calorie fats, such as fried foods, alcohol, or candy. *Vitamins and minerals* are important; most can and should be obtained through a healthy diet, rather than supplements.

Nutrition also is affected by factors such as inconvenience and effort of food shopping, storage, and preparation. The older person often is not hungry, because taste perception is reduced and he or she is not physically active. Poorly fitting dentures often limit a patient's ability to eat. Perhaps, the patient feels rushed during meals or does not like to eat at the times meals are served (see Chapter 27 for suggestions).

Weight control is harder as we age. The body's overall metabolic rate is reduced; fat is harder to eliminate than in younger years. Excess weight can become a serious problem, both from a self-esteem or esthetic point of view and also as related to health. Disorders such as diabetes mellitus, hypertension, myocardial infarction, stroke, back and joint pains, and falling are influenced by obesity. To help control weight, a low-fat, low-calorie, nutrient-dense diet may be recommended. Increasing metabolic rate by regular exercises greatly helps to control weight.

Assessment of Nutritional Status

Assessing nutritional status includes not only observing the person's food or fluid intake, but also understanding availability of food and amounts of specific nutrients needed and consumed. The nurse should encourage patients to eat. However, rather than forcing a patient to eat, try to determine *why* the individual does not want to eat. Perhaps the person has food preferences or has difficulty chewing or swallowing.

Special Considerations

Teeth and Chewing. Tooth loss is not a normal event of aging, but many older people wear dentures or have few or no teeth. They must adapt food so they can chew and eat it. Oral care and denture care by the nurse can facilitate the eating success of **edentulous** (without teeth) patients. Food that is adapted (chopped, pureed, liquid) must be nutritionally balanced and attractively served (see Chapter 28).

Swallowing Difficulties. The older person may have an impaired swallowing mechanism. Make certain food provided is in a consistency the patient can swallow. Semisolid food may be better tolerated than liquids. Elevate the head of the bed, or if possible, have the patient up in a chair for meals. Food should be cut into edible bites so that it can be easily chewed. This also helps prevent choking. It may be advisable to have a suction apparatus available at meals. Special techniques can be used with the patient who has great difficulty swallowing or who refuses to eat. Small, frequent feedings are usually better tolerated than larger, less frequent meals.

Medications and Supplements. Older people may be assisted to take medications by crushing tablets or by putting medicine into custard, cereal, applesauce, or ice cream to aid in swallowing the pills or pill fragments. The nurse must be aware of drug–food interactions, contraindications of mixing drugs and foods, and side effects seen when mixing drugs with certain foods. (Enteric-coated tablets should not be crushed because they are not meant to be digested in the stomach.)

It is illegal to "trick" the person into taking drugs by hiding them in food. Every person has the right to refuse medications unless there is a specific court order.

Supplementation with vitamins and minerals is an area of continuing research. Vitamin deficiencies can greatly affect nutritional status in older adults. However, excessive quantities of vitamins and minerals can be harmful and expensive. Calcium supplementation is often combined with exercise and estrogen as part of postmenopausal therapy in women. Self-administration of supplements is common in seniors. More research is needed to determine benefits (or dangers) of vitamin and mineral supplements. Table 85-1 describes implications of geriatric drug administration as related to body changes. Teaching is an important nursing consideration in the use of medications and supplements.

Water. Water is one substance that frequently must be encouraged in the older adult. Many seniors do not experience thirst as strongly as younger people. Immobile adults often do not drink adequate fluids. *Dehydration* is a serious and frequently overlooked problem in the elderly. A variety of fluids should be offered.

Table 85-1. Changes in Aging as Related to Medication Administration

Factor	*Nursing Implications*
Decreased sense of thirst, dry oral mucosa	Difficulty swallowing meds; decreased absorption
Decreased total body fluid volume or percentage	Higher concentration of water-soluble drugs in blood
Decreased muscle tissue	Slower or decreased absorption of IM medications, shorter needle may be needed
Increased percentage of fatty tissue	Accumulation of fat-soluble drugs; more difficulty locating site for IM injection
Decreased general circulation	Slowed absorption; slowed transport of drugs to cells; slowed removal of drugs or wastes from cells
Decreased circulation to colon, vagina	Slower melting of suppositories
Decreased blood flow to liver and kidneys; decreased liver enzymes	Slowed metabolism and absorption; slowed excretion
Fewer functioning (kidney) nephrons; decreased tubular reabsorption	Slowed or faulty excretion; retention of drugs in body for longer time
Decreased stomach acids and other digestive fluids; lower stomach pH	Slowed absorption
Confusion, forgetfulness	Noncompliance with medication program

Supplementing Oral Intake

In many cases, the older person, particularly one who is ill, cannot eat and drink enough to maintain adequate nutritional status. In this event, an alternate means of supplying nutrients is needed to supplement or replace oral intake. The first choice involves oral supplements, such as Ensure or Resource. If this is not possible, other means must be used. Three major types of mechanical nutrient supplementation are commonly used: intravenous therapy, total parenteral nutrition (TPN), and tube feedings. These are discussed in Chapters 28 and 57.

Personal Hygiene Needs

Skin Care. Changes in the skin and circulatory system may cause the older patient to be more susceptible to skin breakdown or pressure areas than the younger person. Because aging skin has fewer oils, daily bathing is not always necessary. However, daily hygiene measures remain important. Bed baths or a sponge bath at the sink can be alternative hygiene measures. To promote circulation and a sense of independence, seniors should be encouraged to do as much of their own hygiene as possible. Care can progress through the stages of dependent bed bath, sitting in a chair at the sink, assisted shower or bath, and finally self-care. This is a therapeutic method to increase activity and promote self-esteem.

If a patient is incontinent, the skin must be kept clean and dry to prevent skin irritation and breakdown. An older person's skin can become very dry, thin, and **friable** (easily broken). Lotion may be applied to keep skin soft and promote peripheral circulation. Special bath oils are available to keep skin supple; soap is often avoided. Accessory devices may be provided for the inactive patient. These can minimize dermal irritation and pressure and prevent skin breakdown.

> **Key Concepts**
>
> When bath oil is used, the tub may become slippery. Be careful to prevent falls.

Oral Hygiene. The patient must be encouraged to care for the mouth to prevent dental difficulties and **halitosis** (bad breath). Due to arthritis, cerebrovascular accidents, or other difficulties, the nurse frequently must provide assistance. The client may be embarrassed or unable to ask for assistance; therefore, the nurse must actively provide the opportunity for oral hygiene. It also is important to make sure the confused person does not lose his or her dentures.

> **Nursing Alert**
>
> The nurse should encourage older people with dentures to check the condition of their gums regularly. Irritation can result from poorly fitting dentures. Cancer of the mouth sometimes occurs and may go undetected.

Hair Care. Shampoos should be given as needed to promote comfort and cleanliness. Because the older person's hair is often dry and brittle, shampoos should not be given too often. However, a fresh hairdo or haircut may give the patient a more positive self-image and improve self-esteem.

> **Key Concept**
>
> Self-care of the hair is an excellent opportunity for active range-of-motion exercise.

Nail and Foot Care. The fingernails of older adults grow more slowly and are more brittle than in younger years.

Toenails often become hard and thick. Often a podiatrist must trim and care for them. Nails should be cut straight across; corns and calluses can be soaked in warm water but never cut. The nurse also must encourage wearing of proper-fitting flat or low-heeled shoes and panty hose that is not too tight. Feet should be washed, thoroughly dried, and inspected daily. Injuries and discolored areas should be documented and reported to the physician. Even in healthy seniors, infection is possible, and wound healing is often slow in the extremities.

> **Nursing Alert**
>
> Most healthcare facilities do not allow nurses to cut toenails or fingernails of diabetic patients.

Shaving. It is important to maintain self-concept in the older man by encouraging him to shave regularly. Allow the patient to do as much for himself as possible. Be sure he is safe and responsible. Assist when needed, remembering an older man's skin may be more sensitive than that of a younger man. Be careful to prevent cuts. Specific techniques for assisting a male to shave are discussed in Chapter 45. Postmenopausal women may occasionally have facial hair (hirsutism) that needs to be shaved.

Clothing. Choice of clothing depends on physical limitations of the senior and on the environment. Aging adults often need more clothing to maintain internal warmth; layering of clothing is common. The nursing home resident should be allowed to wear his or her own clothes. Patients should be encouraged to dress in street clothes each day. Their efforts to appear clean and well groomed should be complimented. Sometimes a new shirt or dress can greatly enhance the client's morale. Women should be encouraged to apply cosmetics, if this has been part of their daily routine.

Elimination Needs

Difficulties with elimination have many causes. Peristalsis slows. Many people exercise less and avoid proper nutrition. Eating foods such as whole grains, fruits and vegetables provides needed fiber, complex carbohydrates, vitamins, and minerals. Generally, the elderly do not take in enough fluids. Fluid intake may be deliberately reduced as problems with voiding and defecation develop. Foods that once were tolerated now may be irritating.

Constipation. Older people are frequently preoccupied with bowel function. Excessive use of laxatives or enemas should be discouraged, because the normal urge to defecate can be disturbed or even eliminated.

Encourage the elderly to answer the urge to defecate as soon as possible. Changes in fluid and food intake can often eliminate constipation. Prune juice, bran flakes, oatmeal, or applesauce are good alternatives to laxatives. However, sometimes a laxative or mild stool softener (such as docusate sodium—Colace) may be required. Three or more days without a stool may indicate constipation, impaction, or infarction of the bowel. Nursing care in acute and long-term facilities requires daily monitoring of gastrointestinal function. A daily bowel movement is *not* necessary.

Bladder or Bowel Incontinence. The older person may have difficulty controlling bladder and bowel functions. To overcome this problem, he or she can be retrained by following a regular schedule. Such a bladder or bowel retraining program is eagerly accepted by most patients because it can alleviate embarrassment. Specific techniques for bowel and bladder retraining are discussed in Chapter 46.

Because catheters can be a means of introducing organisms into the urinary tract, they are not the treatment of choice for urinary incontinence. If the patient is incontinent, he or she should be cleaned as quickly as possible because this is obviously an embarrassing situation. He or she should never be chided or scolded for incontinence. Effective garments can be purchased today, so the incontinent or partially incontinent person can lead a normal life.

Difficulty in Voiding. Anatomic changes in the aging male and female may cause difficulties with normal voiding. Incontinence is not uncommon. Fecal impaction is a common cause of urinary retention. Accurate intake and output records may be required to monitor excretory status.

Many older people have difficulty voiding because the prostate gland enlarges and obstructs urinary flow. This problem can be painful and embarrassing. Surgery may be necessary in some cases.

Special Concerns of the Aging Adults

Aging adults have needs and concerns unique to their stage in the life cycle.

Communication

Because of physiologic changes in aging, the senses are not as acute as in younger people. Many older people have difficulty with communication. These may be due to poor communication techniques or lack of understanding on the part of the listener.

Age barriers may add to the difficulties of making oneself understood. Feelings of isolation and rejection can be avoided if the older person has someone with whom to talk on a regular basis. It is usually better to place the older patient in a double room; this helps prevent isolation and provides more environmental stimulation. The senior should be encouraged to participate in social events.

Communication is a two-way process. Therapeutic and social communication have different approaches. Be aware of the meanings of touch and body language. Several suggestions that can be used for communication between the older person and the nurse are given in Chapter 36. It is important to show respect; sit down so you do not appear rushed. Make appropriate eye contact and show genuine interest when visiting with the older person, as with any person. Encourage visits from family, friends, and family pets.

Communication and Visual Impairment. Although many older people have difficulty seeing because of cataracts or other eye disorders, they should be encouraged to participate in things they are able to do. Aids for the visually impaired, such as large numbers on the telephone and calendar or magnifying glasses for reading should be provided. Removing obstacles that could cause falls is essential. These patients must be protected from falling because they may not realize their vision is significantly impaired. They can be taught what hazards exist and how to avoid them.

Presbyopia is the specific name for impaired vision that results from normal aging. Presbyopia is caused by a loss of elasticity in the lens of the eye, which makes it difficult to focus light rays on the retina (see Chapter 73). As the person ages, the lens becomes more inflexible and therefore does not become convex enough to focus on nearby objects. The first symptom often is an inability to read the telephone book. This condition can usually be corrected by eyeglasses. Bifocals will probably be needed to allow for far and near vision.

The older person will find that more light is required for reading because the pupils of the eyes cannot adapt as well. As a rule, illumination (footcandle level) must double for each added 13 years of age beyond 40. Night blindness also increases with age. A night light in the patient's room helps prevent injury.

Sjögren's syndrome is a condition that is also common in older people. It causes a drying of the mucous membranes, including the eyes. Eye drops, such as artificial tears (Hypotears, Isopto Alkaline, Liquifilm Forte, Refresh) are often prescribed.

> **Key Concept**
>
> Glasses should be cleaned daily with a soft, dry cloth. Avoid using paper products to clean, because they may scratch the lenses.

Keys to Patient/Family Teaching
Safety Precautions for the Aging Adult

Patient and family teaching in safety measures for the older adult includes the following:

In the Home

- Movement should be cautious, especially on stairs and at curbs.
- Stand up slowly to avoid postural hypotension or dizziness.
- Safe-proof house. Cover cords that might cause falls. Place furniture where it will not be tripped over. Grab bars should be placed on tubs, showers, toilets, stairways.
- Ensure adequate lighting in all living areas. Night-lights must be used at night in bedroom, bathroom, and stairs.
- Use ambulatory devices (canes, walkers, wheel-chairs).
- Follow good housekeeping practices. Clean clutter and spills.
- Establish an emergency calling system with family and friends, neighbors, and local emergency medical services.
- Place a telephone near bed for night emergencies.
- Place a fire extinguisher in the kitchen, and know how to use it. Know how to use smoke detectors, and check batteries regularly. Do not smoke in bed.
- A list of medications should be carried with the person. Understand use of medications and side effects. Review use of medications periodically. Do not drive while taking medications.
- Wear suitable and safe clothing: Avoid flowing robes and nightgowns, flowing sleeves, floppy slippers, long shoelaces.
- Understand problems with loss in proprioception.
- Help with banking, especially of social security check. Ensure safety on the street when coming from the bank, going to the mail box, and so forth.
- Prevent scams. Caution the patient about financial "deals," especially from strangers. Bank can establish an "alert" if a great amount of money is withdrawn or if more than a certain amount is withdrawn.

In the Hospital

- Use call lights and ask for assistance, especially if getting out of bed at night to go to bathroom.
- Keep beds in low position.
- Use a transfer belt when assisting an unsteady person to walk (see Chapter 43).

Communication and Hearing Loss. A specific hearing disorder of aging (**presbycusis**) begins at approximately 40 years and progresses with age. The patient who has a hearing loss should be evaluated to determine if a mechanical hearing aid would compensate for the hearing loss. If so, the nurse should encourage the patient to wear the hearing aid, even if the patient is reluctant to do so. Special devices are available for telephones and televisions to enable the hearing-impaired person to hear better.

The patient should be questioned to make certain that messages are understood. If not understood, different words should be used, and distracting background noises eliminated. If hearing is totally lost, communication can be written or signed. Newspapers and magazines will help keep the hearing-impaired patient aware of current events (see Chapter 73).

Communication and Speech Impairment. Aphasia is the inability to use or understand speech. It is often a mixture of deficits, such as slow speech, incorrect speech, or use of incorrect words and sounds. Aphasia often accompanies a cerebrovascular accident. The patient may not be aware of the communication problem. He or she may not be able to understand speech or writing or may have trouble naming objects. The nurse should remember to converse with the patient, even if the patient is unable to speak. It is important to encourage the patient to communicate in other ways (gestures, picture boards, diagrams, writing). Speech therapy is often helpful. Patience is necessary when communicating with aphasic people. They are probably frustrated, and hurrying makes it even more difficult.

Key Concepts

Talk to the person, not about the person. Often, the person with aphasia has clear thinking processes.

Safety

Statistically, the elderly have fewer accidents than younger people. However, accidental injuries are more likely to be fatal. Accidents are a leading cause of disability and death after age 65. The greatest dangers are falls, fire, suffocation, and poisoning. The most common locations are the person's bedroom, bathroom, or kitchen. The majority of accidents are preventable, although violence against the **vulnerable** older population also is a concern. Fear for one's safety leads to increased psychological stress.

Older people may be unsteady on their feet or may misjudge physical capabilities. Medications or age-related changes can contribute to orthostatic (postural) hypotension. The patient may become dizzy and fall when getting out of a bed or chair. Visual acuity and depth perception changes disturb the person's ability to judge distance.

Educate the older adult and family about home hazards. Safety teaching is important. Some subjects to be taught are listed in the accompanying box. Be sure all people on the staff of the healthcare facility know about these safety measures. Staff members and families also need to be taught about the dangers of using restraints.

Loss of Proprioception. Proprioception is the awareness of posture, movement, and changes in equilibrium in relation to other objects. As we age, the sense of proprioception may be altered or lost. Many older people are not sure where they are stepping, especially if they are walking on dark floors, bare ground, or a dark paved area. The person has more difficulty staying erect without looking. The older person with a loss of proprioception may lose his or her balance when hyperextending the neck to look up at a clock or a high shelf. When balance is lost, it is hard to regain. The nurse can help by teaching the person about obstacles and uneven ground. When walking with an older person, allow him or her to take your arm; do not push or pull. Also, avoid quick turns, so the person does not lose balance.

> **Nursing Alert**
>
> Many older people are afraid of falling and may grab either the nurse or the furniture when lifted or moved. The person must never be rushed or frightened.

Safety Devices. Numerous safety devices for home and hospital are available. Bathtubs and showers can be equipped with antislip surfaces, hand bars, and rails. Night lights are essential for bathrooms and bedrooms. Adaptive devices that make getting on and off the toilet more safely are available. To assist with balance, the older person may use a cane, walker, or other assistive device.

> **Nursing Alert**
>
> Thorough familiarity with operation and safety factors is required whenever a mechanical lift is used to assist the patient into the tub or in and out of bed.

Restraints (Patient Safety Devices). The person should not be restrained by physical or chemical means (medications) unless absolutely necessary. The physically restrained patient will often exert much energy in an attempt to get out. A chemically restrained person often becomes more confused and loses mental capacity. Frequent reminders to the patient to ask for assistance and reassurance that someone is available and willing to assist can replace the use of restraint in many situations. A nurse call light must always be within reach. Generally, a physician's order is needed before applying a restraint. Proper application and frequent monitoring

are necessary to prevent patient injury. (See Chapter 87 for guidelines in using restraints.)

Side rails should be up on the beds of many older patients, especially at bedtime. People tend to become more confused at night. The patient should be instructed to ask for assistance to go to the bathroom. All beds must be in the low position when the patient is alone, day or night. Hospital beds also are available for home use.

> **Nursing Alert**
>
> In some situations, the patient will be in *more danger* with the side rails of the bed up. In the case of the person who continually climbs over the side rails, a physician's order may be written to leave side rails down, even at night. If the bed is in low position, this is safer than taking the chance of the patient falling out of bed *over* the side rails.

Physical Activity and Exercise

Physical activity is an important part of a total health program for the elderly. It is vital to keep moving and exercise; to maintain circulation, muscle tone, and general health; and to prevent disuse deformities. The patient should participate in exercise that compliments his or her lifestyle. The ambulatory person can walk, stretch, swim, or join competitive activities. Exercises may be modified to suit individual needs. Any age patient should be encouraged to participate in active range-of-motion exercises; if this not possible, the nurse must provide passive range of motion.

Inactivity is a known killer of the elderly. The dangers of prolonged bed rest and lengthy sitting include contractures, dermal ulcers, constipation, renal and pulmonary complications (especially pneumonia), cardiovascular disorders, and psychological isolation. Osteoporosis is common. Physical activities promote physical and mental stimulation.

> **Key Concept**
>
> Almost everyone can walk. Walking is the single most highly recommended exercise for the elderly.

Osteoporosis

Osteoporosis is a common disorder of bone metabolism in which the mass of bone is decreased. This reduction in bone density occurs in approximately one-fourth of all elderly people, most commonly in women between the ages of 50 and 70. In this disorder, bone resorption (assimilation) occurs faster than bone formation over a prolonged period.

Osteoporosis is most likely to occur in people in the following situations:

♦ Limited exercise
♦ Prolonged immobilization
♦ Decreased concentration of blood estrogen
♦ Catabolic hormone excess
♦ Long-term administration of high amounts of corticosteriods
♦ Other disorders

Osteoporosis is most common in fair-skinned, lightweight, postmenopausal women. Diagnosis of osteoporosis is made with radiologic examination of bone. Laboratory studies, such as measurement of blood calcium, phosphorus, and phosphatase, are usually normal.

Symptoms may include pain in weight-bearing vertebrae. Radiologic examination may detect loss of bone density, fractures, or loss of vertebral height (Fig. 85-2). Because involved bone tissue loses density and strength, fractures may occur, causing **kyphosis** (curvature of the spine) and a typical hump-backed appearance ("widow's hump").

Treatment is not extensive, beyond prevention of further osteoporotic damage. Appropriate diet, increased calcium intake, supplementary vitamin D, and fluoride may be helpful. Postmenopausal women may be treated with cyclic estrogen administration.

Physical exercise, activity, and a well-balanced diet may be the best preventive measures for osteoporosis. There is no known means to completely control or prevent the osteoporotic process itself.

Sexual Activities

The older adult generally maintains the ability and desire to engage in sexual intercourse. The physical changes that occur with aging may require some modifications of sexual activity. Menopause has no effect on sexual desire (libido; see Chapter 25). Physical acts of affection, with or without intercourse, are important for an individual's physical and emotional well-being. The physical closeness of hugging and holding hands can alleviate feelings of loneliness. Therapeutic touch is beneficial at any age. The nurse must recognize the value of physical contact

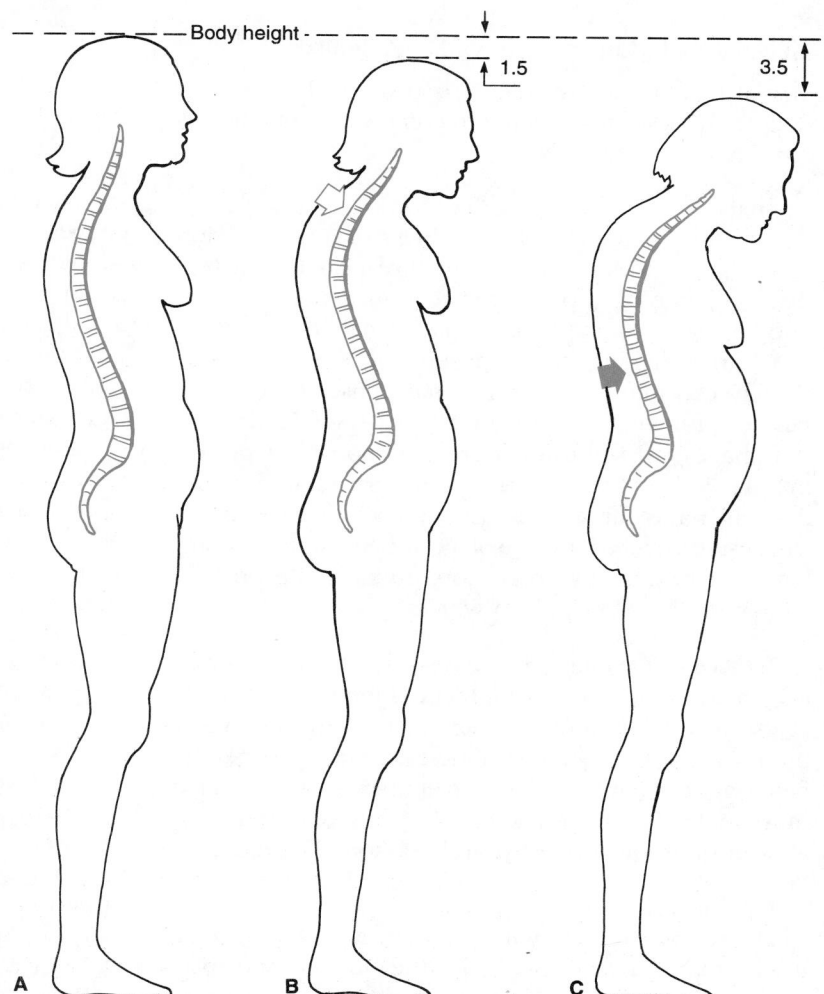

Figure 85-2. Typical loss of height associated with osteoporosis and aging. **(A)** Loss at 10 years postmenopause. **(B)** Loss at 15 years postmenopause: 1.5 inches. **(C)** Loss at 25 years postmenopause: 3.5 inches.

for the older patient. During recuperation from any disease, sexual activity, as with any physical activity, should be discussed with the physician.

Helping the Older Adult Meet Emotional Needs

Psychological health is just as important as physical health. Because the aging person often has had cumulative losses (physical, financial, social), mental health problems are common. Depression, anxiety, suicide, and chemical dependency are often overlooked in the elderly population. The accompanying box identifies signs of stress evidenced in the elderly.

The patient should be encouraged to remain self-sufficient and mentally active. Unless the mind is kept active, the person begins to have feelings of boredom and depression. It is important for the senior to maintain as much independence as is possible. When planning care for an elderly adult, consult the patient, and give the person the opportunity to participate in decision-making.

Mental Health Concerns in Older Patients

Mental health and psychiatric issues are discussed in Chapter 87. Discussed here are common mental health concerns for the elderly.

Anxiety

Anxiety is a feeling of uneasiness or apprehension as a response to some threat. The threat can be real (eg, disease pathology) or perceived (eg, fear of the unknown). Some limited anxiety is normal and can stimulate an individual to purposeful actions. Excessive anxiety can interfere with rational thinking and independent functioning. For an aging person, threats to self-image and self-esteem are common. The person may be faced with loss of health, independence, the familiar home, family contracts, and life itself. Anxiety can result in withdrawal, isolation, confusion, or combative or maladaptive behaviors. Anxiety is especially evident in the older person who is physically ill.

Treatment. Treatment first assesses the level of anxiety (mild, moderate, panic) and identifies available physical and emotional defense mechanisms. Many times, stress is reduced with increased knowledge; the fear is gone because it is no longer unknown. The nurse must remain calm, provide outlets for excess energy, answer questions honestly, and reassure the patient.

Depression

Depression is extremely common in older citizens. It is estimated that 10% to 50% of the elderly population have some symptoms of depression. Cumulative losses

Physical, Emotional, and Mental Signs of Stress in the Aging Adult

- Elevated blood pressure
- Urinary frequency
- Diarrhea
- Increased heart rate
- Dyspnea
- Insomnia
- Fatigue
- Lack of attention to details
- Lack of concentration
- Lack of interest
- Lack of awareness to external stimuli
- Living in the past
- Forgetfulness
- Tearfulness
- Withdrawal
- Paranoia
- Depression
- Irritability
- Feelings of worthlessness

Source: Farrell J. Nursing Care of the Older Person. Philadelphia, J.B. Lippincott, 1990.

and numerous changes, most of which are beyond a person's control, lead to depression. However, most people are reluctant to admit they are depressed. The stigma attached to psychiatric diagnoses is of much concern to the older person; they may assume they should be able to solve their own problems. They may presume that depression, fear, and loneliness are normal aspects of aging.

Clinical depression is often not diagnosed in the senior. Symptoms of depression can manifest as side effects of medications, disease processes, or adjustment to life cycle changes. It is important to differentiate clinical depression from organic brain syndromes. Chapter 86 deals with dementias, which often contain an element of depression. Depression also can be a symptom of long-standing chemical dependency. Symptoms of depression include lack of interest in the surroundings and in self-care, lack of energy and appetite, and altered sleep patterns; as well as suicidal ideation. Depression may be precipitated by a specific event but usually results from a combination of factors, including the following:

- Chemical imbalance, poor nutrition
- Financial difficulties, poverty level subsistence
- Loss of spouse, friends, roles (eg, no longer wife or mother)
- Serious, chronic illness; debilitating disease
- Lack of mental or physical exercise
- Medical side effects, oversedation
- Drug or alcohol abuse

Treatment. Treatment for geriatric depression is often hindered by the patient's reluctance to seek assistance. The lack of medical professionals who specialize in geriatric mental health also limits therapy. The goal of therapy is aimed at increasing self-esteem. Participation in social, recreational, and cultural events is remotivating. Participation in volunteer services and caring for a pet are often helpful. When the causes are understood, it follows that avoiding them can help prevent the disorder. Many of the general suggestions for stress relief also relate to the treatment of depression. The senior is encouraged to get adequate exercise and eat a well-balanced diet. General physical problems are treated. The accompanying box gives suggestions for patient teaching. Various antidepressant medications also may be helpful (see Chapters 56 and 87).

Suicide. Suicide is a serious result of depression. Seniors are the most at-risk group for suicide. The nurse must always take threats or gestures of suicide seriously.

> **Nursing Alert**
>
> It is vital for the nurse to observe for side effects when giving drugs. The dose of an antidepressant given to a younger person is often *toxic* to the elderly person. In addition, *any drug* given to the older person may cause the *opposite effect* than in a younger person (paradoxical effect).

Substance Abuse

Substance abuse is a special problem in the older person. Many factors contribute to geriatric chemical dependency. Among them, loneliness and depression are significant.

Self-Esteem and Substance Abuse. The older person is often a widow or widower and no longer has a regular job; there is "nothing to do." The person's self-esteem suffers from a feeling of worthlessness and lack of purpose. A convenient means of trying to deal with these feelings for some people is chemical overuse, most often in the form of alcoholism or abuse of prescription drugs. Geriatric clients often think of substance abuse as a problem of the young. They then deny that they have a chemical dependency problem.

Alcohol Abuse

Alcoholism in the older person may be difficult to detect. Family and friends may not be aware of their loved one's situation or may live far away. Often, they do not see the person regularly. It is easy to cover up chemical dependency during occasional visits.

> **Keys to Patient/Family Teaching**
> ### Prevention of Depression in the Older Person
>
> Patient and family teaching regarding prevention of depression includes the following:
> - Pursue an active social life with people of all ages. The place of worship usually has social gatherings. Senior citizen centers offer appropriate activities and encourage people to meet other people.
> - Go back to school. The Elderhostel (Elder College) program offers educational programs throughout the United States and other countries. These programs stimulate the mind and offer opportunities for socializing.
> - Join a support group. Share concerns, and gain insight from others in the group.
> - Volunteer at the local hospital or civic organization. Some communities have babysitting services or day-care centers run by older people.
> - Provide consulting service by joining a group such as SCORE (Service Corps of Retired Executives)
> - Acquire a pet. This builds a sense of being needed and provides companionship.
> - Go back to work. Many companies are encouraging retired people to come back to work. The older worker is reliable and dependable. It is also therapeutic for the person to have a place to go and the responsibility and pride in having a job.

Relatives may think the person is "just confused," when in fact he or she is under the influence of alcohol or drugs. If the person is widowed, the spouse may have been covering and enabling the substance abuse for a long time. The family often cannot believe their parent is an alcoholic because there was no difficulty in earlier years. The situation often does not get out of control until the person is alone or retired.

Abuse of Prescription Drugs

Approximately 40% of all adverse drug reactions occur in people older than 65 years; this is approximately five times that of younger people. One-sixth of all hospital admissions of people older than 70 relate to medication complications. There are several contributing factors. Medications react differently in an older person. Many individuals have little knowledge of medication interactions. Some seniors see no harm in sharing medications with a friend or spouse or in using medications after the expiration date. Often, medications are mixed in the same container. Over-the-counter medications are often used inappropriately or misused. The person may not remember how many pills he or she has had or even if they have been taken. The older person may be using chemicals as self-medication and taking doses larger than those prescribed. Confusion occurs when some of the patient's medication labels are stated in generic names, while others use brand names. Some seniors have several physicians who prescribe separate, and often conflicting, medications. Individuals also may deliberately search out several physicians to obtain added prescriptions.

Treatment. Treatment is equally difficult. The older person may be even more resistant than younger chemically dependent people. Seniors feel they have earned the right to live as they wish. They resent younger people, especially their own children, telling them what to do. Denial of the problem is common. Before treatment can begin, the individual must accept help and be prepared to change lifestyle patterns. Substance abuse is discussed further in Chapter 88.

Key Concept

Geriatric confusion should be evaluated for organic pathologies and substance abuse.

Therapies Aimed at Emotional and Psychological Support

Remotivation Techniques. Remotivation is an important adjunct to therapy. This *reality orientation* attempts to focus attention on the present, calling on memories from the patient's past (reminiscence). Participation is encouraged by sharing memories. Reminiscence and reality orientation are useful strategies to promote mental stimulation and validation of life's past events.

Recreation. Recreation is important at any age. In a long-term care facility, an activity or recreation director plans and directs events. These activities are designed to be creative and to motivate seniors to use physical and mental capabilities.

Learning. Intelligence does not normally decline with age. Therefore, learning is possible at any age. While short-term memory loss is common, long-term memory remains good. This implies that a senior will remember skills from long ago. New skills can be acquired but may take longer to learn. Physical limitations also must be considered. Motivation and readiness to learn are just as important in a senior as in anyone else. Lack of direction and decreased stimulation contribute to decreased mental alertness and comprehension.

Social Life and Activities. The patient should be encouraged to carry on a normal social life and to engage in as many previous activities as possible. The family should be included in the care plan and should be encouraged to visit and take the older person with them on trips and outings.

Older people naturally love to see grandchildren and other children. The older person is interested in young people and will enjoy sharing his or her own youthful recollections. Often, nursing students are a favorite among residents of nursing homes.

Pet Therapy. Pets are welcome to many older people. They can provide companionship, stimulate the sense of touch, and encourage a sense of responsibility. Many confused residents will respond to an animal, even though they do not respond to other people. Pet therapy has proven very beneficial in geriatrics and is an accepted activity in many nursing homes (see Fig. 87-1).

Religious Support. The patient should be encouraged to carry on religious practices. Allow the patient privacy when a member of the clergy comes to visit. Many hospitals and nursing homes have visiting clergy who conduct religious services; residents should be encouraged to attend. If it is impossible for a person to attend, tape recordings can be made.

Use of Volunteers

Most community organizations for the aging, nursing homes, and retirement centers have a corps of volunteers who assist in the activity program of the agency. These volunteers are essential, and their participation should be encouraged by nursing staff. They provide many services to patients, such as visiting patients who do not have other visitors, taking residents on outings, helping with craft activities, providing parties and entertainment, and assisting with reading or writing letters.

Church groups or service clubs often work with nursing home residents as a special service. Because the nursing home resident especially enjoys the company of younger people, teens should be encouraged to assist in activities of local nursing homes. Not only is this meaningful to the residents, but it is also a rewarding experience for the young people.

A staff member should coordinate the duties of volunteers to make certain they are helping residents. Volunteers must be encouraged to keep confidences and treat patients with respect. If a volunteer makes a commitment to be at the residence on a certain day, it is important that this obligation be met. The residents rely on and look forward to visits of the volunteers and become upset when volunteers do not keep the schedule. Volunteers should be taught to have empathy for older people. They must develop patience to help the resident perform independently; it is not helpful just to do things for them.

Warning Signs of Abuse

- ♦ Frequent trips to healthcare facility
- ♦ History of unexplained injuries
- ♦ Untreated conditions or wounds
- ♦ Malnutrition or weight loss
- ♦ Poor grooming
- ♦ Inability to perform activities of daily living
- ♦ Inappropriate medication administration
- ♦ Depression, withdrawal, substance abuse
- ♦ Excessive fear
- ♦ Spending or donating large sums of money

Crimes Against the Elderly: Abuse

Elder abuse is the emotional, physical, sexual, or financial exploitation of an aging person. Abuse or neglect may relate to health status and care, personal freedom, property, or income. Any action that places a person in jeopardy may be considered abuse or neglect. Abuse may take many forms. For instance, sales gimmicks, medical quackery, fear tactics, and "con games" are considered elderly exploitation. Many older people are considered **vulnerable adults** and are protected by law; abuse of vulnerable people is a crime and punishable by law. This applies to family members as well as healthcare workers.

Abuse may be at the hand of an individual or an organization. The exhaustion and frustration of daily obligations related to care of an older person can be overwhelming and may lead to mistreatment. The most common abusers are, in descending order, adult children, other relatives, spouse, service provider, friends or neighbors, grandchildren, and siblings. An organization, such as an insurance company, a mail order sales company, or a religious organization, may defraud the elder intentionally or accidentally. Abuse is most often not reported; witnesses are difficult to obtain. Warning signs of abuse are listed in the accompanying box.

Key Concept

The nurse must be observant and aware of the possibility of elder abuse. In most states, it is *illegal for a medical professional not to report abuse.*

Prevention of Abuse

Prevention of abuse begins with recognition of high-risk families. These include families with recent disruption in lifestyle or living arrangements, those with financial problems, those with alcoholism or substance abuse, and those with mental illness. The greater the number of risk factors, the greater the tendency toward abuse. It is important to address the needs of the caregiver as well as those of the individual. Caregivers need to know what resources are available; a respite from daily care can offer relief. Community resources include social service agencies (such as Adult Protection), the police, home healthcare and homemaker services, and "Meals on Wheels."

Keys for Review

Key Questions for Critical Thinking

1. A family for which you provide care has an elderly father who spends 2 days a week in adult day care. Describe the advantages for him, for his adult children with whom he lives, and for the grandchildren in his home.
2. Discuss obesity and its problems as it relates to aging.
3. Describe some of the changes in aging and their implications for medication administration.

Key Questions for Critical Thinking

(continued)

4. Describe ways to increase safety for older people in the home, in a senior day care center, and in a nursing home.
5. Compare adolescents and the elderly in the following: changes in the body and resulting adjustments, employment, lack of independence, decision making, privacy, abuse.

Key Readings

Atchley RC. Social Forces and Aging. An Introduction to Social Gerontology. Belmont, CA, Wadsworth, 1991

Birchenall JM, Streight ME. Care of the Older Adult, Ed 3. Philadelphia, J.B. Lippincott, 1993

Burke MM, Walsh MB. Gerontologic Nursing: Care of the Frail Elderly. St. Louis, Mosby-Yearbook, 1992.

Carnevali DL. Nursing Management for the Elderly, Ed 3. Philadelphia, J.B. Lippincott, 1992

Eliopoulous C. Caring for the Elderly in Diverse Care Settings. Philadelphia, J.B. Lippincott, 1990

Farrell J. Nursing Care of the Older Person. Philadelphia, J.B. Lippincott, 1990

Hogstel MO. Nursing Care of the Older Adult, Ed 3. Albany, NY, Delmar, 1993

Loftis PA, Glover TL. Decision-Making in Gerontologic Nursing. St. Louis, Mosby-Yearbook, 1993

Murray R, Zentner J. Nursing Assessment and Health Promotion Strategies Through the Life Span. East Norwalk, CT, Appleton & Lange, 1993

Smeltzer SC, Bare BG. Brunner & Suddarth's Textbook of Medical-Surgical Nursing, Ed. 7. Philadelphia, J.B. Lippincott, 1992

Enrichment Keys

Cerrato PL. "Piecing together the osteoporosis puzzle." RN 53(4):77–82, 1990

Eliopoulos C. Gerontological Nursing, Ed 3. Philadelphia, J.B. Lippincott, 1993

Keys To Learning More

Chapter 86: dementia and Alzheimer's disease
Chapter 87: psychiatric disorders
Chapter 88: substance abuse

Keys To Learning More (continued)

Chapter 89: rehabilitation techniques
Unit Seventeen: death and dying and hospice care
Chapter 93: career opportunities (Many LPNs and RNs work in extended-care facilities and nursing homes.)

Key Resources

ACTION
    806 Connecticut Avenue, NW
    Washington, DC 20525
    202/254-7310
Administration on Aging
    Department of Health and Human Services
    200 Independence Avenue, SW
    Washington, DC 20201
    202/245-0724
American Association of Retired Persons (AARP)
    601 E Street, NW
    Washington, DC 20049
    202/434-2277
Asociacion Nacional por Personas Mayores
(for Hispanic Seniors)
    3325 Wilshire Boulevard, Suite 800
    Los Angeles, CA 90010
Elderhostel International
    75 Federal Street
    Boston, MA 02110
    617/426-8056
National Indian Council on Aging
    PO Box 2088
    Albuquerque, NM 87103
National Pacific/Asian Resource Association
    2033 6th Avenue, Suite 410
    Seattle, WA 98121
Service Corps of Retired Executives (SCORE)
    1825 Connecticut Avenue, NW, Suite 503
    Washington, DC 20009

86 Dementia-Type Disorders

Keys for Learning

Learning Objectives

♦ Differentiate between confusion, delirium, and dementia.
♦ List components of dementia as defined in the DSM-III-R classification.
♦ Define primary degenerative and secondary dementias.
♦ Briefly describe Alzheimer's disease, the physiologic changes, and theories about its cause.
♦ Describe stages of Alzheimer's disease, and list common behaviors and their probable cause.
♦ Describe laboratory tests, physical examination, and psychometric testing in dementias.
♦ Discuss the use of medications in dementia, and state two adverse reactions to medications that occur in the elderly.
♦ Describe functional assessment, and state danger signs that require the person to have a caregiver.
♦ Describe nursing management of the person with dementia.

Key Terms

ambiguous loss	dementia
aphasia	labile
apraxia	organic brain syndrome
confabulation	primary degenerative dementia
confusion	secondary dementia
delirium	

Keys to Understanding This Chapter

Chapter 3: human care services available for seniors
Chapter 5: basic human needs
Chapter 6: optimum health
Chapter 12: lifestyle changes and developmental tasks of aging
Unit Four: physical changes in normal aging
Unit Five: nutrition and diet therapy
Unit Six: safety
Chapter 36: therapeutic communication

Keys to Understanding This Chapter
(continued)

Unit Nine: basic patient care skills
Unit Eleven: pharmacology and medication administration
Unit Fourteen: disorders of adults
Chapter 85: geriatric nursing

Key Points

♦ There are many reversible causes of confusion and delirium, including physical illness, metabolic disturbances, drug or alcohol toxicity, malnutrition, and sensory deprivation.
♦ Although confusion and delirium can occur at any age, the older adult is more vulnerable because of decreased physiologic reserve and the variety of medications taken.
♦ Primary degenerative dementias include Alzheimer's disease, Pick's disease, Creutzfeldt-Jakob disease, and acquired immunodeficiency syndrome dementia.
♦ Secondary dementias include multi-infarct dementia, Wernicke-Korsakoff syndrome, and metabolic dementias.
♦ Diagnosis of dementia is often difficult; usually only brain tissue biopsy of autopsy can confirm the diagnosis. Other tests are helpful in ruling out treatable causes of dementia.
♦ Alzheimer's disease develops in stages, beginning with memory difficulty and progressing to increasing difficulties with memory, language, and movement. In the final stage, the patient is no longer able to perform activities of daily living.
♦ Treatment for Alzheimer's is palliative; there is no known cure.
♦ Nursing assessment of physical and mental abilities, needs, and resources is integral in the treatment of dementia.
♦ One nursing goal is assessment of the patient's abilities in performing basic and complex activities of daily living.
♦ Respite care and support services are necessary for caregivers.

Key Learning Activities

◆ Visit an Alzheimer's disease support group. What concerns were expressed by caregivers? What solutions were proposed?
◆ Read three recent articles regarding Alzheimer's disease, and develop a report.
◆ Visit a locked Alzheimer's unit. What precautions are taken to maintain residents' safety?

Previous chapters have discussed normal changes associated with aging and problems often associated with the aging process. This chapter looks at some forms of dementia and discusses nursing implications associated with dementia. **Dementia** literally means "mind away." Several types of dementia occur.

Key Concept

The American Psychiatric Association states that classification of dementia is based on the reversibility of the problem and its underlying pathology.

Confusion, Delirium, and Dementia

Confusion. Confusion is the state of not being aware of or oriented to time, place, situation, or personhood. The person may lack orderly thought and be unable to act decisively. Confusion may be a symptom of severe emotional stress or of an organic mental disorder. Severe confusion may be called delirium.

Delirium. Delirium begins with confusion and progresses to incoherence, anxiety, delusions, hallucinations, or fear. Delirium has a sudden onset (often hours or days) and is often reversible. Commonly, delirium occurs in unfamiliar settings, as in a hospital environment. Delirium has been referred to as *acute brain syndrome.* Causes of delirium include physical illness, diabetic reaction, drug or alcohol toxicity, dehydration, malnutrition, head trauma, sensory deprivation or overload, systemic infections, and electrolyte disturbances.

Although delirium can occur at any age, the older adult is more vulnerable to occasional confusion or delirium. The geriatric client has more physical and metabolic difficulties due to deterioration of physical systems. In addition, the older person, as a result of his or her medications, may have periods of confusion, electrolyte imbalances, or dehydration.

Dementia. Dementia is a progressive, chronic state of confusion with loss of memory and cognitive abilities. It is characterized by deterioration of intellect, memory, judgment, and ability to function independently. There are more than 60 causes of dementia. *Reversible* causes of dementia include drug intoxication, benign brain tumors, endocrine dysfunction, and depression. The most common types of *irreversible* dementia are Alzheimer's disease (AD) and multi-infarct dementia.

Organic Brain Syndrome. Organic brain syndrome (OBS) is a general term that refers to a set of mental disorders found in specific *organic* mental conditions, as opposed to those for which no identifiable physical causes can be found. There is actually an organic or physical cause for the dementia, such as AIDS dementia. OBS is characterized by losses in mental, intellectual, and judgment abilities and unstable (**labile**) emotional states. Chronic OBSs are irreversible and include the dementias.

Dementias

Often, the individual or family may not notice the signs and symptoms of dementia in early stages (impaired judgment and abstract thinking). The changes are insidious (gradual and cumulative). As the person has increasing difficulty with social interactions and functional skills, memory loss becomes obvious. Personality changes occur; exaggerated emotions are common. AD accounts for approximately 50% to 60% of dementia.

Multi-infarct dementia accounts for approximately 10% to 20% of the cases; some patients have both disorders.

Types of Dementias

Two main categories of dementias exist: *primary* degenerative dementias and *secondary* dementias. The primary dementias are a disease unto themselves; no other causative agent has been found. Disorders or diseases of secondary dementias are the following:

♦ Multi-infarct disorder (many cerebrovascular accidents [CVA] or strokes)
♦ Multiple transient ischemic attacks ([TIA], causing reduced circulation to the brain)
♦ Wernicke-Korsakoff syndrome (alcohol-related)
♦ Metabolic disorders (such as diabetes mellitus or end-stage renal disease [ESRD])
♦ Drug overdose (toxic dementia)
♦ Crack-related dementia; dementias caused by other illegal drugs
♦ Acquired immunodeficiency syndrome (AIDS) dementia
♦ Dementia of tertiary syphilis (Bayle's disease)

Disorders of primary degenerative dementias follow:

♦ Alzheimer's disease (AD)
♦ Pick's disease
♦ Creutzfeldt-Jakob disease

Before a person can be diagnosed as having an irreversible condition causing dementia, other possible causes of the symptoms must be ruled out. If the dementia is reversible, it can be treated. See the accompanying box for identification factors.

Secondary Dementia

If dementia is caused by a force external to the brain or nerve cells, it is referred to as **secondary dementia**. Some secondary dementias are reversible; some can be arrested. It is important to rule out and treat secondary causes of dementia to stop the progression or alleviate the disorder if possible.

Multi-infarct Dementia

Vascular disease is the second most common cause of dementia. Older people who have a series of small strokes can lose mental abilities as nerve cells die from lack of oxygen and nutrients. *Multi-infarct dementia* can be distinguished from AD in the following ways:

♦ It has an abrupt onset.
♦ It progresses in a stepwise fashion (not gradually and continuously).
♦ It usually coexists with other conditions (diabetes,

Identification of Dementia

♦ Short-term and long-term memory impairment
♦ At least one of the following: impairment of abstract thinking; impairment of judgment; disturbances of higher cortical functioning (such as aphasia or apraxia); or personality change
♦ Above disturbances significantly interfere with work, social activities, or relationships with others
♦ Absence of delirium or intoxication (which could cause the same symptoms)
♦ Insidious onset with progressive deterioration

Exclusion of other causes of the symptoms

♦ Rule out other causes, such as stroke and brain tumors.
♦ Determine if the patient has abnormal blood tests, including serum folate and serum B_{12}.
♦ CT scan shows cerebral atrophy only (no other disorders).
♦ EEG shows slow wave activity only (no other disorders).

Adapted from Diagnostic Criteria from DSM-III-R. American Psychiatric Association, 1987

high blood pressure, cardiac disease, previous strokes).

Small strokes usually can be detected by magnetic resonance imaging (MRI). If detected early, *treatment* is available to prevent future strokes and to keep underlying diseases under control.

Wernicke-Korsakoff Syndrome

This syndrome is the most common type of alcohol-related dementia. It is thought to be caused by direct damage to the brain by alcohol. It may be caused by nutritional factors, or it may be an indirect result of liver damage. Short-term memory is most impaired, although people with this syndrome also may demonstrate poor judgment, lack of insight, diminished attention, and slowed thinking. (They may not have the language problems or perceptual problems of AD.) The characteristic belligerent behavior patterns of some patients with Wernicke-Korsakoff make them difficult management problems.

Acquired Immunodeficiency Syndrome Dementia. The patient in the later stages of acquired immunodeficiency syndrome (AIDS) may become demented. The pathology and exact mechanisms of AIDS dementia are being researched. Dementia does not occur in all cases of AIDS, and in some patients with AIDS dementia, periods of lucidity are possible until late in the disease. AIDS dementia is now the most common dementia caused by infection.

Other Secondary Dementias

Brain injury can occur from numerous physical disorders and can cause dementia. *Toxic dementia* is related to drug overdose. *Metabolic dementias* can occur following untreated end-stage renal disease (uremia), hypoglycemia or hyperglycemia, hypothyroidism or hyperthyroidism, or hepatic (liver) failure. Organic dementias also can be caused by closed head trauma or brain tumors, or by organic disorders such as temporal lobe epilepsy or Huntington's disease.

Crack-Related Dementia

A form of dementia that is becoming more common is related to the abuse of cocaine, particularly "crack cocaine." Relatively little is known about crack-related dementia, but it seems to occur more commonly in young, healthy African American males. It is believed to be irreversible. In addition to the confusion, memory loss, and speech disorders common to other dementias, people with crack-related dementia often are violent.

Primary Degenerative Dementias

Some dementias affect nerve or brain cells and cannot be arrested or reversed. These are the **primary degenerative dementias,** sometimes referred to as age-associated memory impairment (AAMI).

Alzheimer's Disease

AD (sometimes called senile dementia of the Alzheimer's type; SDAT) is a progressive, irreversible, fatal neurologic disorder that affects an estimated 4 million American adults. It is estimated by 2040, approximately 14 million Americans will be diagnosed with AD. Approximately 9% of the population older than 55 years and 20% of those older than 85 years have AD. The duration of AD averages 2 to 10 years but can be up to 20 years. By 1992, AD was the fourth leading cause of death among adults (more than 100,000 American deaths per year). It is projected that the number of people with AD will triple in the next 50 years. This epidemic of dementia is not confined to sex, race, social, or economic class. The public knows this disorder as "senility," although the term Alzheimer's is becoming more common. (It is important to allow the patient and family to use terminology with which they are comfortable.)

> **Key Concept**
>
> Although AD affects a large number of American adults, this number represents only 10% of the total older adult population. Therefore 90% of all older adults never suffer from any type of dementia or AD.

Reflections on Alzheimer's Disease

> "My mind goes to an empty and horrible place. When I come back, I'm in a room full of strangers. I feel so lost and afraid." Stated by a 61-year-old woman in early stages of Alzheimer's disease. These sentiments are echoed by many Alzheimer's patients. The disease is frightening and disabling.
>
> *Quote from Hasselbring "Alzheimer's disease." Medical Self-Care 53-57, January–February, 1986*

Other Primary Dementias

Pick's Disease. Pick's disease, which is rare, can only be differentiated from AD by autopsy. AD brain tissue shows plaques and tangles, but in Pick's the nerve cells are pale and swollen and contain globules of protein (Pick's bodies). The brain looks spongy, due to the increase of non-nerve supporting cells. The symptoms are similar to AD. Pick's disease involves primarily the frontal and temporal lobes of the brain and therefore presents as behavioral or language problems. Pick's has an earlier onset than AD (most commonly between ages 40 and 50). The average survival is approximately 7 years.

Creutzfeldt-Jakob Disease. This rare dementia is caused by a virus and is one of several infectious dementias called *transmissible dementia*. This dementia is rapid in its course; death almost always occurs within 2 years of onset.

> **Key Concept**
>
> More that 50% of all nursing home residents are diagnosed as having AD or another dementia. The cost of institutional care for people with dementia has been estimated to exceed $25 billion per year in the United States.

Diagnosis of Dementia

Although there are some differences between the dementias, the majority of this material is applicable to AD as well as to other dementias.

History. The specific mental and physical changes reported by the individual and the family are extremely important in determining possible causes of cognitive decline in a patient. The physician needs to know the age at which changes began, exact functions lost, whether changes were associated with other medical or emotional events, and what medications the patient was and is taking. This history determines which tests will be performed to rule out specific diseases and alerts the physician to look for specific signs on the examination.

Physical and Neurologic Examination. A physical examination is done to determine the patient's basic general health. The neurologic examination is an important component. The physician generally asks the patient to perform maneuvers or answer questions that are designed to gain information about functioning of specific parts of the brain. This includes tests of vision, eye movement, muscle tone and strength, reflexes, and mental status. Psychiatric assessment is an important part of the overall patient examination. A psychiatric assessment may determine the presence of underlying factors that may exacerbate memory loss, including some forms of depression. The findings of the physician's history and physical examination help to differentiate between types of dementia.

Key Concept

The physician must perform a comprehensive physical and psychological workup to determine if the person has AD or another condition which can be reversed. Definite diagnosis of AD can only be made by biopsy or autopsy, but a thorough examination can rule out other, more treatable, disorders.

Laboratory Tests. Laboratory tests, such as those listed in Table 86-1, are performed to rule out and treat reversible causes of dementia. They are helpful in identifying risk factors associated with some forms of dementia. (AD patients usually have normal laboratory studies.)

Computed Tomography, Magnetic Resonance Imaging, Positron Emission Tomography, and Electroencephalograph Testing. *Computed tomography* and MRI provide a visualization of brain anatomy, which will sometimes demonstrate progressive atrophy of the brain beyond that of normal aging. They are helpful in excluding conditions such as cerebrovascular accidents, results of closed head trauma, hydrocephalus, vascular disease, tumors, and hematomas, but they are not reliable in confirming any diagnosis of dementia. Atrophy of the hippocampus in the brain is one of the first signs seen in AD. (The hippocampus is the area of the brain associated with short-term memory and consolidation of short- and long-term memory.) *Positron emission tomography* may show decreased metabolism in some areas. A newer scan called the *single positron emission computerized tomography* is helpful in evaluating blood perfusion to the brain and the metabolic activity of the brain.

The *electroencephalograph* (EEG) records the electrical activity of the brain. This test is not always performed but may rule out seizure disorders or other brain pathology. In AD, the EEG shows a generalized slowing of brain wave activity. Distinctive EEG changes are seen in Creutzfeldt-Jakob disease.

Psychometric Testing. Usually a brief mental status examination is performed by the physician. An example is the Folstein Mini-Mental State Exam. This examination tests the patient's orientation to time and place; ability to register and recall information; attention, concentration, and calculation ability; and language skills. In AD, the first functions to be lost are memory of recent events, abstract reasoning, mathematic calculations, and the ability to concentrate and follow through on complex tasks. More comprehensive psychometric testing can be completed by a psychologist. This could include standardized intelligence scales, memory scales, testing for judgment and planning abilities, and more comprehensive language testing. (Results of these tests are compared with unimpaired people in the same age group.)

Psychiatric testing also is done, using a scale such as the Brief Psychiatric Rating Scale (BPRS), to rule out psychoses.

Functional Assessment. A functional assessment is part of the diagnostic workup for dementias. The patient is evaluated for his or her ability to perform basic skills required for daily functioning (ADLs). Included in this assessment are abilities to do instrumental activities of daily living (IADLs): meal preparation, shopping, telephone use, and transportation. Functional assessment also is discussed in detail later in this chapter and in Chapter 89.

Key Concept

There is no way to predict which skills will be lost in any patient. One part of the brain may be affected but not another. Therefore, some patients retain specific skills until late in the disease. A thorough evaluation is needed to determine the extent and progression of the disease.

Alzheimer's Disease

Theories of Causes

Scientists have identified one cause of AD, although various hypotheses have been tested. Some of the theories are well supported by research; others are controversial. Several causes have been *hypothesized*:

Table 86-1. Laboratory Studies and Causes of Dementia

Test	Possible Cause of Problem	Rationale
Complete blood count	Anemia	Lack of oxygen (ischemia) in brain causes confusion.
Chemistry screening	Toxicity	Metabolic disturbances, kidney disease, and liver disease cause toxic, confused states.
Fasting blood sugar and other tests for insulin-dependent diabetes mellitus	Diabetes mellitus	Excessively high or low blood sugar levels can cause mental disturbances; nutritional disorders also can contribute to delirium and dementia.
VDRL, RPR, MHA-TP, or FTA-ABS	Syphilis	Tertiary syphilis causes dementia.
Erythrocyte sedimentation rate	Infection, immune disorders	Infectious agents can lead to toxicity; chronic inflammation can lead to ischemia.
Urinalysis	Urinary tract disorders	Uremia, infections, and toxicity can lead to dementia.
Thyroid panel	Hyperthyroidism, hypothyroidism	Confusion and depression can occur with abnormal thyroid levels.
Vitamin B_{12} and folate	Anemias	Inability to make or use red blood cells can cause ischemia to brain; also folate and B_{12} are low in chronic alcoholism.
Cerebrospinal fluid assay	Alzheimer's disease	Low levels of proteus nixon (PN) have been associated with Alzheimer's.
Autoimmune testing	Vasculitis	Elevated in some cases of multi-infarct dementias.

Tests for HIV
   HIV-1 antigen (P24)
   HIV-1 antibody
	Acquired immunodeficiency syndrome (AIDS)	Later stages of AIDS can cause dementia.

Alcohol (ETOH); other chemical screening	Drug or Alcohol-related dementia	Rule out Wernicke-Korsikoff syndrome, crack-related dementias, other chemical toxicities.
Electrolyte levels	Electrolyte imbalance	Excess or deficiency of some electrolytes can cause dementia.

◆ *Genetic.* There may be a familial tendency, possibly related to a defective chromosome. (Approximately 85% of people with Down syndrome develop AD in midlife.)

◆ *Viral.* Other dementias (kuru, Creutzfeldt-Jakob) are caused by viruses. A slow virus (one that remains inactive in the body for a long time) hypothesis is being tested.

◆ *Toxic.* Aluminum has received publicity as a possible cause of dementia; however, aluminum deposits in the brain may be a result rather than a cause. Other toxins (poisons) can cause dementia.

◆ *Immunologic.* Autoimmune processes ("antibrain antibodies") have been identified.

◆ *Trauma.* Tissue injury from serious head injury has been studied.

◆ *Biochemical.* Neurotransmitter deficiency caused by degeneration is under investigation.

◆ *Nutritional.* Malnutrition may play a role in predisposing to AD.

Physiologic Changes Seen in Alzheimer's Disease

The microscopic changes seen in the brain (cerebral cortex) of an AD patient have a distinct appearance. The pathophysiology of AD is based on biochemical morphologic studies of brain tissue obtained by biopsy or autopsy. Three major changes are seen in the brain:

◆ Cerebral cortex atrophy
◆ Loss of neurons
◆ Changes in brain cells

Brain cell changes include the following:

◆ Abnormal neurons, arranged in filaments called *neurofibrillary tangles*—delicate abnormal fibers or threads of proteins

◆ *Senile (neuritic) plaques*—round or ovoid clusters of destroyed synapses, embedded in a central amyloid core

◆ *Granulovascuolar degeneration*—the inside of the cell, crowded with fluid-filled vacuoles and granular material

A significant decrease in the brain's ability to make *acetylcholine*, a vital neurotransmitter, also occurs. Risk factors for AD are summarized in the accompanying box.

Description of Alzheimer's Disease

Behavioral, intellectual, and emotional changes occurring in AD patients develop in fairly regular patterns. Symptoms are always progressive, but the rate of change varies greatly. The individualization of the disease is caused by the random manner in which the process affects brain tissue. A few cases show rapid decline, but more commonly, there may be several months with little change. The general patterns are described in four stages and are introduced below and further illustrated in the accompanying box.

> ### Key Concept
>
> In AD, intelligence often remains intact during much of the progression of the disease. However, the mental functioning is impaired. Thus, the person may test high on a general intelligence test but may not be able to manage his or her ADLs.

Stage I (Early). Intermittent symptoms develop that may or may not be recognized; minor symptoms are often disregarded. The person may have trouble with numbers, language patterns, or handwriting. Examples of behaviors include neglecting to turn off the oven, misplacing things, taking longer to complete routine chores, repeating questions, and unprecedented mis-

Risk Factors for Alzheimer's Disease

- *Age*—Prevalence:
  - Less than 1% in ages 65–85
  - More than 15% in age 85+
  - Greatest incidence over age 90
- *Sex*—Seems more frequent in women; research inconclusive
- *Serious head injuries*—15% to 20% of patients have had serious head injury (up to 35 years before onset)
- *History of thyroid disorders*—Some increase in incidence noted, rationale uncertain
- *Genetics*—Evidence suggests autosomal dominant inheritance; not proven
- *Age of onset*—Varies (even in identical twins)
- *Metabolic or environmental factors*—Suspected, not proven
- *Chromosomal abnormalities*—Alzheimer's seen in approximately 85% of Down syndrome adults over age 40; other chromosomal abnormalities reported

Stages of Primary Degenerative Dementia of the Alzheimer's Type

Stage I: Early

- Short-term memory loss
- Gradual lack of interest in life
- Can't remember nouns, other words
- Vague
- Indifferent to social courtesies
- Isolative
- Indecisive
- Decreased reaction time
- Difficulty in learning
- Uncomfortable in new situations

Stage II: Middle/Advanced

- Significant decline in memory
- Difficulty with familiar tasks
- Confuses day and night; insomnia
- Responds slowly
- May complain of neglect
- May deny problems
- Loses things
- Has trouble with directions
- Inability to care for self; poor ADLs
- Apraxia
- Increasing aphasia
- Outbursts of anger; aggressiveness (in some people)
- More withdrawn and passive (in some people)
- Changes in personal relationships
- Loss of balance; gait changes
- Inability to make decisions

Stage III: Later

- Loss of sense of time
- Disoriented to place, person; unable to recognize family (sometimes)
- Insomnia
- Rambling speech incoherent
- Motor ability deteriorates
- Paranoid
- Confused; memory deteriorates more, remembers only distant past
- Wanders, gets lost
- Unable to perform some ADLs

Stage IV: Final/Terminal

- Total memory loss
- Unable to recognize family, friends
- Ataxia (unable to walk)
- Incontinent of stool and urine
- Mute or speech unrecognizable
- Extreme physical decline
- Death

Adapted from Farrell J. Nursing Care of the Older Person. Philadelphia, J.B. Lippincott, 1990; updated 1994.

management of money. **Confabulation** (fabricating of details of events) may occur as a cover-up for lack of memory.

Stage II (Middle). As the disease progresses, **apraxia** (problems carrying out purposeful movements) and **aphasia** (problems with language) worsen. Concentration, orientation, judgment, and planning abilities are affected. The families become increasingly aware that a problem exists.

State III (Later). During this period, people with dementia may have sudden mood shifts (emotional lability) or become depressed, suspicious (paranoid), fearful, or violent. The behavior may become abusive, causing difficulties for caregivers.

Stage IV (Final). In the last stages of the disease, the person becomes incontinent, unable to walk, and must have all basic care managed by others. Many patients become semicomatose before death. Some remain in the fetal position.

Key Concept

The specific and most common losses in AD are:

◆ Loss of short-term memory
◆ Loss of ability to learn new things
◆ Loss of judgment and planning skills
◆ Personality and mood changes
◆ Loss of reasoning and abstract thinking skills
◆ Loss of language skills
◆ Loss of ability to care for self

Medical Treatment of Alzheimer's Disease

Several medications that effect the transmission of chemicals across synapses are under study. No known medication will stop the progression of the disease. Tacrine HCl (Cognex), approved by the Food and Drug Administration in December of 1993, seems to slow the progression of memory impairment. Tacrine has the ability to increase neurotransmissions in the brain by acting on specific enzymes. While it does not cure AD, it seems to help the patient and family by enhancing the patient's memory capabilities, although this improvement is temporary.

Nursing Considerations. Side effects of this drug include bradycardia, nausea, vomiting, diarrhea, ulcers, jaundice, and rash, which can be troublesome and dangerous. The stool may change color and become light or very dark. Abrupt changes in dosage, either up or down, can cause serious side effects.

Tacrine requires regular monitoring of enzymes such as ALT (alanine aminotransferase), also known as SGPT

(serum glutamic-pyruvic transaminase), to prevent liver damage. It must be used cautiously when patients have surgery, because it potentiates the action of muscle relaxants. Patients with pre-existing heart or liver disorders must be carefully managed and frequently assessed.

Other medications are available to help manage difficult symptoms and behaviors (see box). Female hormones have seemed helpful in some cases. Medication therapy is generally palliative rather than curative. All medications must be used with caution in older people, because medications are not metabolized as well and may have opposite effects than those desired (paradoxical effects). Some drugs increase confusion.

Nursing Alert

Nursing staff should be aware that medication control should be a *last resort* in managing behavior problems in AD because of the numerous side effects of these medications. Nursing management approaches to these problems should be attempted *before* chemicals are tried.

❖ Nursing Process

Data Collection

The nurse's role in establishing baseline data for AD or any other dementia is important. By comparing with this baseline, the physician can identify deterioration trends in the patient. An assessment of the patient's support systems (family, friends, finances) also is imperative.

Physical Assessment

Behaviors and symptoms in early stages of AD can be mistaken for numerous other disorders. The physician must perform a thorough history and physical, and

---

Key Medications
for Alzheimer's disease

◆ Slows memory impairment: tacrine hydrochloride (Cognex)
◆ *Tranquilizers:* haloperidol (Haldol); thiothixene (Navane); thioridazine hydrochloride (Mellaril); and chlorpromazine hydrochloride (Thorazine)
◆ *Antidepressants:* trazodone hydrochloride (Desyrel) and fluoxetine HCl (Prozac)
◆ *Sedatives:* diphenhydramine (Benadryl); triazolam (Halcion); flurazepam (Dalmane); and chloral hydrate (Noctec)

James Swift is a 66-year-old married African American man with a history of Alzheimer's disease, admitted to the hospital for surgical repair of benign prostatic hyperplasia. He is scheduled for an intravenous pyelogram and cystography and transurethral resection of the prostate (TURP). Mr. Swift has been living at home but is already in the second stage of Alzheimer's disease, when problems of memory, reasoning, judgment, and social interaction become more pronounced. His wife reports that at times he gets lost, loses coordination, and frequently roams and paces about the house. Night awakenings are a special problem. His ability to speak and write has been deteriorating. He requires verbal instructions for self-care activities and supervision at mealtimes because of swallowing problems. She explains that he is now often depressed and irritable. A plan of care is designed to facilitate Mr. Swift's preparation for and recovery from surgery. The plan is responsive to the special needs stemming from his Alzheimer's disease. Three priority diagnoses are highlighted below.

Nursing Diagnoses: *Self-care Deficit: Activities of Daily Living, related to altered thought processes (secondary to neuronal degeneration, as evidenced by his neglect of himself and frustration and irritability when pressured to perform self-care*

Goal: Whenever observed, Mr. Swift will participate in self-care activities to the extent that he is able without becoming visibly frustrated—with verbal instruction and encouragement.

Nursing Actions (assess/do/teach)	Rationale	Evaluative Statement
1. Determine, in consultation with his wife, Mr. Swift's routine of care and ability to participate in own care. Keep hospital care as similar to home care as possible, and encourage his independence. Assign the same nurse to care for him consistently. Label items, such as the urinal and bathroom, if this proves helpful.	A predictable routine is essential to his sense of well-being. His transition back home will be easier if he is not allowed to regress in self-care abilities during his hospitalization.	12/5, Goal partially met; patient participates in usual routines of care but becomes visibly agitated with anything new (eg, need to provide a urine specimen). Revision: Continue to support.
2. Explain each nursing intervention, test, or treatment simply and patiently, clearly stating what is expected of him; use a calm and reassuring tone of voice.	Decreasing fright will help Mr. Swift cooperate.	

Nursing Diagnosis: *High Risk for Injury related to impaired memory, judgment, reasoning, as evidenced by tendency to roam and inability to process instructions and warnings.*

Goal: At discharge, patient is free of accident and injury.

(continued)

the nurse does a complete nursing assessment. Basic information, such as the patient's immunizations, particularly flu shots and Pneumovax 23 (protection against pneumococcal pneumonia), should be included on the patient's chart. A variety of other areas also should be assessed, particularly sensory deficits. Often, the nurse is responsible for obtaining substantial information about the patient. The following information from the patient or family aids in the overall picture.[1]

[1] Much of the material in this chapter has been adapted from a workshop conducted on May 5, 1989, by Karen Feldt, RN, MS, a Clinical Nurse Specialist at St. Paul Ramsey Medical Center, St. Paul, Minnesota. Used with permission.

Nursing Actions (assess/do/teach)	Rationale	Evaluative Statement
1. Carefully assess the patient's risk for injury, and institute the appropriate safeguards; orient the patient to his room, and reorient as often as necessary; place him in a single room close to the nurse's station for observation; ensure that he has limited access to stairwells and elevators. If not able to control roaming, use one-on-one observation (nursing, volunteer, family member), and if this is not possible, evaluate the use of a safety belt; try to anticipate his needs, because he may not be able to express them.	The patient with Alzheimer's disease is unable to meet his own safety and security needs. This person is disturbing to a room mate.	12/9, Goal met; patient free of injury at discharge.

Nursing Diagnosis: *Ineffective Disabling Family Coping, related to prolonged demands on family and exhausted personal resources, as evidenced by the family's obvious fatigue and sense of being overwhelmed*

Goal: Family uses the patient's hospitalization and nursing care to tend to their own needs without guilt.

Nursing Actions (assess/do/teach)	Rationale	Evaluative Statement
1. Continue to explore the impact Mr. Swift's illness is having on his family; look for signs of caretaker burnout; give family members "permission" to trust the nurses sufficiently to use the patient's time in the hospital to tend to their own needs.	Some families may fear "abandoning" the patient and require "permission" to meet their own needs.	12/6, Goal met; family members have decreased time spent in the hospital and appear more rested; expressed gratitude for sensitivity to their needs.
2. Explore resources available to the family, including adult day care, Alzheimer's Disease and Related Disorders Association (ADRDA), or the Alzheimer's Support Group, as well as written materials; refer for counseling if appropriate.	The family may be unaware of local resources.	12/7, Family members attended support group and received written information. 12/8, Social service referral done. Patient will be attending adult day care 1 afternoon per week.

VISUAL ACUITY EXAMINATION. Find out when the last vision examination occurred, if there were recent checks for glaucoma or cataracts, and whether glasses are worn. People with AD often have neglected personal healthcare. It is common for them to have perceptual problems. (They often believe something is wrong with their glasses and refuse to wear them.) Glasses are frequently lost or broken. They may find it difficult to place themselves in space and misperceive the edges of chairs or stairs. (This causes frequent falls.)

AUDIOMETRIC TESTING. Find out if hearing has been evaluated. Determine whether the patient has had a hearing aid prescribed and whether he or she wears it. Also find out if it works. (Limited or misinterpreted stimuli may contribute to confusion.)

NUTRITIONAL STATUS. Discuss the history of weight gain or loss and the time frame in which this occurred. Patients may forget to eat or may forget they just ate. Ask about ability to chew and swallow, particularly in later stages of the disease.

SLEEP PATTERN DISTURBANCES. Ask about the total number of hours of rest at night and during the day. Ask if the person gets up during the night and if so, how many times. Determine if this is disruptive to the caregiver.

SKIN CARE. Evaluate skin condition. Check for dryness, bruises, sores, pressure areas, and cracked heels. Check fingernails and toenails.

ORAL CARE. Assess whether the patient is able to brush the teeth or care for dentures. Ask if dentures fit properly, if they are worn regularly, and if gums have been checked recently for sores or irritated areas.

Psychological Assessment

Psychological assessment in AD includes identification of past and present behaviors. Identification of behavior problems is an important component of nursing assessment. This assessment allows the healthcare team to develop a realistic nursing care plan, which includes family education. Behaviors are often responses to environmental cues; the AD patient may be confused by these cues or may easily misinterpret them. The following information includes some common behaviors seen in AD.

AGGRESSION OR AGITATION. Some patients undergo personality changes. A previously mild-mannered person may become loud, begin to curse and swear, and strike out at people. The most common aggressive behavior in community-dwelling patients is verbal abuse, such as hostile language, cursing, or verbal threats.[2] Patients also can be physically aggressive, especially with strangers who have invaded their personal space (eg, healthcare workers). Many hostile behaviors are responses to situations that the confused patient perceives as threatening.

Key Concept

When the confused person says, "I want to go home," do not try to convince him or her that this is his or her home. It is not. You can make statements, such as "You are staying here. You are safe here. It is all paid for."

---

[2] Ryden M. "Aggressive behavior in persons with dementia who live in the community." Alzheimer's Disease and Associated Disorders 2(4): 342-355, 1988.

ANXIETY OR PARANOIA. As patients lose short-term memory and time orientation, they cannot understand what has recently happened and what will happen next. Anxiety may be evidenced by rummaging through drawers, wringing hands, pacing, or displaying worried looks. As things are misplaced, the person may believe they have been stolen. Paranoia may lead to accusing others. Some patients may cover windows and move furniture in front of the door because they are afraid. In nursing facilities, patients may be frightened by simple tasks, such as bathing or the shower, because they cannot understand what is happening.

HALLUCINATIONS AND DELUSIONS. Hallucinations may be misinterpretation of reality (eg, believing that people on television are actually in the room) or they may be visions that the patient believes he or she sees (eg, seeing his or her own reflection and thinking someone else is there or actually having auditory or visual hallucinations). Delusions may cause confused ideas, such as the person's believing that the bank has confiscated all his or her money or that a spouse is going to kill him or her. These symptoms usually are related to organic changes in the brain; trying to reason with the patient does not work.

WITHDRAWAL AND DEPRESSION. In early stages, AD patients who retain insight into their losses may become depressed. Feelings of worthlessness are signs of depression and should be reported to the physician. Suicide (accidental or intentional) is a danger. Some patients respond to antidepressant medications. In many patients, depression seems to lessen spontaneously as the disease progresses and the patient loses insight.

Assessment of Functional Activities of Daily Living

An important part of assessment is determining the patient's ability to carry out basic daily tasks. Components of functional assessment include evaluation of basic ADLs.

DRESSING, BATHING, AND GROOMING. Determine if the patient is able to dress appropriately. Danger signs include soiled clothes worn repeatedly and clothes put on in incorrect sequence (eg, the patient may wear two dresses or underwear on the outside). Determine whether the patient bathes. *Danger signs* include inability to set water temperature or lack of grooming. Assessment includes asking about the ability to shave, comb hair, brush teeth, or use makeup and to ask if these abilities have changed recently. (Solutions for meeting basic ADLs are discussed later in this chapter.)

TOILETING: BOWEL AND BLADDER CONTROL. Evaluate whether the patient is able to remain continent, locate and use the bathroom independently, properly sequence the task, and accomplish basic hygiene practices. If incontinence exists, determine if it can be managed by scheduled toileting.

AMBULATION AND TRANSFER. Does the patient walk without assistance? Can he or she use a cane or walker correctly? *Danger signs* include a history of falls or unsteady gait, wandering off and getting lost, unexplained cuts and bruises, or several falls within the last year.

The family and nursing home also should have a recent photo of the person, in case the person becomes lost and police need to assist in the search. (A photo will help with identification.) A program called "Safe Return" is sponsored by the Alzheimer's Association. For a nominal fee, an ID bracelet and clothing labels are provided.

EATING. Determine whether the patient can use utensils and cut food. If the patient needs to be fed, assess whether he or she is cooperative and can chew and remember to swallow. Danger signs include a history of choking, confusion with utensils, and refusal to eat.

Drugs such as haloperidol (Haldol) can cause urinary retention. Reducing the Haldol dose may help prevent overflow incontinence. Regular toileting is important.

COMMUNICATION SKILLS. Although it varies, language skills are gradually lost as dementia progresses. To assess communication skills, ask if the patient is repeating questions or stories, if he or she is having difficulty finding words or naming objects, and if he or she is making up nonsense words or speaking phrases that do not make sense. Skills deteriorate at different times. For example, some people lose the ability to speak but understand written language; others lose the ability to understand written language early. Music and social skills tend to remain intact until late in the process. Eventually all language skills are lost.

Assessment of Complex or Instrumental Activities of Daily Living

MANAGEMENT OF FINANCES. Find out if the person is able to handle a checkbook, pay bills, and make change. (The demented patient may pay bills more than once or believe they were already paid. He or she may make large contributions to charity because requests look like bills. He or she also may become victims of con artists.) They may hide or lose checks. Danger signs include many unpaid bills, utilities disconnected, or misplacing or donating large amounts of money. (The solution is to have Social Security checks direct deposited; have bills sent to a family member or guardian, or require a cosigner for all checks.)

DRIVING. Determine if the patient is able to drive safely. Is he or she having accidents, getting lost, or trying to get out of a moving car? Danger signs include near misses, accidents, or signs of poor judgment. (The solution is to install door locks controlled by the driver. Request the state to remove the driver's license or have the person retested. In some cases, the person's car must be sold. Vocational rehabilitation and the Veteran's Administration have driving evaluations.)

PUBLIC TRANSPORTATION. Evaluate whether the person can take a bus or train without getting lost, make correct change, and get transfers.

FOOD PREPARATION. Determine whether the patient is able to follow recipes. Check if burners are left on, if there are burned pots or pans, and if food is stored safely. Danger signs include spoiled foods, evidence of fires or burned pans, or hoarding of large amounts of food. (The solution is to contact Meals on Wheels for assistance or disconnect the stove.)

SHOPPING, HOUSEKEEPING, AND LAUNDRY. Determine whether the patient can find items in a store. Has he or she changed from previous patterns of cleaning? Can he or she figure out how to set the washing machine, load detergent, and load clothes? Danger signs include large amounts of the same items in the house, items stored in the wrong place (such as frozen foods in the cupboard), messy home environment (in a previously neat home), washing everything by hand, and soiled clothing in closets or drawers. (The solution is for family members to do or supervise these tasks, or arrange for help through homemaker services.)

TELEPHONE USE. Is the patient able to dial a number, and does he or she know emergency numbers? Danger signs include inability to dial the phone, repeated calls, or calls in the middle of the night to others. (The solution is to keep a list of numbers near the phone. Install a computer dialing device, and have family members or friends call often to check on the patient and caregiver.)

SAFETY IN THE COMMUNITY. Is the patient safe and secure? Determine whether the patient can take measures to ensure his or her own safety. Danger signs include opening doors to strangers, giving strangers or neighbors money, and becoming victims of scams. The person with AD also may be a problem in the neighborhood by walking into other people's houses, or hitchhiking, or requesting money from the neighbors.

Assessment of Support Systems

THE FAMILY. AD and other dementias are overwhelming to the family. Often it is stated that there are two victims: the patient and the family. An important part of assessing the person with dementia includes an understanding of needs of the family or caregiver. Sometimes, the family is not the primary caregiver; instead, a complex network of friends and neighbors may provide necessary supervision or care. Family or caregiver teaching is vital (see accompanying box).

AD has been called the "dementia from which the patient dies twice": first in mind and then in body. Caring for a person with dementia in early stages interferes with a caregiver's recreational time. In later stages, the caregiver spends a majority of time managing the wandering, confused, emotional patient. It is important for

---

Keys to Family Teaching
Provision of a Safe Environment for People with Cognitive Dysfunction

Family teaching to provide safety includes the following:

- Do not allow the person to drive (remove keys, disable car, revoke license).
- Remove guns and ammunition from the house.
- Supervise smoking; lock up supplies; use only ashtrays that will not tip or melt.
- Disable stove or supervise cooking.
- Supervise use of knives and forks; lock up utensils.
- Turn down temperature of water heater.
- Remove dangerous power tools; supervise use of small power tools.
- Supervise use of razors (allow *only* an electric razor) and supervise use of electrical appliances; do not allow appliance use around water; do not allow use of dangerous appliances (food processor, garbage disposal).
- Supervise use of electric fans or air conditioners.
- Lock up all medications, over-the-counter remedies, poisons, paints, cleaning solutions. Make sure primary caregiver knows how and when to administer medications; do not leave with patient to take.
- Supervise use of china and glass dishes to prevent injury from breakage.
- Put a control on thermostat or disable it to prevent the person from constantly adjusting temperature.
- Reduce potential for falls by keeping floors clear of debris (but not highly polished), wipe up spills, do not use throw rugs. Have good railings on stairways. See that the person's shoes fit well. Have halls and stairs well-lighted.
- Install safety locks and buzzers on doors (in case person wanders). Make sure person has identification at all times. Many patients can get through locks and dismantle doors. Fence yard; control access to dangerous areas (swimming pool, beach, highway).
- Keep emergency numbers next to each phone; a preprogrammed phone is a good idea.
- Find a good home for pets, if this person is no longer able to safely care for a pet.

---

caregivers to balance caregiving with activities of their own lives.

FEMALE CAREGIVERS OR AGING CAREGIVERS. Many caregivers are women. Conflicts can arise between demanding roles as caregiver, wife, mother, employee, and homemaker. Spouses of people with dementias are often older themselves and may be unable to handle the physical and psychological demands necessary to manage the constantly increasing level of care needed.

SUPPORT GROUPS.   Support groups for families of patients with AD and other dementias are available. The most prominent is the Alzheimer's Disease and Related Disorders Association, Inc.

Support for patients and family members can be obtained from many areas. The nurse must first identify needs and then be open to adaptations for individual situations. Some needs are educational; for example, what does the family need to know to care for the patient? Practical solutions, such as transportation assistance, legal assistance, insurance and Medicare advice, medical equipment, and meal service are available in most locations. The family as a unit may need counseling because the situation is overwhelming.

RESPITE CARE.   Respite for the family is vital. The patient is cared for by others, so caregivers can have some time to themselves. They need a respite from the constant responsibility of caring for their loved one. A resource for families is called "Homes of Help," sponsored by the Alzheimer's Association.

Assisting With Daily Care

BATHING.   Bathing is frightening in dementia. The following are nursing hints: Be calm. Give the bath at the patient's preferred time. (A rested patient is more cooperative than an overtired patient.) Use low water levels, and have everything prepared before the patient gets in the bathtub. Avoid the noise and confusion of a whirlpool or shower with an easily agitated patient. Pad the walls to reduce echoing (overstimulation). Use positive reinforcement ("You look so handsome"). Use gestures; do not shout to be heard.

DRESSING.   Dressing becomes complicated in dementia. The following are nursing hints: Lay out clean clothes, and remove dirty clothes (to prevent confusion). Offer clothing in sequence; do not give verbal commands at the same time (it is confusing). Use simple clothing (Velcro, elastic waistbands). Suggest using cardigan type shirts or blouses rather than those put on over the head (covering the head is frightening). The person may not be able to manage buttons without help.

PAIN CONTROL.   Pain control is important because many demented people have pain but cannot find the words to express it. Older people often have arthritis or other physical disorders. Give aspirin or other pain medications before doing nursing care, such as bathing or dressing.

NUTRITION AND HYDRATION.   Nutrition and hydration must be maintained. As people age, the sense of thirst becomes less acute. Many older people tend to forget to drink or eat. The following are nursing hints: Offer a small amount of fluid each time you interact; include liquids in all activities. Vary the choices; do not give plain water all the time. Avoid very hot liquids (people with poor judgment are easily burned). Limit the variety of foods to prevent confusion. Cut meats to appropriate sizes to prevent choking. Place patients near people they should mimic. If the patient is fed, place the spoon (forks may be dangerous) in the patient's hand to help him or her understand. Give finger foods if the person cannot manage the utensil.

> **Nursing Alert**
>
> Monitor the person's weight. If weight loss is evident, the person is probably forgetting to eat. Agitation and pacing also take a great deal of energy. Remind the person to chew and swallow. Observe for choking.

The person living at home is in danger from the stove. Gas is particularly dangerous. Remove the knobs or install a master shut-off for either electric or gas stoves.

BLADDER AND BOWEL MANAGEMENT.   Bladder and bowel management becomes a necessity because incontinence is common in later stages. The following are nursing hints: Daytime incontinence can often be avoided by regular toileting. Label the bathroom; give one-step instructions, and make each instruction simple, with one activity identified for each instruction. ("Come with me. Pull down your pants. Sit down.") Families need education in the use of incontinence products at home. Document bowel movements; be alert for constipation or impaction. If the patient develops diarrhea, check for lactose intolerance, constipation, or drug reactions. Blood electrolyte levels may be ordered if diarrhea continues.

> **Nursing Alert**
>
> It is important to increase fluids in the demented person to prevent urinary tract infections and allow the bladder (which is a muscle) to contract properly. Some drugs promote urinary retention; therefore, the patient taking these medications should be monitored closely. Check for edema; assess skin turgor.

SAFETY.   Safety is important in the home and health-care facility. Some safety measures have been described previously.

Nursing Diagnosis

A number of nursing diagnoses for the patient, family, or caregiver may result from information gathered on the database. Examples of some nursing diagnoses that may be seen on nursing care plans for the patient with dementia include the following.

♦ Bowel Incontinence; Constipation; or Diarrhea
♦ Impaired Verbal Communication
♦ Disabling, Ineffective Family Coping
♦ Hopelessness
♦ High Risk for Injury (falls, wandering away)
♦ Knowledge Deficit regarding disease and its treatment
♦ Self-care Deficit (ADLs)
♦ Altered Urinary Elimination

Planning and Implementation

Nursing management of the person with AD includes an understanding of basic communication and behavior management techniques. Nurses can teach caregivers and serve as role models. Assisting the patient to perform ADLs will be a major action of the nurse. Special skills in communication are used and can be taught to the family and caregiver. A routine that is followed daily helps the person with AD adjust in behavior. The family and caregiver need a great deal of support. The nurse should listen to their concerns and be aware of problems that are arising. The accompanying nursing care plan gives examples of how some nursing diagnoses may be addressed and implemented by the nurse who is caring for a patient with AD.

Assisting With Communication

The nurse uses all the communication skills he or she has learned. The accompanying box gives skills specific to caring for a person with dementia.

Your verbal and nonverbal communication has a great influence on how that person will act. If you remain calm, this will have a calming effect on the patient. If you are quiet and gentle, the person will be more likely to cooperate with you. However, do not forget that if you are agitated and rushed, the patient will likely become upset and belligerent.

Assisting With Behavior Management

ANXIETY. Anxiety is common in dementia patients. Often, they acquire frustrating behaviors, which help them to feel more in control. These behaviors include pacing or rummaging through closets or drawers. The following are nursing hints: Reassure the person. Keep commands simple, and reward successes. Work in small groups, and encourage family members to visit one or two at a time. Keep the environment and daily

---

Nursing Skill Guidelines
Communicating With the Person Who Has Dementia

♦ Identify yourself—do not make the patient guess; he or she may not be able to read your name tag.
♦ Tell the person what you are going to do in simple language.
♦ Maintain direct eye contact. (The person can often respond to nonverbal cues after speech is lost.) Stay at the patient's eye level. If the person is in a wheelchair, kneel or sit.
♦ Use a low-pitched voice; speak slowly. (The patient will mirror an angry or tense tone of voice.)
♦ Eliminate background noise. (Avoid overstimulating the confused patient; make sure he or she can hear you.)
♦ Use short, simple sentences; give one-step commands.
♦ Avoid using questions, such as "Why did you . . . ?" or "What do you want?" (These require complex reasoning and memory.)
♦ Label the environment if the patient can read ("John's closet," "bathroom").
♦ Give the person "reassurance cards" ("Your wife is coming at 3 PM"). The patient can refer to these cards if anxious.
♦ Post a simple daily schedule to structure the day. Post the day and date. Have a clock visible.
♦ Be aware of nonverbal language: smile, nod your head, approach the patient from the front, avoid restraining the person, gently touch the person (unless this is frightening to him or her).
♦ Use gestures, such as waving goodbye.

---

routines consistent; assign the same caregivers daily. Allow the person to move around. (This helps reduce anxiety.) Eliminate caffeine and limit sugar in the diet. Avoid overstimulation.

BALKING. Balking, refusal to do things, often occurs when the patient does not understand what is expected. The following are nursing hints: Go away briefly, and come back later with a pleasant tone of voice. Model expected behavior, or have the patient mimic others (eg, eating at a table with others).

PARANOIA. Paranoia or fearfulness is common. The following are nursing hints: Keep the environment calm and predictable; remove excess stimulation. Medications may be helpful. Do not try to reason with the person, but reassure the person that he or she is safe.

AGGRESSIVENESS. Aggressiveness can be physical (striking out), verbal (name calling, cursing), or sexual. The following are nursing hints: Use a calm approach.

Do not confront or try to reason with the patient; scolding aggravates aggressiveness. If necessary, remove the person from the group (to avoid upsetting other patients). Validate feelings ("You seem angry or frightened"). Give reassurance ("You are safe"). If the person was striking out because you were performing nursing care, go away temporarily; allow the person to calm down, and then return. Remember that your tone of voice can either calm or aggravate the patient.

Assisting Caregivers

Social scientist Pauline Boss has coined the term **ambiguous loss** to describe the "debilitating confusion (of the family) about whether their living loved one is still with them or is gone." The patient is "physically present, but psychologically absent." Boss feels that ambiguous loss is the main source of stress for caregivers of AD patients. The reason for this is that "the patient is unable to emotionally interact with—or later even to recognize—the caregiver."[3]

RESPITE CARE. Caregivers of AD patients need breaks to maintain their own mental and physical health. Community alternatives exist, including senior volunteers, home health services, and adult day care. (The patient may live at home and go to adult day care.) Sometimes caregivers feel guilty about not providing care or assistance or cannot afford to provide it. A referral to social service may be needed. Caregivers may be willing to try a supplemental service on a temporary basis. Once they find how helpful it is, they may be less reluctant to seek help in the future.

[3] Alzheimer's and the family: Scientist studies how people cope with "loss" of living loved-one. News, University of Minnesota, College of Home Economics, August/September 1988.

SUPPORT AND EDUCATION. The healthcare team helps with a plan for the family. Document all teaching. The Alzheimer's Association has a newsletter for caregivers and professionals and support groups throughout the United States that are helpful to caregivers. They provide education and group support.

FAMILY DYNAMICS. Boss, cited previously, states that the family must be assisted to go through a "premature grieving process." The person they knew is really gone, and a childlike person has replaced their loved one. The family needs assistance in some areas:

◆ *Identify problems,* and realize the ambiguity of the situation. (The adult is now like a child; the decision-maker is no longer able to make decisions.)
◆ *Validate their perceptions.* (Verify their feelings and perceptions to make sure they correctly understand the situation.)
◆ *Clarify* their perceptions and feelings (to make sure you understand how they are feeling).
◆ *Devise solutions* with the family to problems presented.
◆ *Test* your solutions.
◆ *Evaluate,* reassess, and revise the care plan.

This procedure parallels the nursing process.

Nursing Alert

Someone should be enlisted to check on the primary caregiver of the demented person, particularly if the caregiver also is an older person. A neighbor or relative should call at least twice a day to make sure everything is alright. Otherwise, if something happens to the primary caregiver, the demented person may not know what to do.

Keys For Review

Key Questions for Critical Thinking

1. Compare primary and secondary dementias. Give examples of each. Discuss prognosis and treatment of each.
2. List three changes that occur in the brain cells in the person with AD. Discuss how they are caused and the results of these changes.
3. List at least three characteristics of each of the four stages of AD. Identify nursing care and teaching needed for each.

Key Questions for Critical Thinking
(continued)

4. Differentiate between functional and instrumental ADLs.
5. Describe teaching points for the caregiver who must maintain the safety of a person with AD.

Key Readings

Barry PD. Mental Health and Mental Illness, Ed 5. Philadelphia, J.B. Lippincott, 1994

Birchenall JM, Streight ME. Care of the Older Adult, Ed 3. Philadelphia, J.B. Lippincott, 1993

Carnevali DL. Nursing Management for the Elderly, Ed 3. Philadelphia, J.B. Lippincott, 1992

Erickson EH. The life Cycle Completed. New York, Norton, 1982

Hogstel MO. Nursing Care of the Older Adult, Ed 3. Albany, NY, Delmar, 1993

Murray R, Zentner J. Nursing Assessment and Health promotion Strategies Through the Life Span. East Norwalk, CT, Appleton & Lange, 1993

Nussbaum JF. Communications and Aging. New York, Harper Collins College, 1990

Shives LR. Basic Concepts of Psychiatric-Mental Health Nursing, Ed 3. Philadelphia, J.B. Lippincott, 1994

Enrichment Keys

Atchley RC Social Forces and Aging: An Introduction to Social Gerontology, Belmont, CA, Wadsworth Publishing, 1991

"Geriatric update '94." Nursing '94, 24(3): 59-61, March 1994

Keys to Learning More

Chapter 87: psychiatric disorders
Chapter 88: substance abuse and interventions
Chapter 89: rehabilitation techniques
Chapters 90–91: dying and hospice nursing

Key Resources

Alzheimer's Disease and Related Disorders Association, Inc.
  70 East Lake Street
  Chicago, IL 60601-5997
Alzheimer's Association
  919 N. Michigan Ave., Suite 1000
  Chicago, IL 60611
Alzheimer's Disease Education and Referral Center (A Service of the National Institute on the Aging)
  PO Box 8250
  Silver Spring, MD 20907-8250
National Alzheimer's toll free referral and information service
  1-800-272-3900 (Monday–Friday)

Unit *16* Meeting Special Needs

87 Mental Health and Psychiatric Nursing

Keys for Learning

Learning Objectives

- Define terms relating to mental health and its deviations.
- Describe inpatient and outpatient facilities.
- Describe tardive dyskenesia and its relationship to antipsychotic medications.
- Discuss patient rights in mental health.
- Explore approaches to dealing with the aggressive patient and related nursing care.
- Describe nursing process in the psychiatric setting.
- Discuss nursing responsibilities working with overactive, withdrawn, depressed, hypomanic, regressed, or self-injuring patients.
- Define nursing care of the long-term patient in a mental health unit.

Key Terms

anxiety
delusions
dysthymia
hallucinations
hypomanic
hysteria
labile
milieu
psychiatrist
psychologist
psychosis
reactive disorder
regression

Keys to Understanding This Chapter

Chapter 4: legal and ethical aspects
Chapter 5: basic needs
Chapter 7: community health
Unit Three: development of the individual
Chapter 36: therapeutic communication
Chapter 37: documentation and reporting
Chapter 38: signs and symptoms of illness
Chapter 39: transcultural considerations
Chapter 56: classifications of medicines
Chapter 67: the person with special needs

Keys to Understanding This Chapter
(continued)

Chapter 71: nervous system disorders
Chapter 78: HIV and AIDS
Chapter 86: Alzheimer's disease and dementias

Key Points

- The patient must always be treated with respect and kindness.
- People on mental health units have the same rights as any other patient.
- Occasionally, for his or her own safety or the safety of others, a court order will supersede a patient's wishes.
- The patient must be protected from injury and from injuring other patients or staff.
- People may be brought to the mental health unit because they are dangerous to themselves or to others.
- Medications given in psychiatry often have unpleasant side effects but are taken because the person wishes to control the disorder.
- With the use of medications, many psychiatric patients are now able to live outside the hospital setting.
- The nurse must be careful with the use of restraints to avoid injuring the patient or the staff.
- If a patient is unable to perform activities of daily living independently, the nurse should assist.
- Patients on the mental health unit are considered vulnerable adults.

Key Topics Outline

Mental Health Versus Mental Illness
  Mental Health
  Mental Illness
  Diagnostic and Statistical Manual, Fourth Edition
Psychiatric-Mental Health Practice
  The Mental Healthcare Team
  Treatment Centers and Resources
  Methods of Psychiatric Therapy

Key Learning Activities

♦ Interview a psychiatric nurse. What type of patients are seen most often in his or her unit? What special workshops or training has the nurse had? What suggestions would this nurse make for people considering working in psychiatric nursing?

Key Learning Activities (continued)

♦ Make a list of mental health resources in your community. They may be for evaluation, therapy, or support.
♦ Visit a state or county psychiatric hospital. Observe the patients. Observe security and activities.
♦ Interview a nurse who works in a medical–surgical area. What type of mental health problems does he or she see there?
♦ Visit a group home. What services and facilities are present or absent in the community?

Basic principles of mental health nursing apply to the care of *any patient.* There are psychological aspects inherent in any illness, and *all patients* have basic needs that must be met, whether they are in the mental health unit or not. Many patients with physical illnesses also have emotional or psychiatric problems; often these problems interfere with or influence recovery.

If a mental health problem is present, it does not necessarily mean that a patient needs care in a mental health unit, but it may mean that the stress and influence it has on the body are having a definite effect on the patient's progress toward recovery. If the result is erratic or dangerous behavior, the person's mental health (and possibly, the safety of others) is threatened. To help the person with a mental health problem, the nurse must first understand what mental health is.

Mental Health Versus Mental Illness

Mental Health

There are many definitions of mental health. The World Health Organization's definition of mental health is "a state of physical and mental well-being." Following are other definitions of a mentally healthy person:

♦ One who is responsible for his or her own behavior
♦ One who is able to adjust to new situations and handle personal problems without severe discomfort yet who still has enough energy to be a constructive member of society
♦ One who has intellectual insight into his or her strengths and weaknesses; the person is able to accept weaknesses and use strengths positively
♦ One who is able to accept frustration without re-

sorting to harmful, self-defeating, or endangering behaviors

Mental Illness

Mental illness is a difference in *degree* of behavior, rather than a distinct difference in behavior. We all have some feelings or behaviors that we must learn to control or handle. To deal with stress, people react in certain ways. In the early 1900s, Sigmund Freud named these methods of reacting *defense mechanisms.* Defense mechanisms can be used to resolve a mental conflict, reduce **anxiety** or fear, protect one's self-esteem, or protect one's sense of security. Common examples of defense mechanisms include suppression, repression, rationalization, reaction-formation, displacement, denial, projection, sublimation, and intellectualization. We all use defense mechanisms; it is when they are used to *extreme* that they threaten mental health.

Key Concept

Be aware of your own feelings and reactions. Correct those that are detrimental to delivery of good nursing care. At the same time, recognize the use of defense mechanisms in your patients, so you can plan nursing care to be most effective.

In certain instances, the following behavior patterns may be interpreted as symptoms of a mental disorder:

♦ Sudden change in behavior, such as deep depression or inappropriate overexcitement
♦ Sudden lack of concern about appearance
♦ Physical symptoms, without apparent medically related cause

♦ Overuse of mental defense mechanisms or use of defense mechanisms to an inappropriate degree
♦ Overdependency on drugs or other medications
♦ Loss of contact with reality
♦ Morbid fascination with death or talk of wanting to die or of committing suicide

Diagnostic and Statistical Manual, Fourth Edition

When making a medical diagnosis about a psychiatric problem, the physician uses a specific taxonomy from the *Diagnostic and Statistical Manual,* fourth edition (DSM-IV) of the American Psychiatric Association. This taxonomy is a system consisting of five axes. Each axis addresses a specific category and includes criteria that, when combined, allow the physician to develop a complete psychiatric diagnosis. The multiaxial system is listed in the box.

The person who is hospitalized because of a marked deviation from normal behavior should be assisted in managing his or her feelings so that behavior becomes socially acceptable and nonthreatening again. The goal is to help the person to function effectively and safely outside the hospital.

Degrees of Mental Illness

Mental illness varies considerably in degree or intensity. Clinical diagnosis often is stated as mild, moderate, severe, in partial or full remission, or as prior history. There are certain broad psychiatric diagnoses that the nurse should understand.

Reactive Disorders. Some minor abnormalities that do not completely incapacitate a person are classified as **reactive disorders**, the symptoms of which seem to be connected to anxiety and an inability to develop effective coping skills to deal with life situations. However, because this person often suffers acutely, these should be classified as actual illnesses. Common reactive disorders follow:

♦ **Dysthymia:** depressed mood, decreased interest in life, appetite and sleep changes
♦ **Hysteria:** lack of emotional control or actions (sometimes called *somatization disorder*)
♦ **Phobias:** unreasonable fear of generally harmless things

Personality Disorders. All of us have certain personality traits that define and mold our personalities. When a trait becomes dysfunctional, it can lead to problems with mental health. Common personality disorders follow:

♦ *Obsessive/compulsive disorders:* recurrent thoughts about something, with an irresistible urge to act in a certain way

The Multiaxial System of Psychiatric Diagnoses

Axis I	Clinical syndromes
Axis II	Personality disorders or developmental disorders
Axis III	Physical disorders and conditions
Axis IV	Psychosocial stressors
Axis V	Highest level of adaptive functioning

♦ *Antisocial disorder:* disregard for rights of others, interest only in pleasing self, no remorse for action
♦ *Borderline personality disorder:* pattern of unstable or intense relationships, impulsivity, inappropriate anger, depression; display of self-destructive or self-injurious behavior
♦ *Lack of impulse control:* compulsive gambling, stealing, substance abuse, inappropriate sexual conduct, violence

Mood Disorders. Everyone has a depressed or elated mood occasionally, but when a mood change lasts for a long time and renders the person incapable of total functioning, the condition is known as a mood disorder. An estimated 20 million people in the United States have severe depression. Over the life span, a person's chances of requiring medical treatment for depression are one in four. Clinical depression alters sleep and eating habits and is often accompanied by *somatic* (physical) complaints. Frequently, clinical depression shows a familial pattern, much like diabetes or heart disease. Common mood disorders follow:

♦ *Major depression disorder:* lengthy, depressed mood; weight changes; severe lack of interest or joy in life; severe sleep difficulties (often includes suicidal ideation)
♦ *Bipolar affective disorder:* mood swings, characterized by broad variations in mood from extreme elation to mania to severe, incapacitating depression (**labile** behavior)

Psychosis. Marked deviations from normal behavior and seriously inappropriate conduct usually indicate a psychosis. A **psychosis** is a thought disorder. The psychotic person has poor contact with reality and frequently is disoriented (unable to identify time, place, or people). In psychosis, behavior is unusual, and thinking processes are disturbed. A psychosis can result from a physical cause and is called *organic* (syphilis, brain tumor, infection), or it can be *functional,* in which there is no identifiable physical cause. Common psychoses follow:

◆ *Toxic psychoses:* caused by consumption of alcohol or certain drugs or chemicals (eg, lead, poisons). This is an example of an *organic brain syndrome* or disorder that can be traced to a physical cause.

◆ *Paranoia:* characterized by a well-organized system of **delusions** (false beliefs) about persecution, grandeur, or both. These patients can become very dangerous to others.

◆ *Schizophrenia:* a group of disorders in which there is marked deviation from knowing what is real and what is not. The person may have various accompanying disturbances, including *affective* disturbances (showing no emotion); *behavioral* disturbances (acting in bizarre ways); and *intellectual* disorders (hallucinations—hearing or seeing things that are not there).

◆ *Disruptions related to aging:* more common in seniors or related to the physiologic changes associated with aging, age-associated memory impairment (dementia, Alzheimer's disease, Pick's disease) (see Chapter 86)

Psychiatric-Mental Health Practice

The Mental Healthcare Team

The Physician or Psychiatrist. A **psychiatrist** is a physician who has received special training in treatment of mental disorders. However, physicians usually use a holistic approach to patients and consider mental, phys-

ical, and emotional aspects. Psychiatric difficulties can arise from a person's everyday problems, external conditions, or actual brain disorders. The physician is ultimately responsible for care of the total patient, in addition to coordinating efforts of other members of the healthcare team.

The Nurse. The nurse functions as a member of the mental health team. By creating a therapeutic environment, the nurse assists people, whether inpatients or outpatients, to return to as nearly normal functioning as possible in the shortest time. The nurse must adopt a holistic approach to patients while maintaining an awareness of patient rights. The RN can receive special certification in Psychiatric and Mental Health Nursing.

Other Team Members. Many people are involved in assisting the person experiencing a threat to his or her mental health. The psychiatric technician, mental health worker, or human service worker deals directly with people on the mental health unit. The psychologist is not a physician, although he or she usually has a PhD in psychology. The psychologist provides the patient with psychological testing and counseling or therapy. The occupational therapist, recreational therapist, and music therapist provide diversionary activities, instruction in activities of daily living (ADLs), and job retraining or employment skills. Vocational rehabilitation teachers and veteran's services are often available to make it possible for the person to attend school. The social worker prepares and assists people to plan for

Key Abbreviations and Acronyms for Mental Health Issues

AAMI	Age-associated memory impairment	NOS	Not otherwise specified
AP	Assault precautions (attack)	OBD	Organic brain disorder
AWOL	Absent without leave	OBS	Organic brain syndrome
BPAD	Bipolar affective disorder	OD	Overdose
CD	Chemical dependency	OCD	Obsessive–compulsive disorder
ECT	Electroconvulsive therapy	S/A	Suicide attempt
EP	Escape precautions (elopement)	S/G	Suicide gesture
EPSE	Extrapyramidal side effects	SP or GP	Suicide precautions, general precautions
ETOH W/D	Alcohol withdrawal		
HI	Homicidal ideation	SI	Suicidal ideation
II	Intellectually impaired	SIB	Self-injurious behavior
MDD	Major depressive disorder	S/M	Sadomasochism
MI	Mental illness	SX	Sexual precautions
MI-CD	Mentally ill and chemically dependent	SZ P	Seizure precautions
MI & D	Mentally ill and dangerous	TD	Tardive dyskinesia
MH	Mental health	TR	Therapeutic recreation
MPD	Multiple personality disorder	Vol	Voluntarily admitted

These are examples. They may differ slightly in your area.

discharge and is usually the liaison with interested family members or friends. The social worker may be involved in finding a place for the person to live or obtaining financial assistance for the person.

Treatment Centers and Resources

Mental illness is recognized as being like any other illness; people go to hospitals voluntarily for treatment, just as they might go to a general hospital for an appendectomy. Early hospitalization helps prevent escalation of the illness because the person is removed from emotional stress often found in daily life. In such instances, the hospital provides a more suitable, healthy, and safe environment.

In many cases, hospitalization is not necessary. A person with minor disruptions in mental health may go to an outpatient clinic for treatment. Some psychiatric hospitals have established a service whereby a patient may spend nights at the hospital and carry on a regular job in the daytime. This plan assures the person of needed treatment and removes him or her from a possibly disturbing home environment. In other cases, the person lives at home and attends a day treatment center. Certainly, people who are potentially dangerous to themselves or others must be hospitalized.

Changing attitudes toward mental illness and the development of effective psychotropic drugs have encouraged community hospitals to provide treatment and care for patients with mental health problems.

Third-party payors (insurance companies and health maintenance organizations) sometimes cover the cost of mental healthcare, including the cost of care related to chemical dependency. However, the requirements for inpatient care are becoming more stringent. The inpatient hospital stay is usually short, covering the crisis period only. After discharge, the person is followed on an outpatient basis and often lives in a halfway house or board-and-care home. If a person requires long-term hospitalization, this is often at a state facility.

Emergency Services

Many hospitals and medical centers offer special emergency services to people with disruptions in mental health.

Mental Health Clinic. The emergency mental health clinic or crisis center is part of the hospital's emergency unit. People who reach a point where anything and everything is beyond their coping ability may come to this clinic where they can find assistance. Treatment may include prescribing antidepressants, suggesting a stay in the hospital's mental health unit, or advising periodic visits to a mental health clinic.

The outpatient mental health clinic or community clinic provides ongoing therapy for people who do not need to be hospitalized. Home visits may be included.

Telephone Services. Telephone services are available for people to call and talk to a trained person about problems. Telephone services have proven particularly effective in crisis intervention, such as suicide prevention, drug counseling, and rape counseling. The advantages of the telephone service are its immediate accessibility any time of the day or night and anonymity if the caller does not wish to reveal his or her identity.

Acute Care Mental Health Centers

If a person cannot be helped on an outpatient basis, he or she may be admitted to a mental health unit of a hospital. The terms of admission to a mental health facility vary among states and provinces or even within a state or province. There are several types of admission:

- *Voluntary* admission ("vol")
- *Emergency hold*, placed by a physician, for 72 hours for evaluation of the patient who is dangerous to himself or herself or others ("72 h hold, 72° hold")
- *Transportation hold*, placed by the police, to bring the person to the hospital ("T-Hold")
- *District court hold*, placed by a judge after a preliminary commitment hearing (DCH)
- *Assessment hold* placed by the court to assess a person to determine if they are competent to stand trial for a crime
- Court *commitment* (usually to a state, veteran's administration, or county hospital) for treatment
- *Mentally ill and dangerous*, commitment to a security hospital (*MI&D*)

Although many state hospitals admit people voluntarily, sometimes for special treatment (such as chemical dependency), more people are admitted involuntarily (commitment). Commitment is done through the court system and often follows a lengthy hospitalization in a private or county facility. Many patients in state hospitals are supported by public funds.

Discharge. It is in the interest of the patient and the hospital to prepare the person for discharge as soon as possible. However, the hospital cannot ignore certain responsibilities in this respect. The person and the community must have reasonable security. No one can be absolutely certain whether or not a person will have a relapse, yet everything possible must be done to help him or her adjust on discharge.

The care and treatment of the convalescent person should be planned, keeping the goal of discharge and recovery in mind. Convalescence should be thought of as a new beginning, and the former patient should be encouraged to live as normal and healthy a life as possible. The aim is to involve the person in normal activities that can lead to normal adjustment.

The nursing care plan is designed to prepare the person for discharge. From the moment he or she is admitted, each person should be encouraged to be as independent as possible. Chronically mentally ill people often are discharged to a board-and-care home, halfway house, foster home, or group home.

Chronic Patients in Continued Treatment Services

Mental health institutions of the state hospital type have patients classified in the continued treatment group, although many of these people are discharged into the community. These people have passed the acute stages of illness with little improvement. They still may be confused. Some have senile dementia; some who have been able to respond fairly well to life within the hospital have difficulty adjusting to the outside world. Various programs are available to assist them.

Community Resources

Many community resources are available to help the person who is discharged from the mental health unit or hospital. The nurse and social worker should be aware of these resources so that he or she may offer assistance in providing proper referrals.

Day Clinics. Often a person will benefit from living at home in the evening and coming into the clinic during the day. Activities for the patient include therapy groups, occupational therapy, and recreational therapy. Patients also are taught about their medications.

Respite Care. If the person is difficult or confused, he or she may be placed in an inpatient setting for a few days to give the family some time to themselves and allow them the chance to regroup. This is called *respite care*; it gives the family a respite, or break, from the responsibilities of living with a person with chronic mental health problems.

Outpatient and Community Mental Health Centers. Many people receive counseling from a mental health center on a daily or weekly basis or less often if they wish. They receive guidance that helps them meet the demands of life so that they can function normally on their own the rest of the time. In the case of chemically dependent people, group therapy after discharge from the acute treatment center is vital and often continues for some time.

Halfway Houses and Sheltered Workshops. A person may be able to function outside the formal hospital setting if a semistructured living setting is available. In other instances, the work situation also is included. The halfway house and sheltered workshop act as stepping stones that allow the person to make the transition from the hospital to the everyday world gradually.

Vocational Rehabilitation. The discharged person must become as self-supporting as possible. He or she may need to be vocationally retrained to get a job. Many agencies evaluate, train, and find employment for such people. They also may need to encourage employers to hire people who have been discharged from a mental health unit. If people are to successfully put illnesses behind them, they need encouragement. To help in this endeavor, the employer should be encouraged to work closely with the vocational rehabilitation counselor.

Methods of Psychiatric Therapy

The goal of all therapy is to alleviate or modify the behavior of the person so that he or she will be able to better meet the demands of life and return to their individual optimum level of wellness. Therapy is based on the specific behavior problems and the person's needs in meeting ADLs. Because the therapist and nurse follow many of the same guidelines, the nurse must be aware of the therapeutic goals so that the therapy can be incorporated in nursing care. The therapies discussed below are of specific value in dealing with certain types of behavior.

Individual Psychotherapy. Individual psychotherapy depends of the personal relationship between patient and therapist. The aim of psychotherapy is to relieve symptoms and eventually resolve the disabling conflicts that caused the symptoms. Treatment encourages the person to tell his or her story, discuss problems, and devise ways of dealing with issues with an impartial advisor. Hypnosis and psychoanalysis are among the methods that may be used to achieve this end.

Group Psychotherapy. Group psychotherapy involves more than one patient and provides an opportunity for everyone to participate in discussing individual problems. Thus, the person is able to focus outside of himself or herself by becoming concerned about another person. He or she is drawn out of the private world to become a part of the larger world. The patients often have keen insight into their own behavior and the behavior of others, and they can express feelings and confront others about their behavior. Patients are often more likely to accept suggestions and constructive criticism from other patients than from hospital staff. Group therapy is especially effective for dealing with addictive behaviors and for grief counseling.

Behavior Modification. Also known as *behavior shaping,* this method is used to deal with emotionally disturbed patients and mentally disabled children and adolescents. It is based on the theory that when a person receives a *positive* reward for a task well done, this will reinforce wanting to perform that activity again to win another reward. To be effective, the task or behavior expected of the person must be geared to his or her ability so that success can be achieved.

An effective form of positive reinforcement is food or other forms of physical gratification, although almost any other reward can be reinforcing if used correctly. What is rewarding to one patient may not necessarily be rewarding to another.

Negative reinforcement (punishment) is not effective because it does not promote positive behavior. It does not inform the person of what to do, only what *not* to do. Thus, it is much more effective to reward good behavior and ignore bad behavior.

When using this method, you should show the person what you want to be accomplished, help them accomplish it, then reward him or her for a job well done. The reward is most effective if given immediately. Gradually let the person assume more responsibility for doing the task alone. Consistency is important.

> **Key Concept**
>
> Giving attention to a person is a powerful modifier of behavior.

Remotivation. Many mental health and geriatric units use a special method called remotivation technique or *reality orientation* to reorient people to reality. Patients are placed in a group situation structured so they can discuss things that are meaningful to them. To stimulate conversation, such things as poems or scrapbooks filled with pictures of familiar items can be helpful. (Newspapers or pictures of recent events can spur a discussion.)

Everyone is included in the discussion, and all are encouraged to participate. The method and direction of the discussion are based on the abilities of the group at hand. For example, in a group of severely regressed people, the discussion would be simple, and the leader would need to ask many questions to maintain a discussion.

> **Key Concept**
>
> Everyone needs to know *who* they are, *where* they are, who *other people* are, and *what day* it is to be comfortable.

Reality Therapy. The goal of reality therapy is to help a person face reality, reject irresponsible behavior, and learn new and more socially acceptable ways of behaving. Every person has a need to love and be loved and to feel worthwhile as a human being to himself or her-

self (*self-esteem*) and to others (*acceptance*). If a person is unable to meet these needs in a socially acceptable way, he or she may act inappropriately. Reality therapy attempts to get the patient to meet the demands of life and meet individual needs within the framework of reality and within the context of what is considered acceptable behavior.

Reality therapy does not necessarily accept the traditional approach to mental illness. It differs from conventional psychotherapy by concentrating on the present, rather than on what happened in the past. It is not as important to understand the reasons *why* a person thinks and acts in a certain way; it is important to help him or her understand and solve immediate problems or deal with *behaviors*. The reality therapist deals with *behaviors* as they occur rather than examining feelings or underlying causes.

Transactional Analysis. All interactions between people have meaning and are based on the way the people involved feel at the moment. The goal of transactional analysis is to teach people to react in ways that will produce positive responses in other people rather than hostile ones.

Transactional analysis is based on the concept that all people react, at different times, as either the *child,* the *parent,* or the *adult.* At any particular time, one of the three predominates. Two of these, parent and child, are actually from your past. As a parent, you will often react as your own parents did, and as child, you will often react as you did when you were a child. The goal is to react like a *reasonable adult* in as many situations as possible.

Electroconvulsive Therapy. Electroconvulsive therapy (ECT), also referred to as electroshock therapy, causes a seizure by sending an electric current through the brain. In some unexplained way, this treatment improves the emotional condition of the person. A convulsant drug also can be given intravenously to cause a seizure. It is believed that the seizure affects the level of neurotransmitters in the brain, which affects the person's mood and thoughts.

Current practice tends to restrict the use of ECT to a limited group of patients. It is most commonly used to treat depression in middle-aged and older patients. When successful, ECT can radically alter a person's behavior. The disadvantage of this type of therapy is the person's fear before the treatment and the brief period of intense anxiety and distress between the moment of administration of the premedication and loss of consciousness.

Routine preoperative preparations are carried out. The procedure is often done in the recovery room (PAR). Make sure the person voids before the treatment because incontinence is common. Explain what will happen during the procedure. Make sure the person understands that respiration will be supported, and he or she will not suffocate. This is a common fear. Prevent injury during and after the treatment. Report deviations. Monitor vital signs and allow the person to sleep after the treatment.

The person may be given a cognitive task or test before and after ECT to determine and assess any deterioration of brain function.

One-to-One Therapy. The one-to-one setting provides a therapeutic relationship that is nonthreatening to most people. Patients are encouraged to express concerns and feelings and to indicate how staff can be most helpful. Many people are willing to reveal thoughts and feelings on a one-to-one basis that they would not have the courage to share in group setting. Guidelines for therapeutic communication are detailed in Chapter 36.

Psychodrama. The use of role playing or acting out one's feelings offers many people, especially children and adolescents, an opportunity to release emotions. Many people are able to act out situations in their lives that they are not able to verbalize, such as relationships with a spouse or parents. Close observation of the psychodrama enables staff to plan the most effective measures for treatment and nursing care for each person.

Occupational Therapy. Not only is occupational therapy highly therapeutic, it also acts as a source of enjoyment and gratification for many people. They are able to become active in creative projects, such as arts and crafts, while having the opportunity to socialize with staff or other patients who are working on cooperative projects. Through the creative process, the depressed person has the pleasure of seeing the results of his or her own efforts and gains a sense of success. The overactive person is able to release some energy while working on a project. The occupational therapy department also evaluates concentration ability, the ability to plan, and provides vocational guidance and rehabilitation in many hospitals.

Recreational Therapy. Through planned recreational activities, the person in a mental health unit is helped to reenter the outside world. A group of people may go bowling, to a movie, or out to eat. In this way, they can begin to adapt to normal activities of life, gradually becoming reaccustomed to interacting with society.

Music Therapy. Music is a universal language. Because many nonverbal people enjoy music, they will often enthusiastically join in by playing a rhythm instrument. In this way, the person is helped to become communicative and develop social skills with others without

being forced to speak. Music also is a great source of gratification and fun.

Pet Therapy. Many hospitals and nursing homes are having immense success with the use of animals (Fig. 87-1). Even the most regressed person will usually respond positively to a kitten or puppy. It is often easier for a person with an emotional disturbance to relate first to an animal, which does not impose as much threat as another person. This will prepare a person for human interaction in the future.

Play Therapy. There are two types of play therapy. The first is used to assist children with disruptions in mental health. All children need to play; it is a part of the maturation process. However, some children who are severely disturbed are unable to play. The play therapist guides the behavior of these young patients, slowly helping them to socialize with others and adjust to the outside world. The therapist also can learn about the child and origins of the mental disorder by observing his or her play.

The second type of play therapy is used with adults. One example is the "new games" approach. Games are

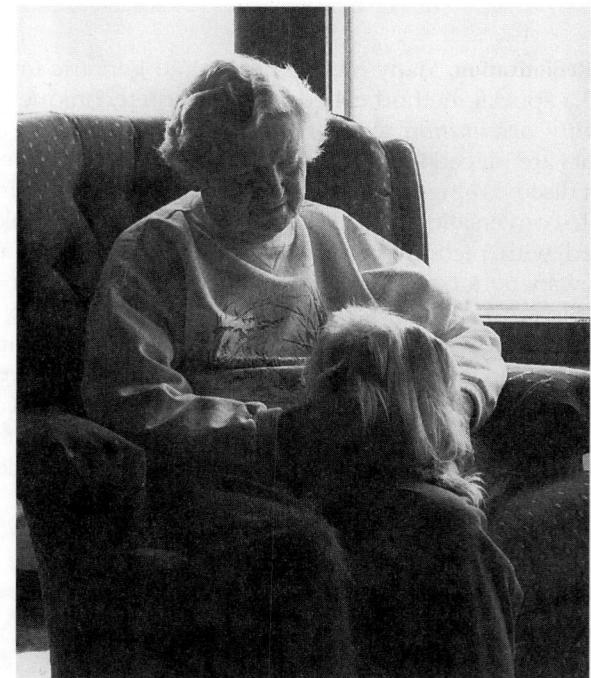

Figure 87-1. Pet therapy is used as an adjunct to treatment in many patient care areas. The depressed, psychotic, or confused person often relates earlier and more comfortably to a fuzzy, friendly animal than to other people. Pet therapy can be used to reorient a person to reality or just to lift one's spirits. In addition, the ability to care for a pet is an important component in assessing a person's level of functioning and ability to perform activities of daily living. (Photo by Kimberly Malcolm.)

designed for various numbers of people and at various activity levels. Many of these games are incorporated in the activity plans for patients in the mental health unit and for those in rehabilitation, geriatric, and chemical dependency units.

The games are played using rules that can be applied to the real world. They are designed to teach people to take psychological and physical risks, to develop trust and a sense of community, to realize that winning is not as important as effort, and to emphasize challenge rather than competition. Imagery and ritual are used to promote a sense of freedom and decrease inhibition.

It is important for staff members to be flexible and feel free to change to another game if the one chosen is not therapeutic.[1]

Hydrotherapy. Most large mental health units have hydrotherapy facilities or a swimming pool. Most patients enjoy swimming and can work off frustrations or relax in the pool. Always closely supervise patients while they are swimming.

Medication Therapy

Antipsychotic medications introduced in the 1950s brought about revolutionary changes in the treatment of mental disorders. Certain drugs can arrest or greatly alleviate adverse symptoms of many mental disorders to the point that the person can function in the community. As a result of antipsychotic medications, the number of long-term patients now able to be discharged from mental health units is greatly increasing. The nurse must follow good nursing practice in administration of medications. The accompanying box summarizes nursing skills in medication therapy. Table 87-1 gives drugs, their actions and uses, and nursing considerations.

Tardive Dyskinesia. This condition occasionally results from long-term use of antipsychotic medications. It also can result, although rarely, from the antidepressant amoxapine (Asendin) or the gastric drug metoclopramide (Reglan). Tardive dyskinesia (TD) is most often mild and does not interfere with the person's life. However, TD can be upsetting to patients, and in some cases, involuntary muscle movements can be disabling. TD usually starts with abnormal tongue movements, which can progress to rhythmic movements of the tongue, lips, eyes, or face. Sometimes this seems to be a chewing movement. Tongue movements include intermittent darting in and out of the mouth, "tongue in cheek," tongue tremor, or a stationary, protruding tongue. The syndrome may extend to include involuntary athetoid (writhing) movements of fingers, toes, extremities, and back and sideways head jerks, usually to one side.

TD may be temporary or permanent. Sometimes the symptoms disappear within a few weeks or months after discontinuation of the drug; in other cases, the disorder persists. If no other drug can be found, the patient may opt to continue a lower dose to control psychotic symptoms. The TD may be lessened or controlled by drugs, such as trihexyphenidyl (Artane), benztropine (Cogentin), or diphenhydramine (Benadryl).

Several evaluation scales are used to assess the presence or absence and severity of TD. These scales are designed to determine if the following types of abnormal movements, which indicate TD, are present:

- Facial tics, grimaces
- Chewing or sucking movements
- Excessive blinking or bursts of blinking
- Abnormal tongue movements (including tremor)
- Abnormal twisting or jerking movements of fingers or arms (not including tremor)
- Abnormal toe or foot movements
- Abnormal head or neck movements or jerking

Many psychiatric patients have other involuntary movements, including arm or hand tremors, pacing, rocking, abnormal verbalizations, or leg jerking, which are not specific signs of TD. Special training is required to perform accurate TD assessment. Fear of TD is the most common reason given by patients for refusal to take medications.

Neuroleptic Malignant Syndrome. This is a potentially fatal condition that can be a result of taking neuroleptic medications. The symptoms include the following:

- Altered level of consciousness
- Autonomic nervous system disturbances (hyperthermia, tachypnea, tachycardia, fluctuating blood pressure)
- Dystonia (impaired muscle tone)
- Akathisia (motor restlessness, inability to sit still)
- Poor response to anticholinergic drugs, given for side effects
- Sleep disturbance
- Abnormal laboratory values: elevated white blood cells, elevated creatine phosphokinase (CPK) (indicating muscle damage from rigidity), and myoglobin in urine (also indicates muscle damage).

The nurse must maintain the airway, monitor vital signs and level of consciousness, hold medications, monitor I & O and nutritional status, and measure daily weight.

The Patient in an Inpatient Setting

Although this chapter is geared primarily to the inpatient care of the person with a mental health or adjustment problem, many of the skills learned here also ap-

[1] New Games Foundation, P.O. Box 7901, San Francisco, CA 94120

Nursing Skill Guidelines
Applying Medication Therapy in the Mental Health Unit

◆ Follow the "five rights" for correct medication administration (see Chapter 57).

◆ It is often helpful to leave the medications in their packages if the unit-dose system is used. (*Rationale: This allows the paranoid person to see you open the package or to open it himself or herself; medication need not be wasted if it is refused, and you can more easily identify and teach about medications.*)

◆ Identify the person before giving any medication. Always check the person's name band. (*Rationale: The person may be confused or may deliberately try to mislead you.*) If the person does not have a name band, ask him or her to tell you his or her name; confirm with another nurse if there is any question. Do not ask, "Are you Mr. Jones?" Many patients will answer "yes," even if this is incorrect.

◆ Assess and document effectiveness of drugs. Drugs are given in mental health for several reasons. Desired effects include the following:

Lessening episodes of *hallucinations* (perceiving something that is not there). These hallucinations are usually *auditory* (hearing voices) or *visual* (seeing things). Less common are *gustatory* (taste), *olfactory* (smell), or *tactile* (touch) hallucinations.

Decreasing *delusional* thinking (false beliefs that cannot be changed by reasoning).

Diminishing *distortions* in the thought process.

Lessening of *destructive behavior* to self or others.

◆ Observe and document the resident's willingness to take medications. If the person refuses, the nurse must document this and the reasons the person gives for refusing. The person has a right to refuse medications and many do. (*Exception:* If the resident has been committed by the court and directed to take medications, he or she must do so. This is called a "Jarvis" order in many states.)

◆ Assess and document side effects. Note exactly what the side effect was and how it progressed. Part of the documentation includes steps taken to alleviate side effects. Common side effects of antipsychotic medications are dry mouth, constipation, hypotension or hypertension, blurred vision, drowsiness, muscle cramping, drooling, and the urge to pace. (*Rationale: A major reason for refusal is the fear of undesirable side effects, especially tardive dyskenesia, a potentially disabling side effect.*)

◆ Teach the resident and family about medications, the importance of following administration times and dosages, possible side effects, and what to do if these occur.

◆ Assess for more severe side effects. These often are extrapyramidal (response of the autonomic nervous system to the medications), such as the following:

Dystonia: Involuntary and irregular movements of the muscles of the trunk and extremities

Akathisia: Extreme inability to sit still, motor restlessness, or muscle quivering tremors

Parkinsonian syndrome: Symptoms similar to Parkinson's disease

Tardive Dyskinesia syndrome: Impairment of voluntary movements, specifically caused by drugs

Neuroleptic malignant syndrome: A potentially fatal disorder also caused by drugs

---

ply to patients in other areas. As a nurse, you will encounter people who are experiencing a threat to mental health in all areas of the hospital or healthcare facility, as well as in daily life.

Key Concept

People who are ill or injured often respond to threats to their health in manners that are not typical of their usual behavior. You may find symptoms of a mental health disorder in many general medical–surgical patients. Often, the undesirable behavior disappears once the medical problem is under control.

The Therapeutic Environment

A therapeutic environment (**milieu** therapy) is one in which all aspects of the person's surroundings, physical and social, are designed to promote health and enable him or her to cope with demands of life in such a way that he or she can live in the community after discharge from the hospital. The therapeutic environment is a community within the hospital in which people are encouraged to interact with one another and to improve their interpersonal relationships. It is hoped they will gain insight into their actions and will change undesirable behavior. The patients form a "government" and, with the help of staff, set up rules and regulations. In this way, they are able to test ways of coping with life. The therapeutic environment can fulfill its function only

Table 87-1. Key Medications: Psychotherapeutic Agents

Drug Class and Examples	Action/Uses	Nursing Considerations
Antipsychotics		
◆ chlorpromazine HCl (Thorazine) ◆ fluphenazine HCl* (Prolixin) ◆ haloperidol* (Haldol) ◆ thioridazine HCl (Mellaril) ◆ thiothixene HCl (Navane) ◆ trifluoperazine HCl (Stelazine) ◆ mesoridazine (Serentil) ◆ molindone (Moban) ◆ loxapine (Loxitane) ◆ perphenazine (Trilafon) ◆ risperidone (Risperidal)	◆ Used in thought disorders and psychosis ◆ Most affect dopamine receptors in brain, controlling agitation, delusions, and hallucinations ◆ Help control psychotic signs and symptoms ◆ Newest agent available	◆ Assess emotional status frequently ◆ Provide hard candy, ice chips, or gum to minimize dry mouth; monitor fluid intake and output (urine retention possible) ◆ Give stool softeners as ordered for constipation ◆ Monitor for postural (orthostatic) hypotension, hypertension, or BP lability, and tachycardia ◆ Assess for possible sedation ◆ Teach patient to avoid alcohol and other central nervous system (CNS) depressants ◆ Teach patient not to change dosage or stop taking medication without notifying physician. Do not stop taking suddenly, taper dose ◆ Instruct patient to avoid direct sunlight for extended periods or wear sunscreen ◆ Monitor for extrapyramidal side effects and TD ◆ Monitor for seizures in all patients, especially those with seizure history (drug lowers seizure threshhold) ◆ NMS potential
◆ clozapine (Clozaril)	◆ Used to treat chronic schizophrenia when tardive dyskinesia is a risk and when other drugs have not been effective	◆ Has all same side effects as other antipsychotics (except TD) PLUS ◆ Watch for severe leukopenia and other blood disorders ◆ Monitor weekly white blood cell counts (required) ◆ Patients with seizure history must be on strict seizure precautions ◆ Warn patients not to take with any other medications without specific physician's orders ◆ Patients must be registered with government
Drugs Given to Offset Extrapyramidal Side Effects		
ANTICHOLINERGIC/ANTIPARKINSON AGENTS		
◆ trihexyphenidyl HCl (Artane) ◆ benztropine mesylate (Cogentin) ◆ biperiden (Akineton) ◆ amantadine (Symmetrel) ◆ diphenhydramine HCl (Benadryl) ◆ propranolol (Inderal)	◆ Block cholinergic receptors, offset dystonic reactions ◆ Transmitted by dopamine ◆ Prevents effects of histamine on smooth muscles ◆ Beta blocker	◆ Do not discontinue abruptly ◆ Monitor vital signs; intake and output (sometimes) ◆ May cause constipation, dry mouth ◆ May cause drowsiness, hypotension; weight gain may be a problem ◆ Causes drowsiness. May be used as night time sleep aid ◆ Watch for worsening of psychosis (anticholinergic delirium), especially with amantadine
Mood Stabilizer		
◆ lithium (Eskalith [slow release], lithium carbonate; liquid form-lithium citrate)	◆ Exact action unknown ◆ Helps prevent or control manic episodes of bipolar and other disorders ◆ Helps "level out" behavior	◆ Administer with or after meals to decrease gastric irritation ◆ Monitor serum lithium levels frequently ◆ Assess for changes in behavior ◆ Maintain salt/fluid level because of the possibility of dehydration; monitor for polydispsia, polyuria ◆ Lithium can cause liver damage, excess weight gain, hand tremor, hypothyroidism ◆ Instruct the patient to avoid taking other medications, such as NSAIDS, which may not be excreted or which can accentuate liver damage

(continued)

Table 87-1 (continued)

Drug Class and Examples	Action/Uses	Nursing Considerations
Antidepressants		
CYCLIC ANTIDEPRESSANTS (CYCLICS) ◆ amitriptyline HCl (Elavil) ◆ clomipramine HCl (Anafranil) ◆ desipramine HCl (Norpramin) ◆ imipramine HCl (Tofranil) ◆ nortriptyline HCl (Pamelor) ◆ doxepin (Sinequan) ◆ trimipramine (Surmontil) ◆ amoxapine (Asendin) ◆ protriptyline (Vivactil)	◆ Stimulate the limbic system affecting norepinephrine and serotonin, increasing their action, with resultant excitatory behavior	◆ Warn patient to avoid alcohol, which is potentiated by drug (sedation effect) ◆ Monitor for signs and symptoms of anticholinergic side effects, such as dry mouth and constipation ◆ Assess for possible sedation ◆ Monitor for orthostatic hypotension; check orthostatic blood pressure frequently ◆ Cannot be stopped abruptly, dose must be tapered
MONOAMINE OXIDASE INHIBITORS (MAO INHIBITORS) ◆ phenelzine SO₄ (Nardil) ◆ tranylcypromine SO₄ (Parnate) ◆ isocarboxyzid (Marplan)	◆ Prevent the metabolism of epinephrine, norepinephrine, and serotonin, increasing psychomotor activity	◆ Instruct in diet restrictions—patient must be on a tyramine-free diet (avoid foods such as aged cheese, beer, chocolate, soy sauce, processed meats) ◆ Teach patient to avoid over-the-counter cold medications, which may cause serious adverse reactions ◆ Avoid alcohol or other depressants ◆ Side effect is hypertensive crisis. Specific antidote is phentolamine (Regitine)
OTHER DRUGS USED TO TREAT DEPRESSION ◆ bupropion HCl (Wellbutrin) ◆ fluoxetine HCl (Prozac) ◆ paroxetine HCl (Paxil) ◆ sertraline HCl (Zoloft) ◆ trazodone HCl (Desyrel) ◆ vanlafaxine (Effexor)	◆ Some are serotonin reuptake inhibitors (Prozac, Paxil, Zoloft)	◆ May cause anxiety, restlessness, insomnia ◆ Give in morning, usually ◆ Trazodone may be given at bedtime; may cause priapism ◆ Few side effects (Prozac, Paxil, Zoloft, Effexor)
Antianxiety Drugs ◆ lorazepam (Ativan) ◆ diazepam (Valium) ◆ chlordiazepoxide (Librium) ◆ chlorazepate (Tranxene) ◆ clonazepam (Klonopin) ◆ flurazepam (Dalmane) ◆ alprazolam (Xanax) ◆ temazepam (Restoril) ◆ buspirone (BuSpar) ◆ not benzodiazepine	◆ Depress the CNS at the limbic and subcortical levels ◆ Reduce hyperactivity without impairing consciousness ◆ Decrease irritability ◆ Sometimes used to control seizures ◆ May be used to control agitated behavior ◆ Fewer side effects	◆ Warn patient to avoid alcohol; it potentiates the action of the drug ◆ Do not discontinue abruptly—severe withdrawal may occur ◆ Administer daily dose close to bedtime to promote sleep ◆ Caution patients to avoid driving if drowsiness occurs ◆ Monitor carefully for signs of dependency ◆ Warn patient that side effects include drowsiness and sedation ◆ Monitor blood pressure (drugs can cause hypotension) ◆ May cause coma

* *Note:* Some of these drugs (Prolixin, Haldol) can be given in *decanoate* or *enanthate* form. These are given IM and only must be repeated every 1 to 6 weeks.

if people are encouraged to live in such a way as to prepare them for eventual discharge.

Rights of the Patient

Civil Rights Legislation. Civil rights laws, including the law that gives a person the right to refuse treatment, have done much to ensure effective treatment of psychiatric problems. The patient's civil rights cannot be violated, even though he or she might be committed by law to the mental health unit. For example, mail can be sent and received by people in a mental health unit without being censored. The person has the right to see friends and relatives, unless the physician orders otherwise. If these rights are violated, the person has sufficient grounds for legal action.

Vulnerable Adult Legislation. Legislation has been passed that protects those who cannot protect themselves. This law is called the *vulnerable adult* law and protects intellectually impaired people and those with disruptions in mental health that are severe enough to render them incompetent or unable to protect themselves. It is illegal to physically, sexually, or verbally abuse or neglect any person.

Advocacy. Most hospital and other healthcare institutions employ counselors or advocates who advise people about their civil rights. These advocates act as effective "watchdogs" against personnel who might be abusive or thoughtless. Any abuse must be reported, or the observer, in addition to the person who was abusive, can be prosecuted.

Security. The mentally disturbed person needs a secure environment, self-protection, and protection from other patients, from hurting other people, and from the outside world. It is the hospital's responsibility to provide this protection. Generally people in the mental health unit are not dangerous. Nevertheless, in any hospital, there are certain patients who are dangerous. The nurse has a duty to prevent injuries to nursing personnel, other employees, and other patients. Some patients are likely to attempt actions of self-mutilation, such as scratching, cutting, biting, or beating themselves. In a unit where people may become violent, the nurse may carry an electronic signal that can be used if assistance is needed. (Let the patients know you have the device. This will usually prevent violence.)

Restraints and Patient Safety Devices. Restraints may be necessary in the psychiatric unit to keep a patient from hurting himself or herself or others or from destroying property. Civil rights laws are intended to prevent the use of undue restraint. Except in the most extreme circumstances, restraints should not be used. *Always* use the *least restrictive* controls. If restraint becomes necessary to keep a person from hurting themselves or someone else or from removing a dressing or interfering with a surgical treatment, certain precautions should be taken (see box). Substitutes for restraint are therapeutic treatments, such as drug therapy, diversion, or as a last resort, seclusion.

Seclusion. Sometimes the person can bring undesirable behavior under control if he or she is placed into a room alone. This is called *seclusion*. Seclusion must be used with care. No patient should be secluded without the written order of the physician.

The person in seclusion must be observed carefully; when the condition permits, he or she should be released. The room temperature should be comfortable; fresh air should be circulating. Frequently give water or juice while in seclusion. The person should have exercise and frequent opportunities for toileting. The number of hours a person spends in seclusion in a 24-hour period should be documented. The person is secluded alone—never with another person. When seclusion is necessary, it should be carried out with every conscientious consideration for the person.

Prevention of Dehumanization

A hospital, particularly a mental health unit, is representative of a total institution. Life is controlled. The larger group must live and perform according to rules set up by the smaller group. As with any form of institutionalized living, measures must be taken to prevent occurrence of a dehumanizing atmosphere. It is vital that the patient maintain his or her individuality and be treated with dignity. Some skills in preventing dehumanization are presented in the box on p. 1385.

The Patient's Visitors

It is to the nurse's advantage to gain the good will and cooperation of visitors. This will help alleviate many problems. The person's relatives and other visitors are often greatly distressed by the person's illness. Frequently they are unable to appreciate his or her condition. They may have been dealing with this person's unpredictable or difficult behavior for many years. They may exaggerate little things. It is helpful to reassure the visitors.

To avoid overwhelming surprise, the patient should be told of the impending visit. He or she should be clean and neat and fully dressed, if possible. All requests for information about the person's condition should be referred to the charge nurse or team leader. The patient must also give permission.

Nursing skill guidelines for observation of supervised visits follow:

- ◆ See that the vulnerable patient does not sign any papers.
- ◆ See that packages are opened in your presence.
- ◆ Permit no smoking except in designated areas.
- ◆ Watch for suicide attempts or efforts to leave without permission.
- ◆ Terminate the visit if the patient becomes disturbed.
- ◆ Document the patient's reaction to the visit. Document interaction with visitors, noting who the visitors were if possible.

The Patient on Outings

Make sure the person understands the rules that apply to outings before he or she leaves the mental health unit. Usually, patients must sign out and indicate where they are going and with whom. The person may be allowed to leave only with staff or may be given an

Nursing Skill Guidelines
Using Patient Safety Devices for the Mentally Ill

- Wear gloves during a restraint. Wear eye goggles if the patient is likely to spit. Be careful you are not bitten.
- Residents in restraints are vulnerable to abuse and should be under constant observation. Usually they are in a locked seclusion room for their own protection, because they become vulnerable when restrained. The person must be checked at least every 15 minutes and is often under constant camera surveillance.
- You must have a specific written order to use restraints. This order can only be written for 24 hours at a time. The application of restraints and observation of the resident must be carefully documented.
- When restraining the arms and legs, be careful not to make the device too tight. Stockinette or soft bandage should be used under the safety device (to prevent injury).
- Some facilities require the use of a waist restraint if the limbs are to be restrained.
- Restraints on psychiatry are usually locked. Every nurse must have a key available, so the patient can be released in an emergency.
- One type of locked restraint has a tiny knob or catch, which must be depressed to lock the buckle. Be sure you know how to manipulate the restraints used in your facility.
- When applying restraints, check the buckle to make sure it is locked.
- If the person is out of control, medications may be forced (intramuscular injection), unless the person agrees to take them orally.
- Offer the opportunity to use the urinal or bedpan or go to the bathroom at least every 1 to 2 hours.
- Offer fluids frequently.
- Do not fasten the arms and legs in an uncomfortable position. If a person must be placed in such a position to prevent injury to others, change the position as soon as possible. Remove the safety device every hour, and allow the patient to exercise.

- If it can be avoided, do not apply a safety device over the chest. This can cause the person to panic. A waist restraint may be needed.
- Never restrain only one side of the body. Even if you feel it is unnecessary to restrain both hands or both feet, restrain the hand and foot on the opposite side, too. When releasing the person from restraints, release one extremity at a time, and alternate "corners." Do not release both extremities on the same side at the same time. Some facilities do not allow only two limbs to be restrained.
- Frequently feel the pulse of the person who is struggling against a safety device, and watch his or her general condition carefully. Death can result from exhaustion. The person also can work down in the bed and strangle on a restraint.
- Be aware that the person may try to do destructive things while restrained, such as tearing the bed linens or biting holes in the mattress.
- The person also may try to harm himself or herself. He or she must be kept safe. For example, if the person in full restraints bites their shoulder, a cervical collar ("whiplash" collar) can be used.
- When restraints are released, give the person a back rub to reduce fatigue.
- Whenever a patient is placed in seclusion or restraints, they must be *thoroughly searched* for any dangerous objects. This includes matches, plastic tableware, plastic bags, pens, pencils, paper clips, staples, and so forth.
- If a patient is out of control, do not attempt to carry out a restraint without assistance. Sometimes, a "show of force" is sufficient. However, the team must be prepared for violence on the part of the patient. The team must be ready to apply involuntary restraints if needed for patient safety and to maintain the safety of others on the unit.
- If a staff member or patient is injured during a restraint, report it immediately and file an incident report. Tests for infectious diseases may be required.

independent pass. The person is informed of the curfew time and what the consequences will be if he or she is late in returning. A physician's order is required before the patient can leave the hospital on a pass; make sure the order is written and signed. The patient signs a "pass waiver" promising to return and releasing the hospital of liability. You are responsible if you allow a person to leave without an order or without signing out against medical advice (AMA).

When the person returns from an outing, note whether he or she is on time. Identify who was with the person. Ask what the person did and how the outing went. Ask if he or she brought anything back from the outing. Chart the person's comments, nonverbal behavior, physical appearance, and any unusual reactions. Be sure to note, for example, if you can detect alcohol on the breath or if the person seems more agitated or depressed.

Nursing Care of the Long-Term Patient

Nursing assessment is discussed later in the chapter. Observation of patients ties the therapy together. The program of nursing care for the long-term patient is threefold: physical care, habit training, and occupation.

Physical Care

Patients should be encouraged to bathe regularly, and suitable clothing should be provided. Even the most deteriorated people often respond in a positive manner to a treatment at the beauty parlor or barber shop or to a pretty, bright dress or a new shirt and trousers. Disregard for personal appearance hastens disorganization; therefore, attention should be given to helping these people keep themselves presentable as much as possible.

The nurse should pay daily attention to caring for fingernails and toenails, combing hair, and brushing teeth. People must be encouraged to do these things for themselves, but the nurse is responsible for seeing that they are carried out; the nurse performs these activities for the person only if he or she cannot do them.

Because some people will be unable to care for their own physical needs, soiling can be a problem. At regular intervals, they should be taken to the bathroom; they should be treated with respect and consideration. The person who refuses or who cannot get out of bed may need skin care to prevent skin breakdown.

Habit Training

Feeding may be a problem. Many patients eat too much and too rapidly; others eat insufficient food. They should have a normal, well-balanced diet, with attention given to eating habits and table manners. Patients should not be expected to eat only with a spoon unless there is a safety consideration.

Behavior modification techniques are often used with this type of person; usually retraining in many ADLs is successful. The long-term patient often benefits from remotivation therapy and from contacts with other people.

The value of recreation and activity to this group is incalculable. An entire ward of patients can enjoy simple activities, such as walks, games, and crafts. Such activities also tend to lessen combative and destructive behavior; tensions are worked off in a healthy manner.

Employment or Occupation

The person in a long-term care facility will benefit from exposure to the world of work, if this is possible. A job or duty in the unit itself, such as keeping one's own living quarters neat, may be attempted by the person first. As this is mastered, the person may progress to a job in the laundry, kitchen, coffee shop, garden, or gift shop within the healthcare facility.

As a person is rehabilitated, he or she may be able to work during the day in a sheltered workshop setting. The feeling of having a job and earning some money adds to any person's self-esteem. Before discharge, most people will need vocational rehabilitation to train them for employment.

Mental Health Nursing Skills

Mental health skills and skills in dealing with undesired behavior are needed in any field of nursing. However, care of the psychiatric patient provides a challenging opportunity for the nurse to use these abilities to the utmost. Working closely with the person day by day, the nurse becomes a source of stability and consistency; he or she is always available, will always listen, is always kind, does not condemn or punish, and believes in and gives the person hope.

The nurse in a mental health setting must demonstrate the ability to carry out specific nursing skills.

Some of these are the same as in any other area of the hospital. Others are specific to mental health nursing. The nurse carefully documents all assessments and care given.

Key Concept

Common orders for precautions include the following:

◆ AP: assault precautions
◆ EP: escape (elopement) precautions
◆ GP/SP: general (suicide) precautions
◆ Sx: sexual precautions
◆ Sz: seizure precautions
◆ W/D (ETOH W/D): withdrawal or alcohol withdrawal

Physical Care

The following are some aspects of physical care that the nurse provides:

◆ Assist with ADLs that the person cannot perform alone; teach and supervise ADLs. Make sure the person maintains adequate nutritional and hydration status. Some patients are *polydipsic* (drink excess amounts) and are on a fluid restriction.
◆ Handle inappropriate or dangerous behaviors exhibited by the patient, sometimes in emergency situations. The nurse must be able to protect himself or herself, without injuring the patient. A special behavior control class is usually provided for staff.
◆ Administer prescribed medications, and observe for side effects; teach the patient about medications. Offer as-needed (PRN) medications for side effects.
◆ Administer physical treatments as ordered.

Emotional Support

The patient and family need the nurse's emotional support, which is given in the following ways:

◆ Establish rapport (a harmonious relationship; see the accompanying box).
◆ Create a therapeutic relationship within the mental health setting.
◆ Provide emotional support to the patient and family.
◆ Provide leadership in socialization activities with one person or a group of patients.
◆ Aid in group therapy sessions.
◆ Conduct remotivation sessions.
◆ Assist the patient to find other needed resources, such as Alcoholics Anonymous or a community social worker.

Other Skills

The nurse functions not only as a nurse, but also as a counselor, teacher, and a surrogate parent or friend.

◆ As a *socializing agent*, the nurse helps patients to

The Nurse-Client Relationship

To establish a good relationship with any person, the nurse should do the following:

◆ Be polite, tactful, and friendly to everyone.
◆ Be truthful but not brutally so. Avoid answering questions evasively.
◆ Be even-tempered and uncritical; sometimes this is difficult, but remember that the person is ill.
◆ Have poise—it gives you confidence in yourself and lets the resident have confidence in you.
◆ Be an *interested* listener; this is always a desirable quality.
◆ Have empathy, an essential characteristic of effective interpersonal relationships. It is not enough to imagine how *you* would feel in the person's situation; you must try to understand how *he* or *she feels*.
◆ Concentrate on the person's strengths and not on the weaknesses.
◆ Be consistent. Tell the truth.
◆ Set appropriate limits.
◆ Remember the "Patient's Bill of Rights."

participate in group activities and interact normally with others.

◆ As a *counselor*, the nurse listens to the person and encourages him or her to work through the problem at hand.
◆ As a *teacher*, he or she helps guide people into socially acceptable activities and teaches about medications.
◆ As a *surrogate parent or friend*, the nurse provides physical and emotional care as needed, while encouraging people to face reality independently.

Nursing Alert

It is inappropriate and unethical to have social contact with a discharged psychiatric patient; this person is considered a vulnerable adult. Always set limits.

Nursing Assessment

Assessments that are documented carefully, objectively, and accurately can be of great help to the therapist or physician working with the person (see box).

The purpose of the ward observations and notes is to record intermittently the condition of the patient. They are mainly descriptions of conduct and behavior and are sometimes made without the person's knowledge. In many settings, the patient is allowed to read the chart or document feelings, thoughts, and activities for the benefit of the healthcare team. The person often has more insight into his or her behavior than the nurses or others. The factors listed below and in the accompanying box can be considered when assessing, planning, and documenting behavior.

Observation. The nurse should observe the patient in the following ways:

◆ Carefully and accurately observe the patient's behaviors while in the unit and while engaging in activities outside the unit or outside the hospital.

◆ Observe the patient's attention to personal appearance and grooming as well as other ADLs.

◆ Observe and record the patient's physical symptoms.

◆ Carefully observe and document the patient's interactions with other people. Note if there are differences in interactions with other patients, staff, and family members.

◆ Assess vital signs at least daily.

Appearance. Assess whether the person is neat and clean or dirty and untidy. Check the clothes to be sure they are appropriate for the situation and activity. Check makeup and hair.

Sociability. Determine whether the patient associates freely with others or prefers to be alone. Document if the person associates only with staff or only with peers.

Behavior. Behavior should be assessed to determine if the person is orderly or disorderly, still or restless, quiet or noisy, friendly or indifferent, interested or uninterested, cooperative or destructive. Determine how time is spent, if there is reluctance to get out of bed, if conduct is always the same, and if the person carries out assigned tasks and takes medications.

Emotional Reactions. Notice if and how the person expresses emotions, such as anxiety, depression, fear, suspicion, happiness, sadness, loneliness, and anger. Observe if the person is irritable, hostile, or excited or has sudden impulsive actions, unprovoked outbreaks of excitement, temper tantrums, or assaultive tendencies. Assess the overall emotional state, and determine if the emotions are relatively constant. Be specific in your assessment and documentation.

Speech. Assessment of speech involves determining the answers to the following questions:

◆ Does speech seem natural? Is it flighty, rapid, loose, disorganized and disconnected, or slow and retarded?

◆ Does speech indicate that the person understands what is said or what is requested? Does the patient repeat words or phrases or use rhyming words? Does the person repeat someone else's words (*echolalia*)? Does he or she coin new words that are not really words (*neologisms*)?

◆ Are there any particular speech defects, such as stuttering, lisping, or stammering? Is the person able to hear?

◆ How much does the person talk? Does he or she talk voluntarily or only when questioned? Does the person talk constantly?

◆ Is the person noisy (with words, singing, or just sounds), or does the person not speak (*mutism*)? Does the person stop talking halfway through a sentence and seem unable to continue (*blocking*)?

◆ Does the conversation make sense? Does he or she dwell on one subject or always return to the same subject? Is the patient able to concentrate on a topic; is speech tangential and loose? What does the person talk about? Do meaningless *word salad* sentences occur? Does the person use profanity? Are his or her responses relevant and coherent? Does the conversation pass from one subject to another without order or apparent connection (*flight of ideas*)?

◆ Does the person remember things? Is the person oriented to time and place?

Nonverbal Behavior. What the patient does not say is often more important than what he or she says. Posture, facial expression, and personal hygiene indicate a great deal about a person's self-image and how he or she views the world. Sometimes a patient may react differently when you are not there, compared with when you are observing or when you or other staff members are approaching. Assess whether the person does inappropriate things, such as smear feces or food or write on the walls. Document any characteristic and repeated gestures or mannerisms. Determine if the person looks at you when talking and if there is *eye contact.* (The nurse must take cultural values into consideration. For example, in many Native American and Asian cultures, looking a person directly in the eye is an act of defiance; it is considered polite to look down when talking to another person.) Describe the patient's *affect* (external expression of emotions). Is it flat, blunted, bright?

Body Complaints. Document if the person complains of pain or discomfort.

Movements. Check if the person is coordinated, shaky, or quick; check if his or her gait is even and controlled. Does he or she sit in one position for long periods? Does the person seem to get "stuck" in one position (*catatonia*)? If you move the person's arm, will he or she maintain that position (*waxy flexibility*)? Is there unusual posturing (eg, ritualistic movement, karate stances)?

Physical Condition. Note the person's general physical condition. Physically ill patients will have orders for medication and treatment in addition to psychiatric orders.

Sleep. Determine the person's pattern of sleep. Is it normal or disturbed? Does he or she talk or cry out during sleep? Does the person sleep walk or talk in his or her sleep? Does the person want to stay in bed all day? Is he or she afraid at night? Is the person sleep-deprived?

Appetite. Document the person's attitude toward food. Does he or she eat willingly, or must he or she be urged and coaxed? Note any peculiar habits in relation to food or eating. Assess the person's table manners (or lack thereof). Does the person eat or drink constantly? Does he or she have a fluid restriction? Does he or she follow dietary orders?

Excretions. Observe the excretory functions. Document menstruation in female patients of reproductive age. Make sure a pregnancy test is *negative* before psychotropic medications are given.

Other Observations. Any unusual occurrences, such as injuries or altercations between patients, should be documented, along with names of witnesses. Overnight visits and long visits outside the hospital also should be documented.

> **Key Concept**
>
> The ability to make a meaningful nursing assessment is an art that can be cultivated. Excellent observation and assessment skills are needed in mental health nursing.

Nursing Care in Specific Behaviors

Although previously in this chapter, broad psychiatric diagnoses are presented, people cannot always be categorized. Therefore, nursing care involves dealing with behaviors exhibited by the person. The following behaviors and approaches are specific to mental health nursing but can be adapted to other areas. These are only guidelines and need to be adapted to fit each person and situation.

The Suicidal Person

From a nursing standpoint, suicidal ideation (SI) and suicide attempts (SA) are perhaps the problems most commonly seen on the inpatient mental health unit. People who have attempted suicide present a challenge for nursing. Any mental health resident presents a potential risk, but certain types of patients are more likely to attempt suicide than others. Refer to the accompanying box for types of people who need close observation. Some of the reasons for suicidal tendencies include a feeling that the illness is a disgrace, ideas of guilt or unworthiness, thoughts of developing imaginary diseases, a lingering or malignant disease, an overwhelming sense of failure, loss of a motivating goal in life, break up of a significant relationship, loss of a job, death of a loved one, chemical dependency, auditory hallucinations, and attention seeking.

Any attempt at suicide should be considered serious: *The nurse must report every attempt, however minor it seems.* Conversations that express the uselessness of life, the desire to die, and similar feelings should be documented and reported. The approach to this problem is to win the person's confidence and maintain a consistently hopeful attitude about his or her recovery. The way to prevent suicide is to give constant and effective supervision and continuous, undemanding emotional support.

Suicide Attempts. People may attempt suicide in the hospital using articles or materials that are readily available. Nurses should watch people closely while they are working in occupational therapy shops to prevent them from securing tools, bits of metal and glass, or

Nursing Skill Guidelines
Suicide Prevention

Types of People Who Need Close Observation

◆ New residents on the mental health unit
◆ Residents who have agitated depression
◆ Depressed people, especially those in early and late stages
◆ People suffering from insomnia/sleep deprivation
◆ Acute alcoholics or those with chemical dependencies
◆ People with ideas of persecution, of being disgraced, of having an incurable disease and those responding to nonexistent voices
◆ Confused people, especially as a result of a drug misuse reaction
◆ People with sudden changes in mood
◆ People undergoing special treatments
◆ Hypochondriacs, particularly when they have a fixed idea about one organ or system
◆ People who have made previous suicidal attempts
◆ People who talk about suicide and express the wish to die

Suicide Methods in the Hospital

◆ Cutting arteries with glass or sharp instruments
◆ Hanging by sheets, blankets, belts, electric cords, ties, or other items
◆ Standing on high places and falling on the ground
◆ Banging the head on such things as the floor or furniture
◆ Tipping over backward in chairs while sitting in them, in hope of breaking the neck
◆ Drinking poison from dressing trays, cleaning solutions, or sterilizing solutions; saving up medications and taking them all at once
◆ Biting and swallowing thermometers, glass, needles, and nails
◆ Bribing privileged patients to obtain destructive articles
◆ Drowning in the bathtub or swimming pool
◆ Setting fires

Preventive Measures

◆ Know whereabouts and condition of each resident at all times; 15-minute checks are a minimum.
◆ Provide a sense of security that encourages confidence.
◆ All residents should have a regularly scheduled "one-to-one" conference with the primary nurse several times a week and should be given a conference whenever they request one.

◆ Most residents must be supervised when smoking. You may have to keep matches; the resident probably is not allowed to have them. If the institution is smoke free, provide supervision if the patient is permitted to smoke outdoors. Make sure the person understands the limits of the area.
◆ Keep medications under lock and key.
◆ Because suicidal people are often integrated into the general hospital population, sharp and dangerous objects are often removed from *all* people on the unit.
◆ Keep elevator doors and dumbwaiters locked.
◆ When possible, express doubt about strange and bizarre ideas, fears, delusions, or hallucinations, but do not ridicule the person or argue.

Care of "Specialed" Residents

◆ Watch carefully every movement of the resident. The nurse must stay at arm's length.
◆ Permit no strings, belts, or ties on the person's clothing. No shoelaces.
◆ Supervise the person *very* closely while he or she is using sharp objects, electrical appliances, and other dangerous items.
◆ The person *must* get out of bed and get dressed each day. Encourage him or her to be independent.
◆ Do not leave the person alone when reporting off duty; wait until relief arrives.
◆ Supervise bathroom use. Leave the door ajar. Listen carefully. Usually tub baths are not allowed, but showers are required.
◆ Occupy the person with suitable games where possible. Encourage reading, but do not read to him or her. Inspire the person to accomplish things.
◆ Anticipate behavior by being aware of mood changes. Occasionally, people will pretend improvement to gain an opportunity for suicide.
◆ Be sure that the person is given any prescribed medication intended to help his or her condition.
◆ Find out if remotivation techniques have been recommended; they often benefit suicidal people.
◆ This person usually is not allowed to leave the unit.

---

similar objects (see Nursing Skill Guidelines box). Any type of cord or rope can be dangerous (electric cords, bathrobe ties, shoelaces, belts), as can plastic bags. Medications must always be kept under lock and key.

When patients injure themselves or others with such articles, they may have been advanced too fast. People also can attempt suicide or deliberate self-injury in other ways, such as diving to the floor from a window ledge or ramming their head into a wall. The early morning hours are a crucial time for depressed people because they dread facing another day. Deeply depressed people are usually not alert enough to carry out a suicide attempt or even try. However, as they begin to recover and regain their willpower, they become more alert and therefore more likely to attempt suicide. The depressed person who is recovering appears so much more optimistic than before that he or she may not be watched closely. The optimism may be because he person has come up with a plan for suicide. People should be observed for signs of suicidal attempts during the early stages of illness, during convalescence, and when the nursing shift changes.

Actively suicidal patients should be "specialed" (given a special nurse who takes care of one person exclusively) 24 hours a day. This type of specialing is different from that in a general hospital. A person specialed in a mental health unit is *never* left alone. The nurse stays within arm's reach of the patient, even when the person is in the bathroom. Refer to the Nursing Skills Guidelines box for care of specialed patients.

Suicide Prevention Centers. In some large cities, suicide prevention centers and telephone hotlines have been established to help people who contemplate suicide. The person who calls the center to say that he or she is going to commit suicide can talk to a trained person who is able to listen and discuss the situation with him or her; the counselor tries to persuade the person to delay acting. Some centers try to rush help out to prevent the suicide threat from being car-ried out.

It is not known how many suicides are prevented by calls to the crisis intervention center; many callers remain anonymous. However, it is believed that just having someone with whom to talk when the crisis is most severe is enough to keep many people from taking their own lives.

The Overactive Person

Activity is a normal characteristic of all forms of life. Certain people are by nature more animated and more forceful than others. Other factors, such as medications, can influence a person's activity level. Just as the degree of activity varies among normal people, so does the overactive behavior of mentally disturbed people. Activity ranges from slightly agitated to an extreme state of frenzy.

The nursing care for different types of people is not the same. Also, marked changes may arise in the same person from time to time, and nursing care has to be adjusted accordingly. A quiet atmosphere is important. Use a calm voice, and avoid long discussions. Do not force issues, but set limits, be consistent, and prevent harm and injury. Involve the person in activities that require the large muscles (running, basketball, tumbling, and dancing). Medications may be required.

The Hypomanic or Manic Person

The person who is more active than normal but able to function falls into the **hypomanic** group; this disorder is sometimes called a *manic episode.* There are three levels of mania: *hypomania, acute mania,* and *delirious mania.* The latter two fall into the *manic* diagnosis. Hypomanic and manic people can be more difficult than the more acutely disturbed. Often they are witty, breezy, and enterprising; because of their keen memory and quick repartee, they are sometimes not recognized as truly disturbed. This type of person also is apt to be interfering (intrusive), domineering, and irritable, with rapid mood swings (lability). He or she rarely accepts hospitalization willingly; as a rule, he or she makes many unreasonable demands. This person is always busy, and the chief problem in nursing care is how to channel this activity. This person is not delusional and is oriented to time and place. He or she often is unable or unwilling to sleep. As the person becomes more sleep deprived, he or she often becomes more irritable, intrusive, and possibly assaultive.

The nurse should be firm but kind, avoid familiarity, avoid arguments, keep the person from irritating others, and keep him or her occupied. If he or she is not permitted to participate in activities off the ward, writing or reading material can be supplied for use on the ward. The hypomanic person often benefits from a competitive game, such as badminton, but it must be carefully controlled. Contact sports should be avoided. This person may enjoy using a punching bag or a stationary bike.

There usually will be an active program of treatment, such as tranquilizing drug therapy and group psychotherapy. Care should be taken to supply extra nourishment and fluids to an overactive person who expends much energy and requires extra calories.

The Highly Disturbed Person

Management and nursing care of the highly disturbed person include physical protection of the person and others. Active people should be allowed a wide scope of activity to work off their surplus energy. Seclusion should be used only for a stated period on written order from the physician. Tranquilizing and sedative drugs can usually control the manic person, although often the person refuses them.

Every attempt should be made to direct the activities of the overactive person toward useful ends. They should be encouraged to bathe frequently. Every measure to keep them clothed should be attempted. An abundance of fluids should be given along with an adequate diet. Care of the mouth and skin is important. Injuries, such as abrasions of the skin, may become infected if not given attention.

In general, neuroleptic drugs are the best treatment for the disturbed person; this provides an opportunity for a much needed rest. Insomnia is usually a problem; warm milk may help. Benadryl, an antihistamine with side effects that include sleepiness, is often given to aid sleep; it also combats medication side effects. Sedatives are not used unless absolutely necessary. Severely disturbed people should be kept away from overstimulation. When possible, they should be taken for walks or allowed to play outdoor games with adequate supervision. It is important when giving any treatment to a highly disturbed person to have adequate assistance at hand. Set firm limits on behavior.

The Hostile or Combative Person. The hostile person may threaten to injure the nurse or others and may become physically violent. This person is on assault precautions (AP). Your documentation may describe homicidal ideation (HI) if the person threatens to kill others.

In a verbal confrontation, the nurse's first impulse may be self-defense; however, to respond with defensive behavior is not effective. *It is dangerous.* An effective response is one that recognizes the person's feelings without becoming judgmental; the person should not be belittled. He or she must be allowed to talk and express feelings. A firm but understanding approach can often prevent a hostile person from displaying physical acts of aggression. He or she should be spoken to in a calm and quiet manner (see accompanying box.)

The violent person is usually happy to have a punching bag available. Provide other socially acceptable, destructive means of venting aggression, such as tearing rags for rugs. Many violent people are controlled by the use of tranquilizing drugs. In a unit where people may become violent, cooperative protection measures must be set up by the staff, all working together to maintain safety. De-escalation of dangerous behavior is vital.

The Confused or Demented Person

The person who is confused needs a calm, quiet environment regulated by routine and free from danger and anxiety (see Chapter 86). Because disorientation to time and place is common, the nurse can help by providing a calendar and clock, and as a further reinforcement, each day can be marked off on the calendar. The person can be reminded by the nurse about holidays or visiting days. To avoid further confusion, the nurse should speak in clear, simple sentences and have the person repeat them if necessary. Question the patient's statements for clarity.

The Delusional or Hallucinative Person

People may have false beliefs (**delusions**) or may perceive false sensory stimuli (**hallucinations**). Hallucinations are not based on fact and may take the form of odors, sounds or voices, tastes, sights, or the sensation of being touched. These hallucinations are described in charting as auditory or visual hallucinations (or olfactory, gustatory, or tactile). Delusions and hallucinations often occur simultaneously in a patient.

When caring for a hallucinative person the nurse does not reinforce the hallucination or delusion. How-

Guidelines for Dealing With a Combative Resident

- ♦ Understand the resident.
- ♦ Anticipate what you are going to do.
- ♦ Avoid becoming excited; speak in a calm and level manner.
- ♦ Do not make statements that can be interpreted as a challenge.
- ♦ Do not allow the person to move behind you.
- ♦ Protect yourself physically.
- ♦ If your facility has an electronic alarm system, carry your electronic signaling device with you at all times, and let the residents know you have it.
- ♦ Call for assistance; have someone clear the area of other residents.
- ♦ Be careful not to injure a resident in any way.
- ♦ Do not retaliate. Remember, the resident is not responsible for his or her actions.
- ♦ Seclusion and restraints may be needed to prevent injury to staff or peers.
- ♦ If a person attacks you, use nonpainful methods to protect yourself and others. Call for assistance.

ever, do not become argumentative; say, for example, that you do not see the dog or hear the music. Build trust in these people by always being consistent. Use a calm and soothing voice. Document exactly what the person says; determine the content of hallucinations if possible. If this person has a fixed delusion about another person, for example, the psychiatrist may need to warn the other person.

Delusional patients may harass and *stalk* love objects. Any threats against government officials require the healthcare professional to notify the U.S. Secret Service.

The Underactive Person

Underactive people are of two main types: those who are withdrawn from reality and apparently unemotional and those who are depressed and think and act in a sluggish manner.

The Withdrawn Person

People who are withdrawn appear to be content to be left alone to think and dwell on private concerns and fantasies. Matters of major concern to other people are completely unimportant to withdrawn people. For example, food and toilet habits are of no concern. Also, conversations with other people hold no interest; they do not interact with peers. Documentation often describes this person as *isolative.* Autism, an extreme form of withdrawal, is discussed in Chapter 67.

The major goal in treatment is to reorient the person to reality; attempts are made to stimulate the person to take an active interest in life. Although he or she can

❖ *Overview of the Nursing Process*
Caring for Depressed Patients

Assessment Priorities

Nursing History

Expressions of feeling sad, unhappy, blue, "down in the dumps"

Loss of interest or pleasure in usual activities

Anxiety

Feelings of inadequacy, helplessness, inability to make decisions

Feelings of fatigue, lassitude

Pessimism, hopelessness

Feelings of worthlessness, self-reproach, or excessive or inappropriate guilt

Complaints of sleep disturbances, gastrointestinal disturbances, decreased libido (sexual drive), extreme weight changes, aches and pains

Physical Examination

Psychomotor agitation or retardation

Stooped posture

Poor personal hygiene

Excessive tearfulness

Nursing Alert

Assess potential for suicide.

Intensity of anger, guilt, and feelings of worthlessness may precipitate suicidal thoughts, feelings, and gestures.

Verbalizes suicidal ideation with plan or intent

Sudden change in activity level—becomes hyperactive or if highly agitated, suddenly becomes calm

Possible Nursing Diagnoses

Impaired Adjustment

Anxiety

Ineffective Individual Coping

Dysfunctional Grieving

Altered Health Maintenance

Hopelessness

Altered Nutrition: Less than Body Requirements

Powerlessness

Self-Care Deficit

Self-Esteem Disturbance

Sexual Dysfunction

Sleep Pattern Disturbance

Social Isolation

Spiritual Distress

Altered Thought Processes

High Risk for Self-Directed Violence

Planning

The nurse designs a plan of care with the resident (and family) to achieve the following resident goals.

The person's physiologic needs are met, as evidenced by the fact that he or she 1) maintains weight (specify range); 2) has lungs clear to auscultation; and 3) maintains muscle tone and strength.

The person's safety needs are met, as evidenced by the absence of any self-inflicted harm.

The person verbalizes emotions appropriate to the situation.

The person begins to show interest in everyday concerns, beginning with personal hygiene.

The person resumes independent self-care activities.

The person describes (demonstrates the use of) adequate coping strategies.

The person expresses new sense of control over his or her goals and future (decreased expression of negative thoughts, helplessness, pessimism).

The person expresses increased self-esteem (decreased expression of worthlessness or guilt).

Implementation

The nurse's first priority is to maintain a safe environment for the resident: 1) observe closely (specify); 2) remove all potentially harmful objects from the room of any resident with self-destructive behaviors; 3) make a contract with the suicidal resident that he or she agree *not* to act on suicidal thought until first contacting the nurse.

Ensure that the resident's physiologic needs are met; encourage the resident's maximal participation in self-care.

Allow the person to express his or her feelings.

Redirect the resident's self-preoccupation to interests in the outside world: 1) involve the person in meaningful, productive tasks and activities; 2) increase the resident's level of socialization.

Promote the resident's increased self-esteem: 1) identify significant others he or she trusts, and facilitate healthy interpersonal relationships; 2) identify and reinforce the person's strengths; 3) encourage good hygiene and grooming.

Overview of the Nursing Process
Caring for Depressed Patients (continued)

Implementation (continued)

Assist the person to replace maladaptive coping mechanisms with healthy coping mechanisms; mobilize social support systems he or she can tap (family and community); and initiate referrals if appropriate.

Administer prescribed antidepressants, and teach the person about the pharmacologic management of depression.

Assist with other treatment modalities, such as electroconvulsive therapy (ECT).

Support the family during the person's treatment and help them to get answers for their questions.

Ask for a clinical nurse specialist or liaison consultation.

Evaluation

The adequacy of the plan of care is determined by evaluating the resident's achievement of the above goals. If he or she is unable to meet key goals, the plan must be modified. Key evaluative criteria include:

Healthy resolution of depression with a return to independent, meaningful living

Absence of self-inflicted harm

Verbalization of goals and plans for the future

---

be encouraged to participate and to converse with others, socialization should not be forced.

Nursing care includes helping the person to maintain good grooming habits, such as bathing regularly, combing hair, and keeping nails trimmed. An adequate diet should be provided; make sure the person eats. Offer nutritional supplements, such as Resource. An intravenous line or feeding tube may be needed. Most physicians believe that the patient must participate in self-care. The nurse can encourage the person to eat by having a cup of coffee or a snack with him or her; the physician should be notified if the person does not eat. This person should be weighed at designated intervals. An exercise routine, preferably outdoor, should be followed. The person should be checked for incontinence; menstrual regularity is checked in women. Participation in remotivation sessions and other groups is encouraged.

The Depressed Person

In dysthymic disorder, the inactive depressed person has some of the problems of the withdrawn person, in addition to other problems. If the person is extremely depressed, the condition is known as *major depressive disorder.* Depression is sometimes described as anger turned inward against the self. In the case of a depressed person, the main objective in treatment is to prevent suicide; thus, this person requires constant observation. The period when the person begins to improve but still has periods of returning depression is most dangerous. The box, Overview of the Nursing Process, shows how the nursing process can be used with the depressed person.

Nursing care is essentially the same for all inactive people. Feeding is important, including nourishment between meals and at night. Because all body processes are slowed, watch for constipation. These people also should

be observed for symptoms of physical disease, because they rarely complain of pain.

Provide a cheerful, sunny room, but do not put depressed people with groups of exuberant people in an effort to cheer them up; this usually has the opposite effect, and tends to make them more conscious of their own unhappiness.

Firmly encourage a depressed person into participating in activities. Although occupational therapy is of great value, it should be kept simple and brief, because these patients tire quickly. This person should be introduced to *one other person* at a time, not to large groups of people. As convalescence progresses, reading, games, and amusements are helpful. Indecision is typical, so give the person only a few choices. Depression, as it relates to chronic pain, is discussed in Chapter 52. Mood-elevating drugs, such as amitriptyline (Elavil), are often helpful.

The Person Who Alternates Between Overactive and Underactive Behavior

In some disorders, the person's behavior alternates between overactivity (mania) and underactivity (depression). A *cyclothymic disorder* is a milder form; the more severe form is known as a *bipolar disorder* or bipolar affective disorder (BPAD). The bipolar disorder was formerly known as *manic-depressive disorder,* an alternation between mania and depression. Both extremes are treated symptomatically. Medications, such as lithium, are often helpful, although the person may independently discontinue the medication after leaving the hospital, causing a relapse.

The Regressive Person

Regression is a return to infantile or childish behavior, such as eating with the hands, urinating on the floor, soiling clothing instead of using the toilet, masturbating openly, or making overt sexual advances.

It takes infinite patience to teach adults basic social skills. It also requires many people to provide enough services for such patients—teaching them proper eating habits at every meal or taking them to the bathroom at regular intervals throughout the day and night. Remotivation and behavior modification techniques are useful for the regressed person.

The most important duty of the nurse in relation to the regressed person's mental state is to get him or her to focus on reality, stimulate interest in practical affairs, and help the person keep in contact with surroundings. To do this, the nurse encourages self-respect and strives to gain the person's confidence. The person should not be reprimanded if he or she soils or behaves inappropriately. Often these people are extremely sensitive, in spite of seeming oblivious to everything. For example, an appropriate bathroom schedule should be set up; reward and praise the person for success.

Try to give the person interesting activities. Use every opportunity to bring this person into stimulating contact with others. Initiate games, and participate in them along with the patients. Be alert for outbursts of violence and for suicide attempts. Encourage the person to verbalize. Accept any verbalization, no matter how minimal. If the person uses profanity, gently guide him or her to more acceptable forms of verbalization.

Today, patients are rarely bed ridden. The patient *must* be up and out of bed and should be dressed for the day, unless physically ill.

> ### Key Concept
>
> Psychiatry offers you the opportunity to combine your interviewing skills with keen nursing assessment skills.

Keys for Review

Key Questions for Critical Thinking

1. Describe the difference between mental health and mental illness. Discuss how nursing care differs between the two.
2. State the patient's rights in a mental health unit or hospital. Explain how the nurse serves as an advocate for these rights. State nursing care that ensures these rights.
3. Define the term "vulnerable adult." Describe who might be considered a vulnerable adult in the mental health unit and why. Discuss ways family members or other people might take advantage of this person. Identify nursing actions to protect this patient.
4. The patient for whom you are responsible on the unit is suicidal. Discuss specific nursing care of this patient as specifically as you can.

Key Readings

American Psychiatric Association. Diagnostic and Statistical Manual of Mental Disorders, Ed. 4. Washington, DC, APA, 1994
Johnson BS. Psychiatric Mental-Health Nursing: Adaptation and Growth, Ed 3. Philadelphia, J.B. Lippincott, 1993
McFarland GK, Thomas MD. Psychiatric Mental Health Nursing: Application of the Nursing Process. Philadelphia, J.B. Lippincott, 1991
McFarland GK, Wasli EL, Gerety EK. Nursing Diagnoses and Process in Psychiatric Mental Health Nursing, Ed 2. Philadelphia, J.B. Lippincott, 1992

Key Readings (continued)

Rawlins RP, Williams SR, Beck CK. Mental Health—Psychiatric Nursing: A Holistic Life-Cycle Approach, Ed 3. St. Louis, Mosby Year Book, 1993
Varcarolis. Foundations of Psychiatric Mental Health Nursing. Philadelphia, W.B. Saunders, 1990

Enrichment Keys

Johnson BS. Child, Adolescent, and Family Psychiatric Nursing. Philadelphia, J.B. Lippincott, 1994
Lippincott's Review Series: Mental Health and Psychiatric Nursing. Philadelphia, J.B. Lippincott, 1992
Shives LR. Basic Concepts of Psychiatric-Mental Health Nursing, Ed 3. Philadelphia, J.B. Lippincott, 1994

Keys To Learning More

Chapter 88: substance abuse
Chapter 89: rehabilitation and ambulatory nursing

Key Resources

American Psychiatric Nurses' Association
  6900 Grove Road
  Thorofare, NJ 08086
Canadian Federation of Mental Health Nurses
  331 Montgomery Avenue
  Winnipeg, Manitoba R3L 1T6
National Mental Health Association
  1021 Prince Street
  Alexandria, VA 22314-2971

88 Substance Abuse

Learning Objectives

♦ Describe signs on routine hospital admission that might indicate substance abuse, including characteristic behavior changes and physical signs.
♦ Describe stages of alcoholism, and discuss the impact on a person's life, his or her family, and society.
♦ Describe nursing measures in working with alcoholics and other substance abusers.
♦ Describe the types of treatment facilities and disulfiram (Antabuse) maintenance and programs for substance abuse.
♦ Describe methadone maintenance.
♦ Define the term over-the-counter drugs; describe problems related to their use.
♦ Describe special abusers and their care.
♦ Describe signs of substance abuse.

Key Terms

alcoholism
blackouts
chemical dependency
co-dependent
delirium tremens
detoxification
enabler
substance abuse
withdrawal

Keys to Understanding This Chapter

Chapter 5: basic human needs, which the substance abuser often is not able to meet sufficiently

Chapter 7: community health and substance abuse's effect on it

Unit Four: normal body structure and function, which may be affected by substance abuse

Chapter 31: emergency treatment in drug abuse

Unit Seven: nursing process

Unit Eight: communication and documentation skills used in substance abuse

Unit Nine: basic patient skills

Keys to Understanding This Chapter
(continued)

Chapter 56: information on drugs, many of them abused

Chapter 61: complications related to pregnancy and childbirth, sometimes complicated by substance abuse

Chapter 62: disorders of the neonate, some complicated by substance abuse

Chapter 66: adolescent chemical dependency

Chapter 85: substance abuse among the elderly

Chapter 87: mental illness, sometimes compounded by substance abuse

Key Points

♦ Substance abuse and chemical dependency are serious problems; they cost thousands of dollars and take many lives.
♦ It is possible to become dependent on many substances, including legal and illegal drugs, alcohol, nicotine, and caffeine or other food substances. Many people abuse more than one substance.
♦ Major precipitating factors include low self-esteem and stress.
♦ Management of substance abuse involves recognition, intervention, treatment, and recovery.
♦ The person with a dual disorder, such as mental illness and chemical dependency, may have more difficulty in achieving successful treatment.
♦ The enabler is a key person in substance abuse.
♦ Many patients admitted to the general hospital may be substance abusers.
♦ Nurses are more likely to abuse substances than the general population.
♦ Care of the patient during detoxification requires excellent assessment and nursing skills.
♦ Most patients require aftercare following intensive treatment.

Individuals respond to stress in numerous ways. One way is through substance abuse. Besides stress, another factor closely related to substance abuse is low self-esteem. Substance abuse is not restricted on the basis of race, creed, sex, or age. The recognition and care of the substance-abusing patient requires high-level nursing assessment, implementation, and patience.

Substance Abuse and Chemical Dependence as a Disease

Substance abuse is the prolonged use of drugs that cause physical and mental impairment. This includes alcohol and marijuana. **Chemical dependency** involves a psychic craving for a drug; the craving may be accompanied by a physiologic need for that chemical.

Substance abuse and chemical dependency are complex and progressive and can be fatal if not treated. Many people consider them to be diseases. The health-care community is just beginning to learn how to deal with these diseases.

A person is considered to be a substance abuser in the following situations:[1]

◆ Drugs that affect the central nervous system (mood-altering drugs) are used regularly.
◆ A behavioral change occurs when using the drugs.

◆ The abuse is following a pathologic course.
◆ The abuse impairs job or social functioning.
◆ The situation lasts at least 1 month.

A person is considered to be chemically dependent in the following situations:

◆ Cannot control use of the substance
◆ Has withdrawal symptoms when use stops or is reduced
◆ Must use drugs to achieve pleasure

The following concepts are basic to the management of all dependencies:

◆ *Recognition.* The condition first must be recognized by someone. It usually is someone other than the chemically dependent person.
◆ *Intervention.* Active intervention must take place. If no one intervenes in the process, it may continue.
◆ *Treatment.* Chemical dependency is a habit that often responds to structured therapies. A particular milieu is sometimes needed to gain control of the habit. In some cases, it may be controlled by the person's ability to see the price of the destructive behavior and deciding to stop the practice. Treatment should address such issues as malnutrition, heart dysfunction, liver disease, general health, social changes, and family issues.
◆ *Recovery.* If treatment is the classroom where the abuser learns how to retake control of his or her life, then life is the laboratory where these theories are put to work. Many therapies assist people to have a successful life after chemicals. Many programs use a 12-step approach or a modification,

[1] "Psychiatric Problems" in Nurse Review. Springhouse, PA, Springhouse, 1989 (updated annually), p. 111.

and many apply principles of behavior modification. Some of these programs are briefly described in this chapter.

Dual Disorders

Many chemically dependent people also have a coexisting disorder that complicates both disorders. A common dual disorder is mental illness combined with chemical dependency. For example, the mentally ill person may not be organized enough to work through a chemical dependency therapy program. Internal voices (auditory hallucinations) may tell the person to use certain chemicals. Many mentally ill people are depressed and use chemicals in an attempt to ease depression or to attempt suicide. In addition, these people often have difficulty locating a therapy or support group where other members understand the need to continue taking neuroleptic and other medications, while discontinuing use of addictive chemical substances.

Causes of Substance Abuse and Chemical Dependency

Despite all that has been written about the causes of substance abuse, no one has yet identified a sole causative factor.

Physical Factors Theory. Excessive consumption of substances (mood-altering chemicals, or "recreational drugs") is the most immediate cause of substance abuse. For example, investigators believe there is a *nutritional* deficiency that alcoholics remedy by drinking alcohol. Research is being conducted to learn whether there is an *endocrine* factor in alcoholism similar to the situation in diabetes. Another theory is that ingestion of alcohol and certain other drugs brings about an *allergic* response, an altered reaction of body tissues to a specific substance (alcohol), which would not produce the same effect in nonsensitive people. Many people use substances "just to feel better."

Genetic Theory. The theory of genetic determination has been the subject of considerable research. It has yet to be determined whether alcoholism and other substance abuse is based on direct biologic transmission or is a learned behavior in children who constantly interact with an alcoholic or substance-abusing parent(s). The genetic theory also would lend credence to the fact that the rate of alcoholism, for example, is higher in some racial groups.

Emotional and Psychological Theories. One can make some generalizations about the substance abuser's personality. It is characterized by difficulties in interpersonal relations, general uneasiness and dissatisfaction with life, low self-esteem, low tolerance for frustration, and a tendency toward excessive and self-destructive acts. As with most exclusively psychological theories, it is unclear whether these characteristics are typical of the potential substance abuser or are the result of the abuse.

Psychological explanations of substance abuse vary in detail but generally are in agreement that a person drinks alcohol or uses drugs to escape stress. Low self-esteem is perhaps the most potent precipitating factor in substance abuse. The dependent person needs the drug to feel good about life and self. The stress theory is compatible with this idea, because stress can be caused by low self-worth; the person continuously tries to be good enough to satisfy his or her own personal ideals.

Theory of Rational Emotive Therapy. Rational emotive therapy or rational recovery is built on the premise that an individual's values and beliefs control behavior. Many beliefs and assumptions are illogical and irrational, but people use them to evaluate themselves anyway. For example, the substance abuser might say, "I am weak; I am worthless; I do not deserve to be happy." The person then convinces himself or herself that these feelings are true. Rational recovery asks the

Key Abbreviations and Acronyms in Substance Abuse and Chemical Dependency

AA	Alcoholics Anonymous
Al-Anon	
CA	Cocaine Anonymous
CD	Chemical dependency
Detox	Detoxification
DTs	Delerium tremens
DUI	Driving under the influence
DWI	Driving while intoxicated
ETOH	Alcohol
LSD	Lysergic acid diethylamide
MAC	Mood-altering chemicals
MADD	Mothers Against Drunk Driving
MI-CD	Mentally ill and chemically dependent
MJ	Marijuana
MVA	Motor vehicle accident
NA	Narcotics Anonymous
OTC	Over-the-counter (drugs)
PCP	Phencyclidine HCl
RET	Rational Emotive Therapy
W/D	Withdrawal

question, "Why do I keep doing the same thing over and over when I know what the result is going to be, and I know I won't like it?"[2]

The Cycle of Depression

Depression is a common characteristic of the substance abuser, and the substance supplies relief. The cyclic nature of this type of depression may be viewed in one of three ways:

◆ *The initial stimulus.* To self-medicate intolerable depression, the substance-abuser "prescribes" increasingly high doses of the drug of choice.
◆ *A result of excessive chemical use.* The substance abuser becomes superficially aware that his or her behavior is socially unacceptable. Relationships with others are deteriorating, and the depression deepens.
◆ *A reason to continue.* To decrease and mask depression, the substance abuser seeks to blunt awareness of problems by alcohol or drug use. The more attempts to mask it, the deeper the depression becomes.

The Nature of Substance Abuse and Chemical Dependency

Progressive Nature. The progressive nature of the disease corresponds to the psychological cause. Generally, as the disease progresses, people cite the different reasons for drinking alcohol or using other drugs:

◆ "I use it to feel better." In the earlier stages of the disease, the chemical alleviates feelings of low self-worth and stress. Therefore, the person uses it to escape and feels better when using.
◆ "I use it to keep from feeling bad." As the disease progresses, the person must increase amounts of the substance in an effort not to feel sick or depressed. It becomes necessary to use the substance to keep from feeling bad, but the person never really feels good.
◆ "I'm losing control." The person now finds that a small amount of the chemical will cause illness or severe intoxication. **Blackouts** (periods of total amnesia) often begin to occur with excessive alcohol use and with some other drugs. At this point, immediate intervention is vital, often to save the person's life.

Defense Mechanisms. Of the many defense mechanisms people use, three deserve emphasis when dis-

cussing substance abuse: *denial, rationalization,* and *projection.* The substance abuser will deny any difficulty in controlling intake long after those around him or her have identified the problem. If the alcoholic does admit to drinking, for example, he or she most likely will blame others. A typical complaint would be that of being saddled with family problems: "If you were a better wife, I would not have to drink."

The Enabler or Co-dependent. The nature of alcoholism as a family disease is precisely what causes it be so complex. It is almost impossible to be an alcoholic without having a co-dependent. The **co-dependent**, also called **enabler**, is the spouse or child who calls work and says the person cannot come in because he or she is sick. The co-dependent is the person who tries to keep the family together, fends off the creditors, and drives the drunk person home after a party. The co-dependent tells the children that "mother can't cook tonight because she has a headache." The co-dependent, however, is often also blamed by the alcoholic for the entire problem, and the co-dependent accepts that blame. They say, "Maybe if I took better care of myself and looked better, the person wouldn't drink." In abuse of many other mood-altering chemicals, the enabler does not always play such an important role.

Nursing Care of the Person With Substance Abuse

Many patients admitted to the general hospital units may be alcoholic or otherwise chemically dependent. Many insurance plans no longer cover inpatient chemical dependency treatment. However, many people are admitted under a diagnosis that is either associated with or is a direct result of alcoholism or abuse of another substance.

Up to 45% of general medical–surgical patients may have an underlying substance abuse problem; 20% to 25% of these are alcoholics. The use of defense mechanisms is strong in the substance abusing person. These people will often convince the physician or nurse that the cause of a medical disorder is another problem; thus, the chemical problem goes undetected.

Nursing Alert
Be alert for signs and symptoms of chemical dependence or withdrawal in *all* of your patients.

General Admission History

Although the licensed practical nurse (LPN) or nursing student does not obtain a formal admission history or make a nursing diagnosis in the hospital, it is im-

[2] Adapted from Intervention Modes, Behavioral Approaches. In Johnson BS. Psychiatric-Mental Health Nursing: Adaptation and Growth, Ed 3. Philadelphia, J.B. Lippincott, 1993.

portant to know the items that are to be included. Often, the LPN will assist with the admission and will talk with the patient and family. Any nurse must report pertinent observations to the person doing the written admission.

Substance Use Assessment. An initial assessment of the patient's use of mood-altering chemicals can be incorporated naturally into every nursing history by asking how often, how, and how much.

The person should be asked, "Do you drink alcohol or use other drugs?" If the answer is yes, he or she should be asked, "Tell me about your drinking or using habits."

The nurse may need to probe further by asking specific questions:

◆ How often do you drink or use chemicals?
◆ Do you drink or use chemicals alone or with others? Are you usually at home or in a bar?
◆ What type of beverages do you drink? Do you combine alcohol and other drugs? Do you drink at work?
◆ How much of each chemical (alcohol, marijuana, cocaine, or other chemicals) do you use in a day? How much do you use in a week? How much does it cost you?

Key Concept

The questions listed above assume greater significance for patients being prepared for surgery or delivery.

Dealing With an Intoxicated Person in the Hospital

Nurses may have occasion to assist in the admission of an intoxicated person, either in the chemical dependency unit, the emergency room, the mental health unit, or in the general hospital. The accompanying box lists nursing care skills in the emergency room. Remember the following general points:

◆ A thorough history is required for safety during detoxification and in the event of complications related to chemical abuse, detoxification, or withdrawal.
◆ All information must be carefully documented.
◆ The physician often orders blood alcohol testing or urine toxicology. This patient is usually screened for all drugs, legal and illegal.

The physician writes orders for the patient based on the physical examination, the patient's history, the admission nursing history and diagnosis, and laboratory tests.

Some visitors may enter the hospital in an intoxicated state. It is usually unwise to allow them to visit patients. You can call your nursing supervisor, charge nurse, or hospital security if you do not know what to do. The intoxicated person, whether using drugs or alcohol, may be excitable. Do not attempt to force an intoxicated person to leave unless you have assistance.

Detoxification

Detoxification is the process of removing a drug or substance's physiologic effects from an addicted person.[3]

Goals in management of the detoxifying client are to give proper sedation and emotional support so that the patient can rest and recover to prevent injury or exhaustion. Treatment will depend in part on the specific substance in the body.

Nursing Alert

Clients in the early stages of withdrawal often show signs of anxiety, uncontrollable fear, tremor, irritability, agitation, hyperactive reflexes, hypertension, gastrointestinal disturbances, diaphoresis, and insomnia. This stage must be managed carefully and correctly. *(Rationale: If not managed properly, this state may lead to another stage that includes visual, tactile, olfactory, and auditory hallucinations. These hallucinations are terrifying to the patient. Seizures also may occur. The person may lose consciousness.)*

Some of the medications used in detoxification are listed in the accompanying box.

Withdrawal Symptoms

Withdrawal is the cessation of alcohol or a drug to which the person has become addicted. Withdrawal symptoms depend on the type of drug used. Various drugs and withdrawal symptoms are discussed in the last section of this chapter.

The person experiencing withdrawal presents many immediate potential nursing problems. The person who is addicted is in psychological and medical jeopardy when withdrawing from the substance. **Detoxification** from alcohol and certain other drugs is a serious medical problem; the process can be *fatal*. Table 88-1 lists specific signs and symptoms during withdrawal and nursing considerations for selected drugs.

---

[3] Based on "Recognition, Management, Safety, Dignity of the Detoxifying Patient," a module developed for Anoka Practical Nursing Program, Anoka, MN, by Josephine Schmer, BS, RN, HE.

Nursing Skill Guidelines
Caring for the Drug-Dependent Person in the Emergency Room

◆ Maintain an open airway in a life-threatening situation.
◆ Monitor the cardiac status; arrhythmias are common.
◆ Remain with the patient at all times during emergency treatment.
◆ Provide a quiet, calm environment. Speak softly.
◆ Tell the patient frequently where he or she is, because the person might be disoriented.
◆ Assure the person of your concern.
◆ Remove harmful objects from the immediate environment. *(Rationale: In a confused and agitated state, the patient might not recognize certain familiar objects and might injure himself or herself or another person.)*
◆ Do not touch the patient unless he or she understands your motive. *(Rationale: The person may react violently to physical contact.)*
◆ Be calm, quiet, and accepting. *(Rationale: If you are afraid, the patient will sense your fear.)*

Delirium Tremens. The acute detoxification period from alcohol is usually considered to be 72 hours. **Delirium tremens** (DTs, alcoholic hallucinosis) is an acute toxic state that can occur during withdrawal in severe alcoholism. The person may experience auditory or visual hallucinations. The person is usually frightened because he or she usually does not lose consciousness. DTs also can be precipitated in an alcoholic by an acute injury or infection. The occurrence of DTs is a serious complication and is considered a medical emergency. The most serious complications of DTs are peripheral circulatory collapse and hyperthermia.

Nursing Alert

The nurse on the medical–surgical unit of the hospital must be aware of the possibility of DTs in a patient who is admitted for an acute infection or severe injury. All people who have been involved in serious motor vehicle accidents should be evaluated for possible drug use.

Nursing Care During the Acute Phase of Detoxification

Following are some of the components of the nursing protocol for withdrawal from alcohol. Most of these procedures are the same as those for withdrawal from other drugs.

◆ An individual nursing care plan should be developed. Observation for several hours (usually 72) is needed to make a comprehensive plan.
◆ A detoxification protocol is followed. This includes careful patient observation and assessment according to the specific hospital protocol.
◆ The usual interval for observations for at least the first 12 hours is *every 15 minutes*, then every 30 minutes for 12 hours. *(Rationale: The person's condition can change rapidly. Detoxification can be life-threatening.)* Follow the protocol in your agency.
◆ Provide a quiet atmosphere. Remove or turn off TV or radio during intense period. Provide subdued lighting. *(Rationale: Stress and stimuli should be reduced.)*
◆ Stay with the client as much as possible. In some cases, family or a friend may be available to assist. The person is carefully observed. *(Rationale: The condition can change rapidly.)*
◆ Nursing assessment is important. *(Rationale: Medications, such as diazepam [Valium], are given PRN based on nursing judgment.)*
◆ Vital signs are closely monitored. Pedal pulses are taken. Tachycardia, dilated pupils, and diaphoresis often occur. All vital signs are usually evaluated. Attempts are made to control hypertension as much as possible but *not to lower the blood pressure too fast. (Rationale: Hypertension is caused by hyperactivity of the autonomic nervous system. Peripheral circulatory collapse may occur.)*
◆ Intravenous fluids may be given. Electrolytes are

Key Medications
for Detoxification

◆ Control or prevention of seizures: diazepam (Valium), chlordiazepoxide (Librium), phenytoin (Dilantin), magnesium sulfate ($MgSO_4$)
◆ Blood pressure control: antihypertensives
◆ Supplemental vitamins: vitamin C, thiamin, folate-folic acid, and a multivitamin (often with added iron)

Nursing Considerations

◆ Supplemental vitamins are used, especially with alcoholics.
◆ Antiseizure medications often help to promote relaxation and sleep.
◆ These drugs must be used very cautiously because of CNS depressant properties. Monitor vital signs carefully.
◆ The drugs may be given IV if necessary.
◆ Some of these drugs have the potential for habituation, especially in the substance-abusing patient.

Table 88-1. Withdrawal Pointers for Selected Drugs

Signs and Symptoms During Withdrawal	Nursing Considerations
Alcohol	
Acute detoxification about 72 hours	Carefully observe vital signs and level of consciousness.
High risk for suicide, clinical depression	Follow detoxification protocol of agency.
Alcohol often combined with other drugs	Patients is worked up for other health problems, such as malnutrition, liver damage, cardiac malfunction, infections, tuberculosis.
Tremors (hands first, then entire body), agitation	
Diaphoresis	
Confusion, disorientation, coma	Follow seizure precautions.
Blackouts, memory loss	Monitor blood sugar levels.
Cardiac arrest	Encourage food and fluids; monitor intake and output.
Delusions, hallucinations (auditory and visual—delirium tremens)	Follow suicide precautions.
Elevated pulse, hypertension	Manage nausea and vomiting.
Nausea, vomiting, anorexia	
Tonic–clonic seizures	
Hypoglycemia, electrolyte imbalance	
Dilated pupils	
Barbiturates	
May range from delerium to loss of consciousness	Follow specific protocol of facility.
Tonic–clonic seizures	Follow seizure precautions.
Sleep disorders, insomnia	Reorient patient as needed.
Confusion	Assess vital signs and level of consciousness often.
Tremor	Keep from hurting self or others.
EEG changes	Maintain patent airway.
Slowed or absent reflexes	
Respiratory changes, apnea	
Abnormal lung sounds	
Heroin	
Nausea, vomiting	Follow protocol of facility.
Diarrhea	Frequently assess vital signs and level of consciousness.
Tearing, runny nose, sore throat	This is most dangerous if patient has concurrent medical disorder, such as heart disease, lung disease, or diabetes.
Dilated pupils	
Tremors, weakness	Patient often is malnourished.
Diaphoresis, chills	Patient may have infections, abscesses, and so forth from injections.
Gooseflesh (hair on extremities stands on end)	
Depression to loss of consciousness or irritability and hyperactivity	Sexual dysfunction is common.
Confusion, disorientation	Follow seizure precautions.
Delusions, hallucinations	
Muscle and joint pain	
Yawning	
Insomnia, sleep disturbances	
Mild hypertension	
Lowered temperature (in some cases, temperature rises)	
Fast, weak, irregular pulse	
Slowed respirations	

(continued)

Table 88-1 *(continued)*

Signs and Symptoms During Withdrawal	Nursing Considerations
Cocaine	Follow protocol of specific facility.
Acute detoxification is 4–5 wk	Treat specific symptoms.
Depression or irritability	Maintain quiet environment with minimum stimulation.
Extreme mood swings (lability)	Seizure precautions often are used.
Lack of feeling (anhedonia)	Assess level of consciousness and vital signs frequently; control hypertension.
Pressured speech, grandiosity, hyperactivity, intrusiveness	Assess mental status and orientation.
Anxiety, paranoia, crying jags	Keep from hurting self or others.
Confusion, poor memory	Carefully observe vital signs.
Tactile hallucinations ("cocaine bugs")	Encourage adequate nutrition and fluid intake.
Sleep disturbances, nightmares	Assess urinary output.
Gastrointestinal symptoms, nausea, vomiting, difficulties with digestion	Assess sleeping habits.
Low urine output (oliguria)	Reorient as needed.
Headache, bone pain, muscle cramps	Particularly dangerous to mother and fetus when used by a pregnant woman.
Runny nose, nasal congestion, eyes tearing	Monitor intake and output; report oliguria.
Dilated pupils	Manage nausea and vomiting.
Respiratory depression	
Sudden increase in temperature	
Extreme hypertension	
Increased pulse rate	
Approximately fourth week—intense craving (high risk for relapse)	
Possible organic mental disorder (brain damage)	

carefully monitored. Encourage fluids. *(Rationale: Dehydration and electrolyte imbalances often occur as a result of diaphoresis and hyperactivity.)*

♦ Temperature is carefully monitored. *(Rationale: Life-threatening hyperthermia is possible.)*

♦ Supplemental vitamin therapy and a high-protein diet are often prescribed. *(Rationale: Many chemically dependent people are undernourished and vitamin deficient.)*

♦ Intake and output, calorie count, and daily weight should be recorded, and fluids are often encouraged. *(Rationale: Restoring fluid and electrolyte balance improves nutritional status.)*

♦ Frequent small feedings are often more palatable than large meals. *(Rationale: The client usually has a decreased appetite.)*

♦ Blood sugar is monitored carefully. The person may receive intravenous dextrose or oral supplement drinks. *(Rationale: Hypoglycemia may occur during withdrawal, because alcohol depletes the glycogen stored in the liver. Alcoholism also impairs glycogenesis, because it damages the liver, as in cirrhosis.)*

♦ Vital signs are assessed often, usually every 30 minutes to 1 hour or more often for the first 24 hours, then less often but at least every 4 hours for

72 hours in acute withdrawal. Include neurologic eye signs if the patient is confused or unconscious. *(Rationale: Drug dosage is often based on vital signs. The client's condition can change rapidly.)*

♦ The client usually is not restrained. Side rails should be up when the person is in bed. *(Rationale: Restraints could agitate the person further. The absence of restraints is another reason for close observation of the client.)*

♦ The client's respiratory, hepatic, and cardiovascular systems are monitored carefully. Report any distress immediately. Monitor results of blood tests. *(Rationale: Complications of detoxification and alcoholism include respiratory distress, pneumonia, liver damage and disease, and cardiac failure.)* An electrocardiogram is often done.

♦ Turn and position the client every 2 hours. *(Rationale: It is important to prevent injuries or difficulties related to inactivity; the person may be confused or unconscious.)*

♦ If the person is nauseated or vomiting, position him or her on the side. *(Rationale: You must prevent aspiration.)*

♦ Seizure precautions are followed. *(Rationale: Seizures are a common complication if detoxification is not successfully managed.)*

- Anticonvulsant drugs are prescribed. *(Rationale: Most of the time, this will prevent seizures.)*
- Other symptoms may occur. Treatment is symptomatic.

> **Key Concept**
>
> Nursing care in detoxification is basically the same no matter what the drug.

Care After Detoxification

The period following detoxification also is important. Usually the client remembers vividly the hallucinations and extreme discomfort experienced and may be willing to enter treatment. The nurse's role includes discussing with the attending physician the possibility of a chemical dependency evaluation. The person may be diagnosed as alcoholic, chemically dependent, polysubstance dependent, co-dependent, or all four. Many alcoholics or chemically dependent people are also co-dependent, living with another person who is a user of alcohol or other drugs.

> **Key Concept**
>
> The patient's general physical condition is assessed following withdrawal. Included are liver function tests, evaluation of gastrointestinal function and conditions, and assessment of general nutritional status. Coexisting conditions, such as injuries, skin rashes, and diabetes, also are diagnosed and treated.

Long-Term Inpatient or Outpatient Treatment

After the initial detoxification period, the person who abuses substances will almost always need some sort of follow-up treatment. Treatment can be on an inpatient basis in a treatment center or on an outpatient basis. The person's attitude, the attitudes of the family, insurance coverage, and the person's work and personal situation often determine what type of follow-up care is recommended. Treatment centers base their treatment on one or more of the following programs:

- The 12-step program based on Alcoholic Anonymous and other groups
- Albert Ellis' Rational Emotional Therapy
- Milton Cudney's Self-Defeating Behavior Theory
- Personal and group counseling
- Improving nutritional and general health
- Client and family education about the disease
- Family counseling

Some alcoholic patients are allowed to take disulfiram (Antabuse), which causes great discomfort when combined with alcohol.

12-Step Programs. The 12-step groups, such as Alcoholics Anonymous and Narcotics Anonymous, teach that untreated chemical dependency is progressive, and the disease is incurable. The disease of chemical dependency is considered to be *arrested or in remission* when the person is not using. The 12-step programs do not actually sponsor or endorse any particular treatment program. The 12-steps are based on admitting powerlessness over chemicals and admitting that one's life has become unmanageable. The person then accepts that a higher power exists, determines whom they have harmed and makes amends, turns their lives over to their higher power, and assists other people. The premise of the 12-step program is, "I have a disease, and it's not my fault. I need assistance to stop using . . ."

Rational Recovery. The premise of rational recovery is based on Milton Cudney's theory of self-defeating behavior and Albert Ellis' rational emotive therapy. The premise of this program is, "I abuse chemicals because I choose to do so, and I quit because I no longer choose to do so."

Nutritional and General Health. All therapy programs offer counseling to the individual at a personal level or in a group setting or to a family. The issues of nutrition and general health must be addressed. The person needs care or a follow-up plan after treatment, and this aftercare is often more important than the intensive phase of treatment. The support and understanding of a counselor or group are an important part of any treatment program.

Family Counseling. The family and the patient need intensive counseling. It is not enough just to treat the substance abuser. Modern treatment centers include an intensive treatment program for the family that is conducted simultaneously with the patient's treatment.

The person and family must realize that they will probably need some follow-up care. *Follow-up care is vital.* They will need encouragement and support to deal with the stresses of any normal family, plus the added challenges that must be met by the recovering family. It is important to note that a person is much less likely to progress in recovery if the family is not also in the recovery mode.

> **Key Concept**
>
> The family and patient may require a social service referral to assist in obtaining employment, financial assistance, or housing.

Treatment Facilities

There are several reasons for the substance abuser to seek treatment. The person may really *want to stop* and may realize that job, loved ones, health, and freedom of action are in jeopardy if the habit continues.

The user may *want to phase out reliance on the drug.* As tolerance to the drug increases, so does the need for money to support the habit; thus, the person might try to find ways to reduce dependence. This is more likely to be seen with heroin and cocaine users than with others.

> **Nursing Alert**
>
> A problem encountered when a person reduces intake of drugs, such as barbiturates or cocaine, is that there may be a greater possibility of overdose. If the drug is stopped, tolerance to it is reduced; if the user then injects or snorts the customary pretreatment dose, it could be equivalent to an *overdose.*

A person might seek treatment in response to a *court order.* In many states, a person apprehended for a crime associated with drug use or involved in an auto accident while intoxicated will be sent by the judge to a treatment facility. When the person enters the treatment facility, the motivation and desire to succeed are often not very strong. However, an underlying rationale for this treatment is that the person is committed for a certain length of time and may begin to participate in the treatment program (sometimes without being truly aware of it). The choice between a treatment facility and jail is a strong reason for some people to enter a drug treatment program.

Components of Treatment Programs

Treatment programs often include general group therapy, women's issues, men's issues, referrals to sexual assault groups, violence anonymous groups, and grief issues. Many treatment facilities have developed special groups within their own programs. Programs developed include women's programs, adolescent programs, senior programs, outpatient day or evening programs, and midday programs. Groups for the chemically dependent mentally ill are becoming more common.

> **Key Concept**
>
> Many substance abusers have low self-esteem and thus a strong unconscious need to fail. Therefore, the nurse helps the patient set realistic goals.

Detoxification Centers

Substance abusers may begin the long road to withdrawal and recovery in detoxification centers. Here, the person withdraws from the substance under medical supervision. The emphasis in a crisis intervention or detoxification center is on supportive care and making plans for long-term therapy to deal with the underlying motivations that led to the dependent behavior patterns. Family therapy also might be planned for the person undergoing treatment. (See previous discussion of detoxification.)

The Therapeutic Community

In a therapeutic community, the person is isolated from the substance-oriented environment. The person's lifestyle is changed in basic ways; he or she is shown ways to cope with life without using drugs. Most of these programs are organized and administered by recovering drug abusers or alcoholics.

Once a person is admitted to this type of program, he or she undergoes detoxification. Close supervision is required. After the acute withdrawal symptoms have passed, the person is given work assignments. The purpose of the work assignment is to help the person to acquire habits of responsibility.

Basically, the goal of treatment is to assist the substance-dependent person to achieve complete detoxification. At the same time, the physical problems associated with abuse are treated. The facility helps the person understand the cycle of dependence.

> **Key Concept**
>
> The substance abuser needs follow-up care, such as Alcoholics Anonymous or Rational Recovery, for at least 2 years after the intensive treatment stage is completed. Some people need this support for life.

Alcoholism

Alcoholism, as substance abuse, is defined as a disease by the American Psychiatric Association in its *Diagnostic and Statistical Manual of Mental Disorders, Fourth Edition, Revised.* The APA definition states: "Substance abuse is a pattern of pathological use and impairment in social or occupational functioning due to substance abuse, minimal duration of at least one month."

Alcoholism is said to be the third major health problem in the United States. Estimates indicate that as many as 15 million people in this country may be alcoholics or problem drinkers. An estimated 60% to 70% of identified alcoholics are male, although the number of known female alcoholics is rising. The number of young people who abuse alcohol is rising also at an alarming rate. Abuse of alcohol and other substances is a factor in a high percentage of automobile accidents.

Family Programs. The people most affected by alcoholism are the spouse and children. The young person who has been raised in an alcoholic family has special problems. These include low self-esteem and feelings of failure, as well as the feeling that they must take care of others because it is their responsibility. These people are often clinically depressed or suicidal and often become alcoholic or chemically dependent themselves.

Al-Anon, Al-A-Tot, and Al-A-Teen, sponsored by Alcoholics Anonymous, offer support and encouragement to the families of alcoholics. Al-Anon is usually for the spouse or adult significant other of the alcoholic, and Al-A-Tot and Al-A-Teen are attended by the children of the alcoholic. A program in St. Paul, Minnesota, called "Children are People" encourages active intervention and therapy with the children in a family. This may begin as early as age 3 to 4 years.

It is important to attend some sort of group regularly for support and education. Often, when the co-dependent person gets help and stops the enabling behavior, the alcoholic can no longer continue the cycle because there is no one to blame for the problems but himself or herself, and that is too painful.

Legislation. Some states have adopted the *implied consent law.* This allows law enforcement officers to require an alcohol test when they have reason to believe a person is driving while intoxicated or when a driver is involved in an auto accident. If a person refuses, they automatically lose their driver's license. Some states now have a "dram shop law," which makes it possible to sue the bar or liquor store that sells liquor to a person who is intoxicated and later causes an accident. In some cases, this law also applies to private house parties.

An organization called Mothers Against Drunk Drivers (MADD) has been successful in getting legislation passed that imposes severe penalties on drivers who are driving while intoxicated or driving while under the influence. This law also includes driving boats and snowmobiles in many states.

Abuse of Other Drugs

While the chemical characteristics of drugs determine their effects on individuals, cultural norms dictate the circumstances under which various drugs are used. A typical American family's medicine cabinet or ordinary advertising on television shows how our culture contributes directly and indirectly to drug dependence. Re-

view the nursing process as related to substance abuse in the accompanying box.

> **Key Concept**
>
> A large percentage of substance abusers overuse more than one substance. Alcohol is often combined with other mood-altering chemicals, especially cocaine. Many of the characteristics of the alcoholic also apply to the polysubstance abuser.

Causes of Drug Abuse

As with alcohol, there is no single common personality disorder or physical condition that causes drug abuse. Attempts to categorize the drug-dependent personality have been inconclusive. Drug abuse is not exclusively a problem of any one group.

The abuser of alcohol and some other drugs is usually a person with a history of social inadequacy and low self-esteem. This person is often immature, searching for some means of escape from reality. Drug abuse also may reflect deep-seated, unsatisfied emotional needs and rebelliousness. Although the attention given the abuser is often negative and punitive, still it is attention.

Drugs, such as cocaine, cut across a much wider representation of the total population. A highly developed ability to manipulate others also is present, and intelligence and ability are often of a high order. The person has learned to survive, by whatever means, sometimes including criminal actions. (For example, stealing often is used to support the habit.)

One of the most compelling reasons for continued drug dependence is the associated physiologic dependence and in some cases, physical dependence.

Treatment of Drug Abuse

Much of the counseling and other psychological treatment of the person who is dependent on drugs is the same or similar to the treatment of the person who is dependent on alcohol. Much of the physical care also is similar. Check your agency's protocol.

Sedative-Hypnotics

The sedative-hypnotic group of drugs is large and includes the barbiturates and minor tranquilizers. Examples are pentobarbital (Nembutal), secobarbital (Seconal, "reds"), and phenobarbital. The drug tables in Chapter 56 contain a more complete listing of various drugs and their effects. All have a potential for physical and psychological dependence and induce tolerance, leading to an ever-increasing dosage.

In acute ("cold turkey") withdrawal, seizures are possible. Withdrawal must be gradual. Overdose and

Overview of the Nursing Process
Substance Abuse

Assessment Priorities

Behavior Changes

Erratic or inappropriate behavior
Sudden changes in mood
Poor school or job attendance or performance
Antisocial acts, such as stealing, embezzling, prostitution, or selling drugs
Declining social status or an incongruent economic situation
Frequent visits to an emergency department for depression or suicide threats

Physical Signs

Needle tracks, often covered by long sleeves
Chronic nasal congestion and cold symptoms with drug snorting; after heavy use, the septum may perforate
Dilated pupils, often masked by sunglasses
Unkempt appearance
Unexplained weight loss
If you suspect substance abuse in a person who presents in the emergency department, ask the physician to order a toxicology screening.

Complications With Overdose

Cerebrovascular spasm as shown by hemorrhage, seizures, hypertensive crisis; angina; myocardial infarction; dysrhythmias; abnormal respirations (Cheyne-Stokes); and hyperthermia

Possible Nursing Diagnoses

Impaired Adjustment
Anxiety
Ineffective Individual Coping
Fear
Altered Growth and Development (fetal)
Altered Health Maintenance
High risk for infection
High risk for injury
Knowledge Deficit
Noncompliance (specify)
Altered Nutrition: Less than Body Requirements
Altered Parenting
Personal Identity Disturbance
Powerlessness
Altered Role Performance
Self-Care Deficit
Self-Esteem Disturbance
Sensory/Perceptual Alterations
Impaired Social Interaction
Altered Thought Processes
High Risk for violence: Self-Directed or Directed at Others

Planning

The nurse designs a plan of care with the client to achieve the following general patient goals:
The person admits that substance abuse has hurt him or her.
The person admits that he or she needs help to stop using the drug.
The person agrees to participate in a substance abuse program.
The person's behavior and physical signs demonstrate decreased or discontinued substance abuse.
The person tests drug free (urine tests, toxicology screening).

Implementation

Refer the client to a psychiatric liaison nurse or a drug abuse counselor.
If a known substance abuser denies abuse, do not withdraw from the case or become angry; continue to break down the denial by pointing out how the addiction has contributed to the person's medical, social, or legal problems.
If all else fails, provide the person with information about getting help; write down a hotline number or other community resource.
Support the family of the substance abuser if they are present, and respond honestly to their questions; the family may be enlisted to encourage the client to seek help (intervention).
For emergency room nursing care of the drug-dependent person, see the box early in this chapter.

Evaluation

The adequacy of the plan of care is determined by evaluating the client's achievement of the above goals. If the person is unable to meet key goals, the plan must be modified. Key evaluative criteria include the following:
The client is drug free.
The client returns to presubstance abuse role performance.
The client seeks and continues treatment and participates in continued follow-up (such as attendance at AA).

acute withdrawal constitute medical emergencies requiring hospitalization. A particular danger is *respiratory depression*.

Marijuana

Marijuana can induce psychological dependence. Research has now shown that physical dependence and negative effects can result from continued use of marijuana. The most common effect of marijuana is a dreamy state, characterized by euphoria; perception of space and time may be distorted.

A panic reaction can occur from a few moments to an hour or more after smoking. The person might experience anxiety, palpitations, rapid pulse, nausea, dyspnea, and a feeling of choking or suffocation. Restlessness is acute, and the person might make pleading appeals for help. There is no evidence that smoking marijuana directly leads to the use of opiates or other drugs. However, most people who use the "harder" drugs smoked marijuana first.

Narcotics

The narcotics group includes opium, heroin, morphine, meperidine, codeine, methadone, and other drugs. With the exception of codeine, all of these drugs are highly addictive and rapidly induce tolerance, physical dependence, and psychological dependence. A specific antidote for narcotic overdose is naloxone HCl (Narcan).

Narcotic withdrawal, although quite uncomfortable, is not as dangerous as is barbiturate withdrawal. Symptoms of narcotic withdrawal resemble those of a cold or an allergic response, with sore throat, rhinorrhea (runny nose), lacrimation (tearing of eyes), and diaphoresis (sweating). In more severe cases, the person appears ill, with dilated pupils, joint pains, and insomnia.

> **Nursing Alert**
>
> Heroin and methadone overdoses are life-threatening emergencies that require immediate medical attention.

Methadone Maintenance

Methadone maintenance is one of the most widely publicized treatment programs for heroin-dependent individuals. Programs using this method substitute methadone for heroine, because methadone does not produce the high that is associated with heroin. Some physicians are reluctant to use methadone because it is addicting, and withdrawal is physically dangerous.

Once the drug-dependent person has reached a maintenance dose of methadone, he or she can be discharged from a detoxification facility and receive meth-adone as an outpatient. Any dose more than 120 mg per day requires state and federal preapproval. For maintenance of narcotic abstinence, *oral administration is required* by law. The powder form is mixed in at least 120 mL of orange juice or powdered citrus drink to mask the bitter taste and the amount of the dose. Tablets are also available. (The drug, given orally, is half as potent as it is when injected.)

Several times a week or daily, supervised urine specimens are required. They are analyzed to determine whether the person has taken opiates, barbiturates, or other drugs while on methadone. Repeated evidence that the person has taken such drugs might result in dismissal from the program.

Many methadone maintenance programs also require the drug-dependent person to participate in some form of group therapy. It is hoped that through the group process, the drug-dependent person will find new ways of problem solving in an environment free of recreational drugs. Some programs make an effort to structure educational programs around health and occupational issues as well.

Central Nervous System Stimulants

These include cocaine and the amphetamines. These drugs induce tolerance and psychological dependence.

Amphetamines

Some trade names for amphetamines are Benzedrine, Dexedrine, and Methedrine. They are mood elevators and appetite depressants, and they combat drowsiness and simple fatigue. Many of these drugs are not sold legally in the United States.

Withdrawal from amphetamines usually causes depression and in some cases, a paranoid psychosis that requires hospitalization. The behavior of people on amphetamines is highly unpredictable, and they require careful, consistent nursing care. Amphetamine abusers often combine amphetamines with sedatives, such as barbiturates and alcohol. Many take sedatives to "even out" the high and avoid the "crash" of stimulant withdrawal.

> **Key Concept**
>
> When a person is withdrawing from amphetamines, prevention from injury to self and others is important.

Cocaine

Cocaine became one of the most widely used drugs in the United States during the 1980s. Dependence on cocaine *quickly occurs*. The cocaine derivative "crack," or "freebase" cocaine is even more dangerous and addicting. New derivatives are still emerging. Cocaine can be absorbed from all mucous surfaces, injected intravenously, or smoked. Because cocaine is often snorted, the user may have a severe chronic inflammation of the nasal mucous membranes. The use of cocaine and its derivatives is particularly dangerous in pregnancy and leads to damage and illness in the fetus. Cardiac arrest can occur from cocaine overdose.

Key Concept

Cocaine can cause irreversible organic brain damage, even in small amounts.

If the person also is using heroin, the general procedure is to give naloxone as a prophylactic measure. During withdrawal from cocaine, vital signs must be monitored continuously, and hypertension must be controlled. Intake and output are monitored. Oliguria, a serious sign, should be reported. Respiratory depression may occur and must be monitored. Respiratory stimulants might be needed. The patient in severe withdrawal usually needs to be in an intensive care unit or have a special duty nurse. There is a high potential for the patient to return to the use of cocaine, because it is so addicting.

Hallucinogens

Hallucinogenic drugs are not believed to cause actual physical dependence, but they do produce psychological dependence and mild tolerance. This group of drugs includes lysergic acid diethylamide (LSD), mescaline, and psilocybin ("mushrooms"). Tolerance to these drugs is highly variable. Their most characteristic effects are intense visual hallucinations of vivid colors and auditory hallucinations. Medications are not usually given to assist in the detoxification of this patient.

The major problems associated with hallucinogenics are acute panic reactions and flashbacks sometimes years later. The user also may be injured by thinking that he or she can fly, walk on water, or stop traffic on a busy freeway. Providing a safe environment is essential. Care for the person on a "bad trip" requires speaking calmly and giving sustained reassurance. This person can also have permanent brain damage, especially if several drugs were combined.

Phencyclidine Hydrochloride

Phencyclidine hydrochloride (PCP or angel dust) has been abused since the late 1970s because of its low cost and easy availability. PCP is a hallucinogen that was originally developed as an anesthetic.

Because PCP has a simple chemical structure, it is believed that most PCP now on the streets is illegally manufactured in the home. Its effects are similar to those of the hallucinogens and central nervous system stimulants. Some believe that PCP prevents the individual from filtering out irrelevant sensory input, so the person becomes overwhelmed by environmental stimuli. The most characteristic effect of the drug is an alteration in body image, frequently accompanied by uncomfortable feelings of unreality. A second effect in some individuals is a feeling of loneliness and isolation.

The most effective way of treating a person who has taken PCP and is experiencing difficulty is to provide as quiet an environment as possible, with as little stimulation as possible. The person on PCP does not benefit from verbal reassurance. It is better for the nurse not to talk at all, an approach that differs from that used to treat a person having a bad trip from one of the other hallucinogens. Permanent brain damage can also result from using this drug.

Nursing Alert

Do not touch this person without warning him or her. You may be seriously injured.

Volatile Substances

Volatile substances are chemical preparations that when inhaled, produce altered states of consciousness and varying degrees of intoxication. They are considered central nervous system depressants. Generally, the abused volatile substances cause slurring of speech, loss of coordination, lessening of inhibitions, and dizziness. Hallucinations, hazy euphoria, marked behavioral and personality changes, and impaired perception and judgment also are likely.

Reports of glue sniffing, gasoline sniffing, and inhaling the vapor from aerosol cans are frequent; inhaling these substances also causes serious damage to lung tissue. (Continual inhalation of hair sprays also can cause respiratory damage.)

Other Abused Substances

Nicotine

Nicotine is a substance contributing to cancer, heart and blood vessel disorders, and many other physical disorders. The United States Federal Trade Commission requires that cigarette packs carry a warning such as "SURGEON GENERAL'S WARNING: Smoking causes lung cancer, heart disease, emphysema, and may complicate pregnancy" or "Smoking by pregnant women may result in fetal injury, premature birth, and low birth weight."

Smoking causes constriction of the blood vessels in the skin, along with a decrease in skin temperature and an increase in blood pressure. Cigarette smoke contains approximately 1% carbon monoxide; this combines with the hemoglobin in the blood to diminish the blood's capacity to carry oxygen. Over time, this can cause damage to tissue, especially heart and lung tissue.

There are many local and national self-help programs that are free or low in cost; their aim is to get the smoker to quit smoking. You can help smokers to find the one best suited to their personal requirements—often several programs have to be tried. The American Cancer Society and the American Lung Association are resources for information.

Caffeine

Caffeine is found not only in coffee, but also in tea, cola drinks, and some other types of soft drinks, and chocolate. As a mild stimulant, it has few peers. There is considerable evidence that 200 to 300 mg of caffeine will partially offset fatigue; the caffeine appears to enhance a person's capacity to perform physically exhausting work well beyond the normal limit. Caffeine also seems to assuage boredom and increase one's attention span.

Two cups of coffee taken close together contain approximately 200 mg of caffeine. In a person whose tolerance to caffeine is limited, even that amount will make it harder to fall asleep and will interfere with normal sleep patterns. Caffeine also is a major component of medications, such as Excedrin and No Doz.

Caffeine acts directly on the vascular muscles, causing them to dilate. At levels of 500 mg of caffeine or higher, the heart rate will increase, and with high blood levels of caffeine, the heartbeat may become irregular. Other related disorders include development or aggravation of cystic breast disease and aggravation of some types of migraine headaches.

Dependence on caffeine is a physical reality. A notable withdrawal symptom is the headache habitual users have after a caffeine-free day. Research is being conducted on the total side effects of caffeine use.

Over-the-Counter Drugs

Over-the-counter drugs can be purchased without a prescription. Yearly, billions of dollars are spent by people who medicate themselves. The kinds of pills that can be purchased at the local drugstore without a prescription are numerous.

Adequate nutrition, with vitamin supplementation if needed and attention to proper rest, sleep, and activity,

Signs of Substance Abuse in a Nurse

- ◆ Consistently signs out more controlled drugs than other staff members
- ◆ Consistently wants to be a medication nurse
- ◆ Opens medication cabinet only when alone
- ◆ Frequently breaks or spills drugs and has to dispose of them
- ◆ Makes many medication errors
- ◆ Spends a great deal of time in the bathroom
- ◆ Wears long sleeves
- ◆ Spends a great deal of time on the unit when not on duty; "hangs around"
- ◆ Noticeable discrepancies as to relief gained by medications occur between reports of patients assigned to this nurse and reports of patients assigned to other staff members
- ◆ Incorrect medication count when this nurse gives medications
- ◆ Medication vials appear altered; medication appears different from normal
- ◆ Behavior that might indicate substance use: illogical or unreadable charting, often comes to work late, extreme mood swings, defensiveness, frequent absences, overuse of sick leave

is often all that is needed to correct minor discomforts. As a nurse, you have many opportunities to teach people about the dangers of self-medication.

Special Abusers

The Pregnant Woman. The pregnant substance abuser can have a complicated labor and delivery with profound effects on her and the baby. Babies of alcohol- and drug-abusing mothers are often of low birth weight. Heroin withdrawal symptoms in a newborn may occur within hours after delivery, and most affected babies demonstrate symptoms within the first 24 hours. The number of cocaine- and crack-addicted babies is increasing in the United States. Not only do these babies have many physical problems, but their mothers often lack parenting skills as well. Chapter 62 describes disorders in newborns caused by maternal drug use.

The Elderly. Often a multiplicity of drugs is taken by older people. As worries about financial status or growing social isolation loom, many elderly people become dependent on alcohol, sedatives, tranquilizers, cathartics, antacids, and sleeping pills. It is not unusual for the person to increase or decrease the medication dosage on personal initiative. In your interactions with older patients, remember that an accurate drug history is an important part of assessment (see Chapter 85).

The Adolescent. Substance abuse is rapidly becoming a serious problem among adolescents and even among younger children. Peer pressure is strong among young people, and self-esteem is often low. These are potent forces toward the use of chemicals. Adolescent chemical dependency is discussed in more detail in Chapter 66.

The Nurse. Drugs are available in the healthcare facility, and it is possible for the nurse to become a substance abuser (see box). Nurses are 50% more likely to become chemically dependent than the general population.[4]

You are bound by law, your code of ethics, and the pledge that you take in nursing to report any staff person who you suspect is abusing drugs or alcohol. This is to protect the patients with whom this nurse might come in contact. The safe care of those patients might rest in your hands.

[4] *Nurse Review*, "Psychiatric Problems," Springhouse, PA, Springhouse, 1989; revised 1994, page 111

Keys for Review

Key Questions for Critical Thinking

1. Describe alcoholism. State its consequences on the individual, family, and community. Describe the enabler and implications related to alcoholism. Identify programs available for the alcoholic person and family.
2. You are examining a pregnant adolescent whom you suspect of using cocaine. Identify the signs and symptoms. Determine your actions. Describe her newborn if she does not stop using cocaine. Discuss what can be expected of her parenting skills. Be as specific as possible.
3. You suspect one of your coworkers to be a substance abuser. State the signs for which you should look. State your responsibilities. Outline what actions you should take.

Key Readings

American Psychiatric Association. Diagnostic and Statistical Manual of Mental Disorders, Ed. 4. Washington, DC, APA, 1994

Black C. Double Duty—Chemically Dependent. Denver, CO, MAC Publishing, 1990

Cudney MR, Hardy RE. Self-Defeating Behaviors: Free yourself from the Habits, Compulsions, Feelings and Attitudes That Hold You Back. San Francisco, Harper SF, a division of Harper-Collins, 1991

Ellis A. When AA Doesn't Work for You: A Rational Guide to Quitting Alcohol. New York, Barricade, 1992

Johnson BS. Psychiatric-Mental Health Nursing: Adaptation and Growth, Ed 3. Philadelphia, J.B. Lippincott, 1993

Shives LR. Basic Concepts of Psychiatric-Mental Health Nursing, Ed 3. Philadelphia, J.B. Lippincott, 1994

Enrichment Keys

Green P. "The Chemically Dependent Nurse." Nursing Clinics of North America, 24(1):81–94, 1989

Thobaben M, Anderson L, Campbell HG. Chemical dependency in home healthcare nurses. Home Healthcare Nurs, Vol. 12 #3, May/June, 1994, 67–69

Keys To Learning More

As you graduate and become employed, you may encounter patients or coworkers who abuse substances or are chemically dependent. This chapter will assist you to more effectively work with these people.

Key Resources

Alcoholics Anonymous
 468 Park Avenue South
 New York, NY 19916
 212/686-1100

Al-Anon Family Group Headquarters
 P.O. Box 182
 Madison Square Station
 New York, NY 10159

National Clearinghouse for Drug Abuse Information
 P.O. Box 2345
 11400 Rockville Pike
 Rockville, MD 20852
 1-800/729-6686

National Council on Alcoholism
 12 West 21st Street
 New York, NY 10010

National Institute on Alcohol Abuse and Alcoholism
 National Institute on Drug Abuse (NIDA)
 5600 Fishers Lane
 Rockville, MD 20857

89 Rehabilitation, Ambulatory, and Home Care Nursing

Keys for Learning

Learning Objectives

- Define rehabilitation, and state its goals.
- List members of the rehabilitation team and their roles.
- Describe community resources for people with disabilities.
- Describe adaptations for homemakers with disabilities and for vocational rehabilitation of workers.
- Describe nursing activities in the physician's office.
- Describe ambulatory surgery and day surgery, and describe nursing responsibilities.
- Describe home nursing.
- Describe the role of the licensed practical nurse in home care nursing.

Key Terms

activities of daily living
Credé's maneuver
hemiplegic
mainstreaming
rehabilitation

paralysis
paraplegic
physiatrist
quadriplegic

Keys to Understanding This Chapter

Chapter 3: the healthcare delivery system
Chapter 5: basic human needs
Chapter 6: public health goals, including maximum wellness for all people
Chapter 7: introduction to the concept of public health
Unit Nine: nursing skills applicable to public health and home care, rehabilitation, and ambulatory nursing
Unit Thirteen: children with a physical dysfunction who may need rehabilitation, ambulatory care, or home care

Keys to Understanding This Chapter
(continued)

Unit Fourteen: adults with a physical dysfunction
Unit Fifteen: care of the elderly adult, many of whom receive home care and rehabilitation

Key Points

- Rehabilitation aims to restore a person to a fully functioning status or to maximize remaining abilities.
- All clients or patients are people first and "clients" next.
- Many different disciplines function as a part of the rehabilitation or home care team.
- Many community resources are available to assist people with disabilities or diseases.
- Adaptive materials are available to assist the person with a disability to perform activities of daily living.
- More healthcare today is being carried out in an ambulatory setting; more surgery is done in day surgery.
- Home care is the fastest growing area of healthcare.
- Many people prefer care in the home.

Key Topics Outline

Rehabilitation Care
  Community Resources
  Nursing Considerations
Ambulatory Nursing
  The Physician's Office or Clinic
  The Emergency Room or Emergi-Center
  The Day Surgery Center or Ambulatory Surgery Center
Home Nursing
  Types of Agencies and Services
  Home Nursing Care

Most of your training so far has been in the hospital or in the nursing home. This textbook presents the variety of services available to individuals. This chapter looks specifically at three services: rehabilitation, ambulatory care, and home care. It discusses the types of care and nursing responsibilities in this care. All of these locations offer employment for graduate nurses. You may need to make minor modifications in procedures to adapt to a specific situation. However, basic principles, such as asepsis, universal precautions, nursing care planning, interpersonal communications, and safety still prevail.

Rehabilitation Care

Rehabilitation is restoration of a person with a disability to his or her former abilities or if complete restoration is not possible, helping the person *adjust* to a disability or physical challenge. The principles of rehabilitation center around early recognition and individualized planning for each client.

An extensive discussion of rehabilitation nursing is beyond the scope of this book, but this introduction shows that principles and purposes of rehabilitation remain the same, regardless of the person's condition.

The goal of all rehabilitation nursing is to assist clients to approach normal functioning as much as possible. *Minimize the person's limitations* and *maximize capabilities* for quality of life (see the accompanying box).

The Client as a Person

The person with a disability has the same needs, feelings, desires, and problems as anyone else and generally does not want to be treated as "special." The person wishes to be as independent as possible.

A client is likely to meet the problem of a disability in the same spirit as when faced with other problems. He or she may be resentful, despairing, or disbelieving or may face a disability with determination to do everything possible to overcome it.

Stages of Adjustment. During adjustment to a disability, a person usually experiences reactions similar to those of any grief process. The first reaction may be *denial.* The person may be confident of recovery, and therefore his or her demands are often childlike. The patient often becomes *angry,* asking "Why me?" Eventually, the client must face reality and may experience depression or *mourning* for his or her lost ability. Hopefully, the client will come to *acceptance* of the limitation and become active in developing realistic long-range goals. Some people do not attain the stage of acceptance. In some cases, psychiatric assistance and counseling for the person and family is an essential part of rehabilitation.

The Rehabilitation Team

The rehabilitation team includes the nurse, therapists (physical, occupational, music, recreation), speech pathologist, vocational counselor, social worker, psychologist, and physicians who specialize in physical medi-

Goals Set Forth by the United Nations Proclamation of 1981 as the ''International Year of the Disabled'' *

1. Help people with disabilities in their physical and psychological adjustment to society.
2. Promote all national and international efforts to provide them with proper assistance, training, care, and guidance to make available opportunities for suitable work and to ensure full integration into society.
3. Encourage study and research projects designed to facilitate practical participation in daily life, such as improving access to public buildings and transportation.
4. Educate and inform the public of the rights of all people to participate in and contribute to various aspects of economic, social, and political life.
5. Promote effective measures for prevention of disabilities and rehabilitation of people who are disabled.

* *These are appropriate goals for any rehabilitation program.*

Key Terminology in Rehabilitation*

DO NOT USE the following words:

- ◆ *Handicapped.* The person may or may not be disabled, but in the person's eye, this disability is not a handicap. Refer to the *person* first—"the person with a disability."
- ◆ *Victim.* This word has a negative connotation. Say "the person who has a head injury."
- ◆ *Crippled.* This term gives a negative impression.
- ◆ *Afflicted.* It would be better to say "affected by" or who "has cerebral palsy."
- ◆ *Disease.* "Disorder" or "condition" is a better term.
- ◆ *Invalid.* Say "a person whose legs are paralyzed."

Remember

- ◆ It is better to refer to a person as, for example, "someone who has had a stroke" than to refer to the person as "the stroke," which sounds dehumanizing, as if he or she is an inanimate object.
- ◆ The person in a rehabilitation unit is usually referred to as a *client* or a *resident,* rather than a patient.
- ◆ Emphasize *abilities.* Do not underestimate what the person can do. Give him or her a chance to try.

* Some information from About Being Sensitive to People with Disabilities. S. Deerfield, MA, Channing Bete, 1992.

trols, respiratory aids, and artificial limbs, can be obtained for the person with a disability. Almost every person can regain a certain amount of function by using special devices and aids. Occupational therapy in the home is particularly helpful in making these adaptations.

The U.S. Division of Vocational Rehabilitation provides testing and counseling services and financial aid for those interested in education and training programs.

Government policies emphasize the need to make public buildings accessible and safe for all people. All new construction must include ramps for wheelchairs, pneumatic doors, and elevators. This reduction of *architectural barriers* has made it possible for many people with disabilities to become employed and lead more productive lives.

Special parking permits are issued, and certain areas must be designated as parking for the disabled. These areas must have ramps over the curbs and extra space so wheelchairs and scooters can maneuver.

Airlines will reserve special seats for people with disabilities.

> **Nursing Alert**
>
> It is illegal for any person to park in a designated "disabled" parking spot, even for a minute, if they do not have a physical disability.

Most young people with disabilities attend regular classes in schools. This is called **mainstreaming**. These young people participate in school activities and have the opportunity to mingle with people their own ages.

cine and rehabilitation, as well as the client and family. Team conferences are held regularly so that all members of the team will be working toward the same goals. Physicians in the area of rehabilitation are sometimes called **physiatrists** or physical medicine and rehabilitation specialists.

Community Resources

The nurse and other members of the rehabilitation team must explore community resources and with the client and family, make a discharge plan. The public health nurse can be involved in preparing the client for home care, for which client and family will need complete instructions. The family should have actively participated in care while the client was in the rehabilitation center, so when he or she is discharged, they have a clear understanding of the person's limitations and capabilities. Public health nursing and home care services are available to assist. Available home care services include nursing, home health aide or homemaker, social work, and physical, occupational, and speech therapy.

Various health agencies and private equipment companies have equipment, such as hospital beds or wheelchairs, available to loan, rent, or purchase. Many rehabilitative aids, such as braces and splints, adaptive devices for the homemaker, special automobile con-

Nursing Considerations

Rehabilitation from injury or illness begins with treatment to halt destructive processes and repair body damage. It continues with preventing further injury and then restoring normal functions when possible.

Rehabilitation nursing provides the client with physical and emotional support. The most important asset of the rehabilitation nurse is *empathy.* The nurse must be sensitive and offer encouragement and assistance.

The nurse also encourages the person to become independent. One of the nurse's functions in rehabilitation is giving physical care and assisting the client with self-care, while encouraging the client to perform as much self-care as possible.

It may take patience and perseverance to interest the client in making an effort to improve the situation and to convince him or her that this is not hopeless. The client and family also must understand the extent of the disability and how it is possible to regain some—perhaps all—normal functions. Even in illnesses that grow progressively worse, the client should be encouraged in self-care as long as possible.

Certain specialized nursing care is important in the care of the person with a disability. Most of these are described with basic procedures in Unit Nine. The index will help you find specific information. **Activities of daily living** (ADLs) are paramount in rehabilitation. Key terminology in rehabilitation is described in the accompanying box. Abbreviations and acronyms are listed in another box.

Activities of Daily Living

When the rehabilitation team has thoroughly evaluated the client and determined what functional capacity is realistic, a program of ADLs can be initiated.

Basic Functional ADLs. These include dressing, bathing, toileting and continence, eating, and transfer and mobility. Skills such as sensory and communication level (hearing, vision, speech) also are evaluated. Because of the disability, adaptations may be necessary so that the client can perform even simple self-care activities. The nurse must teach and guide the client and yet be flexible in the approach to self-care. An assessment of ADLs is listed in the box.

Instrumental ADLs. More complex living skills such as food preparation and money management may or may not be achievable by an individual client. These are called *instrumental* ADLs.

Often a record of ADLs is maintained by nursing staff. This informs all nurses of activities the person is able to do and those being attempted. Nursing care plans are continually updated.

The Homemaker With a Disability. Many homemakers encounter some sort of disabling condition. Devices have been designed to assist them in caring for themselves, their homes, and their families. Some simple adaptations include a board with nails driven through to hold vegetables for peeling and a one-handed can opener, egg beater, or rolling pin. There also is a board with a hole cut in it for holding a mixing bowl. The

Key Abbreviations and Acronyms in Rehabilitation and Home Care

ADL	Activities of daily living
APHA	American Public Health Association
CHHA	Certified Home Health Aide
IADL	Instrumental activities of daily living
JCAHO	Joint Commission on Accreditation of Healthcare Organizations
NAHC	National Association for Home Care
VNAA	Visiting Nurse Association of America

Keys to Nursing Assessment
Examples of ADLs

Functional ADLs

- Dressing skills and assistance needed
- Cleanliness and self-care (bathing, grooming, care of teeth, nails, hair)
- Elimination (toileting skills, continence level)
- Taking of food and fluids (self-feeding, ability to chew and swallow). Ability to prepare meals.
- Communication. Ability to talk.
- Activity and mobility level (walking and transfers, use of walker or wheelchair, skin condition)

Instrumental ADLs

- ADL skills needed at home or work (homemaking, laundry, vocational rehabilitation/retraining)
- Ability to use the telephone
- Ability to shop for groceries and essentials.
- Management of money (paying bills, writing checks, and so forth)
- Ability to drive or use public transportation
- Ability to read and write

level of the stove and sink can be lowered for the person in a wheelchair or scooter. Most wheelchairs have lapboards attached for the occupant to carry things.

Modified Equipment and Adaptive Devices. Modification of equipment is often needed for the person with a disability. Occupational therapists can assist the nurse in improvising equipment. Some common devices are long-handled combs and shoe horns, automatic toothbrushes, large molded handles on eating utensils, prism eyeglasses, a scrub brush mounted with suction cups inside the sink, an adjustable telephone, and other equipment that allows the patient to perform ADLs without needing to use highly developed motor skills (Fig. 89-1).

Adaptive Clothing. A few changes or adjustments made to regular clothing can often allow the person to dress alone or to be more comfortable. Simple clothing modifications include Velcro fasteners instead of buttons, elastic waist bands, large rings on zippers, bras that hook in front or do not have hooks at all, stocking pull-ons, gowns that fasten at the shoulder, instead of in back, and slips with a front zipper.

The person with a disability also can be taught how to dress most easily. For instance, the **hemiplegic** client (a person who is paralyzed on one side of the body) is taught to place clothing on the affected arm or leg first but to undress the unaffected arm or leg first. Patients are taught to put on socks before pants so the toenails will not catch on the pants.

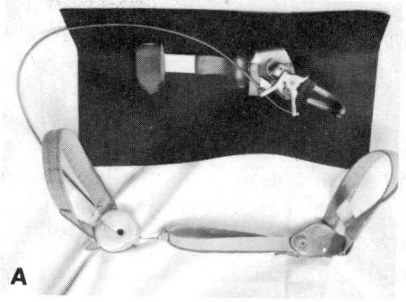
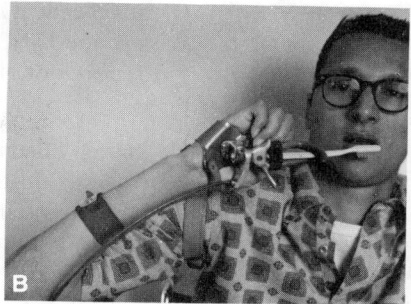
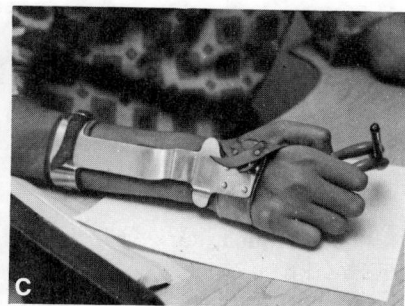

Figure 89-1. Handhooks are developed to do a variety of activities for the person with an amputated hand or arm. **A,** Handhook showing shoulder straps and cable-activated clamp (hook). **B,** Handhook used in holding a toothbrush. **C,** Handhook used in holding a pencil also acts as a splint.

Diversion

Any person who is hospitalized for an extended time needs to find activities to occupy free time and to increase the feeling of self-worth. The occupational and physical therapy staff will not only assist clients to find activities of interest, but will also initiate exercises for muscles that need exercise to prevent deformities. They also will help the client move around and thus prevent such difficulties as hypostatic pneumonia, pressure areas, thrombophlebitis, and constipation. The therapy departments also help the person to find appropriate job retraining and employment.

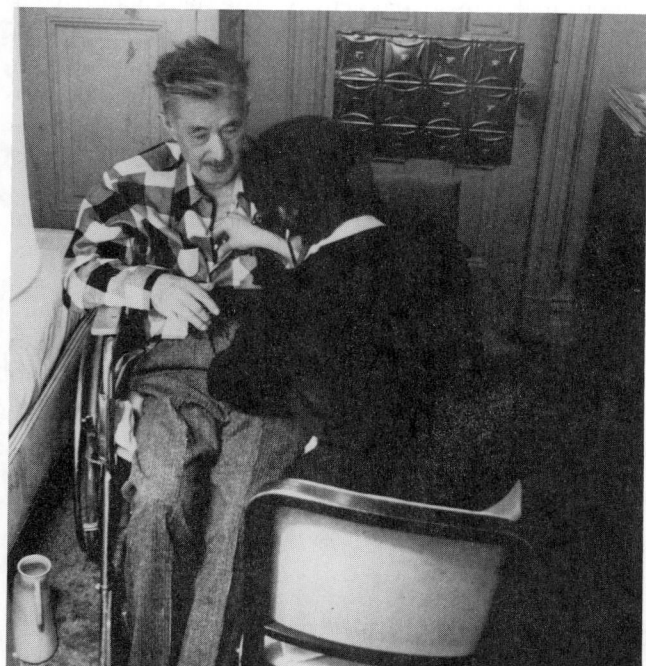

Figure 89-2. The nurse in home care is responsible for providing the best and safest care possible in the patient's own home. The nurse can make suggestions on how to improve the home environment for safe and sanitary care. Courtesy of Visiting Nurse Service of New York.

Recreational Activities. Many games have been adapted for use by people with various disabilities. Examples include checkers with loops so they can be picked up easily, braille playing cards, or a magnetic playing board for the person with spasticity. The occupational or recreation therapist will have other suggestions for diversional activities. Some of these have a specific goal in mind, for example, improvement of fine motor skills and eye–hand coordination by tying flies for fishing or crocheting.

The Person Who is Paralyzed

When a client faces permanent **paralysis** (inability to move a part of the body), some serious physical complications can occur. The major complications include contracted muscles, pressure points that may ulcerate, and bladder and bowel malfunctions. Every nursing measure should be used to prevent these complications.

Skin Care. Measures for preventing pressure areas have been emphasized throughout this book and include the following:

♦ Keep skin dry.
♦ Do not use drying agents, such as alcohol (use lotion).
♦ Keep bedding free of wrinkles.
♦ Change bed or clothing immediately if wet or soiled.
♦ Turn and reposition the person at least every 2 hours.
♦ Keep crumbs out of bed.
♦ Give backrubs; massage bony prominences.
♦ Provide padding or floatation.
♦ Use special devices for assistance (such as the hydraulic patient lift).
♦ Supply a high-protein diet and plenty of fluids.

Special skin or wound care is often ordered to prevent breakdown. Chapter 45 describes skin care in detail.

Range of Motion. Range-of-motion exercises must be performed to move all naturally moving joints. This is done to prevent joint stiffness and muscle shortening. The range-of-motion exercises are passive (done by the nurse) or active (done by the client), depending on the disability. The continuous passive motion (CPM) machine also may be used. The client should be informed that exercise is important to build muscle strength, maintain joint mobility, and build endurance (see Chapter 43). The patient may become hypotensive when moved to a standing position. This adjustment may be done gradually using a tilt table.

Mobility. The patient is first taught basic bed movements and transfers from bed to chair, onto the toilet, and into the bathtub or shower. Ambulation is encouraged to enhance the person's maximum potential. This may involve the use of a walker or cane (see Chapter 43).

Many people use a wheelchair or scooter for mobility. Motorized wheelchairs and scooters are available for the person with limited hand or arm strength. Special wheelchairs are available for racing and sports, as are wheelchairs with various adaptive devices. A standing wheelchair, although expensive, allows the person to meet people at eye level and provides additional mobility and self-esteem for some people. Adaptive lifts and hand controls are available for cars, so the person can maintain independence in transportation.

Braces and Splints. Special braces or splints may be needed to support affected limbs or maintain the correct position.

Splints are available in two forms: *resting splints,* which keep the hand from becoming contracted, and *dynamic* hand splints, which enable the patient to function better than would be possible without the splint (see Figure 89-1).

Braces are often applied to the legs to give support. This might be the case in a **paraplegic** (lower limb paralysis) or hemiplegic. The physical therapist teaches the patient to apply and remove the brace; nursing personnel reinforce this teaching. If the patient is **quadriplegic** (all four extremities and possibly the trunk paralyzed), a neck or back brace also may be needed. A type of inflatable trousers (exoskeleton) may be used to maintain the person in an upright position and to prevent vascular collapse.

Independent Elimination. The person who is paralyzed often needs bowel or bladder retraining to reestablish independent elimination patterns (see Chapter 46).

Bowel Elimination. Fecal impaction can become a problem, although some people manually disimpact themselves daily as part of their bowel program. It is important to eat a well-balanced diet and establish regular times for bowel elimination.

Bladder Elimination. The care of the person with a neurogenic bladder is complex. Fluid intake is often encouraged to approximately 3,000 mL per day. A regular pattern of voiding is established, beginning approximately every 2 hours and gradually increasing the time. Manual pressure over the suprapubic area (**Credé's maneuver**) or self-catheterization may be undertaken. As the program is being established, the person may be awakened during the night to void.

Sexuality

Sexual activity is an important concern for any person with a disability. It may not be considered a top physical priority in rehabilitation, but it is important to the client and merits discussion. The client should be encouraged to ask questions and express concerns.

Many people with varying degrees of paralysis are able to maintain sexual activity. The man may have a penile implant (see Chapter 83); positioning may facilitate intercourse. The woman who is paralyzed can have sexual intercourse, become pregnant, and deliver a normal child. The delivery is sometimes accomplished by cesarean delivery; sometimes delivery is vaginal. A woman with limited mobility and sensation may be concerned about vaginal or bladder infection. Frequent examinations by the physician will usually detect the presence of an infection before it becomes a serious problem.

Some counselors are skilled in dealing with human sexuality. Workshops and seminars are conducted to discuss specific sexual problems of the paralyzed person.

Ambulatory Nursing

The Physician's Office or Clinic

In the physician's office or clinic, the nurse has an opportunity to use many skills learned in the acute care setting. In addition to routine nursing care, the clinic nurse often performs other duties or performs certain duties much more often than in the acute setting. Examples include the following:

◆ Assigning patients to rooms, setting up schedules
◆ Autoclaving supplies
◆ Preparing and collecting specimens and slides
◆ Taking patients' vital signs, height, and weight
◆ Record keeping, such as billing, making appointments, and filing laboratory reports and patient records
◆ Assisting with examinations, including gynecologic, general physical, and neurologic examinations
◆ Assisting with sterile procedures and minor surgical procedures
◆ Special, non-nursing techniques, such as laboratory procedures for electrocardiograms
◆ Cleaning and restocking rooms

The nurse is likely to work with people of all ages and with varying disease conditions every day, unless the clinic is specialized.

The Emergency Room or Emergi-Center

Most hospitals have an emergency room, although free-standing emergi-centers, urgi-centers, or walk-in clinics not attached to a hospital have become common. Many are in shopping malls. Hospitals may have an area of the emergency room specifically reserved for pediatric patients.

Many of the free-standing clinics are open longer hours than a physician's office; sometimes they are open 24 hours a day. The free-standing clinics may treat noncritical ("vertical") patients only; they refer the more critically ill or injured patients to the hospital emergency room.

The Emergency Room

The acute emergency room differs from the general hospital in respect to nursing care. Most often, the person working in the emergency room is a registered nurse (RN), although some rural and small hospitals employ licensed practical or vocational nurses and emergency medical technicians (EMTs) as well. In addition to many routine nursing techniques, the staff in the emergency room is trained to do the following:

◆ Provide crisis support and counseling to families.
◆ Use specialized emergency equipment, such as the endotracheal airway or hand-held ventilating bag.

◆ Assist in cardioversion (defibrillation) or other emergency procedures.
◆ Take primary responsibility for starting and monitoring intravenous lines (after specialized training).
◆ Call the patient's family and appropriate clergy members.
◆ Continuously monitor critically ill patients while they are being examined; it is the nurse's responsibility to notify the appropriate person if difficulties arise.
◆ Perform triage in the event of multiple admissions at one time to determine which patients should be seen first.
◆ Keep an accurate record of emergency procedures performed and medications given, by whom, and at what time.
◆ Assist in taking the patient to x-ray or other diagnostic areas.
◆ Assist in drawing blood or obtaining other specimens for laboratory analysis.
◆ Obtain an electrocardiogram on a patient for evaluation by the physician.
◆ Communicate with ambulance and rescue personnel, and set up the examination and treatment area appropriately to receive the patient when the ambulance arrives.
◆ Coordinate transcription of physician's orders (see Chapter 92); make out requests, or enter information on computer for laboratory tests, x-rays, and other procedures.
◆ Make arrangements for admission to the hospital.
◆ Make arrangements with the operating room for emergency surgery.
◆ Assist in nonsterile procedures, such as cast and traction application.
◆ Assist in emergency sterile procedures, such as suturing, removal of foreign objects from body orifices, or catheterization.
◆ Apply cold packs, and perform other noninvasive procedures
◆ Notify appropriate medical and paramedical personnel in preparation for arrival of the patient.

The Free-Standing Walk-in Clinic
The nurse in the free-standing nonemergency walk-in center performs many routine procedures:

◆ Ensure that patients are seen quickly, efficiently, and with a minimum of paperwork and red tape.
◆ Do initial assessment of all patients. (In some states, this must be done by an RN.)
◆ Assist in providing education to the patient and family.
◆ Call in medication prescriptions to the pharmacy, following the physician, osteopath, dentist, or nurse practitioner's orders. (In some states, such phone calls can be made only by an RN.)

In community-based nursing centers, nurse practitioners provide primary care to people of all ages.

The Day Surgery Center or Ambulatory Surgery Center

Patients come to the day surgery center for many procedures that formerly required hospitalization. Coming into the center just for surgery and recovering at home are much more comfortable and conducive to relaxation than being hospitalized. This reduces stress for the patient and family.

Examples of outpatient procedures are tonsillectomy, carpal tunnel release, débridement, open reduction of some fractures, biopsies, dilation and curettage, and polyp removal. More extensive procedures, such as herniorrhaphy, are sometimes done in the day surgery center. Patients chosen for ambulatory surgery usually do not have any underlying disorders that could contribute to postoperative complications (see Chapter 53).

Criteria have been established to assist in determining patients appropriate for outpatient surgery. Class I patients are those in whom no underlying organic, physiologic, biochemical, or psychiatric disturbance exists. In these people, the condition for which surgery is to be performed is localized (and not systemic). Class II and other classes involve patients with increasing levels of systemic disturbances. Most patients in class I and some patients in class II are candidates for outpatient surgery if the procedure is appropriate for ambulatory surgery.

The day surgery clinic is often in the operating room area of a hospital or is managed by the operating room. Nursing responsibilities and related factors include the following:

◆ Provide preoperative patient teaching and preparation. The patient or family will need to perform much of the preoperative preparation at home. For example, a special diet the night before surgery, nothing by mouth after midnight, pHisoHex scrub, or enemas in the evening must be done at home.
◆ Give instructions verbally and in writing. The written instructions can reinforce the verbal instructions. Document all teaching.
◆ Instruct patients to call if there is any change in physical status. It may be necessary to cancel surgery or do it on an inpatient basis.
◆ Perform specific preparations, such as preoperative scrub and shaving or drawing of blood, the morning of the procedure. The nurse in day surgery will often be expected to carry out these procedures.
◆ Provide family teaching. Explain how to care for the person, and describe untoward symptoms that might occur postoperatively.

◆ The patient is usually not allowed to drive; make sure arrangements have been made for him or her to get home.
◆ Make sure the operative permit is signed before any medications are given. Double-check about allergies.
◆ The preoperative nurse may scrub for surgical procedures in the day surgery center.
◆ Support and remain with the patient during induction, if the procedure is done under general anesthesia, and for the entire procedure, if it is done locally.
◆ Stay with the patient until he or she is awake. Observe for any complications.
◆ Telephone the patient on the first postoperative day. It is important to determine if the patient is having any complications. The nurse must know what questions to ask. This phone call also is an excellent public relations gesture.
◆ Referrals may be made for public health nursing or home care services.
◆ The patient and family must be comfortable with the idea of ambulatory surgery; they must be convinced that it is as safe as inpatient surgery. The relaxed, friendly atmosphere of day surgery centers is conducive to relaxation and recovery. Preoperative medication often is not needed because of the relaxed atmosphere; the patient can walk into the operating room and feel more in control. Many patients have a faster postoperative recovery with fewer complications if less medication is given. The patient also is able to ambulate sooner after surgery; this helps prevent complications. The patient must be strongly motivated to recover and cooperate to do well following ambulatory surgery.

> ### Key Concept
> Most patients are admitted for surgery on the morning of their surgery. Many of the points previously listed apply to these patients too, even if they will be admitted to the hospital following surgery (see Chapter 53).

Home Nursing

The fastest growing field of nursing is home care (Figs. 89-2 and 89-3). Fewer people are being admitted to hospitals, and they are being discharged sooner with more needs for special care.

People are being discharged with drainage tubes, heparin locks, and other complicated equipment. Some ventilator-dependent children are discharged to home. The patient and family are taught to operate all equip-

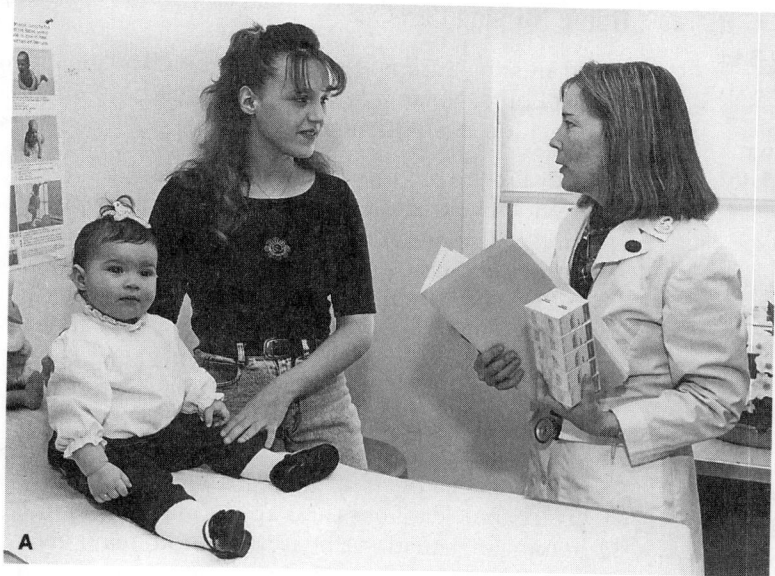
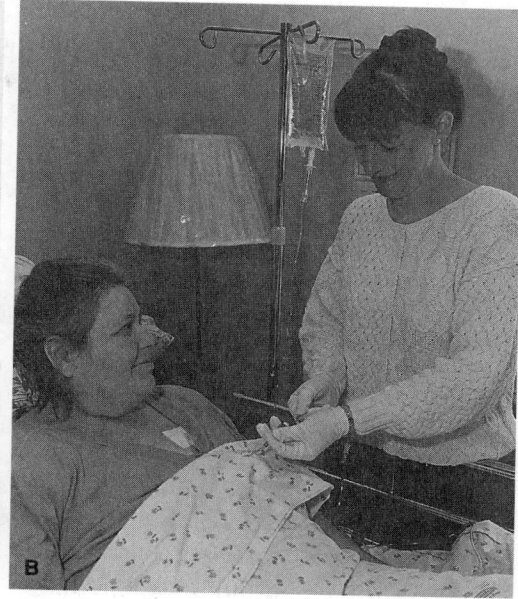

Figure 89-3. Examples of short-term home care. **A,** The visiting nurse explains immunization programs and requirements to a WIC client. **B,** IV therapy can be provided in the home. Photos courtesy of MCOSS Inc., RED Bank, NJ.

ment. The visiting nurse teaches the patient and family and supervises and documents this treatment. In some cases, 24-hour nursing care is provided in the home.

The following are reasons for home care:

◆ Continuous care is provided from hospital to home until recovery or death.
◆ Third-party payors force early discharge from the hospital. Thus, patients are being discharged from the hospital sicker than in the past. They need more total care and assistance with self-care activities and ADLs.
◆ Home care is less expensive than hospital care.
◆ Some people are not admitted to the hospital but receive their entire care at home.
◆ The general population is increasing in age. With more elderly people, more care is needed to manage chronic illness or comorbidity (coexisting disorders).
◆ Family structure may have changed, or a client may not have family members available or be able to provide care.
◆ Many people prefer to receive care in their home.
◆ Sophisticated electronic equipment allows the client to receive care at home. The equipment is self-contained and electronically controlled and therefore can be managed by the family. Procedures such as electroencephalograms and electrocardiograms can be transmitted by phone or computer to the hospital for interpretation.
◆ Many clients prefer to die at home. Hospice care can be provided.

◆ Many clients and families experience less emotional strain at home. This avoids separation from family members, pets, and familiar surroundings.

Types of Agencies and Services

There are several types of home care agencies. These include hospital-based, and private-for-profit, nonprofit voluntary, temporary staffing, and Medicare-certified agencies. Agencies have different credentials. Some maintain JCAHO certification; others are licensed by the Department of Health of the state.

Home care services may be long term, short term, or intermittent. *Long-term care* may be needed for an elderly person with a chronic disease or disabling condition. Services may include periodic assessment or evaluation by the nurse, with personal care services provided by a home health aide. The nurse may assist with "restorative nursing," for example, facilitating maintenance of muscle integrity as much as possible.

Some patients receive long-term care 24 hours a day. Staffing or proprietary agencies provide nursing care in the home for three 8-hour or two 12-hour shifts. In some cases, the family participates by providing care during the day, with nurses on duty at night, so they can rest. Third-party payors usually pay for care provided by aides and licensed practical nurses (LPNs) in catastrophic illness.

In *short-term services or intermittent care,* nursing care is provided periodically. Examples include the following:

◆ A home visit two to three times a week
◆ A home visit to assist a new mother (Fig. 89-3**A**)
◆ Dressing changes twice a day for 1 to 2 weeks
◆ A home visit daily (to assess the patient)
◆ Medication setups (the person takes their own medications after the nurse places them in daily "slots")
◆ Administration of intravenous medications (see Fig. 89-3**B**)
◆ Drawing of blood for various tests

The RN is the case manager of services provided by all disciplines in the home (LPN, home health aide, social workers, therapists [physical, occupational, speech]). Federal Medicare regulations for home care identify standard duties of the LPN or licensed vocational nurse as "furnishing services in accordance with agency policies, prepares clinical and progress notes, assists the physician and RN in performing specialized procedures, prepares equipment and materials for treatments, observing aseptic technique as required, and assists the patient in learning appropriate self-care techniques."[1]

State guidelines generally indicate that LPNs practice within the guidelines of the state's nursing practice legislation and according to specified agency policies. The LPN or home health aide practices under the supervision of and as a team member with the RN. The standards of an accrediting body will guide the agency and the nurse. These define the role of the LPN as "supplemental" and in accordance with agency policies.

Key Concept

In the home setting, the nurse is working in a more independent and isolated role than in the hospital or nursing home. Therefore, it is important to know state and agency policies.

---

[1] "Rules and regulations." Federal Register 54(155):, August 14, 1989.

Home Nursing Care

Good nursing care is essential for the client receiving care at home. Nursing activities and skills used in home care include the following:

◆ Coordinate with hospital and medical staff.
◆ Provide client and family teaching, such as procedures, recognition of symptoms, and how to report to the physician. The nurse provides, evaluates, and documents the teaching on an ongoing basis.
◆ Counsel the patient or client. The nurse is the liaison with the healthcare system.
◆ Accurately assess the client. The nurse is to report untoward symptoms to the physician.
◆ Evaluate the client's total home situation. The nurse is in a special position to assess the care being given, the cleanliness and appropriateness of the home-care situation, the type of food being given the client, the administration of medications, and diversionary activities being provided. The implications for the patient's family must be evaluated as well.
◆ Evaluate the safety of the home for the client. The nurse must suggest equipment needed or changes to be made to help make the home safer.
◆ The nurse must have a knowledge of and be able to suggest community resources. Sometimes the physician must be consulted before referrals are made.
◆ Carefully document all nursing care and teaching.
◆ Reassure the client on the telephone. On days when visits are not scheduled, the nurse may need to call and give support or answer questions.

Key Concept

Members of the home care team plan care. There are many different members of the home care team, as in rehabilitation care. Not all members will serve on all cases.

Keys for Review

Key Questions for Critical Thinking

1. Describe ways the client can adapt ADLs in the home. Determine how the nurse can teach about these devices and activities.
2. Your paralyzed female patient has questions about her sexuality. Suggest what questions she might ask. Formulate your answers.
3. Contrast nursing in the physician's office with nursing in the acute care setting.
4. List potential members of the home healthcare team. Describe how each person and the nurse will relate their activities.

Key Readings

DeLisa JA, Gans BM. Rehabilitation Medicine: Principles and Practice, Ed 2. Philadelphia, J.B. Lippincott, 1993
Flarey D. Redesigning Nursing Care Delivery. Philadelphia, J.B. Lippincott, 1995
Fyke LD. "Caring begins at home." The Canadian Nurse 90(2):26-28, 1994
Garrison SJ. Handbook of Physical Medicine and Rehabilitation Basics. Philadelphia, J.B. Lippincott, 1994
United States Department of Health and Human Services. Healthy People 2000: National Health Promotion and Disease Prevention Objectives (PH Services Publication #91-50212). Boston, Jones & Bartlett, 1992
Wearing J. "The new emphasis of home care." The Canadian Nurse 90(2):22-26, 1994

Enrichment Keys

Hoole AJ. Patient Care Guidelines for Nurse Practitioners, Ed 4. Philadelphia, J.B. Lippincott, 1994
Spradley BW. Readings in Community Health Nursing, Ed 4. Philadelphia, Scott-Foresman/Little-Brown, 1991

Keys to Learning More

Chapter 90: death and dying

Chapter 91: hospice nursing, which is often done in the patient's home

Chapter 93: career opportunities for nurses, often in home care

Key Resources

American Public Health Association (APHA)
   1015-15th Street, NW
   Washington, DC 20005
American Spinal Injury Association
   2020 Peachtree Road NW
   Atlanta, GA 30309
Community Health Nurses Association of Canada
   1049 Flintlock Court
   London, Ontario M6H 4M3
National Association for Home Care (NAHC)
   510 C Street NE
   Stanton Park
   Washington, DC 20002
Visiting Nurse Association of America (VNAA)
   3801 E. Florida Avenue
   Suite 900
   Denver, CO 80210

Unit *17* Assisting the Dying Person and the Family

90 Death and Dying

Learning Objectives

- Define "living will" and "do not resuscitate" orders
- List and define the six stages of coping with a terminal illness. Discuss interactions that might occur with the patient or the family during each stage.
- Describe the total nursing care of the dying person.
- Describe how you might best assist the patient's family to cope with the death of their loved one.
- Describe the care of the body after death.
- Identify the role of the healthcare team in requests for tissue donation.

Key Terms

advance directive

apnea

autopsy

biologic death

Cheyne-Stokes respiration

hyperpnea

Kussmaul's breathing

living will

postmortem examination

preparatory depression

reactive depression

Keys to Understanding This Chapter

This entire book has been concerned with helping people meet their basic needs. During the time of dying, which is a part of the total life process, the patient and family need the nurse's help with basic physical needs and with many emotional and psychological needs.

Key Points

- Death is a normal part of the total life process.
- It is up to the nursing and medical staff to ask the family if they would like to donate organs or tissues when their loved one dies.

Key Points (continued)

- Most people, if they do not die suddenly, pass through definite stages during the dying process. The goal is acceptance.
- The nurse assists the patient and family meet their physical and emotional needs.

Key Topics Outline

Death
Terminal Illness
   Kubler-Ross's Stages of Dying
   The Role of Hope
Care of the Dying Person
Care of the Patient's Family
When Death Occurs
   The Process of Death
   Helping the Family
   Care of the Body

Key Learning Activities

- Write a paper on your feelings about death. Take time to think them through. What do you know about death? List your fears. Have you been around dying people before? How do you think you will feel working with a dying person and family? What are your special strengths that you can use?
- Visit or make a telephone call to your state's eye bank. Ask for information. What are the criteria for tissue and organ donation? What is the role of the nurse? Ask them to send you additional information.
- Read some books or journals about transcultural aspects related to death and dying. If you have friends from other religions or cultures, ask them about their beliefs.

Despite great advances in technology, medical science cannot cure every illness. You may find yourself caring for a dying patient. You will assist patients with the dying experience in various situations, including the hospital, hospice, nursing home, or their own home.

Death

Death is one of the most profound emotional experiences you will encounter as a nurse. Because health-care personnel are constantly preoccupied with preserving life, it is difficult to admit that a patient cannot be cured. It may be difficult for a nurse to resolve the fact of death.

Before a nurse can be helpful to the dying patient and the family, he or she must effectively examine and resolve his or her own feelings about death. It is also helpful to consider the care of a dying patient and the family as a nursing opportunity and privilege.

Death is part of life, an extension of birth. Unfortunately, many people develop a fear of dying. Our attitudes are further shaped by our cultural and religious beliefs. In addition, most think of themselves as immortal. While people can imagine other people dying, they often cannot imagine their own death.

Key Concept

Death is a natural part of life. How you feel about it will influence how helpful you are to dying patients and their families. *Death with dignity* is the goal.

The Living Will

Nearly all states have a **living will** law. This also is known as an **advance directive** and is discussed in Chapter 4. The specifics may vary, but the purpose is the same. The person who signs a living will requests that extraordinary measures not be taken to save his or her life if he or she becomes terminally ill. This usually includes measures such as cardiopulmonary resuscitation (CPR), intubation, tracheotomy and mechanical ventilation, or cardiostimulant drugs. In some states, tube feedings, intravenous lines, and oxygen may be included.

In some situations, the family is allowed to make a decision not to resuscitate, but this may be legally more difficult than using the patient's advance directive. In addition, recent court cases have proven how difficult it is to discontinue life-saving measures once they have been started.

Codes

A person may have a do not resuscitate (DNR), do not intubate (DNI), or both orders on the Kardex. The nursing staff knows that if this person goes into cardi-opulmonary arrest, a "code blue" (or the code name for arrest in that facility) will not be called. The person will be allowed to die naturally, without mechanical or chemical intervention. The person will be kept as comfortable as possible and given emotional support. In the nursing home, you may see a do not hospitalize (DNH) order as well.

Some patients with terminal illnesses are on *full code*. This means that the CPR team is to be called in case of cardiopulmonary arrest, even though death is imminent. It is the nurse's responsibility to know which patients on the unit are DNR and which are full code.

Key Concept

It is not up to the nurse to determine whether or not a code should be called; the patient, the physician, or the patient's family has made this decision. *If any patient does not have a specific DNR order, a code is to be called if they arrest.*

Organ and Tissue Donation

Many people designate that their organs (liver, kidney, heart, lung) and tissues (cornea, bone, skin) are to be donated after their death. Their decision is often recorded on their driver's license, but after death, the family must give permission in most states. Some extraordinary measures may be necessary to preserve organs long enough to be recovered; this is not usually the case with tissues.

Nursing Alert

Even though a person has designated himself or herself as a donor, the family gains custody of the body at death. Most states have a law requiring the hospital to approach each family regarding donation of organs or tissues. (This is called the *Uniform Anatomical Gift Act.*)

Terminal Illness

Kübler-Ross's Stages of Dying

Dr. Elisabeth Kübler-Ross, among other authors, has described certain phases through which a patient may pass in an attempt to cope with impending death. All patients pass through at least some of these stages, except when death is instantaneous or when the patient is unable to resolve conflicts. The family, to complete the grieving process, also may pass through the same basic stages. These stages can overlap, and a person can go back and forth from one stage to another. Table 90-1 reviews these steps in dealing with death.

Denial and Isolation. In this stage, the person does not believe that the diagnosis is correct. ("This can't be happening to me!") This is the stage during which the patient may seek the advice of several doctors, hoping that one of them will offer a more acceptable prognosis.

Anger and Rage. In this stage, the person asks, "Why did this happen to me? Why now?" Often, the patient envies the person who is young and healthy; he or she may strike out at the nursing staff. In some cases, the patient *is* young. The nurse must understand that this is a phase of the illness; the anger being expressed is directed at the situation and not at the nurse as a person. The person is rebelling against the feeling of sudden helplessness.

Bargaining and Developing Awareness. During this stage, which may be very short or entirely absent, patients

Table 90-1. Stages of Dealing With Death

Stage		Suggested Nursing Actions
Denial Shock, often followed by a feeling of isolation	"No, not me!"	Answer questions honestly. Allow person to talk to physician. Encourage family support. Do not argue.
Anger Rage	"Why me?"	Listen. Do not take the patient's anger personally. Do not get angry yourself.
Bargaining Guilt	"Yes me, but . . ." "If I could just live until . . ."	Try to assist in patient's wishes. Encourage family support. Offer spiritual assistance from clergy or support groups.
Depression Grief (Verbal stage)	"Yes, me."	Be there. Listen. Offer counseling or social service assistance. Offer encouragement.
(Nonverbal stage)		Encouragement is not helpful. Allow patient to rest.
Acceptance Self-reliance	"My time is close, and it's OK"	Provide physical care. Be there. Encourage family to be there. Keep room lighted. Support the family.
Detachment Decathexis	No communication	Continue to include patient in conversation (patient may be able to hear). Allow patient to detach. Provide physical care. Try not to leave patient alone. Support the family.

Based, for the most part, on the work of Dr. Elisabeth Kübler-Ross.

make deals with God or with themselves. "If I could just live 2 more weeks, I could see my boy get married." When the time has passed, the patient often feels like making another bargain, postponing death indefinitely. You also may meet patients who seem to make up their minds to live through a certain event, such as a birthday and then die quickly once it is over.

Depression. The patient realizes that he or she is going to die and there is nothing that can be done to stop it. The patient may feel a severe sense of loss concerning his or her job, the money spent on medical bills, the children and other loved ones, and the greatest loss of all, life itself.

Depression often involves two stages: *verbal and nonverbal.* During the verbal stage, also called **reactive depression**, the patients concentrate on past losses. They can be reassured and encouraged. Some people find comfort in writing the story of their life. Later, during the nonverbal stage, also called **preparatory depression**, the patients realize the impact of loss. during this phase, encouragement is not meaningful because patients realize that they will be leaving behind everything they have known. Patients may wish to plan for life after death or for their family after they die, or they may daydream or sleep a great deal in an effort to escape reality. The nurse can be most helpful by being present. Just a touch of the hand or a kind word will be more helpful than meaningless chatter. Let patients know you care and are available, but do not push yourself on them.

Acceptance and Peace. As patients resolve emotional conflicts about death, they enter the stage where they realize and accept the inevitability of death. To reach this point, patients usually must have had time and assistance in working through the earlier stages. While they may sleep a great deal, sleep is no longer a means of escape but is necessary because of weakness and fatigue. As dying patients resign themselves to death, they may seem to be devoid of all feeling. This is a particularly difficult time for the family, who may interpret the patient's acceptance of death as a rejection of life and of them. They must be assisted to understand that the patient will not be able to die comfortably unless he or she has been helped to give up everything associated with life and that although the patient is often unable or unwilling to communicate, he or she usually will appreciate short visits or the presence of a family member.

Detachment. The final stage of dying is detachment, when patients gradually separate themselves from the world so a two-way communication no longer exists between them and the people around them. Because patients may be unresponsive during this time, nursing care is primarily directed toward physical needs. However, patients may hear what is being said, even though they do not respond.

The Role of Hope

Patients may cling to hope and not give up until the very end, when they finally reach acceptance. Until then, the patient should be allowed to hope. However, the nurse should not give any false hope. Dr. Kübler-Ross states that a good response is, "To my knowledge, I have done everything I can to help you. I will continue, however, to keep you as comfortable as possible."

Care of the Dying Person

Once the actual physical process of dying has begun, the nurse's main task is to assist in the supportive and sympathetic care of patients. Allow dying patients to maintain their self-esteem and personal dignity; never do things for patients that they can do themselves.

Care of the Mouth, Nose, and Eyes. The mouth should be swabbed with mouthwash as often as necessary to keep it clean; mineral oil and lemon juice should be applied to the tongue and inside the cheeks. If there is an excess of secretion in the mouth, as happens sometimes, turn the patient on the side to make drainage easier. The nostrils should be freed of crust and moistened and soothed with applications of mineral oil. The eyes may be kept clean by wiping them with wipes or cotton balls moistened in normal saline. The tongue may be dry and should be moistened with a water-soluble lubricant so that it does not stick to the roof of the mouth. Be sure the airway is kept open.

Change of Position. Turn dying patients frequently to make them more comfortable. They may not be able to tell you that they would like a change of position. Support patients with pillows when they are lying on the side. Do not leave them lying on their backs, because this may precipitate choking.

Breathing Difficulties. Kussmaul's breathing often occurs if the patient goes into acidosis as a result of an electrolyte imbalance. This type of breathing is fast (above 20/min), labored, and deep but can rapidly turn into Cheyne-Stokes breathing as heart failure occurs. **Cheyne-Stokes respiration** (periodic breathing) is characterized by alternating periods of **apnea** (absence of breathing) and **hyperpnea** (rapid breathing). Gradually, the apneic periods lengthen.

Respiratory difficulties are less distressing if the patient can be turned onto the side or propped up in a partly sitting position. Always preserve good posture and provide enough support. Make certain that the tongue does not drop back and obstruct the airway. If it does, pull the tongue forward with gauze, and turn the patient onto the side with the head elevated to prevent a recurrence. The collection of mucus and secretions causes the "death rattle" as the patient breathes. Gentle suctioning or a change in position may relieve this. The physician also may order atropine to dry up secretions. The physician may order oxygen to increase the patient's comfort.

Incontinence. The patient may be incontinent of urine or stool, or the bladder may become distended. Keep the patient dry and clean. Notify the physician if the patient does not void for 8 hours or as specified in the patient's care plan. (In some cases, minimal urine is produced because of kidney failure and electrolyte imbalance.)

Diarrhea and Constipation. The patient may have diarrhea or constipation as a result of slowing body processes, lack of oral intake, and immobility. These are handled according to the physician's orders, often depending on how soon the patient is expected to die.

Nutrition and Hydration. The person usually is not interested in eating or taking fluids. The physician, together with the patient and family, determines what course of action to take. Nausea and vomiting are common problems in the terminally ill patient. In some cases tube feeding or total parenteral nutrition is instituted.

Self-Esteem. The person who is dying needs to feel like a worthwhile member of society and of the family. Fixing the person's hair or helping to write a letter can provide some comfort. Many patients wish to help plan their own funeral or write a will. It is important to keep the person clean and comfortable without emphasizing it.. The person may feel inadequate when he or she is no longer able to perform ADLs without assistance.

Odor Control. There may be foul-smelling drainage or discharge or incontinence. It is important for the patient and for the family to keep this under control. Keep the dressings clean and dry and drainage bags emptied. Subtle deodorizers may be helpful.

Pain Relief. Medication, including narcotics, is often given to relieve pain. Some authorities say that dying patients, even though not actually in pain, should have some drugs for distress and exhaustion to make them comfortable and to make dying easier. Large doses of narcotics may be given; the physician is no longer worried about the possibility of addiction. Opiates may be taken intravenously and controlled by the patient. Chapter 91 lists some of the medications used to assist dying patients. Just before death, pain usually disappears; death is now impending.

> **Key Concept**
>
> The patient who has been confused or unconscious up to now may abruptly become lucid and alert. If possible, the family should be called at this time so that the patient has a chance to say a final goodbye.

Failing Circulation. As the circulation fails, the body becomes cold and is frequently covered with perspiration. Heavy blankets may make the person restless. Provide light covering, and keep it loose over the feet, using a bed cradle if necessary.

Ventilation and Lighting. The room should be kept well ventilated. Although air should be allowed to circulate, be sure that it is not blowing on the patient. Oxygen may or may not be helpful at this stage, although it may make breathing slightly easier.

It is usually helpful to keep a light on in the room. Darkness is frightening to many people. Patients are usually more uncomfortable and afraid if it is dark.

Failing Senses. Most patients can hear until the final moment. Speak distinctly, and do not whisper or talk about the patient to someone else. The dying patient is likely to feel a sense of increasing darkness as vision begins to fail and often turns toward a window or other source of light.

Care of the Patient's Family

Often the patient's family feels the stress of this period more keenly than the patient. They feel the sense of loss yet feel they must try to appear as though everything were normal. This attitude can be confusing to the patient, because in the patient's life, *everything* is happening. The person cannot understand why others do not seem sad.

> **Key Concept**
>
> The family must realize that it is acceptable for them to cry or to be sad in front of the patient. It is often therapeutic, because otherwise the patient feels that nobody cares.

If the patient is suffering, you can explain to the family how they can make death easier by taking turns staying with the patient. Encourage the family to keep their family life on as even a keel as possible. Explain the need for rest and nourishment. In the hospital, it is a kindness to a patient's family to offer them a cup of tea or coffee when their waiting period has been long and exhausting. If possible, the family should have a place where they can be alone. If the waiting period is likely to be long, encourage the family to go out for meals and rest, assuring them that they will be called if any change occurs.

Everyday problems also will confront a family at this time. The nurse, social worker, chaplain, and other members of the healthcare team can assist in such matters as advising about financial difficulties; arranging for babysitting and transportation to and from the hospital; indicating where to find temporary housing for out-of-town relatives; and offering information about whom to consult about questions and problems.

Because dying patients can offer comfort to their families by sharing feeling and thoughts, the nurse should encourage such communication. The sooner that patients share their prognosis with their families, the longer they will have to work out the situation together. It is a difficult situation, and the family should feel free to share this time and feelings with the patient. Support groups also are available to assist patients and family members. Many hospitals employ nurses who specialize in assisting dying patients.

Often families seek advice regarding how to handle death when there are children in the family. Although very young children may not be able to verbalize their thoughts clearly, they do grieve and need to be part of the family's grief processing. Nurses should encourage adults to talk honestly and clearly with children about the patient's illness and death when it occurs. Children should be allowed to see the body and/or attend the funeral *if they wish to do so*. If it is a child who is dying, they should be told the truth and be allowed to ask questions.

When Death Occurs

Clinical death occurs when respiration and heartbeat have stopped, unless the patient is being maintained on a ventilator or cardiac pacemaker. Note the exact time when the respiration stops (usually before the heartbeat stops) and when the heart stops beating. The physician should have been notified prior to this. Signs of approaching death are listed in the accompanying box.

Signs of Approaching Death

- Loss of control over urine and bowels may occur.
- Intake of food and drink will diminish, and general nutritional requirements are less.
- Urination may diminish or stop.
- The extremities will feel cooler to the touch as circulation slows down.
- Increased fatigue and difficulty waking up.
- Recognition of familiar people, places, or objects is decreased, and visions of people or things that do not exist are increased.
- Occasionally restlessness is increased.
- Dry mouth and accumulation of thick secretions in the back of the throat occurs.
- Noisy breathing due to secretions in the mouth or chest is common.
- The pattern of breathing changes, such as rapid breathing, followed by periods where the breathing is slow or even absent for as long as 15 seconds.

At the point of death,

- Breathing, heartbeat, and pulse stop entirely.
- The person is entirely unresponsive to shaking or shouting.
- The eyelids may be open or closed, and the pupils are dilated and fixed in one direction.
- Loss of urine and bowel control occurs.
- There is no particular order to these changes.
- These changes may or may not occur.
  NOTE: Not all these changes occur in each death.

Courtesy of Abbott-Northwestern Home Care, Hospice Unit, St. Louis Park, MN.

The Process of Death

The dying process proceeds from the distal portions of the body inward. Therefore, the legs and then the arms lose sensation and the ability to move before the internal organs. Peripheral circulation diminishes first and then stops; the patient often experiences diaphoresis (sweating) or elevated temperature, and then the body cools. The sense of touch is usually diminished, although the person can feel pressure.

Biologic Death

The patient's vital functions may be maintained by mechanical or chemical means even after brain death has occurred. Therefore, there are standards for determining "brain death." These are made under carefully controlled conditions so that in certain situations, a patient may be removed from a respirator, or certain of his or her organs may be removed for transplant procedures. **Biologic death** or *brain death* is formally defined as "irreversible cessation of total brain function, determined by clinical examination." Its determination is based on slightly different criteria in different states.

As a nurse, you may be asked to prepare the patient for an electroencephalogram, control his or her surroundings during the recording, or give support and explanations to the patient's family.

The determination of death while the patient is being maintained on a respirator is difficult for the family. They need to fully understand and accept the fact that even though the patient appears to be breathing, the machine is actually doing the breathing.

Helping the Family

The family must be given assistance as they work through their grief. After death, prepare the body so the family can see it if they wish. Be sure that the body is clean. Place a clean sheet over the patient, but do not cover the face. Remove nasogastric tubes, intravenous lines, and so forth, and turn off monitors. The patient should look comfortable. The family should be allowed to be alone in the room as long as they wish, knowing that the nurse is available if needed. Muted lighting is comforting. Offer to call the chaplain.

If the physician asks to perform an **autopsy (postmortem examination)**, the family may have questions about it. After the family leaves, the nurse is responsible for preparing the body for transportation to the morgue.

Key Concept

A family must make three major decisions before leaving the hospital when a loved one dies:

◆ Whether or not to have an autopsy performed
◆ Whether or not to donate organs or tissues
◆ Choice of funeral home or crematorium

The nurse will often be involved in assisting the family.

Care of the Body

The physician pronounces that the patient is dead and signs the death certificate. After the family has left the room, the nurse prepares the body for transportation to the morgue or pickup by the funeral director.

The following are used in care of the body after death:

◆ Wash your hands and wear gloves. (*Rationale: You will be handling body drainage.*)
◆ Straighten the body, and place a pillow under the head. (*Rationale: This position will be assumed in the casket.*)
◆ If the eyes are to be donated, close them, and place a small ice pack on each eye. A glove with a few ice chips works well. (*Rationale: The ice helps to prevent swelling and discoloration.*)
◆ Remove jewelry. If there is a specific order, a wedding ring may be taped in place. Carefully document this.
◆ List all personal belongings, and have the family sign for them and take them. Make sure to check the closet, the dresser, and the hospital safe. (*Rationale: The family will wish to sort through the patient's belongings.*)
◆ Send all flowers and cards home with the family. (*Rationale: The family may wish to write thank you notes.*)
◆ Close the patient's mouth by placing a rolled towel under the chin. (*Rationale: This provides support.*)
◆ Remove all intravenous lines, monitors, and other equipment form the patient.
◆ Remove all extra equipment from the room; remove all top bed linens but the sheet that covers the patient. (*Rationale: The equipment is not needed and will be in the way.*)
◆ Bathe any part of the body that has been soiled with discharges.
◆ Remove soiled dressings, and replace them with clean ones. Pad the wrists and ankles, and tie them loosely together. (*Rationale: This procedure make handling the body easier and prevents the arms and legs from falling down.*)
◆ Give the patient's dentures and glasses to the funeral director. Most funeral directors prefer to place dentures in the patient's mouth themselves. The patient's glasses may be taken to the funeral home by the family. (*Rationale: Dentures may be broken when being placed in the mouth. Glasses are important so that the person looks natural; the family can make sure they do not get lost en route.*)
◆ Wrap the body before it is taken to the morgue. Every hospital has its own procedure. Usually a shroud or zippered bag is provided.
◆ Attach two tags to the body: one tied to the foot (usually the big toe) and the other to the hand or wrist. Another may be attached to the covering sheet. These tags are stamped with the addressograph, and the diagnosis and date and time of death are added. (*Rationale: The patient must be correctly identified.*)

Overview of the Nursing Process
Care of the Dying Person

Assessment Priorities

Patient and family's understanding of medical condition and prognosis

Patient and family's attitude toward death

Patient's preferences concerning death: desire to be at home or in a hospital or hospice setting; decisions concerning resuscitation, aggressive forms of treatment, advanced life support, organ donation

For the incompetent patient: existence of advance directives, durable power of attorney. It is critical that the authorized decision-maker be known to all members of the health team.

Religious beliefs

Cultural influences

Stage of grief and death reaction (denial and isolation, anger, bargaining, depression, acceptance)

Adequacy of coping behaviors

Adequacy of resources available to the patient and family

Physiologic needs of the patient: personal hygiene, pain control, nutritional and fluid needs, movement, elimination, and respiratory needs

Psychological needs of the patient and family: fear of the unknown, pain, separation, leaving loved ones, loss of dignity, unfinished business; powerlessness

Spiritual needs of the patient and family: need for meaning and purpose, for love and relatedness, for forgiveness, for hope

Possible Nursing Diagnoses

Anxiety

Decisional Conflict

Ineffective Coping

Ineffective Denial

Altered Family Processes

Grieving

Hoplessness

Pain

Powerlessness

Self-Care Deficit

Social Isolation

Spiritual Distress

Other diagnoses will depend on the physiologic responses of the patient to the underlying disease process.

Planning

The nurse designs a plan of care with the dying patient and family to achieve the following general patient goals:

The patient and family verbalize that they feel free to express their needs, fears, emotions.

The patient's preferences concerning death are known and documented.

The patient reports sufficient relief of pain to interact meaningfully with family and to attend to everyday concerns.

The long-term goal is death with dignity, which leaves the family unit intact.

Implementation

Establish a supportive and trusting relationship with the patient and family. (*Note:* In hospice nursing, the family is the primary unit of care.)

Express warmth, care, and concern in interactions with the patient and family; do not be afraid to cry.

Explain the patient's condition and treatment to the patient and family.

Keep the lines of communication open between the medical staff and the patient and family, as well as between the patient and family.

Ensure that the patient's physiologic needs are met. Be especially attentive to the patient's comfort needs.

Talk with the patient when providing care—even more so if the patient is comatose. Provide simple explanations of what is being done and what is to be expected.

Support the patient and family as they work through the stages of grief and dying; refrain from being judgmental.

Encourage the patient and family to take an active role in planning and providing care.

Arrange for the patient's spiritual advisor to visit if the patient so requests. Talk with the patient about his or her beliefs; pray with the patient if asked.

Encourage family members to be open about their needs and to take necessary time for themselves.

Help members of the family to understand the emotions and needs of the dying patient.

When the patient dies, the nurse is responsible for care of the body, including placement of identification tags, care of the family, and ensuring that the death certificate has been signed by the physician. Other nursing responsibilities may include answering family questions about autopsy, offering the opportunity for organ and tissue donation, and meeting the needs of other patients.

Evaluation

The adequacy of the plan of care is determined by evaluating the patient's achievement of the above goals. If the patient or the family is unable to meet key goals, modify the plan. The following are key evaluative criteria:

Death with dignity

Intact family progressing through stages of grief

◆ If the patient had a known communicable disease, note this on the shroud or covering. *(Rationale: Special precautions may need to be taken with the body.)*

◆ Carefully dispose of all dressings, intravenous lines, and so forth according to the contaminated materials procedures of your hospital. *(Rationale: Universal Precautions and Body Substance Isolation apply.)*

◆ Wash your hands.

◆ Complete the patient's chart with documentation of the exact time of death and any pertinent observations.

Key Concept

One of the greatest challenges you will have as a nurse is providing care for a dying person.

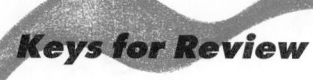

Keys for Review

Key Questions for Critical Thinking

1. You are caring for a patient who is going through the six stages of dying, as described by Kübler-Ross. Discuss each stage and the care you will provide for the patient during each stage. Compare the patient's stages with stages experienced by other members of the family.
2. Identify experiences you have had with death in your family. To your best recollection, outline your experiences, as compared to the stages as outlined by Kübler-Ross. Identify what others said that was helpful to you. Relate your experiences to your nursing career.
3. Review Maslow's hierarchy. Discuss how the needs of the dying person relate to Maslow's basic needs.
4. Identify legal rights of the patient and family during death and dying. State the legal responsibilities of the nurse.

Key Readings

Barbus A. "The dying patient's bill of rights." American Journal of Nursing 99, Vol. 75, No. 1, January, 1975

Castiglia PT, Harbin RE. Child Health Care: Process and Practice. Philadelphia, J.B. Lippincott, 1992

Carven RF, Hirnle CJ. Fundamentals of Nursing: Human Health and Function. Philadelphia, J.B. Lippincott, 1992

Kübler-Ross E. The Final Stage of Growth. New York/ Touchstone, 1986

Key Readings *(continued)*

Kübler-Ross E. On Death and Dying. New York, Macmillan, 1969

Miles A. Caring for the family left behind. AJN December 1993, 34–36

Schuster CS, Ashburn SS. The Process of Human Development: A Holistic Life-Span Approach, Ed 3. Philadelphia, J.B. Lippincott, 1992

Taylor C, Lillis C, LeMone P. Fundamentals of Nursing: The Art and science of Nursing Care, Ed 2. Philadelphia, J.B. Lippincott, 1993

Enrichment Keys

Kübler-Ross E. To Live Until We Say Good-bye. Englewood Cliffs, NJ, Prentice-Hall, 1978

Taylor PB, Ferszt GG. "Letting go of a loved one." Nursing 94 24(1):55-56, January, 1994

Key to Learning More

Chapter 91: hospice nursing

Key Resources

Association for Death Education and Counseling
638 Prospect Avenue
Hartford, CT 60105-4298
National Foundation for Sudden Infant Death
1501 Broadway
New York, NY 10036
Verble, Worth, and Verble
771 Sherwood Drive
Lexington, KY 40502

91 Hospice Nursing

Learning Objectives

- Define hospice and respite care.
- List the four areas of human needs, which are the focus of hospice care.
- List at least seven specific characteristics that must be available in a program for it to be officially classified as a hospice.
- List at least three criteria for admission to a hospice program.
- Define interdisciplinary care as it applies to hospice care, and list some of the disciplines involved.
- Describe bereavement care for the family.
- Discuss the emotional support needed in the hospice for the client, family, and staff.
- Describe nursing measures used in the terminally ill for: anorexia, constipation, diarrhea, respiratory distress, skin breakdown, and pain.

Key Terms

bereavement	primary caregiver
hospice	respite
intractable pain	unremitting pain
pain medication titration	

Keys to Understanding This Chapter

All of the chapters from this textbook have prepared you to assist the hospice patient in meeting basic physical needs. Your knowledge and understanding of the patient and family will help you in assisting them meet emotional and spiritual needs as well.

Key Points

- The hospice program is designed for people who are terminally ill.
- Hospice care focuses on physical, psychological, social, and spiritual needs.
- Respite care may be necessary for family members to assist them to get some needed rest.
- Hospice programs assist the patient *and* the family.
- Many hospice programs follow families for up to 1 year after the person's death to assist the family with bereavement.
- The focus of hospice nursing is twofold: both patient and family need assessment and support.
- Education of families is a major nursing goal.
- The goal of pain and symptom management is relief without side effects.

Key Topics Outline

Characteristics of Hospice
Role of the Hospice Nurse
  Symptom Control

Key Learning Activities

- Interview a hospice nurse. What services are provided to patients and families? What services are offered to the nurses employed there?
- Visit an inpatient hospice unit. Compare and contrast this facility with a traditional medical-surgical unit.
- Interview a chaplain. How do they assist dying patients and their families? Are there differences between working with the person in the hospital and the person in a hospice program?

The term **hospice** is derived from a medieval word that meant "to provide shelter for travelers on difficult journeys." Currently, hospice is not a place but rather a philosophy of care where the terminally ill person can be cared for with dignity, with as much relief of pain as possible, and with relief and control of physical and emotional suffering. The nurse who works with hospice patients will have an opportunity to use skills learned during an entire nursing program.

Hospice care focuses on four human needs:

◆ Physical
◆ Psychological or emotional
◆ Social
◆ Spiritual

Characteristics of Hospice

The first U.S. hospice for healthcare was opened in 1974 in New Haven, Connecticut. The hospice model used in the United States is based on home care with supportive backup inpatient services in case they become necessary.

To be legitimately called a hospice, an agency must have certain characteristics:[1]

◆ The hospice is an autonomous program centrally administered, usually with inpatient and outpatient services. The hospice is "primarily concerned with home care, with back-up inpatient services when home care is not feasible."
◆ The primary unit of care is the client and the family.
◆ Symptom control, not curative measures, is the goal.
◆ Interdisciplinary care is practiced under the direction of a qualified physician.
◆ Specially trained volunteers are available.
◆ Services are available on call 24 hours a day.
◆ Support is available for the staff.
◆ Hospice services are extended to the family during the time of bereavement.
◆ Hospice services are based on physical need, not on financial resources.

The accompanying box lists criteria for admission to a hospice.

Service Coordination. In the hospice program, the client receives care in the home for as long as possible. Today, most hospices are home based and have contracts with inpatient hospices or acute care inpatient

---

[1] Markel S. The Hospice Concept. Atlanta, GA, American Cancer Society, 1978.

Sample Criteria for Admission to a Hospice*

◆ A diagnosis of progressive, terminal illness is confirmed. The physician, client, and family agree that control of symptoms is the primary goal, after determining that no curative treatment is available or desirable.
◆ Life expectancy is usually no more than 6 months from date of admission.
◆ A person (people) agrees to be primary caregiver(s) (responsible for care 24 hours a day).
◆ The patient and family have agreed on DNR/DNI status.
◆ Hospice care can be discontinued with the agreement of the client, family, and attending physician.
◆ Admission can be directed primarily toward meeting the needs of the family.

* Courtesy of Good Samaritan Hospice Care, Kellogg Community College, Battle Creek, MI and Abbott-Northwestern Home Care, Hospice Unit, St. Louis Park, MN.

---

facilities that provide hospice care. Few hospices have their own inpatient units. Some clients choose to die at home, even though a hospice unit may be available. Each family and client must be assisted in making these decisions. If the client is to receive care at home, **primary caregivers** (family, in most cases) must be willing to assume responsibility for the care. The hospice staff meets with the client and the designated caregivers to determine whether this is feasible.

Key Concept

Hospice care does not speed death, nor does it prolong life.

Respite Care. Caring for a dying person at home is exhausting. The term **respite** simply means that the family or other caregivers can occasionally obtain a rest from this care.

This can be accomplished by admitting the client to an inpatient hospice, hospital, or nursing home for a few days or arranging for supplemental care in the home. Some hospices have contracts with hospitals, nursing homes, or healthcare agencies that agree to provide beds and services for hospice clients to provide family respite.

Client and Family as Primary Unit. The client and family decide what type of care will be most comfortable for them. The hospice team works with them in planning this care. A home visit is often made when the person applies for hospice care to assess the physical setup and the family situation. This initial visit is usually made by a specially trained nurse. Later visits are often made by other members of the team.

Symptom Control. The dying person has many physical symptoms that must be handled. Some of these symptoms are discussed in Chapter 90; however, the symptoms involved in hospice care are often managed for a longer time than the symptoms seen in the hospitalized terminal patient. Symptom control is discussed at the end of this chapter.

> **Key Concept**
>
> One of the philosophies of hospice care is that suffering should not be prolonged without extending hope. Symptoms are managed in as noninvasive a manner as possible.

Interdisciplinary Care. The interdisciplinary team consists of nurses, social workers, physicians, therapists (occupational, physical, speech, or respiratory), clergy, and dieticians. Although physician-directed services are required legally, the patient is the center of the care, and the interdisciplinary team responds to the patient's needs. In most cases, radiation therapy and chemotherapy must be discontinued before the client can be admitted to the hospice program.

The client's family (the primary caregiver) is vital in the care. They can identify changes in the client's condition that might not be noticeable to other people. The family can suggest approaches to care that meet with everyone's approval.

Specially Trained Volunteers. An integral part of any hospice program is their specially trained group of volunteers, who are mostly unpaid lay people. Volunteers perform a variety of tasks to assist and support the patient and family. They can provide emotional support, run errands, assist with physical care, provide short periods of respite, and help with child care or household tasks.

Volunteers are often the "unconditional presence" needed for patients and caregivers to share their feelings. Many volunteers are people who have been primary caregivers in their own family.

On-Call Services. The services of the hospice staff are available 24 hours a day. Questions or concerns are met with reassurance or assistance. A home visit may be made at any time to help the family deal with a physical or emotional problem. If the family knows that this service is available, they are likely to be able to keep the person at home for a longer time. In many cases, the hospice client is allowed to die at home, with the on call assistance of the hospice staff.

Emotional Support. Kind and thoughtful communication with the hospice client cannot be overemphasized. This person is dying and knows it. Pain and other symptoms make the situation even more difficult. Many times, nonverbal communication is the most helpful. The client is tired and may have pain. He or she needs to know that someone is there who cares.

The family may be more distressed than the client, so they also need the nurse's support. They need to talk about their concerns, and to feel that others are concerned. You can listen and refer them to the chaplain or social services staff.

Bereavement Care. Bereavement or grieving is part of the process of dealing with the death of a loved one. Often, a member or several members of the hospice staff attend the funeral services. The family is urged to talk to the hospice staff and to work out their grief. The client's family also is encouraged to attend a grief support group for a time after the death of the loved one. Sometimes one or two home visits are made after the death to evaluate and assist in the family's adjustment. Bereavement follow-up usually continues for 1 year following the death of the client.

Support for Hospice Staff. Nurses need emotional support when working with dying people. It is important for the healthcare team to have a regular hospice support group or other means of therapy available so that they can deal with the loss of these people with whom they have spent time, become close, and provided care. It is normal and acceptable to grieve when a client dies. It is also acceptable to let the client and family know of your grief.

Role of the Hospice Nurse

The role of the hospice nurse is one of assessment, support, and education. Hospice nurses do minimal direct patient care. Instead, they focus on identifying patient and family needs and respond to them by teaching skills and coordinating supportive services to assist families to care for their loved ones. This gives the family a sense of confidence and competency and discourages overdependence on the nurse. Some keys to patient teaching are given in the box. Other nursing care is summarized in the next box.

When the Patient Dies at Home[2]

Family teaching in preparation for the patient's death at home includes the following:

- Call the hospice nurse. Have the phone number handy.
- Have information ready:
  - Time of death
  - Last medications administered, dosage, time given
  - Patient's condition during last 8 hours
  - Name, address, and phone number of funeral home
  - Name, address, and phone number of next of kin
  - When patient was last seen by a registered nurse

Symptom Control

Most patients have several different physical symptoms at the same time. It is important to address all of the patient's symptoms while determining which are the most problematic.

Anorexia

Many terminally ill people are unable to eat because of fatigue, pain, anxiety, depression, odors, dehydration, nausea, and general discomfort. It is important to assist the client to eat to preserve strength and quality of life.

The nurse should administer drugs as ordered. Vitamins, tranquilizers, antidepressants, or alcohol may help the person to eat. Pain medication, antiemetics, or tranquilizers approximately one-half hour before meals help the person relax and eat. Some drugs stimulate appetite.

Serve small amounts, and serve meals more frequently than usual. Reassure the client and family that a large intake of food is not necessary. The nurse should check dislikes or specific difficulty with certain foods, offer foods that the person prefers, and season food according to his or her taste. Give soft foods. The nurse can help make mealtime as pleasant as possible by eliminating unpleasant odors and sights and socializing with the client when food is served.

The nurse instructs the caregiver, family, volunteers, or aides regarding the ways to encourage patients to

eat (see Chapter 27). The hospice nurse will often enlist the aid of a dietician. The hospice nurse usually does not feed patients.

Give good mouth care before and after meals. Give supplements as ordered. They provide nourishment without great volume.

Give ice chips because these provide liquid and numb the mouth. Iced drinks, such as iced tea and lemonade, are often taken well. Clear liquids are usually more appealing than creamed liquid milk products or sweetened items, such as ice cream. Popsicles or water ice can be offered.

The nurse should assess for and report dehydration. Dehydration cannot always be avoided. For example, when the client is in the last stages of illness, some dehydration may be beneficial, because it can dry secretions and reduce choking, ascites, pulmonary edema, and difficulty in breathing. The physician must determine whether dehydration is to be treated.

Nausea and Vomiting

The terminally ill person often experiences nausea and vomiting as a result of anorexia; tumor invasion; radiation therapy or chemotherapy; reaction to narcotics, such as opioids; or increased intracranial pressure.

To alleviate the discomfort of nausea and vomiting, the nurse should use many of the same procedures suggested for anorexia. The nurse should assess the patient's nausea for any pattern and remove the cause of nausea if possible. Position the person on the right side. Relaxation techniques are often effective, as are drugs prescribed by the physician. Antiemetics or other antinausea drugs should be given approximately one-half hour before meals (see Key Medications box). Carbonated beverages and dry foods, such as popcorn, also

Providing Care in Hospice Nursing

- Do not try to predict the exact time of death.
- Do not get involved in family disputes.
- Allow the client and family to express their spiritual feelings in the way they desire.
- Maintain your sense of humor.
- Allow the client to be alone or stay with the person, depending on what he or she desires.
- Realize that irrational behavior on the part of the family and the hospice client is a normal part of the grieving process.
- Be honest.
- When in doubt, be quiet.
- Allow the client and family to maintain hope at whatever level.

[2] Guidelines for Hospice Care. St. Louis Park, MN, Abbott-Northwestern Home Care.

Key Medications
for Symptom Control in Hospice Care

- Nausea: prochlorperazine (Compazine); trimethobenzamide (Tigan); chlorpromazine (Thorazine); thiethylperazine (Torecan); haloperidol (Haldol), less sedating for elderly patients; lorazepam HCl (Ativan); metoclopramide HCl (Reglan)
- Diarrhea: loperamide HCl (Imodium), diphenoxylate HCl (Lomotil, Lonox), kaolin and pectin mixtures (Kaopectate, Donnagel-MB), opium tincture (Paregoric)
- Constipation: milk of magnesia; docusate sodium (Colace), stool softener; senna concentrate (Senokot); bisacodyl (Dulcolax) tablets or suppositories; docusate calcium (Surfak); mineral oil
- Pain management: morphine sulfate (MS Contin, Roxanol); hydromorphine HCl (Dilaudid); levorphanol (Levo-Dromoran); oxycodone and ASA (Percodan); oxycodone and acetaminophen (Percocet); codeine; fentanyl (Sublimaze); methadone; meperidine HCl (Demerol), Dexamethasone (Decadron), Cyclobenzaprine (Flexaril)
- Depression: sertraline HCl (Zoloft); imipramine hydrochloride (Tofranil); amitriptyline (Elavil); trimipramine maleate (Surmontil); doxepin (Sinequan)
- Anxiety: buspirone HCl (BuSpar); diazepam (Valium); alprazolam (Xanax); lorazepam (Ativan); chlorpromazine (Thorazine); haloperidol (Haldol); fluphenazine (Prolixin)
- Insomnia: temazepam (Restoril); triazolam (Halcion); estazolam (ProSom); diphenhydramine (Benadryl); amobarbital and secobarbital (Tuinal)

can be given. Wear gloves when giving care if the person is vomiting.

Diarrhea

The terminally ill person may develop diarrhea as a result of a fecal impaction or as a side effect of chemotherapy, radiation therapy, or any medication the patient is taking. The person also might have a bowel obstruction or infection. Wear gloves when handling any body substances.

Follow the physician's order for specific treatment after determining the cause of diarrhea. Use a low-residue diet to lessen stimulation, and eliminate specific foods that cause gas and cramps. The person often knows what foods are not well tolerated. The nurse should encourage the person to drink fluids (not necessarily plain water). Key medications for diarrhea are listed in the Key Medications box.

The nurse also should check electrolyte levels in the blood, because diarrhea can cause serious electrolyte imbalances and life-threatening difficulty. Give good skin care around the rectum. Wear gloves.

Constipation

Many terminally ill people are constipated because of inactivity, low food intake, or a low-residue diet. Constipation also might be a side effect of medications or a result of the disease's invasion of the digestive tract.

If a person suffers from constipation, the diet should be adjusted to include high-residue foods that help increase the frequency of bowel movements (unless a bowel obstruction exists).

A stool softener or routine laxative can be given. Many hospice clients routinely receive a laxative, such as magnesium hydroxide (Milk of Magnesia) or docusate sodium (Peri-Colace). Suppositories also encourage peristalsis. Key medications for constipation are also listed in the box.

The nurse should check for dehydration, because if the person is dehydrated, fluid will be retained, and the feces will become hard and impacted. This can be a serious complication. The nurse should help the person understand that he or she might have a bowel movement only every 2 or 3 days as a result of eating little and not moving around. If the person is not uncomfortable, a bowel movement every 2 or 3 days is not a problem.

Skin Breakdown

A serious problem in terminally ill clients is that of skin breakdown and pressure sores. The person is not moving and is often lying in one position. The nutritional status may be inadequate for reasons previously mentioned. The disease process may have made the skin fragile and easily broken down. Chapter 45 describes skin and wound care in detail. The nurse should stress the importance of pressure points and turning when teaching caregivers skin care of dying patients.

The nurse should wear gloves when giving care if the client's skin is not intact. The person should be given good skin care, and the skin should be clean and dry at all times. The nurse should try to get the person out of bed and relieve pressure as much as possible. Special mattresses may be used to help prevent skin breakdown. It may be necessary to give pain medication to get the clients to move or change positions. The physician should be consulted for specific treatments. The person's disease condition may also warrant particular treatment.

Respiratory Distress

Many terminally ill people have difficulty breathing as a result of the disease process or because of complications of the disease process. Additional oxygen may be needed because of fever, anxiety, infection, or discomfort. The oxygen concentrator is used more in home care than the oxygen tank.

The nurse should keep the hospice client's environment calm and quiet to reduce anxiety and position him or her for maximum comfort to conserve energy. Portable fans to circulate room air are helpful for dyspnea.

Vital signs and the level of consciousness should be assessed. The person may be losing consciousness and thus the ability to breathe adequately without assistance.

Give supplemental oxygen and other treatments as ordered or as needed. Thoracentesis may relieve pressure, medications may lessen secretions and improve respiration, postural drainage may help to eliminate secretions from the lungs, and surgery may be needed to relieve an obstruction. The patient also may benefit from an aerosolized inhaler, cough medicine, decongestant, or low-dose morphine.

Pain

Probably the most common problem in hospice care is the management of chronic and severe pain. The **unremitting pain** (also called **intractable pain**) or **total pain** of terminal disease is different from occasional and temporary pain caused by other conditions. This type of pain is constant and unrelenting. The nurse assesses the pain and its level of interference with activities, rest, and general comfort. The goal is pain prevention and relief, with a minimum of side effects.

As much as possible, the client in the hospice program manages his or her own pain. A patient-controlled analgesia (PCA) pump may be used. Attempts are made to manage with a minimum of medication for as long as possible. Modalities such as heat and massage are used. The client is distracted as much as possible by visiting with family and friends, reading, watching television, and visiting outside the hospice or away from home. Such modalities as biofeedback, massage, acupuncture, and acupressure also may be used.

Sometimes applying ice on the contralateral side (opposite side from the pain) helps.

> **Key Concept**
>
> Sometimes the experience of pain is associated in the patient's mind with life. This attitude may lead to patients refusing adequate pain control. This is often difficult for nurses and caregivers, but it is important to assess the psychological benefits that pain may offer.

Oral Medications. Give medications orally for as long as possible. This helps to maintain the dignity of the client and prevents possible infection and the discomfort of an injection. The client should be involved in self-medication. The nurse should assess and evaluate pain. An assessment tool (see Chapter 52) should be used so that the physician can determine the most effective medications and dosage.

Some oral medications may be effective in less severe pain. Commonly used is codeine or Percodan. When oral medications will no longer control the pain,

intramuscular or intravenous medications are given. A heparin lock is often in place to allow intravenous medications to be given without repeated venipuncture.

Pain Medication Titration. Hospices advocate for **pain medication titration**. Patients often require lower doses for a longer time when taking medications around the clock versus giving medication as needed for existing pain. Twelve-hour pain medication taken once every 12 hours can be effective and easier for families or the patient to manage. Families must be taught the value of titrating pain medications. Give medication *before pain occurs or before it increases.*

> **Key Concept**
>
> If the patient can regulate his or her own medication, usually less will be used. This also adds to the person's self-esteem and adds dignity to his or her care.

Commonly Used Medications. Morphine is often the drug of choice for pain. Whenever administering morphine, assessment of the patient's respiratory status and level of consciousness is essential. Prior to the use of morphine, Brompton's cocktail (a mixture of narcotics, alcohol, a central nervous system stimulant, and other ingredients to enhance the taste) and heroin were used. These are seldom used today. In some cases, patients are allowed to use marijuana for symptom control. Commonly used pain medications also are listed in the Key Medications box.

> **Key Concept**
>
> Certain types of pain require combinations of drugs, and not just one drug, such as morphine, alone.[3] These types of pain and the recommended medications include:
>
> ◆ bone pain (NSAIDs and corticosteroids)
> ◆ smooth muscle pain (belladonna and atropine)
> ◆ nerve pain (Elavil)
> ◆ headache caused by increased intracranial pressure (*aggravated* by morphine or codeine; use Decadron, Elavil, and Prolixin)
> ◆ striated muscle spasm pain (Flexaril)
>
> In some of these situations, morphine will be used in addition, for coexisting pain.

Intravenous Medications. Equipment such as the intravenous infusion pump controller may be regulated by

[3] Hospice Guidelines, Abbott-Northwestern Home Care, St. Louis Park, MN.

the patient or family, either in the hospice unit or in their own home. They are taught to regulate the flow, what to do when the alarm sounds, and when to call for assistance. The home care nurse usually adds the medications to the solution and leaves them for the family to hang. In the hospital, the intraspinal or intrathecal routes also may be used for medication administration.

Key Concept

People who smoke, abuse substances, or are athletic will often require more medication to achieve comfort because of their individual altered endorphin production.

Management of Odor

The greatest aesthetic problem in caring for some clients with cancer is the disagreeable odor. Odor is embarrassing to the client and bothersome to the family. Some of the means for controlling odor are presented in Chapter 90. Another device that may be used in hospice care is the charcoal filter dressing. This allows odors to pass through a charcoal filter before entering the atmosphere. These dressings are expensive and are not usually used unless the odor is very disturbing.

Key Concept

The goal of hospice care is death with dignity. The client is helped to remain active and to make decisions about his or her life for as long as possible.

Depression

The patient may need treatment for depression. If the patient is experiencing a reactive depression, the nurse can intervene with empathetic listening and validating of the patient's feelings. Clinical depression requires drug therapy. This is a sad situation, but clinical depression should be prevented if possible (see Key Medications box).

Anxiety

The patient may be afraid of dying or may be worried about what will happen to his or her loved ones after the death. The patient also may become agitated. The nurse can listen and offer reassurance. Sometimes tranquilizers are prescribed. Key medications for anxiety also are listed in the box. Some of these medications help to control other symptoms, such as nausea, as well.

Insomnia

It is important for the patient to rest and obtain sleep to prevent acceleration of the disease process. The nurse can provide comfort measures, such as fresh bedding and a back rub; soft music or relaxation tapes also may be helpful. Medications may be prescribed. Key medications used in insomnia also are listed in the box.

Key Concept

Nursing functions if a patient dies at home include the following:

◆ Allow family time alone with the deceased.
◆ Prepare the body for transportation to the funeral home.
◆ Remove all equipment.
◆ Count narcotics and dispose of them as per agency policy.
◆ Listen to and validate the families' need to talk about their loved one's final moments and hours.
◆ Document all information.
◆ Make sure the physician and coroner have been notified. (The coroner is not required to come to the home of a registered hospice patient.)

Keys for Review

Key Questions for Critical Thinking

1. Discuss the characteristics and requirements of hospice.
2. Discuss the concept of total pain and how it is treated. Include pharmacology therapy, nonpharmacology therapy, alternatives to medication, and emotional and spiritual support.

Key Readings

Craven RF, Hirnle CJ. Fundamentals of Nursing: Human Health and Function. Philadelphia, J.B. Lippincott, 1992

Key Readings (continued)

Nursing '94 Drug Handbook. Springhouse, PA, Springhouse, 1994
Samarel N. Caring for Life and Death. New York, Hemisphere (Taylor & Francis), 1991
Taylor C, Lillis C, LeMone P. Fundamentals of Nursing: The Art and Science of Nursing Care, Ed 2. Philadelphia, J.B. Lippincott, 1993

Enrichment Keys

Amenta MO, Lippert C. Hospice is a concept, not a place. Home Healthcare Nurse, Vol. 12 #3, May/June 1994, 71–72

Keys to Learning More

As you practice nursing, you will meet people who are working through the death experience. Your own life experiences will help you assist patients and families.

Key Resources

Hospice Action
    PO Box 32331
    Washington, DC 20007
National Hospice Organization
    765 Prospect Street
    New Haven, CT 06511
Concern for Dying
    250 W. 57th Street
    New York, NY 10107
    212/246-6962

Part D Personal Responsibilities of the Graduate Nurse

Unit *18* The Transition From Student to Graduate Nurse

92 Trends in Nursing and Leadership Skills

Keys for Learning

Learning Objectives

- Describe the role of the licensed practical and licensed vocational nurse as a team leader.
- State the duties of the charge nurse or team leader.
- List the guidelines for evening and night shifts.
- Discuss the expanded role of the practical nurse as described in your state's Nurse Practice Act.
- List some computer applications in nursing.
- State the procedure for transcribing orders.
- Relate the responsibilities regarding telephone orders.

Key Terms

autocratic leader

bureaucratic leader

democratic leader

laissez faire

Keys to Understanding This Chapter

This entire book has been designed to prepare you for a career in nursing. Your education has been built on the following:

Part A: basic scientific information

Part B: basic nursing skills

Part C: recognition of deviations from normal and nursing interventions to assist patients of all ages to meet basic needs

Key Points

- The role of the nurse, including the practical nurse, is expanding.
- As a new graduate of a nursing program, you should have additional education and experience to assume leadership roles.
- There are several leadership styles. There is no right or wrong style; any of the styles can work effectively.

Key Points (continued)

- Transcribing or checking a physician's orders is a vital leadership function that must be carried out accurately.
- The nurse is responsible for continuity of patient care 24 hours a day.

Key Topics Outline

The Nursing Team
    The Graduate Nurse
    The Team Leader or Charge Nurse
The Nurse and Leadership Styles
Transcribing Orders
    The Drug Order
    Operative Orders
    Orders for Other Procedures
    Telephone or Verbal Orders

Key Learning Activities

- Interview a licensed practical nurse or registered nurse who works charge. What suggestions would this person have to prepare a new graduate for charge responsibilities?
- Collect brochures regarding continuing education for nurses. What types of programs are available in your area? Are there courses related to nursing leadership?
- Visit a hospital after 9 PM. Describe the differences from the daytime hours.
- Gather employment advertisements for nurses from your local paper, nursing journals, the state JOBS service, and your school's placement office. Compare benefits, salaries, and working conditions. In which positions are you most interested?

In this era of healthcare reform, the licensed practical nurse (LPN) and licensed vocational nurse (LVN) are being used extensively in leadership roles. Effective leadership skills are invaluable. To be a competent leader, the nurse needs to have the ability to direct and influence the actions of others. Leadership styles are described later in this chapter.

The Nursing Team

The total nursing team is made up of several types of nurses. All of these team members work together under the direction of the physician to help the patient return to optimum function as soon as possible.

The registered nurse (RN) has more formal education than the practical nurse. Therefore, he or she is more likely to be the team leader or charge nurse in a hospital. Many RNs give direct patient care, as do LPNs. In a complex nursing situation, the LPN is expected to assist. The nursing assistant also is a valuable member of the nursing team.

The Graduate Nurse

Organizing your work

As a graduate, you will be caring for more patients and probably for more hours than you did as a student. Whatever the situation, you must learn to organize your work so that you are able to give efficient care to all of your patients. This comes with experience, but your team leader will be willing to assist you.

The most important things for the new graduate to remember are the following:

◆ When in doubt about a technique or procedure, ask.
◆ Know when and to whom to report significant symptoms.
◆ Know where to find information about drugs and treatments.
◆ Be thoroughly knowledgeable about the institution's emergency, fire, and disaster regulations and procedures.

Nursing Around the Clock

Nursing goes on around the clock. As a student, you may not have been on duty during the evening or night tours of duty, or you may not have been in the hospital during a full shift. Remember when you leave the hospital, the patient stays there.

In many hospitals, 12-hour shifts are available. This means you could have more days off. However, working the longer shifts may be difficult for you.

The Team Leader or Charge Nurse

The practical nurse may be asked to be a team leader or charge nurse, especially in nursing homes, extended care facilities, and medical clinics.

The National Federation of Licensed Practical Nurses (NFLPN) Revised Statement of Functions and Qualifications of the Licensed Practical Nurse states:

◆ The LPN, with additional preparation in specialized areas and under direction of autonomous health professionals, is qualified to do the following:
  ◆ Supervise other nursing and health-related personnel
  ◆ Coordinate and make assignments of other nursing and health-related personnel and patients
  ◆ Serve as a team leader
  ◆ Serve as a charge nurse[1]
◆ To serve as team leader or charge nurse, the NFLPN Specialized Nursing Practice Standards state that the LPN or LVN must do the following:
  ◆ Have at least 1 year's experience in nursing at the staff level
  ◆ Present personal qualifications that indicate potential abilities for practice in the chosen specialized nursing area
  ◆ Present evidence of completion of a program or course that is approved by an appropriate agency to provide the knowledge and skills necessary for effective nursing services in the specialized field
  ◆ Meet all the standards of practice as set forth by the NFLPN

Besides the special postgraduate training in the skills these posts require, you also need other knowledge and attributes. If you are asked to work as a charge nurse, you need to decide if you are ready to take on that much responsibility.

You will need to study to gain the needed information about legislation, such as Medicare. You may need assistance in planning and implementing patient care and in coordinating and directing the activities of other staff members. You must be able to evaluate the nursing care being given and your own leadership abilities, and you should have someone to whom you can freely go for qualified assistance. You will usually be responsible to the department supervisor, an RN who provides guidance and assistance.

The functions of the charge nurse are listed in the accompanying box. These specific functions are discussed in several books that train LPNs or new graduates to work

[1] The Licensed Practical Nurse as Charge Nurse, U.S. Department of Health, Education, Welfare, Public Health Service. Washington, DC, 1972, p 65.

Functions of the Charge Nurse

Plans Patient Care

- ♦ Demonstrates awareness of the comprehensive nature of long-term care
- ♦ Understands the condition, needs, and therapeutic goals of each patient
- ♦ Receives and interprets verbal and written reports about patient care
- ♦ Makes nursing rounds to observe and determine patient needs
- ♦ Assists the physician with examinations, and treatments
- ♦ Discusses patient care goals with physician, nursing supervisor, and staff
- ♦ Develops or assists other nurses to develop nursing care plans for individual patients
- ♦ May triage to determine which unit or which bed a new patient will occupy

Coordinates Staff Activities

- ♦ Exhibits an understanding of basic human behavior
- ♦ Demonstrates fundamental leadership techniques
- ♦ Uses management principles and procedures
- ♦ Communicates; listens, speaks, reads, writes, gestures effectively
- ♦ Motivates staff to give skilled nursing care to all patients

Implements Patient Care

- ♦ Develops plans to meet needs of all patients
- ♦ Develops plans for common types of emergency situations
- ♦ Assigns personnel in terms of patient needs and staff proficiencies
- ♦ Helps staff care for patients with special needs, the patient with mental illness, the dying patient
- ♦ Coordinates work with that of other departments, such as dietary, housekeeping, physical and occupational therapy, social service
- ♦ Seeks guidance and assistance when problems are beyond scope of practice
- ♦ Prepares and gives verbal and written reports about patients: conferences, nurses' notes, tour of duty, and special reports

Evaluates Patient Care

- ♦ Applies basic principles of evaluation
- ♦ Makes nursing rounds to observe and assess patient care and needs
- ♦ Assesses patient care plans and modifies as necessary
- ♦ Assesses patient care given by staff and guides appropriate changes
- ♦ Appraises self-performance and plans improvement
- ♦ Follows through on quality assurance plans

as team leaders or charge nurses. Many of these functions also have been discussed elsewhere in this book.

- ♦ Establish and update nursing procedures.
- ♦ Establish training protocols and programs.

> **Key Concept**
>
> Note that the role of the team leader or charge nurse parallels the steps in the nursing process.

> **Key Concept**
>
> Not every LPN or RN has the ability to be a charge nurse or team leader. Do not feel inadequate if you are unable or unwilling to work as a charge nurse.

The charge nurse must have leadership and administrative abilities, a thorough knowledge of nursing, and an intuitive understanding of people's behaviors. The practical nurse or new RN should not attempt to be a team leader or work charge without further education and experience beyond the basic nursing program.

The Team Leader in a Medical Clinic. In addition to many of the functions listed previously, the nurse in a medical clinic also is expected to do the following:

- ♦ Schedule patients, trace quality assurance, train other staff, and resolve conflicts.
- ♦ Attend team leader meetings.
- ♦ Write policies.
- ♦ Monitor staffing and dismissal from positions.

The Team Leader in the Extended Care Facility. A standard for a charge nurse in the skilled nursing extended care facility has been established by the U.S. government. This standard states that at least one RN or LPN must be on duty and in charge at all times.

It is desirable that the nurse in charge of each tour of duty be trained or experienced in areas such as nursing administration and supervision and rehabilitation, psychiatric, or geriatric nursing. The charge nurse should have the ability to recognize significant changes in the condition of patients and to take necessary action. The charge nurse should be responsible for the total nursing care of patients during the tour of duty.[2]

[2] The Licensed Practical Nurse as a Charge Nurse, ibid.

Additional duties of the team leader in an extended care facility include:

◆ Receiving reports on assigned patients.
◆ Making patient assignments for team members.
◆ Making rounds, and assessing patients.
◆ Reporting to team members on assigned patients.
◆ Directing administration of medications and treatments.
◆ Conferring with team members regularly throughout the shift.

Making Staff Assignments. If you are functioning as a charge nurse, you will probably be expected to assign duties to other members of the nursing team. You must know your patients; making rounds is usually the first thing you will do, either immediately before or after the change-of-shift report. You also need to know your staff members; each person has special abilities that you can use to the patient's greatest advantage.

It is your responsibility to explain procedures to staff members and to assist them to plan their workload so that all patients receive optimum care. You also must check periodically with your staff to make sure there are no problems with their assignments.

Computer Use in Healthcare. Today's nurse must learn to interact comfortably with various kinds of computerized and electronic equipment. Some of these items are familiar to you by now; the electronic thermometer, the ultrasound, the computed tomography scan, the computerized infusion pump, and the apnea monitor all are household words to you and your classmates.

During your nursing career, you will encounter many new pieces of electronic equipment. Do not be overwhelmed by this. Look up information, or ask questions if you do not know how a particular piece of equipment operates. The scientific advances improve patient care by ensuring greater accuracy of diagnoses and treatment and greater efficiency in delivery of care.

Computers are used in a variety of ways in modern healthcare facilities:

◆ Monitor the patient's condition
◆ Store medical records
◆ Maintain bookkeeping and business records
◆ Regulate specialized machines
◆ Assist physicians in the diagnosis of disease
◆ Conduct quality assurance research
◆ Teach medical and nursing students
◆ Assist in developing a nursing care plan
◆ Supply information on medication dosages, side effects, and times of administration
◆ Order supplies
◆ Make appointments for x-rays and tests

◆ Call up laboratory results
◆ Schedule the operating room
◆ Schedule the nursing staff

If you are not familiar with the use of computers, you may be able to register for a short course at your nursing school. Remember that the operation manuals for new equipment are usually kept on file.

The Nurse and Leadership Styles

Nurses need to develop leadership skills to supervise others effectively. You have developed organizational skills in daily patient care; as a graduate, you may wish to develop additional leadership skills. The varied situations in healthcare will dictate the most appropriate leadership style, but a strong knowledge base is essential to all styles.[3]

Autocratic. Autocratic leaders are self-directed; this style calls for little or no input from staff. In its extreme form, autocratic leadership may be compared with dictatorship, where the leader makes decisions, and the group is expected to carry out orders. In certain situations, such as a code or other emergency, this style may be effective. New graduates may feel more comfortable with an autocratic leader until they gain confidence.

Bureaucratic. Bureaucratic leadership is policy minded. Bureaucratic leaders rely on established protocol for decision-making. The Policy and Procedure Manual offers step-by-step instructions; a bureaucratic leader will consider them as "rules." This style is often helpful for new graduates who need detailed instructions. In addition, some procedures require strict guidelines.

Democratic. The **democratic leader** is people oriented and tries to guide staff in the right direction. Nursing approaches such as team nursing benefit from democratic leadership by fostering team spirit in an atmosphere of mutual respect and shared responsibility. These leaders use group input but will make final decisions when there is no consensus. This style allows for a free flow of ideas, plans, and information between leader and followers.

Laissez faire. The leadership style with the least structure is **laissez faire**. This leader has loosely structured goals with no firm guidelines. The followers are encouraged to choose their own goals and plans for implementation. While leaders that continuously use this style may be well liked, goals may not be accomplished. However, this leader encourages creativity and

[3] Submitted by Frances Stoner.

independence and allows people to try new things without fear of mistakes.

Blended Leadership. Often the most effective leader blends styles. A successful leader can move from one style to another as the situation dictates.

Transcribing Orders

The nurse may be expected to transcribe the physician's orders. In some hospitals, unit managers, hospital unit coordinators, or hospital station secretaries do this, but in many nursing homes, there are no desk workers. This means that the nurse reads the physician's order sheet and carries out the necessary actions, so the patient receives the benefit of the prescribed medical regimen. The practical nurse and RN must know how to transcribe the physician's orders, even though they may not often be asked to do so. The nurse in charge also must know about transcribing orders so that the work of the others can be double-checked for accuracy.

The Drug Order[4]

The following are guidelines for transcribing the physician's orders:

♦ Read all orders. Always do "stat" orders first.
♦ Order the medication from the pharmacy, giving the name of the drug, dose, administration, and frequency of administration.
♦ Write the information on the Kardex, the med card (if used), and the medication administration record (MAR). (Most institutions have a policy that all antibiotics, anticoagulants, hypnotics, and narcotics must be reordered every 48 hours.) You must pencil in the date of the reorder on the Kardex.
♦ Make out an MAR. (Stat orders may be written on a special form.) Enter the patient's name and room number. Enter the name of medication (generic and trade names), dosage, and route of administration. Enter the times (for example, q.i.d. 8-12-4-8 or 0800, 1200, 1600, 2000). Enter the date of the order and the date to be discontinued, if known.
♦ Notify the person giving medications or flag the order.
♦ Make appropriate notations on the doctor's order sheet signifying that you have transcribed the order. Generally, a line is drawn in red under the last order and the physician's signature, and the nurse signs

and writes the date and time on the order sheet. (The nurse in charge of the patient may countersign.)
♦ In some hospitals, a carbon copy of the physician's order sheet is sent directly to the pharmacy. In other institutions, orders are entered on a computer that interacts with the computer in the pharmacy. Sometimes individual prescriptions are written.
♦ When the patient's individual medications arrive from the pharmacy, check them against the physician's orders before putting them in the patient's drawer or medication chart.
♦ If you have any questions, **ask**.

When the medication is discontinued, the nurse should do the following:

♦ Cross out the item on the Kardex or MAR. (Sometimes a yellow or pink highlighter is used.) The information must still be readable after you have crossed it off.
♦ Notify the nurse involved.
♦ Make out a drug credit if there are remaining medications. Send leftover medications back to the pharmacy.
♦ Mark "dc" (for discontinued) on the medication sheet or MAR.
♦ Mark appropriate notations on the doctor's order sheet.

Nursing Alert

Whenever a part of a medication order is changed, such as the dose or the frequency of administration, discontinue the old order and transcribe an entirely new order. This will help to prevent errors or confusion. This is the reason that all medication orders should be written in ink, crossed out, and rewritten if they are changed, rather than erasing, which might be illegible.

The nurse in charge should check all drug orders that you have transcribed until you are a graduate and have become experienced.

The Kardex and MAR become part of the patient's permanent record. Therefore, where orders are crossed out, they should still be legible. Correction fluid and erasures are not to be used in the Kardex, MAR, or chart.

Operative Orders[5]

Each hospital has its own routines for transcribing operative orders; however, the following are some general points. Most patients are admitted the morning of surgery, unless it is an emergency or they are in the hos-

[4] Originally developed by Josephine M. Schmer, BS, RN, HE and the Practical Nursing faculty for Project Opportunity, Anoka Practical Nursing Program, Anoka MN.

[5] Originally developed by Josephine M. Schmer, BS, RN, HE for Project Opportunity, Anoka Practical Nursing Program, Anoka, MN.

pital for another reason. The instructions below apply to the nurse or the family.

Preoperative Orders. Some physicians have routine orders for their patients. Be sure to check off each item. Common elements include the following:

◆ Diet. No food or fluid for at least 12 hours before surgery. Other special diets may be ordered before surgery. The patient is often kept "nothing by mouth" (NPO) after midnight.
◆ Enema. If surgery involves an abdominal cavity, an enema will usually be ordered. (An emergency appendectomy patient will not have an enema.)
◆ Operative consent. The patient must sign the permit before any sedative is given. If this is not done, the next of kin must give permission.
◆ Sedative. These are given to relieve anxiety and tension. A sleeping pill may be given the night before, and preoperative hypo or intravenous medication is given in the morning.
◆ Preparation of operative site. When surgery involves an incision, the skin must be shaved and cleaned where the incision is made. This is referred to as a surgical prep. In many hospitals, the prep is done in the operating room area immediately before surgery.

All of these orders are noted on the Kardex if the patient is in the hospital.

Other Orders. Special laboratory and x-ray examinations may be ordered for the patient in the hospital. All of these must be noted on the Kardex and on the appropriate request forms. Some procedures must be scheduled with the x-ray department.

Morning Admit Patients. Most patients are admitted on the morning of surgery. They are often asked to come to the hospital or clinic the day before surgery for blood work, electrocardiograms, or x-rays.

Preoperative patient and family teaching is necessary. The patient and family must understand diet orders, know the medications to take the evening before admission, and learn how to perform any preparation, such as self-administration of enemas. Document all patient/family teaching.

Postoperative Orders. Some doctors have certain routine orders to which they add individualized orders for each patient. All of these are noted on the Kardex, the appropriate request forms, medication sheets, or blood slips, and the nurse assigned to the patient is told that the orders are checked off and what they are. Be sure to sign your name and draw a red line under the transcribed orders. Common elements include the following:

◆ Canceling preoperative orders. Postoperatively, all preoperative orders are automatically canceled. This includes medications, diet, and activity level. Thus, even if these were routine orders, they must be rewritten after surgery.
◆ Vital signs. After the patient returns from the recovery room, vital signs are taken more often at first and then are usually taken every 4 hours for 48 hours. The person bringing the patient from the post-anesthesia room (PAR) will report the patient's vital sign status and how often the vital signs are to be taken.
◆ Wound checks. Most orders will include assessment of the operative site at certain intervals to make sure that any bleeding is noted before a severe loss of blood has occurred. Note specific orders on the Kardex.
◆ Special tubes and suction. Many patients will have an indwelling catheter in the bladder. A tube may be in the stomach or operative site, to which a suction machine or Hemo-Vac may be connected. This usually lasts approximately 48 hours. Orders will include a notation of the tubes on the Kardex, along with special irrigating instructions.
◆ Intake and output. After major surgery, it is necessary to assess all intake, usually intravenous and oral fluids, and output for several hours. This includes urine, emesis, and wound drainage. This is noted on the Kardex, and an intake and output sheet is made out and placed in the patient's room.
◆ Diet. Food and fluids will gradually be changed according to the patient's stage of healing and location of the incision. These progressive orders are noted on the Kardex and the diet sheet, and the dietary department is notified.
◆ Sedatives and hypnotics. Patients will have special orders for pain and discomfort during the first 24 to 48 hours, which is usually the period of greatest discomfort. Narcotics must have a specific order and must be kept double locked. These orders are transcribed as are any drug orders.
◆ Activity. The patient will gradually increase activity according to condition and progress. The orders for progressive activity must be noted on the Kardex. If the patient is on bed rest, a tag is often placed on the door or bed. If the bed is to be kept lying flat, the electric bed controls are locked.

Orders for Other Procedures

X-ray or Diagnostic Test Orders[6]

X-ray orders include those for special diagnostic procedures and for x-ray or cobalt therapy. Be sure to look up x-ray procedures in the hospital's procedure book so that all routine orders will be carried out.

---

[6] Originally developed for Donna Richardson, BA, MA, RN for Project Opportunity, Anoka MN.

- Record the orders on the Kardex, noting any food or fluid restriction and any special medication. In some cases, other special instructions apply (such as not washing off site markings for radiation therapy).
- Make out the appropriate x-ray order form.
- Telephone the x-ray department for an appointment whenever necessary. In a few cases, the operating room also must be notified, either because the procedure is done in the operating room or because operating room personnel must assist with the procedure (Table 92-1).
- Obtain any bedside signs required, such as "NPO" or "hold breakfast."
- Obtain the information leaflet describing the test for the nurse to give to the patient.
- Notify the patient's nurse of any new order so that he or she can explain the test, put up any bedside sign, and review the information leaflet with the patient. Document all teaching.

Nursing Alert

- In case of error, the wrong test could be done, or the wrong patient could be tested.
- If the patient has not been properly prepared, a procedure may have to be cancelled.
- A hospital day could be wasted by the patient if he or she does not have the correct test at the right time because of a mistake.
- Whenever you do not know about a test or procedure, about the correct form, or about the preparation of the patient, ask.
- Always write legibly to guard against error. Use standard abbreviations only.

Laboratory Orders.[7] Laboratory orders include urinalysis (UA) orders (routine UA, UA for ova and parasites, u-tox); hematology orders (complete blood count, red cell count, white blood cell count); blood or urine chemistry orders (electrolytes, serum enzymes); microbiology (culture and sensitivity determinations); pathology, cytology, and histology (biopsy specimens and fluids to be examined for abnormal cells or for cancer cells); and blood bank orders (requests for blood, packed cells, or other blood constituents or for a type and crossmatch). Some tests may be sent out (such as HIV antibody). These usually require a special form. All laboratory orders must be checked carefully to ensure accuracy.

- Record the order on the Kardex, noting any food or fluid restrictions or special timing regarding a specimen, such as a 12-hour specimen. Also note

[7] Originally developed by Project Opportunity, Anoka, MN.

special procedures, such as "clean catch" or "store on ice in brown bottle."
- Prepare the appropriate laboratory form.
- Follow the procedure as to where the form is sent. The request is often kept on the station if blood is to be drawn there. The form later accompanies the specimen to the laboratory. Stamp all forms and labels with the patient's name plate.
- Call the laboratory if you have any questions regarding an examination or a form. If there is a laboratory manual on the nursing station, always check this first.
- Order a disposable tray for procedures such as lumbar puncture, sternal puncture, thoracentesis, or paracentesis. Fill out the appropriate patient charge slips, or punch the information into the computer.
- Obtain any necessary bedside signs, such as "hold breakfast," "save all urine," "stool specimen," or "sputum specimen."
- Obtain an information leaflet describing the test so that the patient may be informed about the procedure. Notify the patient's nurse of any new order so that the test can be explained. The nurse then puts up any bedside sign, reviews the information leaflet with the patient, and documents the teaching.

Key Concept

The patient must give permission, in writing, for a human immunodeficiency virus test to be done. The physician also must sign the permission, verifying that teaching about the test has been done.

Dietary Orders. Transcribing diet orders includes the following:

- All diet and fluid orders are indicated on the Kardex.
- A diet form is sent to the diet kitchen periodically to keep the dietary staff up-to-date on changes; special instructions, such as NPO; and special diets.
- Intake and output orders are indicated on both forms (Kardex and diet list); bedside signs further instruct the staff to measure intake and output. A bedside sign also indicates if the patient is NPO.

Other Orders. Routine admission orders are used in most units or hospitals, with modifications for individual patients. The physician may write orders that differ from the routine as well. When a new patient is admitted, be sure he or she has orders, especially for activity, diet, medications, and special treatments.

Other orders may be written for treatments, such as "warm moist packs" or "passive range of motion." Orders are written for activity levels, such as ambulation, "bathroom privileges," or "up in chair." Orders may be written for such things as "encourage to visit with fam-

Table 92-1. Common Orders

Examination	Purpose	Preparation†	Appointment Required
X-Ray Orders			
Gastrointestinal series (GI series)	Visualize esophagus, stomach, small intestine	NPO after midnight; hold breakfast	Yes
Colon x-ray (lower GI series)	Visualize large intestine (colon)	NPO; hold breakfast; enemas and laxatives	Yes
Gallbladder ultrasound	Visualize gallbladder and ducts	Fat-free supper; NPO; hold breakfast; special medication	Yes
Intravenous pyelogram (IVP)	Visualize kidneys, ureters, bladder by injecting dye IV	Laxative day before test; NPO after supper; hold breakfast	Yes
Angiogram	Visualize a blood vessel by injecting dye into that vessel (usually aorta or cerebral artery)	Sedation; no foods or fluids several hours before test	Yes, both OR and x-ray
Isotope studies	Radioactive studies done on the brain, kidney, liver, lung, bones, thyroid, heart; include iodine and thyroid uptake	Radioactive dyes may be given in advance; special diets or NPO may be ordered	Yes
Radiation therapy	Treatment with deep x-ray therapy or cobalt; done to treat cancerous disorders	(See Chapter 76)	Yes
Other tests			
Cardiac catheterization	Determines status of heart and blood vessels	NPO after midnight empty bladder	Yes
Colonoscopy	Visualize and/or remove growths from large intestine	Laxative bowel prep, light supper, NPO after midnight	Yes
Computed tomography scan	Visualize nearly any part of body, especially brain and spinal cord	Sedation possible	Yes
Magnetic resonance imaging		Prep depends on part of body to be examined; contrast possible (see Chapter 71 for contraindications)	
Ultrasound	Determine status of fetus (or other internal area of body)	Tell mother *not* to empty bladder	Yes
Amniocentesis	Determine status of fetus	Empty bladder	Yes

* Originally developed by Donna Richardson, BA, MA, RN, for Project Opportunity, Anoka, MN.
† See Chapter 50 for precautions when dye is used.

ily" or "no visitors except wife," and precautions may be written by the doctor, such as "no weight bearing on left leg" or "side rails up at night." If you do not know where to write these, ask for instructions.

Telephone or Verbal Orders

Healthcare facilities vary in their policies regarding who may take telephone orders. The LPN may take telephone or verbal orders only if it is clearly defined in the policies of the institution in which he or she is working. This is because verbal or telephone orders are subject to errors. If the person taking the orders is unfamiliar with drugs and dosages, the likelihood of error is greater. Ideally, all orders should be in writing. In emergency situations, verbal orders often must be taken because there is no time for the physician to write out the order. Each nurse

is responsible for his or her own actions, and if an error occurs, that individual is legally liable.

Key Concept

If you take a telephone or verbal order, write the order in the physician's order sheet. Indicate verbal order or telephone order, the physician's name, the date and time, and your signature. Flag the order for the doctor to sign.

Telephone or verbal orders are potentially dangerous because there is no evidence of the order as given by the physician. Verbal orders *are legal*, however. All telephone or verbal orders are to be signed by the physician at the first possible opportunity. The nursing student or other nonlicensed person *never* takes verbal or telephone orders.

Keys for Review

Key Questions for Critical Thinking

1. Compare patient care in the clinical facility during the day, in the evening, and at night.
2. Describe some functions of the charge nurse in addition to those of the staff nurse.
3. Identify four leadership styles. Give instances when each could be used. Determine with which of the four you are most comfortable as a leader. Identify the one with which you are least comfortable.
4. Formulate your personal philosophy of life as it relates to your employment. Determine in what ways you have changed since you began your course as a PN or VN student.

Key Readings

Cole G. Basic Nursing Skills and Concepts. St. Louis, Mosby-Yearbook, 1991

Deloughery G. Issues and Trends in Nursing. St. Louis, Mosby-Yearbook, 1991

Hill SS, Howlett HA. Success in Practical Nursing: Personal and Vocational Issues, Ed 2. Philadelphia, W.B. Saunders, 1993

Leddy S, Pepper MJ. Conceptual Bases of Professional Nursing, Ed 3. Philadelphia, J.B. Lippincott, 1993

Oklahoma CIMC. Nursing Concepts. Stillwater, OK, Oklahoma Department of Vocational and Technical Education, 1992

Key Readings *(continued)*

Purtillo R. Ethical Dimensions in the Health Professions, Ed 2. Philadelphia, W.B. Saunders, 1993

Enrichment Keys

Borycki EM, Stewart-Archer LA. Nurses can influence health system. Registered Nurse Vol. 6 #3, June/July 1994, 30

Ellis JR, Hartley CL. Nursing in Today's World: Challenges, Issues, and Trends, Ed 4. Philadelphia, J.B. Lippincott, 1992

Harrington CS. Supporting each other. Nursing 94. 62–64

Hein EC, Nicholson MJ. Contemporary Leadership Behavior: Selected Readings, Ed 4. Philadelphia, J.B. Lippincott, 1994

Karnes NJ. "Reflections from a 20th anniversary grad." Imprint 41(1):29, January 1994

Kurzen CR. Contemporary Practical/Vocational Nursing, Ed 2. Philadelphia, J.B. Lippincott, 1993

Timby BK, Scherer JC. Lippincott's Review for NCLEX-PN, Ed 4. Philadelphia, J.B. Lippincott, 1994

Keys to Learning More

Chapter 93: employment opportunities and job-seeking skills

93 Career Opportunities and Job-Seeking Skills

Learning Objectives

- List at least 10 types of healthcare facilities or agencies in which the nurse might seek employment.
- Describe the function of a placement service or registry.
- List items to be included in a resume. Describe the letter of application and application form.
- Describe the protocol for a job interview.
- Describe the value of continuing education, and describe some educational opportunities.
- Describe the advantages of membership in professional organizations.
- Describe the procedure for obtaining a nursing license.

Key Terms

internship

interview

resumé

Keys to Understanding This Chapter

This entire book has helped to prepare you for work in the world of nursing. A review of all the chapters will help to prepare you for the licensure examination.

Key Points

- Multiple employment opportunities exist in nursing.
- Interviewing and completing a resume are an integral part of the job search.
- Frequently, continuing education is financed by employers.

Key Topics Outline

Employment
    Employment Opportunities
    Specialized Employment Opportunities
    Other Opportunities
How to Find Employment
    Job-Seeking Skills
    Resigning From a Position
Further Education
    Postgraduate Study
    Keeping Current
State and National Nursing Associations
Nursing Licensure
    The Nursing Examination
    The Nursing License
Your Personal Life

Key Learning Activities

- Write a resume describing your qualifications: education, paid employment, and volunteer experience.
- Observe nurses in at least three different types of healthcare positions. Compare and contrast their duties.
- Interview the inservice director of your hospital or other health facility. What orientation is available for new graduates? What continuing education is offered?
- Obtain a copy of nursing salary scales from your local area. What differences are there in salaries and benefits?

Rosdahl CB: Textbook of Basic Nursing, 6th ed. © 1995 J.B. Lippincott Company

As you prepare to graduate from your basic nursing program, one of the decisions you must make concerns your future career plans. This chapter describes some of the many opportunities available to you and the skills you will need to seek employment.

Employment

When you accept a position, you are entering into an agreement; therefore, it is important that you be fully informed of and understand the personnel policies of the healthcare facility.

Every institution establishes its own policies; these vary somewhat from one place to another. Salaries may vary according to the size, type, and location of the institution. They are usually higher in large cities and in certain areas of the country. Government hospitals (such as the Veteran's Administration, county and state hospitals, and university hospitals) often have a higher pay scale than private hospitals. Larger facilities may offer career mobility in the form of compensation for advanced training or education. Also, they may offer career ladders that pay additional money and give responsibility based on education and service time.

In some cases, a nurse is paid less until he or she has taken the licensure examination required by the state that authorizes practice as a registered nurse (RN) or a licensed practical nurse (LPN). Until the results of the examination are determined, you are called a graduate nurse or graduate practical nurse. With the advent of computerized licensure examinations, you may be required to practice as a nursing assistant until you are fully licensed. If you do not pass the examination on the first writing, your salary is usually cut back, and you are then required to practice as a nursing assistant until you are licensed.

Employment Opportunities

There are many opportunities for employment, and there is a demand for nurses in most areas.

Hospitals. Most RNs find positions in hospitals as staff nurses who give bedside care and who are supervisors of various nursing services. LPNs also work in hospitals. The practical nurse, as a member of the nursing team, works under the supervision of the RNs. Consideration may be given to an applicant's preference for a specific service, such as pediatrics or obstetrics.

Nursing Homes and Long-term Care Facilities. Many staff positions are available in nursing homes. Many practical nurses work in long-term care facilities. A well-run nursing home establishes policies for employment and salaries similar to those of hospitals. You will have an opportunity to use many of your medical–surgical nursing skills.

Public Health Nursing and Home Care. A growing number of nurses are employed in public health nursing or home care. The certified public health nurses are RNs with a baccalaureate degree. They will generally act as supervisor of the agency and of the other nurses and nursing assistants employed there. Most funding agencies require that case managers be RNs.

The major requirements for a position in public health nursing or home nursing are graduation from an approved school and state licensure. In addition, an applicant is selected on the basis of nursing skills, ability to get along with people, and level of maturity. The visiting nurse makes scheduled home visits to the patients assigned to his or her care. Nursing treatment is performed as ordered. The nurse may need to instruct the patient or family. The public health nurse (PHN) will often make an initial evaluation visit to set up a home care program. The PHN then assists the home care nurses who carry out the nursing care plan. The PHN is the supervisor and makes occasional updating home visits and revises the nursing care plan. Home care nurses perform and document care and participate in team conferences.

Two advantages of home care include the ability to choose which shifts you can work and the opportunity for independence. Benefits, such as insurance and paid vacation, are often available to full-time employees. Salaries are competitive. The home care nurse wears washable street clothes and a name tag and is responsible for providing his or her own transportation.

Hospice Nursing. Hospice care involves the care of terminally ill clients in the hospital or in the client's home. You will help the client and family work through the process of dying. The goal of hospice nursing is to help the client die with dignity.

Chemical Dependency Nursing. Chemical dependency nursing involves the assistance and rehabilitation of people who are alcoholic or otherwise chemically dependent. Working in a hospital or private treatment center or in detox, the chemical dependency nurse wears street clothes and a name tag bearing his or her first name.

Mental Health. Psychiatric settings include psychiatric acute care units housed in acute care facilities or free-standing psychiatric hospitals that treat children through adults. Some long-term care facilities also have specialized units for the geriatric mentally impaired client.

Physicians' Offices. A nurse may be employed in a physician's office to assist with physical examinations, dressings, and other procedures. Duties also may include answering the telephone, making appointments with patients, and serving as a receptionist.

Day Surgery Clinics. Many patients go to day surgery clinics rather than hospitals for minor surgical procedures. Nurses perform routine preoperative and postoperative care and assist during surgical procedures.

Private Duty. The private practitioner takes care of an individual in his or her home, in an institution, or when the patient is traveling. The nurse may be paid by the patient or family. Private duty gives the nurse an opportunity to practice basic bedside and teaching skills and to meet the total needs of one patient. Because it often includes the care of patients with long-term illnesses or patients who are wholly or partially disabled, private duty nursing offers steady employment on a long-term basis.

Occupational Health and Industrial Nursing. Positive health maintenance is a goal of many industries, and the nurse is the wellness coordinator. The nurse teaches preventive health maintenance. In many industries, the nurse is responsible for safety and the Occupational Safety and Health Act regulations. First aid is used in case of an accident. The nurse often has a safety committee and an employee assistance program, including chemical dependency education and prevention. Home visits may also be included in the duties.

Armed Forces. There are opportunities in the Armed Forces for LPNs and RNs. After basic training, the licensed person enters the armed forces at a level higher than that of the usual enlisted person. Usually, the nurse is assigned to a hospital or clinic.

Schools. Some school systems employ certified school nurses and school health aids. LPNs are often employed in an assisting capacity in school systems. The school often has a public health nurse or an RN as well. The assistant nurse or health aide in a school assists with vision and hearing screening, immunization clinics, and athletic physical examinations. He or she also performs routine first aid measures for students or faculty who become ill or who are injured at school. The LPN or RN may assist disabled students in school or on buses.

Volunteers in Service to America. This group gives care and education on a volunteer basis to people in the United States who need it.

Peace Corps. To nurses who qualify, the Peace Corps offers an opportunity to volunteer for human services that are needed in many parts of the world.

Headstart. Headstart employs LPNs and RNs as school nurses or as assistant instructors in their programs.

Camp Nursing. Most camps are required to employ a nurse. This nurse has many of the functions of the school nurse, although many of the illnesses and disorders encountered are different. Campers often suffer from poison ivy or poison oak, insect or snake bites, fractures, lacerations, and various infections. A camper may be sunburned, windburned, or burned in connection with a campfire. The camp nurse also must help with homesickness and often teaches wilderness safety and first aid.

Specialized Employment Opportunities

Some positions are available for LPNs or RNs with special qualifications and the ability to meet the demands of a specialized job. Most of these positions require specialized education beyond the basic nursing program.

Practical Nursing Programs. Some practical nursing programs employ an LPN or nondegreed RN to assist with the clinical supervision of practical nursing students. In some states, however, this is not legal. Qualifications include a sound educational background, proficiency in nursing skills, and ability to get along with people. Previous teaching experience is an asset.

Operating Rooms. Many hospitals now employ LPNs and newly graduated RNs in the operating room. With special training, they may assist in the operation of equipment, such as the heart–lung pump, or serve as surgical scrub nurses. The nurse is prepared for these functions by on-the-job training in the employing hospital or by a postgraduate course in operating room techniques. In most cases, the circulating nurse must be an RN.

Dialysis. Many nurses are specifically trained to work in hospital dialysis units or on mobile dialysis teams that administer dialysis to patients in their own homes. Some clients have an in-home dialysis unit. The nurse will assist and teach the client and family how to operate the machine. In some cases, the nurses operate the dialysis machines. They must understand thoroughly the complications and emergency treatment associated with dialysis.

Hyperbaric Medicine. The nurse may be trained to work in the hyperbaric chamber or with the supporting team outside the chamber. Ex-Navy divers also have found this a good career opportunity.

Veterinary Clinics. More nurses are being employed to work with veterinarians. Nursing techniques are useful in veterinary medicine.

Chiropractic Clinics and Acupuncture Centers. These areas often employ nurses as assistants. In some cases, you would be trained to perform some of the treatments.

Dental and Ophthalmology Clinics. Nurses are employed by dentists or by eye specialists, particularly those who perform surgery.

Emergency Rescue and Emergency Nursing. Some nurses wish to work with injured or critically ill patients. You will usually be required to take an emergency rescue course to be employed in an emergency room or in a ground or air rescue service. Employment in rescue requires quick thinking and accurate decisions. You would use your medical–surgical skills and high technology equipment. Specialized education as a paramedic is required to work with a helicopter or ambulance service. In some areas, an emergency medical technician course may adequately prepare you for this position.

Other Opportunities

The following positions do not require additional education.

Travel. Nurses can be employed as traveling companions or nursing attendants for critically or chronically ill people. Some nurses are employed by cruise lines and serve under the supervision of the attending physician. The traveling nurse must be resourceful, because an emergency may occur when the nurse and patient are inaccessible to a physician or a hospital.

Working Overseas. In many foreign countries, the nurse educated in the United States or Canada is in demand. Sometimes, the government of the host country will pay moving and living expenses, as well as a high salary. This has been the case in Saudi Arabia, for example. The nurse anticipating employment in another country could benefit from learning a language other than English.

Volunteer Service. The graduate nurse must become involved in community affairs. The nurse can be helpful by teaching others about healthcare or by assisting in times of disaster. The nurse also may become involved in expectant parents' classes at local hospitals or adult education classes.

The American Red Cross is the largest national program that uses nursing volunteers to assist in well-baby clinics, children's immunization clinics, and blood donor collection days for the Red Cross blood banks. Nurses also can volunteer to perform emergency first aid during community events, such as festivals and parades. All major and minor league stadiums have a cadre of first aid volunteers who work during games.

> **Key Concept**
>
> Analyze yourself and your strengths. Analyze available jobs, and attempt to match the two.

How to Find Employment

A medical pool registry recruits nurses to work in facilities that need extra help for special duty patients, extra busy periods, or vacation coverage. Nurses register with this agency, which then calls them when a job becomes available. The nurse has the option of declining—an advantage for those who do not wish to work full time. However, you must be available. If you decline too often, the agency will probably stop calling you. A good agency often offers insurance, vacation pay, and inservice education to its employees.

The state JOBS or employment service in each state is affiliated with government. This agency provides free job information. The employment opportunities are on a computer, so positions in many areas are accessible. This agency also has access to government positions. Call your local courthouse to find out how to access the state employment service.

Develop a plan for your job search. Ideas for such a plan are listed in the accompanying box.

Job-Seeking Skills

You need to evaluate your personal requirements before you decide on what type of employment to seek. Such factors as geographic location, shift rotation, ba-

Developing a Job-Search Plan

- ◆ Decide what types of jobs you would like in relation to what is available.
- ◆ Evaluate yourself: What are your greatest skills and assets? Where do you best fit?
- ◆ Spend at least 5 hours a day in your job search, finding a job is your "job" now.
- ◆ Set a goal for the number of contacts per day.
- ◆ Be sure your resume and cover letter are neatly typed and error free.
- ◆ Prepare for interviews. Be sure to plan answers for difficult questions, and dress appropriately.
- ◆ Emphasize the positive: yourself, your education and all former positions.
- ◆ Use "networking" skills to find the unadvertised positions.
- ◆ Arrange factors such as transportation and day care ahead of time.

bysitting, travel, and housing need to be given consideration as you make career decisions.

If you are unwilling to compromise about where or during what hours you wish to work, you may have difficulty obtaining a job. Your first job is important. It sets the pace for future job opportunities. If you perform well the first time, you will leave with good references that will be advantageous in a acquiring the next job.

Writing a Letter of Application

The value of the letter of application, sometimes referred to as the cover letter (if it accompanies a resume), cannot be overestimated. The letter is usually the first thing an employer will see, and if it does not have a positive impact on him or her, your application may not be considered. Remember that your aim is to convince the employer that you are an excellent candidate for the job. The letter should be informative and concise. It should first state the position for which you are applying and how you found out about it. Tell briefly why you feel you are qualified for it. Describe job experiences, skills, and educational background that are applicable. Conclude the letter by informing the employer when you would be available for a personal interview and how you can most easily be contacted. Type the letter neatly on conservative stationery, and enclose it along with an up-to-date personal resume.

Application Forms

When filling out a standard application form, have with you your social security number, your resume, and your license, if you have received it. A favorable impression is conveyed by properly worded responses and careful, neat handwriting or printing in ink.

The employer often uses the way in which you complete the written application as one of the criteria for evaluating you as a prospective employee. Think before you write.

Be prepared to give references for the potential employer to contact. Have addresses and phone numbers, and always contact your references in advance to ask permission before using them.

> **Key Concept**
>
> How you write or print often indicates how you will chart in the future.

Personal Resume

There are two types of **resumes**, one that emphasizes strengths and abilities and one that lists experience chronologically. When seeking a first nursing position, you will usually use the latter type. This lists your education, previous employment, and relevant experience. In stating information on education, list schools, addresses, diplomas or degrees received (most recent first), and licenses held (and in what states). Dates are often not used. List work experience with the most recent position first (name of facility, dates employed, title of position, and name, address, and phone number of supervisor). Identify special skills and special training or honors received, and list references. Be sure to include volunteer positions (see box).

The Personal Interview

Routine procedure usually includes a personal interview with the prospective employer. When you go to an **interview**, wear tailored, conservative clothes and simple jewelry. Be sure your shoes are polished. Avoid extremes in makeup and nail polish. Clean and neatly styled hair and clean short nails are essential to make a good impression. Men should be sure that moustaches or beards are clean and neatly trimmed. Some hospitals prefer to hire male nurses who have relatively short hair and a minimum of facial hair. Remember: The first impression is made in just a few seconds.

You may wish to bring your nursing transcript with you. If it is in a narrative form, you may have to interpret it to the interviewer. You will be asked to sign a release that permits the potential employer to contact your references. (It is illegal for schools or people to release information about you without your written consent.) Be honest about your reasons for leaving previous jobs.

> **Key Concept**
>
> Keep your comments positive. Do *not* "bad mouth" your previous employer.

A prospective employer is interested in knowing about your past employment and school record, punctuality and attendance records, ability to work with others, willingness to accept assignments, and reactions in emergency situations. Guidelines for the job interview are given in the accompanying box. Questions you should be prepared to answer include the following: "What shift will you work?" "Will you work part-time?" "What are your rotation choices (for example, day-night, day-afternoon)?"

> **Key Concept**
>
> Arrive at least 5 minutes early for the interview. If you do not know how to get to the place, make a practice run the day before or get good instructions. Coming late to an interview almost guarantees that you will not get the position.

Aptitude Tests

You may be asked to take aptitude tests. If you relax and try not to succumb to anxiety, you will score better. Generally, it is best not to change an answer once you have written it down. If you are taking a timed test, go through the entire test as quickly as you can, and answer the questions you know. Go back and work on the questions you are unsure about. Do not spend too much time on any one item.

Orientation Programs

Most hospitals have orientation programs for new employees. Discuss with the instructor any procedures in which you feel you need more practice; the instructor will help you to gain this extra knowledge and experience. Also, most hospitals require a medication test and a math test for licensed nurses.

Internship

In some states, recent graduates are required to serve a period of **internship** before being considered full-fledged LPNs or RNs. The internship provides an opportunity to practice nursing skills and helps you complete the transition from student to graduate. Your title in these cases may be *nurse resident* or *nurse intern*; this gives you added help in transferring learned skills to the workplace.

Resigning from a Position

When resigning from a position, give your employer advance notice—at least 2 weeks and preferably 1 month. This gives the agency adequate time to find a replacement when you leave. An advance notice requirement is sometimes stated in personnel policies. Customarily, if you leave before the designated time or leave without notice, you will be paid up to the time of your departure only.

You will not receive a good reference if you leave a job without giving proper notice. It is much easier to find a new job if you depart from the previous one on friendly terms.

Further Education

Postgraduate Study

Specialty Areas. In a number of centers, approved postgraduate courses in nursing specialties are available. Information about approved courses can be obtained by writing to the National Association for Practical Nurse Education and Service, the American Nurses Association, or the National League for Nursing.

Guidelines for Writing A Resume*

- Be positive. Don't emphasize your shortcomings.
- Be specific.
- Be accurate. Make sure there are no errors in dates of employment or school; make sure there are no "typos" or spelling errors.
- Be creative.
- Be brief. Keep to one page, if possible.
- *Type* neatly. A handwritten resume will eliminate you from consideration. Space your resume so it looks attractive. Do not make carbon copies; use a good quality copy machine. Use white bond paper.

Special Tips

- State your career objective.
- Briefly state special circumstances while you were in school (worked 20 hours per week, commuted 50 miles, perfect attendance, grade point average, special awards, activities).
- Put the most emphasis on the last 5 years.
- Include non-nursing and volunteer positions as well.
- List memberships in organizations and offices held; include nursing and community organizations (a limited number).
- List special interests and skills. State your career goal.
- You usually do not need to list your references on the initial resume.
- Do not list personal data, such as married or single, number of children, age, sex, religion. (A professional-looking photograph may be included but is usually not recommended. It is illegal for prospective employers to require a photo.)
- Have another person read and react to your resume before you send it.
- Your nursing program will be able to give you guidelines as to what is included in a good resume. They also may have typing services available to new graduates.

* Excerpted from Responsibilities of the LPN—Career Planning, a module developed for the Anoka Practical Nursing Program, Anoka, MN, by Bette J. Struck, BA, MA, RN.

Many hospitals and nursing homes also have specialty courses for their employees. This is becoming more common, especially in nursing homes.

Licensed Practical Nurse to Registered Nurse Mobility Programs

Many community colleges and private schools have programs that enroll LPNs and offer a specialized program leading to RN licensure. These programs usually last approximately 1 year and build on the education received in the practical nursing program. In other

Guidelines for the Job Interview

◆ Dress neatly and conservatively. Wear a minimum of jewelry, especially if you are a man. Make sure your fingernails are clean.

◆ Write down your questions, and review them ahead of time.

◆ Be sure to arrive a few minutes *early*.

◆ Do your homework on the agency before going. Be able to ask intelligent questions.

◆ Know in advance how you will handle difficult questions, such as "What can you offer us?" "What are your strengths?" "What are your weaknesses?" "What was your biggest mistake?" "What are your long-term career goals?"

◆ Most interviewers will offer to shake your hand. Make sure your handshake is *firm* but not crushing. Use your whole hand, *not* just your fingertips.

◆ Let the person indicate where you should sit. Wait to sit until they have been seated.

◆ Put your purse or briefcase on the floor—not on the interviewer's desk. (Do *not* bring both purse and briefcase; you will be overburdened.)

◆ Sit up straight. Keep your hands folded on your lap or on the table in front of you.

◆ If possible, leave your coat outside the interview room. Then, you will not have to go through taking it off and finding a place to put it during the interview.

◆ Do not smoke or chew gum.

◆ It is usually best not to accept coffee or food.

◆ Look at the person when you speak.

◆ Listen carefully to the questions, and *think* before you talk.

◆ Do not act as though you are desparate for the job.

◆ Inform the interviewer what your special skills and preferences are, but do not exaggerate.

◆ Do not talk too much; when you finish an answer, stop and let the interviewer resume with further questioning.

◆ Some questions to ask may include the specific job description, as well as evaluation policies and available inservice education.

◆ If you do not know what the salary and benefits are, ask these questions *last*.

◆ Do not complain about previous employers. Speak of the previous position in the most positive way possible.

◆ Avoid the use of negative terms in your responses. Speak of "challenges" and "opportunities" instead of problems.

◆ Thank the interviewer for his or her time. Use the person's name, with Mr. or Ms. *Never* use the interviewer's first name.

◆ You may wish to follow up the interview with a letter thanking the person for his or her time and stating that you are interested in the position. Restate your qualifications briefly. Be sure that this letter is just as neatly typed as your letter of application.

◆ Bring your nursing license, school transcript, record of tuberculin test, driver's license, birth certificate, CPR card, and social security card, in case you need them.

◆ If you have written evaluations from previous employment (even if not nursing-related), bring *copies* of them to leave with the interviewer. It is good to show that you have a good previous work history, whether in nursing-related jobs or not.

◆ If possible, have letters of reference already written to leave with the interviewer. This will save them the time of contacting your references.

◆ Have a list of names, addresses, and phone numbers of references with you to leave with the interviewer.

◆ You may be interviewed by a committee, or your interview may be tape-recorded. Do not let this "throw" you.

cases, LPNs are enrolled in a generic RN program but are exempted or tested out of certain courses.

Baccalaureate Degree to Registered Nurse Programs

Some nursing programs enroll people with a baccalaureate degree in majors other than nursing. In these programs, the person is eligible to take the nursing licensure examination in an accelerated time, because general education courses have already been obtained. These courses last approximately 2 years.

Keeping Current

Healthcare Development. Sources of current care information are all around you. Books and magazine articles will help keep you informed about scientific discover-

ies that are improving the treatment of disease. Nursing journals, new textbooks, radio, and television programs discuss health problems. Workshops, conferences, and conventions are available to teach you how to improve your care of patients. Healthcare facilities maintain ongoing inservice education programs for employees. Nurses should take advantage of these opportunities to improve methods and knowledge. Nursing journals also keep you informed about new techniques and procedures.

Continuing Education (Inservice Education). Some states require you to have a certain number of hours or units of continuing education for your nursing license to be renewed. Look on this as an opportunity and a challenge, rather as a problem. This requirement was implemented to improve the quality of nursing care. Take advantage of these classes to improve your own nursing skills. Many facilities offer these educational opportunities free of charge or for a nominal fee.

State and National Nursing Associations

Every nurse has an obligation to support and participate in the activities of national and state nursing associations. You can join through the local division in your residential area. By working collectively, a group can get things done that one person alone could never accomplish. A representative of the local association may be given an opportunity to come and speak to students about the function and activities of the association and how they can join. Your instructors also will have this information.

National Association for Practical Nurse Eeducation and Service, National Federation of Licensed Practical Nurses, National League for Nursing, and American Nurses Association. The National Association for Practical Nurse Education and Service, National Federation of Licensed Practical Nurses, and National League for Nursing are the national organizations with special interests in education and activities of practical nurses. Practical nurses are eligible for membership in these organizations. The state and American Nurses Associations are available to RN graduates, as well as the NLN.

Alumnae Associations. Many schools have alumnae associations. Among their activities are student recruitment programs, scholarship and loan funds, and fundraising events to purchase needed educational equipment for the school.

Nursing Licensure

In Chapters 2 and 4 you were introduced to licensure of nurses, differences in licensing laws, and legal aspects of licensure. Now you have completed your course and are ready to apply for your license.

The Nursing Examination

After graduation, you will be required to pass the National Council Licensure Examination (NCLEX) licensing examination to become licensed as an RN, LPN, or LVN. As of 1994, the test is a computer adaptive test (CAT) rather than a paper-and-pencil test.

Your school must send your application, transcript of your records, and the required fee to the State Board of Nursing, the authority responsible for giving the examination. Licensing examinations are usually given twice a year, but may be more accessible with computer use.

The NCLEX examination is aimed at measuring *entry-level competencies* in nursing. The test[1] "requires basic knowledge of 1) nursing process; 2) coordination of safe, effective care; 3) client's physiological needs; 4) client's psychosocial needs; and 5) maintenance and promotion of health." The examination is strongly based on nursing process and client needs; it requires a knowledge of all the courses you have studied while in your nursing program.

Your nursing program should have prepared you for the examination. The best way to ensure doing well on the examination is to study throughout your basic nursing program. If you master the material as you go along, you should have little difficulty in passing the examination.

The Nursing License

After passing the examination, the newly licensed nurse can use the title LPN, LVN, or RN. If an applicant fails, he or she is given a chance to repeat the examination a limited number of times within a specified period as stated by the law. Many states require refresher or upgrading courses if the student does not pass the examination after two or three attempts. After receiving the license, the nurse is responsible for renewing it according to regulations and for keeping the Board informed about any changes in name, address, or employment status.

If a nurse obtains licensure by waiver, or "grandfather clause," it may not be transferrable to another state. If you have any questions about the requirements for practicing as an LPN or an RN in another state, contact the Board of Nursing in that state.

Maintenance of Your Nursing License
It is your responsibility to keep your license current if you are practicing nursing. It also is your responsibility to practice within the rules and regulations of your state's nurse practice act.

Revocation or Suspension of a Nursing License. In most states, territories, and Canada, the Board of Nursing or another authority has the right to revoke or suspend a nurse's license for just cause. Some of these just causes include the following:

◆ Conviction of a felony
◆ Conviction of other crimes, such as child abuse

---

[1] Adapted from NCLEX-PN, "Test plan for the National Council Licensure Examination for Practical Nurses." Chicago, National Council of State Boards of Nursing, Inc., 1989.

◆ Chemical dependency (until it is controlled)
◆ Stealing medications
◆ Mental incompetence
◆ Fraudulently obtaining a nursing license
◆ Violation of the state nurse practice act (such as practicing nursing without a license)
◆ Suspended or revoked license in another state
◆ Willful neglect or abuse of a patient
◆ Proven negligence in nursing practice

The nurse must be notified before action is taken to suspend or revoke a license. The nurse will be given the opportunity to present his or her case at a hearing. Other actions that may be taken include denial of license renewal, denial of first license, letter of reprimand, suspension of license, or placement of the nurse on formal probation with specific conditions for reinstatement.

Transferring Licensure From One State to Another

After you become licensed, you may wish to move and transfer your licensure to another state. This procedure has several terms, depending on the state. For example, transfer of licensure between states may be called interstate endorsement, reciprocity, or licensure without examination.

To become licensed in another state, you must apply with the state regulating agency of the new state. You will be required to complete an application and pay a fee. If your school meets the new state's educational requirements, and your scores on the licensing examination were adequate, you will be able to become licensed in most states without taking the NCLEX examination again. It will take 4 to 6 weeks to receive your new license, so be sure to plan ahead.

To locate the proper agency, look in the telephone book of the state or territorial capitol city. In many states, this agency is called the *State Board of Nursing.* Other names include the following:

◆ State Board of Nurse Examiners
◆ Department of Professional Regulations (Florida)
◆ Bureau of Professional and Occupational Regulations (Michigan)
◆ Board of Examiners (Connecticut)

You also may get their name, address, and phone number from your local licensing agency. In Canada, contact the Canadian Nurses' Association in Ottawa.

Your Personal Life

Your work life and personal life are related. Plan outside interests; develop lifelong hobbies. Make a plan for financial security. Plan a personal budget. Be realistic—money never goes as far as one thinks it will. Annuities and retirement plans can be budgeted during your best earning years. Invest in a health examination once a year; it is cheaper than being sick or dysfunctional. Get hospitalization and medical insurance with a reliable group plan. All this is insurance for a safer and happier life.

Key Concept

No matter what you choose to do in the future, your nursing background will prove a valuable asset. You can work part time or full time, days or nights; you can use your nursing skills in raising a family and dealing successfully with other people. Good luck! Enjoy your future!

Keys for Review

Key Questions for Critical Thinking

1. Develop a list of your skills, assets, and interests. Discuss which of your experiences you especially enjoyed during your education. Identify the job for which you are best suited, considering the above.
2. Formulate your thoughts about further education. Outline what plans you can make for further education. Determine how this will affect your employment opportunities. Develop a plan of how you can explain this in your employment interview.

Key Questions for Critical Thinking
(continued)

3. Discuss how professional organizations will relate to your career. Think about how much you want to be involved in a professional organization and determine steps to make this happen.

Key Readings

Becker BG, Fenderley DT. Vocational and Personal Adjustments in Practical Nursing, Ed 6. St. Louis, C.V. Mosby, 1990

Clark M. Practical Nursing, Ed 4. Philadelphia, W.B. Saunders (Baillere-Tindall), 1991

Ellis JR, Hartley CL. Nursing in Today's World: Challenges, Issues, and Trends, Ed 4. Philadelphia, J.B. Lippincott, 1992

Kurzen CR. Contemporary Practical/ Vocational Nursing, Ed 2. Philadelphia, J.B. Lippincott, 1993

Enrichment Keys

Adams-Ender CL. "The future of minorities in nursing." Imprint 40(5):51-53, November-December, 1993

Beare PG. Davis' NCLEX-PN Review. Philadelphia, FA Davis, 1994

Enrichment Keys (continued)

Davidhizar R. "Ten tips to help your self-confidence." Imprint 41:23-25, January 1994

Leddy S, Pepper MJ. Conceptual Bases of Professional Nursing, Ed 3. Philadelphia, J.B. Lippincott, 1993

Timby BK, Scherer JC. Lippincott's Review for NCLEX-PN, Ed 4. Philadelphia, J.B. Lippincott, 1994

Walsh KC. "Projecting your best professional image." Imprint 40(5):46-49, November-December, 1993

Wheeler I. "Success in your first interview." Imprint 41(1):20, 37, January 1994

Keys to Learning More

Your education has just begun. That is why we call graduation "commencement." You will continue learning and growing throughout your nursing career.

GLOSSARY

abdomen (ab′do-men): that portion of the body lying between the chest and the pelvis. **Abdominal**: pertaining to the abdomen.

abdominal thrust: the force exerted by a rescuer when treating obstructed airway (*Heimlich maneuver*).

abduct (ab-dukt′): to move away from the center line, as to abduct (raise) the arm. (noun: **abduction**)

ablatio (ab-la′she-o): abnormal detachment, as *ablatio of the retina*.

abnormal (ab-nor′mal): not normal; contrary to the usual structure, condition, or behavior; a malformation or malfunction.

abort (ah-bort′): the premature stopping of a developmental process, as to *abort a pregnancy*.

abrasion (ab-ra′zhun): a scraping or rubbing off of the skin, such as a skinned knee.

abruptio (ab-rup′she-o): separation, as *abruptio placentae*.

abscess (ab′ses): a local collection of pus in a cavity.

absence (ahb′sanz): seizure with momentary loss of consciousness; formerly called *petit mal*.

absorb (ab-sorb′): to take in or incorporate other substances.

acceleration (ak-sel-er-a′shun): a quickening of rate, as of the pulse or respiration.

accommodation (ah-kom-o-da′shun): adjustment, as the *accommodation of the lens* of the eye.

accreditation (ah-kred-i-ta′shun): attaining standards approved by a recognized authority, as *accreditation of a nursing program*.

achalasia (ak-ah-la′ze-ah): failure of the smooth muscles of the gastrointestinal tract to relax at a junction, especially the lower esophagus.

ache (ake): continuous dull or throbbing pain.

achlorhydria (a-klor-hi′dre-ah): absence of hydrochloric acid, as in pernicious anemia or stomach cancer.

acholia (a-ko′le-ah): lack of bile secretion.

acid (as′id): a chemical compound having properties opposed to those of the alkalis; with a pH below 7; sour.

acidosis (as-i-do′sis): a pathologic condition resulting from an accumulation of acid or a depletion of alkali (bases).

acme (ak′me): critical stage of a disease (**crisis**).

acne (ak′ne): disorder of the skin characterized by papules or pustules, such as *acne vulgaris*, which is common in adolescence.

acoustic (ah-koos′tik): pertaining to sound, as the *acoustic nerve*.

acromegaly (ak-ro-meg′ah-le): a condition resulting from overproduction of a pituitary hormone.

activities of daily living (ADL): functioning in normal activities, such as eating, dressing, walking, bathing, (*instrumental activities of daily living, IADL*); more complex ADLs such as cooking or managing money

acuity (ah-ku′i-te): clearness, as in *visual acuity*.

acute (ah-kute′): of short duration, but with severe symptoms; sharp, as an acute pain or disorder.

addiction (ah-dik′shun): emotional or physical dependence, as addiction to a chemical substance.

adduct (a-dukt′): to draw toward the center, as to adduct (lower) the arm. (noun: **adduction**)

adenitis (ad-e-ni′tis): inflammation of a gland.

adenocarcinoma (ad-e-no-kar-si-no′mah): a malignant tumor that is derived from glandular tissue.

adenoids (ad′en-oids): glandular growths at the back of the nose and behind the palate (*pharyngeal tonsil*).

adenoma (ad-e-no′mah): a benign epithelial tumor.

adhesion (ad-he′zhun): the abnormal joining of tissues by a fibrous band, usually resulting from inflammation or injury or following surgery.

adipose (ad′i-pose): fatty, as adipose tissue.

adjuvant (ad′joo-vant): assisting or enhancing therapy given, especially in cancer, to prevent further growth, preventive treatment.

adnexa (ad-nek′sah): accessory organs. (The liver is part of the adnexa of the digestive system.)

adolescence (ad-o-les′ens): the time between onset of puberty and cessation of physical growth, in general about ages 11–19. (adj: **adolescent**)

adrenal (ah-dre′nal): near or above the kidney, as the *adrenal glands*, **suprarenal**.

adulteration (ah-dul-ter-a′shun): addition of impure ingredients, as *adulteration of a drug*.

advance directive: written instructions given in advance about types of health care desired if the patient cannot decide for him/herself. (A *living will* is one type of advance directive.)

adventitia (ad-ven-tish′e-ah): outer coat of a structure, as the *adventitia of an artery*.

advocate (ad′va-kit): a person who works to gain or preserve the rights of others, a defender (as in *patient advocate*). (verb: ad′vo-kat—to work for the rights of others, to assist)

aerobe (a′er-ob): a microorganism that must have oxygen to live, *obligate aerobe*. (Some organisms can live in the presence or absence of oxygen. They are called *facultative aerobes*.)

afebrile (a-feb′ril): without fever.

affect (af′ekt): emotional tone, feeling.

afferent (af′er-ent): conducting toward the center, as *afferent nerves*.

afterbirth (af′ter-berth): a mass of tissue, consisting of the membranes and the *placenta* with the attached umbilical cord, that is cast off after the expulsion of the fetus.

after-pains: abdominal discomfort or cramping after delivery caused by contraction of the uterus to its nonpregnant state, may be intensified by nursing of the infant.

ageism (aj′izm): prejudice against people because they are older.

aging (aj′ing): the process of growing older; sometimes denotes degenerative changes occurring as a result of growing older.

aglutition (ag-loo-tish′un): inability to swallow.

Rosdahl CB: Textbook of Basic Nursing, 6th ed. © 1995 J.B. Lippincott Company

agonist (ag'o-nist): a muscle that contracts to move a body part and is opposed by another muscle (the antagonist).

agranulocytosis (a-gran-u-lo-si-to'sus): an acute disorder, often caused by drug toxicity, in which granulocyte (granular leukocyte) production greatly decreases. This causes neutropenia and renders the body defenseless against bacterial infections. (Also called **malignant neutropenia**.)

AIDS: acquired immunodeficiency syndrome; an autoimmune disorder, caused by the human immunodeficiency virus (HIV).

akathisia (ak-ah-thez'e-ah): constant motor activity, inability to sit down or relax, twitching (a common side effect of neuroleptic drugs—those that modify psychotic behavior).

albumin (al-bu'min): a protein substance found in animal and vegetable tissues.

alcoholism (al'ko-hol-izm): abuse of or dependence on alcohol as a mood-altering substance.

alignment (a-lin'ment): arrangement in a straight line, bringing into line or order, as in *body alignment*.

alimentary canal (al-im-en'ta-re kan-al'): the passage leading from the mouth to the stomach and the intestines, to the outer opening of the rectum; also known as the **digestive tract** or **gastrointestinal tract**.

alkali (al'ka-li): a compound that neutralizes acids (bitter); having a pH above 7; a **base**.

alkalosis (al-kah-lo'sis): a serious condition caused by accumulation of base or loss of acids, a decrease in hydrogen ion concentration (pH) (opposite of acidosis). *Metabolic alkalosis* can be caused by vomiting or excess voiding.

allergen (al'er-jen): a substance capable of producing hypersensitivity (allergy).

allergy (al'er-je): a state in which the body is hypersensitive to a substance, usually a protein.

alleviate (a-le'vi-ate): to lessen or make easier to endure.

allogeneic (al-o-je-ne'ik): persons who are not genetically related (see **allograft**).

allograft (al'o-graft): a graft between individuals of the same species (as in two unrelated persons).

alopecia (al-o-pe'she-ah): abnormal loss of hair, or **baldness**, as in alopecia resulting from cancer chemotherapy.

alveoli (al-ve'o-li): small hollow, as the socket of a tooth or the thin-walled sacs within the lungs, where gas exchange occurs.

Alzheimer's disease (alz'hi-murs dis-es'): a form of dementia, most often in older people.

ambulatory (am'bu-la-to-re): walking or able to walk. (noun: **ambulation**)

amenorrhea (ah-men-o-re'ah): absence or abnormal stoppage of menses (menstruation).

amnesia (am-ne'zhi-ah): pathologic loss of memory.

amniocentesis (am-ne-o-sen-te'sis): perforation of the amniotic sac through the abdomen of a pregnant woman to obtain a sample of amniotic fluid.

amnion (am'ne-on): the inner membrane and the fluid surrounding a fetus ("bag of waters").

amniotomy (am-ne-ot'o-me): surgical rupture of fetal membranes, *artificial rupture of membranes* (AROM).

amplitude (am'pli-tood): fullness; volume, as the *amplitude of the heartbeat*.

ampule (am'pul): small, glass-sealed flask, often containing medication.

ampulla (am-pul'ah): the flasklike dilation of the ends of the semicircular canals in the ear.

amputation (am-pu-ta'shun): removal of a limb or other part of the body.

anabolism (ah-nab'o-lizm): the *constructive* phase of metabolism.

anaerobe (an-a'er-ob): a microorganism that lives in the absence of oxygen. An *obligate anaerobe* cannot live if any oxygen is present. A *facultative anaerobe* can adjust to the presence of oxygen.

analgesic (an-al-je'sik): an agent that relieves pain without causing loss of consciousness, as an *analgesic drug*.

anaphylaxis (an-ah-fi-lak'sis): serious state of shock brought about by hypersensitivity to an allergen (formerly called *anaphylactic shock*).

anasarca (an-ah-sar'kah): massive generalized edema.

anastomosis (ah-nas-ta-mo'sis): the joining together of two normally distinct spaces or organs, as the anastamosis of two ends of bowel after a section has been removed.

anatomy (ah-nat'o-me): the science dealing with the *structure* of the body.

androgen (an'dro-jen): a hormone that stimulates male characteristics (**steroid**).

anemia (ah-ne'me-ah): a deficiency of the blood in quality or quantity; reduction in hemoglobin.

anencephaly (an-en-sef'ah-le): congenital absence of skull and brain.

anergic (an-er'jik): lack of ability to respond to antigens by producing antibodies; weakness, lack of energy (**asthenia**).

anesthetic (an-es-thet'ik): a substance that produces loss of feeling or sensation, used so surgery can be performed.

aneurysm (an'u-rizm): a dilatation of the wall of a vessel that causes the formation of a sac, a life-threatening situation, as an *aortic aneurysm*.

angina (an'ji-nah): a spasmodic, severe attack or pain, as *angina pectoris*.

angiocardiogram (an-je-o-kar'de-o-gram): x-ray of cardiac blood vessels, *coronary arteriography*. (Sometimes called simply **angiogram**.)

angiogram (an'je-o-gram): an x-ray of any blood vessel.

angioedema (an-je-o-e-de'mah): localized edema deep within or under the skin, producing giant wheals (lumps).

angioma (an-je-o'mah): a benign tumor composed of blood (*hemangioma*) or lymph (*lymphangioma*).

angioplasty (an'je-o-plas-te): surgical repair of a blood or lymph vessel; often refers to repair of coronary vessels.

angiospasm (an'je-o-spazm): a sudden contraction of a blood vessel.

anion (an'i-on): a negatively charged ion.

anisuria (an-i-su're-ah): a condition in which polyuria and oliguria alternate with each other.

ankylosis (ang-ki-lo'sis): abnormal consolidation of a joint that causes immobility.

anomaly (a-nom'ah-le): a marked deviation from normal.

anorexia (an-o-rek'se-ah): lack or loss of appetite for food, refusal to eat.

anorexia nervosa (an-o-reks'e-ah ner-vos'ah): a condition in which the person (usually female) refuses to eat because he or she wants to be thin, although he or she is already very thin.

anoxia (an-ok'se-ah): absence of oxygen in body tissue (often used interchangeably with **hypoxia** to mean a decrease of oxygen below the normal level).

antacid (ant-as'id): an agent that counteracts acidity, as in antacid medications.

antagonist (an-tag'o-nist): a muscle that exerts an action opposite that of another muscle; a drug that blocks or reverses the action of another drug.

anteflexion (an-te-flek'shun): a bending forward of an organ, as in an *anteflexed uterus*.

antepartal (an-te-par-tal): occurring before childbirth (in reference to the mother).

anterior (an-te'ri-er): toward the front; the nose is on the anterior part of the head.

anthelmintic (ant-hel-min'tik): an agent or drug that destroys parasitic worms.

antiarrhythmic (an-ti' a-rith'mic): a drug that helps regulate the rhythm of irregular heartbeats.

antibiotic (an-te-bi-ot′ic): a substance produced by a living organism that can destroy (*biocidal*) or weaken (*biostatic*) other organisms. (A well-known antibiotic is *penicillin*.)

antibody (an′ti-bode-e): a specific protein that neutralizes foreign antigens (essential to the immune response). (pl: **antibodies**)

anticoagulant (an-ti-ko-ag′u-lant): a substance that prevents coagulation or clotting, usually of blood.

anticonvulsant (an-te-cun-vul′sent): a drug that reduces, controls or stops seizure activity. (A common anticonvulsant is *Dilantin*.)

antidote (an′ti-dote): an agent that will counteract the effects of a poison or a drug, as an antidote to a particular snake venom.

antiemetic (an-ti-e-met′ik): an agent that prevents or relieves vomiting. (A common antiemetic is *compazine*.)

antigen (an′ti-gen): a substance that stimulates the production of antibodies.

antilithic (an-ti-lith′ik): an agent that prevents calculus (stone) formation. (The presence of stones is called *lithiasis*.)

antineoplastic (an-ti-ne-o-plas′tik): inhibiting the growth of malignant cells. (Cancer is also known as a *neoplasm*.)

antipruritic (an-ti-proo-rit′ik): an agent that prevents or relieves itching (*pruritus*).

antipyretic (an-ti-pi-ret′ik): an agent that relieves or reduces fever. (Common antipyretics are aspirin and Tylenol.)

antiseptic (an-ti-sep′tik): a substance that inhibits the growth of microorganisms without destroying them.

antispasmodic (an-ti-spas-mod′ik): an agent that relieves muscular spasm.

antitoxin (an-te-tok′sin): a particular antibody that is produced to counteract the harmful effect of a toxin.

antitussive (an-ti-tus′iv): an agent that reduces coughing.

antrum (an′trum): cavity or chamber, as the *mastoid antrum*.

anuresis (an-u-re′sis): retention of urine in the bladder; sometimes used interchangeably with **anuria.**

anuria (an-u′re-ah): complete suppression of urine secretion in the kidney.

anus (a′nus): the outer opening or outlet of the rectum. (Adj: **anal**)

anxiety (ang-zi′e-te): apprehensive uneasiness or dread (may be marked by physiologic signs, such as sweating, tension, or increased pulse).

apepsia (ah-pep′se-ah): cessation of digestive function.

apex (a′peks): narrowed or pointed end, as the *apex of the heart*.

Apgar score (ap′gar skor): a method of determining an infant's condition at birth.

aphagia (ah-fa′je-ah): inability to swallow.

aphakia (ah-fa′ke-ah): absence of the lens of the eye, as after cataract removal.

aphasia (ah-fa′ze-ah): inability to express oneself by speech or writing.

aphonia (ah-fo′ne-ah): loss of voice.

aplastic (a-plas′tik): relating to defective development of new tissue, as *aplastic anemia*.

apnea (ap′ne-ah): cessation of breathing.

apogee (ap′o-je): the state of greatest severity of a disease.

apoplexy (ap′o-plek-se): a common name for **stroke**; a **cerebrovascular accident**; extravasation of blood into an organ.

appendage (ah-pen′dij): an outgrowth; a less important portion of an organ.

appendix (ah-pen′diks): a slender, wormlike tube connected to the large intestine at the lower end of the cecum, the *vermiform appendix*.

apprehension (ap-re-hen′shun): anxiety or fear; understanding.

apraxia (ah-prak′se-ah): inability to carry out familiar movements; without sensory or motor impairment, as occurs in Alzheimer's disease.

apyretic (ah-pi-ret′ik): without fever, **afebrile.**

aqueous (a′kwe-us): pertaining to water, as *aqueous zephirin*.

areola (ah-re′o-lah): a narrow zone surrounding a central area, as the areola surrounding the nipple of the breast.

arrector (ah-rek′tor): a muscle that raises a structure, such as the muscles around the hair follicles on the skin.

arrhythmia (ah-rith′me-ah): absence of rhythm, particularly in relation to an abnormality in the rhythm of the heart.

arteriosclerosis (ar-ter-e-oh-skle-ro′sis): a condition of the arteries that produces an abnormal loss of elasticity and a hardening of the arterial walls, especially in the middle layer; formerly called *hardening of the arteries*.

artery (ar′ter-e): any one of the vessels through which the blood passes from the heart to all parts of the body.

arthritis (ar-thri′tis): inflammation of a joint.

arthroplasty (ar-thro-plas′ti): repair of a joint.

arthroscope (ar-thro-skop′): an endoscope used to examine or do surgery within a joint (*arthroscopy*).

articular (ar-tik′u-lar): pertaining to a joint.

articulate (ar-tik′u-late): to unite or join by means of joints; **articulation:** joint, place of joining; enunciation of words, to speak clearly. (Ar-tik′u-lit): able to express oneself clearly with verbal communication, as *the patient was articulate*).

artificial (ar-ti-fish′al): not natural, often man-made.

ascites (ah-si′tez): abnormal collection of fluid in the peritoneal cavity.

aseptic (a-sep′tik): free from germs that can cause infection or disease. (**Medical asepsis** refers to the destruction of pathogens *after* they leave the body, "*clean*"; **surgical asepsis** is destruction of pathogens *before* they enter the body, "*sterile*".)

asexual (a-sek′shoo-al): without sex, a person who has no interest in sex.

asphyxia (as-fix′e-ah): **suffocation;** deficiency of oxygen.

aspiration (as-pi-ra′shun): withdrawal of fluid or gas from a cavity by means of suction; the act of inhaling (pathologic drawing of fluids into the lungs), often causing aspiration pneumonia, as in the case of *meconium aspiration*.

assault (a-salt′): a violent act, either physical or verbal, as in *sexual assault*.

assessment (ah-ses′ment): in the nursing process, the systematic and continuous analysis and evaluation of data about a patient.

astasia (as-ta′ze-ah): inability to stand.

astigmatism (ah-stig′mah-tizm): distorted vision caused by irregular shape of the cornea or lens of the eye.

asthma (az′mah): a disease marked by difficulty in breathing, caused by spasmodic contractions of the bronchial tubes, *bronchial asthma*.

asymptomatic (a-sim-to-mat′ik): without symptoms.

asystole (a-sis′to-le): **cardiac arrest;** absence of heartbeat.

ataxia (ah-tak′se-ah): failure or irregularity of muscle coordination, often a chronic condition; inability to walk.

atelectasis (at-e-lak′tah-sis): collapse of all or part of a lung.

atherosclerosis (ath-er-o-skle-ro′sis): a type of arteriosclerosis characterized by deposits of cholesterol, fatty acids, or plaques on the inner wall of the artery.

athetosis (ath-e-to′sis): slow, repetitive, involuntary writhing movements.

atocia (ah-to′se-ah): female sterility.

atom (at′om): the smallest particle of an element that retains the original properties of that element.

atonic (ah-ton′ik): lacking normal tone or strength, as an *atonic uterus*.

atresia (ah-tre′ze-ah): a closing or congenital absence of a normal anatomic opening, as *esophageal atresia*.

atrium (a′tre-um): entrance (usually refers to upper chambers of the heart). (pl: **atria**)

atrophy (a′tro-fe): a decrease in size or wasting away of a cell, tissue, organ, or part, as atrophy of muscles in paralysis.

audiology (aw-de-ol′o-je): measurement and evaluation of hearing.

aura (aw'rah): a subjective sensation experienced by a person prior to a seizure, such as an epileptic attack or prior to another disorder, such as the migraine headache, a warning.

auricle (aw'ri-kl): flap of cartilage and skin comprising the outer ear; or a portion of the atrium of the heart. (Sometimes used to refer to entire atrium.) External ear, **pinna**.

auscultation (aw-skul-ta'shun): the act of externally listening to sounds from within the body to determine abnormal conditions, as auscultation of blood pressure with a stethoscope.

autism (aw'tizm): preoccupation with inner thoughts, withdrawn from the outside world, as *autistic disorder.*

autoclave (ot-oh-klav'): a pressure steam sterilizer.

autograft (aw'to-graft): a graft that is transplanted from one place to another on the same person's body.

autoimmune (aw-to-i-mun'): allergic response of one's own body to cells or organs within the body, inability of the body to differentiate between "self" and "non self."

autolesion (aw-to-le'zhun): self-inflicted injury, *self-injurious behavior.*

autologous (aw-tol'o-gus): related to self, pertaining to the same person or organism, as an autologous skin graft from another place on one's own body.

autonomic (aw-to-nom'ik): not subject to voluntary control, as the autonomic nervous system, "automatic."

autonomic dysreflexia, AD (aw-to-nom'ik dis-re-flex'e-ah): hyperreflexia or exaggerated autonomic nervous system reflexes occurring, for example, in patients with a spinal cord injury, especially injury above T-6 (the 6th thoracic vertebra).

autopsy (aw'top-se): examination of the body after death; **postmortem** or **necropsy.**

auxiliary (awk-sil'e-a-re): that which assists or helps; extra.

avulsion (ah-vul'shun): the tearing away of a structure or part, as in *traumatic avulsion* of a part.

axilla (ak-sil'ah): the armpit, as in *axillary* temperature.

axon (ak'son): outgrowth of the body of a nerve cell that conducts impulses *away* from the cell body.

Babinski (buh-bin'ski) **reflex**: a reflex caused by scraping the sole of the foot (normal in infant; sign of neurologic damage in adult).

bacteremia (bak-ter-e'me-ah): the presence of bacteria in the blood.

bacteria (bak-te're-ah): microorganisms; some types are disease-causing; common forms are staphylococci, streptococci, bacilli, and spirochetes.

bactericidal (bak-ter-i-si'dal): a substance that *kills bacteria;* to destroy bacteria.

bacteriophage (bak-te're-o-faj): virus that destroys bacteria by lysis.

bacteriostatic (bak-te-re-o-stat'ik): to slow/inhibit growth and development of bacteria, a substance that arrests growth of bacteria.

ballottement (bah-lot'maw): a specific palpation to test for a floating object, such as a fetus.

bandage (ban'dij): a strip of material (gauze, tape, cloth, etc.) used to cover a wound or hold a dressing in place, to give support or to apply pressure. (Verb: to apply a bandage, to bandage)

bariatrics (bar-e-at'riks): the study of obesity.

basal metabolism (ba'sal me-tab'o-lizm): minimum amount of energy used by the body at rest.

baseline (bas'line): a known value used to compare to an unknown, as a baseline blood pressure, to evaluate progress of a disease.

basic (ba'sik): having alkaline properties; able to neutralize acids.

battery (bat'er-e): physical striking or beating, as *assault and battery.*

bedsore (bed'sor): see **pressure ulcer.**

belching (bel'ching): burping, eructation.

benign (be-nine'): harmless, not malignant.

bereavement (be-rev'ment): the normal period of mourning or grieving following the death of a loved one. Follow-up bereavement care is an important component of hospice nursing.

bicuspid (bi-kus'pid): having two cusps or flaps, as the **mitral** (bicuspid) valve of the heart; a premolar tooth with two cusps.

bifid (bi'fid): cleft, split in two (**bifurcated**).

bilateral (bi-lat'er-al): on both sides, as in *bilateral hearing loss.*

bile (bil): fluid produced by the liver and stored in the gallbladder that aids in fat digestion.

biliary (bil'e-a-re): pertaining to bile, the liver, the gallbladder, and the associated ducts, the *biliary system.*

binocular (bin-ok'u-lar): relating to both eyes, as *binocular vision.*

biofeedback (bi-o-fed'bak): a method used to enable a person to have voluntary control over body functions by furnishing that person with information about the current physiologic status of that particular function.

biologic death: permanent and irreversible cessation of the body's physical and chemical processes and failure of body cells.

bionomics (bi-o-nom'iks): ecology, the study of the environment and its relationship to living things.

biopsy (bi'op-se): removal of a piece of body tissue for diagnostic examination, usually microscopic; most often used to look for the presence of cancer.

biotherapy (bi-o-ther'ah-pe): the use of biologic response modifiers (BRM) in cancer treatment.

bisexual (bi-sek'shoo-al): sexual attraction to persons of both sexes, exhibiting both heterosexuality and homosexuality.

blackout (blak'owt): temporary loss of vision and consciousness due to lack of blood supply to the brain and retina (can occur in aviation); sometimes refers to fainting. *Alcoholic blackout:* amnesia experienced by an alcoholic, which is a serious symptom of brain damage.

bladder (blad'er): a membranous muscular sac, as the *gall-* or *urinary bladder.*

bleb (bleb): blister, flaccid vesicle, **bulla.**

blended family: the family that results when two people who already have children marry, the blending of two families into one.

blepharitis (blef-ah-ri'tis): inflammation of the eyelid.

blood pressure (blud presh'ur): the pressure of the blood on the walls of the blood vessels, expressed as *systolic* (contraction phase) over *diastolic* (relaxation phase).

body language: impressions one conveys through body movements and posture, eye contact, and other nonverbal means.

body mechanics: use of safe and efficient methods of moving and lifting.

bolus (bo'lus): a rounded mass, as an amount of food in the intestine, a pill, or a rounded pad. A dose of IV medication given quickly, as a *bolus dose.*

bonding (bon'ding): the development of a close emotional tie, as bonding between a mother and her infant.

botulism (boch'u-lizm): severe form of food poisoning.

bougie (boo'zhe): a long instrument inserted into the body for dilation, also called a **sound.**

brachial (bra'ke-al): pertaining to the arm, as in brachial artery.

bradycardia (brad-e-kar'de-ah): abnormally slow heart action; slow pulse.

bradypnea (brad-ip'ne-ah, brad-e-ne'ah): very slow, regular respirations. Sign of drug overdose; normal during sleep. (If hypoventilation results, also called **oligopnea.**)

braille (bral): an alphabet system for the nonsighted, with raised dots that can be felt with the fingers.

brain death: irreversible cessation of brain and brain stem function to the extent that cardiopulmonary function must be mechanically maintained. The criteria for determination may vary slightly between states. (Also called **cerebral death,** *irreversible coma,* and *persistent vegetative state*).

Braxton–Hicks contractions (braks'tun-hiks kun-trak' shuns): naturally occurring tightening and relaxing of uterine muscles during pregnancy in preparation for labor and delivery; usually irregular and painless.

bronchi (brong'ki): tubular-shaped air passages that connect the trachea and lungs. (sing: **bronchus**)

bronchiectasis (brong-ke-ek'tah-sis): chronic dilation of the bronchi of the lungs, with large amounts of sputum production. (May be genetic ciliary dysfunction.)

bronchiolitis (brong-ke-o-li'tis): inflammation of the bronchioles of the lungs.

bronchitis (brong-ki'tis): inflammation of the bronchi of the lungs.

bronchodilator (brong-ko-di'la-ter): a drug that causes air passages (bronchioles) of the lungs to expand (dilate), thus improving respirations. A common bronchodilator is *epinephrine*.

bronchoscope (brong'ko-skope): a lighted instrument used for the examination of the interior of the bronchi (*bronchoscopy*).

bruit (brwe, broot): an abnormal sound, especially of the heart; the sound normally heard in a shunt for hemodialysis.

brush border (brush): a specialization of the surface of a cell with many microvilli, greatly increasing the surface area.

Brushfield's spots (brush'feeldz): tiny light-colored spots on the iris of the eye in the child with Down syndrome.

bruxism (bruk'sizm): grinding or clenching the teeth, usually during sleep.

buccal (buk'al): pertaining to the cheek or mouth, as the *buccal mucosa*.

bulimia (bu-lim'e-ah): a condition in which the person (usually female) eats huge amounts of food and then causes herself to vomit or uses large amounts of laxatives (*binge–purge syndrome*).

bursa (ber'sah): a small, fluid-filled sac that prevents friction, as in bursae of the shoulder or knee. (pl: **bursae**)

bursitis (ber-si'tis): inflammation of a bursa. Bursitis often affects the shoulder joint.

buttocks (but'oks): the prominence of muscle and fat on the posterior part of the body at the hip line.

cachexia (kah-kek'se-ah): severe ill health and malnutrition; *debilitated state*.

cadaver (kah-dav'er): a dead body.

cafe coronary: slang term for a person who dies by choking while eating, often after rushing out of a restaurant to avoid embarrassment.

calcium (kal'si-um): a mineral element that is the most abundant in the body; found especially in bones and teeth.

calculus (kal'ku-lus): an abnormal concretion usually composed of mineral salts, occurring in the hollow organs of the body; a "**stone**," as a calculus in the kidney or gallbladder. (pl: **calculi**); deposit on the teeth (**tartar**).

callus (kal'us): a hard, thickened portion of the skin; the bony material that makes the union between the ends of fractured bones (also **callous**).

calorie (kal'o-re): the amount of heat required to raise the temperature of 1 kg of pure water 1°C, at a specific exterior air temperature; used to determine energy values of foods (1 kilocalorie = 1000 calories).

cancer (kan'ser): a malignant growth, **neoplasm, carcinoma.**

canker (kang'ker): a sore or ulceration, usually of the oral mucosa or lip.

cannula (kan'u-lah): a tubular instrument for insertion into the body, as the cannula of a tracheostomy tube.

canthus (kan'thus): junction of the eyelids at the corners.

caplet (cap'let): a tablet in the shape of a capsule, making it easier to swallow.

capsule (kap'sul): a small gelatinous case for holding a dose of medicine; a membranous structure enclosing another structure in the body, as the *articular capsule* in a joint.

caput (kap'ut): pertaining to the head, as *caput succedaneum*.

carbohydrate (kar-bo-hi'drat): most widely used source of energy in the world; found mostly in sugars and starches. (Made up of carbon, hydrogen, and oxygen [CHO].)

carbon dioxide (kar'bon di-ok'side): a colorless gas that is exhaled in respiration (CO_2).

carbon monoxide (kar'bon mon-ok'sid): a colorless gas found in automobile exhaust that renders the hemoglobin in the blood incapable of carrying oxygen (CO).

carbuncle (kar'bung-kl): a cluster of boils (*furuncles*).

carcinogen (kar-sin'o-jen): something that causes cancer.

carcinoma (kar-sin-o'mah): cancer, a malignant neoplasm (new growth).

cardiac (kar'de-ak): pertaining to the heart; as in *cardiac arrest*.

cardiac life support: rescue efforts using CPR (*basic cardiac life support*—BCLS) or more advanced means such as intubation, defibrillation, or intravenous fluid administration (*advanced cardiac life support*—ACLS); the initials also refer to persons trained in these areas.

cardinal signs (kar'de-nal): signs of life, functions necessary to life, vital signs (temperature, pulse, respiration, and blood pressure), also called **cardinal symptoms.**

cardiograph (kar'de-o-graf): an instrument for recording the electrical stimulation of the heart, also called **electrocardiograph (ECG).**

cardiology (kar-de-ol'o-je): the study of the heart and heart function.

cardiopulmonary resuscitation (CPR) (car-de-o-pul'mon-ar-e re-sus-i-ta'shun): a combination of external cardiac massage and artificial ventilation.

cardioversion (kar'de-o-ver-zhun): delivery of an electric shock to the heart to restore normal rhythm; counter shock; precordial shock; sometimes called **defibrillation.**

caries (ka're-ez): decay of teeth or bones, as *dental caries*.

carotene (kar'o-teen): yellow or red pigment contained in many foods such as squash, carrots, and green, leafy vegetables; converted to vitamin A in the body.

carpal (kar'pal): pertaining to the wrist (carpus).

carpopedal (kar-po-pe'dal): affecting the wrist and hand or ankle and foot, as in *carpopedal spasm*.

carrier (kar'e-er): an individual who harbors (in the body) the specific organisms of a disease without manifesting its symptoms, thus acting as a distributor or transmitter of the infection.

cartilage (kar'ti-lij): fibrous connective tissue in joints.

cast (kast): an appliance used to render immovable displaced or injured parts, as a cast applied to a fractured leg; a fatty, waxy, or epithelial substance formed in the urinary system and found (abnormally) in urine; a mold or impression, as of the jaw, used to make braces or dentures.

castrate (kas'trat): to remove the gonads (sex organs).

catabolism (kah-tab'o-lizm): the destructive phase of metabolism; breaking down.

cataplexy (kat'ah-plek-se): abrupt attacks of muscular weakness and decreased strength, often associated with narcolepsy (uncontrollable desire to sleep).

cataract (kat'ah-rakt): an opacity of the lens of the eye or its capsule.

cathartic (kath-ar'tik): a medicine that causes the evacuation of the bowels, **laxative, purgative**.

catheter (kath'e-ter): a flexible tube that is passed into the body, usually through body channels, for the withdrawal or instillation of fluids; most often refers to urinary catheter.

catheterization (kath-e-ter-e-za'shun): procedure to insert a catheter into the patient's body, as in *urinary* or *cardiac catheterization*. (verb: to catheterize)

cation (kat'i-on): an ion that carries a positive electrical charge.

caustic (kaws'tik): burning; destructive to tissues.

cavity (kav'it-e): a hollow space within the body or within one of its organs.

celiac (se'le-ak): pertaining to the abdomen, as in *celiac disease*, a malabsorption syndrome.

cell (sel): the minute protoplasmic building unit of living matter; the basic structural unit of the body.

cellulitis (sel-u-li'tis): diffuse inflammation of the soft or connective tissues caused by infection; inflammatory process characterized by edema, redness, and pain.

Celsius (sel'se-us): temperature scale in which water boils at 100° and freezes at 0° (formerly called centigrade).

center of gravity: the center of one's weight; half of one's body weight is below and half above and half to the left and half to the right of the center of gravity. This concept is important in *body mechanics*.

central pain: pain within the central nervous system (may have physical and psychological components).

cephalalgia (sef-al-al'je-ah): head pain. **headache**.

cephalic (se-fal'ik): pertaining to the head.

cephalocaudal (sef-a-lo-caw'dal): literally, "head to toe" (used to denote head-to-toe progression of development in infants).

cephalopelvic disproportion (sef-ah-lo-pel'vik dis-pro-por'shun): the fetal head is too large for vaginal delivery, in relationship to the maternal pelvis.

cerclage (ser-klahzh'): encircling with a ring or loop of suture, used to hold the cervix closed or to hold fractured bone fragments together.

cerebellum (ser-a-bel'um): the part of the brain located on the back of the brain stem. It has three lobes, one median (*vermis*) and two lateral (*hemispheres*).

cerebral (ser'e-bral or se-re'bral): pertaining to the main portion of the brain, as in *cerebral palsy*, a motor disorder usually caused by brain damage.

cerebral death (se-re'bral): irreversible cessation of brain function, **brain death**.

cerumen (se-roo'men): the waxy substance, secreted by the ceruminous glands, that collects in the outer ear canal; **ear wax**.

cervical (ser'vi-kal): pertaining to the neck or cervix of any structure; the uterine cervix is known as the **cervix uteri;** the cervical vertebrae are in the neck area.

cervicitis (ser-vi-si'tus): inflammation of the uterine cervix.

cesarean (se-sa're-an) **delivery**: surgical procedure to deliver a baby through an incision in the abdomen and uterus.

chafe (chaf): to irritate the skin by friction.

chalazion (kah-la'ze-on): a small mass on the eyelid caused by inflammation of a meibomian gland (a sebaceous gland on the eyelid which secretes sebum), **meibomian cyst.**

chancre (shang'ker): the primary lesion of syphilis (*not* a canker sore).

chelation (ke-la'shun): a process for treating poisoning with a metal such as lead (plumbism), in which the chelating agent and the metal combine, become soluble and can be eliminated. (Also used to remove excess iron in sickle cell anemia.)

chemical name: the name of a drug that describes its chemical composition (often same as *generic name*).

chemosis (ke-mo'sis): edema of the conjunctive of the eye. (Adj.: chemotic.)

chemotherapy (ke-mo-ther'ah-pe): the use of chemical agents to treat disease; drug therapy as it relates to treatment of cancer.

chest (chest): the thorax; the part of the body that lies between the neck and the abdominal cavity.

Cheyne-Stokes respiration (chan stoks res-pir-a'shun): respirations characterized by deep breathing alternating with very slow breathing or apnea; indicative of brain damage; often precedes death.

chiropodist (ki-ra'po-dist): foot doctor, **podiatrist.**

chloasma (klo-az'mah): hyperpigmentation (darker coloration) in particular areas of the skin, such as the "mask of pregnancy" or the linea nigra in pregnancy (*chloasma gravidarum*). (Also called **melasma**.)

cholecystic (ko-le-sis'tik): pertaining to the gallbladder. *cholecep-titis* is inflammation of the gallbladder.

cholesterol (ko-les'ter-ol): a steroid alcohol found only in animal tissues; it is needed to produce hormones, vitamin D, and bile acids, but has been connected with atherosclerotic disease. LDL—low-density lipoprotein ("bad" cholesterol) and HDL—high-density lipo-protein ("good" cholesterol) must be balanced to maintain health.

chorea (ko-re'ah): a nerve disorder characterized by involuntary, jerky muscular movements, as *Huntington's chorea.*

choriocarcinoma (ko-re-o-kar-si-no'ma): an epithelial malignancy that develops in trophoblastic cells from the products of conception, usually a hydatiform mole, although it may also develop from an abortion or pregnancy. Choriocarcinoma also rarely develops in male testicular cells.

chorion (ko're-on): the outermost fetal membrane.

chromosome (kro'mo-som): body in the nucleus of a cell that carries genetic factors.

chronic (kron'ik): a condition that remains for a length of time, may be progressive.

chyme (kime): partially digested food as it enters the duodenum.

cicatrix (sik'ah-trik, si-ka'trik): scar.

ciliated (sil'e-a-ted): provided with a fringe of hairlike processes, as in the small intestine (cilia).

circumcise (ser'kum-siz): usually refers to surgical removal of the foreskin (prepuce) of the penis. (Male circumcision is a Jewish religious ritual.) Female circumcision is practiced in some parts of the world. The classification of female circumcision varies, depending on the structural removal (ranges from the clitoris, prepuce, to the labia minora and majora).

circumduction (ser-cum-duct'shun): circular movement of a limb or the eye.

circumoral (ser-kum-o'rel): around the mouth, **perioral**.

cirrhosis (sir-ro'sis): chronic inflammation and degeneration of an organ, especially *cirrhosis of the liver.*

clavicle (klav'i-kal): the collar bone.

clean (klen'): in *medical asepsis,* devoid of all gross contamination and free of *many* microorganisms (mechanical cleansing is sufficient for this purpose).

cleft (kleft): fissure or longitudinal opening, as in *cleft lip.*

client: term sometimes used to refer to patients, especially in the person's own home, a nursing home, outpatient clinic, mental health unit, or chemical dependency unit.

climacteric (kli-mak'ter-ik): cessation of reproductive function in the female (**menopause**), and decreasing testicular activity in the male.

clinical (klin'ik-al): pertaining to instruction at the bedside or actual treatment of the patient (as distinguished from theoretic, experimental, or classroom instruction).

clinical death (klin'a-kl): absence of heartbeat and cessation of breathing, can sometimes be reversed by CPR or other means.

clitoris (klit'or-is): small structure of erectile tissue in the female at the anterior junction of the labia that is stimulated by sexual excitement.

clonus (klo'nus): rapidly alternating involuntary muscle contraction and relaxation, as a *clonic seizure.*

closed questions: questions that can usually be answered by one word, such as "yes" or "no." Closed questions do not promote in-depth therapeutic communication.

clot (klot): semisolid mass, as a *blood clot.*

clubfoot (klub'foot): condition in which one or both feet turn out of normal position. Also called **talipes.**

clysis (kli'sis): administration of fluids for replacement, cleansing, or nourishment by a route other than the oral, as *hypodermoclysis.*

coagulation (ko-ag-u-la'shun): the changing of a liquid to thickened, curdlike form, as *coagulation of blood.*

coarctation (ko-ark-ta'shun): stricture or narrowing, as in *coarctation of the aorta.*

coccus (kok'us): spherical (round) bacterium, as *staphylococcus* or *streptococcus*.

coccyx (kok'siks): tailbone.

cochlea (kok'le-ah): snail-shaped organ of inner ear, the essential organ of hearing, as in *cochlear implant*.

cognitive (kog'ni-tiv): involving knowledge, understanding, and perception; in the mind.

colic (kol'ik): acute abdominal pain; pertaining to the colon; abdominal pain in infants, most common during first 3 months of life.

colitis (ko-li'tis): inflammation of the colon.

cogwheeling (cog'wheel-ing): abnormal muscular rigor that manifests as jerky movements when the muscle is passively stretched, can be a side effect of psychotropic medications (**cogwheel rigidity**).

collagen (kol'ah-jen): white, fibrous structural protein found in tendons, bone cartilage, skin and other connective tissues, as well as in the vitreous humor of the eye.

collateral (kol-lat'er-al): secondary, alternative or accessory, as in *collateral circulation*, established following a heart attack.

colon (kol'lon): the main part of the large intestine, extending from the cecum to the rectum.

colonoscopy (ko-lon-os'ko-pe): examination of the colon with an endoscope.

colostomy (ko-los'to-me): an artificial opening from the colon to the outside of the body by way of a stoma.

colostrum (ko-los'trum): the first fluid secreted by the mammary (breast) glands just before or after childbirth.

coma (ko'mah): profound lack of responsiveness, due to disease or injury; nonresponsiveness, *loss of consciousness, unconsciousness*.

comatose (ko'mah-tos): the state of being in a coma.

communicable disease (ko-mun'ni-ka-bl dis-eze'): a disease that can be transmitted from one person to another; infectious, such as influenza.

communication (kom-myoon-i-ka'shun): giving, receiving, and interpretation of information (may be verbal or nonverbal); a message or letter.

compartment (kom-part'ment): space occupied by a group of muscles circumscribed by tight fibrous structures, especially in the leg and upper arm. *Compartmental syndrome* is a result of swelling in these areas.

compensated (kom'pen-sa-ted): adjustment by the body to heart and circulatory disorders to prevent distress; mechanisms used include tachycardia, cardiac hypertrophy, corollary circulation, and electrolyte adjustments. In mental health, the patient compensates with behaviors designed to cover up thought disturbances or other psychiatric symptoms.

compound (kom'pownd): substance composed of two or more elements united according to chemical weights; they undergo chemical change (elements lose their original characteristics). Table salt is a compound of sodium and chloride (NaCl). (Verb: *to compound*—to make up drug preparations.)

compress (kom'pres): a dressing used to apply pressure, heat, cold, or medication to a local area; (verb: kom-pres'—to push on or squeeze together)

concentrated (kon'sen-tra-ted): made stronger, as a concentrated solution.

concurrent (kon-kur'ent): happening at the same time, as in two concurrent infections.

concussion (kon-kush'un): violent jar or shock, or the injury that results, as a *brain concussion*.

conduction (kon-duk'shun): carrying or conveying of energy such as heat, electricity, or sound.

condyloma acuminatum (kon-di-lo'mah ah-kum-i-na'tum): an elevated wartlike or nipplelike (papilloma) lesion, usually in the genital area. (pl: **condylomata acuminata**) (Also called **venereal warts, genital warts**).

confabulation (kon-fab-u-la'shun): unconscious filling in of memory gaps with made-up information, often seen in organic dementias and psychoses.

confidentiality (kon fa-dench'e-al-i-tee): privacy of information shared by a client with a professional person, expecting the information to remain with that person alone.

congenital (kon-jen'i-tal): existing at birth (may be genetic/inherited or acquired).

congestion (kon-jest'yun): an abnormal accumulation of blood or other fluids in a body part, as *nasal congestion*.

conjunctiva (kon-junk'ti-vah): transparent mucous membrane covering the anterior eye (front).

conscious (kon'shus): capable of responding to stimuli and subjective reactions.

consistency (kon-sis'ten-se): degree of firmness or stiffness.

constipation (kon-stip-a'shun): difficult or infrequent movement of the bowels.

contagious (kon-ta'jus): able to be transmitted from one person to another, **infectious.**

contaminate (kon-tam'i-nate): to make unsterile or unclean.

continuous passive motion (**CPM**): machine that provides exercise for a limb without active participation by patient or nurse.

contraceptive (kon-trah-sep'tiv): an agent that diminishes the likelihood of pregnancy, *birth control device*, as in contraceptive foam.

contracture (kon-trak'tur): abnormal shortening of muscles with resultant deformity.

contraindication (kon-trah-in-di-ka'shun): any situation that makes a form of treatment undesirable, as a medication which is *contraindicated*.

contralateral (kon-trah-lat'er-al): pertaining to the opposite side, as the contralateral crutch in crutchwalking.

contusion (kon-tu'zhun): injury without breaking the skin; a *bruise*.

convalescence (kon-val-es'ens): recovery.

convection (kon-vek'shun): spreading/transmission of heat in a liquid or gas by circulation of heated particles.

convulsions (kon-vul'shuns): involuntary contractions of the voluntary muscles; **seizures.**

co-pay: amount paid for health care by a patient for whom insurance or a health maintenance organization pays the rest.

copulation (kope-u-la'shun): *sexual intercourse* between male and female.

corium (kor'e-um): the dermis, "true skin," the fibrous inner layer of skin just under the epidermis.

cornea (kor'ne-ah): the transparent front covering of the eye, as in *corneal transplant*.

coronary (kor'o-na-re): circular, crownlike; the blood vessels surrounding the heart are *coronary arteries*.

corrosive (ko-ro'siv): destructive to tissue.

cortex (kor'teks): outer layer, as the *adrenal cortex*.

crackle (krak'l): an abnormal, nonmusical respiratory sound heard on auscultation; also called **rale.** *Coarse crackles* sound moist (gurgling); the sound being like Velcro when pulled apart (moist rales). *Fine crackles* sound like rubbing hair on the skin in front of your ear.

cradle (kra'dl): a curved, framelike bed accessory placed over a patient's limb; keeps bedding off the limb, sometimes contains a heat source.

cranial (kra'ne-al): pertaining to the skull, as *cranial nerves*.

craniotomy (kra-ne-ah'to-me): any operation into the cranium (skull), "brain surgery."

Crede's maneuver (kra'daz), Crede's technique: a technique used in bladder rehabilitation (retraining) in which the hands are held flat against the abdomen just below the umbilicus, with firm downward strokes applied toward the bladder, followed by pressure on the bladder itself, to manually express urine.

cretinism (kre'ti-nizm): arrested physical/mental development resulting from congenital thyroid hormone deficiency.

crime: (krim): an illegal act, a felony or misdemeanor, an offense which is against the law.

crisis (kri′sis): the turning point of a disease; sudden intensification of symptoms.

crossmatch (kros′match): testing of donor blood against the recipient's blood to determine compatibility, as a *type and crossmatch*.

crowning (krown′ing): in childbirth, the appearance of the top of the baby's head at the vaginal introitus (entrance, opening).

cryosurgery (kri-o-ser′jer-e): destruction of tissue by the application of extreme cold.

cryptorchidism (krip-tor′ki-dizm): undescended testicles.

crystalluria (krys-tah-lu′re-ah): crystals in the urine.

cubitus (ku′bi-tus): the forearm; the elbow, as in *antecubital space*.

cul-de-sac (kul-de-sak′): a blind pouch.

culdoscopy (kul-dos′ko-pe): examination of the (internal) female viscera by means of an endoscope inserted through the posterior vaginal fornix (a cul-de-sac).

culture (kul′chur): the growing of microorganisms in specific media; the product of culture growth; or the concepts, habits, skills, and institutions of a given group of people (civilization).

curettage (ku-re-tahzh′): scraping of a diseased surface, as *dilation and curettage* of the uterus. (**suction** or **vacuum curettage**: curettage performed with suction through a hollow curet; used to perform abortion.)

curie (ku′re): unit of radioactivity (named for Marie Curie).

cusp (kusp): a pointed projection, as the cusp of a tooth.

cutis (ku′tis): skin, (Adj.: cutaneous).

cyanosis (si-an-o′sis): blueness or duskiness of the skin caused by the deficiency of oxygen and the excess of carbon dioxide in the blood.

cyclothymic (si-klo-thi′mik): a mood disorder characterized by alternating periods of extreme elation and sadness; similar to bipolar disorder, but less extreme. (**Cyclothymia,** *cyclothymic personality*.)

cylindruria (sil-in-droo′re-ah): cylinders (*casts*) in the urine.

cyst (sist): a sac containing liquid or soft material, as a *sebaceous cyst*.

cystalgia (sis-tal′je-ah): pain in the bladder.

cystitis (sis-ti′tus): inflammation of any bladder (most often refers to urinary bladder). (*Cholecystitis* is inflammation of the gallbladder.)

cystocele (sis′to-sel): herniation of the urinary bladder into the vagina.

cytapheresis (sit-ah-fe-re′sis): process by which blood elements are removed, treated, and retransfused back into the person. Sometimes, not all removed cells are replaced.

cytology (si-tol′o-je): the study of cells.

cytomegalovirus, CMV (si-to-meg-ah-lo-vi′rus): a group of host-specific herpesviruses, causing many different symptoms. Particularly dangerous to infants and immunosuppressed persons.

dangle foot, dropfoot: a condition in which the foot hangs in the plantar flexed position as a result of a peroneal nerve disorder.

debility (de-bil′i-te): loss or lack of strength; *weakness*.

debridement (da-brede′-maw): to remove foreign, dead, and contaminated material from a wound, so as to expose the healthy underlying tissue, as *debridement of a burn*.

debris (de-bre′): accumulated or foreign matter.

decalcify (de-kal′si-fi): to deprive of calcium, as the *decalcification of bones*.

deciduous (de-sid′u-us): denoting that which falls off or is shed, as *deciduous teeth*.

decompensated (de-kom′pen-sa-ted): inability of the heart to maintain adequate circulation; inability of defense mechanisms or medications to mask schizophrenia or other psychiatric disorders.

decompose (de-kom-poze′): to decay; rot.

decubitus ulcer (de-ku′bi-tus ul′ser): more correctly called **pressure ulcer** or pressure area.

defecation (def-e-ka′shun): the discharge of solid waste matter (feces) from the intestines; **bowel movement.**

defect (de′fect): an imperfection or flaw, as a *birth defect*.

defibrillate (de-fib′ri-late): to stop rapid, irregular, and ineffective heart activity, usually with electric shock; **cardioversion.**

degeneration (de-jen-er-a′shun): deterioration from a higher to a lower form, as the degeneration of bone tissue.

deglutition (deg-loo-tish′un): swallowing.

dehumanize (de-hu′mah-niz): to make a person/patient feel like an object, to remove one's dignity.

dehydration (de-hi-dra′shun): the removal of water; lack of fluid/water in the body.

delirium (de-lir′e-um): a mental disturbance, usually temporary, marked by wandering speech, delusions, excitement, and at times, hallucinations, as *delirium tremens*.

delusion (de-lu′zhun): a false belief that cannot be corrected by reason; deceit.

dementia (de-men′she-ah): organic loss of intellectual function, as *senile dementia*.

demographics (dem-o-graf′iks): the study of population trends, including births, deaths, and diseases.

dendrite (den′drite): nerve branch that conducts impulses toward the body of the cell.

dentia (den′she-ah): relating to teeth.

denture (den′tur): usually, an artificial set of teeth.

deodorant (de-o′der-ant): an agent that destroys unpleasant odors; *disinfectant*.

deoxyribonucleic acid (DNA) (de-ok″se-ri″bo-new-kla′ik a-sid): a complex nucleic acid occurring in the nucleus of all cells, which is the basic structure of genes and carries the genetic code.

depilatory (de-pil′at-o-re): a preparation for removing hair.

depression (de-presh′un): lowered mental and physical activity; morbid sadness.

dermal (der′mal): relating to the skin, as *dermal abrasion, dermabrasion*.

dermatitis (derm-ah-ti′tis): inflammation of the skin; **rash.**

dermatology (durm-a-tol′o-ji): study of diseases of the skin.

dermis (der′mis): the true skin, **corium.**

descent (de-sent′): moving from a higher to a lower place, as the descent of the fetus within the uterus before birth.

desquamation (des-kwa-ma′shun): the shedding or scaling of the skin or cuticle; *peeling*.

detoxification (de-toks-i-fi-ca′shun): process of removing a toxin (e.g., alcohol) or the effect of the toxin from a patient.

development (di-vel′op-ment): change in body function.

deviation (de-ve-a′shun): turning aside; varying from normal.

dextroversion (dek-stro-ver′shun): turning to the right; located on the right side, as *dextroversion of the eyes*.

diabetes (di-ah-be′tez): a disease characterized by great increase in urinary discharge and increased blood glucose; usually refers to **diabetes mellitus;** may also refer to **diabetes insipidus.** (Diabetes mellitus is classified as insulin-dependent diabetes mellitus [IDDM], which represents about 5% to 10% of all cases, and non-insulin-dependent diabetes mellitus [NIDDM].)

diagnosis (di-ag-no′sis): **Medical diagnosis:** the recognition of a disease by its signs and symptoms, made by a physician. **Nursing diagnosis:** a statement about the patient's actual or potential health concerns that can be managed through independent nursing intervention.

diagnosis-related group (DRG): grouping of medical diagnoses to determine level of payment by an agency such as Medicare.

dialysis (di-al′i-sis): diffusion of dissolved molecules through a semipermeable membrane (most often refers to treatment given to remove waste products from the blood of a patient who suffers from renal failure). **Peritoneal dialysis** is done by way of the peritoneum; **extracorporeal dialysis (hemodialysis)** uses the artificial kidney through a blood vessel shunt.

diaphoresis (di-ah-fo-re′sis): perspiration or sweating, particularly profuse perspiration. (**Sudoresis** also means profuse perspiration.)

diaphragm (di′a-fram): the muscular partition between the thoracic and the abdominal cavities, important in breathing; a type of female contraceptive device; a part of a stethoscope.

diaphysis (di-af′i-sis): the middle portion of a long bone; the shaft of a bone.

diarrhea (di-ar-e′ah): abnormal frequency and fluidity of discharge from the bowels.

diastolic (di-as-tol′ik): the pressure of the blood against the arterial walls when the heart is *at rest* between beats (the bottom number recorded in a blood pressure reading).

diathermy (di′ah-ther-me): the use of high-frequency electrical current in physical therapy or surgery to heat body tissues.

dietetics (di-e-tet′iks): the study of nutrition and therapeutic diets.

diffusion (di-fu′zhun): the state of being widely spaced; the process whereby molecules move in an effort to equalize the concentration of a liquid or gas.

digestion (di-jest′yun): the process of converting food into chemical substances that can be assimilated and absorbed by body tissues.

digit (dij′it): finger or toe.

dilation (di-la′shun): the action of expanding, as in *dilation and curettage* or dilation of blood vessels, *vasodilation*. (*Dilation* and **dilatation** are often used interchangeably.)

diluent (dil′u-ent): a substance that dilutes, thins, or makes another less potent. (When preparing a powdered medication for parenteral administration, the liquid used is the diluent. When giving liquid medication in juice, the juice is the diluent.)

dilute (di-lute′): to thin or weaken or make more fluid by adding another fluid, especially water.

diplopia (di-plo′pe-ah): double vision.

dipsia (dip′se-ah): thirst.

disability (dis-ah-bil′i-te): incapacity; a physical or mental inability to function normally, physical or intellectual challenge.

disarticulation (dis-ar-tik-u-la′shun): separation or amputation of connecting bones at a joint, may refer to *dislocation*, as of a shoulder.

disc (disk): circular or flat plate, as *intervertebral disc* (may also be called **disk**).

discharge planning: process by which a patient is prepared for continuation of care after going home.

disease (dis-eze′): a deviation or departure from normal structure or function of a part or a system of the body that is characterized by certain signs and symptoms; the cause and prognosis may be known or unknown.

disinfectant (dis-in-fek′tant): an agent that frees (a surface) from infection by *destroying germs;* not always effective against spores; often too strong to be used on living tissues.

dislocation (dis-lo-ka-shun′): displacement of a bone from a joint, as *dislocation of the shoulder*.

dismember (dis-mem′ber): to *amputate* a limb or part of a limb.

disorientation (dis-o-re-en-ta′shun): a state of *mental confusion* or loss of bearings.

dissect (di-sekt′): to cut up an organism for study; to separate tissues in surgery.

disseminate (di-sem′i-nate): to scatter or distribute, as in *disseminated intravascular coagulation* (DIC).

dissociation (dis-so-she-a′shun): in psychology, defense mechanism allowing unconscious separation of harmful/painful thoughts and memories from usual consciousness.

distal (dis′tal): remote; farthest from any point of reference, such as from the center or midline. The hand is distal to the shoulder.

distention (dis-ten′shun): the state of being enlarged; stretching, as in *abdominal distention*.

diuresis (di-u-re′sis): increased excretion of urine.

divergence (di-ver′jens): a spreading apart or deviation from the normal course, as *divergence of the eyes* in strabismus.

diverticulitis (di-ver-tik-u-li′tis): inflammation of a diverticulum (outpouching or sac in a mucous membrane), often referring to the colon. (*pl:* **diverticula**)

diverticulosis (di-ver-tik-u-lo′sis): the condition of having diverticula, without inflammation.

diverticulum (di-ver-tik′u-lum): a pouch or sac of variable size occurring either normally or as a herniation through the muscle, as in *Meckel's diverticulum*.

donor (do′ner): a person who furnishes a tissue or organ for transplantation into or grafting onto the body of another.

Doppler (dop′ler) **effect:** the relationship of the frequency of waves, as of sound, to the relative motion of the source of the waves and the observer, with the frequency increasing as they move closer together, as in *Doppler ultrasound*.

dorsal (dor′sal): pertaining to the back, behind. The vertebral column is dorsal to the lungs.

douche (doosh): a stream of water or other fluid directed against a part of a body or into a body cavity, as in *vaginal douche*.

Down syndrome (down′sin′drome): congenital abnormality characterized by specific physical defects and by varying degrees of intellectual impairment. (Formerly called mongolism; also called *Down's* syndrome.)

drug (drug′): substance other than food used to prevent disease, to aid in the diagnosis and treatment of disease, and to restore or maintain functions in body tissues. Also called **medication.**

duct (dukt): canal for fluids; tube, as in *bile duct*.

duodenum (du-o-de′num): proximal (first) portion of the small intestine.

dyscrasia (dis-kra′ze-ah): disease condition that involves an imbalance of component elements, as a *blood dyscrasia*.

dysentery (dis′en-ter-e): a term given to a number of disorders marked by inflammation of the intestines, especially of the colon, which is marked by diarrhea (may be caused by bacteria, chemical agents, or parasitic worms). (A common type in foreign travelers is *amoebic dysentery*.)

dysfunction (dis-fungk′shun): not functioning or operating properly, as a *sexual* or *endocrine dysfunction*.

dyslalia (dis-la′le-ah): impairment of speech ability, usually because of abnormal external speech organs.

dyslexia (dis-lek′se-ah): an inability to read with comprehension due to a central nervous system (CNS) defect, may include symbol reversal.

dysmaturity (dis-mah-tur′i-te): the state of being small or immature for gestational age.

dysmenorrhea (dis-men-o-re′ah): difficult or painful menstruation.

dyspepsia (dis-pep′se-ah): indigestion.

dysphagia (dis-fa′je-ah): difficulty in swallowing.

dysplasia (dis-pla′ze-ah): abnormal development, as in congenital *hip dysplasia*.

dyspnea (disp′ne-ah): difficulty in breathing.

dysrhythmia (dis-rith′me-ah): lacking rhythm, without rhythm, as in an *irregular heartbeat*.

dysthymia (dis-thy-me-ah): depressive disorder, *chronic clinical depression* over a long period of time.

dystocia (dis-tos′e-ah): difficult labor.

dystrophy (dis′tro-fe): any disorder arising from defective nutrition; usually refers to progressive atrophy and weakness of the muscles without nervous system involvement, as *muscular dystrophy*.

dysuria (dis-u′re-ah): difficult or painful urination or voiding.

ear wax: cerumen.

ecchymosis (ek-i-mo′sis): bleeding into the tissues under the skin, leaving small bruises.

echocardiography (ek-o-kar-de-og′rah-fe): recording of activity and location of the heart by means of ultrasound.

echolalia (ek-o-la′le-ah): automatic repeating by a patient of what has been said to him or her.

echopraxia (ek-o-prak′se-ah): involuntary imitation of the movements of other people.

echovirus (eko-vi′-rus): a group of viruses, acronym for *"enteric cytopathogenic human orphan"* (ECHO) *virus.*

eclampsia (e-klamp′se-ah): seizure disorder with high blood pressure, usually related to a complication of pregnancy, *pregnancy-induced hypertension* (PIH).

ecology (i-kol′o-je): the study of the interrelationship of organisms and their environment.

ECT (also EST), electroconvulsive therapy (e-lec-tro-kon-vul′siv ther′ah-pe): used in mental health; administration of an electric shock to induce convulsions (seizures) as a treatment, usually for clinical depression.

ectopic (ek-top′ik): situated in other than the normal location, as *ectopic pregnancy.*

ectropion (ek-tro′pe-on): turning outward (eversion) of an edge, as *ectropion of the eyelid.*

eczema (ek′ze-mah): an inflammatory skin rash, characterized by itching, redness, weeping, oozing, and crusting, and later by scaling.

edema (e-de′mah): abnormal accumulation of fluid in the intercellular tissue spaces of the body; puffiness; *pitting* e.: leaving dents when pressed; **brawny** e.: hard edema.

edentia (e-den′she-ah): absence of teeth. (adj: **edentulous**)

effacement (e-fas′ment): thinning of the cervix in preparation for delivery.

effector (ef-fek′tor): a chemical agent, organ, cell, or muscle group that produces a specific act or effect.

efferent (ef′er-ent): conducting *away* from the center, as an *efferent nerve.*

effleurage (ef-loo-rahzh′): stroking movement in backrub or massage.

effusion (e-fu′zhun): escape of fluid into a part or tissue, as an exudation, such as *pleural effusion.*

egg-crate mattress: a foam pad, shaped like an egg carton, which is used on top of a regular bed mattress to provide comfort and prevent pressure areas.

electrocardiogram (ECG, EKG) (e-lek-tro-kar′deo-gram): recording of electrical activity of heartbeats for baseline or pathology readings.

electrocerebral silence (e-lek-tro-sir-e′brul si′lens): **brain death;** absence of electrical activity in the brain.

electroencephalogram (EEG) (e-lek-tro-en-sef′ah-lo-gram): recording of electrical activity of the brain.

electrolysis (e-lek-trol′i-sis): destruction by use of an electric current, as in removal of hair from the body.

electrolyte (e-lek′tro-lit): a chemical substance that dissociates into electrically charged ions (positive ions are called *cations;* negative ions are called *anions*) when melted or in solution (becomes capable of conducting electricity).

electromyogram (EMG) (e-lek-tro-mi′o-gram): recording of electrical activity of muscles in response to stimuli.

element (el′a-ment): a chemical substance made up of atoms that cannot be further divided without losing the characteristics of the substance; the physical and chemical properties of a particular element are always the same.

elimination (e-lim-in-a′shun): the act of expelling wastes from the body, *voiding* and *defecation.*

emaciation (e-ma-se-a′shun): a wasting away of the flesh, causing extreme leanness, **starvation.** (adj: **emaciated**)

embolus (em′bol-us): a foreign substance, blood clot, fat globule, piece of tissue, or air bubble carried in a blood vessel, which partially or completely obstructs the flow of blood, as a *pulmonary embolus* (**embolism;** pleural **emboli**).

embryo (em′bre-o): a new organism in the first stage of development.

emesis (em′e-sis): the act of vomiting; the product of vomiting, **vomitus.**

emetic (e-met′ik): an agent that causes vomiting, such as *Ipecac.*

emollient (e-mol′e-ent): a soothing medicine, as an *emollient cream.*

empathy (em′pah-the): intellectual understanding and entering into the feelings of another person.

emphysema (em-fi-se′mah): an inflation or swelling of tissues due to the presence of air; usually refers to *chronic pulmonary emphysema,* a severe lung disorder.

empyema (em-pi-e′mah): accumulation of pus in a body cavity, often the pleural (lung) cavity.

enabler (en-ab′ler): a person who covers for and assists another, enabling the individual to continue in a chemical abuse lifestyle.

encephalalgia (en-sef-ah-lal′je-ah): pain in the head; **headache, cephalalgia.**

encephalitis (en-sef-ah-li′tis): inflammation of the brain and the meninges (covering of the brain and spinal cord); also called **sleeping sickness.**

encopresis (en-ko-pre′sis): incontinence of feces not caused by age, disease, or physical disorder.

end-stage renal disease (ESRD): **uremia.**

endemic (en-dem′ik): a disease that is constantly present in a human community but is active in only a few cases.

endocarditis (en-do-kar-di′tis): inflammation of the inner lining of the heart (the *endocardium*).

endocardium (en-do-kar′de-um): the endothelial (inner) lining of the heart and connective tissue bed around the heart.

endocrine (en′do-krin): pertaining to internal secretions (not into ducts or tubes); applies to organs, such as *endocrine glands.*

endocytosis (en-do-si-to′sis): taking material that is too large to pass through the cell wall into a cell by phagocytosis or pinocytosis; *engulfing.*

endogenous (en-doj′en-us): normally occurring or existing within the body or in the community, as in the *endogenous microorganisms* in the body.

endometriosis (en-do-me-tri-o′sis): presence of endometrial tissue in places where it is not normally found.

endorphin (en-dor′fin): a naturally occurring analgesic that the body produces in response to exercise and other stimuli.

endoscope (en′do-skop): a tube-shaped, lighted device used to visualize or operate on hollow organs or within body cavities. Specialized endoscopes include the gastroscope, bronchoscope, and proctoscope. (The procedure is called *endoscopy*).

endotoxin (en-do-tok′sin): a heat-stable toxin (poison) that is released when a bacterial cell is disrupted (less potent than exotoxins).

enema (en′e-mah): an injection of fluid into the rectum, usually to induce evacuation of the bowel.

engagement (en-gaj′ment): the entrance of the fetal head (or presenting part) into the upper part of the pelvic opening.

engorgement (en-gorj′ment): local congestion or distention with fluids, as in *engorgement of the breasts* during pregnancy and lactation.

enteral (en′ter-al): within the intestine.

enteric (en′ter-ik): pertaining to the small intestine. *Enteric-coated* tablets are covered with a substance that prevents their digestion in the stomach.

enteritis (en-ter-i′tis): inflammation of the intestines.

entropion (en-tro′pe-on): inversion, turning inward, as the turning under of the eyelid.

enucleate (e-nu′kle-at): to remove whole and clean; often refers to *removal of an eye.*

enuresis (en-u-re′sis): involuntary discharge of urine, usually referring to discharge of urine occurring during sleep; *bedwetting.*

environment (en-vi′ron-ment): one's surroundings, the situation in which a person lives (as opposed to heredity).

enzyme (en′zim): a protein produced in a cell that activates or speeds up a chemical reaction.

ephelis (e-fe′lis): freckle.

epicardium (ep-i-kar'de-um): the inner layer of the pericardium, which is in contact with the heart.

epicutaneous (ep-e-ku-ta'ne-us): on the skin.

epidemic (ep-i-dem'ik): widespread disease in a certain geographical region.

epidermis (ep-i-der'mis): the outermost layer of the skin.

epididymitis (ep-i-did-i-mi'tis): inflammation of the epididymis (coiled, cordlike structures in the testes through which spermatozoa are carried).

epiglottis (ep-i-glot'is): cartilage that covers the entrance to the larynx.

epilepsy (ep'il-ep-se): a chronic disease marked by attacks of convulsions; a convulsive or **seizure disorder.**

epiphysis (e-pif'i-sis): the end of a long bone.

episiotomy (e-piz-e-ot'o-me): surgical incision into the perineum and vagina, usually during childbirth.

epispadias (ep-i-spa'de-as): absence of the upper wall of the urethra resulting in an abnormal location of the urethral opening, usually occurring in the male; the urethral meatus in epispadias may be located anywhere on the dorsum (upper side) of the penis.

epistaxis (ep-e-stak'is): nosebleed.

equilibrium (e-kwi-lib're-um): state of being in balance (emotional, physical, or chemical); **homeostasis.**

eructation (e-ruk-ta'shun): forceful expulsion of air from the stomach; *belching, burping.*

eruption (e-rup'shun): breaking out of or through the skin; as eruption of teeth or a rash.

erythema (er-i-the'mah): redness of the skin produced by congestion of the capillaries, as may follow a tuberculin test; bright red color associated with capillary dilation, can indicate fever or infection (*not* to be confused with ruddy).

erythrocyte (e-rith'ro-sit): red blood cell.

eschar (es'kar): dead skin and tissue that slough off after a chemical or thermal burn.

escharotomy (es-kah-rot'o-me): surgical incision into eschar and superficial fascia, particularly in a circumferentially burned limb (all the way around), to relieve pressure, thus restoring blood flow to distal unburned tissue.

esophagus (e-sof'ah-gus): passageway for digestion that extends from pharynx to stomach.

estriol (es'tre-ol): an estrogen (female hormone) found in high concentrations in urine.

ethanol (eth'an-nol): alcohol (ethyl or grain alcohol).

ethics (eth'iks): code or rules of behavior for a profession.

ethnic (eth'nik): pertaining to a social group that shares cultural bonds or racial physical traits.

etiology (e-te-ol'o-je): factors that cause a disease, as a disease of "unknown etiology."

euphoria (u-fo're-ah): a general feeling of comfort and well-being; may be exaggerated in mental disorders.

eupnea (yoop-ne'ah): normal respiration.

eustachian tube (u-sta'she-an tube): the passage from the throat to the middle ear; **auditory tube.**

euthanasia (u-thah-na'ze-ah, u-sta'she-an): an easy or painless death (may be induced), often referred to as mercy death or *mercy killing;* deliberate ending of life of a person who has an incurable or painful disease.

evaluation (e-val-yoo-a'shun): in nursing process, measuring the effectiveness of the assessing, diagnosing, planning, and implementing steps.

evaporation (e-vahp-er-a'shun): the process of changing a liquid or solid into a vapor (gas); to give off moisture. Evaporation of sweat helps cool the body.

eversion (e-ver'zhun): turning inside out; turning outward, as eversion of the foot.

evisceration (e-vis-er-a'shun): the protrusion of the intestines through an abdominal wound; removal of the internal contents of a body (as the eyeball).

evulsion (e-vul'shun): extraction by force.

exacerbation (eg-zas-er-ba'shun): increase in severity of a disease or of a single symptom, as in exacerbation of leukemia (as opposed to remission).

exanthum (eg-zan'them): any disease marked by skin eruptions or fever, as *exanthum subitum.*

excise (ek-siz'): to remove by cutting, as a *surgical excision.*

excoriation (eks-ko-re-a'shun): the removal of pieces of skin as a result of scratching or scraping, such as a "skinned" knee.

excreta (eks-kre'tah): waste products discharged from the body, such as feces and urine.

excreted (eks-kre'ted): thrown off or eliminated as waste matter by a normal discharge, as urine, feces, or perspiration.

exhaustion (eg-zawst'yun): extreme tiredness.

exocrine (ek'so-krin): secreting externally through a duct (as opposed to endocrine). *Tears* are an exocrine secretion.

exocytosis (ek-so-si-to'sis): the opposite of endocytosis; discharging material from a cell that is too large to pass through the cell wall.

exogenous (ek-soj'en-us): referring to organisms that enter from outside the body and cause infection.

exophthalmos (ek-sof-thal'mos): abnormal protrusion of the eyes, most often caused by hyperthyroidism (**exophthalmia**).

exotoxin (ek-so-tok'sin): a potent toxin (poison) formed by a bacteria, which can cause severe illness. (Exotoxins change when exposed to heat.)

expectoration (eks-pek-to-ra'shun): *spitting out* and coughing up mucus or other fluid from the lungs and the throat; sputum.

expiration (eks-pi-ra'shun): the exhalation of air from the lungs; sometimes used to refer to death.

exsanguinate (eks-sang'gwin-at): excessive blood loss due to hemorrhage, to "bleed to death."

exstrophy (ek'stro-fe): the turning inside out of an organ, as exstrophy of the bladder.

extended family: one's family beyond that of parents and siblings, (eg, aunts, uncles, cousins, grandparents).

extension (ek-sten'shun): the straightening of a flexed limb (opposite of flexion).

extracellular (ek-strah-sel'u-lar): outside the cell wall, as *extracellular fluid.*

extracorporeal (ek-strah-kor-po're-al): outside the body, as *extracorporeal circulation.*

extravasation (eks-trav-ah-za'shun): discharge or escape, as of blood, from a vessel into the tissues.

exudate (eks'u-date): material that has escaped from blood vessels and is deposited in the tissues or on tissue surfaces, usually contains protein substances; **drainage.**

eye contact: looking another person in the eye, as in "making eye contact" (not staring). "Correct" eye contact is *culturally influenced.*

Fahrenheit (far'en-hite): a temperature scale in which the boiling point of water is 212° and the freezing point is 32°.

failure to thrive (FTT): a condition in which an infant or young child demonstrates inadequate physical growth and other symptoms. (can result from neglect or physical disorders.) **marasmus.**

faint (faint): temporary loss of consciousness due to insufficient blood in the brain; **syncope.**

fascia (fash'e-ah): band or sheet of tissue covering and connecting muscles.

fat (fat): a component of foods that is composed of fatty or greasy material and that yields the highest caloric value per gram; **lipid** material; **adipose** tissue.

fatal (fa'tal): causing death; **lethal.**

fatigue (fah-tig'): weariness resulting from overexertion, extreme tiredness.

febrile (fe'bril): pertaining to a fever.

fecal (fe'kal): pertaining to feces.

feces (fe'seze): the residue, consisting of bacteria, secretions, chiefly of the liver, and a small amount of food residue which is discharged from the intestines: **stool, bowel movement.**

feedback (fed'bak): the receipt of external stimuli as a result of output (can be verbal, nonverbal, and emotional). (Physical feedback is involved in the self-regulation of hormones and electrolytes within the body.)

felony (fel'ah-ne): a crime more serious than a misdemeanor, usually punishable by imprisonment for more than a year. Felonies include murder, euthanasia, kidnapping, and blackmail.

femoral (fem'o-ral): pertaining to the femur (thigh bone) or to the thigh.

ferric (fer'ik): pertaining to iron.

fetal alcohol syndrome (fe'tal al'ko-hol sin'drom): a severe physical and mental birth defect caused by the mother's drinking alcohol during pregnancy.

fetid (fe'tid): having a disagreeable odor, rank, putrid.

fetus (fe'tus): the unborn offspring in the postembryonic (7–8 weeks after fertilization) period, which develops in the uterus.

fever (fe'ver): abnormally high body temperature.

fibrillation (fi-bri-la'shun): small, local, involuntary muscle contractions; not productive, as in *ventricular fibrillation* of the heart.

fibrin (fi'brin): most often formed in the liver and vital to blood clotting, threads of fibrin form a meshwork that provides the foundation for a blood clot.

fibrinogen (fi-brin'o-jen): a protein in blood plasma that is converted into fibrin by the action of thrombin. (Also called **clotting factor I.**)

fibrous (fi'brus): composed of or containing fibers, as in fibrous muscle bands in blood vessels.

fight-or-flight reaction: the automatic reaction, enhanced by the action of hormones such as adrenalin, which enables a person to escape or to deal with danger by fighting or running away.

filtration (fil-tra'shun): the passage or nonpassage of molecules through a filter (sieve), depending on the size of each molecule, as in *filtration of fluids by the kidney* to form urine.

fimbriated (fim'bre-at-ed): fringed, as the *fimbriated end of the ovarian (uterine) tube.*

fissure (fish'er): a narrow furrow or cleft, as a *fissure in the brain.*

fistula (fis'tu-lah): an abnormal tubelike passage, as an *anal fistula.*

flaccid (flak'sid): weak, lax, or lacking muscle tone; **flabby.**

flatus (fla'tus): gas in the intestines or stomach; gas expelled through the anus.

flex (fleks): to bend, as to flex the leg. (noun: **flexion**)

flow sheet: a form used to document patient care (often contains check-off spaces for assessments/review of systems and nursing care items such as bath/shower, oral hygiene, ambulation, wound care and bowel movements, as well as spaces to record items such as IV fluids, vital signs and weight, fluid intake, urine volume and specific gravity, blood glucose tests and patient teaching).

fluoridation (floo-or-i-da'shun): the addition of fluoride to drinking water in an attempt to prevent or reduce dental caries (decay), particularly in children.

fluoroscope (floo'or-o-skōp): a device that allows visualization by means of x-rays; used to examine the form and movement of deep body structures, as *fluoroscopy of the large bowel.*

focus charting: a type of nursing documentation in which the narrative portion is expanded to focus more on the patient's problems and their resolution.

follicle (fol'i-kl): a sac; pouchlike depression or cavity, as the *graafian follicle* of the ovary or the *hair follicle* in the skin.

folliculitis (fo-lik-u-li'tus): the inflammation of a follicle.

fontanel (fon-tah-nel'): a soft spot in the skull of a baby.

footdrop: contracture deformity preventing the patient from putting the heel on the floor, which occurs as a result of improper positioning; can also occur as a result of anterior leg muscle paralysis.

foramen (fo-ra'men): a natural opening or passage, as the *foramen ovale* in the fetal heart.

forceps (for'seps): a two-pronged surgical instrument for grasping or clamping tissues.

foreign body (for'in bod'e): any substance lodged in a place in which it does not belong. (A bean in the child's nose is a foreign body.)

foreskin (for'skin): a loose fold of skin covering the glans penis (removed in circumcision), also called **prepuce.**

formula (for'mu-lah): a prescribed method of preparation (such as infant formula); a symbolic expression of a compound (such as H_2O for water).

fracture (frak'tur): a break, as in a bone.

fraud (frod): dishonesty, cheating, deceit, misrepresentation.

freckle (frek'l): brown or tan macule-type spot on sun-exposed skin, most often in children and in those of certain skin tones. (Also called **ephelis** or **lentigo.**)

frenulum (fren'u-lum): a small fold that limits the movement of an organ or part, as the *frenulum linguae* (frenulum of the tongue, located under the tongue).

frequency (fre'kwen-se): the regularity with which an event occurs; voiding unusually often.

friable (fri'a-bl): **fragile,** easily broken, as *friable skin.*

friction (frik'shun): the act of rubbing.

frontal (frun'tal): pertaining to the forehead; pertaining to the front, anterior, or ventral portion of the body when divided longitudinally from side to side, as the *frontal plane.*

frostbite (frost'bit): freezing of tissue caused by exposure to cold.

function (funk'shun): the normal action of a part or organ.

functional (funk'shun-al): affecting the function, but not the structure, such as a functional disease (one for which no organic basis can be found); also called **ideopathic.**

fundus (fun'dus): bottom or base; the part of a hollow organ farthest from its mouth, as the *fundus of the uterus.*

furuncle (fyur-un'kl): painful, localized, pus-filled skin infection originating in a gland or hair follicle (**boil**).

fusion (fu'zhun): the joining together of two adjacent parts or bodies, as a fusion of vertebrae (*spinal fusion*).

gait (gate): a manner or style of walking.

galactosemia (gah-lak-to-se'me-ah): a genetic disorder in which the enzyme necessary for metabolizing galactose is absent.

gall (gawl): the **bile;** bile helps to digest fats and is stored in the gallbladder.

gallbladder (gahl'blad-er): muscular sac on the undersurface of the liver (it stores and releases bile).

ganglion (gang'gle-on): a knotlike mass, as a *nerve ganglion.*

gangrene (gang'green): the infection and death of a part or a tissue, caused by inadequate circulation.

gastric (gas'trik): pertaining to the stomach, as in gastric analysis (study of gastric fluids).

gastritis (gas-tri'tis): inflammation of the stomach lining.

gastrostomy (gas-tros'to-me): creation of an artificial opening into the stomach for the instillation of food and fluids.

gatch (gach): (verb) to adjust the hospital bed; (noun) the typical hospital bed, with a joint (gatch) in the middle and at the knee, which allows the patient to be placed into various therapeutic positions.

gavage (gah-vahzh'): passing food into the stomach through a tube; forced feeding; hyperalimentation (*not* total parenteral nutrition).

gay (ga): homosexual, sexually attracted to the same sex.

gene (jeen): a unit of heredity within a chromosome.

generalized: existing throughout a system (as opposed to localized).

generic name (je-ner'ik): the name assigned by the first manufacturer of a drug (often the chemical name).

genetics (je-net'iks): the study of *heredity* or inherited characteristics.

genital (jen'i-tal): pertaining to reproduction or to the reproductive organs (genitalia).

geriatrics (jer-e-at'riks): the branch of medicine that deals with aging and its related disorders.

germicidal (jer-mi-si'dal): destructive to pathogens.

gerontology (jer-on-tol'o-je): the study of aging.

gestation (jes-ta'shun): the period of development of the individual from fertilization to birth.

gingiva (jin-ji'vah): **gums,** the fleshy structure around the teeth.

gingivitis (jin-ji-vit'is): inflammation of the gingiva (gums).

gland (gland): an organ that secretes or excretes materials—*endocrine* (ductless) glands secrete hormones; *exocrine* glands secrete substances such as bile, saliva, oil, tears, and sweat into ducts.

glans penis (glanz pe'nis): smooth cap of the penis.

glaucoma (glaw-ko'mah): disease of the eye characterized by increased intraocular pressure.

globulin (glob'u-lin): proteins that are insoluble in water or highly concentrated saline solution, but which dissolve in isotonic (normal) saline. This category includes all plasma proteins, such as clotting factors and immunoglobulins, except albumin and prealbumin.

glomerulus (glo-mer'u-lus): small, twisted mass of capillaries, as the *glomerulus of the kidney.*

glossitis (glos-it'is): inflammation of the tongue.

glucose (gloo'kose): simple sugar, **dextrose;** it is the end product of carbohydrate metabolism and the primary source of energy for living organisms, found in the normal blood of all animals.

gluteal (gloo'te-al): pertaining to the buttocks.

glycogen (gli'ko-gen): a multiple sugar (polysaccharide) that is stored in the body; animal starch.

glycosuria (gli-ko-su're-ah): the abnormal presence of glucose (sugar) in the urine.

goiter (goi'ter): an enlargement of the thyroid gland, causing a swelling in the front part of the neck.

gonad (go'nad): a sex gland or organ.

gonorrhea (gon-o-re'ah): a sexually transmitted disease that is very contagious (and one that is now epidemic in the United States).

gout (gowt): a painful disease of the joints caused by excess uric acid in the blood.

graduate (grad'u-it): pitcher-shaped vessel used for measuring liquids, such as urine; person who has received a degree from a university or college or who has completed a nursing program.

graft (graft): a piece of skin or other tissue from one part of the body (or from another person's body) that is implanted into another body location.

gram (gram): metric unit of weight; abbreviated **g** (1 g = 15 grains = 1/30 oz).

granulation (gran-u-la'shun): the formation of fleshy tissue in healing wounds. Wounds heal best if they granulate from the inside outward.

Graves' disease (gravz): a condition that includes goiter, thyrotoxicosis, exophthalmos, and sometimes skin changes.

gravid (grav'id): pregnant; containing a developing child, as a *gravid uterus.*

gravida (grav'i-dah): a pregnant woman. (*multigravida:* a woman who is pregnant for at least the third time.)

gravital plane (grav'it-al plan): the line of gravity, as in driving an imaginary line through the top of your head, through the center of gravity, and through the base of your support.

gravity (grav'i-te): tendency toward the center of the earth. (**Specific gravity** is the weight of a substance as compared with that of another substance of equal volume, as of urine compared to water.)

groin (groin): the lowest part of the abdominal wall, at which point it joins the thigh, in the area of the external genitalia.

growth (groth'): change in body structure or size; formation of abnormal tissue, such as a tumor.

guaiac (gwi'ak): a test for occult (hidden) blood in body secretions or wastes, most often feces (stool).

gurney (gur'ne): four-wheeled cart. Also called **litter** and **wheeled stretcher.**

gums (gumz): fleshy part of the jaws that hold the teeth, **gingiva.**

gynecology (gin-e-kol'o-je): the branch of medicine that treats diseases of the genital tract in women.

habituation (hah-bit-u-a'shun): acquired tolerance due to repeated use or exposure, as *habituation to a drug.*

hallucination (ha-lu-si-na'shun): seeing, hearing, smelling, tasting, or feeling something when there is no objective stimulus. (Visual, auditory, olfactory, gustatory, or tactile hallucination, respectively.)

hallux (hal'uks): the big toe (digit) of the foot.

headache (hed'ak): pain in the head, **cephalalgia,** encephalalgia

health (helth'): optimum functioning of body, mind, and spirit; absence of disease.

health maintenance organization (**HMO**): an agency that provides prepaid health care, as needed, to members (as opposed to fee paid as service is given). The emphasis is on *prevention.*

heartburn (hart'burn): a burning sensation in the lower esophagus, not related to a heart disorder, **pyrosis.**

helminth (hel'minth): a parasitic worm.

hemangioma (he-man-je-o'mah): a benign tumor composed of blood vessels, usually present at birth; *large birthmark.*

hematemesis (he-mah-tem'e-sis): vomiting of blood.

hematocrit (he-mat'o-krit): the volume percentage of red blood cells in whole blood.

hematology (he-mah-tol'o-je): the study of blood and blood-forming tissues.

hematoma (he-mah-to'mah): a mass of coagulated blood (internal or under the skin) due to a break in the wall of a blood vessel; a mild form is a black eye or a bruise.

hematopoiesis (hem-ah-to-poy-e'sis): process of manufacturing blood cells, mostly occurring in the bone marrow.

hematuria (he-mah-tu're-ah): blood in the urine.

hemiplegia (hem-i-ple'je-ah): paralysis on one side of the body.

hemisphere (hem'i-sfer): usually refers to half of a spherical structure or organ, as the *hemispheres of the brain,* divided from front to back.

Hemoccult (hem'o-kult): a test for occult (hidden) blood in stool or body secretions.

hemodialysis (he-mo-di-al'i-sis): dialysis by way of an arterial shunt and using an artificial kidney (see also **dialysis**); used to remove toxic wastes from the blood in kidney disorders.

hemoglobin (he-mo-glo'bin): the oxygen-carrying pigment in blood that gives blood its red color.

hemolysis (he-mol'i-sis): destruction of red blood cells.

hemophilia (he-mo-fil'e-ah): a congenital condition characterized by spontaneous or traumatic bleeding.

hemoptysis (he-mop'ti-sis): expectoration (spitting) of blood or of blood-stained sputum.

hemorrhage (hem'or-aje): excessive bleeding (internal or external).

hemorrhoid (hem'or-oid): a dilation of the veins (varicose veins) of the anal region (may be internal or external).

hemostasis (he-mo-sta'sis): stoppage of bleeding (naturally, by clotting; or artificially, by tying off, compression, or removal of blood supply).

hemothorax (hem-o-tho'raks): presence of blood in the pleural (chest) cavity.

hepatic (he-pat'ik): pertaining to the liver.

hepatitis (hep-ah-ti'tis): inflammation of the liver. There are several types (A, B, C, D, E), some of which can be transmitted via blood or body secretions.

hereditary (he-red'i-ter-e): genetically determined, transmitted from parent to child, **inherited** (not acquired).

heredity (he-red'it-e): the genetic transmission of physical or mental characteristics from parent to offspring.

hermaphroditism (her-maf'ro-di-tizm): a rare condition characterized by the presence of both ovarian and testicular tissue and ambiguous sexual determination.

hernia (her'ne-ah): abnormal protrusion of an organ or tissue through the structure usually containing it, as an *inguinal hernia* or *hiatal hernia*, **rupture**.

herpes (her'peze): an inflammatory skin disease characterized by the formation of small vesicles in clusters (caused by a virus). (*Herpes simplex* causes fever blisters and canker sores in the mouth; *herpesvirus II* [herpesvirus genitalis] causes genital lesions; *herpes zoster* is also known as *shingles*.)

hesitancy (hez'ah-tan-se): inability to start the stream of urine.

heterograft (het'er-o-graft): a graft obtained from an animal and received by a person; also called **xenograft**.

heterosexual (het-er-o-seks'u-al): pertaining to different sexes; sexually attracted to the opposite sex.

hiatal (hi-a'tal): pertaining to an opening or gap, as a *hiatal hernia*.

hiccup (hik'up): an involuntary, spasmodic contraction of the diaphragm caused by the irritation of the phrenic nerve, which produces a sharp, inspiratory cough; **hiccough**.

hierarchy of needs (hi'er-ar-ke): established by Maslow, the hierarchy categorizes human needs from the most basic vital needs, survival needs (necessary to life), up through higher-level needs such as beauty, love, and learning.

hirsutism (her'sut-izm): abnormal hairiness, particularly in women.

histamine (his'tah-men): an amine found in all body tissues that stimulates dilation of small blood vessels and production of gastric juice. It is involved in inflammation and plays a major role in allergic reactions.

histology (his-tol'o-je): microscopic study of tissues.

histoplasmosis (his-to-plaz-mo'sis): fungal disease caused by repeated inhalation of contaminated dust.

hives (hivz): itching and burning eruptions of the skin; **urticaria**.

holistic (ho-lis'tik): considering man as a functioning whole; encompassing a totality, as in holistic health or high-level wellness. (noun: **Holism**—the state of wellness).

Homan's sign (ho'manz): a test for thrombophlebitis in which pain occurs behind the knee when the foot is hyperflexed upward (dorsiflexion).

homeostasis (ho-me-o-sta'sis): stability, balance, or **equilibrium** in normal body states.

homograft (ho'mo-graft): a graft from one person to another; also called **allograft**.

homosexual (ho-mo-seks'u-al): a person who is sexually attracted to members of the same sex, gay.

hordeolum (hor-de'o-lum): inflammation of the eyelid, **sty**.

hormone (hor'mon): a chemical substance that is secreted, usually from a ductless gland; regulates body processes.

hospice (hos'pis): a facility or program of care that is specifically designed to provide emotional and physical support to terminally ill patients and their families.

host (host): a plant or animal that harbors or nourishes another organism.

human immunodeficiency virus (HIV) (im-u-no-de-fish'en-se): virus that lowers normal immune response, rendering the person susceptible to otherwise harmless (opportunistic) organisms. HIV is the causative organism in acquired immunodeficiency syndrome (AIDS).

humidity (hu-mid'it-e): moisture in the atmosphere. (*Relative humidity* is expressed as a percentage.)

humor (hu'mor): fluid or semifluid substance in the body, as *aqueous humor* of the eye.

hyaline membrane disease (hi'a-lin): a respiratory disorder of newborns, **respiratory distress syndrome**.

hydramnios (hi-dram'ne-os): excessive amniotic fluid surrounding a fetus. **Polyhydramnios**.

hydration (hi-dra'shun): absorption of water, the balance of fluids in the body, as the *patient's hydration level*.

hydrocele (hi'dro-seel): painless swelling of the scrotum caused by a collection of fluid.

hydrocephalus (hi-dro-sef'ah-lus): accumulation of fluid in the skull; it is typically characterized by enlargement of the head if a shunt is not successful; also called **water on the brain**.

hydrometer (hi-drom'et-er): **urinometer** (used to measure specific gravity of a liquid, such as urine).

hydronephrosis (hi-dro-ne-fro'sis): distention of the pelvis and calices of the kidney with urine as a result of obstruction of the ureter or other urinary structure.

hydrotherapy (hi-dro-ther'ap-e): the use of water in the treatment of disease or injury.

hydrothorax (hi-dro-tho'raks): collection of noninfectious watery fluid in the pleural (chest) cavity.

hymen (hi'men): a fold of membrane sometimes found at the external opening of the vagina.

hyoid (hi'oid): shaped like a horseshoe, as the *hyoid bone* at the base of the tongue.

hyperalgesia (hi-per-al-je'ze-ah): increased sensitivity to pain.

hyperalimentation (hi-per-al-i-men-ta'shun): ingestion into the stomach by nasogastric tube of fairly large quantities of food and fluids (an incorrect term for total parenteral nutrition).

hyperbaric (hi-per-bar'ik): greater than normal pressure; *hyperbaric oxygenation* is provided within the hyperbaric chamber and allows the body to absorb more oxygen than at atmospheric pressure.

hypercapnia (hi-per-kap'ne-ah): excess of carbon dioxide in the blood.

hypercarbia (hi-per-kar'be-ah): hypercapnia.

hyperemesis (hi-per-em'e-sis): excessive vomiting. (**Hyperemesis gravidarum** is characterized by pernicious vomiting in pregnancy.)

hyperesthesia (hi-per-es-the'ze-ah): increased sensitivity to stimuli, as to pain.

hyperglycemia (hi-per-gli-se'me-ah): abnormally high blood sugar.

hyperopia (hi-per-oh'pe-ah): light rays focus behind the retina, **far-sightedness**.

hyperplasia (hi-per-pla'ze-ah): abnormal increase in size of a tissue or organ, caused by the excessive growth of new normal cells, as *benign prostatic hyperplasia*.

hyperpnea (hi-perp-ne'ah): abnormal increase in rate and depth of respirations.

hypersomnia (hi-per-som'ne-ah): excessive sleep.

hypertension (hi-per-ten'shun): elevation of blood pressure; also called **high blood pressure**.

hyperthyroidism (hi-per-thi'roi-dizm): excessive function of the thyroid gland, excessive thyroid hormone in the body.

hypertrophy (hi-per'trof-e): an abnormal enlargement of a part or organ, caused by enlargement of existing cells.

hyperventilation (hi-per-ven-ti-la'shun): abnormally fast and deep breathing, usually caused by anxiety, resulting in reduction of carbon dioxide and an increase in oxygen.

hypervolemia (hi-per-vo-le'me-ah): abnormal increase in volume of circulating fluid in the body.

hyphema (hi-fe'mah): hemorrhage into the anterior chamber of the eye.

hypnosis (hip-no'sis): an artifically induced passive state, in which there is increased responsiveness to suggestions and commands; the person appears trancelike.

hypnotic (hip-not'ik): a drug or agent that induces sleep.

hypochondriac (hi-po-kon'dre-ak): morbid anxiety about one's health.

hypodermic (hi-po-der'mik): under the skin; **subcutaneous**.

hypodermoclysis (hi-po-der-mo'kli-sis): introduction of large quantities of fluids into subcutaneous tissues.

hypoesthesia (hi-po-es-the′ze-ah): diminished sensitivity to stimuli.

hypogastric (hi-po-gas′trik): under the stomach, pertaining to the lower middle abdomen.

hypoglycemia (hi-po-gli-se′me-ah): abnormally low blood sugar.

hypomania (hi-po-ma′ne-ah): a mood disorder resembling mania, but of lesser degree; hyperactivity, expansive mood.

hypophysis (hi-pof′i-sis): the **hypophysis cerebri;** the pituitary gland.

hypoplasia (hi-po-pla′ze-ah): incomplete development of an organ or tissue.

hyporeflexia (hi-po-re-flek′se-ah): diminished reflexes.

hypospadias (hi-po-spa′de-as): abnormal development in the male in which the urethra opens on the underside of the penis or onto the perineum.

hypostatic (hi-po-stat′ik): stagnant, due to immobility, as **hypostatic pneumonia.**

hypotension (hi-po-ten′shun): chronic depression in blood pressure; abnormally *low blood pressure.*

hypothalamus (hi-po-thal′am-us): a tiny but complex portion of the brain (believed to be the "master controller" of the hormones).

hypothermia (hi-po-ther′me-ah): low body temperature; also a syndrome (*accidental* hypothermia), caused by exposure to cold, which may be fatal. Hypothermia may also be *induced* for therapeutic purposes such as surgery or *pathologic* as a result of faulty thermoregulation (temperature control). *Hypothermic blanket*: cooling blanket.

hypovolemia (hy-po-vo-le′me-ah): abnormal decrease in volume of circulating blood (plasma) in the body.

hypoxia (hi-pok′se-ah): reduction of oxygen in the tissues; also called **hypoxemia.**

hysterectomy (his-ter-ek′to-me): surgical removal of the uterus.

hysteria (his-ter′e-ah): psychoneurosis characterized by lack of emotional control or physical actions.

iatrogenic (i-at-ro-jen′ik): resulting from the activities of a physician (usually refers to an adverse condition in a patient that occurs as a result of treatment).

icterus (ik′ter-us): yellowing of the skin, also called **jaundice,** as in *icterus gravis.*

idiopathic (id-e-o-path′ik): occurring without known cause, **functional.**

idiosyncrasy (id-e-o-sin′krah-se): an individual peculiarity, *habit.*

ileitis (il-e-i′tis): inflammation of the ileum (lower portion of the small intestine).

ileostomy (il-e-os′to-me): surgical opening of the ileum onto the abdomen by means of a stoma.

ileum (il′e-um): distal portion of the small intestine. (adj: **ileal**)

ileus (il′e-us): intestinal obstruction, usually as a result of inadequate peristalsis.

illness (il′nes): pronounced deviation from the normal healthy state.

imagery (im′aj-re): suggestions to relieve pain or stress, given during self-hypnosis or relaxation.

immobilize (im-mo′bil-ize): to prevent motion, as with a cast or splint.

immunity (i-mu′ni-te): the condition of being nonsusceptible to a certain disease.

immunization (im-u-niz-a′shun): the process of providing protection against infection from a particular disease; **vaccination, inoculation.**

immunogen (im′u-no-jen): a substance capable of initiating or stimulating an immune response.

immunosuppressive (im-yoo-no-su-pres′iv): referring to deliberate suppression of the natural immune system, as in chemotherapy for cancer. (adj: **immunosuppression**)

impaction (im-pak′shun): a condition in which the feces are so tightly fixed in the rectum or colon that the patient cannot expel them. (*fecal impaction*). Wisdom teeth can also become impacted.

impairment (im-par′ment): a defect or disability, as *intellectual impairment.*

imperforate (im-per′fo-rit): lacking a normal opening, sealed, as an *imperforate anus* in the newborn.

impetigo (im-pe-ti′go): bacterial infection of the skin.

implementation (im-ple-men-ta′shun): in nursing process, the carrying out of nursing care plans; also called **interventions.**

impotence (im′po-tens): inability of the male to achieve an adequate erection for sexual intercourse.

incentive spirometer (in-sen′tiv spi-rom′i-ter): a device used to promote full inflation and oxygenation of the lungs, used particularly after surgery and in lung disorders such as pneumonia.

incest (in′sest): sexual activity between close relatives.

incise (in-size′): to cut; to make a surgical incision. (Noun: **incision.**)

incontinence (in-kon′tin-ens): inability to control urination or defecation, (*incontinent*).

incubation (in-ku-ba′shun): the period of a disease between exposure to a microorganism and the manifestation of the clinical symptoms of the disease, the *incubation period.*

incus (ing′kus): one of the bones (ossicles) of the middle ear, the *anvil.*

induction (in-duk′shun): causing to occur, as in causing labor to begin or causing unconsciousness for surgery.

induration (in-du-ra′shun): a hardened place, a lump, as in the skin in a positive reaction to a tuberculin test.

infarct (in′farkt): a localized area of tissue death (necrosis) caused by inadequate circulation, as a *myocardial infarction.*

infection (in-fek′shun): the invasion and multiplication of infective agents in body tissues with a resultant reaction to their presence and their toxins.

infertility (in-fer-til′i-te): inability to produce offspring; lack of fertility or productivity, *barren.*

infiltration (in-fil-tra′shun): the diffusion or accumulation in the tissues or cells of substances not normally present or not normally present in those amounts, as *infiltration of an IV.*

inflammation (in-flah-ma′shun): a condition resulting from irritation in any part of the body, marked by pain, heat, redness, and swelling.

influenza (in-floo-en′zah): an acute viral respiratory infection occurring in epidemics and traced to different viruses. (Also called **flu,** *grippe.*)

informed consent: giving full information and making sure the patient understands before the patient consents to surgery or other medical procedure.

infrared (in-frah-red′): radiation with a wavelength longer than the red end of the spectrum, used therapeutically to provide deep heat.

infusion (in-fu′zhun): slow induction of fluids (not blood) into a vein, as an *intravenous (IV) infusion* of a solution.

ingestion (in-jes′chun): the taking in of food or other substances by mouth, eating.

inguinal (ing′gwi-nal): pertaining to the groin, as an *inguinal hernia.*

inhalation (in-hah-la′shun): the drawing of air, vapor, or fumes into the lungs.

inhibition (in-hi-bish′un): the partial or complete restraint of any process (to inhibit).

injection (in-jek′shun): forcing a liquid into a part of the body or into a body cavity (usually refers to medication passed into a muscle or under the skin by means of a needle and syringe).

inoculation (in-ok-u-la′shun): introduction of a minute amount of a virus or disease-producing microorganism into the body to give protection against certain diseases; **vaccination, immunization.**

inoperable (in-op'er-ah-b'l): denoting a situation in which surgery would not be effective as treatment, as in *inoperable* or far-advanced *cancer*.

insanity (in-san'i-te): the legal or lay term referring to a severe mental disorder; **psychosis.**

insidious (in-sid'e-us): coming on gradually; of subtle or unnoticeable development, sneaky, as the insidious development of a cancer.

in situ (in si'tu): confined to the site of origin, as a *cancer in situ.*

insomnia (in-som'ne-ah): sleeplessness; chronic inability to sleep.

inspiration (in-spi-ra'shun): **inhalation,** drawing of air into the lungs.

instillation (in-sti-la'shun): administration of a liquid one drop at a time, as the instillation of eyedrops.

insufflation (in-su-fla'shun): expansion of a body cavity by blowing up with gas, air, or powder (used to facilitate examination of laparoscopic surgery); "snorting" of a drug such as cocaine.

insulin (in'su-lin): a hormone secreted by the islets of Langerhans of the pancreas which is vital in carbohydrate metabolism. Parenteral insulin is often required in diabetes mellitus.

integument (in-teg'u-ment): the **skin,** the *integumentary system.*

integumentary (in-teg-u-men'tar-e): denoting a covering.

intercellular (in-ter-sel'u-lar): situated between the cells.

intercom (in'ter-kom): the intercommunication system between the patient room and the central nursing station; also the paging system of the hospital.

interdependent (in-ter-de-pen'dent): depending on one another; one action occurs because of another. Activities of various organ systems are interdependent; for example, the nerves, muscles, and bones are interdependent on each other. Interdependent nursing actions are those that occur in cooperation with the physician and other members of the team.

interferon (in-ter-fer'on): a substance released by cells in response to a virus (and some other agents) that results in the decrease of viral multiplication. Interferon is a biologic response modifier used in cancer treatment.

intermittent (in-ter-mit'ent): occurring at intervals; having *alternating* periods of activity and inactivity, as an intermittent fever.

interneuron (in-ter-nu'ron): a neuron between the first afferent neuron and the last motor neuron; neurons whose processes are all in a specific area, such as the olfactory lobe.

interoceptor (in-ter-o-sep'ter): a sensory nerve terminal that transmits impulses *from* the viscera (internal organs).

interstitial (in-ter-stish'al): situated in the interspaces of tissue, as in interstitial or extracellular fluid (not blood or lymph).

intervention (in-ter-ven'shun): to interrupt or intervene in a disease process, as in **nursing** or **surgical intervention**; in nursing process, also called **implementation.**

intima (in'ti-mah): the innermost lining of a blood vessel; also called **tunica intima.**

intracellular (in-trah-sel'u-lar): within the cells, as in *intracellular fluid.*

intracranial (in-trah-kra'ne-al): within the skull (cranium).

intracranial pressure, ICP: the pressure of subarachnoidal fluid in the space between the skull and the brain. Elevated, increased intracranial pressure (IICP) is a significant sign in determining neurologic disorders.

intractable (in-trak'ta-bl): that which cannot be relieved, continuous, unrelentless, as in *intractable pain.*

intradermal (in-trah-der'mal): within the substance of the skin (dermis), **intracutaneous,** as an intradermal tuberculin or allergy test.

intramedullary (in-trah-med'u-lar-re): into the spinal cord or spinal cavity, as *intramedullary injection;* the medulla oblongata; within the marrow of the bones.

intramuscular (in-trah-mus'ku-lar): within the muscle substance, as an *intramuscular injection.*

intraoperative (in-trah-op'er-a-tiv): occurring during a surgical operation.

intrapartum (in-trah-par'tum): occurring during childbirth.

intrathecal (in-trah-the'kal): through the theca of the spinal cord into the subarachnoid space, as insertion of a spinal needle or giving a drug intrathecally.

intravenous (in-trah-ve'nus): within a vein, as *intravenous infusion.*

intrusive (in-tru'siv): in psychiatry, a patient who interrupts or constantly interferes with others or who invades others' personal space.

intubation (in-tu-ba'shun): the insertion of a tube, as into the larynx for breathing.

intussusception (in-tus-sus-sep'shun): the telescoping or prolapsing of one part of the intestine into an adjacent part.

in utero (u'ter-o): within the uterus.

invasive (in-va'siv): term used to describe surgery and some diagnostic tests that involve an incision or puncture through the skin, insertion of an instrument (such as an endoscope), or injection of a foreign substance (such as dye) into the body; quickly spread widely throughout the body, such as *invasive cancer.*

inversion (in-ver'zhun): turning inside out; reversal.

in vitro (ve'tro): in a test tube or artificial environment, as *in vitro fertilization* of an ovum.

in vivo (ve'vo): in the human body.

involuntary (in-vol'un-ta-re): not performed under the control of the will, as *involuntary muscle.*

involution (in-vo-lu'shun): turning inward; a retrograde change of the entire body or in a particular organ, as *involution of the uterus* after childbirth.

ion (i'on): an atom with an electrical charge; positive (**cation**), negative (**anion**). Substances forming ions are called *electrolytes.*

irradiation (i-ra-de-a'shun): exposure to radiant energy; usually refers to x-ray or radioactive energy.

irrigation (ir-i-ga'shun): washing out by a stream of water or solution, as irrigation of the urinary bladder or emergency irrigation of the eye after exposure to a caustic substance.

iris (i'rus): pigmented section over the front of the eyeball that gives the eye its color.

irritant (ir'i-tant): an agent that causes irritation, stimulation, or undue sensitivity to any part of the body.

ischemia (is-ke'me-ah): decrease or lack of blood supply to a body part as a result of the obstruction or constriction of blood vessels.

isograft (i'so-graft): a graft between genetically identical people, as in identical twins.

isolation (i-so-la'shun): the state of being isolated or separated from others; separation of people with infectious diseases from others. *Body substance isolation*: isolation based on universal body substance precautions *plus* precautions against contact and enteric routes of transmission ("stop sign" isolation). *Category-specific isolation*: isolation based on type of hazard present (respiratory, contact, enteric, wound). *Disease-specific isolation*: isolation based on specific hazards of a particular disease. *Protective/neutropenic (reverse) isolation*: isolation that protects the patient from organisms outside the room, used for immunocompromised patients.

isometric (i-so-met'rik): having the same length or dimensions, as isometric exercises (pushing against stable resistance); also called **muscle setting.**

isotonic (i-so-ton'ik): of equal tension; *normal,* as *isotonic saline* that is the same tonicity as body fluids; exercise that shortens the muscle but does not change the force of contraction.

jaundice (jawn'dis): a yellowish discoloration of the skin due to excess bile, **icterus.**

jejunectomy (je-joo-nek'to-me): excision of part or all of the *jejunum* (the part of the small intestine between the duodenum and the ileum).

juvenile (joo've-nil): pertaining to childhood or immaturity; youth.

juxtaposition (juks-tah-po-zish'un): very close together; apposition, adjoining.

Kaposi's sarcoma (kap′o-sez): an opportunistic malignancy that is associated with AIDS and primarily affects the skin.

keloid (ke′loid): a sharply elevated scar on the skin consisting of dense tissue; found most often following a cut or burn and most common in African Americans.

keratin (ker′ah-tin): a protein that is a major component of hair, nails, and the epidermis and is the organic matrix of tooth enamel. (Keratin is sometimes used as the coating for enteric-coated tablets.)

keratitis (ker-a-ti′tis): inflammation of the cornea of the eye.

keratoconus (ker-ah-to-ko′nus): abnormal cone-shaped growth of the cornea, causing severe astigmatism and often blindness; a common indication for corneal transplant.

keratoma (ker-ah-to′ma): **keratosis;** any horny growth, such as a wart or a callous.

keratoplasty (ker′ah-to-plas-te): plastic surgery of the cornea of the eye, **corneal grafting,** corneal transplantation.

kernicterus (ker-nik′ter-us): a condition in the newborn characterized by high levels of bilirubin in the blood, which causes severe neurologic symptoms.

ketosis (ke-to′sis): an increase in ketone bodies in the body tissues and fluids; also called **ketoacidosis.**

kidneys (kid′nees): two bean-shaped organs located at the small of the back at the lower edge of the ribs on either side of the vertebral column. Urine is formed in the kidneys and levels of many electrolytes are regulated by the kidneys. Blood pressure is greatly influenced by the kidneys.

kilocalorie (kil′o-cal-or-e): unit of measurement that specifies the heat energy in a particular amount of food (1 kilocalorie = 1000 calories).

kinesiology (ki-ne-se-ol′o-je): study of body movements.

Koplik's spots (kop′liks spots): small, bright red spots in the mouth and throat found in the early stages of measles (rubeola).

Korotkoff's sounds (ko-rot′kofs): sounds heard during blood pressure measurement with a stethoscope (auscultation).

Kussmaul's respiration (koos′mowlz): severe paroxysmal dyspnea, as in diabetic acidosis and coma; also called **air hunger.**

kyphosis (ki-fo′sis): an abnormal increase in the thoracic curvature of the spine, giving a *hunchback* appearance, commonly a result of osteoporosis.

labia (la′be-ah): literally means lip, as the *labia minora* and *labia majora* of the external female genitalia.

labile (la′bil): unstable; fluctuating, as a labile fever. In psychiatry: rapid mood swings and marked behavior changes.

labor (la′bor): the process by which the uterus contracts and expels the fetus.

labyrinth (lab′i-rinth): the inner ear, including the vestibule, cochlea and semicircular canals.

laceration (las-er-a′shun): a wound produced by tearing or ripping (as opposed to an incision made in surgery).

lacrimal (lak′ri-mal): pertaining to tears, as the lacrimal glands of the eyes, which produce tears.

lactation (lak-ta′shun): secretion of milk by the mammary glands (breasts).

lactose (lak′tose): a sugar found in milk; commonly called **milk sugar.**

lactose intolerance (lak′tos): a genetic absence of the enzyme necessary for metabolizing lactose in milk and dairy products (lactase).

Lamaze method (lah-maz′): a method of natural childbirth.

laminectomy (lam-i-nek′to-me): surgical removal of a posterior arch of a vertebra, more correctly called *lumbar decompression.*

lance (lans): to cut, incise or drain.

lancet (lans-et′): small sterile device used for puncturing the skin to obtain a small sample of blood, as for a blood glucose test.

lanugo (lah-nu′go): fine, downy hair covering the body of a fetus.

laparoscope (lap′ah-ro-skop): endoscope used to examine the peritoneal cavity (laparoscopy).

laryngectomy (lar-in-jek′to-me): surgical removal of the larynx (voice box); the person is then called a **laryngectomee.**

laryngitis (lar-in-ji′tis): inflammation of the larynx, often causing hoarseness or loss of voice.

laryngopharynx (lahr-ing′go-far-inks): lowest segment of the pharynx or throat.

larynx (lahr′inks): boxlike structure of cartilage in the midline of the neck; also called **voice box.**

laser (la′zer): a specific type of intense light that is capable of producing immense heat and power (sometimes used in surgery or in diagnosis).

latent (la′tent): a condition that is concealed or not manifest but is still present, hidden, as *latent syphilis.*

lateral (lat′er-al): pertaining to a side; away from the midline.

lavage (lah-vahzh′): washing out of an organ, such as the stomach or bowel; **irrigation.**

laxative (laks′ah-tiv): a mild **cathartic** that acts to promote evacuation of the bowel.

lens (lenz): a transparent, crystalline structure in the eye that converges or scatters light rays before they focus images on the retina.

lentigo (len-ti′go): a small, brown, pigmented area on the skin due to an increased amount of melanin, commonly known as a **freckle.**

lesbian (lez′be-an): a female homosexual.

lesion (le′zhun): a break in the body tissue, such as a sore or a wound; loss of function of a body part.

let-down: a sensation in the breasts of the lactating woman when she hears or thinks about her baby. *Let-down reflex:* the flowing of milk into the breasts when the mother begins to nurse (*milk-ejection reflex*).

lethal (le′thal): deadly, causing death, **fatal.**

lethargy (leth′ar-je): a condition of sluggishness or mental dullness; indifference.

leukemia (loo-ke′me-ah): a malignant disease of blood-forming organs; may be classified as acute or chronic and also in relationship to the specific blood cell affected, as acute lymphoid (lymphocytic), myelocytic, or granulocytic leukemia.

leukocyte (loo′ko-sit): white blood cell (**WBC).**

leukopenia (loo-ko-pe′ne-ah): decrease in the number of leukocytes in the blood (5000 per cubic millimeter or less).

leukoplakia (loo-ko-pla′ke-ah): a disorder characterized by white patches on the mucous membrane of the cheeks, gums, or tongue that cannot be rubbed off, as *leukoplakia buccalis.*

leukorrhea (lu-ko-re ah): a whitish or yellowish viscid discharge from the vagina or uterus.

liability (li-ah-bil′a-te): something one is required to do, an obligation, often financial; being found guilty of inappropriate or illegal acts.

libel (li′bl): a false or damaging written statement or photograph.

libido (li-be′do): sexual desire.

lie (li): relationship between the long part of the fetus in utero to that of the mother, **presentation, position.**

ligament (lig′ah-ment): a fibrous band connecting bones or cartilages.

ligate (li′gate): to bind or tie with a ligature, as in surgery (such as a *tubal ligation*).

lightening (lit′en-ing): the feeling of decreased abdominal distention caused by the descent of the pregnant uterus deeper into the pelvis, usually 2 to 3 weeks before delivery.

linea (lin′e-ah): a narrow ridge or line. *Linea alba* (al′bah): a white line, the vertical line in the center of the abdomen. *Linea nigra* (ni′grah): black line, the linea alba when it is darkly pigmented during pregnancy.

lingua (ling′gwah): tongue.

lipemia (li-pe′me-ah): fat, **hyperlipemia;** an excess of lipids (fats) in the blood.

lipid (lip′id):   fat.

lipoma (li-po′mah):   a benign tumor composed of fatty tissues.

lithiasis (li-thi′ah-sis):   the condition of having stones (calculi), as in *cholelithiasis* (stones in the gall bladder).

lithotomy (li-thot′o-me):   incision into a duct or organ for the purpose of removing calculi (stones), as a *ureterolithotomy* (removal of kidney stones from the ureter).

lithotripsy (lith′o-trip-se):   the crushing or breaking up of stones (calculi) in the urinary tract or gallbladder. *Extracorporeal shock wave lithotripsy, ESWL:* noninvasive breaking up of stones by means of shock waves directed onto the outside of the body.

litmus paper (lit′mus):   strips of paper used to indicate acidity or alkalinity (pH) of a solution.

litter (lit′er):   four-wheeled cart; also called **gurney, stretcher.** A *litter scale* is used to weigh patients who cannot stand.

liver (liv′er):   largest glandular organ in the body; it plays an important part in many bodily functions.

living will (liv′ing wil):   legal form signed by a person requesting that no extraordinary measures be taken to save his or her life in terminal illness, a form of *advance directive*.

lobe (lob):   defined portions of an organ or gland, such as the lung, liver, ear, brain or tooth.

local (lo′kal):   limited to one part or place; not general, as *local anesthesia* or *localized pain*.

lochia (lo′ke-ah):   the vaginal discharge occurring for 1 or 2 weeks following childbirth.

locus (lo′kus):   place or site.

lordosis (lor-do′sis):   an abnormal increase in the lumbar curvature of the spine; sometimes called **swayback.**

lumbar region (lum′bar re′jun):   that part of the back between the sacrum and the thorax.

lumen (lu′men):   a tube or channel within a tube, as the lumen of a catheter or a needle.

lumpectomy (lump-ek′to-me):   removal of a tumor, leaving associated tissue intact, as a *breast lumpectomy*.

lung (lung):   one of two cone-shaped organs that fills the chest cavity, the organ of respiration.

luxation (luk-sa′shun):   **dislocation.** (*Subluxation* is incomplete dislocation.)

lymph (limf):   transparent fluid that circulates throughout the body tissues and that can be a means by which a malignancy is spread; *lymph nodes* remove bacteria and toxins from the blood and may assist in the formation of antibodies.

lymphocyte (lim′fo-sit):   a particular type of leukocyte that is formed in lymphoid tissue and participates in cell-mediated immunity, as in T cells or T lymphocytes.

lymphoma (lim-fo′mah):   a malignant condition of lymphoid tissue.

lysis (li′sis):   destruction due to a specific agent, as lysis of red blood cells; also a *gradual recovery* from disease (as opposed to crisis).

maceration (mas-e-ra′shun):   the softening of a solid due to soaking, until connective tissue fibers are dissolved, such as maceration of the skin under a cast or bandage.

macrophage (mak′ro-faj):   a large cell derived from a monocyte.

macula (mak′u-la):   a flat discolored spot on the skin; a dense scar of the cornea that can be seen without optical aids.

mainstreaming (man′strem-ing):   bringing physically and intellectually challenged people into school or activities involving nonchallenged people their own age.

malaise (mă′laz):   feeling of illness, general bodily discomfort.

malformation (mal-for-ma′shun):   deformity, incorrect formation.

malignant (ma-lig′nant):   deadly; tending to become progressively worse, as a *malignant tumor;* cancer.

malingering (mah-ling′ger-ing):   a deliberate feigning or exaggeration of the symptoms of illness or injury.

malleus (mal′e-us):   *hammer;* one of three bones (stapes) of the inner ear.

malnutrition (mal-nu-trish′un):   poor intake or inadequate use of food by the body, faulty nourishment.

malocclusion (mal-o-kloo′zhun):   incorrect positioning of the teeth, often corrected by *orthodontia*.

malpractice (mal-prak′tis):   injurious or faulty treatment, professional misconduct.

mammary (mam′ar-e):   pertaining to the mammary gland (**breast**).

mammography (mam-og′ra-fe):   x-ray examination of the breasts, capable of detecting some breast cancers.

mammoplasty (mam′o-plas-te):   plastic surgery of the breast. *Augmentation* m.: enlargement or uplifting of the breast. *Reconstruction* m.: repair following mastectomy or injury. *Reduction* m.: decreasing the size of the breast.

mania (man′ne-ah):   a disordered mental state of extreme excitement; extreme and exhaggerated hyperactivity as a phase of bipolar disorder, expansiveness, increased speed of speech and thoughts, grandiosity. As a combining form: obsessive preoccupation, such as *pyromania* (preoccupation with fire).

marasmus (mah-raz′mus):   a particular form of malnutrition usually seen in infants; also called **failure-to-thrive,** often due to a protein deficiency.

margin (mar′jin):   a boundary line, edge.

marrow (mar′o):   the spongelike material in the hollow cavities in bones. (The red bone marrow produces many blood cells.)

mastectomy (mas-tek′to-me):   surgical removal of all or part of the breast, total mastectomy or partial mastectomy. (Removal of only a lump is called *lumpectomy*).

masticate (mas′ti-kate):   to chew.

mastitis (mas-ti′tis):   inflammation of the breast, as in *chronic cystic mastitis*.

mastoiditis (mas-toid-i′tis):   inflammation of the mastoid process (the projection at the base of the mastoid portion of the temporal bone).

masturbation (mas-tur-ba′shun):   the handling of the genitals to obtain erotic stimulation.

maturation (mat-u-ra′shun):   the process of ripening or becoming fully developed, "growing up."

meatus (me-a′tus):   opening or passage, as of the urinary or *auditory meatus,* **orifice.**

meconium (me-ko′ne-um):   the dark green or black fecal substance in the intestines of the fully grown fetus or newborn infant, passed as the first one or two stools after birth.

media (me′de-ah):   center, middle as *otitis media*, an infection of the middle ear; also substances on which cultures of specific microorganisms are grown, such as agar.

medication (med′i-ka′shun):   a substance other than food used to prevent disease, to aid in diagnosis and treatment of disease, and to restore or maintain functions in body tissues; also called **drug.**

medulla (me-dul′ah):   inner portion of an organ, as the *medulla oblongata* (a center portion of the hindbrain) or the *medulla of the kidney* (as opposed to cortex).

megacolon (meg-ah-ko′lon):   dilation or stretching of the colon, giant colon.

meibomian cyst (mi-bo′me-un):   **chalazion.**

melanin (mel′ah-nin):   a dark pigment that may be present in a tumor (**melanoma**) or may be excreted in the urine (**melanuria**).

melasma (me-laz′mah):   **chloasma.**

melena (mĕ-le′nah):   the passage of dark-colored stools because of partially or fully digested blood; also used to mean abnormal blood in stool or vomitus.

membrane (mem′brane):   a thin layer of tissue covering a surface (as cell or *plasma membrane*), covering a body part or lining a body cavity (as *mucous membrane*). **Drum membrane:** tympanic membrane, (*ear drum*). **Fetal membranes:** membranes that protect the embryo, "bag of waters."

menarche (me-nar′ke):   the establishment of menstruation, the first menses.

Meniere's disease (men-e-arz'): a disorder of the labyrinth of the inner ear, causing vertigo, headache, tinnitus, and hearing loss.

meninges (men-in'jeze): the membranes that cover the brain and spinal cord. (dura mater, arachnoid, pia mater).

meningitis (men-in-ji'tis): inflammation of the meninges.

meningomyelocele (me-ning-go-mi'e-lo-sel): herniation of a portion of the spinal cord, meninges, spinal fluid, and nerves through a defect in the spinal column.

meniscus (me-nis'kus): a crescent-shaped structure, as the crescent-shaped surface of a liquid or a fibrous cartilage within a joint, especially of the knee. (The shape of the meniscus must be considered when measuring liquid medications.)

menopause (men'o-pawz): cessation of menstruation in the female; also called **climacteric, change-of-life.**

menorrhagia (men-o-ra'je-ah): abnormally profuse menstrual flow.

menstruation (men-stroo-a'shun): periodic vaginal discharge of blood and tissues from the nonpregnant uterus; also called **period, menses.**

mental (men'tal): pertaining to the mind and thought processes.

mesentery (mes'en-ter-e): a membranous fold of tissue that attaches internal organs to the body wall.

metabolism (me-tăb'o-lizm): the sum of all chemical and physical processes in building up (*anabolism*) and breaking down (*catabolism*) of protoplasm in living cells. (*Basal metabolism:* the minimum amount of energy used by the body at rest.)

metastasis (me-tas'tah-sis): transfer of disease organisms or cells from one organ or body part to another not directly connected with it; often refers to cancer cells or tuberculosis.

metrorrhagia (mē-tro-ra'je-ah): uterine bleeding occurring at completely irregular intervals and sometimes for a prolonged length of time.

microbe (mi'crobe): a minute or tiny organism (**microorganism**); often refers to pathogenic (harmful) bacteria.

microbiology (mi-'kro-bi-ol'o-je): study of microorganisms.

microencephaly (mi-kro-en-seph'a-le): congenitally small skull and small amount of brain tissue.

micron (mī'kron): micrometer, one thousandth millimeter or one millionth meter; symbol for micron is μm.

microorganism (mi-kro-or'gah-nizm): an organism that cannot be seen by the naked eye, but can be seen with a microscope (such as bacteria, viruses, fungi, and protozoa).

microsurgery (mi-kro-ser'jer-e): performance of very minute (tiny) and exacting surgery using an *operating microscope,* such as eye surgery.

micturition (mik-tu-rish'un): the passage of urine from the urinary bladder; also called **voiding, urinating.**

midline (mid'line): an imaginary line dividing the body into right and left halves, as a *midline incision.*

midwife (mid'wife): a person (not a physician) who is specially trained to assist in prenatal care and the delivery of babies, usually a registered nurse.

migraine (mī'grane): severe periodic headaches, frequently unilateral, and often accompanied by nausea, vomiting, and sensory disturbances.

milia (mil'e-ah): tiny, whitish nodules on the skin, **whiteheads;** when present in neonates, usually appear on the nose and disappear within a few weeks (sing: **milium**).

miliary (mil'e-er-e): having to do with many small ("travelling") lesions, as in *miliary tuberculosis.*

milieu (mē-lyuh'): environment, surroundings, as *therapeutic milieu* in mental health units.

mineral (min'er-al): a nonorganic chemical element or compound vital for building bones and teeth, maintaining muscle tone, regulating body process, and maintaining acid-base balance. Common minerals in the body include calcium and iron.

miosis (mī-o'sis): extreme contraction of the pupil of the eye.

misdemeanor (mis-de-me'ner): a crime less serious than a felony, usually punishable by a fine or imprisonment for less than a year.

mitered (mi'terd): the type of beveled corners used when making a hospital bed.

mitosis (mī-to'sis): cell division.

mitral (mī'tral): shaped like a bishop's miter (a two-sided hat), as relating to the mitral valve of the heart (bicuspid).

mittelschmerz (mit'el-shmertz): "middle pain," pain on ovulation or midway between menstrual periods.

molding (mold'ing): shaping of the fetal head in adjustment to the size and shape of the birth canal.

mole (mol): see **nevus.**

molecule (mol'e-kul): the smallest division of a substance that still possesses the characteristics of that substance; if divided further, breaks down into its individual chemical elements (atoms).

mongolian spot (mon-gol'e-an): a smooth brown or gray nevus (mole) in the sacral area, present at birth.

monocular (mon-ok'u-lar): with only one eye, as *monocular vision.*

monocyte (mon'o-sīt): a particular type of white blood cell that has one nucleus.

mononucleosis (mon-o-nu-kle-o'sis): excess of circulating monocytes, as in *acute infectious mononucleosis.*

mons (mons): a raised area, prominence, as the *mons pubis.*

morbid (mor'bid): inducing disease or having a disease; thoughts of death or severe disease, as *morbid thoughts.*

morgue (morg): a place where dead bodies are kept temporarily until identified and autopsy (postmortem) is done or the body claimed by relatives.

mortal (mor'tal): terminating in death, as a *mortal wound.*

mottled (mah'tld): irregular discoloration, as *mottled skin.*

mucosa (mu-ko'sah): **mucous membrane.**

mucus (mu'kus): the viscid secretion of the mucous glands.

multipara (mul-tip'ah-rah): a woman who has had two or more pregnancies resulting in a live birth; **grand multipara,** a woman who has had many pregnancies.

mumps: a communicable disease that causes swelling of the parotid glands, **epidemic parotitis.** Most common in children, dangerous in adults, preventable by immunization.

muscular dystrophy (MD) (mus'kyoo-lar dis'tro-fe): a group of genetic disorders having symptoms involving progressive wasting of muscles.

mutation (mu-ta'shun): a permanent change in genetic material, as a mutation in a pathogenic organism in response to an antibiotic which results in penicillin-resistant staphylococcus, for example.

mutism (mu'tizm): refusal or inability to speak.

myasthenia (mi-as-the'ne-ah): muscle weakness, as *myasthenia gravis.*

mycosis (mi-ko'sis): disease caused by a fungus, such as *opportunistic mycosis,* a disorder that can occur in a person with a compromised immune system, such as in AIDS or *mycosis fungoides,* a form of cutaneous T-cell lymphoma.

mydriatic (mid-re-at'ik): a drug that dilates the pupil of the eye.

myelin (mi'e-lin): covering of some nerve fibers, as the *myelin sheath.*

myelitis (mi-e-li'tis): inflammation of the spinal cord (**poliomyelitis**) or bone and bone marrow (**osteomyelitis**).

myelocele (mi'e-lo-sēl): herniation of the spinal cord through a defect in the vertebral column.

myelogram (mi'e-lo-gram): a radiograph showing the differential count of various cells in the bone marrow.

myeloma (mi-e-lo'mah): a malignant tumor of cells resembling those found in bone marrow, as *multiple myeloma* or giant-cell tumor.

myocardial (mi-o-kar'de-al): pertaining to the myocardium, as in *myocardial infarction,* ("heart attack").

myocardium (mi-o-kar'de-um): the middle and thickest layer of the heart wall, the muscular layer.

myoclonic (mi-o-klon′ik): severe muscular contractions, as in a seizure.

myogram (mi′o-gram): graph of the electrical activity of muscles.

myopathy (mi-op′ah-thy): any disease of the muscle tissue.

myopia (mi-o′pe-ah): **nearsightedness,** light rays focus in front of the retina.

myositis (mi-o-si′tis): inflammation of a voluntary muscle.

myringotomy (mir-ing-got′o-me): incision into the tympanic membrane (eardrum), usually to relieve pressure or to drain fluid.

myxedema (mik-se-de′mah): condition caused by hypothyroidism (lack of the hormone thyroxine). (This is the adult form of *cretinism.*)

narcolepsy (nar′ko-lep-se): uncontrollable desire to sleep.

narcotics (nar-kot′iks): drugs that produce sleep or stupor and relieve pain at the same time; most narcotics are addictive and are covered by the controlled substances act ("schedule" drugs).

nasal (na′zal): pertaining to the nose, as in *nasal mucosa.*

nasopharynx (na-so-pahr′inks): section of pharynx behind the nose.

natal (na′tal): pertaining to birth.

nausea (naw′se-ah): an unpleasant, sick sensation in the stomach that often leads to vomiting (*nauseous*).

navel (na′vel): **umbilicus,** the scar left by the umbilical cord attachment.

necropsy (nek′rop-se): postmortem examination, **autopsy.**

necrosis (ne-kro′sis): death of tissues.

negligence (neg′li-jens): harm done to a person because of failure to do something that a responsible person would do, neglect; doing something a responsible person would not do, irresponsible care.

neonatal (ne-o-na′tal): relating to the first few weeks after birth. The newborn is called a **neonate.**

neoplasm (ne′o-plazm): tumor, new growth (may be benign or malignant); often refers to cancer. (adj: **Neoplastic**)

nephrectomy (ne-frek′to-me): removal of a kidney.

nephritis (ne-fri′tis): inflammation of the kidney; sometimes called **Bright's disease, pyelitis.**

nephrology (ne-frol′o-je): the branch of medicine dealing with kidney disorders and their treatment.

nephron (nef′ron): the functional unit of the kidney.

nephrosis (ne-fro′sis): any kidney disease, especially one that is degenerative; **the nephrotic syndrome.**

nephrotoxic (nef-ro-tok′sik): destructive to the kidneys; some medications are nephrotoxic.

nerve (nerv): a macroscopic cordlike structure containing individual nerve fibers that carry impulses within the body. The *nervous system* consists of the brain and spinal cord (central nervous system), as well as the peripheral and autonomic nervous systems. Sensory (*afferent*) nerves carry information to the brain; motor (*efferent*) nerves carry impulses from the brain to muscles. Some nerves are *mixed* sensory and motor.

neuralgia (nu-ral′je-ah): pain that extends along one or more nerves, as *trigeminal neuralgia* (tic douloureux).

neurasthenia (nu-ras-the′ne-ah): nervous exhaustion characterized by chronic depression, extreme fatigue and lack of energy; *nervous prostration.*

neurilemma (nu-ri-lem′ah): the plasma membrane that forms the sheath of a Schwann (peripheral) nerve cell.

neuritis (nu-ri′tis): inflammation of a nerve.

neuroglia (noo-ro′gle-a): supporting structure of nerve tissue; also called *glia.*

neurology (nu-rol′o-je): medical specialty related to the brain and nervous system.

neurons (noo′rons): cells making up nervous tissue.

neurosis (nu-ro′sis): a mental or psychiatric disorder characterized by fears, anxieties, and compulsions; considered to be less severe than psychosis.

neutropenia (nu-tro-pe′ne-ah): decreased neutrophils in the blood. **Malignant neutropenia: agranulocytosis**.

nevus (ne′vus): a congenital, circumscribed, discolored area of the skin, either vascular or nonvascular; **mole.** (pl: **nevi**).

nits (nits): the eggs of lice.

nociceptor (no-se-sep′tor): pain receptor, which is stimulated by injury.

nocturia (nok-tu′re-ah): excessive voiding (urination) during the night.

node (nōd): a small mass of tissue, *knot,* swelling (may be benign or malignant).

nonproductive (non-pro-duk′tiv): term used to describe a dry cough in which the person does not cough up any sputum or other material.

nonunion (non-un′yun): failure of segments of a fractured bone to reunite.

nonverbal communication: conveying information or messages without speaking or writing. Components include items such as therapeutic touch, gestures, body language, facial expression, and eye contact.

nosocomial (nos-o-ko′me-al): originating in a hospital, as a *nosocomial infection.*

noxious (nok′shus): harmful, hurtful, disagreeable, as a *noxious stimulus.*

nuclear medicine (nu′kle-ar): diagnosis and treatment of body disorders using radioactivity (includes x-ray, scintillation scan, and radiation therapy).

nucleus (nu′kle-us): the body within the cell that contains chromosomes (sometimes referred to as the regulator).

nulligravida (nul-li-grav′i-dah): a woman who has never been pregnant.

nullipara (nu-lip′ar-rah): a woman who has never borne a live child.

nursing process: systematic method in which the nurse and patient work together to plan and carry out effective nursing care. (The five steps include assessment, nursing diagnosis, planning, implementation, and evaluation.)

nutrition (nu-trish′un): the process of using food for growth and development; the study of foods, nutrients, and diet.

nystagmus (nis-tag′mus): rapid, repetitive involuntary movement of the eyeball, may be horizontal, rotating, vertical, or combinations.

obese (o-bese′): overweight; **morbid obesity** or gross obesity is usually considered to be more than 100 pounds overweight or twice normal weight.

objective (ob-jek′tiv): able to be perceived by another person by means of the senses (a rash is an *objective sign,* as opposed to subjective); a goal or criterion (as objectives for each book chapter); a test item that has a definite answer (open to only one interpretation).

obligate (ob′li-gāt): necessary, compulsory, as an *obligate aerobe* (microorganism that *must* have oxygen).

obstetrics (ob-stet′riks): the branch of medicine that deals with pregnancy, labor, delivery, and the puerperium. (An **obstetrician** is a physician who specializes in this field.)

obstipation (ob-sti-pa′shun): incurable constipation; absence of bowel movements.

obturator (ob-tu-ra′tor): a disc or plate that closes an opening, as the obturator inserted within a tracheostomy tube (used for insertion of the tube and then removed).

occipital (ok-sip′i-tal): pertaining to the back of the head, as the *occipital bone.*

occult (o-kult′): obscure, **hidden,** as *occult blood* in the stool. (Also refers to witchcraft.)

occupational therapy (OT): the department that rehabilitates patients so they can perform activities of daily living (ADLs) and return to work and leisure following an injury or illness.

ocular (ok′u-lar): pertaining to the eye.

oculist (ok'u-list): **ophthalmologist,** a physician who specializes in eye disorders.

ointment (oint'ment): a greasy, semisolid preparation for external use on the body, **unction, unguent.**

olecranon (o-lek'rah-non): the bony projection at the elbow.

olfactory (ol-fak'to-re): pertaining to the sense of smell, as the *olfactory nerve.*

oligopnea (ol-i-gop'ne-ah): hypoventilation, sometimes used interchangeably with *bradypnea.*

oliguria (oli-ig-u're-ah): deficient urinary secretion or infrequent urination.

omphalic (om-fal'ik): pertaining to the umbilicus (navel), as an *omphalocele.*

oncogene (ong'ko-gene): a gene found in tumor cells whose activation converts normal cells into cancer cells. (adj: **oncogenic**—promoting development of a neoplasm)

oncology (ong-kol'o-je): the study of tumors; the study of cancer, as *oncologic nursing.*

onset (on'set): the beginning of an illness, when the first symptoms of disease appear.

onychia (o-nik'e-ah): inflammation of the nailbed (fingernail or toenail), resulting in the loss of the nail.

oophorectomy (oo-fo-rek'to-me): the surgical removal of an ovary or the ovaries; **ovariectomy.**

open-ended questions: questions used in therapeutic communication and interviews that promote in-depth answers and encourage patients to talk about themselves and their concerns.

operable (op'er-ah-bl): appropriate for surgical removal.

ophthalmia (of-thal'me-ah): severe inflammation of the eye and its deeper structures, as *sympathetic ophthalmia.*

ophthalmologist (op-thal-mol'o-jist): a physician who specializes in the treatment of disorders of the eye.

ophthalmoscope (of-thal'mo-skop): a lighted instrument used to inspect the eye.

opiate (o'pe-ate): a drug containing or derived from opium, a sedative or narcotic.

opisthotonos (o-pis-thot'o-nos): a spasm in which the head and heels are close together and the body bowed forward.

opportunistic (op-or-too-nis'tik): a microorganism that usually does not cause disease but that does so under certain circumstances; for example, as AIDS renders the immune system ineffective, opportunistic diseases can infect the person.

optic (op'tik): pertaining to the eye, as the *optic nerve.*

optician (op-ti'shun): one who grinds lenses and fits eyeglasses.

optimum (op'tim-um): the most favorable condition.

optometrist (op-tom'i-trist): a person licensed to test eyes and prescribe eyeglasses and contact lenses. This person is a Doctor of Optometry (OD) but is *not* a physician (MD) and cannot perform surgery or prescribe drugs.

oral (o'ral): pertaining to the mouth, as *oral medications.*

orchitis (or-ki'tis): inflammation of the testicles.

orchiectomy (or-ke-ek'to-me): removal of one or both testes.

orchiopexy (or'ke-o-pek"se): surgical fixation of an undescended testicle so it remains in the scrotum.

organ (or'gan): a group of body tissues having a particular function.

organic (or-gan'ik): pertaining to an organ; an *organic disease* is one that has its origin in a systemic/organic disorder and can be identified by objective means (as opposed to a functional disease).

organ-specific (or'gan): having an effect only on a particular organ, as certain autoimmune disorders.

orgasm (or'gazm): climax of sexual excitement near the end of coitus.

orifice (or'i-fis): opening into a body cavity; any foramen or **meatus.**

orthodontia (or-tho-don'she-ah): the branch of dentistry that deals with malocclusion (misplaced teeth) and other jaw and facial deformities.

orthopedic (or-tho-pe'dik): pertaining to the correction of deformities of the musculoskeletal system, as *orthopedic nursing.*

orthopnea (or-thop'ne-ah): difficult breathing, relieved by sitting or standing erect.

orthotics (or-thot'iks): the practice dealing with the application of braces or appliances to the body—closely related to *prosthetics* (the science that deals with the fabrication of braces and other orthopedic devices).

os (os): opening, any body orifice. Used specifically to refer to the *mouth* and the cervical opening (*cervical os*).

oscillation (os-i-la'shun): extremely fast back and forth movements, a **vibration,** as the movement of the ossicles (bones) of the middle ear, caused by vibrations of sound waves. (An *oscilloscope* measures oscillation of sound waves.)

osmosis (oz-mo'sis): the passage of a solvent from one side of a selectively permeable membrane to the other, due to the relative pressures on both sides.

osseous (os'e-us): bonelike, pertaining to bone.

ossicle (os'i-kl): small bone, particularly those of the middle ear.

ossify (os'i-fi): to change or develop into bone, sometimes an abnormal situation. (noun: **ossification**—the process of bone formation.)

osteoarthritis (os-te-o-ar-thri'tis): a chronic, degenerative form of inflammatory joint disease.

osteoblast (os'te-o-blast): a cell that is associated with bone production; a "bone cell."

osteoclast (os'te-o-klast): a particular type of large multi-nuclear bone cell.

osteogenesis (os-te-o-jen'e-sis): the formation of bone tissue.

osteoma (os-te-o'mah): a tumor made up of bony tissue; may be benign or malignant.

osteomalacia (os-te-o-mah-la'she-a): softening of bones, due to impaired mineralization (often loss of or improper metabolism of calcium).

osteomyelitis (os-te-o-mi-e-li'tis): inflammation of bone caused by a pyogenic (pus-forming) infection. Can cause bone deformity and death.

osteopath (os'te-o-path): a practitioner of osteopathy, which follows generally accepted medical practices and emphasizes normal body mechanics and manipulation of faulty structure. (**DO:** Doctor of Osteopathy [os-te-ah'pa-the].)

osteoporosis (os-te-o-po-ro'sis): a chronic bone disorder caused by a loss of minerals, especially calcium, in the bone (often occurs in aging).

ostomate (os'to-mate): one who has a stoma on the outside of the abdomen to drain feces or urine.

otitis (o-ti'tis): inflammation of the ear, as *otitis media.* Otitis media: inflammation of the middle ear, *tympanitis.*

otology (o-tol'o-je): a study of the anatomy and physiology of the ear and related disorders.

otosclerosis (o-to-skle-ro'sis): an abnormal spongy bone formation in the labyrinth of the ear (often causes hearing loss because the ossicles become fixed and unable to transmit sound waves).

otoscope (o'to-skop): a lighted instrument used to inspect the ear.

outcomes: in nursing process, patient behaviors or clinical manifestations that represent resolution or progress toward resolution. Also called **objectives** or **goals.**

oviducts (ov-i-duks'): passageway for the ovum between the ovary and the uterus. Also called **ovarian tubes, uterine tubes** (formerly called *fallopian tubes*).

ovulation (ov-yoo-la'shun): the process by which an ovum (egg cell) ruptures the surface of the ovary and is expelled into the pelvic cavity.

oxidize (ok'si-dize): to combine or bring about the combination with oxygen, or removal of hydrogen. (One form of oxidation is the rusting of iron; another is the burning of wood.)

oximeter (ok-sim′e-ter): a photoelectric device that measures oxygen concentration/saturation in the blood, as *pulse oximeter,* which is placed on the finger or ear lobe.

oxygen (ok′si-jen): a colorless, odorless gas that is essential to all life and makes up about one fifth of the atmospheric air; also an essential element in water (H_2O) and carbohydrates (CHO).

oxytocic (ok-si-to′sik): an agent that promotes contraction of the uterus, a drug used to induce labor.

pacemaker (pas′mak-er): a stimulus that sets the pace at which something occurs (usually refers to the electronic *cardiac pacemaker* that regulates heartbeat).

pachyderma (pak-i-der′mah): abnormal thickening of the skin ("elephant skin").

pain (pan′): sensation of distress, suffering, or discomfort; the body's way of signalling that something is wrong. (*Acute pain* results from injury or serious disorders. *Chronic pain* continues beyond initial phase of healing. *Intractable pain* is pain which is severe, constant, or unrelenting.)

palate (pal′at): roof of the mouth.

palliative (pal′e-a-tiv): giving relief, but not curative (as chemotherapy is palliative for some types of advanced cancer).

pallor (pal′or): absence of skin pigment, *paleness.*

palpation (pal-pa′shun): the act of feeling with the hand, placing the fingers on the skin to determine the condition of underlying parts.

palpitation (pal-pi-ta′shun): an unduly rapid or throbbing heartbeat that can be sensed by the patient.

palsy (pawl′ze): loss of motion; paralysis (as *Bell's palsy* of the face).

pancarditis (pan-kar-di′tis): widespread, general inflammation of the heart.

pancreas (pan′kre-us): a glandular organ behind the stomach that secretes digestive enzymes vital for digestion. (The islets of Langerhans in the pancreas secrete *insulin,* which is vital in carbohydrate metabolism.)

pandemic (pan-dem′ik): widespread epidemic of disease (as sexually transmitted diseases are often pandemic in many parts of the world).

papilla (pah-pil′ah): small projection or elevation, as the papillae of the tongue. (pl: **papillae**)

papule (pap′ule): a small, solid, circumscribed elevation of the skin, less than 0.5–1.0 cm in diameter.

paracentesis (par-ah-sen-te′sis): a surgical puncture of a body cavity for the aspiration of fluid (often refers to abdominal paracentesis). (The puncture of the thoracic cavity is often called **thoracentesis**).

paradoxical (pa-ra-dox′e-kl): having an effect opposite that desired, as the paradoxical effect of a drug in the elderly.

paralysis (par-al′i-sis): loss of motion or impairment of sensation in a body part.

paranoia (par-ah-noi′ah): mental disorder in which one has delusions of persecution or thinks others will harm him/her. Also may include delusions of grandeur.

paraplegia (par-ah-ple′je-ah): paralysis of the legs and sometimes the lower part of the body.

parasites (par′ah sites): plants or animals that live on or within another organism, taking something from that other organism.

parathyroid (par-a-thi-royd′): small glands lying on either side of the undersurface of the thyroid gland.

parenchyma (pah-reng′ki-mah): the functional elements of an organ, as opposed to its framework.

parenteral (pah-ren′ter-al): administered into the body in a way other than through the alimentary canal (subcutaneous, intravenous, intramuscular), as *parenteral medications.*

parenting (par′ent-ing): providing a safe, healthy, and nurturing environment that encourages optimum growth and development of children.

paresis (pah-re′sis): slight or incomplete paralysis or loss of sensation.

paresthesia (par-es-the′ze-ah): abnormal sensations, such as tingling, burning, etc.

parietal (pah-ri′e-tal): pertaining to the walls of a cavity or organ, as the *parietal pleura;* pertaining to the parietal bone (the bones that form the sides and roof of the cranium [skull]).

parity (par′i-te): the condition of a woman in respect to her having borne live infants.

paroxysm (par-ok′sizm): a sudden periodic attack or recurrence of symptoms of a disease; spasm or seizure.

parturition (par-tu-rish′un): the act of giving birth.

passive (pas′iv): submissive, or not produced by active efforts, as *passive range-of-motion* exercises.

pasteurization (pas′tur-i-za-shun): the destruction of pathogenic bacteria and inhibition in the growth of others by heating a solution without altering the chemical composition of the substance to any extent, such as pasteurization of milk.

patella (pah-tel′ah): **kneecap.**

patent (pā′tent): unobstructed, **open,** as a *patent drainage tube* or *patent airway.*

pathogen (path′o-jen): a disease-producing agent or organism. (Adj: **pathogenic**)

pathology (pah-thol′o-je): the study of changes in body tissues or organs as a result of disease; also used to mean a disease process. (The physician who specializes in this field is a **pathologist.**)

patient record: the chart, Kardex, nursing care plan, and other documents used to maintain patient information and promote continuity of care. Patient records are kept indefinitely and can be referenced in subsequent hospitalizations.

payer, payor (pay′er): term referring to third-party payors, agencies other than the patient (such as insurance companies) that pay for health care.

patient safety device: restraint.

pectoral (pek′tor-al): pertaining to the chest or breast (pectus), as the *pectoral muscles.*

pedal (pēd′al): pertaining to the feet, as the *pedal pulse.*

pediatrics (pe-de-at′rix): the branch of medicine concerned with disorders of children. (**Pediatrician:** physician who treats children.)

pedicle (ped′i-kl): narrow structure, stemlike, such as a *pedicle tissue graft.*

pediculi (pe-dik′u-li): lice. (**Pediculosis:** infested with lice.)

peer (pere) **group**: contemporaries, friends, group of people with whom one associated. (Peer group influence or peer pressure is particularly powerful during adolescence. Observation of peer interaction is important in mental health nursing.)

pellagra (pel-lag′rah): a deficiency disease or syndrome caused by the lack of niacin.

pelvimetry (pel-vim′e-ă-tre): measurements taken of the pelvis, usually during or before pregnancy.

pendulous (pen′du-lus): hanging down loosely, as a *pendulous breast.*

penile (pen′nil): relating to the penis, the male organ of reproduction.

peptic (pep′tik): pertaining to digestion, as a *peptic ulcer.*

percussion (per-kush′un): tapping a part of the body with short sharp blows to elicit sounds or vibrations that aid in diagnosis; often refers to the use of a percussion hammer to elicit a reflex.

percutaneous (per-ku-ta′ne-us): a procedure performed through the skin, as in *percutaneous transluminal coronary angioplasty* (PTCA).

perforation (per-fo-ra′shun): an abnormal hole or break in the walls or membranes of an organ or cavity, as a *perforated ulcer.*

perfusion (per-fu′zhun): the act of pouring through or over, as perfusion of chemotherapeutic agents through the liver's blood vessels as a palliative treatment for cancer.

pericarditis (per-i-kar-di′tis): inflammation of the *pericardium* (the sac enclosing the heart and the roots of some of the great vessels).

perinatal (per-i-na'tal):   the period just before, during, and just after birth.

perineum (per-i-ne'um):   the pelvic floor and associated structures (from the symphysis pubis to the coccyx).

perioperative (per-e-op'er-ah-tiv):   the period of time surrounding surgery, including the preoperative, intraoperative, and postoperative periods.

perioral (per-e-o'ral):   around the mouth, **circumoral.**

periosteum (per-e-os'te-um):   the specialized connective tissue that covers all bones. Periosteum is able to form bone in some cases.

peripheral (pe-rif'er-al):   pertaining to the outward part of surface; further from the center, as *peripheral nervous system.*

peristalsis (per-is-tal'sis):   the wavelike contractions of the intestines by which they propel their contents.

peritoneum (per-i-to-ne'um):   the serous membrane lining the walls of body cavities and enclosing viscera (large interior organs). **Peritonitis** is inflammation of the peritoneum. A structure that lies behind the peritoneum is referred to as *retroperitoneal.*

peritonitis (per-it-o-ni'tis):   inflammation of the peritoneum.

permeable (per'me-a-b'l):   allowing passage of a substance, as a *permeable membrane.*

pernicious (per-nish'us):   tending to be fatal unless treated, as *pernicious anemia.*

personal space: an invisible, mutually understood area/zone around a person that is considered inappropriate for strangers to violate (*varies between cultures*). If a person invades another's personal space (comes too close), it may cause discomfort. Much nursing care must occur within the patients' personal space.

pertussis (per-tus'is):   whooping cough, preventable by immunization.

petechiae (pe-te'ke-i):   small, nonraised, round hemorrhagic areas on the skin that occur during some severe fevers.

petit mal (pe-te' mahl):   former name for *absence seizures.*

petrolatum (pet-ro-la'tum):   a purified, semisolid mixture of hydrocarbons from petroleum used as a lubricant and a base for ointments, as *petroleum jelly* or Vaseline.

pH: symbol for hydrogen ion concentration (use of the symbol with a number denotes whether a substance is acidic [below 7.0] or basic [above 7.0]).

phagocyte (fag'o-sit):   a cell that ingests or engulfs other cells, microorganisms, or foreign particles. This process is called **phagocytosis.**

phalanx (fa'langks):   bone of the finger or toe.

phantom pain (fan'tom):   pain that is perceived or "felt" in a limb after amputation, caused by nerve damage and nerve stimulation.

pharmaceutical (fahr-mah-su'ti-kal):   pertaining to pharmacy or drugs.

pharmacology (fahr'ma-kol-o-je):   the study of chemicals (drugs) and their effect on the body.

pharyngitis (far-in-ji'tis):   inflammation of the *pharynx* (throat).

phenylketonuria (**PKU**) (fen-il-ke-to-nu're-ah):   a congenital disease caused by a defect in metabolism of phenylalanine (an essential amino acid) that if not treated, leads to intellectual impairment.

phimosis (fi-mo'sis):   constriction in the foreskin or prepuce so that it cannot be drawn back over the glans penis.

phlebitis (fle-bi'tis):   inflammation of a vein. (**Thrombophlebitis** is inflammation *and* blood clots.)

phlebotomy (fle-bot'o-me):   incision into a vein, a **cutdown, venisection.** (Sometimes refers to venipuncture, particularly for the purpose of drawing blood.)

phlegm (flem):   viscous mucus secreted by the mucous membranes of the nose and mouth in unusually large quantities, forces the person to cough or clear the throat.

phobia (fo'be-ah):   a persistent, abnormal fear or dread. (**Claustrophobia,** fear of small, enclosed places.)

phosphorus (fos'for-us):   an important mineral found in every body cell.

photophobia (fo-to-fo'be-ah):   abnormal intolerance or sensitivity to light, avoidance of light.

phototherapy (fo-to-ther'ah-pe):   treatment with light, as in physiologic, nonhemolytic jaundice of the newborn.

phrenic (fren'ik):   pertaining to the diaphragm, as the *phrenic nerve;* pertaining to the mind.

physiatrics (fiz-e-ah'triks):   the branch of medicine involved with physical medicine, physical therapy, and rehabilitation.

physical (fiz'ik-al):   pertaining to the body.

physical therapy, PT: the department that rehabilitates patients with limited physical mobility, using physical modalities, exercises, and assistive devices. *Chest physiotherapy* is a form of respiratory therapy that uses percussion and postural drainage to loosen and drain secretions from the lungs.

physiologic (fiz-e-oh-loj'i-k):   pertaining to physiology, the function of the body; normal. *Physiologic needs* are those required to sustain life such as oxygen, food, water, and elimination; survival needs.

physiology (fiz-e-ol'o-je):   the science that deals with the *functions* of the body.

pica (pi'kah):   a craving to eat inedible items or unnatural food items, as *pica in pregnancy.*

pile (pil):   a **hemorrhoid.**

pilonidal (pi-lo-ni'dal):   having a group of hairs, as in *pilonidal cyst* or sinus tract.

pineal (pin'e-al):   shaped like a pine cone, as the pineal body within the brain, or the *pineal gland.*

pinna (pin'ah):   external ear, **auricle.**

pitting (pit'ing):   formation of a small depression, as in *pitting edema.*

pituitary (pi-tu'i-tar-e):   a tiny gland located at the base of the brain that secretes or releases several hormones, including growth hormone; called the *master gland.*

placebo (plah-se'bo):   an inactive or nonmedical substance given in place of a medication to gratify a patient without his or her knowledge of its actual lack of therapeutic value.

placenta (plah-sen'tah):   an organ joining mother and child during pregnancy in human beings and other mammals. The placental blood furnishes nutrients, oxygen, hormones, and other substances to the fetus and carries away wastes. (Also called **afterbirth.**)

placenta previa (plah-sen'tah pre've-ah):   low implantation of the placenta so that it partially or completely covers the cervical os.

planning: in nursing process, developing goals to prevent, reduce, or eliminate problems and identification of nursing interventions that will assist in meeting these goals.

plantar (plan'tar):   pertaining to the sole of the foot, as a *plantar wart.*

plaque (plak):   a patch or flat area (can refer to *dental plaque* [deposit on the teeth] or the fatty deposit on the walls of blood vessels in *atherosclerosis*). *Senile plaques* occur in the cerebral cortex of the person with Alzheimer's disease.

plasma (plaz'mah):   the fluid portion of the blood.

platelet (plat'let):   smallest formed element of the blood; also called **thrombocyte.**

pledget (pled'jet):   a small tuft, as of cotton or lamb's wool.

pleura (ploo'rah):   membrane covering the lungs and lining the walls of the chest cavity, as the *parietal pleura.*

pleurisy (ploo'ri-se):   inflammation of the pleura.

plexus (plek'sus):   a network or tangle, as of veins or nerves.

plication (pli-ka'shun):   surgical pleating or taking of tucks to shorten a structure, as in treatment of retinal detachment.

plumbism (plum'bizm):   chronic lead poisoning.

pneumatic (nu-mat'ik):   pertaining to air or respiration.

Pneumocystis carinii **pneumonia** (no-mo-sis'tis kah-rin'e-i):   an interstitial plasma cell pneumonia, one of the most common opportunistic diseases of AIDS.

pneumonia (nu-mo′ne-ah): inflammation of the lung, with consolidation and drainage. (*Walking pneumonia:* a condition in which the person is ill, but does not remain in bed.)

pneumothorax (no-mo-tho′raks): collapse of a lung, due to air or gas in the chest cavity.

podiatrist (po-di′ah-trist): one who diagnoses and treats foot disorders; also called **chiropodist.**

poison (poy′sun): any substance that affects health or threatens life when absorbed into the body or when in contact with the body surface.

poliomyelitis (pol-i-o-mi-el-i′tis): commonly called **polio;** a condition in which a virus attacks neurons and the myelin sheath, affecting motor nerves and sometimes resulting in paralysis. Preventable by vaccine.

pollution (po-lu′shun): the act of contamination or making impure by noxious substances; may refer to air, food, water or noise contamination.

polycythemia (pol-e-si-the′me-ah): increase in the total cell mass of the blood, ("too many cells").

polydactylism (pol-e-dak′til-izm): having more than the normal number of fingers or toes.

polydipsia (pol-e-dip′se-ah): excessive thirst.

polyneuritis (pol-e-nu-ri′tis): inflammation of many nerves.

polyp (pol′ip): a growth or mass protruding from a mucous membrane. **Pedunculated polyp:** a polyp on a thin stalk; **sessile polyp:** a polyp with a broad base. (May be an overgrowth of normal tissue or may be a true tumor—new growth). They are usually benign, but may later become malignant.

polyphagia (pol-e-fa′je-ah): an abnormal craving for all kinds of food.

polyuria (pol-e-u′re-ah): the voiding of an excessive amount of urine.

popliteal (pop-li-te′al): the space behind the knee.

pore (por): a small opening, as the pores of the skin.

position (po-zish′un): body posture or placement; relationship between the bodies of fetus and mother, **lie, presentation.** *Anatomic p.:* the body stands erect, with palms facing forward. *Lithotomy p.:* the patient lies on the back, with legs separated, thighs acutely flexed on the abdomen, and legs on the thighs (for pelvic examination). *Sims′ p.:* the patient lies on the left side with left thigh slightly flexed and right thigh acutely flexed on the abdomen (for enema). *Trendelenburg′s p.:* the patient lies on the back, with head lowered and legs raised (to treat shock).

post- (prefix): behind, after.

posterior (pos-ter′e-or): located on the back (opposite of anterior).

post mortem (post mor′tem): after death, as post mortem examination (**autopsy**), "post."

postnatal (post-na′tal): after birth.

postoperative (post-op′er-ah-tiv): after surgery.

postpartum (post-par′tum): after childbirth or delivery (refers to the mother).

potassium (po-tas′i-um): chemical element that plays a major role in the acid–base and water balance in the body, a major ion in the intracellular fluid, symbol is K^+.

potentiation (po-ten-she-a′shun): enhancement of one agent by another, so that the combined action is greater than the sum of the two (e.g., alcohol and valium potentiate each other), **synergism.**

prandial (pran′de-al): pertaining to a meal, as a *postprandial* medication or test.

pre- (prefix): before.

precipitate (pre-sip′i-tat): occurring unusually quickly, as in *precipitate labor* and delivery; to settle out, to precipitate.

precursor (pre-ker′sor): something that precedes; a sign or symptom that precedes another, or heralds the onset a disease, see **aura.**

pregnancy (preg′nan-se): the state of having a developing embryo or fetus within the uterus, being with child, *gravid.*

pregnancy-induced hypertension, PIH: an abnormal complication of pregnancy, and for a short time following delivery, characterized by hypertension (high blood pressure), edema, and proteinunia. Seizures may occur if not successfully treated. Also called **gestosis, toxemia of pregnancy** and *pre-eclanepsia-eclampsia syndrome.* May be fatal to mother and/or infant.

premature (pre-mah-tur′): before the proper time, before maturity, as *premature birth.*

premenstrual syndrome (pre-men-stroo′al sin′drom) **(PMS)**: symptoms that are cyclic in nature, occurring 7 to 14 days before the menstrual period.

prenatal (pre-na′tal): before birth, as in *prenatal care,* also called **antenatal.**

preoperative (pre-op′er-a-tiv): before surgery.

prepuce (pre′pus): **foreskin** of the penis (removed in circumcision).

presbycusis (pres-bi-ku′sis): hearing loss occurring with aging.

presbyopia (pres-bi-oh′pe-ah): farsightedness occurring with aging.

prescription (pre-skrip′shun): a written direction for the preparation and use of a medicine (sometimes also refers to a prescribed treatment). abbreviated **Rx**

presentation (prez-en-ta′shun): the relationship of the long axis of a fetus to that of its mother; **position; lie.**

pressure ulcer, pressure sore (*pressure area*): ulcerated sore often caused by prolonged pressure on a bony prominence or other area, especially if the patient is allowed to lie in one position for an extended period of time. Also called *decubitus ulcer,* (formerly called "bedsore").

priapism (pri′ah-piz-um): persistent, painful, abnormal penile erection.

primary (pri′mar-e): first, most important. *Primary needs* are those that must be satisfied before attempting to meet other needs (such as oxygen, food, water, and elimination).

primigravida (pri-mi-grav′i-dah): a woman pregnant for the first time.

primipara (pri-mip′ah-rah): a woman who has had one live birth (often used interchangeably with **primigravida**).

problem-oriented medical record (POMR): the type of nursing/medical documentation that focuses on patient problems, nursing care plan, and problem resolution. Usually used with SOAP or SOAPIER documentation. (Also called *Patient-Oriented Medical Record, Problem-Solving Medical Record.*)

process (pros′es): a prominence or projection, as of the end of a bone. **Nursing Process:** a systematic method of planning, implementing, and evaluating nursing care.

proctoscope (prok′to-skope): a lighted instrument used for inspecting the rectum.

prodromal (pro-drom′al): the period before actual symptoms occur; may involve a *premonition* that a disease is about to occur. Some disorders, such as genital herpesvirus, are more contagious during the prodromal period.

prognosis (prog-no′sis): judging in advance the probable duration, course, and termination of a disease or disorder.

prolapse (pro′laps): falling down, downward displacement of an organ, as the abnormal *prolapse of the uterus.*

proliferation (pro-lif-e-ra′shun): reproduction or multiplication, as of cells.

prone (prōn): lying face downward; lying flat on the ventral surface (front) of the body.

prophylaxis (pro-fi-lak′sis): prevention of disease; *prophylactic* is another name for a condom.

proprietary (pro-pri′e-ter-e) **medicine**: a medication that is copyrighted, trademarked, or patented; a **brand name** (as opposed to generic). A **proprietary hospital:** a health care facility that makes a profit (not a nonprofit agency).

proprioception (pro-pre-o-sep'shun): the sensation of body position in space. (Older people often lose proprioception.)

pro re nata (pro-ra-nah'tah) (**PRN**): as needed; as the situation demands.

prospective (pro-spek'tiv): predetermined, before the fact. *Prospective payment* or reimbursement for health care is made by third-party payors according to a formula or average and does not reimburse actual costs per case.

prostaglandins (pros-ta-glan'dins): fatty acids that are widespread in body tissues and that generally stimulate contraction or relaxation of smooth muscles.

prostate (pros'tat): a doughnut-shaped gland lying just below the bladder in the male; swelling of the prostate (hyperplasia) may cause urinary disorders.

prostatectomy (pros-tah-tek'to-me): removal of the prostate. *Transurethral p.:* removal through the urethra (*TURP*).

prosthesis (pros-the'sis): the replacement of a missing part by an artificial substitute (e.g., an artificial eye, arm or leg is a prosthesis). **Prosthetics** is the manufacture of prostheses, splints, and braces for limbs and the back.

prostration (pros-tra'shun): extreme exhaustion.

protein (pro'ten): groups of amino acids in complex compounds that are vital to life. Protein foods are essential to building and repairing all body tissues and include meat, eggs, fish, legumes and dairy products.

prothrombin (pro-throm'bin): a plasma protein that is converted to thrombin during blood clotting. (Also called **clotting factor II**).

protocol (pro-to-kal): proper procedure, plan, as in *nursing protocol.*

protoplasm (pro'to-plazm): the essential component of the living cell.

proud flesh: soft, edematous granulation tissue that develops in the healing process, especially of large wounds.

proximal (prok'si-mal): nearest to the midline or center, or nearest to the point of origin. The elbow is proximal to the hand.

proximodistal (prok-si-mo-dis'tal): from the center or core outward. (Refers to the pattern of development and achievement of motor control of the infant.)

pruritus (proo-ri'tus): itching.

pseudo-: (prefix) false.

pseudomenstruation (su-do-men-stru-a'shun): small amount of vaginal bleeding in neonates, caused by maternal hormones.

psoriasis (so-ri'ah-sis): a chronic skin disorder that involves red macules and patches covered with flakes or silvery scales. It is believed to have a hereditary or autoimmune origin in some cases.

psyche (si'ke): the mind.

psychiatrist (si-ki'ah-trist): a physician who specializes in the treatment of mental disorders.

psychogenic (si-ko-jen'ik): psychological in origin, not having a physical basis. (A psychogenic disorder is also called **psychosomatic, functional,** or **somatoform,** although it may later develop into an organic disorder. A *conversion disorder* or conversion hysteria is a serious psychogenic mental illness with physical symptoms that cannot be objectively identified.

psychological (si-ko-loge'i-kal): relating to the mind, behavior or thoughts, rather than to the physical body.

psychologist (si-kol'oh-gist): a person trained to treat mental and emotional disorders (not a physician).

psychosis (si-ko'sis): a mental disturbance in which there is a personality disintegration and an escape into unreality (more serious than neurosis).

psychosomatic (si-ko-so-mat'ik): a physical illness that can be traced to an emotional cause, **psychogenic.** Often, no objective signs can be identified.

ptosis (to'sis): a drooping or sagging of an organ or part from its normal position (usually refers to eyelid).

puberty (pu'ber-te): the period in life when a person becomes sexually able to reproduce.

puerperium (pu-er-pe're-um): the period immediately after childbirth, continuing through involution (return of the uterus to its nonpregnant state).

pulmonary (pul'mo-ner-e): pertaining to the lungs, as in *pulmonary tuberculosis.*

pulse (puls): the heartbeat as felt through the walls of the arteries and the skin or as heard at the apex of the heart with a stethoscope.

puncture (punk'tur): a hole made by a pointed object; penetration.

pupil (pyoo'pahl): black center of the eye that regulates the amount of light entering the eye.

purgative (per'gah-tiv): **cathartic; laxative.**

purpura (per'pu-rah): a bleeding disorder that causes small hemorrhages under the skin (*petechiae*) and bruises (*ecchymoses*). *Thrombocytopenic purpura* is characterized by a decrease in platelets.

purulent (pur'u-lent): consisting of or secreting pus.

pus (pus): a yellowish secretion formed in certain kinds of inflammation, consisting of albuminous substances, a thin fluid, leukocytes and their waste products. May also contain pathogenic organisms.

pustule (pus'tule): a small elevation of the skin filled with pus or lymph.

putrefaction (pu-tre-fak'shun): **decomposition;** becoming rotten.

pyelitis (pi-e-li'tis): inflammation of the pelvis of the kidney.

pyelonephritis (pi-el-o-ne-fri'tis): inflammation of the kidney and renal (kidney) pelvis. (Also called **pyelitis, nephritis** and **nephropyelitis.**)

pyemia (pi-e'me-ah): the presence of pus-forming organisms in the blood; a *generalized septicemia.*

pyloric (pi-lor'ik): pertaining to the last portion of the stomach, as the *pyloric sphincter.*

pylorus (pi-lor'us): the bottom (distal) end of the stomach, opening into the duodenum (first part of the small intestine). The term pylorus can denote the pyloric canal, antrum, or sphincter (muscle).

pyogenic (pi-o-jen'ik): producing pus.

pyorrhea (pi-o-re'ah): copious discharge of pus. **Pyorrhea alveolaris,** a purulent infection of the mouth.

pyrexia (pi-rek'se-ah): **fever.**

pyrosis (pi-ro'sis): a burning sensation in the stomach and the esophagus; commonly known as **heartburn.**

pyuria (pi-u're-ah): pus in the urine.

quack (kwak): one who misrepresents medical skill and knowledge of remedies, **charlatan.**

quadrant (kwad'rant): one of four corresponding quarters, as of the abdomen or buttock. For example, the appendix is in the lower right quadrant of the abdomen.

quadriplegia (kwod-ri-ple'je-ah): paralysis of both arms and both legs; also called **tetraplegia.**

quality assurance: standards of care representing acceptable, expected levels of performance by nursing staff and other health care members. (The Quality Assurance Committee sets these standards.)

quickening (kwik'en-ing): the first movements of the fetus felt by the mother in pregnancy, signs of life.

rabies (ra'bes): an acute infectious disease of the central nervous system that can be transmitted by an animal bite.

radial (ra'de-al): pertaining to the radius of the arm (the bone on the thumb side of the forearm). The pulse is often measured in the radial artery.

radiate (ra'de-ate): to diverge or spread from a common central point, as a pain that radiates outward from its source.

radiography (ra-de-og'ra-fe): the process by which a film record (radiograph) is made of structures within the body by exposure of film specially sensitized to gamma rays or **x-rays.**

radioisotope (ra-de-o-i'so-top): a radioactive form of an element. A commonly used radioisotope is I_{131} (radioactive iodine).

radiologist (ra-de-ol'o-jist): a physician who specializes in radiology (therapeutic and diagnostic).

radiopaque (ra-de-o-pāk): a substance that obstructs radiant energy (the radiopaque area appears light on the x-ray). A commonly used radiopaque substance is barium, used for diagnostic x-rays of the GI tract.

radium (ra'de-um): a radioactive element that gives off rays used in treating malignancies, especially of the cervix or tongue.

rale (rahl): an abnormal respiratory sound more descriptively called **crackle** (see description of crackle).

range of motion: ability to move various joints and structures of the body. The patient may be able to move without assistance (*active range of motion*—AROM) or may need physical assistance (*passive range of motion*—PROM).

rapport (rah-por'): a state of harmony or good relationship between two individuals, particularly emphasized in mental health.

rash (rash): a superficial eruption of the skin, as *diaper rash*, **dermatitis**.

rate (rate): the frequency with which an action occurs (as in *pulse rate* or *respiratory rate*). These rates are usually reported as number of times per minute.

reaction (re-ak'shun): action in response to some influence or force, as in *insulin reaction*.

reagent (re-a'jent): a substance used to produce a chemical reaction.

reality orientation: a technique used to assist persons who are confused or disoriented to return to reality; **remotivation therapy.**

receptor (re-sep'tor): a sensory nerve ending that responds to stimuli.

recessive (re-ses'iv): in genetics, a trait that is not manifested unless carried by both chromosomes in a pair.

recovery position: used in emergency rescue; the person is rolled to the side so the head, shoulders, and torso move simultaneously, without twisting.

rectocele (rek'to-sel): herniation of part of the rectum into the vagina.

rectum (rek'tum): the distal portion of the large intestine between the sigmoid colon and the anal canal. (adj: **rectal**—Temperature is taken and some medications are administered rectally.)

recumbent (re-kum'bent): lying down, as *dorsal recumbent* position (lying on the back).

recuperate (re-ku'per-ate): to recover health or gain strength after an illness.

recurrence (re-kur'ence): the return of symptoms after their remission.

reduce (re-dus'): to put back into its normal place, as to reduce a fracture or a hernia; to decrease in weight or size.

referred (re-ferd'): (referring to pain)—pain that is felt at a location other than its origination; when one physician sends (refers) a patient to another physician or specialist.

reflex (re'fleks): an *automatic movement* in response to a particular stimulus, as the knee jerk in response to a tap below the kneecap.

reflux (re'fluks): backward flow (usually refers to blood, urine, or stomach contents), as in *gastric reflux*.

refraction (re-frak'shun): to determine the refractive errors of the eye and to write a prescription for eyeglasses (corrective lenses).

regimen (rej'i-men): a plan of treatment.

regression (re-gresh'un): return to a former state, as a child regresses when ill. Regression of a disease process refers to its relief or subsiding.

regurgitation (re-gur-ji-ta'shun): the return of food from the stomach soon after eating, without the ordinary efforts of vomiting, and often without nausea.

rehabilitation (re-hah-bil-i-ta'shun): the restoration of a person to as normal as possible body structure and/or function after an injury or illness.

reinfection (re-in-fek'shun): a second infection by the same agent.

rejection (re-jek'shun): the immune reaction of a recipient to foreign tissues after transplantation or grafting, as the rejection of a transplanted kidney.

relapse (re-laps'): recurrence of former symptoms during convalescence.

relax (re-laks'): to loosen up or to make less stiff, as to relax a muscle.

remission (re-mish'un): the lessening in severity or subsiding of the symptoms of an illness (as opposed to exacerbation).

remittent (re-mit'ent): periods of **remission** (becoming better) and **exacerbation** (becoming worse).

renal (re'nal): pertaining to the kidney, as *renal failure*.

repression (re-presh'un): the act of restraining or holding back; a mental health term for one of the defense mechanisms.

rescue breathing: one component of CPR, that of blowing breaths into the victim who has stopped breathing.

resection (re-sek'shun): excision of a portion of an organ or structure, as a *gastric (stomach) resection*.

resident: term used to refer to the patient, particularly in a nursing home or other long-term facility; term used to refer to a physician who is studying in a medical specialty.

residual (re-zid'u-al): amount remaining or left behind, as *residual urine*.

resistance (re-zis'tans): the power of the body to overcome the ill effects of injurious agents, such as pathogenic microorganisms, poisons, or irritants; counteracting force, as resistance of a muscle, the air passages, or blood vessels.

resolution (rez-o-lu'shun): lessening of a pathogenic state or disappearance of a disorder; the healing of a wound.

respiration (res-pi-ra'shun): the total process of the exchange of oxygen and carbon dioxide between the air and the cells of the body. (**External respiration** denotes the exchange of gases in the lungs; **internal respiration** denotes exchange of gases between the blood and body cells.)

respiratory distress syndrome (res'pi-ra-tor-e dis-tres' sin'drom) **(RDS)**: leading cause of death in premature newborns in which the lungs have not fully developed and do not expand for adequate breathing. Also called **hyaline membrane disease.**

respiratory therapy (RT) (respiratory care): the department concerned with treatment, management, and care of patients with respiratory disorders through use of oxygen and other gases and assistive devices for breathing and maintenance of ventilation.

respite (res'pit): rest, care provided for long-term or chronic patients so family caregivers can have some time off (a respite).

restraint (re-strant'): means of forcible control; a protective device for a patient (can be chemical, physical, or in a special room). A physical restraint is also called a **patient safety device** (such as a *Posey belt*).

resuscitation (re-sus-i-ta'shun): restoration to life or consciousness of a person who was apparently dead or who had stopped breathing or whose heartbeat had ceased.

retention (re-ten'shun): the holding or keeping within the body of something that is usually expelled, as *retention of urine*.

reticular (re-tik'u-lar): resembling a net, as certain nervous system cells.

reticulocyte (re-tik'u-lo-sit): a young erythrocyte.

retina (ret'i-nah): the innermost tunic of the eyeball, contains rods and cones and is the origin of the optic nerve. Light rays focus at the retina in normal vision.

retinitis (ret-i-ni'tis): inflammation of the retina, as *retinitis pigmentosa*.

retinopathy (re-ti-nop'ah-the): a noninflammatory disorder of the retina of the eye, as *diabetic retinopathy* (which may lead to blindness).

retinoplasty (ret'in-o-plas-te): surgical repair of the retina.

retro- (prefix): backward, behind, as a *retroflexed uterus*.

retroperitoneal (ret-ro-per-i-to-nee′ahl): behind the peritoneum. The kidneys are located retroperitoneally.

retrospective (ret-ro-spek′tiv): after the fact. *Retrospective payment* or *direct reimbursement* by a third-party payor is based on actual costs incurred by the hospital for that particular patient (as opposed to prospective payment).

retrovirus (ret-ro-vi′rus): a large group of RNA-based viruses that tend to infect immunocompromised persons.

resumé (rez′oo-may): a summary of one's educational and employment experience, also called **curriculum vitae.**

rhinitis (ri-ni′tis): inflammation of the mucous membrane lining the nasal cavity.

rhinoplasty (ri′no-plas-te): plastic surgery/repair of the nose.

rhonchi (rong′ki): continuous, low-pitched dry rattling sounds in lungs and breathing passages caused by obstruction and heard on auscultation. Can often be cleared by coughing. (sing: **rhonchus**)

rhythm (rith′m): the pattern or group of intervals at which an event occurs (as in *respiratory* or *cardiac rhythm*). Often documented as regular or irregular, unless there is a particular irregular pattern that can be described. Also a term used to denote the *fertility control method* based on the woman's menstrual cycle.

rickets (rik′ets): a condition in children caused by lack of vitamin D.

rigor mortis (ri′gor mor′tis): the stiffening of the muscles after death. This process takes several hours; its progress can help to determine time of death.

roentgen (rent′gen): unit of x-radiation; **roentgenogram**: an x-ray film.

roseola (ro-se-o′lah): rose-colored rash. *Roseola infantum,* an acute viral disease that usually occurs in infants under age 2 and disappears suddenly, *exanthem subitem.*

rotation (ro-ta′shun): the process of turning about an axis, as rotation of the hand or of the fetus in preparation for delivery.

rubella (roo-bel′ah): mild disease with fever and a mild rash, **German measles** (in English), **3-day measles.**

rubeola (ru-be-oh′lah): **measles** (in English); German measles (in French and Spanish). Preventable by immunization.

ruber, rubor (roo′bor), **rubrum**: redness, a cardinal sign of inflammation.

ruddy (rud′e): dark red or red-purple color associated with stagnant or poorly-oxygenated blood. Circulation must be restored or tissue necrosis will occur. (*Not* to be confused with erythema.)

rupture (rup′tur): **hernia;** to tear, as a ruptured appendix.

rugae (roó je) (*sing*. **ruga**): folds of the stomach when it is empty (they allow the stomach to distend when food is eaten).

sac (sak): a baglike organ or structure; a pouch.

sacral (sa′kral): pertaining to the sacrum (fused vertebrae at the base of the spine).

sagittal (saj′i-tal): an imaginary vertical plane dividing the body into right and left sides, from top-to-bottom. The *midsagittal plane* divides the body into equal, symmetrical halves. (Also means shaped like an arrow, as the coccyx or xiphoid process of the sternum.)

saline solution (sa′lin): solution of salt in water. (**Normal [physiologic] saline** is a 0.9% solution that is *isotonic*—the same concentration as of the serum in the blood. A solution of 0.45% saline is called *half-normal saline.* Both solutions are commonly used for IVs.)

saliva (sah-li′vah): enzyme-containing secretion of the salivary glands of the mouth.

salpingectomy (sal-pin-jek′to-me): surgical removal of an ovarian (uterine) tube.

salt (sawlt): any compound of a base or an acid; table salt (sodium chloride); a purgative, as Epsom salt.

sanguine (sang′gwin): bloody, as *serosanguineous* drainage (blood and serum).

saprophyte (sap′ro-fit): an organism that lives on dead and decaying material.

sarcoma (sar-ko′mah): connective tissue tumor, often malignant, as *Kaposi's sarcoma.*

saturated (sat′u-ra-ted): pertaining to a solution in which no more of a substance can be dissolved, as a *saturated solution of potassium iodide* (SSKI).

scab (skab): the crust formed on a superficial wound, composed of blood cells caught in a fibrin net and combining with other substances.

scabies (ska′bez): contagious skin disorder caused by the itch mite. Often sexually transmitted.

scanography (scan-og′rah-fe): a method of taking radiographs in which all the rays pass through the target at the same angle.

scapula (skap′u-lah): **shoulder blade.**

scar (skar): a mark left after the healing of a wound, **cicatrix.**

scintiscan (sin′ti-skan): a two-dimensional map demonstrating the concentration of projected gamma rays from a radioisotope in a specific organ or tissue.

sclera (skle′rah): the outer coating of the eyeball.

scleroderma (skle-ro-der′mah): chronic hardening and shrinking of the connective tissues of any organ of the body; often refers to thickened, hard, and darkened skin.

sclerosis (skle-ro′sis): hardening; induration (usually applies to the nervous system, as *multiple sclerosis, lateral sclerosis,* or to the blood vessels—*arteriosclerosis*).

scoliosis (sko-le-os′is): a lateral curvature of the normally straight, vertical line of the spine, sometimes is S-shaped ("*curvature of the spine*").

scurvy (skur′ve): a condition caused by a lack of vitamin C.

sebaceous (se-ba′shus): pertaining to sebum (the oily, fatty secretion of the sebaceous gland).

seborrhea (seb-o-re′ah): an increase in the secretion of the sebaceous glands, causing an oily skin, greasy scales, or cheesy plugs. (**Seborrheic dermatitis** is called dandruff.)

sebum (se′bum): the oily secretion of the sebaceous (oil) glands that is composed of fat and dead skin and that is released into the hair follicles.

secondary: not primary, not vital. *Secondary needs,* according to Maslow, are those not necessary to sustain life, but that enhance the quality of life (such as beauty, learning, and love). Primary needs must be met before secondary needs will be attempted.

secrete (se-krete′): to manufacture and release a substance, usually liquid.

secretion (se-kre′shun): a substance secreted, as urine secreted by the kidneys or hormones by the glands.

section (sek′shun): to **cut** or **incise**, as a *cesarean section* (delivery of a fetus through the abdominal wall) or a *frozen section* (a specimen cut out for examination by microscope, usually for cancer detection).

sedative (sed′ah-tiv): a remedy that has a quieting effect, producing sleep.

sediment (sed′i-ment): a precipitate; a substance that settles to the bottom (erythrocyte sedimentation rate is a blood test).

seizure (se′zhur): a sudden attack or recurrence of a disease, as in epilepsy (cerebral seizure), formerly called *convulsion.*

self-actualized: according to Maslow, the person who is fulfilled, complete, having reached one's full potential.

self-esteem: how one feels about oneself, self-respect, self-worth, self-image. The person with *positive self-esteem* feels worthy to receive good things and has a positive self-image.

semen (se′men): fluid carrying spermatazoa that are manufactured in the testes of the male.

seminoma (sem-i-no′mah): malignancy of the testis.

semis (se′mis): half (abbreviated $\overline{ss}$).

senescence (sen-es′ens): the process of growing old.

senile (se′nile): lay term referring to the loss of mental and sometimes physical powers, due to the aging process, often used interchangeably with *dementia.*

sensitization (sen-si-ti-za'shun): the initial exposure to a specific antigen that causes an immune response; if the body is exposed again, a severe allergic reaction may result.

sepsis (sep'sis): the presence of pathogens or their toxins, usually in the blood (condition: **septic, septicemic**).

septum (sep'tum): a dividing wall between two cavities, as the *nasal septum* or the *septa* (pl.) between the chambers of the heart.

sequela (se-kwel'lah): a morbid condition that occurs as a result of another condition; for example, an infection following an injury (pl: **sequelae**).

sequestration (se-kwes-tra'shun): abnormal separation of a part from the whole, as a part of a bone.

serosanguineous (se-ro-sang-gwin'e-us): composed of serum and blood, as *serosanguineous drainage*.

serum (se'rum): the clear liquid that separates from the blood after clotting.

sexually transmitted disease (STD): a disease that can be (and most often is) transmitted by sexual intercourse or other intimate contact, formerly known as *venereal disease*.

shaft (shaft): long, slender portion, as the shaft of a bone or the penis.

sheath (sheth): tubular case or envelope, as the *myelin sheath* surrounding some nerve fibers.

shingles (shing'glz): acute viral disease caused by *herpes zoster*, which attacks the nerve endings and is very painful.

shock (shok): depression of the body functions due to the failure of the circulation or loss of blood.

show (sho): discharge of blood, usually as a beginning sign of labor (**bloody show**).

shunt (shunt): to bypass, to turn aside, to divert; a passage abnormally occurring or surgically placed between two natural channels, as an *arterial-venous shunt* for dialysis or the shunt created to treat hydrocephalus.

sibling (sib'ling): one's brother or sister.

sickle cell (sik'l): an abnormal crescent-shaped erythrocyte. (**Sickle-cell anemia** is a genetic blood defect that is most commonly found in African Americans, also known as **sicklemia.**)

side effect: a result other than that which was intended from a therapeutic agent (often refers to the result of a prescribed drug).

sigmoid (sig'moid): shaped like the letter "C" or "S" (usually refers to the *sigmoid colon* [the last part of the colon before the rectum]).

sign (sin'): objective evidence of disease that can be noted by an observer (as opposed to *symptom,* which can only be described by the patient).

silicosis (sil-i-ko'sis): a lung condition caused by prolonged exposure to silica dust.

sinus (si'nus): a cavity or channel, often refers to the *paranasal sinuses;* may also refer to *fistula* (a sinus tract).

sitz bath (sits): immersion in water of the hips, buttocks, and genital areas to provide heat, without immersing the remainder of the patient's body.

Sjögren's syndrome (sho'grenz): a complex combination of symptoms, usually occurring in middle-aged women. Symptoms include dry eyes and mucous membranes, conjunctivitis, and connective tissue disorders such as rheumatoid arthritis, systemic lupus erythematosus, or scleroderma.

skin (skin): the outer covering of the body, **integument**.

slander (slan'der): malicious verbal statements that are false.

slough (sluf): to *shed,* to cast off; (noun: **slough**—a mass of dead tissue.)

smear (smere): a specimen for microscopic study made by spreading material on a slide.

smegma (smeg'mah): sebaceous gland secretion found under the foreskin of the penis.

sodium (so'di-um): a chemical element that is a major ion in extracellular fluids (common table salt is composed of sodium [Na^+] and chloride).

soluble (sol'u-bul): capable of being dissolved in a liquid.

soma (so'mah): the *body* (as opposed to the mind—psyche).

somnambulism (som-nam'bu-lizm): sleepwalking.

somniloquism (som-nil'o-kwizm): sleep talking.

sonography (so-nog'rah-fe): recording by means of ultrasound.

sordes (sor'deze): foul, dark matter that collects around the teeth and lips in low-grade fevers.

souffle (soo'fl): soft, blowing sound, as the *uterine souffle* in pregnancy.

sound (sown'd): **bougie**.

spasm (spazm): a sudden muscular contraction. (adj: **spastic**)

specific gravity (spe-sif'ik grav'ah-te): the weight of a substance, when compared with another. Fluids, such as urine, are compared to pure water, which has a specific gravity of 1.000.

specimen (spes'i-men): sample.

speculum (spek'u-lum): an instrument used to open a body orifice for examination, as a *vaginal speculum*.

spermatazoa (sper-mah-ta-zo'ah): sperm cells, male reproductive cells.

sphincter (sfingk'ter): a ringlike muscle surrounding and closing an opening, as the *sphincter muscle* of the rectum.

sphincterotomy (sfink-ter-ot'o-mi): incision into a sphincter to release a stricture (abnormal tightness).

sphygmomanometer (sfig-mo-mah-nom'e-ter): an instrument used for measuring arterial blood pressure (may be *mercurial* [containing mercury] or *aneroid* [using a gauge]).

spina bifida (spi'nah bif'id-ah): congenital anomaly in which the vertebral spaces fail to close.

spirometer (spi-rom'e-ter): an instrument that measures air taken into and expelled from the lungs; a piece of the equipment used in a pulmonary function test. **Incentive spirometer**: device used to enhance lung expansion following surgery or in lung disorders, such as pneumonia.

spirometry: the measurement of breathing capacity.

splenectomy (sple-nek'to-me): surgical removal of the **spleen** (a large glandlike organ under the ribs).

splenic: pertaining to the spleen.

splint (splint): an appliance, either rigid or flexible, that holds body parts in place, as an arm splint. (verb: **splint**—to provide firm support with the hands or a pillow so the postoperative patient can cough and deep-breathe more comfortably.)

spondylitis (spon-di-li'tis): inflammation of the vertebrae.

sporadic (spo-rad'ik): widely scattered, not epidemic or endemic, as a *sporadic case* of measles.

spore (spor): reproductive element of some organisms; resting stage of some organisms that is resistant to environmental changes, and is thus very difficult to kill.

sprain (sprān): twisting of a joint with rupture of ligaments (not a fracture) and possibly other damage to blood vessels, tendons, or nerves.

sprue (sproo): a chronic malabsorption syndrome, may be tropical or nontropical.

spur (sper): a projecting body, as a *bone spur*.

sputum (spu'tum): mucous secretion from the lungs, bronchi, or trachea, ejected from the respiratory tract through the mouth (as opposed to saliva).

squamous (skwa'mus): scaly, platelike, as *squamous epithelium*.

stapedectomy (sta-pe-dek'to-me): surgical removal of the *stapes* (stirrup) bone of the middle ear and replacement with a prosthesis. Used to treat deafness caused by *otosclerosis* (fixation of the ossicles-bones of the middle ear).

stasis (sta'sis): a stoppage or stagnation of the flow of fluids, as *venous stasis* (stoppage of blood flow in the veins).

station (sta'shun): the location of the presenting part of the fetus in the birth canal; a nursing/patient unit, as a *nursing station*.

steatorrhea (ste-ah-to-re'ah): excess fat in the feces, as in malabsorption syndromes or a deficiency of the pancreatic enzymes.

stellate (stel'āt): shaped like a star, in rosettes, as a *stellate ganglion*.

stenosis (sten-no'sis): narrowing or constriction of an opening or tube, as *aortic stenosis* or *pyloric stenosis*.

sterile (ster'il): free of microorganisms, **aseptic;** unable to bear children, infertile, barren.

sternal (ster'nal): pertaining to the **sternum** (breast bone), as a *sternal puncture*.

steroid (ste'roid): a class of hormones including the sex hormones and cortisone.

stertorous (ster'to-rus): characterized by a snoring sound, as *stertorous breathing*.

stethoscope (steth'o-skope): an instrument used to amplify internal body sounds, often used to listen to the heartbeat.

stillborn (stil'born): born dead.

stimulant (stim'u-lant): any agent that produces an increase in the activity of the body or one of its parts **(stimulus).**

stoma (sto'mah): an opening on a free surface, such as a pore; an artifically created opening between a body cavity and the body's surface, such as the stoma of a *colostomy, ileostomy* or *tracheostomy*.

stomatitis (sto-mah-ti'tis): inflammation of the mucous membrane of the mouth (includes *gingivitis*—inflammation of the gums and *glossitis*—inflammation of the tongue).

stool (stool): **feces,** discharge from the bowels.

stopcock (stop'cok): a valve that can be turned to regulate the flow within a tube, such as the stopcock on the IV tube that is turned to measure central venous pressure.

strabismus (strah-biz'mus): a deviation of the eye, **squint.** (Convergent strabismus is called **cross-eye;** divergent strabismus is called **exotropia** or *walleye*. Other types include cyclotropia, esotropia, hypertropia, and hypotropia.)

strain (strān): overextension of a muscle.

strangulated (strang'u-lat-ed): closed because of constriction, as a *strangulated hernia*.

stratiform (strat'i-form): arranged in layers.

stress (stres): pressure; reaction to adverse stimulus, as emotional stress or as physical stress placed upon the body by injury, pregnancy, chemicals, or disease, as a *stress fracture*. **Stressor:** an agent that produces stress and disrupts homeostasis.

striated (stri'at-ed): having stripes, as *striated (voluntary) muscle*.

stricture (strik'tur): an abnormal narrowing of a muscle ring, passage, duct, or tube, as an *esophageal stricture*.

stricturotomy: incision into a stricture for the purpose of opening or releasing it.

stridor (stri'dor): a shrill and harsh sound (usually refers to the inspiratory sound made when the larynx is obstructed).

stroke (strok): a sudden attack, often causing paralysis of one or more parts of the body, also known as **apoplexy** or **cerebrovascular accident (CVA),** caused by rupture or blockage of a blood vessel in the brain.

Stryker frame (stri'ker): an apparatus used to turn patients who have a spinal cord injury.

stump (stump): the portion of a leg or arm remaining after an amputation.

stupor (stu'por): reduced responsiveness or partial unconsciousness.

sty, stye (sti): inflammation of one or more sebaceous glands of the eyelid; also called **hordeolum.**

stylet (sti'let): a slender probe; an insert placed in a catheter to make it stiff; a **stylus.**

subacute (sub-ah-kute'): between an acute or chronic state, with some acute features.

subclinical (sub-klin'i-kal): the presence of a disease without any clinical signs, a very mild case of the disease.

subcutaneous (sub-ku-ta'ne-us): beneath the skin, as a *subcutaneous injection*.

subdural (sub-du'ral): between the dura mater and the arachnoid layers of the brain, as a *subdural hematoma*.

subjective (sub-jek'tiv): perceived only by the affected individual (pain is a subjective sign); also referring to a test item that requires judgment and interpretation as to the correct answer, open to more than one interpretation.

subliminal (sub-lim'i-nal): referring to a stimulus that is below the threshold of consciousness.

sublingual (sub-ling'gwal): under the tongue; (nitroglycerin is a drug that is administered sublingually).

subluxation (sub-luk-sa'shun): partial dislocation.

sudden death (sud'n deth'): a situation in which breathing and heartbeat stop; also called **cardiopulmonary arrest.**

sudden infant death syndrome (SIDS): crib death, cot death, infantile apnea syndrome. Thought to be a result of untreated prolonged infantile apnea (PIA) or "near miss."

sudoresis (soo-do-re'sis): profuse sweating, **diaphoresis.**

sudoriferous (su-do-rif'er-us): conveying or transmitting sweat. (*Sudoriparous* soo-do-rip'ah-rus: secreting or producing sweat.)

suffocation (suf-o-ka'shun): stoppage of breathing; **asphyxia.**

superficial (soo-per-fish'al): on or near the surface, not deep, as a superficial burn or cut.

superior (soo-per'e-or): above (**supra:** above).

superlethal (soo-per-le'thal): more than enough to cause death, as a *superlethal* dose of a drug.

supination (su-pin-a'shun): the act of turning to the *supine position;* turning the hand so the palm is upward.

supine (soo'pin): lying on the back with the face upward.

suppository (sup-oz'i-to-re): a conical mass to be introduced into the vagina, rectum, or urethra, usually containing medication (easily melted).

suppression (su-presh'un): stoppage of a normal secretion or discharge, as *suppression of urine*.

suppuration (sup-u-ra'shun): formation or discharge of pus. (adj: **suppurative)**

suprarenal (soo-prah-re'nal): **adrenal,** above the kidney.

surfactant (ser-fak'tant): surface-active agent, such as soap; a mixture of phospholipids (mostly lecithin and sphingomyelin) in the respiratory passages, used as a test for maturity of a fetus.

survival needs: according to Maslow, those needs that are vital to sustain life, **primary needs.**

susceptible (sus-sep'ti-bul): having little resistance, as susceptible to a disease.

suture (su'tur): a surgical stitch; line of union of skull bones.

swallowing (swa'lo-ing): moving food from the mouth through the esophagus, **deglutition.**

symbiosis (sim-bi-o'sis): the relationship between two individuals who mutually reinforce each other and are dependent, two organisms living together to the benefit of each.

sympathectomy (sim-pah-thek'to-me): interruption of stimuli in a portion of the sympathetic nervous system.

sympathy (sim'pa-the): emotional compassion for another's grief or loss; an influence on one organ or part by a disorder of another part, as *sympathetic ophthalmia*.

symptoms (simp'tums): functional evidence of a disease or of the patient's condition perceived by the patient (as opposed to signs, which are perceived by the examiner).

synapse (sin'aps): the functional junction between two neurons (nerve cells) at which point the impulse is transmitted.

synarthrosis (sin-ar-thro'sis): a fused joint, a *fibrous joint*.

syncope (sin'co-pe): a temporary state of unconsciousness, commonly known as **fainting.**

syndrome (sin'drom): a group of symptoms that often occur together, as *Down syndrome*.

synergism (sin'er-jism): joint action of agents in which combined effect is greater than the sum of the individual parts (synergistic drugs enhance the action of each other), **potentiation.**

synovial (si-no've-al): a joint in which there is free movement, due to secretion of synovial fluid. (Also called **diarthrosis.)**

synthesis (sin'the-sis): an artificial or natural production of a compound.

syringectomy (sir-in-jek'to-me): surgical removal of a fistula.

systemic (sis-tem'ik): pertaining to the entire body, general, total (as opposed to local).

systole (sis'to-le): contraction of the heart; systolic blood pressure is the pressure of the blood against the walls of the arteries when the *heart beats* (the top number in the blood pressure reading).

tabes (ta'bez): wasting or progressive atrophy of the body, as *tabes dorsalis* (caused by syphilis).

tachycardia (tak-e-kar'de-ah): abnormally fast heart rate.

tachypnea (tak-ip-ne'ah): very rapid rate of respiration, as seen in high fever.

tactile (tak'til): pertaining to touch.

talipes (tal'i-pez): **clubfoot.**

tamponade (tam-po-nad'): abnormal compression of a part, as in *cardiac tamponade* (due to fluid in the pericardial sac).

tapotement (tah-pot-maw'): tapping movement in backrub or massage.

tarsal (tar'sal): pertaining to the edge of an eyelid or to the instep of the foot.

tartar (tar'tar): deposits on the teeth, **dental calculus.**

taut (tawt): tightly drawn.

telangiectasia (tel-an-je-ek-ta'ze-ah): vascular lesion formed by the dilation of small blood vessels, as *spider telangiectasia.*

temperature (tem'per-a-tur): the degree of hotness or coldness of a substance, as *body temperature.*

temporal (tem'po-ral): pertaining to the temple on the side of the head, as the *temporal lobe* of the brain.

tenacious (te-na'shus): adhesive, sticky, as *tenacious sputum.*

tendinitis (ten-di-ni'tis): inflammation of the tendons, often associated with a buildup of calcium in the shoulder; also called **tendonitis, tenonitis, tenontitis, tenositis.**

tenosynovitis (ten-o-sin-o-vi'tis): inflammation of a tendon sheath.

tepid (tep'id): moderately warm; also called **tepor.**

teratogen (ter'ah-to-gen): an agent or factor that causes defects in a developing embryo, such as a drug taken by the mother during pregnancy.

teratoid (ter'ah-toid): resembling a monster.

terminal (ter'min-al): at the end; also refers to a patient who is dying.

testes (tes'tis): the male gonad (*sing:* **testis.**)

testicular (tes-tik'u-lar): pertaining to the testes.

testosterone (tes-tos'ter-on): major male hormone.

tetanus (tet'ah-nus): a highly fatal disease characterized by muscle spasms and seizures ("**lock-jaw**"). Can be prevented by immunization.

tetany (tet'ah-ne): continuous contraction of one or more muscles; a syndrome in which the wrist or ankle joints are sharply flexed (**carpopedal spasm**).

therapeutic communication: communication (usually verbal) with a patient that is helpful and beneficial; creating a healing, curative, and safe milieu by using communication.

therapy (ther'ap-e): the treatment of disease (**therapeutic**).

thermal (ther'mal): pertaining to heat, as a *thermal burn.*

thermolysis (ther-mol'i-sis): chemical destruction by means of heat, as in thermolysis of pathogenic organisms.

thermoregulation (ther-mo-reg-u-la'shun): *heat regulation,* heat control.

third-party payor: an organization that pays for health care, rather than the patient paying for his/her own care, such as an insurance company or health maintenance organization.

thoracentesis (tho-rah-sen-te'sis): surgical puncture and drainage of the thoracic (chest) cavity.

thoracotomy (tho-rah-kot'o-me): a surgical incision of the wall of the thoracic (chest) cavity.

thorax (tho'raks): the chest.

thrill (thril): a vibration felt upon palpation.

thromboangiitis (throm-bo-an-je-i'tis): inflammation of a blood vessel, with thrombosis. *T. obliterans* (ob-lit'er-ans): disease of medium-sized blood vessels, particularly in the legs.

thrombocytopenia (throm-bo-si-to-pe'ne-ah): decrease in the number of platelets (*thrombocytes*) in the circulation.

thrombophlebitis (throm-bo-fleb-i'tis): formation of a blood clot in a vein, with inflammation.

thrombosis (throm-bo'sis): the formation of blood clots (**thrombi**) in the circulatory system.

thrush: fungus infection of the oral mucous membrane, occurs most frequently in infants and immunosuppressed adults.

thymus (thi'mus): small gland in the upper chest that functions as an endocrine gland.

thyroid (thi'royd): resembling a shield. The thyroid gland, located in the neck, is the largest endocrine gland. It secretes hormones vital to growth and metabolism.

tic (tik): involuntary, spasmodic twitching, as a *facial tic.*

tincture (tingk'tur): an alcoholic solution of a drug or chemical, as *tincture of iodine.*

tinea (tin'e-ah): a name used for many different fungal infections of the skin; **tinea capitis,** ringworm of the scalp; **tinea corporis,** ringworm of the skin; **tinea pedis,** athlete's foot.

tinnitus (ti-ni'tus): ringing or buzzing in the ears; may sometimes be heard by another person.

tissue (tish'u): a group of similar, specialized cells united to perform a specific function, as *epithelial tissue.*

tolerance (tol'er-ans): the ability to endure the continued use of a substance, such as a drug; sometimes refers to increased dosage needed to achieve the desired effect.

tomography (tom-mog'rah-fe): body section or plane roentgenography (*radiographic studies*) with the x-ray tube usually moved in an arc. The images are of single planes of tissue.

tone (tōn): normal vigor and tension, as muscle tone. **Tonicity:** in body fluid, osmotic pressure.

tonic–clonic (to-nik'; claw-nik') **seizures**: seizures characterized by loss of consciousness and alternating periods of muscular contraction and relaxation. Formerly called *grand mal* seizures.

tonometer (to-nom'e-ter): an instrument for measuring tension or pressure (usually intraocular pressure within the eyeball). **Tonograph:** the recording from a tonometer.

tonus (to'nus): tone; the slight, continuous contraction of muscles.

topical (top'e-kal): pertaining to an external or local spot, as a *topical medication* applied to the skin.

torsion (tor'shun): twisting. **Torque:** twisting force.

tort: a wrong or injury for which the injured person has a right to sue. Includes situations such as breach of confidentiality, slander or neglect of duty.

torticollis (tor-ti-kol'is): torsion (twisting) of the neck, **"wry neck."**

total parenteral nutrition: method of nutrition in which a catheter is inserted into a large blood vessel and nutrient solution is administered by continuous drip (**TPN**).

tourniquet (toor'ni-ket): a device used to inhibit bleeding.

toxic (tok'sik): pertaining to a poison or toxin.

toxin (tok'sin): poison, especially refers to protein poisons produced by pathogenic bacteria and some animals and plants.

toxoplasmosis (tok-so-plaz-mo'sis): a congenital or acquired disease that can cause lesions in most body systems. It is particularly dangerous to pregnant women and can be prevented by careful cooking of meat and avoidance of handling cat litter.

tracheostomy (tra-ke-os'to-me): artificial opening through the neck into the *trachea* (the "windpipe") through which the person breathes (may be temporary or permanent).

tracheotomy (tra-ke-ot'o-me): incision into the trachea.

trachoma (trah-ko'mah): a chronic infectious disease of the cornea and conjunctiva of the eye.

traction (trak'shun): exertion of a pulling force, as traction on a fractured bone.

trade name: the copyrighted *brand name* of a drug assigned by its manufacturer. (A drug with the same generic/chemical name can have several trade or **proprietary** names.)

tranquilizer (tran'kwi-li-zer): a drug used to relax or calm an agitated or anxious patient.

transcription (tran-skrip'shun): writing, copying, as in *transcription of physician's orders* into the Kardex.

transcultural nursing (trans-kul'chur-al): the unbiased care of persons from all races, religions, or ethnic groups.

transcutaneous (trans-ku-ta'ne-us): through the skin, **transdermal**.

transdermal (trans-der'mal): through the skin, a substance absorbed into the body after being placed on the skin, as *transdermal administration* of medication by ointment or patch, **transcutaneous.**

transection (tran-sek'shun): cross section; cutting across, as *accidental transection* of the spinal cord causing paralysis.

transfusion (trans-fu'zhun): injection of blood, blood components, or blood substitutes into the circulation of the patient.

transmit (trans-mit'): to pass on, *transfer,* as to transmit inherited characteristics by means of the genes.

transplantation (trans-plan-ta'shun): the transfer of organs or body tissues from one person or animal to another. Some organs/tissues are obtained from *living donors* (kidney); others from *cadaver donors* (kidney, heart, corneas, skin, heart valves, bone).

transposition (trans-po-zish'un): abnormal displacement to the opposite side, as *transposition of the great (blood) vessels.*

transurethral (trans-u-re'thral): through the urethra, as *transurethral resection of the prostrate gland (TURP).*

transverse (trans-vers'): from side to side, **crosswise.**

trauma (traw'mah): a wound or injury, especially from an external source.

tremor (trem'or): trembling, often associated with Parkinson's disease (adj.: **tremulous**).

triage (tre-ahzh'): sorting out of victims of disaster to determine the priority of treatment.

tricuspid (tri-kus'pid): with three cusps or points, as the tricuspid valve of the heart, between the right atrium and ventricle.

triglyceride (tri-glis'er-id): a compound consisting of three molecules of fatty acids and one molecule of glycerol, which is the usual form of fat storage in the body.

trimester (tri-mes'ter): 3 months, as a *trimester in pregnancy.*

triplegia (tri-ple'je-ah): paralysis of three extremities.

trisomy (tri'some-e): the presence of a third chromosome of one type (normally, there are two of each), as *trisomy-21,* a genetic disorder.

trocar (tro'kar): a sharp, pointed instrument inside a cannula used for puncturing the wall of a body cavity.

troche (tro'ke): a lozenge-type medication to be dissolved in the mouth, usually for cough.

truss (trus): a device used to maintain a hernia within the abdominal cavity, not commonly used today.

tuberculosis (too-berk-yoo-lo'sis) **(TB)**: a communicable disease caused by the tubercle bacillus (any organ may be affected but it primarily affects the lung in human beings).

tumescence (too-mes'ens): swollen, **tumid.**

tumor (tu'mor): an abnormal new growth of tissue having no physiologic use, which grows independent of its surrounding structures and may be benign or malignant.

turbid (tur'bid): cloudy.

turgid (tur'jid): congested, swollen, as *turgid extremities* in edema.

turgor (tur'ger): the condition of being turgid; normal or abnormal fullness, as *turgor of the skin.*

tympanic membrane (tim-pan'ik); **tympanum:** eardrum. **Tympanus:** the cavity of the middle ear, just medial to the tympanic membrane.

tympanitis (tim-pah-ni'tis): otitis media, an inflammation of the middle ear.

tympanous (tim'pah-nus): distended with gas, as a *tympanous abdomen.* (drumlike).

ulcer (ul'ser): an open sore on an external or internal surface of the body that causes the gradual disintegration of the tissues, often an ulcer of the stomach (*peptic ulcer*) or a pressure sore (*decubitus ulcer*).

ultrasound (ul'trah-sownd): means by which deep structures of the body can be visualized by the reflection of ultrasonic radiant energy waves. (Ultrasonic energy can also be used to break up undesired objects, such as gallstones.)

umbilicus (um-bil-i'kus (um-bil'ah-kus)): a small scar on the abdomen that marks the former attachment of the umbilical cord to the fetus; also called **navel,** ("belly button").

unconscious (un-kon'shus): a lack of awareness of the environment with an inability to react to sensory stimuli, **comatose.**

unction, unguent (ungk'shun, ung'gwent): **ointment,** salve.

undulation (un-du-la'shun): wavelike motion.

unguinal, ungual (ung'gwi-nal, ung'gwal): pertaining to a fingernail or toenail (*unguis*).

unilateral (u-ni-lat'er-al): on one side only.

universal body substance (secretion) precautions: precautions established by Centers for Disease Control and Prevention in an effort to control the spread of diseases.

unremitting (un-re-mit'ting): relentless, constant, as in *unremitting pain.*

urea (u-re'ah): the end product of protein metabolism in the body and the chief nitrogenous substance in the urine.

uremia (u-re'me-ah): retention of substances in the blood that are usually eliminated in urine; a common blood test for kidney disorders is the BUN (blood urea nitrogen). Uremia is more correctly called **end-stage renal disease (ESRD)** in its later stages.

ureter (yoo-re'ter): the narrow tube that carries urine from the kidney to the urinary bladder.

urethra (yoo-re'thrah): tube through which urine passes from the urinary bladder to the outside of the body.

urgency (ur'jen-se): inability to wait to void.

uric (u'rik): pertaining to urine, as *uric acid.*

urinalysis (ur-in-al'is-is): examination of urine.

urination (u-ri-na'shun): passing of urine from the urinary bladder to outside, **voiding, micturition.**

urinometer (u-ri-nom'e-ter): an instrument that determines specific gravity of urine; also called **urometer, hydrometer.**

urology (u-rol'o-je): the study of urinary disorders in the female and genitourinary disorders in the male. A **urologist** is the physician who specializes in this area.

urticaria (ur-ti-ka're-ah): an allergic reaction of the skin characterized by superficial wheals and often accompanied by severe itching; also called **hives.**

uterine (u'ter-in): pertaining to the uterus, as *uterine tube.*

uterus (yoo'ter-us): hollow, pear-shaped organ in the female pelvis where the fetus develops and grows; also called **womb.**

vaccination (vak-sin-a'shun): the injection of killed or modified live microorganisms for the purpose of treating or producing immunity to certain infectious diseases; also called **inoculation, immunization.**

vagina (vah-jin'ah): muscular canal between the uterus and outside of body. Female organ of sexual intercourse and birth canal.

vaginal (vaj'i-nal): pertaining to the vagina or to any sheath.

vaginitis (vaj-in-i'tus): inflammation of the vagina; sometimes includes inflammation of the vulva.

vagotomy (va-got'o-me): surgical interruption of impulses carried by the vagus nerve (the tenth cranial nerve).

valgus (val'gus): twisted, bent outward, as in *talipes valgus* (a form of clubfoot).

Valsalva's maneuver (val-sal′vahz): forcible exhalation against a closed glottis, causing increased pressure in the thorax, as in straining to defecate.

values clarification: deciding, after contemplation, things that are most important to oneself, assessment of personal ideals.

valve (valv): a membranous structure in an orifice or passage that allows the passage of contents in one direction only, as a *valve of the heart* or in the leg veins.

varicocele (var′i-ko-seel): scrotal swelling caused by varicosities in the spermatic blood vessels (described as feeling like a "bag of worms").

varicose veins (var′i-kose vanes): distended and twisted veins, usually occurring in the legs or as hemorrhoids.

varus (va′rus): bent inward, as in *talipes varus* (a form of clubfoot).

vas (vas): vessel, as *vas deferens*.

vasectomy (vah-sek′to-me): excision of the vas deferens, rendering a male sterile.

vasoconstriction (vas-o-kon-strik′shun): lessening in the circumference of a blood vessel.

vasoconstrictor (vas-o-con-strik′ter): drug that raises blood pressure by causing the lumina (caliber) of blood vessels to become smaller, used to *treat hemorrhage* (excessive bleeding).

vasodilation (vas-o-di-la′shun): increase in the caliber (circumference) of a blood vessel.

vasodilator (vas-o-di′la-ter): drug that lowers blood pressure by causing dilation (enlargement of lumina) of blood vessels, used to *treat hypertension* (high blood pressure).

vasopressor (vas-o-pres′or): agent or activity that stimulates contraction of the capillaries and arteries, as a *vasopressor drug*.

vector (vek′tor): carrier, especially of a disease organism.

vegan (vej′an): a vegetarian who does not eat any animal-originated foods. (A **lacto-vegetarian** eats milk and dairy products; an **ovo-vegetarian** eats eggs.)

vein (van): blood vessels that carry blood back to the heart from the body (in most cases, deoxygenated blood).

venesection (ven-i-sek′shun): an incision into a vein; also called **phlebotomy** or **cutdown.**

venipuncture (ven-i-punk′tur): puncture of a vein, usually with a needle. May be used to obtain a blood specimen or to start an intravenous infusion (IV).

ventilation (ven-til-a′shun): supplying of oxygen to the body through the lungs, *breathing*. A machine called a *ventilator* mechanically supplies oxygen and forces breathing.

ventral (ven′tral): pertaining to the abdomen (opposite of dorsal.)

ventricles (ven′tri-kls): two lower chambers of heart (pump blood to the body and lungs).

ventricular (ven-trik′u-lar): pertaining to a ventricle, as in the heart, as a *ventricular septal defect.*

vermiform (ver′mi-form): shaped like a worm, as the *vermiform appendix.*

verbal communication: the giving of information, news, or messages by speaking or writing.

vernix (ver′niks): (Latin) varnish. **Vernix caseosa:** the substance covering the fetus before and at birth.

verucca (ve-roo′kah): wart, as *verucca plantaris* (plantar's wart).

version (ver′zhun): turning, as of the fetus during normal delivery.

vertigo (ver′ti-go): sensation of rotation or movement of self (*subjective vertigo*) or surroundings (*objective vertigo*). (Not all dizziness is true vertigo.)

vesicle (ves′i-kl): small sac containing liquid, *small blister.*

vesicovaginal (ves-i-ko-vaj′i-nal): pertaining to the bladder and vagina.

vestibule (ves′ti-bul): space at the entrance to another structure, as the vestibule to the vagina or in the inner ear.

vestige (ves′tij): remnant of a structure from a previous stage of development, as a patent ductus arteriosus (which should close at birth).

viable (vi′ah-bl): able to live after birth; **living.**

vial (vi′al): small bottle, usually containing a medication.

villi (vil′i): fingerlike projections in the small intestine that provide absorption area for nutrients to enter into the bloodstream. (sing: **villus**)

viral (vi′ral): caused by or pertaining to a virus, as *viral pneumonia.*

virile (vir′il): possessing masculine traits, especially the ability to perform as a male in sexual intercourse.

virulence (vir′u-lens): ability of a microorganism to cause disease; *strength*, potency.

virus (vi′rus): a very small class of infectious agents made up of genetic material (either DNA or RNA), which can only multiply within a host cell.

viscera (vis′er-ah): large internal body organs, particularly those in the abdominal cavity.

viscid (vis′id): sticky, tenacious, as *viscid sputum.*

vital signs (vi′tal sins′): measurements of functions necessary to sustain life; as temperature, pulse, respiration (TPR), and blood pressure (BP).

vitamin (vit′ah-min): various organic substances essential to life (includes the *fat-soluble vitamins*—A, D, E, and K and the *water-soluble vitamins*—B-complex, C, and others).

vitiligo (vit-l-li′go): a skin condition characterized by white patches, which often become larger.

void (void): to cast out wastes, as to **urinate, micturate.**

voluntary (vol′un-tar-re): controlled by the will, as a *voluntary muscle.*

volvulus (vol′vu-lus): twisting of a loop of intestine; may or may not strangulate.

vomitus (vom′i-tus): matter forcibly expelled from the stomach through the mouth by vomiting; **emesis.**

vulva (vul′vah): the external parts of the female genital organs. (**vulvitis:** inflammation of the vulva.)

wart (wort): a tumor of the skin caused by a virus, **verucca.**

wean (ween): to substitute another method of feeding for breast (or bottle) feeding of an infant.

wellness (well′ness): a state of physical and emotional well being; *optimum health;* **homeostasis.**

wheal (wheel): a smooth, slightly elevated area on the skin, usually pale in the center with a reddened periphery, often accompanied by severe itching.

wheeze (hweez): a whistling respiratory sound, typical of asthma.

withdrawal (with-drawl′): discontinuance of use of a drug.

womb (woom): the **uterus.**

wound (woond): an injury to any body structure caused by physical means; such as a *stab wound* or a *surgical wound.*

wry neck: torticollis

xanthosis (zan-tho′sis): a yellowish pigmentation of the skin (*xanthic:* yellow).

xenograft (zen′o-graft): a graft of tissue between animals of different species, as in the grafting of pigskin onto a human in burn treatment; also called **heterograft.**

xeroderma (ze-ro-der′ma): excessive dryness of the skin.

xiphoid (zi′foid, zif′oid): sword-shaped (usually refers to the *xiphoid process,* the pointed piece of cartilage on the lower end of the sternum).

x-ray (eks′ra): a ray used to make photographic plates of parts of the body and to treat disease; also called **roentgenograms.**

zoster (zos′ter): a viral disease, as *herpes zoster.*

Z-plasty (ze′plas-te): repair of a skin defect by transposing two triangular flaps of adjacent skin; relaxes the contracture caused by a scar.

Z-track: a method of injection of a caustic drug, such as iron.

zygote (zi′gote): the cell resulting from the fusion of two mature germ cells, as an unfertilized egg and a mature sperm cell.

A
Key English-to-Spanish Healthcare Phrases

Phrases that Will Help the Nurse Care for Persons Who Are Spanish Speaking

Although English is the major language spoken in North America, a variety of languages are heard. Prominent among them is Spanish, representing Spain, the Caribbean Islands, Central and South America, and the Philippines. Rapport can be more easily established and the patient and family will be at ease and feel more relaxed if someone on the staff speaks their language. Some healthcare facilities, especially in areas with a large population of Spanish-speaking people, provide interpreters. In smaller hospitals or smaller communities this may not be possible.

It is to your advantage to learn the second language apparent in your community. For this reason the following table of English-to-Spanish has been prepared. Instructions for using it are simple. You look for the phrase in English in the first column of this table. The second column gives the phrase in Spanish. You can write this or point to it. The third column gives a phonetic pronunciation. The syllable in each word to be accented is printed in italic type. Even if you are not proficient in English-to-Spanish, your Spanish-speaking patients will appreciate your trying to converse in their language. Begin with "Buenos dias. ¿Como se siente?" And remember "por favor."*

INTRODUCTORY PHRASES

English	Spanish	Pronunciation
Please*	Por favór	Por fah-*vor*
Thank you	Grácias	*Grah*-see-ahs
Good morning	Buénos días	*Bway*-nos *dee*-ahs
Good afternoon	Buénas tárdes	*Bway*-nas *tar*-days
Good evening	Buénas nóches	*Bway*-nas *Noh*-chays
My name is	Mi nómbre es	Me *nohm*-bray ays
Yes/No	Si/No	See/No
I am a student nurse.	Soy estudiénte enferméra	Soy ays-stoo-dee-*ayn*-tay ayn-fay-*may*-rah
What is your name?	¿Cómo se llama?	¿*koh*-moh say *jah*-mah?
How old are you?	¿Cuántos años tienes?	¿*kwan*-tohs ahn-yos tee-*ayn*-ays?
Do you understand me?	¿Me entiende?	¿Me ayn-tee-*ayn*-day?
Speak slower.	Habla más despacio	*Ah*-blah mahs days-*pah*-see-oh
Say it once again.	Repítalo, por favor	Ray-*pee*-tah-loh, por fah-*vor*
How do you feel?	¿Cómo se siente?	¿*Koh*-moh say see-*ayn*-tay?
Good	Bien	bee-ayn
Bad	Mal	*mah*l
Physician	Medico	*May*-dee-koh
Hospital	Hospital	*Ooh*-spee-tall
Midwife	Comadre	Koh-*mah*-dray
Native Healer	Curandero	Ku-ren-*day*-roh

* You should begin or end any request with the word PLEASE (POR FAVOR).

Rosdahl CB: Textbook of Basic Nursing, 6th ed. © 1995 J.B. Lippincott Company

GENERAL

Zero	Cero	*Se*-roh
One	uno	*oo*-noh
Two	dos	dohs
Three	tres	trays
Four	cuatro	*kwah*-troh
Five	cinco	*sin*-koh
Six	seis	says
Seven	siete	see-*ay*-tay
Eight	ocho	oh-choh
Nine	nueve	new-*ay*-vay
Ten	diez	*dee*-ays
Hundred	ciento, cien	see-*en*-toh, see-*en*
Hundred and one	ciento uno	see-*en*-toh *oo*-noh
Sunday	domingo	doh-*ming*-goh
Monday	lunes	*loo*-nays
Tuesday	martes	*mar*-tays
Wednesday	miercoles	mee-*er*-cohl-ays
Thursday	jueves	*hway*-vays
Friday	viernes	vee-*ayr*-nays
Saturday	sabado	*sah*-bah-doh
Right	derecha	day-*ray*-chah
Left	izqierda	ees-kee-*ayr*-dah
Early in the morning	temprano por la mañana	tehm-*prah*-noh por lah mah-*nyah*-na
In the daytime	en el día	ayn el *dee*-ah
At noon	a mediodía	ah meh-dee-oh-*dee*-ah
At bedtime	al acostarse	al ah-kos-*tar*-say
At night	por la noche	por la *noh*-chay
Today	Hoy	oy
Tomorrow	Mañana	mah-*nyah*-nah
Yesterday	Ayer	ai-*yer*
Week	Semana	say-*mah*-nah
Month	mes	mace

PARTS OF THE BODY

The head	la cabeza	lah kah-*bay*-sah
The eye	el ojo	el *o*-hoh
The ears	los oídos	lohs o-*ee*-dohs
The nose	la nariz	lah nah-*reez*
The mouth	la boca	lah *boh*-kah
The tongue	la lengua	lah *len*-gwah
The neck	el cuello	el koo-*eh*-joh
The throat	la garganta	lah gar-*gan*-tah
The skin	la piel	lah pee-el
The bones	los huesos	lohs hoo-*ay*-sos
The muscles	los músculos	lohs *moos*-koo-lohs
The nerves	los nervios	lohs *nayhr*-vee-ohs
The shoulder blades	las paletillas	lahs pah-lay-*tee*-jahs
The arm	el brazo	el *brah*-soh

The elbow	el codo	el *koh*-doh
The wrist	la muñeca	lah moon-*yeh*-kah
The hand	la mano	lah *mah*-noh
The chest	el pecho	el *pay*-choh
The lungs	los pulmones	lohs *puhl*-moh-nays
The heart	el corazón	el koh-rah-*son*
The ribs	las costillas	lahs kohs-*tee*-jahs
The side	el flanco	el *flahn*-koh
The back	la espalda	lah ays-*pahl*-dah
The abdomen	el abdomen	el *ahb*-doh-men
The stomach	el estómago	el ays-*toh*-mah-goh
The leg	la pierna	lah pee-ehr-nah
The thigh	el muslo	el *moos*-loh
The ankle	el tobillo	el toh-bee-joh
The foot	el pie	el *pee*-ay
Urine	urino	u-*re*-noh

DISEASES

Allergy	Alergia	Ah-*layr*-hee-ah
Anemia	Anemia	ah-*nay*-mee-ah
Cancer	Cancer	Kahn-sayr
Chicken pox	Varicela	Vah-ree-*say*-lah
Diabetes	Diabetes	Dee-ah-bay-tees
Diphtheria	Difteria	Deef-*tay*-ree-ah
German measles	Rubéola	Roo-*bay*-oh-lah
Gonorrhea	Gonorrea	Gun-noh-*ree*-ah
Heart disease	Enfermedad del corazón	Ayn-*fayr*-may-*dahd* dayl koh-rah-*sohn*
High blood pressure	Presión alta	Pray-see-*ohn al*-ta
Influenza	Gripe	*Gree*-pay
Lead poisoning	Envenenamiento con plomo	Ayn-vay-nay-nah-mee-*ayn*-toh kohn *ploh*-moh
Liver disease	Enfermedad del hígado	Ayn-*fayr* may-dahd del ee-*gah*-doh
Measles	Sarampion	Sah-rahm-pee-*ohn*
German measles	Rubeola	roo-be-*oh*-lah
Mumps	Paperas	Pah-*pay*-rahs
Nervous disease	Enfermedades nerviosa	Ayn-fayr-may-*dahd*-days nayr-vee-*oh*-sah
Pleurisy	Pleuresía	Play-oo-ray-*see*-ah
Pneumonia	Pulmonia	Pool-*moh*-nee-ah
Rheumatic fever	Reumatismo (fiebre reumatica)	Ray-oo-mah-*tees*-moh (fee-*ay*-bray ray-oo-*mah*-tee-kah)
Scarlet fever	Escarlatina	Ays-kahr-lah-*tee*-nah
Syphilis	Sifilis	See-fee-lees
Tuberculosis	Tuberculosis	Too-*bayr*-koo-lohs-sees

FAMILY HISTORY

| Are you married? | ¿Es udsted casado? | ¿ays ood-*stayd* kah-*sah*-doh? |
| A widower? | ¿Viudo? | ¿vee-*oo*-doh? |

A widow?	¿Viuda?	¿vee-*oo*-dah?
Do you have children?	¿Tiene udsted hijos?	¿tee-*ayn*-nay ood-*stayd* ee-hohs?
Are they still living?	¿Viven todavia?	¿*vee*-vehn toh-dah-*vee*-ah?
Do you have sisters?	¿Tiene hermanas?	¿tee-*ay*-nay er-*mah*-nahs?
Do you have brothers?	¿Tiene hermanos?	¿tee-*ay*-nay er-*mah*-nohs?
Of what did your mother die?	¿De que murio tu madre?	¿day kay *moo*-ree-oh too *mah*-dray?
And your father?	¿y su padre?	¿ee soo *pah*-dray?
Your grandmother?	¿su abuela?	¿soo ah-boo-*ay*-lah?
Your grandfather?	¿su abuelo?	¿soo ah-boo-*ay*-loh?

QUESTIONS TO BEGIN PHRASES

Do you have . . . ?	¿Tiene . . . ?	¿tee-*ay*-nay?
Are you . . . ?	¿tiene . . . ?	¿tee-*ay*-nay?
How long . . . ?	¿Hace cúanto?	¿*Ah*-say *kwahn*-toh?
How much . . . ?	¿Cúanto?	¿*Kwahn*-toh?
How . . . ?	¿Como?	¿*Ko*-mo?

SIGNS AND SYMPTOMS

Do you have stomach cramps?	¿Tiene calambres en el estómago?	¿Tee-*ay*-nay kah-*lahm*-brays ayn el ays-*toh*-mah-goh?
Chills?	Escalofrios	Ays-kah-loh-*free*-ohs
An attack of fever?	Un ataque de fiebre	Oon ah-*tah*-kay day fee-*ay*-bray
Hemorrhage?	Hemoragia	Ay-moh-*rah*-hee-ah
Nosebleeds?	Hemoragia por la nariz	Ay-moh-*rah*-hee-ah por-lah nah-*rees*
Unusual vaginal bleeding?	Hemoragia vaginal fuera de los periodos	Ay-moh-*rah*-hee-ah *vah*-hee-nahl foo-*ay*-rah day lohs pay-ree-*oh*-dohs
Hoarseness?	Ronquera	Rohn-*kay*-rah
A sore throat?	¿Le duele la garganta?	¿Lay doo-*ay*-lay lah gahr-gahn-tah?
Does it hurt to swallow?	¿Le duele al tragar?	¿Lay doo-ay-lay ahl trah-gar?
Have you any difficulty in breathing?	¿Tiene difficultad al respirar?	¿Tee-*ay*-nay dee-fee-kool-*tahd* ahl rays-*pee*-rahr?
Does it pain you to breathe?	¿Le duele al respirar?	¿Lay doo-*ay*-lay ahl rays-*pee*-rahr?
How does your head feel?	¿Cómo siente la cabeza?	¿*Koh*-moh see-*ayn*-tay lah Kah-*bay*-sah?
Is your memory good?	¿Es buena su memoria?	¿Ays *bway*-nah soo may-moh-*ree*-ah?
Have you any pain in the head?	¿Le duele la cabeza?	¿Lay doo-*ay*-lay lah Kah-*bay*-sah?
Do you feel dizzy?	¿Tiene udsted vértigo?	¿Tee-*ay*-nay ood-*stayd vehr*-tee-goh?
Are you tired?	¿Está udsted cansado?	¿Ay-*stah* ood-*stayd* kahn-*sah*-doh?
Can you eat?	¿Puede comer?	¿*pway*-day koh-*mer*?
Have you a good appetite?	¿Tiene udsted buen apetito?	¿Tee-*ay*-nay ood-*stayd* bwayn ah-pay-*tee*-toh?
How are your stools?	¿Cómo son sus heces fecales?	¿*Koh*-moh sohn soos *hay*-says fay-*kal*-ays?
Are they regular?	¿Son regulares?	¿Sohn ray-goo-*lah*-rays?
Are you constipated?	¿Está estreñido?	¿Ay-*stah* ays-trayn-*yee*-do?
Do you have diarrhea?	¿Tiene diarrea?	¿Tee-*ay*-nay dee-ah-*ray*-ah?
Have you any difficulty passing water?	¿Tiene dificultad en orinar?	¿Tee-*ay*-nay dee-fee-kool-*tahd* ayn oh-ree-*nahr*?
Do you pass water involuntarily?	¿Orina sin querer?	¿Oh-*ree*-nah seen kay-rayr?

How long have you felt this way?	¿Desde cuándo se siente así?	*Days*-day *Kwan*-doh say see-*ayn*-tay ah-see?
What diseases have you had?	¿Qué enfermedades ha tenido?	¿Kay ayn-fer-may-*dah*-days hah tay-*nee*-doh?
Do you hear voices?	¿Tiene los voces?	¿Tee-*ay*-nay los *vo*-ses?

EXAMINATION

Remove your clothing	Quítese su ropa	*Key*-tay-say soo *roh*-pah
Put on this gown	Pongáse la bata	Pohn-*gah*-say lah *bah*-tah
Need a urine specimen	Es necesário una muéstra de su orina	Ays nay-say-*sar*-ee-oh oo-nah moo-*ay*-strah day oh-*ree*-nah
Be seated	Siéntese	See-*ayn*-tay-say
Recline	Acuestése	Ah-cways-*tay*-say
Sit up	Siéntese	See-*ayn*-tay-say
Stand	Parése	Pah-*ray*-say
Bend your knees	Dóble las rodíllas	*Doh*-blay lahs roh-*dee*-yahs
Relax your muscles	Reláje los músculos	Ray-*lah*-hay lohs *moos*-koo-lohs
Try to	Aténte	Ah-*tayn*-tay
Try again	Aténte ótra vez	Ah-*tayn*-tay *oh*-tra vays
Do not move	No se muéva	Noh say moo-*ay*-vah
Turn on (or to) your left side	Voltése a su ládo izquiérdo	Vohl-*tay*-say ah soo *lah*-doh is-key-*ayr*-doh
Turn on (or to) your right side	Voltése a su ládo derécho	Vohl-*tay*-say ah soo *lah*-doh day-*ray*-choh
Take a deep breath	Respíra profúndo	Ray-*speer*-rah pro-*foon*-doh
Hold your breath	Deténga su respiración	Day-*tayn*-gah soo ray-speer-ah-see-*ohn*
Don't hold your breath	No deténga su respiración	Noh day-*tayn*-gah soo ray-speer-ah-see-*ohn*
Cough	Tosa	*toh*-sah
Open your mouth	Abra la boca	*ah*-brah lah *boh*-kah
Show me . . .	Enséñeme . . .	ayn-*sayn*-yay-may
Here There	Aquí Allí	Ah-kee ah-jee
Which side?	¿En qué lado?	Ayn kay *lah*-doh?
Let me see your hand	Enséñeme la mano	Ayn-*sehn*-yay-may lah *mah*-noh
Grasp my hand	Apriete mi mano	Ah-*pree*-it-tay mee *mah*-noh
Raise your arm	Levante el brazo	Lay-*vahn*-tay el *brah*-soh
Raise it more	Más alto	Mahs *ahl*-toh
Now the other	Ahora el otro	Ah-*oh*-rah el *oh*-troh

TREATMENT

It is necessary	Es necesario	ays neh-say-*sah*-ree-oh
An operation is necessary	Una operación es necesaria	oo-nah oh-peh-rah-see-*ohn* ays neh-say-*sah*-ree-ah
A prescription	una receta	*oo*-na ray-*say*-tah
Use it regularly	tómelo con regularidad	*toh*-may-loh kohn ray-goo-*lah*-ree-dad
Take one teaspoonful three times daily (in water)	Tome una cucharadita tres veces al dia, con agua	*Toh*-may oo-na koo-chah-rah-*dee*-tah trays *vay*-says ahl *dee*-ah, kohn ah-gwah

Gargle	Haga gargaras	*Ah*-gah gar-*gah*-rahs
Use injection	use una inyección	*oo*-say *oo*-nah in-*yek*-see-ohn
Oral contraceptives	una pildora	*oo*-nah peel-*doh*-rah
A pill	una pastilla	*oo*-nah pahs-*tee*-yah
A powder	un polvo	oon *pohl*-voh
Before meals	antes de las comidas	*ahn*-tays day lahs koh-*mee*-dahs
After meals	despues de las comidas	*days*-poo-ehs day lahs koh-mee-dahs
Every day	todos los dia	*toh*-dohs lohs *dee*-ah
Every hour	cada hora	*kah*-dah *oh*-rah
Breathe slowly—like this (in this manner)	respire despacio—asi	rays-*pee*-ray days-*pah*-see-oh—ah-*see*
This is oxygen	este oxigéno	*ays*-tay oh-see-*hay*-noh
Remain on a diet	estar a dieta	ays-*tar* a dee-*ay*-tah
You may eat . . .	puede comer	*pway*-day koh-*mer*
You may drink icewater	puede tomar agua con hielo	*pway*-day toh-*mahr ah*-gwah kohn hee-*yeh*-lo
Milk	leche	*leh*-chay
Tea	té	tay
Coffee	café	kah-*fay*
Chocolate	chocolate	choh-koh-*lah*-tay
Beef bouillon	caldo de carne	*kahl*-doh day *kahr*-nay

BEDSIDE CARE

How do you feel?	¿Como se siénte?	¿*Koh*-moh say see-*ayn*-tay?
Have you slept well?	¿Ha dormido bien?	¿ah dohr-*mee*-doh bee-*ayn*?
Are you warm?	¿Tiéne calór?	¿Tee-*ay*-nay kahl-*or*?
Are you warm enough?	¿Esta suficiénte calór?	¿*Ay*-stah soo-fee-see-*ayn*-tay ka-*lor*?
Are you cold?	¿Tiéne frío?	¿Tee-*ay*-nay *free*-oh?
Do you have pain?	¿Tiéne dolór?	¿Tee-*ay*-nay doh-*lorh*?
Where is the pain?	¿Adónde es el dolór?	¿Ah-*dohn*-day ays ayl doh-*lorh*?
Do you want medication for your pain?	¿Quiére medicación para su dolór?	¿Key-*ay*-ray may-dee-kah see-*ohn pak*-rah soo doh-*lorh*?
Are you comfortable?	¿Está comfortáble?	¿*Ay*-*stah* kohm-for-*tah*-blay?
Are you hungry?	¿Tiéne hámbre?	¿Tee-*ay*-nay *ahm*-bray?
Is the (coffee, tea) hot enough?	¿Esta (café, té) suficiénte caliénte?	¿*Ay*-stah (Kah-*fay*, tay) soo-fee-see-*ayn*-tay kahl-ee-*ayn*-tay?
Are you thirsty?	¿Tiéne sed?	¿Tee-*ay*-nay sayd?
You may not eat/drink	No cóma/béba	Noh *koh*-mah/bay-*bah*
You can only drink water	Solo puéde tomár água	Soh-loh *pway*-day toh-mar *ah*-gwah
You can only take ice chips	Solo puéde tomár pedazítos de hiélo	Soh-loh *pway*-day toh-*marh* pay-dah-*zee*-tohs day eee-*ay*-loh
Take a bath	Tome un baño	*Toh*-may oon *bahn*-yoh
A sponge bath	Un baño de esponja	oon *bahn*-yoh day ays-*pohn*-ha
Apply bandage to . . .	Ponga una vendaje a . . .	*pohn*-gah *oo*-nah vehn-*dah*-hay ah . . .
Apply ointment	Aplíquese unguento	ah-*plee*-kay-say oon-goo-*ayn*-toh
Keep very quiet	Estése muy quieto	ays-*tay*-say moo-ay key-*ay*-toh
You must not speak	No debe hablar	noh *day*-bay ha-*blahr*
Swallow small pieces of ice	Trague pedacitos de hielo	*trah*-gay peh-dah-*see*-tohs day hee-*yay*-lo

It will be uncomfortable	Séra incomódo	*Say*-rah een-koh-*moh*-doh
It will sting	Va ardér	Vah ahr-*dayr*
You will feel pressure	Vá a sentír presión	Vah ah sayn-*teer* pray-see-*ohn*
I am going to:	Voy a:	Voy ah
Count (take) your pulse	Tomár su púlso	Toh-*marh* soo *pool*-soh
Take your temperature	Tomár su temperatúra	Toh-*marh* soo taym-pay-rah-*too*-rah
Take your blood pressure	Tomar su presión	Toh-*marh* soo pray-see-*ohn*
Start an IV line	Comensár una intravenósa	Koh-mayn-*sarh* oo-nah een-trah-vayn-*oh*-sah
Give you pain medicine	Dárle medicación para dolór	*Darh*-lay may-dee-kah-see-*ohn* pah-rah doh-*lohr*
Empty your bladder with a small tube	Vaciár su vejíga con una túbo pequeño	Vah-see-*arh* soo vee-*hee*-gah kohn oo-nah *too*-boh pay-*kay*-nyoh
Give you an enema	Dárle un lavádo	*Darh*-lay oon lah-*vah*-doh
You should (try to):	Tráte de:	*Trah*-tay day:
Call for help/assistance	Llamár para asisténcia	Yah-*marh* pah-rah ah-sees-*tayn*-see-ah
Empty your bladder	Orínar	Oh-*ree*-narh
Do you still feel very weak?	¿Se siente muy débil todavía?	Say see-*ayn*-tay moo-ee *day*-beel toh-dah-*vee*-ah
It is important to:	Es importánte de:	Ays eem-por-*tahn*-tay day
Walk (ambulate)	Caminár	Kah-mee-*narh*
Drink fluids	Bebér líquidos	Bay-*bayr* lee-key-dohs

Sources of Further Information

Bongiovanni GL. Medical Spanish, Ed 2. New York, McGraw-Hill, 1991

Gonzalez-Lee T, Simon HJ. Medical Spanish. Englewood Cliffs, NJ, Prentice Hall, 1990

Hart TL. Speedy Spanish for Nursing Personnel, Santa Barbara, CA, Baja Books, 1988

Harvey WC. Spanish for Health Care Professionals. Hauppage, NY, Barron, 1994

Perez-Sabido J. Spanish-English Handbook for Medical Professionals, Ed 4. Los Angeles, CA, Practice Management Information, 1993

Wilbur CJ, Lister S. Medical Spanish. Stoneham, MA, Butterworth-Heinemann, 1990

Thanks to Eugene Gomez, MHW and Carmen Diverti, MD, Hennepin County Medical Center, Minneapolis, MN, for proofreading and making suggestions for Appendix A.

B

Key Abbreviations and Acronymns Used in Healthcare*

AA	Alcoholics Anonymous; African American
AALPN	American Association of Licensed Practical Nurses
AAMI	age-associated memory impairment
AARP	American Association of Retired Persons
ABG	arterial blood gases
ABO	A, B, AB and O (blood groupings)
ACE	angiotensin-converting enzyme inhibitor (medication); all-cotton elastic (roller bandage)
ACLS	advanced cardiac life support
ACS	American Cancer Society
ACT	activated clotting time (test)
ACTH	adrenocorticotropic hormone (corticotropin)
ACU	acute coronary unit
AD	autonomic dysreflexia; Alzheimer's disease
ADA	American Diabetes Association
ADD	attention deficit disorder
ADH	antidiuretic hormone (vasopressin)
ADL	activities of daily living
AEA	above elbow amputation
AEB	as evidenced by (in nursing diagnosis)
AGA	appropriate for gestational age
AHA	American Hospital Association; American Heart Association
AI	artificial insemination
AIDS	acquired immunodeficiency syndrome
AKA	above knee amputation; also known as (alias)
ALL	acute lymphocytic leukemia
ALS	amyotrophic lateral sclerosis
ALT	alanine aminotransferase, serum (liver function test)
AM	morning
AMA	against medical advice; American Medical Association
AML	acute myelogenous leukemia
ANA	American Nurses Association
ANS	autonomic nervous system
AP	apical pulse; anteroposterior (repair); assault precautions; antepartum
APHA	American Public Health Association
APTT	activated partial thromboplastin time (test)
A-R	apical–radial (pulse)
ARDS	adult respiratory distress syndrome
AROM	active (assistive) range of motion; artificial rupture of membranes
ARRP	anatomic retropubic radical prostatectomy
ASA	acetylsalicylic acid (aspirin)
ASAP	as soon as possible
ASCP	American Society of Clinical Pathologists
ASHD	arteriosclerotic heart disease
AST	aspartate aminotransferase, serum (formerly SGOT)
ATN	acute tubular necrosis
AV	atrioventricular (valves—tricuspid and mitral)
A&W	alive and well
Ax	axillary (temperature)
AZT	zidovudine (medication, now called ZDU)
Ba	barium
BBP	blood-borne pathogen
BBT	basal body temperature
BCLS	basic cardiac life support
BE	barium enema (x-ray)

* Consider the context in which an acronym is used because the same initials may have more than one meaning.

BEA	below elbow amputation
BKA	below knee amputation
BLS	basic life support
BM	bowel movement
BP	blood pressure
BPAD	bipolar affective disorder
BPH	benign prostatic hyperplasia (hypertrophy)
BPM	beats per minute
BPRS	brief psychiatric rating scale
BRAT	bananas, rice, applesauce, toast (diet)
BRM	biologic response modifiers
BRP	bathroom privileges
BSE	breast self-examination
BSI	body substance isolation
BUN	blood urea nitrogen
BW	birth weight
Bx	biopsy
C	Celsius, centigrade (temperature); calorie
CA	cancer; carcinoma; Cocaine Anonymous
C&S	culture and sensitivity
CAD	coronary artery disease
CAF	cytoxan, Adriamycin, fluorouracil
CAPD	continuous ambulatory peritoneal dialysis
CAT	computerized axial tomography; computer assisted (adaptive, aided) testing
CBC	complete blood count
CC	chief complaint
CCFA	Crohn's and Colitis Foundation of America
CCU	coronary (cardiac) care unit
CD	chemically dependent; chemical dependency
CDC	Centers for Disease Control and Prevention
CDU	chemical dependency unit
CEA	carcinoembryonic antigen
CEU	continuing education unit
CF	cystic fibrosis
CHF	congestive heart failure
CHHA	certified home health aide
CHO	carbohydrate
CLL	chronic lymphocytic leukemia
CMF	cytoxan, methotrexate, fluorouracil
CMG	cystometrogram (voiding test)
CML	chronic myelogenous leukemia
CMS	color, motion, and sensitivity; circulation, mobility, and sensation (of extremity)
CMV	cytomegalovirus
CNS	central nervous system
C/O	complains (complaints) of
COLD	chronic obstructive lung disease
COPD	chronic obstructive pulmonary disease
CP	cerebral palsy

CPAP	continuous positive airway pressure
CPD	cephalopelvic dysproportion
CPM	continuous passive motion
CPR	cardiopulmonary resuscitation, computer-based patient record
CPT	chest physiotherapy
Cr	creatinine
CRNA	Certified Registered Nurse Anesthetist
Cryo	cryoprecipitate (test)
CS	completed stroke, cardiac sphincter
C & S	culture and sensitivity
CSF	cerebrospinal fluid, colony-stimulating factor
CSR	central supply room; central service room
CSS	central sterile supply, central service supply
CT	computerized (computed) tomography (CT scan)
CUC	chronic ulcerative colitis
CV	cardiovascular
CVA	cerebrovascular accident ("stroke")
CVP	central venous pressure
CXR	chest x-ray
db	decibel
D&C	dilation and curettage
D/C	discontinue
DCH	district court hold
DDS	Doctor of Dental Surgery
DDST	Denver Developmental Screening Test
DEA	Drug Enforcement Agency
DEP	Department of Environmental Protection
DES	diethylstilbestrol
Detox	detoxification
DIC	disseminated intravascular coagulation
Diff	differential count (of white blood cells)
DJD	degenerative joint disease
DMD	Duchenne muscular dystrophy
DNA	deoxyribonucleic acid
DNH	do not hospitalize
DNI	do not intubate
DNR	do not resuscitate
DO	Doctor of Osteopathy
DOA	dead on arrival (admission)
DOB	date of birth
DOE	dyspnea on exertion
DOH	Department of Health
DPAHC	durable power of attorney for healthcare
DPAHD	durable power of attorney for healthcare decisions
DRF	drip rate factor (for IVs)
DRG	diagnosis-related groups
DSM IV	Diagnostic and Statistical Manual of Mental Disorders, 4th Edition

DT	diphtheria and tetanus toxoids	FBS	fasting blood sugar (glucose)
DTAD	drain tube attachment device	FDA	Food and Drug Administration
DTs	delerium tremens	5-FU	5-Fluorouracil (medication)
DTP	diphtheria and tetanus toxoids with pertussis vaccine	FF	force fluids
		FFP	fresh frozen plasma
DTR	deep tendon reflex	FH	family history
DUI	driving under the influence (of chemicals)	FHR	fetal heart rate
DVM	Doctor of Veterinary Medicine	FHT	fetal heart tones
DVT	deep vein thrombosis	FR	fluid restriction
DWI	driving while intoxicated	FSH	follicle-stimulating hormone
Dx	diagnosis	FTND	full-term normal delivery
EC	enteric-coated (tablets)	FTT	failure to thrive
ECF	extended care facility; extracellular fluid	FUO	fever of unknown origin
ECG	electrocardiogram; cardiogram	FVD	fluid volume deficit
ECT	electroconvulsive therapy	FVE	fluid volume excess
EDD	estimated date of delivery	Fx	fracture
EDR	electrodermal response	G	gravida (number of pregnancies)
EEG	electroencephalogram (brain wave graph)	GB	gallbladder
EENT	eyes, ears, nose, and throat	GC	gonococcus (causes gonorrhea)
EER	electroencephalographic response	GDM	gestational diabetes mellitus
EGD	esophagogastroduodenoscopy	GH	growth hormone
e-IPV	enhanced-potency inactivated poliovirus vaccine	GI	gastrointestinal (digestive)
		G tube	gastric tube; gastrostomy tube (into stomach)
EKG	electrocardiogram	GTT	glucose tolerance test
ELISA	enzyme-linked immunosorbent assay	GU	genitourinary
EMG	electromyogram (muscle activity)	GYN	gynecology
EMS	emergency medical services	HAV	hepatitis A virus
EMT	emergency medical technician	HBO	hyperbaric oxygenation
EOM	extraocular movement	HBV	hepatitis B virus; hepatitis B vaccine
EP	escape precautions	HCG	human chorionic gonadotropin
EPA	Environmental Protection Agency	Hct	hematocrit
EPS	electrophysiology studies	HCV	hepatitis C virus
EPSE	extrapyramidal side effects (of psychotropic medications)	HD	Huntington's disease; hemodialysis
		HDV	hepatitis D virus
ER	emergency room; endoplasmic reticulum	HELLP	hemolysis, elevated liver enzymes, low platelet count
ERCP	endoscopic cholangiopancreatography (x-ray)	HEV	hepatitis E virus
ERG	electroretinogram (electrical activity of retina)	Hgb, Hg	hemoglobin
		HI	homicidal ideation
ERT	estrogen replacement therapy	Hib	heomophilus influenzae type B conjugate vaccine
ESADDI	estimated safe and adequate daily dietary intake	HMO	health maintenance organization
ESR	erythrocyte sedimentation rate ("sed rate")	HIV	human immunodeficiency virus
ESRD	end-stage renal disease	H&P	history and physical (examination)
EST	electroshock therapy	HPV	human papillomavirus
ESWL	extracorporeal shock wave lithotripsy	HR	heart rate
ET	enterostomal therapist; endotracheal tube	HRA	Health Resources Administration
ETOH	ethyl alcohol (ethanol)	HS	hour of sleep (at bedtime)
ETOH W/D	alcohol withdrawal	HSA	Health Services Administration
F	Fahrenheit (temperature)	HSV	herpes simplex virus
FAS	fetal alcohol syndrome		
FAT	fetal activity test		

HTLV-I	human T-cell leukemia (lymphotropic) virus, type I	LH	luteinizing hormone (male)
HTN	hypertension	LLL	left lower lobe (of lung)
HUC	health unit coordinator	LLQ	left lower quadrant (of abdomen)
HUS	hemolytic uremic syndrome	LMP	last menstrual period
Hx	history	LOA	left occiput anterior (position of fetus)
IADL	instrumental activities of daily living	LOC	level of consciousness
I&D	incision and drainage (incise and drain)	LOP	left occiput posterior (position of fetus)
I&O	intake and output	LP	lumbar puncture (spinal tap)
IBD	inflammatory bowel disease	LPM	liters per minute (of oxygen)
IBS	irritable bowel syndrome	LPN	Licensed Practical Nurse
ICF	intermediate care facility; intracellular fluid	LTB	laryngotracheobronchitis
ICP	intracranial pressure	LUQ	left upper quadrant (of abdomen)
ICSH	interstitial cell-stimulating hormone (female)	LVN	Licensed Vocational Nurse
ICU	intensive care unit	L&W	living and well
IDDM	insulin-dependent diabetes mellitus	MA	medical assistance (financial assistance)
IFN	interferon	MAC	mood-altering chemicals
IG	immune globulin	MADD	Mothers Against Drunk Driving
IGT	impaired glucose tolerance	MAO	monoamine oxidase inhibitor (medication)
II	intellectually impaired	MAP	mean arterial pressure
IICP	increased intracranial pressure	MAR	medication administration record
IM	intramuscular	MAST	medical antishock trousers
INH	isoniazid (medication)	MD	Doctor of Medicine (medical doctor); muscular dystrophy
IOL	intraocular lens (implant)	MDD	major depressive disorder
IOP	intraocular pressure	mEq	milliequivalent
IPPB	intermittent positive-pressure breathing	MG	myasthenia gravis
IQ	intelligence quotient	MH	mental health; marital history
ITP	idiopathic thrombocytopenia purpura	MHU	mental health unit
IU	international unit	MI	myocardial infarction; mentally ill
IUD	intrauterine device	MI-CD	mentally ill and chemically dependent
IV	intravenous	MI&D	mentally ill and dangerous
IVD	intervertebral disk	MJ	marijuana
IVF	in vitro fertilization	mm Hg	millimeters of mercury
IVIG	intravenous immune globulin	MMPI	Minnesota Multiphasic Personality Inventory
IVP	intravenous pyelogram (x-ray)	MMR	measles, mumps, and rubella virus combined vaccine
IVPB	intravenous piggy back	MOM	milk of magnesia
JCAHO	Joint Commission on Accreditation of Healthcare Organizations	MPD	multiple personality disorder
JRA	juvenile rheumatoid arthritis	MRI	magnetic (resonance) imaging
J tube	jejunostomy tube (into jejunum)	MS	multiple sclerosis; mitral stenosis
KUB	kidney-ureters-bladder (x-ray)	MSDS	material safety data sheet
KVO	keep vein open	MSH	melanocyte-stimulating hormone
L&D	labor and delivery	MT	music therapy
LBW	low birth weight	MVA	motor vehicle accident
LDS	Church of Jesus Christ of the Latter Day Saints (Mormon)	NA	narcotics anonymous; Native American
LE	lower extremity; lupus erythematosus	NAD	no acute distress
LES	lower esophageal sphincter	NAHC	National Association of Home Care
LFT	liver function test(s)	NANDA	North American Nursing Diagnosis Association
LGA	large for gestational age	NAPNES	National Association for Practical Nursing Education and Service

NCLEX	National Council Licensing Examination (-PN: for Practical Nurses; -RN: for Registered Nurses)	PASS	pull (pin), aim (nozzle), squeeze (handle), sweep (from side-to-side) when fighting fires
NCP	nursing care plan	PCA	patient-controlled analgesia (pump); personal care attendant
Neuro	neurology (nervous system disorders)	PCP	*Pneumocystis carinii* pneumonia; phencyclidine HCl
NF	neurofibromatosis		
NFLPN	National Federation of Licensed Practical Nurses	PDA	patent ductus arteriosus
		PDR	Physician's Desk Reference
NG	nasogastric tube (through nose into stomach)	PE	polyethylene (tubes); physical examination; pulmonary embolism
NGC	nongonococcal cervicitis	Peds	pediatrics (care of children)
NGU	nongonococcal urethritis	PEG	percutaneous endoscopic gastrostomy (tube)
NICU	neonatal intensive care unit		
NIDDM	non–insulin-dependent diabetes mellitus	PERRLA	pupils equal, round, react to light, accomodation OK
NIH	National Institutes of Health	PET, PETT	positron emission (transaxial) tomography (scan)
NKDA	no known (drug) allergies		
NLN	National League for Nursing	PH	past history
NOS	no other symptoms, not otherwise specified	PI	present illness
		PIA	prolonged infantile apnea
NRM	non-rebreathing mask	PIC, PICC	percutaneous intravenous (central) catheter (PICC line)
NS, NSS	normal saline (isotonic saline) solution		
NSAID	nonsteroidal anti-inflammatory drug	PID	pelvic inflammatory disease
NSVD	normal spontaneous vaginal delivery	PIH	pregnancy-induced hypertension
NWB	non–weight-bearing	PKU	phenylketonuria
O&P	ova (eggs) and parasites	PM	afternoon
OB	obstetrics	PMH	past medical history
OBD	organic brain disorder	PMN	polymorphonuclear (lymphocytes)
OBS	organic brain syndrome	PM&R	physical medicine and rehabilitation
OCD	obsessive–compulsive disorder	PMS	premenstrual syndrome
OCT	oxytocic challenge test	PNS	peripheral nervous system
OD	Doctor of Optometry; right eye (oculus dexter); overdose	POC	plan of care
		POMR	problem-oriented medical record; patient-oriented medical record
OFC	occipital–frontal circumference		
OH	oral hygiene	PP	postpartum; postprandial (after a meal)
OOB	out of bed	PPD	purified protein derivative (tuberculin test); postpartum day (1st, 2nd, etc.)
OPD	outpatient department		
OPV	(live) oral poliovirus vaccine	PPE	personal protective equipment
OR	operating room	PPF	plasma protein fraction
ORIF	open reduction, internal fixation (orthopedics)	PPG	postprandial (after a meal) glucose (test)
		PPO	preferred provider organization
ORS	oral rehydration solution	PR	per rectum (rectally)
Ortho	orthopedics (musculoskeletal disorders)	PRL	prolactin (hormone)
OS	left eye (oculus sinister)	PRM	partial-rebreathing mask
OSHA	Occupational Safety and Health Act/Administration	Procto	proctology, proctoscopy (rectal exam)
		PROM	passive range of motion; premature rupture of membranes
OT	occupational therapy		
OTC	over-the-counter (medication)	PSA	prostate specific antigen
OU	both eyes, each eye (oculi uterque)	PSDA	Patient Self-Determination Act
PA	pernicious anemia; physician's assistant	PSI	pounds per square inch (pressure)
P&A	percussion and auscultation	PSMR	problem-solving medical record
Pap	Papanicolaou test (Pap smear)	PSV	pressure support ventilation
PAR	postanesthesia recovery		

Psych	psychiatry
PT	physical therapy; prothrombin time (pro-time test); preterm (pregnancy)
PTCA	percutaneous transluminal coronary angioplasty
PTH	parathyroid hormone (parahormone)
PTSD	post-traumatic stress disorder
PTT	partial thromboplastin time
PUS	prostate ultrasound
PVC	premature ventricular contraction
PWB	partial weight-bearing
QA	quality assurance
qd	every day
QI	quality improvement
qod	every other day
R	rectal (by rectum); respirations
RA	rheumatoid arthritis
RACE	rescue, alarm, confine, extinguish (fire fighting)
RAI	radioimmunoassay; radioactive iodine uptake (test)
RBC	red blood cell (erythrocyte)
RC	Roman Catholic; respiratory care
RDA	recommended daily allowance
RDS	respiratory distress syndrome
Rehab	rehabilitation
REM	rapid eye movement
RET	rational emotive therapy
RGP	rigid gas permeable (contact lens)
RHD	rheumatic heart disease
RIA	radioimmunoassay
RIND	reversible ischemic neurologic deficit
RLE	right lower extremity (leg)
RLQ	right lower quadrant (of abdomen)
RN	Registered Nurse
RNA	ribonucleic acid
R/O	rule out
ROA	right occiput anterior (position of fetus)
ROM	range of motion
ROS	review of systems
RPh	Registered Pharmacist
RPR	rapid plasma reagin
RR	recovery room; respiratory rate
RRA	Registered Record Administrator
RSV	respiratory synctial virus
R/T	related to (in nursing diagnosis)
RT	respiratory therapy
RUE	right upper extremity (arm)
RUG	resource utilization group
RUQ	right upper quadrant (of abdomen)
Rx	treatment, give as follows. . .

SA	suicide attempt
SBE	subacute bacterial endocarditis
SBFT	small bowel follow-through (x-ray)
SCORE	Service Corps of Retired Executives
SDAT	senile dementia of the Alzheimer's type
SG	suicide gesture
SGA	small for gestational age
SGOT	serum glutamic-oxaloacetic transaminase (now called AST)
SI	suicidal ideation
SIADH	syndrome of inappropriate antidiuretic hormone
SIB	self-injurious behavior
SIDS	sudden infant death syndrome
SIE	stroke in evolution
SIMV	synchronized intermittent mandatory ventilation
SL	sublingual
SLD	specific learning disability; special learning disability
SLE	systemic lupus erythematosus
S/M	sadomasochism
SNF	skilled nursing facility
SOAP	subjective, objective, assessment, plan
SOAPIER	subjective, objective, assessment, plan, implementation, evaluation, reassessment
SOB	shortness of breath
S/P	status post
SP/GP	suicide precautions/general precautions
Sp Gr	specific gravity
SROM	spontaneous rupture of membranes
SSE	soap suds enema
SSKI	saturated solution of potassium iodide
STD	sexually transmitted disease
STH	somatotrophic hormone (somatotropin)
SubQ	subcutaneous (under the skin)
SVE	sterile vaginal examination
Sx	symptoms
SxP	sexual precautions
T	tympanic (by eardrum)
TAC	time, amount, characteristics (stool, sputum, emesis)
T&A	tonsillectomy and adenoidectomy
TB	tuberculosis
TCDB	turn, cough, and deep breathe
TCH	turn, cough, and hyperventilate
TD	tardive dyskinesia; transdermal
TED	thromboembolytic disease (sox)
TENS	transcutaneous electrical nerve stimulation
TFT	thyroid function test(s)
THA	total hip arthroplasty (replacement)
TIA	transient ischemic attack

TKA	total knee arthroplasty (replacement)
TKO	to keep open (IV)
TLSO	thoracolumbar sacro-orthosis
TMJ	temporomandibular joint (disorder)
TO	telephone order
t-PA	tissue plasminogen activator
TPA	total parenteral alimentation
TPN	total parenteral nutrition
TPR	temperature, pulse, and respiration
TR	therapeutic recreation
Trach	tracheostomy
TSE	testicular self-examination
TSH	thyroid-stimulating hormone
TSS	toxic shock syndrome
TURBT	transurethral resection of a bladder tumor
TURP	transurethral resection of the prostate
TWE	tap water enema
Tx	treatment
UA	urinalysis
UNOS	United Network of Organ Sharing
UPP	urethral pressure profile (voiding test)
URI	upper respiratory infection
US	ultrasound (examination)
USDHHS	United States Department of Health and Human Services
USP(NF)	United States Pharmacopeia and National Formulary
USPHS	United States Public Health Service
UTI	urinary tract infection
VA	Veteran's Administration
VD	venereal disease (sexually transmitted disease)
VDRL	Venereal Disease Research Laboratory (test)
VNA	Visiting Nurse Association
VNAA	Visiting Nurse Association of America
VO	verbal order
Vol	voluntarily admitted
Vol & spec	volume and specific gravity
VS	vital signs
WBC	white blood cell (leukocyte); white blood count
W/D	withdrawal
WD/WN	well-developed, well-nourished
WHO	World Health Organization
WIC	Women, Infants, and Children (agency)
WISC-R	Weschler Intelligence Scale (for children)-Revised
WNL	within normal limits
ZDU	zidovudine (medication used in HIV and AIDS)

C
Normal Values and Reference Tables

Table C-1. Blood Chemistries

Determination	Specimen	Age/Sex	Normal Value	
Albumin (see Protein electrophoresis)				
Aldolase	Serum	Newborn	4 × adult value	
		Adult	<11 IU/L	
Amylase	Serum	Newborn	5–65 U/L	
		>1 y	25–125	
Ascorbic acid	Serum		0.6–2.0 mg/dL	
Bicarbonate	Serum	Arterial	21–28 mmol/L	
		Venous	22–29	

			Premature (mg/dL)	Full-term (mg/dL)
Bilirubin, total	Serum	Cord	<2	<2
		0–1 d	<8	<6
		1–2 d	<12	<8
		2–5 d	<16	<12
		Adult		0.2–1.0
		Pregnancy	Unchanged	

Determination	Specimen	Age/Sex	Normal Value
Bilirubin, direct (conjugated)	Serum		0.8–0.4 mg/dL
Calcium, ionized	Serum, plasma, whole blood	Cord, newborn	5.5 ± 0.3 mg/dL
		Infant	4.0–5.1
		Adult	4.48–5.25
Calcium, total	Serum	Cord, newborn	9–11.5 mg/dL
		Infant	9–10.9
		Adult	8.4–10.2
		Pregnancy	7.8–9.3
Carbon dioxide, partial pressure ($Paco_2$)	Whole blood, arterial	Newborn	27–40 mm Hg
		Infant	27–40
		Pregnancy	27–32
		Female adult	32–45
Carbon monoxide	Whole blood		0.5–1.5% saturation of Hgb (children and nonsmokers); symptoms >20%
Chloride	Serum or plasma	Cord	96–104 mmol/L
		Newborn	97–110
		Adult	98–106
		Pregnancy	Slight elevation
	Sweat	Normal	0–35 mmol/L
		Marginal	30–60
		Cystic fibrosis	60–200

Table C-1 (continued)

Determination	Specimen	Age/Sex	Normal Value
Cholesterol, total	Serum	Adult	140–200
Creatinine kinase, CK (creatine phosphokinase, CPK; 30°C)	Serum	Adult: M	12–70
		F	10–55
			(higher after exercise)
Creatinine	Serum or plasma	Infant	0.2–0.4 mg/dL
		Adult: M	0.6–1.2
		F	0.5–1.0
		Pregnancy	(0.47–0.7)
Creatinine clearance (endogenous)	Serum or plasma and timed urine	Newborn	40–65 mL/min/1.73 m²
		Under 40 y	
		M	97–137
		F	88–128
			(decreases 6.5 mL/min/decade)
Ethanol	Blood		0.0%
			Toxic: 50–100 mg/dL; CNS depression: >100 mg/dL
Fatty acids, free	Serum or plasma	Adults	8–25 mg/dL
		Children and obese adults	<31
Fibrinogen	Whole blood	Newborn	125–300 mg/dL
		Adult	200–400
		Pregnancy	450
Folate	Serum	Newborn	7–32 ng/mL
		Adult	1.8–9 ng/mL
		Pregnancy	1.9–14
Glucose	Serum	Adult	70–105 (fasting)
	Blood	Adult	65–95
	Urine		70–125 (non-fasting)
			<0.5 g/d

Glucose tolerance Dosages: Child 1.75 g/kg of ideal weight, (maximum 75 g) Adult 75 g total dose	Serum		

Time	Normal	Diabetic
Fasting	70–105	>115
60 min	120–170	≥200
90 min	100–140	≥200
120 min	70–120	≥140

Determination	Specimen	Age/Sex	Normal Value
Insulin, (12 h, fasting)	Serum, plasma	Newborn	3–20 mcIU/mL
		Adult	7–24
Iron-binding capacity (TIBC)	Serum	Infant	100–400 μg/dL
		Adult	250–400
		Pregnancy	300–450
Iron	Serum	Newborn	100–250 μg/dL
		Infant	40–100
		Adult: M	50–160
		F	40–150
		Pregnancy	Decreased
Lactate	Whole blood, venous		4.5–19.8 mg/dL
Lactate dehydrogenase (LDH)	Serum	Newborn	160–450 U/L
		Infant	100–250
		Adult	60–170
Lead	Whole blood	Child	<30 μg/dL
		Adult	<40
		Acceptable for industrial exposure	<60
		Toxic	≥100

Table C-1 (continued)

Determination	Specimen	Age/Sex	Normal Value
Lipase (Tietz method; 37°C)	Serum		0.1–1.0 U/mL
		Child	1–6 mIU/mL
		Adult:	4–14
		F, premenopause	4–25
		F, midcycle	25–250
		F, postmenopause	25–200
Magnesium	Serum	Newborn	1.2–1.8 mEq/L
		Adult	1.3–2.1
Oxygen capacity	Whole blood, arterial		1.34 mL/g hemoglobin
Oxygen, partial pressure	Whole blood, arterial	Birth	8–24 mm Hg
		5–10 min	33–75
		30 min	31–85
		>1 h	55–80
		1 d	54–95
		Adult	83–108 decreases with age
Oxygen, % saturation	Whole blood, arterial	Newborn	40–90%
		Thereafter	95–99%
Phenylalanine	Serum	Full-term newborn	1.2–3.4
		Adult	0.8–1.8
Phosphatase, acid prostatic, 37°C	Serum		<3.0 ng/mL
			0.11–0.60 U/L
Phosphatase, alkaline SKI method		Adult	20–70
		Pregnancy >50% rise	
Phospholipids (lipids P × 25)	Serum and plasma	Adult	125–275
Phosphorus, inorganic	Serum	Adult	3.0–4.5
		Pregnancy	Unchanged
Potassium	Serum	Infant	4.1–5.3
		Adult	3.5–5.1
Protein, total	Serum	Adult, recumbent–0.5 g higher in ambulatory patients	6.0–7.8
Protein, electrophoresis, (cellulose acetate)	Serum	Total	
Salicylates	Serum, plasma		Negative: <2.0 mg/dL
			Therapeutic: 15–30
			Toxic: >30
Sodium	Serum	Adult	136–146
Testosterone	Serum	Adult: M	572 ± 135
		F	37 ± 10
Thiamine (vitamin B$_1$)	Serum		2.0 mcg/dL

Triglycerides (TG)	Serum, after 12-h fast		*mg/dL*	
			Male	Female
		12–15 y	36–138	41–138
		16–19 y	40–163	40–128
		20–29 y	44–185	40–128
		Recommended (desirable) levels for adults:	Male 40–160	
			Female 35–135	

Urea nitrogen	Serum/plasma	Cord	21–40 mg/dL
		Newborn	3–12
		Adult	7–18
Uric acid	Serum	Child	2.0–5.5 mg/dL
		Adult: M	3.5–7.2
		F	2.6–6.0
Vitamin A	Serum	Adult	30–65 mcg/dL
Vitamin B$_{12}$	Serum	Newborn	175–800 pg/mL
		Adult	140–700

Table C-1 *(continued)*

Determination	Specimen	Age/Sex	Normal Value
Vitamin C	Plasma		0.6–2.0 mg/mL
Vitamin E	Serum		5–20 mcg/mL
Volume	Whole blood	Adult	72–100
	Plasma	Adult	49–59

† Higher in African Americans.

These values may vary slightly, depending on the particular laboratory performing the tests. The figures stated here are considered to be "within normal range" values.

Table C-2. Urine Chemistries

Determination	Age/Sex	Normal Value
Catecholamines (24 h)	Infant	
	Norepinephrine	0–10 µg/d
	Epinephrine	0–2.5
	Adult	
	Norepinephrine	15–80
	Epinephrine	0.5–20
Chloride (24 h)	Infant	2–10 mmol/d
	Adult (varies greatly with Cl intake)	110–250
Creatinine	Infant	8–20 mg/kg/d
	Adult	14–26
	Pregnancy	Elevated
Lead (24 h)		<80 µg/L
Osmolality (random)		50–1400 mOsmol/kg H₂O depending on fluid intake. After 12 h fluid restriction >850 mOsmol/kg H₂O
Protein, total 24 h		50–80 mg/d (at rest) <250 mg/d after intense exercise <150 mg/dL (as glucose)
Reducing substances		
Specific gravity		
Random void		1.002–1.030
After 12-h fluid restriction		>1.025
24 h		1.015–1.025
Vanillylmandelic acid VMA (24 h)	Newborn	>1.0 mg/d
	Infant	>2.0
	Adult	2–7

Source: Adapted from Fischbach F. A Manual of Laboratory and Diagnostic Tests, Ed 4. Philadelphia, J. B. Lippincott, 1992.

g/dL = grams per deciliter.

10³/mm³ = thousand per cubic meter.

IU = International Unit.

mmol/L = millimole per liter.

mL/min/1.73 m² = milliliter per minute per 1.73 square meter of body surface area.

(meq) µ/dL = micrograms per deciliter.

meq = milliequivalents.

mg/mL = nanogram per milliliter.

D
Exchange Lists for Meal Planning

The reason for dividing food into six different groups is that foods vary in their carbohydrate, protein, fat, and calorie content. Each exchange list contains foods that are alike—each choice contains about the same amount of carbohydrate, protein, fat, and calories.

The following chart shows the amount of these nutrients in one serving from each exchange list.

Exchange List	Carbohydate (g)	Protein (g)	Fat (g)	Calories
Starch/Bread	15	3	trace	80
Meat				
Lean	—	7	3	55
Medium-fat	—	7	5	75
High-fat	—	7	8	100
Vegetable	5	2	—	25
Fruit	15	—	—	60
Milk				
Skim	12	8	trace	90
Low-fat	12	8	5	120
Whole	12	8	8	150
Fat	—	—	5	45

As you read the exchange lists, you will notice that one choice often is a larger amount of food than another choice from the same list. Because foods are so different, each food is measured or weighed so the amount of carbohydrate, protein, fat, and calories is the same in each choice.

You will notice symbols on some foods in the exchange groups. Foods that are high in fiber (3 g or more per exchange) appear in boldface. High-fiber foods are good for you. It is important to eat more of these foods.

Foods that are high in sodium (400 mg) or more of sodium per exchange) have a *; foods that have 400 mg or more of sodium if two or more exchanges are eaten have a ** symbol. It's a good idea to limit your intake of high-salt foods, especially if you have high blood pressure.

1. Starch/Bread List

Each item in this list contains approximately 15 g carbohydrate, 3 g protein, a trace of fat, and 80 calories. Whole grain products average about 2 g fiber per exchange. Some foods

are higher in fiber. Those foods that contain 3 g or more of fiber per exchange appear in **boldface.**

CEREALS/GRAINS/PASTA

Bran cereals, concentrated (such as Bran Buds®, All Bran®)	1/3 cup
Bran cereals, flaked	1/2 cup
Bulgur (cooked)	1/2 cup
Cooked cereals	1/2 cup
Cornmeal (dry)	2 1/2 Tbsp.
Grape-Nuts®	3 Tbsp.
Grits (cooked)	1/2 cup
Other ready-to-eat unsweetened cereals	3/4 cup
Pasta (cooked)	1/2 cup
Puffed cereal	1 1/2 cup
Rice, white or brown (cooked)	1/3 cup
Shredded wheat	1/2 cup
Wheat germ	3 Tbsp.

DRIED BEANS/PEAS/LENTILS

Beans and peas (cooked) (such as kidney, white, split, blackeye)	1/3 cup
Lentils (cooked)	1/3 cup
Baked beans	1/4 cup

STARCHY VEGETABLES

Corn	1/2 cup
Corn on cob, 6 in. long	1
Lima beans	1/2 cup
Peas, green (canned or frozen)	1/2 cup
Plantain	1/2 cup
Potato, baked	1 small (3 oz.)

Rosdahl CB: Textbook of Basic Nursing, 6th ed. © 1995 J.B. Lippincott Company

Potato, mashed	1/2 cup
Squash, winter (acorn, butternut)	1 cup
Yam, sweet potato, plain	1/3 cup

BREAD

Bagel	1/2 (1 oz.)
Bread sticks, crisp, 4 in. long × 1/2 in.	2 (2/3 oz.)
Croutons, low fat	1 cup
English muffin	1/2
Frankfurter or hamburger bun	1/2 (1 oz.)
Pita, 6 in. across	1/2
Plain roll, small	1 (1 oz.)
Raisin, unfrosted	1 slice (1 oz.)
Rye, pumpernickel	1 slice (1 oz.)
Tortilla, 6 in. across	1
White (including French, Italian)	1 slice (1 oz.)
Whole wheat	1 slice (1 oz.)

CRACKERS/SNACKS

Animal crackers	8
Graham crackers, 2 1/2 in. square	3
Matzoh	3/4 oz.
Melba toast	5 slices
Oyster crackers	24
Popcorn (popped, no fat added)	3 cups
Pretzels	3/4 oz.
Rye crisp, 2 in. × 3 1/2 in.	4
Saltine-type crackers	6
Whole-wheat crackers, no fat added (crisp breads, such as Finn®, Kavli®, Wasa®)	2–4 slices (3/4 oz.)

STARCH FOODS PREPARED WITH FAT

(Count as 1 starch/bread exchange, plus 1 fat exchange.)

Biscuit, 2 1/2 in. across	1
Chow mein noodles	1/2 cup
Corn bread, 2 in. cube	1 (2 oz.)
Cracker, round butter type	6
French fried potatoes, 2 in. to 3 1/2 in. long	10 (1 1/2 oz.)
Muffin, plain, small	1
Pancake, 4 in. across	2
Stuffing, bread (prepared)	1/4 cup
Taco shell, 6 in. across	2

Waffle, 4 1/2 in. square	1
Whole-wheat crackers, fat added (such as Triscuit®)	4–6 (1 oz.)

2. Meat List

Each serving of meat and substitutes on this list contains about 7 g protein. The amount of fat and number of calories varies, depending on what kind of meat or substitute you choose. The list is divided into three parts based on the amount of fat and calories: lean meat, medium-fat meat, and high-fat meat. One ounce (one meat exchange) of each of these includes:

	Carbohydrate (g)	*Protein (g)*	*Fat (g)*	*Calories*
Lean	0	7	3	55
Medium-fat	0	7	5	75
High-fat	0	7	8	100

LEAN MEAT AND SUBSTITUTES

(One exchange is equal to any one of the following items.)

Beef:	USDA Select or Choice grades of lean beef, such as round, sirloin, and flank steak; tenderloin; and chipped beef*	1 oz.
Pork:	Lean pork, such as fresh ham; canned, cured or boiled ham*; Canadian bacon*, tenderloin.	1 oz.
Veal:	All cuts are lean except for veal cutlets (ground or cubed). Examples of lean veal are chops and roasts.	1 oz.
Poultry:	Chicken, turkey, Cornish hen (without skin)	1 oz.
Fish:	All fresh and frozen fish	1 oz.
	Crab, lobster, scallops, shrimp, clams (fresh or canned in water)	2 oz.
	Oysters	6 medium
	Tuna** (canned in water)	1/4 cup
	Herring** (uncreamed or smoked)	1 oz.
	Sardines (canned)	2 medium
Wild Game:	Venison, rabbit, squirrel	1 oz.
	Pheasant, duck, goose (without skin)	1 oz.
Cheese:	Any cottage cheese**	1/4 cup
	Grated parmesan	2 Tbsp.

	Diet cheeses* (with less than 55 calories per ounce)	1 oz.
Other:	95% fat-free luncheon meat*	1 1/2 oz.
	Egg whites	3 whites
	Egg substitutes with less than 55 calories per 1/2 cup	1/2 cup

* 40 mg or more of sodium per exchange.
** 400 mg or more of sodium if two or more exchanges are eaten.

MEDIUM-FAT MEAT AND SUBSTITUTES

(One exchange is equal to any one of the following items.)

Beef:	Most beef products fall into this category. Examples are: all ground beef, roast (rib, chuck, rump), steak (cubed, Porterhouse, T-bone), and meatloaf.	1 oz.
Pork:	Most pork products fall into this category. Examples are: chops, loin roast, Boston butt, cutlets.	1 oz.
Lamb:	Most lamb products fall into this category. Examples are: chops, leg, and roast.	1 oz.
Veal:	Cutlet (ground or cubed, unbreaded)	1 oz.
Poultry:	Chicken (with skin), domestic duck or goose (well drained of fat), ground turkey	1 oz.
Fish:	Tuna** (canned in oil and drained)	1/4 cup
	Salmon** (canned)	1/4 cup
Cheese:	Skim or part-skim milk cheeses, such as:	
	Ricotta	1/4 cup
	Mozzarella	1 oz.
	Diet cheeses* (with 56–80 calories per ounce)	1 oz.
Other:	86% fat-free luncheon meat**	1 oz.
	Egg (high in cholesterol, limit to 3/wk)	1
	Egg substitutes with 56–80 calories per 1/4 cup	1/4 cup
	Tofu (2 1/2 in. × 2 3/4 in. × 1 in.)	4 oz.
	Liver, heart, kidney, sweetbreads (high in cholesterol)	1 oz.

* 400 mg or more of sodium per exchange.
** 400 mg or more of sodium if two or more exchanges are eaten.

HIGH-FAT MEAT AND SUBSTITUTES

Remember, these items are high in saturated fat, cholesterol, and calories, and should be used only three (3) times per week.
(One exchange is equal to any one of the following items.)

Beef:	Most USDA Prime cuts of beef, such as ribs, corned beef**	1 oz.
Pork:	Spareribs, ground pork, pork sausage* (patty or link)	1 oz.
Lamb:	Patties (ground lamb)	1 oz.
Fish:	Any fried fish product	1 oz.
Cheese:	All regular cheeses, such as American*, Blue*, Cheddar**, Monterey Jack**, Swiss	1 oz.
Other:	Luncheon meat*, such as bologna, salami, pimento loaf	1 oz.
	Sausage*, such as Polish, Italian smoked	1 oz.
	Knockwurst*	1 oz.
	Bratwurst**	1 oz.
	Frankfurter* (turkey or chicken)	1 frank (10/lb.)
	Peanut butter (contains unsaturated fat)	1 Tbsp.

Count as one high-fat meat plus one fat exchange:

	Frankfurter* (beef, pork, or combination)	1 frank (10/lb.)

* 400 mg or more of sodium per exchange.
** 400 mg or more of sodium if two or more exchanges are eaten.

3. Vegetable List

Each vegetable serving on this list contains about 5 g carbohydrate, 2 g protein, and 25 calories. Vegetables contain 2–3 g dietary fiber. Vegetables that contain 400 mg or more of sodium per exchange are identified with an asterisk *.

Unless otherwise noted, the serving size for vegetables (one vegetable exchange) is:

1/2 cup of cooked vegetables or vegetable juice
1 cup of raw vegetables

Artichoke (1/2 medium)
Asparagus
Beans (green, wax, Italian)
Bean sprouts
Beets
Broccoli
Brussels sprouts
Cabbage, cooked
Carrots
Cauliflower
Eggplant
Greens (collard, mustard, turnip)
Kohlrabi
Leeks

Mushrooms, cooked
Okra
Onions
Pea pods
Peppers (green)
Rutabaga
Sauerkraut*
Spinach, cooked
Summer squash (crookneck)
Tomato (one large)
Tomato/vegetable juice*
Turnips
Water chestnuts
Zucchini, cooked

Starchy vegetables such as corn, peas, and potatoes are found on the Starch/Bread List.

For free vegetables, see Free Food List at the end of Appendix D.

4. Fruit List

Each item on this list contains about 15 g carbohydrate and 60 calories. Fresh, frozen, and dried fruits have about 2 g fiber per exchange. Fruits that have 3 g or more of fiber per excahnge appear in **boldface**. Fruit juices contain very little dietary fiber.

The carbohydrate and calorie content for a fruit exchange are based on the usual serving of the most commonly eaten fruits. Use fresh fruits or fruits frozen or canned without sugar added. Whole fruit is more filling than fruit juice and may be a better choice for those who are trying to lose weight. Unless otherwise noted, the serving size for one fruit exchange is:

1/2 cup of fresh fruit or fruit juice
1/4 cup of dried fruit

FRESH, FROZEN, AND UNSWEETENED CANNED FRUIT

Apple (raw, 2 in. across)	1 apple
Applesauce (unsweetened)	1/2 cup
Apricots (medium, raw)	4 apricots
Apricots (canned)	1/2 cup, or 4 halves
Banana (9 in. long)	1/2 banana
Blackberries (raw)	3/4 cup
Blueberries (raw)	3/4 cup
Cantaloupe (5 in. across) (cubes)	1/3 melon 1 cup
Cherries (large, raw)	12 cherries
Cherries (canned)	1/2 cup
Figs (raw, 2 in. across)	2 figs
Fruit cocktail (canned)	1/2 cup

Grapefruit (medium)	1/2 grapefruit
Grapefruit (segments)	3/4 cup
Grapes (small)	15 grapes
Honeydew melon (medium) (cubes)	1/8 melon 1 cup
Kiwi (large)	1 kiwi
Mandarin oranges	3/4 cup
Mango (small)	1/2 mango
Nectarine (2 1/2 in. across)	1 nectarine
Orange (2 1/2 in. across)	1 orange
Papaya	1 cup
Peach (2 3/4 in. across)	1 peach, or 3/4 cup
Peaches (canned)	1/2 cup or 2 halves
Pear	1/2 large, or 1 small
Pears (canned)	1/2 cup, or 2 halves
Persimmon (medium, native)	2 persimmons
Pineapple (raw)	3/4 cup
Pineapple (canned)	1/3 cup
Plum (raw, 2 in. across)	2 plums
Pomegranate	1/2 pomegranate
Raspberries (raw)	1 cup
Strawberries (raw, whole)	1 1/4 cup
Tangerine (2 1/2 in. across)	2 tangerines
Watermelon (cubes)	1 1/4 cup

DRIED FRUIT

Apples	4 rings
Apricots	7 halves
Dates	2 1/2 medium
Figs	1 1/2
Prunes	3 medium
Raisins	2 Tbsp.

FRUIT JUICE

Apple juice/cider	1/2 cup
Cranberry juice cocktail	1/3 cup
Grapefruit juice	1/2 cup
Grape juice	1/3 cup
Orange juice	1/2 cup
Pineapple juice	1/2 cup
Prune juice	1/3 cup

5. Milk List

Each serving of milk or milk products on this list contains about 12 g carbohydrate and 8 g protein. The amount of fat in milk is measured in percent (%) of butterfat. The calories vary, depending on what kind of milk you choose. The list is divided into three parts based on the amount of fat and calories: skim/very low-fat milk, low-fat milk, and whole milk. One serving (one milk exchange) of each of these includes:

	Carbohydrate (g)	Protein (g)	Fat (g)	Calories
Skim/Very Low-fat	12	8	trace	90
Low-fat	12	8	5	120
Whole	12	8	8	150

Milk is the body's main source of calcium, the mineral needed for growth and repair of bones. Yogurt is also a good source of calcium. Yogurt and many dry or powdered milk products have different amounts of fat. If you have questions about a particular item, read the label to find out the fat and calorie content.

Milk is good to drink, but it can also be added to cereal, and to other foods. Many tasty dishes such as sugar-free pudding are made with milk (see the Combination Foods list). Add life to plain yogurt by adding one of your fruit exchanges to it.

SKIM AND VERY LOW-FAT MILK

skim milk	1 cup
1/2% milk	1 cup
1% milk	1 cup
low-fat buttermilk	1 cup
evaporated skim milk	1/2 cup
dry nonfat milk	1/3 cup
plain nonfat yogurt	8 oz.

LOW-FAT MILK

2% milk	1 cup fluid
plain low-fat yogurt (with added nonfat milk solids)	8 oz.

WHOLE MILK

The whole milk group has much more fat per serving than the skim and low-fat groups. Whole milk has more than 3 1/4% butterfat. Try to limit your choices from the whole milk group as much as possible.

whole milk	1 cup
evaporated whole milk	1/2 cup
whole plain yogurt	8 oz.

6. Fat List

Each serving on the fat list contains about 5 g fat and 45 calories. The foods on the fat list contain mostly fat, although some items may also contain a small amount of protein. All fats are high in calories and should be carefully measured. Everyone should modify fat intake by eating unsaturated fats instead of saturated fats. The sodium content of these foods varies widely. Check the label for sodium information.

UNSATURATED FATS

Avocado	1/8 medium
Margarine	1 tsp.
Margarine, diet**	1 Tbsp.
Mayonnaise	1 tsp.
Mayonnaise, reduced-calorie**	1 Tbsp.
Nuts and Seeds:	
Almonds, dry roasted	6 whole
Cashews, dry roasted	1 Tbsp.
Pecans	2 whole
Peanuts	20 small or 10 large
Walnuts	2 whole
Other nuts	1 Tbsp.
Seeds, pine nuts, sunflower (without shells)	1 Tbsp.
Pumpkin seeds	2 tsp.
Oil (corn, cottonseed, safflower, soybean, sunflower, olive, peanut)	1 tsp.
Olives**	10 small or 5 large
Salad dressing, mayonnaise-type	2 tsp.
Salad dressing, mayonnaise-type, reduced-calorie	1 Tbsp.
Salad dressing (oil varieties)*	1 Tbsp.
Salad dressing, reduced-calorie*	2 Tbsp.

(Two tablespoons of low-calorie salad dressing is a free food.)

SATURATED FATS

Butter	1 tsp.
Bacon**	1 slice
Chitterlings	1/2 ounce
Coconut, shredded	2 Tbsp.
Coffee whitener, liquid	2 Tbsp.
Coffee whitener, powder	4 tsp.
Cream (light, coffee, table)	2 Tbsp.
Cream, sour	2 Tbsp.
Cream (heavy, whipping)	1 Tbsp.
Cream cheese	1 Tbsp.
Salt pork**	1/4 ounce

* 400 mg or more of sodium per exchange.
** 400 mg or more of sodium if two or more exchanges are eaten.

Free Foods

A *free food* is any food or drink that contains less than 20 calories per serving. You can eat as much as you want of those items that have no serving size specified. You may eat two or three servings per day of those items that have a specific serving size. Be sure to spread them out through the day.

Drinks

Bouillon* or broth without fat
Bouillon, low-sodium
Carbonated drinks, sugar-free
Carbonated water
Club soda
Cocoa powder, unsweetened
  (1 Tbsp.)
Coffee/Tea
Drink mixes, sugar-free
Tonic water, sugar-free

Nonstick pan spray

Salad greens

Endive
Escarole
Lettuce
Romaine
Spinach

Sweet Substitutes

Candy, hard, sugar-free
Gelatin, sugar-free
Gum, sugar-free
Jam/Jelly, sugar-free
  (less than 20 cal./2 tsp.)
Pancake syrup, sugar-free
  (1–2 Tbsp.)
Sugar substitutes
  (saccharin, aspartame)
Whipped topping
  (2 Tbsp.)

Fruit

Cranberries, unsweetened
  (1/2 cup)
Rhubarb, unsweetened
  (1/2 cup)

Vegetables

(raw, 1 cup)
Cabbage
Celery
Chinese cabbage
Cucumber
Green onion
Hot peppers
Mushrooms
Radishes
Zucchini

Condiments

Catsup (1 Tbsp.)
Horseradish
Mustard
Pickles, dill, unsweetened
Salad dressing, low-calorie
  (2 Tbsp.)
Taco sauce (3 Tbsp.)
Vinegar

Seasonings can be very helpful in making food taste better. Be careful of how much sodium you use. Read the label, and choose those seasonings that do not contain sodium or salt.

Basil (fresh)
Celery seeds
Chili powder
Chives
Cinnamon
Curry
Dill
Flavoring extracts
  (vanilla, almond,
  walnut, peppermint,
  butter, lemon, etc.)
Garlic
Garlic powder
Herbs
Hot pepper sauce
Lemon
Lemon juice
Lemon pepper
Lime
Lime juice
Mint
Onion powder
Oregano
Paprika
Pepper
Pimento
Spices
Soy sauce
Soy sauce, low-sodium
  ("lite")
Wine, used in cooking
  (1/4 cup)
Worcestershire sauce

Combination Foods

Much of the food we eat is mixed together in various combinations. These combination foods do not fit into only one exchange list. It can be quite hard to tell what is in a certain casserole dish or baked food item. This is a list of average values for some typical combination foods. This table will help you fit these foods into your meal plan.

Food	*Amount*	*Exchanges*
Casseroles, homemade	1 cup (8 oz.)	2 starch, 2 medium-fat meat, 1 fat
Cheese pizza*, thin crust	1/4 of 15 oz. or 1/4 of 10″	2 starch, 1 medium-fat meat, 1 fat
Chili with beans (commercial)*	1 cup (8 oz.)	2 starch, 2 medium-fat meat, 2 fat
Chow mein* (without noodles or rice)	2 cups (16 oz.)	1 starch, 2 vegetable, 2 lean meat
Macaroni and cheese*	1 cup (8 oz.)	2 starch, 1 medium-fat meat, 2 fat
Soup		
Bean*	1 cup (8 oz.)	1 starch, 1 vegetable, 1 lean meat
Chunky, all varieties*	10-3/4 oz. can	1 starch, 1 vegetable, 1 medium-fat meat
Cream* (made with water)	1 cup (8 oz.)	1 starch, 1 fat
Vegetable* or broth-type*	1 cup (8 oz.)	1 starch
Spaghetti and meatballs* (canned)	1 cup (8 oz.)	2 starch, 1 medium-fat meat, 1 fat
Sugar-free pudding (made with skim milk)	1/2 cup	1 starch
Beans Used as Meat Substitute		
Dried beans, peas, lentils	1 cup (cooked)	2 starch, 1 lean meat

3 grams or more of fiber per exchange.
* 400 mg or more of sodium per exchange.

The exchange lists are the basis of a meal planning system designed by a committee of the American Diabetes Association and the American Dietetic Association. Although designed primarily for people with diabetes and others who must follow special diets, the exchange lists are based on principles of good nutrition that apply to everyone. © 1989 American Diabetes Association, American Dietetic Association.

Index

Page numbers followed by *f* indicate illustrations; *t* following a page number indicates tabular material.

Nursing Diagnoses, North American Nursing Diagnosis Association, 1994

Activity Intolerance
Activity Intolerance, High Risk for
Adjustment, Impaired
Airway Clearance, Ineffective
Anxiety
Aspiration, High Risk for
Body Image Disturbance
Body Temperature, High Risk for Altered
Breastfeeding, Effective
Breastfeeding, Ineffective
Breastfeeding, Interrupted
Breathing Pattern, Ineffective
Cardiac Output, Decreased
Caregiver Role Strain
Caregiver Role Strain, High Risk for
Communication, Impaired Verbal
Constipation
Constipation, Colonic
Constipation, Perceived
Coping, Defensive
Coping, Ineffective Individual
Decisional Conflict (Specify)
Denial, Ineffective
Diarrhea
Disuse Syndrome, High Risk for
Diversional Activity Deficit
Dysreflexia
Family Coping: Compromised, Ineffective
Family Coping: Disabling, Ineffective
Family Coping: Potential for Growth
Family Processes, Altered
Fatigue
Fear
Fluid Volume Deficit
Fluid Volume Deficit, High Risk for
Fluid Volume Excess
Gas Exchange, Impaired
Grieving, Anticipatory
Grieving, Dysfunctional
Growth and Development, Altered
Health Maintenance, Altered
Health-Seeking Behaviors (Specify)
Home Maintenance Management, Impaired
Hopelessness
Hyperthermia
Hypothermia
Incontinence, Bowel
Incontinence, Functional
Incontinence, Reflex
Incontinence, Stress
Incontinence, Total
Incontinence, Urge
Infant Feeding Pattern, Ineffective
Infection, High Risk for
Injury, High Risk for
Knowledge Deficit (Specify)
Noncompliance (Specify)

Nutrition, Altered: Less than Body Requirements
Nutrition, Altered: More than Body Requirements
Nutrition, Altered: Potential for More than Body
    Requirements
Oral Mucous Membrane, Altered
Pain
Pain, Chronic
Parental Role Conflict
Parenting, Altered
Parenting, High Risk for Altered
Peripheral Neurovascular Dysfunction, High Risk for
Personal Identity Disturbance
Physical Mobility, Impaired
Poisoning, High Risk for
Post-Trauma Response
Powerlessness
Protection, Altered
Rape Trauma Syndrome
Rape Trauma Syndrome: Compound Reaction
Rape Trauma Syndrome: Silent Reaction
Relocation Stress Syndrome
Role Performance, Altered
Self-Care Deficit
    Bathing/Hygiene
    Feeding
    Dressing/Grooming
    Toileting
Self-Esteem, Chronic Low
Self-Esteem, Situational Low
Self-Esteem, Disturbance
Self-Mutilation, High Risk for
Sensory-Perceptual Alterations (Specify) (visual, auditory,
    kinesthetic, gustatory, tactile, olfactory)
Sexual Dysfunction
Sexuality Patterns, Altered
Skin Integrity, High Risk for Impaired
Skin Integrity, Impaired
Sleep Pattern Disturbance
Social Interaction, Impaired
Social Isolation
Spiritual Distress
Suffocation, High Risk for
Swallowing, Impaired
Therapeutic Regimen, Ineffective Management of
Thermoregulation, Ineffective
Thought Processes, Altered
Tissue Integrity, Impaired
Tissue Perfusion, Altered (Specify Type) (renal, cerebral,
    cardiopulmonary, gastrointestinal, peripheral)
Trauma, High Risk for
Unilateral Neglect
Urinary Elimination, Altered
Urinary Retention
Ventilation, Inability to Sustain Spontaneous
Ventilatory Weaning Response, Dysfunctional
Violence, High Risk for: Self-Directed or Directed at Others